The Headaches

SECOND EDITION

The Headaches

SECOND EDITION

Edited by

Jes Olesen, M.D.
Professor and Chairman
Department of Neurology
Glostrup Hospital
University of Copenhagen
Glostrup, Copenhagen, Denmark

Peer Tfelt-Hansen, M.D.
Associate Professor
Department of Neurology
Glostrup Hospital
University of Copenhagen
Glostrup, Copenhagen, Denmark

K. Michael A. Welch, M.D.
Senior Associate Dean for Research in Graduate Studies
Department of Neurology
University of Kansas School of Medicine
University of Kansas Medical Center
Kansas City, Kansas

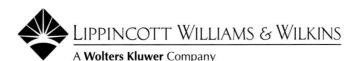

LIPPINCOTT WILLIAMS & WILKINS
A **Wolters Kluwer** Company
Philadelphia · Baltimore · New York · London
Buenos Aires · Hong Kong · Sydney · Tokyo

Acquisitions Editor: Anne M. Sydor
Developmental Editor: Joanne Husovski
Production Editor: Robin E. Cook
Manufacturing Manager: Tim Reynolds
Cover Designer: Patricia Gast
Compositor: Lippincott Williams & Wilkins Desktop Division
Printer: Courier Westford

©2000 by LIPPINCOTT WILLIAMS & WILKINS
227 East Washington Square
Philadelphia, PA 19106-3780 USA
www.LWW.com

Printed in the USA

Library of Congress Cataloging-in-Publication Data

The headaches / edited by Jes Olesen, Peer Tfelt-Hansen, K. Michael A. Welch.
  — 2nd ed.
        p. cm.
  Includes bibliographical references and index.
  ISBN 0-7817-1597-0
     1. Headache. I. Olesen, Jes. II. Tfelt-Hansen, Peer.
  III. Welch, K. M. A. (K. Michael A.)
     [DNLM: 1. Headache. WL 342 H4329 1999]
  RB128.H445 1999
  616.8′491—dc21
  DNLM/DLC   99-21427
  For Library of Congress   CIP

Care has been taken to confirm the accuracy of the information presented and to describe generally accepted practices. However, the authors, editors, and publisher are not responsible for errors or omissions or for any consequences from application of the information in this book and make no warranty, expressed or implied, with respect to the currency, completeness, or accuracy of the contents of the publication. Application of this information in a particular situation remains the professional responsibility of the practitioner.

The authors, editors, and publisher have exerted every effort to ensure that drug selection and dosage set forth in this text are in accordance with current recommendations and practice at the time of publication. However, in view of ongoing research, changes in government regulations, and the constant flow of information relating to drug therapy and drug reactions, the reader is urged to check the package insert for each drug for any change in indications and dosage and for added warnings and precautions. This is particularly important when the recommended agent is a new or infrequently employed drug.

Some drugs and medical devices presented in this publication have Food and Drug Administration (FDA) clearance for limited use in restricted research settings. It is the responsibility of the health care provider to ascertain the FDA status of each drug or device planned for use in their clinical practice.

10 9 8 7 6 5 4 3 2 1

Contents

III. The Migraines

Migraine: Clinical Features

Migraine: Management

Migraine: Acute Drug Treatment of the Attack

Migraine: Prophylactic Drug Management

Migraine: Special Types and Complications

IV. Tension-Type Headache, Cluster Headache, and Miscellaneous Primary Headaches

Tension-Type Headache: Pathophysiology

Tension-Type Headache: Clinical Features

Tension-Type Headache: Management

Headache Associated with Head Trauma

Headache Associated with Vascular Disorders

Headache Associated with Nonvascular Intracranial Disorders

Headache Associated with Substances or Their Withdrawal

Headache Associated with Systemic Disorders

Headache of Facial Pain Associated with Disorders of the Skull and Cervical Spine

Cranial Neuralgias, Nerve Trunk Pain, and Deafferentation Pain

VI. Special Problems in the Headaches and Their Management

Contributors

Ishaq Abu-Arafeh, M.D.
Department of Paediatrics
Stirling Royal Infirmary
Livilands
Stirling FK8 2AU
United Kingdom

Frank Andrasik, M.D.
Behavioral Medicine Laboratory
University of West Florida
11000 University Parkway
Pensacola, Florida 32514-5751

Guy Arnold, M.D.
Universitätsklinikum Charité
Medizinische Fakultät der Humboldt-
*   Universität zu Berlin*
Universitätsklinik und Piloklinik für Neurologie
Schumannstrasse 20-21
10117 Berlin, Germany

Messoud Ashina, M.D.
Department of Neurology
Glostrup Hospital
University of Copenhagen
DK-2600 Glostrup, Copenhagen
Denmark

Taruna K. Aurora, M.D.
Department of Emergency Medicine
Henry Ford Hospital
2799 West Grand Boulevard
Detroit, Michigan 48202

Flemming W. Bach, M.D.
Department of Neurology
University of Århus
Århus Kommunehospital
Norrebrogade
DK-8000 Århus
Denmark

Robert W. Baloh, M.D.
Department of Neurology/Head and Neck
*   Surgery*
U.C.L.A. Medical School, and
Division of Neurotology
Department of Neurology
U.C.L.A. Hospital
710 Westwood Plaza
Los Angeles, California 90095-1769

Lars Bendtsen, M.D.
Department of Neurology
Glostrup Hospital
University of Copenhagen
DK-2600 Glostrup, Copenhagen
Denmark

Valérie Biousse, M.D.
Department of Neurology
Hôpital Lariboisière
2 rue Ambroise Paré
75475 Paris
France

Nikolai Bogduk, M.D.
Department of Anatomy and Musculoskeletal
*   Medicine*
University of Newcastle, and
Newcastle Bone and Joint Institute
Royal Newcastle Hospital
Newcastle, New South Wales 2300
Australia

Jörgen Boivie, M.D.
Department of Neurology
University Hospital
S-581 85 Linköping
Sweden

Marie-Germaine Bousser, M.D.
Department of Neurology
Lariboisière Medical Faculty
Paris VII University, and
Department of Neurology
Hôpital Lariboisière
2 rue Ambroise Parè
75475 Paris
France

Jannick Brennum, M.D.
Department of Neurosurgery
University Hospital of
*   Copenhagen–Rigshospitalet*
Blegoamsvie 29
DK-2100 Copenhagen
Denmark

Dennis E. Bulman, Ph.D.
Division of Neurology
Department of Medicine
University of Ottowa, and
Research Scientist
Ottawa General Hospital Research Institute
The Ottowa Hospital—General Campus
501 Smyth Road
Ottawa, Ontario K1H 8L6
Canada

Rami Burstein, M.D.
Department of Neurobiology
Harvard Medical School,
Assistant Professor and Vice-Chairman
Department of Anesthesia and Critical Care
Beth Israel Deaconess Medical Center, and
Harvard Institutes of Medicine
77 Avenue Louis Pasteur, Room 830
Boston, Massachusetts 02115

Gennaro Bussone, M.D.
Third Department of Clinical Neurology
Istituto Nazionale Neurologico
"Carlo Besta"
Via Celoria 11
20133 Milan, Italy

J. Keith Campbell, M.D.
Department of Neurology
Mayo Clinic and Mayo Medical School
200 First Street SW
Rochester, Minnesota 55905

Jane Y. Carlsson, Ph.D.
Department of Rehabilitation
College of Health and Caring Sciences
Göteborg University
Box 111
S-405 30 Göteborg, Sweden

Kenneth L. Casey, M.D.
Department of Neurology
University of Michigan, and
Department of Neurology
Veteran's Affairs Medical Center
2215 Fuller Road
Ann Arbor, Michigan 48105

James John Corbett, M.D.
University of Mississippi School of Medicine, and
Department of Neurology
University of Mississippi Medical Center
2500 North State Street
Jackson, Mississippi 39216-4505

F. Michael Cutrer, M.D.
Department of Neurology
Harvard Medical School, and
Director, Partners Headache Center
Massachusetts General Hospital/Brigham and
*   Women's Hospital*
15 Parkman Street, VBK-905
Boston, Massachusetts 02114-3117

Giovanni D'Andrea, M.D.
Neurophysiopathology Service
Headache and Cerebrovascular Diseases Center
San Bortolo Hospital
Viale Ridolfi
36100 Viceza
Italy

Erik Dahl
Department of Anatomy
Odontologisk Institutt
University of Oslo
Blindern
P.O. Box 1052
0316 Oslo 3
Norway

Carl G. H. Dahlöf, M.D.
Department of Clinical Pharmacology
Sahlgrenska University Hospital, and
Gothenburg Migraine Clinic
Sociala Huset, Uppg D
S-41117 Göteborg
Sweden

Jaqueline deBelleroche, M.D.
Division of Neuroscience and Psychological
*   Medicine*
Department of Neuromuscular Diseases
Imperial College School of Medicine
Charing Cross Hospital
Fulham Palace Road
London W6 8RF
United Kingdom

Milena De Marinis, M.D.
Department of Neurological Sciences
University of Rome "La Sapienza"
00185 Rome
Italy

Hans-Christoph Diener, M.D.
Department of Neurology
University of Essen, and
Department of Neurology
University Hospital Essen
Hufelandstrasse 55
D-45122 Essen
Germany

Jonathan O. Dostrovsky, M.D.
Department of Physiology
Program in Neurosciences
University of Toronto
Medical Sciences Building #3305
Toronto, Ontario M5S 1A8
Canada

Peter D. Drummond, Ph.D.
Department of Psychology
Murdoch University
South Street
Perth, Western Australia 6150
Australia

Anne Ducros, M.D.
Laboratoire de Pathologie de l'Immunité
Faculté de Médecine Necker-Enfants Malades
156, rue de Vaugirard
75730 Paris Cedex 15
France

John G. Edmeads, M.D.
Department of Medicine
Sunnybrook Health Science Center
University of Toronto
2075 Bayview Avenue
Toronto, Ontario M4N 3M5
Canada

Lars Edvinsson, M.D.
Department of Internal Medicine
University Hospital of Lund
S-221 85 Lund
Sweden

Karl Einhäupl, M.D.
Department of Neurology
Universtätsklinikum Charité
Schumannstrasse 20/21
D-10117 Berlin
Germany

Karl Ekbom, M.D.
Department of Neurology
Huddinge University Hospital at the Karolinska
* Institute*
S-14186 Huddinge
Sweden

Marcello Fanciullacci, M.D.
Institute of Internal Medicine and
* Therapeutics IV*
Headache Centre
University of Florence School of Medicine
Viale Pieraccini 18
50139 Florence
Italy

Markus Färkkilä, M.D.
Department of Neurology
University of Helsinki, and
Department of Neurology
Meilahti Hospital
Haartmaninkatu 4
00290 Helsinki
Finland

Michel D. Ferrari, M.D.
Associate Professor, Department of Neurology
Leiden University Medical Centre
P.O. Box 9600
NL-2300 RC Leiden
The Netherlands

Heli Forssell, D.D.S.
Department of Oral Surgery
Turku University, and
Department of Oral Diseases
Turku Universtiy Central Hospital
Lemminkäisenaktu 2
SF-20520 Turku
Finland

Peter A. Forsyth, M.D.
Departments of Neurosciences and Oncology
University of Calgary and Tom Baker Cancer
* Centre, and*
Department of Clinical Neurosciences
Foothills Hospital
1331 29th Street N.W.
Calgary, Alberta T2N 4N2
Canada

Peter J. Goadsby, M.D.
The National Hospital for Neurology and
* Neurosurgery*
Queen Square
London WC1N 3BG
United Kingdom

Hartmuth Göbel, M.D.
Kiel Pain Clinic
University of Kiel
Heikendorfer Weg 9-27
D-24149 Kiel
Germany

Philip B. Gorelick, M.D.
Department of Neurological Sciences
Rush University Medical College, and
Center for Stroke Research
1645 West Jackson Boulevard, Suite 400
Chicago, Illinois 60612

Richard H. Gracely, M.D.
Clinical Measurement and Mechanisms Unit
Pain and Neurosensory Branch
National Institute of Dental Research
National Institutes of Health
Building 10, Room 3C-403
Bethesda, Maryland 20892

Steven B. Graff-Radford, M.D.
Department of Diagnostic Sciences
U.C.L.A., and
Director, The Pain Center
Cedars-Sinai Medical Center
444 South San Vicente Boulevard #1101
Los Angeles, California 90048

Mirja Hämäläinen, M.D.
Department of Pediatric Neurology
University of Helsinki, and
Specialist, Department of Pediatric Neurology
Hospital for Children and Adolescents
P.O. Box 280
FIN-00029 HYKS Heksinki
Finland

Edith Hamel, Ph.D.
Department of Neurology and Neurosurgery
Montréal Neurological Institute
McGill University
3801 University Street
Montréal, Québec H3A 2B4
Canada

Jan Erik Hardebo, M.D.
Neurologic Institution
University Hospital of Lund
S-22185 Lund
Sweden

Patrick Henry, M.D.
Service de Neurologie
Hôpital Pellegrin
Place Amélie Raba Léon
33076 Bordeaux
France

Rachel Hering-Hanit, M.D.
Sackler School of Medicine
Tel Aviv University
Ramat Aviv 69978, and
Headache Unit
Department of Neurology
Meir General Hospital
Kfar-Sava 44281
Israel

Kenneth A. Holroyd, M.D.
Department of Psychology
Ohio University
Athens, Ohio 45201-2979

Masamitsu Iino, M.D.
Department of Pharmacology
Faculty of Medicine
The University of Tokyo
Hongo, Bunkyo-ku
Tokyo 113-0033
Japan

Hansruedi Isler, M.D.
Neurologische Klinik
Universitäts Spital Zürich
Frauenklinikstrasse 26
CH-8091 Zürich
Switzerland

Inger Jansen-Olesen, M.D.
Department of Pharmocology
The Royal Danish School of
*   Pharmacy*
Universitetsparken 2
DK-2100 Copenhagen Ø
Denmark

Kai Jensen, M.D.
Department of Neurology
Hilleroed Hospital
DK-3400 Hilleroed
Denmark

Rigmor Jensen, M.D.
Department of Neurology
Glostrup Hospital
University of Copenhagen
DK-2600 Glostrup, Copenhagen
Denmark

Troels Staehelin Jensen, M.D., Ph.D.
Department of Neurology F
Århus Kommunehospital
Noerrebragade 44
DK-8000 Århus C
Denmark

Rajiv Joseph, M.D., PhD
Department of Neurology
Baylor Medical Center
621 Clara Barton, Suite 104
Garland, Texas 75042

Karin Jurkat-Rott, M.D.
Department of Applied Physiology
University of Ulm
Albert-Einstein-Allee 11
D-89069 Ulm
Germany

Holger Kaube, M.D.
Department of Neurology
University of Essen
D-45122 Essen
Germany

Matthias Keidel, M.D.
Department of Neurology
University of Essen
Hufelandstrasse 55
D-45122 Essen
Germany

James W. Lance, M.D.
Department of Neurology
University of New South Wales, and
Institute of Neurological Sciences
Prince of Wales Hospital
High Street, Randwick
Sydney, New South Wales 2031
Australia

Michael Langemark, M.D.
Department of Neurology
Hilleroed Hospital
Helsevej 2
DK-3400 Hilleroed
Denmark

Martin Lauritzen, M.D.
Department of Clinical Neurophysiology
Glostrup Hospital
University of Copenhagen
DK-2600 Glostrup, Copenhagen
Denmark

Frank Lehmann-Horn, M.D.
Department of Applied Physiology
University of Ulm
Albert-Einstein-Allee 11
89069 Ulm
Germany

Richard B. Lipton, M.D.
Departments of Neurology, Epidemiology, and
* Social Medicine*
Albert Einstein College of Medicine,
* and*
Staff Neurologist
Headache Unit
Montefiore Medical Center
1300 Morris Park Avenue
Bronx, New York 10467

Gian Camillo Manzoni, M.D.
Department of Neurology
University of Parma
Strada Del Quartiere 4
43100 Parma
Italy

Paul R. Martin, PhD
Department of Psychology
University of New England
Armidale, New South Wales 2351
Australia

Timothy J. Martin, M.D.
Department of Ophthalmology
Wake Forest University School of
* Medicine*
Medical Center Boulevard
Winston-Salem, North Carolina 27157-1033

Hélène Massiou, M.D.
Department of Neurology
Hôpital Lariboisiére
2 rue Ambroise Paré
75475 Paris
France

Ninan T. Mathew, M.D.
Houston Headache Clinic
1213 Hermann Drive, Suite 350
Houston, Texas 77004

Arne May, M.D.
Klinik für Psychiatrie und Psychotherapie
Station P2
Virchowstr. 174
D-45147 Essen
Germany

John McEwen, M.D.
Department of Clinical Pharmacology and
* Therapeutics*
Ninewells Hospital and Medical School
Dundee DD1 9SY
United Kingdom

Patrick McGrath, M.D.
Department of Psychology
Dalhouise University
Halifax, Nova Scotia B3H 4J1
Canada

Kathleen Ries Merikangas, M.D.
Department of Epidemiology and Public Health
Genetic Epidemiology Research Unit
Yale University School of Medicine
40 Temple Street, Suite 7B
New Haven, Connecticut 06510-3223

Harold Merskey, M.D.
Department of Psychiatry
University of Western Ontario, and
Department of Psychiatry
London Health Sciences Centre
University Campus
339 Windermere Road
London, Ontario N6A 5A5
Canada

Karl Messlinger, M.D.
Department of Physiology and Experimental
*   Pathophysiology*
University of Erlangen-Nürnberg
Universitätsstrasse 17
D-91054 Erlangen
Germany

Philippe Michel, M.D.
Department of Neurology and Biostatistics
Hospital Pellegrin
Place Amelie Raba Leon
33076 Bordeaux
France

Panayiotis Mitsias, M.D.
Department of Neurology
Case Western Reserve University
Cleveland, Ohio 44109, and
Acute Stroke Unit
Department of Neurology
Henry Ford Hospital
2799 West Grand Boulevard
Detroit, Michigan 48202

José M. Pereira Monteiro, M.D.
Department of Neurology
Instituto de Ciencias Biomedicas Abel Salazar
Porto University, and
Department of Neurology
Hospital Santo Antonio
Largo Prof. Abel Salazar, 3
4050 Porto
Portugal

Michael A. Moskowitz, M.D.
Massachusetts General Hospital
Harvard Medical School
149 13th Street, Room 6403
Charlestown, Massachusetts 02129

Ewan J. Mylecharane, M.D.
Department of Pharmacology
University of Sydney
Sydney, New South Wales 2006
Australia

Giuseppe Nappi, M.D.
Department of Neurology
University of Rome La Sapienza
00185 Rome, and
C. Mondino Foundation
Via Palestro 3
27100 Pavia
Italy

Jes Olesen, M.D.
Department of Neurology
Glostrup Hospital
University of Copenhagen
DK-2600 Glostrup, Copenhagen
Denmark

John R. Østergaard, M.D.
Department of Pediatrics
University Hospital of Århus, and
Department of Pediatrics A
Skejby Hospital
Brendstrupgaardsvej
DK-8200 Århus N
Denmark

Teresa Paiva, M.D.
Laboratory EEG/ SLEEP
Centro de Estudos Egas Moniz
Hospital Santa Maria
1600 Lisbon
Portugal

Jan Passchier
Department of Medical Psychology and
*   Psychotherapy*
Erasmus University
3000 DR Rotterdam
The Netherlands

Richard C. Peatfield, M.D.
Charing Cross Hospital
Fulham Palace Road
London W6 8RF
United Kingdom

Olaf Pongs, M.D.
Universität Hamburg
Universitats-Krankenhaus Eppendorf
Zentrum fur Molekulare Neurobiologie
Institut fur Neurale Signalverabeitung
Martinistrs. 52
D-20246 Hamburg
Germany

Jerome B. Posner, M.D.
Department of Neurology
Cornell University Medical College,
* and*
Department of Neurology
Memorial Sloan-Kettering Cancer Center
1275 York Avenue
New York, New York 10021

André Pradalier, M.D.
Xavier Bichat Paris VII University
16 Rue Henri Huchard
75018 Paris, and
Chief, Service Médecine Interne 4
Hôpital Louis Mourier
178, rue des Renouillers
92700 Colombes Cedex
France

Antonio Prusinski, M.D.
Department of Neurology
Medical Academy
22 Kopcinskiego Street
90-153 Lodz
Poland

Nabih M. Ramadan, M.D.
Eli Lilly and Company
Indianapolis, Indiana 46285

Birthe Krogh Rasmussen, M.D.
Department of Neurology
Hilleroed Hospital
DK-3400 Hilleroed
Denmark

Povl Riis, M.D.
Den Centrale Videnskabstetiske Komité
Bredgade 43
DK-1260 K benhavn K

F. Clifford Rose, M.D.
London Neurological Centre
110 Harley Street
London W1N 1AF
United Kingdom

David Russell, M.D.
Department of Neurology
The National Hospital University of Oslo
Pilestredet 32
N-0027 Oslo
Norway

Michael Bjørn Russell, M.D.
Department of Neurology
Glostrup Hospital
University of Copenhagen
DK-2600 Glostrup, Copenhagen
Denmark

Fumihiko Sakai, M.D.
Department of Medicine
Kitasato University
1-15-1 Kitasato, Sagamihara
228 Kanagawa
Japan

Margarita Sanchez del Rio, M.D.
Massachusetts General Hospital
Harvard Medical School
149 13th Street, CNY-6403
Charlestown, Massachusetts 02129

Jürgen Sandkühler, M.D.
II. Physiologisches Institut
University of Heidelberg
Im Neuenheimer Feld 326
69120 Heidelberg
Germany

Giorgio Sandrini, M.D.
Department of Neurological Sciences
University of Pavia, and
Assistant Coordinator
Department of Neurological Rehabilitation
IRCC C. Mondino Foundation
Via Palestro 3
27100 Pavia
Italy

Joel R. Saper, M.D.
Michigan Head Pain and Neurological Institute
3120 Professional Drive
Ann Arbor, Michigan 48104-5199

Pramod R. Saxena, M.D.
Department of Pharmacology
Erasmus University
P.O. Box 1738
3000 DR Rotterdam
The Netherlands

Jean Schoenen, M.D.
University Department of Neurology
CHR Citadelle
Boulevard du 12eme de Ligne 1, and
University of Liège
Place du XX Aout
B-4000 Liège
Belgium

Robin G. Shanks, M.D.
Department of Therapeutics and Pharmacology
Queen's University of Belfast
The Whitla Medical Building
97 Lisburn Road
Belfast BT9 7BL
United Kingdom

Fred D. Sheftell, M.D.
Department of Psychiatry
New York Medical College
Valhalla, New York 10595, and
New England Center for Headache
778 Long Ridge Road
Stamford, Connecticut 06902

Stephen D. Silberstein, M.D.
Department of Neurology
Thomas Jefferson University, and
Department of Neurology
Jefferson Headache Center
Thomas Jefferson University Hospital
111 South 11th Street, Suite #8130
Philadelphia, Pennsylvania 19107-5092

Glen D. Solomon, M.D.
Merck & Co., Inc.
30125 Bolingbrook Road
Pepper Pike, Ohio 44124

Seymour Solomon, M.D.
Department of Neurology
Albert Einstein College of Medicine, and
Headache Unit
Department of Neurology
Montefiore Medical Center
111 East 210th Street
Bronx, New York 10467

Marjolijn J. Sorbi
Associate Professor
Department of Health Psychology
Utrecht University
3508 TC Utrecht
The Netherlands

Per Soelberg Sørensen, M.D., D.MSc.
University of Copenhagen
Department of Neurology
Copenhagen University Hospital
Rigshospitalet
DK-2100 Copenhagen
Denmark

Timothy J. Steiner, M.B., L.L.M., Ph.D.
Reader, Division of Neuroscience
Imperial College School of Medicine
Charing Cross Campus
Fulham Palace Road
London W6 8RP
United Kingdom

Walter F. Stewart, M.D.
Department of Epidemiology
School of Hygiene and Public Health
The Johns Hopkins University
615 North Wolfe Street
Baltimore, Maryland 21205

Svend Strandgaard, M.D.
Department of Nephrology
Herlev Hospital
DK-2730 Herlev
Denmark

Andrew M. Strassman, M.D.
Department of Anesthesia
Harvard Medical School, and
Assistant in Anesthesia
Department of Anesthesia and Critical Care,
DANA-717
Beth Israel Deaconess Medical
Center
330 Brookline Avenue
Boston, Massachusetts 02215

Pawan Suri, M.D.
Department of Emergency Medicine
Henry Ford Hospital
2799 West Grand Boulevard
Detroit, Michigan 48202

Norihiro Suzuki, M.D.
Department of Neurology
Kitasato University
1-15-1 Kitasato
Sagamihara, Kanagawa 228-8555
Japan

Peter Svensson, D.D.S.
Center for Sensory-Motor Interaction
Aalborg University
Frederik Bajers Vej 7D
DK-9220 Aalborg E, and
Clinical Associate
Royal Dental College
University of Århus
Vennelyst Boulevard
DK-8000 Århus C
Denmark

Christopher F. Terrence, M.D.
Department of Neuroscience
New Jersey Medical School
185 South Orange Avenue
Newark, New Jersey 07102, and
VA New Jersey Health Care System
385 Tremont Avenue
East Orange, New Jersey 07019-1095

Peer Tfelt-Hansen, M.D.
Department of Neurology
Glostrup Hospital
University of Copenhagen
DK-2600, Glostrup, Copenhagen
Denmark

Lars Lykke Thomsen, M.D.
Department of Neurology
Glostrup Hospital
University of Copenhagen
DK-2600 Glostrup, Copenhagen
Denmark

Noboru Toda, M.D.
Department of Pharmacology
School of Medicine
Shiga University of Medical Sciences
Seta, Ohtsu 520-2192
Japan

B. Todd Troost, M.D.
Department of Neurology
Wake Forest University School of Medicine
Medical Center Boulevard
Winston-Salem, North Carolina 27157-1078

Steinar Vilming, M.D.
Department of Neurology
Ullevaal Hospital, University of Oslo
Kirkevn. 166
0407 Oslo
Norway

Maurice Vincent, M.D.
Department of Neurology
Faculdade de Medicina
Universidade Federale do Rio de Janeiro, and
Headache Sector
Servico de Neurologia
Hospital Universitário Clementino Fraga Filho
Av. Brig. Trompowski, S/N
Rio de Janeiro, RJ 21949-590
Brazil

Elisabet Waldenlind, M.D.
Department of Neurology
Karolinska Institute, and
Department of Neurology
Huddinge University Hospital
S-14186 Huddinge
Sweden

Michael Wall, M.D.
Departments of Neurology, Ophthalmology, and
  Visual Sciences
University of Iowa
200 Hawkins Drive
Iowa City, Iowa 52242

K. Michael A. Welch, M.D.
Department of Neurology
University of Kansas School of Medicine
University of Kansas Medical Center
3023 Murphy
3901 Rainbow Boulevard
Kansas City, Kansas 66106

Clifford J. Woolf, M.D.
Department of Anesthesiology and Critical Care
Harvard Medical School
240 Longwood Avenue
Boston, Massachusetts 02115, and
Neural Plasticity Research Group
Department of Anesthesiology and Critical Care
Massachusetts General Hospital
149 13th Street, Room 4309
Charlestown, Massachusetts 02129

Alessandro S. Zagami, M.D.
Department of Medicine
University of New South Wales, and
Senior Staff Specialist in Neurology
Institute of Neurological Sciences
Prince of Wales Hospital
High Street
Randwick
Sydney, New South Wales 2031
Australia

Preface to the First Edition

Many factors prompted us to prepare this book at this time. Headache has always been important clinically, but only within the last decade has a body of solid, research-based evidence grown enough to justify a comprehensive, reference-type volume devoted exclusively to the headaches. The possibilities for diagnosing and classifying headaches greatly improved upon publication of the headache classification and operational diagnositic criteria of the International Headache Society in 1988. This book faithfully adheres to the new classification concerning terminology, diagnostic criteria, and order of presentation.

Our aim has been to include, in one volume, the scientific foundations, the diagnosis, and the management of all headaches. Each chapter is based on a critical evaluation of the published literature, and all contributors have been scientifically active within the topics that they cover. In the field of headache, many important new research findings have been made in centers around the world. For this reason, we have tried to present an internationally useful and accepted volume. Many of the chapters have been written by collaborators from different centers; often, an author from North America together with an author from outside North America. We feel that this has assured international representation. The involvement of many authors and the principle of joint authorship have made it difficult to achieve homogeneity across chapters. Although we have attempted to eliminate this problem, it is inevitably not always with complete success. We hope that the scientific expertise and personal involvement of the authors make up for any inconsistencies.

Jes Olesen, M.D.
Peer Tfelt-Hansen, M.D.
K.M.A. Welch, M.D.

Preface

The first edition of this book was in many ways an experiment. Was the scientific body of evidence sufficient to justify an extensive reference volume? Were the many clinicians who work with headache patients ready for an encyclopedia of headaches? And was it possible to produce a volume that could satisfy the needs on both sides of the Atlantic and in the rest of the world? We are pleased that the book did indeed prove successful and that it has established itself as the primary source of reference in the headache field.

Since the first edition, headache research has progressed at an ever-accelerating pace. The mechanisms have been elucidated by the demonstration of the first headache gene, which codes for a voltage-gated calcium channel and in which mutations cause familial hemiplegic migraine. PET studies have demonstrated a brain stem center possibly generating the migraine attack as well as hypothalamic activation cluster headache. New insights have been gained into the molecular mechanisms of migraine pain incriminating, in particular, nitric oxide as an offending molecule. Therapy has advanced equally with the advent of several new treatments for acute migraine attacks and cluster headache. Tension-type headache is a new field of investigation, which is still in its infancy. Nevertheless, much has been learned about its mechanisms and treatment since the first edition. These and many more advances have made a new edition necessary.

We have not made radical changes in the highly successful format of the first edition, but we do believe that we have managed to organize the material in a somewhat more logical and coherent fashion. We have kept the system of shared authorship for most chapters. The necessity for change varies widely in the individual chapters a few contain just minor revisions but the majority has been extensively revised and several have been completely rewritten. We have also deleted some chapters and added a few new ones for example, the chapter on the relation between sleep and headache and chapters on serotonin.

Headache patients constitute the largest group of patients in neurological practice and the huge need for better diagnosis and treatment of headache patients has become better recognized during the last six years. Also, headache research has taken its place as one of the leading fields of neurological progress and headache has been a major theme at most of the important recent neurological congresses. Unfortunately, complicated headache patients still have to wait for organized, multidisciplinary headache clinics at referrals and university departments. A goal for the next six years is to create major improvements in the availability and quality of headache treatment.

We hope that the present volume will contribute to further manifest headache as a core discipline of neurology and that it will be a stimulus to develop better service for headache patients.

Jes Olesen, M.D.
K. Michael A. Welch, M.D.
Peer Tfelt-Hansen, M.D.

The Headaches, Second Edition, edited by
J. Olesen, P. Tfelt-Hansen, and K.M.A. Welch.
Lippincott Williams & Wilkins, Philadelphia © 2000.

General Aspects of the Headaches

CHAPTER 1

Historical Background

Hansruedi Isler and F. Clifford Rose

MESOPOTAMIA, EGYPT, GREECE, ROME: FROM MYTHOLOGY TO MEDICINE

> Headache roameth over the desert, blowing like the wind,
> Flashing like lightning, it is loosed above and below;
> It cutteth off him who feareth not his god like a reed,
> like a stalk of henna it slitteth his thews.

These Assyrio-Babylonian translations for the library at Niniveh from the 7th century B.C. (36) describe various severe internal diseases under the heading of headache; it would be wrong to interpret "flashing like lightning" (or "like a star" or "eyes full of cloud") as visual migraine aura; the context suggests a cachectic fever, and malaria or infections are much more likely explanations. Such headache was believed to be caused by demons and was treated by incantations and a wide variety of healing materials fastened on the head. The same can be said of Egyptian descriptions, but the one-sided appearance of severe headache is often quite impressive, especially when the gods Horus and Seth are both complaining about their headaches, or when the god Horus invokes the goddesses Isis and Nyphthys, begging them to let down a spare head on him from the sky as he cannot stand his one-sided headache any longer (2). The word for this, *ges tep,* appears in three papyri from 1500 B.C. to 250 A.D. (Rosalind Park, personal communication, 1996). It has been translated as "migraine," but this one-sided headache without other known migraine symptoms might as well have been cluster headache, trigeminal neuralgia, local infection or infestation, or a result of neoplastic

lesions. Similarly, prehistorical trepanned skulls found in Egypt have been explained as relics of brain surgery for headache, but no further evidence supports this claim, although scraping the forehead down to the bone to make it bleed was a headache remedy among the fellahin up until the twentieth century.

The Greeks regarded headache as a serious complaint. In the Hippocratic books it appears as a symptom of dangerous disease, along with fever, nausea, vomiting, bleeding from the nose, convulsions, and various sensory disturbances (38). Even Zeus, the supreme god, complained of insupportable headache for which he forced Vulcan to split his head with an axe, thus giving birth from his head to Pallas Athene, goddess of learning and strategy (11) (Fig. 1). Plato's dialogue "Charmides" has Socrates promise a headache drug to the hero provided he first undergoes Socrates' psychotherapy—for you cannot treat the eyes without curing the head, the head without treating the body, nor the body without treating the soul (23).

In Rome, in the first century A.D., the Greek physician Aretaeus of Cappadocia (Fig. 2) wrote a textbook of neurologic diseases including headache, epilepsy, and hysteria (1). He set the pattern for such textbooks up to the nineteenth century, and his division of headaches into heterocrania (migraine), cephalalgia (mild or infrequent headache), and cephalea (frequent or chronic severe headache) survived together with his textbook pattern. Ultimately, it provided the roots of the 1988 international classification of the International Headache Society (IHS), where the distinction of migraine from tension-type headache (cephalea) was pivotal (9).

In the second century A.D., Galen of Pergamon (Fig. 3), another Greek doctor in Rome, established the foundation of future Islamic and European medicine up to the seventeenth century. Dependant on Aretaeus, he enriched

H. Isler: Neurologische Klinik, Universitäts Spital Zürich, CH-8091 Zürich, Switzerland.

F. C. Rose: London Neurological Centre, London, W1N 1AF, United Kingdom.

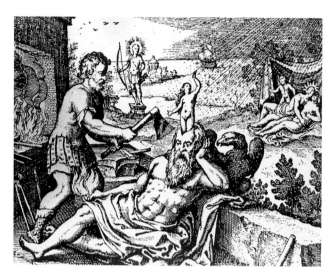

FIG. 1. Zeus and Vulcan, from an eighteenth century illustration.

the clinical descriptions and pathophysiologic theories (22): migraine is caused by yellow bile irritating intracranial structures, but the noxious matter is held back by the falx cerebri, therefore affecting only half of the brain and meninges. Throbbing pain originates from the blood vessels, tension pain (Greek *tonôdes*) from tendons or nerves. Today's tension headache is a late echo of this. Our word "migraine" came from Galen's hemicrania by way of France, where the sixteenth century novelist-

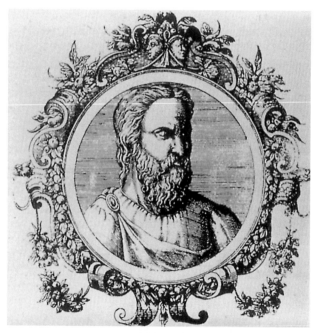

FIG. 2. Aretaeus, or Aretaios the Cappadocian, first century A.D. He gave the first unequivocal description of migraine. His classification of cephalalgia, cephalaea, and migraine is the root of modern classifications of headache.

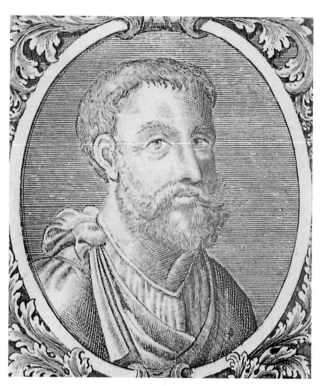

FIG. 3. Galen of Pergamon, second century A.D. He first used the term "hemicrania" and explained the headaches by assorted traditional pathophysiologic theories.

physician Rabelais used migraine as a term for a fire grenade (19). Galen's idea of yellow bile from the liver causing migraine survives to this day in France as a residue from the alcohol-prone colonial times: *migraine hépatique*. Another Greek idea lasted up to the middle ages. Aretaeus and Galen described what they called scotoma in Greek, but vertigo in Latin, mainly consisting of typical vestibular vertigo and oscillopsia. This was a disorder migraine could evolve into, but it was much more severe and dangerous than migraine itself. Greek scotoma is often mistaken for visual migraine aura, which more recently also has been referred to as scotoma ("dark eye"), whereas ancient Greek and Roman scotoma had nothing in common with migraine aura.

MEDIEVAL MEDICINE: BYZANTINE, MUSLIM, AND EUROPEAN HEIRS OF GALEN

The Greek medical heritage was kept alive in the Byzantine empire and was revived in the Islamic countries. In the sixth century, Alexander of Tralleis in Byzantium gave a detailed account of the headaches based on Aretaeus and Galen, as well as on his own practical experience (30). In the tenth century, the Persian physician Avicenna used Alexander's writings when he brought Galenic medicine and Aristotelian philosophy together. Avicenna observed that many headaches were not associated with brain damage or noxious substances because the senses were not dulled, but rather so acute that any sound, light, or smell would trigger a headache (32). He established a putative pathogenetic classification of *soda* (an Arabic word taken from the Persian *sar dard*, headache). A table of this classification was published in Latin and German in the sixteenth century (17), shortly before Paracelsus burned Avicenna's books in the marketplace.

European medieval teachings included Islamic concepts, combining various mystical ideas of the many headache saints with clinical impressions, such as Hildegard von Bingen's understanding of migraine comorbidity with melancholy (21) and the experimental natural science of Albert the Great and his fellow thirteenth century scientists. Hildegard had her own mystical visions, which have been interpreted as visual aura of migraine, with ornamental elements of illustrations suggestive of the zigzag contours of the aura. But her visions are far too structured for mere aura phenomena, and similar zigzag frames occur in other illuminated books of her time. Hildegard, a skilled clinical observer, had a striking explanation of the unilaterality of migraine: nobody could survive the atrocious pain if it were on both sides of the head.

RENAISSANCE MEDICINE: A GALENIC BASIS OF A MEDICAL REVOLUTION

In fifteenth and sixteenth century Galenic medicine (15), pulsatile and tensionlike pain are clearly attributed to blood vessels and nerves (nerves or tendons), respectively. This relic of Galen's pathophysiology is still extant in two current classification criteria: throbbing pain in migraine and tensionlike pain in tension type headache (9). The academic argumentation of Galenic textbooks of this period [e.g., Houllier and Fernel (15)] set the stage for the new medicine of the scientific revolution in the seventeenth century, when researchers such as Harvey and Willis strove to incorporate their new findings into the successful Galenic patterns.

THE SEVENTEENTH CENTURY NEUROLOGIST: CLASSIC DESCRIPTIONS OF HEADACHE

Charles Le Pois of Pont-à-Mousson (Fig. 4), Lorraine, explained epilepsy, hysteria, and migraine as intracranial diseases. He wrote of his own migraine with premonitory symptoms ("febricula," "a little fever"), attributing it to the stress and deprivations he had to sustain as a poor student. He described *hemicraniae insultus*, attacks of migraine with features of stroke, in a girl whom he observed from ages 12 to 17. At 12 she experienced a severe left temporal headache followed by bilious vomiting. The headache was preceded by a sense of numbness,

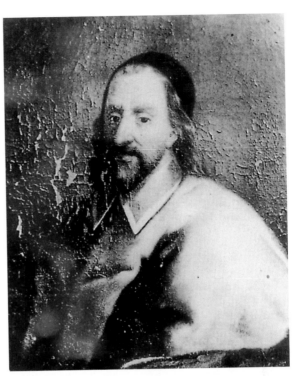

FIG. 4. Charles Le Pois, Latinized. Carolus Piso, 1563–1633, Pont-à-Mousson (Lorraine). He gave the first clear description of migraine with aura and of premonitory symptoms (1618) and explained migraine, epilepsy, and hysteria as cerebral disorders.

stiffness, and a sensation resembling the movement of ants crawling from her left little finger, across her other fingers and hand, and up the arm a*urae cujusdam instar ascendentis*, like an ascending breeze. Later attacks occurred in the temples and were often triggered by pleasant smells, such as musk, and associated with a numbness in her left limbs (25).

Thomas Willis of Oxford and London initiated systematic brain research with some highly qualified teams. He launched the term "neurology" in 1664, together with attempted localization of cerebral functions by human and animal dissections with intravenous dye injections. At least two of his localizations still prevail: he identified the gray cortex as the source, and tracts of white matter as the pathways of cerebral activity. In 1672, he wrote a textbook of neurophysiology and nervous diseases in which two chapters were devoted to headache (13). Among his many pathophysiologic assumptions is a hypothesis linking intracranial vasoconstriction with subsequent dilatation, not far beyond the old Galenic explanations but already nearly identical with Wolf's twentieth century vascular hypothesis of migraine. He described premonitory symptoms of migraine (*fames canina*, ravenous hunger) and the slow proximal spreading of some symptoms (nerve spasms), as well as seasonal accumulation of attacks. Willis found people of all constitutions, ages, and social standings among the headache sufferers.

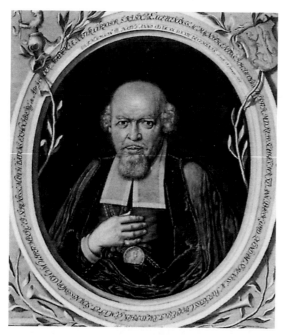

FIG. 5. Johann Jakob Wepfer, 1620–1695, Schaffhausen. He corrected the traditional ignorance concerning the cerebrovascular system and provided the first descriptions of subdural hematoma, trigeminal neuralgia, basilar migraine, migrainous stroke, and visual aura.

He said that headache was so little known that even the knowledge of quacks and old women might be useful; he had gained medical knowledge as a poor arts student, helping a canon's wife in the preparation of herbal drugs. His many remedies included at least one that would have worked: the newly introduced *potus cophey*, coffee.

Johann Jakob Wepfer (Fig. 5) of Schaffhausen on the Rhine reformed the knowledge of the cerebrovascular system. His book on stroke was cited by Willis, whom Wepfer held in great esteem. Wepfer launched the field of experimental toxicology, working with many associates who tried out drugs on all kinds of animals. His descriptions of trigeminal neuralgia, subdural hematoma, basilar migraine, and migrainous stroke are classic (12), and his clinical work on migraine reappeared in French and German textbooks of the eighteenth century. A case of transient hemianopia published in 1723 by Vater is usually mistaken for the first report of visual migraine aura. In this dissertation by J.C. Heinicke (10), the hemianopia appeared only once, without any associated migraine symptom. Wepfer's account of visual aura of 1727 (18), cited by Tissot, was based on a seventeenth century case and may be the earliest.

A NEW ART OF OBSERVATION: THE GREAT TEXTBOOKS OF THE EIGHTEENTH CENTURY

Herman Boerhaave in Leiden, the "teacher of Europe," and his star student van Swieten, who founded the Vienna School of Medicine, wrote a commentary to Hippocrates' aphorisms, the most influential medical textbook of the century. They managed to give a complete account of episodic cluster headache (16), the first known to us up to now. Robert Whytt, a Scottish student of Boerhaave, wrote a book on nervous diseases in 1764 (39). He explained them as results of sympathy between various parts of the body. The brain and the spinal cord were the sources of sympathy, and the soul, extending through the whole body by the nerves, was its mover. Altered sensitivity of disturbed nerves often caused irregular vascular reactions to various agents: "sudden changes of weather, errors in diet, fatigue of body, strong passions, suppression of ordinary evacuations … In migraine, the blood vessels are either affected with continual spasm, or agitated with uncommon alternate contractions and relaxations in consequence of which the patient feels a pain, fullness, and pulsation about the forehead and the temples." Carl Linné, one of Boerhaave's Scandinavian students, classified diseases according to his botanical methods. François Boissier de Sauvages in Montpellier did the

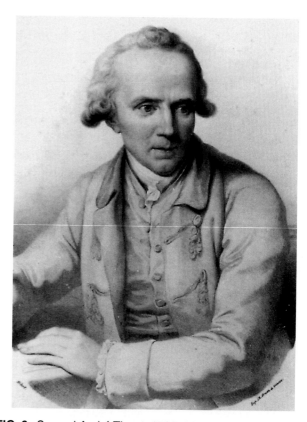

FIG. 6. Samuel André Tissot, 1728–1797, Lausanne. Author of medical bestsellers of the late eighteenth century. His *Traité des Nerfs*, the leading textbook on neurology in his time, contains a comprehensive account of migraine, which prepared the ground for new observations up until the middle of the nineteenth century.

same, including headache and migraine "from the moon" and "from insects." Samuel Auguste Tissot (Fig. 6) from Lausanne and Pavia, a student of Sauvages, wrote a textbook of neurologic diseases, *Traité des Nerfs et de leurs Maladies* (37), which provided the groundwork for the Parisian neurologists of the nineteenth century. When L. Thomas corrected the views of Paris neurologists on ophthalmic migraine in his book of 1887 (35), his main source of the eighteenth and earlier centuries was still Tissot's *Traité des Nerfs*. Tissot's friend Albrecht von Haller, who lost his migraine when he abstained from wine, confirmed that migraine was due to irritation of the stomach inducing a reaction in the supraorbital nerve. The *Traité des Nerfs* contains a detailed defense of the origin of migraine from the stomach. Tissot describes premonitory symptoms as well as the visual aura of migraine, including a hemianopic form, and, citing Wepfer, "flashes of light, scintillating false images."

John Fothergill (1712–1780), who made trigeminal neuralgia so well known that his name was used as an eponym, also introduced the term "fortification" for visual migraine aura: objects appear "surrounded with luminous angels like those of fortifications. A singular glimmering in the sight." He suffered personally from migraine, and his paper of 1778 (7) on "sick headache" was to make the complaint easily distinguished. It was a masterpiece.

A HARVEST OF MIGRAINE THEORIES IN NINETEENTH CENTURY EUROPE

Scientists (20) such as Wollaston, Wheatstone, and leading astronomers, John Herschel, Sir David Brewster, Sir George Biddell Airy, and Sir George's son, Dr. Hubert Airy, precisely drew and described their visual migraine aura, creating a need for better understanding of this puzzling symptom. "Ophthalmic migraine" became a popular term, and a group of physicians in Paris with an interest in neurology concluded that this form of migraine must be completely different from common migraine, a new disease entity in its own right. A neuralgia of the iris was discussed. The whole concept was rejected by L. Thomas in his book on migraine (35) of 1887, for which he was awarded a prize by the Paris faculty of medicine. He pointed out that most arguments for an isolated entity of ophthalmic migraine did not account for the nature of the aura; edema of the eyelid, conjunctival injection, and other peripheral eye symptoms were used as criteria for ophthalmic migraine, whereas visual aura all too often appeared in migraine patients who usually experienced migraine without aura.

The relationship of migraine and epilepsy became a central subject in England when E.H. Sieveking, who had published tables of the headache syndromes, wrote his book on epilepsy in 1858 (33). He found that 66% of his epileptic patients had headache with their seizures. Sieveking's views had considerable impact because he was involved with the introduction of bromide, the first effective anticonvulsant. In 1873, E. Liveing (26) described migraine as a "nerve-storm" raging within the brain, from the thalami to the centers governing the sympathetic system. John Hughlings Jackson (18) said in 1888, "I should class migraine, epilepsy proper, and epileptiform seizures as epilepsies, on the basis that in each there is a discharging lesion of some part of the cerebral cortex... but in so classifying them... I no more overlook their vast differences... than I confound whales, bats, and hedgehogs when I say that all these animals are mammals." Similarly, P.J. Moebius in Germany introduced his status migrainosus in analogy with "status epilepticus" at the end of the century (27). And W.R. Gowers wrote in 1907 (8), "Some surprise may be felt that migraine is given a place in the borderland of epilepsy, but the position is justified by many relations." This position was still kept by Wilder Penfield and Jasper in 1954 (31), and even longer by the pediatric neurologists who treated migraine with anticonvulsants up to the 1970s, 25 years before valproate and gabapentin were shown to be effective migraine prophylactics.

When Emile Du Bois-Reymond in Berlin developed experimental electrophysiology around the middle of the century, he also developed his migraine theory. He was pale when he had migraine. He concluded that migraine was caused by sympathetic hyperactivity inducing vasospasm (3). Möllendorf, a general practitioner in Berlin, reported on patients whose faces became red during migraine attacks. He thought that migraine was due to paralysis of the sympathetic system (28). These contrasting views have remained imprinted on the vascular theories of migraine until the present time. Möllendorf's paper was misunderstood for 125 years as an early description of cluster headache (34). Eulenburg in Germany in 1871 (4) and Latham in England in 1887 (24) sought to reconcile the antagonistic theories by placing them in a more comprehensive context. Eulenburg accepted both forms of migraine (4), reporting successful treatment of the red, angioparalytic form of migraine by subcutaneous ergotamine injections in 1883 (5); oral ergot had been used for migraine at least since 1862 (29). Autonomic vasomotor theories dominated migraine for more than a century, accompanied by a fringe of divergent ideas. Perhaps the most important of these was the group of neuralgia theories, although Romberg's neuralgia of the brain was denounced by Eulenburg as a mere tautology. Trigeminal, nasal, cervical, muscular, dural, glandular, cortical, and neurotoxic theories linked ancient Galenic tenets with the ideas prevailing now, at the end of the twentieth century. Flatau (Fig. 7) (6) summed up the situation at the end of the nineteenth century, concluding that none of them can elucidate all phenomena of the disorder.

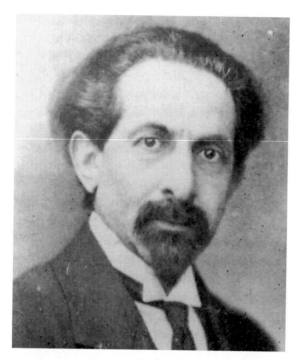

FIG. 7. Edward Flatau, 1868–1932, Warsaw, founder of Polish neurology. His unique monograph of 1912, *Die Migräne*, contains a thoroughly structured survey of most earlier authors, precise clinical observations, a critical evaluation of pathophysiology, and uncritical opinions on treatment, including arsenic cures.

TWENTIETH CENTURY, FIRST HALF: A NEW ERGOT TRIGGERS MIGRAINE RESEARCH

It was again ergotamine, this time in pure form (1916), that motivated clinical research on migraine from 1919 and onward in Switzerland, Germany, and the United States. In 1928, ergotamine was compared with placebo, an early approach to the scientific methodology of drug trials of the 1990s. Among the secondary effects of the new drug were the classic 1948 book by H.G. Wolf, *Headache and Other Head Pain,* based on clinical and experimental data (40), and the ad hoc classification of headaches in 1956. Ergotamine also led to recognition of drug-induced chronic headache in the United States by Bayard C. Horton, at first attributed to the "ergot cycle," but the same is found in any other instant relief-type drugs that stop migraine attacks.

TWENTIETH CENTURY, SECOND HALF: MIGRAINE CLINICS AND THE TRIPTANS

After World War II, the development of pain clinics induced the design of migraine clinics in the United States and Europe (e.g., London, Copenhagen, Florence, Zurich) and of a small international community of headache specialists, many of whom are among the authors of the present book. One of their achievements is

the first international classification of headaches in 1988 (9).

Pathophysiologic research in Florence and Sydney presented evidence for a special role of serotonin in the course and control of migraine attacks, eventually leading to the development of prophylactic serotonin antagonists. Specific serotonin receptor agonists for the acute treatment of the migraine attack were then developed in the United Kingdom, amounting to an entirely new pathophysiologic and pharmacologic research system.

REFERENCES

1. Adams F, editor and translator. *the extant works of Aretaeus, the Cappadocian.* London: New Sydenham Society, 1856.
2. Borghouts JF. *The magical texts of papyrus Leiden I 348.* Leiden: E.J. Brill, 1971:15–24.
3. Du Bois-Reymond E. Zur Kenntniss der Hemikranie. *Arch Anat Physiol Wissensch Med* 1860;461–468.
4. Eulenburg A. *Lehrbuch der functionellen Nervenkrankheiten.* Berlin: August Hirschwald, 1871
5. Eulenburg A. Subcutane Injectionen von Ergotinin- (Tanret) = Ergotininum citricum solutum (Gehe). *Deutsche Med Wochenschr* 1883;9:636–640.
6. Flatau E. *Die migräne.* Berlin: Verlag Julius Springer, 1912.
7. Fothergill J. Remarks on that complaint … under the name of the sick headache. *Med Observe Inquiry* 1777–1784;6:103–107, London.
8. Gowers WR. *The Border-land of epilepsy.* London: J & A Churchill: 1907.
9. Headache Classification Committee of the International Headache Society. Classification and diagnostic criteria for headache disorders, cranial neuralgias and facial pain. *Cephalalgia* 1988;8[Suppl. 7]:1–96.
10. Heinicke JC. (mostly wrongly cited as "Vater") *Dissertatio inauguralis medica qua visus vitia duo rarissima, alterum duplicati, alterum dimidiati.* Wittenbergae: Litteris Viduae Gerdesiae, 1723.
11. Hemsterhuis T, ed. *Luciani Samosatensis* colloquia selecta. Hephaistos kai Zeus. Amstelaedami: apud Wetstenios, 1708:67.
12. Isler H. Johann Jakob Wepfer (1620–1695): discoveries in headache. *Cephalalgia* 1985;[Suppl. 3]:424–425. Main source: Wepfer *J. Obs de Affectibus Capitis.* Scaphusiae: Ziegler, 1727.
13. Isler H. Thomas Willis' chapters on headache of 1672. *Headache* 1986; 26:95–98.
14. Isler H. The origins of neurology in the 17th century. In: Rose FC, ed. *Neuroscience across the centuries.* London: Smith-Gordon Nishimura, 1989:79–86.
15. Isler H. The Galenic tradition and migraine. *J Hist Neurosci* 1992;1:227–233.
16. Isler H. Episodic cluster headache from a textbook of 1745: Van Swieten's classic description. *Cephalalgia* 1993;13:172–174. Primary source: Van Swieten G. *Commentaria in Hermanni Boerhaave aphorismos de cognoscendis et curandis morbis.* Vol. II. Lugduni Batavorum: Apud Johannem et Hermanum Verbeek, 1745:534.
17. Isler H, Agarwalla P, Jagella C. Differential diagnosis of headaches in the 16th century: Bouhahylyha Byngezla's system. In print. *Cephalalgia* 1998;18. Source: Bouhahylyha Byngezla. *Tacuini Aegritudinum.* Strasbourg: Argentorati, 1532.
18. Jackson JH. Remarks on the diagnosis and treatment of diseases of the brain. *Br Med J* 1888;2:59–63, 111–117.
19. Jaquet C. *Joyce et Rabelais.* Paris: Didier, 1972. Source: Sainéan L. *La langue de Rabelais.* Paris: E. de Boccard, 1922:342. (cf. Joyce J. Finnegans wake. p. 4. Malachus Micgranes.)
20. Jarcho S. Migraine in astronomers and "natural philosophers." *Bull NY Acad Med* 1968;44:886–891.
21. Kaiser P, ed. *Hildegardis causae et curae.* Lipsiae: Aedibus B.G. Teubneri, 1903:90.
22. Kuehn CG, ed. *Claudii Galeni opera omnia.* Vol. XII. De locis affectis. Leipzig: Officina Car. Cnoblochii, 1826.
23. Lamb WRM, editor and translator. *Plato, Charmides etc.* Loeb Classical Library. London: William Heinemann, 1977:18–21.
24. Latham PW. *On nervous or sick headache, its varieties and treatment.* Cambridge, England: Deighton, Bell & Company, 1873.

25. Le Pois Ch. (Piso, Carolus). *Selectiorum observationum et consiliorum de praeteritis hactenus morbis, effectibusque praeter naturam ab aqua, seu serosa colluvie et diluvie, ortis liber singularis.* Lugduni Batavorum 1733 (Ponti ad Monticulum: 1618).

26. Liveing E. *On megrim, sick-headache, and some allied disorders.* London: J. and A. Churchill, 1873.

27. Möbius PJ. *Die Migräne.* Vienna: Alfred Hölder, 1898.

28. Möllendorf W. Ueber Hemikranie. *Virchows Arch Pathol Anat Klin Med* 1867;41:285–295.

29. Moretti E. Storia di una cefalalgia scorbutica guarita mediante l'uso interno dell'estratto di segale cornuto. *Giorn Med Mil* 1862;10: 392–394.

30. Patsioti I. Alexander of Tralleis on headache. In print. *Cephalalgia* 1998:18.

31. Penfield W, Jasper H. *Epilepsy and the functional anatomy of the human brain.* Boston: Little, Brown & Company: 1954.

32. Rolfinck W. *Ordo et methodus medicinae commentatoriae, hos en eidei cognoscendi et curandi dolorem capitis.* Jena: Johannes Nisius, 1671.

33. Sieveking EH. *On epilepsy and epileptiform seizures.* London: John Churchill, 1858.

34. Sjaastad O. *Cluster headache syndrome.* London: WB Saunders, 1992:9.

35. Thomas L. *La migraine.* Paris, 1887 (Prix Civrieux 1886).

36. Thompson RC. *The devils and evil spirits of Babylonia.* London: Luzac and Co., 1904. The Ninth Tablet (65 f.).

37. Tissot SA. (Weber FA, translator.) *Abhandlung von den Nerven und ihren Krankheiten.* Vierter Band: Ueber die Natur und Heilung einiger wichtiger Nervenkrankheiten (migraine, epilepsy, among others). Königsberg: CG Dengel, 1783:94–159.

38. Van der Linden JA, ed. *Magni Hippocratis Coi opera omnia Graece & Latine.* 2 vols. Lugduni Batavorum: apud Danielem, Abrahamum & Adrianum à Gaasbeeck, 1665.

39. Whytt R. *Observations on the nature, causes and cure of those diseases which are commonly called nervous, hypochondriac or hysteric; to which are prefixed some remarks on the sympathy of the nerves.* London: Becket, Du Hondt/Edinburgh: Balfour, 1765.

40. Wolff HG. *Headache and other head pain.* New York: Oxford University Press, 1948.

The Headaches, Second Edition,
edited by J. Olesen, P. Tfelt-Hansen, and K.M.A. Welch.
Lippincott Williams & Wilkins, Philadelphia © 2000.

General Aspects of the Headaches

CHAPTER 2

Classification of Headache

Jes Olesen

Classification may sound like a boring topic, but it is essential to everything a practicing physician does. We all diagnose and treat on the basis of some sort of classification and diagnostic criteria, often without knowing it. Formal disease classification and diagnostic criteria are difficult to remember and are often difficult to apply in routine clinical practice. It is important, however, that routine diagnosis be a reflection of a consistent classification system and a set of scientifically derived diagnostic criteria.

The ideal disease classification makes order out of chaos. It specifies how many different disorders should be recognized within a particular field and subclassifies these disorders. All available evidence, including that derived from complicated and experimental procedures, is used. Disease taxonomy often varies from country to country, but it should be international. In the past, so-called disease definitions were popular. These were brief descriptions of the diseases without specific requirements regarding number, duration, and severity of symptoms and signs or laboratory findings. In recent years, it has been realized that operational diagnostic criteria, that is, diagnostic criteria by which all requirements are quantitatively specified, must replace nonoperational definitions of all diseases.

The classification of headache disorders has followed the general trend. No internationally accepted classification or diagnostic criteria existed until the 1960s. In 1963 an ad hoc committee of the United States National Institutes of Health produced a classification of headache disorders that, at the time, represented a major step forward

(1). Unfortunately its so-called definitions were open to interpretation. Migraine, for example, was defined as "recurrent attacks of headache, widely varied in intensity, frequency, and duration. The attacks are commonly unilateral in onset; are usually associated with anorexia, and sometimes with nausea and vomiting; and some are preceded by, or associated with, conspicuous sensory, motor, and mood disturbances; and are often familial." Cluster headache was regarded as a subform of migraine but was later documented to be unrelated to migraine.

Some attempts were made to operationalize previous diagnostic criteria so that readers of scientific papers would be able to judge which type of patients had been studied (21,33). These criteria gained some support but were never internationally accepted. In 1985 the International Headache Society (IHS) formed a headache classification committee, which in 1988 published the first international headache classification that included operational diagnostic criteria for all headache disorders (9) (Table 1). This classification was endorsed by all national headache societies represented in the IHS and also by the World Federation of Neurology. The complete international headache classification has been translated into German (30), French (11), Italian (5), Spanish (36), Turkish (4), and many other languages. The World Health Organization (WHO) accepted the major principles of the new classification, which have been used in the International Classification of Diseases 10 (ICD 10) (37). A more extensive use of the IHS classification was made in ICD 10 neurological adaptation (38), and recently the WHO guide to headache diagnosis provided a crossway between ICD 10 NA and the IHS classification (13). An example is given in Table 2. It can be said with confidence that the IHS classification has been universally accepted and that no competing classification exists.

J. Olesen: Department of Neurology, Glostrup Hospital, University of Copenhagen, DK-2600 Glostrup, Copenhagen, Denmark.

TABLE 1. *Classification of headache disorders, cranial neuralgias, and facial pain (9)*

1. Migraine
1.1 Migraine without aura
1.2 Migraine with aura
    1.2.1 Migraine with typical aura
    1.2.2 Migraine with prolonged aura
    1.2.3 Familial hemiplegic migraine
    1.2.4 Basilar migraine
    1.2.5 Migraine aura without headache
    1.2.6 Migraine with acute onset aura
1.3 Ophthalmoplegic migraine
1.4 Retinal migraine
1.5 Childhood periodic syndromes that may be precursors to or associated with migraine
    1.5.1 Benign paroxysmal vertigo of childhood
    1.5.2 Alternating hemiplegia of childhood
1.6 Complications of migraine
    1.6.1 Status migrainosus
    1.6.2 Migrainous infarction
1.7 Migrainous disorder not fulfilling above criteria

2. Tension-type headache
2.1 Episodic tension-type headache
    2.1.1 Episodic tension-type headache associated with disorder of pericranial muscles
    2.1.2 Episodic tension-type headache unassociated with disorder of pericranial muscles
2.2 Chronic tension-type headache
    2.2.1 Chronic tension-type headache associated with disorder of pericranial muscles
    2.2.2 Chronic tension-type headache unassociated with disorder of pericranial muscles
2.3 Headache of the tension-type not fulfilling above criteria

3. Cluster headache and chronic paroxysmal hemicrania
3.1 Cluster headache
    3.1.1 Cluster headache periodicity undetermined
    3.1.2 Episodic cluster headache
    3.1.3 Chronic cluster headache
        3.1.3.1 Unremitting from onset
        3.1.3.2 Evolved from episodic
3.2 Chronic paroxysmal hemicrania
3.3 Cluster headache-like disorder not fulfilling above criteria

4. Miscellaneous headaches unassociated with structural lesion
4.1 Idiopathic stabbing headache
4.2 External compression headache
4.3 Cold stimulus headache
    4.3.1 External application of a cold stimulus
    4.3.2 Ingestion of a cold stimulus
4.4 Benign cough headache
4.5 Benign exertional headache
4.6 Headaches associated with sexual activity
    4.6.1 Dull type
    4.6.2 Explosive type
    4.6.3 Postural type

5. Headache associated with head trauma
5.1 Acute posttraumatic headache
    5.1.1 With significant head trauma and/or confirmatory signs
    5.1.2 With minor head trauma and no confirmatory signs
5.2 Chronic posttraumatic headache
    5.2.1 With significant head trauma and/or confirmatory signs
    5.2.2 With minor head trauma and no confirmatory signs

6. Headache associated with vascular disorders
6.1 Acute ischemic cerebrovascular disease
    6.1.1 Transient ischemic attack (TIA)
    6.1.2 Thromboembolic stroke
6.2 Intracranial hematoma
    6.2.1 Intracerebral hematoma
    6.2.2 Subdural hematoma
    6.2.3 Epidural hematoma
6.3 Subarachnoid hemorrhage
6.4 Unruptured vascular malformation
    6.4.1 Arteriovenous malformation
    6.4.2 Saccular aneurysm
6.5 Arteritis
    6.5.1 Giant cell arteritis
    6.5.2 Other systemic arteritides
    6.5.3 Primary intracranial arteritis
6.6 Carotid or vertebral artery pain
    6.6.1 Carotid or vertebral dissection
    6.6.2 Carotidynia (idiopathic)
    6.6.3 Post endarterectomy headache
6.7 Venous thrombosis
6.8 Arterial hypertension
    6.8.1 Acute pressor response to exogenous agent
    6.8.2 Pheochromocytoma
    6.8.3 Malignant (accelerated) hypertension
    6.8.4 Preeclampsia and eclampsia
6.9 Headache associated with other vascular disorder

7. Headache associated with nonvascular intracranial disorder
7.1 High cerebrospinal fluid pressure
    7.1.1 Benign intracranial hypertension
    7.1.2 High-pressure hydrocephalus
7.2 Low cerebrospinal fluid pressure
    7.2.1 Postlumbar puncture headache
    7.2.2 Cerebrospinal fluid fistula headache
7.3 Intracranial infection
7.4 Intracranial sarcoidosis and other non-infectious inflammatory diseases
7.5 Headache related to intrathecal injections
    7.5.1 Direct effect
    7.5.2 Due to chemical meningitis
7.6 Intracranial neoplasm
7.7 Headache associated with other intracranial disorder

8. Headache associated with substances or their withdrawal
8.1 Headache induced by acute substance use or exposure
    8.1.1 Nitrate/nitrite induced headache
    8.1.2 Monosodium glutamate induced headache
    8.1.3 Carbon monoxide induced headache
    8.1.4 Alcohol-induced headache
    8.1.5 Other substances
8.2 Headache induced by chronic substance use or exposure
    8.2.1 Ergotamine induced headache
    8.2.2 Analgesics abuse headache
    8.2.3 Other substances

TABLE 1. *Continued.*

8.3 Headache from substance withdrawal (acute use)
  8.3.1 Alcohol withdrawal headache (hangover)
  8.3.2 Other substances
8.4 Headache from substance withdrawal (chronic use)
  8.4.1 Ergotamine withdrawal headache
  8.4.2 Caffeine withdrawal headache
  8.4.3 Narcotics abstinence headache
  8.4.4 Other substances
8.5 Headache associated with substances but with uncertain mechanism
  8.5.1 Birth control pills or estrogens
  8.5.2 Other substances

9. Headache associated with noncephalic infection
9.1 Viral infection
  9.1.1 Focal noncephalic
  9.1.2 Systemic
9.2 Bacterial infection
  9.2.1 Focal noncephalic
  9.2.2 Systemic (septicemia)
9.3 Headache related to other infection

10. Headache associated with metabolic disorder
10.1 Hypoxia
  10.1.1 High-altitude headache
  10.1.2 Hypoxic headache (low-pressure environment, pulmonary disease causing hypoxia)
  10.1.3 Sleep apnea headache
10.2 Hypercapnia
10.3 Mixed hypoxia and hypercapnia
10.4 Hypoglycemia
10.5 Dialysis
10.6 Headache related to other metabolic abnormality

11. Headache or facial pain associated with disorder of cranium, neck, eyes, ears, nose, sinuses, teeth, mouth or other facial or cranial structures
11.1 Cranial bone
11.2 Neck
  11.2.1 Cervical spine
  11.2.2 Retropharyngeal tendinitis
11.3 Eyes
  11.3.1 Acute glaucoma
  11.3.2 Refractive errors
  11.3.3 Heterophoria or heterotropia
11.4 Ears
11.5 Nose and sinuses
  11.5.1 Acute sinus headache
  11.5.2 Other diseases of nose or sinuses
11.6 Teeth, jaws and related structures
11.7 Temporomandibular joint disease (functional disorders are coded to group 2)

12. Cranial neuralgias, nerve trunk pain, and deafferentation pain
12.1 Persistent (in contrast to tic-like) pain of cranial nerve origin
  12.1.1 Compression or distortion of cranial nerves and second or third cervical roots
  12.1.2 Demyelination of cranial nerves
    12.1.2.1 Optic neuritis (retrobulbar neuritis)
  12.1.3 Infarction of cranial nerves
    12.1.3.1 Diabetic neuritis
  12.1.4 Inflammation of cranial nerves
    12.1.4.1 Herpes zoster
    12.1.4.2 Chronic postherpetic neuralgia
  12.1.5 Tolosa-Hunt syndrome
  12.1.6 Neck-tongue syndrome
  12.1.7 Other causes of persistent pain of cranial nerve origin
12.2 Trigeminal neuralgia
  12.2.1 Idiopathic trigeminal neuralgia
  12.2.2 Symptomatic trigeminal neuralgia
    12.2.2.1 Compression of trigeminal root or ganglion
    12.2.2.2 Central lesions
12.3 Glossopharyngeal neuralgia
  12.3.1 Idiopathic glossopharyngeal neuralgia
  12.3.2 Symptomatic glossopharyngeal neuralgia
12.4 Nervus intermedius neuralgia
12.5 Superior laryngeal neuralgia
12.6 Occipital neuralgia
12.7 Central causes of head and facial pain other than tic douloureux
  12.7.1 Anaesthesia dolorosa
  12.7.2 Thalamic pain
12.8 Facial pain not fulfilling criteria in groups 11 and 12

13. Headache not classifiable

TABLE 2. *Conversion table between the codes of the IHS Classification and ICD-10, ICD-NA*

IHS code	
Etiological code	Headache code
1. Migraine	G43
1.1 Migraine without aura	G43.0
1.2 Migraine with aura	G43.1
1.2.1 Migraine with typical aura	G43.10
1.2.2 Migraine with prolonged aura	G43.11
1.2.3 Familial hemiplegic migraine	G43.1 × 5′
1.2.4 Basilar migraine	G43.1 × 3′
1.2.5 Migraine aura without headache	G43.1 × 4′
1.2.6 Migraine with acute onset aura	G43.12
1.3 Ophthalmoplegic migraine	G43.80
1.4 Retinal migraine	G43.81
1.5 Childhood periodic syndromes that may be precursors to or associated with migraine	G43.82
1.5.1 Benign paroxysmal vertigo of childhood	G43.821
1.5.2 Alternating hemiplegia of childhood	G43.822
1.6 Complications of migraine	G43.3
1.6.1 Status migrainosus	G43.2
1.6.2 Migrainous infarction	G43.3
1.7 Migrainous disorder not fulfilling above criteria	G43.9

IHS, International Headache Society; ICD, International Classification of Diseases; NA, neurological adaptation.

THE INTERNATIONAL CLASSIFICATION OF HEADACHE DISORDERS

All headache disorders are organized into 13 major groups (Table 1). Groups 1 through 4 cover the primary headaches; groups 5 through 11 cover the secondary headaches; group 12 covers the cranial neurologias and facial pain; and group 13 is "headache not classifiable." Within each group, diagnoses are ordered in a hierarchic system using up to four digits, giving it universal applicability, because in general practice, for instance, doctors can classify to the first or second digit, whereas in specialist practice, the third and sometimes the fourth digits can be used. For some types of research, it is necessary to classify patients to the fourth digit. Although the original publication of the headache classification committee is a small book of almost 100 pages, essentials of the new classification, including diagnostic criteria, can be contained in a small pocket folder (10).

TAXONOMY AND PREVIOUSLY USED TERMS

The classification given in Table 1 includes the new taxonomy. In the past, headache taxonomy was bewildering. Many old terms have remained in use despite lack of agreement about their exact meaning. Examples are vidian neuralgia, Sluder's neuralgia, and erythromelalgia of the head. Much more serious, however, is that similar confusion prevailed regarding important forms of migraine, even within the English-speaking world. For example, the terms *classic* and *classical* migraine were used interchangeably and both with variable meaning. Some used the terms only for patients with a visual aura, and others included patients who also had aura symptoms from the extremities. Hemiplegic migraine was used to describe patients with hemiparesis by some, but more often the term also was used for patients with hemisensory symptoms. Nonexperts often confused the words *classical* and *typical*, so that a patient could have a classical common migraine. In the non-English-speaking world, discrepancies were even more pronounced. The committee decided, therefore, to create new terms when absolutely necessary and to indicate a translation into customary usage by listing previously used terms. This also will be done in the present volume. Among the more important changes are that common migraine became migraine without aura and classic/classical migraine became migraine with aura. The latter now includes the following previously used terms: migraine accompagné, hemiplegic, complicated, ophthalmic, hemisensory, aphasic, basilar, and confusional migraine. The previously used terms *muscle contraction headache* and *tension headache* also were abandoned in favor of the term *tension-type headache*. This term acknowledged our ignorance about the pathophysiology of the disorder while keeping open the possibility that a muscular factor is important as well as a central nervous system factor.

OPERATIONAL DIAGNOSTIC CRITERIA

The difficulty with an operational headache diagnosis is the lack of abnormalities in routine laboratory investigations. Sophisticated measurement techniques such as regional cerebral blood flow and transcranial Doppler cannot be used because the equipment is unavailable to most physicians when the diagnosis is made. The criteria of the IHS, therefore, depend largely on the headache history and the exclusion of organicity by physical and neurologic examinations and necessary laboratory tests. The IHS has used the system developed by the American Psychiatric Society for the operational diagnostic criteria of psychiatric disorders (7). The operational diagnostic criteria for migraine without aura are given in Table 3. The scheme consists of a number of letter headings: A, B, C, and so on. Each of the requirements under these letter headings has to be fulfilled to diagnose migraine without aura. Each letter heading may, however, cover several characteristics, not all of which need to be fulfilled. Therefore, features present in, for example, 50% of patients can be included. These criteria pertain to the characteristics of both headache and its associated symptoms. Note that, under C, it is required only that pain characteristics fulfill two of the four criteria. We have all seen typical migraine patients whose pain was bilateral or whose pain was not pulsating. Such patients can be accommodated easily in these operational diagnostic criteria if two of the other features fulfill criterion C. A similar situation is true for criterion D. Although most patients have nausea or vomiting or both during migraine

TABLE 3. *Diagnostic criteria for migraine without aura*

A. At least five attacks fulfilling B–D
B. Headache attacks lasting 4–72 h (untreated or unsuccessfully treated)
C. Headache has at least two of the following characteristics:
   1. Unilateral location
   2. Pulsating quality
   3. Moderate or severe intensity (inhibits or prohibits daily activities)
   4. Aggravation by walking stairs or similar routine physical activity
D. During headache at least one of the following:
   1. Nausea and/or vomiting
   2. Photophobia and phonophobia
E. At least one of the following:
   1. History and/or physical and/or neurological examinations do not suggest one of the disorders listed in groups 5–11
   2. History and/or physical and/or neurological examinations do suggest such disorder, but it is ruled out by appropriate investigations
   3. Such disorder is present, but migraine attacks do not occur for the first time in close temporal relation to the disorder

From ref. 9, with permission.

attacks, an occasional patient will have absolutely typical migraine but without nausea, which is possible if the patient has photophobia as well as phonophobia. The purpose of the rather complicated criterion E is to indicate that laboratory investigations are not necessary to exclude organic disorder in the great majority of headache patients.

Although the operational diagnostic criteria are by far the most important, the headache classification also provides the necessary definitions, that is, short descriptions of the disorders in normal language. These criteria are intended for use in textbooks and teaching purposes, and they are more readable. As an example, the short description of migraine without aura reads as follows: "idiopathic, recurring headache disorder manifesting in attacks lasting 4 to 72 hours. Typical characteristics of headache are unilateral location, pulsating quality, moderate or severe intensity, aggravation by routine physical activity, and association with nausea, photophobia, and phonophobia" (9).

HOW TO USE THE IHS CLASSIFICATION

The IHS classifies headaches, not patients. This situation is difficult to understand for the practicing physician facing the individual patient. This problem is similar to the classification of epilepsy. Attacks are easy to classify, but it is difficult to classify patients. The difficulties arise from the coexistence of different disorders and from changes in headache diagnosis over the years. Each discrete form of headache in a patient must be diagnosed. Some patients indicate that they have many different forms of headache, even if they are all varieties of a single form of headache according to the IHS classification. Other patients believe their different forms of headache are variations of the same diagnosis. The patient's history must be taken carefully, and it must be evaluated how many different forms of headache the patient has and which criteria are fulfilled. The diagnosis of *combination headache* has been abandoned; these patients are now classified as having migraine without aura and tension-type headache. Subforms of tension-type headache and cluster headache are mutually exclusive, but subforms of migraine are not. Thus, a patient can have more than one migraine diagnosis, for example, migraine without aura and migraine with aura.

If a patient receives two diagnoses, which is the more important, and how can the severity of the headache disorder be determined? It is recommended that physicians indicate the estimated number of headache days per year in brackets after each diagnosis, thereby adding a quantitative aspect to headache diagnosis. Not all headache episodes experienced by a patient can or should be diagnosed. Atypical episodes are frequent because of early treatment, lack of ability to remember symptoms exactly,

and other factors. The patient should be asked to describe typical untreated or unsuccessfully treated episodes. It should be decided which set of diagnostic criteria these episodes fulfill and whether the required number of episodes has been experienced. Then the number of days per year when the patient has this type of headache should be estimated, adding treated attacks and less typical attacks believed to be of the same type. In unclear cases, it is recommended that physicians ask the patient to keep a diagnostic headache diary (27). Prospective recording of symptoms usually makes the diagnostic process much more precise. If a particular form of headache fulfills two sets of criteria, the diagnosis mentioned first in the classification should be coded.

SCIENTIFIC EVALUATION OF THE IHS HEADACHE CLASSIFICATION

The ideal classification should be sensitive, specific, and exhaustive. Sensitivity is maximal if all patients with a particular form of headache are diagnosed as such. Specificity is maximal if only patients with a particular kind of headache receive the diagnosis, not patients with other kinds of headaches. It is difficult to evaluate these characteristics, however, because there is no "gold standard" with which to compare. Before the IHS classification was implemented, a study was conducted to compare patients diagnosed as usual with patients diagnosed according to the IHS criteria (15). Using for comparison the traditional method of diagnosing, the new criteria had good sensitivity and specificity.

The primary headaches constitute disease entities characterized by a clustering of specific combinations of symptoms. It is intuitively evident that the explicit diagnostic criteria for all headache disorders of the IHS (9) represent a substantial improvement over previous diagnostic systems. Nevertheless, the criteria require systematic field testing. Some fundamental requirements of a classification exist, one of which is that it should be *generalizable*, which means that it should be applicable in diverse settings (headache clinics, general practices, general populations, and others). The IHS criteria are derived from expert consensus. As such, they are based primarily on experience with highly selected migraine patients. Thus, the criteria might be expected to be most relevant in a specialist practice or in a hospital setting; however, in recent years, the IHS criteria have been used in several epidemiological studies from the general population and have been found to be highly applicable (19,23,24). Other basic requirements to the ideal classification are those of exhaustiveness, reliability, and validity. These aspects of the classification have been addressed in several studies (8,12,15–17,19,23,25).

Exhaustiveness indicates that it is possible to classify all headaches according to the diagnostic criteria (12,23), which was shown to be the case in a large Danish population-based study (23). *Reliability* encompasses low interobserver variability and repeatability and has been found to be quite good (8,16,27). *Validity* means that the diagnosis reflects the underlying biological disorder. Unfortunately, it is difficult to evaluate the validity because no gold standard exists. Nonetheless, different approaches have been used to study the validity of the classification. Some have compared the IHS diagnoses with the diagnoses of expert clinicians (12,17). Others (15,19) have validated the criteria by comparing with diagnoses obtained using the former Ad Hoc Committee classification of headache (1). Somewhat diverging results are reported mainly as a result of various methodological limitations in some studies.

In recent years, the IHS criteria have been used worldwide in several large multicenter, multinational, double-blind drug trials (31,34,35) (see also Chap. 52). These studies have shown remarkably consistent response rates to the triptans, reflecting the homogeneity of the defined migraine group. The validity also is reflected in consistent epidemiologic profiles and homogeneous nosologic entities of the various headache types that have been found in several epidemiological studies all using the IHS diagnostic criteria (2,6,12,18,24,28,31,32).

With the aim of assessing and improving the reliability and validity of the IHS criteria, future work should focus on continued field testing in various settings. More precise operationalization, including more explicit behavior-oriented criteria to define each individual feature, may improve the reliability, sensitivity, and specificity of the IHS diagnostic criteria.

CRITIQUE OF THE IHS CLASSIFICATION AND NEED FOR REVISION

Compared with other disease classifications, the IHS classification has received only modest critique. Most persistent has been the request for recognition of something called *chronic daily headache*, which of course is a step backward because it lumps together several different types of headache (22). The IHS approach to diagnose all discrete types of headaches is in line with WHO recommendations (37,38) and stimulates a stringent diagnostic approach, which helps in planning treatment. Several adjustments, however, are well argued: Sudden-onset chronic tension-type headache, SUNCT, hypnic headache, and perhaps hemicrania continua need to be recognized. A further digit should probably code for the most likely causative factor for migraine, as done for tension-type headache. Aggravation by excessive use of symptomatic medication is particularly important. Genetic coding of inherited syndromes needs to be worked into the classification. The second edition of the IHS classification is expected to be published in 2002.

RESEARCH OPPORTUNITIES OFFERED BY THE IHS CLASSIFICATION

One of the major advantages of operational diagnostic criteria is that they force us to think systematically and logically about clinical problems; it therefore exposes our ignorance and has led to renewed interest in questions such as, Is it true that migraine attacks last 4 to 72 hours? How often and among which age groups do they not? What is the interobserver variation of headache diagnosis? Can or should migraine without aura be subdivided into menstrual and nonmenstrual forms? In migraine with aura, does the headache always follow the aura? Can one migrainous aura symptom be shorter than 5 min or longer than 60 min and, if so, how often does this happen? Do different aura symptoms always occur in succession? The number of questions that can and should be answered by scientific studies is almost endless. As our knowledge of nosographic details improves, it will be easy to change the operational diagnostic criteria in future revisions of the headache classification. The operational diagnostic criteria make it possible to search for experimental models of migraine. Does nitroglycerine-induced headache really fulfill the criteria for migraine? Does histamine-induced headache fulfill them? These questions already have been answered positively, but there are many more. New treatments, such as (serotonin) 5HT1 receptor agonists, can be used to adjust the criteria. Do people respond to these drugs only if their headache fulfills migraine criteria, or do borderline patients also respond? Studies of the biochemistry and physiology of headaches also benefit from the classification. It is now possible to characterize precisely the headache episodes during which blood samples were drawn for analysis, for example, of platelet aggregation or serotonin content. It is also more clear whether different results in different studies are due to differences in patient material or methods.

USE OF THE HEADACHE CLASSIFICATION IN THIS VOLUME

The headache classification is used in several different ways in this volume. The book follows the sequence of the international headache classification and applies its taxonomy and operational diagnostic criteria. Each chapter begins with the IHS classification and then gives the short descriptions, operational diagnostic criteria, and previously used terms as listed in the IHS classification (9). The chapters describing the headache disorders present the material in the same sequence according to a general scheme: IHS and WHO code numbers; short description; other terms; epidemiology; genetics; anatomy and pathology; pathophysiology; clinical features, including operational diagnostic criteria prognosis; and management.

REFERENCES

1. Ad Hoc Committee on Classification of Headache. Classification of headache. *JAMA* 1962;179:717–718.

2. Breslau N, Davis GC, Andreski P. Migraine, psychiatric disorders, and suicide attempts: An epidemiologic study of young adults. *Psychiatry Res* 1991;37:11–23.

3. Cady RK, Wendt JK, Kirchner JR, Sargent JD, Rothrock JF, Skoggs H Jr. Treatment of acute migraine with subcutaneous sumatriptan. *JAMA* 1991;265:2831–2835.

4. Çelebi A, Özcan H. *Basarilari, kranial nevraljiler ve yüz a ?rilarinin siniflanmasi ve tani kriterleri.* Istanbul: Sandoz Ürünleri, 1990:1–113.

5. Commissione per la Classificazione delle Cefalee dell' International Headache Society. Classificazione e criteri diagnostici delle cefalee, delle nevralgie craniche e dei dolori facciali. In: Bussone G, Nappi G, Rossi F, eds. *Informatica e Cefalee.* Roma: Cluster Press, 1988:1–96.

6. Edmeads J, Findlay H, Tugwell P, Pryse-Philips W, Nelson RF, Murray TJ. Impact of migraine and tension-type headache on life-style, consulting behaviour, and medication use: a Canadian population survey. *Can J Neurol Sci* 1993;20:131–137.

7. *Diagnostic and Statistical Manual of Mental Disorders (DSM) IV.* Washington, DC: American Psychiatric Association, 1995.

8. Granella F, D Alessandro R, Manzoni GC, et al. International Headache Society classification: interobserver reliability in the diagnosis of primary headaches. *Cephalalgia* 1994;14:16–20.

9. Headache Classification Committee of the International Headache Society. Classification and diagnostic criteria for headache disorders, cranial neuralgias and facial pain. *Cephalalgia* 1988;8(Suppl 7):1–96.

10. Headache Classification Committee of the International Headache Society. Classification of headache disorders, cranial neuralgias and facial pain; and diagnostic criteria for primary headaches disorders. Pocket version. Cophenhagen: Headache Classification Committee (c/o Jes Olesen), 1989:1–16.

11. Henry P. Céphalées, nevralgies craniennes, douleurs de la face: classification et critères diagnostiques. *Rev Prat* 1990;5:416–444.

12. Henry P, Michel P, Brochet B, Dartiques JF, Tison S, Salamon R. A nationwide survey of migraine in France: prevalence and clinical features in adult. *Cephalalgia* 1992;12:229–237.

13. ICD-10 guide for headaches. *Cephalalgia* 1997;17(Suppl 19):1–82.

14. Isler H. *Klassifikation der Kopfschmerzen, Kopfneuralgien und Gesichtsschmerzen: diagnostische Kriterien für primäre Kopfwehsyndrome.* Baar: Janssen Pharmaceutica, 1990:1–35.

15. Iversen HK, Langemark M, Andersson PG, Hansen PE, Olesen J. Clinical characteristics of migraine and episodic tension-type headache in relation to old and new diagnostic criteria. *Headache* 1990;30:514–519.

16. Leone M, Filippini G, D'Amico D, Farinotti M, Bussone G. Assessment of International Headache Society diagnostic criteria: a reliability study. *Cephalalgia* 1994;14:280–284.

17. Michel P, Dartigues JF, Henry P, et al. Validity of the International Headache Society Criteria for Migraine. *Neuroepidemiology* 1993;12:51–57.

18. Michel P, Pariente P, Duru G, Dreyfuss J-P, Chabriat H, Henry P. Mig

19. Merikangas KR, Whitaker AE, Angst J. Validation of diagnostic criteria for migraine in the Zürich longitudinal cohort study. *Cephalalgia* 1993;13(Suppl 12):47–53.

20. Olesen J. The International Headache Society classification and diagnostic criteria are valid and extremely useful. *Cephalalgia* 1996;16:293–295.

21. Olesen J, Krabbe AAE, Tfelt-Hansen P. Methodological aspects of prophylactic drug trials in migraine. *Cephalalgia* 1981;1:127–141.

22. Olesen J, Rasmussen BK. The International Headache Society classification of chronic daily and near-daily headaches: a critique of the criticism. *Cephalalgia* 1996;16:407–411.

23. Rasmussen BK, Jensen R, Olesen J. A population-based analysis of the diagnostic criteria of the International Headache Society. *Cephalalgia* 1991;11:129–134.

24. Rasmussen BK, Jensen R, Schroll M, Olesen J. Epidemiology of headache in a general population—a prevalence study. *J Clin Epidemiol* 1991;44:1147–1157.

25. Rasmussen BK, Jensen R, Olesen J. Questionnaire versus clinical interview in the diagnosis of headache. *Headache* 1991;31:290–295.

26. Ravnik IM. Merila za razvr ?anje in diagnostiko glavobolov, nevralgij mo ganskih ivcev in obraznih bole in. Derevi *Pediatrini Dnevi* 1989;11:119–140.

27. Russell MB, Rasmussen BK, Brennum J, Iversen HK, Jensen R, Olesen J. Presentation of a new instrument: the diagnostic headache diary. *Cephalalgia* 1992;12:369–374.

28. Russell MB, Rasmussen BK, Thorvaldsen P, Olesen J. Prevalence and sex-ratio of the subtypes of migraine. *Int J Epidemiol* 1995;24:612–618.

29. Sakai F. *Jpn J Headache* 1991;18:91–103.

30. Soyka D, Lungershausen E. Klassifikation und diagnostische Kriterien f;auur Kopfschmerzerkrankungen, Kopfneuralgien und Gesichtsschmerz. *Nervenheilkunde* 1989;8:161–203.

31. Stewart WF, Lipton R, Celentano DD, Reed ML. Prevalence of migraine headache in the United States. *JAMA* 1992;267:64–69.

32. Stewart WF, Lipton RB, Liberman J. Variation in migraine prevalence by race. *Neurology* 1996;47:52–59.

33. Tfelt-Hansen P, Olesen J. Methodological aspects of drug trials in migraine. *Neuroepidemiology* 1985;4:204–226.

34. The Subcutaneous Sumatriptan International Study Group. Treatment of migraine attacks with sumatriptan. *N Engl J Med* 1991;325:316–321.

35. The Oral Sumatriptan Dose-Defining Study Group. Sumatriptan: an oral dose-defining study. *Eur Neurol* 1991;31:300–305.

36. Titus F, Targa C, Martinez-Lage JM, eds. *Classificasion y criterios diagnosticos de los cephalias, los neurolgias craneales y el dolor facial.* Barcelona: Editorial MCR, 1–107.

37. World Health Organization. *The International Statistical Classification of Diseases and Related Health Problems.* 10th rev. Geneva: World Health Organization, 1992–1994.

38. World Health Organization. *Application of the International Classification of Diseases to Neurology.* 2nd ed. Geneva: World Health Organization, 1997.

The Headaches, Second Edition,
edited by J. Olesen, P. Tfelt-Hansen, and K.M.A. Welch.
Lippincott Williams & Wilkins, Philadelphia © 2000.

General Aspects of the Headaches

CHAPTER 3

Epidemiology of Headache

Birthe Krogh Rasmussen and Richard B. Lipton

Epidemiologic studies are generally conducted in samples that are representative of a definable population such as a city, a country, or a school (16,40). These studies have contributed to our understanding of headache disorders from a number of perspectives. They have helped to clarify the demarcation among primary headache disorders and to assess the reliability, validity, and generalizability of various case definitions for various types of headache. Studies of headache prevalence have clarified the scope and distribution of the public health problem posed by migraine and tension-type headache among other disorders. Examination of sociodemographic, familial, and environmental risk factors help identify the groups at greatest risk for disease. Population-based studies also have demonstrated clinically important comorbidities, particularly for migraine. Burden of disease studies have shown that headache disorders have a profound impact on individual headache sufferers and on society as measured by quality of life, indirect costs, and patterns of health care utilization.

In this chapter we review some epidemiologic terms, discuss the importance of case definition in epidemiologic research, and consider some of the methodologic issues in headache epidemiologic research. We close by reviewing studies of headache prevalence overall; the epidemiology of specific headache disorders is discussed in other chapters.

B. K. Rasmussen: Department of Neurology, Hilleroed Hospital, DK-3400 Hilleroed, Denmark.

R. B. Lipton: Departments of Neurology, Epidemiology, and Social Medicine, Albert Einstein College of Medicine, and Headache Unit, Montefiore Medical Center, Bronx, New York 10467.

METHODOLOGIC ASPECTS

Headache Case Definitions

For clinical practice and epidemiologic research, it is important to have reliable and valid case definitions (18, 34). In this context, reliability requires that independent diagnostic evaluations yield consistent diagnostic results. Because headache diagnosis is symptom based, reliability is a function of the diagnostic criteria, the procedures used to collect diagnostic information, and the application of the information to the criteria. On the other hand, validity refers to the relationship between the assigned diagnosis and the underlying biology of the disorder. Because there is no true diagnostic gold standard for the primary headache disorders, validity is difficult to study. Validity is supported when our diagnostic groups include members with consistent epidemiologic profiles: common risk factors, natural histories, treatment response profiles, and biological or genetic markers.

Many case definitions for migraine and other headache disorders have been proposed. Although different definitions have emphasized different features, many criteria are poorly specified. For example, the criteria of the Ad Hoc Committee on Classification of Headache (1962) (2) do not specify the features or combinations of features required to establish or exclude a diagnosis, but only which features are usually present. Such a lack of clarity in case definition will invariably lead to unreliability in diagnosis both in epidemiologic research and in clinical practice.

Some researchers have included family history as a defining feature of migraine. Information provided by a patient about headache in relatives is often inaccurate (35). In addition, some studies have included family history as part of the migraine definition and then investigated the prevalence of headache in first-degree relatives of migraine sufferers, inescapably overestimating familial aggregation. Family history, in our view, should be a confirmatory, not a diagnostic, criterion.

Empirical approaches have been used to clarify the symptom features that distinguish migraine from tension-type headache. This work is sometimes interpreted to test the spectrum or continuum concept, the idea that migraine and tension-type headache exist as polar ends on a continuum of severity, varying more in degree than in kind. The alternative model views migraine and tension-type headache as distinct entities that differ in severity. Waters examined the associations between his three key features of migraine (warning, unilateral pain, and nausea or vomiting) in population-based samples and found that as headache intensity increased, migrainous symptoms occurred together more frequently (55,56,58). He concluded that "the distribution of the headache severity extends as a continuous spectrum from mild attacks, which usually have neither unilateral distribution nor warning nor nausea, to severe headaches which are frequently accompanied by the three migraine features." Other researchers have made similar arguments for the continuum concept.

In our view, these data do not distinguish the opposing models. These results are also compatible with the hypothesis that migraine and tension-type headache are distinct nosologic entities that differ in severity. Differences in epidemiologic profiles, patterns of family transmission, and treatment response suggest that migraine and tension-type headache are distinct (41). If the continuum concept is correct, the current literature on migraine describes the epidemiology of the upper tail of a distribution of severity rather than the epidemiology of a distinct disorder.

To improve the classification of headache disorders, in 1988 the International Headache Society (IHS) published its criteria for a broad range of headache disorders (12). The criteria, based on international expert consensus, are much more explicit than the prior consensus criteria. They clearly indicate the features that are required to confirm or exclude particular headache diagnoses. Empirical assessment of the criteria is an area of active research. In one study, four clinicians reviewed videotapes of structured interviews and then assigned diagnoses based on IHS criteria. High overall levels of agreement are reflected by the kappa statistic of 0.74 (11). Other studies also have examined the performance of the IHS criteria. Conflicting results have been obtained with respect to the comprehensiveness of the criteria. Analysis of several population-based studies revealed the criteria to be comprehensive in that virtually all headache types can be classified (13,22,42,44); however, in some clinic-based studies, substantial numbers of patients could not be classified (20,23,51). Particularly problematic for the IHS criteria is the classification of very frequent headaches

with migrainous features (33). Revisions to the IHS criteria for frequent headaches have been proposed and applied to epidemiologic studies (48,50). As data emerge, the IHS criteria will be reviewed and may be revised. The IHS criteria represent a seminal advance in headache classification and have provided a critical foundation for epidemiologic studies over the past decade.

Epidemiologic Terms

Many epidemiologic studies have examined headache prevalence. *Prevalence* refers to the proportion of a given population that has a disease over a defined period of time. The *lifetime prevalence* indicates how many subjects who have ever, during any period of their lives, had headache. *Period prevalence* refers to the proportion of individuals who have the disorder over some defined interval, usually 1 year. Period prevalence increases as the period selected for study increases. Prevalence is an important measure of the burden of disease.

Incidence refers to the onset of new cases of a disease in a defined population over a given period of time. To conduct a headache incidence study, one must first eliminate from study anyone in the population who has a headache disorder. Headache-free individuals are then followed over time to determine the rate of development of new cases.

There is a mathematical relationship between incidence and prevalence. Prevalence is determined by the product of average incidence and average duration of disease. In a given population, the prevalence of a headache disorder may increase because either incidence or duration of disease is increasing. Prevalent cases include a mixture of both incidence (new) cases and prevalence (old) cases with persistence of disease. Problems of recall may influence the results, particularly in regard to lifetime prevalences and particularly in the less severe and less frequent types of headache.

Population Sources

The source and the representativeness of the study samples are critical issues in epidemiologic research. Epidemiologic studies of headache have used several sources. Most often, studies sample from a defined community such as a country or a city. Some studies sample from schools or registries (i.e., health, twin, birth, or voter registries). The population of potentially eligible individuals for a study is referred to as the source population. The results of a well conducted study should apply to the source population and, ideally, to broader groups as well. Studies of headaches in samples from headache clinics or even from general practice may not give generalizable results; patients in such series may have more severe, more frequent, or more complex types of headache than the general population and may also be different in other respects. About half of subjects with migraine and more than 80% of subjects with tension-type headache have never consulted a general practitioner because of their headache, and even fewer consult a specialist (17,19,43,58). Such individuals may differ from those who seek medical attention, resulting in selection bias. Even when a control group is included in such selected populations, the risk of bias persists. If the consultation rates of exposed and unexposed cases and controls differ, their relative odds of exposure to the putative cause will be distorted in clinic- or hospital-based studies (Berkson's paradox) (3). An example of this referral bias could be a study in a headache clinic searching for a possible association between migraine and allergic conditions using patients with tension-type headache as controls. If patients with coexisting migraine and allergy are more likely to seek treatment than are, for example, subjects with coexisting tension-type headache and allergy, this study may lead to the finding of a spurious relationship between migraine and allergy. The best way to avoid such problems is to study random samples from the general population.

Sampling Methods

Several alternative methods of selecting samples from a source population have been used. In the complete ascertainment strategy, all eligible members of a source population (i.e., 6-year-olds in a school or residents of a small town) are included. Using random sampling, eligible individuals are selected at random using random digit dialing or other methods. Sometimes households rather than individuals are selected at random. In systematic sampling, individuals are ordered and selected; for example, every fourth person in a birth registry may be targeted. Some studies use stratified sampling to ensure that the study population resembles the source population in terms of key features such as gender or age. Other schema—outside the scope of this chapter—include cluster and quota sampling.

Regardless of the sampling method, high rates of participation are desirable. Participation rate is defined as the proportion of targeted and eligible individuals who actually participate in the study. As participation rates decrease, the opportunity for bias increases. For example, if individuals with headache are more likely to participate in a headache prevalence study, prevalence might be overestimated. If well-educated headache sufferers are more likely to participate, the association between headache status and education can be distorted.

Case Ascertainment

Once the study sample is identified, case status is determined using a range of methods. Some studies have used medical records or self-reported physician diagnosis to identify headache sufferers. This method is problematic for several reasons. A substantial proportion of headache sufferers do not ever consult doctors for headache, and of those who do consult, many may not receive a specific medical diagnosis. Even if a diagnosis is assigned, diagnostic criteria will be uncertain. As a consequence, methods that rely on consultation and diagnosis substantially underestimate rates of disease.

In epidemiologic studies, headache histories should be systematically ascertained. There are no precise objective diagnostic tests for primary headaches. Headache is subjective, and the diagnosis of headache depends on the subject's description of his or her symptoms. Headache diagnoses should be based on a headache history, a physical and neurologic examination, and the selected application of diagnostic tests to exclude secondary causes of headache, when indicated. For research purposes, the history should be based on a semistructured questionnaire, administered by an experienced clinician. A semistructured questionnaire ensures that critical diagnostic features are captured and allows the clinician to probe to obtain information of maximal accuracy. This constitutes the current gold standard assessment for headache diagnosis. Unfortunately, these methods are virtually cost prohibitive for large-scale studies in geographically dispersed populations. A few excellent studies have rigorously used these methods (44,46).

Many epidemiologic studies have used self-administered questionnaires or structured diagnostic interviews (by telephone or in person). Often, general medical and neurologic examinations are not obtained for reasons of cost and convenience. Fortunately, secondary headaches detected by examination are rare in the general population. When structured interviews or questionnaires are used, they should be validated in the setting of intended use, with gold standard clinical assessments.

Episodic Attacks that Vary Over Time

The primary headache disorders are usually characterized by discrete, episodic attacks and headache-free intervals. Any single type of headache may vary from attack to attack within the individual and from one period of time to another. The extent and nature of headache evolution over time has not been clearly established because of the paucity of long-term follow-up studies (4,5,57,60). It is extremely important to define the time period for prevalence estimates. In several previous clinical and population-based studies, the time period for defining a case simply was not defined.

Because of the episodic nature of headache disorders, the sufferers are usually in an interictal state at the time of a clinical assessment or research interview. Thus, diagnosis is based on patients recall of prior attacks. Because the attacks of a given person vary, recall on any particular day may be influenced by the characteristics of the most recent or most severe attacks or the time interval between the most recent attack and the interview. These issues influence clinical assessments as well as epidemiologic research.

Comorbidity

Another epidemiologic issue in headache research is comorbidity. Comorbidity refers to the cooccurrence of two conditions in the same individual with greater than chance frequency. Comorbidity must be studied in population samples to avoid distortion by referral bias in clinically treated samples. Also when searching for factors or conditions associated with headache, the time period for defining a case is important. A late look at those affected early may miss short episodes, mild cases, and cases in which the exposure disappears or changes with disease onset (prevalence-incidence bias) (27). The prevalence-incidence bias may distort relative odds in both upward and downward directions (47).

Coexisting Headaches

Subjects frequently suffer from more than one form of headache at a given point in time and over a lifetime. At one point in the individuals life one form may predominate, but later it may be another. Many suffer from more than one type of headache in the same period of time (e.g., migraine without aura and episodic tension-type headache). Nevertheless, in most previously published scientific studies the current practice has been to categorize patients as having either migraine or tension-type headache. The Headache Classification Committee of the IHS (12) recommends that patients receive a separate diagnosis for each type of headache. The purpose is to classify the major types of headache experienced by each person, not to classify the individual into a single category.

PREVALENCE OF HEADACHE

All the difficulties described in the preceding section must be compounded when evaluating previous studies of

TABLE 1. *Some prevalence studies of headache in industrialized countries*

Study	Sample source	Study method	Respondents (No.)	Age (yr)	Time period prevalence	Headache (%) Males	Females	All
Crisp et al., 1977, U.K. (6)	General population	Questionnaire	727	adults	Lifetime	69	94	
D'Alessandro et al., 1988, Italy (7)	General population	Interview	1144	>7	One-year	57	85	
Göbel et al., 1994, Germany (10)	General population	Questionnaire	4061	>18	Lifetime			71
Linet et al., 1989, U.S.A. (15)	General population	Lay telephone interview	10,169	12–29	Lifetime	91	95	
Michel et al., 1995, France (24)	General population	Questionnaire	9411	≥18	3-month	39	58	
Mitsikostas et al., 1995, Greece (25)	General population	Lay interview	3501	15–75	One-year	19	40	
Newland et al., 1978, U.K. (26)	General population	Questionnaire	2066	>18	One-year	73	81	
Nikiforow, 1981, Finland (28)	General population	Clinical interview	200	>15	Lifetime One-year	69	83	91 77
Nikiforow and Hokkanen, 1978, Finland (29)	General population	Questionnaire	3067	>15	One-year	58	73	66
O'Brien et al., 1994, Canada (30)	General population	Lay telephone interview	2922	>18	One-year	84	91	
Philips, 1977, U.K. (36)	General practice	Questionnaire	597	16–60	Six-months	74	89	
Post and Gubbels, 1985, Netherland (37)	General practice	Questionnaire	2252	16–65	One-year	64	84	74
Rasmussen et al., 1991, Denmark (43)	General population	Clinical interview & examination	740	25–64	Lifetime Point	93 11	99 22	96 16
Waters, 1974, U.K. (56)	General population	Questionnaire	1718	>21	One-year	64	78	
Ziegler et al., 1977, U.S.A. (61)	Church congregations	Questionnaire	1809	>15	Lifetime	83	84	

the prevalence of headache. Varying diagnostic criteria and methodologies may contribute to the strikingly different findings of previous reports. Several such reports from America and Western Europe are summarized in Table 1. Some of these surveys also provide data on the prevalence of specific headache types, which will be discussed later. Although the overall headache prevalence figures vary, in most studies headache prevalence is over 70%. In most studies the term "headache" has not been defined; in others it is clearly stated that headache includes all forms of headache (migraine, tension-type headache, symptomatic headaches, mild and severe types, etc.) (44,61). Minor differences in how the questions are phrased also may have major influence on the results. Some ask, "Do you suffer from headache?" Others ask, "Do you have headache?" It seems that the words "suffer from" gives a lower prevalence than the word "have."

In 1985, a national epidemiologic survey on the prevalence of headache and six other painful conditions was conducted in the United States (N=1,254; Nuprin Pain Report) (52). Prevalence of headache was 78% among the adult women and 68% among men. In a large-scale epidemiologic health survey in Denmark in 1987 (N=4,753), 19% had headache within the current 14 days (45). Headache was one of the most frequently reported symptoms in the adult general population, even more frequent than the common cold. In 1971, Wadsworth et al. (53), in their survey of symptoms in the community, found complaints of headache in 21% during a 14-day period. In two population-based studies including a clinical interview of all participants, the lifetime prevalence of headache was over 90% (28,44) (see Table 1).

Only a few studies of the prevalence of headache in areas remote from the United States and Western Europe have been conducted. In a community health survey in Jerusalem, in a population mainly comprising Jewish immigrants and their offspring, headache prevalence was 76% (71% in men, 81% in women) (1). A survey in an urban population in Zimbabwe found a prevalence of headache of 20%, but subjects with rare episodes of headache were not included in the figure (14). A prevalence study among Nigerian University students reported a prevalence of recurrent headaches of about 60% (32). Variation in headache prevalence in various populations may result from methodologic differences among studies, cultural differences in symptom reporting, or differences in either constitutional (genetic) or environmental risk factors.

SEX AND AGE DISTRIBUTION

The prevalence of headache is higher in women than in men (see Table 1) partly due to the high female preponderance of migraine. However, tension-type headache and several other types of headache also are more common in women than in men (44,49). The female prepon-

derance of the headache disorders has been attributed to a possible influence of female hormones (39,59).

In cross-sectional studies the prevalence of headache decreases after middle age, probably because many subjects become headache free with increasing age (26,29, 36,44,56,61). Drawing longitudinal conclusions from cross-sectional data can be problematic. The lifetime age and gender-specific prevalences of headache have been reported in a study of a nonclinic population in the United States (61) and in a Danish population study (44). The data from these two studies are illustrated in Figure 1. Because these data represent lifetime prevalences, absent profound cohort effects, lifetime prevalence should increase with increasing age. In the U.S. study, and among men in the Danish study, the lifetime prevalence of headache in the older age groups decreased relative to younger ages. To account for this seemingly paradoxical finding, Ziegler suggested that older age groups may forget headaches that remitted at earlier ages. Increased headache incidence among the younger age groups or increased mortality among the older subjects with headache also might account for lower prevalence with advanced age, although there is no evidence for these effects (57).

Data on the 1-year period prevalence of headache by age in four European studies are presented in Figure 2 (women) and Figure 3 (men). In aggregate, these data show lower 1-year prevalence in the older versus younger age groups, which is most likely explained by remissions

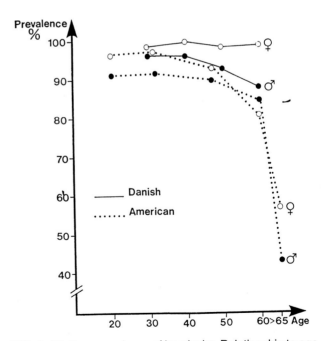

FIG. 1. Lifetime prevalence of headache. Relationship to age and sex. Data are from a Danish population study (44) and an American study of a nonclinic population (61). The median age was taken from the age groups given in the original articles.

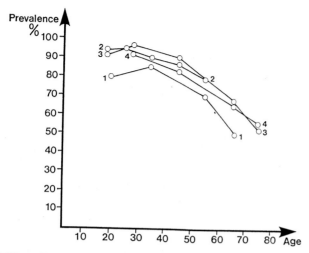

FIG. 2. Prevalence of headache in the previous year among women according to age in four European studies. *1,* Nikiforow and Hokkanen, 1978 (29) (approximate figures of urban population derived from graphs of the original article); *2,* Philips, 1977 (36) (prevalence in previous 6 months); *3,* Newland et al., 1978 (26). *4,* Waters, 1974 (56). Median ages were taken from the age groups given in the original articles.

of headaches with increasing age. More effective treatment due to higher consultation rates or recall bias in the elderly also may contribute to the decrease. Small longitudinal studies show that certain groups of headache sufferers remit before reaching older age (5,9,60). In addition, data on age of onset show that onset of headache is low after middle age, adding few new cases to the headache pool (39,61). The preponderance of evidence suggests that prevalence decreases with increasing age due to

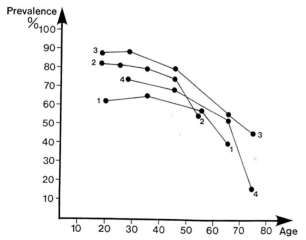

FIG. 3. Prevalence of headache in the previous year among men according to age in four European studies. *1,* Nikiforow and Hokkanen, 1978 (29) (approximate figures of urban population derived from graphs of the original article); *2,* Philips, 1977 (36) (prevalence in previous 6-months); *3,* Newland et al., 1978 (26); *4,* Waters, 1974 (56). Median age was taken from the age groups given in the original articles.

remission, but whether the incidence differs in different age cohorts due to exposure to different risk factors cannot be assessed from these studies. Additional longitudinal studies are required to distinguish a real effect of aging from cohort or period effects.

RELATIONSHIP TO SOCIODEMOGRAPHIC FACTORS

A number of demographic factors besides sex and age have been explored in relation to headache. The variation in headache prevalence with socioeconomic status has long been a subject of research. Most previous hypotheses have been based on clinical impressions in consulting samples. They only express the psychosocial status of headache sufferers consulting a clinic and cannot be confirmed in population-based studies. Several population-based studies have attested to the fairly uniform prevalence of headache in various social groups (8,26,29, 38,54). In these analyses it is important to control for the effects of age, gender, and race. Possible associations between headache and either educational background or marital status also have been studied, but again the results are confounded by problems of definition and population selection. In the Nuprin Pain Report (52) college graduates (77%) tended to report headache more frequently than did those with only some high school education (68%). Ogden (31) found higher prevalence of headache in educated individuals, and Nikiforow and Hokkanen (29) reported from a Finish population study correspondingly lower prevalence among the less educated. In the Finnish study it was pointed out that, when excluding the pensioners from the analyses, the correlation between headache and education disappeared. Subjects who had only attended primary school were overrepresented among the older subjects of the sample; thus, the association actually found between low headache prevalence and lower education may reflect the lower prevalence among the older. These data emphasize the importance of controlling for the effect of age when analyzing possible associations between headache and various sociodemographic variables.

In Finland, headache was found to be most common among married individuals and least common in widowers (29). Ogden (31) found a significantly higher prevalence of headache among single people and a lower prevalence among married and widowed people, but he noted that single persons are generally younger and thus in general have more headaches. Again, age may be an important confounder. Adjustments for the effects of age were included in a recent Danish study of headache and psychosocial factors. No relationships were found between the primary headaches and employment status, category of industry, education, or marital status (38). However, a specific design is required to clarify whether headache is overrepresented in any specific industrial category. Effects of education and social class have been reported in studies of migraine (16) and tension-type headache (49) in the United States. Because these effects run in opposite directions, it is possible that in a sample of mixed headache types, the effects cannot be detected.

Some studies have found no difference in prevalence rates of headache according to race (21,31), whereas others have found higher prevalence in whites compared with blacks (52). Comparing the prevalence of headache in urban and rural areas, no significant difference has been reported in the literature (38,52). In one study, however, a significantly higher prevalence of headache among young men in the town area compared with the rural areas was found, indicating an earlier spread of the headache complaint in urban environments (29).

REFERENCES

1. Abramson JH, Hopp C, Epstein LM. Migraine and non-migrainous headaches. A community survey in Jerusalem. *J Epidemiol Commun Health* 1980;34:188–193.
2. Ad hoc committee on classification of headache. Classification of headache. *JAMA* 1962;179:717–718.
3. Berkson J. Limitations of the application of fourfold table analysis to hospital data. *Biometrics Bull* 1946;2:47–53.
4. Bille B. Migraine in childhood and its prognosis. *Cephalalgia* 1981;1: 71–75.
5. Bille B. A 40-year follow-up of school children with migraine. *Cephalalgia* 1997;17:488–491.
6. Crisp AH, Kalucy RS, McGuinness B, Ralph PC, Harris G. Some clinical, social and psychological characteristics of migraine subjects in the general population. *Postgrad Med J* 1977;53:691–697.
7. D'Alessandro R, Benassi G, Lenzi PL, et al. Epidemiology of headache in the Republic of San Marino. *J Neurol Neurosurg Psychiatry* 1988; 51:21–27.
8. Duckro PN, Tait RC, Margolis RB. Prevalence of very severe headache in a large US metropolitan area. *Cephalalgia* 1989;9:199–205.
9. Fry J. *Profiles of disease*. Edinburgh: Livingstone, 1966.
10. Göbel H, Petersen-Braun M, Soyka D. The epidemiology of headache in Germany: a nationwide survey of a representative sample on the basis of the headache classification of the International Headache Society. *Cephalalgia* 1994;14:97–106.
11. Granella F, D'Alessandro R, Manzoni GC, et al. International Headache Society classification: interobserver reliability in the diagnosis of primary headaches. *Cephalalgia* 1994;14:16–20.
12. Headache Classification Committee of the International Headache Society. Classification and diagnostic criteria for headache disorders, cranial neuralgias and facial pain. *Cephalalgia* 1988;8[suppl 7]:1–96.
13. Henry P, Michel P, Brochet B, et al. A nationwide survey of migraine in France: prevalence and clinical features in adults. *Cephalalgia* 1992; 12:229–237.
14. Levy LM. An epidemiological study of headache in an urban population in Zimbabwe. *Headache* 1983;23:2–9.
15. Linet MS, Stewart WF, Celentano DD, Ziegler D, Sprecher M. An epidemiologic study of headache among adolescents and young adults. *JAMA* 1989;261:2211–2216.
16. Lipton RB, Stewart WF. Epidemiology and comorbidity of migraine. In: Goadsby PJ, Silberstein SD, eds. *Headache: blue books of neurology*, Vol. 17. London: Butterworth-Heinemann, 1997:75–96.
17. Lipton RB, Stewart WF, Celentano DD, Reed M. Undiagnosed migraine: a comparison of symptom-based and physician diagnosis. *Arch Intern Med* 1992;152:1273–1278.
18. Lipton RB, Stewart WF, Merikangas KR. Reliability in headache diagnosis. *Cephalalgia* 1993;13[suppl 12]:29–33.
19. Lipton RB, Stewart WF, Simon D. Medical consultation for migraine: results from the American Migraine Study. *Headache* 1998;38:87–96.
20. Manzoni GC, Granella F, Sandrini G, Cavallini A, Zanferrari C, Nappi G. Classification of chronic daily headache by International Headache Society Criteria: limits and proposals. *Cephalalgia* 1995;15:37–43.
21. Markush RE, Herbert RK, Heyman A, O'Fallon WM. Epidemiologic study of migraine symptoms in young women. *Neurology* 1975;25: 430–435.
22. Merikangas KR, Whitaker AE, Angst J. Validation of diagnostic criteria for migraine in the Zürich longitudinal cohort study. *Cephalalgia* 1993;13[suppl 12]:47–53.
23. Messinger HB, Spierings ELH, Vincent AJP. Overlap of migraine and tension-type headache in the International Headache Society classification. *Cephalalgia* 1991;11:233–237.
24. Michel P, Pariente P, Duru G, Dreyfuss J-P, Chabriat H, Henry P. Mig access: a population-based, nationwide, comparative survey of access to care in migraine in France. *Cephalalgia* 1996;16:50–55.
25. Mitsikostas DD, Tsaklalidou D, Athanasiadis N, Thomas A. The prevalence of headache in Greece: correlations to latitude and climatological factors. *Headache* 1996;36:168–173.
26. Newland CA, Illis LS, Robinson PK, Batchelor BG, Waters WE. A survey of headache in an English City. *Res Clin Stud Headache* 1978;5: 1–20.
27. Neyman J. Statistics—servant of all sciences. *Science* 1955;122: 401–406.
28. Nikiforow R. Headache in a random sample of 200 persons: a clinical study of a population in Northern Finland. *Cephalalgia* 1981;1: 99–107.
29. Nikiforow R, Hokkanen E. An epidemiological study of headache in an urban and a rural population in Northern Finland. *Headache* 1978;18: 137–145.
30. O'Brien B, Goeree R, Streiner D. Prevalence of migraine headache in Canada: a population-based survey. *Int J Epidemiol* 1994;23: 1020–1026.
31. Ogden H. Headache studies, statistical data. *J Allergy* 1952;23:58–75.
32. Ogunyemi AO. Prevalence of headache among Nigerian University students. *Headache* 1984;24:127–130.
33. Olesen J, Rasmussen BK. The International Headache Society classification of chronic daily headaches: a critique of the criticism. *Cephalalgia* 1996;16:407–411.
34. Olesen J, Rasmussen BK. Classification of migraine. In: Goadsby, Silberstein, eds. *Headache: blue books of neurology*, Vol. 17. London: Butterworth-Heinemann, 1997:97–105.
35. Ottman R, Hong S, Lipton RB. Validity of family history data on severe headache and migraine. *Neurology* 1993;43:1954–1960.
36. Philips C. Headache in general practice. *Headache* 1977;16:322–329.
37. Post D, Gubbels JW. Headache: an epidemiological survey in a Dutch rural general practice. *Headache* 1986;26:122–125.
38. Rasmussen BK. Migraine and tension-type headache in a general population: psychosocial factors. *Int J Epidemiol* 1992;21:1138–1143.
39. Rasmussen BK. Migraine and tension-type headache in a general population: precipitating factors, female hormones, sleep pattern and relation to lifestyle. *Pain* 1993;53:65–72.
40. Rasmussen BK. Epidemiology of headache [Thesis]. *Cephalalgia* 1995;15:48–68.
41. Rasmussen BK. Migraine and tension-type headache are separate disorders. *Cephalalgia* 1996;16:217–223.
42. Rasmussen BK, Jensen R, Olesen J. A population-based analysis of the diagnostic criteria of the International Headache Society. *Cephalalgia* 1991;11:129–134.
43. Rasmussen BK, Jensen R, Olesen J. Impact of headache on sickness absence and utilisation of medical services. A Danish population study. *J Epidemiol Commun Health* 1992;46:443–446.
44. Rasmussen BK, Jensen R, Schroll M, Olesen J. Epidemiology of headache in a general population—a prevalence study. *J Clin Epidemiol* 1991;44:1147–1157.
45. Rasmussen NK, Groth MV, Bredkjær SR, Madsen M, Kamper-Jørgensen F. *Sundhed & Sygelighed i Danmark*. Copenhagen: Dansk Institut for Klinisk Epidemiologi, 1987.
46. Russell MB, Rasmussen BK, Thorvaldsen P, Olesen J. Prevalence and sex-ratio of the subtypes of migraine. *Int J Epidemiol* 1995;24: 612–618.
47. Sackett DL. Bias in analytic research. *J Chron Dis* 1979;32:51–63.
48. Scher AL, Stewart WF, Liberman J, Lipton RB. Prevalence of frequent headache in a population sample. *Headache* 1998;38:497–506.
49. Schwartz BS, Stewart WF, Simon D, Lipton RB. Epidemiology of tension-type headache. *JAMA* 1998;279:381–383.
50. Silberstein SD, Lipton RB, Sliwinski M. Classification of daily and near-daily headache: a field study of revised IHS criteria. *Neurology* 1996;871–875.

51. Solomon S, Lipton RB, Newman LC. Evaluation of chronic daily headache—comparison to criteria for chronic tension-type headache. *Cephalalgia* 1992;12:365–368..

52. Taylor H, ed. *The Nuprin pain report.* New York: Louis Harris & Associates, 1985.

53. Wadsworth MEJ, Butterfield WJH, Blaney R. Health and sickness. The choice of treatment. In: *Perception of illness and use of services in an urban community.* London: Tavistock, 1971.

54. Waters WE. Migraine: intelligence, social class, and familial prevalence. *Br Med J* 1971;2:77–81.

55. Waters WE. The epidemiological engima of migraine. *Int J Epidemiol* 1973;2:189–194.

56. Waters WE. The Pontypridd headache survey. *Headache* 1974;14:81–90.

57. Waters WE, Campbell MJ, Elwood PC. Migraine, headache, and survival in women. *Br Med J* 1983;287:1442–1443.

58. Waters WE, O'Connor PJ. Epidemiology of headache and migraine in women. *J Neurol Neurosurg Psychiatry* 1971;34:148–153.

59. Welch KMA, Darnley D, Simkins RT. The role of estrogen in migraine: a review and hypothesis. *Cephalalgia* 1984;4:227–236.

60. Whitty CWM, Hockaday JM. Migraine: a follow-up study of 92 patients. *Br Med J* 1968;1:735–736.

61. Ziegler DK, Hassanein RS, Couch JR. Characteristics of life headache histories in a nonclinic population. *Neurology* 1977;27:265–269.

The Headaches, Second Edition,
edited by J. Olesen, P. Tfelt-Hansen, and K.M.A. Welch.
Lippincott Williams & Wilkins, Philadelphia © 2000.

General Aspects of the Headaches

CHAPTER 4

Impact of Headache on the Individual Sufferer

Glen D. Solomon and Carl G. H. Dahlöf

Migraine is a highly prevalent chronic disease that normally affects people during their most productive years (47). Despite the magnitude of direct costs, the indirect costs of the migraine disease are greater. The primary sources of indirect costs are the inability to perform normal tasks at home, school, or the workplace.

IMPACT OF MIGRAINE ON THE FAMILY

Data are available describing the effects of migraine on family or social functioning. Edmeads et al. (16) conducted an interview study on a subset of over 100 migraine sufferers included in the study of Pryse-Phillips et al. (33). Aspects that were addressed by the interview included sufferers' attitudes toward their condition, the effect of headache on their lives, and their incentive to seek medical attention. Thirty-five percent of patients believed that migraine headache influenced social plans, roughly 40% admitted to being worried about the possible occurrence of headache at a future event, and approximately 45% worried about driving because of headache. About 50% of the subjects believed that their headaches had an effect on their families. Data from those who completed 3-month diary records showed that cancellation of social activities and family activities was necessary with 17% of migraine headaches (16).

Smith (38) has looked in detail at the impact of migraine on the family in a national sample of 4,000 households in the United States. Results from 350 migraine sufferers with children and 77 nonsufferer spouses showed that migraine affects other members of the family as well as the sufferer and may have serious effects on spousal relationships and particularly on younger children. Sixty-one percent of migraine sufferers felt that migraine impacted on family. Twenty-one percent of interviewees rated the impact of migraine on the family as very or extremely serious. One third felt that migraine negatively affected their relationship with their children. Seventy-three percent missed activities with children due to migraine. Thirty-six percent of those interviewed felt that migraine negatively affected their relationship with their spouse. The author concluded that the impact of migraine on the family may add to migraine suffering (38).

Osterhaus (31) reported that migraine can seriously impair leisure activities. Migraine sufferers lost an average of 5.6 leisure days per year due to migraine. In addition, they had 11.1 leisure days per year with limited participation due to migraine.

IMPACT ON GENERAL WELL-BEING

The disruptive effect of migraine is not confined to the duration of the attack. Dahlöf and Dimenäs (11) compared the general well-being between attacks of 138 migraine patients with that of an age- and sex-matched control group. Three self-administered questionnaires were used to assess subtle changes in subjective symptoms, frequently reported subjective symptoms, and changes in sense of well-being. Compared with control subjects, migraine sufferers reported disturbed contentment, vitality, and sleep, and perceived more symptoms and greater emotional distress. Further evidence for the

G. D. Solomon: Merck & Co., Inc., Pepper Pike, Ohio 44124.

C. G. H. Dahlöf: Department of Clinical Pharmacology, Sahlgrenska University Hospital, and Gothenburg Migraine Clinic, S-41117 Göteborg, Sweden.

long-term effects of migraine were obtained in a questionnaire survey of employees of a National Health Service (NHS) trust hospital in the United Kingdom, in which migraine sufferers were consulted about the impact of their migraine both during and between attacks (6). During attacks, 76% of sufferers always had to lie down, 90% postponed their household tasks, and 50% generally had to miss work. Between attacks, around half of the sufferers reported difficulties in interacting with family, friends, or work colleagues (7). It has been suggested that it is the unpredictability of migraine that leads to difficulties in organizing a normal family life (11,41).

Migraine may impart a burden of fear and anxiety on the sufferer. In one study, which interviewed 75 outpatients attending a neurologic clinic, 50 admitted that they had experienced fear because of their migraine. The three most common fears expressed by these patients were of having a tumor, loss of work, and the severity of their pain (3).

The combination of the impact of migraine and the fear associated with it may lead migraine sufferers to modify their behavior. In a study by Edmeads et al. (16), many migraine sufferers reported that they sought to avoid headache-triggering factors such as smoke, noise, and emotional pressure. Many also sought to avoid certain activities and said that being a migraine sufferer affected job decisions. These findings are in agreement with the anecdotal accounts given by migraine sufferers of the coping strategies that they adopt and the restrictions that such strategies impose (21).

QUALITY OF LIFE MEASURES

To evaluate the impact of headache and headache therapies on the individual sufferer, outcomes research is emerging as an important tool. Outcome measures in headache include clinical evaluations, economic assessments, and humanistic measures. In the primary headache disorders, the traditional clinical outcome measures used in other disease states, such as mortality, physical markers, blood tests, or diagnostic images, are not relevant. The important clinical measures in headache therapy are headache frequency, severity, time to relief of pain, and the presence and relief of associated symptoms. Of increasing importance is the impact of these clinical measures on patient-perceived quality of life (QOL), work performance, and economic cost (23).

The increasing awareness of the burden of headache and the lack of traditional clinical measures have made the humanistic evaluation of headache more important. One of these humanistic measures is QOL. The World Health Organization defines QOL as individuals' perceptions of their position in life in the context of the culture and value systems in which they live, and in relation to their goals, expectations, standards, and concerns (48). This multidimensional construct encompasses the person's physical and psychological domains, level of independence, social relationships, environment, and personal beliefs. Health-related quality of life (HRQOL) represents the net effect of an illness and its consequent therapy on a patient's perception of his or her ability to live a useful and fulfilling life. For the purposes of this chapter, HRQOL and QOL will be used interchangeably.

In headache, the measurement and reporting of QOL has not been widely standardized. Many studies report well-being, disability, or QOL in general terms, using nonvalidated instruments, which prohibit comparison with other studies. To evaluate the appropriateness of QOL assessments and to apply the results in various clinical and research settings, instruments must be scientifically developed and standardized. QOL is assessed using health scales or questionnaires that combine a subjective perception of the sufferer's life situation and an objective assessment of health factors. Development of these instruments involves patient focus groups, literature review, and input from health-care professionals. The science of assessing the measurement characteristics of a scale, referred to as psychometrics, is derived from the social sciences, specifically psychology, where abstract concepts such as personality and intelligence are objectively measured. HRQOL instruments measure concepts such as pain and vitality, which are not otherwise directly measurable (35). To be scientifically robust measures of outcome, the questionnaires need to be reliable, validated, and sensitive to clinically relevant changes (10). These properties are defined as follows (18):

1. The instrument must be reliable; it must provide results that are accurate, consistent, and stable over time. Reliability issues of internal consistency, test-retest, inter-rater and intra-rater agreement, and parallel forms of the instrument must be statistically and critically analyzed.
2. The instrument must be valid; it must measure the concept it purports to measure. Three factors assessed in validating an instrument are content validity, criterion validity, and construct validity, which includes convergent and discriminate correlations.
3. The instrument must be responsive; it must detect clinical changes as well as statistical differences over time or after an intervention. These changes must be clinically meaningful to the patient and physician.

Quality of life can be measured with a variety of generic and specific instruments. Generic questionnaires are generally chosen for comparisons between study populations and different diseases, whereas disease-specific questionnaires are designed to assess problems associated with a single disease or treatment.

GENERIC QOL INSTRUMENTS

Generic instruments address a broad range of life aspects related to health. These instruments can be used for many diseases and allow for comparison with healthy controls and other disease populations. However, in some diseases the generic instruments are often too general and the questions too broad based to be responsive to changes.

The Medical Outcomes Study (MOS) Short Form (developed by the Rand Corporation, Santa Monica, CA), was originally developed as a 20-item questionnaire (the SF-20) (46); a more extensive version containing 36 items (the SF-36) (28) was developed later. The SF-20 assesses six domains: physical functioning, role functioning, social functioning, mental health, health perceptions, and pain. The SF-36 domains also include vitality and distinguishes role functioning impairments resulting from physical and emotional aspects of health. Both instruments have been validated in chronic headache and migraine patients.

A major advantage of using the SF-36 in headache evaluation is the wealth of data accumulated with the questionnaire. Data have been obtained from headache patients from tertiary care headache centers (26) and from the workplace (24), as well as from migraine patients enrolled in multiple clinical trials in the United States and Europe (40). The SF-36 has been analyzed to determine minimal change scores for each domain in chronic headache patients (25). This allows users to determine the clinical significance of changes within a domain after an intervention.

Other generic health scales used in migraine are the Sickness Index Profile (14) and the Nottingham Health Profile (NHP) (27), which measure behavior and perceived health status, concepts that are similar but distinct from QOL. The Psychological General Well-Being (PGWB) index assesses changes in a patient's sense of well-being (11). Well-being is exclusively an expression of the individual's subjective perception and describes his or her own qualitative evaluation of general well-being in relation to a disorder treatment or both. This subjective variable comprises the individual's global judgement of what is positive and negative in their life and is based on the person's own knowledge and values. A high general well-being is characterized by a positive balance between what the individual perceives as good and bad (15). A high general well-being therefore does not necessarily mean absence of negative events, merely that the positive components outweigh them (4).

The Minor Symptoms Evaluation Profile (MSEP) questionnaire is designed to assess subjective central nervous system–related symptoms that might affect a patient's well-being (8,12). The instrument uses a visual analogue scale. Low values on the visual analogue scale indicate positive feelings, whereas high values indicate negative ones. The MSEP consists of 24 items. All items of the MSEP, with the exception of the sleep variables, refer to the patient's current feelings (i.e. at the time of filling in the scale). Sleep items, however, reflect the patient's recollection of the previous night. The items have been categorized into three separate dimensions:

1. Contentment (seven items: happiness, tranquility, self-control, decisiveness, self-confidence, mental fatigue, and general well-being)
2. Vitality (five items: enthusiasm, initiative, endurance, concentration, and responsiveness)
3. Sleep (three items: nocturnal sleep, quality of sleep, and insomnia)

The use of dimensions as primary variables for evaluation of subjective symptoms apparently reduces the variability in response and helps to avoid a multiple test situation. In addition, construct validity has been established by calculating the correlation coefficients between dimensions of the MSEP and those of other questionnaires (e.g., the NHP and the PGWB). Compared with the equivalent dimensions of the other questionnaires for measurement of HQL, the dimensions of the MSEP were found to be most relevant.

DISEASE-SPECIFIC QOL INSTRUMENTS

Disease-specific instruments can address diseases, symptoms, treatments, or populations. These instruments address in-depth issues more focused to patients concerns. However, a new measure must be developed for each disease, and different diseases cannot be directly compared. However, the specific instruments are more likely to be responsive to therapeutic interventions in a particular disease.

The Henry Ford Headache Disability Inventory (19) is a reliable, validated, disease-specific instrument used to measure the degree of disability caused by chronic headache. Unlike most other disease-specific instruments, it is not limited to migraine. It measures patient-perceived disability in physical and emotional domains, rather than HRQOL. The concept of disability has not been clearly distinguished from that of QOL and, thus, these two types of scales may similarly determine the nonmedical impact of disease on a patient.

Migraine-specific QOL questionnaires have been developed and tested for reliability and validity. Some of these instruments are proprietary and are used by pharmaceutical companies in clinical trials of new medications. This population of patients is often subject to bias because of their attendance at a specialty clinic and their willingness to participate in clinical trials. The 24-Hour Migraine-Specific Quality of Life Questionnaire has been developed to assess QOL in the 24-hour period after an acute migraine attack (17,34). The 15 questions across five domains measure work functioning, social function, energy, concerns, and symptoms. The instrument has good internal consistency, construct, and discriminant validity and is responsive to variations in acute migraine attacks. The 24-Hour Migraine-Specific Quality of Life

Questionnaire is a composite evaluation of a patient's day with migraine and of the impact of acute therapy. Another instrument, the Migraine-Specific Quality of Life measure, a reliable and validated 25-item questionnaire, is designed to assess the long-term QOL effects from migraine. This Migraine-Specific Quality of Life questionnaire measures psychological well-being more so than functional status (50). A third specific instrument, also known as the Migraine-Specific Quality of Life Questionnaire, is a 16-item instrument that assesses aspects of health believed to be particularly affected by migraine. There are three domains: role-function restrictive (degree to which performance of normal activities is restricted by migraine), role-function preventive (degree to which performance of normal activities is prevented by migraine), and emotional function (1). The questionnaire is reliable and valid (29).

QOL IN CHRONIC HEADACHE

Solomon et al. (43) administered the SF-20 to 208 consecutive patients attending a headache clinic and found that chronic headache disorders were associated with statistically significant limitations in all six health categories of patient well-being and functioning. They confirmed that the MOS survey was a reliable and valid measure of QOL for patients with chronic headache disorder. Headache patients' data were compared with published data from a healthy population and from groups of patients with other chronic medical conditions. The patients with chronic headache showed significant impairment on all six domains of the SF-20 compared with the healthy population. Patients with chronic headache functioned less well than did patients with arthritis, diabetes, depression, or back problems (43). Based on published information, the only chronic conditions having similar levels of functional impairment to chronic headache were myocardial infarction within the past year and congestive heart failure (45).

Further analysis of the SF-20 data by headache diagnoses revealed specific patterns for cluster, chronic tension-type, and migraine headache (44). Cluster headache patients had marked pain scores and limitations in social functioning with generally well preserved physical functioning and health perceptions. Chronic tension-type headache patients had lower mental health scores than migraine patients. Patients with chronic tension-type headache reported more pain than did patients with migraine, although these reports may reflect the frequency and chronicity of the headache rather than the severity of a given headache attack. Physical functioning, role functioning, and social functioning were all markedly impaired in chronic tension-type headache patients. These scores reflect the clinical perception that patients with chronic tension-type headache have more depression and anxiety than other patients with headache.

Migraine patients reported the least amount of pain compared with other headache sufferers; however, their pain was still much worse than that reported in other studies of patients with back pain or arthritis. In migraine patients, role functioning, a measure of the ability to work, was more impaired than either physical or social functioning.

QOL IN MIGRAINE

Osterhaus et al. reported results using the SF-36 in migraine patients (32). The scores of 825 migraine sufferers, adjusted for comorbid conditions, were compared with a general population of comparable age and gender with no reported chronic disease. The scores from the migraine group were significantly lower. The most profoundly impaired domains were bodily pain and role functioning related to physical health. The migraine sufferers' scores were also compared with those of patients with other chronic diseases. Migraine scores were significantly lower than hypertension scores in all domains except general health perception. The scores of migraine patients were significantly lower than those of patients with diabetes in all domains except general health perceptions and physical functioning. Scores for bodily pain, social functioning, role disability secondary to emotional problems, and mental health were significantly lower for migraine patients than for osteoarthritis patients. In comparison with clinical depression, migraine sufferers had lower scores for bodily pain, but higher scores for general health perception, role disability secondary to emotional problems, and mental health. Patients who reported their migraine headaches as moderate, severe, or very severe all scored significantly below the general population on measures of bodily pain, social functioning, role function secondary to physical health, physical functioning, and mental health.

Using the PGWB, MSEP, and the Subjective Symptoms Assessment Profile (SSAP), Dahlöf demonstrated that migraine patients experience poorer subjective well-being and QOL, even between attacks (11).

IMPACT OF THERAPY ON QOL

Despite the prevalence and impact of headache, there is a limited, but growing, body of data on the effects of headache therapy on QOL. The absence of these data hinders our ability to compare prophylactic with abortive therapies and to compare outcomes among different therapeutic agents.

Acute changes in patient well-being related to treatment of migraine were first reported by Dahlöf and Bjorkman using the MSEP (10). Patients evaluated with the MSEP after abortive migraine treatment with diclofenac potassium, a nonsteroidal antiinflammatory drug, reported significantly greater improvement in well-being than did those receiving placebo. Although this study demonstrates that changes in patients' perceptions of well-being can be altered using drug therapy for migraine, the long-term effect of diclofenac potassium on QOL was not addressed.

In a study of patients with chronic headache, Skobieranda et al. (37) used the SF-20 and a pain scale to determine changes in QOL after the first 6 months of treatment at an outpatient tertiary care headache center. Treatment was individualized and included abortive therapy (before the introduction of sumatriptan) and, where appropriate, prophylactic treatment. Although there were no significant improvements in the SF-20 scores after 6 months of treatment, 52% of patients reported an improvement in pain scores. These researchers recognized that the SF-20 may not have been responsive to change after treatment in a sample of patients with headaches of various types, even though a majority of patients with chronic headache did achieve traditional clinical endpoints (improvement in pain). The researchers believed that these observations supported the need for longer treatment of chronic headache before assessing changes in QOL and that headache impacted QOL in dimensions other than pain alone.

Dahlöf also studied QOL during 6 months' treatment of migraine in a headache clinic (9). Information about patient well-being and subjective symptoms were obtained by means of three self-administered standardized questionnaires: the MSEP, SSAP, and PGWB. He reported that treatment reduced the number of days per month with migraine, absenteeism from work, and migraine-associated symptoms, but did not significantly improve general well-being between attacks. Thus, the impaired general well-being/QOL of the migraine patient between the attacks might be attributable to factors other than the migraine attacks. It might be that the personal characteristics of the migraine patients contribute to their impaired general well-being between attacks.

Mannix (26) studied QOL and headache-related disability during 12 months' treatment of headache in a headache clinic. Treatment was individualized and included abortive therapy, prophylactic treatment, patient education, and follow-up care. She reported improvement in QOL and disability, measured by the SF-36 and the HDI, beginning as early as 1 month and continuing for 1 year. The improvements in QOL and disability correlated with an improvement in global assessment, headache frequency, and headache severity.

Information on the impact on QOL using prophylactic treatment for migraine is also limited. Dahlöf (7) used the MSEP to compare the effects of prophylaxis with flunarizine (a calcium antagonist) and propranolol (a betablocker) with placebo. He found that the prophylactic treatments were perceived by the patients to be essentially equivalent and did not differ from placebo. Solomon and Kunkel (39) used the SF-20 to evaluate QOL during long-term (7-month) prophylactic migraine therapy with flur-

biprofen, a nonsteroidal antiinflammatory drug. They reported improved role functioning (headache interfered less with work) that corresponded with reductions in headache frequency and intensity and a beneficial effect on QOL, which was sustained over the 7 months of the study. This 15-patient, unblinded study suggested that the beneficial effects of prophylactic therapy could be quantified by both standard headache measurements and general QOL scales. Whether changes in QOL reflected the effect of medication or a regression of these scores toward population means could not be answered with this study design.

In patients with chronic tension-type headache, guided imagery, a relaxation technique based on visualizing pleasant images and body awareness, has been evaluated as an adjunct to individualized pharmacotherapy (22). Guided imagery has been shown to improve QOL, as measured by the SF-36, and to improve patients' global assessment of their headaches.

Documentation of the long-term impact on QOL using abortive medication for migraine exists for sumatriptan and the newer 5-hydroxytryptamine 1D (5-HT$_{1D}$) agonists. Studies using either general health status, migraine-specific, or pain-specific instruments have examined the effects of sumatriptan on migraine sufferers' HRQOL in the absence of a migraine attack (1,2,5,13,20,30,40,42). Results of these eight studies consistently indicate that sumatriptan, administered orally or subcutaneously, significantly enhanced key dimensions of QOL. Across studies using the SF-36, social functioning scores most consistently improved with sumatriptan, although health perception, vitality, pain, mental health, and role functioning scores also were increased. Sumatriptan treatment also has been associated with improvements in each of the three domains of the Migraine-Specific Quality of Life Questionnaire: role-function preventive, role-function restrictive, and emotional function (1,20). In the social domain of pain-specific questionnaires, sumatriptan treatment has been associated with improvements in the ability to work and to move about and with enjoyment of life (42). The QOL studies involving migraine sufferers treated with sumatriptan revealed that improvement in QOL occurs within 3 months and that the benefits are sustained for at least a year (43).

The striking consistency of these findings across studies provides important convergent evidence that treatment of migraine with sumatriptan is associated with improvements in multiple dimensions in patients' perceptions of their QOL. QOL studies using the SF-36 and specific instruments also have been conducted in clinical trials with rizatriptan, zolmetriptan, and other 5-HT$_{1D}$ agonists. Preliminary data from the rizatriptan studies, presented only in abstract form at meetings, suggest improvements in QOL at least as great as those of sumatriptan.

Educational programs, individually or as part of comprehensive treatment programs, also have detectable effects on patients' sense of well-being. An evaluation of the Comprehensive Migraine Treatment Program on 30 patients with migraine or mixed headache found that comprehensive care contributed positively to patients' knowledge about their illness and confidence in their ability to manage it (36). Other researchers have confirmed that enhanced self-efficacy through education about headache and headache treatments resulted in patients' ratings of such program's benefits that were equal to or higher than preventive or abortive treatments in contributing to treatment success (49).

The impact of a workplace education program also has been measured using the SF-36 and the HDI (24). Components of the program included education on headache types, trigger factors, prevention, and treatment techniques. The program consisted of a slide presentation, participant worksheet, and handouts. Compared with baseline, 1 month after the program a significantly higher percentage of participants used nonmedication techniques for managing headaches (proper diet, exercise, headache diary, breathing/relaxation exercises). One month after the program, SF-36 scores significantly improved on all domains except physical functioning. The largest improvements were in the domains of role-physical and role-emotional. Disability due to headache also decreased after the program.

CLINICAL ROLE OF QOL INSTRUMENTS

Standardized instruments for measuring HRQOL are becoming widely accepted in migraine. The results have provided information on the burden and impact of migraine. Dissemination of such information may lead to improved patient access to health care and management of headache patients that is designed to better meet their physical and psychological needs. Both generic and specific instruments complement clinical trials of medications or interventions by assessing the impact of disease and therapy on patients' functioning and well-being. In addition to relieving the personal suffering of headache patients, improved QOL also may reduce the socioeconomic burden of migraine.

Results to date have focused on group means; the interpretation of QOL changes for individual patients are not yet available. Therefore, application for clinical practice apart from the clinical trial setting, has not been fully appreciated. In addition to pharmaceutical interventions, the specific components of headache therapy must eventually be analyzed to determine their impact on QOL. Some of these components include physician experience, patient education, nursing care, and nonpharmacologic therapy.

No single instrument has been recognized as the gold standard in migraine QOL assessment. Many different QOL instruments and combinations of QOL instruments and clinical outcomes have been reported. The future of

QOL research may see the evolution of combined generic and specific instruments. Patient preferences, expectations, and satisfaction also will need to be addressed for a comprehensive view of migraine impact and treatment outcome. Ultimately, the headache community must decide which outcome measure or measures are most valuable. This decision will be influenced by the experience of medical professionals in the field of headache, the assessment and satisfaction of headache patients, and economic pressures. The impact of changes over time, for whatever reason, has to be controlled in future clinical trials. Based on current QOL research and its future applications, QOL may represent the final common pathway of all the physiologic, psychological, and social inputs into the therapeutic process.

REFERENCES

1. Adelman JU, Sharfinan M, Johnson R, et al. Impact of oral sumatriptan on workplace productivity, health related QoL, healthcare use and patient satisfaction with medication in nurses with migraine. *Am J Managed Care* 1996;2:1407–1416.
2. Beall D, Cohen J, Miller D. An interim analysis of the use of subcutaneous sumatriptan in a managed care setting: effects on health-related quality of life, impact on health care resource use, and clinical efficacy [Abstract]. *Pharmacotherapy* 1995;15:385.
3. Blau JN. Fears aroused in patients by migraine. *Br Med J* 1984; 288:1126.
4. Bradburn NM. *The structure of physiological well-being.* Chicago: Aldine, 1969
5. Bullinger M, Bruggenjurgen B. Quality of life assessment among migraine sufferers under current treatment and after three months treatment with sumatriptan. Poster presented at the European Federation of Neurological Societies, Berlin, 1993.
6. Clarke CE, MacMillan L, Sondhi S, Wells NEJ. Economic and social impact of migraine. *Q J Med* 1996;89:77–84.
7. Dahlöf C. Flunarizine versus long-acting propranolol in the prophylactic treatment of migraine: a double blind parallel group study. In: Rose FC, ed. *New advances in headache research.* London: Smith-Gordon, 1989:281–289.
8. Dahlöf C. Minor Symptoms Evaluation (MSE) Profile—a questionnaire for assessment of subjective CNSq-related symptoms. *Scand J Prim Health Care* 1990;1:19–25
9. Dahlöf C. Health-related quality of life under six months treatment of migraine—an open clinic-based longitudinal study. *Cephalalgia* 1995;15:414–422.
10. Dahlöf C, Bjorkman R. Diclofenac-K (50 and 100 mg) and placebo in the acute treatment of migraine. *Cephalalgia* 1993;13:117–123.
11. Dahlöf C, Dimenäs E. Migraine patients experience poorer subjective well being/quality of life even between attacks. *Cephalalgia* 1995;15: 31–36.
12. Dahlöf C, Dimenäs E, Olofsson B. Documentation of an instrument for assessment of subjective CNS-related symptoms during cardiovascular pharmacotherapy. *Cardiovasc Drugs Ther* 1989;3(6)919–27.
13. D'allens H, Richard A, Bertin L. Responsiveness assessment of a specific quality of life questionnaire for migraine sufferers (QVM) [Abstract]. *Qual Life Res* 1994;3:72.
14. Damiano AM. The Sickness Impact Profile. In: Spilker B, ed. *Quality of life and pharmacoeconomics in clinical trials,* 2nd ed. Philadelphia: Lippincott-Raven, 1996:347–354.
15. Diener E. Subjective well-being. *Psychol Bull* 1984;95:542–575.
16. Edmeads J, Findlay H, Tugwell P, Pryse-Phillips W, Nelson RF, Murray TJ. Impact of migraine and tension-type headache on life-style, consulting behaviour, and medication use: a Canadian population survey. *Can J Neurol Sci* 1993;20:131–137.
17. Hartmaier SL, Santanello NC, Epstein RS, Silberstein SD. Development of a brief 24-hour migraine-specific quality of life questionnaire. *Headache* 1995;35:320–329.

18. Hobart JC, Lamping DL, Thompson AJ. Evaluating neurological outcome measures: the bare essentials. *J Neurol Neurosurg Psychiatry* 1996;60:127–130.

19. Jacobson GP, Ramadan NM, Aggarwal SK, Newman CW. The Henry Ford Hospital Headache Disability Inventory (HDI). *Neurology* 1994; 44:837–842.

20. Jhingran P, Cady RK, Rubino J, Miller D, Grice RB, Guttennan DL. Improvements in health-related quality of life with sumatriptan treatment for migraine. *J Fam Pract* 1996;42:36–42.

21. Liddell J. Migraine: the patient's perspective. *Rev Contemp Pharmacother* 1994;5:253–257.

22. Mannix LK, Chandurkar RS, Rybicki LA, Tusek DL, Solomon GD. Effect of guided imagery on quality of life for patients with chronic tension-type headache. Presented at the American Association for the Study of Headache, San Francisco, June 1998.

23. Mannix LK, Solomon GD. Quality of life in migraine. *Clin Neurosci* 1998;5:38–42.

24. Mannix LK, Solomon GD, Kippes C. Impact of headache education program in the workplace. Presented at the Migraine Trust, London, September 1998.

25. Mannix LK, Solomon GD, Pathak DS, Rybicki LA. Magnitude of SF-36 score changes based on patient assessment changes in headache. *Cephalalgia* 1997;17:321.

26. Mannix LK, Solomon GD, Rybicki LA. Long-term patient-reported outcomes in a specialty headache clinic. Poster presented at the American Academy of Neurology, Minneapolis, April 1998.

27. McEwen J, McKenna SP. Nottingham Health Profile. In: Spilker B, ed. *Quality of Life and Pharmacoeconomics in Clinical Trials*, 2nd ed. Philadelphia: Lippincott-Raven, 1996:281–286.

28. McHomey CA, Ware JE, Raczek AE. The MOS 36-item short form health survey (SF-36): II. Psychometric and clinical tests of validity in measuring physical and mental health constructs. *Med Care* 1993;31:247–263.

29. Miller DW, Kirchdoerfer LJ, Shepherd MD, Osterhaus JT, Jhingran PJ. A disease-specific questionnaire to measure quality of life effects attributable to migraine. Poster presented at the 10th annual meeting of the Health Services Research Association, Washington, DC, 1993.

30. Mushet GR, Miller D, Clements B. Impact of sumatriptan on workplace productivity, nonwork activities, and health related quality of life among hospital employees with migraine. *Headache* 1996;36:137–143.

31. Osterhaus JT, Gutterman DL, Plachetka JR. Healthcare resource and lost labour costs of migraine headaches in the US. *Pharmacoeconomics* 1992;2:67–76.

32. Osterhaus JT, Townsend RJ, Gandek B, Ware JE. Measuring the functional status and well-being of patients with migraine headache. *Headache* 1994;34:337–343.

33. Pryse-Phillips W, Findlay H, Tugwell P, Edmeads J, Murray TJ, Nelson RF. A Canadian population survey on the clinical, epidemiologic and societal impact of migraine and tension-type headache. *Can J Neurol Sci* 1992;19:333–339.

34. Santanello NC, Hartmaier SL, Epstein RS, Silberstein SD. Validation of a new quality of life questionnaire for acute migraine headache. *Headache* 1995;35:330–337.

35. Schipper H, Clinch JJ, Olweny, CLM. Quality of life studies: definitions and conceptual issues. In: Spilker B, ed. *Quality of life and pharmacoeconomics in clinical trials*, 2nd ed. Philadelphia: Lippincott-Raven, 1996:11–24.

36. Scopp AL, Peters KS. Patient rating of trigger elimination effectiveness in comprehensive migraine treatment program [Abstract]. *Headache* 1992;32:269.

37. Skobieranda FG, Solomon GD, Gragg LA. Quality of life changes in headache patients following six months of outpatient treatment: use of the Medical Outcomes Study Instrument [Abstract]. *Headache* 1993; 33:283.

38. Smith R. Impact of migraine on the family. *Headache* 1996;36:278.

39. Solomon GD, Kunkel RS. Long-term use of flurbiprofen in migraine prophylaxis [abstract]. *Headache* 1992;32:269–270.

40. Solomon GD, Nielson K, Miller D. The effects of sumatriptan on migraine: Health related quality of life. *Med Interface* 1995;8:134–141.

41. Solomon GD, Price KL. Burden of migraine: a review of its socioeconomic impact. *Pharmacoeconomics* 1997;11[Suppl. 1]:1–10.

42. Solomon GD, Skobieranda FG, Genzen JR. Quality of life assessment among migraine patients treated with sumatriptan. *Headache* 1995; 35:449–454.

43. Solomon GD, Skobieranda FG, Gragg LA. Quality of life and well-being of headache patients: measurement by the Medical Outcomes Study Instrument. *Headache* 1993;33:351–358.

44. Solomon GD, Skobieranda FG, Gragg LA. Does quality of life differ among headache diagnoses? Analysis using the Medical Outcomes Study Instrument.*Headache* 1994;34:143–147.

45. Stewart AL, Greenfield S, Hays RD. Functional status and well-being of patients with chronic conditions. Results from the Medical Outcomes Study. *JAMA* 1989;262:907–913.

46. Stewart AL, Hays RD, Ware JE. The MOS short-form general health survey. Reliability and validity in a patient population. *Med Care* 1988;26:724–735.

47. Stewart WF, Lipton RB, Celentano DD. Prevalence of migraine headache in the United States, *JAMA* 1992;267:64–69.

48. Szabo S. The World Health Organization Quality of Life (WHOQOL) Assessment Instrument. In: Spilker B, ed. *Quality of life and pharmacoeconomics in clinical trials*, 2nd ed. Philadelphia: Lippincott-Raven, 1996:355–362.

49. VandenBree MB, Passchier J, Emmen HH. Influence of quality of life and stress coping behaviour on headaches in adolescent male students: an explorative study. *Headache* 1990;30:165–168.

50. Wagner THJ, Patrick DL, Galer BS, Berzon RA. A new instrument to assess the long-term quality of life effects from migraine: development and psychometric testing of the MSQOL. *Headache* 1996;36: 484–492.

The Headaches, Second Edition,
edited by J. Olesen, P. Tfelt-Hansen, and K.M.A. Welch.
Lippincott Williams & Wilkins, Philadelphia © 2000.

General Aspects of the Headaches

CHAPTER 5

Socioeconomic Costs of Headache

Philippe Michel

Cost-of-illness and economic evaluation methods are used to assess the socioeconomic aspects of migraine. Their aims are different, however. The first approach aims to measure all patterns of health care resources used for medical migraine management, production losses, and intangible consequences (quality of life). Because education, screening, and rehabilitation are nonrelevant areas in migraine, studies of migraine focus on the burden related to diagnosis and treatment. Cost-of-illness studies of migraine have been quite popular over the years. The aim of these studies is to argue for more resources to be devoted to the disease by pointing out the economic consequences of allowing the disease to take its course and to provide estimates for economic evaluation studies. More studies have been undertaken and published on the topic of migraine than on most diseases, although the relevance of some studies can be questioned (10). Studies on other types of headaches are rare. [For tension-type headaches, see Rasmussen (27) and for headaches in general, see Benassi et al. (1) and Stewart et al. (34).]

Economic evaluation or *efficiency* evaluation (the two terms are synonymous here) studies aim to compare the costs and results of different alternatives (e.g., education versus curative treatment, screening severe migraineurs for treatment versus no screening, prophylactic versus acute treatment). In this type of evaluation, the following questions are asked:

- Is the health procedure, service, or program worth doing compared with other things that could be done with the same resources?
- Are we satisfied that health care resources (i.e., those required to make the procedure, service, or program

available to those who could benefit from it) should be spent in this way rather than some other way?

It is imperative to note that although economic evaluation provides important information to decision makers, it addresses only one dimension of health care program decision (10). Economic evaluation is most useful and appropriate when preceded by three other types of evaluation that address the questions of efficacy (can it work?), effectiveness (does it work?), and others, such as availability and acceptability. Because these last types of evaluation have been applied only to curative treatment, it is not surprising that the economic evaluation of interventions in migraine only concerns this aspect of care.

COST-OF-ILLNESS STUDIES

Definition and Methods

Cost-of-illness studies consist of three components:

- *Direct costs*, incurred mainly by the health care system in diagnosing and treating the disease
- *Indirect costs*, in terms of lost production owing to lost working days, diminished productivity resulting from illness or disability, or losses incidental to premature death
- Intangible costs such as pain, suffering, or reduction in quality of life of sufferers

The last component relates to quality-of-life approaches and is developed more fully in another chapter.

Two approaches may be used. The *prevalence approach* estimates the direct and indirect costs of disease in a specific year. This approach is the only one used in the field of migraine. It is appropriate, however, in helping decision makers choose the priorities for funding research. It is appropriate to prioritize between interven-

P. Michel: Department of Neurology and Biostatistics, Hospital Pellegrin, 33076 Bordeaux, France.

tions only if the full effects of these interventions are likely to be experienced within a single year. If not, the *incidence approach* is relevant: It estimates the lifetime costs of cases first diagnosed in a given year. It has not been used because it requires estimates to be made of disease progression and of methods of future care.

The estimates of costs were assessed using two methods: the *top-down* and the *bottom-up methods*. The first method consists of computing the costs from a national database. Its accuracy depends on the current codification system of the disease (i.e., the 9th International Classification of Disease diagnostic category 346) and on the quality of the available data, which were not collected for this purpose. The second method relates to costs measured by *ad hoc* questionnaires in a sample of migraine sufferers. Accuracy depends mainly on the representativeness of the sample because the cost is extrapolated from the sample to the total population.

Estimation of Health Care Resources Related to Migraine (Direct Costs)

The first estimates of medical consumption were published nearly 30 years ago: Waters and O'Connor observed that 46% of women in South Wales had never consulted a doctor for their headaches (41). Since then, the definition of migraine, the epidemiologic methods,

and the definition of health care resources have been refined. Herein only the results of cross-sectional, general population-based studies using criteria of International Headache Society (IHS) are used (3,12,17,18, 27–29,32,37). Studies conducted on a subsample of the general population also were excluded from this review (Table 1).

Most studies present the results of resources used instead of costs or charges. These estimates are more useful because the format allows comparison between studies to be done more easily than cost data. The results are rather variable, and therefore the health care resources consumed for migraine cannot be determined precisely at present.

These results cannot provide information for decision makers about whether more resources should be devoted to treating migraine. In fact, the reverse hypothesis is proposed by the economists: Resource utilization depends mainly on the availability of treatment options, their costs, and their effectiveness (i.e., resources previously devoted to the treatment of migraine) (11). Also, these results do not help in setting medical research priorities. Because no standardized medical consumption measurement method is available, the results are sparse and do not provide a baseline against which new interventions could be assessed. They highlight the importance of migraine, in addition to and not in place of the more usual estimates of morbidity (frequency of attacks, length of the disease).

TABLE 1. *Patterns of resources utilization related to migraine: results of the IHS criteria, general population-based studies (%)[a]*

Type of resource	Study	Men	Women	Total
Primary care physicians ever consulted for migraine	Edmeads et al. (n = 2.905)			81
	Stang and Osterhaus (n = ?)	77	85	
	Lipton et al. (n = 1,720)	57	68	66
	Rasmussen et al. (n = 740)	43	61	56
	Van Roijen et al. (n = 434)			70
	Michel et al. (n = 340)			56
	Sakai and Igarashi (n = 338)			30
	Roh et al. (n = 320)			24
Specialist consulted during previous year	Edmeads (n = 2.905)			41
	Rasmussen et al. (n = 740)	17	16	16
Specialist consulted during previous 6 mo	Michel et al. (n = 340)			20
Medication used during previous year (yes)	Rasmussen et al. (n = 740)	35	56	49
Ratio (% migraineurs using only OTC/ % migraineurs using prescribed medication)	Celentano et al. (n = 20.468)	67/28	57/40	
	Edmeads et al. (n = 2.905)			91/44
	Sakai and Igarashi (n = 338)			57/24
Ever hospitalized for headaches	Stang and Osterhaus (n = ?)	6	8	7
Hospitalized during previous year	Rasmussen et al. (n = 740)	3	1	2
Complementary examinations during previous year	Rasmussen et al. (n = 740)			3
Complementary examinations during previous 6 mo	Michel (n = 340)			51
Emergency room visit	Celentano et al. (n = 2.905)	13	13	13
	Edmeads (n = 2.905)		14	

IHS, International Headache Society; OTC, over-the-counter.
[a]Point estimates (most studies do not provide information on confidence interval). The sample size used for estimation is indicated into brackets in the second column.

All studies report that a large percentage of migraineurs never consult a physician for migraine. The concept in fact should be refined and split into categories of "ever consulted," "current consulters," and "lapsed consulters" (12). Population-based studies in Western countries report similar results (12,17,18,27,32,39). In Asia, this proportion is lower (28,29). The proportion of sufferers who "ever consulted" is not a direct measurement of nonquality of care because many migraineurs adopt effective coping strategies against pain and do not need care; however, some of them are in need of care. In Canada, Edmeads studied the reasons why 65% of patients did not return to their primary care physician or neurologist: 55% were satisfied with the treatment and did not need to consult again; however, 17% did not return because of problems with the medication; and 38% were "turned off" by their doctors; that is, they felt that they were not taken seriously, they were not given enough consultation, or the doctor was not knowledgeable or able to communicate (13). About 20 years ago, Packard showed that, in a highly selected sample of military personnel and their dependents, 50% of patients wanted an explanation and reassurance first, whereas two-thirds of doctors viewed pain relief as the most important aim of management (25). In France, 43% of migraineurs thought that nothing could be done for migraine (19), 35% were not satisfied with their primary care physician's service, and 52% believed that orthodox medicine was not effective (18). This last article analyzed the factors associated with a demand for care using a multivariate logistic regression model. The independent variable was whether the patient had ever consulted a doctor for headache. Factors associated with consultation were belief in the effectiveness of medical care [95% confidence interval (CI) of adjusted odds ratio (OR), 0.9–22.1, almost reaching the significance level], pain intensity (95% CI of adjusted OR, 1.5–4.7), frequency of attacks (95% CI of adjusted OR, 1.1–1.8), length of the disease (95% CI of adjusted OR, 1.01–1.06 per year), and social insurance (95% CI of adjusted OR, 1.3– 5.3). The income, duration of attacks, and handicap were not associated with a demand for care (18). Recently, Lipton and associates found that, in women, ever consulting was associated with pain intensity, the number of migraine symptoms, attack frequency, duration, and disability. For men, none of the variables reached statistical significance. They performed separate analyses, although gender did not seem to be an effect modifier (17).

The therapeutic inadequacies are another concern. The extensive use of over-the-counter (OTC) drugs is well documented. Moreover, in France, 15% of migraineurs used drugs given by family or friends. In this population-based study, only 17% of the migraineurs reported that they knew at least one drug by name from a list of all antimigraine drugs, and only 10% had actually tried one of these drugs. Moreover, 59% of those who viewed migraine as a severe headache preferred nonspecific analgesic medication (19).

Von Korff and associates (39) conducted a 2-year cohort study that included three interviews at 1-year intervals in 662 headache patients from a primary care setting. They defined *chronic* or *frequent users* of medications as using for 14 or more days in the prior month for two of the three interviews and *chronic* or frequent polypharmacy as chronic or frequent use of two or more classes of headache medications. They identified 21% as chronic or frequent users and 2.6% as chronic or frequent polypharmacy users. Chronic or frequent use of OTC medications was twice as common as chronic or frequent use of prescription drugs. The following were the risk factors for frequent or chronic use of headache medication (39):

- Frequency of attacks (strongest association)
- Type of headache
- Age
- Pain intensity

Gender, education, depressive symptoms, and pain-low focused coping were not factors for medication use. Prevalence studies found that between 6% and 12% of migraineurs have had a prophylactic treatment (12).

Sparse data about medical consumption in other sectors of health care are available. Among the 20% to 40% of migraineurs who consult specialists during a 1-year period, the rate of neurologist consultation is less than 10%; the most frequently consulted specialists in France and the Netherlands were ophthalmologists and homeopaths (19,37). Use of the emergency department (ED) also reflects inefficiencies. A large proportion of migraineurs visiting the ED are regular ED users. In a health maintenance organization setting, 36% of 152 migraineurs had repeated visits (mean, 4.2) during the 5-month study period (15); in an urban teaching hospital in the United States, 11% of 185 migraineurs accounted for 42.5% of visits (30). The use of laboratory examinations seems to be variable, and the rate of hospitalization is less than 10%. Do these results indicate poor quality of care? To answer this question, measurement of both process and outcome data (e.g., satisfaction of the migraine sufferers or objective assessment of the effectiveness of these treatment strategies) is required.

The relationship between these inadequacies and their consequences in terms of inappropriate medical consumption illustrates the presence of two populations of migraineurs (Fig 1): on the one hand, migraineurs whose treatment is not appropriate and, on the other hand, migraineurs in need of care who do not seek it. The last concern is, indeed, about demand for care. Stewart and colleagues observed in a population-based sample of headache sufferers that, among subjects absent from work during the week preceding the interview, only 31% of women and 18% of men had consulted a physician during the previous 12 months (34). Therefore, the concept of severe migraine was promoted to single out a homogeneous group of sufferers most in need of care.

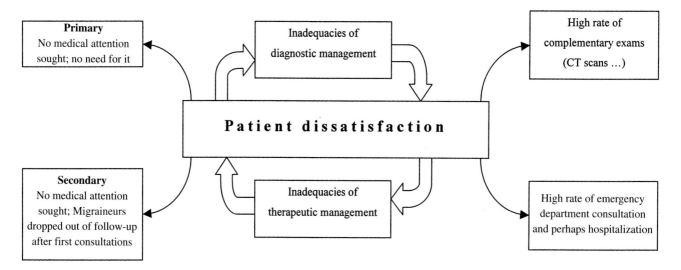

FIG. 1. The vicious circle resulting from inadequacies of management and its socioeconomic consequences.

Estimates of the total health care expenditures from Blau and Drummond indicated that "the total cost of treating migraine is relatively modest at about £23 million (1990) per annum," or 0.1% of total National Health Service (NHS) expenditures, using a top-down method (2). In France, the total direct cost was 4.88 billion francs (1990) (95% CI, 3.13–6.62) (or U.S.$156 per migraineur per year) and 1% of the total health care costs using a bottom-up method. Hospitalization was the greatest source of expenditure. The distribution of consumption costs was highly skewed: More than 25% of migraineurs had an annual total direct cost lower than 15 francs (nearly U.S.$3), and 10% of migraineurs were responsible for 70% of all expenditures (4). In a U.S. bottom-up study, a cost of $940 (1989) per migraineur was calculated (the study was, however, part of a randomized control trial and used a selected sample) (24). A U.S. top-down estimate, that is, based on national databases, was $382 per migraineur (5). These U.S. studies were not population based. In the Netherlands, the direct costs amounted to 134 million Netherlands guilders (1988) (U.S.$80 million), or 0.3% of total health care costs using a top-down method. The authors found that the costs of alternative practitioners (e.g., homeopaths) were responsible for a considerable part (80%) of the direct costs and that only 6% ever consulted a neurologist. They concluded that migraine patients often are not satisfied with the outcome of orthodox health care (37).

Estimation of Production Loss Due to Migraine (Indirect Costs)

Indirect costs of migraine include the production losses that can be attributed to migraine. The production loss is traditionally measured as the lost income related to the number of workdays missed (*human capital method*). For paid labor, hours lost are valued by the average value added per worker by age and gender, which is assumed to be proportional to gross labor income. Three types of production loss are measured: absenteeism, reduced productivity at work, and household productivity.

Absenteeism

Absenteeism in migraine has been studied extensively. Using either bottom-up or top-down design, estimates of the number of workdays lost were calculated in samples of migraine sufferers from the general population (4,7,24,27,35,37,40). Despite the differences in employment and economic contexts, the results are rather consistent (Table 2). Among these, two estimates are higher than the others: Those by Stewart and colleagues (35) and those by Osterhaus and associates (24) are likely to be overestimated because the former focused on the most severe attacks and the latter used a selected sample. Von Korff and colleagues conducted the only prospective assessment of absenteeism: Using a 3-month diary survey in 122 migraineurs from the general population, the mean annual number of workdays lost was 4.4 (40).

More recent studies, however, suggested that this cost assessment method had a basic limitation (22,23): The causal relationship between migraine and absenteeism may be biased by comorbidities (31). In the case of migraine, these comorbidities are mainly general symptoms related to pain, psychological disturbances, or psychosomatic diseases (5,19,36,38), which sometimes occur concomitantly with headaches, and migraineurs may not be able to identify precisely whether the sick leave was due to headache; therefore, the number of lost workdays may be overestimated. Whether this bias is

TABLE 2. *Estimates of absenteeism in migraine*

Study	Assessment of absenteeism (sample size)	Period	Definition of migraine	Mean annual number of missed workdays		
				Men	Women	Total
Chicoye et al. (France, 1992)	Retrospective (n = 340)	6 mo	IHS			4.0
Cull et al. (UK, 1992)	Retrospective (n = 374)	3 mo 12 mo	IHS	1.5	2.1	1.9
Rasmussen et al. (Denmark, 1992)	Retrospective (n = 67)	12 mo	IHS	1.6	2.3	2.0
Van Roijen et al. (The Netherlands, 1995)	Retrospective (n = 436)	2 wk	IHS	1.0	3.9	3.2
To et al. (Canada, 1995)	Retrospective (n = 14,400)	2 wk	ICD9			2.3*
Stewart et al. (USA, 1996)	Retrospective (n = 1,663)	1 wk 1 mo 12 mo	IHS severe	3.8	8.3	7.4
Von Korff et al. (USA, 1998)	Prospective (n = 122)	3 mo	IHS			4.4
Michel (France, 1999)	Prospective and comparative (n = 231)	3 mo	IHS			2.18 (incremental 1.68)

ICD, International Classification of Diseases; IHS, International Headache Society.

important never was assessed. Therefore, we introduced a comparison group in the study design and calculated the incremental costs.

The principle of the incremental absenteeism cost approach, recently used in cost-of-illness studies, is the use of a comparison group. The hypothesis is that the number of losses common in migraineurs and controls cannot be related to migraine and reflects the losses attributable to causes other than migraine. The remaining portion of absenteeism is the part attributable to migraine. Three studies were conducted in employee settings. The comparison group comprised low back pain sufferers, another common neurologic disease with similar consequences in terms of deficiencies, disabilities, and handicap (8). The two other studies included subjects who are not susceptible to headaches, and both concluded that there was no difference of absenteeism between migraineurs and controls (22,23). Michel and associates assessed the incremental amount of headache-related absenteeism in a general population-based setting (20). We found that the higher absenteeism rate for migraine sufferers compared with that of members of the comparison group is not due to headaches but to other health problems. This surprising result was related to the fact that migraineurs avoided sick leave during the days with headache. These results must be confirmed in other countries because national differences may play a role. For example, in Denmark, people seem to stay at home because of migraine attack.

The proportion of migraineurs with workdays lost during days with headache was low in the two prospective studies (60% and 88% respectively) (20,40). Again, a small number of migraineurs accounted for the greater part of losses. Von Korff and associates reported that the most disabled 20% of the participants accounted for 77% of the lost workdays (40).

A limitation of all these studies is the use of the *human capital method*, according to which production losses are valued by using the average earnings, whereas the actual loss for society may be much smaller (10). Migraine leads to short-term absences that may not result in production loss; that is, the work may be covered by others or "made up" by the migraineur on return to work. Van Roijen and colleagues indicated that the elasticity for annual labor time versus labor productivity has been estimated at between 0.6 and 0.9 (37). Two alternative approaches are available, the *friction cost* and the *willingness-to-pay* methods. The first method states that the amount of production lost because of disease depends on the delay needed by the organization to restore its initial production. This method is appropriate for long-term absences (with replacement of the worker) but may lead to similar results for migraine. The willingness-to-pay method is based on the preference of patients who state the amount they agree to spend to increase a probability of result, for example, to avoid migraine attacks. In practice, the willingness-to-pay method has been difficult to implement and has not been published, to our knowledge, in cost-of-illness studies on migraine.

Reduced Productivity at Work

Because migraineurs may avoid sick leave for migraine, a large part of production losses may be related to reduced productivity at work. Reduced productivity is measured using four methods:

- Patients' estimates of the number of workdays in which migraine symptoms were present in the previous month multiplied by the self-assessed level of performance affected by migraine (24)
- Patients' estimates of the number of hours worked with migraine symptoms each time a migraine attack occurred multiplied by the number of attacks per month and by the self-assessed level of performance affected by migraine (24)
- Patients' estimates of additional hours they should have worked in the past 2 weeks to make up productivity losses on days when they attended work despite experiencing migraine (37)
- Patient estimates of the portion of the day worked (either a full or a half day) were multiplied by the self-assessed percent of reduced effectiveness, the method used in a prospective design (40).

The mean annual number of days lost due to reduced productivity, according to the method, was, respectively, 9, 13.3, 4, and 5.6 (24, 37,40). The indirect costs are higher than the direct costs (Table 3). The ratio of indirect to direct costs is 1.1 (20), 4 (37), 8 (24), and 9 (2). A part of this variability is due to methodologic differences. The results consistently showed that productivity is reduced by 40% to 60% during work with migraine. Again, 40% of subjects accounted for 75% of the total reduced productivity (40).

Interestingly, Van Roijen and colleagues compared the results for each of the three first methods to investigate their feasibility and validity (37). Between 10% and 17% of data were missing. They found little correlation between the answers obtained using the third method and the two first methods ($r = 0.37$ and $r = 0.33$). The estimated costs according to the two first methods were about four to five times higher than those calculated using the third method. According to the method used, the ratio-reduced productivity costs to absenteeism was

between 1 and 6. This variability outlines the need for a valid measurement of reduced productivity at work.

Unpaid Productivity

Van Roijen and colleagues studied the unpaid productivity losses using a comparative approach. They compared the retrospectively self-assessed number of hours of household productivity lost between migraine and control subjects who did not have migraines, matched by age, gender, and labor force participation. They did not find significant differences between the two groups in time spent on household work and concluded that their method was probably too unrefined to measure small differences (37). Again, more valid methods are needed. Given the relative importance of indirect costs, economic analyses of medical interventions for migraine that are conducted from a societal perspective should focus on the reduction of work productivity losses resulting from migraine.

Economic Evaluation in Migraine

This last aspect of the socioeconomic approach to migraine is the most relevant for decision makers. We have few data, almost all of which concern pharmacoeconomic studies. Most of these data examined the economics of treatment with triptans. Clinical endpoints are efficacy, onset of action, percentage of patients who become pain free with treatment, recurrence of symptoms, and adverse events or side effects. Unfortunately, the conclusions of most of these studies are limited by the absence of blinding and parallel control groups. Few economic data are available from direct comparisons of the triptans with other antimigraine agents. Other limitations are discussed in a review (6). Finally, a full analysis should take into account the extent to which the availability of new and extremely effective treatments might alter demand, clinical practice, and the impact of ineffective or inappropriate use of treatments (33). A single cost-benefit analysis compared the direct costs (i.e., only drug

TABLE 3. *Societal perspective of the burden of migraine (in US$ per migraineur)*

	Van Roijen et al. (1988 estimates)	Osterhaus et al. (1989 estimates)	Blau and Drummond (1991 estimates)	Michel et al. (1990 and 1995 estimates)
Direct costs (healthcare costs)	80	817		156
Absence from work	160	3,744 to 4,128 for men	3	225–300
		2,088 to 2,484 for women	27	
Reduced productivity	165			

The variations are mainly due to differences of methods of data collection ("top-down" in Osterhaus et al. and Blau and Drummond studies and "bottom-up" in Van Roijen et al. and Michel et al. studies). The clinical trial sample of Osterhaus et al. is certainly responsible for the higher estimates. Other differences also exist (e.g., study design, type of healthcare sectors taken into account, method of valuation). This table illustrates the urgent need for standardization of the cost-of-illness method (11).

costs) and the indirect costs between sumatriptan and customary treatment and showed a net reduction in the cost of migraine to society of £125 (1996) per patient per year (14).

CONCLUSION

Methodologically sound evaluation studies should cover two areas: management of migraine and education and knowledge dissemination.

Management of Migraine

What is the most effective and efficient secondary care organization?

Few studies deal with this health service research question. A descriptive study compared the treatment of headaches between a dedicated outpatient center, a walk-in urgent-care center, and a traditional hospital emergency trauma unit (16). Such studies using experimental designs may be useful.

Is the screening of severe migraine sufferers efficient?

Much of the literature has focused on the definition of severe migraine and assessment of its prevalence. Clinical severity is associated with a higher rate of disability, greater medical consumption, and more frequent absenteeism from work. For these reasons, the screening of severe cases among the general population may be a cost-effective intervention, although this remains to be demonstrated because a screening tool is not sufficient to warrant a cost-effective intervention, which depends also on the ability of the care system to use this tool, the prevalence of severe migraineurs, the willingness of the screened subjects to seek curative care, and he accessibility of care. Moreover, we recently questioned the accuracy of the definition of severity, arguing that the severe attack concept should be split into two components: *severe attack* and *severe migraine sufferer*. The former may be valid for acute treatment strategies, whereas the latter should be preferred for determining the need for prophylactic treatment (21).

Education and Knowledge Dissemination

What are the most effective and efficient methods to reach the migraineurs in need of care who do not seek it? By improving the level of knowledge and attention from physicians, including the publication of guidelines in general medical reviews (9,26) is one such method. Moreover, these guidelines should rely on evidence-based data, which nowadays are largely missing. Communicating the relevance of scientific progress in migraine to primary care physicians and specialists involved in the treatment of migraine should be a priority as well as calling attention to the patient's expectation of treatment (13). Raising the awareness of patients about the efficacy of new treatments should be a priority. From an economic viewpoint, the methods of education and the impact of related interventions should be studied more precisely and could be the most cost-effective intervention for improving the management of migraine.

REFERENCES

1. Benassi G, d'Allessandro R, Lenzi PL, Manzaroli D, Baldrati A, Lugaresi E. The economic burden of headache: an epidemiological study in the republic of San Marino. *Headache* 1986;26:457–459.
2. Blau JN, Drummond MF. *Migraine*. London: Office of Health Economics, 1991:1–42.
3. Celentano DD, Stewart WF, Lipton RB, Reed ML. Medication use and disability among migraineurs: a national probability sample. *Headache* 1992;32:223–228.
4. Chicoye A, Auray JP, Duru G, et al. The burden of migraine in France. In: Chytil MK, ed. *Proceedings of the Fifth International Conference on System Science in Health Care.* Prague: Omnipress, 1992; 1554–1559.
5. Clouse JC, Osterhaus JT. Healthcare resource use and costs associated with migraine in a managed healthcare setting. *Pharmacoeconomics* 1994;28:659–664.
6. Coukell Aj, Lamb HM. Sumatriptan: a pharmacoeconomic review of its use in migraine. *Pharmacoeconomics* 1997;11:473–490.
7. Cull RE, Wells NEJ, Miocevich ML. The economic cost of migraine. *British Journal of Medical Economics* 1992;2:103–115.
8. Dartigues JF, Michel P, Lindoulsi A, Dubroca B, Henry P. Comparative view of the socio-economic impact of migraine versus low back pain. *Cephalalgia* 1998;18(Suppl 21):26–29.
9. Goadsby PJ, Olesen J. Diagnosis and management of migraine. *BMJ* 1996;312:1279–1283.
10. Drummond MF, Stoddart GL, Torrance GW. *Methods for the economic evaluation of health programmes.* Oxford: Oxford University Press, 1990:1–182.
11. Drummond MF. Cost of illness studies: a major headache? *Pharmacoeconomics* 1992;2:1–4.
12. Edmeads J, Findlay H, Tugwell P, Pryse-Philipps W, Nelson RF, Murray TJ. Impact of migraine and tension-type headache on life-style, consulting behaviour, and medication use: a Canadian population survey. *Can J Neurol Sci* 1993;20:131–137.
13. Edmeads J. Why is migraine so common? *Cephalalgia* 1998;18: (Suppl)22:2–7.
14. Gross MLP, Dowson AJ, Deavy L. Impact of oral sumatriptan 50mg on work productivity and quality of life in migraineurs. *British Journal of Medical Economics* 1996;10:231–246.
15. Kaa KA, Carlson JA, Osterhaus JT. Emergency department resource use by patients with migraine and asthma in a health maintenance organization. *Ann Pharmacother* 1995;29:251–256.
16. Linbo L, Bartleson JD, Morgan-Thompson D, Greff L, Naessens JM. Acute treatment of periodic severe headache: comparison of three outpatient care facilities. *Headache* 1998;38:105–111.
17. Lipton, RB, Stewart WF, Simon D. Medical consultation for migraine: results from the American Migraine Study. *Headache* 1998;38:87–96.
18. Michel P, Auray JP, Chicoye A, et al. Le GRIM: prise en charge des migraineux en France: coût et recours aux soins. *J Econ Med* 1993;11: 71–80.
19. Michel P, Pariente P, Duru G, et al. Mig-Access: a population-based, nationwide, comparative survey of access to care in migraine in France: *Cephalalgia* 1996;16:50–55.
20. Michel P, Dartigues JF, Durv G, Moreau J, Salamon R, Henry P. Incremental absenteeism due to headaches in migraine: Results from the Mig-Access French National Cohort. *Cephalalgia* 1999;19:503–510.
21. Michel P, Dubroca B, Dartigues JF, El Hasanaoui A, Henry P. Frequency of severe attacks in migraine sufferers of the Gazel cohort. *Cephalalgia* 1997;17:863–866.
22. Michel P, Dartigues JF, Lindoulsi A, et al. Loss of productivity and quality of life in migraine sufferers among French workers: results from the Gazel cohort. *Headache* 1997;37:71–78.
23. Mounstephen AH, Harrison RK. A study of migraine and its effects in a working population. *Occup Med* 1995;45:311–317.
24. Osterhaus JT, Gutterman DL, Plachetka JR. Healthcare resource and labor costs of migraine in the US. *Pharmacoeconomics* 1992;2:67–76.

25. Packard R. What does the patient want? *Headache* 1979;19:370–374.
26. Pryse-Philipps WEM, Dodick DW, Edmeads JG, et al. Guidelines for the diagnosis and management of migraine in clinical practice. *Can Med Assoc J* 1997;156:1273–1287.
27. Rasmussen BK, Jensen R, Olesen J. Impact of headache on sickness absence and utilisation of medical services: a Danish population study. *J Epidemiol Commun Health* 1992;46:443–446.
28. Roh JK, Kim JS, Ahn YO. Epidemiologic and clinical characteristics of migraine and tension-type headache in Korea. *Headache* 1998;38:356–365.
29. Sakai F, Igarashi H. Prevalence of migraine in Japan: a nationwide survey. *Cephalalgia* 1997;17:15–22.
30. Salomone III JA, Thomas RW, Althoff JR, Watson WA. An evaluation of the role of the ED in the management of migraine headaches. *Am J Emerg Med* 1994;12:134–137.
31. Schwartz M, Iezzoni LI, Moskowitz MA et al. The importance of comorbidities in explaining differences in patient costs. *Med Care* 1996;34:767–782.
32. Stang P, Osterhaus J. Impact of migraine in the United States: data from the National Health Interview Survey. *Headache* 1993;33:29–35.
33. Steiner TJ. Long-term cost-benefit assessment of anti-migraine drugs. *Cephalalgia* 1995;(Suppl)15:37–40.
34. Stewart WF, Cenetano DD, Linet MS. Disability, physician consultation, and use of prescription medications in a population-based study of headache. *Biomed Parmacother* 1989;43:711–718.
35. Stewart WF, Lipton RB, Simon D. Work-related disability: results from the American migraine study. *Cephalalgia* 1996;16:231–238.
36. To T, Wu KW. Health Care utilization and disability of migraine: the Ontario Health Survey. *Can J Publ Health* 1995;86:195–199.
37. Van Roijen L, Essink-Bot ML, Koopmanshap MA, Michel BC, Rutten FFH. Societal perspective on the burden of migraine in the Netherlands. *Pharmacoeconomics* 1995;7:170–179.
38. Von Korff M, Ormel J, Dworkin SF. Grading the severity of chronic pain. *Pain* 1992;50:133–149.
39. Von Korff M, Galer BS, Stang P. Chronic use of symptomatic headache medications. *Pain* 1995;62:179–186.
40. Von Korff M, Stewart F, Simon DJ, Lipton RB. Migraine and reduced work performance. A population-based diary study. *Neurology* 1998;50:1741–1745.
41. Waters WE, O'Connor PJ. Epidemiology of headache and migraine in women. *J Neurol Neurosurg Psychiatr* 1971;34:148–153.

The Headaches, Second Edition,
edited by J. Olesen, P. Tfelt-Hansen, and K.M.A. Welch.
Lippincott Williams & Wilkins, Philadelphia © 2000.

General Aspects of the Headaches

CHAPTER 6

Clinical Approach to the Headache Patient

Peter J. Goadsby and Ninan T. Mathew

When all is said in this volume on the neurobiology of headache, the problem remains consumately that of the clinician. The clinical approach to the headache patient is characterized by care, attention to detail, and a willingness to be flexible about the symptom interpretation while information is being gleaned. Headache diagnosis can be a daunting task given the myriad clinical problems that are seen daily. None of us can always be completely confident or complacent about the clinical process. Headache is an excellent illustration of the basic principles of good medicine, and most headaches can be confidently diagnosed after certain basic information is collected. In this chapter we will attempt to cover in outline what one might ask and look for in taking a headache history. The reader is referred elsewhere for a more detailed account (2,6).

BASIC NOSOLOGY: PRIMARY AND SECONDARY HEADACHE

It is useful to have a simple nosology when approaching headache patients, and we would suggest the basic differentiation of primary versus secondary headache. The common causes of secondary headache are listed in Table 1. These population-based data give some insight into the likelihood of confronting many of the syndromes that we dread. The clinician must remain vigilant concerning secondary headache and alert to the warnings that are offered (Table 2). Perhaps the most useful question that can be asked is how long the patient has had headache. A long history will demand time to sift,

whereas a short accelerating history demands action. Features such as development of new headache, change in character, marked increase in frequency or severity or associated features, such as fever or neurologic symptoms (including weakness, clumsiness, balance disturbance, or altered cognitive function), all direct the clinician to seek a cause.

HISTORY

The two most important questions in the history are how long has the patient had the current type of headache and how often do they have attacks. The length of the history is a good guide to whether it is benign and the frequency a good guide as to tractability to treatment, with notable exceptions. It can be difficult to establish what is going on, and to this end a headache diary can be very useful (5). Some of the questions that need to be addressed are listed as follows:

1. How does the headache comes on, sudden or slow, and at what time?
2. Are there warning signs, premonitory symptoms (yawning, polyuria, mood change), or frank aura symptoms?
3. Concerning the pain, what is its site, radiation, and quality?
4. What are the associated symptoms—nausea and vomiting, photophobia, phonophobia, osmophobia, diarrhea, or aggravation by movement?
5. Are there any clear trigger factors—coughing, exertion, sexual activity?
6. What makes the headache worse—bending, straining, or better, lying down or rest?
7. What do you currently use and, in detail, what has already been used for both attacks and prevention?

P.J. Goadsby: The National Hospital for Neurology and Neurosurgery, London, WC1N 3BG, United Kingdom.
N.T. Mathew: Houston Headache Clinic, Houston, Texas 77004.

TABLE 1. *Common causes of headache*

Primary headache		Secondary headache	
Type	Prevalence (%)	Type	Prevalence (%)
Migraine	16	Systemic infection	63
Tension-type	69	Head injury	4
Idiopathic stabbing	2	Vascular disorders	1
Exertional	1	Subarachnoid hemorrhage	<1
Cluster headache	0.1	Brain tumor	0.1

Data from Rassmussen (4).

TABLE 2. *Warning signs in headache*

Sudden onset pain
Fever
Marked change in pain character or timing
Neck stiffness
Pain associated with cognitive dysfunction
Pain associated with neurologic disturbance, such as clumsiness or weakness
Pain associated with local tenderness, such as of the temporal artery.

Data from Goadsby and Olesen (1).

8. How does the headache effect your daily work and home life?
9. Is there any other past or current medical history of note?
10. Is there a family history?
11. In the personal history are there any significant factors, such as occupation or emotional issues?

Although this list is not comprehensive, it serves as a starting point upon which one might build the useful questions to provide a good history.

PHYSICAL EXAMINATION

One must exclude by careful physical examination clinical signs, such as papilledema, diplopia, facial weakness, limb incoordination or weakness, or gait disturbances, as well as fever or other signs of systemic illness. This is best done by a complete neurologic examination, including the cranial nerves, limbs, and gait. It is useful to palpate the cranium for lumps or localized tenderness and to examine the temporal arteries. Frequently, the greater occipital nerves will be tender to palpation in patients with frequent headache, but whether this represents true cervical or occipital pathology is doubtful. One should record the blood pressure as a minimum in terms of general information because it impacts on many treatments used in primary headache syndromes if it is not well controlled.

INVESTIGATION

A suspicion of secondary headache must be pursued by appropriate investigations such as brain imaging with computed tomography (CT) or magnetic resonance (MR) scan, blood biochemistry, and blood count, including an erythrocyte sedimentation rate in the those patients over 50 years of age, in whom the possibility of giant cell arteritis must never be overlooked. For patients with a clear history of migraine and normal neurologic examination CT scanning is an extremely low-yield investigation, with some 0.4% of patients having some lesion (3). Investigation often can be apparently fruitless, but one should never underestimate the importance of impressing upon the patient the fact that we are interested in their problems and in pursuing what is important to them. To a certain extent what is studied is subject to local disease and societal pressures.

CONCLUSION

Headache management starts with diagnosis and this begins with a good history and physical examination. This clinical process provides clear information for the physician and sets patients at ease in the knowledge that the doctor is interested in their problem. A good clinical approach is a powerful tool that can never be underestimated in the management of headache.

REFERENCES

1. Goadsby PJ, Olesen J. Diagnosis and management of migraine. *Br Med J* 1996;312:1279–1282.
2. Lance JW, Goadsby PJ. *Mechanism and management of headache.* London: Butterworth-Heinemann, 1998.
3. Quality Standards Subcommittee of the American Academy of Neurology. The utility of neuroimaging in the evaluation of headache patients with normal neurologic examinations. *Neurology* 1994;44:1353–1354.
4. Rassmussen BK. Epidemology of headache. *Cephalalgia* 1995;15:45–68.
5. Russell MB, Rassmussen BK, Brennum J, Iversen HK, Jensen RA, Olesen J. Presentation of a new instrument: the diagnostic headache diary. *Cephalalgia* 1992;12:369–374.
6. Silberstein SD, Lipton RB, Goadsby PJ. *Headache in clinical practice.* Oxford: ISIS Medical Media, 1998.

The Headaches, Second Edition,
edited by J. Olesen, P. Tfelt-Hansen, and K.M.A. Welch.
Lippincott Williams & Wilkins, Philadelphia © 2000.

General Aspects of the Headaches

CHAPTER 7

Clinical Pharmacology and Randomized Controlled Clinical Trials in Headache

Carl G. H. Dahlöf and Peer Tfelt-Hansen

The clinical pharmacology of a drug includes both pharmacokinetics—what the body does to the drug—and pharmacodynamics—what the drug does to the body. In this chapter only a brief account of those aspects of clinical pharmacology relevant to migraine and its treatment will be given, which should help the reader to understand the expressions used in later chapters addressing headache therapy. This chapter also includes a section on the evaluation of the quality of the methods and results in randomized controlled clinical trials in migraine.

PHARMACOKINETICS

Pharmacokinetics is that aspect of clinical pharmacology dealing with the degree of drug absorption, the time taken to achieve a peak plasma concentration, the degree of binding to plasma proteins, its distribution from plasma to tissue site of action, the extent of its metabolism, and the pattern of excretion. The absorption, distribution, biotransformation, and excretion of a drug all involve its passage across cell membranes (1). Important characteristics of a drug are its molecular size and shape, solubility at the site of its absorption, degree of ionization, and relative lipid solubility of its ionized and nonionized forms.

C.G.H. Dahlöf: Department of Clinical Pharmacology, Sahlgrenska University Hospital, and Gothenburg Migraine Clinic, S-41117 Göteborg, Sweden.

P. Tfelt-Hansen: Department of Neurology, Glostrup Hospital, University of Copenhagen, DK-2600 Glostrup, Copenhagen, Denmark.

Absorption

The degree of absorption of a drug depends on its route of administration: oral, sublingual, subcutaneous, rectal, or inhalational. Absorption from the gastrointestinal tract is governed by factors that are generally applicable, such as surface area for absorption, blood flow to the site of absorption, physical state of the drug, and its concentration at the site of absorption. Any factor that accelerates gastric emptying will be likely to increase the rate of drug absorption, whereas any factor that delays gastric emptying will probably have the opposite effect, regardless of the characteristics of the drug. During migraine attacks, gastrointestinal stasis may impair the absorption of aspirin and tolfenamic acid, and the absorption can be normalized by administering the antiemetic metoclopramide, which promotes gastrointestinal motility (3,14,15), but the neuroleptic-type antiemetic thiethylperazine does not have this effect (16).

The bioavailability of a drug is an estimate of the amount of intact drug entering the systemic circulation after administration by the intended route and therefore is a function of absorption, excretion, and metabolism. If the metabolic or excretory capacity of the gut and liver, the first-pass metabolism, for a given agent is great, bioavailability will be low. The bioavailability after a certain route of administration is calculated by comparing the area under the curve (AUC) with that of the AUC after intravenous administration, expressed as a percentage. That bioavailability is not the same as the amount of a drug absorbed can be exemplified by ergotamine. Sixty-six percent of ergotamine is absorbed after oral administration, but the bioavailability is less than 1%, as a result of extensive first-pass metabolism in the liver (see Chapter 51). If the concentration of a drug in plasma is plotted against time after administration, a curve is outlined, the peak height (C_{max}) and the time taken to reach the peak (t_{max}) of which are measures of the rate of availability.

Drug Distribution

Patterns of drug distribution reflect certain physiologic factors and physicochemical properties of drugs. An initial phase of distribution may be distinguished that reflects cardiac output and regional blood flow. The most important facet of a drug's distribution is its movement into bodily tissues, especially whether or not the drug is able to cross the blood–brain barrier. Cerebral blood flow is the only limitation to penetration into the central nervous system (CNS) by highly lipid-soluble drugs. The rate of diffusion of drugs with increasing polarity into the CNS is proportional to the lipid solubility of the nonionized molecules.

The apparent space in the body available to contain the drug is called the volume of distribution. Dividing the amount of drug in the body by the plasma concentration yields a volume of distribution. A large volume of distribution indicates that little of the drug is left in the central compartment and that most of the drug has been distributed to other peripheral compartments.

Metabolism and Excretion

Generally, the aim of biotransformation is to turn lipophilic drugs into more hydrophilic metabolites that are readily excreted from the body. Many drugs are in this way inactivated by the liver metabolism, although formation of active metabolites can take place as an intermediate step of biotransformation.

Clearance is a measure of the body's ability to eliminate drug. The kidney is the most important organ for elimination of drugs and their metabolites. The elimination half-life ($t_{1/2}$) of a drug from plasma (time taken for plasma concentration of a drug to halve) is important as a guide for estimating times for elimination of drugs from the body and, during multiple dosing, as a guide for calculating the rate of accumulation of the drug. A large volume of distribution means that little of the drug is available for metabolism/excretion in the central compartment, and this generally explains the longer elimination half-life of the drug.

Plasma Concentration Measurements

If we could measure the concentrations of a drug at its site of action, the more likely we would be able to link those concentrations to a clinical response; but this is not possible in migraine. The next best alternative is to try to relate plasma drug concentrations with clinical or pharmacologic effects; but so far this approach has not been successful in migraine either, even when the concentrations of active metabolites also have been taken into account (2).

PHARMACODYNAMICS

Pharmacodynamics is the term applied to the study of pharmacologic effects and mechanisms of action once a drug has reached its site(s) of action from the blood stream after absorption.

Mode of Drug Action

Most drugs act specifically as agonists or antagonists of receptors, as uptake inhibitors, ion channel modifiers, or enzyme inhibitors. The particular mechanisms relevant to drug action in headache therapy will be addressed in those sections of this book dealing with individual drugs. Suffice it to say that nearly all of the drugs used in the treatment or prevention of migraine act on specific receptors, especially those that are the natural receptors for neurotransmitters released by serotonergic, adrenergic, and dopaminergic neurons. These receptors are located not only on structures in the head, brain, vessels, and other tissues, but in peripheral structures, including blood vessels throughout the body, the heart, and organs containing smooth muscle, such as the gastrointestinal tract, tracheobronchial tree, and bladder. It follows, therefore, that a drug action directed at a particular specific receptor in the head also will affect those peripheral structures possessing the same receptor species. Neurotransmitter pharmacology is complicated even more by the fact that several specific receptor subtypes exist for the same endogenous transmitter substance [at least 14, for instance, have been claimed in the case of 5-hydroxytryptamine (5-HT)] (5,6,11,13). Furthermore, receptors for entirely different substances sometimes possess significant structural homology, which explains why certain drugs affect (stimulate or block) more than one type of receptor. Ergotamine, for example, is a powerful agonist on 5-HT$_{1A}$, 5-HT$_{1B}$, 5-HT$_{1C}$, 5-HT$_{1D}$, 5-HT$_{2A}$, and 5-HT$_{2C}$ receptors and dopamine receptors. In addition to that, ergotamine also has a mixed agonist/antagonist pharmacology at the α_1- and α_2-adrenoceptors (Richard Hargreaves, personal communication).

Dose-Response Relationship

The animal pharmacologist may be able to observe changes in the magnitude of a drug response over a wide range of drug concentrations to determine the complete dose-response relationship. If the response, expressed as a percentage of the maximal response that an agonist drug is capable of inducing, is plotted against the logarithm of the dose (concentration), a sigmoid curve usually results, with points between 20% and 80% falling on a straight line. However, not all agonist drugs that act on the same receptors can elicit the same maximal response. Such differences have been explained as the drugs possessing different intrinsic activities (or efficacies). Thus, a drug (X) with high intrinsic activity capable of causing the maximal possible tissue response is termed a full agonist, whereas one (Y) with low intrinsic activity that can induce a less than maximal response, even with the highest doses possible when acting on the same receptor as drug X, is termed a partial agonist (Fig. 1A). Because it occupies receptors that would otherwise be free for activation by a full agonist, a partial agonist behaves as a partial antagonist in the presence of a full agonist.

When antagonists occupy receptors, they induce no response and therefore have no intrinsic activity. They merely prevent agonists from inducing their responses. In the presence of a competitive antagonist, the log dose-response curve to the agonist is displaced in a parallel manner to the right of the curve in its absence (Fig. 1B). An antagonist that acts noncompetitively binds irreversibly to receptors, and the maximal response of the tissue to the corresponding agonist can no longer be achieved (Fig. 1C) unless the tissue possesses excess or spare receptors. In this case a full agonist can cause a maximal response by stimulating only a small proportion of the total number of receptors and will induce a maximal tissue response even in the presence of a noncompetitive antagonist until the latter leaves too few receptors to enable the agonist to cause a maximal response.

EVALUATION OF THERAPEUTIC TRIALS IN MIGRAINE

A randomized controlled trial of a drug intended for use in migraine and other headaches often forms the basis for both pathophysiologic theories and further development of new drugs. Furthermore, in migraine, randomized controlled trials should, as for any other disease, form the basis for therapeutic decisions. Such studies should therefore be of high quality, which has not always been the case. A committee of the International Headache Society has formulated guidelines for controlled trials of drugs in migraine (7), and these should be consulted for

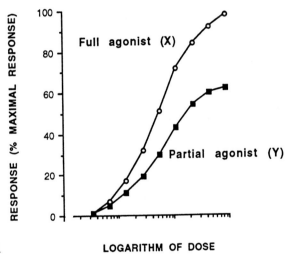

A

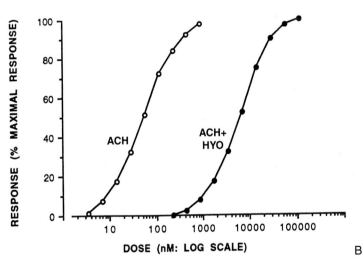

B

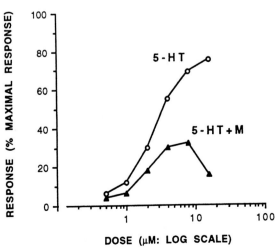

C

FIG. 1. A: Log dose-response curves to full *(X)* and partial *(Y)* agonists. The ordinate is the percentage maximal response. **B:** Competitive antagonism. The example shown is of a full log dose–contractile response curve to acetylcholine on the guinea pig isolated ileum in the absence *(ACH)* and presence *(ACH+HYO)* of the muscarinic cholinoceptor antagonist hyoscine (0.33 μM). The ordinate is the percentage maximal response to acetylcholine. **C:** Noncompetitive antagonism. The example shown is of a full log dose–contractile response curve to 5-HT on the guinea pig isolated ileum in the absence *(5-HT)* and presence *(5-HT+M)* of the nicotinic cholinoceptor antagonist mecanylamine (25 μM). The ordinate is the percentage maximal response to acetylcholine, from which it can be seen that maximal 5-HT receptor activation leads to a smaller response of the ileum than maximal acetylcholine receptor activation.

details. Similar guidelines have been published for tension-type headache (8) and cluster headache (9). In the following paragraphs, a brief indication is given of how to judge the quality of published results of controlled trials in migraine (Table 1).

Aim of the Study

Often the aim of the study is stated vaguely, for example, "We wanted to compare A and B." If a new drug is compared with placebo, then the aim of the study is clearly to demonstrate superiority with regard to efficacy or safety over placebo. When a new drug is compared with a standard drug and placebo is included, then the aim is probably to demonstrate that both active drugs are comparable in efficacy (and/or safety) and superior to placebo. If placebo is not included, there is no way of knowing, unless explicitly stated, whether the investigator intended to demonstrate superiority of the new drug over the standard drug or comparability, which, in any case, requires inclusion of placebo. To use a standard drug for comparison without placebo is similar to using historical controls, a method not to be recommended for controlled drug trials. If the stated aim of the study is to demonstrate that a new drug is better than a standard drug, then the standard drug will take the place of placebo.

Design of the Study

A placebo control is needed in most cases. The subjective nature of the response measured in migraine trials and the variable and sometimes high placebo response necessitate the use of the double-blind technique. However, maintaining blindness is not always easy; it may be broken by the emergence of characteristic pharmacologic effects. For example, the beta-blockers are difficult sub-

TABLE 1. *Checklist to assist with the evaluation of a controlled trial in migraine*

Aim of study
  a. New drug better than placebo?
  b. New drug better than standard drug?
  c. New drug comparable with standard drug?
Design of study
  a. Double-blind?
  b. Placebo controlled?
  c. Parallel or cross-over comparison?
Efficacy parameters
  a. Acute treatment trials
    1. Simple efficacy parameter?
    2. Side effects?
  b. Prophylactic trials
    1. Migraine attack frequency?
    2. Headache index?
    3. Side effects?
Presentation of results and statistics?
  a. Confidence intervals?

jects for crossover comparison with placebo because of the pulse-slowing effect, particularly during physical exercise.

Either crossover or parallel group comparisons can be used in drug trials in migraine. Opinion is divided as to their relative merits and the practical consequences of the drawbacks (e.g., carryover effect, problems with blinding, etc.) of the crossover trial (7). The main advantage of the crossover trial is its power, the probability of detecting a certain difference between treatments with regard to the likely variability in response to treatment within the population sample. Furthermore, this design is often more powerful in detecting significant differences in adverse events, and one can ask for the patient's preference with this design. The trend in acute treatment trials has been to use parallel group comparison (10–12), but this design demands inclusion of several hundred patients in each treatment group if comparability is to be demonstrated with narrow confidence limits.

Efficacy Parameters

Acute Treatment Trials

Simple efficacy parameters such as the proportion of headaches resolved within 2 hours of taking the drug (7) or a clinically relevant decrease of headache on a simple verbal scale after, for example, 2 hours (10) should be used. Only then can the clinician judge whether a clinically relevant effect has been observed.

Prophylactic Trials

Migraine attack frequency should be used as the main parameter; indeed, most trials of active drugs have shown that efficacy is related to this parameter. The number of days the patient has migraine over a given time is also an acceptable efficacy parameter and is simpler for the patients to record. In contrast, elaborate headache indices—either frequency×severity or frequency×severity×duration—are difficult to interpret clinically and have inherent statistical problems (7). Thus, the results of a trial should not be judged on the basis of changes in headache indices. Side effects are especially important in prophylactic trials because many patients stop such treatment because of them. So if the report of such a trial indicates that active drug and placebo give rise to similar side effect incidences, the result should be treated with caution because it is probably attributable either to the trial including too few patients or to an inadequate adverse events reporting system.

Presentation of Results and Statistics

Preferably, the results of all the objectives stated in the study protocol should be presented in a subsequent publication. The most fair and informative way of presenting the results is to give confidence intervals, usually a 95% interval (4). The reader can then judge whether what he or she considers to be a clinically relevant effect falls within the confidence interval. Furthermore, when comparability of two active drugs is claimed, this should be evidenced by narrow confidence intervals.

REFERENCES

1. Benet LZ, Kroetz DL, Sheiner LB. Pharmacokinetics: the dynamics of drug absorption, distribution, and elimination. In: Hardman JG, Limbird RW, eds. *Goodman and Gilman's the pharmacological basis of therapeutics,* 9th ed. New York: McGraw-Hill, 1996.
2. Cortelli P, Sacquegna T, Albani F, et al. Propranolol plasma levels and relief of migraine. Relationship between plasma propranolol and 5-hydroxy-propranolol concentrations and clinical effects. *Arch Neurol* 1985;42:46–48.
3. Dahlöf CGH, Hargreaves RJ. Pathophysiology and pharmacology of migraine: is there a place for anti-emetics in future treatment strategies? *Cephalalgia* 1998;18:593–604.
4. Gardner MJ, Altman DG. Confidence intervals rather than P values: estimation rather than hypothesis testing. *Br Med J* 1986;292:746–750.
5. Gerhardt CC, van Heerikhuizen H. Functional characteristics of heterologously expressed 5-HT receptors. *Eur J Pharmacol* 1997;334:1–23.
6. Hoyer D, Martin G. 5-HT receptor classification and nomenclature: towards a harmonization with the human genome. *Neuropharmacology* 1997;36:419–428.
7. International Headache Society Committee on Clinical Trials in Migraine. Guidelines for controlled trials of drugs in migraine. First edition. *Cephalalgia* 1991;11:1–12.
8. International Headache Society Committee on Clinical Trials (Schoenen J, Chairman). Guidelines for trials of drug treatments in tension-type headache. First edition. *Cephalalgia* 1995;15:165–179.
9. International Headache Society Committee on Clinical Trials in Cluster Headache (Solomon S, chairman). Guidelines for controlled trials in cluster headache. First edition. *Cephalalgia* 1995;15:452–461.
10. Pilgrim AJ. Methodology of clinical trials of sumatriptan in migraine and cluster headache. *Eur Neurol* 1991;31:295–299.
11. Saxena PR, De Vries P, Villalon CM. 5-HT1-like receptors: a time to bid goodbye. *Trends Pharmacol Sci* 1998;19:311–316.
12. Tfelt-Hansen P. Efficacy and adverse events of subcutaneous, oral and intranasal sumatriptan used for migraine treatment: a systematic review based on number needed to treat. *Cephalalgia* 1998;18:532–538.
13. TiPS 1998 Receptor and Ion Channel Nomenclature Supplement. *Trends Pharmacol Sci* 1998;19:45–47.
14. Tokola Ra, Neuvonen PJ. Effects of migraine attacks and metoclopramide on the absorption of of tolfenamic acid. *Br J Clin Pharmacol* 1984;17:67–85.
15. Volans GN. The effect of metoclopramide on the absorption of effervescent aspirin in migraine. *Br J Clin Pharmacol* 1975;2:57–63.
16. Wainscott G, Kaspi T, Volans GN. The influence of thiethylperazine on the absorption of effervescent aspirin in migraine. *Br J Clin Pharmacol* 1976;3:1015.

The Headaches, Second Edition,
edited by J. Olesen, P. Tfelt-Hansen, and K.M.A. Welch.
Lippincott Williams & Wilkins, Philadelphia © 2000.

General Aspects of the Headaches

CHAPTER 8

Ethical Issues in Headache Research and Management

Timothy J. Steiner and Povl Riis

Medical research is the means to a better understanding of etiologic and pathogenetic mechanisms, and to progress in classifying, diagnosing, treating, and preventing human disease. Headache research can ultimately be performed only in humans: the peculiarly symptomatic nature of headache syndromes—pain, nausea, hyperesthesia, debility—and the changes that occur with therapy require subjective description and cognitive interpretation. Headache research, whether on patients or volunteers, is strongly conditioned by good research ethics. It shares a number of fundamental ethical demands with other biomedical studies having humans as subjects, but also presents various special demands (30).

ETHICAL PRINCIPLES

Practical ethics are concerned much less with the idea that final solutions to ethical problems exist as discernible truths than with the perception of tensions, to be resolved by applying generally accepted principles. A number of ethical principles are established in medical practice and declared in guidelines. They include autonomy of patients, justice—with particular reference to resource allocation in a context of limited resources (distributive justice), nonmaleficence, and beneficence (2)—together with the medical professional ethical principles of veracity (truthtelling) (37), fidelity (the keeping of promises), and confidentiality. Recent challenges to the notion of principalism—the view that the approach to medical ethics should be on the basis of a set of ethical principles (2)—favor a more general approach in care and research based on the needs of patients, the responsibilities of doctors, the good of society as a whole, and deserts.

The term "needs of patients" is not the same as the "needs of the patient." Participation in clinical research is not always in the direct interests of the subject, whereas, to be ethically justified, it must potentially serve the good of society as a whole (46). This more general approach to determining what is ethical creates a more comfortable climate in which to propose clinical research (30) and is apparent in long-established ethical doctrine. The Declaration of Helsinki (52) enjoins physicians that "The health of my patient will be my first consideration," but it opens with, "It is the mission of the physician to safeguard the health of *the people*" (emphasis added).

ISSUES IN HEADACHE RESEARCH

Ethical research involving humans has necessary features that independent research ethics committees will look to and consider in the light of accepted generic or specific guidelines on research ethics:

1. Originality of the idea and methodology above a high minimum standard
2. Respect for the safety of patients or human volunteers who are the subjects of the research, and for their rights to information and autonomy
3. Respect for fundamental human values of a given society
4. Scientific honesty, including full disclosure of economic conflicts of interest

T.J. Steiner: Division of Neuroscience, Imperial College School of Medicine, Charing Cross Campus, London W6 8RP, United Kingdom.

P. Riis: Den Centrale Videnskabstetiske Komité, DK-1260, Copenhagen K, Denmark.

AUTONOMY OF SUBJECTS OF RESEARCH

The basic Kantian principal (31) is that people should not be used as the means to someone else's ends. Medical research, it was said, is a means to better future care, usually of individuals other than the research subjects. Many tensions in research are the expression of conflict between competing human needs, wants, values, ambitions, and objectives, which gives rise to what are termed people's agendas (30). The several parties involved in clinical trials, for example, have different agendas. If the patient's agenda is guided by his or her need or want to be well, the physician may share this objective through a desire to help the patient as a good doctor, but each will have other agenda items. The physician-trialist tempers his or her wish to help the patient because he or she wants also to be a good investigator, and the first objective of the trial is not the good of the individual patient (even though it should have it much in mind). The tension is resolved if the patient adds to his or her agenda a wish to help the doctor, or future patients. This, in an informed, competent, and autonomous patient, is what is meant by consent.

The consent of human subjects is required for whatever is done to them, in treatment and other interventions or research. This principle, stated explicitly or implicitly in virtually all codes of ethics and documents of guidance on ethical practice since the Nuremberg trials (34), pervades medical ethics and should underpin the practice of modern medicine. It upholds autonomy, or the right to self-determination and the notion of respect for persons (31), against paternalism, the view that doctors know far more than patients and therefore know best, without need to consult them (4,17,23). It stands against utilitarian arguments, flawed but seductive, that the good brought to many by medical research sufficiently justifies harm done to a few on the way.

Nevertheless, circumstances may erode autonomy (12,18,20), particularly that of dependent patients. Autonomy is affected, for example, in a given society, by limited availability of treatment. Offers of free or improved care (21) are an inducement to consent, casting doubt on how voluntary it is ["consent or be discharged" (46)]. There is no doubt that this occurs in headache trials, and it happens because access to health care is limited or new treatments are haphazardly or systematically restricted. Where there is no state-supported health care, the only means of obtaining treatment for some individuals is to enter a clinical trial. Although it does happen, this trade is not openly discussed between investigator and patient.

CONFIDENTIALITY

Support for the principle of medical confidentiality, set out in the Hippocratic Oath, is common to virtually all ethical guidance to doctors throughout history and across the civilized world (16). It is deeply rooted in pragmatism. Mutual trust and respect are essential ingredients in the doctor-patient relationship: patients who are not assured of confidentiality and therefore fail to disclose relevant details may not receive optimal treatment.

In research, confidentiality is commonly breached. This is especially true of trials monitored as part of the quality assurance of good clinical practice. The sudden expansion of interest in headache makes this particularly relevant. Controls have difficulty in keeping pace with so many sponsored clinical trails currently underway, as well as their spread to parts of the world where medical confidentiality may not be protected by law. The increasing use of third-party monitors, some with lesser professional qualifications, widens the range of people having direct access to patients' medical records. Breach of confidentiality itself requires consent. "Subjects should be told of the limits to the investigator's ability to safeguard confidentiality and of the anticipated consequences of breaches of confidentiality" (7).

CHOICES IN RESEARCH

One of the most important current ethical concerns in headache research relates to what actually gets done. It is not obvious who makes choices, according to what agenda(s), with respect to what research is needed and what is undertaken. What the public needs (and, to a lesser extent, what the public wants) should be decisive but, except in those few countries with legally based systems of research ethics control having strong lay representation, public opinion in these matters has no clear means for coherent expression. Least likely to be involved in choice making are people with headache.

Doctors aware of deficiencies in health care and interested in undertaking research to repair them are frequently unable to secure financial support for it. Government-supported research into the better management of headache often has low priority. Public finance of research is available to a limited extent from charitable and patient-led organizations set up with support for research into headache as one of their objectives. Although these sources of support are of significant potential benefit to headache sufferers, there is no oversight to ensure justice, in the sense of leading to a distribution of fair shares to all in need (8). The pharmaceutical industry has the means to support research across most therapeutic areas, but is market-driven in its choices, and it is not at all evident that market forces are just. For example, massive pharmaceutical investment in drug development recently is bringing undoubted benefits to those with migraine, who comprise barely one fifth of all sufferers from headache. The majority, those with tension-type headache, and the most disabled, those with chronic daily headache, have little current expectation from research in the pharmaceutical industry.

ACHIEVING THE RIGHT BALANCE IN DRUG DEVELOPMENT

Ethically, the number of people exposed to an unproven drug (or to a placebo) should be not excessive, but enough to demonstrate efficacy and safety. Proof of efficacy in headache conditions requires relatively large numbers because endpoints are subjective, whereas placebo-response rates are commonly high. Efficacy is proved only if endpoints, as well as being statistically sensitive, are clinically relevant and respect patients' values (46). There is no agreement on what are the best measures of efficacy in headache trials, although thoughtful recommendations exist (27–29).

Efficacy and safety of new drugs for headache may need to be evaluated for multiple dosages in children, adults, and the elderly, in specialist clinics and in primary care. The clinical characteristics of headache (including the need for and response to drug treatment) as well as safety of treatments may differ between these groups. It is necessary to establish the minimum effective dose, and sometimes the maximum tolerated dose. Full evaluation of headache therapy may require testing within several permutations of these circumstances. If this calls on the participation of many patients, it has to be so.

Where pharmaceutical companies compete for clinical trials resources, as they currently do in migraine, every trial undertaken has an opportunity cost-affecting other planned trials. Studies whose aim is solely to support marketing, if they direct resources away from trials properly investigating safety or efficacy, are *unethical* and in stringent national control systems will be treated accordingly.

THE USE OF PLACEBO IN STUDIES OF HEADACHE

The use of placebos in clinical trials is still debated generally (6). In headache, unlike some other therapeutic areas, the ethical use of placebo does not depend on whether or not there are better standard treatments. The Declaration of Helsinki (52) states, "In any medical study, every patient—including those of a control group, if any—should be assured of the best proven diagnostic and therapeutic method." Because standard treatments do exist for both acute and prophylactic treatment of headache, this appears to rule placebo unethical (39).

But central to acceptable deliberate use of treatments less efficacious than standard treatments is autonomous patients' consent voluntarily to forego the latter. Details of these treatment options that will be foregone are part of the information to potential subjects. Headache occurs transiently, and the consensual withholding of best therapy will not lead to any significant or long-term harm, especially with professional surveillance and rescue medications available (46). Whereas the International Headache Society (IHS) Ethics Subcommittee (30) found that

the use of placebo requires justification in all cases, they expressly rejected the argument, for headache trials, that "even informed patients may not be disinterested enough to decide rationally whether it is tolerable to be deprived of an accepted treatment" (39). Use of placebo is more problematic in long-term studies because consent must be continuing, but the issues are similar.

As for justification, placebo controls may be demanded by regulatory authorities as proof of drug efficacy, but this is not an ethical argument. On the other hand, patients may be fruitlessly exposed to risk if a trial produces equivocal results because of inappropriate control. Comparison with placebo reduces the exposure to an unknown drug needed to establish its efficacy. In a particular group of patients in a trial, if a new drug and an active comparator evoke similar responses without placebo control, it is not known in that group if either has improved outcome over natural history (45) (previous evaluations of the comparator against placebo are historical). Comparison with active agents can come later if prescribers wish to know what advantage a new treatment offers over alternatives (22,24), but patients can establish this for themselves by trying each one—a reasonable proposal at least for acute therapy. With prophylactic drugs the situation is different in that many currently available are not themselves reliably superior to placebo.

The real ethical concern over use of placebo arises through the principle of truth-telling and the difference between what is said to the patient and what he or she understands (46). Placebo is known to be associated with some therapeutic effect: to call it a dummy or inactive substance tells but may not impart the truth. Placebos are commonly used not only as a comparator with a trial treatment, but also during a run-in period to establish a baseline and/or identify placebo responders or noncompliers. Objections to the second use rest in part on the partial deceit needed to foil patients' presumptions as to when they might be receiving placebo (42).

PAYMENTS TO INVESTIGATORS

At a time of unprecedented activity among pharmaceutical companies developing antimigraine drugs and a shortage of experienced clinical trials facilities, few trials are conducted primarily for academic interest. Many are conducted as contract research. Investigators have little input into the protocol or prospect of authorship of publications, and conduct them for financial reward.

Questions must arise about research performed principally for payment. Paying investigators for their time spent in work under contract is not itself exceptional; the unease is about selling patients (46). In the United Kingdom in 1990, the Royal College of Physicians of London (40) held that "payments made on a per capita basis...are unethical." This was vigorously challenged by the Association of the British Pharmaceutical Industry, and the guideline was soon after amended to recommend payments to practices or departments that related to workload (41). Because workload depends on the numbers of patients recruited, whether this amounts to pressure to recruit inappropriately is not certain, but the presumption does tend to arise.

The response in some countries is a national system of rigorous oversight by research ethics committees. This requires a sound legal structure. In Denmark, for example, where such a system is in place, the Research Councils demand that payments be collected in a publicly controlled local fund (10).

QUALIFICATIONS OF INVESTIGATORS IN CLINICAL RESEARCH

Good clinical practice and, sometimes, legal statutes (49) require sponsors to ensure that appropriate skills and experience are possessed by investigators contracted to conduct their clinical trials. In many countries, no similar control applies to academic research, but investigators should be well qualified in the condition to be studied (5,48,52) because patients expect and are entitled to be appropriately managed, and this is at the heart of the professional duty of care. Whether investigators are qualified as researchers is a separate question.

Every investigator, whether involved in trials or other forms of clinical research, should meet the approval of a research ethics committee. The IHS Ethics Subcommittee considers it unethical for investigators, unless appropriately supervised, to undertake clinical research without reasonable competence in the condition being studied and, in the case of sponsored clinical trials of drugs, in good clinical practice (30). Equally, it is unethical for sponsors to put clinical research in the hands of investigators who do not have reasonable competence (30,49). But physicians are not, by virtue of their medical training, necessarily competent in research. Furthermore, it must be judged case by case what exactly are reasonable skills and qualifications for investigators, whereas it is unclear how they are acquired. Pharmaceutical companies base their choice of investigators on expectations of enrolling sufficient numbers of subjects (5).

Headache is managed far more in primary care than by specialists; research, especially trials, should be conducted in both settings, subject to the provisos regarding competence. An investigator who is not primarily responsible for a patient-subject's management has a professional duty to keep informed those who are.

QUALITY OF HEADACHE RESEARCH AND GOOD CLINICAL PRACTICE GUIDELINES

Poor-quality clinical research is unethical because it puts patients at risk and consumes resources, with opportunity cost, without possibility of benefit to anyone (30).

Data from such studies may be worthless or, worse, misleading. Clinical research undertaken to support drug registration, particularly clinical trials, is subject to well-developed codes of external quality assurance usually referred to as good clinical practice (25). Clinicians involved in drug development research have a duty (often reinforced in contract) to be familiar with good clinical practice and comply fully with its principles and practice.

Good clinical practice has been seminal in the ethical conduct of drug trials not so much because of the standards it promotes, but because it introduces audit and quality assurance. It has done much to prevent or uncover fraud (50). Nevertheless, it has little effect in promoting good scientific (as opposed to administrative) methods, nor does it stand in the way of studies with a poor rationale. The codified approach of good clinical practice alters investigators' intellectual involvement (46). Cookbook clinical trials stifle intelligent thought and, conducted according to protocols written not by investigators but by sponsor companies, deprive the former of claim to the property in a trial. This raises issues about who does own (and control) the property.

In many countries, no comparable formal codes of practice protect the quality of nonsponsored or academic clinical research, which then rests only on a combination of academic competence, diligence, and integrity. It is not evident that this is sufficient (1): studies of general and specialist medical journals have shown that researchers commonly use wrong techniques, or the right techniques wrongly, misinterpret their results or report them selectively, and draw unjustified conclusions. The IHS Clinical Trials Subcommittee identified the poor quality of many published trials in headache as a reason for the formulation of guidelines (29). One cause has been identified: "...much poor research arises because researchers feel compelled for career reasons to carry out research that they are ill-equipped to perform, and nobody stops them" (1). This remains true, even though some jurisdictions, in the Nordic countries, for example, have taken an effective stand against it.

RIGHTS OF OWNERSHIP OF DATA AND RESTRICTIONS ON INFORMATION FLOW

It is commonplace that sponsored drug trial and some other research protocols provide that all data produced by the research are the property of the sponsor. Ethically, the issues arise not over ownership as such, but over control (19). In multicenter studies, individual investigators without access to the whole of the data cannot judge whether they have been analyzed appropriately. Furthermore, whoever has control of data can publish them in a particular way or place, or not at all (33,35,36).

Whether or not these are problems in reality, there are legitimate concerns that they might be (3,13). With the sudden expansion of interest in headache, large numbers of sponsored multicenter studies are underway or being planned, the emphasis often on rapid completion. Such controls as there are have difficulty keeping pace. Investigators move on to new studies unmindful of those completed. Wheatley (51) placed the responsibility for ensuring proper data handling and analysis on the investigators, who should agree with sponsors about data management of multicenter trials, and about analysis policies, in the protocol, which is part of the contract between them and the sponsor. The IHS Ethics Subcommittee agreed (30), and they also wondered if a headache trial registry could help to answer the problem of nondissemination (14,32,43,44). The new headache subgroup within the International Cochrane Collaboration (47) is welcomed, and some countries have found solutions at a national level (9,38).

ISSUES IN HEADACHE DIAGNOSIS AND MANAGEMENT

Diagnostic methods in the management of headache patients must be based on scientific evidence of safety and accuracy, but seen in the light of costs. The marketing of diagnostic equipment before reliable evidence of these qualities has been collected is unethical. So is the use of diagnostic procedures that are sham, unnecessary, or covertly experimental. Sometimes the costs of these are passed on to patients.

Because the diagnosis of most headache conditions (certainly the common ones) is based on history and examination rather than on diagnostic tests, the clinical skills these require cannot be circumvented. The IHS classification of headache (26) has clarified the diagnostic criteria for many headache types, although not without some criticism, but these are a tool for the educated, whereas the underlying problem is lack of education. In headache, ignorance is widespread: in the general population as to nature, cause, treatment, and prognosis; among captains of industry and governments as to prevalence, consequent disability, and the economic burden; and among doctors at all levels (who receive little training in this field) as to mechanisms, diagnosis, and management. It is an unfortunate truth that although headache is common both in primary care and in neurologic clinics, interest in it is not. Whatever may be patients' rights to timely and correct diagnosis as a prelude to timely and correct treatment (53) (see Chapter 135), the reality is often a shortfall.

Therapeutic methods applied to headache patients must likewise be based on reliable evidence of effect, evaluated relative to side effects and cost. Marketing of new treatments without such evidence is unethical, whereas the use of many standard treatments is based on so-called clinical experience rather than more formally adduced evidence. This has to be acceptable: the alternative would be "a state of paralysis until some piece of research is done" (11).*

HEADACHE AWARENESS AND IMPACT OF PUBLIC OPINION

Competition for limited resources in most countries means that patients with some illnesses are less likely to receive treatment than those with others. Distributive justice calls for fair shares to all who need them, but the public perception of headache is unsophisticated, regarding it as not a disease at all or as benign and therefore deserving low priority. Such views are not justifiable in the light of the high cost of working days and productivity lost through headache, which pleads forcefully for a larger slice of the health-care cake than it currently receives in many countries. In some countries, people may receive no treatment for headache, resorting instead to self-treatment that is inappropriate, or using untested alternative methods. They are endangered by misleading advertising of proprietary treatments for headache (15), or may be induced to enter clinical trials or other research that they would not otherwise have undertaken. Of course, restricting treatment for headache frees resources for other conditions, but there is a question of balance, which at present does not appear to be right.

THE NEED TO UNDERSTAND COST EFFECTIVENESS

Premium pricing of a new treatment may mean that many people have little real opportunity to benefit from it. (One ethical issue, beyond the scope of this chapter, is whether research to develop such treatments should be conducted in populations where this is so.) But important relationships between cost and effect in medical management occur not only at the level of individual patients, but raise serious issues in distributional ethics. In countries with reimbursable health care costs, whatever is expended on diagnostic or treatment methods that are ineffective is wasted and not available for others (opportunity cost).

Equally, it is self-evident that the appearance in the market of new, highly effective, but very expensive treatments will cause serious perturbations in health-care budgets if the target population is large, as with headache. There is a predictability about this. Failure to assess cost implications of this sort during a drug development program denies prescribers an ethical basis for rationing the treatment if simple economics dictate that it cannot be prescribed to all who might benefit.

---

*"Descartes saw the opportunity of acting would not infrequently pass away before we could free ourselves of doubt. That in order to seek truth, it is necessary to doubt . . . that we ought also to consider as false all that is doubtful . . . that we ought not meanwhile to make use of doubt in the context of life" (11).

REFERENCES

1. Altman DG. The scandal of poor medical research [Editorial]. *Br Med J* 1994;308:283–284.
2. Beauchamp TL, Childress JF. *Principles of biomedical ethics,* 3rd ed. New York: Oxford University Press, 1989.
3. Braithwaite J. *Corporate crime in the pharmaceutical industry.* London: Routledge & Kegan Paul, 1984 (reprinted 1986).
4. Chalmers I. What do I want from health research and researchers when I am a patient?*Br Med J* 1995;310:1315–1318.
5. Cocchetto DM, Wallace JR. Qualifications of investigators for clinical investigations conducted under an IND: a discussion paper. *Drug Inform J* 1992;26:167–173.
6. Collier J. Confusion over use of placebos in clinical trials [Editorial]. *Br Med J* 1995;311:821–822.
7. Council for International Organizations of Medical Sciences. *International ethical guidelines for biomedical research involving human subjects.* Geneva: Croms, 1993.
8. Crisp R, Hope T, Ebbs D. The Asbury draft policy on ethical use of resources (and following commentaries). *Br Med J* 1996;312: 1528–1533.
9. Danish Central Scientific-Ethical Committee. *Collection of annexes.* Copenhagen: The Danish Research Councils, 1994.
10. Danish Committee on Scientific Dishonesty. *Annual report 1996.* Copenhagen: The Danish Research Councils, 1997.
11. Descartes R. Principles of human knowledge [Translator Veitch J]. In: The meditations and selections from the principles. Illinois: Open Court 1901 repr 1988, p 130.
12. Doyal L. Journals should not publish research to which patients have not given fully informed consent—with three exceptions. *Br Med J* 1997;314:1107–1111.
13. Dukes MNG, Swartz B. *Responsibility for drug-induced injury.* Amsterdam: Elsevier, 1988.
14. Easterbrook PJ. Directory of registries of clinical trials. *Stat Med* 1992: 11:345–423.
15. European Federation of Pharmaceutical Industries Associations. EC Directive on the advertising of medicinal products. A reading of the current texts (a note by the legal department). Brussels: EFPIA, 1992.
16. General Medical Council. *Professional guidance and fitness to practice.* London: General Medical Council, 1994.
17. Goodare H, Smith R. The rights of patients in research [Editorial]. *Br Med J* 1995;310:1277–1278.
18. Green R. Method in bioethics: a troubled assessment. *J Med Philos* 1990;15:179–197.
19. Hampton JR, Julian DG. Role of the pharmaceutical industry in major clinical trials. *Lancet* 1987;2:1258–1259.
20. Harris J. *The value of life: an introduction to medical ethics.* London: Routledge, Kegan & Paul, 1985.
21. Hart JT. Recruitment to randomised controlled trials [Letter]. *Lancet* 1993;341:1539.
22. Henry D, Hill S. Comparing treatments [Editorial]. *Br Med J* 1995;310: 1279.
23. Herxheimer A. The rights of the patient in clinical research. *Lancet* 1988;2:1128–1130.
24. Hill AB. Medical ethics and controlled trials. *Br Med J* 1963;1: 1043–1049.
25. International Conference on Harmonisation. ICH harmonised tripartite guideline for good clinical practice. *Good Clin Pract J* 1996;3[Suppl]: 2–27.
26. International Headache Society Classification Committee. Classification and diagnostic criteria for headache disorders, cranial neuralgias and facial pain. *Cephalalgia* 1988;8[Suppl 7]:13–96.
27. International Headache Society Committee on Clinical Trials. Guidelines for trials of drug treatment sin tension-type headache, 1st ed. *Cephalalgia* 1995;15:452–462.
28. International Headache Society Committee on Clinical Trials in Cluster Headache. Guidelines for controlled trials of drugs in cluster headache. *Cephalalgia* 1995;15:452–462.

29. International Headache Society Committee on Clinical Trials in Migraine. Guidelines for controlled trials of drugs in migraine, 1st ed. *Cephalalgia* 1991;11:1–12 (revision expected 1999).
30. International Headache Society Ethics Subcommittee. Ethical issues in headache research and management: report and recommendations. *Cephalalgia* 1998;18:505–529.
31. Kant I. *Groundwork of metaphysics of morals.* New York: Harper & Row, 1958.
32. Levy G. Publication bias: its implications for clinical pharmacology. *Clin Pharmacol Ther* 1992;52:115–119.
33. Munro AJ. Publishing the findings of clinical research. *Br Med J* 1993; 307:1340–1341.
34. Nuremberg Code (forming part of the judgment in United States vs Karl Brandt). *Trials of war criminals before the Nuremberg Military Tribunals under Control Council Law No. 10.* Vols. 1 and 2: The medical case. Military Tribunal I, 1947. Washington, DC: US Government Printing Office, 1948–1949.
35. Pearn J. Publication: an ethical imperative. *Br Med J* 1995;310: 1313–1315.
36. Rennie D. Thyroid storm. *JAMA* 1997;277:1238–1243.
37. Riis P. Fraud in medical research: the Danish scene. In: Lock S, Wells F, eds. *Fraud and misconduct in medical research.* London: British Medical Journal Publishing Group, 1993.
38. Riis P, Nielsen L, Almind G, Pedersen NS. *Health science information banks-biobanks.* Copenhagen: The Danish Scientific-Ethical Committee, the Danish Medical Research Council, the Danish Council of Ethics, 1996.
39. Rothman KJ, Michels KB. Sounding board. The continuing unethical use of placebo controls. *N Engl J Med* 1994;331:394–398.
40. Royal College of Physicians of London. *Guidelines on the practice of ethics committees in medical research involving human subjects.* London: Royal College of Physicians, 1990.
41. Royal College of Physicians of London. Addition to guidelines on the practice of ethics committees in medical research involving human subjects, section 17. London: Royal College of Physicians, April 8, 1992.
42. Senn S. Are placebo run ins justified? *Br Med J* 1997;314:1191–1193.
43. Simes RJ. Publication bias: the case for an international registry of clinical trials. *J Clin Oncol* 1986;4:1529–1541.
44. Spilker B. *Guide to clinical trials.* New York: Raven, 1991:816–819.
45. Spriet A, Dupin-Spriet T, Simon P. Choice of the comparator: placebo or active drug? In: Spriet A, Dupin-Spriet T, Simon P, eds. *Methodology of clinical drug trials,* 2nd ed. New York: Karger, 1994.
46. Steiner TJ. Ethical aspects of headache treatment trials. In: Olesen J, Tfelt-Hansen, eds. *Headache treatment: trial methodology and new drugs.* Philadelphia: Lippincott-Raven, 1997:71–78.
47. Steiner TJ. Treating headache from an evidence base: the Cochrane Collaboration. *Cephalalgia* 1998;18[Suppl 21]:63–65.
48. United States Food and Drug Administration. *General considerations for the clinical evaluation of drugs.* Washington, DC: US Government Printing Office, 1977.
49. United States Government. *Title 21, Code of Federal Regulations, part 312.50.* Washington, DC: US Government Printing Office, 1990.
50. Various authors. The problem of unreliable data and fraud in clinical research. *Good Clin Pract J* 1994;1(3):4–27.
51. Wheatley D. Clinical trial results: whose responsibility? Report of meeting of Royal Society of Medicine Forum on Clinical Pharmacology and Therapeutics, 18th March 1991. *J R Soc Med* 1992;85: 242–244.
52. World Medical Assembly. Declaration of Helsinki: recommendations guiding medical doctors in biomedical research involving human subjects. Helsinki, Finland, 18th World Medical Assembly, 1964. Revised Tokyo, Japan, 29th World Medical Assembly, 1975; Venice, Italy, 35th World Medical Assembly, 1983; Hong Kong, 41st World Medical Assembly, 1989; Somerset West, South Africa, 48th World Medical Assembly, 1996.
53. World Medical Assembly. Declaration of Lisbon: The rights of the patient. Lisbon, 33rd World Medical Assembly, 1981.

The Headaches, Second Edition,
edited by J. Olesen, P. Tfelt-Hansen, and K.M.A. Welch.
Lippincott Williams & Wilkins, Philadelphia © 2000.

Basic Science Aspects of the Headaches

CHAPTER 9

Anatomy of Muscles, Tendons, Joints, Blood Vessels, and Meninges

Lars Edvinsson and Erik Dahl

The skeletal system provides rigidity, support, protection, muscle attachment, and leverage. Most of the structures of the body are soft, pliable, and compressible. Muscles are firm only when contracting, and various forms of connective tissue (other than cartilage and bone) are stiff only when resisting physical forces. The other elements of the body would clump together in a shapeless mass if a rigid framework was not present. The skeletal system provides an internal mechanism of rigidity upon which other systems can act or be aligned.

Vital organs of the body are encased by the skeletal system, either completely or in association with elements of connective tissue and the muscular system. The brain is completely surrounded by the bones of the skull. The spinal cord is almost completely protected by bony parts of the vertebrae, although some apertures are filled by strong connective membranes or ligaments. The contraction of a muscle would be ineffectual if one end were not firmly attached to the fixed portion of the skeletal system and the other end equally firmly attached to the skeletal member of the body part to be moved.

THE SKULL

The skull bones may be divided into two groups: those forming the cranium (the "brain box") and those forming the face. The cranial bones enclose the cranial cavity, which is divided into anterior, middle, and posterior portions. The bones of the face form mainly the anterior part

of the skull. The primary function of the skull is to protect the brain and its associated sense organs for vision, hearing, taste, and smell. It also provides attachment for many of the muscles of the head and neck.

Although it is thought of as a single bone, the skull is composed of 28 separate bones. Many of these bones are flat, consisting of two thin plates of compact bones enclosing a narrow layer of cancellous bone. In terms of shape, however, the bones are far from flat and can show pronounced curvatures. The term *diploé* is used to describe the cancellous bone within the flat bones of the skull.

One may also subdivide the skull into neurocranium and viscerocranium. In humans, the neurocranium is extraordinarily large. The very size and dominance of the human brain emphasizes the skull's cerebral function, overshadowing others. Even in this limited role, the cranium cannot be considered merely protective. Sporadic protection of the brain from external impacts is of undoubted value; the need for a barrier against stresses due to the play of powerful masticatory and axial musculature is less obvious but is continual. In addition to these extraneous forces, the rigid cranial walls provide continuous isolation for the cerebral circulation. Moreover, the reputed buffering by meninges, subarachnoid space, and contained fluid could be effective only within a rigid container.

The brain's dependence on uninterrupted blood flow is well known; independence of cerebral arterial pressure from extracranial variations, due to some form of autoregulation the basic nature of which is still unidentified, is also well established. It appears likely that localization of a brain in a rigidly maintained space is a factor in such mechanisms, despite lack of precise evidence. However, the cranial cavity is not closed. Cerebrospinal

L. Edvinsson: Department of Internal Medicine, University Hospital of Lund, S-221 85 Lund, Sweden.

E. Dahl: Department of Anatomy, Odontologisk Institutt, Universitiy of Oslo, 0316 Oslo 3, Norway.

fluid passes freely through the foramen magnum, displaceable in either direction. Variability in volume of fluid in the cerebral ventricular system and numerous connections between intra- and extracerebral veins add to the complexity of the fluid circulation. Nevertheless, it appears undeniable that enclosure of the brain in an otherwise invariable space must be a crucial factor in the control of the cerebral circulation.

THE CERVICAL VERTEBRAE

This part of the vertebral column is extremely flexible, permitting a wide range of movements of the head and neck. The seven cervical vertebrae are smaller than those lower in the column, but the main distinguishing characteristic is the presence of three foramina instead of only one. In addition to the usual vertebral foramen, there is an

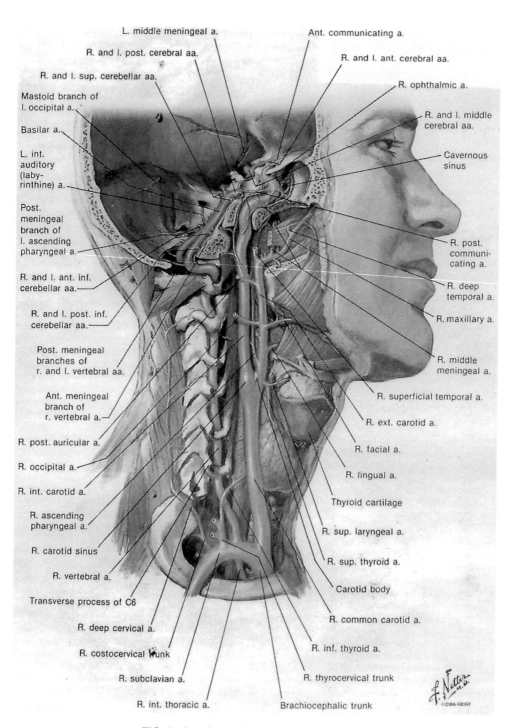

FIG. 1. Arteries to the brain and meninges.

opening in each transverse process called the transverse foramen (Fig. 1), through which pass the vertebral arteries on their way to the brain.

The first two cervical vertebrae have additional distinctive features and have been given specific names. The atlas, or the first cervical vertebra, supports the head. Having no body or spinous process, it is little more than a bony ring, which receives, on its superior articular surface, the condyles of the occipital bone. By means of this joint, one is able to rock the skull back and forth, as in nodding agreement. The second cervical vertebra is called the axis, and it is easily identified by the presence of the odontoid process, which arises from the body. This process fits up into the anterior part of the atlas and forms the axis of rotation. The seventh cervical vertebra has a very prominent spinous process, which can be felt at the nape of the neck.

THE JOINTS OF THE CERVICAL VERTEBRAE

The joints of the cervical vertebra, with the exception of the specialized joints between atlas and axis, are arranged on a common plane (Fig. 2). The vertebral bod-

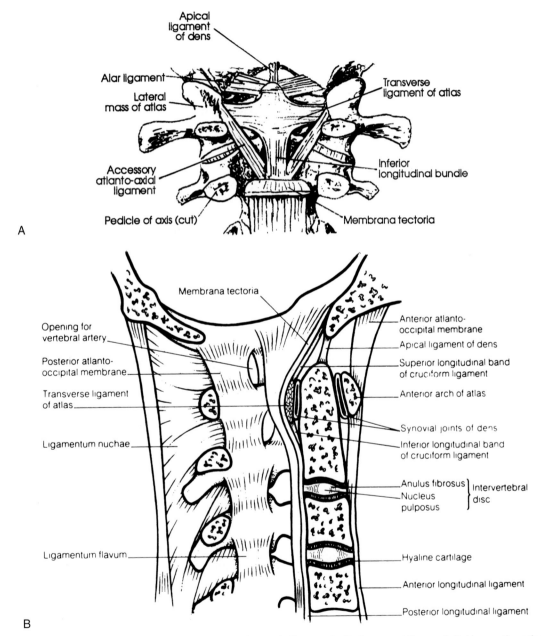

FIG. 2. A: Dissection from behind to show the main ligaments that connect the occipital bone, the atlas, and the axis. **B:** Median sagittal section through the base of the skull and the upper cervical vertebrae to illustrate some of the vertebral joints and ligaments.

ies, united by intervertebral fibrocartilaginous discs, form a series of nonsynovial, cartilagenous joints. The intervertebral discs, because of their pliability, provide flexibility to the vertebral column and function as shock absorbers. The disc consists of a tough outer fibrocartilaginous ring, the annulus fibrosus, and inside a gelatinous mass, the nucleus pulposus. The amount of movement at a single joint is not great, but the range of movement in the entire series is considerable. Gliding movement also occurs at each of the synovial joints between articular processes of adjacent vertebrae.

The joints are strengthened by anterior and posterior ligaments (see Fig. 2). These run in the midline along the anterior and posterior surfaces of the bodies of the vertebrae. They are attached to the intervertebral discs. The anterior longitudinal ligament is stronger and is attached above to the anterior tubercle of the atlas and to the basilar part of the occipital bone. The posterior longitudinal ligament runs inside the vertebral canal and is attached above to the body of the axis.

THE JOINTS BETWEEN THE VERTEBRAE

The articular facets of adjacent vertebrae are united by synovial joints (see Fig. 2). Concerning the ligaments associated with the vertebral arches passing between adjacent laminae is the ligamentum flavum. This is composed primarily of elastic fibers. Whereas the tips of the spinous processes in other parts of the vertebral column are joined by interspinous and supraspinous ligaments, these are poorly developed in the cervical region, and the ligamentum nuchae is present. This is a triangular, fibroelastic septum lying between the postvertebral muscles in the midline. Its posterior border extends from the external occipital protuberance to the spinal aspect of the seventh cervical vertebra. Its anterior border is attached to the spines of the cervical vertebrae and to the posterior tubercle of the atlas. Its superior border is attached to the external occipital crest. The movements of the vertebral column are described as flexion, extension, lateral flexion, and rotation.

ATLANTOOCCIPITAL JOINTS

The two atlantooccipital joints between the occipital condyles and the superior articular facets of the atlas are uniaxial synovial joints placed on either side of the foramen magnum (see Fig. 2). The anterior and posterior atlantooccipital membranes, attached to the edge of the foramen magnum superiorly and to the arch of the atlas inferiorly, strengthen the joints. Movement, occurring around a transverse axis, results in nodding or flexion and extension of the head.

ATLANTOAXIAL JOINTS

The atlantoaxial joints are a pair of synovial joints between the articular processes of the first and second cervical vertebrae (atlas and axis, respectively) and two median synovial joints formed by the articulation of the dens of the axis anteriorly with the anterior arch of the atlas and posteriorly with the transverse ligament. The transverse ligament of the atlas is a stout band of connective tissue that passes posterior to the dens and attaches to the medial aspect of the lateral masses of the atlas. From the middle of the transverse ligament, longitudinal fibers pass superiorly to insert into the anterior edge of the foramen magnum and inferiorly to attach to the posterior surface of the body of the axis. These longitudinal bands, together with the transverse ligament, form the cruciate ligament of the atlas. The axis is directly attached to the occipital bone by the apical and alar ligaments, which arise from the tip and either side of the dens, respectively.

Rotary movements of the head occur between the atlas and axis. Movement is free. However, the alar ligaments limit rotation of the skull and atlas upon the axis, and the apical ligament tightens during extension.

MUSCLES OF THE HEAD AND NECK

The head is balanced atop the axial skeleton in the erect anatomic position. It is held in this balanced position partly by its own weight pressing down on the atlantooccipital joint and partly by the coordinated action of the muscles that approach the base of the skull from all directions. The action of antagonists is important in movements of the head and neck because frequently a movement, once started, is largely completed by gravity. The antagonists then have the role of regulating the gravity movement and checking it at the appropriate point. For example, when the head and the neck are bent forward in flexion, the muscles extend and control the forward fall of the head produced by gravity. If the body is in the supine position, however, the gravity tends to resist flexion of the head, which then can be performed only by active concentration of muscles that can produce flexion.

The mobility of the cervical part of the vertebral column greatly extends the range of motion of the head. It will be found that many of the muscles that produce movements of the neck also move the head either by direct attachments to the skull or because the head is carried along as the neck is moved in various directions.

Muscles Moving the Head Alone

The head alone can be moved without accompanying movements of the neck. Several small short muscles under the base of the skull are grouped together as the suboccipital muscles. There are also several other muscles that run longer, independent courses to move the head.

Suboccipital Muscles

Suboccipital muscles are clustered together in a ring formation immediately below the base of the skull (Fig. 3).

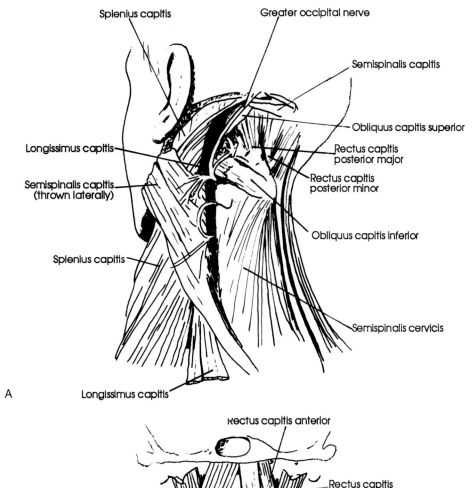

Splenius capitis

Greater occipital nerve

Semispinalis capitis

Obliquus capitis superior

Rectus capitis posterior major

Rectus capitis posterior minor

Longissimus capitis

Semispinalis capitis (thrown laterally)

Obliquus capitis inferior

Splenius capitis

Semispinalis cervicis

Longissimus capitis

A

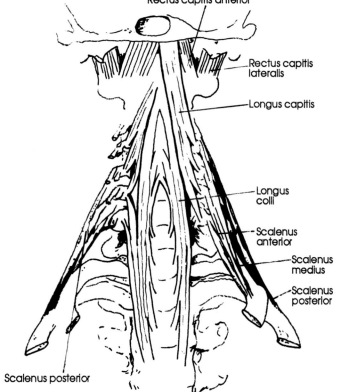

Rectus capitis anterior

Rectus capitis lateralis

Longus capitis

Longus colli

Scalenus anterior

Scalenus medius

Scalenus posterior

B   Scalenus posterior

FIG. 3. A: Suboccipital triangle of the left side. **B:** Prevertebral and scalene muscles.

They run a short course from attachments on the atlas or axis to the occipital bone of the skull or, in one case, from the axis to the atlas. These muscles usually work together to extend or flex the skull by a rocking motion of the occipital condyles on the atlas or to rotate the skull and atlas together around the pivot joint with the axis. The short, quick, almost automatic movements of the head in following movements of the eyes are largely the function of these muscles.

Sternocleidomastoid Muscle

A long, straplike muscle crosses the neck obliquely from origins on both the anterior surface of the manubrium and the medial one third of the clavicle as it ascends to insert upon the mastoid process of the skull. The sternocleidomastoid muscle has the effect of dividing the neck into two geographic areas: a superior and medial anterior triangle and a posterior and lateral posterior triangle.

The triangles of the neck are convenient for designating the location of structures in the neck. The action of the sternocleidomastoid muscle is to pull the skull downward on the same side and to draw it forward. The result is that the head is tilted to the same side and, at the same time, the face is rotated toward the opposite side. The tendinous origin of the two muscles can be felt diverging at the base of the neck above the sternum where they outline the suprasternal fossa. When one's head is turned to the right, the taut borders of the muscle on the left can be followed obliquely upward to its insertion. If both muscles act at the same time, there can be no turning of the head because the muscles oppose each other. Flexion of the head will result instead, particularly when the body is supine and it is necessary to raise the head, as from a pillow, against the resistance of gravity.

Associated Muscles

A long series of deep muscles, closely related to the vertebral column, exists to produce movement of the axial skeleton. The most superior of these deep muscles extend between the cervical vertebrae and the skull. Although their parent muscle masses are concerned with movements of the vertebral column, the following compartments move the head in company with those movements. It should be remembered that, when they act, other muscles are producing movements of the neck or the entire back.

Anterior Muscles

The longus capitis is a thin muscle that arises from the transverse process of the third to the sixth cervical vertebrae. It runs upward along the front and sides of the upper cervical vertebrae to insert upon the base of the skull in front of the rectus capitis anterior. Its action, similar to that of its suboccipital companion, is that of flexion of the head.

Posterior Muscles

Posteriorly located along the vertebral column are the superior portions of the deep back muscles. The longissimus capitis and the semispinalis capitis continue the long column of muscles upward to the skull, where they attach to the posterior aspect of the base of the skull, overlapping the posterior suboccipital muscle (see Fig. 3A). The splenius muscle, which runs from the thoracic spinous processes to the cervical transverse processes, has a part, the splenius capitis, that extends from the ligamentum nuchae of the cervical vertebrae upward and laterally to attach behind the sternocleidomastoid muscle on the mastoid process. All these muscles control the forward fall of the head with gravity in flexion and, as the head extends, bring it back from the flexed position to its normal attitude.

Muscles that Move the Neck

The neck is moved by muscles located anterior or posterior to the bodies of the cervical vertebrae. These muscles have their lower attachments to the axial skeleton below the neck.

Scalene Muscles

Three slender fusiform muscles descend obliquely laterally from attachments to the anterior surface of the transverse processes of the cervical vertebrae to the first or second rib (see Fig. 3B). The scalenus muscles have an anteroposterior relationship to each other and thus are named the scalenus anterior, medius, and posterior. They are active in lateral flexion of the neck but, combining forward in their descent, can also contribute to forward bending. It should be noted, however, that the sternocleidomastoid muscle, while pulling on the head, is powerful in lateral flexion of the neck. The two sternocleidomastoid muscles acting together are stronger in flexion of the head and neck than the scalenes.

The longissimus cervicis is primarily a flexor muscle of the neck. It is a flat muscle, running along the sides and the front of the cervical vertebrae.

Associated Muscles

The long posterior muscle masses of the deep back muscles have attachments to the back of the neck. Cervical portions of the longissimus, semispinalis, and splenius muscles described with the head muscles form a group of posterior cervical muscles. These act with the muscles of the back to control flexion of the neck and to return the flexed neck and the head to the upright position.

Two sets of muscles are related to the hyoid bone, which is unarticulated to the rest of the skeleton and is located in the neck between the mandible and the larynx. The muscles that attach to the hyoid bone are called the suprahyoid and the infrahyoid muscles because of their positional relationship to the bone. The infrahyoid muscles anchor the hyoid bone against the pull of the suprahyoid muscles, which use the bone for their lower attachment. The suprahyoid muscles form or shape the floor of the mouth. All use the hyoid bone for their lower attachment and, therefore, depend on the contraction of the infrahyoid muscles to provide a fixator action on the hyoid bone.

Facial Muscles

Facial muscles are the muscles of facial expression. Their contractions move the fleshy parts of the face for speech and cause the various expressions associated with emotions and feelings. Some of the facial muscles are listed as follows:

Orbicularis oculi encircles the eye and closes or winks the eye.
Orbicularis oris encircles the mouth and closes and protrudes the lips.
Levator labii superioris elevates the upper lip to give an expression of contempt.
Zygomaticus draws the corners of the mouth up and back, as in smiling.
Risorius draws the corners of the mouth directly sideways, as in a grimace.
Triangularis draws the corners of the mouth down and back to create an expression of sadness.
Depressor labii inferioris depresses the lower lip.
Mentalis elevates the lower lip and protrudes it, as in pointing.
Buccinator lies beneath the muscles listed above and compresses the cheek. It is sometimes called the trumpeter's muscle because it is used intensively in playing a brass musical instrument like a trumpet.
Corrugator produces frown lines in the central forehead.

Cranial Muscles

The cranial muscles lie on the forehead, on the back of the head, and around the ears. The epicranius is the only cranial muscle. It is divided into an occipitofrontal group consisting of an anterior frontalis and posterior occipitalis and a temporoparietal group consisting of the auricular muscles. The occipitalis and frontalis attach to a broad, flat tendon (galea aponeurotica) over the top of the skull. The frontalis pulls the scalp forward, and the occipitalis draws the scalp backward.

MUSCLES OF MASTICATION

The muscles of mastication are the muscles acting on the temporomandibular joint to close the jaws. The masticatory muscles are intensely strong. They produce the major power to forcibly close the jaws, to clench the teeth, and to grind food. These muscles protrude and retract the mandible and move it from side to side. In contrast to the action of the masticatory muscles, opening of the jaws is largely the result of gravity during inhibition of masticatory muscle action, assisted by the contraction of the suprahyoid and platysma muscles.

Four muscles are most important in mastication. The temporalis fills a depression on the side of the skull and elevates the mandible, closing the mouth. The masseter covering the ramus of the mandible is the most powerful jaw-closing muscle. Both temporalis and masseter can be felt contracting with clenching of the jaws and feeling the skull in the appropriate area. The medial pterygoid is internal to the mandibular ramus and elevates the jaw; the lateral pterygoid lies between the medial pterygoid and the ramus and depresses the mandible, opening the jaw (mouth). The pterygoids also move the mandible laterally.

Muscles Associated with the Hyoid Bone

These muscles may be grouped according to their position relative to the hyoid bone. Most are named by their origin and insertion and contribute to the movements that occur when we swallow. The suprahyoid muscles (above the hyoid bone) include the digasticus, consisting of two portions or bellies. The posterior belly draws the hyoid backward; the anterior belly draws it forward. The stylohyoid draws the hyoid bone up and back. The myelohyoid forms the floor of the mouth. It lies between the limbs of the mandibular body and raises the hyoid bone and tongue. The infrahyoid muscles (below the hyoid bone) are listed as follows:

Sternohyoid draws the hyoid downward.
Sternothyroid draws the larynx downward.
Thyreohyoid draws the larynx upward if the hyoid is fixed.
Omohyoid draws the hyoid downward.

Neck Muscles

The muscles of the neck consist of two superficial muscles on the anterior neck and a number of deep muscles that attach to the vertebrae and the skull.

Superficial Muscles

The platysma is a broad sheet covering the inner side of the shoulder and lateral neck and mandible. It draws the corners of the mouth down and sideways as in screaming or in an expression of horror. The sternocleidomastoid flexes the neck if the muscles are operating together and, operating singly, rotates the head to the opposite side while pointing the chin upward.

Deep Muscles

These may be divided into anterior, lateral, and posterior groups. The anterior group includes the longus colli, longus capitis, and rectus capitis, all of which flex the neck on the chest. The lateral group includes the three scalenes, which bend the neck to the side and help to elevate the ribs if the neck is fixed. The posterior group includes the semispinalis, longissimus, and splenius, which extend the neck and raise the chin.

Movements Possible

The column may be flexed or bent forward, extended or bent backward, abducted or bent to the side, adducted or returned to the midline, and rotated or twisted. Some of the muscles responsible for these actions also have other functions in the overall movement of the spinal column, but they are not described in detail in this chapter.

MUSCLES PROVIDING FACIAL EXPRESSION

A group of thin muscles that are closely applied to the scalp and to the face have developed primarily to move the scalp or to guard the opening of the skull. The contraction of these muscles also produces characteristic movements of the face in the display of emotion. The many small muscles beneath the skin of the scalp and face, particularly around the eyes and mouth, alter facial expression, a very important means of communication.

The epicranius (occipitofrontalis) is a broad musculofibrous sheet that covers the top and the sides of the skull. It is composed of two muscular portions, the frontalis and the occipitals, connected by a fibrous sheet called the epicranial aponeurosis or galea aponeurotica. The frontal fibers of the muscle extend over the forehead to insert by blending of these fibers with facial muscles that encircle the orbits or cover the root of the nose. The occipital fibers draw the scalp backward; the frontal fibers draw it forward. The frontal portion also wrinkles the forehead and raises the eyebrows.

Facial movements and the variety of facial expressions are largely the by-products of the action of muscles that exist primarily to guard the orifices of the orbits, nose, and mouth. The muscles responsible for the protection of these openings act as sphincters or dilators to control the degree of opening or closing of the eyelids, nostrils, or lips.

The orbicularis oculi keeps the lid closely applied to the eyeball, closes the eyes, and draws down the eyebrow. The orbicularis oris lies within the lips and is the sphincter of the mouth. The other muscles associated with the lips have been variously named and subdivided but are not described in this chapter.

The buccinator muscle arises from the side of the maxilla superiorly, from the inner surface of the mandible inferiorly, and from the pterygomandibular raphe, which is a dense band of the deep fascia of the pharynx. The buccinator thus constitutes the essential muscular coat of the cheek and is inserted into the corner of the mouth. The buccinator aids in chewing movements by keeping the cheek more firmly in contact with the teeth, preventing food from being pocketed between teeth and cheek.

All the muscles of the scalp and of facial expression are innervated by the seventh cranial nerve, the facial nerve, except for the levator palpebrae superior. Since the facial nerve is the sole nerve supply of many facial muscles, disease or injury affecting it will have widespread effects that are disastrous to the individual.

NERVE SUPPLY TO THE HEAD AND NECK

Nerves of the Face

Both motor and sensory nerves are found on the face. The motor nerves are derived from the facial nerve (cranial nerve VII). The sensory innervation is primarily from the three divisions of the trigeminal nerve, with a small contribution from the cervical plexus via the great auricular nerve. The brain gives rise to 12 pairs of cranial nerves, which supply motor and sensory fibers to structures in the head, neck, and shoulder regions. Each cranial nerve varies in the components it carries, depending on the structures innervated.

Several of the cranial nerves, specifically the fourth, sixth, eleventh, and twelfth, although supplying striated muscles, do not contain any demonstrable sensory fibers. It is generally accepted that sensory fibers from these muscles are conveyed to the central nervous system by branches of the fifth, the trigeminal nerve. Because of its widespread sensory distribution, both superficial and deep, the trigeminal nerve is often described as the great sensory nerve of the head. The trigeminal nerve is the largest cranial nerve. It supplies sensory fibers to the anterior cranium and face and motor fibers to the chewing muscles. Ophthalmic, maxillary, and mandibular branches form the nerve and supply sensory fibers to all structures within their distribution (Fig. 4).

The trigeminal nerve has two roots, a sensory root and a motor root, attached close together to the side of the pons. On the sensory root, as it passes laterally into the middle fossa of the skull, there is a large ganglion, the trigeminal (gasserian) ganglion. There are three large sensory branches bringing fibers into this ganglion: (a) the ophthalmic, bringing sensory impressions from the orbit, upper eyelid, bridge of the nose, and scalp as far as the crown of the head; (b) the maxillary, bringing sensory impressions from the lower eyelid, lower portions of the

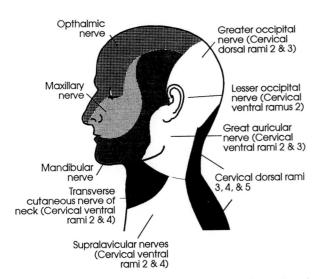

FIG. 4. Cutaneous nerve supply of the face, scalp, and neck.

nose, upper cheek, upper lip, jaw, and palate; and (c) the mandibular, bringing sensory impressions from the lower lip and jaw, tongue, lower part of the face and cheek, and front of the ear. The ophthalmic nerve passes through the superior orbital fissure, the maxillary through the foramen rotundum, and the mandibular through the foramen ovale. The motor root of the trigeminal nerve lies beneath the trigeminal ganglion and continues into the mandibular nerve as it emerges through the foramen ovale. The motor fibers go to the muscles of mastication, namely, the medial and the lateral pterygoid muscles, the masseter muscle, and the temporal muscle. For this reason, the motor part of the trigeminal is frequently called the masticator nerve. The motor root also supplies two muscles in the neck, the anterior belly of the digastric and the mylohyoid, and the tensor veli palatini and tensor tympani muscles. The tensor veli palatini and tensor tympani muscles are supplied by fibers from the branch going to the medial pterygoid muscle. The fifth nerve carries sensory fibers for heat, cold, pain, and touch but not for taste.

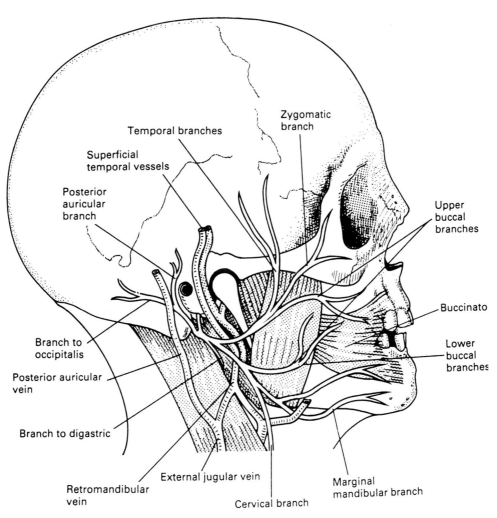

FIG. 5. Facial nerve.

Facial Nerve

The facial nerve (Fig. 5) arises from the side of the brain stem just behind the pons, very close to the eighth nerve. Together with the eighth nerve, the seventh nerve enters the internal acoustic meatus. It then continues through the facial canal, passes over the inner ear, changes its direction to course downward in the mastoid process, and emerges to course downward in the mastoid process and then emerges through the stylomastoid foramen. Its fibers are then distributed to the muscles of facial expression. Within its sheath, the facial nerve, essentially motor, also carries sensory fibers from the taste buds of the anterior two thirds of the tongue. These sensory fibers have their nuclei in the geniculate ganglion, which is a small, oval swelling present on the facial nerve in the facial canal. The facial nerve carries sensory fibers from the muscles of facial expression. The facial nerve, in addition, contains secretory fibers (cranial autonomic outflow) to the submandibular and sublingual salivary glands, and there are other secretory fibers that reach the lacrimal gland by a complicated pathway. As for the functions of the other cranial nerves, they are easily assessed by simple proceedings, and these form an important part of a neurologic examination.

NEUROVASCULAR STRUCTURES OF THE NECK

On either side of the midline tubes (the larynx and trachea in front and pharynx behind) are several ascending and descending neurovascular structures:

1. The carotid tree
2. The subclavian tree
3. The internal jugular vein
4. The subclavius vein
5. The glossopharyngeal, vagus, accessory, and hypoglossal nerves in the neck.

Carotid Tree

The right and left common carotid arteries enter the neck behind their respective sternoclavicular joints (see Fig. 1). The right artery begins at the bifurcation of the brachiocephalic trunk, but the left artery is a direct branch of the aortic arch. Variations in origin do occur, however. The common carotid artery is surrounded in the neck by a sheath of loose connective tissue, and this also invests the internal jugular vein and the vagus nerve. The artery ends at the upper border of the thyroid cartilage of the larynx by dividing into the external and the internal carotid arteries. The common carotid is dilated at the point where it bifurcates to form the carotid sinus, and specialized endings in the wall of this sinus are sensitive to changes in arterial blood pressure. A small chemoreceptor called the carotid body is located just behind the point of division of the common carotid. The internal carotid artery may be traced upward from its origin to the carotid foramen in the base of the skull. Its intracranial course is described elsewhere. As with the common carotid, it is also closely related to the internal jugular vein and vagus nerve and is enclosed with these structures in the carotid sheath. The external carotid artery ascends to a point behind the neck of the mandible, and here, within the substance of the parotid gland, it divides into its terminal branches, the superficial temporal and maxillary arteries. Apart from these two terminal branches, it usually has six other branches, which are not described in detail here (superior thyroid artery, ascending pharyngeal artery, lingual artery, facial artery, and occipital and posterior auricular arteries).

Subclavian Tree

The subclavian artery arises from the brachiocephalic trunk on the right and directly from the aortic arch on the left. Speaking descriptively, the artery is divided into three parts by the scalenus anterior muscle. The first part is the section of the artery between its origin and the medial border of the scalenus anterior. The second part lies behind the muscle, and the third part extends from the lateral border of the muscle to the outer border of the first rib. Several important nervous structures are related to the subclavian arteries as they pass between the thorax and the neck. The vagus nerve crosses the front of the first part of the artery on both sides. Tiny cardiac branches of both parasympathetic and sympathetic systems also stream over the front of the artery. On the left side, the phrenic nerve also lies close to the first part of the artery. The sympathetic trunk is located behind the first part of the subclavian artery on each side. A loop of sympathetic tissue, the ansa subclavia, loops around the first part of the artery from the middle ganglion to the inferior or stellate ganglion.

Internal Jugular Vein

The internal jugular vein begins in the jugular notch as a continuation of the sigmoid sinus and here is dilated as the superior bulb of the jugular vein (Fig. 6). It descends in the carotid sheath accompanied by the internal and common carotids and the vagus nerve. The internal jugular vein receives various tributaries in the neck.

Subclavian Vein

The subclavian vein starts at the outer border of the first rib in front of its corresponding artery and in front of the scalenus anterior. It does not therefore pass through the scalene triangle. It ends by uniting with the internal jugular vein.

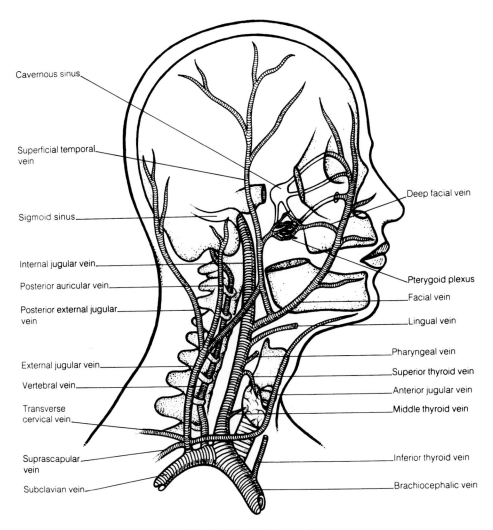

Cavernous sinus

Superficial temporal vein

Sigmoid sinus

Internal jugular vein

Posterior auricular vein

Posterior external jugular vein

External jugular vein

Vertebral vein

Transverse cervical vein

Suprascapular vein

Subclavian vein

Deep facial vein

Pterygoid plexus

Facial vein

Lingual vein

Pharyngeal vein

Superior thyroid vein

Anterior jugular vein

Middle thyroid vein

Inferior thyroid vein

Brachiocephalic vein

FIG. 6. Veins of the neck.

Glossopharyngeal, Vagus, Accessory, and Hypoglossal Nerves in the Neck

The ninth, tenth, and eleventh cranial nerves supply structures in the neck, but the twelfth cranial nerve is a nerve of passage destined for the musculature of the tongue. In the neck, however, fibers from the first cervical ventral ramus hitchhike along the hypoglossal nerve and leave it to supply musculature in front of the neck.

The glossopharyngeal nerve enters the neck through the central part of the jugular foramen. The nerve has superior and inferior sensory ganglia at its exit from the skull. Sensory fibers for general sensation and taste have their cell bodies in these two ganglia. The glossopharyngeal nerve has branches communicating with the superior cervical sympathetic ganglion of the sympathetic trunk, with the vagus, and with the auricular branch of the vagus. It also communicates with the facial nerve. In the neck, the glossopharyngeal nerve gives off a carotid branch, which descends on the internal carotid artery to the carotid sinus and carotid body. During its descent, the nerve also receives vagal fibers. It also sends out pharyngeal and lingual branches.

The vagus nerve leaves the skull through the middle part of the jugular foramen. It bears a superior and an inferior ganglion. Both ganglia contain sensory cell bodies, and the superior gives off a meningeal branch. The vagus nerve has several communicating branches to the glossopharyngeal nerve and the sympathetic trunk, the facial nerve, the inferior ganglion, the sympathetic trunk, and the hypoglossal nerve. The vagus gives off pharyngeal and laryngeal nerves.

The accessory nerve supplies the sternocleidomastoideus and trapezius. The hypoglossal nerve supplies motor fibers to the tongue.

The facial nerve leaves the skull through the stylomastoid foramen and enters the face. It lies in very close proximity to the parotid gland, and its course takes it into the substance of the gland. Here it divides into branches, which lie superficial to the external carotid artery. Although there are five named branches, there are frequent communications between the branches themselves and between the branches and the sensory branches of the trigeminal nerve to the face.

AUTONOMIC NERVOUS SYSTEM IN THE NECK

The occurrence of blood vessels and glandular tissue in the neck indicates the necessity for the presence of the autonomic system in this region. The autonomic system has two complementary parts, parasympathetic and sympathetic, which differ in structure and function. Parasympathetic preganglionic efferent fibers emerge through certain cranial nerves, whereas sympathetic preganglionic fibers emerge through thoracic spinal nerves. The somata of parasympathetic postganglionic neurons are peripheral, sited distant from the central nerve system in discrete ganglia near the structures innervated. The somata of sympathetic postganglionic neurons are located mostly in ganglia of the sympathetic trunk or ganglia in more peripheral plexus, but they are almost always closer to the spinal cord than the effector innervated.

Parasympathetic Nervous System

Preganglionic parasympathetic axons are myelinated and occur in the oculomotor, facial, glossopharyngeal, vagal, and accessory cranial nerves. Along with the cranial nerves, the following four parasympathetic ganglia are located in the head:

1. The ciliary ganglion of the third nerve sends visceral motor fibers to the ciliary muscle and the sphincter muscle of the iris.
2. The ptergopalatine (sphenopalatine) ganglion of the seventh nerve sends visceral motor fibers to the lacrimal gland and to glands located in the nasal and pharyngeal mucosa.
3. The otic ganglion of the ninth nerve sends visceral motor fibers to the parotid gland.
4. The submandibular (submaxillary) ganglion of the seventh nerve sends visceral motor fibers to the submandibular and sublingual salivary glands.

Sensory fibers of the trigeminal nerve pass through the above-mentioned ganglia, therefore, they are frequently described along with the fifth nerve, although functionally they are not part of it. Sensory fibers pass through the ciliary ganglion to join the ophthalmic branch. Sensory fibers from the submandibular and sublingual salivary glands pass through the submandibular ganglion to the lingual branch of the mandibular division. Fibers from the superior cervical ganglion also pass through these ganglia. Only the fibers of the parasympathetic system synapse in the ganglia. The autonomic fibers of the vagus have a widespread distribution of autonomic fibers but do not have any influence in the anatomic area discussed.

Sympathetic Nervous System

The sympathetic system, which is the larger autonomic division, includes the two ganglionated trunks and their branches, plexuses, and subsidiary ganglia.

Cranial Part of the Sympathetic System

The cranial part begins on each side as the internal carotid nerve, a branch of the superior cervical ganglion containing the postganglionic fibers of its neurons. Ascending behind the internal carotid artery, it divides in the carotid canal into branches, a lateral and a medial, which give off filaments to the artery and form the medial part of the internal carotid plexus. The internal carotid plexus is prolonged around the anterior and the middle cerebral arteries and the ophthalmic arteries, reaching the pia mater along the cerebral vessels. The source of the sympathetic vasoconstrictor fibers is the internal carotid and vertebral plexus, but their precise distribution from each is unresolved.

Cervical Part of the Sympathetic Trunk

The cervical part consists of three (occasionally two or rarely four) cervical sympathetic ganglia, united by long, slender, interganglionic rami. It has no white rami communications but gives gray rami communications to all the cervical ventral rami. This part of the trunk lies on the prevertebral muscles, posterior to the carotid sheath. It continues superiorly into the cranium as the internal carotid nerve, which ascends with the internal carotid artery and branches up into the internal carotid plexus on it. Inferiorly, the cervical part is continuous with the thoracic part anterior to the neck of the first rib, and here the trunk turns backward to follow the vertebral curvature.

The superior cervical ganglion is a fusiform structure 2.5 cm or more in length. It lies on the fascia covering the longus capitus muscle posterior to the internal carotid artery, the internal jugular vein, and the last four cranial nerves. It represents the fused upper four cervical segmental ganglia and hence gives off gray rami to the first four cervical nerves.

The middle cervical ganglion is the smallest and most variable of the cervical ganglia. It usually lies on the inferior thyroid artery, but it may lie further inferiorly on the vertebral artery. The ganglion represents the fifth and sixth cervical ganglia and sends gray rami to the corresponding nerves.

The cervicothoracic (stellate) ganglion is large and irregular in shape. It is formed by fusion of the inferior cervical ganglion (sometimes the middle) with the first thoracic ganglion (sometimes the second). The cervicothoracic ganglion lies at the junction of the cervical and thoracic parts of the sympathetic trunk. The superior part of the ganglion may lie anterior to the vertebral artery, the ganglion vertebrale. It is then often fused with the middle cervical ganglion and united with the remainder by strands encircling the artery. The middle cervical and cervicothoracic ganglia are united by an interganglionic ramus (commonly multiple) and by a connection that loops around the subclavian artery, the ansa subclavia. When the two ganglia are fused, the ansa unites the upper and lower parts of the common ganglionic mass.

ANATOMIC ORGANIZATION OF CEREBRAL AND EXTRACEREBRAL VASCULATURE

Extensive observations of patients have identified cranial vessels from which pain or discomfort can be referred. Ray and Wolff (9) elicited pain by stimulation of both extra- and intracranial vessels (superficial temporal, supratrochlear, frontal, middle meningeal arteries; superior sagittal sinus; and sylvian vein).

The vascularization of the head is composed of three major systems: (a) branches of the external carotid other than to the scalp, (b) the scalp, and (c) the cerebral circulation. Because the first group comprises principally the intrinsic arteries of the face, which we find less important in the scope of this book, our survey concentrates mainly on the other two. The mode of innervation of the different types of vessels is described in a separate chapter.

Blood Vessels of the Scalp

Arteries

The arterial supply to the scalp is derived from the superficial temporal artery, the posterior auricular artery, and the occipital artery, all branches of the external carotid artery (see Fig. 1). In addition, the scalp also receives contributions from the supraorbital and supratrochlear (frontal) branches of the ophthalmic artery; the latter is a subdivision of the internal carotid arterial system. The terminal ramifications of these arteries freely anastomose with each other as well as with their counterparts on the contralateral side.

From a clinical point of view, the superficial temporal artery is probably the most important of these vessels (arteria temporalis). It provides the main blood supply to the scalp and is one of the two terminal branches of the external carotid artery. Its branches supply the scalp over the frontoparietal convexity, with its different underlying structures. The middle temporal artery, the posterior auricular artery, and the occipital artery, which also supply different structures of the scalp, do not have the same clinical importance.

Veins

The veins of the scalp have multiple connections with the diploic veins (see Fig. 6). The scalp veins also connect with the superior sagittal sinus via the posterior parietal emissary veins and with the transverse sinus via the mastoid emissary veins. Both the multiple occipital veins and the superficial temporal veins finally drain into the external jugular vein.

Blood Vessels of the Meninges

Arteries

The blood supply to the meninges is derived from branches of the main trunks to the head, that is, the external and internal carotid and the vertebral arteries. These branches pass through various foramina of the cranium to course between the dura mater and the adjacent calvaria. The middle meningeal artery is the largest of the meningeal arteries and provides the major blood supply to the dura mater (Fig. 7). It arises from the maxillary artery, enters the calvarium through the foramen spinosum, and ramifies into frontal and parietal branches. Meningeal branches from the internal carotid artery arise from the cavernous segment, whereas meningeal branches of the ophthalmic artery are issued after it has entered the orbit supplying meninges of the anterior and middle parts of the cranium, to the remaining part of the skull through the foramen magnum, and supply the falx cerebelli and the posteromedial portion of the dura and the posterior fossa (see Fig. 7). The arteries supplying the meninges anastomose freely ipsilaterally and contralaterally.

Diploic and Meningeal Veins

Diploic veins are anastomosing spaces lined with endothelium in the narrow cavity (diploe) of the flat bones of the skull (Fig. 8). They may be seen in radiographs, especially of older individuals. There are usually at least four different vessels on each side: the frontal, anterior temporal, posterior temporal, and occipital diploic veins.

The meningeal veins arise from the diploe and from plexuses in the fused dura mater and periosteum (see Fig. 8). Some terminate in cranial venous sinuses, whereas others run with the meningeal arteries and end in the extracranial veins. Those that accompany the middle meningeal artery separate that vessel from the bone and are readily torn when the bone is fractured due to a skull trauma. The meningeal veins leave the skull through the foramen ovale or the foramen spinosum and end in the pterygoid plexus.

Blood Vessels to the Brain

Arterial Supply

The arterial supply to the brain is derived from two pairs of trunk arteries, the vertebral arteries and the inter-

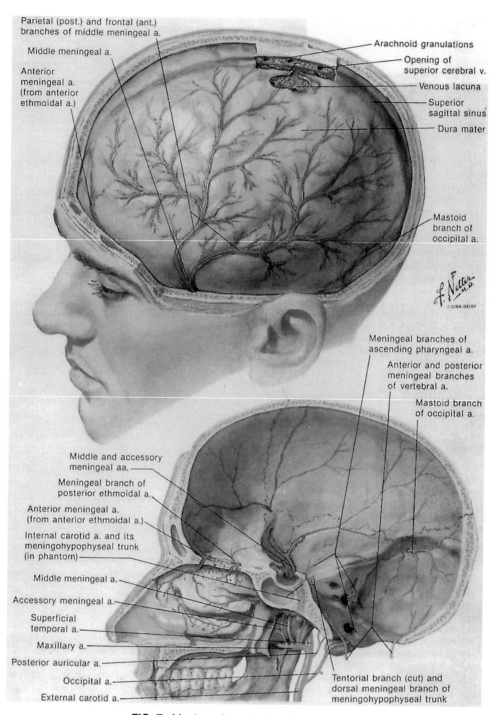

FIG. 7. Meningeal arteries and dura mater.

nal carotid arteries, located at the base of the brain (Fig. 9). The blood flowing through the branches of these arteries supplies the different parts of the brain. Each branch has a rather marked area of distribution, reflected by regional territories that are of great functional significance. It should be emphasized, however, that there is considerable individual variation in the different cerebral vessels and their ramifications. Thus a certain degree of diversity of the individual vascular pattern seems to be the rule and not the exception, something resembling a cerebrovascular fingerprint.

Generally, the branches derived from the internal carotid arteries supply the anterior half of the thalamus; the corpus striatum; practically the entire internal capsule; and the frontal, parietal, and lateral portions of the brain (see Fig. 9). The vertebral arteries supply the caudal

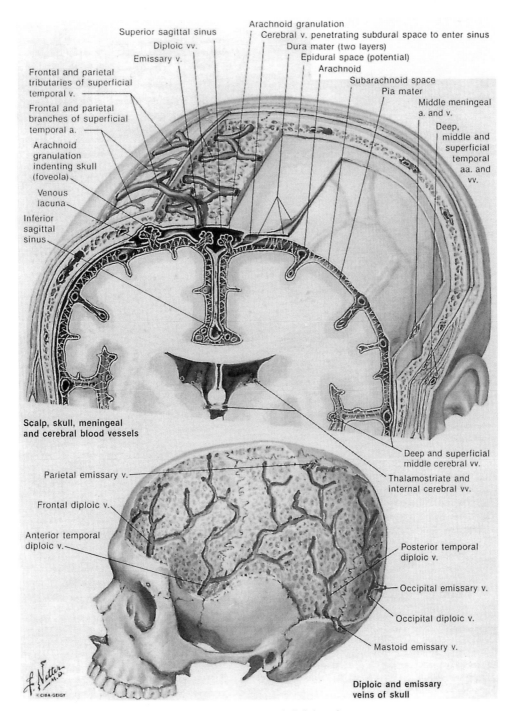

Superior sagittal sinus
Diploic vv.
Emissary v.
Arachnoid granulation
Cerebral v. penetrating subdural space to enter sinus
Dura mater (two layers)
Epidural space (potential)
Arachnoid
Subarachnoid space
Pia mater
Middle meningeal a. and v.
Frontal and parietal tributaries of superficial temporal v.
Frontal and parietal branches of superficial temporal a.
Arachnoid granulation indenting skull (foveola)
Venous lacuna
Inferior sagittal sinus
Deep, middle and superficial temporal aa. and vv.
Scalp, skull, meningeal and cerebral blood vessels
Deep and superficial middle cerebral vv.
Thalamostriate and internal cerebral vv.
Parietal emissary v.
Frontal diploic v.
Anterior temporal diploic v.
Posterior temporal diploic v.
Occipital emissary v.
Occipital diploic v.
Mastoid emissary v.
Diploic and emissary veins of skull

FIG. 8. Meninges and diploic veins.

half of the brain, including the hindbrain, the midbrain, the caudal half of the thalamus, the occipital lobes, and the basal portion of the temporal lobes.

The internal carotid arteries constitute the major arterial supply to the brain and other intracranial and orbital structures, each contributing about 40% of the total perfusion of the brain. The internal carotid arteries enter the carotid canal at the base of the skull and turns through the petrosal portion of the temporal bone just anterior to the middle ear. The vessel follows a sinusoidal course, as it rises through the foramen lacerum and crosses the cavernous sinus next to the sphenoid bone and the pituitary fossa. It enters the cranial cavity by a sharp upward bend, where it gives off branches to the tympanic cavity and the pituitary gland. It then successively gives off the following branches to the brain and the eye: anterior choroidal, ophthalmic, posterior communicating, anterior cerebral, and middle cerebral arteries.

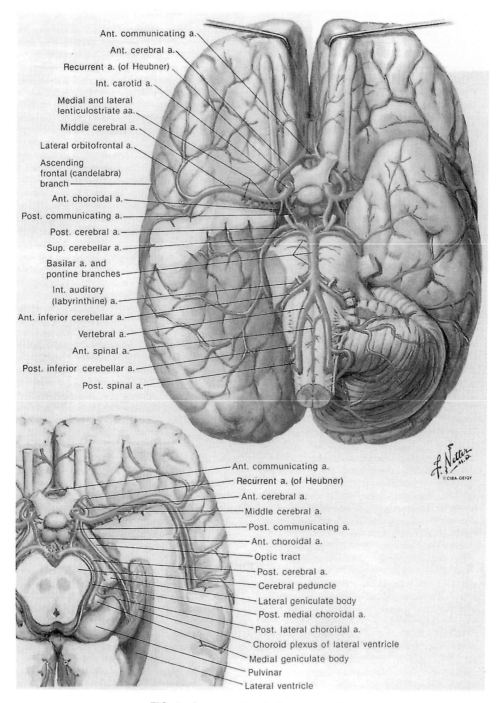

FIG. 9. Arteries of brain (basal views).

Each vertebral artery arises from the subclavian artery, enters the cranium through the foramen magnum, and gives off an anterior spinal artery and the posterior inferior cerebellar artery. The two vertebral arteries unite at the junction of the pons and the medulla to form the basilar artery (see Fig. 9), which at the level of the pons gives off the anterior inferior cerebellar artery and the internal auditory artery and at the midbrain level the superior cerebellar artery. The basilar artery then divides into the two posterior cerebral arteries, which supply, via large surface branches, the inferior temporal and medial occipital lobes and the posterior corpus callosum and via smaller penetrating branches of the thalamus and the subthalamic nuclei as well as parts of the midbrain.

On the basal surface of the brain, four main arterial trunks form an anastomosing and equalizing distribution known as the arterial circle of Willis (see Fig. 9). Under normal circumstances (especially in young people), such an arrangement would permit an adequate perfusion of all parts of the brain tissue despite an occlusion or obstruction of one of the four vital arteries. Anteriorly, this circle is formed by the horizontal portion of the anterior cerebral branches of the internal carotid artery and their interconnecting vessel, the anterior communicating artery (see Fig. 9). Laterally and posteriorly, it is formed by the posterior communicating branches of the internal carotid arteries and their connections with the respective posterior cerebral arterial branches of the basilar artery (see Fig. 9).

From the circle of Willis and the main cerebral arteries (anterior, middle, and posterior), two types of branches originate: the paramedian or central (also known as the ganglionic) and the circumferential or cortical. The central and cortical arteries are not connected with each other but form two distinct systems.

The central arteries arise from the circle of Willis and the proximal portion of the three cerebral arteries; dip perpendicularly into the brain substance; and irrigate the diencephalon, corpus striatum, and internal capsule (Fig. 10A). They are terminal arteries; that is, the branches of one artery do not anastomose with those of the others, so

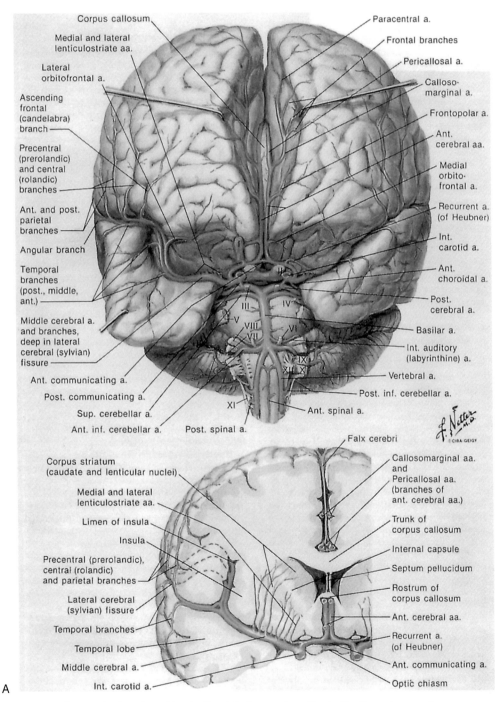

FIG. 10. A: Arteries of brain (frontal view and section). *Continued on next page.*

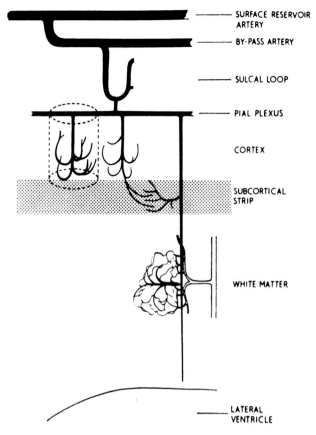

SURFACE RESERVOIR ARTERY

BY-PASS ARTERY

SULCAL LOOP

PIAL PLEXUS

CORTEX

SUBCORTICAL STRIP

WHITE MATTER

LATERAL VENTRICLE

B

FIG. 10. *Continued.* **B:** Pictorial summary of the anatomic patterns of the circulations of the cerebral hemispheres.

occlusion of these vessels will produce a softening of the area deprived of its blood supply. The anterior and posterior choroidal arteries and branches of the middle and posterior cerebral arteries may be included in this group.

The large cortical branches of each cerebral artery enter the pia mater, where they form a superficial plexus of more or less freely anastomosing vessels, in some places continuous with the plexus derived from other main arteries. From this plexus arises the smaller terminal arteries, which enter the brain substance at right angles and run a variable distance, the shorter ones arborizing in the cortex, the longer ones supplying the medullary substance of the hemispheres (see Fig. 10B). Due to anastomosis of the larger cortical branches, the occlusion of one of these vessels is compensated for to a variable extent by the blood supply from neighboring branches, although such collateral circulation is rarely sufficient for optimal nutrition of the deprived area; that is, an impaired function is seen clinically.

Venous Drainage of the Brain

The venous drainage of the brain stem and the cerebellum roughly parallel the arterial supply. On the other hand, the venous subdivisions in the cerebellum do not parallel the arterial ramifications. In general, the venous trunks have short, stocky branches that come off at right angles, resembling the silhouette of an oak tree.

The cerebral veins are classified as a superficial (external surface) cerebral group and as a deep cerebral group. Rich anastomoses occur between the two groups through the vascular network within the brain substance. Blood from the cerebral cortex on the upper lateral and medial aspects drains into the superior sagittal (dural) sinus, which drains blood into the occipital (confluence of the sinuses) and then to the right lateral and sigmoid sinuses into the right internal jugular vein. Blood from the other regions of the cerebral cortex drains into the other dural sinuses in the vicinity of the veins and finally into the internal jugular veins. The deep cerebral veins drain toward the region of the foramen of Monro to form the two internal cerebral veins located in the region (velum interpositum) just above the choroid plexus of the third ventricle. These vessels join in the vicinity of the pineal body to form the vein of Galen (see Fig. 9). Blood from the superficial veins tends to drain through the right jugular vein, and blood from the deep cerebral veins drains through the left jugular vein in the neck.

The veins of the brain all empty into a system of intercommunicating, endothelium-lined channels, the sinuses of the dura mater between the meningeal and periosteal layers of the dura. The walls of these sinuses, unlike those of other veins, are composed of the fibrous tissue of the dura; hence they exhibit a greater tautness and do not collapse when sectioned. Their walls contain no muscular tissue, but their lumina are lined with endothelium. They receive blood from the brain, meninges, and diploe and communicate through emissary channels with veins outside the skull.

FEATURES OF THE CRANIAL VASCULATURE

The blood vessels of the brain are much more than merely passive elements. Measurements of intraluminal pressure have demonstrated that half of the aortic pressure is lost just after blood leaves the major cerebral arteries. In pial vessels, a further 25% of the pressure is lost (12). Because the cerebral circulation seems to be devoid of precapillary sphincters, the regulation of resistance across this vascular bed lies mainly in the arterial and arteriolar segments. In comparison with the peripheral circulations that are well endowed with precapillary sphincters, this arterial system of resistance seems to be unique to the brain. It is therefore important to define and understand the morphologic structures and the factors that control metabolism and reactivity of cerebrovascular smooth muscle cells, the barrier mechanisms that exist to gases and nutrients, and the interaction of metabolic end products with the smooth muscle cells. One must consider that the plumbing is there to supply the neuronal elements with oxygen and glucose and that the vasculature accordingly acts in concert with these basic needs. In addition, it is of great significance to recognize how the metabolic activity of brain neurons transmits information to the blood vessels, causing them to increase or decrease in diameter, therefore altering the supply of glucose and oxygen to meet the changes in neuronal cell requirements.

Arteries

Arteries are generally characterized according to their size as large, medium, and small, to which are added the smallest of all, the arterioles. A more functional classification of arterial vessels is provided in the following sections.

Conducting Arteries

These are the largest arteries, characterized by a large lumen and thick fibromuscular walls in which the elastic component is prominent (the carotid and vertebral arteries).

Distributing Arteries

Names are given to these vessels according to the region the arteries traverse or the part of the body they supply with blood (e.g., A. cerebri media).

Small Arteries

These are vessels that branch repeatedly within the organ and ultimately are not visible to the eye as they pass into the microscopic zone.

Arterioles

Arterioles are microscopic vessels that ramify amid the tissue components of an organ (see Fig. 10). They are the smallest arterial vessels to possess smooth muscle cells. Because the walls are thin, the contraction of smooth muscle can shut off the arterial circulation into the capillary network beyond. In this way the amount of blood supplied, and thus the degree of function of the structures dependent on an arteriole or group of arterioles, can be controlled.

Capillaries

This is the simplest form of a blood vessel, and it is in fact an endothelial tube. The number and density of capillaries vary from tissue to tissue in direct proportion to the metabolic activity of the tissue and in brain, even depending on local conditions. There is a direct correlation between the local metabolism and the regional density of capillaries (7). Tissues with high metabolic rates and the greatest need for oxygen may have one capillary for each functioning unit. For example, each nerve cell in the brain is considered to be located within the loop of one capillary so that it may be considered to be bathed in or from a pool of blood separated only by the thin endothelial membrane of the same capillary.

End Arteries, Collateral Circulation, and Arterial Boundary Zones

There are three major possibilities for collateral perfusion of the different brain regions: extracerebral arterial anastomoses, extra-intracranial anastomoses, and intracerebral anastomoses. Extra-intracranial anastomoses are a feature of many species, but they do not exist in the human brain. In certain regions of the body there are arteries that have no anastomoses with their neighbors (end arteries). If an artery of this type is occluded, serious nutritional disturbances resulting in cell death (necrosis) will occur within the area supplied by the affected vessel. The central artery of the retina is the best example of an end artery, and its occlusion is followed by permanent blindness. A specific feature of the cortical vasculature, first noted by Heubner (6) is the extensive anastomotic link that exists between arterioles and venules on the cortical surface, as opposed to the minimal intraarteriolar connections within the cortex, if there are any.

Although the large arteries at the base of the brain form effective anastomoses (the circle of Willis), the central arteries (intraparenchymal) communicate with each other only through the capillary bed. They are functionally considered as end arteries owing to their inherent deficiency in establishing an effective collateral circulation.

Morphologic Organization of Cerebral Vessels

Generally, all the cerebral vessels are similar in structure and are composed of the usual three coaxial coats: the tunica interna, the tunica media, and the tunica externa (adventitia). However, there are some differences in the archetype of the extra- and intracerebral arterioles, especially regarding the adventitia, which are described in some detail below.

Extraparenchymal Cerebral Arteries

Tunica Intima

The lumen is lined by a single layer of endothelial cells without fenestrations. The internal elastic lamina appears to be made up of a homogeneous matrix or ground substance in which the elastic tissue is deposited.

Tunica Media

The tunica media is built up of several layers of smooth muscle cells. As the vessels diminish in size, the muscular coat is reduced, until finally, in the small arterioles, it has only a single layer of muscle cells. In all vessels, membrane-to-membrane contacts between smooth muscle cells are seen regularly. Moreover, in the arterioles, processes of the endothelial and smooth muscle cells penetrate the remnants of the elastic membrane and the basement membrane and constitute membranous contacts with each other as myoendothelial junctions.

Tunica Externa (Adventitia)

The tunica externa is built up of bundles of collagen, which for the most part run longitudinally or circumferentially. The outer border of the vessel wall has a sharply defined boundary of thin cellular processes from fibrocytes. Where the vessels enter the cerebral cortex (see Fig. 10), there seems to be a membranous junction between this outer lining of the vessel wall and the cytoplasmic processes of the pia.

Traditionally, many researchers have separated the major arteries at the base of the brain and the pial vessels (together called extraparenchymal vessels) from those that penetrate into the brain tissue (intraparenchymal vessels). Morphologic observations (10,11) and functional studies (8) have not provided support for this subdivision apart from the obvious difference in vessel size. It is now possible to study the penetrating arterioles *in vitro,* and indeed the evidence so far suggests that these arterioles in many respects react just as the smaller pial vessels do (1).

Light microscopy has not given any indication of pronounced differences in the morphologic organization between vessels of the brain and those in other vascular beds. However, electron microscopy and specific staining methods have revealed certain differences, including (a) the tightness of endothelial junctions, (b) relative paucity of pinocytotic vesicles, and (c) localization of specific enzymes in the microvessel wall.

In the adult, the major cerebral arteries have a much thinner wall than do peripheral arteries of the same caliber. The probable reason for this is that, for intracranial arteries, the arterial pressure pulse is damped by the surrounding cerebrospinal fluid being enclosed within the rigid skull. This hypothesis is illustrated splendidly by the somewhat neglected experiments of Hassler (5), who showed that, in rabbits, trepanation at birth resulted in a marked hypertrophy of the medial layer. Whereas under normal circumstances cerebral arteries function correctly with a relatively thin medial layer, this fact might explain the predisposition of intracranial vessels to the development of aneurysms.

The large distributing vessels most frequently lie free in the subarachnoid space, whereas their penetrating branches make contact with the cortical surface. It is apparent that some of the vessels that enter the brain substance arise from the distributing vessels at an angle of 90 degrees, whereas others may enter more obliquely. At the point of entering, the outer boundary of the penetrating blood vessel and the pia come into very close contact, and no clear perivascular space can be observed along the intraparenchymal course of the vessels.

Intraparenchymal Cerebral Vessels

The vascular endothelium forms a completely continuous layer without fenestrations. A thick basement membrane and a fragmented layer of elastic tissue separate the intima from the tunica media. The media is composed of one to three layers of smooth muscle cells and contributes most of the thickness of the arteriolar wall. The outer layer of the intracerebral arterioles is thin and differs to some extent from the adventitial coat of the extraparenchymal vessels. From the point of entry of an arteriole in the cortical parenchyma, the adventitia usually contains a single layer of cellular elements, which apparently are extensions of the leptomeningeal sheath of the penetrating vessel. These cellular processes are separated from the neural tissue by a small amount of collagen and a distinct basement membrane, which is continuous with the basement membrane covering the surface of the brain. Collagen fibers are also found between the cytoplasmic processes of the adventitia and the smooth muscle cells of the tunica media. Thus, it seems as though the leptomeningeal cytoplasmic processes at least in some places separate the different components of the adventitial coat into a pial layer (the cerebral basement membrane, collagen fibers, and pial processes) and an epipial layer (collagen between the pial processes and the smooth muscle cell layer). Within this epipial area, foamy cells resembling macrophages are occasionally encountered. A well-defined space separating the penetrating vessel from the surrounding cerebral tissue, limited on the one side by a distinct outer boundary of the vessel wall and on the other side by the pial covering of the neuropil, does not seem to be present within the cerebral cortex.

At regular intervals, endothelial processes penetrate the basement membrane and the elastic lamina and come in close contact with the smooth muscle cells to form myoendothelial junctions. Similarly, processes of smooth muscle cells of the media break through the basement membrane and establish contacts with the endothelial cells. Different kinds of such myoendothelial junctions are seen. Serial sections indicate that there may be an accumulation of fibrillary material within the endothelial cells adjacent to the junctions. Occasionally, condensations of several membranelike structures are observed at the myoendothelial junctions. Lateral membrane-to-membrane contacts between smooth muscle cells are commonly seen (2,3). As the arterioles become smaller, the thickness of the outer coat and the number of smooth muscle cells are gradually reduced. These cell layers finally disappear at the capillary levels, where only the fused vascular and parenchymal basement membranes separate the neuropil from the endothelium.

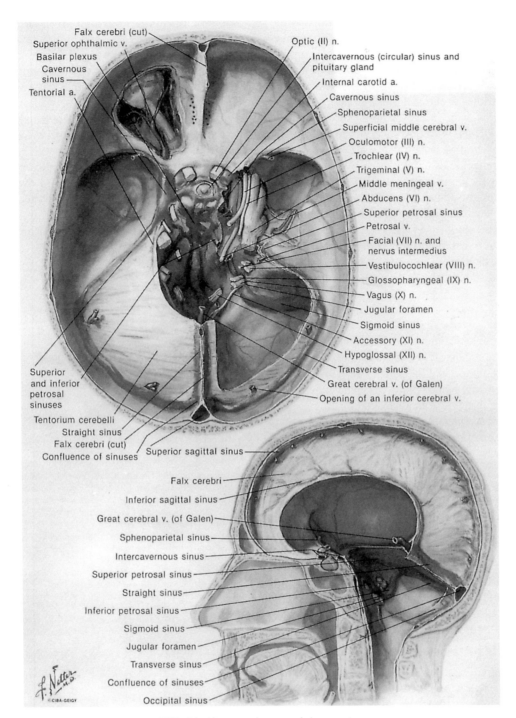

FIG. 11. Venous sinuses of dura mater.

Capillaries

As in the arterioles, the endothelium of the capillaries forms a completely continuous layer with no fenestrations. The walls of capillaries close to arteriolar origins may contain pericytes surrounded by basement membrane. Membranous contacts between cytoplasmic processes of the pericytes or astrocytes and endothelium, similar to the myoendothelial junctions of the arterioles,

are rarely seen. In capillaries without pericytes, the basement membrane is the only structure that separates the endothelium from the surrounding cortical parenchyma.

Topography of Cortical Microvasculature

The cortical microvasculature has two major features. Arterioles penetrate the cortex at right angles to the surface and give rise to capillaries at all laminae (see Fig.

10*B*). The columnal organization of the cortical vasculature is but one of many such vertical anatomic arrangements in the cerebral cortex, each of which has circulatory and metabolic correlates. The vertical arteriolar organization produces minute boundary zones between penetrating arterioles at the distal end of capillaries; the columnar patterns seen in the cerebral cortex in local blood flow, NADH/NAD⁺ redox state, or glucose metabolism during hypoxia or ischemia are a consequence of the vascular architectonics.

Capillary density in the brain is altered by a number of conditions. During postnatal maturation in humans, capillary density (which at birth is approximately one third of the adult level) doubles in the first year of life and achieves the adult level by the end of the fourth year (4). In the rat, there is a rapid increase in capillary density between days 10 and 20 after birth (13).

CONCLUSIONS

The human brain constitutes only 2% of the total weight of the body, but it receives 15% of the cardiac output, and its oxygen consumption is 20% of that of the entire body. The brain receives its blood supply through two vascular systems, those of the carotid and the vertebral arteries. The two carotid arteries enter the skull via the carotid canal, branch (into the anterior and middle cerebral arteries), and communicate with each other through the anterior communicating artery that connects the two anterior cerebral arteries. The two vertebral arteries enter the foramen magnum, join at the level of the junction of pons and medulla to form the basilar artery, and pass anteriorly to divide at the level of the midbrain into the two posterior cerebral arteries. The carotid arteries communicate with the vertebral artery system through the posterior communicating arteries, thus forming a remarkable anastomosis, the circulus arteriosus or the circle of Willis.

The arteries that supply the brain parenchyma are the origin of two systems of vessels. One of these is the central system, and its vessels supply the thalami and corpora striata. The other is the cortical system, and its vessels ramify in the pia mater and supply the cortex and the subadjacent brain substance.

The venous drainage of the brain can be divided into an internal group of vessels emptying into the vein of Galen and the straight sinus and an external group of veins that lie over the surface of the hemispheres and drain through the superior sagittal sinus and the lateral basal sinuses (Fig. 11).

Generally, all the cerebral vessels are similar in structure and are composed of the usual three coaxial coats: the tunica interna, media, and externa (adventitia). However, there are some differences in the archetype of the extra- and intracerebral arterioles, especially regarding the adventitia.

Arterioles penetrate the cortex at right angles to the surface and give rise to capillaries at all laminae. The distribution of capillaries within the brain is heterogeneous, and they seem to be structurally organized and paralleled to the number of synapses in the region.

As in the arterioles, the endothelium of the capillaries forms a completely continuous layer with no fenestrations. Membranous contacts between cytoplasmic processes of pericytes or astrocytes and endothelium, similar to the myoendothelial junctions of the arterioles, are also present.

Blood flow to the brain is highly protected, yet the brain remains highly susceptible to disturbances of the blood supply, and this is reflected in the high incidence of symptomatic cerebral vascular disease in the population at large. Diseases of the blood vessels are among the most frequent serious neurologic disorders.

REFERENCES

1. Dacey RG Jr, Duling BR. Effect of norepinephrine on penetrating arterioles of rat cerebral cortex. *Am J Physiol* 1984;246:H380–H385.
2. Dahl E. The fine structure of intracerebral vessels. *Z Zellforsch* 1973;145:577–586.
3. Dahl E. The innervation of the cerebral arteries. *J Anat* 1973;115:53–63.
4. Diemer K. Capillarisation and oxygen supply to the brain. In: Lubbers DW, Luft UC, Thews G, Witzel E, eds. *Oxygen transport in blood and tissue.* Stuttgart: Thieme, 1968:118–123.
5. Hassler O. Morphological studies on the large cerebral arteries, with reference to the etiology of subarachnoid hemorrhage. *Acta Psychiatr Neurol Scand* 1961;[Suppl 154]:1–145.
6. Heubner O. *Die luetische Erkrankung der Hirnarterien.* Leipzig: Ebende, 1874.
7. Kuschinsky W. Physiology and general pathophysiology of the cerebral circulation. In: Olesen J, Edvinsson L, eds. *Basic mechanisms of headache.* Amsterdam: Elsevier Science Publishers BV, 1988.
8. McCulloch J, Edvinsson L. Cerebrovascular smooth muscle reactivity: a critical appraisal of *in vitro* and *in situ* techniques. *J Cereb Blood Flow Metab* 1984;4:129–139.
9. Ray BS, Wolff HG. Experimental studies on headache. Pain sensitive structures of the head and their significance in headache. *Arch Surg* 1940;41:813–856.
10. Rhodin JAG. The ultrastructure of mammalian arterioles and precapillary sphincters. *J Ultrastruct Res* 1967;18:181–223.
11. Samarasinghe DD. The innervation of the cerebral arteries in the rat: an electron microscope study. *J Anat* 1965;99:815–828.
12. Stromberg DD, Fox JR. Pressures in the pial arterioles microcirculation of the cat during changes in systemic arterial blood pressure. *Circ Res* 1972;31:229–239.
13. Zeman W, Innes JRM. *Craigie's neuroanatomy of the rat.* New York: Academic Press, 1963.

SUGGESTED READING

Berkovitz BKB, Moxham BJ. *A textbook of head and neck anatomy.* London: Wolfe Medical Publications, 1988.

Dahl E, Edvinsson L. Anatomical organization of cerebral and extracerebral vasculature. In: Olesen J, Edvinsson L, eds. *Basic mechanisms of headache.* Amsterdam: Elsevier, 1988:27–47.

Edvinsson L, MacKenzie ET, McCulloch J. *Cerebral blood flow and metabolism.* New York: Raven, 1993.

Kandel ER, Schwartz JH. *Principles of neural science.* Amsterdam: Elsevier, 1991.

Pegington J. The head and neck. In: *Clinical anatomy in action,* 2nd ed. Edinburgh: Churchill Livingstone, 1986.

Romanes GJ. *Cunningham's textbook of anatomy,* 12th ed. Oxford: Oxford University Press, 1981.

Williams PL, Warwick R, Dyson U, Bannister LH. *Gray's anatomy,* 37th ed. Edinburgh: Churchill Livingstone, 1989.

The Headaches, Second Edition,
edited by J. Olesen, P. Tfelt-Hansen, and K.M.A. Welch.
Lippincott Williams & Wilkins, Philadelphia © 2000.

Basic Science Aspects of the Headaches

CHAPTER 10

Anatomy of Central Nervous System Pathways Related to Head Pain

Karl Messlinger and Rami Burstein

It is generally assumed that primary headaches result from nociceptive processes that involve the cranial meninges, particularly perivascular compartments of the dura mater encephali and large cerebral arteries. This conclusion has originally been derived from the classical intraoperative experiments by Ray and Wolff (80), followed by supplementary studies of other investigators, who demonstrated that headachelike pain can be elicited by mechanical and electrical stimulation of dural blood vessels and basal arteries but not of other meningeal structures (16). These pain-sensitive compartments are richly supplied by nerve fibers immunoreactive to the neuropeptides substance P and calcitonin gene-related peptide (CGRP) (66,71), which may be indicative for nociceptive afferents. The distribution of these peptidergic fibers within the cranial meninges and hence the presumptive meningeal nociceptive innervation fit very well the experimental data of Ray and Wolff's studies. Central pathways related to head pain should therefore be considered with regard to the central projection of meningeal afferents, particularly the afferent innervation of the dura mater encephali and basal arteries. Neurohistologic or functional studies addressing this topic, however, are remarkably rare. This overview is therefore substantially based on studies that focused on central pathways related

to nociceptive input from other trigeminal tissues, which will be compared with the limited work about meningeal representation in the central nervous system.

CENTRAL TRIGEMINAL PATHWAYS

Meningeal Representation in the Trigeminal Ganglion

The fifth cranial nerve arising from the trigeminal ganglion, also referred to as the semilunar or Gasserian ganglion, conveys sensory information from most parts of the head, including intracranial structures, to the central nervous system. The trigeminal ganglion belongs to the peripheral trigeminal system but is mentioned in this chapter because attempts have been made to map meningeal representation in the ganglion using retrograde tracing techniques. Mayberg et al. (62) applied horseradish peroxidase (HRP) to meningeal structures such as the middle meningeal artery in the cat and found projections predominantly to the ophthalmic division (V1) of the ipsilateral trigeminal ganglion, although a few neurons in the maxillar (V2) and mandibular (V3) divisions also were stained. The basal dura mater in the middle cranial fossa was represented mainly in the third division of the trigeminal ganglion (92). The finding that all three divisions of the trigeminal nerve contribute to the innervation of the meninges (though not equally) is in accordance with old anatomic observations in primates (63). Remarkably, retrograde labeling of nerve fibers around basal arteries, from which head pain can be provoked in humans (80), was found not only in the trigeminal ganglion but also in the first and second spinal ganglia in the rat (1).

K. Messlinger: Department of Physiology and Experimental Pathophysiology, University of Erlangen-Nürnberg, D-91054 Erlangen, Germany.

R. Burstein: Department of Neurobiology, Harvard Medical School, Department of Anesthesia and Critical Care, Beth Israel Deaconess Medical Center, and Harvard Institutes of Medicine, Boston, Massachusetts 02115.

Organization of the Trigeminal Brain Stem

The central processes of trigeminal primary afferents forming the sensory root of the trigeminal nerve enter the brain stem at the pontine level and terminate in sensory nuclei, which as a whole are called the trigeminal brain stem nuclear complex (TBNC). The TBNC is composed of the principal sensory nucleus (Vp) and the spinal trigeminal nucleus (Vsp), as shown in Fig. 1. A major part of the trigeminal nerve terminates in the Vp, whereas the other fibers descend, making up the spinal trigeminal tract. The descending axons give rise to collaterals that extend into the Vsp, which is subdivided into three subnuclei (72) (see Fig. 1): a rostral subnucleus oralis (Vo), a middle subnucleus interpolaris (Vi), and a caudal subnucleus caudalis (Vc). The Vc is often referred to as the medullary dorsal horn (MDH) because of its anatomic and physiologic similarities to the spinal dorsal horn. Olszewski (72) identified three histologically different regions in the MDH: an outer marginal region, the substantia gelatinosa, and a deep magnocellular region. Later Gobel et al. (29) proposed a laminar subdivision of the MDH similar to Rexed's nomenclature of the spinal dorsal horn (82), in which lamina I corresponds to the marginal layer, lamina II to the substantia gelatinosa, and laminae III and IV to the magnocellular region. Despite the large number of studies that used the term "lamina V" to describe the location of deep neurons in Vc, the boundaries of this lamina have not been defined. Histologically, they are clearly demarcated laterally and dorsally by the less reticulated appearance of lamina IV but poorly demarcated medially and ventrally, as lamina V merges with the medullary reticular formation (70). Based on single-unit recording of deep Vc neurons that receive exclusive trigeminal input, the ventral border of lamina V seems to extend about 400 μm below the ventral border of lamina IV in the rat (41). Adjacent to the rostral Vsp, groups of neurons are found intermingled in the spinal trigeminal tract down to the transition of Vi and Vc (see Fig. 1). These cells are referred to as the interstitial islands of Cajal, or as the paratrigeminal or interstitial nucleus (77). The interstitial nucleus cells have been suggested to be functional homologues to neurons in laminae I and II of the Vc, because both tend to be nociceptive specific and have restricted receptive fields (e.g. in the tooth pulp or the cranial dura mater) (23,90).

Numerous anatomic and electrophysiologic studies (89,95) have demonstrated that the Vp, the spinal trigeminal tract, and the subnuclei of the Vsp are topographically organized in a ventrodorsal direction. Mandibular afferents terminate in the dorsal aspect of each trigeminal subnucleus (dorsomedial in the MDH), ophthalmic afferent terminals are ventral (ventrolateral in MDH), and maxillary terminals are interposed. The rostrocaudal organization of the TBNC is less clear. The results of early anatomic (97) and neurophysiologic (51) studies suggested that each subnucleus receives information

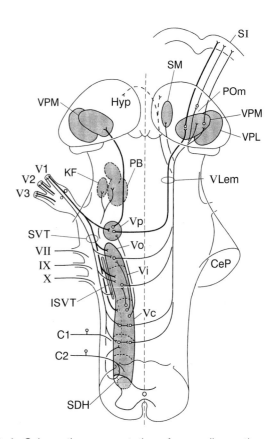

FIG. 1. Schematic representation of ascending pathways of the central trigeminal system with priority to nociception. The figure is based on a representation of the human trigeminal system by Nieuwenhuys et al. (69) but includes trigeminal structures found in other species, which may differ in part from the trigeminal system of primates. Contours of nuclei are simplified, symbols for single cell bodies and nerve fibers represent populations of neurons. The trigeminal brain stem nuclear complex (*TBNC*) includes subnucleus principalis (*Vp*) and the spinal trigeminal nucleus, which consists of subnuclei oralis (*Vo*), interpolaris (*Vi*), and caudalis (*Vc*). Primary afferents from the trigeminal divisions (V1–3) project to all subnuclei of the TBNC, thick myelinated fibers mainly to Vp, and thin A and C fibers preferentially to caudal subnuclei and the first spinal segments (C1–2). Minor projections to the spinal trigeminal nucleus run through nerves VII, IX, and X (not further described). Inter-subnuclear connections are shown originating from Vc but may connect all subnuclei of the TBNC. Neurons from Vp ascend to the ipsilateral and to the contralateral thalamus, forming the trigeminal lemniscus (*VLem*). Trigeminothalamic neurons involved in nociception project via a crossed pathway mainly to the ventroposteromedial nucleus (*VPM*), the medial region of the posterior complex (*POm*), and the nucleus submedius (*SM*) in the medial thalamus. There is also a significant projection from the TBNC to the hypothalamus (*Hyp*) and to the pontine parabrachial (*PB*) and Kölliker-Fuse (*KF*) nuclei. CeP, cerebellar pedunculus; SDH, spinal dorsal horn; SI, primary somatosensory cortex; SVT, spinal trigeminal tract; ISVT, interstitial nucleus of the SVT; VPL, ventroposterolateral thalamic nucleus.

from all parts of the head. Jacquin et al. (44) labeled various mandibular nerves in the rat with HRP and found that they projected to all trigeminal subnuclei, although the anterior oral afferents tended to terminate most heavily in the rostral TBNC, whereas the posterior perioral-auricular afferents terminated preferentially in the caudal aspect of the complex. It is yet unknown if a similar somatotopic distribution in ventrodorsal and rostrocaudal directions exists for intracranial trigeminal structures. Taking into account that meningeal afferents predominantly arise from the ophthalmic division within the trigeminal ganglion, they can be expected to project mainly to ventral parts of the Vsp. Recent electrophysiologic experiments are consistent with this idea, showing that neurons in the Vsp of the rat with input from the supratentorial dura mater are preferentially located in the ventrolateral part of the nucleus (10,86).

Concluded from clinical observations, it has long been assumed that the Vc is responsible for processing nociceptive and temperature information from the face and head, whereas the Vp is responsible for tactile information. Isolated lesions of the Vc caused ipsilaterally complete or partial loss of pain and temperature sensation, whereas tactile sensations remained nearly intact (54). This clinical experience led Sjoqvist (91) to develop the method of trigeminal tractotomy for the relief of facial pain, in which the spinal trigeminal tract at the level of the obex was transected. The clinical data were supplemented and extended with a large body of neurophysiologic evidence demonstrating the necessity of the Vc in the perception of pain in trigeminal tissues. On the other hand, more recent data suggest that all subnuclei in the spinal trigeminal tract contribute to facial and cranial nociception (19,23).

Terminations of Trigeminal Afferents in Subnuclei of the TBNC

The distribution of nociceptive afferent terminals in the trigeminal brain stem has been studied by axonal tracing and by immunohistochemistry using antibodies directed against "sensory" neuropeptides such as substance P and CGRP.

Hayashi (33) and Jacquin et al. (46,47) injected HRP into functionally identified facial primary afferents in the Vsp of the cat and the rat, respectively, to examine the central terminations of these labeled axons. They found high-threshold mechanoreceptive (nociceptive) A-delta afferents forming extensive terminal arbors in the superficial Vi and, most pronounced, in the substantia gelatinosa of Vc (33). In the rat, a second termination area was localized in laminae III to V of Vc (46). The extensive arbor pattern exhibited by nociceptive afferents could be readily distinguished from most low-threshold afferent terminals in both subnuclei. In line with the above findings, the sensory projection from the cornea, which is thought to be mainly nociceptive, was shown to be focused in the outer laminae of Vsp (73). In contrast, neurons with nociceptive

input from the masseter muscle, the tooth pulp, and the cranial dura mater were preferentially located in deeper laminae of the Vsp (10,23,34). Apart from the heavy projection of nociceptive primary afferents to the caudal subnuclei, a sparse projection of corneal and tooth pulp afferents also was shown in Vp and Vo (73,100).

Corresponding to the distribution of nociceptive afferent terminals in the Vsp visualized by the HRP technique, substance P and CGRP immunoreactive nerve fibers have been demonstrated in different species preferentially around the substantia gelatinosa of Vi and Vc (4,74,96). In the ferret, substance P and CGRP immunoreactivity was most dense in outer laminae of Vc and in the caudal part of Vi (4), although immunoreactivity to these neuropeptides was also present in Vo and in the main sensory nucleus (Vp). Trigeminal rhizotomy in the cat caused disappearance of most of the CGRP immunoreactive fibers throughout the TBNC, whereas a considerable number of substance P immunoreactive fibers remained intact (38,96), indicating that nearly all CGRP-positive fibers in the TBNC are trigeminal primary afferents, whereas a proportion of substance P–positive fibers has a central origin. Electron microscopic immunocytochemistry in the cat Vsp has revealed CGRP immunoreactivity within the substantia gelatinosa in axon terminals, which formed synaptic contacts onto dendritic profiles on the one hand, and on the other hand received presynaptic contacts (39). Substance P in particular has been implicated in the nociceptive processing within the Vsp. Henry et al. (37) have found that iontophoretic administration of substance P activated selectively nociceptive neurons in Vc of the cat. It may be significant with regard to the pathophysiology of headaches that stimulation of the rat dura mater with acidic solution provoked release of immunoreactive substance P in the medullary trigeminal brain stem (85).

Representation of Meningeal and Corneal Nociceptors in the Spinal Trigeminal Nucleus

Electrophysiologic studies in the cat and the rat have shown that the cranial meninges are well represented in Vc (20,94) but also in Vi and Vo (23). In the rat, the majority of neurons that could be activated by electrical stimulation of dural sites (sinus transversus or parietal dura mater) were found in the caudal Vc (10,86), but there was another peak in the distribution of recording sites around the obex level corresponding to the transition of Vi and Vc (86). Interestingly, most of these neurons had convergent cutaneous input, and their facial receptive fields were preferentially located in periorbital, frontal or parietal areas, that is, the same areas in which the patients of Ray and Wolff (80) felt head pain elicited by stimulation of supratentorial dural structures. In a study in the cat nearly all Vc neurons with meningeal input had facial receptive fields located in the ophthalmic division, whereas a considerable proportion of neurons in Vo and Vi had facial receptive fields in maxillary and mandibular areas (23).

The interpretation of these findings with regard to the central mechanisms involved in headache is yet open but may implicate similar mechanisms as in corneal nociception, the morphologic and functional basis of which has been studied in more detail. Similarly to the cranial dura, the cornea may be innervated mainly, if not exclusively, by nociceptive afferents. Transganglionic tracing studies of corneal afferents in monkeys have shown a moderate projection to the caudal Vc but a heavy projection to the transition region between Vi and Vc (58). Accordingly, neurons in the rat Vsp activated by corneal stimulation were preferentially found at two sites: in the region between Vc and the first cervical segment (C1), and at the Vi/Vc region, respectively (65). Neurons recorded at the Vc/C1 transition had periorbitally localized facial receptive fields and were either wide dynamic range (WDR) or nociceptive specific (NS) according to their responses to cutaneous stimulation. Neurons at the Vi/Vc transition, many of which had no facial receptive field or were low threshold, showed properties suggestive of an indirect excitatory input from the Vc/C1 region (65). It has been assumed that the transition region of Vc/C1 is most important in processing nociceptive information from primary afferents to mediate the sensory-discriminative aspect of pain, whereas the Vi/Vc region may be involved in the recruitment of descending control pathways (64).

Connections between Subnuclei of the TBNC

The nociceptive information processed in the subnuclei of the TBNC does not simply reflect the primary afferent input. Rather there are connections between the various subnuclei that allow information transfer within the trigeminal system (see Fig. 1). Anatomic studies using degeneration techniques have shown projections from Vc to more rostral nuclei of the TBNC (93), which was confirmed by physiologic experiments showing antidromic activation of Vc neurons from Vo (42). Jacquin et al. (45) used anterograde tracing to demonstrate ascending connections between each of the TBNC subnuclei in the rat, as well as a weak projection to the contralateral Vsp. Retrograde tracing from Vp labeled cell bodies in all laminae of the more caudal subnuclei (45). It appears likely, therefore, that the MDH transmits information to all rostral components of the TBNC, but it remains to be determined whether this pathway is an essential source of nociceptive input to the rostral subnuclei. Hallas and Jacquin (31) described that the number of Vi neurons responsive to noxious facial stimuli does not change following surgical interruption of the ascending projection from Vc. In contrast, Greenwood and Sessle (30) showed that the responses of neurons in Vo and Vp to noxious stimuli were reversibly depressed by cold block of the ascending input from Vc. Considerable evidence for a modulation of the activity of neurons in more rostral subnuclei by Vc in the cat also was collected by

other experimenters (21). In a recent examination, Dallel et al. (18) have shown that morphine microinjection into the substantia gelatinosa of Vc produces inhibition of the C fiber–evoked responses of Vo neurons, whereas injection of morphine directly into the Vo was not effective, suggesting that (systemic) morphine acts antinociceptive through blocking the C fiber inputs in Vc. It is yet unknown if this intersubnuclear system plays a significant role in headaches.

Projections from Trigeminal Brain Stem to Thalamic Nuclei

The rat thalamus has been shown to receive direct contralateral input from each of the TBNC subnuclei (49,57). The majority of the TBNC neurons projecting to the contralateral thalamus was found in Vp, the remaining neurons were located in Vi, with smaller contributions from Vo and Vc (49). The contralateral fibers from Vp ascend with the medial lemniscus and are often referred to as the trigeminal lemniscus (see Fig. 1), but there is also a marked ipsilateral projection from Vp in cat and monkey, which appears to be absent in rodents (49,57,60). The spinal trigeminal subnuclei in cat and monkey project to the thalamus via a crossed pathway that joins the contralateral spinothalamic tract (11). The trigeminothalamic projections terminate preferentially in the medial subnucleus of the thalamic ventroposterior complex (VPM) (see Fig. 1). Rodent trigeminothalamic axons terminate in the corresponding thalamic ventrobasal complex (VB). Peschanski et al. (76) have shown that the VPM/VB projections from Vp overlap those from the remainder of TBNC.

Most neurons in primate VPM respond to low-threshold stimuli (53), whereas a small percentage of these cells has WDR characteristics responding more vigorously to noxious stimuli. Nociceptive-specific VPM neurons have been identified in the cat, and most of these were located in the "shell" region of VPM (102). Interestingly, Yokota and Matsumoto (101) have reported that the responses of nociceptive VPM neurons can be inhibited by reversibly cooling the caudal TBNC or transecting the spinal trigeminal tract at the level of the obex. This suggests that the nociceptive projection to the VPM is derived from the caudal TBNC. The results of other studies indicate that the issue is still unresolved, however. For example, Raboisson et al. (79) found that responses of VB neurons to orofacial noxious stimulation in the rat were not abolished following large trigeminal tractotomy, and Broton and Rosenfeld (7) reported that only rostral cuts of the TBNC resulted in significant deficits in facial nociception in the rat. It is yet unknown whether this (nociceptive) pathway from the rostral TBNC to the thalamus is limited to mediation of orofacial pain.

For the central pathways involved in headache it is significant that neurons in laminae I and V of Vc that responded to electrical, mechanical and chemical stimulation of the dura mater and received convergent input from the skin projected directly to VPM and adjacent thalamic areas in the rat (10). Because these neurons were sensitized by brief chemical stimulation of the dura, that is, responded to intra- and extracranial stimulation that previously induced minimal or no responses, they are likely to signal intra- and extracranial hypersensitivity, which may also occur during migraine. Similarly in the cat, neurons responding to electrical and mechanical stimulation of dural structures (the medial meningeal artery and/or the superior sagittal sinus) were located in and around the VPM (22,106). Thalamic NS and WDR neurons as well as neurons excited by chemical noxious stimuli (bradykinin or capsaicin) applied to the craniovascular receptive fields were typically located in the periphery of the VPM and, as a second location, in the medial part of the posterior complex (POm) in the cat (28,106) (see Fig. 1). These results were confirmed with the 2-desoxyglucose method, which revealed increased metabolic activity following stimulation of the superior sagittal sinus in both VPM and POm of the cat (28). The functional studies mentioned are in accordance with projections of the caudal TBNC not only to VPM but also to the posterior thalamus in rat and cat (75,88).

In addition, a projection from the caudal TBNC to a further thalamic region associated with pain, the internal medullary lamina, has been demonstrated in the monkey (27). More important, however, may be another projection to the medial thalamus (see Fig. 1). Using anterograde HRP and autoradiographic techniques, Craig and Burton (17) showed that lamina I cells of the MDH terminate in the caudal aspect of the nucleus submedius in the cat. A similar projection from caudal Vi and rostral Vc was demonstrated in the rat (75,105), suggesting that the trigemino-submedial pathway may be important in nociception. Sessle (87) has suggested that nociceptive neurons of the medial thalamus have properties consistent with a role in the mediation of emotional and motivational aspects of pain. The involvement of this thalamic region in headache needs to be confirmed.

Projections from Trigeminal Brain Stem to other Subcortical Nuclei

In addition to the thalamus, TBNC neurons also project to a number of diencephalic and brain stem areas involved in regulation of autonomic, endocrine, affective and motor functions. For example, all TBNC subnuclei contain neurons that project directly to the hypothalamus (56). The majority of these neurons were found bilaterally in laminae I, II, and V of C1–2 and Vc, in the transition zone between Vc and Vi, and in the paratrigeminal nucleus, thus suggesting a role in nociception. In fact, trigeminohypothalamic tract neurons in C1–2 and Vc responded preferentially or exclusively to noxious mechanical and thermal stimulation of the facial skin and to electrical, mechanical, and chemical stimulation of the dura mater encephali (10). Within the hypothalamus, these ascending neurons project to the lateral preoptic, anterior, lateral, perifornical, and caudal nuclei. Because neurons in these hypothalamic nuclei integrate complex physiologic functions and behaviors, and because disruption of emotional, endocrine, autonomic, and other physiologic functions are frequently associated with migraine attacks, trigeminohypothalamic tract neurons may provide the afferent limb for the initiation of these symptoms.

Important bilateral projection from the TBNC to the parabrachial and Kölliker-Fuse nuclei also have been identified (2,25,35). Neurons in the caudal spinal trigeminal complex, including those in the superficial laminae of the MDH, send axons to the external portion of the lateral parabrachial area (see Fig. 1). Hayashi and Tabata (35) have shown that a large percentage of somatosensory neurons in the parabrachial nuclei respond exclusively to noxious stimuli. Bernard et al. (2) have postulated that this projection is part of a trigeminopontoamygdaloid pathway that may be involved in the affective, behavioral, and autonomic reactions to noxious events, which also may apply to severe headaches such as migraine. Conversely, direct descending projections from the parabrachial nucleus to the TBNC have been suggested to be involved in the control of trigeminal nociception.

Tract tracing studies also have demonstrated trigeminal afferent and TBNC projections to a number of other brain stem nuclei (59). The superior colliculus, for example, receives projections from the entire TBNC (8). The TBNC subnuclei, especially Vi, exhibit a robust projection to the ipsilateral cerebellum (57) and to the contralateral inferior olive (44). The TBNC also has been shown to project to the nucleus of the solitary tract (59). This pathway may be important in the coordination of somatic and visceral reflexes. Numerous investigators have demonstrated that neurons in the TBNC project to the adjacent reticular formation (81), providing another possible substrate for the processing of nociceptive information.

Trigeminal Projections to the Cerebral Cortex

The role of the cerebral cortex in trigeminal nociception has been studied by Kenshalo and collaborators (15,50), demonstrating that some primate cortical neurons in the SI region respond to noxious stimuli applied to the facial skin. This group has identified two populations of cortical nociceptive neurons, both of which are capable of encoding the intensity of painful stimuli. One population had restricted, contralateral receptive fields. The researchers suggested that these neurons may play a role in the sensory-discriminative aspect of pain. The small receptive fields presumably would facilitate the spatial localization of a painful stimulus. The second population of cortical nociceptive neurons possessed large, whole-body receptive fields. The response characteristics of these neurons would not permit them to localize a noxious stimulus but would signal the occurrence and intensity of the event. It was suggested that these neurons may play a role in cortical arousal.

Recently radiologic and electroencephalographic methods have been introduced to localize areas in the human brain that are likely to be involved in processing of pain evoked in the trigeminal system. May et al. (61), who used positron emission tomography (PET) to detect regions in the brain activated by an experimental painful stimulus (subcutaneous capsaicin injection) to the forehead, found increases in blood flow in the insula and the anterior cingulate cortex, regions that are usually activated when thermal painful stimuli are applied to the body (12). Interestingly, patients examined with PET during spontaneous migraine attacks also showed activation of an area that was related to the brain stem (99). Bromm and Chen (6) recorded long-latency brain potentials evoked by laser stimulation of the forehead and found four generators, which were suggested to correspond to the contra- and ipsilateral secondary somatosensory cortex, the frontal cortex, and a deep midline structure, possibly the cingular gyrus. On the whole, functional neuroimaging in headaches has produced no conclusive results so far.

CENTRAL MODULATION OF TRIGEMINAL NOCICEPTION

The TBNC has been shown to receive monoaminergic, enkephalinergic, and other peptidergic projections from regions known to be important in the modulation of nociceptive systems. Neurochemical and neurophysiologic studies show that interactions in the brain stem involving ascending and descending modulatory systems are exceptionally complex. Because antinociceptive systems are discussed separately (see Chapter 14), this chapter contains only a brief report on this topic with regard to the trigeminal system.

Descending Inhibitory System to the Medullary Dorsal Horn

A neuronal network extending from the frontal cortex and the hypothalamus through the periaqueductal gray matter (PAG) to the rostral ventromedial medulla (RVM) and to the medullary and spinal dorsal horn is probably the most powerful descending inhibitory system (Fig. 2). The RVM includes the nucleus raphe magnus (NRM) and the adjacent reticular formation and projects to the outer laminae of the spinal and medullary dorsal horn (26). Electrical stimulation of the PAG or RVM as well as injection of opioids into these structures has been shown

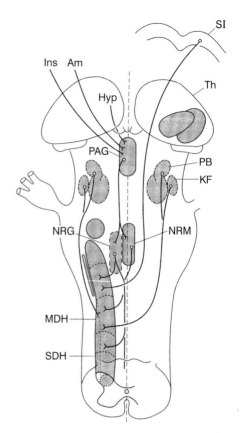

FIG. 2. Schematic representation of descending pathways to the central trigeminal system related to nociception, as far as the structures are mentioned in this chapter. The periaqueductal gray matter (*PAG*) receives input from the insular cortex (*Ins*), the amygdala (*Am*), and the hypothalamus (*Hyp*) and projects to the nucleus raphe magnus (*NRM*) and the adjacent reticular formation, including the nucleus reticularis gigantocellularis (*NRG*) within the rostral ventromedial medulla. From this area 5-HT pathways descend to the medullary (*MDH*) and spinal dorsal horn (*SDH*). Other descending pathways arise bilaterally from the parabrachial (*PB*) and Kölliker-Fuse (*KF*) nuclei, and there is a direct projection from the somatosensory cortex (*SI*) to the subnucleus interpolaris.

to reduce the activity of nociresponsive neurons in the superficial dorsal horn (14,55,68). The PAG receives important projections from parts of the forebrain such as insular cortex and the amygdala. Helmstetter et al. (36) have recently shown that microinjection of opioids into the rat basolateral amygdala causes antinociception through the PAG-RVM system. Descending inhibitory pathways also may originate in specific cortical projection areas. Chiang et al. (13) showed that the jaw-opening reflex induced by orofacial noxious input was inhibited by stimulation of the orofacial region in the somatosensory cortex. Another important source of input to the PAG is the hypothalamus. Stimulation of hypothalamic regions can produce analgesia and has been shown to suppress responses of rat Vc neurons (32,83).

Presumptive Inhibitory Mechanisms in the Medullary Dorsal Horn

The local circuit in the Vsp responsible for nociceptive and antinociceptive mechanisms is not precisely known, but analogous systems to the spinal dorsal horn are likely. As noted above, there is a large body of evidence that nociceptive afferents are terminating in laminae I and II and to a minor extent in laminae III through V in Vc. Whereas lamina I of the dorsal horn is the major source of centrally projecting neurons, most neurons in the substantia gelatinosa (lamina II) are interneurons. A subclass of these neurons (containing excitatory transmitters) is suggested to relay inputs from primary afferents to lamina I but also to deeper laminae. There are dendrites from nociceptive (WDR) cells of deeper laminae (lamina V) in the substantia gelatinosa, and lamina II cells are conversely connected to cells in deeper laminae. Other lamina II interneurons (containing transmitters such as GABA and enkephalin) are likely to act inhibitory on projection neurons (26) but also on glutaminergic terminals of primary afferents in Vsp (43) suggesting presynaptic inhibition of primary afferent input.

Both thalamic relay neurons and local interneurons in the dorsal horn are contacted by axon terminals of the descending pathway from RVM, and there is evidence for modulation of the activity of both rostrally projecting dorsal horn cells and inhibitory interneurons (see references in 26). The inhibitory interneurons in the substantia gelatinosa are likely to receive excitatory input from 5-hydroxytryptamine (5-HT) containing descending neurons from the PAG-RVM system. Morphine has been shown in the rabbit to inhibit the release of substance P and to increase the release of 5-HT in superficial layers of the Vc, which is in agreement with the hypothesis that opioids activate the descending 5-HT pathway to the Vsp (103).

Activity of On and Off Cells in RVM and PAG

Stimulation of the RVM causes antinociceptive effects that can be measured by inhibition of nociceptive reflexes such as the tail flick. Three classes of neurons have been identified in the RVM and the PAG that behave differentially prior to the occurrence of the tail flick (26). "Off cells" pause immediately before the reflex, whereas "on cells" are activated. Neurons of a third class (neutral cells) show no consistent changes in activation (67). A proportion of neutral cells that contains 5-HT is suggested to play a role in the modulation of nociceptive transmission (78).

Injection of opioids into the RVM or PAG causes activation of off cells and inhibition of on cells, whereas nociceptive reflexes are inhibited (67). Thus, off cell activity is related to suppression of nociception, whereas increased on cell activity is accompanied by an increased responsiveness to noxious stimuli. The activity of on and off cells has recently been found to be modulated by agonists of the 5-HT$_1$ receptor (84). The on/off cell concept is particularly interesting with regard to the mechanisms involved in head pain, because 5-HT$_1$ receptor agonists are effective in the treatment of migraine and other severe headaches. Recent interest has focused on binding sites and central actions of 5-HT$_1$ receptor agonists to understand the mechanisms of their antinociceptive activity (e.g., 9,40). So far, however, effects of specific 5-HT receptor agonists (and likewise of endogenous 5-HT) cannot be explained by selective inhibition of a distinct cell type in the trigeminal brain stem or the RVM (84).

Other Descending Antinociceptive Pathways

Nuclei of the parabrachial area, which receive nociceptive input from outer laminae of the Vsp have recently been shown in the rat to project directly and bilaterally to all subnuclei of the TBNC (104). They also may constitute a powerful descending antinociceptive system (see Fig. 2). The projections originating in the ventrolateral parabrachial and the Kölliker-Fuse nuclei terminate mainly in the ventrolateral parts of the TBNC, which are known to receive afferent input from tissues of the ophthalmic division, including meningeal structures. Electrical stimulation of the parabrachial area in the rat caused inhibitory effects on spontaneous and evoked activities of nociceptive neurons in Vc, which were similar to those seen with stimulation of the nucleus raphe magnus (14).

In addition, the Vsp receives direct input from the contralateral somatosensory cortex (see Fig. 2) (48). The corticotrigeminal projection has been shown to contribute to the control of receptive field size, convergence, and responsiveness of low-threshold neurons in Vi (48), and it seems possible that similar mechanisms are involved in the control of nociresponsive neurons in the Vsp.

Diffuse Noxious Inhibitory Controls

The activity of nociceptive spinal and medullary dorsal horn neurons, typically those with WDR characteristics, can be reduced by remote noxious stimulation from all parts of the body outside of their excitatory receptive field (52). This diffuse noxious inhibitory controls (DNIC) system largely survives spinal cord transection and thus is independent from the PAG-RVM descending inhibitory system (5). The neuronal circuits involved in DNIC may include the medullary subnucleus reticularis dorsalis (98). DNIC is also found in a major proportion of WDR neurons in the rat Vsp with convergent afferent input from the face (24) and the cranial dura mater (unpublished results). It is possible that acupuncture, transcutaneous electrical nerve stimulation, and other pain therapy strategies based on peripheral counterirritation, which are frequently applied in headaches, are acting through a mechanism comparable with DNIC (3).

ACKNOWLEDGEMENTS

The authors thank Drs. J. Ellrich, W. Neuhuber and K. Schepelmann for critical comments on the manuscript and K. Burian for preparing the artwork.

REFERENCES

1. Arbab MAR, Wiklund L, Svendgaard NA. Origin and distribution of cerebral vascular innervation from superior cervical, trigeminal and spinal ganglia investigated with retrograde and anterograde WGA-HRP tracing in the rat. *Neuroscience* 1986;19:695–708.
2. Bernard JF, Peschanski M, Besson JM. A possible spino (trigemino)-ponto-amygdaloid pathway for pain. *Neurosci Lett* 1989;100:83–88.
3. Bing Z, Villanueva L, Le Bars D. Acupuncture and diffuse noxious inhibitory controls: naloxone reversible depression of activities of trigeminal convergent neurones. *Neuroscience* 1990;37:809–818.
4. Boissonade FM, Sharkey KA, Lucier GE. Trigeminar nuclear complex of the ferret: anatomical and immunohistochemical studies. *J Comp Neurol* 1993;329:91–312.
5. Bouhassira D, Bing Z, Le Bars D. Studies of the brain structures involved in diffuse noxious inhibitory controls in the rat: the rostral ventromedial medulla. *J Physiol (London)* 1993;463:667–678.
6. Bromm B, Chen ACN. Brain electrical source analysis of laser evoked potentials in response to painful trigeminal nerve stimulation. *Electroencephalogr Clin Neurophysiol* 1995;95:14–26.
7. Broton JG, Rosenfeld JP. Rostral trigeminal projections signal perioral facial pain. *Brain Res* 1982;243:395–400.
8. Bruce LL, McHaffie JG, Stein BE. The organization of trigeminotectal and trigeminothalamic neurons in rodents: a double-labeling study with fluorescent dyes. *J Comp Neurol* 1987;262:315–330.
9. Bruinvels AT, Landwehrmeyer B, Gustafson EL, et al. Localization of 5-HT1B, 5-HT1D alpha, 5-HT1E and 5-HT1F receptor messenger RNA in rodent and primate brain. *Neuropharmacology* 1994;33:367–386.
10. Burstein R, Yamamura H, Malick A, Strassman AM. Chemical stimulation of the intracranial dura induces enhanced responses to facial stimulation in brain stem trigeminal neurons. *J Neurophysiol* 1998;79:964–982.
11. Burton H, Craig AD. Distribution of trigeminothalamic projection cells in cat and monkey. *Brain Res* 1979;161:515–521.
12. Casey KL, Minoshima S, Morrow TJ, Koeppe RA. Comparison of human cerebral activation pattern during cutaneous warmth, heat pain, and deep cold pain. *J Neurophysiol* 1996;76:571–581.
13. Chiang CY, Dostrovsky JO, Sessle BJ. Role of anterior pretectal nucleus in somatosensory cortical descending modulation of jaw-opening reflex in rat. *Brain Res* 1990;515:219–226.
14. Chiang CY, Hu JW, Sessle BJ. Parabrachial area and nucleus raphe magnus-induced modulation of nociceptive and nonnociceptive trigeminal subnucleus caudalis neurons activated by cutaneous or deep inputs. *J Neurophysiol* 1994;71:2430–2445.
15. Chudler EH, Anton F, Dubner R, Kenshalo DR Jr. Responses of nociceptive SI neurons in monkeys and pain sensation in humans elicited by noxious thermal stimulation: effect of interstimulus interval. *J Neurophysiol* 1990;63:559–569.
16. Coffey RJ, Rhoton AL. Pain-sensitive cranial structures. In: Dalessio D, Silberstein S, eds. *Wolff's headache and other head pain*. Oxford: Oxford University Press, 1993:19–41.
17. Craig AD, Burton H. Spinal and medullary lamina I projection to nucleus submedius in medial thalamus: a possible pain center. *J Neurophysiol* 1981;45:443–466.
18. Dallel R, Duale C, Molat JL. Morphine administered in the substantia gelatinosa of the spinal trigeminal nucleus caudalis inhibits nociceptive activities in the spinal trigeminal nucleus oralis. *J Neurosci* 1998;18:3529–3536.
19. Dallel R, Raboisson P, Woda A, Sessle BJ. Properties of nociceptive and non-nociceptive neurons in trigeminal subnucleus oralis of the rat. *Brain Res* 1990;521:95–106.
20. Davis KD, Dostrovsky JO. Activation of trigeminal brainstem nociceptive neurons by dural artery stimulation. *Pain* 1986;25:395–401.
21. Davis KD, Dostrovsky JO. Effect of trigeminal subnucleus caudalis cold block on the cerebrovascular-evoked responses of rostral trigeminal complex neurons. *Neurosci Lett* 1988;94:303–308.
22. Davis KD, Dostrovsky JO. Properties of feline thalamic neurons activated by stimulation of the middle meningeal artery and sagittal sinus. *Brain Res* 1988;454:89–100
23. Davis KD, Dostrovsky JO. Responses of feline trigeminal spinal tract nucleus neurons to stimulation of the middle meningeal artery and sagittal sinus. *J Neurophysiol* 1988;59:648–666.
24. Dickenson AH, Le Bars D, Besson JM. Diffuse noxious inhibitory controls (DNIC). Effects on trigeminal nucleus caudalis neurones in the rat. *Brain Res* 1980;200:293–305.
25. Feil K, Herbert H. Topographical organization of spinal and trigeminal somatosensory pathways to the rat parabrachial and Kölliker-Fuse nuclei. *J Comp Neurol* 1995;353:506–528.
26. Fields HL, Basbaum AI. Central nervous system mechanisms of pain modulation. In: Wall PD, Melzack R, eds. *Textbook of pain*. Edinburgh: Churchill Livingstone, 1994:243–257.
27. Ganchrow D. Intratrigeminal and thalamic projections of nucleus caudalis in the squirrel monkey (*Saimiri sciureus*): a degeneration and autoradiographic study. *J Comp Neurol* 1978;178:281–312.
28. Goadsby PJ, Zagami AS, Lambert GA. Neural processing of craniovascular pain: a synthesis of the central structures involved in migraine. *Headache* 1991;31:365–371.
29. Gobel S, Falls WR, Hockfield S. The division of the dorsal and ventral horns of the mammalian caudal medulla into eight layers using anatomical criteria. In: Anderson DJ, Matthews B, eds. *Pain in the trigeminal region*. New York: Elsevier, 1977:443–453.
30. Greenwood LF, Sessle BJ. Inputs to trigeminal brain stem neurones from facial, oral, tooth pulp and pharyngolaryngeal tissues. II. Role of trigeminal nucleus caudalis in modulating responses to innocuous and noxious stimuli. *Brain Res* 1976;117:227–238.
31. Hallas BH, Jacquin MF. Structure-function relationships in rat brain stem subnucleus interpolaris. IX. Inputs from subnucleus caudalis. *J Neurophysiol* 1990;64:28–45.
32. Hamba M, Hisamitsu H, Muro M. Wind-up of tooth pulp-evoked responses and its suppression in rat trigeminal caudal neurons. *Brain Res Bull* 1992;29:883–889.
33. Hayashi H. Morphology of terminations of small and large myelinated trigeminal primary afferent fibers in the cat. *J Comp Neurol* 1985;240:71–89.
34. Hayashi H, Sumino R, Sessle BJ. Functional organization of trigeminal subnucleus interpolaris: nociceptive and innocuous afferent inputs, projections to thalamus, cerebellum, and spinal cord, and descending modulation from periaqueductal gray. *J Neurophysiol* 1984;51:890–905.
35. Hayashi H, Tabata T. Pulpal and cutaneous inputs to somatosensory neurons in the parabrachial area of the cat. *Brain Res* 1990;511:177–179.
36. Helmstetter FJ, Tershner SA, Poore LH, Bellgowan PSF. Antinociception following opioid stimulation of the basolateral amygdala is expressed through the periaqueductal gray and rostral ventromedial medulla. *Brain Res* 1998;779:104–118.
37. Henry JL, Sessle BJ, Lucier GE, Hu JW. Effects of substance P on nociceptive and non-nociceptive trigeminal brain stem neurons. *Pain* 1980;8:33–45.
38. Henry MA, Johnson LR Nousek-Goebl NA, Westrum LE. Light microscopic localization of calcitonin gene-related peptide in the normal feline trigeminal system and following retrogasserian rhizotomy. *J Comp Neurol* 1996;365:526–540.
39. Henry MA, Nousek-Goebl NA, Westrum LE. Light and electron microscopic localization of calcitonin gene-related peptide immunoreactivity in lamina II of the feline trigeminal pars caudalis/medullary dorsal horn: a qualitative study. *Synapse* 1993;13:99–107.
40. Hoskin KL, Goadsby PJ. Comparison of more and less lipophilic serotonin (5HT1B/1D) agonists in a model of trigeminovascular nociception in cat. *Exp Neurol* 1998;150:45–51.
41. Hu JW. Response properties of nociceptive and non-nociceptive neurons in the rat's trigeminal subnucleus caudalis (medullary dorsal horn) related to cutaneous and deep craniofacial afferent stimulation and modulation by diffuse noxious inhibitory controls. *Pain* 1990;41:331–345.
42. Hu JW, Sessle BJ. Trigeminal nociceptive and non-nociceptive neurones: brain stem intranuclear projections and modulation by orofacial, periaqueductal gray and nucleus raphe magnus stimuli. *Brain Res* 1979;170:547–552.

43. Iliakis B, Anderson NL, Irish PS, Henry MA, Westrum LE. Electron microscopy of immunoreactivity patterns for glutamate and γ-aminobutyric acid in synaptic glomeruli of the feline spinal trigeminal nucleus (subnucleus caudalis). *J Comp Neurol* 1996;366:465–477.

44. Jacquin MF, Barcia M, Rhoades RW. Structure-function relationships in rat brainstem subnucleus interpolaris. IV. Projection neurons. *J Comp Neurol* 1989;282:45–62.

45. Jacquin MF, Chiaia NL, Haring JH, Rhoades RW. Intersubnuclear connections within the rat trigeminal brainstem complex. *Somatosens Motor Res* 1990;7:399–420.

46. Jacquin MF, Renehan WE, Mooney RD, Rhoades RW. Structure-function relationships in rat medullary and cervical dorsal horns. I. trigeminal primary afferents. *J Neurophysiol* 1986;55:1153–1186.

47. Jacquin MF, Stennett RA, Renehan WE, Rhoades RW. Structure-function relationships in the rat brainstem subnucleus interpolaris. II. Low and high threshold trigeminal primary afferents. *J Comp Neurol* 1988; 267:107–130.

48. Jacquin MF, Wiegand MR, Renehan WE. Structure-function relationships in rat brainstem subnucleus interpolaris. VIII. Cortical inputs. *J Neurophysiol* 1990;64:3–45.

49. Kemplay S, Webster KE. A quantitative study of the projections of the gracile, cuneate and trigeminal nuclei and of the medullary reticular formation to the thalamus in the rat. *Neuroscience* 1989;32:153–167.

50. Kenshalo DR, Isensee O. Responses of primate SI cortical neurons to noxious stimuli. *J Neurophysiol* 1983;50:1479–1496.

51. Kruger L, Siminoff R, Witkovsky P. Single neuron analysis of dorsal column nuclei and spinal nucleus of trigeminal in cat. *J Neurophysiol* 1961;24:333–349.

52. Le Bars D, Villanueva L. Electrophysiological evidence for the activation of descending inhibitory controls by nociceptive pathways. In: Fields HL, Besson JM, eds. *Pain modulation, progress in brain research.* Vol. 77. Amsterdam: Elsevier, 1988:275–299.

53. Lenz FA, Dostrovsky JO, Tasker RR, Yamashiro K, Kwan HC, Murphy JT. Single-unit analysis of the human ventral thalamic nuclear group: somatosensory responses. *J Neurophysiol* 1988;59:299–316.

54. Lisney SJW. Some current topics of interest in the physiology of trigeminal pain: a review. *J R Soc Med* 1983;76:292–296.

55. Lovick TA, Wolstencroft JH. Inhibitory effects of nucleus raphe magnus on neuronal responses in the spinal trigeminal nucleus to nociceptive compared with non-nociceptive inputs. *Pain* 1979;7:135–145.

56. Malick A, Burstein R. Cells of origin of the trigeminohypothalamic tract in the rat. *J Comp Neurol* 1998;400:125–144.

57. Mantle St. John LA, Tracey DJ. Somatosensory nuclei in the brainstem of the rat: independent projections to the thalamus and cerebellum. *J Comp Neurol* 1987;255:259–271.

58. Marfurt CF, Echtenkamp SF. Central projections and trigeminal ganglion location of corneal afferent neurons in the monkey, *Macaca fascicularis. J Comp Neurol* 1988;272:370–382.

59. Marfurt CF, Rajchert DM. Trigeminal primary afferent projections to "non-trigeminal" areas of the rat central nervous system. *J Comp Neurol* 1991;303:489–511.

60. Matsushita M, Ikdea M, Okado N. The cells of origin of the trigeminothalamic, trigeminospinal and trigeminocerebellar projections in the cat. *Neuroscience* 1982;7:1439–1454.

61. May A, Kaube H, Buchel C, et al. Experimental cranial pain elicited by capsaicin: a PET study. *Pain* 1998;74:61–66.

62. Mayberg MR, Nicholas TZ, Moskowitz MA. Trigeminal projections to supratentorial pial and dural blood vessels in cats demonstrated by horseradish peroxidase histochemisty. *J Comp Neurol* 1984;223:46–56.

63. McNaughton FL. The innervation of the intracranial blood vessels and dural sinuses. *Assoc Res Nerv Ment Dis* 1938;18:178–200.

64. Meng ID, Hu JW, Bereiter DA. Differential effects of morphine on corneal-responsive neurons in rostral versus caudal regions of spinal trigeminal nucleus in the rat. *J Neurophysiol* 1998;79:2593–2602.

65. Meng ID, Hu JW, Benetti AP, Bereiter DA. Encoding of corneal input in two distinct regions of the spinal trigeminal nucleus in the rat: cutaneaous receptive field properties, responses to thermal and chemical stimulation, modulation by diffuse noxious inhibitory controls, and projections to the parabrachial area. *J Neurophysiol* 1997;77:43–56.

66. Messlinger K, Hanesch U, Baumgärtel M, Trost B, Schmidt RF. Innervation of the dura mater encephali of cat and rat: ultrastructure and calcitonin gene-related peptide-like and substance P-like immunoreactivity. *Anat Embryol* 1993;188:219–237.

67. Morgan MM, Fields HL. Pronounced changes in the activity of noci-

ceptive modulatory neurons in the rostral ventromedial medulla in response to prolonged thermal noxious stimuli. *J Neurophysiol* 1994; 72:1161–1170.

68. Morgan MM, Heinricher MM, Fields LH. Circuitry linking opioid-sensitive nociceptive modulatory system in periaqueductal grey and spinal cord with rostral ventromedial medulla. *Neuroscience* 1992;47:863–871.

69. Nieuwenhuys R, Voogd J, van Huijzen C. *The human central nervous system—a synopsis and atlas.* Berlin: Springer, 1988.

70. Nord SG, Kyler HJ. A single unit analysis of trigeminal projections to bulbar reticular nuclei of the rat. *J Comp Neurol* 1968;134:485–494.

71. Nozaki K, Uemura Y, Okamoto S, Kikuchi H, Mizuno N. Origins and distribution of cerebrovascular nerve fibers showing calcitonin gene-related peptide-like immunoreactivity in the major cerebral artery of the dog. *J Comp Neurol* 1990;297:219–226.

72. Olszewski J. On the anatomical and functional organization of the spinal trigeminal nucleus. *J Comp Neurol* 1950;92:401–409.

73. Panneton WM, Burton H. Corneal and periocular representation within the trigeminal sensory complex in the cat studied with transganglionic transport of horseradish peroxidase. *J Comp Neurol* 1981; 199:327–344.

74. Pearson JC, Jennes L. Localization of serotonin- and substance P-like immunofluorescence in the caudal spinal trigeminal nucleus of the rat. *Neurosci Lett* 1988;88:151–156.

75. Peschanski M. Trigeminal afferents to the diencephalon in the rat. *Neuroscience* 1984;12:465–487.

76. Peschanski M, Roudier F, Ralston HJ III, Besson JM. Ultrastructural analysis of the terminals of various somatosensory pathways in the ventrobasal complex of the rat thalamus: an electron-microscopic study using wheat germ agglutinin conjugated to horseradish peroxidase as an axonal tracer. *Somatosens Res* 1985;3:75–87.

77. Phelan KD, Falls WM. The interstitial system of the spinal trigeminal tract in the rat: anatomical evidence for morphological and functional heterogeneity. *Somatosens Motor Res* 1989;6:367–399.

78. Potrebic SB, Mason P, Fields HL. The density and distribution of serotonergic appositions onto identified neurons in the rat rostral ventromedial medulla. *J Neurosci* 1995;15:3273–3283.

79. Raboisson P, Dallel R, Woda A. Responses of neurones in the ventrobasal complex of the thalamus to orofacial noxious stimulation after large trigeminal tractotomy. *Exp Brain Res* 1989;77:569–576.

80. Ray BS, Wolff HG. Experimental studies on headache: pain sensitive structures of the head and their significance in headache. *Arch Surg* 1940;1:813–856.

81. Renehan WE, Jacquin MF, Mooney RD, Rhoades RW. Structure-function relationships in rat medullary and cervical dorsal horns. II. Medullary dorsal horn cells. *J Neurophysiol* 1986;55:1187–1201.

82. Rexed B. The cytoarchitectonic organization of the spinal cord in the cat. *J Comp Neurol* 1952;96:415–495.

83. Rhodes DL, Liebeskind JC. Analgesia from rostral brain stem stimulation in the rat. *Brain Res* 1978;143:521–532.

84. Roychowdhury SM, Heinricher MM. Effects of iontophoretically applied serotonin on three classes of physiologically characterized putative pain modulating neurons in the rostral ventromedial medulla of lightly anesthetized rat. *Neurosci Lett* 1997;226:136–138.

85. Schaible H-G, Ebersberger A, Peppel P, Beck U, Messlinger K. Release of immunoreactive substance P in the trigeminal brain stem nuclear complex evoked by chemical stimulation of the nasal mucosa and the dura mater encephali—a study with antibody microprobes. *Neuroscience* 1997;76:273–284.

86. Schepelmann K, Ebersberger A, Pawlak M, Oppmann M, Messlinger K. Response properties of trigeminal brain stem neurons with input from the dura mater encephali in the rat. *Neuroscience* 1999;90: 543–544.

87. Sessle BJ. Neurophysiology of orofacial pain. *Dent Clin North Am* 1987;31:595–613.

88. Shigenaga Y, Nakatani Z, Nishimori T, Suemune S, Kuroda R, Matano S. The cells of origin of cat trigeminothalamic-projections: especially in the caudal medulla. *Brain Res* 1983;277:201–222.

89. Shigenaga Y, Okamoto T, Nishimori T, et al. Oral and facial representation in the trigeminal principal and rostral spinal nuclei of the cat. *J Comp Neurol* 1986;244:1–18.

90. Shults RC. Nociceptive neural organization in the trigeminal nuclei. In: Light AR, ed. The initial processing of pain and its descending control: spinal and trigeminal systems. *Pain and Headache.* Vol. 12. Basel: Karger, 1992:178–202.

91. Sjoqvist O. Studies on the pain conduction in the trigeminal nerve. *Acta Psychiatr Neurol Scand* 1938;17[Suppl]:1–139.
92. Steiger HJ, Meakin CJ. The meningeal representation in the trigeminal ganglion—an experimental study in the cat. *Headache* 1984;24: 305–309.
93. Stewart WA, King RB. Fiber projections from the nucleus caudalis of the spinal trigeminal nucleus. *J Comp Neurol* 1963;121:271–286.
94. Strassman AM, Mason P, Moskowitz MA, Maciewicz RJ. Response of brainstem trigeminal neurons to electrical stimulation of the dura. *Brain Res* 1986;379:242–250.
95. Strassman AM, Vos BP. Somatotopic and laminar organization of fos-like immunoreactivity in the medullary and upper cervical dorsal horn induced by noxious facial stimulation in the rat. *J Comp Neurol* 1993; 331:495–516.
96. Tashiro T, Takahashi O, Satoda T, Matsushima R, Uemura-Sumi M, Mizuno N. Distribution of axons showing calcitonin gene-related peptide- and/or substance P-like immunoreactivity in the sensory trigeminal nuclei of the cat. *Neurosci Res* 1991;11:119–133.
97. Torvik A. Afferent connections to the sensory trigeminal nuclei, the nucleus of the solitary tract and adjacent structures: an experimental study in the rat. *J Comp Neurol* 1956;106:51–142.
98. Villanueva L, Bouhassira D, Le Bars D. The medullary subnucleus reticularis dorsalis (SRD) as a key link in both the transmission and modulation of pain signals. *Pain* 1996;67:231–240.
99. Weiller C, May A, Limmroth V, et al. Brain stem activation in spontaneous human migraine attacks. *Nat Med* 1995;1:658–660.
100. Westrum LE, Canfield RC, O'Connor TA. Each canine tooth projects to all brain stem trigeminal nuclei in cat. *Exp Neurol* 1981;74: 787–799.
101. Yokota T, Matsumoto N. Somatotopic distribution of trigeminal nociceptive specific neurons within the caudal somatosensory thalamus of cat. *Neurosci Lett* 1983;39:125–130.
102. Yokota T, Koyama N, Matsumoto N. Somatotopic distribution of trigeminal nociceptive neurons in ventrobasal complex of cat thalamus. *J Neurophysiol* 1985;53:1387–1400.
103. Yonehara N, Shibutani T, Imai Y, Inoki R. Involvement of descending monoaminergic systems in the transmission of dental pain in the trigeminal nucleus caudalis of the rabbit. *Brain Res* 1990;508:234–240.
104. Yoshida A, Chen K, Moritani M, et al. Organization of the descending projections from the parabrachial nucleus to the trigeminal sensory nuclear complex and spinal dorsal horn in the rat. *J Comp Neurol* 1997;383:94–111.
105. Yoshida A, Dostrovsky JO, Sessle BJ, Chiang CY. Trigeminal projections to the nucleus submedius of the thalamus in the rat. *J Comp Neurol* 1991;307:609–625.
106. Zagami AS, Lambert GA. Stimulation of cranial vessels excites nociceptive neurones in several thalamic nuclei of the cat. *Exp Brain Res* 1990;81:552–566.

The Headaches, Second Edition,
edited by J. Olesen, P. Tfelt-Hansen, and K.M.A. Welch.
Lippincott Williams & Wilkins, Philadelphia © 2000.

Basic Science Aspects of the Headaches

CHAPTER 11

Cephalic Neurovascular Transmitters and Receptors

Inger Jansen-Olesen and Lars Edvinsson

Migraine attacks are known to involve alterations or even dysfunction in the regulation of tone in intra- or extracranial blood vessels (62). The nature of these alterations is not clearly established, and a number of candidate neurotransmitters have been discussed (22). Some of these candidates have their origin in sympathetic, parasympathetic, or sensory neurons (Fig. 1); endothelial cells; mast cells; or on blood-borne cells. The anatomy of the innervation is discussed in part elsewhere in this book. An increasing number of perivascular neurotransmitters have been detected and their receptor mechanisms and effects have been elucidated since the 1960s (10). In addition, endothelium-derived relaxing factors have been demonstrated; today these include nitric oxide (NO) prostaglandin I_2 (PGI_2), and endothelium-derived hyperpolarizing factor (EDHF). These agents are released following the stimulation of receptors located on endothelial cells causing relaxation. Thus, a number of mechanisms exist for regulation of tone in cranial blood vessels. Because there are considerable species differences in innervation and receptor types, this chapter focuses on studies of human cranial blood vessels.

THE SYMPATHETIC SYSTEM

The cranial vasculature has been shown to be supplied with sympathetic nerve fibers in which noradren-

I. Jansen-Olesen: Department of Pharmacology, The Royal Danish School of Pharmacy, DK-2100 Copenhagen Ø, Denmark.

L. Edvinsson: Department of Internal Medicine, University Hospital of Lund, S-221 85 Lund, Sweden.

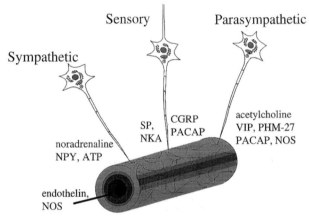

FIG. 1. Schematic illustration showing the putative organization of perivascular nerve fibers in the cranial circulation; sympathetic fibers originate in the superior cervical ganglion (NA, NPY, ATP), sensory fibers in the trigeminal ganglion (SP/NKA, CGRP, PACAP), and parasympathetic fibers in the sphenopalatine and otic ganglia (ACh, VIP/PHM-27, PACAP, NOS).

aline (NA) and the 36–amino acid peptide neuropeptide Y (NPY) coexist (24). Cerebral arteries from laboratory animals are equipped with a well-developed plexus of NA/NPY-containing fibers. Veins are less densely innervated. Smaller arteries and arterioles are innervated by single fibers only. In the human cranial vasculature, a dense network of NA- and NPY-containing nerve fibers has been shown (Table 1) (42). Quantitative measurements of NPY in extracts of human cerebral, middle

TABLE 1. *Relative amounts of peptide-containing fibers in human cerebral, middle meningeal, and temporal arteries graded arbitrarily from rich supply (***) to few fibers (*)*

Peptide	Artery		
	Cerebral	Meningeal	Temporal
NPY	**	**	***
VIP	**	**	**
SP	*	*	*
CGRP	**	**	**

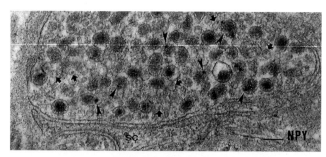

FIG. 2. Electron micrograph demonstrating the ultrastructural localization of NPY immunoreactivity in nerve varicosities of the human superficial temporal artery. The large granular vesicles (*arrowheads*), but not the smaller granular vesicles (*arrows*), display immunogold labeling (15-nm gold particles). SC, Schwann cell. Bar = 150 nm.

meningeal, and superficial temporal arteries revealed higher concentrations of NPY in the superficial temporal artery than in the cerebral and middle meningeal arteries ($p < 0.05$) (Table 2). With immunoelectron microscopy we have in perivascular nerve terminals of the temporal (40) and middle meningeal (18) arteries shown large vesicles containing NPY-immunoreactivity (-ir) (Fig. 2). Small electrolucent vesicles probably store NA. The sympathetic innervation of cortical pial arteries is very dense compared with that of the other nerve fiber systems in these arteries.

In human cerebral and middle meningeal arteries, the administration of NPY elicits concentration-dependent contraction (Table 3). The NPY-induced contraction is somewhat stronger in magnitude than that of NA; however, NPY is markedly more potent than NA (see Table 3). Low concentrations of NPY (10^{-8} M) do not modify the contraction induced by NA (see Table 3). In human temporal arteries, on the other hand, NPY usually does not induce contraction but it potentiates NA-mediated contractions without changing maximum contraction (see Table 3). The response to NA in cerebral and middle meningeal arteries is not modified by NPY. In cerebral, middle meningeal, and temporal arteries, the contractile responses to NA are antagonized by the α_1-adrenoceptor blocker prazosin (74). Neither this antagonist nor the 5-hydroxytryptamine (5-HT) blocker ketanserin cause blockade of contractions or potentiation induced by NPY.

The two different actions of NPY seem to be mediated via different mechanisms. The NPY-induced contractions are markedly reduced by calcium antagonists or by calcium depletion (15). In contrast, the potentiating effect of NPY on peripheral arteries has been shown not to be directly dependent on the extracellular calcium but is attenuated by oubain and is absent in a sodium-free buffer solution (85). Thus, in the human temporal artery the NPY receptor is modulating the level of intracellular Ca^+ or increasing the sensitivity of the contractile apparatus. The NPY contractions in cerebral arteries can be blocked by D-myo-inositol-1.2.6-trisphosphate, an NPY blocker (11), whereas it is unaffected by other antagonists (15). In addition, reverse-transcriptase polymerase chain reaction (RT-PCR) has shown that the NPY Y_1 receptor mRNA and the parallel shift of the NPY contraction by BIBP 3226 clearly establish the presence of the Y_1 receptor in human brain vessels (58). The different mode of action of NPY described above for cerebral and middle meningeal arteries compared with temporal arteries suggests that NPY may participate with NA in maintaining the upper limit of autoregulation in the cerebrovascular bed during acute increases in arterial blood pressure. In temporal arteries, NPY may serve as a modulator of adrenergically mediated responses (43).

Microapplication of NA or NPY *in situ* results in strong concentration-dependent contractions in pial arterioles on the cortical surface in anesthetized cats. The contractions induced by NA are more potent in pial veins than in arterioles, whereas the opposite is found for NPY (16).

TABLE 2. *Concentration of immunoreactive NPY, VIP, SP, and CGRP in different human arteries obtained at autopsy*

Artery	NPY concentration (pmol/g)	VIP concentration (pmol/g)	SP concentration (pmol/g)	CGRP concentration (pmol/g)
Temporal	13.5 ± 2.2	0.5 ± 0.2	0.5 ± 0.2	1.0 ± 0.3
Meningeal	6.5 ± 1.6	1.2 ± 0.4	0.3 ± 0.06	3.9 ± 1.1
Cerebral	3.0 ± 2.4	2.3 ± 0.7	2.3 ± 0.8	1.7 ± 0.3

Patient age >60 years. Values are means ± SEM; n = 5–8 patients.
Adapted from Jansen et al. (42).

TABLE 3. *Effects of NPY and NA on isolated human cerebral, middle meningeal, and temporal arteries in vitro*

Peptide	Cerebral			Meningeal artery			Temporal artery		
	n	E_{max}	pD_2	n	E_{max}	pD_2	n	E_{max}	pD_2
NPY	4	47 ± 13	8.2 ± 0.3	5	69 ± 14	7.5 ± 0.3	—	—	—
NA	4	27 ± 8	6.3 ± 0.5	4	35 ± 9	6.0 ± 0.1	6	96 ± 5	6.2 ± 0.04
NA + NPY	4	39 ± 3	6.4 ± 0.4	4	43 ± 5	5.8 ± 0.4	6	98 ± 5	7.0 ± 0.1

All values are means ± SEM.

n, number of vessels examined; E_{max}, maximum contraction; pD_2, -log concentration eliciting half-maximal relaxation.

Adapted from Jansen et al. (42)

THE PARASYMPATHETIC SYSTEM

Parasympathetic nerve fibers containing vasoactive intestinal polypeptide (VIP) and peptide histidine isoleucine (PHI) have been found around the cerebral arteries in all species studied. A close association of the cholinergic markers choline acetyltransferase (ChAT) and acetylcholinesterase (AChE) and VIP has been observed in nerve fibers around cerebral arteries, and a colocalization of ACh and VIP has been suggested (32,76). However, in a recent study, ChAT and VIP seemed to be located in separate fibers that run in parallel to each other; colocalization occurred in less than 5% of the fibers (56). The AChE-positive VIP/PHI fibers originate not only in the sphenopalatine ganglion but also in the otic ganglion and internal carotid miniganglia (19). Electron microscopic studies have shown that cholinergic nerve terminals are separated from the smooth muscle cells by a distance of 80 to 100 nm. Thus, the criteria for a functional innervation are fulfilled (23). In addition to the immunoelectron microscopy, we have shown VIP-ir in terminals of perivascular nerve fibers innervating the superior temporal artery of humans (40).

Only a sparse to moderate supply of VIP-ir fibers are found in the wall of human cerebral, middle meningeal, and temporal arteries (see Table 1). Quantitative measurements with radioimmunoassay revealed higher concentrations of VIP in the cerebral and middle meningeal arteries than in the temporal arteries (see Table 2).

Acetylcholine (ACh), VIP, and the human counterpart to PHI, peptide histidine methionine 27 (PHM), are potent vasodilators in the human cranial arteries. In the middle meningeal and cerebral arteries (Fig. 3), VIP is consistently more potent than PHM and ACh. A different pattern of potency is seen in the temporal artery, where VIP, PHM, and ACh are equivalent (Table 4). The two peptides relax the vessels by approximately the same amount in the three regions. ACh results in a lower maximum effect in the middle meningeal as compared with cerebral and temporal arteries. Relaxations induced by VIP and PHM are not affected by β-adrenoceptor, histamine H_2, or cholinergic antagonists. The mechanism of action of VIP and PHI/PHM involves an increase in the vessel wall adenylyl cyclase activity and is unrelated to the release of an endothelium-derived relaxing factor through which ACh induces dilatation (17). Previous studies in laboratory animals have shown that low ACh concentrations cause endothelium-dependent relaxation by binding to muscarinic M_3 receptors in the endothelium (30). High concentrations of ACh induce non– endothelium-dependent constriction by binding to muscarinic M_2 receptors, probably located on the vascular smooth muscle.

Other peptides that belong to the family of VIP-related peptides are helodermin, helospectins I and II, pituitary adenylate cyclase-activating peptide (PACAP), glucagon, and secretin. The pattern of parasympathetic innervation is complex, with PACAP, helodermin, and helospectin I and II being costored with VIP in varying subgroups of parasympathetic nerves (82,83). All these peptides induce vasodilation, and their functional importance will be investigated in the near future. The situation is further complicated by recent observations that nitric oxide synthase (NOS)/NADPH diapherase, a marker for NO-con-

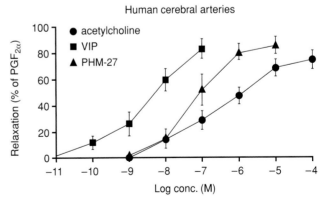

FIG. 3. Concentration-dependent relaxation of isolated human cerebral arteries following administration of acetylcholine, vasoactive intestinal peptide (VIP), and peptide histidine methionine-27 (PHM-27) to vessels precontracted with prostaglandin $F_{2\alpha}$. Mean values ± SEM.

TABLE 4. *Effects of ACh, VIP, and PHM on isolated human cerebral, middle meningeal, and temporal arteries in vitro*

Substance	Cerebral artery			Meningeal artery			Temporal artery		
	n	I_{max}	pD_2	n	I_{max}	pD_2	n	I_{max}	pD_2
ACh	11	76 ± 6	6.5 ± 0.3	9	41 ± 6	5.7 ± 0.5	6	77 ± 11	7.0 ± 0.1
VIP	6	83 ± 7	8.6 ± 0.2	6	62 ± 6	8.0 ± 0.1	6	77 ± 6	7.4 ± 0.1
PHM	6	87 ± 6	7.2 ± 0.2	4	72 ± 5	6.8 ± 0.1	6	76 ± 8	6.9 ± 0.3

All values are means ± SEM.

n, number of vessels examined; I_{max}, maximum relaxation; pD_2, -log concentration eliciting half-maximal relaxation.

Adapted from Jansen et al. (42).

taining nerves, also seems to exist in the wall of cerebral vessels (80). In rat cerebral arteries some of these NOS-containing fibers appear to coexist with VIP (61).

THE SENSORY SYSTEM

Human cranial arteries are supplied with a small amount of substance P– and a moderate amount of calcitonin gene-related peptide (CGRP)-containing nerve fibers located in the adventitia, sometimes in close apposition to the media layer (see Table 1). The concentration of CGRP is in general higher than the concentration of substance P. The level of substance P is higher in the cerebral arteries than in the middle meningeal and temporal arteries. The level of CGRP is higher in the middle meningeal artery than in the cerebral and temporal arteries (see Table 2). Previous studies in laboratory animals have shown a moderate supply of SP– and a rich supply of CGRP-containing nerve fibers around cerebral blood vessels of various mammals. Although several origins for cerebrovascular CGRP, substance P, and neurokinin A (NKA) fibers have been described, the major source is in the trigeminal ganglion, which sends fibers to innervate the circle of Willis and its anterior and caudal branches. Substance P, NKA, and CGRP immunoreactivity are frequently colocalized in the perikarya of neurons of the trigeminal ganglion of all species examined, including humans. With immunoelectron microscopy we have shown CGRP-ir vesicles in terminals of perivascular nerve fibers of the superficial temporal artery of humans (40). The number of CGRP-containing neuronal cell bodies in the trigeminal ganglion exceeds the number of substance P–containing cells (49,81).

Substance P, NKA, and CGRP all act as potent relaxant agents on all arteries examined (Table 5). The middle meningeal artery is more sensitive to substance P compared with both cerebral and temporal arteries. However, the reverse can be seen for CGRP, where the cerebral arterial responses are pronounced, whereas the middle meningeal artery shows the least potent responses of the cranial arteries examined (see Table 5).

Three types of tachykinin receptors have been described: neurokinin 1 (NK-1), neurokinin 2 (NK-2), and neurokinin 3 (NK-3). These have been differentiated on the basis of the order of potency for a series of agonists. At the NK-1 receptor, substance P is the most potent tachykinin, whereas NKA and NKB show high affinity for the NK-2 and NK-3 binding sites, respectively (49,69). The order of agonist potency for substance P and NKA in the human cranial vessels suggests that they are equipped with the NK-1 type of receptor; however, in a study performed on human cerebral arteries in which we included NKB and neuropeptide K (NPK) as agonists, the responses suggested the possibility of a mixed population of NK-1 and NK-2 receptors (35). Furthermore, Spantide, a substance P antagonist that has been suggested to act via the NK-1 and NK-2 receptor subtypes, competitively antagonized the relaxant responses to substance P in human cerebral arteries (35).

In recent years the cDNA encoding human $CGRP_1$ receptors has been cloned (3). CGRP belongs to a family of peptides that comprises five known members: calci-

TABLE 5. *Effects of SP, NKA, and CGRP on isolated human cerebral, middle meningeal, and temporal arteries in vitro*

Substance	Cerebral artery			Meningeal artery			Temporal artery		
	n	I_{max}	pD_2	n	I_{max}	pD_2	n	I_{max}	pD_2
SP	16	68 ± 5	8.7 ± 0.2	9	60 ± 8	9.9 ± 0.4	9	72 ± 4	9.0 ± 0.3
NKA	7	81 ± 10	7.7 ± 0.3	6	43 ± 13	7.6 ± 0.4	9	65 ± 9	8.4 ± 0.3
CGRP	12	91 ± 4	10.0 ± 0.2	6	85 ± 4	8.7 ± 0.2	11	83 ± 6	9.5 ± 0.4

All values are means ± SEM.

n, number of vessels examined; I_{max}, maximum relaxation; pD_2, -log concentration eliciting half-maximal relaxation.

Adapted from Jansen et al. (42).

tonin, amylin, the two CGRP peptides α- and β-CGRP, and adrenomedullin. The peptides in the calcitonin family probably act through seven-transmembrane domain G protein–coupled receptors (55).

A calcitonin receptor–like receptor (CRLR) can function as either a CGRP receptor or an adrenomedullin receptor, depending on the coexpression of a novel family of single transmembrane proteins, which have been called receptor activity modifying proteins (RAMP). RAMPs are required to transport CRLR to the plasma membrane. RAMP1 presents the receptor at the cell surface as a mature glycoprotein and a CGRP receptor. RAMP2-transported receptors are core glycosylated and represent adrenomedullin receptors (Fig. 4) (55).

In isolated cerebral arteries, relaxation induced by human α as well as by human β-CGRP were blocked by the CGRP antagonist human α-CGRP$_{8-37}$. The mean pA$_2$-values to the antagonist towards the two CGRP agonists were close to 6.50 in cerebral and dural arteries (Jansen-Olesen, unpublished observations). It is, however, notable that there are considerable variations in pA$_2$ values between arteries from different patients (4.87–7.58).

The neurotoxic substance capsaicin acts on sensory neurons to release stored substances. It has been used as a tool in studies of primary afferent sensory neurons. In our hands, capsaicin induced a biphasic relaxation of human cerebral arteries (n = 4). Pretreatment with 10^{-6} M human α-CGRP$_{8-37}$ significantly inhibited the first phase but not the second phase of capsaicin-induced relaxation (Fig. 5). Thus, CGRP seems to be the main substance responsible for dilatation due to release of stored substances in sensory neurons (44).

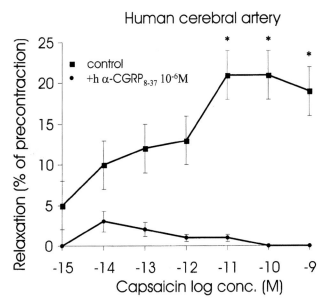

FIG. 5. Relaxant responses, given in percentage of precontraction induced by prostaglandin F$_{2α}$, to capsaicin in absence and presence of human α-CGRP$_{8-37}$, 10^{-6} M in human cerebral arteries. Values are given as means ± SEM. Six experiments from three patients; *Mann-Whitney U-test, $p < 0.05$.

Tachykinins and CGRP exert their relaxant actions via different mechanisms. The vasomotor response to α-CGRP, but not to substance P, occurs concomitantly with the activation of adenylyl cyclase, whereas substance P but not CGRP requires an intact endothelium for relaxant responses (17). In human cerebral arteries, CGRP has been shown to increase cyclic adenosine monophosphate (cAMP) levels concomitant with relaxation. This response is blocked by α-CGRP$_{8-37}$ (41) (Fig. 6). These findings agree well with the demonstration of CGRP$_1$

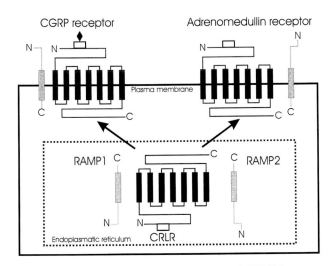

FIG. 4. The role of RAMP1 and RAMP2 and CRLR in generating CGRP and adrenomedullin receptors. ◆ Terminal glycosylation. □ Core glycosylation. Reproduced from McLatchie et al. (55).

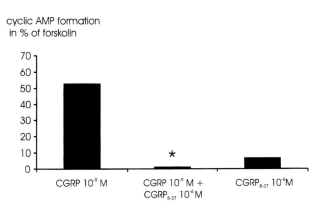

FIG. 6. Increase in cyclic AMP levels induced by 10^{-9} M human α-CGRP, 10^{-9} M human α-CGRP in the presence of 10^{-6} M human α-CGRP$_{8-37}$, and 10^{-6} M human α-CGRP$_{8-37}$ alone in human cerebral arteries. The values are given in percentage relative to the effect induced by 10^{-6} M forskolin. Values are given as means ± SEM. Four to 16 experiments from three to nine patients.

receptor mRNA (13) and RAMP1, as well as RAMP2 and RAMP3 (71), in human brain vessels. Substance P but not α-CGRP has been shown to induce endothelium-dependent relaxation in the human extracranial circulation (40), suggesting that the trigeminal system may modulate responses in intra- and extracranial circulations differently. Substance P may induce an inflammatory response in the middle meningeal artery, whereas such a reaction has not been seen in the cerebral circulation (52). In contrast, CGRP has been found to be involved in a dynamic reflex aimed to protect the brain against excessive vasoconstriction (54). This is further supported by studies in humans, where there is a marked and selective increase in craniovascular levels of the powerful vasodilator peptide CGRP, but not of NPY, VIP, and substance P during the headache phase of migraine both with and without aura (28). The elevation of CGRP is reduced after sumatriptan administration in parallel with amelioration of the headache (27). These findings provide the first direct evidence of a peptidergic involvement in migraine pathophysiology.

ENDOTHELIUM

Endothelial cells participate in the regulation of vascular tone by producing and releasing not only endothelium-relaxing agents (NO, prostacyclin, EDHF), but also contracting substances such as thromboxane A$_2$, superoxide anions, and endothelins.

Nitric Oxide

The relaxant effects of ACh, substance P, and NKA are known to involve the release from vascular endothelial cells of a short-lived relaxant factor (EDRF) (26). Furchgott (26) suggested that EDRF may be NO because endothelium-independent vasodilators such as sodium nitroprusside and nitroglycerine (NTG) are known to generate free NO. The free NO rapidly diffuses to the smooth muscle cells, where it stimulates guanylyl cyclase to produce cyclic guanosine monophosphate (cGMP). Intravenous NTG (which is converted to NO) has for some time been used to induce vascular headache (see elsewhere in this book). Vasodilatation induced by the production of NO can be antagonised by N^G-monomethyl-L-arginine, an inhibitor of NO synthase that converts L-arginine to NO and L-citrulline (66). For the human cranial vascular bed, there is no published report on the role of NO; however, NOS-ir perivascular nerves have been shown in human cerebral vessels (80) and temporal arteries (Gulbenkian, unpublished observations). Although we could not show any perivascular NOS-ir in the middle meningeal artery, there was ample NOS-ir in the endothelium (18) (Fig. 7), and in a still unpublished study we have shown that mRNA for neuronal NOS is present in the human middle meningeal artery (Fig. 8). In preliminary studies of the superficial temporal arteries

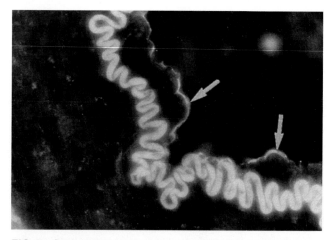

FIG. 7. Cryostat section of a human middle meningeal artery immunostained for nitric oxide synthase (NOS-endothelial form). Endothelial cells display a strong immunofluorescence staining (*arrows*).

we observed that the vasodilator response to ACh, substance P, and NKA is lost after removal of the endothelium and after treatment with the nitric oxide synthase inhibitor. The response is restored after administration of L-arginine (Jansen-Olesen and Edvinsson, unpublished observations).

Endothelin

The endothelins (ET) represent a family of potent endothelium-generated contractile peptides that are

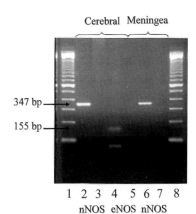

FIG. 8. Electrophoresis of RT-PCR products corresponding to mRNA encoding human constitutive nitric oxide synthase (cNOS) (lanes 2, 3, 6, and 7) and endothelial (e) NOS (lanes 4 and 5). The amplified products were of the predicted size (cNOS 347 base pairs and eNOS 155 base pairs). Lanes 2–4, human cerebral artery; lanes 5–6, human middle meningeal artery. As a negative control, no amplification product occurred when reverse transcriptase was omitted in the first-strand cDNA reaction (lanes 3, 5, and 7). Promega's 100-base pair DNA ladder was run in each of the outside lanes to confirm the molecular size of the amplification product (lanes 1 and 8).

important mediators of endothelium-induced vasoconstrictor activity. Three 21–amino acid ET peptides are known in this family: ET-1, ET-2, and ET-3. To date, two receptor subtypes (ET_A, ET-1-selective; and ET_B, ET-nonselective) have been cloned.

Endothelin is a potent activator of cranial arteries in humans (1,33,57) as well as in goats, cats, and pigs (39). Human, middle meningeal, and superficial temporal arteries and veins contracted after exposure to ET (1). The effect on cerebral arteries is much stronger than that observed in the temporal and middle meningeal arteries. Removal of the endothelium did not affect ET-induced contractions. Nimodipine reduced the maximal responses to ET in all arteries but reduced only slightly the effect in veins (33).

In recent studies we have observed that ET-1 and ET-2 are equipotent, whereas ET-3 hardly induces any contractile effect per se. Together with the observation that FR139317, a selective ET_A antagonist, shifts in parallel the contractile response to ET-1, this clearly demonstrates the existence of ET_A receptors in cranial vessels (2). This was greatly supported by the demonstration that the ET_A receptor mRNA is present (57). We also found that the ET_B receptor agonist sarafotoxin relaxes cerebral arteries, and this response was blocked by an ET_B receptor antagonist (57). The importance of ET in migraine has recently attracted interest. It was observed that there is a significant increase in plasma levels of ET-1 in conjunction with migraine attacks (25). However, in a recent study the ET_A/ET_B blocker bosentan was shown not to be effective in aborting acute migraine attacks (53).

5-HYDROXYTRYPTAMINE

A role for 5-HT in the pathophysiology of migraine has long been suggested based on several lines of evidence: (a) Levels of the main 5-HT breakdown product 5-hydroxyindoleacetic acid (5-HIAA) in the urine are increased during attacks (4); (b) the levels of 5-HT in cubital and external jugular veins are diminished and a 5-HT–releasing factor occurs during the headache phase (4); and intravenous injection of 5-HT alleviates or even abolishes migraine headache (46). This view is supported by the common characteristic of a variety of drugs used in the prophylaxis of migraine: the ability to antagonize various receptor-mediated actions of 5-HT.

Nerve fibers containing 5-HT are numerous around small cortex pial blood vessels (12,14). Substantial concentrations of 5-HT and its metabolite 5-HIAA occur in small pial vessels. The 5-HT–containing nerves on these vessels seem to originate in the median and dorsal raphe nuclei in the brain stem (14,51,70). Two weeks after median and dorsal raphe lesions in rats, the 5-HT concentrations in pial vessels are reduced by 54% and 48%, respectively. Occasional 5-HT–containing cells can be seen in the superior cervical ganglion (84). Sympathec-

tomy causes a reduction in 5-HT levels in the major cerebral arteries of the circle of Willis (52) but only minor or no observable change in the levels in cortex pial arterioles (14). Furthermore, 5-HT can be taken up into perivascular sympathetic nerves and may act as a false neurotransmitter (84).

Microapplication of 5-HT in situ has revealed that arterioles with diameters of less than 70 μm dilate, whereas larger arteries (greater than 200 μm in diameter) constrict (34). The dilator effect can be blocked by propranolol, and the constrictor response by methysergide (20) or ketanserin (78). A broadly similar response is seen in cerebral veins (48).

5-Hydroxytryptamine receptors are characterized according to the order of potency of responses induced by different agonists and the effect of selective 5-HT receptor antagonists. In several peripheral vascular tissues from laboratory animals, it appears that $5-HT_2$ receptors are primarily responsible for 5-HT–induced vasoconstriction. This contrasts with other vessels such as the saphenous vein and the basilar arteries of dogs (38). A considerable number of 5-HT receptors, mainly of the $5-HT_1$ subtypes, have been identified by radioligand binding (72); however, only some of the $5-HT_1$ subtypes have found functional correlates.

Molecular cloning has revealed the existence of at least five different $5-HT_1$ receptor subtypes, namely the 1A, 1B, 1D, 1E, and 1F receptors. Two of these, $5-HT_{1B}$ and $5-HT_{1D}$ receptors, are activated by sumatriptan-like drugs (86).

Agonists

The agonist data for human cerebral, basilar, and middle meningeal arteries have revealed that 5-carboxamidotryptamin (5-CT) is most potent, followed by 5-HT. According to Bradley and colleagues (5), this order of potency is suggestive of activation of the $5-HT_1$ subtype of receptors (38,59,68). In these regions, sumatriptan is slightly less potent than 5-CT and 5-HT. Furthermore, the $5-HT_{1A}$ agonist 8-OH-DPAT induces a strong contraction but with low potency (38,59). Together these data argue against the presence of the $5-HT_{1A}$ subtypes of receptors. Thus, the agonist data suggest the presence in human cerebral, basilar, and middle meningeal arteries of a receptor belonging to the $5-HT_{1B/1D}$ group (Table 6). Previous studies on the human basilar artery (68) and the proximal ramification of the middle cerebral artery (29) have shown the same rank order of potency as we found for fresh cerebral arteries from the temporoparietal cortical region (38). As has been shown for other species, cerebral arteries are more sensitive to 5-HT than peripheral arteries (21). Furthermore, correlation analysis of vasoconstrictor potency in human cerebral arteries with the affinity values (K_D) for brain 5-HT receptors indicate that a receptor site correlating to the $5-HT_{1B}$ and $5-HT_{1D}$

TABLE 6. *Contractions induced by different 5-HT agonists on human cerebral arteries*

Agonist	n	pEC$_{50}$ (M)	E$_{max}$ (% PGF$_{2\alpha}$ contraction)
Avitriptan	13	8.0 ± 0.2	24 ± 5
5-CT	14	7.5 ± 0.2	83 ± 15
DHE	6	7.3 ± 0.5	27 ± 9
Zolmitriptan	6	7.2 ± 0.6	41 ± 7
5-HT	24	7.1 ± 0.1	56 ± 12
183C91	6	7.0 ± 0.2	39 ± 12
Sumatriptan	13	6.8 ± 0.2	50 ± 10
5-me-trypt	6	6.5 ± 0.2	73 ± 16
Tryptamin	6	5.9 ± 0.3	42 ± 9
α-met-5-HT	5	5.6 ± 0.4	50 ± 10
8-OH-DPAT	6	5.2 ± 0.4	61 ± 10
CPP	7	Unobtained	Unobtained
MPP	6	Unobtained	Unobtained

pEC$_{50}$, -log concentration of agonist eliciting half-maximum contraction; E$_{max}$, maximum contraction induced by the agonists tested; n, number of patients studied.

The data are means ± SEM.

5-HT, 5-hydroxytryptamine; 5-CT, 5-carboxamidotryptamine, 5-me-trypt, 5-methoxytryptamine; α-met-5-HT, α-methyl-5-hydroxytryptamine; 8-OH-DPAT, 8-hydroxy DPAT; MPP, 1-(2-methoxyphenyl)piperazine; CPP, 1-(3-chlorophenyl)piperazine.

Adapted from Nilsson et al. (59)

receptor subtypes is responsible for mediating vasoconstriction (59) (Fig. 9).

These findings are supported by studies in which the distribution of mRNA coding for 5-HT$_{1B}$ and 5-HT$_{1D}$ receptors as well as by immunohistochemical studies using selective antibodies for the 5-HT$_{1B}$ and 5-HT$_{1D}$ receptors, have shown expression of the 5-HT$_{1B}$ receptor

but not the 5-HT$_{1D}$ receptor in human cerebral and middle meningeal arteries (31,50,59) (Fig. 10).

The agonist pattern is different in temporal arteries; 5-HT is more potent than 5-CT. Furthermore, the cerebral and middle meningeal arteries are more sensitive to 5-CT than is currently seen in the temporal artery. Tryptamine, CPP, MPP, 8-OH-DPAT, and 2-methyl-5-HT have low potency in all three vascular regions. 5-HT is more potent than 5-CT, indicating the presence of 5-HT$_2$-type receptors in the temporal artery (38).

Sumatriptan, zolmitriptan, and avitriptan are selective 5-HT$_{1B/1D}$ receptor agonists, which are effective in aborting acute attacks of migraine. These agonists all act as strong vasoconstrictor agents in human cerebral arteries (59). In addition, sumatriptan has been shown to induce contraction of the middle meningeal and temporal arteries. In low concentrations (10^{-8} to 10^{-7} M), sumatriptan was found to be a significantly stronger vasoconstrictor of meningeal arteries than of cerebral and temporal arteries (37).

Antagonists

Previous studies of human cerebral and temporal arteries have demonstrated that the contractile effect of 5-HT is antagonized by nonselective 5-HT antagonists, such as methylergometrine (77) and methysergide (21,36,75). Furthermore, methysergide was more potent as a 5-HT antagonist on the cerebral artery (active at 10^{-8} M) than on temporal arteries (not active below 10^{-7} M) (36). These observations suggest that the 5-HT response in the temporal artery is mediated via 5-HT$_2$ receptors. In human cerebral arteries, 5-HT is a potent vasoconstrictor that cannot

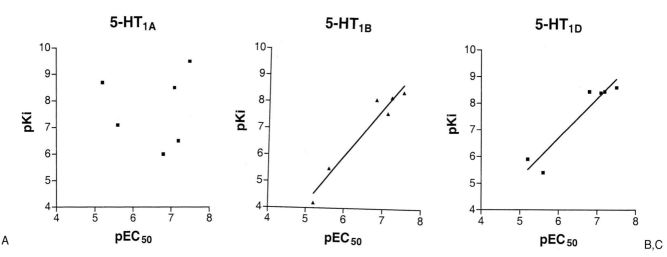

FIG. 9. Correlations between vasoconstrictor potency in human isolated cerebral artery (pEC$_{50}$) with measurements of affinity (pK$_D$) at 5-HT$_{1A}$ **(A)**, 5-HT$_{1B}$ **(B)**, and 5-HT$_{1D}$ receptors **(C)** obtained in binding experiments. Linear regression analysis was performed using Graph Pad Prism. Significant correlation was found between vasoconstrictor potency and 5-HT$_{1B}$ receptor affinity ($r^2 = 0.94$) and 5-HT$_{1D}$ receptor affinity ($r^2 = 0.90$) but not with 5-HT$_{1A}$ receptor affinity ($r^2 = 0.0006$) or 5-HT$_2$ receptor affinity ($r^2 = 0.18$, data not shown).

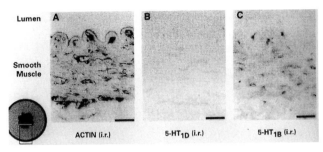

FIG. 10. Representative immunohistochemical findings in the middle meningeal artery. Immunoreactivity (ir) was detected using di-amino benzidine as the chromagen that yields orange/brown immunostaining. Hematoxylin was used as a counterstain to detect cell nuclei. Thin (6–7 μm) cross sections of the artery were obtained, and high-power micrographs of parts of these sections are shown. **A:** The smooth muscle layer of the tunica media as defined using a smooth muscle α-actin antibody. **B:** Little or no 5-HT$_{1D}$-ir was detected within the smooth muscle layer. **C:** Dense 5-HT$_{1B}$-ir within the smooth muscle layer. Scale bar = 20 μm. Reproduced from Longmore et al. (50).

be blocked by ketanserin (38). Because ketanserin is a selective and potent 5-HT$_2$ antagonist, this strongly suggests that there is no significant population of 5-HT$_2$ receptors in cerebral arteries. The rank order of antagonist potency at 5-HT$_1$ receptor subtypes is in concert with this suggestion (67). The response to 5-HT in the middle meningeal artery provides evidence for the existence of two types of 5-HT receptors; ketanserin is active in concentrations causing blockade of 5-HT$_2$ receptors, and 5-CT–induced contractions of human cerebral and middle meningeal arteries were antagonized by methiotepin. Although the effect was not competitive in the middle meningeal arteries, there was no antagonistic effect of methiothepin in the temporal artery (38). For the middle meningeal artery, the response to 5-CT was antagonized at 10^{-8} and 10^{-7} M of methiothepin; thus, the contractile effect in this artery is more sensitive to methiothepin than that seen in cerebral vessels. This suggests that the 5-CT–induced contraction possibly involves two types of receptors, a 5-HT$_1$ receptor subtype comparable with that of cerebral arteries and, as was suggested above, a 5-HT$_2$ receptor site. This suggestion is in agreement with results with the selective agonist sumatriptan (7,37,68), which suggested that 5-HT$_{1B/1D}$ receptors may mediate contractions of canine and human basilar arteries.

Methiothepin and the 5-HT$_{1B/1D}$ receptor antagonist GR 55562 also acted as potent antagonists of sumatriptan-induced contractions in human cerebral arteries (59). For methiothepin, Schild analysis revealed pA$_2$ values of 10.2 and 9.75 in the human cerebral and middle meningeal arteries, respectively. In the temporal artery, methiothepin at higher concentrations (10^{-7} to 10^{-6} M) depressed (noncompetitively) the sumatriptan-induced contractions (38).

MAST CELLS

The role of histamine and other vasoactive amines in headache is still subject to much debate. Experimental headache, caused by infusion of histamine, is in many ways similar to the pulsating headache seen in migraine (65). Therefore, understanding the mechanism of vascular changes caused by endogenous substances such as histamine may greatly increase our understanding of the migraine attack. Moreover, migraine patients seem more susceptible than control patients to histamine-induced headache.

Early studies concluded that experimental histamine-induced headache originates intracranially. Thus, intraspinal saline injection causing increased intracranial pressure diminished the headache (6,73), and infiltration of pericranial tissue with local anesthetics did not change the headache (87). Headache also could be provoked by injection of histamine into the internal carotid artery but was not seen following injection into the external carotid artery (60). On the other hand, Tindall and Greenfield (79) noted that histamine injection caused a more marked increase in blood flow in the external carotid artery than in the internal carotid artery. Krabbe and Olesen (47) demonstrated a small increase in cerebral blood flow (rCBF) after intracarotid histamine. The administration of histamine to cerebral vessels from different species causes either relaxation or contraction. In guinea pigs and rabbits, it causes contraction by activation of H$_1$ receptors. In cats and rats, dilator responses seem to be mediated mainly via histamine H$_2$ receptors.

The administration of histamine to prostaglandin F$_{2\alpha}$-precontracted human middle meningeal arteries induces a concentration-related dilatation. In most other species studied, dilatation of cerebral vessels by histamine is mediated via H$_2$ receptors and contraction is mediated via H$_1$ receptors (63). Studies of human cerebral arteries indicate that the histamine-induced dilatation is mediated by both H$_1$ and H$_2$ receptors, the former being most important (63,64). This conclusion was drawn from experiments in which an H$_1$ receptor antagonist (mepyramine) alone blocked the histamine-induced dilatation, whereas an H$_2$ receptor antagonist (cimetidine) alone did not alter the dilatory response. However, combined treatment with H$_1$ and H$_2$ antagonists unmasked the dilatory effect on H$_2$ receptor stimulation.

Experiments with small human temporal arteries indicate that histamine-induced dilatation is mediated by both H$_1$ and H$_2$ receptors, but here the H$_2$ receptor is predominant (64).

These findings of H$_1$ as well as H$_2$ receptors in the human cranial circulation are supported by studies in which expression of mRNA coding for histamine H$_1$ and H$_2$ receptors have been shown in human cerebral, middle meningeal, and temporal arteries (45).

TABLE 7. *Comparison of histamine-induced relaxations on human cranial arteries precontracted by prostaglandin $F_{2\alpha}$ (3×10^{-6} M)*

Artery	IC_{50} (M)[a]	I_{max} (% $PGF_{2\alpha}$ contraction)[a]
Cerebral	$5.2 \pm 1.6 \times 10^{-8}$	93 ± 5
Meningeal	$1.3 \pm 0.4 \times 10^{-7}$	95 ± 7
Temporal	$2.8 \pm 0.6 \times 10^{-7}$	81 ± 4

Values are means $\pm$ SEM of 10 to 12 experiments.
[a]IC_{50} (histamine concentration eliciting half-maximal response) and I_{max} (maximum effect of histamine) in human cerebral meningeal, and temporal arteries.
Adapted from Ottosson et al. (65).

In cranial arteries without endothelium or in N^G-Nitro-L-Arginine Methyl Ester (L-NAME)–pretreated arteries, histamine-induced relaxation was significantly less potent than in cranial arteries with an intact endothelium without the presence of nitric oxide synthase inhibitor (45). The combined treatment with L-NAME and cimetidine caused a further displacement of the concentration-response curve. Thus, it would appear that the H_1 receptor is located on the endothelium in human cranial arteries and is coupled to the production of nitric oxide (45).

In temporal arteries, cimetidine alone antagonized the histamine response, whereas mepyramine alone was without effect. The combination of H_1 and H_2 receptor antagonists unmasked the dilatory effect of H_1 receptor stimulation in temporal arteries. The pA_2 values calculated were 8.6 for mepyramine and 6.6 for cimetidine (64).

In human meningeal arteries, both cimetidine and mepyramine alone antagonized the histamine-induced dilatation in a competitive way. The combination of both antagonists further reduced the dilatation seen upon histamine administration. Thus, both receptors seem to be of importance for the histamine-induced dilatation of human meningeal arteries, and neither appears to dominate (64). The pA_2 value of 6.3 for cimetidine is in accordance with the results in temporal and cerebral vessels, whereas the value 9.8 for mepyramine is somewhat higher (63,64). A comparison of the IC_{50} values in the three cranial arteries indicates that cerebral arteries are the most sensitive to histamine, followed by meningeal arteries and temporal arteries (Table 7). The findings that H_1 receptor antagonists almost abolished histamine-induced headache in migraine patients, whereas H_2 receptor antagonists are less effective (47), support the hypothesis that experimental histamine-induced headache due to vasodilatation is intracranial in origin.

ACKNOWLEDGMENTS

This work was supported by grants from the Danish Medical Research Council (9601844 and 9702065), the Danish Pharmacist Foundation, the Lundbeck Foundation, Denmark, the Swedish Medical Research Council (5958 and 11238) and the Faculty of Medicine, University Hospital, Lund, Sweden.

REFERENCES

1. Adner M, Jansen I, Edvinsson L. Endothelin-A receptors mediate contraction in human cerebral, meningeal and temporal arteries. *J Auton Nerv Syst* 1994;49[Suppl]:117–121.
2. Adner M, You JP, Edvinsson L. Characterization of endothelin-A receptors in the cerebral circulation. *Neuroreport* 1993;4:441–443.
3. Aiyar N, Rand K, Elshourbagy N, et al. A cDNA encoding the calcitonin gene-related peptide type 1 receptor. *J Biol Chem* 1996;19: 11325–11329.
4. Anthony M, Hinterberger H, Lance JW. The possible relationship of serotonin to the migraine syndrome. In: Friedman AP, ed. *Research and clinical studies in headache.* Vol 1. Basel: Karger, 1969:29–59.
5. Bradley PB, Engel G, Feniuk W, et al. Proposals for the classification and nomenclature of functional receptors for 5-hydroxytryptamine. *Neuropharmacology* 1986;25:563–576.
6. Clark D, Hough H, Wolff HG. Experimental studies on headache: observations on histamine headache. *Arch Neurol Psychiatry* 1936;35: 1054–1070.
7. Connor HE, Feniuk, W. Humphrey, PAA. Characterization of 5-HT receptors mediating contraction of canine and primate basilar artery by use of GR 43175, a selective 5-HT$_1$-like receptor agonist. *Br J Pharmacol* 1989;96:379–387.
8. Dennis T, Fournier A, Cadieux A, et al. HCGRP 8-37, a calcitonin gene-related peptide antagonist revealing calcitonin gene-related peptide heterogenity in brain and periphery. *J Pharmacol Exp Ther* 1990;254:123–128.
9. Donoso VM, Fournier A, St. Pierre S, Huidobro-Toro JP. Pharmacological characterization of CGRP1 receptor subtype in the vascular system in the rat: studies with hCGRP fragments and analogues. *Peptides* 1990;11:885–889.
10. Edvinsson L. Role of perivascular peptides in the control of the cerebral circulation. *Trends Neurosci* 1985;8:126–131.
11. Edvinsson L, Adamsson M, Jansen I. Neuropeptide Y antagonistic properties of D-myo-inositol-1.2.6-triphosphate in guinea pig basilar arteries. *Neuropeptides* 1990;17:99–105.
12. Edvinsson L, Birath E, Uddman R, et al. Indoleaminergic mechanisms in brain vessels; localization, concentration, uptake and *vitro* responses of 5-hydroxytryptamine. *Acta Physiol Scand* 1984;121:291–299.
13. Edvinsson L, Cantera L, Jansen-Olesen I, Uddman R. Expression of calcitonin gene-related peptide$_1$ receptor mRNA in human trigeminal ganglia and cerebral arteries. *Neurosci Lett* 1997;229:209–211.
14. Edvinsson L, Dequeurce A, Duverger D, MacKenzie ET, Scatton B. Central serotonergic nerves project to the pial vessels of the brain. *Nature* 1983;306:55–57
15. Edvinsson L, Emson P, McCulloch J, Tatemoto K, Uddman R. Neuropeptide Y: cerebrovascular innervation and vasomotor effects in the cat. *Neurosci Lett* 1983;43:79–84.
16. Edvinsson L, Emson P, McCulloch J, Tatemoto K, Uddman R. Neuropeptide Y: immunocytochemical localization to and effect upon feline pial arteries and veins *in vitro* and *in situ. Acta Physiol Scand* 1984;122:155–163.
17. Edvinsson L, Fredholm BB, Hamel E, Jansen I, Verrecchia C. Perivascular peptides relax cerebral arteries concomitant with stimulation of cyclic adenosine monophosphate accumulation or release of an endothelium derived relaxing factor in the cat. *Neurosci Lett* 1985;58: 213–217.
18. Edvinsson L, Gulbenkian S, Barroso CP, Jansen-Olesen I, Polak JM. Innervation of the human middle meningeal artery: immunohistochemistry, ultrastructure, and role of endothelium for vasomotility. *Peptides* 1998;19:1213–1225.
19. Edvinsson L, Hara H, Uddman R. Retrograde tracing of nerve fibres to the rat middle cerebral artery with True Blue: co-localization with different peptides. *J Cereb Blood Flow Metab* 1989;9:212–218.
20. Edvinsson L, Hardebo JE, MacKenzie ET, Stewart M. Dual actions of serotonin on pial arterioles *in situ* and the effect of propranolol on the response. *Blood Vessels* 1977;14:366–371.
21. Edvinsson L, Hardebo JE, Owman C. Pharmacological analysis of 5-

hydroxytryptamine receptors in isolated intracranial and extracranial vessels of cat and man. *Circ Res* 1978;42:143–151.

22. Edvinsson L, MacKenzie ET, McCulloch J, Uddman R. Nerve supply and receptor mechanisms in intra- and extracerebral blood vessels. In: Olesen J, Edvinsson L, eds. *Basic mechanisms of headache.* Amsterdam: Elsevier, 1988;129–144.

23. Edvinsson L, Nielsen KC, Owman C, Sporrong B. Cholinergic mechanisms in pial vessels. Histochemistry, electron microscopy and pharmacology. *Z Zellforsch* 1972;131:311–325.

24. Ekblad E, Edvinsson L, Wahlstedt C, Uddman R, Håkanson R, Sundler F. Neuropeptide Y co-exists and co-operates with noradrenaline in perivascular nerve fibres. *Regul Pept* 1984;8:225–235.

25. Färkkilä M, Palo J, Saijonamaa O, Fyhrquist F. Raised plasma endothelin during acute migraine attack. *Cephalalgia* 1992;12:383–384.

26. Furchgott RF. The requirement for endothelial cells in the relaxation of arteries by acetylcholine and some other vasodilators. *Trends Pharmacol Sci* 1984;2:173–176.

27. Goadsby PJ, Edvinsson L. Sumatriptan reverses the changes in calcitonin gene-related peptide seen in the headache phase of migraine. *Cephalalgia* 1991;11[Suppl 11]:3–4.

28. Goadsby PJ, Edvinsson L, Ekman R. Vasoactive peptide release in the extracerebral of human during migraine headache. *Ann Neurol* 1990;28:183–187.

29. Hamel E, Bouchard D. Contractile 5-HT1 receptors in human isolated pial arterioles: correlation with 5-HT$_{1D}$ binding sites. *Br J Pharmacol* 1991;102:227–233.

30. Hamel E, Estrada C. Cholinergic innervation of pial and intracerebral blood vessels: evidence, possible origins and sites of action. In: Seylaz J, Sercombe R, eds. *Neurotransmission and cerebrovascular function II.* Amsterdam: Elsevier, 1989;151–173.

31. Hamel E, Fan E, Linville D, Ting V, Villemure JG, Chia LS. Expression of mRNA for the serotonin 5-hydroxytryptamine$_{1D}$ beta receptor subtype in human and bovine cerebral arteries. *Mol Pharmacol* 1993;44:242–246.

32. Hara H, Hamill GS, Jacobowitz DM. Origin of cholinergic nerves to the rat major cerebral arteries: coexistence with vasoactive intestinal polypeptide. *Brain Res* 1985;14:179–188.

33. Hardeboe JE, Kåhrström J, Owman C, Salford LG. Endothelin is a potent constrictor of human intracranial arteries and veins. *Blood Vessels* 1989;26:249–253.

34. Harper AM, MacKenzie ET. Effects of 5-hydroxytryptamine on pial arteriolar calibre in anaesthetized cats. *J Physiol* 1977;271:735–746.

35. Jansen I, Alafaci C, McCulloch J, Uddman R, Edvinsson L. TAChykinins (substance P, neurokinin A, neuropeptide K, neurokinin B) in the cerebral circulation: vasomotor responses *in vitro* and *in situ*. *J Cereb Blood Flow Metab* 1991;11:567–575.

36. Jansen I, Blackburn T, Dons K, Edvinsson L. Comparison of 5-hydroxytryptamine antagonistic effects of methysergide, ICI 169,369 and ICI 170.809 in human temporal and cerebral arteries. *Pharmacol Toxicol* 1991;68:8–13.

37. Jansen I, Edvinsson L, Mortensen A, Olesen J. Sumatriptan is a potent vasoconstrictor of human dural arteries via a 5-HT$_1$-like receptor. *Cephalalgia* 1992;12:202–205.

38. Jansen I, Edvinsson L, Olesen J. 5-Hydroxytryptamine receptor characterization of human cerebral, middle meningeal and temporal arteries: regional differences. *Acta Physiol Scand* 1993;147:141–150.

39. Jansen I, Fallgren B, Edvinsson L. Mechanisms of action of endothelin on isolated feline cerebral arteries: *in vitro* pharmacology, and electrophysiology. *J Cereb Blood Flow Metab* 1989;9:7463–747.

40. Jansen I, Gulbenkian S, Valenca A, et al. The peptidergic innervation of the human superficial temporal artery: immunocytochemistry, ultrastructure and vasomotility. *Peptides* 1995;16:275–287.

41. Jansen I, Mortensen A, Edvinsson L. Charactetrization of calcitonin gene-related peptide receptors in human cerebral vessels: vasomotor responses and cAMP accumulation. In: Calcitonin gene-related peptide: the first decade of a novel pleitropic neuropeptide. *Ann NY Acad Sci* 1992;657:435–440.

42. Jansen I, Uddman R, Ekman R, Olesen J, Ottosson A, Edvinsson L. Distribution and effects of neuropeptide Y, vasoactive intestinal polypeptide, substance P and calcitonin gene-related peptide in human middle meningeal artery: comparison with cerebral and temporal arteries. *Peptides* 1992;13:527–536.

43. Jansen I, Uddman R, Hocherman M, et al. Localization and effects of neuropeptide Y, vasoactive intestinal polypeptide, substance P, and cal-

citonin gene-related peptide in human temporal arteries. *Ann Neurol* 1986;20:496–501.

44. Jansen-Olesen I, Mortensen A, Edvinsson L. Calcitonin gene-related peptide is released from capsaicin-sensitive nerve fibres and induces vasodilatation of human cerebral arteries concomitant with activation of adenylyl cyclase. *Cephalalgia* 1996;16:310–316.

45. Jansen-Olesen I, Ottosson A, Cantera L, et al. Role of endothelium and nitric oxide for histamine-induced responses in human cranial arteries and detection of mRNA encoding H$_1$- and H$_2$-receptors using RT-PCR. *Br J Pharmacol* 1997;121:41–48.

46. Kimball RW, Friedman MD, Vallejo E. Effect of serotonin in migraine patients. *Neurology* 1960;10:107–111.

47. Krabbe A, Olesen J. Headache provocation by continuous intravenous infusion of histamine. Clinical results and receptor mechanisms. *Pain* 1980;8:253–259.

48. Leber K, Auer LM, Sayama I. *In vitro* effect of serotonin on cat pial veins. In: Auer LM, Low F, eds. *The cerebral veins: an experimental and clinical update.* Vienna: Springer, 1993:277–283.

49. Lee C-M, Campbell NJ, Williams BJ, Iversen LL. Multiple tachykinin binding sites in peripheral tissues and in brain. *Eur J Pharmacol* 1986;130:209–217.

50. Longmore J, Shaw D, Smith D, et al. Differential distribution of 5HT1D- and 5HT1B-immunoreactivity within the human trigemino-cerebrovascular system: implications for the discovery of new antimigraine drugs. *Cephalalgia* 1997;17:833–842.

51. Marco EJ, Balfagon G, Salaices M, Sánchez-Ferrer CF, Marin J. Serotonergic innervation of cat cerebral arteries. *Brain Res* 1985;338:137–139.

52. Markowitz S, Saito K, Moskowitz MA. Neurologically mediated leakage of plasma protein occurs from blood vessels in dura mater but not in brain. *J Neurosci* 1987;4129–4136.

53. May A, Gijsman HJ, Wallnofer A, Jones R, Diener HC, Ferrari MD. Endothelin antagonist bosentan blocks neurogenic inflammation, but is not effective in aborting migraine attacks. *Pain* 1996;67:375–378.

54. McCulloch J, Uddman R, Kingman TA, Edvinsson L. Calcitonin gene-related peptide: functional role in cerebrovascular regulation. *Proc Natl Acad Sci U S A* 1986;83:5741–5745.

55. McLatchie LM, Fraser NJ, Main MJ. RAMPs regulate the transport and ligand specificity of the calcitonin-receptor-like receptor. *Nature* 1998;393:333–339.

56. Miao FJ-P, Lee TJ-F. Cholinergic and VIPergic innervation in cerebral arteries: a sequential double-labelling immunohistochemical study. *J Cereb Blood Flow Metab* 1990;10:32–37.

57. Nilsson T, Cantera L, Adner M, Edvinsson L. Presence of contractile endothelin-A and dilatory endothelin-B receptors in human cerebral arteries. *Neurosurgery* 1997;40:346–351.

58. Nilsson T, Cantera L, Edvinsson L. Presence of neuropeptide Y Y$_1$ receptor mediating vasoconstriction in human cerebral arteries. *Neurosci Lett* 1996;204:145–148.

59. Nilsson T, Longmore J, Shaw D, Jansen-Olesen I, Edvinsson L. Contractile 5-HT$_{1B}$ receptors in human cerebral arteries: pharmacological characterisation and localisation with immunohistochemistry. *Br J Pharmacol* (in press).

60. Northfield DWC. Some observation on headache. *Brain* 1938;61:133–162.

61. Nozaki K, Moskowitz MA, Maynard KI, et al. Possible origins and distribution of immunoreactive nitric oxide synthase-containing nerve fibers in cerebral arteries. *J Cereb Blood Flow Metab* 1993;13:70–79.

62. Olesen J. Cerebral and extracranial circulatory disturbances in migraine: pathophysiology implications. *Cerebrovasc Brain Metab Rev* 1991;3:1–28.

63. Ottosson A, Jansen I, Edvinsson L. Characterization of histamine receptors in isolated human cerebral arteries. *Br J Pharmacol* 1988;94:901–907.

64. Ottosson A, Jansen I, Edvinsson L. Pharmacological characterization of histamine receptors in the human temporal artery. *Br J Clin Pharmacol* 1989;27:139–145.

65. Ottosson A, Jansen I, Langemark M, Olesen J, Edvinsson L. Histamine receptors in the isolated human middle meningeal artery. A comparison with cerebral and temporal arteries. *Cephalalgia* 1991;11:183–188.

66. Palmer RMJ, Ferrige AG, Moncada S. Nitric oxide release accounts for the biological activity of endothelium-derived relaxing factor. *Nature* 1987;327:524–526.

67. Parsons AA. 5-HT receptors in human and animal cerebrovasculature. *Trends Pharmacol Sci* 1991;12:310–315.

68. Parsons AA, Whalley ET, Feniuk W, Connor HE, Humphrey PPA. 5-HT$_1$-like receptors mediate 5-hydroxytryptamine-induced contraction of human isolated basilar artery. *Br J Pharmacol* 1989;96:434–449.

69. Regoli D, Drapeau G, Dion S, D'Orleans-Juste P. Pharmacological receptors for substance P and neurokinins. *Life Sci* 1987;40:109–117.

70. Reinhard JF, Liebmann JE, Schlosberg AJ, Moskowitz MA. Serotonin neurons project to small blood vessels in the brain. *Science* 1979;206:85–87.

71. Sams A, Jansen-Olesen I. Expression of calcitonin receptor-like receptor (CRLR) and receptor activity modifying proteins (RAMPs) in human cranial arteries. *Neurosci Lett* 1998;258:41–44.

72. Saxena PR, Ferrari MA. 5-HT$_1$-like receptor agonists and the pathophysiology of migraine. *Trends Pharmacol Sci* 1989;10:200.

73. Schumacher GA, Wolff HG. Experimental studies on headache. *Arch Neurol Psychiatry* 1941;45:199–214.

74. Skärby T, Andersson KE. Contraction-mediating α-adrenoceptors in isolated human omental, temporal and pial arteries. *J Auton Pharmacol* 1984;4:219–229

75. Skärby T, Tfelt-Hansen P, Gjerris F, Edvinsson L, Olesen J. Characterization of 5-hydroxytryptamine receptors in human temporal arteries: comparison between migraine sufferers and non-sufferers. *Ann Neurol* 1982;12:272–277.

76. Suzuki N, Hardebo JE, Owman C. Origins and pathways of choline acetyltransferaase-positive parasympathetic nerve fibres to cerebral vessels in rat. *J Cereb Blood Flow Metab* 1990;10:399–408.

77. Tfelt-Hansen P, Jansen I, Edvinsson L. Methylergometrine antagonizes 5HT in the temporal artery. *Eur J Clin Pharmacol* 1987;33:77–79.

78. Thompson JA, Wei EP, Kontos HA. Inhibition by ketanserin of serotonin induced cerebral arteriolar constriction. *Stroke* 1984;15:1021–1024.

79. Tindall GT, Greenfield JC. The effects of intra-arterial histamine on blood flow in the internal and external carotid artery in man. *Stroke* 1973;4:46–49.

80. Tomimoto H, Nishimura M, Suenaga T, et al. Distribution of nitric oxide synthase in the human cerebral blood vessels and brain tissues. *J Cereb Blood Flow Metab* 1994;14:930–938.

81. Uddman R, Edvinsson L, Ekman R, McCulloch J, Kingman TA. Innervation of the feline cerebral vasculature by nerve fibres containing gene-related peptide: trigeminal origin and co-existence with substance P. *Neurosci Lett* 1985;62:131–136.

82. Uddman R, Goadsby PJ, Jansen I, Edvinsson L. PACAP, a VIP-like peptide, immunohistochemical localization and effect upon cat pial arteries and cerebral blood flow. *J Cereb Blood Flow Metab* 1993;13:291–297.

83. Uddman R, Goadsby PJ, Jansen I, Edvinsson L. Helospectin-like peptides, immunohistochemical localization and effects on cat pial arteries and cerebral blood flow. *J Cereb Blood Flow Metab* 1999;19:61–67.

84. Verhofstad AAJ, Steinbusch HWM, Penke B, Varga J, Joosten HWJ. Serotonin-immunoreactive cells in the superior cervical ganglion of the rat: evidence for the existence of separate serotonin- and catecholamine-containing small ganglionic cells. *Brain Res* 1981;212:39–49.

85. Wahlestedt C, Edvinsson L, Ekblad E, Håkanson R. Neuropeptide Y potentiates noradrenaline-evoked vasocontriction; mode of action. *J Pharmacol Exp Ther* 1986;234:735–741.

86. Weinshank RL, Zgombick JM, Macchi MJ, Branchek TA, Hartig PR. Human serotonin 1D receptor is encoded by a subfamily of two distinct genes: 5HT$_{1D}$ alpha and 5-HT$_{1D}$ beta. *Proc Natl Acad Sci U S A* 1992;89:3630–3634.

87. Wolff HG. *Headache and other head pain.* Oxford, England: Oxford Univerity Press, 1972.

The Headaches, Second Edition,
edited by J. Olesen, P. Tfelt-Hansen, and K.M.A. Welch.
Lippincott Williams & Wilkins, Philadelphia © 2000.

Basic Science Aspects of the Headaches

CHAPTER 12

Peripheral Activation and Sensitization of Nociceptors

Andrew M. Strassman, Karl Messlinger, and Rami Burstein

PHYSIOLOGY OF PERIPHERAL NOCICEPTORS

Skin, as well as other somatic and visceral tissues, are innervated by a class of small-diameter (Aδ and C) sensory fibers that respond preferentially to intense, potentially damaging stimuli. In the skin, such nociceptors normally exhibit no discharge in the absence of stimulation or injury and have relatively high response thresholds to externally applied mechanical and thermal stimuli (34,41). These characteristics distinguish them from cutaneous low-threshold mechanoreceptive and thermoreceptive primary afferent fibers.

In addition, cutaneous nociceptors are sensitive to endogenous substances such as bradykinin that are produced at sites of tissue injury or inflammation. Such inflammatory mediators not only can evoke discharge in nociceptors, but also can produce sensitization, expressed as a decreased response threshold to mechanical or thermal stimuli, and an increased response to normally suprathreshold stimuli. Sensitization is also often accompanied by the development of ongoing discharge in the absence of externally applied stimuli. Sensitization of peripheral nociceptors is thought to be partly responsible

for the phenomenon of primary hyperalgesia (30,40). Primary hyperalgesia refers to the lowered pain threshold and increased pain to suprathreshold stimuli that develops at a site of injury. (As described in Chapter 15, the secondary hyperalgesia that develops in an area of undamaged tissue surrounding an injury is thought to be mediated by alterations in the properties of central neurons.)

Cutaneous nociceptors have been classified based on their responsiveness to mechanical, thermal, and chemical stimuli (34,41). Mechano-heat nociceptors respond to both noxious mechanical and heat stimuli, with thermal response thresholds that are typically somewhat lower than the usual pain threshold of approximately 45°C. Many of these fibers, which typically conduct in the C and low Aδ range, are also responsive to inflammatory chemicals, and are then called polymodal nociceptors. A second class, called high-threshold mechanoreceptors, display a similar sensitivity to noxious mechanical stimuli but are either insensitive or much less sensitive to heat, with response thresholds that are higher than 50°C prior to sensitization. These fibers are mostly Aδ and usually lack chemosensitivity, based on studies in the rat (31,58), although studies in primates have actually found greater chemosensitivity in these fibers (18,27). Both classes include fibers that respond to noxious cold (6,23,47,57). Fibers that lack mechanosensitivity but respond to noxious heat also have been described (4,31). In addition, some fibers have been found that are initially unresponsive to mechanical stimuli but acquire mechanosensitivity following exposure to inflammatory mediators (18). Such fibers have been described in a variety of somatic and visceral tissues and are thought to be important contributors to inflammatory pain and hyperalgesia (39).

A. Strassman: Department of Anesthesia, Harvard Medical School, and Department of Anesthesia and Critical Care, Beth Israel Deaconess Medical Center, Boston, Massachusetts 02215.

K. Messlinger: Department of Physiology and Experimental Pathophysiology, University of Erlangen-Nürnberg, D-91054 Erlangen, Germany.

R. Burstein: Department of Neurobiology, Harvard Medical School, Department of Anesthesia and Critical Care, Beth Israel Deaconess Medical Center, and Harvard Institutes of Medicine, Boston, Massachusetts 02115.

Visceral tissues receive a sensory innervation from small-diameter (Aδ and C) fibers that share with cutaneous nociceptors a number of anatomic and physiologic properties, including a sensitivity to a wide spectrum of inflammatory mediators (12). However, classification of visceral afferents as nociceptors is complicated by the fact that the criteria used for defining cutaneous nociceptors are not directly applicable to visceral afferents (12). This is true partly because of the fundamentally different roles served by these afferents and the corresponding differences in the nature of the adequate stimuli for visceral and cutaneous pain. For example, direct mechanical trauma such as from cutting, which evokes pain and activates nociceptors in skin, is generally not painful in hollow viscera, although distension can be extremely painful. Conversely, some visceral afferents display a sensitivity to relatively small increases in temperature that would be innocuous in the skin but are potentially harmful to internal organs (1,8). In addition, there is generally far less information available on pain thresholds for visceral tissues than there is for skin.

More important, the existence of a distinct class of visceral afferents that are uniquely responsible for nociceptive function is open to question. Although there exist visceral afferents with high response thresholds, it has been argued that they represent one end of a single population of afferents with response thresholds distributed throughout the physiologic and supraphysiologic range (13,38). Some visceral afferents exhibit a wide dynamic range type of response, in that they respond with increasing discharge frequency to increases in stimulus intensity from the innocuous to the noxious range. This contrasts with cutaneous innervation, in which no wide dynamic range neurons are present peripherally; instead, innocuous and noxious stimuli are detected by separate populations of afferents. Examination of the stimulus-response functions for visceral afferents in a number of tissues indicates that progressive increases in stimulus intensity from the innocuous to the noxious range evoke a progressive increase in the discharge of individual afferents along with the recruitment of increasing numbers of afferents with progressively higher thresholds (38). Such data suggest that visceral nociception may be subserved in part by summation of inputs from afferents with a wide range of response thresholds, rather than (or in addition to) activity in a single population of specific nociceptors.

Until recently, relatively little was known about the transduction mechanisms by which nociceptors become activated in response to noxious stimuli. The fact that mechanical and thermal sensitivity can be modulated independently in individual nociceptors is evidence for the existence of separate, possibly multiple, transduction mechanisms (5,48). Recently, the receptor for capsaicin, the active ingredient in chili peppers, was cloned and identified as a nonselective cation channel (11,65). The cloned receptor is expressed selectively in a population of small-diameter dorsal root ganglion cells, consistent with the selective action of capsaicin *in vivo* on a subpopulation of small-diameter primary afferent nociceptors. The capsaicin receptor is activated by noxious heat and therefore may function as a heat transducer *in vivo*. Another heat-activated nonselective cation current also has been identified in a subpopulation of dorsal root ganglion cells that can be distinguished from the capsaicin-activated current by its lower relative contribution from calcium ions, as well as its insensitivity to ruthenium red (14,51). The heat-activated current is enhanced by bradykinin through a protein kinase C–dependent mechanism, and is also enhanced by prostaglandin E_2 (PGE$_2$). There thus appear to exist multiple transduction pathways for noxious heat. The basis for mechanotransduction in nociceptors remains largely unknown.

INFLAMMATORY MEDIATORS

Sensitivity to inflammatory mediators is common to small-diameter afferents in both somatic and visceral tissues, and is fundamental to their function in signaling the state of the tissue and evoking protective responses. As mentioned above, such agents may both evoke discharge and enhance the neurons' sensitivity to other stimuli. These processes of activation and sensitization may be evoked independently (54,58,60) and are mediated by distinct cellular mechanisms.

The excitatory and sensitizing effects of inflammatory mediators can be mediated either by a direct action on the primary afferent terminals or by an indirect action through the release of other agents from either the neuron itself or from other non-neural tissue elements. For example, bradykinin, which is cleaved from circulating precursor proteins by activated kallikreins at sites of tissue injury, excites peripheral nociceptors by a direct action and also sensitizes them to mechanical and thermal stimuli (20,32). Bradykinin also appears to produce sensitization to heat through a direct action (14). In contrast, PGE$_2$ and other arachidonic acid metabolites generally evoke little or no discharge in most cutaneous and visceral afferents, but produce sensitization to mechanical and thermal stimuli through a direct action on nociceptors (35,42,67). In articular afferents, however, prostaglandins evoke both excitation and sensitization (54,55). Bradykinin exerts its direct excitatory action in part through an increase in sodium conductance that is thought to be dependent on diacylglycerol-induced activation of protein kinase C, whereas PGE$_2$ sensitization is though to involve elevation of cyclic adenosine monophosphate (cAMP) (20,32,49).

Serotonin (5-hydroxytryptamine; 5-HT) is released by activated platelets during inflammation and produces excitation and sensitization of nociceptors, although the sensitizing effect may in some cases require the presence of other inflammatory agents (49). It is thought to activate primary afferents through a direct excitatory action at the 5-HT$_3$ receptor, which is a cation-selective ion channel (26,52). It also produces sensitization by a direct action that appears to be via 5-HT$_1$–like and 5-HT$_2$ receptors through a cAMP-dependent mechanism (26,64). However, an opposing, inhibitory action is exerted on cAMP synthesis via 5-HT$_{1A}$ and 5-HT$_{1D}$ receptors that reduces calcium current and neuropeptide release (9,26). These latter actions are thought to be involved in the antimigraine effect of 5-HT$_{1D}$ agonists such as sumatriptan (see Chapter 16).

Adenosine triphosphate (ATP) is released from cells by tissue damage and excites sensory neurons through an action at the P2X purinoreceptor, which is a nonselective cation channel (49,61). Recently a P2X$_3$ purinoreceptor subtype was identified that is selectively expressed by primary afferent C-fiber neurons (15,17,33). Adenosine is a breakdown product of ATP that produces pain and hyperalgesia through a direct cAMP-dependent action at the A$_2$ adenosine receptor (62). One of the actions of adenosine, as well of 5-HT and PGE$_2$, is to enhance the magnitude of a tetrodotoxin-resistant voltage-gated sodium current that is expressed only in C fibers (2,24,53).

Inflammatory mediators can exhibit synergistic effects when applied in combination. For example, bradykinin-evoked discharge of small-diameter primary afferents is greatly enhanced by 5-HT (25,31). Histamine, which is released by degranulating mast cells, produces only itch sensations when applied alone to skin, but produces pain following a conditioning application of bradykinin (28). This change is paralleled by an increase in the histamine response of C-fiber neurons and in the proportion of histamine-responsive neurons. Acidic pH, which is present in inflamed tissues, not only produces activation and sensitization of C fibers, but also enhances the effects of other inflammatory mediators (59). Concurrent application of an acidic buffer solution (pH 6.1) increased both the amplitude and the duration of the C-fiber response to an inflammatory soup containing bradykinin, 5-HT, histamine, and PGE$_2$. In addition, some neurons that did not respond to either solution alone responded to the combination of the two. The excitatory actions of acidic pH appear to be mediated in part through an H$^+$-gated non-selective cation channel that is expressed in small-diameter neuropeptide-containing sensory neurons (16, 45,66). Acidic pH also potentiates current flow through the capsaicin receptor (11,65).

PHYSIOLOGY OF DURAL AFFERENTS

Anatomic studies in humans and animals have shown that the trigeminal nerve gives rise to a sensory innervation of the intracranial meninges (3,37,44,46). This intracranial trigeminal sensory innervation is most dense around the major blood vessels of the dura and pia,

including the proximal portions of the circle of Willis, the meningeal arteries, and the dural venous sinuses. Stimulation of these meningeal vascular sites in awake neurosurgical patients can evoke painful sensations that are typically referred to the temporal or orbital region (50). As with many visceral tissues, pain was the only sensation that could be evoked by meningeal stimulation, regardless of whether the stimulus was electrical, mechanical, or thermal. These observations indicated that meningeal sensory innervation can evoke painful sensations when stimulated experimentally, and formed the basis for the idea that activation of these sensory fibers may be involved in some types of clinically occurring headaches, possibly including migraine.

Classically it was thought that activation of perivascular meningeal sensory fibers might occur in migraine as a result of stretching produced by arterial vasodilation (36,68). However, most recent studies using modern measurement techniques have either failed to find vasodilation occurring during migraine attacks or have detected amounts that were considered insufficient to account for the headache because greater vasodilation can occur in the absence of headache (22,43,63). One possibility that was raised in the original formulation of the vasodilation theory (68) is that even moderate vasodilation might cause pain if it were accompanied by sensitization of the perivascular sensory fibers. The question then arises of whether moderate vasodilation could itself produce such sensitization, or whether other processes might be involved.

Two such processes that have been the focus of current research are cortical spreading depression (see Chapter 22) and meningeal neurogenic inflammation (see Chapter 17). Cortical spreading depression consists of a slowly propagating depression of neural activity that has been proposed as the basis for the migraine aura. It is accompanied by elevated cortical levels of excitatory agents such as potassium and glutamate that might be capable of activating meningeal sensory fibers. One of the potential consequences of sensory fiber activation is the peripheral release of neuropeptides, which can themselves produce inflammatory effects in the innervated tissue and can induce release of inflammatory mediators from other tissue elements such as mast cells, whose released contents may include histamine and cytokines. Signs of neurogenic inflammation, including vasodilation and plasma extravasation, can be induced in the dura by electrical stimulation of the trigeminal ganglion or the dura itself (29,43). Substance P acting at the neurokinin-1 receptor appears to be responsible for extravasation, whereas calcitonin gene–related peptide mediates the vasodilation (10,29,56). Ebersberger et al. (21) have further shown that trigeminal ganglion stimulation evokes dural release of the sensitizing agent PGE$_2$.

Most of the current theories of migraine headache, as well as a number of other headaches, postulate an activation or sensitization of intracranial sensory fibers by some form of mechanical or chemical stimuli. In order to identify the types of stimuli that can activate meningeal sensory fibers, a number of recent studies have focused on the response properties of primary afferent neurons that innervate the intracranial dura (8,19,60). These studies have recorded discharge of dural afferents in response to electrical, mechanical, thermal, and chemical forms of dural stimulation. Dostrovsky et al. (19) initially identified dural afferent neurons in the trigeminal ganglion of the rat that responded to electrical stimulation of the superior sagittal sinus or the middle meningeal artery at

Aδ- and C-fiber latencies. Some of the cells could be activated by traction applied to the sagittal sinus, and one was also activated by radiant heat. Strassman et al. (60) further examined rat dural afferents for chemosensitivity and sensitization to mechanical stimuli. Neurons were recorded in the trigeminal ganglion that responded to electrical stimulation of the transverse sinus (Fig. 1). Most of the neurons had mechanosensitive receptive fields on the transverse sinus and adjacent dura from which they could be activated by punctate probing or stoking. The neurons also could be activated by chemical

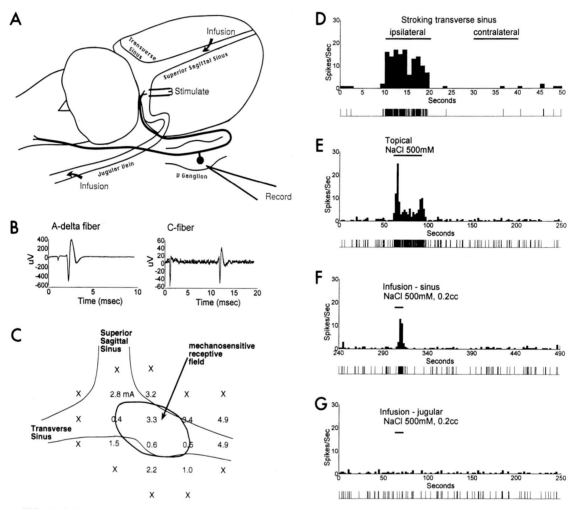

FIG. 1. **A:** Experimental setup for studying the activity of sensory neurons that innervate the dural venous sinuses in anesthetized rats. A primary afferent neuron is shown with its cell body in the trigeminal ganglion. Its central axonal branch exits the ganglion caudally to project to the brain stem, and its peripheral axonal branch exits the ganglion rostrally but then turns back and courses upward to innervate the dural wall of the ipsilateral transverse sinus. **B:** Responses of two trigeminal ganglion cells to single-shock stimulation of the dura overlying the ipsilateral transverse sinus. **C:** Map of the response thresholds (mA) of a trigeminal ganglion cell at dural stimulation sites on and around the ipsilateral transverse sinus. **D:** Response to stroking the dura within the mechanosensitive field outlined in (C). **E–G:** Responses of the same cell to chemical stimulation delivered either by topical application to the dural surface (E) or by infusion into the superior sagittal sinus (F), and absence of response to control infusion delivered into the jugular vein (G). Since the direction of blood flow is from the dural sinuses through the jugular vein to the heart (A), the absence of a response to the jugular infusion provides evidence that the response to sinus infusion was from a site of action between the sinus and the jugular vein. Reprinted from Strassman et al. (60).

stimuli such as hypertonic sodium chloride, applied either topically to the surface of the dura or by intravascular infusion into the sinus. The response to sinus infusion suggests that the neurons may be capable of responding to endogenous substances within the dural sinuses, and thus may be affected by chemical alterations in the cerebral cortex because the sinuses collect venous drainage from the cortex.

In addition to sodium chloride, the neurons also could be activated by dural application of a number of other algesic agents, including potassium chloride, capsaicin, pH-neutral buffer solutions of low or high osmolarity, and an acidic mixture of inflammatory mediators. Besides activating the neurons, chemical stimuli also produced a sensitization to mechanical stimuli, such that the neuron's mechanical response threshold was lowered. Sensitization to mechanical stimuli was observed both in neurons that discharged in response to the sensitizing chemical agent as well as in neurons that did not, indicating that sensitization and activation are at least partially independent processes. Such sensitization of meningeal afferents to mechanical stimuli could be partly responsible for certain types of headache symptoms. For example, in migraine, as well as in meningitis, the pain is increased by normally innocuous activities such as coughing or sudden head movement, symptoms that have been regarded as an indication of exaggerated sensitivity to intracranial mechanical stimuli (7,68). Such sensitization also might contribute to the throbbing pain of migraine, if neuronal response thresholds were lowered sufficiently for the neurons to respond to the normally innocuous elevation in intracranial pressure that accompanies the arterial pulse.

A similar population of dural afferents with mechanosensitive receptive fields on or adjacent to the anterior part of the superior sagittal sinus was recorded by Bove and Moskowitz (8) from the nasociliary nerve of the guinea pig. All of the neurons also could be activated by dural application of one or more of a number of algesic or inflammatory agents. A substantial proportion of the neurons responded to warming or cooling stimuli, and many exhibited thermal response thresholds within the physiologic range (Fig. 2). Many of these neurons, as well as those studied by Strassman et al. (60), responded to intensities of mechanical stimuli that were considerably lower than those required to activate nociceptors or evoke pain when applied to the skin. Although the mechanical and thermal response thresholds were generally lower than those of cutaneous nociceptors, their properties were considered appropriate for meningeal nociceptors because they responded preferentially to intensities of mechanical and thermal stimuli that would be noxious for intracranial tissues, and were also activated by excitatory chemicals that are thought to be specific for nociceptors. Based on their response properties, it was argued that these afferents might be activated under pathologic conditions such as increased intracranial pressure or meningitis.

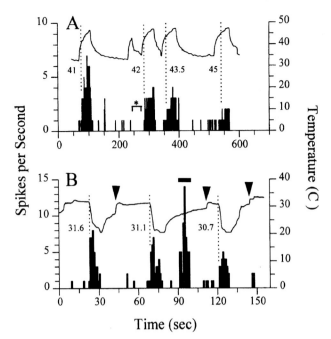

FIG. 2. Responses of dural afferent neurons to thermal stimulation of the dura. **A:** Four consecutive trials of radiant heat. **B:** Three trials of 0°C cold buffer. Arrowheads indicate application of warm buffer. Bar indicates mechanical stimulation. Reprinted from Bove and Moskowitz (8).

Neurophysiologic studies of dural afferent neurons support the idea that some of these neurons serve a nociceptive function and that they may become activated during some types of clinically occurring headaches. Further characterization of the physiologic conditions that are capable of activating neurons, as well as the dural afferent pharmacologic agents that are capable of modulating their activity, may lead to better understanding of headache pathogenesis and treatment.

REFERENCES

1. Adelson DW, Wei JY, Kruger L. Warm-sensitive afferent splanchnic C-fiber units *in vitro*. *J Neurophysiol* 1997;77:2989–3002.
2. Akopian AN, Sivilotti L, Wood JN. A tetrodotoxin-resistant voltage-gated sodium channel expressed by sensory neurons. *Nature* 1996; 379:257–262.
3. Andres KH, von During M, Muszynski K, Schmidt RF. Nerve fibres and their terminals of the dura mater encephali of the rat. *Anat Embryol* 1987;175:289–301.
4. Beck PW, Handwerker HO, Zimmermann M. Nervous outflow from the cat's foot during noxious radiant heat stimulation. *Brain Res* 1974; 67:373–386.
5. Belmonte C, Gallar J, Pozo MA, Rebollo I. Excitation by irritant chemical substances of sensory afferent units in the cat's cornea. *J Physiol* 1991;437:709–725.
6. Bessou P, Perl ER. Response of cutaneous sensory units with unmyelinated fibers to noxious stimuli. *J Neurophysiol* 1969;32:1025–1043.
7. Blau JN, Dexter SL. The site of pain origin during migraine attacks. *Cephalalgia* 1981;1:143–147.
8. Bove GM, Moskowitz MA. Primary afferent neurons innervating guinea pig dura. *J Neurophysiol* 1997;77:299–308.
9. Cardenas CG, DelMar LP, Scroggs RS. Two parallel signaling pathways couple 5HT(1A) receptors to N- and L-type calcium channels in C-like rat dorsal root ganglion cells. *J Neurophysiol* 1997;77:3284–3296.

10. Carmody J, Pawlak M, Messlinger K. Lack of a role for substance P in the control of dural arterial flow. *Exp Brain Res* 1996;111:424–428.

11. Caterina MJ, Schumacher MA, Tominaga M, Rosen TA, Levine JD, Julius D. The capsaicin receptor: a heat-activated ion channel in the pain pathway. *Nature* 1997;389:816–824.

12. Cervero F. Sensory innervation of the viscera: peripheral basis of visceral pain. *Physiol Rev* 1994;74:95–138.

13. Cervero F, Janig W. Visceral nociceptors: a new world order? *Trends Neurosci* 1992;15:374–378.

14. Cesare P, McNaughton P. A novel heat-activated current in nociceptive neurons and its sensitization by bradykinin. *Proc Natl Acad Sci U S A* 1996;93:15435–15439.

15. Chen CC, Akopian AN, Sivilotti L, Colquhoun D, Burnstock G, Wood JN. A P2X purinoceptor expressed by a subset of sensory neurons. *Nature* 1995;377:428–431.

16. Chen CC, England S, Akopian AN, Wood JN. A sensory neuron-specific, proton-gated ion channel. *Proc Natl Acad Sci U S A* 1998;95:10240–10245.

17. Cook SP, Vulchanova L, Hargreaves KM, Elde R, McCleskey EW. Distinct ATP receptors on pain-sensing and stretch-sensing neurons. *Nature* 1997;387:505–508.

18. Davis KD, Meyer RA, Campbell JN. Chemosensitivity and sensitization of nociceptive afferents that innervate the hairy skin of monkey. *J Neurophysiol* 1993;69:1071–1081.

19. Dostrovsky JO, Davis KD, Kawakita K. Central mechanisms of vascular headaches. *Can J Physiol Pharmacol* 1991;69:652–658.

20. Dray A. Kinins and their receptors in hyperalgesia. *Can J Physiol Pharmacol* 1997;75:704–712.

21. Ebersberger A, Averbeck B, Messlinger K, Reeh PW. Release of substance P, calcitonin gene-related peptide and prostaglandin E_2 from rat dura mater encephali following electrical and chemical stimulation, *in vitro*. *Neuroscience* 1999;89:901–907.

22. Friberg L, Olesen J, Iversen HK, Sperling B. Migraine pain associated with middle cerebral artery dilatation: reversal by sumatriptan. *Lancet* 1991;338:13–17.

23. Georgopoulos AP. Functional properties of primary afferent units probably related to pain mechanisms in primate glabrous skin. *J Neurophysiol* 1976;39:71–83.

24. Gold MS, Reichling DB, Shuster MJ, Levine JD. Hyperalgesic agents increase a tetrodotoxin-resistant Na^+ current in nociceptors. *Proc Natl Acad Sci U S A* 1996;93:1108–1112.

25. Handwerker HO, Reeh PW, Steen KH. Effects of 5HT on nociceptors. In: Besson JM, ed. *Serotonin and pain.* New York: Elsevier, 1990:1–15.

26. Hen R. Of mice and flies: commonalities among 5-HT receptors. *Trends Pharmacol Sci* 1992;13:160–165.

27. Khan AA, Raja SN, Manning DC, Campbell JN, Meyer RA. The effects of bradykinin and sequence-related analogs on the response properties of cutaneous nociceptors in monkeys. *Somatosens Motor Res* 1992;9:97–106.

28. Koppert W, Reeh PW, Handwerker HO. Conditioning of histamine by bradykinin alters responses of rat nociceptor and human itch sensation. *Neurosci Lett* 1993;152:117–120.

29. Kurosawa M, Messlinger K, Pawlak M, Schmidt RF. Increase of meningeal blood flow after electrical stimulation of rat dura mater encephali: mediation by calcitonin gene-related peptide. *Br J Pharmacol* 1995;114:1397–1402.

30. LaMotte RH, Thalhammer JG, Torebjork HE, Robinson CJ. Peripheral neural mechanisms of cutaneous hyperalgesia following mild injury by heat. *J Neurosci* 1982;2:765–781.

31. Lang E, Novak A, Reeh PW, Handwerker HO. Chemosensitivity of fine afferents from rat skin *in vitro*. *J Neurophysiol* 1990;63:887–901.

32. Levine JD, Taiwo YO. Inflammatory pain. In: Wall PD, Melzack R, eds. *Textbook of pain.* New York: Churchill Livingstone, 1994:45–56.

33. Lewis C, Neidhart S, Holy C, North RA, Buell G, Surprenant A. Coexpression of P2X2 and P2X3 receptor subunits can account for ATP-gated currents in sensory neurons. *Nature* 1995;377:432–435.

34. Light AR. *The initial processing of pain and its descending control: spinal and trigeminal systems.* New York: Karger, 1992.

35. Martin HA, Basbaum AI, Kwait GC, Goetzl EJ, Levine JD. Leukotriene and prostaglandin sensitization of cutaneous high threshold C- and A-delta mechanonociceptors in the hairy skin of rat hindlimb. *Neuroscience* 1987;22:651–659.

36. Martin JB. Headache. In: Wilson JD, Braunwald E, Isselbacher KJ, et al., eds. *Harrison's principles of internal medicine.* New York: McGraw-Hill, 1991:108–115.

37. Mayberg MR, Zervas NT, Moskowitz MA. Trigeminal projections to supratentorial pial and dural blood vessels in cats demonstrated by horseradish peroxidase histochemistry. *J Comp Neurol* 1984;223:46–56.

38. McMahon, SB. Mechanisms of cutaneous, deep and visceral pain. In: Wall PD, Melzack R, eds. *Textbook of pain.* New York: Churchill Livingstone, 1994:129–152.

39. McMahon SB, Koltzenburg M. Novel classes of nociceptors: beyond Sherrington. *Trends Neurosci* 1990;13:199–201.

40. Meyer RA, Campbell JN. Myelinated nociceptive afferents account for the hyperalgesia that follows a burn to the hand. *Science* 1981;213:1527–1529.

41. Meyer RA, Campbell JN, Raja SN. Peripheral neural mechanisms of nociception. In: Wall PD, Melzack R, eds. *Textbook of pain.* New York: Churchill Livingstone, 1994:13–44.

42. Mizumura K, Minagawa M, Tsujii Y, Kumazawa T. Prostaglandin E2-induced sensitization of the heat response of canine visceral polymodal receptors *in vitro*. *Neurosci Lett* 1993;161:117–119.

43. Moskowitz MA, Macfarlane R. Neurovascular and molecular mechanisms in migraine headaches. *Cerebrovasc Brain Metab Rev* 1993;5:159–177.

44. O'Connor TP, van der Kooy D. Pattern of intracranial and extracranial projections of trigeminal ganglion cells. *J Neurosci* 1986;6:2200–2207.

45. Olson TH, Riedl MS, Vulchanova L, OrtizGonzalez XR, Elde R. An acid sensing ion channel (ASIC) localizes to small primary afferent neurons in rats. *Neuroreport* 1998;9:1109–1113.

46. Penfield W, McNaughton M. Dural headache and innervation of the dura mater. *Arch Neurol Psychiatry* 1940;44:43–75.

47. Perl ER. Myelinated afferent fibres innervating the primate skin and their response to noxious stimuli. *J Physiol* 1968;197:593–615.

48. Pozo MA, Gallego R, Gallar J, Belmonte C. Blockade by calcium antagonists of chemical excitation and sensitization of polymodal nociceptors in the cat's cornea. *J Physiol* 1992;450:179–189.

49. Rang HP, Bevan S, Dray A. Nociceptive peripheral neurons: cellular properties. In: Wall PD, Melzack R, eds. *Textbook of pain.* New York: Churchill Livingstone, 1994:57–78.

50. Ray BS, Wolff HG. Experimental studies on headache: pain-sensitive structures of the head and their significance in headache. *Arch Surg* 1940;41:813–856.

51. Reichling DB, Levine JD. Heat transduction in rat sensory neurons by calcium-dependent activation of a cation channel. *Proc Natl Acad Sci U S A* 1997;94:7006–7011.

52. Robertson B, Bevan S. Properties of 5-hydroxytryptamine3 receptor-gated currents in adult rat dorsal root ganglion neurones. *Br J Pharmacol* 1991;102:272–276.

53. Sangameswaran L, Delgado SG, Fish LM, et al. Structure and function of a novel voltage-gated, tetrodotoxin-resistant sodium channel specific to sensory neurons. *J Biol Chem* 1996;271:5953–5956.

54. Schaible HG, Schmidt RF. Excitation and sensitization of fine articular afferents from cat's knee joint by prostaglandin E_2. *J Physiol* 1988;403:91–104.

55. Schepelmann K, Messlinger K, Schaible HG, Schmidt RF. Inflammatory mediators and nociception in the joint: excitation and sensitization of slowly conducting afferent fibers of cat's knee by prostaglandin I_2. *Neuroscience* 1992;50:237–247.

56. Shepheard SL, Williamson DJ, Hill RG, Hargreaves RJ. The non-peptide neurokinin1 receptor antagonist, RP 67580, blocks neurogenic plasma extravasation in the dura mater of rats. *Br J Pharmacol* 1993;108:11–12.

57. Simone DA, Kajander KC. Responses of cutaneous A-fiber nociceptors to noxious cold. *J Neurophysiol* 1997;77:2049–2060.

58. Steen KH, Reeh PW, Anton F, Handwerker HO. Protons selectively induce lasting excitation and sensitization to mechanical stimulation of nociceptors in rat skin, *in vitro*. *J Neurosci* 1992;12:86–95.

59. Steen KH, Steen AE, Reeh PW. A dominant role of acid pH in inflammatory excitation and sensitization of nociceptors in rat skin, *in vitro*. *J Neurosci* 1995;15:3982–3989.

60. Strassman AM, Raymond SA, Burstein R. Sensitization of meningeal sensory neurons and the origin of headaches. *Nature* 1996;384:560–564.

61. Surprenant A, Buell G, North RA. P2X receptors bring new structure to ligand-gated ion channels. *Trends Neurosci* 1995;18:224–229.

62. Taiwo YO, Levine JD. Direct cutaneous hyperalgesia induced by adenosine. *Neuroscience* 1990;38:757–762.

63. Thomsen LL, Iversen HK, Olesen J. Cerebral blood flow velocities are reduced during attacks of unilateral migraine without aura. *Cephalalgia* 1995;15:109–116.

64. Todorovic S, Anderson EG. 5-HT$_2$ and 5-HT$_3$ receptors mediate two distinct depolarizing responses in rat dorsal root ganglion neurons. *Brain Res* 1990;511:71–79.

65. Tominaga M, Caterina MJ, Malmberg AB et al. The cloned capsaicin receptor integrates multiple pain-producing stimuli. *Neuron* 1998;21: 531–543.

66. Waldmann R, Champigny G, Bassilana F, Heurteaux C, Lazdunski M. A proton-gated cation channel involved in acid-sensing. *Nature* 1997; 386:173–177.

67. White DM, Basbaum AI, Goetzl EJ, Levine JD. The 15-lipoxygenase product, 8R,15S-diHETE, stereospecifically sensitizes C-fiber mechanoheat nociceptors in hairy skin of rat. *J Neurophysiol* 1990;63: 966–970.

68. Wolff HG. *Headache and other head pain.* New York: Oxford University Press, 1963.

The Headaches, Second Edition,
edited by J. Olesen, P. Tfelt-Hansen, and K.M.A. Welch.
Lippincott Williams & Wilkins, Philadelphia © 2000.

Basic Science Aspects of the Headaches

CHAPTER 13

Central Transmission of Cephalic Pain

Jonathan O. Dostrovsky and Andrew M. Strassman

THE TRIGEMINAL COMPLEX

The trigeminal brain stem nuclear complex (TBNC) is the major central termination site of trigeminal primary afferent fibers. It is therefore the major site of entry into the central nervous system of sensory signals underlying orofacial and cranial sensation. Although all subdivisions of the trigeminal complex receive projections from the trigeminal nerve, it is the caudalmost part of the trigeminal complex, the subnucleus caudalis (SNC), that traditionally has been considered to be most critical in the mediation of painful sensations (the anatomic organization and nuclear subdivisions of the TBNC are described in Chapter 10). This inference was initially made from early clinical observations of selective loss of pain and temperature sensation in the ipsilateral trigeminal territory following neurologic lesions that were confined to the caudalmost part of the TBNC (104) or following surgical deafferentation of this region by trigeminal tractotomy near the level of the obex (89). Further evidence for the importance of caudalis in nociception has come from animal studies showing that the caudalis is a major termination site for small-diameter trigeminal primary afferent fibers (37,72), that it contains many neurons with nociceptive response properties, including antidromically identified trigeminothalamic neurons (56,84), and that it is anatomically similar to the spinal dorsal horn (45). However, it has become increasingly clear from recent neurophysiologic studies that rostral parts of the trigeminal complex are also critically involved in nociception, particularly for inputs from the intraoral and perioral regions.

RESPONSE PROPERTIES OF SNC NEURONS

The SNC, often referred to as the medullary dorsal horn (45), is analogous to the spinal dorsal horn in both its anatomic and physiologic organization, and is a direct continuation of the dorsal horn of the upper cervical spinal cord. The majority of neurons that have been recorded in SNC exhibit orofacial receptive fields from which they can be activated by appropriate mechanical or thermal stimulation. The receptive fields of SNC neurons are organized in a somatotopic representation of the trigeminal dermatome that is continuous with the representation of the posterior head and neck region in the upper cervical dorsal horn. The somatotopic organization in the SNC follows that of the primary afferent projections (see Chapter 10), whereby the rostrocaudal axis of the face is represented from rostral to caudal in the SNC, and the dorsoventral axis of the face is represented from ventral to dorsal (or ventromedial to dorsolateral, depending on the species and the rostrocaudal level in the nucleus) (37,72).

As in the spinal dorsal horn, neurons in the SNC can be categorized as low-threshold mechanoreceptive (LTM), thermoreceptive, and nociceptive, according to their preferred modality of stimulation within their cutaneous or mucosal receptive field (55,56,80,84). The nociceptive neurons are further classified as nociceptive-specific (NS) or wide-dynamic-range (WDR), based on their responses to graded intensities of mechanical stimulation. NS neurons respond solely to noxious stimulus intensities, whereas WDR neurons respond with increas-

J. O. Dostrovsky: Department of Physiology, Program in Neurosciences, University of Toronto, Toronto, Ontario M5S 1A8, Canada.

A. M. Strassman: Department of Anesthesia, Harvard Medical School, and Department of Anesthesia and Critical Care, Beth Israel Deaconess Medical Center, Boston, Massachusetts 02215.

ing discharge frequency to increases in mechanical stimulus intensity from the innocuous (brushing) to the noxious (pinch) range (56,74,84,106). Both WDR and NS neurons receive primary afferent input from slowly conducting fibers (Aδ alone or Aδ plus C), whereas WDR neurons also receive input from Aβ fibers, accounting for their tactile sensitivity. The majority of WDR and NS neurons also respond to noxious heat applied to their cutaneous receptive field. A somewhat smaller proportion also respond to noxious cold stimuli (74). Many WDR neurons can respond differentially to changes in thermal stimulus intensity within the noxious range, and their stimulus-response functions match well with those found in human psychophysical studies of noxious thermal discrimination.

Neurons in the SNC show a differential laminar distribution according to response class similar to that found in the spinal dorsal horn, with thermoreceptive neurons in the superficial laminae (I–II), low-threshold mechanoreceptive neurons in the deep laminae (III–IV and V), NS neurons in laminae I–II and V, and WDR neurons primarily in lamina V (3,19,56,58,84,106). Antidromically identified trigeminothalamic neurons are found mostly in laminae I–II and V and include both nociceptive (WDR and NS) and thermoreceptive neurons (in lamina I only), but relatively few LTM neurons. LTM neuron input to the thalamus arises mainly from more rostral parts of the trigeminal complex (37), consistent with the relatively minor effect of SNC lesions on tactile sensation (89,104).

Nociceptive neurons in the SNC commonly receive inputs from noncutaneous tissues as well, including muscle (masseter and temporalis), temporomandibular joint, intranasal mucosa, cornea, tooth pulp, and blood vessels of the intracranial dura (3,11,35,81,87). The convergence of afferent input from separate superficial and deep peripheral tissues is also seen in nociceptive neurons in the spinal cord (10,102), and has been postulated as the basis for the clinical phenomenon of referred pain of deep or visceral origin. As has been found in the spinal cord, SNC neurons that receive inputs from deep tissues generally exhibit a cutaneous receptive field as well and are usually nociceptive in their cutaneous response properties. The large, nociceptive cutaneous receptive fields exhibited by many neurons that receive convergent inputs from deep tissues are consistent with the diffuse, poorly localized, radiating quality that often characterizes pain of deep or visceral origin.

RESPONSE PROPERTIES OF NOCICEPTIVE NEURONS IN ROSTRAL PARTS OF THE TRIGEMINAL NUCLEAR COMPLEX

Evidence for a role in nociception of rostral portions of the trigeminal nuclear complex initially came from observations that the loss of facial pain sensation produced by obex tractotomy was not complete, in most cases at least partially sparing the intraoral and perioral region (68,108). Similarly, reflex or behavioral responsiveness to noxious orofacial stimuli may persist following tractotomy or SNC lesions in animals (12,99); conversely, nociceptive responsiveness may be diminished by more rostral lesions of the trigeminal complex (12,46). Anatomic studies have documented the presence of terminations from small-diameter primary afferent fibers in the oralis (40), and intracellular labeling studies have found that small-diameter nociceptive primary afferents contribute some terminations to the caudal part of the interpolaris, in addition to their heavier projections to the SNC (50,61). Several studies have described nociceptive neurons in the interpolaris and oralis (7,23,39,57,60,85,86), including neurons that receive convergent inputs from tooth pulp, muscle, or dura (29,51).

Many of these neurons had receptive fields that included the intraoral and perioral region, and this correlates well with the neurologic and behavioral studies showing the persistence of oral nociception following SNC lesions.

RESPONSES TO CEREBROVASCULAR INPUTS

The population of SNC neurons that receives input from the intracranial dura has been of particular interest for the understanding of central mechanisms of headache (see Chapters 9 and 17). These neurons were initially identified by their response to electrical stimuli delivered to dural sites overlying the superior sagittal sinus and the middle meningeal artery in anesthetized cats (Fig. 1) (25,90) and subsequently have been described in the rat as well (14,38). Such dura-responsive neurons in almost all cases can also be activated by mechanical stimulation within a facial receptive field that is most typically in the temporal or orbital region, often including the cornea and periorbital skin, and is usually nociceptive (WDR or NS). The distribution of these nociceptive receptive fields largely overlaps the region of referred pain evoked by supratentorial dural stimulation in humans, consistent with a role for these neurons in the mediation of dural pain. The neurons also can be activated by potentially noxious forms of dural stimulation, including traction of dural blood vessels (30) and topical or subarachnoid infusion or intrasinus injection of bradykinin and other algesic or inflammatory agents (14,26,38). Dura-responsive neurons with similar response properties also have been found in the upper cervical dorsal horn and in the lateral cervical nucleus (4,64,69,70).

Immunocytochemical labeling for c-*fos* following electrical and mechanical stimulation of dural blood vessels or chemical stimulation of the subarachnoid space found *fos*-labeled neurons in laminae I and V of the dorsal horn in a widespread rostrocaudal distribution extending from upper cervical to medullary levels (66,79, 83,91). A similar area of activation was found in studies

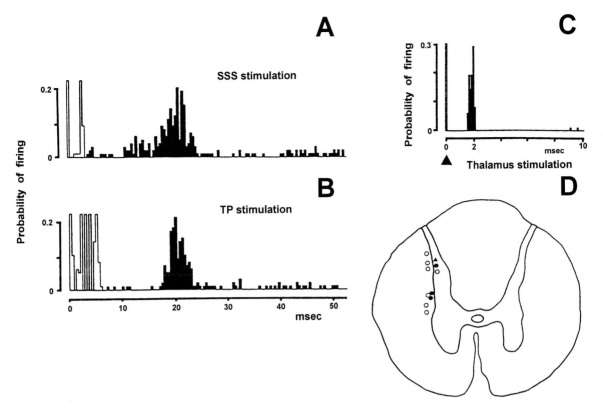

FIG. 1. Responses of a unit in the cervical spinal cord. This unit responded to **(A)** SSS, **(B)** tooth pulp (*TP*), and **(C)** thalamic stimulation. In **(D)**, the location of the unit referred to above is marked by a triangle. In the same line drawing, all the identified units responding to both SSS and TP stimulation (●) and units responding to SSS, but not TP, stimulation (○) are shown. Redrawn from Angus-Leppan et al. (4).

that measured increased regional blood flow and metabolism during electrical stimulation of the superior sagittal sinus (43). Intracellular labeling studies also have confirmed the distribution of dura-responsive neurons in the ventrolateral part of lamina V and have shown further that such neurons give rise to an extensive axonal projection system that arborizes at multiple levels of the SNC and the caudal part of the interpolaris (see Fig. 2) (92). The extensive intratrigeminal projections of dura-responsive neurons may contribute to the diffuse pattern of neuronal activation found in the c-*fos* studies. The *fos* studies also showed a separate region of activation at the border between the SNC and interpolaris, an area that also shows *fos* labeling following corneal stimulation (76,93). This region has been largely unexplored in electrophysiologic studies, but recent unit recording data have indicated that the corneal-responsive neurons in this region differ from those in more caudal parts of the SNC in their receptive field properties and their responses to morphine (77,78).

Further evidence supporting a role in headache for dura-responsive neurons in the SNC and the upper cervical dorsal horn has come from pharmacologic studies of these neurons. Neuronal activity and c-*fos* labeling in these regions induced by electrical stimulation of dural blood vessels were attenuated by systemic administration

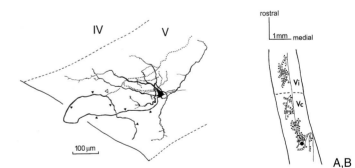

FIG. 2. Anatomic reconstruction of a neuron in lamina V of the trigeminal nucleus caudalis that responded to dural stimulation and was labeled by intracellular injection of horseradish peroxidase. The neuron gave rise to axonal projections within lamina V of the caudalis as well as the caudal part of interpolaris. **A:** Coronal reconstruction showing the soma-dendritic tree, the initial axonal trajectory (▲), and part of an axonal collateral within lamina V (△). **B:** Horizontal diagram of the axonal arborization in the caudalis (Vc) and interpolaris (Vi). The large dot marks the soma and the small dots mark the regions that contain axonal boutons. Modified from Strassman et al. (92).

of agents that are used in the treatment of migraine and other headaches, including ergot alkaloids and serotonin 1B/D receptor agonists (21,42,53,54,65,69). One study also demonstrated suppression of neuronal responses to dural stimulation by ergot compounds when applied iontophoretically through the recording micropipette, raising the possibility that the therapeutic effects of these agents may occur partly through a central site of action (69).

Dura-responsive neurons have also been recorded in the interpolaris and oralis of the cat. They had properties similar to those described in the SNC, although the percentage of non-nociceptive neurons was higher than was found for dura-responsive neurons in SNC (29). Cold block applied to the SNC reduced the responses of nociceptive interpolaris and oralis neurons to facial and dural stimulation, indicating that nociceptive inputs reach the rostral subnuclei in part via a relay in the SNC (27,86). This is further supported by the recent finding that C fiber–evoked responses of oralis neurons can be suppressed by microinjection of morphine into the SNC, but not by microinjection into the oralis (22).

NOCICEPTIVE NEURONS IN OTHER BRAIN STEM REGIONS

A number of brain stem regions outside the trigeminal complex contain neurons that can be activated by noxious facial stimulation, and thus may participate in the processing or modulation of orofacial nociception; although their responses to cerebrovascular inputs have not been examined, there is no reason to doubt that such inputs would also be effective. Because these regions lie outside the main termination zone of trigeminal primary afferents, their trigeminal inputs presumably are relayed primarily via projections from neurons within the trigeminal complex. Two of these regions whose role in nociception has been the subject of recent studies are the parabrachial nuclei and the medullary reticular formation

The parabrachial area is an important target of projections from nociceptive neurons in lamina I of the dorsal horn at both spinal and trigeminal levels (52,59,73). The lateral parts of the parabrachial area (lateral and external subnuclei) contain substantial numbers of neurons that respond to noxious intensities of mechanical or thermal (heat or cold) cutaneous stimulation with receptive fields that typically cover large portions of the body (8,9,75). Many of these neurons project to the ventromedial hypothalamus and the central nucleus of the amygdala.

The lateralmost part of the medullary reticular formation is included within the trigeminal complex as lamina V (or V/VI) of SNC and contains both nociceptive and nonnociceptive neurons with receptive fields that are generally restricted to the ipsilateral trigeminal dermatome. However, deeper parts of the medullary reticular formation, which are outside the main projection area of trigeminal primary afferents, also contain neurons that respond to noxious facial stimulation, but the receptive fields of these neurons are usually larger, often bilateral, and sometimes include the entire body (24,41,82,105). One such population of neurons with large nociceptive receptive fields that has been studied in detail is located in the subnucleus reticularis dorsalis (96–98). Neurons in this region participate in reciprocal anatomic connections with the spinal dorsal horn (2,94,95) and have been postulated to play an important role in diffuse noxious inhibitory control, a form of inhibitory modulation of nociceptive transmission (see Chapter 14). Nociceptive trigeminal neurons undoubtedly also activate other structures in the brain stem, including the periaqueductal gray, nucleus raphe magnus, reticular formation, and various brain stem autonomic nuclei. However, the physiologic properties of these neurons have not been studied in detail, and their functions in nociception have not been elucidated.

THALAMUS

The pain arising from the craniofacial region is mediated primarily if not exclusively by ascending projections that relay in the thalamus and terminate in the cortex. It appears likely that perception of pain occurs as a result of activation of cortical regions. However, in view of the extensive reciprocal connections between the cortex and thalamus, the thalamus likely also plays an essential role in processing nociceptive information and mediating pain sensations. Although some nociceptive neurons in the trigeminal brain stem complex project to the parabrachial area and other regions as mentioned above, these pathways remain poorly studied and understood, and probably do not play an important role in pain perception. These latter pathways and the projections from lamina I SNC neurons to various brain stem autonomic nuclei (17) are likely to be important in mediating some of the other, nonperceptual (e.g., autonomic) effects, elicited by nociceptive stimuli. Nevertheless, the demonstration, at least in the rat, of the existence of a nociceptive pathway that ascends to the amygdala via the parabrachial nucleus (8) bypassing the thalamus, suggests that some aspects of pain sensation could arise without relay in the thalamus.

There are two major thalamic regions that have been implicated in nociception: the lateral thalamus, particularly the ventrobasal complex (VB) and the ventroposteriorly adjacent regions, and the medial thalamus. Portions of both these regions receive projections from the spinothalamic tract (STT) and its trigeminal equivalent originating primarily in the SNC (20,48,100,101). The best studied of these regions is the ventrobasal complex (VB) which receives its major projection from the dorsal column nuclei and the trigeminal main sensory (principalis) nucleus.

LATERAL THALAMUS

The VB contains somatotopically organized neurons relaying tactile information from the face and mouth and the rest of the body to the primary somatosensory cortex. Most of the neurons in this region are non-nociceptive and respond to low threshold mechanical inputs. Neurons in the medial portion of the VB thalamus (the nucleus ventralis posteromedialis, VPM) have orofacial receptive fields (20,37,48,100). In the rat and primate, nociceptive neurons (about 10%) are scattered throughout the VB; in the cat, nociceptive neurons are only found on the edges of the nucleus (20,48,100,107). The nociceptive (48,100) neurons in this region in the primate are of both the WDR and NS type and generally have properties [e.g., localized receptive field (RF), graded responses to noxious mechanical and thermal stimuli, somatotopic organization] consistent with the general view that they are involved in pain localization and discrimination (20,100). However, in the rat VB, most of the nociceptive neurons are NS, and many have a large RF that is frequently bilateral and often involves both orofacial and spinally innervated structures; a well-organized somatotopic arrangement of nociceptive neurons is lacking in the rat (48,49,100).

Posterior or ventroposterior to the VB is another region where nociceptive neurons have consistently been recorded. This poorly defined region probably includes the regions termed PO (posterior nucleus) in the rat and POm in the cat. In the primate this region is more complex and may include a number of separate regions. Many nociceptive-specific neurons have been reported in the ventroposterior inferior nucleus (VPI) (6) and in a separate region that has been termed the posterior ventromedial nucleus (VMpo) (18). The VMpo receives a major input from lamina I of the SNC and the dorsal horn and projects to the SI and insula cortex (20), both regions that have been implicated in nociception in recent imaging studies. The VPI projects to the secondary somatosensory cortex (SII), which also has been shown to be activated by pain stimuli in some studies. Stimulation in the region ventroposterior to the VB in human frequently elicits painful sensations, including sensations in the craniofacial region (36,71). In view of these various findings, it is likely that this region plays an important role in mediating painful sensations.

MEDIAL THALAMUS

The involvement of the medial thalamus in pain was first suggested from the clinical observations of Dejerine and Roussy and Head and Holmes that chronic central pain would frequently develop following destruction of the lateral thalamus or its projections (20). The medial thalamus is a complex collection of separate nuclei whose functions are poorly understood. These nuclei generally have widespread and diffuse inputs and projections (63). The proposed role of some of these nuclei (particularly the centralis lateralis, centre median, parafascicular nucleus, and submedius) in mediating pain results pri-

marily from studies showing that they receive input from the STT, SNC, or reticular formation (20,100) and that they contain nociceptive neurons. The neurons in these regions have large receptive fields. This feature, in conjunction with the suggestions of Head and Holmes, has given rise to the currently held concept that this region mediates the affective-motivational aspects of pain. However, there has been no convincing direct support for this hypothesis in recent years. Of interest is the existence within the medial thalamus of the rat and cat of a region called the submedius, which receives a prominent projection from lamina I of the SNC and which contains nociceptive neurons. In contrast to the other medial thalamic structures mentioned above, this nucleus has a highly focused reciprocal projection with the ventrolateral orbital cortex, a region that in the rat has been shown to contain nociceptive neurons (33). It has been proposed that a functionally equivalent region may exist in the primate in the ventrocaudal part of the medialis dorsalis nucleus. This region has been shown to receive a projection from lamina I of the SNC and spinal cord and to project to the cingulate cortex, a cortical region implicated in pain in recent imaging studies (20).

DEEP/VISCERAL INPUTS TO THE THALAMUS

There have been relatively few studies that have examined the effects of noxious inputs from deep and visceral structures. It has been found that a considerable proportion of the VB neurons with a cutaneous RF in rats, cats, and monkeys receive convergent inputs from noncutaneous afferents, such as deep or visceral inputs (1,13, 20,47,100). It is worth noting that thalamic neurons activated by deep and visceral inputs tend to be much more widespread and frequently are classified as LTM on the basis of their cutaneous RF. Although craniofacial deep inputs have not been systematically studied, extensive convergence of inputs from cranial vessel and pulpal afferents onto VPM neurons with an orofacial RF has been extensively documented, particularly in cats (5,28,35,103,107).

CEREBROVASCULAR INPUTS TO THE THALAMUS

Several studies have specifically examined the effects of craniovascular stimulation on thalamic neurons in the cat. The study of Davis and Dostrovsky (28) reported the existence of neurons that were excited by electrical stimulation of the MMA and SSS. Some also were shown to be activated by mechanical stimulation of the vessels. All had excitatory RFs on the face, but only some were classified as NS on the basis of their cutaneous RFs. The remainder were either LTM neurons or neurons activated by tapping (Fig. 3). They were located mostly dorsal or anterior to the VPM or in the POm. Zagami and Lambert

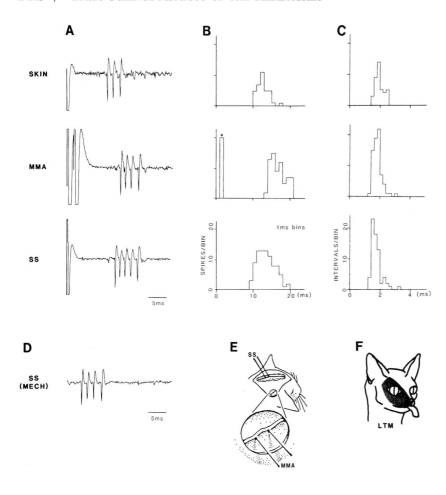

FIG. 3. Responses of an LTM neuron located in the POm excited by stimulation of the MMA and SSS. **A–C:** Typical digitized oscilloscope traces: poststimulus time histograms (PSTHs) **(A and B)** and interspike interval histograms **(C)** of the neuronal responses to electrical stimulation of the skin, MMA, and SSS. **D:** Digitized oscilloscope trace of the neuronal response to mechanically displacing the SSS. **E:** Location of the MMA- and SSS-stimulating electrodes. **F:** The neuron's RF is indicated by the shaded region on the figurine of the cat's head. From Davis and Dostrovsky (28).

(109) also studied the effects of MMA and SSS stimulation on cat thalamic neurons. About 50% of the neurons excited from these structures were found to be in the VPM and 10% in the ventral periphery of the VPM. Almost 50% were LTM and had RFs on the face. Most of the RFs were in the V1 division or included V1. Some

neurons were shown to be excited by bradykinin (Fig. 4). In a later study they also showed that capsaicin applied to the vessels excited many cells in the VPM and POm but, interestingly, only those that had nociceptive receptive fields. Finally, in 1995 Angus-Leppan et al. (5) studied the convergence of SSS and tooth pulp inputs on cat thal-

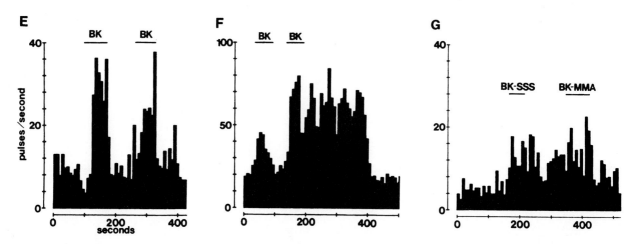

FIG. 4. These PST histograms show the responses of three different cells in the cat thalamus to the application of BK to the MMA (*E*), the SSS (*F*), and both vessels (*G*). Redrawn and modified from Zagami and Lambert (109).

amic cells. Over 50% of the cells were excited by both TP and SSS stimulation and were located in the VB or intralaminar nuclei. However, cells also were found that were activated by only one of these inputs. Goadsby et al. (44) reported that electrical stimulation of the SSS resulted in increased metabolic activity in the VPM and POm, and this finding is consistent with the reports cited above of the existence of neurons in these regions that are excited by cerebrovascular stimulation.

Much less is known about the processing of pain at the cortical level. Stimulation in the cortex rarely evokes pain, and cortical lesions rarely and inconsistently eliminate pain (67,101). Recent functional imaging studies have revealed that painful stimuli result in simultaneous activation of several cortical regions. The regions most consistently activated are the primary and secondary (33) somatosensory cortices and parts of the insula and anterior cingulate cortex (15,16,31,32,62). These are all regions where, as mentioned above, thalamic nuclei implicated in pain have been shown to send projections. In addition, in animal studies nociceptive neurons have been described in all these regions (34,88,101). It would appear that the sensation of pain is dependent on the combined activity in these multiple regions, although it is likely that different aspects of the pain sensation are preferentially mediated by activity in subsets of these regions. There have been no specific studies that have examined the cortical effects of nociceptive deep and visceral inputs other than from the tooth pulp; however, there is no reason to believe that cerebrovascular inputs are processed in different regions.

REFERENCES

1. Al-Chaer ED, Westlund KN, Willis WD. Nucleus gracilis: an integrator for visceral and somatic information. *J Neurophysiol* 1997;78: 521–527.
2. Almeida A, Tavares I, Lima D, Coimbra A. Descending projections from the medullary dorsal reticular nucleus make synaptic contacts with spinal cord lamina I cells projecting to that nucleus: an electron microscopic tracer study in the rat. *Neuroscience* 1993;55:1093–1106.
3. Amano N, Hu JW, Sessle BJ. Responses of neurons in feline trigeminal subnucleus caudalis (medullary dorsal horn) to cutaneous, intraoral, and muscle afferent stimuli. *J Neurophysiol* 1986;55:227–243.
4. Angus-Leppan H, Olausson B, Boers P, Lambert GA. Convergence of afferents from superior sagittal sinus and tooth pulp on cells in the upper cervical spinal cord of the cat. *Neurosci Lett* 1994;182: 275–278.
5. Angus-Leppan H, Olausson B, Boers P, Lambert GA. Convergence of afferents from superior sagittal sinus and tooth pulp on cells in the thalamus of the cat. *Cephalalgia* 1995;15:191–199.
6. Apkarian AV, Shi T. Squirrel monkey lateral thalamus. I. Somatic nociresponsive neurons and their relation to spinothalamic terminals. *J Neurosci* 1994;14:6779–6795.
7. Azerad J, Woda A, Albe-Fessard D. Physiological properties of neurons in different parts of the cat trigeminal sensory complex. *Brain Res* 1982;246:7–21.
8. Bernard JF, Besson JM. The spino(trigemino)pontoamygdaloid pathway: electrophysiological evidence for an involvement in pain processes. *J Neurophysiol* 1990;63:473–490.
9. Bester H, Menendez L, Besson JM, Bernard JF. Spino (trigemino) parabrachiohypothalamic pathway: electrophysiological evidence for an involvement in pain processes. *J Neurophysiol* 1995;73:568–585.
10. Blair RW, Weber RN, Foreman RD. Characteristics of primate spinothalamic tract neurons receiving viscerosomatic convergent inputs in T_3–T_5 segments. *J Neurophysiol* 1981;46:797–811.
11. Broton JG, Hu JW, Sessle BJ. Effects of temporomandibular joint stimulation on nociceptive and nonnociceptive neurons of the cat's trigeminal subnucleus caudalis (medullary dorsal horn). *J Neurophysiol* 1988;59:1575–1589.
12. Broton JG, Rosenfeld P. Cutting rostral trigeminal complex projections preferentially affects perioral nociception in the rat. *Brain Res* 1986;397:1–8.
13. Brüggemann J, Shi T, Apkarian AV. Squirrel monkey lateral thalamus. II. Viscerosomatic convergent representation of urinary bladder, colon, and esophagus. *J Neurosci* 1994;14:6796–6814.
14. Burstein R, Yamamura H, Malick A, Strassman AM. Chemical stimulation of the intracranial dura induces enhanced responses to facial stimulation in brain stem trigeminal neurons. *J Neurophysiol* 1998;79:964–982.
15. Casey KL, Minoshima S, Berger KL, Koeppe RA, Morrow TJ, Frey KA. Positron emission tomographic analysis of cerebral structures activated specifically by repetitive noxious heat stimuli. *J Neurophysiol* 1994;71:802–807.
16. Coghill RC, Talbot JD, Evans AC, Meyer E, Gjedde A, Bushnell MC, Duncan GH. Distributed processing of pain and vibration by the human brain. *J Neurosci* 1994;14:4095–4108.
17. Craig AD. Distribution of brainstem projections from spinal lamina I neurons in the cat and the monkey. *J Comp Neurol* 1995;361:225–248.
18. Craig AD, Bushnell MC, Zhang E-T, Blomqvist A. A thalamic nucleus specific for pain and temperature sensation. *Nature* 1994;372: 770–773.
19. Craig AD, Dostrovsky JO. Thermoreceptive lamina I trigeminothalamic neurons project to the nucleus submedius in the cat. *Exp Brain Res* 1991;85:470–474.
20. Craig AD, Dostrovsky JO. Processing of nociceptive information at supraspinal levels. In: Yaksh TL, Lynch C 3rd, Zapol WM, Maze, M, Biebuyck JF, and Saidman LJ, eds. *Anesthesia: Biologic Foundations*. Philadelphia: Lippincott-Raven, 1997:625–642.
21. Cumberbatch MJ, Hill RG, Hargreaves RJ. Rizatriptan has central antinociceptive effects against durally evoked responses. *Eur J Pharmacol* 1997;328:37–40.
22. Dallel R, Duale C, Molat J-L. Morphine administered in the substantia gelatinosa of the spinal trigeminal nucleus caudalis inhibits nociceptive activities in the spinal trigeminal nucleus oralis. *J Neurosci* 1998;18:3529–3536.
23. Dallel R, Raboisson P, Woda A, Sessle BJ. Properties of nociceptive and non-nociceptive neurons in trigeminal subnucleus oralis of the rat. *Brain Res* 1990;521:95–106.
24. Darian-Smith I, Yokota T. Cortically evoked depolarization of trigeminal cutaneous afferent fibers in the cat. *J Neurophysiol* 1966;29: 170–184.
25. Davis KD, Dostrovsky JO. Activation of trigeminal brain-stem nociceptive neurons by dural artery stimulation. *Pain* 1986;25:395–401.
26. Davis KD, Dostrovsky JO. Cerebrovascular application of bradykinin excites central sensory neurons. *Brain Res* 1988;446:401–406.
27. Davis KD, Dostrovsky JO. Effect of trigeminal subnucleus caudalis cold block on the cerebrovascular-evoked responses of rostral trigeminal complex neurons. *Neurosci Lett* 1988;94:303–308.
28. Davis KD, Dostrovsky JO. Properties of feline thalamic neurons activated by stimulation of the middle meningeal artery and sagittal sinus. *Brain Res* 1988;454:89–100.
29. Davis KD, Dostrovsky JO. Responses of feline trigeminal spinal tract nucleus neurons to stimulation of the middle meningeal artery and sagittal sinus. *J Neurophysiol* 1988;59:648–666.
30. Davis KD, Dostrovsky JO. Responses of feline trigeminal spinal tract nucleus neurons to stimulation of the middle meningeal artery and sagittal sinus. *J Neurophysiol* 1988;59:648–666.
31. Davis KD, Taylor SJ, Crawley AP, Wood ML, Mikulis DJ. Functional MRI of pain- and attention-related activations in the human cingulate cortex. *J Neurophysiol* 1997;77:3370–3380.
32. Davis KD, Wood ML, Crawley AP, Mikulis DJ. fMRI of human somatosensory and cingulate cortex during painful electrical nerve stimulation. *Neuroreport* 1995;7:321–325.
33. Dostrovsky JO, Hutchison WD, Davis KD, Lozano AM. Potential role of orbital and cingulate cortices in nociception. In: Besson JM, Guilbaud G, Ollat H, eds. *Forebrain areas involved in pain processing*. Paris: John Libbey Eurotext, 1995:171–181.

34. Dostrovsky JO, Craig AD. Nociceptive neurons in primate insular cortex [Abstract]. *Soc Neurosci Abstr* 1996;22:111.

35. Dostrovsky JO, Davis KD, Kawakita K. Central mechanisms of vascular headaches. *Can J Physiol Pharmacol* 1991;69:652–658.

36. Dostrovsky JO, Wells FEB, Tasker RR. Pain sensations evoked by stimulation in human thalamus. In: Inoki R, Shigenaga Y, Tohyama M, eds. *Processing and inhibition of nociceptive information, International Congress Series 989*. Amsterdam: Excerpta Medica, Elsevier, 1992:115–120.

37. Dubner R, Sessle BJ, Storey AT. *The neural basis of oral and facial function*. New York: Plenum, 1978.

38. Ebersberger A, Ringkamp M, Reeh PW, Handwerker HO. Recordings from brain stem neurons responding to chemical stimulation of the subarachnoid space. *J Neurophysiol* 1997;77:3122–3133.

39. Eisenman J, Landgren S, Novin D. Functional organization in the main sensory trigeminal nucleus and in the rostral subdivision of the nucleus of the spinal trigeminal tract in the cat. *Acta Physiol Scand* 1963;59[Suppl 214]:5–44.

40. Falls WM, Alban MM. Morphology and synaptic connections of small myelinated primary trigeminal axons arborizing among neurons in the border zone of rat trigeminal nucleus oralis. *Somatosensory Res* 1986;4:97–110.

41. Fujino Y, Koyama N, Yokota T. Differential distribution of three types of nociceptive neurons within the caudal bulbar reticular formation in the cat. *Brain Res* 1996;715:225–229.

42. Goadsby PJ, Hoskin KL. Inhibition of trigeminal neurons by intravenous administration of the serotonin (5HT)1B/D receptor agonist zolmitriptan (311C90): are brain stem sites therapeutic target in migraine? *Pain* 1996;67:355–359.

43. Goadsby PJ, Zagami AS. Stimulation of the superior sagittal sinus increases metabolic activity and blood flow in certain regions of the brainstem and upper cervical spinal cord of the cat. *Brain* 1991;114:1001–1011.

44. Goadsby PJ, Zagami AS, Lambert GA. Neural processing of craniovascular pain: a synthesis of the central structures involved in migraine. *Headache* 1991;31:365–371.

45. Gobel S, Falls WM, Hockfield S. The division of the dorsal and ventral horns of the mammalian caudal medulla into eight layers using anatomical criteria. In: Anderson D, Matthews B, eds. *Pain in the trigeminal region*. New York: Elsevier/North-Holland Biomedical, 1977:443–453.

46. Graham SH, Sharp FR, Dillon W. Intraoral sensation in patients with brainstem lesions: role of the rostral spinal trigeminal nuclei in pons. *Neurology* 1988;38:1529–1533.

47. Guilbaud G, Berkley KJ, Benoist J-M, Gautron M. Responses of neurons in thalamic ventrobasal complex of rats to graded distension of uterus and vagina and to uterine suprafusion with bradykinin and prostaglandin F$_{2\alpha}$. *Brain Res* 1993;614:285–290.

48. Guilbaud G, Bernard JF, Besson JM. Brain areas involved in nociception and pain. In: Wall PD, Melzack R, eds. *Textbook of pain*. Edinburgh: Churchill Livingstone, 1994:113–128.

49. Guilbaud G, Peschanski M, Gautron M, Binder D. Neurones responding to noxious stimulation in VB complex and caudal adjacent regions in the thalamus of the rat. *Pain* 1980;8:303–318.

50. Hayashi H. Morphology of central terminations of intra-axonally stained, large, myelinated primary afferent fibers from facial skin in the rat. *J Comp Neurol* 1985;237:195–215.

51. Hayashi H, Sumino R, Sessle BJ. Functional organization of trigeminal subnucleus interpolaris: nociceptive and innocuous afferent inputs, projections to thalamus, cerebellum, and spinal cord, and descending modulation from periaqueductal gray. *J Neurophysiol* 1984;51:890–905.

52. Hayashi H, Tabata T. Physiological properties of sensory trigeminal neurons projecting to mesencephalic parabrachial area in the cat. *J Neurophysiol* 1989;61:1153–1160.

53. Hoskin KL, Kaube H, Goadsby PJ. Central activation of the trigeminovascular pathway in the cat is inhibited by dihydroergotamine—a c-Fos and electrophysiological study. *Brain* 1996;119:249–256.

54. Hoskin KL, Kaube H, Goadsby PJ. Sumatriptan can inhibit trigeminal afferents by an exclusively neural mechanism. *Brain* 1996;119:1419–1428.

55. Hu JW. Response properties of nociceptive and non-nociceptive neurons in the rat's trigeminal subnucleus caudalis (medullary dorsal horn) related to cutaneous and deep craniofacial afferent stimulation and modulation by diffuse noxious inhibitory controls. *Pain* 1990;41:331–345.

56. Hu JW, Dostrovsky JO, Sessle BJ. Functional properties of neurons in cat trigeminal subnucleus caudalis (medullary dorsal horn). I. Responses to oral-facial noxious and nonnoxious stimuli and projections to thalamus and subnucleus oralis. *J Neurophysiol* 1981;45:173–192.

57. Hu JW, Sessle BJ, Raboisson P, Dallel R, Woda A. Stimulation of craniofacial muscle afferents induces prolonged facilitatory effects in trigeminal nociceptive brain-stem neurones. *Pain* 1992;48:53–60.

58. Hutchison WD, Tsoukatos J, Dostrovsky JO. Quantitative analysis of orofacial thermoreceptive neurons in the superficial medullary dorsal horn of the rat. *J Neurophysiol* 1997;77:3252–3266.

59. Hylden JL, Hayashi H, Bennett GJ, Dubner R. Spinal lamina I neurons projecting to the parabrachial area of the cat midbrain. *Brain Res* 1985;336:195–198.

60. Jacquin MF, Barcia M, Rhoades RW. Structure-function relationships in rat brainstem subnucleus interpolaris: IV. Projection neurons. *J Comp Neurol* 1989;282:45–62.

61. Jacquin MF, Stennett RA, Renehan WE, Rhoades RW. Structure-function relationships in the rat brainstem subnucleus interpolaris: II. Low and high threshold trigeminal primary afferents. *J Comp Neurol* 1988;267:107–130.

62. Jones AKP, Brown WD, Friston KJ, Qi LY, Frackowiak RSJ. Cortical and subcortical localization of response to pain in man using positron emission tomography. *Proc R Soc Lond B Biol Sci* 1991;244:39–44.

63. Jones EG. *The thalamus*. New York: Plenum, 1985.

64. Kaube H, Hoskin KL, Goadsby PJ. Activation of the trigeminovascular system by mechanical distension of the superior sagittal sinus in the cat. *Cephalalgia* 1992;12:133–136.

65. Kaube H, Hoskin KL, Goadsby PJ. Inhibition by sumatriptan of central trigeminal neurones only after blood-brain barrier disruption. *Br J Pharmacol* 1993;109:788–792.

66. Kaube H, Keay KA, Hoskin KL, Bandler R, Goadsby PJ. Expression of c-Fos–like immunoreactivity in the caudal medulla and upper cervical spinal cord following stimulation of the superior sagittal sinus in the cat. *Brain Res* 1993;629:95–102.

67. Kenshalo DR Jr, Willis WD Jr. The role of the cerebral cortex in pain sensation. In: Jones EG, Peters A, eds. *Cerebral cortex*. New York: Plenum, 1991:151–212.

68. Kunc Z. Significant factors pertaining to the results of trigeminal tractotomy. In: Hassler R, Walker AE, eds. *Trigeminal neuralgia*. Philadelphia: WB Saunders, 1970:90–98.

69. Lambert GA, Lowy AJ, Boers PM, Angus-Leppan H, Zagami AS. The spinal cord processing of input from the superior sagittal sinus: pathway and modulation by ergot alkaloids. *Brain Res* 1992;597:321–330.

70. Lambert GA, Zagami AS, Bogduk N, Lance JW. Cervical spinal cord neurons receiving sensory input from the cranial vasculature. *Cephalalgia* 1991;11:75–85.

71. Lenz FA, Dougherty PM. Pain processing in the human thalamus. In: Steriade M, Jones EG, McCormick DA, eds. *Thalamus*. Volume 2. Experimental and clinical aspects. Amsterdam: Elsevier, 1997:617–651.

72. Light AR. *The initial processing of pain and its descending control: spinal and trigeminal systems*. Basel, Switzerland: Karger, 1992.

73. Light AR, Sedivec MJ, Casale EJ, Jones SL. Physiological and morphological characteristics of spinal neurons projecting to the parabrachial region of the cat. *Somatosens Motor Res* 1993;10:309–325.

74. McHaffie JG, Larson MA, Stein BE. Response properties of nociceptive and low-threshold neurons in rat trigeminal pars caudalis. *J Comp Neurol* 1994;347:409–425.

75. Menendez L, Bester H, Besson JM, Bernard JF. Parabrachial area: electrophysiological evidence for an involvement in cold nociception. *J Neurophysiol* 1996;75:2099–2116.

76. Meng ID, Bereiter DA. Differential distribution of Fos-like immunoreactivity in the spinal trigeminal nucleus after noxious and innocuous thermal and chemical stimulation of rat cornea. *Neuroscience* 1996;72:243–254.

77. Meng ID, Hu JW, Benetti AP, Bereiter DA. Morphine produces opposite effects on corneal-responsive neurons in two regions of the spinal trigeminal nucleus [Abstract]. *Abstracts, 8th World Congress on Pain*. Seattle: IASP Press, 1996:149.

78. Meng ID, Hu JW, Benetti AP, Bereiter DA. Encoding of corneal input in two distinct regions of the spinal trigeminal nucleus in the rat: cutaneous receptive field properties, responses to thermal and chemical

stimulation, modulation by diffuse noxious inhibitory controls, and projections to the parabrachial area. *J Neurophysiol* 1997;77:43–56.

79. Moskowitz MA, Nozaki K, Kraig RP. Neocortical spreading depression provokes the expression of c-fos protein–like immunoreactivity within trigeminal nucleus caudalis via trigeminovascular mechanisms. *J Neurosci* 1993;13:1167–1177.

80. Mosso JA, Kruger L. Receptor categories represented in spinal trigeminal nucleus caudalis. *J Neurophysiol* 1973;36:472–488.

81. Nagano S, Myers JA, Hall RD. Representation of the cornea in the brain stem of the rat. *Exp Neurol* 1975;49:653–670.

82. Nord SG, Kyler HJ. A single unit analysis of trigeminal projections to bulbar reticular nuclei of the rat. *J Comp Neurol* 1968;134:485–494.

83. Nozaki K, Boccalini P, Moskowitz MA. Expression of c-fos–like immunoreactivity in brainstem after meningeal irritation by blood in the subarachnoid space. *Neuroscience* 1992;49:669–680.

84. Price DD, Dubner R, Hu JW. Trigeminothalamic neurons in nucleus caudalis responsive to tactile, thermal, and nociceptive stimulation of monkey's face. *J Neurophysiol* 1976;39:936–953.

85. Raboisson P, Dallel R, Clavelou P, Sessle BJ, Woda A. Effects of subcutaneous formalin on the activity of trigeminal brain stem nociceptive neurones in the rat. *J Neurophysiol* 1995;73:496–505.

86. Sessle BJ, Greenwood LF. Inputs to trigeminal brain stem neurones from facial, oral, tooth pulp and pharyngolaryngeal tissues: I. Responses to innocuous and noxious stimuli. *Brain Res* 1976;117:211–226.

87. Sessle BJ, Hu JW, Amano N, Zhong G. Convergence of cutaneous, tooth pulp, visceral, neck and muscle afferents onto nociceptive and non-nociceptive neurones in trigeminal subnucleus caudalis (medullary dorsal horn) and its implications for referred pain. *Pain* 1986;27:219–235.

88. Sikes RW, Vogt BA. Nociceptive neurons in area 24 of rabbit cingulate cortex. *J Neurophysiol* 1992;68:1720–1732.

89. Sjoqvist O. Studies on pain conduction in the trigeminal nerve. A contribution to the surgical treatment of facial pain. *Acta Psychiatr Scand* 1938;17[Suppl]:1–139.

90. Strassman A, Mason P, Moskowitz M, Maciewicz R. Response of brainstem trigeminal neurons to electrical stimulation of the dura. *Brain Res* 1986;379:242–250.

91. Strassman AM, Mineta Y, Vos BP. Distribution of fos-like immunoreactivity in the medullary and upper cervical dorsal horn produced by stimulation of dural blood vessels in the rat. *J Neurosci* 1994;14:3725–3735.

92. Strassman AM, Potrebic S, and Maciewicz RJ Anatomical properties of brainstem trigeminal neurons that respond to electrical stimulation of dural blood vessels. *J Comp Neurol* 1994;346:349–365.

93. Strassman AM, Vos BP. Somatotopic and laminar organization of fos-like immunoreactivity in the medullary and upper cervical dorsal horn induced by noxious facial stimulation in the rat. *J Comp Neurol* 1993;331:495–516.

94. Tavares I, Lima D. Descending projections from the caudal medulla oblongata to the superficial or deep dorsal horn of the rat spinal cord. *Exp Brain Res* 1994;99:455–463.

95. Villanueva L, Bernard JF, Le Bars D. Distribution of spinal cord projections from the medullary subnucleus reticularis dorsalis and the adjacent cuneate nucleus: a Phaseolus vulgaris-leucoagglutinin study in the rat. *J Comp Neurol* 1995;352:11–32.

96. Villanueva L, Bing Z, Bouhassira D, Le Bars D. Encoding of electrical, thermal, and mechanical noxious stimuli by subnucleus reticularis dorsalis neurons in the rat medulla. *J Neurophysiol* 1989;61:391–402.

97. Villanueva L, Bouhassira D, Bing Z, Le Bars D. Convergence of heterotopic nociceptive information onto subnucleus reticularis dorsalis neurons in the rat medulla. *J Neurophysiol* 1988;60:980–1009.

98. Villanueva L, Cliffer KD, Sorkin LS, Le Bars D, Willis WD Jr. Convergence of heterotopic nociceptive information onto neurons of caudal medullary reticular formation in monkey (*Macaca fascicularis*). *J Neurophysiol* 1990;63:1118–1127.

99. Vyklicky L, Keller O, Jastreboff P, Vyklicky L Jr, Butkhuzi S. Spinal trigeminal tractotomy and nociceptive reactions evoked by tooth pulp stimulation in the cat. *J Physiol Paris* 1977;73:379–386.

100. Willis WD Jr. Nociceptive functions of thalamic neurons. In: Steriade M, Jones EG, McCormick DA, eds. *Thalamus*. Vol. II. Experimental and clinical aspects. Oxford, England: Elsevier, 1997:373–424.

101. Willis WD Jr. The pain system. The neural basis of nociceptive transmission in the mammalian nervous system. In: Gildenberg PL, ed. *Pain and headache*. Basel, Switzerland: Karger, 1985:1–346.

102. Willis WD Jr, Coggeshall RE. *Sensory mechanisms of the spinal cord*. New York: Plenum, 1991.

103. Woda A, Azerad J, Guilbaud G, Besson JM. Etude microphysiologique des projections thalamiques de la pulpe dentaire chez le chat. *Brain Res* 1975;89:193–213.

104. Woods AH. Segmental distribution of spinal root nucleus of the trigeminal nerve. *J Nerv Ment Dis* 1913;40:91–101.

105. Yokota T, Koyama N, Nishikawa Y, et al. Trigeminal nociceptive neurons in the subnucleus reticularis ventralis. I. Response properties and afferent connections. *Neurosci Res* 1991;11:1–17.

106. Yokota T, Nishikawa N. Reappraisal of somatotopic tactile representation within trigeminal subnucleus caudalis. *J Neurophysiol* 1980;43:700–712.

107. Yokota T, Nishikawa Y, Koyama N. Tooth pulp input to the shell region of nucleus ventralis posteromedialis of the cat thalamus. *J Neurophysiol* 1986;56:80–98.

108. Young RF. Effect of trigeminal tractotomy on dental sensation in humans. *J Neurosurg* 1982;56:812–818.

109. Zagami AS, Lambert GA. Stimulation of cranial vessels excites nociceptive neurones in several thalamic nuclei of the cat. *Exp Brain Res* 1990;81:552–566.

The Headaches, Second Edition,
edited by J. Olesen, P. Tfelt-Hansen, and K.M.A. Welch.
Lippincott Williams & Wilkins, Philadelphia © 2000.

Basic Science Aspects of the Headaches

CHAPTER 14

Inhibition of Nociception

Jürgen Sandkühler and Troels Staehelin Jensen

The intensity of pain felt by a patient may not always match the level of nociceptor activation. For example, immediately after an accident a severely wounded patient may feel no pain at all for some time, whereas a minor trauma might have evoked intense pain in the same person. In a healthy human subject the intensity of pain induced by identical, repetitive noxious stimuli may vary with a circadian rhythm. In situations of emotional stress, during prolonged body exercise (long-distance runners), and during sexual intercourse the pain threshold may be elevated considerably. This mismatch between the level of nociceptive input and the perceived intensity of pain can now be explained by neuronal circuits in the central nervous system that modulate the transmission of nociceptive information. Neurons in the spinal dorsal horn or in its trigeminal correlate, the trigeminal subnucleus caudalis (medullary dorsal horn), are relay stations that receive nociceptive information from peripheral nociceptors and transmit this information to the brain, which ultimately leads to the sensation of pain. These relay stations are important sites for clinically relevant inhibition (or facilitation) of nociception. All vertebrates investigated so far, including humans, possess powerful endogenous antinociceptive systems that may reduce or even abolish transmission of nociceptive information at spinal or trigeminal relays. Some of the most effective forms of pain therapy known today activate these endogenous mechanisms of antinociception. Since the 1960s, the progress in pain therapy has

benefited considerably from successful interactions between basic sciences and clinical medicine. New discoveries made in basic sciences have often quickly been imported into clinical practice. On the other hand, effective clinical treatments of pain syndromes have guided basic researchers to identify new antinociceptive principles in the nervous system. The neuronal mechanisms of endogenous antinociception and their clinical implications are summarized in this chapter.

Various forms of endogenous antinociception have been identified that can be classified into two major categories: (1) descending inhibition of nociception in the spinal or medullary dorsal horn by systems that originate from brain stem sites and (2) afferent-induced inhibition in the spinal or medullary dorsal horn that is evoked by stimulation of sensory nerve fibers. In any case, the final inhibition takes place at or near the first synapse of the nociceptive pathways. Even though most of the previous work has addressed spinal dorsal horn mechanisms of antinociception, numerous studies have shown that similar or identical mechanisms also apply to the trigeminal subnucleus caudalis (5,28). Evidence suggests that an imbalance in activity between brain stem nuclei mediating antinociception and vascular control may be relevant to the pathogenesis of migraine (18,31).

DESCENDING INHIBITION OF NOCICEPTION

Powerful supraspinal descending systems have been identified that are mainly inhibitory, but facilitatory effects also have been observed. These systems are tonically active and depress spinal nociception under physiologic conditions. In addition, descending inhibition can be activated by environmental stimuli, pharmacologically or by deep brain stimulation.

J. Sandkühler: II. Physiologisches Institut, University of Heidelberg, 69120 Heidelberg, Germany.

T. S. Jensen: Department of Neurology F, Århus Kommunehospital, DK-8000 Århus C, Denmark.

TONIC DESCENDING INHIBITION

The existence of tonic descending inhibition of spinal nociception is now well established. Complete spinalization or circumscribed lesions in the lateral funiculi of the spinal cord invariably and immediately lead to a disinhibition of nociceptive neurons in the spinal dorsal horn caudal to the lesion. Both background activity and stimulus-evoked responses of nociceptive spinal dorsal horn neurons are strongly enhanced and the thresholds for nociceptive behavior are lowered in spinalized animals. This indicates that the transmission of nociceptive information in the spinal cord is subject to tonic descending inhibition from pathways that travel in the lateral funiculi. The supraspinal origins of these descending antinociceptive systems have not been identified with certainty. In the cat, but not in the rat, the medullary *lateral reticular nucleus* may be involved. The spinal mechanisms of tonic descending antinociception are largely unknown. It has been suggested that some forms of chronic, ongoing spontaneous pain and centrally mediated hyperalgesia may result from insufficient activity in these tonic descending antinociceptive pathways. Regular fluctuations of activity in these systems (e.g., during the sleep–wake cycle) may contribute to the circadian rhythm of nociception (4).

DESCENDING ANTINOCICEPTION ACTIVATED FROM BRAIN STEM SITES

Analgesia is often one characteristic feature of complex behavioral response patterns. For example, acute, massive stress is typically accompanied by cardiovascular and respiratory reactions and also by profound analgesia. Nociceptive thresholds also may be elevated during physical exercise and during sexual intercourse. These complex and highly integrated activities are organized at supraspinal levels, suggesting that the corresponding antinociception is also initiated supraspinally. Indeed, Reynolds (23) discovered that electrical stimulation at brain stem sites may induce strong antinociception. This phenomenon was then systematically investigated by numerous groups and, as a consequence, deep brain stimulation was soon introduced into clinical practice as a new therapeutic tool in human pain patients (1,11). Stimulations at numerous sites in the brain stem, diencephalon, and somatosensory cortex were shown to depress or abolish nociceptive neuronal responses in the spinal dorsal horn (Fig. 1) (9). Some of the antinociceptive stimulation sites have direct descending projections to the spinal cord via long serotonergic, adrenergic, or peptidergic nerve fibers that mainly travel in the dorso-

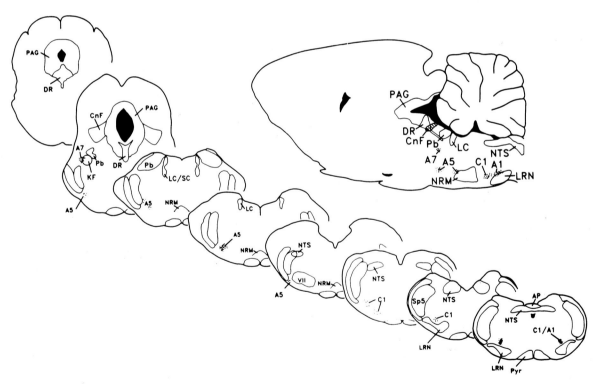

FIG. 1. These parasaggital and coronal sections of the rat brain illustrate the location of brain stem cell groups and anatomic nuclei that are associated with the depression of pain. *A1, A5,* and *A7,* norepinephrine-containing cell groups; *AP,* area postrema; *C1,* epinephrine-containing cell group; *CnF,* nucleus cuneiformis; *DR,* nucleus raphe dorsalis; *KF,* Kölliker-Fuse nucleus; *LC* and *LC/SC,* locus coeruleus/subcoeruleus; *LRN,* lateral reticular nucleus; *NRM,* nucleus raphe magnus; *NTS,* nucleus tractus solitarius; *PAG,* periaqueductal gray; *Pb,* parabrachial area; *Sp5,* spinal trigeminal nerve. Reproduced from Gebhart and Randich (9).

lateral or ventrolateral funiculi. The major antinociceptive stimulation sites that send direct projections to the spinal or medullary dorsal horn are listed from caudal to rostral. Antinociceptive neurons in the lateral reticular nucleus of the caudal ventrolateral medulla are tonically active in some species and can be further activated by focal stimulation. The inhibition involves the release of norepinephrine and activation of α_2-adrenoreceptors in the spinal cord. Because the direct projections from the lateral reticular nucleus to the spinal cord are not adrenergic, an ascending–descending loop via adrenergic cell group A5 may also be involved. The medullary *nucleus raphe magnus* and adjacent reticular formation have strong direct serotonergic projections to the spinal dorsal horn, and stimulation in the nucleus raphe magnus may produce a powerful antinociception with relatively few observable side effects. In the spinal cord the raphe-spinal inhibition is mediated by $5-HT_1$, $GABA_A$, and $GABA_B$ receptors and possibly also by opioid receptors but not by glycine receptors. Some raphe-spinal neurons display discharge patterns that correlate well with the level of vigilance and may be most active during sleep. In the pons the locus coeruleus/subcoeruleus is the major source of direct noradrenergic innervation of the spinal cord in some species, and stimulation in this nucleus also produces a strong antinociception that is mediated by spinal α_2-adrenoreceptors. Neurons in the nucleus locus coeruleus change activity with different levels of vigilance from arousal to the sleep–wake cycle and play a role in vestibulospinal reflexes and spinal motor output. Locus coeruleus neurons also control cerebral circulation and may induce vascular changes similar to those in migraine (2). The *parabrachial area,* including the A7 adrenergic cell group and the *Kölliker-Fuse nucleus* in the midbrain, also sends direct antinociceptive fibers to the spinal cord. In addition, these nuclei project to preganglionic sympathetic neurons in the thoracic intermediolateral column.

Effective antinociceptive stimulation sites are also found in areas of the brain that have no direct projections to the spinal cord. The descending inhibitions evoked from these sites are mediated via synaptic relays in one or more of the above-mentioned brain stem nuclei, from caudal to rostral. Neurons in the *nucleus of the solitary tract* may mediate descending antinociception, probably via a relay in the lateral reticular nucleus. This inhibition can be triggered by sensory stimulation of vagal cardiopulmonary afferents. Acute noxious stimuli may activate a descending inhibition of nociceptive responses in those spinal segments that do not process the conditioning noxious stimulus. This phenomenon has been termed diffuse noxious inhibitory control and appears to be mediated by neurons in the *subnucleus reticularis dorsalis.* In healthy subjects but not in patients with lesions in the retroolivary part of the medulla (Wallenberg syndrome), a diffuse noxious inhibitory control of pain per-

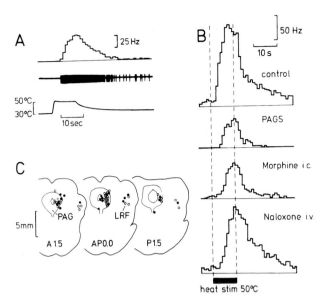

FIG. 2. Inhibition of noxious heat-evoked responses of individual wide–dynamic range neurons in the spinal dorsal horn of the anesthetized cat by morphine microinjection or by focal electrical stimulation at identical sites in the PAG. **A:** (From bottom to top) Skin temperature during noxious skin heating, oscilloscope record of neurons response, and its peristimulus time histogram. **B:** Peristimulus time histograms of heat-evoked responses of another neuron recorded under control conditions, during electrical stimulation in PAG (PAGS), following microinjection of morphine (10 µg in 1 µL intracranially) and following intravenous injection of the µ opioid receptor antagonist naloxone. In **C** stimulation sites (○) and sites where morphine also was microinjected (●). From Gebhart et al. (10).

ception can be elicited (29). Descending inhibition induced by stimulation in various subdivisions of the midbrain *periaqueductal gray* (PAG) and the *nucleus raphe dorsalis* has been intensively studied (Fig. 2). Descending inhibition from the PAG is partly mediated by synaptic relays in the medullary nucleus raphe magnus and adjacent reticular formation (3). However, during focal chemical stimulation at the various subdivisions of the PAG, numerous neurons inside the PAG (27) and in well-defined nuclei of the brain stem are also activated. Thus, focal stimulation of cell bodies at well-defined brain stem sites may activate a large number of nearby and remote nuclei in the brain stem that may act synergistically to produce antinociception and also may serve other functions (e.g., during stress response or defense reaction) (25). Neurons in the *anterior pretectal nucleus* can be activated by electrical stimulation of dorsal column fibers and may mediate a descending inhibition via reticulospinal neurons in the ventrolateral medulla. This may be a mechanism underlying analgesia by electrical stimulation of the dorsal columns. Results obtained by positron emission tomography in patients during a spontaneous migraine attack suggest that pathologic activity in brain stem nuclei regulating antinociception and vascular control may be related to the pathogenesis of this disease (31). Recently a discrete acute sclerotic lesion in the PAG could be identified as the cause for severe headache in a young women.

PHARMACOLOGIC ACTIVATION IN THE BRAIN STEM OF ENDOGENOUS ANTINOCICEPTION

Three families of endogenous opioids have been identified that include dynorphins binding predominantly to κ opioid receptors, enkephalins that bind to δ opioid receptors, and β-endorphins that bind to μ opioid receptors. Opioid receptors are found at numerous sites in the brain and in virtually all of the above-mentioned antinociceptive brain stem sites. Different theories have been advanced to explain the action of morphine in the brain (8,32). There is experimental support to indicate that morphine gives rise to:

- Activation of indirect, descending inhibition in the dorsal horn
- Direct inhibition of nociceptive throughput at brain stem levels
- Activation of indirect inhibition in the brain stem
- Inhibition of ascending nociception in the brain stem
- Direct cortical or thalamic inhibition of nociception

Activation of Indirect, Descending Inhibition in the Dorsal Horn

The microinjection of the μ opioid receptor agonist morphine in microgram doses into the PAG induces an analgesia that is attenuated by transection of spinal pathways, suggesting that morphine acting in the PAG may induce a descending inhibition in the spinal cord. Morphine given systemically or microinjected into brain stem sites modulates spinal reflexes, evokes the release of monoamines from the spinal cord, and reduces nocicep-

tive responses of dorsal horn neurons (Fig. 3; see also Fig. 2). Microinjection of morphine at PAG sites is mimicked by microinjection of excitatory amino acids and by focal electrical stimulation. These supraspinally induced effects are reduced significantly by spinally administered monoamine receptor antagonists (12). Morphine may activate antinociceptive output neurons in the PAG by inhibiting GABAergic interneurons that tonically inhibit output neurons (disinhibition). An activation of descending inhibitory systems by systemic or supraspinal morphine has been observed directly by some researchers, but not by others.

Activation of Indirect Inhibition in the Brain Stem

The transmission of nociceptive information to the brain is subserved by multiple systems, including the spinocervical, spinothalamic, spinoreticular, and spinomesencephalic fiber systems, that project into the brain stem core. There is evidence that experimental excitation at brain stem sites by focal electrical stimulation or by microinjection of excitatory amino acids may result in a behavior similar to that evoked by painful stimuli. Neuronal responses at these nociceptive brain stem sites can be inhibited directly by descending fiber systems originating from the above-mentioned brain stem nuclei. For example, electrical stimulation in the PAG inhibits spontaneous and noxious evoked neuronal activity in the lower brain stem.

Direct Inhibition of Nociceptive Throughput at Brain Stem Levels

The transmission of nociceptive information at brain stem sites can also be inhibited directly by activating opioid receptors that are located presynaptically to nociceptive spinobulbar projections. Opioid receptor binding is present in the brain stem at all levels. Part of this binding

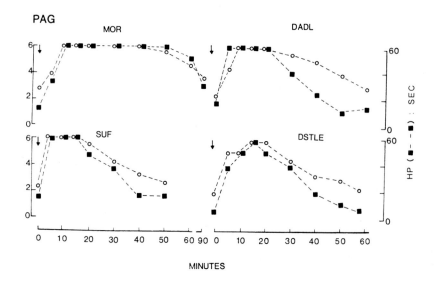

FIG. 3. Illustrates the effects of intracerebral microinjections of opioid ligands given in a volume of 500 nL at time zero (*arrows*) into the PAG on tail-flick (○) and hot plate (■) response latencies. Prolongation of these reflex latencies indicate thermal analgesia. **Top left:** Morphine (μ opioid receptor agonist), 15 nmol. **Bottom left:** Sufentanil (μ opioid receptor agonist), 1.5 nmol. **Top right:** DADL (D-Ala^2-D-Leu^5-enkephalin, δ opioid receptor agonist). **Bottom right:** DSTLE (D-Ser^2-Thr^6-leucine enkephalin, δ opioid receptor agonist). From Jensen and Yaksh (13).

may be located presynaptic to brain stem neurons receiving collateral input from ascending nociceptive fibers from the spinal cord or the trigeminal complex. In addition, the finding that opioids at the cellular level exert an inhibitory effect is consistent with a direct postsysnaptic inhibition of brain stem neurons.

Inhibition of Ascending Nociception in the Brain Stem

Noradrenergic and serotonergic fibers from the locus coeruleus and the dorsal raphe nucleus, respectively, project not only to spinal and medullary dorsal horn but also project strongly to the forebrain, and these ascending projections may depress nociception at forebrain sites. Lesions of both the locus coeruleus and dorsal raphe nucleus are associated with a reduced antinociceptive effect of morphine and a reduction of forebrain serotonin and noradrenaline.

Direct Cortical or Diencephalic Inhibition of Nociception

Given the dense opioid receptor binding in medial and lateral thalamic nuclei and in cortical areas, and given the general hyperpolarizing effect of opioids on neuronal activity, it is likely that part of the antinociceptive effect of opioids may be associated with a direct inhibition of nociceptive neurons in the cortex and diencephalon. However, at this writing the evidence for such an action is limited.

Multiple Opioid Receptors

The predominant opioid receptor in the brain is the κ_3 receptor subtype. There are some notable exceptions from this rule, such as the PAG, where μ receptors predominate even though members of all three opioid families are found within this area together with their respective receptors. Microinjections of μ_1 receptor agonists into the PAG, the nucleus raphe magnus, or the locus coeruleus produce an antinociception, whereas μ_2 receptors in spinal cord appear to mediate spinal opioid analgesia. Analgesia by selective agonists at κ_3 opioid receptors show no cross-tolerance with either morphine or κ_1 opioid receptor agonists; the latter exert their analgesic actions mainly in the spinal cord (19). Selective agonists at the δ_1 opioid receptors are potent analgesics when applied to the spinal cord, whereas agonists at the δ_2 receptor subtype, which is found mainly supraspinally, are less potent.

DEEP BRAIN STIMULATION IN HUMANS FOR PAIN RELIEF

Stimulation of deep brain structures was introduced following the promising experimental observation that focal electrical stimulation in the PAG produces powerful antinociception in animals. In studies on humans, pro-

found and long-lasting analgesia was achieved in some patients, whereas others did not benefit from deep brain stimulation. Stimulation in the thalamus, PAG, mesencephalic reticular formation, and, rarely, hypothalamus have been applied to patients with various chronic nociceptive, neuropathic, or mixed pain conditions. The results differ markedly between centers, but in a recent survey the average success rate was reported to be 50%. The development of tolerance to stimulation of brain sites, cross-tolerance with morphine, and the reversal of stimulation-produced analgesia by naloxone suggest that the analgesic effect of deep brain stimulation is in part mediated by opioids.

In conclusion, antinociceptive neurons have been identified at numerous brain stem sites that are also implicated in a wide variety of nonsensory functions. A dense network of connections exists between these antinociceptive nuclei and other areas of the brain, which is in line with the fact that analgesia and hypoalgesia are often part of complex behavioral patterns such as acute stress responses or sleep-wake cycles. This limits the use of analgesic deep brain stimulation to those sites with few and tolerable side effects.

AFFERENT-INDUCED ANTINOCICEPTION IN THE DORSAL HORN

An effective analgesia can be achieved by some forms of sensory stimulation, for example, by activation of cutaneous warm, cold, or mechanoreceptors during physical therapy, or by excitation of nociceptors during acupuncture. Direct electrical stimulation of sensory nerves, during transcutaneous electrical nerve stimulation, also may be antinociceptive. Fundamentally different forms of spinal antinociception are induced by stimulation of large-diameter sensory nerve fibers that transmit information from low-threshold mechanoreceptors versus stimulation of small-diameter sensory nerve fibers that mainly transmit sensory information from nociceptors and thermoreceptors.

ANTINOCICEPTION BY STIMULATION OF LOW-THRESHOLD SENSORY NERVE FIBERS

It has long been recognized that repetitive, high-frequency stimulation of large-diameter sensory nerve fibers ($A\alpha/\beta$ fibers) may depress nociceptive responses of spinal dorsal horn neurons. The same inhibitory effect can be achieved by electrical stimulation of dorsal columns as axon collaterals of sensory $A\alpha/\beta$ fibers travel within this tract. Thus, dorsal column stimulation may be antinociceptive via two different mechanisms, segmental inhibition and a descending inhibition via the anterior pretectal nucleus. High-frequency stimulation of sensory $A\alpha/\beta$ fibers leads to an excitation of interneurons in the superficial spinal dorsal horn that synaptically release GABA. The GABAergic inhibition reduces the excitability of nociceptive neurons in the spinal dorsal horn by a pre- or postsynaptic mechanism. GABA may act on $GABA_A$ and $GABA_B$ receptors, which are both present on presynaptic terminals of $A\delta$ and C fibers, possibly mediating presynaptic inhibition. Blockade of GABA receptors may reduce the inhibitory effects of dorsal column stimulation, whereas blockade of spinal opioid receptors appears to be ineffective (4). The duration of inhibition is typically limited to the duration of conditioning stimulation. This form of spinal antinociception has been described by Melzack and Wall in their gate-control theory (17), which was quickly followed by the clinical development of transcutaneous electrical nerve stimulation as a new tool for the treatment of pain (30).

Transcutaneous electrical nerve stimulation and dorsal column stimulation is mainly used for neurogenic pain (e.g., phantom pain and post-herpetic neuralgia) but also may be used for mixed nociceptive and neurogenic pain such as low back pain with arachnoiditis and complex regional pain syndromes. The average long-term success rate is similar to that with deep brain stimulation situated around 50%.

LONG-TERM DEPRESSION OF SYNAPTIC STRENGTH IN PRIMARY AFFERENT $A\delta$ AND C FIBERS

When the intensity of conditioning electrical nerve stimulation is raised so that fine, weakly myelinated $A\delta$ fibers are also recruited, prolonged, low-frequency stimulation (approximately 15 minutes at 1 Hz) induces a depression of synaptic strength between primary afferent $A\delta$ or C fibers and higher order neurons in the superficial spinal dorsal horn (Fig. 4) (26). This inhibition always outlasts the duration of conditioning stimulation and is not reversible within the recording periods (up to 3 hours). This long-term depression of synaptic strength in $A\delta$ and C fibers is not mediated by $GABA_A$ or glycine receptors but requires activation of ionotropic glutamate receptors of the NMDA subtype and G protein–coupled metabotropic glutamate receptors.

Synaptic strength between sensory $A\delta$ or C fibers and spinal dorsal horn neurons cannot only be depressed but also can be potentiated for prolonged periods of time. This long-term potentiation is considered to be a synaptic mechanism of central hyperalgesia that may develop after peripheral trauma, inflammation, or nerve injury (20,22,24). The long-term potentiation may be reversed by prolonged low-frequency stimulation of afferent $A\delta$ fibers. The long-term depression of synaptic strength following stimulation of afferent $A\delta$ fibers may be a mechanism that underlies long-lasting analgesia following some forms of needle acupuncture or electroacupuncture.

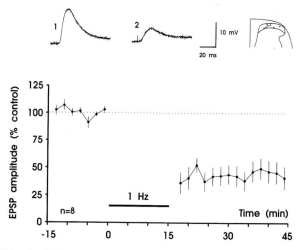

FIG. 4. Robust long-term depression of fast excitatory synaptic transmission in the superficial spinal dorsal horn by low-frequency stimulation of primary afferent $A\delta$ fibers. In a spinal cord–dorsal root slice preparation from a young rat, $A\delta$ fiber–evoked excitatory postsynaptic potentials (*EPSPs*) were elicited in neurons of lamina II by electrical stimulation of dorsal roots. Conditioning stimulation of dorsal roots with 1 Hz for 15 minutes (*horizontal bar*) induced a depression of synaptic strength that always outlasted the period of conditioning stimulation and was not reversible within the recording period of up to 3 hours. From Sandkühler et al. (26).

The relief of pain by stimulation of afferent nerve fibers depends on the intensity, frequency, and duration of stimulation. These stimulation parameters are also critical for the induction of long-term depression of synaptic strength between fine sensory nerve fibers and neurons in the spinal dorsal horn. However, the parameters of conditioning stimulation alone do not predict the change in synaptic efficacy; the activity level in descending antinociceptive systems is also important (14). It is well known that the activity in endogenous antinociceptive systems may vary considerably over time and between patients. This may now explain the clinical observation that identical therapeutic stimulations may have different analgesic effects within and between patients.

Classical chinese acupuncture typically leads to an excitation of nociceptors and to tolerable pain during manual twirling of fine needles inserted at selected points of the skin. Electroacupuncture often uses low-frequency stimulation (around 1–2 Hz, for approximately 20 minutes) that also evokes low-intensity pain. The analgesia that can be achieved by these procedures may outlast the duration of stimulation by many hours or even by days and weeks. A number of studies show that acupuncture stimulation need not be applied at the dedicated acupuncture points. These findings may well be explained by a long-term depression of synaptic strength in nociceptive pathways if the counterstimulation is applied to dermatomes or Head zones that correspond to the painful area. In contrast, a long-lasting activation of propriospinal or supraspinal descending inhibitory pathways may be involved in analgesia that is produced by heterotopic forms of counterstimulation (e.g., by acupuncture-like forms of stimulation at sites remote from the painful areas).

PHARMACOLOGY OF ANTINOCICEPTION IN THE DORSAL HORN

A number of classical neurotransmitters and neuro-modulators and their receptors have been identified that contribute to the inhibition of nociceptive information at the level of the spinal or medullary dorsal horn.

GABA acting on $GABA_A$ and $GABA_B$ receptors may induce pre- or postsynaptic inhibition of nociceptive spinal dorsal horn neurons. GABAergic neurons are abundant in superficial dorsal horn as are GABA receptors. GABAergic inhibition appears to be tonically active in spinal cord and can be further activated by low-threshold afferent stimulation (see earlier section on Antinociception by Stimulation of Low-Threshold Sensory Nerve Fibers) and by descending inhibitory pathways (see earlier section on Descending Antinociception Activated from Brain Stem Sites).

Members of the three opioid families (β-endorphin, enkephalins, dynorphins) and their receptors (μ, δ, and κ subtypes) are expressed in dorsal horn neurons. About 60% to 70% of spinal μ and δ-receptors and about half of the spinal κ opioid receptors are present presynaptically on terminals of Aδ and C fibers. In the superficial dorsal horn, opioids may inhibit release of neurotransmitters from these fine primary afferent nerve fibers. This may be mediated primarily by activation of μ_2, δ_1, δ_2, and κ_1 opioid receptors that are known to depress synaptic transmission in the spinal dorsal horn. The presynaptic location of μ opioid receptors on small-diameter Aδ and C fibers may explain why morphine is highly effective in depressing pain that arises from nociceptors. In contrast, morphine is less effective in depressing some forms of neuropathic pain that are accompanied by loss of opioid receptors on primary afferent terminals or neuropathic pain arising from activation of large-diameter Aβ fibers that do not have opioid receptors on their terminals (15). In addition, opioids also depress spinal nociceptive neurons by a postsynaptic mechanism (34). Although the activation of spinal μ and δ opioid receptors is clearly antinociceptive, the effects of spinal κ receptors are not uniform. Dynorphin, an endogenous ligand of κ opioid receptors, may have antianalgesic effects when released from supraspinal descending pathways and may attenuate morphine analgesia (21). Blockade of spinal κ opioid receptors also may block stress-induced antinociception. Putative pure κ opioid receptor agonists may, however, enhance or depress spinal nociception. Activation of the κ_1 receptor subtype is apparently mainly inhibitory in the spinal dorsal horn (6,15,35). Apparently a profound syn-ergism exists between spinal and supraspinal sites of opioid action. For example, the concomitant injection of morphine both intracerebroventricularly and intrathecally increases the potency of morphine by almost 10-fold (33).

Adrenergic agonists acting on spinal α_2-adrenoreceptors are antinociceptive and may mimic the spinal release of norepinephrine from fibers descending from the nucleus locus coeruleus or A5 cell group. (See earlier in this chapter.) Spinal dorsal root ganglion cells express G protein–coupled α_2 adrenoreceptors that may inhibit presynaptic Ca^{2+} influx and open inward rectifying potassium channels. Subtypes of α_2 adrenoreceptors exist in the mammalian central nervous system, including the human spinal cord, and also may mediate postsynaptic inhibition of nociceptive dorsal horn neurons. In addition, inhibitory α_2 adrenoreceptors are present presynaptically on preganglionic sympathetic fibers. Spinal α_2 adrenoreceptor agonists may therefore induce severe hypotension. An α_2-adrenoreceptor subtype that specifically mediates pure analgesia has not yet been identified.

The excitatory amino acids L-glutamate and L-aspartate are the major excitatory neurotransmitters in the spinal cord. These fast-acting neurotransmitters are released from the terminals of primary nociceptive nerve fibers. Various ionotropic glutamate receptors have been identified, including AMPA and NMDA receptors. There is evidence that the NMDA receptor plays a significant role in centrally mediated hyperalgesia. For instance, long-term potentiation of synaptic strength, wind-up of C fiber–evoked responses of dorsal horn neurons, touch-evoked pain, and aftersensations reflecting hyperexcitability in the nervous system all can be blocked by NMDA receptor antagonists. Combination of NMDA antagonists with opioids or sodium channel blockers may be a new way of obtaining pain relief in chronic pain conditions.

Nitric oxide (NO) is a diffusible gas that acts as a neurotransmitter or neuromodulator at numerous sites in the nervous system, including the nociceptive system of the dorsal horn. NO is produced by the enzyme nitric oxide synthase (NOS), which converts arginine into citruline and NO. The diffusible gas NO increases neuronal excitability both pre- and postsynaptically. NOS-like immunoreactivity is found mainly in the superficial layers of the dorsal horn and is increased in states of chronic nerve injury and prolonged inflammation. NOS inhibitors have been shown to reduce hyperalgesia in neuropathic pain models and the NMDA-induced hyperalgesia when given intrathecally (16).

A number of additional receptor agonists have been identified that induce antinociception in the dorsal horn. Cholinergic agonists acting on postsynaptic M_1 muscarinic receptors but not on presynaptic M_2 muscarinic receptors are antinociceptive. Adenosine acting on spinal presynaptic A_1 receptors reduces neurotransmitter release from primary afferent nerve terminals via G_i protein and mediates postsynaptic inhibition in neurons of the superficial spinal dorsal horn by activating potassium currents. Serotonin (5-hydroxytryptamine; 5-HT) is released from descending raphe spinal fibers. Its antinociception is mediated by spinal 5-HT_{1B} and probably also via activation of 5-HT_{1A} and 5-$HT_{1C/2}$ receptors. The activation of spinal 5-HT_3 receptors may indirectly modulate nociception via the release of GABA.

The antinociceptive effects of these receptor agonists may display complex interactions. The antinociceptive efficacy and dorsal horn mechanisms of action of ketamine are currently being debated. Apparently complex interactions with opioid, monoaminergic, and cholinergic systems and local anesthetic effects are involved. In the spinal cord, α_2 adrenoreceptor agonists may act synergistically with opioids. The antinociceptive effects of spinally released norepinephrine are enhanced by spinal injections of cholinesterase inhibitors, suggesting that release of spinal acetylcholine is important. Because systemic opioids are believed to activate descending inhibitory noradrenergic pathways, it is not surprising that opioid antinociception may be potentiated by spinal coadministration of norepinephrine reuptake and cholinesterase inhibitors (7).

In conclusion, the discoveries of synaptic, cellular, and systemic mechanisms of spinal and trigeminal antinociception provide new targets for the prevention and the treatment of acute and chronic pain states, including headaches.

REFERENCES

1. Adams IE, Hosobuchi Y, Fields HL. Stimulation of internal capsule for relief of chronic pain. *J Neurosurg* 1974;41:740–744.
2. Agnoli A, De Marinis M. Vascular headaches and cerebral circulation: an overview. *Cephalalgia* 1985;5[Suppl 2]:9–15.
3. Basbaum AI, Fields HL. Endogenous pain control mechanisms: review and hypothesis. *Ann Neurol* 1978;4:451–462.
4. Besson J-M, Chaouch A. Peripheral and spinal mechanisms of nociception. *Physiol Rev* 1987;67:67–186.
5. Chiang CY, Sessle BJ, Hu JW. Parabrachial area and nucleus raphe magnus-induced modulation of electrically evoked trigeminal subnucleus caudalis neuronal responses to cutaneous or deep A-fiber and C-fiber inputs in rats. *Pain* 1995;62:61–68.
6. Duggan AW, North RA. Electrophysiology of opioids. *Pharmacol Rev* 1984;35:219–281.
7. Eisenach J. Update on spinal cord pharmacology in pain. *Acta Anaesthesiol Scand Suppl* 1997;110:124–126.
8. Gebhart GF. Opiate and opioid peptide effects on brain stem neurons: relevance to nociception and antinociceptive mechanisms. *Pain* 1982; 12:93–140.
9. Gebhart GF, Randich A. Brainstem modulation of nociception. In: Klemm WR, Vertes RP, eds. Brainstem mechanisms of behavior. New York: John Wiley & Sons, 1990:315–352.
10. Gebhart GF, Sandkühler J, Thalhammer JG, Zimmermann M. Inhibition in spinal cord of nociceptive information by electrical stimulation and morphine microinjection at identical sites in midbrain of the cat. *J Neurophysiol* 1984;51:75–89.
11. Hosobuchi Y, Adams JE, Linchitz R. Pain relief by electrical stimulation of the central gray matter in humans and its reversal by naloxone. *Science* 1977;197:183–186.
12. Jensen TS, Yaksh TL. II. Examination of spinal monoamine receptors through which brainstem opiate-sensitive systems act in the rat. *Brain Res* 1986;363:114–127.
13. Jensen TS, Yaksh TL. III. Comparison of the antinociceptive action of μ and δ opioid receptor ligands in the periaqueductal gray matter, medial and paramedial ventral medulla in the rat as studied by the microinjection technique. *Brain Res* 1986;372:301–312.
14. Liu X-G, Morton CR, Azkue JJ, Zimmermann M, Sandkühler J. Long-term depression of C-fibre–evoked spinal field potentials by stimulation of primary afferent Aδ-fibres in the adult rat. *Eur J Neurosci* 1998;10:3069–3075.
15. Lombard MC, Besse D, Besson J-M. Opioid receptors in the superficial layers of the rat spinal cord: functional implications in pain processing. *Prog Brain Res* 1995;104:77–92.
16. Meller ST, Gebhart GF. Nitric oxide (NO) and nociceptive processing in the spinal cord. *Pain* 1993;52:127–136.
17. Melzack R, Wall PD. Pain mechanisms: a new theory. *Science* 1965; 150:971–979.
18. Micieli G, Tassorelli C, Bosone D, et al. Increased cerebral blood flow velocity induced by cold pressor test in migraine: a possible basis for pathogenesis? *Cephalalgia* 1995;15:494–498.
19. Pasternak GW. Pharmacological mechanisms of opioid analgesics. *Clin Neuropharmacol* 1993;16:1–18.
20. Pockett S. Spinal cord synaptic plasticity and chronic pain. *Anesth Analg* 1995;80:173–179.
21. Rady JJ, Fujimoto JM. Dynorphin A(1-17) mediates midazolam antagonism of morphine antinociception in mice. *Pharmacol Biochem Behav* 1993;46:331–339.
22. Randic M, Jiang MC, Cerne R. Long-term potentiation and long-term depression of primary afferent neurotransmission in the rat spinal cord. *J Neurosci* 1993;13:5228–5241.
23. Reynolds DV. Surgery in the rat during electrical analgesia induced by focal brain stimulation. *Science* 1969;164:444–445.
24. Sandkühler J. Neurobiology of spinal nociception: new concepts. In: Carli G, Zimmermann M, eds. *Progress in brain research*, Vol. 110. Amsterdam: Elsevier, 1996:207–224.
25. Sandkühler J. The organization and function of endogenous antinociceptive systems. *Prog Neurobiol (NY)* 1996;50:49–81.
26. Sandkühler J, Chen JG, Cheng G, Randic M. Low frequency stimulation of afferent Aδ-fibers induces long-term depression of primary afferent synapses with substantia gelatinosa neurons in the rat. *J Neurosci* 1997;17:6483–6491.
27. Sandkühler J, Herdegen T. Distinct pattern of activated neurons throughout the rat midbrain periaqueductal gray induced by chemical stimulation. *J Comp Neurol* 1995;357:546–553.
28. Sessle BJ, Hu JW, Dubner R, Lucier GE. Functional properties of neurons in cat trigeminal subnucleus caudalis (medullary dorsal horn). II. Modulation of responses to noxious and nonnoxious stimuli by periaqueductal gray, nucleus raphe magnus, cerebral cortex, and afferent influences, and effect of naloxone. *J Neurophysiol* 1981;45:193–207.
29. Villanueva L, Le Bars D. The activation of bulbo-spinal controls by peripheral nociceptive inputs: diffuse noxious inhibitory controls. *Biol Res* 1995;28:113–125.
30. Wall PD, Sweet WH. Temporary abolition of pain in man. *Science* 1967;155:108–109.
31. Weiller C, May A, Limmroth V, et al. Brain stem activation in spontaneous human migraine attacks. *Nat Med* 1995;1:658–660.
32. Yaksh TL, Al-Rodhan NRF, Jensen TS, Besson JM. Sites of action of opiates in production of analgesia. In: Fields HL, ed. *Progress in brain research: pain modulation*. New York: Elsevier, 1988:371.
33. Yeung JC, Rudy TA. Multiplicative interaction between narcotic agonisms expressed at spinal and supraspinal sites of antinociceptive action as revealed by concurrent intrathecal and intracerebroventricular injections of morphine. *J Pharmacol Exp Ther* 1980;215:633–642.
34. Yoshimura Y, North RA. Substantia gelatinosa neurones hyperpolarized *in vitro* by enkephalin. *Nature* 1983;305:529–530.
35. Zieglgänsberger W. Central control of nociception. In: Mountcastle VB, Bloom FE, Geiger SR, eds. *Handbook of physiology—the nervous system IV*. Baltimore: Williams & Wilkins, 1986:581–645.

The Headaches, Second Edition,
edited by J. Olesen, P. Tfelt-Hansen, and K.M.A. Welch.
Lippincott Williams & Wilkins, Philadelphia © 2000.

Basic Science Aspects of the Headaches

CHAPTER 15

Central Sensitization and Headache

Rami Burstein and Clifford J. Woolf

Synaptic strength is not fixed. The amplitude of a synaptic contact between one neuron and another may both decrease and increase as a result of presynaptic and postsynaptic mechanisms. This plasticity is fundamental to the normal operation of the nervous system and contributes to long-term changes in neural function, including memory and learning. Such plasticity is not only adaptive, however, but also can contribute to neurologic disease. In particular, it is now clear that *central sensitization,* an activity-dependent change in the excitability and synaptic strength of neurons in the dorsal horn of the spinal cord is responsible for the generation of secondary hyperalgesia and allodynia in acute and chronic pain states (27,48,49). Central sensitization was discovered in 1983 in the rat spinal cord, where it has a role in producing postinjury pain hypersensitivity (47) and now has been documented in many laboratory animal species and in humans (20,24,33,35,43). Changes in somatosensory hypersensitivity in patients after surgical trauma and in human volunteers have been shown to be due to central sensitization, a finding that has opened new opportunities for effective treatment of these conditions (34,41). There is good evidence that central sensitization also can be produced in the trigeminal system and that it has a particular role in the pathogenesis of headache.

This chapter reviews the evidence in favor of a contribution of central sensitization to headache, using, when available, data obtained from the trigeminal system. If such information is not currently available, data from comparable studies on the spinal cord are used, because most indications are that the two systems resemble each other in most, but not all, respects. Some differences relate to the unique innervation by the trigeminal system of the intracranial meningeal and blood vessels, which is likely to have a major bearing on particular features of migraine. Another difference is related to the presence on trigeminal neurons of serotonin (5-HT) receptor subtypes not found on sensory neurons in the rest of the somatosensory system; this too may relate to the specific antimigraine action of 5-HT$_{1B/1D}$ agonists.

Central sensitization has two distinct phases: an *initiation phase* and a *maintenance phase,* each with different mechanisms. First, the mechanisms responsible for these two phases are reviewed, followed by an explanation of how changes in the excitability of neurons they produce manifest to produce some of the key symptoms of headache in general and of migraine in particular. Finally, this chapter discusses the therapeutic implications for headache of the involvement of central sensitization in its pathogenesis.

PHASES OF CENTRAL SENSITIZATION

Initiation Phase

Central sensitization is induced by activity in peripheral C-fibers; and activation of low-threshold A-fibers does not initiate this form of activity-dependent plasticity (51). C-fiber nociceptors can be activated by mechanical, thermal, and chemical stimuli. Normally, intracranial C-fiber nociceptors would not be active, but they begin to fire when exposed to increased levels of potassium and hydrogen ions as well as to the release of inflammatory

R. Burstein: Department of Neurobiology, Harvard Medical School, Department of Anesthesia and Critical Care, Beth Israel Deaconess Medical Center, and Harvard Institutes of Medicine, Boston, Massachusetts 02115.

C. J. Woolf: Department of Anesthesiology and Critical Care, Harvard Medical School, Boston, Massachusetts 02115, and Department of Anesthesiology and Critical Care, Massachusetts General Hospital, Charlestown, Massachusetts 02129.

mediators and growth factors. As part of cortical spreading depression (21), it has been well documented that there is release of K^+ (26) and H^+ (10,36) ions, both of which activate C-fibers. K^+ ions will depolarize the terminals directly, and H^+ ions will cause a depolarization acting on the vallinoid (capsaicin receptor, VR1) (7) and the acid-sensitive ion channel receptor (ASIC) (44). Once the initial activation of meningeal C-fibers nociceptors occurs, a further increase in activity may be generated by the subsequent initiation of neurogenic inflammation (15,30). For example, depolarization of the peripheral terminals and the axon reflex initiated by orthodromic activity will result in the peripheral release of substance P and calcitonin gene-related peptide (CGRP) from C-fiber terminals, both of which are capable of producing plasma extravasation, mast cell degranulation, and platelet aggregation (17,30), which in turn result in the release of histamine, 5-HT, and prostaglandin E_2 (PGE_2) and bradykinin, all chemical mediators found in inflamed tissue that are capable of further activating and sensitizing C-fibers (17,19). A key role of the tetrodotoxin (TTX)–resistant sodium ion channel in the peripheral sensitization of C-fiber terminals was recently found (16). Dural afferents exposed for a short period (several minutes) to an inflammatory soup containing a mixture of these mediators result in alteration in their peripheral sensitivity for up to an hour (40).

Induction Phase

Once C-fibers are activated in the periphery, this will result in the release from their central terminals in the superficial layers of the nucleus caudalis of the trigeminal system of C-fiber transmitters as a result of calcium inflow into the axon terminals. C-fibers, unlike A-fibers, contain multiple transmitters, including the excitatory amino acid glutamate and the neuropeptides substance P and CGRP (45) (Fig. 1). The release of these transmitters can be modulated actively by receptors on the central terminals. The μ-opiate receptor and adenosine receptors, for example, act to decrease transmitter release (53); at least while in the spinal cord, presynaptic N-methyl D-aspartate (NMDA) and $P2_{X3}$ receptors act as positive-feed forward autoreceptors that increase transmitter release (22). Of particular interest to migraine is evidence that the 5-HT_{1B} receptor is located on dural arteries, that 5-$HT_{1B, 1D, and 1F}$ receptors are found in the trigeminal ganglia (4,5,23), and that only 5HT_{1D} receptors are transported from the trigeminal ganglion to their peripheral terminals in the dura and central terminals in nucleus caudalis (23). Agonists to these receptors may act to reduce transmitter release from the fibers and, therefore, the initiation of central sensitization.

In addition to the multiple transmitters in the C-fiber terminal, multiple receptors for these transmitters are located on the postsynaptic neurons with which they

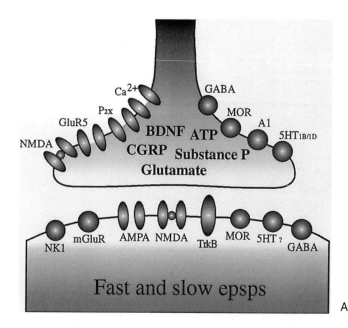

A

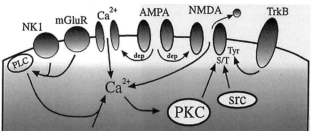

B

FIG. 1. A: A diagrammatic representation of a C-fiber terminal in the nucleus caudalis illustrating the multiple transmitters and neuromodulators in the axon presynaptic terminal and the multiple presynaptic receptors that modulate transmitter release. Those on the *left* augment and those on the *right* depress transmitter release. Also illustrated are the many different postsynaptic receptors on the neurons innervated by C-fibers. This diagram shows that the synaptic connection between nociceptor and central neuron is complex and generates a combination of fast and slow synaptic potentials. **B:** An illustration of the second-messenger signal transduction mechanisms initiated by C-fiber activity in central neurons. A key target of this biochemical processing is the NMDA receptor altering its properties and thereby increasing the excitability of the membrane, which manifests as central sensitization. (Modified from Woolf CJ, Mannion MJ, and Neumann S. Null mutations lacking substance: elucidating pain mechanisms by genetic pharmacology. *Neuron* 1998;20:1063–1066.)

make contact in the nucleus caudalis, including ionotropic and metabotropic receptors (see Fig. 1). The combination of these multiple transmitters and receptors means that C-fibers, unlike A-fibers, elicit long-lasting, slow synaptic potentials in neurons in the spinal cord and nucleus caudalis (29). These slow synaptic potentials are responsible for one windup, a unique property of C-fibers, characterized by a progressive increase in the response elicited by a standard low-frequency repeated

C-fiber input (28). Windup is generated as a result of the summation of the slow synaptic currents; the nonlinear nature of this increase can be explained by recruitment of NMDA receptors through removal of their normal voltage-dependent blockade by magnesium ions (1,38). This form of activity-dependent plasticity manifests only during a C-fiber input and must be clearly differentiated from central sensitization, which is a long- lasting facilitation initiated by C-fiber inputs that can be maintained independent of such inputs. The inputs that generate windup may be sufficient to produce central sensitization but are not necessary.

Maintenance Phase

Two different mechanisms produce prolonged changes in the excitability of dorsal horn neurons after brief C-fiber inputs. Both are contingent on an increase in intracellular calcium in the postsynaptic neuron. Such an increase in calcium ion concentration can occur by calcium entry through ionotropic ion channels, particularly the NMDA receptor; through voltage-dependent calcium ion channels as a result of depolarization of the membrane; and, finally, through the release of calcium from intracellular stores as a result of the activation of G-protein–coupled receptors, such as the glutamate metabotropic mGluR and the substance P Neurokinin 1 (NK1) receptors (1). The increased calcium levels act to activate protein kinase C and nitric oxide synthase (NOS). Protein kinase C will phosphorylate membrane-bound proteins, including serine and threonine residues on the NMDA receptor (8). This action results in a change in the functional properties of the NMDA receptor so that the normal Mg^{2+} ion block of the channel is lost or reduced and the receptor can be activated by glutamate at resting membrane potentials instead of only at depolarized levels (8). As a result, the glutamate sensitivity of neurons in the nucleus caudalis is reduced greatly so that they will respond to any given synaptic input with a much greater response. Activation of NOS will result in the release of nitric oxide synthase (NO), which can act as a retrograde signal from one neuron to another and, through production of cyclic glucose monophosphate (GMP), can augment transmitter release (54). In addition to these two key players, some evidence suggests that activation of cyclooxygenase in central neurons also may play a contributory role in the induction and maintenance of central sensitization and may explain a central action of nonsteroidal antiinflammatory drugs (NSAIDs) (25). Because central sensitization is associated with depolarization of the postsynaptic cell, the summation of slow synaptic potentials, these cells become more susceptible to use-dependent sodium channel blockers, such as lidocaine, which selectively bind to the inactive state of the ion channel. These blockers are found in much greater abundance in cells that are depolarized than in those that are not (31).

As discussed, an increase in excitability can initiate the phenomenon of central sensitization. The phenomenon, however, also can be produced by the removal or reduction of phasic and tonic inhibitory mechanisms, that is, disinhibition, which occurs after the administration of subconvulsant doses of the glycine receptor antagonist strychnine or the γ-aminobuutyric acid (GABA$_A$) receptor antagonist biccuculine (39,52).

MANIFESTATIONS OF CENTRAL SENSITIZATION

Cellular Manifestations

Central sensitization resulting from either an increase in excitability as a change in the properties of the NMDA receptor or from a reduction in inhibitory mechanisms in neurons of nucleus caudalis will result in an increase in synaptic input to these cells. This increase will result in recruitment of previously subthreshold inputs, such that the output of the cell, as detected by recording its action-potential firing pattern will change (9,50). In its simplest form, central sensitization manifests as a change in the gain of the neurons, which can be detected at a single-cell level by recording the receptive field properties of the neurons, and as changes in sensitivity to standard stimuli in patients.

Receptive Field Manifestations

Experimentally, the induction of central sensitization in trigeminal brainstem nuclei can be achieved when those C-fiber nociceptors that innervate deep structures are activated by inflammatory agents (6,18). As in the spinal cord (13), these changes include receptive field expansion, increased responsiveness to noxious stimuli, increased spontaneous activity, and the recruitment of novel low-threshold inputs (18). Such changes closely resemble the tactile allodynia and hyperalgesia seen in capsaicin-induced central sensitization in human subjects.

In the trigeminovascular system, changes in neuronal gain and the recruitment of previously subthreshold inputs were documented recently in laboratory animals after a brief application of endogenous allogenic substances, such as 5-HT, histamine, bradykinin, and prostaglandins to the dura overlying the meningeal sinuses, which are richly innervated by nociceptors (6,14, 40). A brief local chemical stimulus of meningeal nociceptors results in mechanical hypersensitivity of these sensory fibers within 5 minutes; recovery is within 60 to 90 minutes (40). Such chemical stimulation of the dura, and the activity it generates in the nociceptors, also results in sensitization of those nucleus caudalis nociceptive second-order neurons that receive convergent input from the dura (intracranially) and the skin (extracranially). This sensitization outlasts the peripheral sensitization of the nociceptors by many hours (Fig. 2). The following are characteristics of this central sensitization: (a) a reduction in the minimum mechanical force (i.e., threshold) required to induce neuronal activation by indenting their dural receptive fields, (b) an increased neuronal responsiveness to innocuous mechanical stimulation of their cutaneous receptive fields, (c) a reduced threshold and increased responses to heating and cooling their cutaneous receptive fields, (d) expansions of both dural and cutaneous receptive fields, and (e) the development of ongoing neuronal activity (6).

Initiation of the migraine attack may be accompanied by the release of potassium from cortical neurons, which could lead to the further local release of inflammatory mediators, cytokines and growth factors, which will act on meningeal nociceptors. Thus, the peripheral sensitization of meningeal nociceptors may contribute to the intracranial hypersensitivity that develops immediately after the onset of a migraine attack. Activation of these nociceptors also will induce central sensitization in neurons in the trigeminal nuclei of the brainstem. This change within the central nervous system could account for the extracranial and pericranial hypersensitivity and tenderness that develop during the attack and that sometimes last hours after the attack ends.

Clinical Manifestations

Pulsating (or throbbing) pain and its aggravation by routine physical activities (e.g., coughing, holding one's breath, bending over, rotating the head from side to side, climbing stairs, walking) are among the most common symptoms of migraine (3,32). Although not as commonly described by patients, pericranial myofacial tenderness and decreased pain threshold are often present in patients suffering from chronic tension-type headache (2) and migraine attack (12,42,46). One explanation for the intracranial hypersensitivity and the pulsating nature of the pain is sensitization of meningeal C-fiber nociceptors. When these meningeal C-fiber nociceptors become mechanically hypersensitive, they can respond to changes in pressure transferred to the dura during regular physical activities that increase intracranial pressure. Because the intracranial space is closed, any change in intracranial pressure is propagated throughout this space (11) and consequently affects the dura. For example, normal pulsation of arterial pressure that causes small brain movements that press the dura against the bone could be sufficient to activate meningeal C-fiber nociceptors if they are sensitized (i.e., during a migraine attack) and insufficient if they are not sensitized (i.e., during a migraine-free period).

Whereas intracranial hypersensitivity could be mediated by sensitization of meningeal C-fibers, the extracranial hypersensitivity is likely to be mediated exclusively by sensitization of central trigeminal (meningeal-sensitive) nociceptive neurons in the brainstem. Evidence for central sensitization in animal studies includes the development of extracranial cutaneous hypersensitivity in trigeminal nucleus caudalis neurons following a brief and restricted intracranial stimulation (6). Evidence for similar sensitization in clinical studies include the development of tenderness and sensitivity to pain on the scalp but not on the fingers of patients during migraine attacks (12). Because in the animal study cutaneous (extracranial) nociceptors were not affected by the restricted intracranial meningeal stimuli, the presence of extracranial mechanical and thermal allodynia and secondary hyperalgesia suggest that the occurrence of scalp and pericranial tenderness during headaches that have intracranial components (i.e., migraine) require no extracranial pathology. It points instead to the development of central sensitization along the trigeminovascular pathway.

Unlike migraine, tension-type headache often causes an increased sensitivity to pain not only in pericranial locations but also in extracephalic locations, such as the Achilles tendon (37) and the fingers (2). Because meningeal-sensory neurons in nucleus caudalis usually do not process sensory information that originates in these remote locations, it is tempting to speculate that, in

FIG. 2. The development of intracranial and extracranial hypersensitivity following chemical irritation of the dura. Comparisons of physiological responses of a dura-sensitive neuron in lamina V of Vc that projects to the hypothalamus (**A**). The responses of the neuron to a graded increase in the intensity of mechanical indentation of the dura (**B**), mechanical stimulation of the skin (**C**), and slowly heating (**D**) the skin are shown before (*left*) and after (*right*) the irritation of the dura with the low pH buffer. *Black area* in the hypothalamus depicts the low-threshold point for antidromic activation, *black dot* in the brainstem depicts the recording site, *black areas* on the skin and dura depict the sizes and locations of receptive fields before chemical irritation of the dura, and *gray area* on the dura depicts the expanded receptive field after chemical irritation. *Numbers* above the lines in B indicate forces of von Frey hairs, *boxes* in B depict the mechanical threshold, and *numbers* under lines in C indicate the mean number of spikes per second in response to each stimulus. *Arrowheads* in D show the temperature at which a response occurred. Note the drop in the mechanical threshold of the dural receptive field, the exaggerated response to brushing the skin, and the drop in the thresholds for heating the skin. *HYP*, hypothalamus, *Br*, brush, *Pr*, pressure; *Pi*, pinch; *Sq*, squeeze; *VBC*, ventrobasal complex. (Adapted from ref. 6, with permission.)

Projection site
(in the hypothalamus)

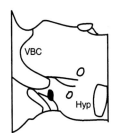

Recording site
(in lamina V)

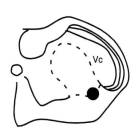

Receptive firelds
(on the dura and skin)

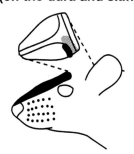

A

Intracranial hypersensitivity - mechanical dural stimulation

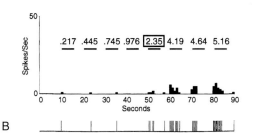

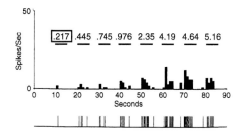

B

Extracranial hypersensitivity - mechanical skin stimulation

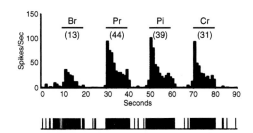

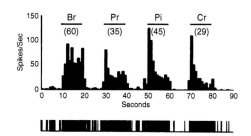

C

Extracranial hypersensitivity - thermal skin stimulation

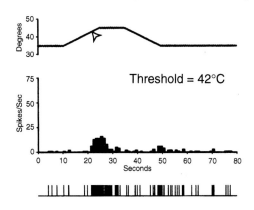

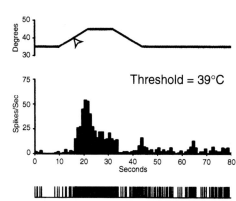

D

Before sensitization

After sensitization

addition to sensitization of neurons in the cervical spinal cord and trigeminal nuclei, sensitization of supraspinal neurons also may occur. Another possibility is that tension-type headache may be a manifestation of abnormally low activity of pain modulatory or inhibitory systems. It is certainly possible to produce central sensitization both by increasing excitability by C-fiber input and by removing inhibitory influences. Although it is not possible to determine whether it is the increased muscular tenderness that causes the headache or vice versa (because they occur simultaneously), the traditional notion proposes that chronic tension of head, neck, and shoulder muscles plays a key role in the initiation of these type of headaches. Theoretically, it is possible that, as in fibromyalgia and other muscle-pain disorders with unknown initiation factors, chronic tenderness of pericranial muscles reflects not abnormal inputs of muscle nociceptors but rather a change in gain in nociceptive spinal and supraspinal neurons. In other words, the pain in the muscles may be a form of hyperalgesia caused by a change in the excitability of central neurons, and the tenderness is a symptom of the neurologic abnormality, not its cause.

THERAPEUTIC IMPLICATIONS FOR THE TREATMENT OF MIGRAINE

Central sensitization has initiation, induction, and maintenance phases. In the trigeminovascular system, the initiation phase appears to be induced by chemical activation and sensitization of meningeal C-fiber nociceptors (40); 30 to 60 minutes after its initiation, central sensitization seems to be maintained independent of incoming inputs from the meningeal C-fibers (6). The therapeutic implications of these results are that (a) drugs that target the initiation phase of central sensitization should be administered immediately at the onset of the migraine attack (i.e., within the first 20 minutes) because they will have a better chance of preventing the activation and sensitization of the meningeal C-fiber nociceptors that lead to the perception of intracranial hypersensitivity and may abort the initiation of central changes; and (b) drugs that target the maintenance phase of central sensitization should be administered if the migraine pain is accompanied by extracranial hypersensitivity and continues for several hours.

Current theories propose that the initiation phase of migraine pain is induced by chemicals such as potassium ions, protons, histamine, 5-HT, bradykinin and PGE_2. Theoretically, to minimize the action of these chemicals on meningeal C-fiber nociceptors, NSAIDs, $5\text{-HT}_{1B/1D}$ agonists, and agents that block the VR1 and ASIC receptors could be used. The induction phase of central sensitization may be mediated by activation of presynaptic NMDA, $P2_{x3}$ and $5\text{-HT}_{1B/1D}$ receptors located on the central terminals of C-fiber nociceptors, which augment

transmitter release. Drugs that act to reduce transmitter release (i.e., μ-opiate and adenosine receptor agonists) should minimize the induction of central sensitization. Finally, prolonged changes in the excitability of dorsal horn neurons after brief C-fiber inputs depend on increased levels of intracellular calcium in the postsynaptic neuron. To prevent the increased calcium level, ionotropic ion channels like the NMDA receptor, voltage-dependent calcium ion channels, and G-protein–coupled receptors such as the substance P NK1 and mGluR must be blocked. The increased calcium acts via kinases to phosphorylate membrane receptors, including the NMDA receptor. A potentially important approach to interfering with the maintenance of a central sensitization state will be the development of new NMDA receptor antagonists. Because the currently clinically available NMDA antagonists (i.e., ketamine, dextrorphan, and memantine) are not potent or selective and have potential psychotropic actions, we must await new classes of such antagonists currently under development, such as NMDA receptor glycine site antagonists. Other possibilities of decreasing central sensitization include inhibition of NOS to prevent release of NO, which is believed to augment transmitter release, and the inhibition of cyclooxygenase in the trigeminal brainstem nuclei.

ACKNOWLEDGMENT

This work was supported by National Institutes of Health Grants DE-10904 and NS-35611-01 and by gifts from the Boston Foundation and the Goldfarb Family.

REFERENCES

1. Baranauskas G, Nistri A. Sensitization of pain pathways in the spinal cord: cellular mechanisms. *Prog Neurobiol* 1998;54:349–365.
2. Bendtsen L, Jensen R, Olesen J. Decreased pain detection and tolerance thresholds in chronic tension-type headache. *Arch Neurol* 1996;53:373–376.
3. Blau JN, Dexter SL. The site of pain origin during migraine attack. *Cephalalgia* 1981;1:143–147.
4. Bonaventure P, Voorn P, Luyten WHML, Leysen JE. 5HT(1B) and 5HT(1D) receptor mRNA differential co-localization with peptide mRNA in the guinea pig trigeminal ganglion. *Neuroreport* 1998;9:641–645.
5. Bouchelet I, Cohen Z, Case B, Seguela P, Hamel E. Differential expression of sumatriptan-sensitive 5-hydroxytryptamine receptors in human trigeminal ganglia and cerebral blood vessels. *Mol Pharmacol* 1996;50:219–223.
6. Burstein R, Yamamura H, Malick A, Strassman AM. Chemical stimulation of the intracranial dura induces enhanced responses to facial stimulation in brainstem trigeminal neurons. *J Neurophysiol* 1998;79:964–982.
7. Caterina MJ, Schumacher MA, Tominaga M, Rosen TA, Levine JD, Julius D. The capsaicin receptor: a heat-activated ion channel in the pain pathway. *Nature* 1997;389:816–824.
8. Chen L, Huang L-YM. Protein kinase C reduces Mg^{2+} block of NMDA-receptor channels as a mechanism of modulation. *Nature* 1992;356:521–523.
9. Cook AJ, Woolf CJ, Wall PD, McMahon SB. Dynamic receptive field plasticity in rat spinal cord dorsal horn following C primary afferent input. *Nature* 1987;325:151–153.
10. Csiba L, Paschen W, Mies G. Regional changes in tissue pH and glu-

cose content during cortical spreading depression in rat brain. *Brain Res* 1985;336:167–170.

11. Daley ML, Pasupathy H, Griffith M, Robertson JT, Leffler CW. Detection of loss of cerebral vascular tone by correlation of arterial and intracranial pressure signals. *IEEE Trans Biomed Eng* 1995;42:420–424.

12. Drummond PD. Scalp tenderness and sensitivity to pain in migraine and tension headache. *Headache* 1987;27:45–50.

13. Dubner R, Basbaum AI. Spinal dorsal horn plasticity following tissue or nerve injury. In: Wall PD, Melzack R, eds. *Textbook of pain.* New York: Churchill-Livingstone, 1994;225–241.

14. Ebersberger A, Ringkamp M, Reeh PW, Handwerker HO. Recordings from brainstem neurons responding to chemical stimulation of the subarachnoid space. *J Neurophysiol* 1997;77:3122–3133.

15. Goadby PJ, Edvinsson L. The trigeminovascular system and migraine: studies characterizing cerebrovascular and neuropeptide changes seen in humans and cats. *Ann Neurol* 1993;33:48–56.

16. Gold MS, Reichling DB, Schuster MJ, Levine JD. Hyperalgesic agents increase a tetrodotoxin-resistant Na^+ current in nociceptors. *Proc Natl Acad Sci USA* 1996;93:1108–1112.

17. Handwerker HO, Reeh PW. Pain and inflammation. In: Bond MR, Charlton JE, Woolf CJ, eds. *Proceedings of the VIth World Congress on Pain.* Amsterdam: Elsevier, 1991:59–70.

18. Hu JW, Sessle BJ, Raboisson P, Dallel R, Woda A. Stimulation of craniofacial muscle afferents induces prolonged facilitatory effects in trigeminal nociceptive brainstem neurons. *Pain* 1992;48:53–60.

19. Kessler W, Kirchhoff C, Reeh PW, Handwerker HO. Excitation of cutaneous afferent nerve endings in vitro by a combination of inflammatory mediators and conditioning effect of substance P. *Exp Brain Res* 1992;91:467–476.

20. Koltzenburg M, Torebjork HE, Wahren LK. Nociceptor modulated central sensitization causes mechanical hyperalgesia in acute chemogenic and chronic neuropathic pain. *Brain* 1994;117:579–591.

21. Lauritzen M. Pathophysiology of migraine aura—the spreading depression theory. *Brain* 1994;117:199–210.

22. Liu H, Mantyh PW, Basbaum AI. NMDA-receptor regulation of substance P release from primary afferent nociceptors. *Nature* 1997;386:721–724.

23. Longmore J, Shaw D, Smith D, et al. Differential distribution of 5HT1D- and 5HT1B-immunoreactivity within the human trigemino-cerebrovascular system: implications for the discovery of new antimigraine drugs. *Cephalalgia* 1997;17:833–842.

24. Magerl W, Wilk SH, Treede RD. Secondary hyperalgesia and perceptual wind-up following intradermal injection of capsaicin in humans. *Pain* 1998;74:257–268.

25. Malmberg AB, Yaksh TL. Hyperalgesia mediated by spinal glutamate or substance P receptor blocked by spinal cyclooxygenase inhibition. *Science* 1992;257:1276–1279.

26. Mayevsky A, Doron A, Manor T, Meilin S, Zarchin N, Ouaknine G. Cortical spreading depression recorded from human brain using a multiparametric monitoring system. *Brain Res* 1996;740:268–274.

27. McMahon SB, Lewin GR, Wall PD. Central hyperexcitability triggered by noxious inputs. *Curr Opin Neurobiol* 1993;3:602–610.

28. Mendell LM. Modifiability of spinal synapses. *Physiol Rev* 1984;64:260–324.

29. Miller BA, Woolf CJ. Glutamate-mediated slow synaptic currents in neonatal rat deep dorsal horn neurons in vitro. *J Neurophysiol* 1996;76:1465–1476.

30. Moskowitz, MA, Macfarlane R. Neurovascular and molecular mechanisms in migraine headache. *Cerebrovasc Brain Metab Rev* 1993;5:159–177.

31. Nagy I, Woolf CJ. Lignocaine selectively reduces C-fibre evoked neuronal activity in rat spinal cord in vitro by decreasing *N*-methyl-D-aspartate and neurokinin receptor mediated post synaptic depolarizations: implications for the development of novel centrally acting analgesics. *Pain* 1996;64:59–70.

32. Rassmussen BK, Jensen R, Olesen J. A population-based analysis of the diagnostic criteria of the International Headache Society. *Cephalalgia* 1991;11:29–34.

33. Ren K, Dubner R. NMDA receptor antagonists attenuate mechanical hyperalgesia in rats with unilateral inflammation of the hindpaw. *Neurosci Lett* 1993;163:22–26.

34. Richmond CE, Bromley LM, Woolf CJ. Preoperative morphine preempts postoperative pain. *Lancet* 1993;342:73–75.

35. Simone DA, Sorkin LS, Oh U, et al. Neurogenic hyperalgesia: central neural correlates in responses of spinothalamic tract neurons. *J Neurophysiol* 1991;66:228–246.

36. Scheller D, Kolb J, Tegtmeier F. Lactate and pH change in close correlation in the extracellular space of the rat brain during cortical spreading depression. *Neurosci Lett* 1992;135:83–86.

37. Schoenen J, Bottin D, Hardy F, Gerard P. Cephalic and extracephalic pressure pain thresholds in chronic tension-type headache. *Pain* 1991;47:145–149.

38. Sivilotti LG, Thompson SWN, Woolf CJ. The rate of rise of the cumulative depolarization evoked by repetitive stimulation of small-calibre afferents is a predictor of action potential windup in rat spinal neurones in vitro. *J Neurophysiol* 1993;69:1621–1631.

39. Sivilotti LG, Woolf CJ. The contribution of $GABA_A$ and glycine receptors to central sensitization: disinhibition and touch-evoked allodynia in the spinal cord. *J Neurophysiol* 1994;72:169–179.

40. Strassman AM, Raymond SA, Burstein R. Sensitization of meningeal sensory neurons and the origin of headaches. *Nature* 1996;384:560–564.

41. Stubhaug A, Breivik H, Eide PK, Kreunen M, Foss A. Mapping of punctuate hyperalgesia around a surgical incision demonstrate that ketamine is a powerful suppressor of central sensitization to pain following surgery. *Acta Anaesthesiol Scand* 1997;41:1124–1132.

42. Tfelt-Hansen P, Lous I, Olesen J. Prevalence and significant of muscle tenderness during common migraine attack. *Headache* 1981;21:49–54.

43. Torebjork HE, Lundberg LER, LaMotte RH. Central changes in processing of mechanoreceptor input in capsaicin-induced sensory hyperalgesia in humans. *J Physiol (Lond)* 1992;448:765–780.

44. Waldmann R, Champigny G, Bassilana F, Heurteaux C, Lazdunski M. A proton-gated cation channel involved in acid-sensing. *Nature* 1997;13;386:173–177

45. Willis WD, Coggeshall RE. Sensory mechanisms of the spinal cord. New York: Plenum Press, 1991,132–148.

46. Wolff HG, Tunis MM, Goodell H. Studies on headache: evidence of tissue damage and changes in pain sensitivity in subjects with vascular headaches of the migraine type. *Arch Intern Med* 1953;92:478–484.

47. Woolf CJ. Evidence for a central component of post-injury pain hypersensitivity. *Nature* 1983;306:686–688.

48. Woolf CJ. Somatic pain—pathogenesis and prevention. *Br J Anaesth* 1995;75:169–176.

49. Woolf CJ, Doubell TP. The pathophysiology of chronic pain—increased sensitivity to low threshold Ab-fibre inputs. *Curr Opin Neurobiol* 1994;4:525–534.

50. Woolf CJ, King AE. Dynamic alterations in the cutaneous mechanoreceptive fields of dorsal horn neurons in the rat spinal cord. *J Neurosci* 1990;10:2717–2726.

51. Woolf CJ, Wall PD. The relative effectiveness of C primary afferent fibres of different origins in evoking a prolonged facilitation of the flexor reflex in the rat. *J Neurosci* 1986;6:1433–1443.

52. Yaksh TL. Behavioural and autonomic correlates of the tactile evoked allodynia produced by spinal glycine inhibition: effect of modulatory receptor systems and excitatory amino acid antagonists. *Pain* 1989;37:111–123.

53. Yaksh TL, Jessell TM, Gamse R, Mudge AW, Leeman SE. Intrathecal morphine inhibits substance P release from mammalian spinal cord in vivo. *Nature* 1980;286:155–157.

54. Zorumski CF, Izumi Y. Nitric oxide and hippocampal synaptic plasticity. *Biochem Pharmacol* 1993;46:777–785.

The Headaches, Second Edition,
edited by J. Olesen, P. Tfelt-Hansen, and K.M.A. Welch.
Lippincott Williams & Wilkins, Philadelphia © 2000.

Basic Science Aspects of the Headaches

CHAPTER 16

Serotonin Receptors

Relevance to Migraine Pathogenesis and Treatment

Edith Hamel

The indoleamine serotonin (5-hydroxytryptamine, 5-HT) is broadly distributed in the nervous system, is found in blood platelets and mast cells, and among its many functions has been implicated in the pathophysiology of migraine headache (see Chapter 39). To exert its actions, 5-HT interacts with multiple receptors localized on the membrane of a variety of cells from different organs, spanning from neurons located in the central and peripheral nervous systems to the endothelial and smooth-muscle cells of blood vessels. The ability of 5-HT or 5-HT-related compounds to induce migraine attacks, prevent them when used in prophylaxis, or acutely abort the migraine-associated symptoms has brought new impetus in the understanding of the role of 5-HT and its receptors in the etiology and treatment of migraine headache. These apparently opposite effects of 5-HT in migraine possibly could be explained by its interaction with distinct 5-HT receptors which, depending on subtype, localization, and time of activation in the migraine process, could lead to different responses. In recent years, research has focused primarily on specific subtypes of the 5-HT$_1$ and 5-HT$_2$ receptor families but also, at least more recently, on the 5-HT$_7$ receptor; and unprecedented progress has been made in the understanding of the neurobiology and treatment of migraine headache. These advances, together with their strengths and weaknesses in view of the current thinking about migraine pathogenesis

and treatment, are highlighted in this chapter. Other recent reviews on this aspect can be consulted (23,37).

SEROTONIN RECEPTORS: MULTIPLICITY AND CLASSIFICATION

The complexity of the 5-HT receptors was first recognized pharmacologically, and the development of new receptor ligands that selectively interact with specific receptors has been of great help in the understanding of the heterogeneity and function of many of the presently known 5-HT receptors. Pharmacologic identification of 5-HT receptors has proven restrictive, however, with regard to species differences and subtle differences in affinity profiles for the ligands that are available. As a result, unequivocal discrimination cannot always be readily achieved between receptors that share similar functional and transductional characteristics (29). In this respect, molecular biology has brought tremendous progress in the field of 5-HT receptors with the cloning of several pharmacologically identified, suspected, and even unsuspected 5-HT receptors (for reviews, see refs. 11,27,28,29,43). Most of all, the advent of gene cloning techniques provided a means to distinguish 5-HT receptors on the basis of their protein primary structure (27,29,37). Currently, as recommended by the International Union of Pharmacology (IUPHAR) (27,29), seven families (5-HT$_1$ to 5-HT$_7$) of 5-HT receptors are recognized. With the exception of the 5-HT$_3$ receptor, which is a ligand-gated ion channel, all others are G-protein–coupled receptors with seven transmembrane domains (Fig. 1). All receptor subtypes

E. Hamel: Department of Neurology and Neurosurgery, Montreal Neurological Institute, McGill Unversity, Montréal, Québec H3A 2B4, Canada.

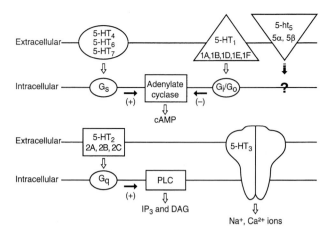

FIG. 1. Schematic representation of the different serotonin (*5-HT*) receptor families and subtypes with their positive (+) and negative (−) coupling to the main transduction systems. Signaling occurs through activation of specific G-proteins and interaction with adenylate cyclase or phospholipase C (*PLC*) for all but the 5-HT$_3$ receptor, which is an ion-gated channel. (Modified from ref. 11, with permission.)

within each family are structurally related and coupled to the same primary effector system. Novel 5-HT receptors and more allelic variants still may be discovered, but so far the 5-HT$_1$ (5-HT$_{1A}$, 5-HT$_{1B}$, 5-HT$_{1D}$, 5-HT$_{1E}$, and 5-HT$_{1F}$) and 5-HT$_2$ (5-HT$_{2A}$, 5-HT$_{2B}$, and 5-HT$_{2C}$) receptor families are the most heterogeneous (see Fig. 1).

SEROTONIN RECEPTORS AND MIGRAINE

5-HT$_{2B}$ Receptors in Migraine Pathogenesis

Although the exact role of 5-HT in the pathogenesis of migraine headache remains unknown, it has been hypothesized that the optimal goal in migraine management may be to stabilize 5-HT neurotransmission (45). It is likely, however, that both neuronal and platelet (58) (see also Chapter 33) stores of 5-HT are mobilized during a migraine episode. Indeed, the current working hypothesis for a role of 5-HT$_2$ receptors in migraine pathogenesis may provide arguments to support a role for 5-HT, irrespective of its neuronal or circulating origin, in the triggering events that culminate in a migraine attack. It is noteworthy that a landmark characteristic of some of the most commonly used compounds in migraine prophylaxis, namely pizotifen, methysergide, cyproheptadine, amitriptyline, mianserin, chlorpromazine, and propranolol, is their antagonistic behavior at specific subtypes of the 5-HT$_2$ receptor family, now known as the 5-HT$_{2B}$/5-HT$_{2C}$ (formerly 5-HT$_{1C}$) receptors (18,20,21, 33,47). This characteristic is also in line with previous observations that the 5-HT$_2$ receptor agonist m-chloro-phenylpiperazine (m-CPP) can trigger typical migraine

attacks in susceptible persons when it is administered at doses that yield plasma concentrations compatible with activation of 5-HT$_{2B/2C}$ receptors (5).

In attempts to discriminate which 5-HT$_2$ receptor is involved in migraine pathogenesis, a prevalent role for 5-HT$_{2B}$ over the 5-HT$_{2C}$ receptor subtype was implied pharmacologically by (a) the lack of clinical efficacy of the 5-HT$_{2A/2C}$ receptor antagonist ketanserin, (b) the preserved antimigraine activity of (+)-propanolol, which exhibits comparable affinity at 5-HT$_{2B}$ but a considerably lower one at 5-HT$_{2C}$ receptors than racemic propranolol (21,33,47), and (b) the similarity in the pharmacologic profile of the m-CPP sensitive 5-HT$_2$ receptor and the 5-HT$_{2B}$ receptor mediating, via release of nitric oxide (NO), the endothelium-dependent dilation of peripheral blood vessels (19). These observations led to the hypothesis that activation of endothelial 5-HT$_{2B}$ receptors in brain vessels is a key factor in the pathogenesis of migraine headache (18,21,33 (Fig. 2).

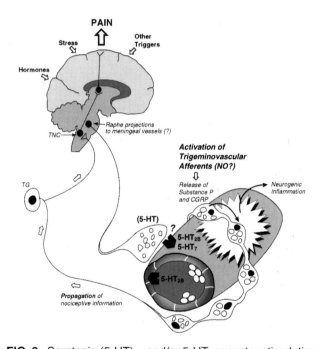

FIG. 2. Serotonin (5-HT)$_{2B}$ and/or 5-HT$_7$ receptor stimulation as an initiating event in migraine headache. The possibility that neurogenic inflammation develops following activation of trigeminovascular afferents by nitric oxide (*NO*) generated from stimulation of endothelial 5-HT$_{2B}$ receptors in brain vessels, which would lead to pain generation and propagation centrally, has received experimental support. 5-HT$_{2B}$ receptors, however, are also present on smooth muscle, and their role remains to be elucidated. 5-HT from both neuronal and platelet (shown in the lumen of the vessel) stores could be mobilized to activate these receptors (see text for details). The 5-HT$_7$ receptor on the smooth muscle also may participate in the dilatation induced by 5-HT in the migraine process (see text for additional details). *TNC*, trigeminalis nucleus caudalis; *TG*, trigeminal ganglion. (Inspired from ref. 20.)

**Endothelial 5-HT$_{2B}$ Receptors in Human Brain
Vessels: the NO Connection**

The aforementioned scenario implies the existence of
an endothelial 5-HT$_{2B}$ receptor mediating vasodilation
via NO synthesis and release in human brain vessels.
Although pharmacologic and functional studies in human
brain vessels to prove this point are lacking, a body of circumstantial evidence tends to support the hypothesis, the
most important being the selective expression of the 5-
HT$_{2B}$ receptor and the corresponding lack of a 5-HT$_{2C}$
receptor message in human brain vessels (4,8,47) and,
more specifically although not exclusively, in human
brain endothelial cells and in smooth-muscle cells (4,8).
In addition, functional studies in the pig anterior cerebral
artery have shown that the 5-HT$_2$ receptor agonist 1-(2,5-
dimethoxy-4-iodophenyl)-2-aminopropane (DOI) induced
a small (about 15% of induced tone) dose-dependent
vasodilation that was sensitive to the nitric oxide synthase
(NOS) inhibitor L-nitroarginine but not to 5-HT$_{2A/2C}$
receptor blockade (47). Because endothelial denuded
vessels were not used in this study, the origin for NO
could not be confirmed. Recently, however, it was shown
that 5-HT can promote the release of NO from human
brain endothelial cell cultures (4), which suggests that an
NO-mediated cerebral vasodilation could possibly occur
in human cerebral blood vessels on activation of endothelial 5-HT receptors. Further investigations with selective
5-HT$_{2B}$ receptor compounds will be required to confirm
that the hypothesis is fully sustainable in human cerebral
blood vessels.

A most interesting aspect of this hypothesis is its ability to unify activation of cerebrovascular 5-HT$_{2B}$ receptors
with the observation that migraine sufferers may be supersensitive to NO (40,41) (see Chapter 40). More specifically, it has been argued that endothelial NO is the
common denominator for spontaneous as well as pharmacologically induced headaches (53). In spontaneous
migraines, in which an increase in serotonin levels may
prevail (45), endothelial 5-HT$_{2B}$ receptors activation could
increase NO production and release and start the process
of vascular neurogenic inflammation thought to be crucial
for the development of migraine headache (17,39) (see
Chapter 17). NO, once released from the endothelial cells,
can diffuse to the smooth muscle layer to induce dilation
and also has the potential to activate trigeminovascular
sensory nerve terminals that contain substance P and calcitonin gene-related peptide (CGRP) (56), both neuropeptides being actively involved in the manifestation and
transmission of head pain (see Fig. 2). The recent success
of a nonselective NOS inhibitor in the treatment of
migraine headache (35) supports this hypothesis even
though the source of NO still needs to be confirmed by
additional studies with selective inhibitors of the endothelial, neuronal, or inducible isoform of NOS.

In conclusion, the possibility that serotonin may be a
contributing factor in the generation of headache pain,
through interaction with a 5-HT$_{2B}$ receptor strategically
located in meningeal blood vessels, is supported by pharmacologic and molecular evidence. The dual localization
of 5-HT$_{2B}$ receptors on cerebrovascular smooth muscle
and endothelial cells may reveal a previously unsuspected
locus of action for 5-HT in migraine initiation, depending
on its site of release and its ability to interact with available receptors. In this respect, endothelial 5-HT$_{2B}$ receptors could be activated by 5-HT released in the blood-
stream after platelet activation, whereas those located on
the smooth muscle would represent a privileged target for
5-HT released from perivascular nerve terminals,
whether of central or peripheral origin (8). Whether a
contributing dysfunction in migraine sufferers resides in
their vascular or trigeminovascular reactions to 5-HT or
NO (49) or, alternatively, in disturbances in 5-HT neurotransmission at the time of an attack (57) still remains a
highly pertinent question. Further, the relatively long
delay (hours) for a migraine to develop after the administration of drugs like m-CPP or nitroglycerin remains
unexplained and may suggest that still unknown mechanisms need to be identified. The development of selective
5-HT$_{2B}$ receptor antagonists will be an essential step in
this effort (16). Their venue may help to identify the
respective roles of the endothelial and muscular 5-HT$_{2B}$
receptors and should increase our overall understanding
of the role of 5-HT in the initiation of a migraine attack.
A potential drawback in this type of compound is that the
5-HT$_{2B}$ receptors appear to be distributed ubiquitously in
human blood vessels; therefore, selectivity of action, if
needed, may be difficult to achieve.

5-HT$_7$ Receptors in Migraine Pathogenesis

Recently, the 5-HT$_7$ receptor was identified as a receptor able to mediate cerebrovascular smooth-muscle dilatation through an endothelium-independent mechanism, as
demonstrated in peripheral blood vessels (12,51). A putative role of the 5-HT$_7$ receptor in the regulation of cerebrovascular tone and migrane has been advanced on the
basis of (a) the ability of 5-HT to produce smooth-muscle
relaxation in dog basilar and middle cerebral arteries
through a receptor with a pharmacologic profile that corresponds closely to that of the 5-HT$_7$ receptor (50); (b) the
relatively high affinity of most of the antimigraine prophylactic 5-HT receptor antagonists at the cloned 5-HT$_7$
receptor (51); and (c) the high expression of 5-HT$_7$ tran-
scripts in both animal (54) and human (8,47) brain vessels
(52). Expression of 5-HT$_7$ receptor mRNA has been
shown together with an increase in cyclic adenosine
monophosphate (cAMP) levels in cultured smooth-muscle cells from human brain vessels (8); it is thus possible
that a similar relaxant mechanism operates in human

brain vessels. Such a mechanism would provide a means by which perivascular serotonergic nerve terminals, which are located at the adventitial–medial border (see Fig. 2), could directly elicit dilatation of meningeal blood vessels without a need for interaction with the endothelial compartment. Interestingly, correlation analyses similar to those reported above for the 5-HT$_{2B}$ receptor also demonstrate a highly significant relationship ($r = 0.99$; $p < 0.005$) between the affinity of several antimigraine prophylactic compounds at the recombinant 5-HT$_7$ receptor and their clinically effective doses (Terron, personal communication). These recent observations may highlight a new role for 5-HT$_7$ receptors in human brain vessels during dysfunction of the neurovascular serotonergic system, if indeed they do occur during a migraine episode (see Chapter 39).

5-HT$_1$ RECEPTORS IN MIGRAINE SYMPTOMATIC TREATMENT

The most spectacular advance in our understanding of the mechanisms underlying migraine headache has been the discovery of the 5-HT$_1$ receptor agonist sumatriptan as a highly effective antimigraine compound (10,30). Although originally developed to induce contraction of putatively distended cranial blood vessels (7,22), sumatriptan also was found to interact presynaptically with receptors on trigeminovascular afferents whose activation has proven particularly important in the development of meningeal neurogenic inflammation and hence migraine pain (6,39) (see Chapter 17). Sumatriptan-sensitive sites of action in the pain-transmitting pathway have been identified centrally and suggested as additional putative antimigraine targets for brain penetrant triptan derivatives (48). Sumatriptan has high affinity for 5-HT$_{1B}$, 5-HT$_{1D}$, and 5-HT$_{1F}$ receptor subtypes (9), and the recent development of 5-HT$_1$ receptor subtype-specific compounds and antibodies has allowed a relatively precise identification of its vascular and neuronal sites of action, thereby providing a basis for a more targeted therapeutic approach (see Fig. 3).

Vascular 5-HT$_{1B}$ Receptors

The 5-HT$_{1B}$ (formerly 5-HT$_{1D\beta}$) receptor originally was identified as the target for sumatriptan in human cerebral blood vessels on the basis of pharmacologic studies showing a stronger positive correlation between the profile of the vascular 5-HT$_1$ receptor mediating cerebral contraction and that of the cloned human 5-HT$_{1B}$, as opposed to the 5-HT$_{1D}$ (then known as 5-HT$_{1D\alpha}$), receptor (9,25,26,34). Additional investigations provided a definite answer in showing expression of 5-HT$_{1B}$, but not 5-HT$_{1D}$, receptor mRNA (2,26) and protein (36) in human brain vessels. In addition to 5-HT$_{1B}$ receptors, mRNA

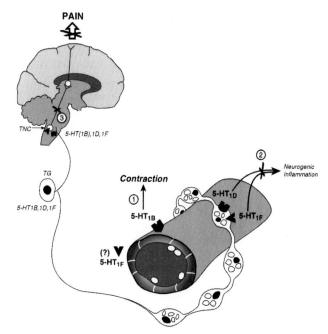

FIG. 3. Schematic representation of the putative sites of action for serotonin (*5-HT*)$_1$ receptor compounds in the symptomatic treatment of migraine headache. Activation of postsynaptic 5-HT$_{1B}$ receptors on vascular smooth muscle will result in contraction of putatively distended blood vessels ①. Presynaptically, activation of 5-HT$_{1D}$ or 5-HT$_{1F}$ receptors on trigeminovascular afferents will block the release of substance P and calcitonin gene-related peptide (*CGRP*) and hence the development of neurogenic inflammation ②, which will block the generation and propagation of pain. In the trigeminalis nucleus caudalis (*TNC*), presynatic and postsynaptic 5-HT$_1$ receptors have been identified and could interrupt the transmission of pain centrally ③; these sites represent additional targets for brain-penetrant compounds. 5-HT$_{1F}$ receptor mRNA is found in isolated human brain vessels, but the role of this receptor, if any (?), remains to be identified. *TG*, trigeminal ganglion (see text for additional details).

expression of sumatriptan-sensitive 5-HT$_{1F}$ receptors was detected in human cerebral vessels (2). This receptor, however, has been excluded from the 5-HT-mediated cerebral vasoconstriction on the basis of correlation analysis (26,34) and, more recently, lack of contractile effect of a selective 5-HT$_{1F}$ receptor agonist in the rabbit saphenous vein (32), a tissue that shares a similar contractile 5-HT receptor as that of human cerebral arteries.

Sumatriptan also can induce contraction of human coronary arteries, an effect most likely mediated by the 5-HT$_{1B}$ receptor, which is expressed (3,31) and functional (see 15) in this artery. Without being the only explanation for some of the undesirable side effects encountered with sumatriptan with respect to the cardiovascular system, the presence of 5-HT$_{1B}$ contractile receptors at this level has surely contributed to recent efforts aimed at developing novel compounds that would be deprived of such activity.

Neuronal 5-HT$_1$ Receptors: Possibility for Peripheral and Central Sites of Action

Peripheral 5-HT$_1$ Receptors on Trigeminovascular Afferents

Moskowitz and colleagues extensively studied the implication of the trigeminovascular system in the manifestation of migraine pain (for additional details, see Chapter 17). Their work contributed significantly to challenging the importance of the vascular effect of sumatriptan while enhancing a possible neuronal locus of action that involves blockade of nociceptive information. They originally reported that sumatriptan, through inhibitory presynaptic 5-HT$_1$ receptors located on trigeminovascular afferents, could block the release of substance P and CGRP, and thus the development of neurogenic inflammation (6). This observation in an animal model gained much credibility when studies in humans provided evidence for the activation of the trigeminovascular system during migraine headache. In addition, the elevated CGRP levels in venous blood were found to normalize in parallel with headache relief after administration of sumatriptan in patients with migraine (24) and cluster headache (14).

The nature of the 5-HT$_1$ receptor(s) mediating the effect of sumatriptan at these presynaptic sites has not been convincingly identified. The presence of both 5-HT$_{1B}$ and 5-HT$_{1D}$ receptor mRNAs (2) and proteins (36) has been demonstrated in human trigeminal ganglia. However, in centrally (trigeminalis nucleus caudalis; see also next section) and peripherally (meningeal blood vessels) located nerve terminals of trigeminal ganglion neurons, only 5-HT$_{1D}$ receptor could be immunocytochemically demonstrated in humans (36). This finding strongly indicates that the 5-HT$_{1D}$ receptor subtype is most likely a presynaptic receptor targeted by sumatriptan in controlling neurogenic inflammation. In the guinea pig, which has been used as a reliable model of human 5-HT$_{1B/1D}$ trigeminovascular receptors, 5-HT$_{1B}$ receptor mRNA is colocalized with substance P and CGRP mRNAs in trigeminal ganglion neurons, whereas 5-HT$_{1D}$ receptor message is colocalized with message for CGRP but not substance P (1). This observation led to the suggestion that if selective 5-HT$_{1D}$ receptor agonists are proven to be effective antimigraine drugs, this finding would lend support for a primary important role of CGRP and its vasodilatory effects in the manifestation of migraine pain.

In addition to 5-HT$_{1B}$ and 5-HT$_{1D}$ receptor subtypes, 5-HT$_{1F}$ receptor mRNA has been detected in human trigeminal ganglia (2). Selective 5-HT$_{1F}$ receptor agonists recently were shown to block effectively the trigeminovascular-mediated neurogenic inflammation in the rat and guinea pig while having no vasocontractile properties in the rabbit shaphenous vein (32,44). Sumatriptan-sensitive 5-HT$_{1F}$ receptors may thus prove to be an interesting new presynaptic target for the acute treatment of migraine headache, because they also should be devoid of any vasocontractile effect at the human 5-HT$_{1B}$ vascular receptor (26,34) and thus reduce cardiovascular side effects. The availability of selective 5-HT$_{1F}$ receptor agonists and the results of clinical trials will be awaited to establish their utility in the treatment of migraine headache. Compounds with relatively low or no affinity for the 5-HT$_{1F}$ receptor (e.g. alniditan, IS-159) have proven to be effective antimigraine compounds in clinical trials, an observation that may suggest that activation of the 5-HT$_{1F}$ receptor may not be an exclusive locus of action for interruption of migraine headache.

Central 5-HT$_1$ Receptors in the Trigeminalis Nucleus Caudalis

An additional level of interest in the acute treatment of migraine headache has been the cells located centrally in the trigeminalis nucleus caudalis that transduce intracranial nociceptive information to higher integrative centers. These cells represent an attractive neuronal therapeutic target that could be dissociated from vascular effects. Interestingly, binding sites that recognize 5-HT$_1$ receptor compounds, such as sumatriptan, have been localized at this level in humans (42) and in guinea pigs, where they have been shown to correspond to 5-HT$_{1B}$, 5-HT$_{1D}$, and 5-HT$_{1F}$ receptor subtypes (55). On the basis of receptor binding sites, proteins, and mRNA localization, it has been argued that 5-HT$_{1B/1D}$ (55), or exclusively 5-HT$_{1D}$ (36), would be primarily presynaptic receptors, whereas 5-HT$_{1F}$ receptors would be located postsynaptically on local neurons (55). In a recent physiological study in the cat, both evoked and spontaneous firing of trigeminalis caudalis neurons could be inhibited by locally delivered triptan derivatives (48). Together, these findings support the view that central presynaptic or postsynaptic 5-HT$_1$ receptors are potential sites of action for the new generation of brain penetrant triptan derivatives (e.g.,naratriptan, zolmitriptan, rizatriptan) (see Chapter 39). Identification of the exact nature of these central receptors will be possible when selective receptor subtype compounds become available. Additional 5-HT$_1$ receptors in the nucleus tractus solitarius and area prostrema (42), regions that are devoid of blood–brain barrier, could be accessible even to non–brain-penetrant compounds such as sumatriptan and potentially explain some of their antiemetic effects.

In conclusion, current evidence indicates that the vasocontractile effect of the triptans is mediated by 5-HT$_{1B}$ receptors, whereas the 5-HT$_1$ receptor located presynaptically on trigeminovascular afferents seem to correspond to a 5-HT$_{1D}$ or 5-HT$_{1F}$ receptor or both (Fig. 3). Exclusion of a presynaptic trigeminovascular 5-HT$_{1B}$ receptor in humans is based on the immunocytochemical demonstration that only 5-HT$_{1D}$ receptors could be found at the peripheral and central projection area of trigeminal ganglion neurons (36). The exact nature of the putative central locus of action of brain-penetrant triptans remains to be determined. The recent and forthcoming development of 5-HT receptor subtype-specific compounds (see Chapter 39) will help to identify which receptor subtype is involved and where it is located and may yield drugs selective for the neuronal sites that are free of vascular actions. The benefit of such drugs as well as of those acting centrally over nonselective and peripherally acting 5-HT$_1$ receptor agonists still remains to be clinically demonstrated. Before prescribing brain-penetrant compounds on a regular basis, it should be considered that 5-HT$_{1B/1D}$ receptors are broadly distributed centrally in the human brain (42) and, more specifically, are also present in human brain intraparenchymal microvessels (8,46), in which 5-HT is able to elicit vasomotor responses (13). Although activation of these central receptors may not be of consideration on an acute basis, it may become relevant in patients who are regular consumers of this type of medication.

ACKNOWLEDGMENT

I thank the Medical Research Council of Canada and the Heart and Stroke Foundation of Québec for supporting the work performed in my laboratory. More specifically, the work and comments of I. Bouchelet, Z. Cohen, and A. Elhusseiny are greatly acknowledged as well as Dr. M. J. Moreno for reviewing the manuscript and Ms L. Michel for preparing it.

REFERENCES

1. Bonaventure P, Voorn P, Luyten WHML, Leysen JE. 5HT$_{1B}$ and 5HT$_{1D}$ receptor mRNA differential co-localization with peptide mRNA in the guinea pig trigeminal ganglion. *Neuroreport* 1998;9:641–645.
2. Bouchelet I, Cohen Z, Case B, Séguéla P, Hamel E. Differential expression of sumatriptan-sensitive 5-hydroxytryptamine receptors in human trigeminal ganglia and cerebral blood vessels. *Mol Pharmacol* 1996;50:219–223.
3. Bouchelet I, Cohen Z, Séguéla P, Hamel E. Differential expression of sumatriptan-sensitive 5-HT$_1$ receptors in human neuronal and vascular tissues. In: Sandler M, Ferrari M, Harnett S, eds. *Migraine: pharmacology and genetics.* New York: Chapman & Hall, 1996;55–66.
4. Bouchelet I, Cohen Z, Stanimirovic D, Hamel E. Endothelial 5-HT$_{2B}$, but not 5-HT$_{2C}$, receptors in human brain vessels: possible role in migraine headache. *J Cereb Blood Flow Metab* 1997;17(Suppl 1): S351.
5. Brewerton TD, Murphy DL, Mueller EA, Jimerson DC. Induction of migraine-like headaches by the serotonin agonist m-chlorophenylpiperazine. *Clin Pharmacol Ther* 1988;43:605–609.
6. Buzzi MG, Moskowitz MA, Peroutka SJ, Byun B. Further characterization of the putative 5-HT receptor which mediates blockade of neurogenic plasma extravasation in rat dura mater. *Br J Pharmacol* 1991;103:1421–1428.
7. Caekebeke JFV, Ferrari MD, Zwetsloot CP, Jansen J, Saxena PR. Antimigraine drug sumatriptan increase blood flow velocity in large cerebral arteries during migraine attacks. *Neurology* 1992;42: 1522–1526.
8. Cohen Z, Bonvento G, Lacombe P, Hamel E. Serotonin in the regulation of brain microcirculation. *Prog Neurobiol* 1996;50:335–362.
9. Connor HE, Beattie DT. 5-Hydroxytryptamine receptor subtypes and

10. Doenicke A, Brand J, Perrin VL. Possible benefit of GR43175, a novel 5-HT$_1$-like receptor agonist, for the acute treatment of severe migraine. *Lancet* 1988;1:1309–1311.
11. Eglen RM. An overview of current 5-hydroxytryptamine receptor research. *ID Research Alerts Serotonin* 1996;1:13–18.
12. Eglen RM, Jasper JR, Chang DJ, Martin GR. The 5-HT$_7$ receptor: orphan found. *Trends Pharmacol Sci* 1997;18:104–107.
13. Elhusseiny A, Hamel E. Vasomotor effects of acetylcholine and serotonin in human and bovine brain intracortical arterioles. *Soc Neurosci Abst* 1998;24:1172(abst 461.9).
14. Fanciullacci M, Alessandri M, Figini M, Geppetti P, Michelacci S. Increase in plasma calcitonin gene-related peptide from the extracerebral circulation during nitroglycerin-induced cluster headache attack. *Pain* 1995;60:119–123.
15. Ferro A, Longmore J, Hill RG, Brown MJ. A comparison of the contractile effects of 5-hydroxytryptamine, sumatriptan and MK-462 on human coronary artery in vitro. *Br J Clin Pharmacol* 1995;40: 245–251.
16. Forbes IT, Ham P, Booth DH, et al. 5-Methyl-1-(3-pyridylcarbamoyl)-1,2,3,5-tetrahydropyrrolo[2,3-f]indole: a novel 5-HT$_{2C}$/5-HT$_{2B}$ receptor antagonist with improved affinity, selectivity, and oral activity. *J Med Chem* 1995;38:2524–2530.
17. Fozard JR. The pharmacological basis of migraine treatment. In: Blau JN, ed. *Migraine: clinical and research aspects.* Baltimore: The Johns Hopkins University Press, 1987;165–184.
18. Fozard JR. 5-HT$_{1C}$ receptor agonism as an initiating event in migraine. In: Olesen J, Saxena PR, eds. *5-Hydroxytryptamine mechanisms in primary headaches.* New York: Raven Press, 1992;200–212.
19. Fozard JR. 5-Hydroxytryptamine and nitric oxide: the causal relationship between two endogenous precipitants of migraine. In: Sandler M, Ferrari M, Harnett S, eds. *Migraine: pharmacology and genetics.* New York: Chapman & Hall, 1996;167–179.
20. Fozard JR, Gray JA. 5-HT$_{1C}$ receptor activation: a key step in the initiation of migraine? *Trends Pharmacol Sci* 1989;10:307–309.
21. Fozard JR, Kalkman HO. 5-Hydroxytryptamine (5-HT) and the initiation of migraine: new perspectives. *Naunyn Schmiedebergs Arch Pharmacol* 1994;350:225–229.
22. Friberg L, Olesen J, Iversen HK, Sperling B. Migraine pain associated with middle cerebral artery dilatation: reversal by sumatriptan. *Lancet* 1991;338:13–17.
23. Goadsby PJ. How do the currently used prophylactic agents work in migraine? *Cephalalgia* 1997;17:85–92.
24. Goadsby PJ, Edvinsson L. The trigeminovascular system and migraine: studies characterizing cerebrovascular and neuropeptide changes seen in humans and cats. *Ann Neurol* 1993;33:48–56.
25. Hamel E, Bouchard D. Contractile 5-HT$_1$ receptors in human isolated pial arterioles: correlation with 5-HT$_{1D}$ binding sites. *Br J Pharmacol* 1991;102:227–233.
26. Hamel E, Fan E, Linville D, Ting V, Villemure J-G, Chia L-S. Expression of mRNA for the serotonin 5-hydroxytryptamine$_{1D\beta}$ receptor subtype in human and bovine cerebral arteries. *Mol Pharmacol* 1993;44: 242–246.
27. Hartig PR, Hoyer D, Humphrey PPA, Martin GR. Alignment of receptor nomenclature with the human genome: classification of 5-HT$_{1B}$ and 5-HT$_{1D}$ receptor subtypes. *Trends Pharmacol Sci* 1996;17:103–105.
28. Hoyer D, Clarke DE, Fozard JR, et al. International union of pharmacology classification of receptors for 5-hydroxytryptamine (serotonin). *Pharmacol Rev* 1994;46:157–203.
29. Hoyer D, Martin GR. Classification and nomenclature of 5-HT receptors: a comment on current issues. *Behav Brain Res* 1996;73:263–268.
30. Humphrey PPA, Feniuk W. Mode of action of the anti-migraine drug sumatriptan. *Trends Pharmacol Sci* 1991;12:444–446.
31. Ishida T, Hirata K, Sakoda T, et al. 5-HT$_{1Dbeta}$ receptor mediates the supersensitivity of isolated coronary artery to serotonin in variant angina. *Chest* 1998;113:243–244.
32. Johnson KW, Schaus JM, Durkin MM, et al. 5-HT$_{1F}$ receptor agonists inhibit neurogenic dural inflammation in guinea pigs. *Neuroreport* 1997;8:2237–2240.
33. Kalkman HO. Is migraine prophylactic activity caused by 5-HT$_{2B}$ or 5-HT$_{2C}$ receptor blockade? *Life Sci* 1994;54:641–644.
34. Kaumann AJ, Parsons AA, Brown AM. Human arterial constrictor serotonin receptors. *Cardiovasc Res* 1993;27:2094–2103.

35. Lassen LH, Ashina M, Christiansen I, et al. Nitric oxide synthase inhibition: a new principle in the treatment of migraine attacks. *Cephalalgia* 1998;18:27–32.
36. Longmore J, Shaw D, Smith D, et al. Differential distribution of 5HT$_{1D}$- and 5HT$_{1B}$- immunoreactivity within the human trigemino-cerebrovascular system: implications for the discovery of new antimigraine drugs. *Cephalalgia* 1997;17:833–842.
37. Martin GR. Serotonin receptor involvement in the pathogenesis and treatment of migraine. In: Silberstein S, Goadsby PJ, eds. *Headache blue books of practical neurology*, Vol 17. Butterworth-Heineman, 1997;25–38.
38. Massen VanDenBrink AM, Bax WA, Ferrari MD, Zijlstra FJ, Bos E, Saxena PR. Augmented contraction of the human isolated coronary artery by sumatriptan: a possible role for endogenous thromboxane. *Br J Pharmacol* 1996;119:855–862.
39. Moskowitz MA. Neurogenic versus vascular mechanisms of sumatriptan and ergot alkaloids in migraine. *Trends Pharmacol Sci* 1992;13:307–311.
40. Olesen J, Iversen HK, Thomsen LL. Nitric oxide supersensitivity: a possible molecular mechanism of migraine pain. *Neuroreport* 1993;4:1027–1030.
41. Olesen J, Thomsen LL, Iversen HK. Nitric oxide is a key molecule in migraine and other vascular headaches. *Trends Pharmacol Sci* 1994;15:149–153.
42. Pascual J, del Arco D, Romon T, del Olmo E, Castro E, Pazos A. Autoradiographic distribution of [^{3}H]sumatriptan-binding sites in postmortem human brain. *Cephalalgia* 1996;16:317–322.
43. Peroutka SJ. Molecular biology of serotonin (5-HT) receptors. *Synapse* 1994;18:241–260.
44. Phebus LA, Johnson KW, Zgombick JM, et al. Characterization of LY344864 as a pharmacological tool to study 5-HT$_{1F}$ receptors: binding affinities, brain penetration and activity in the neurogenic dural inflammation model of migraine. *Life Sci* 1997;61:2117–2126.
45. Raskin NH. Acute and prophylactic treatment of migraine: practical approaches and pharmacologic rationale. *Neurology* 1993;43(Suppl 3):S39–S42.
46. Riad M, Tong X, El Mestikawy S, Hamon M, Hamel E, Descarries L. Endothelial expression of the 5-HT$_{1B}$ antimigraine drug receptor in rat and human brain microvessels. *Neuroscience* 1998;86:1031–1035 .
47. Schmuck K, Ullmer C, Kalkman HO, Probst A, Lubbert H. Activation of meningeal 5-HT$_{2B}$ receptors: an early step in the generation of migraine headache? *Eur J Neurosci* 1996;8:959–967.
48. Storer RJ, Goadsby PJ. Microiontophoretic application of serotonin (5HT)$_{1B/1D}$ agonists inhibits trigeminal cell firing in the cat. *Brain* 1997;120:2171–2177.
49. Strassman AM, Raymond SA, Burstein R. Sensitization of meningeal sensory neurons and the origin of headaches. *Nature* 1996;384:560–564.
50. Terron JA. Evidence for the putative 5-HT$_7$ receptor mediating direct relaxation to 5-hydroxytryptamine in canine cerebral blood vessels. *Ann NY Acad Sci* 1998;861:283.
51. Terron JA. The 5-HT$_7$ receptor: a target for novel therapeutic avenues? *Drugs* 1998;1:302–310.
52. Terron JA. Involvement of the 5-HT$_7$ receptor in cerebrovascular vasodilation: potential impact in migraine. *Proc West Pharmacol Soc* 1998;41:247–251.
53. Thomsen LL, Olesen J. The role of nitric oxide in migraine pain. In: Sandler M, Ferrari M, Harnett S, eds. *Migraine: pharmacology and genetics*. New York: Chapman & Hall, 1996;154–166.
54. Ullmer C, Schmuck K, Kalkman HO, Lubbert H. Expression of serotonin receptor mRNAs in blood vessels. *FEBS Lett* 1995;370:215–221.
55. Waeber C, Moskowitz MA. [^{3}H]sumatriptan labels both 5-HT$_{1D}$ and 5-HT$_{1F}$ receptor binding sites in the guinea pig brain: an autoradiographic study. *Naunyn Schmiedeberg Arch Pharmacol* 1995;352:263–275.
56. Wei EP, Moskowitz MA, Boccalini P, Contos HA. Calcitonin gene-related peptide mediates nitroglycerin and sodium nitroprusside-induced vasodilation in feline cerebral arteries. *Circ Res* 1992;70:1313–1319.
57. Weiller C, May A, Limmroth A, et al. Brain stem activation in spontaneous human migraine attacks. *Nat Med* 1995;1:658–660.
58. Winther K, Hedman C. Platelet function and migraine. In: Olesen J, Edvinsson L, eds. *Basic mechanisms of headache*. London: Elsevier Science Publishers B.V., 1988;301–312.

The Headaches, Second Edition,
edited by J. Olesen, P. Tfelt-Hansen, and K.M.A. Welch.
Lippincott Williams & Wilkins, Philadelphia © 2000.

Basic Science Aspects of the Headaches

CHAPTER 17

The Trigeminal System

Margarita Sanchez del Rio and Michael A. Moskowitz

Headaches, described as throbbing, boring, and often unilateral, constitute an important part of the migraine syndromes (the most troublesome part for most patients). Although extracranial vessels may be involved, it is now acknowledged that most often the pain is transmitted by intracranial perivascular sensory axons. The network of relevant sensory fibers originates in large part from neurons within the trigeminal ganglia and defines the trigeminovascular system, an important substrate and final common pathway for the transmission of vascular headaches. Although the precise cause is unknown, arguments have been advanced that migraine-type headaches develop from multiple causes and signal the presence of real or threatened tissue injury (as in other organs). In headache, the tissues at risk include the brain, the large cephalic blood vessels, and even perivascular nerves themselves.

Sensory fibers exhibit at least two functions: They transmit nociceptive information into brainstem, chiefly the trigeminal nucleus caudalis (TNC), and also promote a sterile inflammatory response within target tissues by releasing vasodilating and permeability-promoting peptides from perivascular nerve endings. In an experimental animal model, one action of the ergot alkaloids, sumatriptan, and the new generation of triptans was identified as blockade of the development of sterile inflammation in the dura mater by inhibiting neuropeptide release. A second effect, perhaps mediated through the same receptor, is to block neural transmission within trigeminovascular fibers. This chapter includes a brief description of the experimental findings leading to these conclusions and their possible importance to headache pathophysiology.

M. Sanchez del Rio and M. A. Moskowitz: Massachusetts General Hospital, Harvard Medical School, Charlestown, Massachusetts 02129.

THE TRIGEMINOVASCULAR SYSTEM

Anatomic tracing (53,54) and immunohistochemistry studies (38) in laboratory animals (including primates and humans) provide unequivocal evidence for the existence of sensory axons innervating cephalic blood vessels. Neuropeptides, such as substance P (SP) (37,54), neurokinin A (NKA) (82), calcitonin gene-related peptide (CGRP) (55), and galanin, are synthesized by messenger RNA and ribosomal mechanisms within trigeminal ganglia cells. The neurons of greatest relevance reside primarily within the ophthalmic division (53,54). Neuropeptides are transported from cells within the first division to a plexus within the adventitial layer of cephalic vessels. At the electron microscopic level, this plexus consists of small-diameter unmyelinated axons characteristic of C-fibers (38,52). Neuropeptide-containing vesicles have been visualized within these axons (19,23,57). Neuropeptide release occurs predominantly from these vesicles by calcium-dependent mechanisms (69). Membrane specializations or synaptic contacts are distinctly unusual.

In all likelihood, trigeminovascular fibers reach the internal carotid artery at the pericarotid plexus within the cavernous sinus and pierce the dura mater to enter the middle cranial fossa along with the carotid artery. Most probably, this plexus is involved to an important extent in cluster headache (68). Within the cranium, trigeminal axons distribute predominantly to the ipsilateral anterior, middle, and posterior cerebral arteries. A few fibers cross to innervate the contralateral anterior cerebral artery. Although single fibers do not send axonal branches to innervate both intracranial and extracranial arteries (64,74), recent studies indicate that trigeminovascular fibers project widely within the cranium so that, for example, the same trigeminal ganglia cell that projects to the middle cerebral artery also sends an axon to innervate the middle meningeal artery (74). The density of sensory axons is greatest along the proximal arteries of the circle of Willis and diminishes considerably over the convexity. The basilar and vertebral arteries contain fibers that arise from the upper cervical ganglia (80); the basilar artery contains sensory fibers that project from the superior vagal ganglia as well (31). Recently, SP- and CGRP-containing neurons were found in a satellite miniganglion located on the carotid artery within the carotid canal. Neurons within this ganglion send axonal projections to innervate large pial arteries (91). This new finding explains why total removal of the trigeminal ganglia in experimental animals does not completely deplete the pial vessels of their sensory neuropeptides. The relationship of this miniganglion to vascular headaches remains to be explored.

Blood vessels of the dura mater, an important pain-sensitive tissue, also receive rich trigeminal and upper cervical projections (17,54,56). All three trigeminal divisions innervate this important brain covering. The middle meningeal artery contains axons primarily from the ipsilateral first trigeminal division, whereas the superior sagittal sinus receives a bilateral innervation. The first and second divisions innervate the dura within the anterior fossa, and the second and third divisions project to the middle cranial fossa, whereas upper cervical nerves as well as vagus and trigeminal ganglia innervate dural structures within the posterior fossa.

Sensory fibers surrounding the middle cerebral and basilar arteries terminate within the trigeminal brainstem nuclear complex, including main sensory nucleus, pars oralis, and pars interpolaris (2). Terminals also are found in the nucleus tractus solitarius, dorsal motor nucleus of the vagus, and ventral periaqueductal gray.

It is important to emphasize that vascular headaches exhibit several features in common with visceral pains originating in other organs, such as the bladder, heart, and bowel. For example, both are poorly localized and diffuse and are referred to superficial organs, such as skin and muscle. Visceral pains and headaches often are accompanied by intense motor and autonomic responses, such as muscle spasms, sweating, and increased heart rate and blood pressure. Furthermore, visceral organs are relatively insensate except for the organ capsule, the meninges providing an example of the brain's capsule. Furthermore, both trigeminovascular and visceral afferents (e.g., lung) possess a multiplicity of axonal receptors, which can block the development of the neurogenic inflammatory response (see the following section).

NEUROGENIC INFLAMMATION

As already noted, vasodilation and plasma extravasation are major components of the inflammatory response that may develop through sensory neurogenic mecha-

nisms. We believe neurogenic inflammation provides a mechanism to explain the changes in blood flow that sometimes develop during the headache phase in patients with classic migraine and to explain the occurrence of hyperalgesia. In the latter instance, sensory nerve fibers become sensitized to previously innocuous stimuli (e.g., vessel pulsations or venous pressure changes). Furthermore, levels of CGRP in venous blood increase in migraine patients and during trigeminal stimulation, probably reflecting neuropeptide release from activated sensory fibers (22) (Fig. 1). It is important to note that neurogenic inflammation is not the cause of migraine headache, nor is it the initiator of pain.

Experimentally, neurogenic inflammation accompanies antidromic electric stimulation of sensory nerves or follows mechanical or chemical stimulation of these same fibers (4,45). This form of sterile inflammation develops independently of central nervous system activity, because the response follows from stimulating the peripheral cut ends of sensory axons. Unmyelinated C-fibers mediate this response. Lewis in 1937 suggested the term *nocifensor system* to recognize the role of neurogenic inflammation as a potent endogenous defense in the early phase of tissue damage. It has been well established that SP (an 11 amino acid-containing peptide), NKA (a decapeptide), and CGRP (a 37 amino acid-containing peptide) released from peripheral sensory axons mediate some or all of neurogenic inflammation (38,84). All three peptides are therefore vasoactive and dilate blood vessels. CGRP is the most potent vasodilator, acting through the activation of receptors on vascular smooth-muscle cells. In addition, SP and NKA, but not CGRP, promote the leakage of albumin from blood vessels, most likely by an action at the postcapillary venule. None of these peptides is capable of disrupting the blood–brain barrier and, because of their size and charge, penetrate the barrier poorly under normal circumstances.

Neurogenic inflammation has been observed in several tissues at portals of entry, including the skin (84), the respiratory tract (41,84), the genitourinary system (42,71), and parts of the gastrointestinal tract (18). It follows that neurogenic inflammation occurs almost exclusively in those tissues possessing neuropeptide-containing fibers innervating blood vessels and can be attenuated by specific receptor blockers (e.g., SP) or by drugs that inhibit the release of neuropeptides from these fibers (95).

Recently, neurogenic inflammation was demonstrated in the dura mater of experimental animals but not in the dura mater of animals in whom C-fibers were previously destroyed (44). As in other tissues, neurogenic inflammation within the dura mater involves the release of vasodilating neuropeptides from capsaicin-sensitive nerve fibers. Released neuropeptides then initiate a cascade of events resulting in the formation of endothelial microvilli, endothelial vesicles, and vacuoles, specifically within postcapillary dural venules; degranulation of

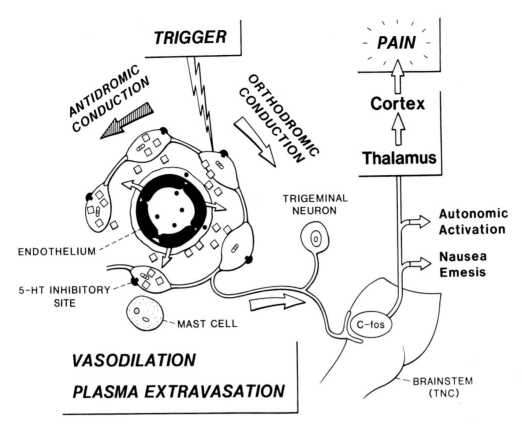

FIG. 1. Pathophysiological mechanism and postulated antinociceptive site for sumatriptan and ergot alkaloids in vascular headaches. The triggers for headache (which remain unknown) activate perivascular trigeminal axons, which release vasoactive neuropeptides to promote neurogenic inflammation (vasodilation, plasma extravasation, mast cell degranulation). Orthodromic and antidromic conduction along trigeminovascular fibers spreads the inflammatory response to adjacent tissues and transmits nociceptive information toward the trigeminal nucleus caudalis and higher brain centers for the registration of pain. Experimental data support the postulation that sumatriptan activates an inhibitory receptor resembling 5-HT$_{1D}$ on perivascular fibers and, in so doing, blocks neuropeptide release and impulse conduction in trigeminovascular neurons, because sumatriptan blocks neurogenic inflammation and inhibits *c-fos* expression within the trigeminal nucleus caudalis, respectively. A receptor site for acute antimigraine drugs, such as sumatriptan, is postulated to reside in the meninges to explain both effects, because sumatriptan penetrates the blood–brain barrier poorly. Molecular studies have confirmed the existence of 5-HT$_{1B/D}$ receptor mRNA within trigeminal ganglion cells. (From ref. 65, with permission.)

mast cells; platelet aggregation and an increase in leakage of plasma from meningeal vessels (14,15). One report documenting that neurogenic edema does not develop in ocular tissues during a migraine or cluster attack in humans supports the conclusion that branches of the trigeminal nerve innervating this organ (and most other trigeminal branches) are not involved in migraine and headache mechanisms (52).

Components of the neurogenic inflammation response develop within the distribution of the trigeminal nerve in humans as well. Local vasodilation was observed in the facial skin of patients during trigeminal ganglion lesion (16,86,92). Numular areas of intense vasodilation develop with thermal or electric stimulation. Furthermore, SP and CGRP levels increase in the jugular veins of patients during thermocoagulation of the trigeminal ganglion (22).

EFFECTS OF ANTIMIGRAINE DRUGS

Recently, the ergot alkaloids [ergotamine tartrate, dihydroergotamine (DHE), chronic methysergide] sumatriptan, zolmitriptan, and rizatriptan were reported to block neurogenic plasma extravasation in the rat and guinea pig dura mater (47,81,96). The fact that all six compounds relieve migraine with and without aura and cluster headaches suggest that they may work at a mechanism common to all headaches. Methysergide, a third ergot derivative, is useful for prophylaxis when chronically administered but is not useful for the acute attack. Pretreatment with a single injection of sumatriptan, zolmitriptan, rizatriptan, ergotamine, or dihydroergotamine, but only chronic administration of methysergide, blocked neurogenic inflammation in dura mater induced either by trigeminal electric stimulation or by capsaicin (45,46,96). Therapeutically relevant doses were sufficient, and the response was selective within intracranial but not extracranial tissues innervated by the trigeminal nerve. Furthermore, blockade of neurogenic plasma extravasation was achieved when drugs were injected 45 minutes after trigeminal stimulation. A recent study documented that blood vessels of the dura mater continue to leak plasma proteins for many minutes following a relatively brief (i.e., 5 minutes) stimulation period. This leakage is dependent on continued neuropeptide release from sensory fibers. As evidence, endopeptidase 24.11, a zinc metallopeptidase ectoenzyme that degrades SP and NKA, inhibits the delayed response when administered intravenously. Endopeptidase 24.11 and sumatriptan exhibited the same time course of activity in this model (26).

We concluded from these findings that ergots and the triptans decrease neurogenic plasma extravasation by a C-fiber-dependent mechanism, perhaps by a mechanism coupled to blocking neuropeptide release from perivascular fibers. The following evidence supports the postulation that sumatriptan and related compounds inhibit neurogenic inflammation through prejunctional mechanisms:

1. Dihydroergotamine or sumatriptan pretreatment attenuated the elevated plasma CGRP levels within draining venous effluent during trigeminal stimulation, presumably reflecting decreased sensory neurotransmitter release (9).

2. Plasma leakage in the dura mater induced by exogenous SP or NKA administration, in contrast to that evoked by nerve stimulation, was not blocked by sumatriptan, dihydroergotamine, ergotamine tartrate, or CP-93,129, a selective $5-HT_{1B}$ receptor agonist (10,12,50, 81). The $5-HT_{1B}$ receptor subtype in rats and mice subserves the same physiologic functions as the $5-HT_{1D}$ receptor subtype in guinea pigs and humans. CP-93,129 blocks neurogenic plasma extravasation selectively in rat but not guinea pig dura mater, whereas sumatriptan is somewhat more potent at the $5-HT_{1D}$ than at the $5-HT_{1B}$ receptor subtype and blocks plasma extravasation in both species (50).

3. Sumatriptan or dihydroergotamine significantly attenuates or abolishes the mast cell, platelet, and endothelial cell changes accompanying neurogenic inflammation. The existence of sumatriptan or dihydroergotamine receptors on each of these cell types seems most unlikely (11).

4. Molecular biology studies confirm that trigeminal ganglion cells possess a gene homologous to the $5-HT_{1B/D}$ receptor family (7,79).

5. Immunohistochemical studies have demonstrated a differential distribution of the $5-HT_{1D}$ and $5-HT_{1B}$ receptors within the human trigeminovascular system. Only $5-HT_{1B}$-receptor protein was detected on dural arteries, whereas only $5-HT_{1D}$-receptor protein was detected on trigeminal sensory neurons, including peripheral and central projections to dural blood vessels and to the medulla (40).

6. $5-HT_{1B/D}$ receptors mediate the inhibition of neurotransmitter release in other regions of the peripheral and central nervous system (58).

7. Sumatriptan, zolmitriptan, and ergometrine were able to inhibit evoked and spontaneous firing of second-order trigeminal neurons by direct local application. These findings demonstrate that the synapse of the trigeminal nucleus in the brainstem and upper cervical cord provide additional sites of action for brain-penetrating antimigraine drugs of the $5-HT_{1B/1D}$ class (90). If sumatriptan does not cross the blood–brain barrier, an argument in favor of a peripheral mechanism of drug action seems likely. Regardless, both receptor binding sites are located on primary afferent axons arising from trigeminal ganglia and support a prejunctional mechanism of action as originally postulated by our group (81).

Prejunctional receptors on trigeminovascular fibers also have been identified for other receptor types: α2-adrenoceptor, histamine H_3 receptors, u-opioid receptors, and somatostatin receptors have been implicated based on the effects of UK-14,304 and idazoxan, R-a-methyl histamine, thiperamide, morphine, naloxone, and octreotide (a synthetic somatostatin analogue) on the dural neuroinflammatory process, respectively. Inhibition of transmitter release mediated by these receptors may explain the anecdotal success of somatostatin, adrenalin, or narcotic analgesics in headache relief and may suggest new avenues for novel treatments (49).

Gamma-aminobutyric acid (GABA) receptors also have been implicated in trigeminovascular pharmacology. Sodium valproate, an effective drug for migraine prophylaxis (25), modulates GABAergic neurotransmission by inhibiting GABA aminotransaminase and activating glutamic acid decarboxylase (39,43). Valproic acid and muscimol ($GABA_A$ agonist) but not baclofen ($GABA_B$ agonist) attenuate meningeal neurogenic inflammation following trigeminal stimulation (35). Moreover, valproate selectively reduces c-fos expression within laminae I and II of the TNC after cephalic noxious stimulation, suggesting the importance of $GABA_A$ receptors to nociception (13). Pharmacologic evidence suggests that the $GABA_A$ receptor complex involved in the attenuation of plasma-protein extravasation does not reside on afferent C-fibers, inasmuch as valproate attenuates SP-induced plasma extravasation in animals neonatally treated with capsaicin (35). The evidence suggests that the receptor complex resides on parasympathetic fibers emanating from the sphenopalatine ganglia. When these projections have been sectioned, the action of drugs such as valproate, muscimol, neurosteroids, and benzodiazepines is abolished.

L-Glutamate (Glu), an excitatory neurotransmitter involved in nociception, coexists in trigeminal unmyelinated C-fibers within the dorsal horn with SP (3). Electron microscopy studies have revealed presynaptic Glu-immnureactive terminals within lamina II of feline TNC (28). Bereiter and Benetti showed that noxious stimulation of the face using microdialysis techniques caused excitation of small trigeminal C-fibers and release of Glu and aspartate within the TNC in rats (5). Glutamate acts through ligand-gated ion channels (ionotropic: NMDA, AMPA, and kainic acid) and G-protein-coupled metabotropic receptors (mGluR). NMDA receptors are located on the presynaptic terminals of afferent fibers (36) and in most dorsal root ganglion neurons (85). Presynaptic NMDA receptors appear to mediate SP release in the spinal cord (49). MK-801, a potent and selective noncompetitive NMDA receptor antagonist, reduces capsaicin-induced c-fos expression, a marker of neuronal activity, within the TNC (62). Therefore, agents that block NMDA receptors might provide a new therapeutic approach for future antimigraine drug development.

THE PREJUNCTIONAL RECEPTOR

5-HT_{1D}- and 5-HT_{1B}-receptor proteins are distributed differentially within the human trigeminovascular system (40). The fact that the 5-HT_{1B}-receptor protein is present exclusively on smooth-muscle cells in meningeal blood vessels confirms the conclusions of previous studies using pharmacologic correlation. These studies show that vasoconstrictor responses to sumatriptan are mediated by the 5-HT_{1B} receptor (8,25,30,93,97). In contrast, 5-HT_{1D} receptor proteins were detected in trigeminal sensory neurons, including peripheral projections to the dura as well as within the TNC and solitary tract. These brainstem regions are known to possess binding sites for sumatriptan and zolmitriptan, as detected by autoradiographic studies in rats and guinea pigs (59,94). Selective 5-HT_{1D} receptor agonists may therefore decrease headache by abrogating neuropeptide release and blocking neurotransmission without the potential side effects mediated through 5-HT_{1B} receptor activation (i.e., coronary and carotid artery vasoconstriction).

A previously unrecognized role of the 5-HT_{1F} receptor may be involved in the blockade of neurogenic dural inflammation by drugs that show high affinity for this receptor subtype. Such is the case for sumatriptan, zolmitriptan, the ergot alkaloids, and LY344864, a highly selective 5-HT_{1F} receptor agonist (48,76). C-fos expression within TNC, a marker of neuronal activation after capsaicin-induced cephalic pain, is decreased significantly after pretreatment with LY344864 (61), demonstrating the probable role of the 5-HT_{1F} receptor in the mediation of pain. Recently, 5-HT_{1F} receptor mRNA was detected in the guinea pig trigeminal ganglion, suggesting a possible role for the receptor protein in the prejunctional inhibition of neuropeptide release (1).

Potent neuronal effects of acute antimigraine drugs do not preclude the possible existence of more than a single mechanism of action. At present, however, there are significant limitations to the published human data supporting the vasoconstrictor theories (65,66). The possibility that therapeutically relevant receptor sites reside within the central nervous system (e.g., the TNC) is being explored, and some evidence has been provided. In the TNC and superficial laminae of the dorsal horn of the C1 and C2 spinal cord, [^{3}H]-dihydroergotamine (21), [^{3}H]-sumatriptan (59), and [^{3}H]-zolmitriptan (20) bind with high affinity. Although sumatriptan is highly polar and therefore would not be expected to cross the blood–brain barrier with ease, the fact that patients report fatigue and mood changes following sumatriptan administration suggests a central action; unfortunately, there is no evidence to suggest disruption of the blood–brain barrier in this condition. On the other hand, animal experiments have shown that sumatriptan is capable of inhibiting spontaneous and induced neuronal firing only after mannitol-induced blood–brain barrier disruption (29,88). Because blood–brain barrier disruption in the brainstem is unlikely in migraine sufferers, these data indicate that the antimigraine action of sumatriptan may be predominately mediated by inhibition of plasma protein extravasation or direct vasoconstriction of large cerebral arteries and dural vessels or blockade of neurotransmission in 5-HT_{1D}-receptor–containing axons. On the other hand, brain-penetrant 5-$HT_{1B/1D}$ agonists, such as zolmitriptan, may access an additional target site on primary afferent brainstem nerve endings (25,78). Unfortunately, brain-penetrant drugs show only incremental improvement in efficacy over sumatriptan. Differences in oral bioavailability and pharmacokinetics, rather than central nervous system penetration per se, may account for these advantages.

How reliable is the model of neurogenic inflammation as a predictor of drug efficacy? Although many drugs do show a correspondence, not all drugs that block neurogenic inflammation in animal models can be expected to work in migraine. First, receptor types and their amino acid sequences may differ in rodents and humans, and mechanisms identified in rodents may not exist in humans, which may explain why the compound CP122,288, which potently blocks neurogenic inflammation in rats and guinea pigs, is inactive in humans. That is, its receptor (or other mechanism of action) in animals remains undiscovered and (despite intense investigation) may not exist in humans. Considering that drugs with identified mechanisms of presumable relevance often do not show clinical efficacy, results with CP122,288 are not unexpected. Second, drugs that block neurogenic inflammation by inhibiting neuropeptide receptors, such as NK1 receptor antagonists, do not block afferent fiber firing or peptide release at central synapses and provide a less satisfactory therapeutic target than prejunctional receptors. Although fraught with major shortcomings largely resulting from poor oral absorption, one clinical trial using LY344864, an NK1 receptor antagonist, showed no therapeutic efficacy in migraine subjects. Explanations for drug failure have been discussed recently (63).

INHIBITION OF *C-FOS* EXPRESSION

C-fos expression is both a spatial and a temporal marker of central nervous system activity and is useful in studying central responses to noxious stimulation (87). Hunt and colleagues found that *c-fos* antigen is expressed by cells in laminae I and II$_O$ (the pain-receiving and -transmitting zones) in the spinal cord and brainstem after delivery of a noxious stimulus to the periphery (27). Presley and colleagues (77) determined in another pain model that the number of *c-fos*-labeled cells in laminae I and II$_O$ was related to stimulus intensity and that morphine reduced the number of expressing cells.

We observed that sumatriptan and related drugs attenuated the expression of *c-fos* within laminae I and II$_0$ caused by noxious chemical stimulation of the meninges (73). Noxious stimulation of the nasal mucosa (topical formalin) was not affected by these drugs. Meningeal stimulation was achieved by injecting an algesic substance, blood, into the subarachnoid space. The number of labeled cells, related to the amount of blood injected, was reduced by morphine administration or chronic surgical or chemical denervation. Effective dosages of sumatriptan and related compounds approximated the amounts required to block neurogenic plasma extravasation within dura mater.

The pattern of expressing cells after blood administration suggests the importance of primary afferent fibers to the site of action of sumatriptan and related compounds (72). If the assumptions concerning the relation between *c-fos* expression and pain are correct, vasodilation cannot be a prerequisite for drug efficacy, nor can vasoconstriction be the primary mechanism of action. Clinical studies support these assertions. Transcranial Doppler studies document that headaches caused by nitroglycerin administration occur when vasodilation is waning (66).

Sumatriptan and related compounds may have broad applications for the treatment of nonmigraine headaches caused by meningeal inflammation. The drugs blocked *c-fos* expression in response to intracisternal potassium or to carageenan, a potent inflammatory agent (73). It has been established that sumatriptan and dihydroergotamine (DHE) decrease headaches with diverse (albeit unknown) pathogeneses and clinical expression (e.g., cluster headache and migraine with and without aura) and that headaches unrelated to migraine or cluster headaches respond as well. In this vein, sumatriptan and related compounds may prove useful for decreasing headache pain associated with meningovascular irritation, such as from acquired immunodeficiency syndrome (AIDS) or other viral and bacterial infections and from subarachnoid hemorrhage. The absence of hypnotic effects and the low addictive potential suggest important advantages to this therapeutic strategy.

NEOCORTEX AS A POTENTIAL MIGRAINE TRIGGER

Recent studies suggest that neurophysiologic events within the cerebral cortex can activate brainstem regions involved in the processing of nociceptive information through trigeminovascular mechanisms (64) (Fig. 2). In these studies, the effects of neocortical spreading depression (SD) were examined on the expression of immunoreactive *c-fos* protein within the superficial laminae of the TNC. To induce recurrent SD, KCl was microinjected repeatedly into the left parietal cortex; SD was detected by electrophysiologic methods within adjacent frontal cortex. In response, *c-fos* protein-LI was visualized in the ventrolateral TNC (corresponding to the ophthalmic division), chiefly in laminae I and II$_0$ and predominantly within spinal segment. SD significantly increased cell staining within ipsilateral TNC. In comparing labeling between the two sides, staining was reduced to an insignificant difference after chronic surgical transection of meningeal afferents and recurrent SD. Pretreatment with sumatriptan attenuated *c-fos* protein-LI in this model as well.

What therefore constitutes an effective stimulus for trigeminovascular activation after recurrent SD? To our knowledge, no detailed reports describe the electrophysiologic properties of primary nociceptors within the meninges. In other tissues, the vast majority of nociceptors are polymodal and respond to noxious, thermal, mechanical, and chemical stimuli (6,33,34). Local release or new synthesis of chemical constituents, such as bradykinin potassium, hydrogen ion, and certain neurotransmitters such as serotonin (35,89), activates or sensitizes primary afferent fibers. Neugebauer and colleagues (70) provided evidence for nociceptor sensitization to passive joint motion following intraarticular bradykinin or prostaglandin injections. Some of the same agents are released into the neocortex during SD. For example, hydrogen ions and potassium concentrations increase within the interstitial space by 5- to 20-fold during a single SD; levels of prostaglandins increase as well. Oxygen free radicals, mediators of tissue injury, are generated during the formation of prostaglandins (32). Cumulative or tonic stimulation by recurrent SDs is required, inasmuch as signals generated by single SDs did not raise the number of stained cells.

In the cerebral cortex, SD may be one of several neurophysiologic events capable of activating nociceptive mechanisms in the cerebral cortex. Generalized seizures activate trigeminovascular fibers and, in so doing, increase blood flow in the neocortex (83). Stimuli injurious to the brain, such as ischemia (67), and to blood ves-

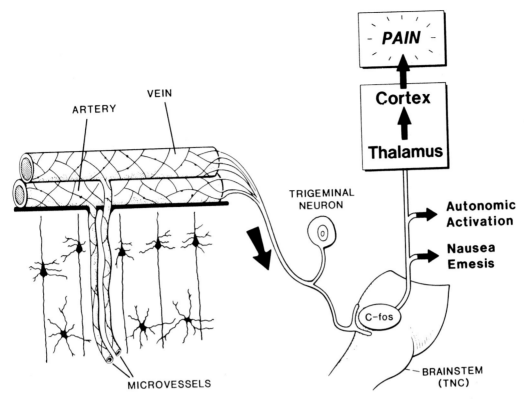

FIG. 2. Diagram depicting the relationship between pial vessels, the trigeminovascular system, and the neocortex. Recent data indicate that neurophysiologic activity within neocortex (i.e., recurrent spreading depression) can activate the ipsilateral trigeminovascular system, as evidenced by induction of the *c-fos* antigen within laminae I and II$_O$ of trigeminal nucleus caudalis. One postulation holds that ions, neurotransmitters, and other biologically active substances released into the extracellular space from neurons and glia may activate innervating nerve fibers after reaching the perivascular space. Of note is that sectioning the trigeminal branch innervating the meninges or systemic administration with sumatriptan can significantly reduce the *c-fos* response.

sels, such as acute, severe hypertension (83), also can activate this system. Pain and headache develop in humans during seizures, ischemia, and severe hypertension. In fact, headache of migraine with aura develops following a focal neurologic event (most often referable to the neocortex), which some have likened to the spreading depression of Leao (60,75).

The findings are consistent with the following formulation: neurophysiologically driven ionic and metabolic mechanisms (e.g., SD) promote the release of nociceptive substances from the neocortex into the interstitial space. Within the perivascular space, released substances activate and sensitize trigeminovascular fibers surrounding pial vessels supplying and draining the neocortex within Virchow–Robin spaces. As a result, impulses are conveyed to the TNC and then to more rostral centers. Pain may ensue. Less likely, products released from cortex may stimulate meningeal vessels, which in turn release nociceptive molecules. We speculate that these findings may be relevant to headache pathophysiology and to the pathogenesis of photophobia and phonophobia accompanying stimulation of meningeal afferents.

Based on the preceding findings, it seems intuitively correct that, despite the lack of exact information regarding headache pathogenesis, headache pain ultimately must activate the trigeminovascular system. Accordingly, the perivascular primary sensory neuron may be viewed as a final common pathway subject to activation or modulation by local factors within the vessel lumen and vessel wall. Elucidating these factors will provide both excitement and challenge for future investigators in this field and possibly therapeutic benefits for patients who suffer from migraine.

REFERENCES

1. Adham N, Bard JA, Zgombick JM, et al. Cloning and characterization of the guinea pig 5HT$_{1F}$ receptor subtype: a comparison of the pharmacological profile to the human species homolog. *Neuropharmacology* 1997;36:569–576.
2. Arbab MA-R, Delgado T, Wiklund L, Svendgaard NA. Brain stem terminations of the trigeminal and upper spinal innervation of the cerebrovascular system: WGA-HRP transganglionic study. *J Cereb Blood Flow Metab* 1988;8:54–63.
3. Battaglia G, Rustioni A. Coexistance of glutamate and substance P in dorsal root ganglion neurons of the rat and monkey. *J Comp Neurol* 1988;277:302–312.

4. Bayliss WM. Further researches on antidromic nerve impulses. *J Physiol* 1902;28:276–299.

5. Bereiter DA, Benetti AP. Excitatory amino release within spinal trigeminal nucleus after mustard oil injection into the temporomandibular joint region of the rat. *Pain* 1996;67:451–459.

6. Bessou P, Perl ER. Response of cutaneous sensory units with unmyelinated fibers to noxious stimuli. *J Neurophysiol* 1969;32:1025–1043.

7. Bruinvels AT, Landwehrmeyer B, Moskowitz MA, Hoyer D. Evidence for the presence of 5-HT1B receptor messenger RNA in neurons of the rat trigeminal ganglia. *Eur J Pharmacol* 1992;227:357–359.

8. Bouchelet I, Cohen Z, Case B, Seguela P, Hamel E. Differential expression of sumatriptan-sensitive 5-hydroxytryptamine receptors in human trigeminal ganglia and cerebral blood vessels. *Mol Pharmacol* 50: 219–223.

9. Buzzi MG, Dimitriadou V, Theoharides TC, Moskowitz MA. 5-Hydroxytryptamine receptor agonists for the abortive treatment of vascular headaches block mast cell, endothelial and platelet activation within dura mater after trigeminal stimulation. *Brain Res* 1992;583: 137–149.

10. Buzzi MG, Moskowitz MA, Peroutka SJ, Byun B. Further characterization of the putative 5-HT receptor which mediates blockade of neurogenic plasma extravasation in rat dura mater. *Br J Pharmacol* 1991; 103:1421–1428.

11. Buzzi MG, Carter WB, Shimizu T, Heath HH 3rd, Moskowitz MA. Dihydroergotamine and sumatriptan attenuate levels of CGRP in plasma in rat superior sagittal sinus during electrical stimulation of the trigeminal ganglion. *Neuropharmacology* 1991;30:1193–1200.

12. Buzzi MG, Moskowitz MA. The antimigraine drug, sumatriptan (GR 43175) specifically blocks neurogenic plasma extravasation from blood vessels in dura mater. *Br J Pharmacol* 1990;99:202–206.

13. Cutrer FM, Limmroth V, Ayata G, Moskowitz MA. Attenuation by valproate of c-fos expression within rat trigemianl nucleus caudalis caused by chemical stimulation of the meninges. *Br J Pharmacol* 1995;116: 3199–3204.

14. Dimitriadou V, Buzzi MG, Theoharides T, Moskowitz MA. Ultrastructural evidence for neurogenically mediated changes in blood vessels of the rat dura mater and tongue following antidromic trigeminal stimulation. *Neuroscience* 1992;48:187–203.

15. Dimitriadou V, Buzzi MG, Moskowitz MA, Theoharides TC. Trigeminal sensory fiber stimulation induces morphological changes in rat dura mater mast cells. *Neuroscience* 1991;44:97–112.

16. Drummond PD, Gonski A, Lance JW. Facial flushing after thermocoagulation of gasserian ganglion. *J Neurol Neurosurg Psychiatry* 1983; 46:611–616.

17. Feindel W, Penfield W, McNaughton F. The tentorial nerves and localization of intracranial pain in man. *Neurology* 1960;10:555–563.

18. Figini M, Emanueli C, Grady EF, et al. Substance P and bradykinin stimulate plasma protein extravasation in the mouse gastrointestinal tract and pancreas. *Am J Physiol* 1997;272:785–793.

19. Gibbins IL, Furness JB, Costa M, MacIntyre I, Hillyard CJ, Girgis S. Co-localization of calcitonin gene-related peptide-like immunoreactivity with substance P in cutaneous, vascular and visceral sensory neurons of guinea pigs. *Neurosci Lett* 1985 57:125–130.

20. Goadsby PJ, Knight YE. Direct evidence for central sites of action of zolmitriptan (311C90): an autoradiographic study in cat. *Cephalalgia* 1997;17:153–158.

21. Goadsby PJ, Gundlach AL. Localization of [3H]-dihydroergotamine binding sites in the cat central nervous system:relevance to migraine. *Ann Neurol* 1991;29:91–94.

22. Goadsby PJ, Edvinsson L, Ekman R. Release of vasoactive peptides in the extracerebral circulation of humans and the cat during activation of the trigeminovascular system. *Ann Neurol* 1988;23:193–196.

23. Gulbenkian S, Merighi A, Wharton J, Varndell IM, Polak JM. Ultrastructural evidence for the coexistence of calcitonin gene-related peptide and substance P in secretory vesicles of peripheral nerves in the guinea pig. *J Neurocytol* 1986;15:535–542.

24. Hering R, Kuritzky A. Sodium valproate in the prophylactic treatment of migraine: a double-blind study versus placebo. *Cephalalgia* 1992; 12:81–84.

25. Hoskin KL, Goadsby PJ. Comparison of more and less lipohilic serotonin (5HT1B/1D) agonists in a model of trigeminovascular nociception in cat. *Exp Neurol* 1998;150:45–51.

26. Huang Z, Byun BJ, Matsubara T, Moskowitz MA. Time-dependent blockade of neurogenic plasma extravasation in dura mater by 5-HT1B/D agonists and endopeptidase 24,11. *Br J Pharmacol* 1993;108:331–335.

27. Hunt SP, Pini A, Evan G. Induction of c-fos-like protein in spinal cord neurons following sensory stimulation. *Nature* 1987;328:632–634.

28. Iliakis B, Anderson NL, Irish PS, Henry MA, Westrum LE. Electron microscopy of immunoreactivity patterns for glutamate and gamma-aminobutyric acid in synaptic glomeruli of the feline spinal trigeminal nucleus (subnucleus caudalis) *J Comp Neurol* 1996;366:465–477.

29. Kaube H, Hoskin KL, Goadsby PJ. Inhibition by sumatriptan of central trigeminal neurones only after blood–brain barrier disruption. *Br J Pharmacol* 1993;109:788–792.

30. Kaumann AJ, Parsons AA, Brown AA. Human arterial constrictor serotonin receptors. *Cardiovasc Res* 1993;27:2094–2103.

31. Keller JT, Beduk A, Saunders MC. Origin of fibres innervating the basilar artery of the cat. *Neurosci Lett* 1985;58:263–268.

32. Kontos HA. Oxygen radicals in CNS damage. *Chem Biol Interact* 1989;72:229–255.

33. Kumazawa K, Mizumura K. Chemical responses of polymodal receptors of the scrotal contents in dogs. *J Physiol (Lond)* 1980;299: 219–231.

34. Lang E, Novak A, Reeh PW, Handwerker HO. Chemosensitivity of fine afferents from rat skin in vitro. *J Neurophysiol* 1990;63:887–901.

35. Lee WS, Limmroth V, Ayata C, et al. Peripheral GABAA receptor mediated effects of sodium valproate on dural plasma extravasation to substance P and trigeminal stimulation. *Br J Pharmacol* 1995;116: 1661–1667.

36. Liu H, Wang H, Sheng M, Jan LY, Jan YN, Basbaum AI. Evidence for presynaptic N-methyl-D-aspartate autoreceptors in the spinal cord dorsal horn. *Proc Natl Acad Sci USA* 1994;8383–8387.

37. Liu-Chen L-Y, Liszczak T, King J, et al. An immunoelectron microscopic study of substance P-containing axons in feline cerebral arteries. *Brain Res* 1986;369:12–20.

38. Liu-Chen L-Y, Mayberg M, Moskowitz MA. Immunohistochemical evidence for a substance P-containing trigeminovascular pathway to pial arteries in cats. *Brain Res* 1983;268:162–166.

39. Loscher W. Valproate induced changes in GABA metabolism at the subcellular level. *Biochem Pharmacol* 1981;30:1364–1366.

40. Longmore J, Shaw D, Smith D, et al. Differential distribution of 5HT1D- and 5HT1B-immunoreactivity within the human trigemino-cerebrovascular system: implications for the discovery of new antimigraine drugs. *Cephalalgia* 1997;17:833–842.

41. Lundberg JM, Brodin E, Hua X, et al. Vascular permeability changes and smooth muscle contraction in relation to capsaicin-sensitive substance P afferents in guinea pig. *Acta Physiol Scand* 1984;120:217–227.

42. Maggi CA. The dual function of capsaicin-sensitive sensory nerves in the bladder and urethra. *Ciba Found Symp* 1990;151:77–83.

43. Maitre M, Ciesielski L, Cash C, Mandel P. Comparison of the structural characteristics of the 4-aminobutyrate:2-oxyglutarate transaminases from cat and himan brain, and of their affinities for certain inhibitors. *Biochem Biophys Acta* 1978;522:385–399.

44. Markowitz S, Saito K, Moskowitz MA. Neurogenically-mediated plasma extravasation in dura mater: effect of ergotalkaloids. *Cephalalgia* 1988;8:83–91.

45. Markowitz S, Saito K, Moskowitz MA. Neurogenically mediated leakage of plasma protein occurs from blood vessels in dura mater but not brain. *J Neurosci* 1987;7:4129–4136.

46. Martin GR. Serotonin receptor involvement in the pathogenesis and treatment of migraine. In: Goadsby PJ, Silberstein SD, eds. *Headache.* Boston: Butterworth-Heinemann, 1997:25–38.

47. Martin GR, Robertson AD, MacLennan SJ, et al. Receptor specificity and trigemino-vascular inhibitory actions of a novel 5-HT1B/1D receptor partial agonist, 311C90 (zolmitriptan). *Br J Pharmacol* 1997;121:157–164.

48. Marvizon JC, Martinez V, Grady EF et al. Neurokin 1 receptor internalization in spinal cord slices induced by dorsal root stimulation is mediated by NMDA receptors. *J Neurosci* 1997;17:8129–8136.

49. Matsubara T, Moskowitz MA, Huang Z. UK-14,304 and r(-)alpha-methyl-histamine and octreotide (SM201-995) block plasma protein leakage within dura mater by prejunctional mechanisms. *Eur J Pharmacol* 1992;224:145–150.

50. Matsubara T, Moskowitz MA, Byun BJ. CP-93,129, a potent and selective 5-HT1B receptor agonist blocks neurogenic plasma extravasation within rat but not guinea-pig dura mater: special report. *Br J Pharmacol* 1991;104:3–4.

51. Matsuyama T, Shiosaka, Wanaka A, et al. Fine structure of peptidergic and catecholaminergic nerve fibers in the anterior cerebral artery and their interrelationship: an immunoelectron microscopic study. *J Comp Neurol* 1985;235:268–276.

52. May A, Shepheard S, Wessing A, et al. Retinal plasma extravasation can be evoked by trigeminal stimulation in rat but does not occur during migraine attacks. *Cephalalgia* 1997;17:240.

53. Mayberg MR, Zervas NT, Moskowitz MA. Trigeminal projections to supratentorial pial and dural blood vessels in cats demonstrated by horseradish peroxidase histochemistry. *J Comp Neurol* 1984;223: 46–56.

54. Mayberg MR, Langer RS, Zervas NT, et al. Perivascular meningeal projections from cat trigeminal ganglia: possible pathway for vascular headache in man. *Science* 1981;213:228–230.

55. McCulloch J, Uddman R, Kingman T, et al. Calcitonin gene-related peptide: functional role in cerebrovascular regulation. *Proc Natl Acad Sci USA* 1986;83:5731–5735.

56. McMahon MD, Norregaard TV, Beyerl BD, et al. Trigeminal afferents to cerebral arteries and forehead are not divergent axon collaterals in cat. *Neurosci Lett* 1985;60:63–68.

57. Messlinger K, Hanesch U, Baumgartel M, Trost B, Schmidt RF. Innervation of the dura mater encephali of cat and rat: ultrastructure and calcitonin gene-related peptide-like and substance P-like immunoreactivity. *Anat Embryol* 1993;188:219–273.

58. Middlemiss D, Hutson PH. The 5HT$_{1B}$ receptors. In: Whitaker-Azmitia PM, Peroutka SJ, eds. *The neuropharmacology of serotonin*. New York: New York Academy of Science, 1990;132–148.

59. Mills A, Martin GR. Autoradiographic mapping of [^{3}H]sumatriptan binding in cat brain stem and spinal cord. *Eur J Pharmacol* 1995;280: 175–178.

60. Milner PM. Note on a possible correspondence between the scotomas of migraine and spreading depression of Leao. *EEG Clin Neurophysiol* 1958;10:705.

61. Mitsikostas DD, Sanchez del Rio M, Waeber C, Moskowitz MA. 5-hydroxytryptamine 1F subtype receptor modulates capsaisin induced c-fos expression within rat trigeminal nucleus candalis. A new target for anti-migraine drugs. *Eur J Pharmacol* 1999. In press.

62. Mitsikostas DD, Sanchez del Rio M, Waeber C, Moskowitz MA, Cutrer FA. The NMDA receptor antagonist MK-801 reduces capsaicin-induced c-fos expression within rat trigeminal nucleus caudalis. *Pain* 1998;76:239–248.

63. Moskowitz MA, Mitsikostas DD. A negative clinical study in the search for a migraine treatment. *Cephalalgia* 1997;17:720–721.

64. Moskowitz MA, Nozaki K, Kraig RP. Neocortical spreading depression provokes the expression of *c-fos* protein-like immunoreactivity within trigeminal nucleus caudalis via trigem-inovascular mechanisms. *J Neurosci* 1993;13:1167–1177.

65. Moskowitz MA. Neurogenic versus vascular mechanisms of sumatriptan and ergot alkaloids in migraine. *Trends Pharmacol Sci* 1992;13:307–311.

66. Moskowitz MA. Interpreting vessel diameter changes in vascular headaches [Guest Editorial]. *Cephalalgia* 1991;12:5–7.

67. Moskowitz MA, Sakas DE, Wei EP, et al. Postocclusive cerebral hyperemia is markedly attenuated by chronic trigeminal ganglionectomy. *Am J Physiol* 1989;257:H1736–H1739.

68. Moskowitz MA. Cluster headache: evidence for a pathophysiologic focus in the superior pericarotid cavernous sinus plexus. *Headache* 1988;28:584–586.

69. Moskowitz MA, Brody M, Liu-Chen L-Y. In vivo release of immunoreactive substance P from putative afferent nerve endings in bovine pia arachnoid. *Neuroscience* 1983;9:809.

70. Neugebauer V, Schaible H-G, Schmidt RF. Sensitization of articular afferents to mechanical stimuli by bradykinin. *Pflugers Arch* 1989;415: 330–335.

71. Nimmo AJ, Whitaker EM, Castairs JR, Morrison JF. The autoradiographic localization of calcitonin gene-related peptide and substance P receptors in human fallopian tube. *Q J Exp Physiol* 1989;74:955–958.

72. Nozaki K, Boccalini P, Moskowitz MA. Expression of *c-fos*-like immunoreactivity in brainstem after meningeal irritation by blood in the subarachnoid space. *Neuroscience* 1992;49:669–680.

73. Nozaki K, Moskowitz MA, Boccalini P. CP-93,129, sumatriptan, dihydroergotamine block *c-fos* expression within rat trigeminal nucleus caudalis caused by chemical stimulation of the meninges. *Br J Pharmacol* 1992;106:409–415.

74. O'Connor TP, van der Kooy D. Pattern of intracranial and extracranial projections of trigeminal ganglion cells. *J Neurosci* 1986;6:2200–2207.

75. Olesen J, Larsen B, Lauritzen M. Focal hyperemia followed by spreading oligemia and impaired activation of rCBF in classic migraine. *Ann Neurol* 1981;9:344–352.

76. Phebus LA, Johnson KW, Zgombick JM, et al. Characterization of LY344864 as a pharmacological tool to study 5-HT1F receptors: binding affinities, brain penetration and activity in the neurogenic dural inflammation model of migraine. *Life Sci* 1997;61:2117–2126.

77. Presley RW, Menetrey D, Levine JD, Basbaum AI. Systemic morphine suppresses noxious stimulus-evoked Fos protein-like immunoreactivity in the rat spinal cord. *J Neurosci* 1990;10:323–335.

78. Proietti-Cecchini A, Afra J, Schoenen J. Intensity dependence of the cortical auditory evoked potentials as a surrogate marker of central nervous system serotonin transmission in man: demonstration of a central effect for the 5HT$_{1B/1D}$ agonist zolmitriptan (311C90, Zomig). *Cephalalgia* 1997;17:849–854.

79. Rebeck GW, Maynard KI, Hyman B, Moskowitz MA. Selective 5-HT$_{1D}$ alpha serotonin receptor gene expression in trigeminal ganglia: implications for antimigraine drug development. *Proc Natl Acad Sci U S A* 1994;91:3666–3669.

80. Saito K, Moskowitz MA. Contributions from the trigeminal and upper cervical ganglia to the feline circle of Willis: effects of lesioning on substance P content in pial vessels. *Stroke* 1989;20:524–526.

81. Saito K, Markowitz S, Moskowitz MA. Ergot alkaloids block neurogenic extravasation in dura mater: proposed action in vascular headaches. *Ann Neurol* 1988;24:732–737.

82. Saito K, Greenberg S, Moskowitz MA. Trigeminal origin of beta-preprotachykinin in feline pial blood vessels. *Neurosci Lett* 1987;76: 69–73.

83. Sakas DE, Moskowitz MA, Wei EP, Kontos HA, Kano M, Ogilvy C. Trigeminovascular fibers increase blood flow in cortical grey matter by axon-dependent mechanisms during acute, severe hypertension or seizures. *Proc Natl Acad Sci U S A* 1989;86:1401–1405.

84. Saria AL, Lundberg J, Skofitsch G, et al. Vascular leakage in various tissues induced by substance P, capsaicin, bradykinin, serotonin, histamine and antigen challenge. *Naunyn Schmiedebergs Arch Pharmacol* 1983;324:212–218.

85. Sato K, Kiyama H, TaePark H, Tohyama M. AMPA, KA and NMDA receptors are expressed in the rat DRG neurons. *Neuroreport* 1993;4: 1263–1265.

86. Schmelz M, Luz O, Averbeck B, Bickel A. Plasma extravasation and neuropeptide release in human skin as measured by intradermal microdialysis. *Neurosci Lett* 1997;18:117–120.

87. Sheng M, Greenberg ME. The regulation and function of *c-fos* and other immediate early genes in the nervous system. Neuron 1990;4: 477–485.

88. Shepheard SL, Williamson DJ, Williams J, Hill RG, Hargreaves RJ. Comparison of the effects of sumatriptan and the NK1 antagonist CP-99,994 on plasma extravasation in dura mater and *c-fos* mRNA expression in trigeminal nucleus caudalis of rats. *Neuropharmacology* 1995; 34:255–261.

89. Steen KH, Reeh PW, Anton F, Handwerker HO. Protons selectively induce lasting excitation and sensitization to mechanical stimulation of nociceptors in rat skin, in vitro. *J Neurosci* 12:86–95.

90. Storer RJ, Goadsby PJ. Microiontophoretic application of serotonin (5HT)$_{1B/1D}$ agonists inhibit trigeminal cell firing in the cat. *Brain* 1997; 120:2171–2177.

91. Suzuki N, Hardebo J-E, Owman C. Origins and pathways of cerebrovascular vasoactive intestinal polypeptide-positive nerves in rat. *J Cereb Blood Flow Metab* 1988;8:697–712.

92. Sweet WH, Wepsic JG. Controlled thermocoagulation of trigeminal ganglion and rootlets for differential destruction of pain fibers. Part I. Trigeminal neuralgia. *J Neurosurg* 1974;40:143–156.

93. Ullmer C, Schmuck K, Kalkman, Lubbert H. Expression of serotonin receptor mRNAs in blood vessels. *FEBS Letts* 1995;370:215–221.

94. Waeber C, Moskowitz MA. [^{3}H]sumatriptan labels both 5HT$_{1D}$ and 5HT$_{1F}$ receptor binding sites in guinea pig brain: an autoradiographic study. *Naunyn Schmiedebergs Arch Pharmacol* 1997;352:263–275.

95. Williamson DJ, Hargreaves RJ, Hill RG, Shepheard SL. Intravital microscope studies on the effects of neurokinin agonists and calcitonin gene-related peptide on dural vessel diameter in the anaesthetized rat. *Cephalalgia* 1997;17:518–524.

96. Williamson DJ, Shepheard SL, Hill RG, Hargreaves RJ. The novel antimigraine agent rizatriptan inhibits neurogenic dural vasodilation and extravasation. *Eur J Pharmacol* 1997;328:61–64.

97. Yu XJ, Waeber C, Castañon N, et al. Knock-out mice lacking 5-HT$_{1B}$ receptors: 5-CT and CP-122,288, but not sumatriptan or CP-93,129, block dural plasma extravasation. *Cephalalgia* 1995;15(Suppl 14):59.

The Headaches, Second Edition,
edited by J. Olesen, P. Tfelt-Hansen, and K.M.A. Welch.
Lippincott Williams & Wilkins, Philadelphia © 2000.

Basic Science Aspects of the Headaches

CHAPTER 18

Classification and Structure of Ion Channels

Olaf Pongs

All eucaryotic cells are surrounded by a plasma membrane. In addition, the cells contain intracellularly a variety of membrane-enclosed organelles, for example, the endoplasmic reticulum, Golgi apparatus, secretory vesicles, mitochondria, lysosomes, and, last but not least, the nucleus. The organelles provide compartments in which different metabolic activities are localized. The communication of signals between the compartments as well as the one between cells and the outside world requires the regulated and effective passage of many charged and uncharged solutes across the lipid bilayer membranes. Thus, transporters, pumps, and ion channels constitute an important class of integral membrane proteins, allowing for regulated intra- and extracellular signal transduction (32). In this review we discuss only ion channels that are expressed in cell plasma membranes.

Ion channels have the general property to form membrane-spanning pores. Along the electrochemical gradient, ions of appropriate size and charge may pass through the channel pores. This facilitates the passive movement of ions across the cell membrane. Thereby, the activity of ion channels may control the electrical potential across the plasma membrane of excitable and nonexcitable cells. As a consequence, ion channel activity is involved in diverse cellular processes, for example, the generation, propagation, and waveform of action potentials; the release of neurotransmitters; the secretion of peptide hormones; the homeostasis of salts and fluids; and cellular proliferation. It is therefore not surprising that an increasing number of mutations in channel genes are being discovered and correlated with heritable human diseases (channelopathies) that may not necessarily be lethal (1,9,10,33,43,47,67), as discussed at the end of this review.

O. Pongs: Universität Hamburg, Universitäts-Krankenhaus Eppendorf, Zentrum fur Molekulare Neurobiologie, Institut fur Neurale Signalverarbeitung, D-20246 Hamburg, Germany.

STRUCTURAL BASIS OF CHANNEL FUNCTION

Three properties of ion channels are central to their function. First, the channel pores allow a rapid movement of ions from one side of the membrane to the other. In general, the flow rate of ions is only about one order of magnitude smaller than the free diffusion rate in water. Thus, millions of ions flow through open channels per second down their respective electrochemical gradient. Second, ion channels may have very selective pores that can recognize the right from the wrong ion. A selectivity filter may endow the channel with the property to let selectively pass only Na^+, K^+, Ca^{2+}, or Cl^- ions. Thus, ion channels are not permanently open, that is, they contain a gate that controls the transition of a closed state into the open state (36). The gating of ion channels can be regulated by physical signals (e.g., pressure, light, temperature, potential) or chemical signals (e.g., second messengers, transmitters, fatty acids, peptides).

SOME SIMPLE BIOPHYSICS

In most mammalian cells, the extracellular concentration of Na^+, Ca^{2+}, and Cl^- is higher than the intracellular one, and, vice versa, the intracellular K^+ concentration is higher than the extracellular one. This has important consequences for the resting membrane potential as well as for the direction of passive ion movement (current) through the channel pores. The current flow, which is determined by the electrochemical gradient, is zero. According to the Nernst equation, the chemical and electrical driving forces for the particular ion cancel each other out. The potential that corresponds to this situation is referred to as the Nernst potential. For a particular ion, the Nernt potential or reversal potential, correlates to the membrane potential where an ion current across the membrane reverses direction. The reversal potentials for

K^+ are in the range of -70 to -100 mV for eucaryotic cells; the ones for Cl^- are in the range of -30 to -65 mV; and the ones for Na^+ are approximately $+50$ mV. At rest, the cellular membrane potential is slightly positive to the K^+ reversal potential (-70 to -30 mV) because the resting membrane potential is predominantly determined by the activity of K^+ or Cl^- channels. As a consequence, the direction of Na^+ and Ca^{2+} currents is usually from outside to inside the cell, and that of K^+ currents the opposite. The direction of Cl^- currents, on the other hand, may be more variable because membrane resting potentials may be encountered that are either negative or positive to the Cl^- reversal potential. Thus, activation of GABA receptors (Cl^- channels) may lead to a depolarizing Cl^- outward current (e.g., during early development of GABA-ergic interneurons) or to a repolarizing Cl^- inward current such as in many adult interneurons (58). Note that any change in the chemical and electrical driving forces (e.g., changes in extracellular K^+ concentration) will affect the respective reversal potential, and accordingly the resting membrane potential. It is important to recognize that the resting membrane potential does not refer to a static situation but to an actively controlled cellular steady state in which the summation of all currents across the membrane is zero. This state is achieved only via high energy consumption, which is necessary to maintain and establish the electrochemical gradients required for cellular signaling.

The flow of ionic current through ion channels may follow Ohm's law. Then, the amount of current (I) that passes through the channel is directly proportional to the membrane voltage (V). In reality, however, the I-V relationships that are encountered are nonlinear (non-ohmic). This behavior is called rectification. It can be outward and/or inward (Fig. 1) depending on whether the slope of the I-V curve is higher in the outward or inward direction. Accordingly, the respective ion channels have been referred to us as inwardly or outwardly rectifying channels.

It has been found that ion channel activity may be affected by membrane voltage. This observation provides a simple rationale for understanding the nonlinear I-V relationships shown in Figure 1A. When the ion channel activity decreases at a more depolarized membrane potential, the respective current is inwardly rectifying; when the ion channel activity increases at a more depolarized membrane potential, the respective current is outwardly rectifying. How can channel activity change with voltage? Unfortunately, there is no simple answer because ion channels can respond to membrane potential changes in many ways. In theoretical terms, the slope of the curve may reflect the number (N) of active ion channels in the plasma membrane that contribute to the current, the open probability (Po) of the ion channels, and the single-channel conductance:

$$I = (N \cdot Po \cdot \gamma) \cdot V \qquad (Eq.\ 1)$$

The open probability Po, that is, the fraction of time a channel spends in the open state, is directly related to its gating behavior. The gating of ion channels represents one of the most important forms for controlling channel activity. The gating of ion channels is best studied using the patch-clamp technique (29), which allows the measurement of single-channel behavior in small membrane patches (Fig. 1B). A typical single-channel recording shows that a channel may switch back and forth between the closed and open state in a repetitive manner. Several parameters can be discerned in ion channel gating. When a single ion channel becomes activated, one may observe the delay or latency of the first opening. Then one may measure the probability of times that the channel will be in open and closed states and determine Po. One also may obtain the single-channel conductance. Gating behavior may be regulated by intrinsic channel structures (e.g., voltage-sensors) or by extrinsic factors (e.g., Ca^{2+}, cyclic nucleotides, spermin/spermidine, inositol phosphate). Channels may then be classified according to their ion selectivity (Na, K, cation, Cl) and the main determinant of their gating behavior (voltage, CA^{2+}, cyclic, nucleotide, etc.). Accordingly, we may have voltage-gated Na channels, cyclic-nucleotide gated cation channels, Ca^{2+}-activated K channels. Sometimes ion channels also may be classified according to the type of macroscopic current that they mediate, for example, inward rectifying and outward rectifying K channels. The gating behavior of ion channels also may be modulated by phosphorylation-

---

FIG. 1. A: Current-voltage relationships for ion channels showing inward rectification and outward rectification. ○, reversal potential E_{rev} for K^+ channel; •, reversal potential for nonselective cation channel; Δ, reversal potential for Na^+ channel. Bell-shaped current voltage relationship may be observed for voltage-activated ion channels, which inactivate more rapidly at depolarized membrane potentials than they activate. **B:** Hypothetical trace of single-channel activity that may be observed in a patch-clamp experiment. Voltage protocol is illustrated by "–" (holding potential) and "+" (test potential). First latency: delay between jump to test potential and first single-channel opening. C: Hydrophobicity plot of a potassium channel α-subunit sequence derived from *Shaker* cDNA. Hydrophobic segments S1 to S6 are indicated. They may traverse the membrane. Accordingly, the derived protein sequence may have a membrane topology as shown in D. **D:** Membrane topology of K^+ channel α subunit with hydrophobic, membrane-spanning segments (depicted as cylinders) and a pore-forming P domain between segments S5 and S6, which dips into the membrane, entering and exiting from the extracellular side. *N*, cytoplasmic amino-terminus; *C*, cytoplasmic carboxy-terminus.

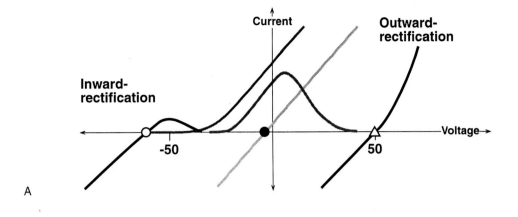

A

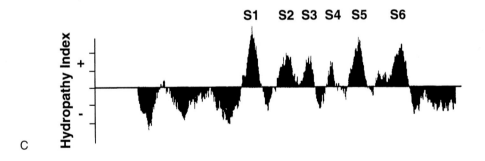

B

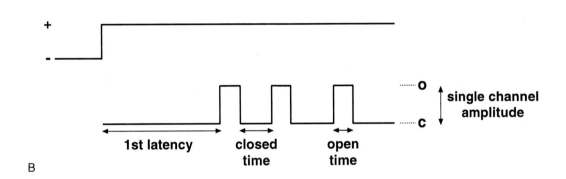

C

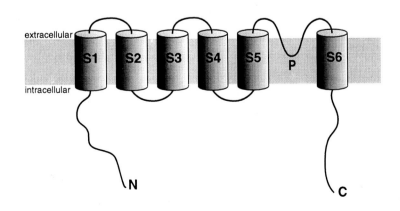

D

dephosphorylation, by interactions with other proteins (e.g., G protein, proteins of the extracellular matrix, and proteins of the cytoskeleton), and by the reversible association-dissociation of auxiliary subunits (14,17,19,35, 41,48,50,55,56,59).

GENERAL STRUCTURAL PRINCIPLES

The combination of molecular biological and electrophysiologic methods has produced in the last decade enormous progress in our knowledge of ion channel

structure and function (14,15,19,27,37,38,48,66). Channel-forming proteins may vary considerably in size, ranging from ~100 to more than 1,000 amino acids. Despite these variations, some common structural principles have emerged. Mammalian channel proteins usually are members of gene superfamilies and may be classified accordingly (15,19,66). Furthermore, all channel proteins contain hydrophobic segments that transverse the lipid bilayer. They may be readily recognized by constructing a hydrophobicity plot (Fig. 1C). The hydrophobicity along the sequence is averaged for each amino acid residue and

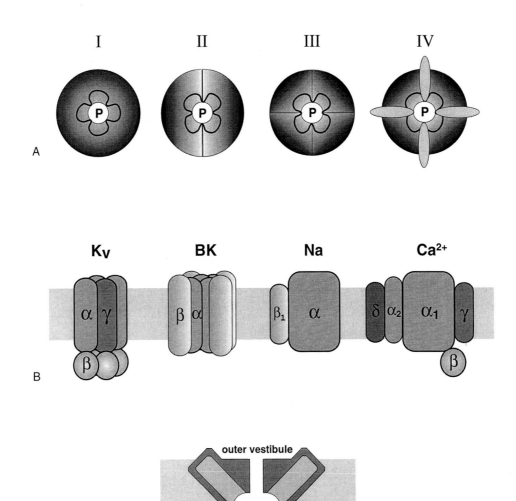

FIG. 2. A: Four P domains may be assembled to form a functional ion channel pore. The four P domains may be encoded in one polypeptide (I) (e.g., like in voltage-gated Na^+ channels and in voltage-gated Ca^{2+} channels). Alternatively, the channel subunits may contain two P domains (II) (e.g., in TWIK-type K^+ channels) or only one P domain (e.g., voltage-gated K^+ channels) (III). Also, the P domains may be formed by more than one type of ion channel subunit (IV) (e.g., Kv LQT1 channels may recruit minK subunits for pore formation). **B:** The topology of the subunits forming the voltage-gated K^+, Ca^{2+}, and Na^+ channels, and the calcium-activated large-conductance K^+ channel. Only the α and α_1 subunits may form by themselves functional channels in heterologous *in vitro* expression systems.

plotted. (The respective algorithms are available with every standard software package for analyzing protein structures.) Hydrophobic sequences of approximately 20 amino acids are likely to transverse the membrane. The detection of hydrophobic sequences may then be used to predict a membrane topology for the respective ion channel protein (Fig. 1D). Ion channels frequently exhibit an additional hydrophobic domain that does not span the membrane, but enters and exits the membrane from the same side and forms a loop (Fig. 1D) (49). Because this loop structure is an important element for ion channel pore formation (24,69,78), it is called the P (pore) domain. Many mutational structure/function studies have been conducted. Generally, the results have lent strong support for the channel protein topologies that were originally predicted on the basis of hydrophobicity plots. Recently the successful crystallization of a small bacterial K channel has provided a first detailed insight into the three-dimensional structure of an ion channel (21) (see below). The derived crystal structure agrees extremely well with the structural models that were made previously on the basis of analyzing the functions of native and mutated ion channel proteins.

Ion channels may consist of one single polypeptide in the form of a homoner. Alternatively, ion channels may be assembled from more than one subunit, for example, as dimers, trimers, tetramers (15,19,37,66). Assembly may involve the association of like subunits (homomers) or of different subunits (heteromers) (Fig. 2A). Commonly, the integral membrane proteins (subunits) that form functional channels in *in vitro* expression systems are called α subunits. Most ion channels probably consist of additional (β, γ, δ) subunits (Fig. 2B). They have various auxiliary functions and may be integral membrane proteins or be associated with cytoplasmic α-subunit structures (14). The auxiliary subunits may influence the gating behavior, the ion conductance through the pore, the cell surface expression, the interaction with extra- and intracellular matrix proteins, and the subunit assembly. Thus, ion channels are most often heteromeric complexes containing more than one subunit.

SIMPLE CHANNEL STRUCTURES

Apparently, the most simple ion channel α subunits are polypeptides with two membrane-spanning domains, M1 and M2, and a P domain linking the M1 and M2 domains (20,38,46,51) (Fig. 3A). These subunits form inwardly rectifying K (K_{IR}) channels. Function K_{IR} channels are formed by assembly of four subunits as homo- or heterotetramers. The pore is built from four P domains with a K-channel signature sequence (GYGD). In addition to the P domain, other residues residing in both the transmembrane and cytoplasmic domains make important contributions to a functional K_{IR}-channel pore. Prominent members of the K_{IR}-channel family are the G protein–

sensitive GIRK channels (45,74) and the ATP-sensitive K_{ATP} channels (4,34,70). GIRK channel activity is regulated by receptor activation (e.g., activation of cardiac muscarine-receptors activates K_{IR}-channels in the heart) (45). Interestingly, GIRK channel activation by G-protein binding is indirect (Fig. 3B). In fact, GIRK channels are activated by the lipid PIP_2 (6). G proteins probably stabilize PIP_2 binding to GIRK channels, and this increases Po. K_{ATP} channels require K_{IR} 6.2 subunits and the sulfonylurea receptor protein (4,34) for their function (see Fig. 3A). The SUR proteins are members of the ATP-binding cassette (ABC) family of proteins (31). The CFTR channel is another member of this family. K_{IR} 6.2 subunits contain in their carboxy-terminus sequences that inhibit their functionality in the absence of SUR receptors (70). However, it is still debated whether the ATP sensitivity of KATP channels is correlated with ATP-binding properties, either of K_{IR} 6.2 channels or SUR receptors or both. The importance of K_{ATP} channels for insulin secretion by pancreatic β cells has made them an important drug target for treating non–insulin-dependent diabetes mellitus (3). It also has been found that individuals with familial persistent hyperinsulinemic hypoglycemia of infancy carry a mutated SUR1 receptor gene (22,34). The mutations probably result in a loss of functional K_{ATP} channels, causing unregulated excessive insulin secretion.

The inward rectification of K_{IR} channels is caused by plugging the internal mouth of the channel pore by polyamines such as spermine, spermidine, and putrescine, and by Mg^{2+} (see Fig. 3B) It has been shown that negatively charged amino acid residues in the M2 segment and in the carboxy-terminus are important for binding spermine/Mg^{2+} and for providing rectifying properties (20,51). The spermine/Mg^{2+} block of K_{IR} channels provides a good explanation for understanding the inwardly rectifying behavior. At negative membrane potentials, K_{IR} channels are open and K^+ ions can freely pass through the pore. More depolarized membrane potentials increase the driving force not only for K^+, but also for spermine and Mg^{2+}. These cations enter the inner vestibule of K_{IR} channels and bind strongly, thereby interfering with the passage of K^+ through the pore. When the membrane potential returns to more negative values (e.g., negative to the K reversal potential), the spermine/Mg^{2+} block is elevated.

THREE DIMENSIONAL STRUCTURE OF A SIMPLE K^+ CHANNEL

Recently, K channel proteins with an M1-P-M2 structural motif have been discovered in bacteria (38,60). This made it possible to express the proteins with high yield in bacterial expression systems (60) and to crystallize a bacterial K^+ channel from *Streptomyces lividans* (KcsA) (21). The crystal structure was solved to a 3.4-Å resolution. At this resolution, the backbone fold of the tetra-

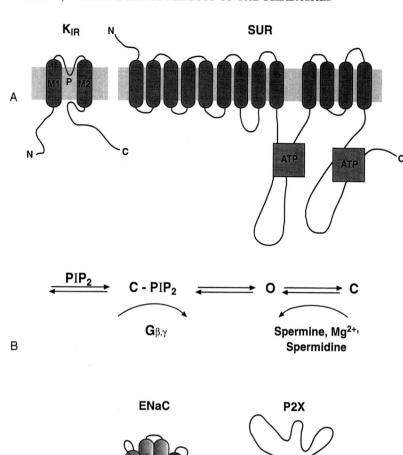

FIG. 3. A: Proposed topology of subunit of inwardly rectifying K+ channels (K_IR) consisting of two membrane-spanning hydrophobic segments M1 and M2, and a P domain inserted into the membrane from the outside. Additionally, a carboxy-terminal cytoplasmic domain may contribute to K_IR pore formation. ATP-sensitive K+ channels (KATP) contain an auxiliary subunit, the sulfonylurea (SUR) receptor, a member of the ATP-binding cassette protein family. **B:** Simplified hypothetical scheme to illustrate transition of closed (C) K_IR channels to the open state (O). The transition is facilitated by PIP_2, which binds to the closed K_IR channel to form a C-PIP_2 complex. The complex may be stabilized by G_{β,γ} protein. Spermine (spermidine, Mg^{2+}) acts as an open channel blocker. **C:** Backbone fold of the tetrameric KcsA channel from *Streptomyces lividans* as revealed by crystallographic analysis. Data are adapted from Doyle et al. (21).

meric KcsA channel is clearly discerned. The subunits are inserted into the tetramer such that the helical M1 membrane-spanning segment faces the lipid membrane and the helical M2 membrane-spanning segment the channel pore. The M2 helices are tilted and slightly linked, so that the subunits open like the petals of a flower facing the extracellular side of the membrane (see Fig. 2C). The pore lining is mainly hydrophobic, except for the selectivity filter. It is lined by polar main chain atoms belonging to the signature sequence amino acids. The main chain atoms create a stack of sequential oxygen rings for coordinating dehydrated K+ ions. These structural details are in excellent agreement with previous structural predictions made from functional and mutagenesis studies on cloned ion channels.

MORE COMPLEX ION CHANNEL STRUCTURES

To date the structures of all known K-channel α subunits seem to be derived from the M1-P-M2 structural motif. K-channel α subunits that assemble to voltage-gated K (Kv) channels consist of six hydrophobic transmembrane segments (S1 to S6) and a P domain located between S5 and S6 (see Fig. 1D). The voltage-sensing domains appear to be located mainly in segments S2 and S4 (53). The S4 segment has attracted particular attention because it contains a regular array (every fourth residue) of positively charged amino acids. They may contribute directly to the gating charges that move across the membrane in response to a change in membrane potential. This gating charge movement apparently results in a conformational change that may be the molecular basis for the voltage-dependent activation of voltage-gated K channels (53). The voltage dependence of activation obviously causes the channels to mediate outwardly rectifying currents that increase nonlinearly with voltage until all available channels have been activated to a maximum Po (see Equation 1). Only then does the Kv channel produce currents with an ohmic behavior. Similarly, the voltage-gated Na+ and Ca^{2+} channels contain positively charged membrane-spanning segments (S4), which may operate as voltage-sensors (2,53,77). Apparently the voltage-sensors of Na⁺, Ca²⁺, and K⁺ channels are made up from similar molecular structures, which operated in these channels through analogous mechanisms. Once activated, many voltage-gated ion channels tend to inactivate (see Fig. 3B). The inactivation time course may be very rapid, lasting a few milliseconds, or may be slow, lasting hundreds to thousands of milliseconds. The inactivated channel needs to recover from inactivation. Recovery pathways may pass through open channel states or directly through closed states. Channels usually are refractory to activation during recovery from inactivation. Distinct segments of amino acids (domains) on ion channel subunits have been identified that may determine the inactivation type (Fig. 4), for example, some Kv^a subunits have an amino-terminal inactivating domain that binds like a tethered ball on a chain to a receptor at or near the inner mouth of the activated Kv channel and thereby plugs the open pore (80). This type of inactivation has been coined N-type inactivation. Other Kv channel subunits have critical carboxy-terminal residues for inactivation in segment S6, which may

cause a C-type inactivation of the open pore (7). For voltage-gated Na⁺ channels, a hinged-lid type of inactivation mechanism has been proposed (23). This mechanism depends critically on a small region between the six-transmembrane segment domains III and IV with a phenylalamine at its center (residue 1489 in rat brain sodium channel type I).

EPISODIC PHENOTYPE OF ION CHANNEL MUTANTS

Approximately 50 different Kv α subunits are known (15). They form Kv channels exhibiting different voltage dependences of activation, different single-channel conductances and different time-scales of activation and, respectively, inactivation. Thus, an enormous diversity is most likely necessary to meet a cell's many needs for controlling and modulating membrane potential. The abundance of Kv channels may reflect some redundancy in the repolarizing capacity of a eucaryotic cell. Thus, a cell may not need the whole set of possible Kv channels under normal circumstances. In addition, cells may compensate for the absence of certain Kv channels by overexpressing others. However, under situations of excessive excitation, the cell may require the activity of all available Kv channels to attenuate or dissipate an excitatory situation that may be stressful and potentially harmful. Most likely, the available battery of K⁺ channels endows a cell with a certain buffering capacity against harmful depolarizing threats. Thus, the loss of Kv channel function may become apparent only under special conditions and may not be apparent under normal circumstances. This proposition may explain the phenotype of some "channellopathies" (ion channel–related diseases) exhibiting episodically recurrent symptoms. Examples are (Table 1) an autosomal-dominant form of ataxia (11), which is caused by mutations in the KCNA1 gene encoding Kv1.1 α subunits; a benign form of a familial juvenile epilepsy, which is caused by mutations in the KCNQ2 gene encoding Kv LQT2 subunits (8,16,63); two types of the LQT syndrome, an episodically occurring heart arrhythmia caused by mutated HERG, Kv LQT1, or minK subunits (5,18,43,59,65).*

The tetramic structure of Kv channels has another important consequence for the genetics of Kv channel mutants. Mutants that effect the gating machinery or the pore structure of Kv channels but still assemble with wild-type Kv α subunits most likely are antimorphs. One mutant subunit may already suffice to render the complete tetrameric channel inactive. Thus, these mutants are dominant, as is observed for many known mutations in

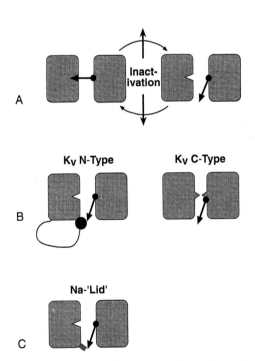

FIG. 4. Different types of inactivation have been discovered in voltage-gated ion channel. **A:** Common to all inactivations is an apparent impairment of ion-channel gate opening or closing. Schematic illustrations do not imply whether the gate is inside or outside the membrane electric field. **B:** Inactivating domains may behave like a tethered ball or a lid. Both structures may close the open pore and, thereby, inactivate the channel. **C:** Alternatively, the channel pore may undergo a conformational change, disabling the gate from swinging back into place. The inactivation illustrated in **B** and **C** has been described for voltage-gated K⁺ and Na⁺ channels.

---

*MinK subunits have only one membrane-spanning segment. They assemble together with Kv LQT1 and thereby may influence Kv LQT1 gating and pore properties. It is still debated whether minK subunits are auxiliary or pore-forming subunits.

TABLE 1. *Channelopathies related to K⁺ channels*

Channel	References	Syndrome
KATP	22	Hyperinsulinemic hyperglycemia
KCNA1	11	Episodic ataxia
KCNQ1	5, 59	LQT1 syndrome
KCNQ2	63	Benign form of juvenile epilepsy
KCNQ3	16	Benign form of juvenile epilepsy
KCNQ4	44	Deafness
HERG	18	LQT2 syndrome
ROMK1	62	Barter syndrome

For descriptions of the various genes and mutants, see text.

K-channel genes in humans and animals. In contrast, mutants that generate assembly-defective Kv α subunits are most likely recessive because the mutant subunit does not assemble with wild-type subunits. Mutations in other Kv-channel genes have been discovered that are correlated with a permanent loss of function, for example, mutations in the DFNA4 (KCNQ4) gene are correlated with deafness (44).

CYCLIC NUCLEOTIDE GATED CATION CHANNELS

The voltage sensors may be regarded as an intrinsic gating mechanism leading to the activation of the channel. Alternatively, channels may be gated by intrinsic or extrinsic factors such as Ca^{2+}, cyclic nucleotides, G proteins, lipids (see PIP_2 in Fig. 3B). Thus, K⁺ channels may be activated by Ca^{2+}. The Ca^{2+} may be bound to a domain residing in the α subunit (12,39) or may bind to an auxiliary subunit like calmodulin in the case of small-conductance K channels (76). Cyclic nucleotide gated (CNG) channels are assembled from α and β subunits (42,79). They contain a six-transmembrane segment structural motif reminiscent of Kv-channel α subunits and a CNG binding domain. The α subunits alone may express functional nonselective ion channels in *in vitro* expression systems. Some CNG channels may have a high Ca^{2+} permeability and may be gated either by cAMP or cGMP (42,79). The CNG-binding domain is located within the cytoplasmic carboxy-terminus. Most likely, binding of CNGs stabilizes the open state of CNG channels. It has been proposed that CNG-dependent gating of CNG channels does not reflect an acceleration of the transition of the closed to the open state, but rather a delay in the backward reaction (i.e., the transition from the open to the closed state) (79). Thereby, CNG binding apparently increases the open probability of CNG channels. The P-domain sequences of CNG and Kv channels revealed near or at the selectivity filter structural differences. They have been shown to be an important determinant of the differing ion selectivities of Kv and CNG channels (30). The experiments emphasize that CNG and Kv channels

belong to the same superfamily of ion channels. Small structural variations may transform CNG channels to Kv channels and vice versa. Indeed, several Kv channels related to the *Drosophila ether-à-go-go* (*eag*) gene have been cloned that also have a carboxy-terminal CNG-binding domain. The function of the CNG domain in *eag*-type channels has not yet been elucidated. A new branch encodes hyperpolarization-activated nonselective voltage-gated cation channels. They mediate in *in vitro* expression system I_f currents (26). These currents may determine the regular firing properties of excitable cells, that is, pacemaker activity. Thus, ion channels of the CNG-channel superfamily are involved in a variety of cellular functions, including photoreceptor signal transduction in rod and cone cells, olfactory responsiveness, and pacemaker activity, for example, in thalamic neurons and in the sinoatrial node.

STRUCTURE OF ENAC-TYPE ION CHANNELS

EnaC stands for amiloride-sensitive epithelial Na⁺ channels. These non–voltage-gated channels are important for transepithelial salt transport. ENaC channels are found in principal cells in the collecting duct of the mammalian kidney, where they provide the aldosterone-regulated Na⁺ entry pathway necessary for salt reabsorption. ENaC channels are assembled from three different subunits (α, β, and γ) (13). Mutations in the β and γ subunit genes cause a heritable form of pseudoaldosteronism (Liddle syndrome) (25,64). The increased activity of the mutant ENaC channels leads to hypertension and to enhanced salt readsorption by the kidney. On the other hand, mutant ENaC channels that are inactivated cause pseudohypoaldosteronism type I (PHAI). This renal disease is a salt-wasting disorder that occurs because Na⁺ uptake in the collecting duct in the kidney has been impaired. ENaC channel subunits have a topology distinct from those encountered in the Ca/Na/K channel superfamily. They may comprise two transmembrane segments that are separated by a large extracellular loop sequence. It has been proposed that part of this loop enters and exits the membrane in a manner similar to the P domain. Unlike the P domains in the Ca/Na/K channel superfamily, the pore-forming structure in the ENaC ion channel family has not been elucidated yet in great detail. So far, a structure like the K-channel signature sequence is not obvious.

Subsequent to the molecular cloning of ENaC channels, channel-forming polypeptides have been discovered that are related in sequence or topology. Several of the related ENaC polypeptides form in *in vitro* expression systems nonselective ion channels that may be gated by changes in intracellular pH or by changes in cell volume and pressure. In the nematode *C. elegans*, certain genes involved in neurodegeneration (degenerins) and mechanosensation (mec) encode proteins homologous to ENaC polypeptides (52,72). Therefore, it is hypothesized that ENaC/mec/degenerin type channels may play some role in the transmission of sensory signals involving pain, touch, inflammation, and pressure (72). P2X receptors appear to have a topology that is similar to the one of ENaC family members, that is, two membrane-spanning hydrophobic segments connected by an extracellular heavily glycosylated large loop (52). P2X receptors bind extracellular ATP, which may serve as a neurotransmitter to bind and open the P2X cation channels. P2X receptors represent an ATP-gated nonselective cation channel family. Note that a role in pain sensation has been proposed for P2X type channels, for pH-regulated mec channels, and for certain tetrodotoxin-insensitive voltage-gated Na^+ channels (68).

THE MIP FAMILY OF CHANNEL PROTEINS

The MIP family received its name from the characterization of the major intrinsic protein (MIP) of the bovine lens fiber cell membrane. Members of this family have been reported to have transmembrane-channel activities for ions, water, decarboxylates, and straight-chain carbon compounds. The most reknowned member of the MIP family is the water channel (aquaporin) (54,73,75). Aquaporins achieve high water transport rates, which are required, for example, in red blood cell function and in the kidney.

The MIP family proteins are highly conserved, containing a duplicated structure that may have arisen by a tandem intragenic duplication. The topology of the MIP proteins reflects this duplication. Although MIP proteins have six membrane-spanning hydrophobic segments like Kv and CNG channels, they are folded into two halves, forming two domains of three transmembrane segments. One aquaporin has been crystallized (75).

CHLORIDE CHANNELS

Chloride channels are permeable to anions, particularly to chloride, the most abundant anion in the body. The Nernst potential for Cl^- is close to the resting membrane potential in many cells. Thus, chloride inward currents may be important to reset the membrane potential upon excitation. Conversely, hyperpolarized cell membranes (i.e., having a membrane potential below the reversal potential for Cl^-) may be depolarized by opening chloride channels. Taking the many diverse roles of chloride channels in excitable and nonexcitable cells into account, it may not be surprising that many structurally different chloride channels are found in mammalian cells. They may be related to the ligand-gated ion channel superfamily (GABA receptors, glycine receptors) (61,71), to the ATP-binding cassette transporter family (CFTR Cl^- channel) (57), to the ClC-Cl^- channel family (40), or to the I_{Cln}-channel family (28). Chloride channel

pore-forming structures are not yet as well understood as those of voltage-gated cation channels. Therefore, they are not discussed here.

The repolarization of action potentials generated upon excitation in mammalian muscle cells is mainly due to the activity of ClC-1 channels. Thus, certain muscle myotonias (recessive generalized myotonia of the Becker type and a dominant myotonia congenita, Thompson disease) are caused by mutations in the ClC-1 gene (40). Also, some inherited forms of nephrolithiasis are due to mutation in the ClC-5 gene. Finally, the CFTR Cl^- channel is an important Cl^- channel because mutations in the CFTR gene are causally related to inherited cystic fibrosis (57).

CONCLUSIONS

Many genes have been discovered that code for ion channel subunits. The α subunits of cation-selective ion channels have related topologies and structural properties. They may have evolved from a common ancestor. Mutations in a few ion channel genes have been correlated with human diseases and therefore have been called channelopathies. They often are episodic in nature, leading to such conditions as migraine (CACNA1), ataxia (KCNA1), and epilepsy (KCNQ2/KCNQ3). Some mutations that lead to loss of ion channel function may be compensated by increased expression and/or activity of other ion channels.

REFERENCES

1. Ackerman MJ, Clapham DE. Ion channels basic science and clinical disease. *N Engl J Med* 1997;336:1575–1586.
2. Armstrong CM, Hille B. Voltage-gated ion channels and electrical excitability. *Neuron* 1998;20:371–380.
3. Ashcroft FM. Sweet news for hypoglycemic babies. *Nature Med* 1996;12:1301–1302.
4. Ashcroft FM, Gribble FM. Correlating structure and function in ATP-sensitive K^+ channels. *TINS* 1998;21:288–294.
5. Barhanin J, Lesage F, Guillemare E, Fink M, Lazdunski M, Romey G. KvLQT1 and IsK (minK) proteins associate to form the IKs cardiac potassium current. *Nature* 1996;384:78–80.
6. Baukrowitz T, Schulte U, Oliver D, et al. PIP2 and PIP as determinants for ATP inhibition of KAPT channels. *Science* 1998;282:1141–1144.
7. Baukrowitz T, Yellen G. Modulation of K^+ current by frequency and external $[K^+]$: a tale of two inactivation mechanisms. *Neuron* 1995;15:951–960.
8. Bievert C, Schroeder BC, Kubisch C, et al. A potassium channel mutation in neonatal human epilepsy. *Science* 1998;279:403–406.
9. Boyden PA, Jeck CD. Ion channel function in disease. *Cardiovasc Res* 1995;29:312–318.
10. Brown AM. Cardiac potassium channels in health and disease. *Trends Cardiovasc Med* 1997;7:118–124.
11. Browne DL, Gancher ST, Nutt JG, et al. Episodic ataxia/myokymia syndrome is associated with point mutations in the human potassium channel gene, KCNA1. *Nat Genet* 1994;8:138–140.
12. Buttler A, Wu A, Baker K, Salkoff. A family of putative potassium channel genes in Drosophila. *Science* 1989;243:943–947.
13. Canessa CM, Schild L, Buell G, et al. Amiloride-sensitive epithorial Na^+ channel is made of three homologous subunits. *Nature* 1994;367:463–467.
14. Catterall WA. Structural and function of voltage-gated ion channels. *Annu Rev Biochem* 1995;64:493–531.

15. Chandy KG, Gutmann GA. Voltage-gated K+ channels. In: *Handbook of receptors and channels.* Boca Raton, FL: CRC Press, 1995.

16. Charlier C, Singh NA, Ryan SG, et al. A pore mutation in a novel KQT-like potassium channel gene in an idiopathic epilepsy family. *Nat Genet* 1998;18:53–55.

17. Craven SE, Bredt DS. PDZ proteins organize synaptic signaling pathways. *Cell* 1998;93:495–498.

18. Curran ME, Splawski I, Timothy KW, Vincent GM, Green ED, Keating MT. A molecular basis for cardiac arrhythmia: HERG mutations cause lon QT syndrome. *Cell* 1995;80:795–803.

19. DeWaard M, Gurnett CA, Campbell KP. Structural and functional diversity of voltage-activated calcium channels. *Ion Channels* 1996;4:41–87.

20. Doupnik CA, Davidson N, Lester HA. The inward rectifier potassium channel family. *Curr Opin Neurobiol* 1995;5:268–277.

21. Doyle DA, Cabral JM, Pfuetzner RA, et al. The structure of the potassium channel: molecular basis of K+ conduction and selectivity. *Science* 1998;280:69–77.

22. Dunne MJ, Kane C, Shepherd RMSJA, et al. Familial persistent hyperinsulinemic hypoglycemia of infancy and mutations in sulfonylurea receptor. *N Engl J Med* 1997;336:703–706.

23. Eaholtz G, Scheuer T, Catterall WA. Restoration of inactivation and block of open sodium channels by an inactivation gate peptide. *Neuron* 1994;12:1041–1048.

24. Ellinor PT, Yang J, Sather WA, Zhang JF, Tsien RW. Ca2+ channel selectivity at a single locus for high-affinity Ca2+ interactions. *Neuron* 1995; 15:1121–1132.

25. Firsov D, Schild L, Gautschi I, Mérillat AM, Schneeberger E, Rossier BC. Cell surface expression of the epithelial Na channel and a mutant causing Liddle syndrome: a quantitative approach. *Proc Natl Acad Sci U S A* 1996;93:15370–15375.

26. Gaus R, Seifert R, Kaupp UB. Molecular identification of an hyperpolarization-activated channel in sea urchin sperm. *Nature* 1998;393:583–587.

27. Goldin AL. Voltage-gated sodium channels. In: *Handbook of receptors and channels.* Boca Raton, FL: CRC Press, 1995.

28. Gschwentner M, Susanna A, Schmarda A, et al. I$_{cln}$: a chloride channel paramount for cell volume regulation. *J Allergy Clin Immunonol* 1996; 98[suppl]:98–101.

29. Hamill OP, Neher ME, Sakmann B, Sigworth F. Improved patch-clamp techniques for high-resolution current recording from cells and cell-free membrane patches. *Pflugers Arch* 1991;391:85–100.

30. Heginbotham L, Abramson T, McKinnon R. A functional connection between the pores of distantly related ion channels as revealed by mutant K– channels. *Science* 1992;258:1152–1155.

31. Higgins DF. The ABC of channel regulation. *Cell* 1995;82:693–696.

32. Hille B. *Ionic channels of excitable membranes,* 2nd ed. Sunderland, MA: Sinauer Associates, 1992.

33. Hoffmann EP. Voltage-gated ion channelopathies: inherited disorders caused by abnormal sodium, chloride, and calcium regulation in skeletal muscle. *Annu Rev Med* 1995;46:431–441.

34. Inagaki N, Gonoi T, Clement JP IV, et al. Reconstitution of IKATP: an Inward Rectifier Subunit Plus the Sulfonylurea Receptor. *Science* 1995; 170:1166–1170.

35. Isom LL, Ragsdale DS, De Jongh KS, et al. Structure and function of the β2 subunit of brain sodium channels, a transmembrane glycoprotein with a CAM motif. *Cell* 1995;83:433–442.

36. Jan LY, Jan YN. Potassium channels and their evolving gates. *Nature* 1994;371:119–122.

37. Jan LY, Jan YN. Cloned potassium channels from eukaryotes and prokaryotes. *Annu Rev Neurosci* 1997;20:91–123.

38. Jan LY, Jan YN. Voltage-gated and inwardly rectifying potassium channels. *J Physiol* 1997;505:267–282.

39. Jan LY, Jan YN. Ways and means for left shifts in the MaxiK channel. *Proc Natl Acad Sci U S A* 1997;84:13383–13385.

40. Jentsch TJ. Chloride channels: a molecular perspective. *Curr Opin Neurobiol* 1996;6:303–310.

41. Jonas EA, Kaczmarek LK. Regulation of potassium channels by protein kinases. *Curr Opin Neurobiol* 1996;6:318–323.

42. Kaupp U. Family of cyclic nucleotide gated ion channels. *Curr Opin Neurobiol* 1995;5:434–442.

43. Keating MT, Sanguinetti MC. Pathophysiology of ion channel mutations. *Curr Opin Genet Dev* 1996;6:326–333.

44. Kubisch C, Schroeder BC, Friedrich T, et al. KCNQ4, a novel potassium channel expressed in sensory outer hair cells, is mutated in dominant deafness. *Cell* 1999;96:1–20.

45. Kunkel MT, Peralta EG. Identification of domains conferring G protein regulation on inward rectifier potassium channels. *Cell* 1995;83:443–449.

46. Lester HA, Dougherty DA. New views of multi-ion channels. *J Gen Physiol* 1998;111:181–183.

47. Lifton RP. Genetic determinants of human hypertension. *Proc Natl Acad Sci U S A* 1995;92:8545–9551.

48. McCleskey EW. Calcium channels: cellular roles and molecular mechanisms. *Curr Opin Neurobiol* 1994;4:304–312.

49. McKinnon R. Pore loops: an emerging theme in ion channel structure. *Neuron* 1995;14:889–892.

50. McPhee JC, Dank YL, Davidson N, Lester HA. Evidence for a functional interaction between integrins and g protein-activated inward rectifier K+ channels. *J Biol Chem* 1998;273:34696–34702.

51. Nichols CG, Lopatin AN. Inward rectifier potassium channels. *Annu Rev Physiol* 1997;59:171–191.

52. North RA. Families of ion channels with two hydrophobic segments. *Curr Opin Cell Biol* 1996;8:474–483.

53. Papazian DM, Bezanilla F. How does an ion channel sense voltage? *News Physiol Sci* 1997;12:203–210.

54. Park JH, Saier MH. Phylogenetic characterization of the MIP family of transmembrane channel proteins. *J Membr Biol* 1996;153:171–180.

55. Pragnell M, De Waard M, Mori Y, Tanabe T, Snutch TP, Campbell KP. Calcium channel β-subunit binds to a conserved motif in the I–II cytoplasmic linker of the α$_1$-subunit. *Nature* 1994;368:67–70.

56. Rettig J, Heinemann SH, Wunder F, Lorra C, Parcej DN, Dolly JO, Pongs O. Inactivation properties of voltage-gated K+ channels altered by presende of β-subunit. *Nature* 1994;26:289–294.

57. Riordan JR. The cystic fibrosis transmembrane conductance regulator. *Annu Rev Physiol* 1993;55:609–630.

58. Rivera C, Voipio J, Payne JA, et al. The K+/Cl– co-transporter KCC2 renders GABA hyperpolarizing during neuronal maturation. *Nature* 1999; 297:251–255.

59. Sanguinetti MC, Curran ME, Zou A, et al. Coassembly of KvLQT1 and minK (IsK) proteins to form cardiac IKs potassium channel. *Nature* 1996;384:80–83.

60. Schrempf H, Schmidt O, Kümmerlen R, et al. A prokaryotic potassium ion channel with two predicted transmembrane segments from *Streptomyces lividans.* *EMBO J* 1995;14:170–178.

61. Sieghart W. Structure and pharmacology of γ-aminobutyric acidA receptor subtypes. *Pharmacol Rev* 1995;47:181–234.

62. Simon DB, Karet FE, Rodriguez-Soriano J, et al. Genetic heterogeneity of Bartter's syndrome revealed by mutations in the K+ channel, ROMK. *Nat Genet* 1996;14:152–156.

63. Singh NA, Charlier C, Stauffer D, et al. A novel potassium channel gene, KCNQ2, is mutated in an inherited epilepsy of newborns. *Nat Genet* 1998;18:25–29.

64. Snyder PM, Price MP, McDonald FJ, et al. Mechanism by which Liddle's syndrome mutations increase activity of a human epithelial Na+ channel. *Cell* 1995;83:969–978.

65. Splawski I, Tristani-Firouzi M, Lehmann MH, Sanguinetti MC, Keating MT. Mutations in the hminK gene cause long QT syndrome and suppress Iks function. *Nat Genet* 1997;17:338–340.

66. Stea A, Soong TW, Snutch TP. Voltage-gated calcium channels. In: *Handbook of receptors and channels.* Boca Raton, FL: CRC Press, 1995.

67. Stoffel M, Jan LY. Epilepsy genes: excitement traced to potassium channels. *Nat Genet* 1998;12:6–8.

68. Tate S, Benn S, Hick C, et al. Two sodium channels contribute to the TTX-R sodium current in primary sensory neurons. *Nature Neuro* 1998; 1:653–655.

69. Terleau H, Heinemann SH, Stühmer W, et al. Mapping the site of block by tetrodotoxin and saxitoxin of sodium channel II. *FEBS Lett* 1991;293: 93–96.

70. Tucker SJ, Gribble FM, Zhao C, Trapp S, Ashcroft FM. Truncation of Kir6.2 produces ATP-sensitive K+ channels in the absence of the sulphonalurea receptor. *Nature* 1997;387:179–183.

71. Tyndale RF, Olsen RW, Tobin AJ. GABAA receptors. In: *Handbook of receptors and channels.* Boca Raton, FL: CRC Press, 1995.

72. Waldmann R, Champigny G, Bassilana F, Heurteaux C, Lazdunski M. A proton-gated cation channel involved in acid-sensing. *Nature* 1997; 386:173–177.

73. Welte W, Nestel U, Wacker T, Diederichs K. Structure and function of the porin channel. *Kidney Int* 1995;48:930–940.

74. Wickman KD, Clapham D. G-protein regulation of ion channels. *Curr Opin Neurobiol* 1995;5:278–285.

75. Wintour EM. Water channels and urea transporters. *Clin Exp Pharmacol Physiol* 1997;24:1–9.

76. Xia XM, Fakler B, Rivard A, et al. Mechanism of calcium gating in small-conductance calcium-activated potassium channels. *Nature* 1998;395:503–507.

77. Yang N, George AL, Horn R. Molecular basis of charge movement in voltage-gated sodium channels. *Neuron* 1996;16:113–122.

78. Yool AJ, Schwartz K. Alternation of ionic selectivity of a K$^+$ channel by mutation of the H5 region. *Nature* 1991;349:700–704.

79. Zagotta WN, Siegelbaum SA. Structure and function of cyclic nucleotide-gated channels. *Ann Rev Neurosci* 1996;19:235–263.

80. Zagotta WN, Hoshi T, Aldrich RW. Restoration of inactivation in mutants of Shaker potassium channels by a peptide derived from ShB. *Science* 1990;250:568–571.

The Headaches, Second Edition,
edited by J. Olesen, P. Tfelt-Hansen, and K.M.A. Welch.
Lippincott Williams & Wilkins, Philadelphia © 2000.

Basic Science Aspects of the Headaches

CHAPTER 19

Physiology of Ion Channels

Frank Lehmann-Horn and Karin Jurkat-Rott

In 1990 the molecular basis for a hereditary disorder in humans was first demonstrated genetically to be impaired ion channel function (6). Since then, more than a dozen diseases, now collectively known as *channelopathies*, have been described (16). These disorders are not at all restricted to excitable tissues; however, because ion channels, and especially the subgroup of voltage-gated channels, are important for muscle and neuron function in mediating excitability, the most striking advances have been made in the field of neurologic research. In addition, certain types of epilepsy, ataxia, and hemiplegic migraine are associated with mutations in a neuronal voltage-gated channel, the P-Q type calcium channel (26). This association indicates that ion channels may play an important role in the pathogenesis of headaches and pain in general, making a short overview of the physiologic function of voltage-gated ion channels worthwhile.

FUNCTION OF VOLTAGE-GATED CHANNELS

Physiologic Channel States

Voltage-gated channels have a transmembraneous pore that is highly selective for only a single type of ion, the conductance of which changes with membrane potential. Depolarization causes channel activation by markedly increasing the open probability until the time-dependent occurrence of channel inactivation during maintained depolarization reduces it, a process that is not intrinsically voltage dependent. Repolarization of the membrane before the process of inactivation will deactivate the

channel (i.e., reverse activation). Inactivated channels cannot reactivate immediately but instead require repolarization and a certain time for recovery from inactivation. Thus, voltage-sensitive cation channels usually have at least one open resting state and two closed states: the resting state from which the channels can activate and the inactivated state. Transitions from any one state into another is possible in both directions, allowing also transition from the resting to the inactivated state at depolarisation as well as recovery from inactivation by way of the open state. Forward and backward rate constants for the transitions determine the likelihood of the various channel states (Fig. 1).

Activation and Deactivation

Activation results from a depolarization-induced conformational change of the protein, leading to opening of the ion-conducting pore. This process can be fully reversed when membrane repolarization occurs before channels inactivate, called *deactivation*. Even when the pore is pharmacologically blocked, activation is associated with measurable charge movements through the membrane voltage field, the so-called gating current. The unusually high density of positive charges in the four transmembrane S4 segments, each containing four to eight positive amino acids, makes them a natural candidate for the voltage sensor. These highly conserved S4 segments carry arginine or lysine at every third position with two nonpolar residues interposed between them and form amphipathic α-helices. Replacing positive charges with neutral or negatively charged ones reduces the steepness of the voltage dependence of activation (39). The S4 segments seem to move in a spiral path ("sliding helix" or "helical screw" model) outward through canaliculi of the

F. Lehmann-Horn and K. Jurkat-Rott: Department of Applied Physiology, University of Ulm, 89069 Ulm, Germany.

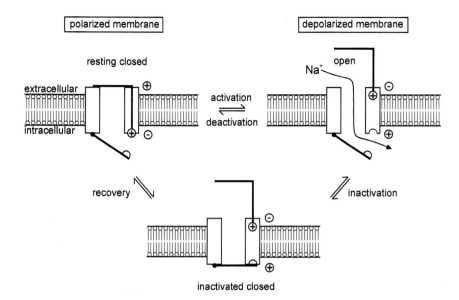

FIG. 1. Scheme of three states of the sodium channel that opens rapidly on depolarization and then closes to a fast inactivated state from which it reopens rarely. Repolarization of the membrane, initiated by the inactivation of the channel, leads to recovery from inactivation (= resting state), from which activation is again possible. Outward movement of the voltage sensor on depolarization results in both opening of the pore and exposure of a docking site for the inactivation gate.

channel protein, the outer charges becoming exposed on the cell surface while the inner charges become buried in the membrane during activation (45). This view, which resulted from mutagenesis experiments, also explains earlier findings that the size and shape of the hydrophobic (neutral) residues are also important for the ability of S4 to move and that neutralization of the outermost charge may have little effect, whereas neutralization of positive residues in turn 2, 3, or 4 of the helix strongly affects the voltage dependence.

Inactivation and Recovery from Inactivation

Voltage-gated channels usually display two modes of inactivation, fast and slow, depending on the duration of the repolarization needed for recovery. These nonconducting inactivated states probably are mediated by different molecular mechanisms. Fast inactivation describes the rapid (milliseconds) and complete decay of currents observed in response to short depolarizations. Slow inactivation occurs when cells are depolarized for seconds or minutes. Recovery from inactivation takes place at membrane repolarization on similar time scales as inactivation itself. The transition from the inactivated closed state to the resting closed state rarely causes reopening of the channel, because closing of the activation gate usually occurs faster than opening of the inactivation gate.

Fast Inactivation

Fast inactivation derives most of its voltage dependence from coupling to activation. The conformational changes resulting from depolarisation-induced activation increase the rate of inactivation. From studies on the intracellular perfusion of the giant axon with the proteolytic enzyme pronase, which abolished sodium channel

inactivation, it has become obvious that the inactivation gate is submembraneous and accessible to cytoplasmic agents. The absence of charge movements during inactivation suggested the location of the inactivation gate outside the membrane voltage field. Based on these studies, Armstrong and Bezanilla (1) proposed a ball-and-chain model in which the ball, tethered to the cytoplasmic side of the channel by the chain, swings into the inner mouth of the pore, where it bounds and blocks ion fluxes. Although originally proposed for the sodium channel, this model has been proved for fast-inactivating potassium channels where the pore-blocking ball is part of or attached to the N-terminus (so-called N-type inactivation) (11). For sodium channels, one or more of the cytoplasmic loops that link the various repeats could be involved in fast inactivation. That the loop between domains III and IV is essential was demonstrated by antibodies that only when directed against this region slowed fast inactivation (40). Mutagenesis experiments confirmed the sodium channel III/IV loop as an inactivation gate. When the mRNA encoding the sodium channel was cleaved, eliminating the III–IV interlinker encoding region and the two parts of the molecule were then coexpressed in *Xenopus* oocytes, inactivation was markedly slowed (39). The inactivation particle itself (i.e. the ball) seems to consist of three consecutive amino acids near the middle of the loop, namely, a phenylalanine and, less important, two other hydrophobic amino acids (43). Functional similarity allows this III/IV loop of the sodium channel even to confer fast inactivation to slowly inactivating potassium channels (27).

Because of the resemblance of this III–IV loop to the hinged lids of allosteric enzymes controlling substrate access, a slight modification of the ball-and-chain model was proposed. According to this hinged-lid model, the inactivation particle acts as a latch of a putative catch to be identified, and one of the hinges consists of a pair of glycines situated in the vicinity of the phenylalanine (27,43). In potassium channels, the S4–S5 interlinkers are adjacent to the intracellular orifice and may act as the acceptor for the N-type inactivation particle (12). Similar but not identical parts of the supposed S4–S5 helices and adjacent amino acids of the transmembrane segments S5 and S6 may form the catch of the sodium channel (18,21).

Slow Inactivation

Slow inactivation (resulting in channel closure), also called C-type (as counterpart to N-type) or core-associated inactivation, is not only kinetically distinct from fast inactivation, but it also involves different structural elements. Present in almost all voltage-gated (cation) channels, it is detectable even when fast inactivation has been destroyed. In potassium channels, it is a process that is influenced by cations of the external solution, which interacts with certain amino acids of the ion-conducting pore (foot-in-the-door model of gating) (7). Another mechanism involves modification of the intracellular vestibule by an auxiliary subunit (25).

Role of Channel Subunits

All voltage-gated sodium and calcium channels and at least the potassium channels of the *Shaker* family show varying composition of proteins copurifying in detergent solutions. Of these, the α-subunit determines the main characteristics of the complex conveying ion specificity and containing ion conducting pores, voltage sensors, gates for different opened and closed channel states, and important binding sites for endogenous and exogenous ligands. The basic motif of this essential subunit is a tetramic association of a series of six transmembrane α-helical segments, numbered S1–S6, connected by both intracellular and extracellular loops, the interlinkers. Channel function is dependent on supplemental subunits that may modify voltage sensitivity, kinetics, expression levels, or membrane localization (8). The auxilliary subunits of the different cation channels do not share homologous structures, indicating a large variety in possible mechanisms of channel modification.

Specific Voltage-Gated Channels

Sodium Channels

Membrane depolarization of excitable cells causes sodium channel activation in a feed-forward mechanism as the resulting increase in sodium conductance of the membrane is associated with further depolarization and activation of surrounding sodium channels, which in turn produces an action potential that rises to a peak close to

the sodium equilibrium potential within about 1 msec. The channel's intrinsic inactivation occurs within a few milliseconds (even at artificially maintained depolarization) and leads under unclamped, that is, natural conditions, to repolarization of the membrane, even in the absence of any voltage-gated potassium channels, a fact often missed in textbooks. After an action potential, the cell membrane is inexcitable for a short period, the so-called refractory period. The duration of this period is regulated by recovery of the channels from inactivation, limiting the firing rate of the cells (Figs. 1 and 2).

Heterologous coexpression of the β1-subunit, together with the α1-skeletal muscle subunit increases functional expression and current amplitude, shifts the steady-state activation and inactivation curves toward more negative potentials, and accelerates recovery from inactivation but does not seem to interact with the cardiac channel (20). At least two intrinsic conformation or gating modes exist, the faster inactivation of which is stabilized by β1 (33).

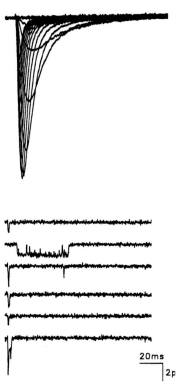

FIG. 2. Activation and inactivation of sodium channels of adult skeletal muscle expressed in *HEK293* cells. The *upper panel* shows families of sodium currents recorded at various test potentials in the whole-cell mode, and the *lower panel* traces of six subsequent single-channel recordings, each obtained by clamping the membrane potential from -90 to -20 mV. The channels open at the beginning of the depolarization step and immediately inactivate; during sustained depolarization, they rarely show reopenings such as bursts (as in trace 2) or short events (as in trace 3). (Modified from ref. 24, with permission.)

Structurally, the extracellular domain is decisive for both inactivation and recovery from inactivation.

Genes associated with diseases in man are *SCN4A* and *SCN5A*. Mutations of these cause *hyperkalemic periodic paralysis*, also in horses, *paramyotonia congenita, potassium-aggravated myotonia*, and *long QT syndrome 3*. Whereas the product of *SCN4A* is the only sodium channel α-subunit detectable in the fully differentiated and innervated skeletal muscle, *SCN5A* is expressed in both cardiac and fetal skeletal muscle. Additionally, *SCN8A* is a candidate gene for an inherited neurodegenerative disease as a deletion in the mouse homologue causes motor endplate disease and ataxia in the mouse. Even in the fruit fly, *Drosophila melanogaster*, mutations in the para locus encoding a neuronal voltage-gated sodium channel that is similar to those of vertebrate sodium channels can cause paralysis.

Calcium Channels

In the synaptic region of dendrites and cell somata of the central nervous system, membranes are depolarized by the opening of three classes of glutamate-gated channels that mediate influx of calcium and monovalent cations: AMPA, kainate, and NMDA receptors. In axon terminals and sarcolemma, calcium influx is mediated along the electrochemical gradient by voltage-gated ion-specific calcium channels. As in sodium channels, membrane depolarization activates them in a feed-forward mechanism and produces a macroscopic action potential with slight overshoot some 100 mV short of the calcium equilibrium potential. In contrast to sodium channels, rate constants for activation and the channel's intrinsic inactivation are slower so that repolarisation of the membrane is delayed (Fig. 3).

Voltage-gated calcium channels are classified into transient (T-type) and long-lasting (L-type) currents according to their inactivation properties, and B (brain), N (neuronal), P (Purkinje cell) and R (resistant) channels are distinguished by their tissue expression pattern. Whereas T-type channels are low-voltage activated, the thresholds for L-type and P-types are high. R-type channels are opened by a depolarization smaller than that needed for high-voltage activated (HVA) channels such as L-type channels and larger than that necessary for low-voltage activated (LVA) channels like the T-type. Especially the cardiac L-type channel can be activated by cyclic adenosine monophosphate (cAMP)-dependent protein kinase A by means of certain G_S-proteins (46). The α1-subunits of N, P, and R channels may be voltage dependently inhibited by other G-proteins by a direct interaction between the Gβγ-complex and the α1-subunit (10). These stimulatory or inhibitory receptor-coupled mechanisms may coexist in synapses of the autonomous nervous system and its effector cells. Mutations in the skeletal muscle channel cause *hypokalemic periodic par-*

alysis and *malignant hyperthermia susceptibility type 5* in humans and *muscular dysgenesis* in mice. Other channel types are considered potential targets for autoantibodies in a subtype of *amyotrophic lateral sclerosis* and the *Lambert–Eaton syndrome*.

Calcium Channel α-Subunits of the Brain

The neuronal $α_{1A}$-channel associated with *familial hemiplegic migraine, episodic ataxia type 2*, and *spinocerebellar atrophy type 6* in humans and *ataxia* and *seizures* in mice (*tottering* and *leaner*) is expressed in the brain, the presynaptical membrane of the neuromuscular junction, axon-associated Schwann cells, and distal kidney convolute tubule. Its subcellular localization, many splice variants (30), variability in coexpression of auxiliary subunits and the N-type channel (47) influence functional characterisitics. The resulting electrophysiologic properties exhibit such different characteristics as the rapidly inactivating Q-type (granular cell-type calcium channel) and the slowly inactivating P-type current (Purkinje cell calcium channel [35]) originally thought to be mediated by two totally different voltage-gated calcium channels.

Additional Subunits of Calcium Channels

Even though the 1 subunits form functional channels by themselves, maximally four additional subunits, α2, β, γ, and δ, copurify. The α2/δ-subunit, which can bind the anticonvulsant drug gabapentin, not only increases α1 expression rates and current density but also accelerates inactivation kinetics and shifts both steady-state inactivation and activation curves in hyperpolarizing directions. Coexpression of any of the four β-subunits with $α_{1A}$ markedly increases the number of channel complexes inserted into the membrane and the current amplitude (2). Coexpression with $α_{1S}$ increased the number of dihydropyridine (DHP)–binding sites and accelerated current activation kinetics, however, without increasing current density (15). Similar effects have been noted for $α_{1C}$ when expressed in oocytes, increasing both the rate of activation and current. The type of β can determine decisively the current characteristics of channel complexes; that is, $β_{2A}$ induces the P-type current, and $β_{1B}$ and $β_3$ induce the Q-type current when coexpressed with $α_{1A}$ (36). β1 is an intracellular acid protein that binds to the loop connecting domains I and II of the α1-subunit, distinct from the consensus site for the G-protein complex (4). β3, on the other hand, is capable of differential modulation of G-protein inhibition of $α_{1A}$- and $α_{1B}$-subunits (29). The subunit is specifically expressed in skeletal muscle.

Coexpression with cardiac α1-subunits in amphibian and mammalian cell systems moderately increased calcium current amplitude and inactivation rate. The main effect is a shift of the voltage dependence of inactivation in the hyperpolarising direction (34,17).

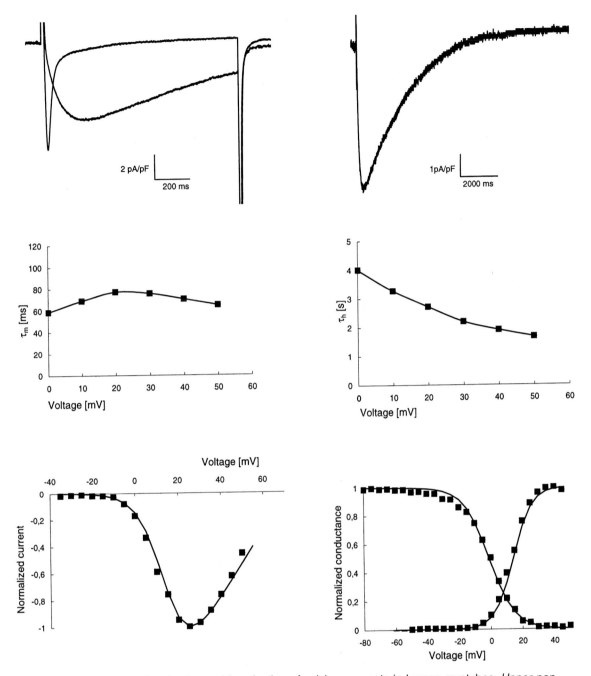

FIG. 3. Parameters of activation and inactivation of calcium currents in human myotubes. *Upper panels* show currents during voltage steps applied from a holding potential of –90 mV to both –20 mV and +25 mV (*left*) and to +20 mV (*right*). Note the fast low-threshold T-type calcium current on the left in addition to the slow high-threshold L-type current. The *middle panels* display the voltage dependence of the activation time constant τm (*left*) and of the inactivation time constant τh (*right*). The lower panels exhibit the average L-type current-voltage relationship (*left*) and the voltage dependence of steady-state activation and inactivation. Curves were calculated with the means of Boltzmann fit parameters. (Modified from ref. 14, with permission.)

Potassium Channels

Membrane depolarization activates voltage-gated potassium channels, which, once opened, conduct potassium ions along the concentration gradient and against the electric gradient. This outward current leads to repolarization or hyperpolarization of the membrane that induces channel deactivation. If depolarization is maintained, potassium channels inactivate with channel-intrinsic kinetics. Besides these voltage-gated channels, a large spectrum of channels are more or less sensitive to membrane potential and are activated or blocked by endogenous ligands. Voltage-insensitive potassium channels convey background conductance and therefore determine the resting membrane potential of cells, both excitable and nonexcitable. They also play a role in transmembrane transport, volume regulation, and signal transduction. Corresponding to their functional diversity and varying electrophysiologic properties, more than 13 subfamilies exisit, eight of which show the typical ion channel structural features of voltage sensor, toxin binding sites, and a single ion-conducting pore.

Classic Voltage-gated α-Subunits: Kv as Human Homologues of Shaker, Shab, Shaw, and Shal

These channels inactivate at different rates and to a varying extent (fast N-type and slow C-type inactivation). The rapidly inactivating A-type Kv channels operate in the subthreshold range of an action potential and play a key role in the generation of presynaptic and postsynaptic signals; the slowly inactivating, delayed rectifying channels repolarize the cell membrane during an action potential and reduce cell excitability. Both types are found in almost all eukaryotic cells of the animal and plant kingdoms and are present not only in nerve or muscle cells but also in lymphocytes, pancreatic islet cells, and others. The α-subunits typically form tetramers containing six transmembrane segments each; therefore, a tetramer corresponds to the already discussed sodium or calcium α-subunits (3). Among the classic voltage-gated potassium channel families, *Shaker/Kv1* (KCNA), *Shab/Kv2* (KCNB), *Shaw/Kv3* (KCNC), and *Shal/Kv4* (KCND), compatibility to aggregate as homotetramers (or within a channel subfamily also as heterotetramer) is conferred by a so-called T1 segment, an α-helical structure within the intracellularly located N-terminus, probably forming the vestibule of the pore as suggested by crystallisation experiments. Such tetramers show fast N-type inactivation if the N-terminus of one of the α subunits carries the inactivation "ball," for example, when Kv1.4 is involved. In the absence of the N-type ball, rapid inactivation can be achieved by the β1-subunit (19), as for Kv1.1; but, in the presence of an N-type inactivation prevention (NIP) as in Kv1.6, fast inactivation cannot be achieved even in heteromultimers with Kv1.4. From the functional point of view, however, the mode of inactivation in Kv channels may not be of major importance as long as channels are already deactivated during the repolarizing phase of a single action potential, thus before inactivation starts. The situation might be different during repetitive stimulation. So far, only mutations in Kv1.1 have been described to be associated with human disease, specifically, *episodic ataxia type 1*.

Voltage-sensitive α-Subunits: SLO or BK, Ikr or HERG, and LQT

These channels do not have an intracellular N-terminus. An aequous N-terminus seems to be completely absent in LQT, whereas that of SLO is located extracellularly. Consequently, SLO possesses an additional transmembrane segment, called S0 (42). SLO, encoded by *KCNMA1*, is known as the large-conductance (>150 pS with symmetric potassium concentrations) calcium-activated channel, or B_K (B for big) channel, that requires massive depolarization for activation in the absence of intracellular calcium. It possesses four additional hydrophobic segments S7–S10, which are thought to be associated with the inner surface of the membrane conveying calcium sensitivity. A subunit, hslo-beta, interacts with SLO and increases its sensitivity to charybdotoxin and intracellular calcium.

Nearly a decade ago, Ikr (r for rapid) was electrophysiologically described as a relatively fast delayed rectifier in cardiac myocytes and was contrasted to the slow delayed rectifying potassium current, Iks (s for slow) (44). Surprisingly, it showed similarity to the *Drosophila* ether-a-go-go (eag) potassium channel, leading to the term human ether-a-go-go related gene (*HERG*). Heterologous expression indeed showed a potassium channel with gating and pharmacologic properties similar to the Ikr current. A unique feature of the voltage-dependent gating of this channel is the relatively fast C-type inactivation resulting from high sensitivity to extracellular cations as well as the slow activation–deactivation compared with rapid inactivation. This combination of gating kinetics produces a novel inward-rectifying behavior of the channel: Inactivation is faster than activation, and so membrane depolarization is not associated with an outward current; recovery from inactivation is faster than deactivation so that repolarization causes a long-lasting tail current (32). *HERG* mutations cause the *long QT syndrome type 2*.

Channels of the LQT family are encoded by *KCNQ1-3*. Heterologous expression of *KCNQ1* cDNA led to currents the kinetics of which were unlike any potassium current. When coexpressed with *KCNE1* cDNA encoding MinK (see the following section), the potassium current density was much greater and was indistinguishable from the slow delayed rectifier current in the heart, Iks, both kinetically and pharmacologically. *KCNQ1* mutations cause the *long QT syndrome type 1*. *KCNQ2/3* mutations cause benign neonatal convulsions.

Definitive and Putative Subunits

Several sequences and structures conduct potassium ions only when associated with one of the above-mentioned α-subunits. Of the β-subunit family interacting with the voltage-gated α-subunit from the cytoplasma, two are known: the β1-subunit encoded by *KCNA1B* that confers N-type inactivation as well as the β2-subunit encoded by *KCNA2B* that increases the expression rate of the channel complex. A structurally different subunit, hslo-beta, which contains two transmembrane segments, interacts with SLO and increases its sensitivity to charybdotoxin (9) and to intracellular calcium concentrations greater than 100 nM, which occur during cellular excitation and functionally couple the two subunits (22). MinK proteins (also called ISK or Isk; encoded by *KCNE1*) containing a single transmembranous domain can conduct slowly activating potassium currents when expressed in oocytes and some cell lines that also may endogenously express interacting proteins like LQT channels. These currents are similar to those recorded in cardiac and some epithelial cells and are modulated following activation of various second- messenger systems. MinK is suggested to act as the subunit of LQT of so far unclear stoichiometry. The C-terminus of MinK is supposed to interact with the pore region of LQT, resulting in prolonged openings and smaller single-channel conductance. Mutations in MinK cause long QT syndrome type 6.

Chloride Channels

Chloride channels are present in the plasma membrane of most cells and play important roles in cell-volume regulation, transepithelial transport, secretion of fluid from secretory glands, and stabilization of membrane potential. They can be activated by extracellular ligands, intracellular calcium, cAMP, G-proteins, cell swelling, mechanical stretch, and transmembrane voltage. As mechanisms of activation may overlap, and expression of a given channel may not be restricted to a certain cell type, the classification is intriguing. Voltage-dependent chloride channels fulfill a variety of functions, depending on their tissue distribution: stabilization of the membrane potential, regulation of cell volume, and concentration of extracellular medium (13). The channels can be found both in plasmalemma and in the lining of internal organelles. In axons, voltage-dependent chloride conductance is so small that it is usually neglected, whereas that of skeletal muscle is even larger than the resting conductance for potassium. Nevertheless, its electrophysiologic identification and characterization at the single channel level turned out to be difficult because of its low single-channel conductance, near 1 pS as estimated from noise analysis (28). The large macroscopic chloride conductance, therefore, must result from a high channel density in the membrane (Fig. 4).

CLC1, the main chloride channel of skeletal muscle, is functional when expressed in *Xenopus* oocytes (37) or human embryonic kidney cells (5,28) without any other subunits. The channel conducts over the entire physiologic voltage range, showing inward rectification in the negative potential range. It is activated on depolarization and deactivated with hyperpolarizing voltage steps to a non-zero steady-state level and has a single-channel conductance of about 1 pS (28). As already known from macroscopic experiments performed in the early 1970s, the channel can be blocked by external I- and by low concentrations of 9-anthracene carboxylic acid.

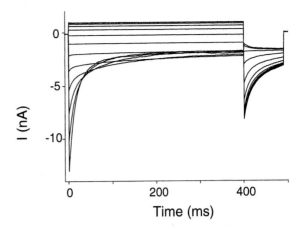

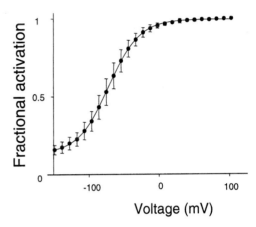

FIG. 4. Behavior of human skeletal muscle CLC-1 channels expressed in a mammalian cell line. *Upper panel*: Macroscopic currents, recorded in the patch-clamp whole-cell mode, were activated from a holding potential of 0 mV by voltage steps to potentials of −145 to +95 mV and deactivated after 400 ms by polarisation to −105 mV. *Lower panel*: Voltage dependence of the relative open probability in the physiologic potential range is shown. (Modified after ref. 41, with permission.)

Topologic arrangement of the putative 13 helical segments is not fully clarified. Currently, two different configurations for ClC1 are accepted, namely, a model that places S4 extracellularly and the hydrophobic core of S9–S12 crosses the membrane several times (31) or, alternatively, a model that places S2 extracellularly (23). Functional CLC channel proteins consist of double-barrelled homodimers with two functional off-axis pores, each with its own independent activation gate but with a slowly inactivating gate in common. Evidence for this model came from coexpression studies of naturally occurring mutations changing the single-channel conductance with wild-type, which resulted in channels with different conductance levels and largely independent pores. Mutations in CLC1 cause dominant or recessive *myotonia congenita*.

Closely related members of the same subfamily may assemble as heterodimers, such as the voltage-dependent skeletal muscle chloride channel CLC1 and the voltage- and volume-sensitive ubiquitously expressed CLC2. The proteins show a typical chloride over iodide specificity, are blockable by unspecific agents only, and can both be inwardly (*CLC1* and *CLC2*) or outwardly rectifying (*CLC5*). The latter conducts noninactivating currents detectable only at voltages more positive than -20 mV (38), mutations of which cause a recessive form of nephrocalcinosis. The other mammalian genes, such as the widely expressed *CLCN3* and *CLCN4*, the kidney-specific genes *CLCNKA* and *CLCKB*, and the ubiquitously expressed *CLCN6* and *CLCN7* genes could not be functionally expressed as Cl-channels or their expression has been controversially discussed. Even coexpression of several evolutionarily closely related genes such as *CLCN3* and *CLCN4* did not yield conducting channels, suggesting lack of adequate environment to function, such as missing auxilliary subunits or secondary processing pathways.

ROLE OF ION CHANNELS IN HUMAN DISEASE

Disease is associated with functional alterations of ion channels. When taking into consideration that ion channels are expressed ubiquitously, possible associations to human disorders to be detected in the future are boundless. Despite the diversity of this class of proteins, the pathophysiology of all known ion channelopathies seem to follow a similar pattern in which membrane depolarization plays the key role, leading to both hyperexcitability and underexcitability, depending on the grade of the disturbance.

Knowledge of structure–function relationships on the molecular level is invaluable in interpreting both genetic findings and electrophysiologic studies. Whereas in the monomers of sodium and calcium channels mainly dominant mutations occur, generating a change of function with dominant-positive (gain of function) or dominant-negative (loss of function) effects, the situation in the multimers of chloride and potassium channels is much more complicated (for review, see 16). Functional consequences of strong mutations may be diluted by coaggregation of mutant with wild-type proteins, making potentially dominant mutations recessive. On the other hand, weak mutations may lead to disease by coaggregation of mutant homomultimers. For hemiplegic migraine, the causative mutations in the P/Q-type calcium monomer are dominant. causing a change of function. This will be of use in developing a therapeutic model as the effect of potential drugs on the disturbed channel function can be determined directly.

REFERENCES

1. Armstrong CM, Bezanilla F. Inactivation of the sodium channel: II. Gating current experiments. *J Gen Physiol* 1977;70:567–590.
2. Brice NL, Berrow NS, Campbell V, et al. Importance of the different beta subunits in the membrane expression of the alpha1A and alpha2 calcium channel subunits: studies using a depolarization-sensitive alpha1A antibody. *Eur J Neurosci* 1997;9:749–759.
3. Chandy KG, Gutman GA. Voltage-gated K- channel genes. In: Nort AR, ed. *Handbook of receptors and channels: ligand- and voltage-gated ion channels*. Boca Raton, FL: CRC Press, 1995;1–71.
4. De Waard M, Liu H, Walker D, Scott VES, Gurnett CA, Campbell KP. Direct binding of G-protein complex to voltage-dependent calcium channels. *Nature* 1997;385:446–450.
5. Fahlke C, Rüdel R, Mitrovic N, Zhou M, George AL Jr. An aspartic acid residue important for voltage-dependent gating of human muscle chloride channels. *Neuron* 1995;15:463–472.
6. Fontaine B, Khurana TS, Hoffman EP, et al. Hyperkalemic periodic paralysis and the adult muscle sodium channel α-subunit gene. *Science* 1990;250:1000–1003.
7. Grissmer S, Cahalan MD. Divalent ion trapping inside potassium channels of human T lymphocytes. *J Gen Physiol* 1989;93:609–630.
8. Gurnett CA, Campbell KP. Transmembrane auxiliary subunits of voltage-dependent ion channels. *J Biol Chem* 1996;271:27975–27978.
9. Hanner M, Schmalhofer WA, Munujos P, Knaus H-G, Kaczorowski GJ, Garcia ML. The subunit of the high-conductance calcium-activated potassium channel contributes to the high-affinity receptor for charybdotoxin. *Proc Natl Acad Sci U S A* 1997;94:2853–2858.
10. Herlitze S, Garcia DE, Mackie K, Hille B, Scheuer T, Catterall WA. Modulation of Ca2- channels by G-protein subunits. *Nature* 1996;380:258–262.
11. Hoshi T, Zagotta WN, Aldrich RW. Biophysical and molecular mechanisms of Shaker potassium channel inactivation. *Science* 1990;250:533–538.
12. Isacoff EY, Jan YN, Jan LY. Putative receptor for the cytoplasmic inactivation gate in the Shaker K- channel. *Nature* 1991;353:86–90.
13. Jentsch TJ, Günther W, Pusch M, Schwappach B. Properties of voltage-gated chloride channels of the ClC gene family. *J Physiol* 1995;482P:19S–25S.
14. Jurkat-Rott K, Uetz U, Pika-Hartlaub U, et al. Calcium currents and transients of native and heterologously expressed mutant skeletal muscle DHP receptor α1 subunits (R528H). *FEBS Letters* 1998;423:198–204.
15. Lacerda AE, Kim HS, Ruth P, et al. Normalization of current kinetics by interaction between the a1 und b subunits of the skeletal muscle dihydropyridine-sensitive Ca2+ channel. *Nature* 1991;352:527–530.
16. Lehmann-Horn F, Jurkat-Rott K. Voltage-gated ion channels and hereditary disease. *Physiol Rev* in press.
17. Lerche H, Klugbauer N, Lehmann-Horn F, Hofmann F, Melzer W. Expression and functional characterization of the cardiac L-type calcium channel carrying a skeletal muscle DHP-receptor mutation causing hypokalaemic periodic. *Pflügers Arch* 1996;431:461–463.
18. Lerche H, Peter W, Fleischhauer R, et al. Role in fast inactivation of the IV/S4-S5 loop of the human muscle Na- channel probed by cysteine mutagenesis. *J Physiol* 1997;505:345–352.
19. MacKinnon R, Aldrich RW, Lee AW. Functional stoichiometry of Shaker potassium channel inactivation. *Science* 1993;262:757–759.
20. Makita N, Bennett PB Jr, George AL Jr. Voltage-gated Na- channel 1 subunit mRNA expressed in adult human skeletal muscle, heart, and brain is encoded by a single gene. *J Biol Chem* 1994;269:7571–7578.
21. McPhee JC, Ragsdale DS, Scheuer T, Catterall WA. A critical role for transmembrane segment IVS6 of the Na+ channel α subunit in fast inactivation. *J Biol Chem* 1995;269:7571–7578.
22. Meera P, Wallner M, Jiang Z, Toro L. A calcium switch for the functional coupling between α(*hslo*) and subunits (K$_{VCa}$) of maxi K channels. *FEBS Lett* 1996;382:84–88.
23. Middleton RE, Pheasant DJ, Miller C. Purification, reconstitution, and subunit composition of a voltage-gated chloride channel from *Torpedo electroplax*. *Biochemistry* 1994;33:1389–1398.
24. Mitrovic N, Lerche H, Heine R, et al. Role in fast inactivation of conserved amino acids in the IV/S4–S5 loop of the human muscle Na+ channel. *Neurosci Lett* 1996;214:9–12.
25. Morales MJ, Wee JO, Wang S, Strauss HC, Rasmusson RL. The N-terminal domain of a K+ channel subunit increases the rate of C-type inactivation from the cytoplasmic side of the channel. *Proc Natl Acad Sci USA* 1996;93:15119–15123.
26. Ophoff RA, Terwindt GM, Vergouwe MN, et al. Familial hemiplegic migraine and episodic ataxia type-2 are caused by mutations in the Ca2+ channel gene CACNL1A4. *Cell* 1996;87:543–552.
27. Patton DE, West JW, Catterall WA, Goldin AL. A peptide segment crit-

ical for sodium channel inactivation functions as an inactivation gate in a potassium channel. *Neuron* 1993;11:967–974.

28. Pusch M, Steinmeyer K, Jentsch TJ. Low single channel conductance of the major skeletal muscle chloride channel, ClC-1. *Biophys J* 1994; 66:149–152.

29. Roche JP, Treistman SN. The Ca^{2+} channel 3 subunit differently modulates G-protein sensivity of $\alpha 1A$ and $\alpha 1B$ Ca^{2+} channels. *J Neurosci* 1998;18:878–886.

30. Sakurai T, Westenbroek RE, Rettig J, Hell J, Catterall WA. Biochemical properties and subcellular distribution of the BI and rbA isoforms of alpha 1A subunits of brain calcium channels. *J Cell Biol* 1996;134: 511–528.

31. Schmidt-Rose T, Jentsch TJ. Transmembrane topology of a CLC chloride channel. *Neurobiology* 1997;94:7633–7638.

32. Schönherr R, Heinemann SH. Molecular determinants for activation and inactivation of HERG, a human inward rectifier potassium channel. *J Physiol* 1996;493:635–641.

33. Schreibmayer W, Wallner M, Lotan I. Mechanism of modulation of single sodium channels from skeletal muscle by the b1-subunit from rat brain. *Pflügers Arch* 1994;426:360–362.

34. Singer D, Biel M, Lotan I, Flockerzi V, Hofmann F, Dascal N. The roles of the subunits in the function of the calcium channel. *Science* 1991;253:1553–1556.

35. Snutch TP, Leonard JP, Gilbert MM, Lester HA, Davidson N. Rat brain expresses a heterogeneous family of calcium channels. *Proc Natl Sci Acad Sci U S A* 1990;87:3391–3395.

36. Stea A, Tomlinson WJ, Soong TW, Bourinet E, Dubel SJ, Vincent SR, Snutch TP. Localization and functional properties of a rat brain $\alpha 1A$ calcium channel reflect similarities to neuronal Q- and P-type channels. *Proc Natl Acad Sci U S A* 1994;91:10576–10580.

37. Steinmeyer K, Ortland C, Jentsch TJ. Primary structure and functional expression of a developmentally regulated skeletal muscle chloride channel. *Nature* 1991;354:301–304.

38. Steinmeyer K, Schwappach B, Bens M, Vandewalle A, Jentsch TJ. Cloning and functional expression of rat CLC-5, a chloride channel related to kidney disease. *J Biol Chem* 1995;270:31172–31177.

39. Stühmer W, Conti F, Suzuki H, et al. Structural parts involved in activation and inactivation of the sodium channel. *Nature* 1989;339:597–603.

40. Vassilev PM, Scheuer T, Catterall WA. Identification of an intracellular peptide segment involved in sodium channel inactivation. *Science* 1988;241:1658–1661.

41. Wagner S, Deymeer F, Kürz LL, et al. The dominant chloride channel mutant G200R causing fluctuating myotonia: clinics, electrophysiology and channel pathology. *Muscle Nerve* 1998;21:1122–1128.

42. Wallner M, Meera P, Toro L. Determinant for β-subunit regulation in high-conductance voltage-activated and Ca^{2+}-sensitive K^{+} channels: an additional transmembrane region at the N terminus. *Proc Natl Acad Sci USA* 1996;93:14922–14927.

43. West JW, Patton DE, Scheuer T, Wang Y, Goldin AL, Catterall WA. A cluster of hydrophobic amino acid residues required for fast Na^{+} channel inactivation. *Proc Natl Acad Sci U S A* 1992;89:10910–10914.

44. Wymore RS, Gintant GA, Wymore RT, Dixon JE, McKinnon D, Cohen IS. Tissue and species distribution of mRNA for the IKr-like K^{+} channel, *erg*. *Circ Res* 1997;80:261–268.

45. Yang N, George AL Jr, Horn R. Molecular basis of charge movements in voltage-gated sodium channels. *Neuron* 1996;16:113–122.

46. Yatani A, Wakamori M, Niidome T, et al. Stable expression and coupling of cardiac L-type Ca^{2+} channels with 1-adrenoceptors. *Circ Res* 1995;76:335–342.

47. Zhuchenko O, Bailey J, Bonnen P, et al. Autosomal dominant cerebellar ataxia (SCA6) associated with small polyglutamine expansions in the α_{1A}-voltage-dependent calcium channel. *Nature Genetics* 1997;15:62–69.

The Headaches, Second Edition,
edited by J. Olesen, P. Tfelt-Hansen, and K.M.A. Welch.
Lippincott Williams & Wilkins, Philadelphia © 2000.

Basic Science Aspects of the Headaches

CHAPTER 20

Channelopathies and Their Possible Relations to Migraine

Dennis E. Bulman

Ion channels are part of a large family of macromolecules whose functions include the control and maintenance of electric potential across cell membranes, secretion, and signal transduction (21). The superfamily of voltage-gated ion channels includes the K^+, Na^+, and Ca^{2+}. These cation channels are related evolutionarily, sharing a fundamental design consisting of a set of six potentially membrane-spanning segments (S1–6). The six segments constitute a domain that is present only once in the K^+ channels but is repeated four times within the α_1-subunit of the Na^+ and Ca^{2+} channels. Segment 4 is thought to function as the voltage sensor and contains basic residues at every third or fourth position (21,24). The amino acid sequence of the individual voltage-gated ion channels are highly conserved across species, with some regions of the channel conserved between humans and *Drosophila*. Generally, a high degree of sequence conservation across species has been considered evidence in favor of strong selective pressure on these channels.

Mutations in these voltage-gated ion channel genes have been shown to cause or have been implicated in a number of episodic disorders, including periodic paralysis, episodic ataxia, familial hemiplegic migraine, long QT syndrome, and paroxysmal dyskinesia. Correlation of the various mutations with the clinical phenotype is providing insight into the pathophysiology of these channel proteins. Interestingly, different mutations within the same ion channel gene may cause quite distinct clinical disorders; conversely, mutations in different ion channel

genes may result in similar phenotypes (genetic heterogeneity). Chromosomal localization of ion channel subunits as well as disorders attributed to mutations in calcium, chloride, sodium, and potassium channels are listed in Tables 1 through 4, respectively. The roles played by ion channels in the pathogenesis of neuromuscular and neurologic disease represent a paradigm for the role of ion channels in other episodic disorders such as migraine.

PERIODIC PARALYSIS

The periodic paralytic disorders of skeletal muscle and the nondystrophic myotonias are diseases that are caused by mutations in voltage-gated ion channel genes. Disease-based phenotypic variation is most pronounced in the gene that encodes the α-subunit of the skeletal muscle sodium channel gene (*SCN4A*). Hyperkalemic periodic paralysis, paramyotonia congenita, combined hyperkalemic periodic paralysis and paramyotonia congenita, acetazolamide-responsive myotonia, and myotonia permanens/fluctuans are all clinically distinct autosomal dominant disorders caused by mutations in the α-subunit of the skeletal muscle sodium channel, SCN4A (20,37,47,48,50,54). All these disorders are inherited in an autosomal dominant manner, although the penetrance may vary.

Hyperkalemic periodic paralysis is characterized by attacks of generalized weakness that usually occur during the first decade of life. Commonly, attacks start in the morning and last 15 minutes to 1 hour and then remit spontaneously. A major factor in the precipitation of a paralytic attack in persons with hyperkalemic periodic paralysis is an increase in extracellular potassium. Resting after strenuous work or potassium intake can provoke

D. Bulman: Division of Neurology, Department of Medicine, University of Ottowa, and Ottawa General Hospital Research Institute, The Ottawa Hospital–General Campus, Ottawa, Ontario K1H 8L6, Canada.

TABLE 1. *Genes encoding calcium channel subunits, their chromosomal location, and status regarding human disease*

Channel type	Gene name	Location	Disease (MIM number)
Calcium			
	CACNA1A	19p13.1	Familial hemiplegic migraine type 1(141500)
			Episodic ataxia type 2 (108500)
			SCA6 (183086)
			Tottering
			Leaner
			Rolling
	CACNA1B	9q34	
	CACNA1C	12p13	
	CACNA1D	3p21.2–p21.3	
	CACNA1E	1q25–q31	
	CACNA1F	Xp11.23	Congenital stationary night blindness (310500)
	CACNA1S	1q31–q32	Hypokalemic periodic paralysis (170400)
			Malignant hyperthermia 5 (601887)
			Muscular dysgenesis
	CACNA2	7q21–q22	
	CACNB1	17q21–22	
	CACNB2	10p12	
	CACNB3	12q13	
	CACNB4	2q22–23	*Lethargic*
	CACNG	17q24	*Stargazer*
	RYR1	19q13.1	Malignant hyperthermia 1 (145600)
			Central core disease (117000)
	RYR2	1q42.1–q43	
	RYR3	15q14	

MIM, mendelian inheritance of man (38).
Corresponding mendelian inheritance in man number given in parentheses; known mouse mutants are given in italics.

an attack of weakness, usually accompanied by a significant increase in serum potassium levels. Rarely does the level of serum potassium rise to a point that can cause cardiac problems. Moderate exercise can hasten recovery, although slight muscle weakness may persist for a couple of days. Interestingly, the frequency of attacks declines after the patient reaches the mid-30s or early 40s, a phe-

nomenon also noted in some families with episodic ataxia and in familial hemiplegic migraine.

Paramyotonia congenita is characterized by muscle stiffness that appears during exercise and worsens with continued exercise or exposure to cold. The myotonia primarily affects the neck, face, and long muscles of the hand. In most cases, muscle weakness occurs after exer-

TABLE 2. *Chloride channel genes, their chromosomal location, and status regarding human disease*

Channel type	Gene name	Location	Disease (MIM number)
Chloride			
	CLCN1	7q32–7qter	Tompsen's disease (160800)
			Becker's myotonia (255700)
			Myotonia Levior (118425.0007)
			adr
	CLCN2	3q27–q28	
	CLCN3	4q32	
	CLCN4	Xp22.3	
	CLCN5	Xp11.22	Dent disease (300009)
			X-linked recessive nephrolithiasis (310468)
			X-linked recessive hypophosphatemic rickets (307800)
	CLCN6	1p36	
	CLCN7	16p13	
	CLCNKA	1p36	
	CLCNKB	1p36	Bartter Syndrome, type 3 (602023)

MIM, mendelian inheritance in man (38).
Corresponding mendelian inheritance in man number given in parentheses; known mouse mutants are given in italics.

TABLE 3. *Genes encoding sodium channel subunits, their chromosomal location, and status regarding human disease[a]*

Channel type	Gene name	Location	Disease (MIM number)
Sodium			
	SCN1A	2q24	
	SCN1B	19q13.1	Generalized epilepsy with febrile seizures + (600235)
	SCN2A1	2q23–q24.1	
	SCN2A2	2q23–24	
	SCN2B	11q22–qter	
	SCN3A	2q24–31	
	SCN4A	17q23.1–q25.3	Hypokalemic periodic paralysis (170400)
			Paramyotonia congenita (168300)
			Combined hyperkalemic periodic paralysis and paramyotonia congenital (170500)
			Myotonia fluctuans/permanens (170500)
			Acetazolamide-responsive myotonia congenita (170500)
			Malignant hypothermia 2 (154275)
	SCN4B		
	SCN5A	3p21	Long QT Syndrome, type 3 (600163)
	SCN6A	2q21–q23	
	SCN7A		
	SCN8A	12q13	*Motor endplate disease*
			Jolting
	SCN9A		
	SCNN1A	12p13	Pseudohypoaldosteronism, type 1 (264350)
	SCNN1B	16p12.1–p12.2	Pseudohypoaldosteronism, type 1 (264350)
	SCNN1D	1p36.2–p36.3.	
	SCNN1G	16p12.1–p12.2	Pseudohypoaldosteronism, type 1 (264350)

MIM, mendelian inheritance of man (38).
[a]Corresponding mendelian inheritance in man number given in parentheses; known mouse mutants are given in italics.

cise or exposure to cold. The symptoms are present at birth and persist throughout life. In cases in which the patient exhibits both paramyotonia congenita and hyperkalemic periodic paralysis, symptoms of the latter usually appear in the second decade of life. The phenotype of paramyotonia congenita without paralysis on exposure to cold represents yet another variant of paramyotonia congenita (32).

Acetazolamide-responsive myotonia (61) has clinical onset in the first decade and resembles Thomsen's disease, a skeletal muscle chloride channel disorder, in appearance, except muscular stiffness is painful (49). Moreover, myotonia is provoked by fasting and oral potassium and can be relieved by carbohydrates, similar to hyperkalemic paralysis, although paralysis is not a feature. Cold only mildly enhances the myotonia. Acetazolamide, a carbonic anhydrase inhibitor, tends to provide dramatic relief.

The sodium channel myotonias, namely, myotonia fluctuans, myotonia permanens, and acetazolamide-responsive myotonia, differ from the nonparalytic paramyotonia variant in that these disorders are potassium, but not cold, sensitive. *Myotonia fluctuans* is a fluctuating myotonic condition that appears during adolescence and spontaneously varies in severity; like hyperkalemic paralysis, it increases markedly following potassium loading. Myotonia is induced by exercise but has a delayed onset (35,52,53). Many patients have

almost constant fibrillation-like activity. *Myotonia permanens* is similar to myotonia fluctuans, except myotonia is permanent and much more severe. There is continuous myotonic activity on electromyelography (EMG) (34,53). Pulmonary compromise can occur as a result of stiffness of the respiratory muscles.

Hypokalemic periodic paralysis (HOKPP) is a disease caused by mutations in the gene encoding the L-type (dihydropyridine sensitive) calcium channel α_1-subunit. HOKPP is an autosomal dominant disorder with complete penetrance in male subjects and approximately 50% penetrance in female subjects. It is characterized by episodic attacks of weakness in association with decreased serum potassium levels. HOKPP was mapped to 1q31 q32 (14); subsequently, three different mutations within the α_1-subunit of the dihydropyridine-sensitive calcium channel CACNA1S were identified (28,49). The *CACNA1S* gene has been excluded in a French kindred with HOKPP, suggesting that HOKPP is a genetically heterogeneous disorder (46).

Myotonia Congenita

Both Thomsen's and Becker's myotonia congenita, which are inherited as autosomal dominant and autosomal recessive disorders, respectively, are due to mutations in the skeletal-muscle voltage-gated chloride channel gene. Although the muscle stiffness is temporary, it is

TABLE 4. *Genes encoding potassium channel subunits, their chromosomal location, and status regarding human disease*

Channel type	Gene name	Location	Disease (MIM number)
Potassium			
	KCNA1	12p13	Episodic ataxia/myokymia (160120)
	KCNA1B	3q26.1	
	KCNA2	12	
	KCNA2B	1p36	
	KCNA3	1p13.3	
	KCNA4	11p14	
	KCNA5	12p13	
	KCNA6	12p13	
	KCNA7	19q13.3	
	KCNA10	1p13.1	
	KCNB1	20q13.2	
	KCNC1	11p15	
	KCNC2	19q13.3–q13.4	
	KCNC3	19q13.3	
	KCNC4	1p21	
	KCND1		
	KCND2		
	KCND3		
	KCNE1	21q22.1–q22.2	Long QT syndrome
	KCNQ1	11p15.5	Long QT syndrome, type 1 (192500)
	KCNQ2	20q13.3	Benign familial neonatal convulsions type 1 (121200)
	KCNQ3	8q24.22–q24.3	Benign familial neonatal convulsions type 2 (121201)
	HERG	7q35–q36	Long QT syndrome, type 2 (152427)
	KCNJ1	11q24	Hyperprostaglandin E syndrome (601678)
	KCNJ2	17	
	KCNJ3	2q24.1	
	KCNJ4	22q13.1	
	KCNJ5	11q24	
	KCNJ6	21q22.1	*Weaver*
	KCNJ7	21q22.1	
	KCNJ8	12p11.23	
	KCNJ10	1q	
	KCNJ11	11p15.1	
	KCNJ12	11p15.1	
	KCNJ15	21q22.2	
	KCNJN1	17p11.1–p11.2	
	KCNK1	1q42–q43	
	KCNK3		
	SUR1	11p15.1	Persistent hyperinsulinemic hypoglycemia of infancy (256450)
	SUR2		

Corresponding mendelian inheritance in man number given in parenthesis, known mouse mutants are given in italics.
MIM, mendelian inheritance in man.
From ref. 38 with permission.

most pronounced when initiating a muscle contraction after a period of rest. Subsequent contractions of the same muscle or muscle group result in a reduction of loss of the myotonia.

Long QT Syndrome

Long QT syndrome (LQTS) derives its name from the patient's electrocardiogram, which shows a prolongation of the Q and T waves as a result of abnormalities of myocardial repolarization. It can cause ventricular arrhythmias, syncope, and sudden death in young, other-wise healthy persons (23). LQTS is a genetically hetero-geneous disorder in which four loci (LQT1 4) have been identified. The LQT loci were first mapped to 11p15.5 (29,30), 7q35 36 (LQT2) (25), 3p21 24 (LQT3) (25), and 4q25 q27 (LQT4) (56). Using a candidate gene approach, mutations in an inwardly rectifying potassium channel gene, *HERG* (for human ether-a-go-go-related gene), were identified as the cause of LQT2 (7). Similarly, mutations in the cardiac sodium channel gene *SCN5A* were found to cause LQT3 (67). Using a positional cloning strategy, mutations in the voltage-gated potas-sium channel gene *KVLQT1* were identified as the cause of LQT1 (55,66). Mutations in the *KLVQT1* gene have been estimated to be responsible for more than 50% of all LQTS (67). Defects in *KLVQT1* also have been shown to be responsible for Jervell and Lange–Nielsen syndrome, a recessively inherited disorder characterized by congenital bilateral deafness associated with LQTS (42).

Paroxysmal Dyskinesia

Familial paroxysmal dyskinesias (FPD) include choreoathetotic, dystonic, and mixed forms and can be classified as either acquired or inherited (18). Both kinesiogenic (movement-induced) and nonkinesiogenic types have been noted (8,11,18,31,41). In addition, both autosomal dominant and autosomal recessive inheritance have been seen. Two groups independently mapped the gene for the nonkinesiogenic form of familial paroxysmal dyskinesia (*FPD1*) to a 10-cM region of chromosme 2q36 (12,15). Coincidentally, the locus for another movement disorder, paroxysmal choreoathetosis with spasticity (CSE), was mapped to a cluster of potassium channel genes on chromosome 1p (1). Voltage- gated or ligand-gated ion channels and glutamate receptors are all potential candidate genes for these disorders.

NEUROTOLOGIC DISORDERS

Neurotologic symptoms commonly occur with migraine, and patients may experience vertigo or hearing loss as their only symptoms (2). Acetazolamide is effective in controlling vertigo and motion sickness in patients with migraine (3) as it has with many of the other episodic disorders that are due to mutations in ion channel genes. We have identified a number of families with acetazolamide-responsive paroxysmal vestibulocerebellar ataxia, all of whom experience severe headaches that commence after attacks of vertigo. Because of the clinical resemblance to episodic ataxia type, there is a strong possibility that these episodic vestibular disorders are also due to mutations in ion channel genes.

FAMILIAL HEMIPLEGIC MIGRAINE AND EPISODIC ATAXIA

The episodic ataxias are a clinically and genetically heterogeneous group of disorders (16) that are inherited as autosomal dominant traits. Patients present with episodes of ataxia that vary in severity and duration, and patients also may have other signs of cerebellar dysfunction (39). Episodic ataxia with myokymia (EA-1) was the first disorder in vertebrates attributable to a mutation in a potassium channel gene (5).

Myokymia is due to spontaneous and repetitive discharges from peripheral nerves and occurs during and between attacks. von Brederlow and colleagues (64) and subsequently others (33,59,62) mapped the second EA

locus to 19p13. The EA-2 locus fell within a previously defined 30-cM region known to contain the gene for familial hemiplegic migraine (FMH) (26). Two years later, mutations in the α_{1A}-subunit of the P/Q-type calcium channel gene, *CACNA1A*, were found to be responsible for both FHM and EA-2 (45). Of the mutations causing FHM, all were shown to be missense mutations resulting in amino acid substitutions. In contrast, the mutations causing EA-2 were shown to shift the translational reading frame, resulting in premature termination of translation (Fig. 1). Both disorders are clinically different, although signs of clinical overlap have been noted. FHM is characterized by periodic, commonly unilateral, pulsatile headaches that may affect infants, children, and adults and includes episodes of unilateral paralysis, which may outlast the headache.

Some patients with FHM have been reported to have a cerebellar disturbance with dysarthria and horizontal nystagmus (44), similar to that seen in patients with EA-2. The search is currently under way for at least one other FHM gene, because a number of families have been described as having this condition not linked to 19p13 (22,27,60). In contrast, persons who have familial EA-2 experience discrete episodes of pancerebellar disturbances with dysarthria, titubations, dysmetric limb movements, severe truncal and gait ataxia; headaches, vertigo, and nausea were reported in a subset of patients (16,19,72). The duration of attacks is usually variable, lasting from minutes to hours, although there are reports (65) of attacks lasting days. The attacks may be precipitated by emotional stress, exercise, alcohol ingestion, carbohydrate ingestion, and onset of menses. Patients with EA-2 may have an associated migraine (nonhemiplegic) after onset of the ataxic symptoms. Interictal examination reveals often persistent nystagmus and residual mild cerebellar incoordination. Atrophy of the cerebellar vermis has been described in some families with EA-2 (63) but not in others (4,9,36,70).

Shortly after identification of the FHM/EA-2 gene defects, the trinucleotide repeat expansion disorder, spinocerebellar ataxia type 6 (SCA6), was found to be due to a CAG expansion within *CACNA1A* (73). SCA6 is a mild but slowly progressive cerebellar ataxia of the limbs and gait. Patients have dysarthria, nystagmus, and mild vibratory and proprioceptive sensory loss (73). The disease progresses for 20 to 30 years, resulting in the patient becoming wheelchair bound. Clinical onset begins in the 40s, with marked signs of cerebellar atrophy and cerebellar Purkinje cell loss, moderate loss of granule cells, and loss of cells in the dentate nucleus and inferior olive (73).

Mutations in the orthologous gene in mice were shown to be responsible for the naturally occurring and recessively inherited tottering (*tg*) and leaner (*tg*^la^) mouse phenotypes (13). The *tg* mutation results in spike and wave discharges, mild ataxia, and periodic convulsions. Spontaneous behavioral arrest is associated with synchronous,

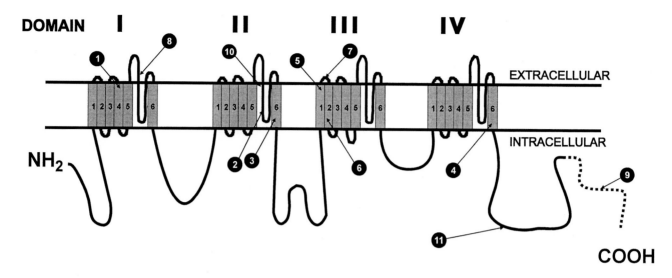

FIG. 1. Schematic representation of the P/Q-type calcium channel, CACNA1A, and the distribution of mutations for familial hemiplegic migraine (45), episodic ataxia (45,70), episodic and progressive ataxia (71), SCA6 (71), tottering (13), and leaner (13) are illustrated. The dashed line at the COOH-tail of the channel signifies the area of the protein that is subject to alternative splicing.

bilateral cortical polyspike discharges, similar to those that occur in patients with absence epilepsy (43). Similar to EA-2, stress appears to trigger the episodic events. The leaner (tg^{la}) mutation, which is allelic to tg, causes profound chronic ataxia associated with Purkinje and granule cell loss within the anterior cerebellum. Whereas spike and wave discharges in the leaner mouse have been detected, paroxysmal convulsions have not been observed. Both the tottering and leaner phenotypes are quite different from that of EA-2 and more complex than FMH. The recessively inherited *lethargic* (*lh*) mouse phenotype, which is associated with ataxia and seizures, was recently found to be due to a four-base insertion within the Ca^{2+} channel β-subunit (6). The neurologic aspects of the phenotype are similar to those of the *tottering* mouse (13), which may not be surprising, given that the β_4- and α_{1A}-subunits interact as part of a functional calcium channel.

Two additional loci for FHM on chromosome 1q31 (17) and chromosome 1q21 q23 (10) have been identified through family studies. The locus at 1q31 has implicated the neuronal calcium channel α_{1E}-subunit gene, which maps to the same region of chromosome 1. If it can be proven that mutations in the α_{1E} gene cause FHM, the link between inherited ion channel disorders and FHM will be firmly established (40). Other than the involvement of *CACNA1A* with FHM, the speculation that migraine may be due to mutations in other ion channel genes is based on the observations that channelopathies tend to present as episodic disorders and triggers such as stress often induce an attack.

Voltage-gated calcium channels regulate a number of biologic functions, including the generation of action potentials in dendrites, allowing calcium entry into the cell, thereby initiating neurotransmitter release and other intracellular regulatory processes, and play a pivotal role in the control of neuronal firing (68). Calcium channel types differ with respect to their voltage dependence, inactivation rate, ionic selectivity, and pharmacology. The kinetics and voltage dependence of inactivation define the specific channel subtype as L, N, P/Q, or R. Each channel is composed of five subunits: α_1, α_2, β, γ, and δ. The α_1-subunit is able to form the structural channel and to confer voltage sensitivity and may be encoded by one of at least six genes (A, B, C, D, E, or S). The complex ramifications of mutations in any one subunit have not been fully appreciated, because the six α_1 and four β-subunits may form different combinations (58,69). In addition, the α_1-subunit has been shown to undergo extensive alternative splicing (51,57). The distribution of the alternatively spliced products and the various subunits within the brain is not known, suggesting that mutations within one of the subunits of the neural calcium channels may have a complex effect.

Ion channel genes are probably expressed in every cell, because they are required to perform a variety of functions, such as the maintenance of membrane electric potential, cell signaling, secretion, and absorption. Only a small proportion of ion channel genes that have been mapped are known to be responsible for heritable disorders. Mutations in genes encoding voltage-gated ion channels are known to cause or have been implicated in a number of episodic neurologic and neuromuscular disorders.

ACKNOWLEDGMENT

This work was supported by grants from the Medical Research Council of Canada. Dr. Bulman is a scholar of the Medical Research Council of Canada.

REFERENCES

1. Auburger G, Ratzlaff T, Lunkes A, et al. A gene for autosomal dominant paroxysmal choreoathetosis/ spasticity (CSE) maps to the vicinity of a potassium channel gene cluster on chromosome 1p, probably within 2 cM between D1S443 and D1S197. *Genomics* 1996;31:90–94.
2. Baloh RW. Neurotology of migraine. *Headache* 1997;37:615–621.
3. Baloh RW, Foster CA, Yue Q, Nelson SF. Familial migraine with vertigo and essential tremor. *Neurology* 1996;46:458–460.
4. Bouchard JP, Roberge C, Vangelder NM, Barbeau A. Familial periodic ataxia responsive to acetazolamide. *Can J Neurol Sci* 1984;11: 550–553.
5. Browne DL, Gancher ST, Nutt JG, et al. Episodic ataxia/myokymia syndrome is associated with point mutations in the human potassium channel gene, *KCNA1*. *Nat Genet* 1994;8:136–140.
6. Burgess DL, Jones JM, Meisler MH, Noebels JL. Mutation of the Ca^{2+} channel beta subunit gene *Cchb4* is associated with ataxia and seizures in the lethargic (lh) mouse. *Cell* 1997;88:385–392.
7. Curran ME, Splawski I, Timothy KW, Vincent GM, Green ED, Keating MT. A molecular basis for cardiac arrhythmia: *HERG* mutations cause long QT syndrome. *Cell* 1995;80:795–803.
8. Demirkiran M, Jankovic J. Paroxysmal dyskinesias: clinical features and classification. *Ann Neurol* 1995;38:571–579.
9. Donat JR, Auger R. Familial periodic ataxia. *Arch Neurol* 1979;36: 568–569.
10. Ducros A, Joutel A, Vahedi K, et al. Mapping of a second locus for familial hemiplegic migraine 1q21 q23 and evidence of further heterogeneity. *Ann Neurol* 1997;42:885–890.
11. Fahn S. The paroxysmal dyskinesia. In: Marsden CD, Fahn S, eds. *Movement disorders.* Oxford: Butterworth Heinemann, 1994:310– 345.
12. Fink JK , Rainier S, Wilkowski J, et al. Paroxysmal dystonic choreoathetosis: tight linkage to chromosome 2q. *Am J Hum Genet* 1996;59: 140–145.
13. Fletcher CF, Lutz CM, O'Sullivan TN, et al. Absence epilepsy in tottering mutant mice is associated with calcium channel defects. *Cell* 1996;87:607–617.
14. Fontaine B, Vale Santos JM, Jurkat-Rott K, et al. Mapping of hypokalaemic periodic paralysis (HypoPP) to chromosome 1q31-q32 in three European families. *Nat Genet* 1994;6:267–272.
15. Fouad GT, Servidei S, Durcan S, Bertini E, Ptacek LJ. A gene for famil-

ial paroxysmal dyskinesia (*FPD1*) maps to chromosome 2q. *Am J Hum Genet* 1996;59:135—139.
16. Gancher ST, Nutt JG. Autosomal dominant episodic ataxia: a heterogeneous syndrome. *Mov Disord* 1986;1:239–253.
17. Gardiner K, Barmada MM, Ptacek LJ, Hoffman EP. A new locus for hemiplegic migraine maps to 1q31. *Neurology* 1997;49:1231–1238.
18. Goodenough DJ, Fariello RG, Annis BL, Chun RWM. Familial and acquired paroxysmal dyskinesias. *Arch Neurol* 1978;35:827–831.
19. Griggs RC, Moxley RT, Lafrance RA, McQuillen J. Hereditary paroxysmal ataxia: response to acetazolamide. *Neurology* 1978;28:1259–1264.
20. Heine R, Pika U, Lehmann-Horn F. A novel *SCN4A* mutation causing myotonia aggravated by cold and potassium. *Hum Mol Genet* 1993; 2:1349–1353.
21. Hille B. *Ion channels of excitable membranes,* 2nd ed. Sunderland, MA: Sinauer Associates, 1992.
22. Hovatta I, Kallela M, Farkkila M, Peltonen L. Familial migraine: exclusion of the susceptibility gene from the reported locus of familial hemiplegic migraine on 19p. *Genomics* 1994;23:707–709.
23. Jackman WM, Friday KJ, Anderson JL, Aliot EM, Clark M, Lazzara R. The long QT syndromes: a critical review, new clinical observations and a unifying hypothesis. *Prog Cardiovasc Dis* 1988;31:115–172.
24. Jan LY, Jan YN. Potassium channels and their evolving gates. *Nature* 1994;371:119–122.
25. Jiang C, Atkinson D, Towbin JA, et al. Two long QT syndrome loci map to chromosomes 3 and 7 with evidence for further heterogeneity. *Nat Genet* 1994;8:141–147.
26. Joutel A, Bousser MG, Biousse V, Labauge P, Chabriat H, Nibbio A. A gene for familial hemiplegic migraine maps to chromosome 19. *Nat Genet* 1993;5:40–45.
27. Joutel A, Ducros A, Vahedi K, et al. Genetic heterogeneity of familial hemiplegic migraine. *Am J Hum Genet* 1994;55:1166–1172.
28. Jurkat-Rott K, Lehmann-Horn F, Elbaz A, et al. A calcium channel mutation causing hypokalemic periodic paralysis. *Hum Mol Genet* 1994;3:1415–1419.
29. Keating M, Atkinson D, Dunn C, Timothy K, Vincent GM, Leppert M. Linkage of a cardiac arrhythmia, the long QT syndrome, and the Harvey *RAS-1* gene. *Science* 1991;252;704–706.
30. Keating M, Dunn C, Atkinson D, Timothy K, Vincent GM, Leppert M. Consistent linkage of the long-QT syndrome to the Harvey *Ras-1* locus on chromosome 11. *Am J Hum Genet* 1991;49:1335–1339.
31. Kertesz A. Paroxysmal kinesigenic choreoathetosis. *Neurology* 1967; 17:680–690.
32. Koch MC, Baumbach K, George AL, Ricker K. Paramyotonia congenita without paralysis on exposure to cold: a novel mutation in the *SCN4A* gene (*Val1293Ile*). *Neuroreport* 1995;6:2001–2004.
33. Kramer PL, Yue Q, Gancher ST, et al. A locus for the nystagmus-associated form of episodic ataxia maps to an 11-cM region on chromosome 19p. *Am J Hum Genet* 1995;57:182–185.
34. Lehman-Horn F, Rüdel R, Ricker K. Workshop report: non-dystrophic myotonias and periodic paralysis. *Neuromuscul Disord* 1993;3: 161–168.
35. Lerche H, Heine R, Pika U, et al. Human sodium channel myotonia: slowed channel inactivation due to substitutions for a glycine within the III–IV linker. *J Physiol* 1993;470:13–22.
36. Margolin DI, Nutt JG, Lovrien EW. Familial periodic ataxia. *Trans Am Neurol Assoc* 1981;106:53–57.
37. McClatchey AI, Van den Bergh P, Pericak-Vance M, et al. Temperature-sensitive mutations in the III–IV cytoplasmic loop region of the skeletal muscle sodium channel gene in paramyotonia congenita. *Cell* 1992;68:769–774.
38. McKusick VA. *Mendelian inheritance in man:* catalogs of human *genes and genetic disorders.* Baltimore: Johns Hopkins University Press, 11th ed., 1994.
39. Moon SL, Koller WC. Hereditary periodic ataxias. In: Vinken PJ, Bruyn GW, Klawans HL, eds. *Handbook of clinical neurology.* New York: Elsevier Science Publishing, 1974:433–443.
40. Moskowitz MA, Cutrer M. Attacking migraine headache from beginning to end. *Neurology* 1997;49:1193–1195.
41. Mount LA, Reback S. Familial paroxysmal choreoathetosis. *Arch Neurol Psychiatry* 1940;44:841–847.
42. Neyroud N, Tesson F, Denjoy I, et al. A novel mutation in the potassium channel gene *KVLQT1* cdauses the Jervell and Lange-Nielsen cardioauditory syndrome. *Nat Genet* 1997;15:186–189.
43. Noebels JL, Sidman RL. Inherited epilepsy: spike-wave and focal

motor seizures in the mutant mouse tottering. *Science* 1979;204: 1334–1336.

44. Ohta M, Araki S, Kuroiwa Y. Familiial occurence of migraine with a hemiplegic syndrome and cerebellar manifestations. *Neurology* 1967; 17:813–817.

45. Ophoff RA, Terwindt GM, Gerbouwe MN, et al. Familial hemiplegic migraine and episodic ataxia type-2 are caused by mutations in the Ca^{2+} channel gene CACNL1A4. *Cell* 1996;87:543–552.

46. Plassart E. Elbaz A, Santos JV, et al. Genetic heterogeneity in hypokalemic periodic paralysis (hypoPP). *Hum Genet* 1994;94:551–556.

47. Ptáček LJ, George AL, Barchi RL, et al. Mutations in an S4 segment of the adult skeletal muscle sodium dchannel cause paramyotonia congenita. *Neuron* 1992;8:891–897.

48. Ptáček LJ, George AL, Griggs RC, et al. Identification of a mutation in the gene causing hyperkalemic periodic paralysis. *Cell* 1991;67: 1021–1027.

49. Ptáček LJ, Tawil R, Griggs RC, et al. Dihydropyridine receptor mutations cause hypokalemic periodic paralysis. *Cell* 1994;77:863–868.

50. Ptáček LJ, Tawil R, Griggs RC, et al. Sodium channel mutations in acetazolamide-responsive myotonia congenita, paramyotonia congenita and hyperkalemic periodic paralysis. *Neurology* 1994;44:1500–1503.

51. Rettig J, Sheng ZH, Kim DK, Hodson CD, Snutch TP, Catterall WA. Isoform-specific interaction of the alpha 1A subunits of brain $Ca2^+$ channels with the presynaptic proteins syntaxin and SNAP-25. *Proc Natl Acad Sci USA* 1996;93:7363–7368.

52. Ricker K, Lehmann-Horn F, Moxley RT. Myotonia fluctuans. *Arch Neurol* 1990;47:268–-272.

53. Ricker KW, Moxley RT, Heine R, Lehmann-Horn F. Myotonia fluctuans, a third type of muscle sodium channel disease. *Arch Neurol* 1994; 51:1095–1102.

54. Rojas CV, Wang J, Schwartz LS, Hoffman EP, Powell BR, Brown RH Jr. A met-to-val mutation in the skeletal muscle Na-channel α-subunit in hyperkalaemic periodic paralysis. *Nature* 1991;354:387–389.

55. Russell MW, Dick M, Collins FS, Brody LC. *KVLQT1* mutations in three families with familial or sporadic long QT syndrome. *Hum Mol Genet* 1996;5:1319–1324.

56. Schott J-J, Charpentier F, Peltier S, et al. Mapping of a gene for long QT syndrome to chromosome 4q25 217. *Am J Hum Genet* 1995;57: 1114–1122.

57. Snutch TP, Tomlinson WJ, Leonard JP, Gilbert MM. Distinct calcium channels are generated by alternative splicing and are differntially expressed in the mammalian CNS. *Neuron* 1991;7:45–57.

58. Tanaka O, Sakagami H, Kondo H. Localization of mRNAs of voltage-dependent Ca(2+)-channels: four subtypes of alpha 1- and beta-subunits in developing and mature rat brain. *Brain Res Mol Brain Res* 1995;30: 1–16.

59. The BT, Silburn P, Lindblad K, Betz R, Boyle R. Familial periodic cerebellar ataxia without myokymia maps to a 19-cM region on 19p13. *Am J Hum Genet* 1995;56:1443–1449.

60. Terwindt GM, Ophoff RA, Haan J, Frants RR, Ferrari MD. Familial hemiplegic migraine: a clinical comparison of families linked and unlinked to chromosome 19. *Cephalalgia* 1996;16:153–155.

61. Trudell RG, Kaiser KK, Griggs RC. Acetzaolamide-responsive myotonia congenita. *Neurology* 1987;37:488–491.

62. Vahedi K, Joutel A, Van Bogaert P, Ducros A. A gene for hereditary paroxysmal cerebellar ataxia maps to chromosome 19p. *Ann Neurol* 1995;37:289–293.

63. Vighetto A, Froment JC, Trillet M, Aimard G. Magnetic resonance imaging in familial paroxysmal ataxia. *Arch Neurol* 1988;45:547–549.

64. Von Brederlow B, Hahn AF, Koopman WJ, Ebers GC, Bulman DE. Mapping the gene for acetazolamide responseive hereditary paroxysmal cerebellar ataxia to the pericentromeric region of chromosome 19. *Hum Mol Genet* 1995;4:279–284.

65. White JC. Familial periodic nystagmus, ertigo, and ataxia. *Arch Neurol* 1969;20:276–280.

66. Want Q, Curren ME, Splawski I, et al. Positional cloning of a novel potassium channel gene: *KVLQT1* mutations cause cardiac arrhythmias. *Nat Genet* 1996;12:17–23.

67. Wang Q, Shen J, Splawski I, et al. *SCN5A* mutations associated with an inherited cardiac arrhythmia, long QT syndrome. *Cell* 1995;80: 805–811.

68. Westenbroek RE, Hell JW, Warner C, Dubel SJ, Snutch TP, Catterall WA. Biochemical preoperties and subcellular distribution of an N-type calcium channel alpha 1 subunit. *Neuron* 1992;9:1099–1115.

69. Williams ME, Marubio LM, Deal CR, et al. Structure and functional characterization of neuronal alpha 1E calcium channel subtypes. *Br J Biol Chem* 1994;269:22347–22357.

70. Yue Q, Jen C, Nelson SF, Baloh RW. Progressive ataxia due to a missense mutation in a calcium-channel gene. *Am J Hum Genet* 1997;5: 1078–1087.

71. Yue Q, Jen C, Thwe MM, Nelson SF, Baloh RW. De novo mutation in CACNA1A caused acetazolamide-responsive episodic ataxia. *Am J Med Genet* 1998;77:298–301.

72. Zasorin NL, Baloh RW, Myers LB. Acetazolamide responsive episodic ataxia syndrome. *Neurology* 1983;33:1212–1214.

73. Zhuchenko O, Bailey J, Bonnen P, et al. Autosomal dominant cerebellar ataxia (SCA6) associated with small polyglutamine expansions in the α_{1A}-voltage-dependent calcium channel. *Nat Genet* 1997;15:62–69.

The Headaches, Second Edition,
edited by J. Olesen, P. Tfelt-Hansen, and K.M.A. Welch.
Lippincott Williams & Wilkins, Philadelphia © 2000.

Basic Science Aspects of the Headaches

CHAPTER 21

Regulation and Function of Intracellular Calcium in Neurons, Vascular Smooth Muscle, and Endothelium

Masamitsu Iino

Changes in intracellular Ca^{2+} concentration ($[Ca^{2+}]_i$) regulate a myriad of cell functions, such as contraction, cell motility, secretion, transmitter release, gene expression, synaptic plasticity, and immune responses. It is astonishing that so simple a molecule as Ca^{2+} regulates a wide repertoire of important cell functions. Recent studies led to the discovery of many of the molecules that are central in the regulation of Ca^{2+} signalling. Furthermore, technological advances in the imaging of $[Ca^{2+}]_i$ has revealed unique spatiotemporal patterns of Ca^{2+} signalling, which seem to explain the versatility of Ca^{2+} signals. This chapter summarizes the basic properties of molecular mechanisms that regulate $[Ca^{2+}]_i$ as well as the roles of Ca^{2+} signalling in the regulation of cell functions, with special reference to neurons, smooth-muscle cells, and endothelial cells.

CA²⁺ MOVEMENT ACROSS THE CELL MEMBRANES

$[Ca^{2-}]_i$ in unstimulated cells remains at or below ~100 nM, which is about 10,000-fold lower than the extracellular Ca^{2+} concentration. Thus, when influx of Ca^{2+} by way of the plasma membrane is allowed, $[Ca^{2+}]_i$ readily increases. To mediate the influx of Ca^{2+}, there are several classes of Ca^{2+} channels in the plasma membrane. Extracellular Ca^{2+} is not the only source for the increase of $[Ca^{2+}]_i$. Membrane-bound intracellular organelles such as

the endoplasmic reticulum (ER) contain high concentrations of Ca^{2+} and therefore function as Ca^{2+} stores. Thus, the flux of Ca^{2+} across the ER membrane by way of the intracellular Ca^{2+} release channels increases the $[Ca^{2+}]_i$. The Ca^{2+} concentration gradient across the cell membrane or the organelle membrane is created by active processes that use the free energy of adenosine triphosphate (ATP). The major mechanisms involved in the regulation of $[Ca^{2+}]_i$ are summarized in Figure 1 and are explained in the following section.

CA²⁺ CHANNELS

Voltage-dependent Ca²⁺ Channel (VDC)

Among the Ca^{2+} channels on the plasma membrane, voltage-dependent Ca^{2+} channels (VDCs) have been studied and characterized most extensively (13,20,52). They are expressed in excitable cells and have several subtypes, such as L, T, N, P and R. They are composed of heteromultimers of α_1, α_2, β, and other subunits. The α_1-subunit contains both an ion channel pore and a voltage sensor. Among the VDCs, the L-type Ca^{2+} channel is often referred to as the dihydropyridine receptor (DHPR), because Ca^{2+} channels of this type bind dihydropyridine Ca^{2+} channel antagonists with high affinity.

VDCs, like voltage-dependent Na^+ channels, are able to participate in action potential generation because of the regenerativity of their activity. Apart from the action potential generation, the prominent function of the VDCs is conversion of membrane potential change to an intracellular Ca^{2+} signal. Thus, VDCs allow the influx of Ca^{2+} by way of

M. Iino: Department of Pharmacology, Faculty of Medicine, The University of Tokyo, Tokyo 113-0033, Japan.

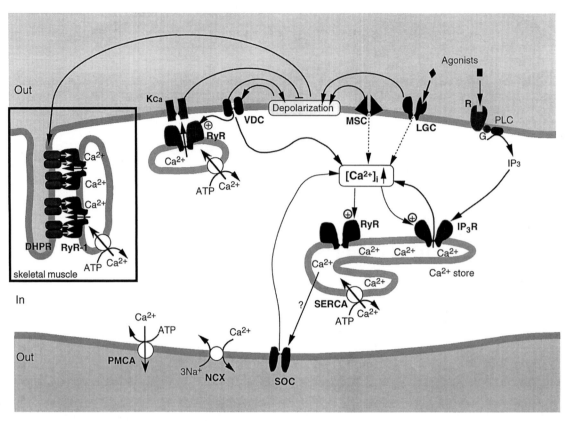

FIG. 1. Schematic diagram of the molecular mechanisms for the regulation of intracellular Ca^{2+} concentration. *VDC*, voltage-dependent Ca^{2+} channel; *DHPR*, dihydropyridine receptor; *LGC*, ligand-gated Ca^{2+} channel; *MSC*, mechanosensitive channel; *SOC*, store-operated Ca^{2+} channel; *RyR*, ryanodine receptor; *IP₃*, inositol 1,4,5-trisphosphate; *IP₃R*, IP_3 receptor; *SERCA*, sarco(endo)plasmic reticulum Ca^{2+} ATPase; *PMCA*, plasma membrane Ca^{2+} ATPase; *NCX*, Na^+-$Ca2^+$ exchange system.

the plasma membrane on depolarization, thereby conveying a membrane voltage signal that is limited within the cell membrane to the entire cytoplasm. The L-type Ca^{2+} channels (i.e., DHPRs) in skeletal muscle cells use a somewhat different mechanism to convert depolarization to $[Ca^{2+}]_i$ increase. Skeletal muscle DHPRs make contact with ryanodine receptors (RyRs) at the T–SR junction, where the transverse-tubule membrane (invaginating plasma membrane) and the sarcoplasmic reticulum (SR) membrane are juxtaposed (Fig. 1, box inset). The dominant role of the DHPR here is to detect the depolarization of the plasma membrane and to transmit the signal to the RyR (see following) on the SR membrane in a direct protein–protein coupling for the release of Ca^{2+} from the SR (63,64). So far, this type of coupling has been demonstrated only in skeletal muscle cells. It is possible that similar coupling will be found in the brain, where RyR-1 is also expressed.

Ligand-gated Ca^{2+} Channel (LGC)

Glutamate Receptor

Subsets of glutamate receptors, that is, *N*-methyl-D-aspartate (NMDA) receptors and some alpha-amino-3-

hydroxy-5-methylisoxazole-4-propionic acid (AMPA) receptors, allow the influx of Ca^{2+} on binding of glutamate. In the case of the NMDA receptor, permeation of Ca^{2+} is inhibited by Mg^{2+} bound to the channel at a resting membrane potential, and a strong depolarization of the plasma membrane is required for the dissociation of Mg^{2+}. Therefore, only on strong synaptic activation that allows sufficient depolarization of the postsynaptic membrane does the NMDA receptor become permeable to Ca^{2+} (7). AMPA receptors are heteromultimers of different subunits (GluR1, GluR2, GluR3, and GluR4). Ca^{2+} permeability of the AMPA receptors depends on the subunits that constitute the channel, and channels without GluR2 (GluRB) have a high permeability to Ca^{2+} (34).

P2X Receptor

Purinoceptive intrinsic ion channel P2X receptors have a multimeric structure. Each subunit has two transmembrane domains with both N- and C-termini located in the cytoplasm. The extracellular loop between the transmembrane domains contains the ATP binding site. Seven subtypes of P2X receptors (P2X₁–P2X₇) derived from different genes have been cloned and display different sensitivities to agonists and antagonists (9,37). They are permeable not only to Ca^{2+} but also to Na^+ and K^+. Therefore, concomitant depolarization by the movement of monovalent cations and the resulting activation of the VDCs are also important for the influx of Ca^{2+}, in addition to the permeation of Ca^{2+} through the P2X receptor itself.

P2X receptors are expressed in smooth-muscle cells with $P2X_1$ as the dominant subtype. Therefore, as a cotransmitter of noradrenaline at the sympathetic nerve endings, ATP induces depolarization of the smooth-muscle cells. P2X receptors also are expressed in sensory neurons, and both $P2X_2$ and $P2X_3$ receptors are implicated in peripheral pain detection at the site of tissue damage (14,39). P2Y receptors, on the other hand, are G-protein-coupled purinergic receptors and mediate the activation of phospholipase C or the inhibition of adenylyl cyclase.

Mechanosensitive Channel (MSC)

In certain cell types, mechanical stress applied to the cell membrane results in an increase in $[Ca^{2+}]_i$ as a result of activation of the mechanosensitive channels. Although mechanosensitive channels themselves may allow influx of Ca^{2+}, they are often more permeable to monovalent cations and produce depolarization, which then induces Ca^{2+} influx by way of the the VDCs.

Mechanosensitive channels were characterized in *Caenorhbaditis elegance* as *mec* family gene products (72). Two of the *mec* family gene products MEC-4 and MEC-10 have some sequence homology with the mammalian amiloride-sensitive epithelial Na^+ channel (ENaC) and P2X receptors. Interestingly, single channel activity of ENaC incorporated in a planar lipid bilayer was shown to have stretch sensitivity (2). It is possible that members of the ENaC family are involved in mechanosensitivity in mammalian tissues.

Store-operated Ca^{2+} Channel (SOC)

Depletion of the Ca^{2+} store induces the influx of Ca^{2+} through putative store-operated Ca^{2+} channels (SOCs) (58). Identification of the molecules responsible for the SOC activity is under way. Genetic studies in *Drosophila melanogaster* led to the discovery of the *Trp* gene product, which functions as the Ca^{2+} influx pathway in photoreceptor cells. Six subtypes (Trp1–Trp6) of mammalian homologues of the *Trp* gene product have been identified (74). HEK cells expressing either Trp4 or Trp5 showed enhanced levels of store-operated inward Ca^{2+} current and were thought to be the SOCs in the brain (Trp5) and peripheral tissues (Trp4) (60,61). In another study, however, Trp5-expressing HEK cells showed agonist-activated Ca^{2+} influx but not store-depletion-activated Ca^{2+} influx (56). Further study is required to confirm whether

Trp4 or Trp5 is sufficient for the function of SOCs. The nature of the signal that is transmitted from the depleted Ca^{2+} store to the SOCs on the plasma membrane is not known.

Ca^{2+} Release Channels

Ryanodine Receptor

Ryanodine receptors (RyRs) are Ca^{2+}-release channels that were first discovered in the skeletal-muscle SR. The functional RyR Ca^{2+} release channel is composed of four subunits, each containing about 5,000 amino acids (48). There are multiple transmembrane-spanning regions near the C-terminus, where the RyR crosses the ER membrane and forms the ion channel (23). The large N-terminal domains of the four subunits form a quatrefoil-shaped cytoplasmic structure with the approximate dimensions $29 \times 29 \times 12$ nm (w × d × h) (62). There are three RyR subtypes (RyR-1, RyR-2, and RyR-3) derived from different genes (29,57,71). RyR-1 and RyR-2 are the dominant subtypes expressed in the skeletal and cardiac muscles, respectively. RyR-3 was first cloned from the brain, but it is also expressed in the skeletal muscle and other cell types, including inexcitable cells (68). In the central nervous system, all three subtypes are expressed with different distributions (24).

RyR is activated by an increase in the cytoplasmic Ca^{2+} concentration to around 1 to 100 μM. Therefore, it functions as the Ca^{2+}-induced Ca^{2+} release (CICR) channel (21). The Ca^{2+} sensitivity depends on the subtype, and the order is likely to be RyR-2 > RyR-1 > RyR-3. In cardiac muscle cells, Ca^{2+} influx through the L-type Ca^{2+} channel (DHPR) triggers Ca^{2+} release from the SR through RyR-2. Therefore, RyR functions as the Ca^{2+} signal amplifier. In skeletal muscle cells, RyR-1 seems to be regulated directly by protein–protein interaction with the DHPR (see the section on VDC and Fig. 1). This type of direct coupling is specific to RyR-1 and is not supported by RyR-2 or RyR-3 (73).

The immunophilin FK506 binding protein (FKBP12) has been implicated in the regulation of RyRs. FKBP12 modulates channel gating of the RyR by increasing the number of channels with full conductance levels (by >400%), decreasing the open probability after caffeine activation and increasing the mean open time. FK506 or rapamycin displaces FKBP12 from the RyR and reverses these stabilizing effects (10).

Inositol 1,4,5-Trisphosphate (IP3) Receptor

Inositol 1,4,5-trisphosphate (IP_3) is a product of cleavage of phosphatidylinositol 4,5-bisphosphate by phospholipase C (PLC). There are three classes of PLC: PLCβ is activated by heterotrimeric G-proteins, whereas PLCγ is activated by tyrosine phosphorylation. The regulatory mechanism of PLCδ is not fully understood. In response to the activation of many cell surface receptors, IP$_3$ serves as the second messenger and binds to the IP$_3$ receptor (IP$_3$R) to induce Ca^{2+} mobilization.

The IP$_3$R is composed of about 2,700 amino acids and has sequence homology with the RyR both in the N-terminus and in the channel-forming regions. There are three IP$_3$R subtypes (IP$_3$R-1, IP$_3$R-2, and IP$_3$R-3) derived from different genes (8,25,69). As with the RyR, they also form channels as tetramers. Unlike the RyR, IP$_3$Rs form heterotetramers (35,51).

The IP$_3$ sensitivity depends on the IP$_3$R subtype. The order of affinity to IP$_3$ is IP$_3$R-2 > IP$_3$R-1 > IP$_3$R-3 (54). IP$_3$R is also sensitive to Ca^{2+} as is the case with RyR (31). Therefore, both Ca^{2+} and IP$_3$ are required for the opening of IP$_3$R expressed in smooth-muscle cells (31,32) and in cerebellar Purkinje cells (6). This Ca^{2+} sensitivity is likely to be responsible for the generation of Ca^{2+} waves (5).

Ca^{2+} Pumps

Sarco(endo)plasmic Reticulum Ca^{2+} ATPase (SERCA)

The SERCA pumps transport Ca^{2+} against the concentration gradient of Ca^{2+} in the ER or the Ca^{2+} stores (43). There are three SERCA genes that are tissue specifically expressed: *SERCA1* in fast-twitch skeletal muscle, *SERCA2* in cardiac and slow-twitch muscles as well as smooth-muscle and nonmuscle tissues, and *SERCA3* in nonmuscle cells, including endothelial cells. There are further subsets within each subtype due to alternative splicing.

Phospholamban regulates the activity of the SERCA in a phosphorylation-dependent manner. Phospholamban binds to the SERCA and inhibits pump activity. On phosphorylation of phospholamban by cyclic AMP- or cyclic guanosine monophosphate (GMP)-dependent protein kinase, it dissociates from the SERCA, and the activity of the SERCA is enhanced (1). This mechanism is important in the positive inotropic effect of β-agonists in cardiac myocytes. Phospholamban is also expressed in smooth-muscle cells and has effects on contraction (38).

Plasma Membrane Ca^{2+} ATPase (PMCA)

PMCA mediates the extrusion of Ca^{2+} by way of the plasma membrane (12). It has an overall structural similarity to SERCA and is derived from four different genes. La^{3+} inhibits the activity of PMCA while it does not do so in SERCA. The activity of PMCA is stimulated by direct binding of calmodulin.

Na$^+$–Ca^{2+} Exchange System (NCX)

There is a Na$^+$ concentration gradient across the plasma membrane that is created by Na$^+$/K$^+$ ATPase. The influx of 3 mole of Na$^+$ along the Na$^+$ concentration gradient is coupled to the extrusion of 1 mole of Ca^{2+} against the Ca^{2+} concentration gradient through the NCX (forward reaction). The reaction is reversible, and the exchanger can work in the reverse direction (*backward reaction*), that is, Na$^+$ extrusion and Ca^{2+} influx. Because the forward reaction moves one net positive charge inward as three Na$^+$ ions are moved for the exchange of one Ca^{2+} ion, the forward reaction is favored when membrane potential is hyperpolarized, and the backward reaction is favored on depolarization. Three different genes encode tissue specifically expressed subtypes of NCX (*NCX1, NCX2,* and *NCX3*) (55). There is no major difference in the functional properties among the different subtypes of NCX (41).

INTRACELLULAR CA^{2+} REGULATION AND CELL FUNCTIONS

Neurons

Exocytosis

Invasion of nerve endings with action potentials triggers the opening of voltage-dependent Ca^{2+} channels in the presynaptic membrane. The resulting Ca^{2+} influx and subsequent binding of Ca^{2+} to the regulatory sites of the membrane fusion machinery initiate the exocytosis of secretory vesicles (75). This is an extremely rapid on–off process, taking less than a fraction of a millisecond. To achieve rapid cessation of the fusion process, the dissociation rate of the Ca^{2+} from the regulatory site must be high. On the other hand, the bimolecular binding rate constant is limited by diffusion. These requirements make the ratio of the dissociation rate constant to the binding rate constant (i.e., the dissociation constant for Ca^{2+}) of the regulatory site large; therefore, a high Ca^{2+} concentration (>100 μM) is required to attain an abrupt initiation of exocytosis. For the huge but brief Ca^{2+} transients required, Ca^{2+} channel pores must reside close to the active zone where exocytosis takes place (65).

Much slower Ca^{2+} transients regulate hormone release from endocrine cells on activation by various hormone-releasing hormones (65). The G-protein–coupled receptors for releasing hormones generate IP$_3$ and repetitive increases in [Ca^{2+}]$_i$ (Ca^{2+} oscillations).

Synaptic Plasticity

Repetitive stimulation of a synapse at a high rate often results in prolonged enhancement or depression of the efficacy of synaptic transmission, and this process is referred to as *long-term potentiation* (LTP), or *long-term depression* (LTD). An increase in postsynaptic [Ca^{2+}]$_i$ is often essential for the formation of synaptic plasticity.

Ca^{2+} influx by way of the NMDA receptor is important for LTP in hippocampal CA1 neurons (7,45). There are some indications that Ca^{2+} release from the intracellular Ca^{2+} stores also participates in the NMDA receptor-mediated LTP. LTP in inhibitory interneuron in vasolateral amygdala, on the other hand, is induced by Ca^{2+} influx through Ca^{2+}-permeable AMPA receptors (44). In certain other types of synapses, different Ca^{2+}-dependent mechanisms are involved in the synaptic plasticity. A cerebellar Purkinje neuron receives synaptic inputs from a climbing fiber and numerous parallel fibers at the dendritic shaft and spines, respectively. At both synapses, glutamate is used as the transmitter and is received by AMPA receptors on the postsynaptic membranes. Simultaneous inputs from both climbing fiber and parallel fiber result in the LTD of the parallel fiber–Purkinje neuron synapse in a Ca^{2+}-dependent process (42). The inward current through the AMPA receptors here is carried predominantly by monovalent cations. Concomitant depolarization activates the voltage-dependent Ca^{2+} channel. On the other hand, Purkinje cells express an extremely high level of IP_3R-1. Metabotropic glutamate receptors (mGluR1) colocalize at the parallel fiber synapses and are expected to generate IP_3. Therefore, Ca^{2+} release from the IP_3-sensitive stores has been suggested to participate in the increase in $[Ca^{2+}]_i$ at the spines of Purkinje cells.

Cell Death

Excessive exposure of neurons to the transmitter glutamate results in cell death and this process, which is termed *excitotoxicity*, is thought to underlie hypoxic–ischemic brain damage (15). Massive Ca^{2+} influx through the NMDA receptor or Ca^{2+}-permeable AMPA receptors is considered a prominent factor leading to neuronal cell death. Secondary release of Ca^{2+} from the stores through the CICR also may be required for neurotoxicity (50). Recently, overload of mitochondria with Ca^{2+} resulting from the influx of Ca^{2+} was implicated in neurotoxicity (67).

OTHER CENTRAL NERVOUS SYSTEM FUNCTIONS

Changes in $[Ca^{2+}]_i$ regulate various other functions of neurons (4,27). In developing neurons or neurites, oscillatory change in $[Ca^{2+}]_i$ has been observed and is essential for cell differentiation (28). Changes in $[Ca^{2+}]_i$ regulates gene expression. For example, Ca^{2+}-dependent protein kinases regulate the activity of transcription factors, such as CREB (66). Mice with a targeted disruption of IP_3R-1 gene suffer from seizures (46). Thus IP_3R-1 may be involved in the suppression of excessive activity of neurons. Ca^{2+} release by way of the RyR-3 seems to be involved in the regulation of locomotor activity (70) and the regulation of the autonomic nervous system. The RyR was implicated in the circadian rhythm in the suprachiasmatic nucleus (18).

Vascular Smooth Muscle

Myogenic Response

Pressurization of the blood vessel, that is, distention of the vascular wall, results in the constriction of the vessel (3). In other words, stretched vascular walls generate active contraction (47). Furthermore, the active contraction often displays a sinusoidal rhythm. Activation of the mechanosensitive ion channel by the distention of the vessel wall and the resulting depolarization and hence activation of VDCs seem important for the increase in $[Ca^{2+}]_i$ and the resulting active contraction. The mechanism for the pace making of rhythmic contractions remains elusive. This myogenic response may be important for the autoregulation of blood flow through organs such as the brain and kidney.

Agonist-Induced Contractions

Depolarization of the plasma membrane is not the sole mechanism for the increase in $[Ca^{2+}]_i$ in vascular smooth-muscle cells. Stimulation by agonists such as noradrenaline and angiotensin II within a certain concentration range results in the increase in $[Ca^{2+}]_i$ without significant depolarization. The receptor activation triggers the activation of phospholipase C through the heterotrimeric G-protein, resulting in the generation of IP_3 and the Ca^{2+} mobilization from the intracellular stores.

The $[Ca^{2+}]_i$ change in the vascular smooth-muscle cells in the rat tail artery was visualized on activation of the perivascular sympathetic nerve (33). The average $[Ca^{2+}]_i$ response took place in three phases. An early phasic response, which started immediately after the initiation of the electric stimulation of the perivascular sympathetic nerve network, subsided within a few seconds. Then a delayed phasic response developed within several seconds and was followed by a tonic $[Ca^{2+}]_i$ increase. The early phasic response was insensitive to prazosin, an α_1-adrenergic antagonist that completely inhibited both delayed phasic and tonic responses. Measurement of $[Ca^{2+}]_i$ within individual smooth-muscle cells using confocal imaging of the smooth-muscle cell layer revealed that the $[Ca^{2+}]_i$ changes displayed oscillatory responses. Because the phase of Ca^{2+} oscillations differed among individual cells, the average $[Ca^{2+}]_i$ response lost the oscillatory features and showed phasic and tonic responses. Furthermore, the spatial distribution of the intracellular $[Ca^{2+}]_i$ change showed a characteristic pattern. In the early phasic response, $[Ca^{2+}]_i$ increased rather homogeneously within the cell. Because this response was inhibited by suramin, a relatively specific purinergic antagonist, it was likely to be due to depolarization by the activation of P2X receptors by ATP, a cotransmitter of noradrenaline at the sympathetic nerve varicosities. During the Ca^{2+} oscillations in the delayed phasic and tonic responses, the $[Ca^{2+}]_i$ increase took the form of a Ca^{2+} wave at a velocity of about 20 m/s.

The reason the Ca^{2+} mobilization takes the form of a Ca^{2+} wave is believed to reside in a property of the IP_3R, that is, the Ca^{2+} dependence of the IP_3-induced Ca^{2+} release (see the section on IP_3R). The Ca^{2+} dependence gives rise to a positive feedback mechanism in the Ca^{2+} mobilization. Thus, Ca^{2+} release from local IP_3Rs successively activates the Ca^{2+} release by means of the adjacent IP_3Rs; this process results in the generation of Ca^{2+} waves (5). On the other hand, the mechanism for the Ca^{2+} oscillation is less well understood. There are two major hypotheses. First, Ca^{2+} oscillation is assumed to take place at a constant IP_3 concentration (5). To generate intermittent Ca^{2+} release at a constant IP_3 concentration, there must be both an inactivation mechanism as well as a time-dependent recovery mechanism from the inactivation in the Ca^{2+} release process; however, the molecular mechanism of the inactivation remains elusive. The second hypothesis postulates oscillatory changes in the IP_3 concentration due to positive feedback effects of Ca^{2+} on the PLC activity (49). The time course of IP_3 concentration change must be elucidated at a single-cell level.

Endothelium-Derived Relaxing Factor

Endothelial cells produce various vasoactive substances, including an endothelium-derived relaxing factor (EDRF). EDRF is nitric oxide (NO) and seems physiologically important for the regulation of blood pressure. Indeed, in mutant mice with a targeted disruption of the gene for the endothelial NO synthase (eNOS), blood pressure was elevated compared with control mice (30). How NO relaxes smooth-muscle cells is now under study. NO activates soluble guanylyl cyclase to increase the cGMP, which then activates cGMP-dependent protein kinase (G-kinase). In mutant mice with a targeted disruption of G-kinase gene, NO failed to relax smooth-muscle cells (59). Signalling processes downstream of the G-kinase remain elusive. One of the effects of NO on the smooth-muscle cells is to decrease $[Ca^{2+}]_i$. NO inhibits the frequency of noradrenaline-induced Ca^{2+} oscillations in vascular smooth-muscle cells (36).

Ca²⁺ Sparks and Spontaneous Transient Outward Current

Ca^{2+} sparks are transient and localized Ca^{2+} increases that result from release of Ca^{2+} from the stores through a single or a few clustered RyRs. They were first observed in cardiac cells and occur either spontaneously or in response to Ca^{2+} influx through the DHPR (11). Similar Ca^{2+} sparks were observed in smooth-muscle cells. The localized Ca^{2+} increase is enough to activate Ca^{2+}-sensitive K^+ channels (K_{Ca} or BK channels) to induce transient outward currents, which may stabilize the membrane potential (53).

Vascular Endothelial Cells

Agonist-Induced Responses

Vascular endothelial cells express a variety of cell surface receptors for agonists such as acetylcholine (muscarinic receptor), bradykinin, ATP (P2Y receptor), and thrombin. Activation of these receptors is coupled to an increase in IP_3 concentration within vascular endothelial cells. Ca^{2+} waves and oscillations are then generated (36), which then would activate Ca^{2+}-calmodulin-dependent eNOS to generate NO. A recent result added further complexity to the eNOS activation mechanism, and recruitment of Hsp90 seems to be required, in addition to Ca^{2+}, to activate eNOS fully (26).

Mechanical Stress and NO Production

Shear stress applied to the endothelial cells is supposed to activate eNOS activity (16). It was proposed that shear stress induces $[Ca^{2+}]_i$ increase. Whether shear stress directly activates $[Ca^{2+}]_i$ increase remains controversial, however. Several studies suggest that the presence of an agonist such as ATP in the perfusate is required for flow-dependent increase in $[Ca^{2+}]_i$. Because ATP is hydrolyzed by the ecto-ATPase, flow over the endothelial cells is expected to facilitate binding of ATP to the cell surface P2Y receptor. Such a mechanism can give rise to an apparent flow dependence of Ca^{2+} mobilization. Furthermore, a Ca^{2+}-independent tyrosine phosphorylation-mediated activation mechanism of eNOS was recently postulated (22). Further work is required to elucidate the relationship between shear stress and NO production.

Versatility of Ca²⁺ Signals

As reviewed here, in neurons, smooth-muscle cells, and endothelial cells, Ca^{2+} is an extremely versatile signalling molecule. One of the characteristics of Ca^{2+} signals is that they can transmit information by altering their spatial distribution. For example, in smooth muscle cells, a $[Ca^{2+}]_i$ increase throughout the cell induces contraction, whereas localized $[Ca^{2+}]_i$ rises (Ca^{2+} sparks) may relax the cells by hyperpolarizing the membrane potential as a result of opening of K_{Ca} channels. In neurons, localized $[Ca^{2+}]_i$ increase is essential for the specificity of synapses that undergo plastic change in LTP or LTD. The temporal pattern of Ca^{2+} signalling is also an important factor in controlling cell functions. It can be brief in the case of transmitter release in presynaptic terminals, or it may be long lasting in, for example, agonist-stimulated smooth-muscle cells and endocrine cells. Ca^{2+} signals often take the form of oscillations. Because Ca^{2+}-mediated activation kinetics of enzyme or gene expression differs depending on different molecules, the frequency of Ca^{2+} oscillation is important in selective activation of enzymes or genes (17,19,40). An understanding of the spatiotemporal regulation of Ca^{2+} signalling is expected to help us elucidate the disorders of Ca^{2+}-regulated cell functions.

REFERENCES

1. Arkin IT, Adams PD, Brunger AT, Smith SO, Engelman DM. Structural perspectives of phospholamban, a helical transmembrane pentamer. *Annu Rev Biophys Biomol Struct* 1997;26:157–179.
2. Awayda MS, Ismailov II, Berdiev BK, Benos DJ. A cloned renal epithelial Na+ channel protein displays stretch activation in planar lipid bilayers. *Am J Phyiol* 1995;268:C1450–C1459.
3. Bayliss W. On the local reaction of the arterial wall to changes of internal pressure. *J Physiol* 1902;28:220–231.
4. Berridge M. Neuronal calcium signaling. *Neuron* 1998;21:13–26.
5. Berridge MJ. Inositol trisphosphate and calcium signalling. *Nature* 1993;361:315–325.
6. Bezprozvanny I, Watras J, Ehrlich BE. Bell-shaped calcium-response curve of Ins(1,4,5)P3- and calcium-gated channels from endoplasmic reticulum of cerebellum. *Nature* 1991;351:751–754.
7. Bliss TV, Collingridge GL. A synaptic model of memory: long-term potentiation in the hippocampus. *Nature* 1993;361:31–39.
8. Blondel O, Takeda J, Janssen H, Seino S, Bell GI. Sequence and functional characterization of a third inositol trisphosphate receptor subtype, IP3R-3, expressed in pancreatic islets, kidney, gastrointestinal tract, and other tissues. *J Biol Chem* 1993;268:11356–11363.
9. Boarder MR, Hourani SM. The regulation of vascular function by P2 receptors: multiple sites and multiple receptors. *TIPS* 1998;19:99–107.
10. Brillantes AB, Ondrias K, Scott A, et al. Stabilization of calcium release channel (ryanodine receptor) function by FK506-binding protein. *Cell* 1994;77:513–523.
11. Cannel M, Soeller C. Sparks of interest in cardiac excitation-contraction coupling. *TIPS* 1998;19:16–20.
12. Carafoli E. The calcium pumping ATPase of the plasma membrane. *Annu Rev Physiol* 1991;53:531–547.
13. Catterall WA. Structure and function of voltage-gated ion channels. *Annu Rev Biochem* 1995;64:493–531.
14. Chen CC, Akopian AN, Sivilotti L, Colquhoun D, Burnstock G, Wood JN. A P2X purinoceptor expressed by a subset of sensory neurons. *Nature* 1995;377:428–431.
15. Choi DW. Calcium-mediated neurotoxicity: relationship to specific channel types and role in ischemic damage. *TINS* 1988;11:465–469.
16. Davies PF. Flow-mediated endothelial mechanotransduction. *Physiol Rev* 1995;75:519–560.
17. De Koninck P, Schulman H. Sensitivity of CaM kinase II to the frequency of Ca^{2+} oscillations. *Science* 1998;279:227–230.
18. Ding J, Buchanan G, Tischkau S, et al. A neuronal ryanodine receptor mediates light-induced phase delays of the circadian clock. *Nature* 1998;394:381–384.
19. Dolmetsch RE, Xu K, Lewis RS. Calcium oscillations increase the efficiency and specificity of gene expression. *Nature* 1998;392:933–936.
20. Dunlap K, Luebke JI, Turner TJ. Exocytotic Ca^{2+} channels in mammalian central neurons. *TINS* 1995;18:89–98.
21. Endo M. Calcium release from the sarcoplasmic reticulum. *Physiol Rev* 1977;57:71–108.
22. Fleming I, Bauersachs J, Fisslthaler B, Busse R. Ca^{2+}-independent activation of the endothelial nitric oxide synthase in response to tyrosine phosphatase inhibitors and fluid shear stress. *Circ Res* 1998;82:686–695.
23. Franzini-Armstrong C, Protasi F. Ryanodine receptors of striated muscles: a complex channel capable of multiple interactions. *Physiol Rev* 1997;77:699–729.
24. Furuichi T, Furutama D, Hakamata Y, Nakai J, Takeshima H, Mikoshiba K. Multiple types of ryanodine receptor/Ca^{2+} release channels are differentially expressed in rabbit brain. *J Neurosci* 1994;14:4794–4805.
25. Furuichi T, Yoshikawa S, Miyawaki A, Wada K, Maeda N, Mikoshiba K. Primary structure and functional expression of the inositol 1,4,5-trisphosphate-binding protein P400. *Nature* 1989;342:32–38.
26. Garcia-Cardena G, Fan R, Shah V, et al. Dynamic activation of endothelial nitric oxide synthase by Hsp90. *Nature* 1998;392:821–824.
27. Ghosh A, Greenberg ME. Calcium signaling in neurons: molecular mechanisms and cellular consequences. *Science* 1995;268:239–247.
28. Gu X, Spitzer NC. Distinct aspects of neuronal differentiation encoded by frequency of spontaneous Ca^{2+} transients. *Nature* 1995;375:784–787.
29. Hakamata Y, Nakai J, Takeshima H, Imoto K. Primary structure and distribution of a novel ryanodine receptor/calcium release channel from rabbit brain. *FEBS Lett* 1992;312:229–235.
30. Huang PL, Huang Z, Mashimo H, et al. Hypertension in mice lacking the gene for endothelial nitric oxide synthase. *Nature* 1995;377:239–242.
31. Iino M. Biphasic Ca^{2+} dependence of inositol 1,4,5-trisphosphate-induced Ca release in smooth muscle cells of the guinea pig taenia caeci. *J Gen Physiol* 1990;95:1103–1122.
32. Iino M, Endo M. Calcium-dependent immediate feedback control of inositol 1,4,5-trisphosphate-induced Ca^{2+} release. *Nature* 1992;360:76–78.
33. Iino M, Kasai H, Yamazawa T. Visualization of neural control of intracellular Ca^{2+} concentration in single vascular smooth muscle cells in situ. *EMBO J* 1994;13:5026—5031.
34. Jonas P, Burnashev N. Molecular mechanisms controlling calcium entry through AMPA-type glutamate receptor channels. *Neuron* 1995;15:987–990.
35. Joseph SK, Lin C, Pierson S, Thomas AP, Maranto AR. Heteroligomers of type-I and type-III inositol trisphosphate receptors in WB rat liver epithelial cells. *J Biol Chem* 1995;270:23310–23316.
36. Kasai Y, Yamazawa T, Sakurai T, Taketani Y, Iino M. Endothelium-dependent frequency modulation of Ca^{2+} signalling in individual vascular smooth muscle cells of the rat. *J Physiol* 1997;504:349–357.
37. Khakh BS, Kennedy C. Adenosine and ATP: progress in their receptors' structures and functions. *TIPS* 1998;19:39–41.
38. Lalli J, Harrer JM, Luo W, Kranias EG, Paul RJ. Targeted ablation of the phospholamban gene is associated with a marked decrease in sensitivity in aortic smooth muscle. *Circ Res* 1997;80:506–513.
39. Lewis C, Neidhart S, Holy C, North RA, Buell G, Surprenant A. Coexpression of P2X2 and P2X3 receptor subunits can account for ATP-gated currents in sensory neurons. *Nature* 1995;377:432–435.
40. Li W, Llopis J, Whitney M, Zlokarnik G, Tsien RY. Cell-permeant caged InsP3 ester shows that Ca^{2+} spike frequency can optimize gene expression. *Nature* 1998;392:936–941.
41. Linck B, Qiu Z, He Z, Tong Q, Hilgemann DW, Philipson KD. Functional comparison of the three isoforms of the Na+/Ca^{2+} exchanger (NCX1, NCX2, NCX3). *Am J Physiol* 1998;274:C415–C423.
42. Linden DJ. Long-term synaptic depression in the mammalian brain. *Neuron* 1994;12:457–472.
43. MacLennan DH, Rice WJ, Green NM. The mechanism of Ca^{2+} transport by sarco(endo)plasmic reticulum Ca^{2+}-ATPases. *J Biol Chem* 1997;272:28815–28818.
44. Mahanty NK, Sah P. Calcium-permeable AMPA receptors mediate long-term potentiation in interneurons in the amygdala. *Nature* 1998;394:683–687.
45. Malenka RC, Nicoll RA. NMDA-receptor-dependent synaptic plasticity: multiple forms and mechanisms. *TINS* 1993;16:521–527.
46. Matsumoto M, Nakagawa T, Inoue T, et al. Ataxia and epileptic seizures in mice lacking type 1 inositol 1,4,5-trisphosphate receptor. *Nature* 1996;379:168–171.
47. Meininger GA, Davis MJ. Cellular mechanisms involved in the vascular myogenic response. *Am J Physiol* 1992;263:H647–659.
48. Meissner G. Ryanodine receptor/Ca^{2+} release channels and their regulation by endogenous effectors. *Annu Rev Physiol* 1994;56:485–508.
49. Meyer T, Stryer L. Calcium spiking. *Annu Rev Biophys Biophys Chem* 1991;20:153–174.
50. Mody I, MacDonald JF. NMDA receptor-dependent excitotoxicity: the role of intracellular Ca^{2+} release. *TIPS* 1995;16:356–359.
51. Monkawa T, Miyawaki A, Sugiyama T, et al. Heterotetrameric complex formation of inositol 1,4,5-trisphosphate receptor subunits. *J Biol Chem* 1995;270:14700–14704.
52. Mori Y, Mikala G, Varadi G, et al. Molecular pharmacology of voltage-dependent calcium channels. *Jpn J Pharmacol* 1996;72:83–109.
53. Nelson MT, Cheng H, Rubart M, Santana LF, Bonev AD, Knot HJ, Lederer WJ. Relaxation of arterial smooth muscle by calcium sparks. *Science* 1995;270:633–637.
54. Newton CL, Mignery GA, Südhof TC. Co-expression in vertebrate tissues and cell lines of multiple inositol 1,4,5-trisphosphate (InsP3) receptors with distinct affinities for InsP3. *J Biol Chem* 1994;269:28613–28619.
55. Nicoll DA, Quednau BD, Qui Z, Xia YR, Lusis AJ, Philipson KD.

Cloning of a third mammalian Na⁺-Ca²⁺ exchanger, NCX3. *J Biol Chem* 1996;271:24914–24921.

56. Okada T, Shimizu S, Wakamori M, at al. Molecular cloning and functional characterization of a novel receptor-activated TRP Ca²⁺ channel from mouse brain. *J Biol Chem* 1998;273:10279–10287.

57. Otsu K, Willard HF, Khanna V, Zorzato F, Green N, MacLennan D. Molecular cloning of cDNA encoding the Ca²⁺ release channel (ryanodine receptor) of rabbit cardiac muscle sarcoplasmic reticulum. *J Biol Chem* 1990;265:13472–13483.

58. Parekh AB, Penner R. Store depletion and calcium influx. *Physiol Rev* 1997;77:901–930.

59. Pfeifer A, Klatt P, Massberg S, et al. Defective smooth muscle regulation in cGMP kinase I-deficient mice. *EMBO J* 1998;17:3045–3051.

60. Philipp S, Cavalie A, Freichel M, et al. A mammalian capacitative calcium entry channel homologous to *Drosophila* TRP and TRPL. *EMBO J* 1996;15:6166–6171.

61. Philipp S, Hambrecht J, Braslavski L, et al. A novel capacitative calcium entry channel expressed in excitable cells. *EMBO J* 1998;17:4274–4282.

62. Radermacher M, Rao V, Grassucci R, et al. Cryo-electron microscopy and three-dimensional reconstruction of the calcium release channel/ryanodine receptor from skeletal muscle. *J Cell Biol* 1994;127:411–423.

63. Ríos E, Pizarro G. Voltage sensor of excitation-contraction coupling in skeletal muscle. *Physiol Rev* 1991;71:849–908.

64. Schneider M. Control of calcium release in functioning skeletal muscle fibers. *Annu Rev Physiol* 1994;56:463–483.

65. Schweizer FE, Betz H, Augustine GJ. From vesicle docking to endocytosis: intermediate reactions of exocytosis. *Neuron* 1995;14:689–696.

66. Silva AJ, Kogan JH, Frankland PW, Kida S. CREB and memory. *Annu Rev Neurosci* 1998;21:127–148.

67. Stout A, Raphael H, Kanterewicz B, Klann E, Reynolds I. Glutamate-induced neuron death requires mitochondrial calcium uptake. *Nature Neuroscience* 1998;1:366–373.

68. Sutko JL, Airey JA. Ryanodine receptor Ca²⁺ release channels: does diversity in form equal diversity in function? *Physiol Rev* 1996;76:1027–1071.

69. Südhof TC, Newton CL, Archer BTD, Ushkaryov YA, Mignery GA. Structure of a novel InsP3 receptor. *EMBO J* 1991;10:3199–3206.

70. Takeshima H, Ikemoto T, Nishi M, et al. Generation and characterization of mutant mice lacking ryanodine receptor type 3. *J Biol Chem* 1996;271:19649–19652.

71. Takeshima H, Nishimura S, Matsumoto T, et al. Primary structure and expression from complementary DNA of skeletal muscle ryanodine receptor. *Nature* 1989;339:439–445.

72. Tavernarakis N, Driscoll M. Molecular modeling of mechanotransduction in the nematode Caenorhabditis elegans. *Annu Rev Physiol* 1997;59:659–689.

73. Yamazawa T, Takeshima H, Sakurai T, Endo M, Iino M. Subtype specificity of the ryanodine receptor for Ca²⁺ signal amplification in excitation-contraction coupling. *EMBO J* 1996;15:6172–6177.

74. Zhu X, Jiang M, Peyton M, et al. *trp*, a novel mammalian gene family essential for agonist-activated capacitative Ca²⁺ entry. *Cell* 1996;85:661–671.

75. Zucker RS. Exocytosis: a molecular and physiological perspective. *Neuron* 1996;17:1049–1055.

The Headaches, Second Edition,
edited by J. Olesen, P. Tfelt-Hansen, and K.M.A. Welch.
Lippincott Williams & Wilkins, Philadelphia © 2000.

Basic Science Aspects of the Headaches

CHAPTER 22

Cortical Spreading Depression

Martin Lauritzen

The characteristic development of sensory disturbances during migraine auras suggests that the underlying mechanism is a disturbance of the cerebral cortex, probably the cortical spreading depression of Leao (CSD) (45). This viewpoint is supported by the finding of unique changes of brain blood flow during attacks of migraine with aura, which have been replicated in animal experiments during CSD (39) (Fig. 1). The literature concerning CSD is overwhelming, and a number of reviews cover most studies (3,8,39,49,64). The possible link between CSD and migraine was reviewed recently (39) and will be described here mainly in relation to newer studies.

DESCRIPTION OF THE PHENOMENON

Neurons and glial cells depolarize during CSD, giving rise to an intense but transient spike activity (seconds). Neuronal silence immediately follows, lasting for a few minutes; evoked potentials usually take 15 to 30 minutes to recover (3). The sequence of brief excitation followed by a short-lasting depression is supposed to be the neurophysiologic basis of the sensory symptoms during migraine auras. CSD is associated with a dramatic failure of brain ion homeostasis, efflux of excitatory amino acids from nerve cells, and enhanced energy metabolism (Fig. 2). CSD has been induced in most gray-matter regions studied so far, for example, in the cortex, the hippocampus, and the cerebellum of a variety of species (3) and in human cortical tissue in vitro (1) and in human hippocampus and striatum in vivo (3). In a series of patients with severe head trauma studied in the intensive care unit,

Mayevsky and colleagues recognized in one patient repetitive cycles of depolarizations associated with large increases of extracellular potassium and depression on the electroencephalogram (EEG) (42). This was the first electrophysiologic recording of CSD in human neocortex in vivo. Thus, human cortical tissue support the development of CSD, but an electric recording of CSD from the human neocortex during migraine in vivo is still missing.

HOW DOES A CSD SPREAD?

Several explanations for the spreading mechanism of CSD have been proposed. Extracellular diffusion of one or more chemical mediators, most likely K^+ and glutamate, is probably involved (49,52). CSD in the neocortex of a variety of species, including humans, is dependent on activation of a single receptor, the NMDA receptor (1), one of the three subtypes of glutamate receptors (40). The calcium influx triggered by NMDA-receptor activation is the proper stimulus for nitric oxide (NO) synthase activity, and part of the cerebrovascular response to CSD is dependent on NO. Several studies have shown that induction of CSD by microdialysis of K^+ or agonists for the NMDA receptor is associated with efflux of glutamate at the site of elicitation (51,60). During propagation of a CSD, the extracellular concentrations of a number of amino acids, including glutamate, glycine, and taurine, increase and extracellular arginine decreases (14). The latter change may be relevant to the increased NO synthesis and release during and following CSD as demonstrated recently (66) by an NO-sensitive miroelectrode (57).

The microdialysis technique could not answer the question of whether the transmitter release occurred before or after the depolarization wave because of the low

M. Lauritzen: Department of Clinical Neurophysiology, Glostrup Hospital, University of Copenhagen, DK-2600 Glostrup, Copenhagen, Denmark.

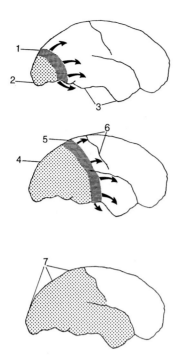

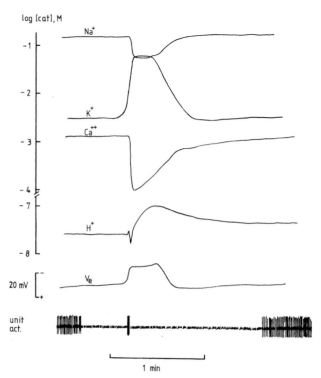

FIG. 2. Electrophysiologic changes accompanying cortical spreading depression (*CSD*) in the rat brain. Interstitial ion concentrations of sodium, potassium, calcium, and hydrogen was measured by ion-selective electrodes. Note that the scale is logarithmic. The extracellular potential (*VE*) and the single unit of activity were measured by single-barrelled potential electrodes. CSD was elicited in frontal cortex, and the electrophysiologic changes were recorded in the parietal cortex. The figure illustrates the dramatic failure of brain ion homeostasis during CSD as sodium and calcium enter the cells while potassium and hydrogen ions enter the extracellular space. The disturbance is self-limiting, and after a few minutes, normal brain ion homeostasis is reestablished. (From ref. 38, with permission.)

FIG. 1. Hypothesis of development of attack of migraine with aura based on aspects of cortical spreading depression (*CSD*) and migraine. The figures represent lateral views of the human brain at different intervals after the beginning of the attack, spaced by approximately 30 minutes. *Dotted area*: Represents the region of reduced cerebral blood flow. *Striped area*: The region of neuronal depolarization during the first minutes of CSD. The direction of propagation of CSD (*arrows*). *1*, Initially during an attack of migraine with aura a CSD is elicited at the occipital pole, spreading anteriorly at the lateral, mesial, and ventral sides of the brain. At the CSD wave front, transient ionic and metabolic disequilibria trigger perturbed neuronal function, cerebral blood flow changes and neurological symptoms. *2*, Following CSD, cortical cerebral blood flow decreases by 20% to 30% for 2 to 6 hours. *3*, Cerebral blood flow in regions not invaded by CSD remains normal until encountered by CSD. *4*, The region of reduced cerebral blood flow expands as the CSD move anteriorly. *5*, Somatosensory symptoms from the extremities appear when the CSD invades the primary sensory cortex at the postcentral gyrus. *6*, CSD usually stops on reaching the central sulcus, but in many patients it does not even propagate this far. The ventral spread of CSD causes activation of pain-sensitive fibers and headache. *7*, Full-scale attack. The CSD has stopped and is now detectable as a persistent reduction of cortical cerebral blood flow. At this time, the patient suffers from headache, but has no focal deficits. (From ref. 38, with permission.).

time resolution, but this problem was addressed using voltammetry, which showed that transmitter release succeeded the onset of the DC shift techniques (46,54). This finding suggests that chemical neurotransmission plays only a secondary role in the spreading mechanism of CSD, and potassium takes center stage as the primary candidate for CSD propagation. High extracellular K^+, by decreasing the resting membrane potential, might take away the voltage-sensitive Mg^{2+} block of the NMDA

receptor, which would make the receptor extremely sensitive to small increases of extracellular glutamate. Receptor activation would trigger further neuronal depolarization and other biochemical events known to be associated with NMDA receptor activation, including potassium release.

The importance of potassium fits well with recent data showing that the susceptibility of the tissue to produce CSD is enhanced when the function of glial cells is hampered (36). Glial cells are major scavengers of extracellular potassium, and deterioration of glial cell function resulting from metabolic toxins leads to neuronal cell death in response to spreading depression (36). Normal function of glial cells is important in preventing CSD initiation and neuronal damage during repeated episodes of CSD, but normal glial cell function is not required for the CSD to spread, because full-blown CSDs can be produced while the glial cells are heavily poisoned, synaptic function being entirely normal (35). The glial depolarization during CSD is related to passive Donnan-like KCl and water fluxes into astrocytes (67), which have only a passive role in CSD. The active repolarizing phase is located in neurons, and the spread of the CSD is not a process that involves glial cells, as suggested previously; only neurons are necessary.

Spreading depression bears a strong resemblance to gap-junction–mediated calcium waves among cultured astrocytes (48), but CSD may propagate in calcium-free media without any change in intracellular calcium (2). Still, the association between propagated calcium waves and CSD is noteworthy. Although calcium waves may not be the mechanism of CSD, increased intracellular calcium will be important when considering the physiological consequences of CSD. Cortical spreading depression elicited in several in vitro preparations have proven to be sensitive to blockers of gap junctions (33,41,48). The effect of these alkyl alcohols on CSD propagation is consistent with the idea that opening gap junctions is required for CSD propagation. Alternatively, interference with the lipid phase of neuron membranes may explain the blocking effect. The development of new nontoxic blockers of gap junctions is interesting in the context of new avenues for migraine therapy.

IS CSD ONE OR SEVERAL PHENOMENA?

Under different experimental conditions, CSD may develop differently, depending on the procedures used to elicit it. CSD usually is recognized by its large change of DC potential or the corresponding change of the extracellular potassium concentration. Microinjection of K^+ into the hippocampus elicited a CSD propagating in the dendritic layer with a faster onset, a lower threshold, a larger amplitude, and a faster propagation velocity than a CSD triggered in the cell-body layer (pyramidal cell-body layer). In some preparations, the direction of spread was in one direction in the dendritic layer and in the opposite direction in the cell-body layer (24). In the rat cerebral cortex, the profiles of DC potential and K^+ shifts changed as a function of depth and the mode of elicitation (needle stab versus KCl). Recurrent CSDs propagating from the site of KCl application had longer duration and lower frequencies in superficial (dendritic) layers than in deeper (cell-body) layers. Potassium-induced CSDs sometimes propagated independently in the superficial and deep layers. In contrast, a CSD elicited by needle stab usually invaded the entire cortex with DC potentials that differed in shape from recurrent KCl-elicited CSDs (58). There appeared to be a barrier for the vertical spread of CSD between a depth of 800 and 1,200 mm. Thus, the electrophysiologic correlates of CSD differ depending on the site of recording and the mode of elicitation. Consequently, caution should be exercised and what is meant by CSD always should be clearly defined when comparing results between groups.

HOW LONG DOES A SPREADING DEPRESSION LAST?

There is no simple answer to this question. The electrophysiologic events last at most 5 to 10 minutes, whereas metabolic and cerebrovascular changes may take 1 to 2 hours to return to normal. Repeated episodes of CSD increase the immunohistochemical staining of glial fibrillary acidic protein in the rat cortex as a result of upregulation of mRNA for that protein in activated glial cells, lasting for up to 4 days (32). The c-fos protooncogene and mRNA for nerve growth factor (NGF) increased for up to 24 hours after repeated CSD episodes (23), as do several other markers for immediate early genes, even after single CSD episodes (30). Recent data suggest that neuronal NO synthase activity in glial cells increases after CSD (5). The number of neuronal NOS (nNOS)—positive cells in the somatosensory cortex was significantly increased at 6 hours and at 3 days after SD, whereas inducible NOS expression remained unchanged. Double-labeling of nNOS and glial fibrillary acidic protein identified these nNOS-positive cells as astrocytes. Other studies have shown increased expression of heat-shock proteins, cyclooxygenase 2, and other growth factors besides those already mentioned (4,29,50,56). Despite the increase in the synthesis of selected proteins, overall protein synthesis is decreased during CSD, probably as a result of the great energy demands related to the regenerative processes in the cortex (43).

Interest in the biochemical impact of CSD is increasing because previous exposure of the brain to CSD protects the nerve cells against brain ischemia (27). The long-lasting changes in brain gene expression and protein synthesis that CSD episodes produce might be useful when looking for new therapeutic strategies against stroke. Conversely, if CSD indeed is the basis of migraine, then it is must be considered that the brain of migraine patients at least to some extent is protected against ischemia by CSD itself.

Thus, the short and transient effect on the electrocorticogram, should not mislead us to believe that CSD is a short-lasting event. Indeed, CSD induces a massive depolarization of the cerebral cortex which has long-lasting effect on brain gene expression and protein synthesis.

BRAIN BLOOD FLOW DURING CSD

Cortical blood flow (CBF) decreases before CSD or during the onset of depolarization, but the vasoconstriction is variable and usually brief (9,38). During return to normal of ionic changes, CBF increases by approximately 100% in anesthetized animals (37,60), simultaneously with the release of lactate to the brain interstitial fluid (61). The cortical flow increase is heterogeneous, small in the upper 250 μm and large at 250 to 500 μm and in deeper layers (12). The increase in flow lasts 1 to 2 minutes and is rapidly succeeded by a 20% to 30% flow reduction resulting from cortical arteriolar vasoconstriction, whereas CBF in noninvaded regions remains constant (9,16,34,37,44,55,62). The hypoperfusion in rats persists about 1 hour. Blood pressure autoregulation of CBF is preserved in the entire brain. In contrast, the vascular responsiveness is markedly impaired after CSD in response to, for example, changes of $PaCO_2$ (34,37,55), basal forebrain stimulation (34), and vasoactive substances applied directly to the pial arterioles (65). At 90 minutes after CSD, cortical CBF increases transiently (15). The well-known CBF changes in CSD was recently reproduced in awake, freely moving animals (63). The changes in CBF associated with CSD are similar to those in patients who have migraine with aura during attacks (38).

Nitric oxide and other vasoactive substances are important for the cerebrovascular changes during CSD (14), as predicted from the finding that brain extracellular L-arginine decreases during CSD and that brain cortical cGMP increases by up to 400% (19). Inhibitors of NO synthase activity appear to be without effect on the CBF increase in rats (10,16). In cats, the cerebrovasodilatation was totally dependent on NO in one study (20), whereas other investigators found more modest reductions in response to NO synthase inhibition (66). In rabbits and cats, the calcitonin-gene–related peptide may contribute as well (6).

L-arginine pretreatment prevents the development of oligemia after CSD and increases the rate of recovery of the cerebrovascular responsiveness to hypercapnia after CSD. Thus, shortage of L-arginine may contribute to the development of reduced CBF after CSD (13). This finding may have clinical importance as well, because it may be possible to treat persistent reduction of CBF in migraine patients with L-arginine.

DOES CSD EXPLAIN MIGRAINE HEADACHE?

The generation of headache from intracranial sources requires activation of pain-sensitive fibers located at the ventral surface of the brain in humans. It has been suggested that CSD activates nociceptive fibers in rats (47), but awake rats do not experience CSD as an aversive stimulus (31), and some data indicate that CSD has no effect on cephalic nociceptors (26). Therefore, the mechanism by which CSD may inflict pain in humans is still not understood.

NEW TECHNIQUES TO IMAGE THE DEVELOPMENT OF CSD IN HUMANS THROUGH THE INTACT SKULL

It is difficult to produce images of CSD when recording variables with a short duration corresponding to the CSD wave front. The massive depolarization during the onset of CSD lasts only about 1 minute and, given a propagation velocity of 3 mm per minute, at most 3 to 6 mm of the cortex will be depolarized at any one time. The possibility of detecting this signal by magnetoencephalographic techniques is still being explored, and the possibility that the outcome of this approach will be positive increases with the development of multichannel equipment. The initial results obtained in the isolated turtle cerebellum suggested that a large signal would be detectable (53), but the subsequent data obtained in the rabbit were ambiguous (17), and the results obtained in humans were inconclusive (68).

There is enormous interest in imaging CSD using magnetic resonance imaging (MRI) (11,18,21,25,28,59) because of the possible involvement of CSD in migraine and the possible relation of CSD to focal ischemia as part of the mechanism of the penumbra. The ultimate goal is to be able to image episodes of CSD in the border zone of acute strokes. CSD has been convincingly demonstrated with diffusion-weighted MRI using both rats with a stroke and rats in which CSD was induced by mechanical or chemical stimulation (21). The images show signals of increased intensity up to 2 mm across, lasting approximately 1 min, and propagating away from the site of elicitation. The recovery time of the signal correlates with the perfusion defect in the affected region, and prolonged recovery times may represent depolarizations in the ischemic penumbra (59). Hyperglycemia delays the initial phases and shortens the recovery time of the intensity changes (11). In a recent study of patients during typical spontaneous migraine auras, no changes in the apparent diffusion coefficient could be observed, but in perfusion-weighted images, indications of a spreading oligemia was observed (7). The detection of CSD in humans by MRI techniques probably will depend on the development of more sensitive methods than the one used in that study (6).

The change of oxygen content in the arterial and venous blood is the basis of infrared spectroscopy, which was applied during CSD in the rat (69). The skull is translucent for infrared light, and the technique is applicable to humans. A multichannel system will be needed for migraine research. Both MRI and infrared spectroscopy image aspects of brain function related to blood flow; the main argument against the spreading depression theory of migraine is that CBF measurements are insufficient as evidence. Still, the results from studies of cerebral blood flow during migraine attacks suggest a CSD in the neocortex of intact humans in vivo, and CSD remains the best explanation for the migraine aura (38). The possible relation between CSD and migraine is still not fully explored, and the framework that CSD provides for understanding migraine has contributed to changes in the view of migraine as an psychogenic condition outside the reach of science to a disorder whose understanding will apply and appeal to many branches of neurobiology.

ACKNOWLEDGMENT

This study was supported by The Friis Foundation, The Danish Medical Research Council, The NOVO Foundation, The Foundation For Experimental Research in Neurology, The Danish Migraine Society, Lykfelds Legat, Fonden af 1870, and The Cool-Sorption Foundation.

REFERENCES

1. Avoli M, Louvel J, Drapeau C, Pumain R, Kurcewicz I. GABAA-mediated inhibition and in vitro epileptogenesis in the human neocortex. *J Neurophysiol* 1995;73:468–484.
2. Basarsky TA, Duffy SN, Andrew RD, MacVicar BA. Imaging spreading depression and associated intracellular calcium waves in brain slices. *J Neurosci* 1998;18:7189–7199.
3. Bures J, Buresova O, Krivanek J. *The mechanism and applications of Leao's spreading depression of electroencephalographic activity.* Prague: Academia, 1974.
4. Caggiano AO, Breder CD, Kraig RP. Long-term elevation of cyclooxygenase-2, but not lipoxygenase, in regions synaptically distant from spreading depression. *J Comp Neurol* 1996;376:447–462.
5. Caggiano AO, Kraig RP. Neuronal nitric oxide synthase expression is induced in neocortical astrocytes after spreading depression. *J Cereb Blood Flow Metab* 1998;18:75–87.
6. Colonna DM, Meng W, Deal DD, Busija DW. Calcitonin gene-related peptide promotes cerebrovascular dilation during cortical spreading depression in rabbits. *Am J Physiol* 1994;266:H1095–H1102
7. Cutrer FM, Sorensen AG, Weisskoff RM, et al. Perfusion-weighted imaging defects during spontaneous migrainous aura. *Ann Neurol* 1998;43:25–31.
8. do Carmo R. *Spreading depression.* Berlin: Springer-Verlag, 1992.
9. Duckrow RB. Regional cerebral blood flow during spreading cortical depression in conscious rats. *J Cereb Blood Flow Metab* 1991;11:150–154.
10. Duckrow RB. A brief hypoperfusion precedes spreading depression if nitric oxide synthesis is inhibited. *Brain Res* 1993;618:190–195.
11. Els T, Rother J, Beaulieu C, de Crespigny A, Moseley M. Hyperglycemia delays terminal depolarization and enhances repolarization after peri-infarct spreading depression as measured by serial diffusion MR mapping. *J Cereb Blood Flow Metab* 1997;17:591–595.
12. Fabricius M, Akgoren N, Dirnagl U, Lauritzen M. Laminar analysis of cerebral blood flow in cortex of rats by laser-Doppler flowmetry: a pilot study. *J Cereb Blood Flow Metab* 1997;17:1326–1336.
13. Fabricius M, Akgoren N, Lauritzen M. Arginine-nitric oxide pathway and cerebrovascular regulation in cortical spreading depression. *Am J Physiol* 1995;269:H23–H29
14. Fabricius M, Jensen JH, Lauritzen M. Microdialysis of interstitial amino acids during spreading depression and anoxic depolarization in rat neocortex. *Brain Res* 1993;612:61–69.
15. Fabricius M, Lauritzen M. Transient hyperemia succeeds oligemia in the wake of cortical spreading depression. *Brain Res* 1992;602:350–353.
16. Fabricius M, Lauritzen M. Examination of the role of nitric oxide for the hypercapnic rise of cerebral blood flow in rats. *Am J Physiol* 1994;266:H1457–H1464.
17. Gardner-Medwin AR, Tepley N, Barkley GL, et al. Magnetic fields associated with spreading depression in anaesthetised rabbits. *Brain Res* 1991;540:153–158.
18. Gardner Medwin AR, van Bruggen N, Williams SR, Ahier RG. Magnetic resonance imaging of propagating waves of spreading depression in the anaesthetised rat. *J Cereb Blood Flow Metab* 1994;14:7–11.
19. Gault LM, Lin CW, LaManna JC, Lust WD. Changes in energy metabolites, cGMP and intracellular pH during cortical spreading depression. *Brain Res* 1994;641:176–180.
20. Goadsby PJ, Kaube H, Hoskin KL. Nitric oxide synthesis couples cerebral blood flow and metabolism. *Brain Res* 1992;595:167–170.
21. Hasegawa Y, Latour LL, Formato JE, Sotak CH, Fisher M. Spreading waves of a reduced diffusion coefficient of water in normal and ischemic rat brain. *J Cereb Blood Flow Metab* 1995;15:179–187.
22. Herdegen T, Sandkuhler J, Gass P, Kiessling M, Bravo R, Zimmermann M. JUN, FOS, KROX, and CREB transcription factor proteins in the rat
cortex—basal expression and induction by spreading depression and epileptic seizures. *J Comp Neurol* 1993;333:271–288.
23. Herrera DG, Maysinger D, Gadient R, Boeckh C, Otten U, Cuello AC. Spreading depression induces *c-fos*-like immunoreactivity and NGF mRNA in the rat cerebral cortex. *Brain Res* 1993;602:99–103.
24. Herreras O, Somjen GG. Propagation of spreading depression among dendrites and somata of the same cell population. *Brain Res* 1993;610:276–282.
25. Hossmann KA. Periinfarct depolarizations [Review]. *Cerebrovasc Brain Metab Rev* 1996;8:195–208.
26. Ingvardsen BK, Laursen H, Olsen UB, Hansen AJ. Possible mechanism of *c-fos* expression in trigeminal nucleus caudalis following cortical spreading depression. *Pain* 1997;72:407–415.
27. Kawahara N, Ruetzler CA, Klatzo I. Protective effect of spreading depression against neuronal damage following cardiac arrest cerebral ischaemia. *Neurol Res* 1995;17:9–16.
28. Kleinschmidt A, Steinmetz H, Sitzer M, Merboldt KD, Frahm J. Magnetic resonance imaging of regional cerebral blood oxygenation changes under acetazolamide in carotid occlusive disease. *Stroke* 1995;26:106–110.
29. Kobayashi S, Harris VA, Welsh FA. Spreading depression induces tolerance of cortical neurons to ischemia in rat brain. *J Cereb Blood Flow Metab* 1995;15:721–727.
30. Kokaia Z, Gido G, Ringstedt T, et al. Rapid increase of BDNF messenger RNA levels in cortical neurons following spreading depression—regulation by glutamatergic mechanisms independent of seizure activity. *Mol Brain Res* 1993;19:277–286.
31. Koroleva VI, Bures J. Rats do not experience cortical or hippocampal spreading depression as aversive. *Neurosci Lett* 1993;149:153–156.
32. Kraig RP, Dong LM, Thisted R, Jaeger CB. Spreading depression increases immunohistochemical staining of glial fibrillary acidic protein. *J Neurosci* 1991;11:2187–2198.
33. Kunkler PE, Kraig RP. Calcium waves precede electrophysiological changes of spreading depression in hippocampal organ cultures. *J Neurosci* 1998;18:3416–3425.
34. Lacombe P, Sercombe R, Correze JL, Springhetti V, Seylaz J. Spreading depression induces prolonged reduction of cortical blood flow reactivity in the rat. *Exp Neurol* 1992;117:278–286.
35. Largo C, Cuevas P, Somjen GG, Martin DR, Herreras O. The effect of depressing glial function in rat brain in situ on ion homeostasis, synaptic transmission, and neuron survival. *J Neurosci* 1996;16:1219–1229.
36. Largo C, Ibarz JM, Herreras O. Effects of the gliotoxin fluorocitrate on spreading depression and glial membrane potential in rat brain in situ. *J Neurophysiol* 1997;78:295–307.
37. Lauritzen M. Cerebral blood flow in migraine and cortical spreading depression. *Acta Neurol Scand Suppl* 1987;113:1–40.
38. Lauritzen M. Cortical spreading depression as a putative migraine mechanism. *Trends Neurosci* 1987;10:8–13.
39. Lauritzen M. Pathophysiology of the migraine aura: the spreading depression theory. *Brain* 1994;117:199–210.
40. Lauritzen M, Hansen AJ. The effect of glutamate receptor blockade on anoxic depolarization and cortical spreading depression. *J Cereb Blood Flow Metab* 1992;12:223–229.
41. Martins-Ferreira H, Ribeiro LJ. Biphasic effects of gap junctional uncoupling agents on the propagation of retinal spreading depression. *Braz J Med Biol Res* 1995;28:991–994.
42. Mayevsky A, Doron A, Manor T, Meilin S, Zarchin N, Ouaknine GE. Cortical spreading depression recorded from the human brain using a multiparametric monitoring system. *Brain Res* 1996;740:268–274.
43. Mies G. Inhibition of protein synthesis during repetitive cortical spreading depression. *J Neurochem* 1993;60:360–363.
44. Mies G, Paschen W. Regional changes of blood flow, glucose, and ATP content determined on brain sections during a single passage of spreading depression in rat brain cortex. *Exp Neurol* 1984;84:249–258.
45. Milner PM. Note on a possible correspondence between the scotomas of migraine and spreading depression of Leao. *Electroencephalogr Clin Neurophysiol* 1959;10:705–705.
46. Moghaddam B, Schenk JO, Stewart WB, Hansen AJ. Temporal relationship between neurotransmitter release and ion flux during spreading depression and anoxia. *Can J Physiol Pharmacol* 1987;65:1105–1110.
47. Moskowitz MA, Nozaki K, Kraig RP. Neocortical spreading depression provokes the expression of *c-fos* protein-like immunoreactivity within trigeminal nucleus caudalis via trigeminovascular mechanisms. *J Neurosci* 1993;13:1167–1177.

48. Nedergaard M, Cooper AJ, Goldman SA. Gap junctions are required for the propagation of spreading depression. *J Neurobiol* 1995;28: 433–444.

49. Nicholson C. Volume transmission and the propagation of spreading depression. In: Lehmenkühler A, ed. *Migraine:* basic mechanisms and treatment, Munich: Urban & Schwarzenberg, 1993:293–308.

50. Nimura T, Weinstein PR, Massa SM, Panter S, Sharp FR. Heme oxygenase-1 (HO-1) protein induction in rat brain following focal ischemia. *Brain Res Mol Brain Res* 1996;37:201–208.

51. Obrenovitch TP. The ischaemic penumbra: twenty years on [Review]. *Cerebrovasc Brain Metab Rev* 1995;7:297–323.

52. Obrenovitch TP, Zilkha E, Urenjak J. Evidence against high extracellular glutamate promoting the elicitation of spreading depression by potassium. *J Cereb Blood Flow Metab* 1996;16:923–931.

53. Okada YC, Lauritzen M, Nicholson C. Magnetic field associated with spreading depression: a model for the detection of migraine. *Brain Res* 1998;442:185–190.

54. Pavlasek J, Haburcak M, Masanova C, Orlicky J. Increase of Catecholamine content in the extracellular space of the rat's brain cortex during spreading depression wave as determined by voltammetry. *Brain Res* 1993;628:145–148.

55. Piper RD, Lambert GA, Duckworth JW. Cortical blood flow changes during spreading depression in cats. *Am J Physiol* 1991;261:H96–102.

56. Plumier JC, David JC, Robertson HA, Currie RW. Cortical application of potassium chloride induces the low-molecular weight heat shock protein (Hsp27) in astrocytes. *J Cereb Blood Flow Metab* 1997;17: 781–790.

57. Read SJ, Smith MI, Hunter AJ, Parsons AA. Enhanced nitric oxide release during cortical spreading depression following infusion of glyceryl trinitrate in the anaesthetized cat. *Cephalalgia* 1997;17:159–165.

58. Richter F, Lehmenkuhler A. Spreading depression can be restricted to distinct depths of the rat cerebral cortex. *Neurosci Lett* 1993;152:65–68.

59. Rother J, de Crespigny AJ, D'Arceuil H, Mosley ME. MR detection of cortical spreading depression immediately after focal ischemia in the rat. *J Cerebral Blood Flow Metabolism* 1996;16:214–220.

60. Scheller D, Heister U, Dengler K, Peters T. Do the excitatory amino acids aspartate and glutamate generate spreading depressions in vivo? In: Krieglstein J, ed. *Pharmacology of cerebral ischemia*, 1990: 205–210.

61. Scheller D, Kolb J, Tegtmeier F. Lactate and pH change in close correlation in the extracellular space of the rat brain during cortical spreading depression. *Neurosci Lett* 1992;135:83–86.

62. Shibata M, Leffler CW, Busija DW. Pial arteriolar constriction following cortical spreading depression is mediated by prostanoids. *Brain Res* 1992;572:190–197.

63. Shimazawa M, Hara H. An experimental model of migraine with aura: cortical hypoperfusion following spreading depression in the awake and freely moving rat. *Clin Exp Pharmacol Physiol* 1996;23:890–892.

64. Somjen GG, Aitken PG, Czeh GL, Herreras O, Jing J, Young JN. Mechanism of spreading depression: a review of recent findings and a hypothesis. *Can J Physiol Pharmacol* 1992;70(Suppl):S248–S254.

65. Wahl M, Lauritzen M, Schilling L. Change of cerebrovascular reactivity after cortical spreading depression in cats and rats. *Brain Res* 1987; 411:72–80.

66. Wahl M, Schilling L, Parsons AA, Kaumann A. Involvement of calcitonin gene-related peptide (CGRP) and nitric oxide (NO) in the pial artery dilatation elicited by cortical spreading depression. *Brain Res* 1994;637:204–210.

67. Walz W. Role of astrocytes in the spreading depression signal between ischemic core and penumbra [Review]. *Neurosci Biobehav Rev* 1997; 21:135–142.

68. Welch KM, Barkley GL, Ramadan NM, D'Andrea G. NMR spectroscopic and magnetoencephalographic studies in migraine with aura: support for the spreading depression hypothesis. *Pathol Biol Paris* 1992;40:349–354.

69. Wolf T, Lindauer U, Obrig H, et al. Systemic nitric oxide synthase inhibition does not affect brain oxygenation during cortical spreading depression in rats: a noninvasive near-infrared spectroscopy and laser-Doppler flowmetry study. *J Cereb Blood Flow Metab* 1996;16: 1100–1107.

The Headaches, Second Edition,
edited by J. Olesen, P. Tfelt-Hansen, and K.M.A. Welch.
Lippincott Williams & Wilkins, Philadelphia © 2000.

Basic Science Aspects of the Headaches

CHAPTER 23

Animal Models of Headache

Peter J. Goadsby and Holger Kaube

In recent years, animal models have made a considerable contribution to our understanding of primary headache syndromes, and entire volumes have been devoted to the subject (12). These model systems have the advantage of being able to control the variables to a greater degree than usually can be done in human studies, but they have the distinct disadvantage of always being an approximation to the problem rather than being a direct measure. Primary headache syndromes in general, and migraine in particular, remain essentially clinical problems. Migraine, defined by the International Headache Society (72) as an episodic disorder that features unilateral, often throbbing pain aggravated by movement and associated with nausea and sensitivity to light and sound, cannot currently be modeled completely, but its constituent parts can be explored to a large degree in experimental animals (Table 1). Animal models can be used to build a picture of the clinical syndrome, which in turn can be tested as new functional imaging methods become available, leading to new questions for experimentalists; thus, the iterative process of understanding headache progresses.

The question of which model should be used is dictated largely by what one wishes to know. The underlying message for model interpreters is that no single model predicts the entire clinical picture, because no model for migraine exists; rather, only models of its constituent parts are available. It follows that every model will work and every model will fail in a certain, partly unpredictable, manner until migraine finally gives up its fundamental secrets. To a large degree, pharmacologic devel-

TABLE 1. *Clinical features and their putative biology*

Clinical feature	Biological explanation
Unilateral distribution of pain	Trigeminal involvement Nerve Nucleus
Throbbing character of pain	Vascular innervation
Aggravation by movement	Neurogenic inflammation
Nausea	Activation of NTS
Photophobia/ phonophobia	Signal noise distortion → locus coeruleus
Episodic nature	?Channelopathy
Overall defect	Aminergic sensory control systems Locus coeruleus Dorsal raphe nucleus/PAG

NTS, nucleus of the tractus solitarius; PAG, periaqueductal grey matter.

opments have driven modeling in recent years. Currently used models are constructed primarily around pain and therefore predict responses to acute-attack therapy and shed light on the pathophysiology of the attack. In general, current models are rather limited in their application to preventive management strategies, although taking advantage of what is now known of the central nervous system sites of interest in migraine and cluster headache will allow development of models of attack initiation and even termination. This chapter discusses primarily models of the acute attack of migraine.

PAIN MODELS

Blood Vessels

The fact that migraine has long been considered a vascular headache has driven much of the clinical work in the field. Our view is that migraine should be considered a neurovascular headache to place the role of the nerves

P. J. Goadsby: The National Hospital for Neurology and Neurosurgery, London WC1N 3BG, United Kingdom.

H. Kaube: Department of Neurology, University of Essen, D-45122 Essen, Germany.

This chapter is modified from ref. 20.

and vessels in perspective. The study of the cranial circulation has been rewarding; indeed, vascular studies, such as those of the arteriovenous anastomoses (AVAs) (66), have been absolutely pivotal to therapeutic advances in the field. Vascular models include studies of the anatomy and neural innervation of the cranial vasculature, studies of cranial vessels (both in vitro and in vivo), and studies of the AVAs (12). The underlying purpose has been one of examining the receptor pharmacology and physiology of the cranial circulation to characterize novel vasoconstrictor mechanisms that would reverse the assumed vasodilatation associated with acute migraine attacks.

Whereas Wolff (75) described migraine as due to vasodilatation, the relationship of vascular change to headache is now hotly debated and much less certain than Wolff had considered. For at least a third of patients, there is no vascular quality to the pain (11), which may reflect the fact that both the vessels and dura mater are pain producing (64); therefore, the description used for pain of dura mater origin may not include throbbing or pounding (15). In some patients, the blood-flow velocity of the large cerebral vessels is reduced, but regional cerebral blood flow is unchanged (16), believed to be due to dilatation of large vessels. Indeed, administration of sumatriptan is associated with an increase in blood-flow velocity in the middle cerebral vessels (4), although the changes in blood-flow velocity may not be temporally related to resolution of the headache (50). The other major drawback of the vascular models has been the safety issue that inherently arises when new drugs are designed to have vascular effects. The issue of cardiovascular safety continues to plague the triptans as a class, and certainly due diligence and care are essential in their use. If both a neural and a vascular action for antimigraine drugs is necessary, perhaps this issue will never be resolved. In the patient's interest, a nonvascular solution should be sought until the underlying pathophysiology is better defined.

Peripheral Neural Activation

Given that pain signals must pass from peripheral structures to the central nervous system, the nociceptive nerve terminal has been the subject of intense study in recent years. Models of peripheral nerve activity have included surrogates, such as plasma protein extravasation (PPE) or neuropeptide release, and direct measurements, such as those of nerve-fiber activity or trigeminal ganglion neuronal activity.

Plasma Protein Extravasation

Moskowitz and Cutrer (57) provided an interesting series of experiments to suggest that the pain of migraine may be a form of sterile neurogenic inflammation. In the rat, neurogenic PPE can be seen during electric stimulation of the trigeminal ganglion (51); PPE can be blocked by ergot alkaloids, indomethacin, acetylsalicylic acid, the serotonin (5-HT)-1 agonists, sumatriptan, almotriptan, alniditan, eletriptan, naratriptan, rizatriptan, zolmitriptan, γ-aminobutyric acid (GABA) agonists, benzodiazepines, neurosteroids, substance P antagonists, and a highly potent analogue of sumatriptan, CP122,288 (8). PPE is a plausible explanation for the aggravation of migraine pain by movement. It is unlikely to be the fundamental element of dysfunction, nor does it explain all aspects of the syndrome. Magnetic resonance imaging (MRI) techniques have not demonstrated this phenomenon in humans (59), nor can it be seen in the retina of patients during acute migraine or cluster headache, despite the fact that it can be demonstrated in the rat retina (54).

As new compounds have been studied, several drugs have been found to be effective in PPE but not in migraine. Bosentan, a potent endothelin antagonist that blocks PPE, was found to be ineffective in a double-blind, placebo-controlled study of acute migraine (53). Similarly, four negative studies of neurokinin-1 (substance P) antagonists have shown that, despite being potent inhibitors of PPE, these agents are ineffective as acute antimigraine agents, whether administered orally (10,32) or intravenously (5,60). Perhaps most difficult to reconcile in terms of a pivotal role for PPE in migraine is the fact that the highly potent blocker of PPE (48), the conformationally restricted analogue of sumatriptan, CP122,288 (35), is ineffective in treating acute migraine attacks (65).

Recently, two additional compounds have been taken into clinical development based on their effect on PPE. The first, the 5-HT$_{1F}$ agonist LY334,370 (63), has been tested on PPE, in addition to other tests, but it is not just a PPE blocker. 5-HT$_{1F}$ receptors are found in the trigeminocervical complex (73); thus, any clinical action of this compound will not resolve specific issues surrounding PPE until it can be studied in other model systems. Indeed, the available data on its vascular effects are limited, and it cannot be concluded that it is devoid of vascular actions until studies in human vessels have been completed, although in the phase I human profile it appears to be rather benign (34). If the compound is successful, it will begin to reveal the sites of action of the current group of triptans; because alniditan was shown to be clinically useful (33) without being a significant 5-HT$_{1F}$ receptor agonist (49), LY334,370 cannot provide exclusive information about the role of the 5-HT$_{1B/1D}$ receptors in treating migraine.

Another compound development is a neurosteroid (ganoxelone), which has been reported to be effective in headache above a particular plasma concentration but not at the primary efficacy endpoint (9). Checking blood levels to make definitive conclusions about drug actions in a condition such as migraine, in which drug absorption can be limited, is crucial, although perhaps a better test of a new concept is the intravenous route, which was used for both substance P (neurokinin-1) (5,60) and CP122,288 (65).

Neuropeptide Release

Studies of cranial venous neuropeptide levels have proved useful in characterizing activation of the trigeminovascular system's involvement in primary neurovascular headaches (13). Stimulation of the trigeminal ganglion in both cats and humans leads to an increase in cranial levels of both substance P and calcitonin gene-related peptide (CGRP) (24). Stimulation of pain-producing intracranial structures, such as the superior sagittal sinus, also results in release of CGRP and but not substance P (76); during trigeminal ganglion stimulation in the rat, CGRP is released within the superior sagittal sinus (3). During migraine, CGRP is elevated in the external jugular vein blood, whereas substance P is not elevated in either adults (25) or adolescents (18). Taken together, these data provide a coherent link between animal modeling and the human condition.

During both spontaneous (21) and provoked (14) acute attacks of cluster headache, CGRP, but not substance P, is elevated and similarly during the pain of chronic paroxysmal hemicrania (22). In terms of understanding the pathophysiology of cluster headaches, it is important to note that vasoactive intestinal polypeptide (VIP), a marker for cranial parasympathetic nerve activation (42), is also elevated in cluster headache and paroxysmal hemicrania (21,22). Treatment with sumatriptan reduces CGRP levels in humans as migraine subsides and in experimental animals during trigeminal ganglion stimulation (23). Treatment with avitriptan, a clinically effective (6) potent $5HT_{1B/1D}$ agonist (67), blocks CGRP release in experimental animals, but it has much less of an effect on PPE than does sumatriptan; administration of the potent blocker of neurogenic PPE, CP122,288, is not effective in blocking CRGP release at doses specific for PPE (47). The release of these peptides offers the prospect of a marker for migraine that can be measured in a venous blood sample and seems highly predictive of antimigraine activity in humans.

Direct Measurement of Peripheral Neuronal Activity

Direct recordings from fibers of the nasociliary branch of the ophthalmic nerve have been used to examine sensitization of primary afferents (1). These studies have shown that lowering pH, application of an inflammatory soup, or capsaicin can sensitise these neurons. Similarly, by recording from trigeminal ganglion neurons, it can be shown that an inflammatory soup will lower the threshold for mechanical stimulation of primary afferent fibres in the dura mater (71). These model systems are ideal for addressing some of the most basic issues in persistent and frequent headache syndromes and give a plausible basis to the common clinical observation of cutaneous sensitivity to light touch that many migraine sufferers describe.

Central Pain Transmission

Trigeminal neurons can be studied directly by recording from them using standard electrophysiological methods, by examining the actions of populations of neurons using either the expression of the protooncogene protein product *Fos* as a marker of perturbation in a neuronal system, or by 2-deoxyglucose metabolic mapping of patterns of neuronal activity. A key feature to the outcome of such studies is that only activity that reflects the applied stimulus can be measured.

We refined the stimulation of the trigeminovascular system by focusing on structures that produce pain in humans. Whereas the trigeminal ganglion is accessible and contains nociceptive neurons, it also transmits all the sensory modalities from the head and as such is unsuitable for studies of nociceptive mechanisms. The intracranial large vessels, great sinuses, and large arteries as well as the dura mater are pain producing (15,55,61,62) and thus provide an ideal, albeit somewhat more challenging, target. Stimulation of the superior sagittal sinus in humans is painful (15,56) and produces activation of neurons in the superficial laminae of the trigeminal nucleus caudalis and the dorsal horns of C_1 and C_2, the trigeminocervical complex. This activation is determined by measuring 2-dexoyglucose metabolism (31), by local synthesis of *Fos* protein (26,46), or by effecting better temporal resolution using extracellular electrophysiology with electrodes placed in the area (38) and with specific spatial resolution for pharmacologic studies that employ microiontophoretic techniques (70). Furthermore, we developed a method of stimulating a vessel in a more physiologic manner by dilating it intraluminally using mechanical means (43); this method has allowed dissociation of prejunctional and postjunctional effects of the triptans (39).

Activation of pain-producing structures, such as the superior sagittal sinus, either by direct electric stimulation or by mechanical stimulation leads to activation of probable pain neurons in experimental animals (26, 38,46). These neurons may be inhibited by a range of compounds that are useful in migraine, such as aspirin (44), dihydroergotamine (38), sumatriptan after blood–brain barrier disruption (45,68), naratriptan (30), rizatriptan (7), zolmitriptan (27), and serotonin (28). Their firing is unaffected by bosentan (Goadsby, unpublished data), which is also ineffective in the clinical treatment of acute migraine (2). Furthermore, the neurokinin-1 antagonists do not effect trigeminocervical complex activation as measured electrophysiologically or by *Fos* activation (29) and also were ineffective in clinical studies of acute migraine in at least two placebo-controlled studies (10,32). Moreover, the highly potent anti-PPE compound CP122,288 (48) does not effect second-order trigemino-cervical activation (37) or CGRP release into the cranial circulation after superior sagittal sinus stimulation (47) and has been shown to be unequivocally ineffective when administered intravenously (65). In contrast, preliminary clinical data indicate a role for glutamatergic (NMDA)-mediated excitatory amino acid transmission in migraine with a report of abolition of headache with ketamine (58); we recently showed involvement of NDMA and AMPA receptors in transmission in the trigeminal nucleus (69).

These systems allow study of the second-order neurons of this pathway that have an obligate involvement in the pain of migraine. Studies can focus on individual groups of neurons using electrophysiologic methods to determine temporal and dynamic relationships or on populations to determine more completely the overall effects of activation or inhibition by other neuronal systems or drugs.

MODELING-ASSOCIATED SYMPTOMS OF MIGRAINE

It has been difficult to model the associated features of migraine, notably nausea, photophobia, and phonophobia. Given that photophobia and phonophobia are subjective symptoms, it may be difficult but probably not impossible to develop inferential models of these symptoms. It is likely that nausea can be modeled in experimental animals in the setting of examining areas of the brainstem that are activated during stimulation of pain-producing intracranial structures. Either electric (46) or mechanical (39) stimulation of the superior sagittal sinus of the cat or electric stimulation in the monkey (26) results in *Fos* expression in the caudal aspect of the medial division of the nucleus of the tractus solitarius. Cells in this region, when stimulated, produce emesis; these subnuclei project to motor and premotor regions considered to be the pattern generator of the emetic act (17). As such, reduced *Fos* expression in this region by intravenous administration of zolmitriptan (36) is consistent with that drug's clinical profile in terminating the pain and associated features of the migraine attack. Expanded focus on these neurons may be rewarding in understanding this sometimes disabling feature of migraine.

COMPARING ANIMAL MODELS—IS IT POSSIBLE?

Although there are several levels for comparison and interpretation of animal models of trigeminovascular nociception, perhaps the only widely meaningful comparison is with clinical outcome. In any such comparison, it must be stressed that errors will occur, because the current models examine parts of the whole rather than the entire picture. A poignant example would be the question of whether neurokinin-1 (substance P) receptor antagonists are ineffective in acute migraine. Do such compounds that have failed acute-attack studies have efficacy in prevention or in early treatment of attacks? When a compound fails an acute-attack study, can we be sure that it failed because the receptor system being tested is not involved? Or is there some simpler explanation? As in the case of ganaxolone, was the drug absorbed sufficiently by the oral route? For the purpose of this section, the assumption is made that the statistically proven result of a clinical trial is clinically correct, although for the reasons just stated, this must be viewed with suitable caution. Another issue is that preclinical models generally do not factor into consideration the pharmacokinetic differences between compounds. These differences may have profound effects on their ultimate clinical efficacy and role. Simple issues, such as maximum time of concentration (T_{max}), may exert a profound effect on clinical outcome; so the results of a clinical study or the effects of model must be integrated with pharmacokinetic data in the final analysis when determining appropriate development compounds (19).

Direct Comparisons of Models with Clinical Outcome

A simple approach to evaluating the currently used models would be to list in a qualitative manner the compounds that work and do not work in humans and to compare this list with their effects in various model systems (Table 2). From these data, messages appear. It seems reasonable to conclude that, in isolation, trigeminal-evoked neurogenic PPE is not a consistent predictor of antimigraine activity. Inhibition of CGRP, which has the virtue of having been carried out in parallel in humans during migraine, remains a good predictor of outcome, whereas inhibition of trigeminocervical complex activity and trigeminovascular effects after stimulation of pain-producing structures also predicts outcome. Although the vascular actions are dissociated in certain compounds, such as acetylsalicylic acid, they are analgesic, and the question of the obligatory role of a vascular action for specific antimigraine compounds remains the burning question of the next decade (41).

TABLE 2. *Comparison of models and clinical outcome*

	Craniovascular	CGRP	PPE	Vn	Clinical
Acetylsalicylic acid	X	✓	✓	✓	✓
Triptans	✓	✓	✓	✓	✓
Bosentan	?	?	✓	X	X
NK-1 antagonist	X	X	✓	X	X
PPE-antagonist[a]	X	X	✓	X	X
Neurosteroid	?	?	✓	?	?

CGRP, calcitonin gene-related peptide; clinical, compound is effective in migraine; PPE, plasma protein extravasation; Vn, trigeminocervical complex inhibition; ✓, compound effective in model; X, compound ineffective in model; ?, outcome in model unclear.
[a]CP122,288. From ref. 35.

CONCLUSION

Migraine is a complex neurobiologic problem. Modeling migraine was simpler when the accepted view was that it was all due to dilated blood vessels and that simply by measuring the diameter of or blood flow in the cranial vessels, all would be revealed. It is noteworthy that by using a simple yet elegant approach to drug development and modeling in migraine, Humphrey and colleagues (40), with the collaboration of Saxena's group (66), propelled the field toward the next millennium and triggered remarkable interest in the field. Which model to choose? If the goal is to develop new medicines that can be differentiated from the triptans, models that cover the basic issues of the craniovascular actions and both peripheral and central neural activity should be used, with emphasis on dissociation of vascular and neuronal mechanisms. If the goal is to understand better the physiology of these systems, the answer is to use models that may contribute to the understanding of the processes and develop new ways of exploring the physiology behind migraine. This goal can be achieved only if an integrated physiologic approach is pursued. We believe this goal can be reached best by using in vivo functional brain imaging in animals. Ultimately, model systems must move to provide information that can be tested more easily in humans, most likely involving the use of functional neuroimaging, which affords the best chance of correlating what is happening in model systems with what we now know is taking place in the brain during acute primary headache syndromes (52,74).

REFERENCES

1. Bove GM, Moskowitz MA. Primary afferent neurons innervating guinea pig dura. *J Neurophysiol* 1997;77:299–308.
2. Brandli P, Loffler B-M, Breu V, Osterwalder R, Maire J-P, Clozel M. Role of endothelin in mediating neurogenic plasma extravasation in rat dura mater. *Pain* 1996;64:315–322.
3. Buzzi MG, Moskowitz MA, Shimizu T, Heath HH. Dihydroergotamine and sumatriptan attenuate levels of CGRP in plasma in rat superior sagittal sinus during electrical stimulation of the trigeminal ganglion. *Neuropharmacology* 1991;30:1193–1200.
4. Caekebeke JF, Ferrari MD, Zwetsloot CP, Jansen J, Saxena PR. Antimigraine drug sumatriptan increases blood flow velocity in large cerebral arteries during migraine attacks. *Neurology* 1992;42:1522–1526.
5. Connor HE, Bertin L, Gillies S, et al. The GR205171 Clinical Study Group: clinical evaluation of a novel, potent, CNS penetrating NK$_1$ receptor antagonist in the acute treatment of migraine. *Cephalalgia* 1998;18:392.
6. Couch JR, Saper J, Meloche JP. Treatment of migraine with BMS180048: response at 2 hours. *Headache* 1996;36:523–530.
7. Cumberbatch MJ, Hill RG, Hargreaves RJ. Rizatriptan has central antinociceptive effects against durally evoked responses. *Eur J Pharmacol* 1997;328:37–40.
8. Cutrer FM, Limmroth V, Waeber C, Yu X, Moskowitz MA. New targets for antimigraine drug development. In: Goadsby PJ, Silberstain SD, eds. *Headache*. Philadelphia: Butterworth-Heinemann, 1997:59–72.
9. Data J, Britch K, Westergaard N, et al. A double-blind study of ganaxolone in the acute treatment of migraine headaches with or without an aura in premenopausal females. *Headache* 1998;38:380.
10. Diener HC. Substance-P antagonist RPR100893-201 is not effective in human migraine attacks. In: Olesen J, Tfelt-Hansen P, eds. *Proceedings of the VIth International Headache Seminar*. New York: Lippincott–Raven, 1996.
11. Drummond PD, Lance JW. Extracranial vascular changes and the source of pain in migraine headache. *Ann Neurol* 1983;13:32–37.
12. Edvinsson L. *Experimental headache models in animals and man*. London: Martin Dunitz, 1998.
13. Edvinsson L, Goadsby PJ. Neuropeptides in headache. *Eur J Neurol* 1998;5:329–341.
14. Fanciullacci M, Alessandri M, Figini M, Geppetti P, Michelacci S. Increases in plasma calcitonin gene-related peptide from extracerebral circulation during nitroglycerin-induced cluster headache attack. *Pain* 1995;60:119–123.
15. Feindel W, Penfield W, McNaughton F. The tentorial nerves and localisation of intracranial pain in man. *Neurology* 1960;10:555–563.
16. Friberg L, Olesen J, Iversen HK, Sperling B. Migraine pain associated with middle cerebral artery dilatation—reversal by sumatriptan. *Lancet* 1991;338:13–17.
17. Fukuda H, Koga T. The Botzinger complex as the pattern generator for retching and vomiting in the dog. *Neurosci Res* 1991;12:471–485.
18. Gallai V, Sarchielli P, Floridi A, et al. Vasoactive peptide levels in the plasma of young migraine patients with and without aura assessed both interictally and ictally. *Cephalalgia* 1995;15:384–390.
19. Goadsby PJ. 5-HT$_{1B/1D}$ agonists in migraine: comparative pharmacology and its therapeutic implications. *CNS Drugs* 1998;10:271–286.
20. Goadsby PJ. Animal models of migraine: which model, why and for what? In: Edvinsson L, ed. *Experimental headache models in animals and man*. London: Martin Dunitz; 1999 (in press).
21. Goadsby PJ, Edvinsson L. Human in vivo evidence for trigeminovascular activation in cluster headache. *Brain* 1994;117:427–434.
22. Goadsby PJ, Edvinsson L. Neuropeptide changes in a case of chronic paroxysmal hemicrania—evidence for trigemino-parasympathetic activation. *Cephalalgia* 1996;16:448–450.
23. Goadsby PJ, Edvinsson L. The trigeminovascular system and migraine: studies characterising cerebrovascular and neuropeptide changes seen in man and cat. *Ann Neurol* 1993;33:48–56.
24. Goadsby PJ, Edvinsson L, Ekman R. Release of vasoactive peptides in

the extracerebral circulation of man and the cat during activation of the trigeminovascular system. *Ann Neurol* 1988;23:193–196.

25. Goadsby PJ, Edvinsson L, Ekman R. Vasoactive peptide release in the extracerebral circulation of humans during migraine headache. *Ann Neurol* 1990;28:183–187.

26. Goadsby PJ, Hoskin KL. The distribution of trigeminovascular afferents in the non-human primate brain macaca nemestrina: a *c-fos* immunocytochemical study. *J Anat* 1997;190:367–375.

27. Goadsby PJ, Hoskin KL. Inhibition of trigeminal neurons by intravenous administration of the serotonin (5HT)-1-D receptor agonist zolmitriptan (311C90): are brain stem sites a therapeutic target in migraine? *Pain* 1996;67:355–359.

28. Goadsby PJ, Hoskin KL. Serotonin inhibits trigeminal nucleus activity evoked by craniovascular stimulation through a 5-HT$_{1B/1D}$ receptor: a central action in migraine? *Ann Neurol* 1998;43:711–718.

29. Goadsby PJ, Hoskin KL, Knight YE. Substance P blockade with the potent and centrally acting antagonist GR205171 does not effect central trigeminal activity with superior sagittal sinus stimulation. *Neuroscience* 1998;86:337–343.

30. Goadsby PJ, Knight YE. Naratriptan inhibits trigeminal neurons after intravenous administration through an action at the serotonin (5HT$_{1B/1D}$) receptors. *Br J Pharmacol* 1997;122:918–922.

31. Goadsby PJ, Zagami AS. Stimulation of the superior sagittal sinus increases metabolic activity and blood flow in certain regions of the brainstem and upper cervical spinal cord of the cat. *Brain* 1991;114: 1001–1011.

32. Goldstein DJ, Wang O, Saper JR, Stoltz R, Silberstein SD, Mathew NT. Ineffectiveness of neurokinin-1 antagonist in acute migraine: a crossover study. *Cephalalgia* 1997;17:785–790.

33. Goldstein J, Dahlof CGH, Diener H-C, et al. Alniditan in the acute treatment of migraine attacks: a subcutaneous dose-finding study. *Cephalalgia* 1996;16:497–502.

34. Gossen D, de Suray J-M, Onkelinx C. First human dose study with LY334370, a selective 5HT$_{1F}$ agonist. *Cephalalgia* 1998;18:413.

35. Gupta P, Brown D, Butler P, et al. The in vivo pharmacological profile of a 5-HT1 receptor agonist, CP122,288, a selective inhibitor of neurogenic inflammation. *Br J Pharmacol* 1995;116:2385–2390.

36. Hoskin KL, Goadsby PJ. A comparison of a hydrophilic and a more lipophilic serotonin (5HT) 1B/1D agonist in a model of trigeminovascular nociception in cat. *Exp Neurol* 1998;150:45–51.

37. Hoskin KL, Goadsby PJ. CP122,288 has no effect on *c-fos* expression in the trigeminal nucleus caudalis after superior sagittal sinus stimulation. *Cephalalgia* 1997;17:402.

38. Hoskin KL, Kaube H, Goadsby PJ. Central activation of the trigeminovascular pathway in the cat is inhibited by dihydroergotamine: a *c-Fos* and electrophysiology study. *Brain* 1996;119:249–256.

39. Hoskin KL, Kaube H, Goadsby PJ. Sumatriptan can inhibit trigeminal afferents by an exclusively neural mechanism. *Brain* 1996;119: 1419–1428.

40. Humphrey PPA, Feniuk W, Marriott AS, Tanner RJN, Jackson MR, Tucker ML. Preclinical studies on the anti-migraine drug, sumatriptan. *Eur Neurol* 1991;31:282–290.

41. Humphrey PPA, Goadsby PJ. Controversies in headache. The mode of action of sumatriptan is vascular? a debate. *Cephalalgia* 1994;14: 401–410.

42. Jansen I, Goadsby PJ, Uddman R, Edvinsson L. Vasoactive intestinal peptide (VIP) like peptides in the cerebral circulation. *J Auton Nerv Syst* 1994;49:S97–S103.

43. Kaube H, Hoskin KL, Goadsby PJ. Activation of the trigeminovascular system by mechanical distension of the superior sagittal sinus in the cat. *Cephalalgia* 1992;12:133–136.

44. Kaube H, Hoskin KL, Goadsby PJ. Intravenous acetylsalicylic acid inhibits central trigeminal neurons in the dorsal horn of the upper cervical spinal cord in the cat. *Headache* 1993;33:541–550.

45. Kaube H, Hoskin KL, Goadsby PJ. Sumatriptan inhibits central trigeminal neurons only after blood–brain barrier disruption. *Cephalalgia* 1993;13:41.

46. Kaube H, Keay K, Hoskin KL, Bandler R, Goadsby PJ. Expression of c-fos-like immunoreactivity in the trigeminal nucleus caudalis and high cervical cord following stimulation of the sagittal sinus in the cat. *Brain Res* 1993;629:95–102.

47. Knight YE, Edvinsson L, Goadsby PJ. Blockade of release of CGRP after superior sagittal sinus stimulation in cat: a comparison of avitriptan and CP122,288. *Cephalalgia* 1997;17:248.

48. Lee WS, Moskowitz MA. Conformationally restricted sumatriptan analogues, CP-122,288 and CP-122,638, exhibit enhanced potency against neurogenic inflammation in dura mater. *Brain Res* 1993;626:303–305.

49. Leysen JE, Gommeren W, Heylen L, et al. Alniditan, a new 5-hydroxytryptamine$_{1D}$ agonist and migraine-abortive agent: ligand-binding properties of human 5-hydroxytryptamine$_{1D\alpha}$, human 5-hydroxytryptamine$_{1D}$, and calf 5-hydroxytryptamine$_{1D}$ receptors investigated with [^{3}H]-5-hydroxytryptamine and [^{3}H]alniditan. *Mol Pharmacol* 1996;50: 1567–1580.

50. Limmroth V, May A, Auerbach P, Wosnitza G, Eppe T, Diener HC. Changes in cerebral blood flow velocity after treatment with sumatriptan or placebo and implications for the pathophysiology of migraine. *J Neurol Sci* 1996;138.

51. Markowitz S, Saito K, Moskowitz MA. Neurogenically mediated leakage of plasma proteins occurs from blood vessels in dura mater but not brain. *J Neurosci* 1987;7:4129–4136.

52. May A, Bahra A, Buchel C, Frackowiak RSJ, Goadsby PJ. Hypothalamic activation in cluster headache attacks. *Lancet* 1998;351:275–278.

53. May A, Gijsman HJ, Wallnoefer A, Jones R, Diener HC, Ferrari MD. Endothelin antagonist bosentan blocks neurogenic inflammation, but is not effective in aborting migraine attacks. *Pain* 1996;67:375–378.

54. May A, Shepheard S, Wessing A, Hargreaves RJ, Goadsby PJ, Diener HC. Retinal plasma extravasation can be evoked by trigeminal stimulation in rat but does not occur during migraine attacks. *Brain* 1998;121: 1231–1237.

55. McNaughton FL. The innervation of the intracranial blood vessels and the dural sinuses. In: Cobb S, Frantz AM, Penfield W, Riley HA, eds. *The circulation of the brain and spinal cord.* New York: Hafner Publishing, 1966:178–200.

56. McNaughton FL, Feindel WH. Innervation of intracranial structures: a reappraisal. In: Rose FC. *Physiological aspects of clinical neurology.* Oxford: Blackwell Scientific Publications; 1977:279–293.

57. Moskowitz MA, Cutrer FM. Sumatriptan: a receptor-targeted treatment for migraine. *Annu Rev Med* 1993;44:145–154.

58. Nicolodi M, Sicuteri F. Relief of migraine attack with N-methyl-D-aspartic acid receptor antagonist ketamine: a double blind comparison with placebo-theoretic implications. *Cephalalgia* 1996;16:372.

59. Nissila M, Parkkola R, Sonninen P, Salonen R. Intracerebral arteries and gadolinium enhancement in migraine without aura. *Cephalalgia* 1996;16:363.

60. Norman B, Panebianco D, Block GA. A placebo-controlled, in-clinic study to explore the preliminary safety and efficacy of intravenous L-758,298 (a prodrug of the NK1 receptor antagonist L-754,030) in the acute treatment of migraine. *Cephalalgia* 1998;18:407.

61. Penfield W. A contribution to the mechanism of intracranial pain. *Proceedings of the Association for Research in Nervous and Mental Disease* 1934;15:399–415.

62. Penfield W, McNaughton FL. Dural headache and the innervation of the dura mater. *Arch Neurol Psychiatry* 1940;44:43–75.

63. Phebus LA, Johnson KW, Zgombick JM, et al. Characterization of LY334370 as a pharmacological tool to study 5HT$_{1F}$ receptors—binding affinities, brain penetration and activity in the neurogenic dural inflammation model of migraine. *Life Sci* 1997;61:2117–2126.

64. Ray BS, Wolff HG. Experimental studies on headache. Pain sensitive structures of the head and their significance in headache. *Arch Surg* 1940;41:813–856.

65. Roon K, Diener HC, Ellis P, et al. CP-122,288 blocks neurogenic inflammation, but is not effective in aborting migraine attacks: results of two controlled clinical studies. *Cephalalgia* 1997;17:245.

66. Saxena PR. 5-HT in migraine—an introduction. *J Neurol* 1991;238: S36–S37.

67. Saxena PR, De Vries P, Wang W, et al. Effects of avitriptan, a new 5-HT$_{1B/1D}$ receptor agonist, in experimental models predictive of antimigraine activity and coronary side-effect potential. *Naunyn Schmiedebergs Arch Pharmacol* 1997;355:295–302.

68. Shepheard SL, Williamson DJ, Williams J, Hill RG, Hargreaves RJ. Comparison of the effects of sumatriptan and the NK1 antagonist CP-99,994 on plasma extravasation in the dura mater and *c-fos* mRNA. expression in the trigeminal nucleus caudalis of rats. *Neuropharmacology* 1995;34:255–261.

69. Storer RJ, Goadsby PJ. Excitatory amino acid transmission in the trigeminocervical complex: a role in migraine? *Cephalalgia* 1998;18: 399–400.

70. Storer RJ, Goadsby PJ. Microiontophoretic application of serotonin

(5HT)$_{1B/1D}$ agonists inhibits trigeminal cell firing in the cat. *Brain* 1997;120:2171–2177.

71. Strassman AM, Raymond SA, Burstein R. Sensitization of meningeal sensory neurons and the origin of headaches. *Nature* 1996;384:560–563.

72. The Headache Classification Committee of The International Headache Society. Classification and diagnostic criteria for headache disorders, cranial neuralgias and facial pain. *Cephalalgia* 1988;8:1–96.

73. Waeber C, Moskowitz MA. [^{3}H]sumatriptan labels both 5-HT1D and 5HT-1F receptor bindings sites in the guinea pig brain: an autoradio-graphic study. *Naunyn-Schmiedebergs Arch Pharmacol* 1995;352: 263–275.

74. Weiller C, May A, Limmroth V, et al. Brain stem activation in spontaneous human migraine attacks. *Nat Med* 1995;1:658–660.

75. Wolff HG. *Headache and other head pain.* New York: Oxford University Press, 1963.

76. Zagami AS, Goadsby PJ, Edvinsson L. Stimulation of the superior sagittal sinus in the cat causes release of vasoactive peptides. *Neuropeptides* 1990;16:69–75.

The Headaches, Second Edition,
edited by J. Olesen, P. Tfelt-Hansen, and K.M.A. Welch.
Lippincott Williams & Wilkins, Philadelphia © 2000.

Basic Science Aspects of the Headaches

CHAPTER 24

Human Models of Headache

Lars Lykke Thomsen and Jes Olesen

WHY HUMAN HEADACHE MODELS

It is difficult to study spontaneous headache attacks. These attacks occur unpredictably, and the often severe pain, which in the case of migraine may be aggravated by physical activity and accompanied by vomiting, is an obstacle to the patient traveling to the hospital to participate in, for example, pathophysiologic studies. Even if patients overcome these obstacles, they often arrive at the laboratory at different times after onset of attacks, complicating interpretation. Thus, pathophysiologic events may change during the course of an attack and, moreover, the causative or triggering factors may precede the headache by several hours or perhaps days and therefore may not be detectable at the time of the study. Good experimental models obviously would allow more controlled conditions. Moreover, experimental headache models represent potential tools in the development of new treatment strategies. Considering the often time-demanding testing of headache drugs, especially prophylactic drugs, in clinical trials, valid models of human headache would facilitate drug development. Furthermore, such models would make toxicologic studies and phase II dose-finding studies easier to perform.

Proper validation of potential models is essential. Introduction of the diagnostic criteria for headache disorders of the International Headache Society (IHS criteria) (20), in combination with increased pathophysiologic understanding, have made it possible to compare clinical and pathophysiologic changes of experimentally induced headaches with spontaneous attacks and thereby to establish the validity of an experimental headache model.

Unfortunately, this validation has been carried out only to a limited extent and only in a few models. The distinct symptoms and the well-characterized vascular changes during spontaneous attacks of migraine and cluster headache (41) have made it comparatively easy to develop and validate models of these disorders. In several models developed so far, sufferers of migraine and cluster headache seem particularly susceptible to regular attacks compared with controls. Using this parameter as an endpoint, models using nitroglycerin and histamine provocation have been validated as potential diagnostic tests for migraine (19,37). The sensitivity, however, was too low (37); nonetheless, the high specificity reported in these studies underline their validity as experimental models (19,37). The pathophysiology of tension-type headache is less well characterized, and good experimental human models of tension-type headache are only in the development phase (42).

EXISTING HUMAN MODELS OF VASCULAR HEADACHE

Nitroglycerin-induced Headache

A suitable headache-inducing compound for experimental studies should be safe, well tolerated, and easy to control. Glyceryl trinitrate (GTN), which has been used safely in the treatment of angina pectoris for more than a century and has a short half-life, fulfills all these criteria.

Recently, the headache-inducing effect of GTN was systematically validated as a potential model of human vascular headache. In this model, intravenous infusion of GTN is used, and headache intensity is scored on a 0- to 10-point verbal rating scale (0–3, mild headache; 4–6, moderate headache; 7–10, severe headache) (21). Using this model, a series of studies demonstrated that the

L. L. Thomsen and J. Olesen: Department of Neurology, Glostrup Hospital, University of Copenhagen, DK-2600 Glostrup, Copenhagen, Denmark.

headache induced during GTN infusion in healthy subjects is mostly bilateral and mild to moderate in intensity (21,24,43). The pain quality is pulsating and the intensity most often aggravated by routine physical activity. The accompanying symptoms characteristic of migraine attacks (photophobia and phonophobia, nausea, vomiting) are, however, rarely present during GTN-induced headache in nonmigraine headaches (21,24,43). The GTN-induced headache shows a fairly low day-to-day variability in both headache intensity and characteristics (21). It is dose dependent up to a dose of 0.5 μg/kg per minute, at which point a reproducible ceiling effect in headache score has been demonstrated (Fig. 1). This maximal effect was not due to rapidly developed tolerance, because headache intensity showed no attenuation during 7 hours infusion of GTN (0.5 μg/kg per minute) (26). By using high-frequency ultrasound, it is possible to measure the luminal diameter of small superficial arteries (40). Using this equipment, the temporal artery responses in relation to nitrate-induced headache was studied in healthy subjects during and after administration of the long-acting nitrate 5-isosorbide-mononitrate (5-ISMN) (25). Both headache and dilatation of the temporal artery were dose dependent and decreased rapidly after cessation of the infusion (25). A combination of blood-velocity measurements with transcranial Doppler ultrasound (TCD) and cerebral blood flow (CBF) measurements using single-photon emission computed tomography (SPECT) showed that blood velocity in the middle cerebral artery (MCA) decreased, whereas regional cerebral blood flow (rCBF) remained constant during and after GTN administration in healthy subjects. This finding suggests dilatation of the MCA (6,22). The

hemodynamic responses during GTN-induced headache in healthy subjects are thus similar to findings during spontaneous migraine (without aura) headache with unchanged rCBF and dilatation of both intracranial and extracranial large arteries (13,23). In contrast to increased plasma levels of the vasodilator peptide calcitonin-gene–related peptide (CGRP) and of the vasoconstrictor peptide endothelin during migraine attacks, plasma levels of these peptides seem unchanged during GTN-induced headache in healthy subjects (12,17,27,52).

Previous studies suggested that subjects with a personal history of migraine or a positive family history of migraine in addition to the nonmigraine headache during GTN administration experience a delayed migraine headache in association with GTN administration (8,19,49). This finding was recently confirmed in a placebo-controlled trial in which the characteristics and accompanying symptoms of a possible delayed headache were prospectively recorded in sufferers of migraine without aura until 12 hours after infusion of GTN (51). These characteristics were compared with those of spontaneous attacks in the same patients. Eighty percent of the patients experienced headache during the GTN infusion, but only one of these headaches satisfied the migraine criteria; however, 80% of the patients developed a regular migraine attack after GTN. Peak migraine headache occurred at a mean of 5.5 hours after the infusion (Fig. 2). The median peak headache intensity in the migraine patients who experienced a postinfusion migraine was 7 on a 0 to 10 scale, and the pain characteristics and accompanying symptoms of the induced migraine attacks were similar to those reported during spontaneous migraine

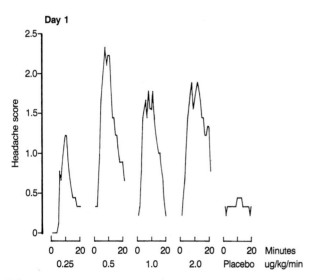

FIG. 1. Average headache scores during glyceryl trinitrate (GTN) infusions and washout periods in healthy subjects. The GTN infusions were discontinued at 10 minutes. (From ref. 21, with permission.)

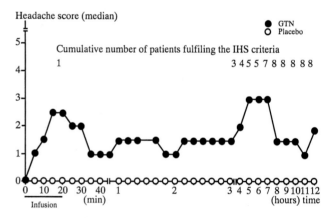

FIG. 2. Median headache intensity over time during and after glyceryl trinitrate (GTN) and placebo infusion in ten sufferers of migraine without aura. Headache was scored on a 10-point verbal scale. The headache intensity reached its peak value at a mean of 5.5 hours (median peak intensity, 7; range, 3–10) in eight patients who experienced a delayed migraine after termination of the nitroglycerin infusion. The cumulative number of patients fulfilling International Headache Society (IHS) criteria for migraine without aura is shown at the top of the figure. (From ref. 51, with permission.)

attacks in the patients (Fig. 3). Another study demonstrated that healthy subjects do not develop a delayed migraine attack, although they may experience delayed nonmigraine headache (43). Sufferers of migraine with aura also experience this delayed migraine headache despite the fact that GTN provocation does not induce aura symptoms (4). The difference between the response to GTN in healthy subjects and migraine sufferers underline the validity of the GTN model. The GTN-induced dilatation of the MCA was observed for a 3-hour period in sufferers of migraine without aura. During this observation period, the time profile of GTN-induced MCA dilatation corresponded well with the headache response (51). After sublingual administration of another nitrate (isosorbide dinitrate), MCA responses were observed for a longer period during nitrate-induced delayed migraine headache in sufferers of migraine without aura (2). Compared with baseline, MCA blood velocities still were reduced at this time (3 to 5 hours after isosorbide dinitrate administration) but only on the side of the usual spontaneous migraine pain (2).

In sufferers of cluster headache, a regular cluster headache attack may be induced after GTN administration but only during cluster periods (7,10). After sublingual GTN, studies showed that characteristic cluster attacks are induced after a relatively constant latency period of 30 to 50 minutes (7,10). Interestingly, cluster headache attacks may not be provoked by GTN for some hours after a previous attack, suggesting that a refractory period occurs (7,10). Blood velocity in the MCA decreased bilaterally during unilateral GTN-induced cluster headache attacks, whereas rCBF remained within normal limits (7). The blood velocity response was, however, more pronounced on the headache side, suggesting bilateral dilatation of the MCA, which is more pronounced on the symptomatic side (7). It has been suggested that release of vasodilating peptides from the trigeminovascular system is responsible for the latter, because CGRP is increased in blood from the external jugular vein during GTN-induced cluster headache (11).

Effect of Specific Drugs in the GTN Model

The GTN model has proven to be sensitive and powerful in intervention studies. This finding was demonstrated initially in a study showing that *N*-acetyl cysteine in combination with GTN significantly induced more headache than placebo and GTN in a double-blind crossover design in ten healthy subjects (24). Because the applicability of an experimental model in any future drug development depends on the response to existing effective drugs, the effect of sumatriptan on GTN-induced headache and large-artery responses was examined in two studies (28,47). In a double-blind crossover study, sumatriptan 6 mg or placebo was injected subcutaneously in ten healthy subjects, followed by a 20-minute infusion of GTN 0.12 µg/kg per minute (28). Sumatriptan significantly decreased the GTN-induced headache. Interestingly, the temporal and radial artery diameter decreased after sumatriptan (28). Another study confirmed the effect of sumatriptan in reducing GTN-induced headache and in addition showed that the combination of GTN and sumatriptan in healthy subjects also prevents GTN-induced dilatation of the MCA (47). These studies suggest that the GTN model of experimental vascular headache in humans may be a valuable tool in the preclinical development of future migraine drugs. More studies, however, are necessary to establish the precise value of the model in this aspect, because a recent study showed no effect of dihydroergotamine on GTN-induced headache in healthy subjects (33). Furthermore, the potential of GTN-induced migraines and cluster headache attacks in acute and prophylactic drug development so far has not been examined systematically, and the other models to be described have not been used systematically to test the efficacy of drugs.

Histamine-Induced Headache

Histamine is another compound that has been known to cause headache of a throbbing nature (5,39,48). Previous studies used intravenous bolus injections or subcutaneous injections (5,39,48). An injection causes a headache that intensifies rapidly, reaches a peak, and then declines. Such a model does not allow repeated scoring of headache characteristics or continuous measurements of hemodynamic parameters. Continuous intravenous infusion of histamine seems more attractive as an experimental model. Using the latter approach, a comparison of headache responses to increasing doses of histamine (0.16, 0.33, 0.66 µg/kg per minute) was done in sufferers of migraine without aura, tension-type headache, and

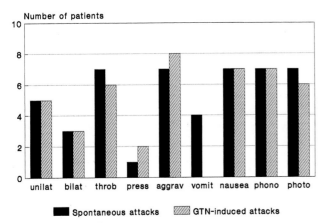

FIG. 3. Clinical characteristics of glyceryl trinitrate (*GTN*)-induced migraine. A comparison between spontaneous and GTN-induced migraine in eight of ten migraine patients who developed migraine after GTN infusion (0.5 mg/kg/min, for 20 min) is illustrated.

nonsufferers from headache (31). In a dose-dependent fashion, headache was experienced by patients with tension-type headache and migraine. The headache was more severe and more pulsating in migraine sufferers (31). Nonsufferers from headache experienced no headache or just a mild pressing sensation. Unfortunately, the higher dose was accompanied by marked flushing and side effects such as heating sensation in the face and palpitations. No serious side effects occurred, however, and it was not necessary to discontinue the test in any patients because of side effects (31). Accompanying symptoms allowing precise classification of the induced headaches (nausea, vomiting, photophobia, and phonophobia) were not reported in the short study period, but in a recent study these data were collected systematically (35). In this latter double-blind 12-hour study, sufferers of migraine without aura were randomized to pretreatment with either mepyramine or placebo before histamine infusion (35). Seven of ten patients who received histamine in combination with placebo experienced a migraine attack fulfilling the diagnostic criteria for migraine without aura. Peak headache intensity was reached at 5.1 hours (mean) after the histamine infusion. The biphasic time profile of the histamine-induced headache was exactly the same as after GTN (Fig. 4 and see Fig. 24-2). rCBF is unchanged during histamine as well as GTN infusions (32). Thus, the prolonged decrease in MCA blood velocity observed throughout a 3-hour observation period after histamine infusion reflects intracranial arterial dilatation (36). Interestingly, H1 receptor blockade by mepyramine not only blocked the histamine-induced headache response in migraineurs but also the histamine-induced decrease in MCA velocity (36). Histamine inhalation has

been validated as a potential diagnostic test for migraine (37). In a double-blind study, 15 migraine sufferers and 15 controls scored headache intensity and characteristics induced by inhalation of increasing doses of histamine. Eleven of the migraine sufferers and eight of the healthy controls experienced headache after the inhalations. These headaches fulfilled the IHS criteria for migraine without aura in six of the migraine patients but in none of the controls. Using this parameter, the specificity of the test was 1, whereas the sensitivity was only 0.4 (37). Thus, this test is too insensitive as a simple diagnostic test, but the high specificity shows its validity as an experimental model.

Headache Induced by Reserpine, Metachlorophenylpiperazine, Fenfluramine, and Prostacyclin

Reserpine given intravenously or intramuscularly in doses ranging from 0.20 to 2.5 mg causes headache with some migrainous features in most migraine patients but not in controls (30,34,44). Reserpine depletes not only platelets but also presynaptic nerve terminals of their content of monoamines. Substances released include serotonin (5-HT). An individually variable time lag occurs between reserpine dosing and headache. Headache onset normally occurs 1.5 to 2 hours after exposure (30,34,44). Reserpine-induced headache has been reported to be identical to the usual migraine of the patients. Thus, the headache is often unilateral, pulsating, and associated with nausea or vomiting (30,34,44). No data concerning photophobia and phonophobia are available. In these rather old studies, the induced headaches were not classified according to the IHS diagnostic criteria. Reserpine induces long-lasting side effects besides headache, which is a limiting factor for its utility as an experimental model (34,44). These side effects include nausea, fatigue, and dizziness for 2 to 5 days after reserpine provocation.

The headache-inducing properties of the 5-HT$_{2B}$ (or a similar receptor) agonist metachlorophenylpiperazine (mCPP), which is a metabolite of the antidepressant trazodone, has been reported (3,15,18). Brewerton and colleagues reported that an oral mCPP dose of 0.5 mg/kg, which induced headache in 28 of 52 subjects. The subjects who had a personal or family history of migraine experienced the most severe headaches. In addition, seven of eight subjects with a personal history of migraine reported headaches that were indistinguishable from their spontaneous migraines (3). The headache response did not occur until 8 to 12 hours after intake of mCPP (3). Gordon and colleagues confirmed that mCPP (0.25 mg/kg orally) induces headache in subjects who suffer from migraines and those who do not. In contrast to the findings of Brewerton and colleagues, no statistical difference in headache response was found between

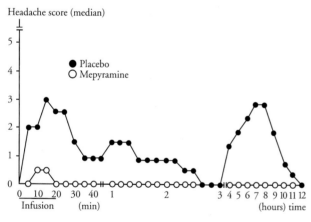

FIG. 4. Median histamine-induced headache over time in ten sufferers of migraine without aura pretreated with the H1 blocker meyramine (0.5 mg/kg administered intravenously) before histamine (0.5 mg/kg/min administered intravenously for 20 min) and in ten migraine patients pretreated with placebo before histamine infusion. Headache was significantly reduced by pretreatment with mepyramine ($p < 0.005$, Mann-Whitney). (From ref. 35, with permission.)

migraine sufferers and controls (18). Both studies found a correlation between the development of headache and the plasma concentration of mCPP (3,18).

A recent randomized, double-blind, three-way crossover study was designed to investigate the pharmacokinetics of mCPP and the induction of migraine after oral (0.5 mg/kg) and intravenous (0.1 mg/kg) administration in 14 healthy subjects (15). Oral mCPP induced headache in all tested subjects and migraine according to the IHS criteria of migraine without aura in four, with a delay from 5.5 to 9.5 hours. Intravenous mCPP induced headache in 11 of 13 tested subjects, but it did not induce migraine headache. mCPP showed large variability in pharmacokinetics after both oral and intravenous administration, and no relation was demonstrated between the area under the curve of mCPP and the induction of migraine (15).

Studies of healthy volunteers and migraine patients undergoing a provocation with fenfluramine, which causes the release of 5-HT, was recently reviewed by Panconesi and Secuteri (45). In migraine sufferers, oral fenfluramine (40 mg) induced or exacerbated headaches similarly to usual attacks after 1 to 3 hours (9). In a subsequent study, fenfluramine (40–60 mg) provoked headaches more frequently than placebo in migraine patients and more often in migraine patients than in controls (50). As part of an ongoing study, fenfluramine was administered to seven migraine patients and four matched controls to examine any difference in headache responses. In migraine patients, fenfluramine induced headache with more features of migraine than in controls (16); however, in neither of the latter studies were the induced headaches classified according to the IHS classification (16,50).

Finally, the headache-inducing properties of the vasodilator prostacyclin was studied during infusion into healthy subjects, migraine sufferers, and cluster headache sufferers (46). All subjects developed bilateral pulsating headaches as well as facial flushing and in some cases also abdominal cramps. No or little nausea was produced, and in no case of either migraine or cluster headache did the headache resemble spontaneous attacks, making this compound less attractive as an experimental model (46).

HUMAN MODELS OF TENSION-TYPE HEADACHE

Psychosocial stress has long been regarded an important trigger factor for tension-type headache. Based on this assumption, headache has been induced experimentally by psychological stress in a few human studies. In one study, subjects suffering from tension-type headache, subjects who suffer from migraine headaches, and non-sufferers from headache were stressed by arithmetic problems for 1 hour. Tension-type headaches were induced in 70% of headache sufferers, with no differences in responses between migraine and tension-type

headache sufferers. Only 25% of the control group experienced headaches (14). In another study, an imaginary electric current was applied through the heads of sufferers of tension-type headache, migraine patients, and a healthy control group. The induced headaches were generally mild, and only slightly more severe headaches were experienced by headache patients compared with the healthy control group (38). Whereas the value of both studies is limited by the lack of proper classification of the induced headaches, they may be suggestive of a causal relationship between central mechanisms (psychological stress) and headache.

Other experimental studies focused on peripheral mechanisms. Thus, hypertonic saline was infused into the sternocleidomastoid muscle for 1 minute in healthy subjects with the induction of a short- lasting nonclassified headache of approximately 4 minutes' duration (1). Others applied pressure to the head by a head screw apparatus (53) to produce a generalized headache, which disappeared when the apparatus was removed. A more promising approach was introduced in a recent controlled study in which headache was induced by voluntary tooth clenching in 58 sufferers of tension-type headache (during a headache-free day) and in 30 age- and sex-matched healthy controls. The participants clenched their molar teeth to a maximum and thereafter to maintain 10% of this maximal contraction for 30 minutes. To ensure that the contraction level was kept constant, a visual feedback system was used. Immediately before and after the clenching procedure, electromographic levels, thermal and mechanical pain thresholds, and pericranial tenderness were recorded. Patients were told that the purpose of the study was to examine whether pain thresholds and pericranial muscles reacted differently to the clenching procedure in the two groups, but subjects were blinded to the risk of developing headache. Within the next 24 hours after clenching, 68% of the tension-type headache sufferers and 16% of the controls experienced a tension-type headache according to IHS criteria (29). After clenching, pericranial tenderness was increased in the participants who experienced headache, whereas tenderness was unchanged in those who did not experience headache. Pain thresholds and EMG levels showed no differences between groups. Further refinement of this model may provide a valid and useful method for the induction of tension-type headache for future studies.

CONCLUSION AND FUTURE MODELS

The reviewed experimental human headache models seem particularly promising for understanding the mechanisms of migraine and perhaps cluster headache. In fact, these models may be of great value with regard to the elucidation of the molecular mechanisms of these disorders, as discussed further in Chapter 40. So far, vascular events, release of peptides, and changes in pain thresholds have been carried out during the immediate headaches induced by substances that induce vascular headache; however, the fact that induction of a regular migraine attack or cluster attack in susceptible persons is delayed compared with exposure to these substances suggests that a cascade of physiologic events occurs. Future studies aiming at elucidating and separating these events individually and studies of events taking place during the full-blown experimentally induced attack no doubt will provide useful information about the development and maintaining mechanisms of spontaneous migraine and cluster headaches. Furthermore, the existing models offer potential possibilities for preclinical testing of new drugs for acute as well as prophylactic treatment of migraine and cluster headache. Good and reliable human models of tension-type headache are still lacking, but they seem to be in their development phase. Future models for different types of headache may be developed as new pathophysiologic knowledge becomes available. Systematic testing of the significance of these findings with regard to the induction of a particular type of headache will follow. As an example, the finding of increased plasma levels of the vasodilator peptide CGRP in jugular venous blood during spontaneous migraine headache (17) encouraged testing of intravenous infusion of this peptide in experimental settings.

REFERENCES

1. Asthon-Miller JN, McGlashen KM, Herzenberg JE, Stohler CS. Cervical muscle myoelectric response to acute experimental sternocleidomastoid pain. *Spine* 1990;15:1006–1012.
2. Bellantonio P, Micieli G, Buzzi MG, et al. Hemodynamic correlates of early and delayed responses to sublingual administration of isosorbide dinitrate in migraine patients: a transcranial Doppler study. *Cephalalgia* 1997;17:183–187.
3. Brewerton TD, Murphy DL, Mueller EA, Jimerson DC. Induction of migraine like headaches by the serotonin agonist m-chlorophenylpiperazine. *Clin Pharmacol Ther* 1988;43:605–609.
4. Christiansen I, Thomsen LL, Daugaard D, Ulrich V, Olesen J. Glyceryltrinitrate induced headache in migraine with aura. Submitted.
5. Clark D, Hough H, Wolff HG. Experimental studies on headache: observations on headache produced by histamine. *Arch Neurol Psychiatry* 1936;35:1054–1069.
6. Dahl A, Russell D, Nyberg-Hansen R, Rootwell K. Effect of nitroglycerin on cerebral circulation measured by transcranial Doppler and SPECT. *Stroke* 1989;20:1733–1736.
7. Dahl A, Russel D, Nyberg-Hansen R, Rootwell K. Cluster headache: transcranial Doppler ultrasound and rCBF studies. *Cephalalgia* 1990;10:87–94.
8. Dalsgaard-Nielsen T. Migraine diagnostics with special reference to pharmacological tests. *Int Arch Allergy Immunol* 1955;7:312–322.
9. Del Bene E, Anselmi B, Del Bianco PL, et al. Fenfluramine headache: a biochemiical and monoamine receptorial human study. In: Sicuteri F, ed. *Headache: new vistas.* Florence: Biomedical Press, 1977:101–109.
10. Ekbom K. Nitroglycerin as a provocative agent in cluster headache. *Arch Nerol* 1968;19:487–493.
11. Fanciullacci M, Alassandr M, Figni M, Geppetti P, Michelacci S. Increase in plasma calcitonin gene-related peptide from the extraerabral circulation during nitroglycerin-induced cluster headache attack. *Pain* 1995;60:119–123.
12. Farkkila M, Palo J, Saijonmaa O, Fyhrquist F. Raised plasma endothelin during acute migraine attack. *Cephalalgia* 1992;12:383–384.
13. Friberg L, Olesen J, Iversen HK, Sperling B. Migraine pain associated with middle cerebral artery dilatation: reversal by sumatriptan. *Lancet* 1991;338:13–17.
14. Gannon LR, Haynes SN, Cuevas J, Chavez R. Psychophysiological correlates of induced headaches. *J Behav Med* 1987;10:411–423.
15. Gijsman HJ, Gerven JMA, Schoemaker RC, Ferrari MD,. Metachlorophenylpiperazin (m-cpp) is no useful tool for migraine provocation. *Cephalalgia* 1997;17:390.
16. Glover V, Ahmed F, Hussein N, Jarman J, Peatfield R. Central 5-Hydroxy-tryptamine supersensitivity in migraine. In: Sandler M, Ferrari M, Harnett S, eds. *Migraine pharmacology and genetics.* London: Chapman & Hall, 1996:117–126.
17. Goadsby PJ, Edvinsson L, Ekman R. Vasoactive peptide release in the extracerebral circulation of humans during migraine headache. *Ann Neurol* 1990;28:183–187.
18. Gordon ML, Lipton RB, Brown S, et al. Headache and cortisol responses to m-chlorophenylpiperazine are highly correlated. *Cephalalgia* 1993;13:400–405
19. Hansen HJ, Drewes VM. The nitroglycerin ointment test: a double-blind examination. *Dan Med Bull* 1970;17:226–229.
20. Headache classification committee of the International Headache Society. Classification and diagnostic criteria for headache disorders, cranial neuralgias and facial pain. *Cephalalgia* 1988;8(Suppl 7):1–92.
21. Iversen HK, Olesen J, Tfelt-Hansen P. Intravenous nitroglycerin as an experimental model of vascular headache. Basic Characteristics. *Pain* 1989a;38:17–24.
22. Iversen HK, Holm S, Friberg L. Intracranial hemodynamics during intravenous nitroglycerin infusion. *Cephalalgia* 1989;9(suppl 10):84–5.
23. Iversen HK, Nielsen TH, Olesen J, Tfelt-Hansen P. Arterial responses during migraine headache. *Lancet* 1990;336:837–839.
24. Iversen HK. N-acetylcysteine enhances nitroglycerin-induced headache and arterial responses. *Clin Pharmacol Ther* 1992;52:125–133.
25. Iversen HK, Nielsen TH, Garre K, Tfelt-Hansen P, Olesen J. Dose-dependent headache response and dilatation of extremity and extracarnial arteries after three doses of 5-isosorbidmononitrate. *Eur J Clin Pharmacol* 1992;42:31–35
26. Iversen HK, Nielsen TH, Tfelt-Hansen P, Olesen J. Lack of tolerance of head ache and radial artery diameter during a 7 hour intravenous infusion of nitroglycerin. *Eur J Clin Pharmacol* 1993;44:47–50.
27. Iversen HK, Jansen I, Edvinsson L, Olesen J. Calcitonin gene-related peptide levels during nitroglycerin-induced headache. *Cephalalgia* 1993;13(Suppl 13):185.
28. Iversen HK, Olesen J. Headache induced by a nitric oxide donor (nitroglycerin) responds to sumatriptan: a human model for development of migraine drugs. *Cephalalgia* 1996;16:412–418.
29. Jensen R, Olesen J. Initiating mechanisms of experimentally induced tension-type headache. *Cephalalgia* 1996:16:175–82.
30. Kimbal Rw, Friedman AP, Vallejo E. Effect of serotonin in migraine patients. *Neurology* 1960;10:107–111.
31. Krabbe AE, Olesen J. Headache provocation by continuous intravenous infusion of histamine: clinical results and receptor mechanisms. *Pain* 1980;8:253–259.
32. Krabbe AE, Olesen J. Effects of histamine on cerebral blood flow in man. *Cephalalgia* 1982;20:15–18.
33. Kruuse C, Thomsen LL, Iversen HK, Olesen J. The effect of DHE on GTN induced headache in healthy subjects. *Cephalalgia* 1997;17:390 (abst).
34. Lance JW. 5-hydroxytryptamine and its role in migraine. *Eur Neurology* 1991;31:279–81.
35. Lassen LH, Thomsen LL, Olesen J. Histamine induces migraine via the H1- receptor: support for the NO-hypothesis of migraine. *Neuroreport* 1995;6:1475–1479.
36. Lassen LH, Thomsen LL, Olesen J. Histamine induces both immediate and delayed headache in migraineurs due to H1-receptor activation: support for the NO hypothesis of migraine. In: Olesen J, Moskowitz MA, eds. *Abstracts of the 5th International Headache Research seminar.* Copenhagen: Notex Press, 1994:69.
37. Lassen LH, Heinig JH, Oestergaard S, Olesen J. Histamine inhalation is a specific but insensitive laboratory test for migraine. *Cephalalgia* 1996;16:550–553.
38. Martin PR, Marie GV, Nathan PR. Psychophysiological mechanisms of chronic headaches: investigation using pain induction and pain reduction procedures. *J Psychosom Res* 1992;36:137–148.

39. Northfield DWC. Some observations on headache. *Brain* 1938;61: 133–162.

40. Nielsen TH, Iversen HK, Tfelt-Hansen P, Olesen J. Small arteries can be accurately studied in-vivo, using high frequency ultrasound. *Ultrasound Med Biol* 1993;19:717–25.

41. Olesen J. Cerebral and extracranial circulatory disturbances in migraine: pathophysiological implications. *Cerebrovasc Brain Metab Rev* 1991;3:1–28.

42. Olesen J, Moskowitz MA, eds. *Experimental headache models.* Philadelphia: Lippincott-Raven Publishers, 1995.

43. Olesen J, Iversen HK, Thomsen LL. Nitric oxide supersensitivity: a possible molecular mechanism of migraine pain. *Neuroreport* 1993;4: 1027–1030.

44. Olesen J, Lassen LH. Experimental headache induced by histamine, metachlorphenylpiperazine, and reserpine. In: Olesen J, Moskowitz MA, eds. *Experimental headache models.* Philadelphia: Lippincott-Raven Publishers, 1995:259–266.

45. Panconesi A, Sicuteri R. Headache induced by serotonergic agonists—a key to the interpretation of migraine pathogenesis? *Cephalalgia* 1997;17:3–14.

46. Peatfield RC, Gawel MJ, Rose FC. The effect of infused prostacyclin in migraine and cluster headache. *Headache* 1981:21:190–5.

47. Schmetterer L, Wolzt M, Krejcy K, et al. Cerebral and ocular hemodynamic effects of sumatriptan in the nitroglycerine headache model. *Clin Pharmcol Ther* 1996;60:199–205.

48. Schumacher GA, Wolff HG. Experimental studies on headache. *Arch Neurol Psychiatry* 1941;45:199–213.

49. Sicuteri F, Del Bene E, Poggioni M, Bonazzi A. Unmasking latent dysnociception in healthy subjects. *Headache* 1987;27:180–185.

50. Sicuteri F, Poggioni M, Panconesi A. Upregulation of pain transmission from deficient analgesia in migraine. In: Paoletti R, Vanhoutte PM, Brunello N, Maggi FM, eds. *Serotonin:* from cell biology *to pharmacology and therapeutics.* Dordrecht: Kluwer Academic, 1990:391–404.

51. Thomsen LL, Kruuse C, Iversen HK, Olesen J. A nitric oxide donor (nitroglycerin) triggers genuine migraine attacks. *Eur J Neurol* 1994;1:73–80.

52. Thomsen LL, Iversen HK, Emmeluth C, Bie P. Venous plasma levels of endothelin-1 are not altered immediately after nitroglycerin infusion in healthy subjects. *Eur J Clin Pharmacol* 1995;48:139–142.

53. Wolff HG. Headache and other head pain: New York: Oxford University Press, 1963:582–616.

The Headaches, Second Edition,
edited by J. Olesen, P. Tfelt-Hansen, and K.M.A. Welch.
Published by Lippincott Williams & Wilkins, Philadelphia, 2000.

Basic Science Aspects of the Headaches

CHAPTER 25

Measurement of Experimental and Clinical Head Pain

Jannick Brennum and Richard H. Gracely

The International Association for the Study of Pain (IASP) defines pain as "an unpleasant sensory and emotional experience associated with actual or potential tissue damage or described in terms of such damage." This definition emphasizes the important fact that it is not possible to observe pain directly or to measure it objectively. Pain is a multidimensional experience, and the purpose of pain measurement is to quantify one or more of these dimensions (e.g., intensity, quality, affective value). Table 1 organizes pain evaluation into six theoretic classes defined by the measurement of either clinical or experimental pain sensations by verbal report, observable behavior, or physiological measures. This chapter focuses on the first row of Table 1, with special consideration to methods and issues relevant to measurement of pain in the head. Full treatment can be found in extensive reviews and books dedicated to this subject (11,13,14,26).

VERBAL REPORTS OF CLINICAL PAIN SENSATION

A variety of pain-rating systems have been developed. The best known are the numeric rating scales, the visual analog scale (VAS), and the verbal descriptor scales. The numeric rating scales quantify the magnitude of pain by requesting a number within a given range, for example,

0–10 or 0–100 (numeric category scale) or from an unlimited range (magnitude estimation). The verbal descriptor scales are categoric scales offering a list of descriptors that may be aimed at differentiating pain intensities (e.g., none, slight, moderate, and strong pain) or affective response to a stimulus or pain condition (e.g. not bad at all, annoying, unpleasant, disagreeable, distressing, intolerable, the most unpleasant imaginable). Using the VAS, the patient indicates the type of pain on a line anchored at its extremes with descriptors such as "no pain" and "unbearable pain" for evaluation of pain intensity or "not bad at all" and "the most unpleasant imaginable" for evaluation of affective value. Categoric measurements often are interpreted literally as providing equidistant subjective units, which is not the case. The usefulness of different rating scales has been compared in several studies, and the overall conclusion seems to be that there is no significant difference between verbal descriptor, visual analog, and numeric rating scales; however, many critical comparisons have not been made. For example, in a recent study examining heat-evoked pain sensations, the VAS showed poor reliability between 4 weekly sessions (30).

The VAS, category, and verbal descriptor scales assess single dimensions of pain magnitude or recognize pain intensity and pain unpleasantness. These scales emphasize features common to all types of pain. Other scales explicitly recognize the differences among different pain syndromes and assess the complexity of this experience. The most widely known is the McGill Pain Questionnaire (MPQ), which presents 20 separate categories with two to six descriptors in each describing (a) the sensory–discriminative qualities of pain, (b) the affective–motivational dimension concerning the emotional and aversive

J. Brennum: Department of Neurosurgery, University Hospital of Copenhagen–Rigshospitalet, DK-2100 Cophenhagen, Denmark.

R. H. Gracely: Clinical Measurement and Mechanisms Unit, Pain and Neurosensory Branch, National Institute of Dental Research, National Institutes of Health, Bethesda, Maryland 20892.

TABLE 1. *Pain measurement*

	Clinical	Experimental
Verbal report	Clinical pain-rating scales	Psychophysics
		Hyperalgesia
Behavior	Observation	Observation
	Medical records	Self-report
	Self-report	Human/animal
Physiology	Syndrome-specific use of experimental stimuli	Nociceptive reflex
		Evoked potentials
	Microneurography	Functional brain imaging

aspects of pain, and (c) the cognitive–evaluative dimension reflecting cognitive evaluations of pain and its consequences (e.g., suffering and impact on the quality of life). Patients choose terms that describe their sensations and feelings and, in addition, indicate their topographic pain distribution on a body map and complete a six-point verbal pain-intensity rating scale and a scale describing temporal pain characteristics.

Several studies examined the validity of the MPQ and generally support the structure, some with minor modifications. The MPQ was sensitive to pain-control interventions. Several studies have used the qualitative measures of the MPQ, or scales derived from it, to test its ability to discriminate between different pain syndromes of the head and face. These studies found differences between migraine and either tension (16) or cluster (22) headaches. Another study showed that the MPQ distinguished between atypical facial pain and trigeminal neuralgia (25). One important issue in these studies is comparison of this discriminative power to that of poorly and well-trained clinicians and whether the use of the MPQ increases the accuracy of conventional diagnostic evaluations. A comparison of VAS, verbal, and MPQ scales found differences that were related more strongly to the type of instrument than to any distinction between sensory and affective dimensions of pain, suggesting that the type of instrument and the repsonse required (marking a line, choosing a qualitative word) heavily influences the result (15).

The MPQ has been used to construct a scale specifically for measurement of headache pain (16). At the headache clinic in Copenhagen, we routinely use a headache diary based on the operational criteria of the International Headache Society (29). In our experience, this diary is a valuable aid in the treatment of headache patients, who often have difficulties recalling symptoms and medications during retrospective clinical interviews. These specialty scales promise to be useful in the analysis of headache mechanisms and evaluation of treatment efficacy.

PAIN PSYCHOPHYSICS: VERBAL REPORT OF EXPERIMENTALLY EVOKED SENSATIONS

Psychophysical procedures describe the relationship between the intensity of a given stimulus and the percep-

tion evoked by that stimulus. In applications to pain research, the stimulus is usually painful. In a variety of pain conditions, however, and as a consequence of many treatments, not only pain perception but also nonpainful somatosensory functions are altered. Psychophysical procedures can be used to quantify such changes in somatosensory functions, for example, hypoesthesia and hyperesthesia for different stimulus modalities (e.g., cold, warm, touch, pressure and vibration), hypoalgesia and hyperalgesia (reduced or increased responses to normally painful stimuli), and allodynia (pain evoked by normally nonpainful stimuli). Psychophysical methods often are divided into threshold and scaling methods. The *threshold methods* determine the minimal stimulus intensity that evokes a specific subjective experience (e.g., detection threshold, pain threshold). The *scaling methods* use a scale of a subjective dimension (e.g., pain intensity) to determine the amount of the subjective dimension evoked by a range of stimulus magnitudes. In pain evaluation, scaling methods usually are used to assess suprathreshold, painful stimuli. Methods that assess pain tolerance, the maximal stimulus intensity tolerated by a subject, are also suprathreshold; however, pain tolerance also can be classified as a threshold procedure because the method determines a stimulus intensity corresponding to a specified subjective level.

The most common threshold method is the *method of limits*, in which patients indicate when the pertinent subjective level is reached during a series of increasing or a series of alternatingly increasing and decreasing stimulus intensities. If the stimulus is continuous, the stimulus duration can be the variable parameter recorded, for example, the duration of submersion of an extremity in ice water (cold pressor test) or the time from occlusion of circulation (tourniquet/ischemic pain test) until the chosen threshold is reached. If the stimulus is controllable, the *method of adjustment* can be used, in which the subject adjusts the stimulus intensity to produce the desired sensation. In *staircase titration* procedures, the subject or patient classifies individual stimuli as being above or below a given desired subjective level, and the next stimulus intensity is chosen to approximate that level. The predictability of a single staircase (i.e., the patient soon learns the relation between his or her response and the intensity of the following stimulation) may be reduced by using several staircases in randomized order.

The major advantage of the methods of limits technique is that it requires only a relatively simple setup and that it is less time consuming. The results obtained with this technique are influenced by the reaction time of the patient if continuously increasing stimulus intensities are used, which may be a problem, especially in investigations of somatosensory functions mediated by the slowest conducting afferents, that is, warmth perception and second pain mediated by unmyelinated C-fibers with conduction velocities in the range of 0.5 to 2 m per second. The use of ascending series also contains errors of anticipation and confounds sensory magnitude with number of trials or elapsed time, which can result in artifactual results. The development of the staircase methods offers a number of advantages, including reduced bias, evaluation of relevant suprathreshold levels, measures of subjective performance, and ability to track pain sensitivity efficiently over time (11).

In the simplest scaling method, a standard stimulus (predetermined intensity and duration) is presented and the response is noted. This method may be useful in some situations where it is important to use a fast procedure, but the method is quite vulnerable to bias because the subject soon learns that only one stimulus intensity is presented, which may either stabilize the responses or bias the response according to the subject's expectations. Increasing the number of stimulus intensities, spacing them closely so that they cannot be identified, and presenting them in random order improves bias control and increases the informative value description of responses to a range of stimulus intensities rather than to a single intensity. Possible responses range from binary, that is, painful–nonpainful, to all the rating scales used for assessment of clinical pain. In addition, unbounded scales have been used in which subjects match their sensations to an unlimited or large response space. The common method of *magnitude estimation* allows use of all possible numbers without restriction. Other methods, termed *cross-modality matching*, require subjects to adjust the intensity of a different stimulus modality, for example, luminance of a lamp or volume of an acoustical tone, to match the sensation magnitude evoked by a pain stimulus. One variation uses cross-modality matching or other procedures to quantify verbal descriptors, which then are used as response choices (13).

If brief painful stimuli are presented, it is often possible for the subject to discriminate two pain sensations, the first pain of short latency mediated by A-delta fibers and the second pain of longer latency mediated by C-fibers. These may be quantified by either direct ratings or by reaction-time latencies (11). This technique may be useful, for example, in discriminating the effects of an analgesic treatment on pain mediated by C- and A-delta fibers. By using repetitive stimuli, it is possible to investigate alterations in temporal summation, which may be a key factor in the pathophysiology of some pain conditions (10) and may be a mechanism of action of some analgesics.

Psychophysical methods are used to address several research issues. A classic goal has been the assessment of analgesia in a controlled laboratory setting. A history of these studies reveals initial success, a period of repeated failure, and, after refinement of the methods, the present routine demonstration of experimental analgesia by a variety of pharmacologic and nonpharmacologic pain-control interventions (6,7,11). Psychophysical methods are not limited to measurements of analgesic efficacy but are used increasingly in investigations of the mechanisms of pain and antinociception to assist in clinical pain assessment and to analyze human reporting behavior. Many of these applications have been described in previously cited reviews (11,13,14,26). Recent examples include analysis of central integration mechanisms involved in morphine analgesia in volunteer subjects (7) and quantitative sensory assessments in patients with reflex sympathetic dystrophy (12), diabetic neuropathy (20), central pain (4), migraine (8), and trigeminal neuralgia (9). Sensitivity to painful mechanical pressure has been evaluated in patients suffering from headache and other syndromes of the head and neck. Studies have compared sensitivity during attacks with that during headache-free periods in the same patients and also with that evaluated in normative samples (1–3,18,19). Pain sensitivity has been shown to correlate reliably with verbal reports of pain from myofascial pain in the head and neck (19). One issue is whether these findings are stimulus or method specific; a recent study comparing normal subjects and patients in chronic pain found differences in only a subset of experimental pain measures (5).

Psychophysical methods also can assist in evaluating the magnitude of clinical pain by using procedures in which patients compare and match their pain to the "known reference" of sensations evoked by an external stimulus. This matching method provides a second independent method of assessing the magnitude of clinical pain. Comparing these two measures provides a means of evaluating the consistency of the reports of an otherwise unobservable stimulus. In studies using experimental orofacial acute (cold spray on exposed dentin) or chronic (myofascial) pain, most subjects and patients can rate accurately both experimental and clinical pain and can match directly the sensations of these types of pain (13).

Models of Hyperalgesia

Nociception may be divided into standard nociception and sensitized nociception. In recent years, it has become increasingly clear that the physiology of nociception under normal conditions and in states of inflammation and hyperalgesia differs markedly in a variety of ways ranging from the types of afferent fibers involved in nociception to changes in the gene expression of central nervous system (CNS) neurons involved in nociception. Hyperalgesia can be due to sensitization of peripheral nociceptors, sensitization of CNS neurons, or a combination of both. Demonstration of hyperalgesia or allodynia or both, however, does not reveal the etiology of sensitized nociception; that is, whether it is due to peripheral, central, or both peripheral and central sensitization. Various human experimental models of hyperalgesia have been developed, which to some extent allow differentiation between peripheral and central sensitization. These models vary mostly in the stimulus used to induce hyperalgesia (e.g., heat, cold, mechanical, chemical). Hyperalgesia occurs not only at the site of injury (*primary hyperalgesia*) but also in normal, undamaged tissue surrounding the injury (*secondary hyperalgesia*). At the site of injury, there is hyperalgesia to both heat and mechanical stimuli; in the area of secondary hyperalgesia, only hyperalgesia to mechanical stimuli is found. The hyperalgesia to heat in the area of primary hyperalgesia reflects peripheral sensitization of nociceptors, whereas the mechanical hyperalgesia in the area of secondary hyperalgesia reflects central sensitization (for review, see 21). Such models of hyperalgesia have been used in studies of physiologic mechanisms of hyperalgesia and in evaluations of analgesics (17,28). More recently, such models have been used to investigate hyperalgesia in clinical pain, as elegantly used by Morris and colleagues in their demonstration of increased hyperalgesia induced by capsaicin in patients with rheumatoid arthritis compared with healthy controls (27).

Factors of Variation in Psychophysics

Various stimulus- and subject-related factors influence psychophysical measurements. The stimulus-related factors include the area of stimulation that within a given range is related to the perception magnitude resulting from spatial summation. The repetition rate, stimulus duration, or rate of change if continuous stimuli are used also may influence the perception magnitude as a result of changes of temporal summation, adaptation, or sensitization. The stimulator–subject interphase (e.g., skin resistance for electric stimuli, skin color for radiant heat stimuli, application pressure for contact thermodes) may introduce marked variations in measurements if not controlled properly. Factors of variation related to the subject include stimulus location, sex, age, time of day, and location in menstrual cycle. Careful control of these factors of variation is essential in psychophysical studies, and detailed description of the control procedures are necessary for comparison and replication of results.

PAIN BEHAVIOR

Informal observation of pain behavior is an intrinsic part of all clinical and experimental work with pain. Nevertheless, with the exception of medication use or patient-controlled analgesia (PCA) protocols, standardized registration of pain behavior has not yet become a widely used tool. Several observational methodologies have been developed. Keefe developed a method targeting key behaviors in low back pain that has been applied to arthritis and pain in the head and neck (23). Also relevant to headache pain are recent studies of pain-specific facial expressions (24).

PHYSIOLOGICAL RESPONSES

Several physiologic responses evoked by experimental stimulation (e.g., cortical responses, nociceptive reflexes) correlate with verbal reports of pain magnitude. Recent advances in functional brain imaging using methods such as positron emission tomography (PET) and functional magnetic resonance imaging (fMRI) reveal a number of supraspinal structures that are likely involved in the sensory discriminative and affective processing of nociceptive input. These physiologic measures may be useful in studies of pain physiology and pharmacology, but it is essential to keep in mind what these techniques measure. They supply measurements of individual factors that contribute to the perception of pain (e.g., transduction, transmission, reflex arcs), which under given circumstances may correlate with some aspects of perceived pain. Extrapolations from these measures to the integrated pain experience always should be made cautiously. Measures may correlate with verbal reports under specific conditions but disassociate under the conditions of interest.

CONCLUSION

Pain is defined through verbal descriptions of a personal experience, and these descriptions are the principal measure used for clinical diagnosis; monitoring of clinical treatment; clinical trials of pain control interventions; and experimental evaluations of the mechanisms of pain, pain control, and human reporting behavior. Behavioral and physiological measures have been developed in part to provide "objective" measures of pain. Although these measures provide a valuable adjunct to verbal assessment, they never can approach the validity and demonstrated utility of verbal pain measures. Clinical verbal measures have been shown to reliably grade pain level; evaluate treatments; and distinguish between pain syndromes, including those in head, face, and neck. Increasingly sophisticated experimental methods have been used to aid in the diagnosis and evaluation of clinical magnitude and in studies of the basic mechanisms of pain and pain control. Present pain-measurement techniques have advanced considerably from those used 30 to 40 years ago. The present methods are the direct result of an integration of psychometrics, psychophysics, linguistics, behaviorism, human physiology, and clinical medicine.

The future promises further significant improvement in the ability to quantify subjective pain experience.

REFERENCES

1. Bendtsen L, Jensen R, Olesen J. Decreased pain detection and tolerance thresholds in chronic tension-type headache. *Arch Neurol* 1996;53: 373–376.
2. Bendtsen L, Jensen R, Olesen J. Qualitatively altered nociception in chronic myofascial pain. *Pain* 1996;65:259–264.
3. Bono G, Antonaci F, Sandrini G, Pucci E, Rossi F, Nappi G. Pain pressure thresholds in cluster headache patients. *Cephalalgia* 1996;16: 62–66.
4. Bovie J, Leijon G, Johansson I. Central post-stroke pain—a study of the mechanisms through analyses of the sensory abnormalities. *Pain* 1989; 37:173–185.
5. Boreau F, Luu M, Doubrere JF. Study of experimental pain measures and nociceptive reflex in chronic pain patients and normal subjects. *Pain* 1991;44:131–138.
6. Brennum J. Quantitative sensory examination of epidural anaesthesia and analgesia in man. *Acta Physiol Scand* 1996;157(Suppl): 634.
7. Brennum J, Arendt-Nielsen L, Horn A, Secher NH, Jensen TS. Quantitative sensory examination during epidural anaesthesia and analgesia in man: effects of morphine. *Pain* 1993;52:75–83.
8. Drummond PD. Photophobia and autonomic responses to facial pain in migraine. *Brain* 1997;120:1857–1864.
9. Dubner R, Sharav Y, Gracely RH, Price DD. Idiopathic trigeminal neuralgia: sensory features and pain mechanisms. *Pain* 1987;31:23–33.
10. Fusco BM, Colantino O, Giacovazzo M. Alteration of central excitation circuits in chronic headache and analgesic misuse. *Headache* 1997;37: 486–491.
11. Gracely RH. Experimental pain models. In: Max M, Portenoy R, Laska E. *Advances in pain reseach and therapy*, vol 18. *The design of analgesic clinical trials*. New York: Raven Press, 1991:33–47.
12. Gracely RH, Lynch SA, Bennett GJ. Painful neuropathy: altered central processing maintained dynamically by peripheral input. *Pain* 1992;5: 175–194.
13. Gracely RH. Methods of testing pain mechanisms in normal man. In: Wall PD, Melzack R, eds. *Textbook of pain*, 3rd ed. London: Churchhill Livingstone, 1994:315–336.
14. Gracely RH, Naliboff BD. Measurement of pain sensation. In: Kruger L, ed. *Handbook of perception and cognition: somatosensory systems*. New York: Raven Press, 1996:243–313.
15. Holroyd KA, Talbot F, Holm JE, Pingel JD, Lake AE, Saper JR. Assessing the dimensions of pain: a multitrait-multimethod evaluation of seven measures. *Pain* 1996;67:259–265.
16. Hunter M. The headache scale: a new approach to the assessment of headache pain based on pain descriptors. *Pain* 1983;16:361–373.
17. Ilkjær S, Petersen KL, Brennum J, Wernberg M, Dahl JB. Effect of systemic *N*-methyl-D-aspartate receptor antagonist (ketamine) on primary and secondary hyperalgesia in humans. *Br J Anaesth* 1996;76:829–834.
18. Jensen K, Tuxen C, Olesen J. Pericranial muscle tenderness and pressure-pain threshold in the temporal region during common migraine. *Pain* 1988;35:65–70.
19. Jensen R, Rasmussen BK, Pedersen B, Lous I, Olesen J. Cephalic muscle tenderness and pressure pain threshold in a general population. *Pain* 1992;48:197–203.
20. Jensen TS, Bach FW, Kastrup AD, Brennum J. Vibratory and thermal thresholds in diabetics with and without clinical neuropathy. *Acta Neurol Scand* 1991;84;326–333.
21. Jensen TS, Brennum J. The relation of thermally and mechanically evoked pain to pathological pain. In: Boivie J, Hansson P, Lindblom U, eds. *Progress in pain research and management:* touch, temperature, and pain in health and disease. Seattle: IASP Press, 1994:373–388.
22. Jerome A, Holoroyd KA, Thefanous AG, Pingel JD, Lake AE, Saper JR. Cluster headache pain vs. other vascular headache pain: differences revealed with two approaches to the McGill Pain Questionaire. *Pain* 1988;4:35–42.
23. Keefe FJ. Behavioral measurement of pain. In: *Advances in pain research and therapy*, vol 12. *Issues in pain measurement.* New York: Raven Press, 1989:405–424.
24. LeReshe L, Dworkin SF. Facial expressions of pain and emotions in chronic TMD patients. *Pain* 1988;35:71–78.
25. Melzack R, Coderre T, Fromm G, Ansel R. Trigeminal neuralgia and atypical facial pain: use of the McGill Pain Questionaire for discrimination and diagnosis. *Pain* 1986;27:302.
26. Melzack R, Katz J. Pain measurement in persons in pain. In: Wall PD, Melzack R, eds. *Textbook of pain,* 3rd ed. London: Churchhill Livingstone, 1994:337–351.
27. Morris VH, Cruwys SC, Kidd BL. Characterization of capsaicin-induced mechanical hyperalgesia as a marker for altered nociceptive processing in patients with rheumatoid arthritis. *Pain* 1997;71:179–186.
28. Petersen KL, Brennum J, Dahl JB. Experimental evaluation of the analgesic effect of ibuprofen on primary and secondary hyperalgesia. *Pain* 1997;70:167–174.
29. Russel M, Rasmussen BK, Brennum J, Iversen H, Jensen R, Olesen J. Presentation of a new instrument: the diagnostic headache diary. *Cephalalgia* 1992;12:369–374.
30. Yarnitsky D, Sprecher E, Zaslansky, Hemli JA. Multiple session experimental pain measurment. Pain 1996;67:327–333.

The Headaches, Second Edition,
edited by J. Olesen, P. Tfelt-Hansen, and K.M.A. Welch.
Lippincott Williams & Wilkins, Philadelphia © 2000.

Basic Science Aspects of the Headaches

CHAPTER 26

Psychological Modulation of Pain

Peter D. Drummond and Kenneth A. Holroyd

It is generally recognized that psychological factors influence the experience of pain. Our working model of this interaction is shown in Figure 1. According to this model, negative emotional states such as depression and anxiety heighten the distress associated with pain, which in turn influences pain intensity and has impact on behavioral responses.

Pain operates at the physiologic level (stimulation of nociceptors, biochemical processes, inhibitory and excitatory pain modulating circuitry), the behavioral level (verbal and physical activity), and the subjective level (thoughts and feelings). Obviously, these levels are not discrete and interact closely with each other. In particular, attitudes and affective states can influence the perception of pain and modify cognitive, emotional, and behavioral responses. At a broader level, individual differences in personality, past experiences, and cultural background affect the experience of pain by influencing beliefs and emotions. Ongoing pain often disrupts normal activities and heightens anxiety and depression. In turn, these psychological disturbances increase the likelihood of pain becoming chronic.

A detailed review of studies investigating the complex relationship between psychological factors and pain is beyond the scope of this chapter. Instead, we have used recently published research to illustrate important aspects of this relationship.

INDIVIDUAL DIFFERENCES

Although cultural and ethnic differences in the response to pain have been recognized for some time, the influence of cultural variables on the experience of chronic pain has only recently been a focus of research attention. In a major study on this subject, Bates et al. (7) investigated 372 patients from six ethnic backgrounds ("Old American," Hispanic, Irish, Italian, French Canadian, and Polish) who presented for treatment of chronic pain in Worcester, Massachusetts. Both the sensory and affective ratings from the McGill Pain Questionnaire differed among groups, with highest scores in Hispanics and Italians. Consistent with this finding, Hispanics and Italians reported that pain interfered more with work and daily activities and caused more distress than people from other ethnic groups. In addition, individual variation in pain scores was influenced by cultural background; within the Hispanic, Italian, and French Canadian groups, patients with an external locus of control gave higher pain ratings than patients with an internal locus of control. These findings suggest that culturally acquired beliefs about pain influence both the style of describing pain and the behavioral response to pain. These beliefs also may affect the perception of pain by influencing the patient's attentional focus and emotional responses; for example, it may be difficult to ignore pain in cultures that encourage an outward emotional expression of pain (7).

Cultural background is thought to affect the treatment of pain by influencing how well medical staff are able to recognize patients' suffering. In addition, patients from certain ethnic groups may seek earlier or more intensive treatment because of their culturally acquired beliefs. To investigate these possibilities, Ng et al. (29) examined the amount of prescribed and self-administered narcotic medication in people from various ethnic backgrounds who were treated with patient-controlled analgesia for postoperative pain. Hispanics were prescribed less narcotic medication in terms of the bolus size and the lockout period before another narcotic bolus could be admin-

P. D. Drummond: Department of Psychology, Murdoch University, Perth, Western Australia 6150, Australia.

K. A. Holroyd: Department of Psychology, Ohio University, Athens, Ohio 45701-2979.

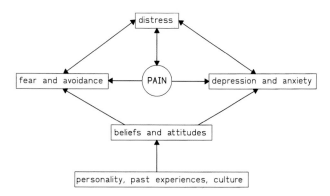

FIG. 1. Psychological factors that may influence the perception of pain. Cultural values, personality traits, and previous experiences (learning history) influence beliefs and attitudes, which in turn may influence levels of anxiety and depression. These negative moods amplify emotional distress, increase the perception of pain, and heighten fear and avoidance of pain-related activities. Conversely, beliefs and attitudes that promote positive coping strategies minimize avoidance of pain-related activities, negative moods, emotional distress, and pain.

istered than were white or black Americans, even after factors such as age, gender, site of surgery, and history of preoperative narcotic use were controlled statistically. In contrast, the amount of self-administered narcotic medication did not differ among the various ethnic groups, indicating that adequate analgesia was achieved with similar doses of medication in the different groups. In sum, these findings suggest that cultural factors influence prescribing practices to a greater extent than the amount of medication required for adequate postoperative analgesia.

Personality traits such as introversion and neuroticism appear to influence the response to transient pain. An early study by Lynn and Eysenck (23) established that neurotic, introverted patients suffered in silence, whereas extroverted patients were more likely to express their pain. Extroverts may be able to attenuate noxious sensory input more easily than introverts, who appear to have a greater physiologic sensitivity than extroverts to any sensory input.

Whether personality traits such as introversion and neuroticism increase the likelihood of pain becoming chronic is controversial; however, the severity of psychological disturbances in chronic pain patients appears to be influenced by preexisting personality traits. For example, a 2-year prospective investigation of psychological variables in patients with whiplash injury indicated that levels of extroversion and neuroticism were similar in patients who recovered fully and those who went on to develop chronic neck pain and headaches (31); however, symptomatic patients reported more persistent distress, with increased nervousness, social withdrawal and aggressiveness, and decreased well-being. BenDebba et al. (8) recently investigated personality factors in relation

to pain and symptoms of psychological distress in a large group of patients who were referred to orthopedic specialists or neurosurgeons for diagnosis and treatment of persistent low-back pain. They identified a modest association between neuroticism and the severity of pain at the outset and at 1 and 2 years' follow-up; they also identified a strong relationship between neuroticism and a general measure of psychological distress at each time point. It seems reasonable to conclude that personality traits influence the severity of pain in some chronic pain conditions, and generally influence the extent of psychological distress.

Individuals with similar pain problems may nonetheless have quite dissimilar ideas about what influences the onset and course of their pain. Those with an internal locus of control hold the belief that the variables that influence their pain are potentially within their control (e.g., dietary triggers or self-imposed work pressure), whereas individuals with an external locus of control believe that these variables are outside their control, that the onset and course of their pain is determined by chance or fate (e.g., hormonal fluctuations, inherited vulnerability) or by the actions of health professionals. Also, some individuals perceive themselves as capable of taking actions necessary to affect the onset and course of pain (e.g., successfully avoiding pain triggers or more effectively managing work stress); that is, they believe themselves to be efficacious in their efforts to influence their pain, whereas others believe they are incapable of influencing the onset and course of their pain. Social learning theory postulates that these loci of control and self-efficacy beliefs play a central role in shaping not only the individual's experience of pain, but also psychological and biological responses to pain (4).

ATTENTION AND ANXIETY

Like any other sensation, the perception of pain depends largely on the focus of attention. Many laboratory studies have confirmed that distraction increases pain threshold and tolerance (24), although distraction may be more effective for mild than intense pain. In fact, focusing on the sensations of pain might reduce emotional reactions to intensely painful stimuli, and may thus be more effective than distraction for reducing distress (24). In general, the effect of distraction on perception of pain is likely to be influenced by many factors, including stimulus predictability and duration, the possibility of harmful consequences, the extent of control over the painful stimulus, and the situational context.

Laboratory studies have uncovered an interesting interaction between short-term anxiety and pain (Fig. 2). If anxiety directs attention toward painful stimulation, pain responses generally increase. Pain-related anxiety (e.g., dental fears) may focus attention on pain and thus increase pain responses. Thus, generally anxious subjects

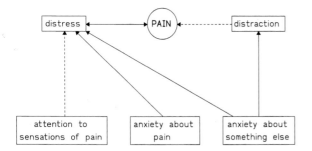

FIG. 2. Interaction between anxiety and pain sensitivity. An increase in anxiety about pain increases emotional distress and painful sensations; conversely, focusing attention on the sensory features of pain reduces distress (*dotted line*) and pain. Anxiety about something other than pain could act as a distraction and reduce painful sensations (*dotted line*), or could increase emotional distress and ultimately amplify pain.

may anticipate aversive consequences more readily than less anxious subjects, and may have difficulty diverting their attention away from pain. Conversely, pain-irrelevant anxiety could act as a distraction and reduce pain responses.

To investigate the mechanism of analgesia associated with shifts in attention, Janssen and Arntz (19) administered the opioid antagonist naltrexone or placebo before subjects received mildly painful electrical stimulation. The level of anxiety associated with the distracting stimulus was manipulated by asking subjects to watch an innocuous video or a live spider (people who were frightened of spiders were selected as subjects); in addition, the subjects were asked to attend to or ignore the electrical stimulus. Pain ratings were lower when subjects ignored than when they attended to the painful stimulus. Pain ratings were also lower in high- than low-anxiety conditions, possibly because of the distracting effect of anxiety. Whether opiate receptors mediate the analgesic effect of distraction is uncertain because a low dose of naltrexone inhibited analgesia, whereas a higher dose did not.

Release of endogenous opioids during acute psychological stress inhibits sensations of pain. Paradoxically, however, increases in physiological activity during stress may enhance sensitivity to pain during subsequent pain induction. For example, Caceres and Burns (10) identified an association between cardiovascular reactivity during stressful mental arithmetic and decreased pain thresholds and tolerance during subsequent pain induction; interestingly, this association did not hold when pain induction preceded the stressful task, suggesting that hyperalgesia developed in response to stress. The mechanism of this hyperalgesic response is uncertain.

Persistent pain often interferes with concentration on other activities. For example, Eccleston et al. (12) reported recently that performance on a cognitive task was impaired in patients with high-intensity pain who

also scored highly on a measure of awareness of diffuse somatic complaints. This subgroup of patients were also more anxious and depressed than other patients. Thus, a hypervigilance toward pain cues might interfere with concentration on other activities and contribute to psychological distress. In addition, a tendency to fear pain and avoid pain-related activities could compromise treatment in some patients (2).

MOOD DISTURBANCES

There is a high rate of depression in chronic pain patients. Depression is often associated with increased reports of pain and disability, decreased activity levels, a poor pain prognosis, and premature termination of treatment. Predictors of depression include age, gender, educational level, marital status, work status, and involvement in litigation. For example, Averill et al. (3) recently reported that depression in chronic pain patients was high in younger women and older men and was associated with a lower educational level, being unmarried, being employed but planning litigation, or being unemployed but not planning litigation.

Prospective studies have confirmed an association between undesirable daily events, mood disturbances, and pain intensity in patients with chronic pain syndromes. For example, in rheumatoid arthritis patients with active signs of inflammation, joint pain increased on the day of and the day after undesirable events (1). Similarly, pain intensity was associated with mood disturbances in 57 chronic pain patients who rated their pain intensity, mood, and activity level eight times per day over 6 consecutive days (34). These findings suggest that pain contributes to mood disturbances but, additionally, that mood disturbances also impact on pain. Regardless of the direction of causality, mood disturbances such as depression are an important component of chronic pain syndromes and often require medical or psychological treatment in their own right.

The development of chronic pain after an accident is sometimes complicated by symptoms of posttraumatic stress disorder. Pain, psychological distress, and functional disability are often elevated in such cases. For example, Geisser et al. (16) investigated affective distress, disability, and symptoms of posttraumatic stress disorder in 241 patients who presented for treatment of chronic pain. Patients with pain resulting from an accident who reported significant symptoms of posttraumatic stress disorder also reported more anxiety, depression, pain, and functional disturbances than patients with fewer symptoms of posttraumatic stress disorder and those whose pain had not started after an accident. Similarly, Difede et al. (11) noted a close relationship between general distress and pain levels in burn victims; in addition, symptoms of posttraumatic stress disorder involving avoidance were associated with elevated pain reports in female patients.

COPING WITH PAIN

The perception that one's pain problems are potentially within the individual's control and the perception that one can take actions to influence pain have been associated with adaptive psychological responses to pain in experimental and clinical situations (17,22,26). For example, at comparable levels of headache activity, individuals who perceive their headaches as having an internal locus of control use less medication and report less affective distress (anxiety, depression, and somatic complaints) than individuals who perceive their headaches as having primarily an external locus of control (28). The perception that one is capable of taking action to influence headaches is similarly associated with lower levels of affective distress and less reliance on passive methods of coping with their headaches (27). Psychological adaptation to headaches thus appears to be determined by the individual's beliefs about their ability to influence the onset and course of headaches, as well as by the frequency and severity of headaches themselves. This suggests that physician–patient interactions might do well to encourage the development of a sense of personal efficacy in patients, with efforts to enhance self-efficacy becoming an integral part of the therapeutic contact.

Self-efficacy beliefs have been associated not only with adaptive psychological responses to pain, but also with important psychophysiologic responses. Stress-induced analgesia (SIA) is an adaptive, endogenous, opioid-mediated analgesic response evoked by pain or other acute stress (13). In an elegant series of experiments, Maier and colleagues (25) demonstrated that painful electric shock fails to evoke SIA in animals who can exert control over the shock, but the identical (uncontrollable) shocks administered to yoked control animals do evoke this opioid-mediated analgesic response. It is thus not pain per se that triggers SIA, but only pain that is experienced as uncontrollable. Similarly, difficult cognitive tasks fail to evoke SIA in humans if the pace of work is controlled by the subject; however, the same cognitive tasks evoke SIA when the pace of work cannot be controlled (5). Whether or not pain evokes SIA may depend on the individual's perceived self-efficacy. Thus, an intervention that enhances perceived self-efficacy enables subjects to cope with cold pressor pain without mobilizing SIA, whereas an intervention that lowers perceived self-efficacy makes mobilization of SIA likely (5). The finding that effective cognitive coping skills enable subjects to tolerate experimental pain even under opiate blockade provides additional evidence that perceived coping efficacy enables individuals to cope with pain without mobilizing emergency opioid pain modulation systems (6,9). On the basis of these findings, we might speculate that individuals who perceive themselves as incapable of coping successfully with their headaches would repeatedly mobilize emergency pain control systems during headache episodes, possibly eventually exhausting this pain control system; in contrast, individuals who are confident in their coping abilities would be less likely to mobilize these pain control systems, and thus better retain endogenous pain modulation capabilities. This admittedly speculative hypothesis offers a biologic link whereby perceived coping inefficacy might contribute to the development of chronic headache disorders.

Patients who catastrophize about their pain and believe that the severity of pain is largely out of their hands understandably report high levels of psychological distress (20), and this psychological distress may be what triggers the SIA response (13). In a recent study of patients attending a pain management center, patients who were using passive coping strategies (e.g., hoping and praying or catastrophizing) reported higher levels of depression, lower levels of activity, and more general distress than patients who were using active coping strategies (e.g., doing or thinking about something else to divert attention away from the pain) (32). Cognitive behavioral treatments that explicitly or implicitly attempt to enhance coping effectiveness also decrease levels of psychological distress and disability in chronic pain syndromes, including headache (33). Biofeedback training also produces reductions in pain largely by altering the locus of control and self-efficacy beliefs rather than by directly altering the physiologic responses that are the focus of training (see Chapter 84). Finally, placebos, which by definition control pain through psychological mechanisms, may reduce pain by enhancing self-efficacy beliefs, at least under some conditions: perceived self-efficacy to endure pain thus predicted pain tolerance following placebo administration in one study ($r = 0.61$) (6). Placebo-induced analgesia appears to be context dependent, involving opioid-mediated analgesia under some conditions and nonopioid mechanisms under other conditions; thus, no single psychological or biological mechanism seems to account for placebo effects observed in all contexts (13,14). Nonetheless, the expectation that one will be able to control or tolerate pain appears to have important psychological and physiologic consequences (13,21).

Like every other human behavior, learning processes underlie psychological and behavioral responses to chronic pain (15). Pain-related behavior is reinforced not only by the patient's own way of coping with pain (e.g., to decrease activity), but also by the social environment (e.g., responsibilities are taken over). Furthermore, pain expression and tolerance may be influenced by observing the reaction of others. Operant treatment procedures are promising methods of counteracting such operantly conditioned behavioral problems.

CONCLUSIONS

The studies discussed here illustrate some of the ways that psychological factors can influence the perceptions of acute pain and maintain or exacerbate chronic pain.

Many of these psychological influences and outcomes are familiar to clinicians treating patients for complaints of headache. For example, psychological distress is clearly related to the frequency and chronicity of headaches (30). Furthermore, pain management techniques that promote a sense of control over headache activity are of proven benefit (18). Like other pain syndromes, the interaction between psychological factors and the perception of headache intensity is a two-way process. Emotional responses that focus attention on headache are likely to amplify painful sensations; conversely, psychological techniques such as meditation and relaxation aim to shift sensations of head pain out of conscious awareness. Addressing personality traits, cultural values, and psychological disturbances that modulate each patient's response to headache should increase the therapeutic benefits flowing from psychologically oriented pain management programs.

Maladaptive pain reactions can be learned, reinforced, and modified. Problems such as noncompliance with treatment or drug dependence often stem from anxiety, depression, or incorrect assumptions by the patient. Careful exploration of the patient's psychological and social situation, and appropriate psychological intervention, is sometimes more useful than prescribing drugs for complaints of pain.

REFERENCES

1. Affleck G, Tennen H, Urrows S, Higgins P. Person and contextual features of daily stress reactivity: individual differences in relations of undesirable daily events with mood disturbance and chronic pain intensity. *J Pers Soc Psychol* 1994;66:329–340.
2. Asmundson GJG, Norton GR, Allerdings MD. Fear and avoidance in dysfunctional chronic back pain patients. *Pain* 1997;69:231–236.
3. Averill PM, Novy DM, Nelson DV, Berry LA. Correlates of depression in chronic pain patients: a comprehensive examination. *Pain* 1996;65:93–100.
4. Bandura A. *Self-efficacy: the exercise of control.* New York: WH Freeman, 1997.
5. Bandura A, Cioffi D, Taylor CB, Brouillard ME. Perceived self-efficacy in coping with cognitive stressors and opioid activation. *J Pers Soc Psychol* 1988;55:479–488.
6. Bandura A, O'Leary A, Taylor CB, Gauthier J, Gossard D. Perceived self-efficacy and pain control: opioid and nonopioid mechanisms. *J Pers Soc Psychol* 1987;53:563–571.
7. Bates MS, Edwards WT, Anderson KO. Ethnocultural influences on variation in chronic pain perception. *Pain* 1993;52:101–112.
8. BenDebba M, Torgerson WS, Long DM. Personality traits, pain duration and severity, functional impairment, and psychological distress in patients with persistent low back pain. *Pain* 1997;72:115–125.
9. Bruehl S, Carlson CC, Wilson JF, et al. Psychological coping with acute pain: an examination of the role of endogenous opioid mechanisms. *J Behav Med* 1996;19:129–142.
10. Caceres C, Burns JW. Cardiovascular reactivity to psychological stress may enhance subsequent pain sensitivity. *Pain* 1997;69:237–244.
11. Difede J, Jaffe AB, Musngi G, Perry S, Yurt R. Determinants of pain expression in hospitalized burn patients. *Pain* 1997;72:245–251.
12. Eccleston C, Crombez G, Aldrich S, Stannard C. Attention and somatic awareness in chronic pain. *Pain* 1997;72:209–215.
13. Fields HL. Pain modulation and headache. In: Goadsby PJ, Silberstein SD, eds. *Headache.* Boston: Butterworth-Heinemann, 1997:39–58.
14. Fields HL, Price DD. Toward a neurobiology of placebo analgesia. In: Harrington A, ed. *The placebo effect: an interdisciplinary exploration.* Cambridge, MA: Harvard University Press, 1997:93–116.
15. Fordyce WE. Pain and suffering: a reappraisal. *Am Psychol* 1988;43:276–283.
16. Geisser ME, Roth RS, Bachman JE, Eckert TA. The relationship between symptoms of posttraumatic stress disorder and pain, affective disturbance and disability among patients with accident and non-accident related pain. *Pain* 1996;66:207–214.
17. Holman H, Lorig K. Perceived self-efficacy in self-management of chronic disease. In: Schwarzer R, ed. *Self-efficacy: thought control of action.* Washington, DC: Hemisphere, 1992.
18. Holroyd KA, Penzien DB. Pharmacological versus non-pharmacological prophylaxis of recurrent migraine headache: a meta-analytic review of clinical trials. *Pain* 1990;42:1–13.
19. Janssen SA, Arntz A. Anxiety and pain: attentional and endorphinergic influences. *Pain* 1996;66:145–150.
20. Jensen MP, Turner JA, Romano JM, Karoly P. Coping with chronic pain: a critical review of the literature. *Pain* 1991;47:249–283.
21. Kirsch I. Specifying nonspecifics: psychological mechanisms of placebo effects. In: Harrington A, ed. *The placebo effect: an interdisciplinary exploration.* Cambridge, MA: Harvard University Press, 1997:166–186.
22. Litt MD. Self-efficacy and perceived control: cognitive mediators of pain tolerance. *J Pers Soc Psychol* 1988;54:149–160.
23. Lynn R, Eysenck JH. Tolerance for pain, extraversion and neuroticism. *Percept Mot Skills* 1961;12:161–162.
24. McCaul KD, Malott JM. Distraction and coping with pain. *Psychol Bull* 1984;95:516–533.
25. Maier SF. Stressor controllability and stress-induced analgesia. *Annals of the New York Academy of Sciences* 1986;467:55–72.
26. Manning MM, Wright TL. Self-efficacy expectancies, outcome expectancies, and the persistence of pain control in childbirth. *J Pers Soc Psychol* 1983;45:421–431.
27. Martin N, Holroyd K, Rokiki L. The headache self-efficacy scale: adaptation to recurrent headaches. *Headache* 1993;33:244–248.
28. Martin NJ, Holroyd KA, Penzien DB. The headache-specific locus of control scale: adaptation to recurrent headaches. *Headache* 1990;30:729–734.
29. Ng B, Dimsdale JE, Rollnik JD, Shapiro H. The effect of ethnicity on prescriptions for patient-controlled analgesia for post-operative pain. *Pain* 1996;66:9–12.
30. Philips HC, Jahanashahi M. The effects of persistent pain: the chronic headache sufferer. *Pain* 1985;21:163–176.
31. Radanov BP, Begre S, Sturzenegger M, Augustiny KF. Course of psychological variables in whiplash injury—a 2-year follow-up with age, gender and education pair-matched patients. *Pain* 1996;64:429–434.
32. Snow-Turek AL, Norris MP, Tan G. Active and passive coping strategies in chronic pain patients. *Pain* 1996;64:455–462.
33. TerKuile MM, Spinhoven P, Linssen ACG, van Houwelingen HC. Cognitive coping and appraisal processes in the treatment of chronic headaches. *Pain* 1995;74:257–264.
34. Vendrig AA, Lousberg R. Within-person relationships among pain intensity, mood and physical activity in chronic pain: a naturalistic approach. *Pain* 1997;73:71–76.

The Headaches, Second Edition,
edited by J. Olesen, P. Tfelt-Hansen, and K.M.A. Welch.
Lippincott Williams & Wilkins, Philadelphia © 2000.

The Migraines

CHAPTER 27

The Migraines: Introduction

Jes Olesen

Migraine is an important and fascinating disorder. The importance is due to its high prevalence and disabling severity. The total sum of suffering caused by migraine is probably higher than that of any other kind of headache. The fascination stems from its rich and varied symptomatology, which, especially in migraine with aura, is a window into certain aspects of the function of the human brain. Furthermore, after many years during which migraine mechanisms seemed elusive, the understanding of this disease is now rapidly increasing, and a coherent model of its mechanisms has been proposed (see Chapter 33). The neurobiological nature of migraine can no longer be doubted.

Migraine was not clearly defined or classified until 1988 (6), and its subforms have only in recent years been studied individually. The greater part of our knowledge about migraine therefore still originates from studies in which patients suffering from migraine without aura (MO) and migraine with aura (MA) (previously common and classic migraine) were mixed. Consequently it is still not possible to cover the epidemiology, pathophysiology, clinical picture, treatment, etc., for migraine without aura and migraine with aura separately. In this book, we have instead adopted the approach of discussing them together and, whenever solid knowledge was available about each form separately, to specify that. We subsequently discuss the rarer and even more distinct subforms of migraine separately. The international classification of migraine (6) is given in Table 1.

J. Olesen: Department of Neurology, Glostrup Hospital, University of Copenhagen, DK-2600 Glostrup, Copenhagen, Denmark.

INTERRELATIONSHIPS BETWEEN MIGRAINE WITH AND WITHOUT AURA

To what extent are migraines with and without aura interrelated? The great majority of patients who suffer from migraine without aura have never had an attack of migraine with aura. On the other hand, among patients who have attacks of migraine with aura, it is very common to also have attacks of migraine without aura. In population-based studies, having both migraine with and without aura was not more frequent than expected than by chance. However, sufferers of frequent migraine with aura had significantly more frequent attacks of migraine without aura than did the general population (13,14). It is a common clinical observation, though never scientifi-

TABLE 1. *International classification of migraine*

1. Migraine
   1.1 Migraine without aura
   1.2 Migraine with aura
      1.2.1 Migraine with typical aura
      1.2.2 Migraine with prolonged aura
      1.2.3 Familial hemiplegic migraine
      1.2.4 Basilar migraine
      1.2.5 Migraine aura without headache
      1.2.6 Migraine with acute-onset aura
   1.3 Ophthalmoplegic migraine
   1.4 Retinal migraine
   1.5 Childhood periodic syndromes that may be precursors to or associated with migraine
      1.5.1 Benign paroxysmal vertigo of childhood
      1.5.2 Alternating hemiplegia of childhood
   1.6 Complications of migraine
      1.6.1 Status migrainosus
      1.6.2 Migrainous infarction
   1.7 Migrainous disorder not fulfilling above criteria

From Headache Classification Committee (6).

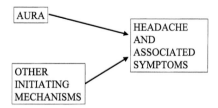

FIG. 1. Different initiating mechanisms and the shared pain mechanisms of migraine with and without aura.

cally documented, that migraine without aura may change into migraine with aura and vice versa. A person may for years suffer exclusively from one form and then later from the other form or from both forms. Migraines with and without aura respond equally well to 5-hydroxytrypt-amine (5-HT$_1$) receptor agonists (see Chapter 52). It is a generally accepted clinical experience that the two forms of migraine also respond equally well to ergot prepara-tions, but this has never been scientifically documented. A methodologically sound and reasonably powerful dou-ble-blind trial of metoprolol in the prophylactic treatment of migraine with aura showed an effect quite similar to the effect in several trials of migraine without aura (9). It thus looks as if the two forms of migraine generally respond to the same treatments. Recent pathophysiologic studies indicate that dilatation of large intra- and extra-cranial arteries occurs in both forms of migraine during an attack but that regional cerebral blood flow changes other than those secondary to pain itself are present only in migraine with aura (see Chapter 35).

Genetic epidermologic studies and twin studies strong-ly suggest that migraines with and without aura are inher-ited differently (Chapter 30). Finally, it was shown that glycerol trinitrate does not provoke an aura but does pro-voke an attack of migraine without aura in patients suf-fering exclusively from migraine with aura. The most rea-sonable interpretation of these interrelationships is that the painful phase and its associated nausea and other symptoms are shared by the two forms of migraine. Migraine with aura is initiated by the cerebral disturbance causing the aura (probably cortical spreading depres-sion), whereas migraine without aura is triggered by other (largely unknown) mechanisms (Fig. 1).

INTERRELATIONSHIPS BETWEEN MIGRAINE AND OTHER HEADACHE SYNDROMES

In the previously used headache classification of the ad hoc committee of the U.S. National Institutes of Health (1), subforms of migraine were not clearly distinguished, and cluster headache was grouped as a subform of migraine. The most extreme version of this tendency to lump separate headache disorders is the so-called contin-uum severity model. It suggests that all headaches form a continuum, with tension-type headache representing the

mildest end of the spectrum, then migraine without aura, migraine with aura, and with cluster headache at the severest end of the spectrum (2,17). In fact, there is no clinically significant overlap between migraine with and without aura (3,4). Furthermore, the former does not rep-resent the severest end of the migraine spectrum because pain and associated symptoms are less pronounced in migraine with aura than in migraine without aura (13,14). The previously mentioned differences in regional cere-bral blood flow between migraine with and without aura contradict the idea of a continuum of headaches, and so do several studies of the genetics of headache (see Chap-ter 30). The great majority of patients with tension-type headache never have migraine, and the great majority of migraine sufferers experience no more tension-type head-ache than the normal population (12,16). Migraine with-out aura and tension-type headache have different sex and age distributions, and they differ with regard to a number of biochemical parameters and platelet abnormalities as discussed elsewhere in this volume. Pericranial muscle tenderness is increased in tension-type headache but not in migraine outside an attack (8). In conclusion, the con-tinuum severity model is an artifact produced by the use of questionnaires, which just compare parts of the symp-tomatology and ignore the differences.

Having dismissed the continuum severity model, it must be acknowledged, however, that patients with fre-quent migraine attacks experience more days with ten-sion-type headache than the normal population and that patients with chronic tension-type headache probably have migrainous episodes more frequently than the nor-mal population. Overlap at the severe end of the spectrum of each disease can, however, be explained by conver-gence of pain-conducting fibers from cranial blood ves-sels and cranial myofascial tissues upon the same neurons in the nucleus of the trigeminal tract in the brainstem and by further convergence upon neurons in the thalamus and higher centers (10) (Fig. 2). A barrage of incoming noci-

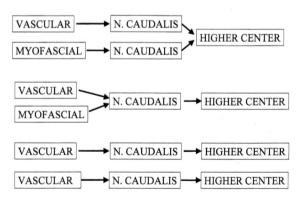

FIG. 2. Partially shared cerebral pain pathways may explain some similarities between migraine and tension-type headache.

ceptive impulses from muscle could, according to this model, assist vascular input in firing neurons. Conversely, increased vascular input in migraineurs may sensitize neurons in the brainstem to incoming impulses from myofascial tissues and thereby increase the likelihood of episodes of tension-type headache. Added to these mechanisms is the propensity of afferent neurons in the brainstem to become sensitized by nociceptor input (see Chapter 15).

In the present book, we adopt the view that migraine with aura and migraine without aura are distinct subforms of migraine that share nociceptive mechanisms and that migraine and tension-type headache are distinct diseases that do not share etiology or peripheral pain mechanisms. Their association is probably caused by partially shared central nervous system afferent pain pathways.

REFERENCES

1. Ad hoc Committee on Classification of Headache. Classification of headache. *JAMA* 1962;179:717–718.
2. Bakal DA, Kaganov JA. Symptom characteristics of chronic and nonchronic headache sufferers. *Headache* 1979;19:285–289.
3. Drummond PD, Lance JW. Clinical diagnosis and computer analysis of headache symptoms. *J Neurol Neurosurg Psychiatry* 1984;47:128–133.
4. Ekbom K. A clinical comparison of cluster headache and migraine. *Acta Neurol Scand* 1970;46[suppl 41]:1–48.
5. Friberg L, Olesen J, Iversen HK, Sperling B. Migraine pain associated with middle cerebral dilatation: reversal by sumatriptan. *Lancet* 1991; 338:13–17.
6. Headache Classification Committee of the International Headache Society. Classification and diagnostic criteria for headache disorders, cranial neuralgias and facial pain. *Cephalalgia* 1988;8[suppl 7]:1–96.
7. Iversen HK, Langemark M, Andersson PG, Hansen PE, Olesen J. Clinical characteristics of migraine and episodic tension-type headache in relation to old and new diagnostic criteria. *Headache* 1990;30:514–519.
8. Jensen R, Rasmussen BK, Pedersen B, Olesen J. Cephalic muscle tenderness and pressure pain threshold in headache. A population study. *Pain* 1993;52:193–199.
9. Kangasniemi P, Andersen AR, Andersson PG. Classic migraine: effective prophylaxis with metoprolol. *Cephalalgia* 1987;7:231–238.
10. Olesen J. Clinical and pathophysiological observations in migraine and tension-type headache explained by integration of vascular, supraspinal and myofascial inputs. *Pain* 1991;46:125–132.
11. Olesen J, ed. *Migraine and other headaches: the vascular mechanisms.* New York: Raven, 1991.
12. Rasmussen BK, Jensen R, Schroll M, Olesen J. Interrelations between migraine and tension-type headache in the general population. *Arch Neurol* 1992;49:914–918.
13. Rasmussen BK, Olesen J. Migraine with aura and migraine without aura. An epidemiological study. *Cephalalgia* 1992;12:221–228.
14. Russell MB, Rasmussen BK, Fenger K, Olesen J. Migraine without aura and migraine with aura are distinct clinical entities: a study of 484 male and female migraineurs from the general population. *Cephalalgia* 1996;16:239–245.
15. Subcutaneous Sumatriptan International Study Group. Treatment of migraine attacks with sumatriptan. *N Engl J Med* 1991;325:316–321.
16. Ulrich V, Russell MB, Jensen R, Olesen J. A comparison of tension-type headache in migraineurs and non-migraineurs: a population based study. *Pain* 1996;67:501–506.
17. Waters WE. The epidemiological enigma of migraine. *Int J Epidemiol* 1973;2:189–194.

The Headaches, Second Edition,
edited by J. Olesen, P. Tfelt-Hansen, and K.M.A. Welch.
Lippincott Williams & Wilkins, Philadelphia © 2000.

The Migraines

CHAPTER 28

Epidemiology of Migraine

Birthe Krogh Rasmussen and Walter F. Stewart

The public health significance of migraine is often overlooked, probably because of its episodic nature and the lack of mortality attributed to the disorder. Migraine is, however, often incapacitating, with considerable impact on social activities and work, and may lead to significant consumption of drugs.

Most previous knowledge of migraine has been based on studies conducted in selected groups of patients, for example, from hospitals, clinics, or general practitioners. Clinical samples comprise more severe and chronic cases, and referral patterns vary considerably across settings, so results cannot be extrapolated to the general population. Several studies have documented that about half of all migraine sufferers had never consulted a doctor for their headache (15,20,25,26,28,39,59). Such individuals may differ from those who seek medical attention. Patients who attend neurology or migraine clinics are even more highly selected. It is therefore essential to understand the spectrum and heterogeneity of migraine that studies are conducted in representative samples of the general population.

The main problem in any study of the epidemiology of migraine has been that of defining the disease entity because there is no laboratory correlate or other objective marker. Previous classification systems lacked precision, included ambiguous expressions, and were nonoperational, which resulted in vague criteria. With the promulgation of explicit diagnostic criteria for all headache disorders by the Headache Classification Committee of the

International Headache Society (IHS) (17) in 1988, significant advances were made in describing the epidemiology of migraine. In a metaanalysis of population-based prevalence studies, it was reported that the case definition used accounts for most of the variation when comparing prevalence estimates between studies (54). In the past 10 years, numerous studies have used IHS criteria to describe the epidemiology of migraine. The variation among these studies is considerably less than among studies published before 1988.

INCIDENCE OF MIGRAINE

There is a general lack of population-based data on the incidence of migraine. However, two epidemiologic studies have assessed retrospectively (based on the reported age of migraine onset) the incidence of migraine in the United States and Denmark. Stewart et al. conducted a population-based telephone survey of over 10,000 people 12 to 29 years of age in Washington County, Maryland (51). Among the 1,410 respondents defined as migraineurs, the onset of migraine peaked in childhood and adolescence, then declined over time. Incidence peaked earlier for boys than for girls, a result that is confirmed in another American study (7). The overall incidence rates for migraine were 601 per 100,000 female person-years and 222 per 100,000 male person-years.

In a study of a representative sample of 25- to 64-year old Danes with clinically confirmed migraine meeting IHS diagnostic criteria, the age-adjusted annual incidence of migraine was estimated to be 370 per 100,000 person-years—580 per 100,000 person-years in women and 160 per 100,000 person-years in men (37). Incidence rates for subjects less than 30 years of age were comparable in these studies (Table 1).

B. K. Rasmussen: Department of Neurology, Hilleroed Hospital, DK-3400 Hilleroed, Denmark.

W. F. Stewart: Department of Epidemiology, School of Hygiene and Public Health, The Johns Hopkins University, Baltimore, Maryland 21205.

TABLE 1. *Incidence rates for migraine in the United States and Denmark*

	Incidence rate per 1000 person-years	
	Males	Females
United States	2.2	6.0
Denmark	1.8	6.5

Subjects were under 30 years of age.
Data from Stewart et al. (51) and Rasmussen (37).

PREVALENCE OF MIGRAINE

Previous estimates of the prevalence of migraine range from 3% to about 35% (8,27). As well as differences in the definitions employed, differing methodologies are also used, and these may be largely responsible for the variation in prevalence estimates. Some studies are community surveys; others are clinical series or studies of more or less selected populations. Age and sex differences across samples influence the prevalence results. Differing methods of ascertainment of cases also have been used. In population-based screening studies, self-administered headache questionnaires or interviewers without clinical experience have been used extensively. If questionnaires or lay interviews are to be useful tools for diagnosing headache disorders, the validity and reliability of the measurements must be assessed, but this aspect has been ignored in most previous studies. Due to the episodic nature of most of the headaches and the frequent coexistence of different types of headache, skillful validation of the information obtained is necessary to distinguish between relevant and irrelevant information (38).

Because of the episodic nature of headache disorders, it is important to assess the period of time under consideration when studying the prevalence and distribution of the disorders in the population. Different surveys have used different time periods: often 1 year, sometimes 2 years, or a lifetime prevalence. The lifetime prevalence indicates how many subjects who have ever, during any period of their lives, had the particular type of headache. The proportion of subjects with headache in the year immediately preceding the survey may be indicated as 1-year period prevalence. The number of new cases in a year (incidence rate) requires follow-up of a cohort to be established. In several previous clinical and population-based studies the time factor used for defining a case is not stated. All these methodologic difficulties are compounded when evaluating previous studies on the epidemiology of migraine.

The results of several recent prevalence studies from the industrialized part of the world are shown in Table 2. Several recent population-based studies have shown similar prevalence rates (14,18,25,40,46,52,53). Four European studies (18,25,40,46) and four U.S. studies (7,14,33,52,53), all using the operational diagnostic criteria of the IHS (17) have reported congruent prevalence figures for migraine in adults (Table 2). In Denmark, a random sample of 1,000 men and women 25 to 64 years of age was drawn from the National Central Person Registry of all Danish residents. Headaches were classified according to a physician-conducted diagnostic interview and a neurologic examination using the IHS diagnostic criteria. The participation rate was 76%, and information about a further 20% was obtained by telephone interview (40). The survey showed, in agreement with another recent Danish epidemiologic study (46), a lifetime prevalence of migraine of 16%—8% in men and 25% in women, a male:female incidence ratio of 1:3. The 1-year period prevalence of migraine was 10%—6% in men and 15% in women (40). The 1-year period prevalence of migraine without aura (previously called common migraine) was 6%, with a male:female incidence ratio of 1:5. The prevalence of migraine with aura (previously called classic migraine) was 4%, with a male:female incidence ratio of 2:3 (41,42). Sex-related factors seem to be of even more importance in migraine without aura than in migraine with aura.

In France, Henry et al. conducted a national migraine survey using IHS criteria (18). To study a representative sample of the French population with regard to age, gender, occupational category, and place of residence, a quota sampling survey was performed by a national public opinion poll agency in which subjects were asked specific questions about their headaches and associated symptoms. Using a diagnostic algorithm based on the IHS criteria (including borderline migraine cases), the prevalence (previous few years) was 12%—6% among men and 18% among women. These results are quite similar to those of the Danish studies and to those of another French study (25). In a U.S. migraine prevalence study, questionnaires were sent to 15,000 households selected to be representative of the U.S. population. The overall response rate was 63.4%, yielding 20,468 respondents 12 to 80 years of age. The self-administered questionnaires using modified IHS criteria yielded a 1-year period prevalence of migraine of 6% in males and 18% in females (52). These results are consistent with another large U.S. population study (53).

In summary, mutually confirmed prevalence data from recent population-based studies in Denmark (40,46), France (18,25), the United States (52,53), and Canada (14,28), all using the IHS diagnostic criteria, have shown a homogeneous picture regarding migraine prevalence. A reasonable estimate of the 1-year prevalence of migraine in adults is 10% to 12%—6% among men and 15% to 18% among women.

TABLE 2. *Some prevalence studies of migraine in industrialized countries*

Study	Sample source	Study method	Respondents (n)	Age (yr)	Time period prevalence	Migraine		
						Males (%)	Females (%)	All (%)
Breslau et al., 1991, U.S.A. (7)	Health maintenance organization	Lay interview	1,007	21–30	Lifetime	7	16	13
					One-year	3	13	
D'Alessandro et al., 1988, Italy (11)	General population	Interview	1,144	>7	One-year	9	18	16
Edmeads et al., 1993, Canada (14)	General population	Lay telephone interview	2,737	>15	Lifetime	9	23	16
Göbel et al., 1994, Germany (16)	General population	Questionnaire	4,061	>18	Lifetime	22	32	27
Henry et al., 1992, France (18)	General population	Lay interview	4,204	>15	Few year	6	18	12
Linet et al., 1989, U.S.A. (19)	General population	Lay telephone interview	10,169	12–29	One-month	3	7	
Michel et al., 1995, France (25)	General population	Questionnaire	1,003	≥18	Three-month	8	18	13
O'Brien et al., 1994, Canada (28)	General population	Lay telephone interview	2,922	≥18	Lifetime	8	25	17
					One-year	7	22	15
Rasmussen et al., 1991, Denmark (40)	General population	Clinical interview and examination	740	25–64	Lifetime	8	25	16
					One-year	6	15	10
Russell et al., 1995, Denmark (46)	General population	Interview and examination	3,471	40	Lifetime	12	24	18
Stewart et al., 1992, U.S.A. (52)	General population	Questionnaire	20,468	12–80	One-year	6	18	12
Stewart et al., 1996, U.S.A. (53)	General population	Lay telephone interview	12,328	18–65	One-year	8	19	

GEOGRAPHIC DIFFERENCES AND RACE

Recent prevalence studies from Africa and Asia exhibit a somewhat consistent picture. In general, studies in these continents that have used IHS criteria show a considerably lower prevalence of migraine in both women and men than studies in Western countries. Specifically, some surveys of migraine prevalence in Africa have yielded results fairly similar to those reported in the Western literature (4,21,29,31,47), whereas others have confirmed generally lower prevalence figures (1,55,61,62). Migraine has been estimated to affect 1.5% of people in Hong Kong (61), 2.6% in Saudi Arabia (1), and 3% in Ethiopia (55). Prevalence rates in Japan and Malaysia are nearer to those found in Western countries, with rates of 8.4% and 9.0%. respectively (4,47). Cross-cultural differences might reflect differences in diagnostic criteria and field methods; they might also reflect real differences in constitutional factors or risk factors. Two studies in the United States have reported equal rates of migraine in blacks and whites (7,23). However, one study found a lower migraine prevalence in black men than in white men, but no racial difference in women (52). In this study, black men reported less frequent disability from their severe headaches than did white men, which may reflect a culturally determined difference in illness behavior. To investigate the basis of these international variations in migraine prevalence, Stewart et al. (53) compared the prevalence of migraine among whites, African Americans and Asian Americans living in the United States. Migraine prevalence was significantly higher in whites (20.4%) than in African Americans (16.2%) or Asian Americans (9.2%). However, migraine was common in all races in this study. These data suggest that cultural or environmental differences may contribute to international differences in migraine prevalence, but race-related differences in genetic vulnerability to migraine may be important.

FREQUENCY OF MIGRAINE

The frequency of migraine, that is, the average number of days with migraine (or number of attacks) per year. Studies in general populations agree that many migraineurs have fewer than one attack per month (19,27,28,33,40,53), but in clinical samples the frequency is somewhat higher (22,48). This would be expected because high frequency is a compelling reason for referral. In a nonselected sample, 62% of subjects with migraine in the previous year had it on fewer than 8 days per year, 24% had it on 8 to 14 days a year, and 14% had migraine on more than 14 days a year (40) (Fig. 1). The percentage with frequent migraine is probably a minimum value because 7% of the migraineurs received prophylactic treatment (39). In a clinic population, 68% of the patients had less than four attacks a month and 32% had more than 4 attacks a month (48).

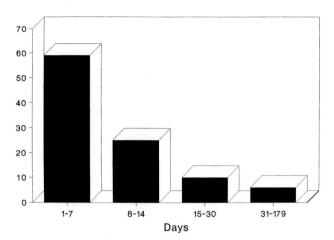

FIG. 1. Number of days with migraine in the previous year. Data from the Danish population study of Rasmussen et al. (40).

SEX AND AGE DISTRIBUTION

Migraine has been found consistently to be more prevalent in women than in men, with a male:female ratio of about 1:2 to 1:3 (7,8,24,32,48,52,53,58,60,64). In the past, it has been suggested that the female preponderance might be due to a more frequent use of medical services by women (30). This hypothesis has been disproven by studies of community samples in which the female preponderance is clearly established (see Table 2). In schoolchildren, the prevalence of migraine increases steadily with age (3,6), and a reversal of the sex distribution in favor of female preponderance occurs at about the age of 12 (3,6). The reason for the preponderance in women is still unexplained, but increasing incidence around the time of menarche, menstrual precipitation, and improvement during pregnancy and at the age of menopause suggest some relationship to female hormones.

The prevalence of migraine increases with age until peak prevalence is reached during the fourth or fifth decade of life and decreases with increasing age thereafter (6,27,33,49,52) (Fig. 2). The prevalence appears to remain higher in women than in men, even after the age of menopause (18,52). Data on age of onset contribute to the explanation of the observed lower prevalence, with advancing age showing that onset of migraine is low after middle age, adding few new cases to the headache pool. The most common age at onset of migraine is in the second and third decades of life (6,27,36,37,51). Migraine may be self-limiting, resulting in decreasing prevalence with increasing age, but whether the incidence differs in different age cohorts due to exposure to different risk factors cannot be assessed from these studies. Distinguishing a real effect of aging from cohort or period effects requires longitudinal follow-up studies.

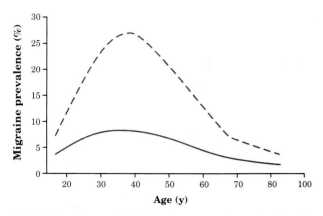

FIG. 2. Prevalence of migraine by age and gender (females, broken line; males, solid line). Data from the U.S. migraine study of Stewart et al. (52).

SOCIODEMOGRAPHIC FACTORS

A number of demographic factors besides sex and age have been explored in relation to migraine. The social distribution of migraine has long been a subject of speculation. A long-held hypothesis that migraine is more common in persons with higher intelligence and in persons with professional backgrounds has been based on experience with clinic patients, but data from samples of the general population do not support this view. Population studies do not reveal increased prevalence in the more privileged or educated (6,11,13,27,33,35,37). Indeed, recent studies from the United States have reported increased risk for migraine in less-educated (7,50) or lower-income groups (50,52). Waters (57), reporting on the Pontypridd epidemiologic survey, found no evidence that individuals with migraine were more intelligent or of higher social class. However, Waters did find that the more intelligent migraine sufferers and those in the higher social classes were more likely to consult a doctor. Likewise Lipton et al. (20) found in a population-based study a significantly higher prevalence of physician-diagnosed migraine in high-income groups compared with low-income groups and concluded that low income may be a barrier to diagnosis and treatment. The social difference in consultation behavior, where the privileged are most likely to seek help, may explain previous claims (based on clinical samples) that migraine was more common among the highly educated.

MIGRAINE WITH AURA AND MIGRAINE WITHOUT AURA

Despite the IHS criteria (17) being used increasingly in recent epidemiologic studies, few studies have described the migraine subforms. Previous studies that have estimated the specific prevalences of migraine with aura (classic migraine) and migraine without aura (common migraine) agree that the prevalence of migraine with aura is lower than that of migraine without aura. Inaccuracy in the diagnosis of aura symptoms may be an important problem. The aura symptoms may be extremely difficult to describe. The difficulties in diagnosing aura symptoms by means of a questionnaire and in a headache diary also have been described (38,43,44).

Prevalence studies of migraine with aura in the United States and Western Europe are shown in Table 3. In a study of an unselected Finnish population, the 1-year prevalence of migraine with aura was 5.5% (2% in men and 8% in women) (27). In a study of a representative sample of the general population in Denmark, the 1-year prevalence of migraine with aura was 4% (3% in men and 5% in women) (41,42). In a study of young adults (27- to 28-year-olds) in Zurich, a 1-year prevalence of 4.6% was reported (24). In a U.S. study of young adults (21- to 30-year-olds), a 1-year prevalence of 1.3% in men and 6.0% in women was found (7). In a Jerusalem population sample the prevalence of migraine with aura was 2.1% (2). Levy (21) reported in a study of 5,028 individuals in Zimbabwe that none had features of classical migraine, whereas Ogunyemi (29) found in a study among Nigerian University students that migraine with aura occurred in 5.1% of the female students and 3.4% of the male students.

The variation in prevalence of migraine with aura in previous studies may be real or due to differences in the

TABLE 3. *Some prevalence studies of migraine with aura in the United States and Western Europe*

Study	Sample source	Respondents (n)	Age	Time period prevalence	Migraine with aura	
					Males (%)	Females (%)
Breslau et al., 1991, U.S.A. (7)	Members of a health maintenance organization	1,007	21–30	Lifetime	3.4	7.4
				One-year	1.3	6.0
D'Alessandro et al., 1988, Italy (11)	General population	1,144	>7	One-year	0.6	0.9
Nikiforow, 1981, Finland (27)	General population	200	>15	One-year	2	8
Philips, 1977, U.K. (32)	General practice	597	16–60	Six-months	0.5	2.5
Rasmussen et al., 1992, Denmark (42)	General population	740	25–64	Lifetime	4	9
				One-year	3	5
Russell et al., 1995, Denmark (46)	General population	3,471	40	Lifetime	4	8

definition used, variation in the method of case ascertainment, and age and sex differences across samples. Based on the most recent studies, a 1-year period prevalence of around 4% seems most likely (Table 3).

In specific studies of migraine without aura, the prevalence varies strikingly from about 2% to more than 15% (8,15,27,32,59). Taking the previously discussed methodologic limitations into account and assuming that the 1-year period prevalence of unspecified migraine is about 10% to 12% and that of migraine with aura presumably 4%, it seems likely that the prevalence of migraine without aura is around 6% to 8%.

Both migraine with and without aura show female preponderance. The overrepresentation of women seems more clear-cut in migraine without aura (9–11,19,42). In men the two major subtypes of migraine have been found to be nearly equally common, whereas in women the prevalence of migraine without aura is clearly higher than that of migraine with aura (7,42). These sex differences may reflect an influence of female hormones, which may be even more important in migraine without aura than in migraine with aura. It has been shown that clinical factors related to female hormones (such as menarche, menstruation, pregnancy, use of oral contraceptives, menopause) are clearly more strongly associated with migraine without aura than in migraine with aura (42,45). The ages at onset of migraine without aura and migraine with aura also differ, and varying risk factor profiles may be identified (37,42,45,51).

COEXISTING MIGRAINE WITH AND WITHOUT AURA

Some clinical studies have found a high percentage of subjects having both migraine with aura and migraine without aura (12,34,63), whereas other studies (both clinical and population based) do not confirm such frequent coexistence (22,42,45,46,48,56). Only a proportion of all migraineurs consult doctors about their headaches (14,15,26,39,59). The clinical impression of frequent cooccurrence may be a result of unrepresentative cases due to selection (Berkson's fallacy) (5). Subjects with more than one disease may be more likely to consult a physician than subjects with only one disease. Thus, spuriously high proportions of subjects with both migraine with aura and migraine without aura may be expected in headache-prone populations. In a Danish study of a representative general population, migraine with and without aura are studied separately (42). In this study it was found that the lifetime prevalence of migraine with aura was 6% and migraine without aura was 9%. Only 1% to 2% of the population had migraine both with and without aura. Among subjects with migraine (with or without aura), 36% had migraine with aura, 55% had migraine without aura, and 9% had both. No significant association of these disorders emerged, that is, coexisting

migraine with aura and migraine without aura is not more common than expected by chance (42). This result has recently been confirmed in another large Danish epidemiologic study (45,46). Besides selection bias in clinical series, several problems of classifying migraine subforms exist and may contribute to explain the apparent overrepresentation of cases of migraine both with and without aura. Early morning attacks of migraine may mimic migraine without aura if the aura phase has occurred during sleep. Thus, migraine present at awakening may wrongly be classified as migraine without aura. Similar problems may arise if the aura emerges from "silent areas" of the brain or if it is unnoticed for one or another reason. Patients with such attacks and who usually have pure attacks of migraine with aura will spuriously be taken to suffer from migraine without aura in addition.

In conclusion, additional descriptive and analytical population-based epidemiologic studies as well as longitudinal follow-up studies are needed to further elucidate the natural history of migraine and its subtypes.

REFERENCES

1. Abduljabbar M, Ogunniyi A, al Balla S, al-Dalaan A. Prevalence of primary headache syndrome in adults in the Qassim region of Saudi Arabia. *Headache* 1996;36:385–388.
2. Abramson JH, Hopp C, Epstein LM. Migraine and non-migrainous headaches. A community survey in Jerusalem. *J Epidemiol Community Health* 1980;34:188–193.
3. Abu-Arefeh I, Russell G. Prevalence of headache and migraine in schoolchildren. *BMJ* 1994;309:765–769.
4. Alders EEA, Hentzen A, Tan CT. A community-based prevalence study on headache in Malaysia. *Headache* 1996;36:379–384.
5. Berkson J. Limitations of the application of fourfold table analysis to hospital data. *Biometrics Bull* 1946;2:47–53.
6. Bille B. Migraine in school children. *Acta Paediatrica* 1962;51[Suppl 136]:1–151.
7. Breslau N, Davis GC, Andreski P. Migraine, psychiatric disorders, and suicide attempts: an epidemiologic study of young adults. *Psychiatry Res* 1991;37:11–23.
8. Brewis M, Poskanzer DC, Rolland C, et al. Neurological disease in an English city. *Acta Neurol Scand* 1966;42[Suppl 24]:1–89.
9. Celentano DD, Stewart WF, Linet MS. The relationship of headache symptoms with severity and duration of attacks. *J Clin Epidemiol* 1990;43:983–994.
10. Crisp AH, Kalucy RS, McGuinness B, Ralph PC, Harris G. Some clinical, social and psychological characteristics of migraine subjects in the general population. *Postgrad Med J* 1977;53:691–697.
11. D'Alessandro R, Benassi G, Lenzi PL, et al. Epidemiology of headache in the Republic of San Marino. *J Neurol Neurosurg Psychiatry* 1988;51:21–27.
12. Davies PTG, Peatfield RC, Steiner TJ, Bond RA, Rose FC. Some clinical comparisons between common and classical migraine: a questionnaire-based study. *Cephalalgia* 1991;11:223–227.
13. Duckro PN, Tait RC, Margolis RB. Prevalence of very severe headache in a large US metropolitan area. *Cephalalgia* 1989;9:199–205.
14. Edmeads J, Findlay H, Tugwell P, Pryse-Phillips W, Nelson RF, Murray TJ. Impact of migraine and tension-type headache on life-style, consulting behaviour, and medication use: a Canadian population survey. *Can J Neurol Sci* 1993;20:131–137.
15. Ekbom K, Ahlborg B, Schèle R. Prevalence of migraine and cluster headache in Swedish men of 18. *Headache* 1978;18:9–19.
16. Göbel H, Petersen-Braun M, Soyka D. The epidemiology of headache in Germany: a nationwide survey of a representative sample on the basis of the headache classification of the International Headache Society. *Cephalalgia* 1994;14:97–106.

17. Headache Classification Committee of the International Headache Society. Classification and diagnostic criteria for headache disorders, cranial neuralgias and facial pain. *Cephalalgia* 1988;8[Suppl 7]:1–96.

18. Henry P, Michel P, Brochet B, et al. A nationwide survey of migraine in France: prevalence and clinical features in adults. *Cephalalgia* 1992; 12:229–237.

19. Linet MS, Stewart WF, Celentano DD, Ziegler D, Sprecher M. An epidemiologic study of headache among adolescents and young adults. *JAMA* 1989;261:2211–2216.

20. Lipton RB, Stewart WF, Celentano DD, Reed ML. Undiagnosed migraine headaches. A comparison of symptom-based and reported physician diagnosis. *Arch Intern Med* 1992;152:1273–1278.

21. Levy LM. An epidemiological study of headache in an urban population in Zimbabwe. *Headache* 1983;23:2–9.

22. Manzoni GC, Farina S, Granella F, Alfieri M, Bisi M. Classic and common migraine. Suggestive clinical evidence of two separate entities. *Funct Neurol* 1986;1:112–122.

23. Markush RE, Herbert RK, Heyman A, O'Fallon WM. Epidemiologic study of migraine symptoms in young women. *Neurology* 1975;25: 430–435.

24. Merikangas KR, Angst J, Isler H. Migraine and psychopathology. *Arch Gen Psychiatry* 1990;47:849–853.

25. Michel P, Pariente P, Duru G, Dreyfuss J-P, Chabriat H, Henry P. Mig access: a population-based, nationwide, comparative survey of access to care in migraine in France. *Cephalalgia* 1996;16:50–55.

26. Newland CA, Illis LS, Robinson PK, Batchelor BG, Waters WE. A survey of headache in an English city. *Res Clin Stud Headache* 1978;5: 1–20.

27. Nikiforow R. Headache in a random sample of 200 persons: a clinical study of a population in Northern Finland. *Cephalalgia* 1981;1: 99–107.

28. O'Brien B, Goeree R, Streiner D. Prevalence of migraine headache in Canada: a population-based survey. *Int J Epidemiol* 1994;23: 1020–1026.

29. Ogunyemi AO. Prevalence of headache among Nigerian university students. *Headache* 1984;24:127–130.

30. Ostfeld AM. The natural history and epidemiology of migraine and muscle contraction headache. *Neurology* 1963;13:11–15.

31. Osuntokun BO, Schoenberg BS, Nottidge V, et al. Migraine headache in a rural community in Nigeria: results of a pilot study. *Neuroepidemiology* 1982;1:31–39.

32. Philips C. Headache in general practice. *Headache* 1977;16:322–329.

33. Pryse-Phillips W, Findlay H, Tugwell P, Edmeads J, Murray TJ, Nelson RF. A Canadian population survey on the clinical, epidemiologic and societal impact of migraine and tension-type headache. *Can J Neurol Sci* 1992;19:333–339.

34. Ranson R, Igarashi H, MacGregor EA, Wilkinson M. The similarities and differences of migraine with aura and migraine without aura: a preliminary study. *Cephalalgia* 1991;11:189–192.

35. Rasmussen BK. Migraine and tension-type headache in a general population: psychosocial factors. *Int J Epidemiol* 1992;21:1138–1143.

36. Rasmussen BK. Migraine and tension-type headache in a general population: precipitating factors, female hormones, sleep pattern and relation to lifestyle. *Pain* 1993;53:65–72.

37. Rasmussen BK. Epidemiology of headache [Thesis]. *Cephalalgia* 1995;15:48–68.

38. Rasmussen BK, Jensen R, Olesen J. Questionnaire versus clinical interview in the diagnosis of headache. *Headache* 1991;31:290–295.

39. Rasmussen BK, Jensen R, Olesen J. Impact of headache on sickness absence and utilisation of medical services. A Danish population study. *J Epidemiol Commun Health* 1992;46:443–446.

40. Rasmussen BK, Jensen R, Schroll M, Olesen J. Epidemiology of headache in a general population—a prevalence study. *J Clin Epidemiol* 1991;44:1147–1157.

41. Rasmussen BK, Jensen R, Schroll M, Olesen J. Interrelations between migraine and tension-type headache in the general population. *Arch Neurol* 1992;49:914–918.

42. Rasmussen BK, Olesen J. Migraine with aura and migraine without aura: an epidemiological study. *Cephalalgia* 1992;12:221–228.

43. Russell MB, Iversen HK, Olesen J. Improved description of the migraine aura by a diagnostic aura diary. *Cephalalgia* 1994;14: 107–117.

44. Russell MB, Rasmussen BK, Brennum J, Iversen HK, Jensen R, Olesen J. Presentation of a new instrument: the diagnostic headache diary. *Cephalalgia* 1992;12:369–374.

45. Russell MB, Rasmussen BK, Olesen J. Migraine without aura and migraine with aura are distinct clinical entities: a study of 484 male and female migraineurs from the general population. *Cephalalgia* 1996; 16:239–245.

46. Russell MB, Rasmussen BK, Thorvaldsen P, Olesen J. Prevalence and sex-ratio of the subtypes of migraine. *Int J Epidemiol* 1995;24: 612–618.

47. Sakai F, Igarashi H. Epidemiology of migraine in Japan: a nationwide survey. *Cephalalgia* 1997;17:15–22.

48. Selby G, Lance WJ. Observations on 500 cases of migraine and allied vascular headache. *J Neurol Neurosurg Psychiatry* 1960;23:23–32.

49. Sillanpää M. Changes in the prevalence of migraine and other headaches during the first seven school years. *Headache* 1983:23: 15–19.

50. Stang PE, Osterhaus JT. Impact of migraine in the United States: data from the National Health Interview Survey. *Headache* 1993;33:29–35.

51. Stewart WF, Linet MS, Celentano DD, Van Natta M, Ziegler D. Age-and sex-specific incidence rates of migraine with and without visual aura. *Am J Epidemiol* 1991;134:1111–1120.

52. Stewart WF, Lipton R, Celentano DD, Reed ML. Prevalence of migraine headache in the United States. *JAMA* 1992;267:64–69.

53. Stewart WF, Lipton RB, Liberman J. Variation in migraine prevalence by race. *Neurology* 1996;47:52–59.

54. Stewart WF, Simon D, Schechter A, Lipton RB. Population variation in migraine prevalence: a meta-analysis. *J Clin Epidemiol* 1995;48: 269–280.

55. Tekle Haimanot R, Seraw B, Forsgren L, Ekbom K, Ekstedt J. Migraine, chronic tension-type headache, and cluster headache in an Ethiopian rural community. *Cephalalgia* 1995;15:482–488.

56. Van den Bergh V, Amery WK, Waelkens J. Trigger factors in migraine: a study conducted by the Belgian Migraine Society. *Headache* 1987;27:191–196.

57. Waters WE. Migraine: intelligence, social class, and familial prevalence. *BMJ* 1971;2:77–81.

58. Waters WE. *The epidemiology of migraine.* Bracknell, Berkshire: Boehringer Ingelheim, Bracknell, 1974.

59. Waters WE, O'Connor PJ. Epidemiology of headache and migraine in women. *J Neurol Neurosurg Psychiatry* 1971;34:148–153.

60. Waters WE, O'Connor PJ. Prevalence of migraine. *J Neurol Neurosurg Psychiatry* 1975;38:613–616.

61. Wong TW, Wong KS, Yu TS, Kay R. Prevalence of migraine and other headaches in Hong Kong. *Neuroepidemiology* 1995;14:82–91.

62. Zhao F, Tsay J-Y, Cheng X-M, et al. Epidemiology of migraine: a survey in 21 provinces of the People's Republic of China, 1985. *Headache* 1988;28:558–565.

63. Ziegler DK, Hassanein RS. Specific headache phenomena: their frequency and coincidence. *Headache* 1990;30:152–156.

64. Ziegler DK, Hassanein RS, Couch JR. Characteristics of life headache histories in a nonclinic population. *Neurology* 1977;27:265–269.

The Headaches, Second Edition,
edited by J. Olesen, P. Tfelt-Hansen, and K.M.A. Welch.
Lippincott Williams & Wilkins, Philadelphia © 2000.

The Migraines

CHAPTER 29

Migraine Comorbidity

Kathleen Ries Merikangas and Birthe Krogh Rasmussen

The term "comorbidity" refers to the coexistence of two conditions within the same individual (19). Failure to classify and analyze comorbid diseases can create misleading medical statistics and may cause spurious comparisons during the planning and evaluation of treatment for patients. Comorbid disorders may alter the clinical course of illness by affecting time of detection, prognostics, treatment, and outcome of illness (26). Possible explanations for comorbidity include (a) shared risk factors; (b) one condition causing the other condition; and (c) random cooccurrence of the two disorders.

Nonrandom cooccurrence of two conditions may be attributable to several methodologic artifacts: samples selected from clinical settings that are nonrepresentative of persons with the index disease in the general population [i.e., Berkson's paradox (1)]; assessment bias, in which the cooccurrence of two conditions is an artifact of overlap in the diagnostic criteria or in the assessments used to ascertain the criteria; and the lack of an appropriate comparison group to control for factors that confound the association between the two conditions.

Aside from identification of bias, investigation of patterns of comorbidity is important for several reasons. First, differential patterns of comorbidity among subtypes of a particular index disorder may indicate a different form of the condition. Second, differential associations between particular pairs of diseases may yield clues regarding the pathogenesis of the index disease. If two conditions emanate from the same underlying etiologic factors, investigations of their etiology can be targeted to risk factors that are common to both conditions. Finally, if the comorbid disorders are a consequence of the index disease, interventions can be developed to prevent the development of the secondary conditions.

Associations between migraine and a variety of somatic and psychiatric conditions have been reported in the literature since it was first described as a discrete syndrome. Because most of the early descriptions of such associations were based on clinical case series, empirical evidence was lacking. Several factors complicate the investigation of comorbidity of migraine and other conditions: discrimination from "migraine equivalents," defined as alternate manifestations of migraine that occur in an attacklike fashion, including abdominal pain, dizziness or vertigo, or visual symptoms; lack of specificity of symptom expression or constellations within individuals over time; and the involvement of several systems in migraine, including the cerebrovascular, gastrointestinal, and sensory systems, as well as the central nervous system.

There is dramatic variability in the methodology of studies of comorbidity and migraine, which limits their conclusiveness. Studies of comorbidity require valid definitions and reliable ascertainment of each of the disorders under consideration. The majority of studies of comorbidity of migraine, which were conducted prior to the introduction of the diagnostic criteria of the International Headache Society (25), used idiosyncratic definitions of migraine ranging from recurrent headaches to classical migraine with neurologic prodromes. Moreover, standardized definitions of both disorders were included in few of the clinical or epidemiologic studies of comorbidity and migraine. In general, clinical series and case-control studies have used the most thorough clinical evaluations of the subjects. In contrast, epidemiologic studies

K.R. Merikangas: Department of Epidemiology and Public Health, Genetic Epidemiology Research Unit, Yale University School of Medicine, New Haven, Connecticut 06510-3223.

B.K. Rasmussen: Department of Neurology, Hilleroed Hospital, DK-3400 Hilleroed, Denmark.

tended to apply less rigorous definitions of the disorders because collection of extensive diagnostic information on both conditions was precluded by the sheer magnitude of the studies.

Epidemiologic studies generally have sufficient statistical power to detect associations between migraine and rare diseases; however, the smaller sample sizes of clinical and case-control studies may prohibit significant findings. The absence of comorbid relationships may be a result of type 2 statistical error due to small sample size rather than a true lack of association between migraine and other diseases. Another methodologic limitation of the majority of studies of migraine comorbidity is the failure to incorporate confounding risk factors, which could explain the association between several diseases and migraine. In addition, the interrelationships between the comorbid disorders themselves are often not established in multivariate analyses, thereby yielding spurious associations. Finally, as noted above, the samples of both the clinical series and case-control studies may be biased with respect to the increased probability that persons with two or more conditions are represented in clinical samples (i.e., Berkson's paradox). Thus, the epidemiologic studies are necessary to identify such biases in clinical samples. Case-control studies and cross-sectional epidemiologic studies mainly generate hypotheses about possible associations, and longitudinal population-based studies are necessary to test the hypotheses and reliably identify comorbidities.

COMORBIDITY OF MIGRAINE AND MEDICAL DISORDERS

Comorbidity of migraine and several other disorders has been reported in clinical series, case-control studies, and epidemiologic surveys. Merikangas and Fenton investigated migraine comorbidity using data from a large-scale epidemiologic study in the U.S. adult population (35). After controlling for confounding factors, sig-

nificant associations were found between migraine and cardiovascular disorders, hypotension, stroke, epilepsy, and gastrointestinal and respiratory disorders (Table 1). The following discussion focuses on associations between migraine and selected somatic conditions for which evidence has been presented in the literature.

Cardio- and Cerebrovascular Disorders

Comorbidity between migraine and cardio- and cerebrovascular conditions, such as hypertension, numerous manifestations of heart disease, and stroke, have been the most widely studied of all classes of somatic conditions. It is likely that the focus on these conditions derives from concern regarding migraine-induced stroke and the role of underlying vascular disease in triggering attacks of migraine.

Hypertension

Nearly all case-control studies examining the association between migraine and hypertension have reported a positive association. Controlled studies of migraine patients have found higher levels of systolic blood pressure (49), as well as overall blood pressure (22). Likewise, an increased risk of migraine has been reported among hypertensives as compared with controls (31). Research also has shown that relatives of migraine patients are more likely to be hypertensive (11). In contrast, the results of community-based surveys that have examined comorbidity between hypertension and migraine have not confirmed an association between hypertension and migraine (10,43–45,50,51).

Heart Disease

Heart diseases including mitral valve prolapse, coronary artery disease, ischemic heart disease, angina, and the arrhythmias also have been associated with migraine.

TABLE 1. *Medical disorders associated with migraine in the NHANES follow-up study*

Disorder	Migraine (%)	No migraine (%)	Odds ratio	95% confidence interval
Allergy	36.1	23.4	1.7	1.5–1.9
Angina	7.5	5.2	2.1	1.6–2.8
Asthma/bronchitis	24.3	15.0	2.0	1.7–2.3
Colitis	8.7	3.4	2.3	1.8–2.9
Epilepsy	1.7	0.7	2.4	1.4–4.1
Heart attack	10.1	9.2	2.2	1.6–2.9
Hypotension	18.6	10.7	1.8	1.5–2.1
Stroke	4.1	3.4	1.6	1.2–2.3
Ulcer	20.6	12.5	2.2	1.9–2.6

Covariates included in models: sex, age, heart condition, history of smoking, diabetes, hypertension, heart murmur, and regular exercise.
Data from Madans et al. (30) and Merikangas and Fenton (35).

The only one of these phenomena that has been studied extensively is mitral valve prolapse. Although there are several negative reports from uncontrolled clinical series, most of these studies lacked sufficient power to test this association adequately. The results of several controlled studies have found a two- to fourfold risk of mitral valve prolapse in young women with migraine compared to those without migraine (21). However, Featherstone (17) did not detect this association in his case-control study of 200 cases of recurrent headache compared with 200 age- and sex-matched controls. Likewise, Chen et al. (10) found that the association between heart attacks and migraine was no longer significant after controlling for smoking. Inconsistent measures of mitral valve prolapse and varying definitions of migraine or recurrent headache across these studies are likely reasons for these inconsistent findings.

Family study findings also have not confirmed a strong relationship between heart disease and migraine in relatives. Although a number of previous studies have suggested comorbid heart attacks within relatives of subjects with migraine (11,20,28), Sternfeld et al. (46) determined that only chest pain, and not myocardial infarction, was related to migraine. Other studies have confirmed no association between migraine and cardiovascular diseases (43). Although there appears to be some comorbidity, the inconsistent methods and findings, as well as the limited number of studies, suggest no strong relationship between heart disease and migraine at this time. The increase in risk for cardiovascular disease may also be due to the independent effects of migraine medications.

Cerebrovascular Disorders

Large-scale community studies in the United States have shown that the risk of stroke is a twofold greater in migraine sufferers than in people without migraine (6,37). In examining this association, it is critical to discriminate between migraine-induced stroke (migrainous infarction) and stroke that occurs among individuals with migraine as well as migraine with onset secondary to stroke. Recent reviews by Featherstone (18) and Welch and Levine (52) discuss the diagnostic criteria for migrainous cerebral infarction. In a study of U.S. male physicians 40 to 84 years of age (6), the risk of stroke was twofold higher in migraine sufferers than in people without migraine. Two recent case-control studies have confirmed an increased stroke risk, particularly in young women with migraine with aura who were currently smoking or using oral contraceptives (7,48). Thus, as reviewed elsewhere in this text, evidence from epidemiologic studies suggests that there is a significant relationship between migraine and stroke.

Epilepsy

A large family study of epilepsy (40) reported that there was a twofold increase in migraine among both epileptic probands and their relatives (29). In contrast to earlier epidemiologic studies (2,14,15), the results indicated a strong association between migraine and epilepsy, which was independent of seizure type (29). It was suggested that the comorbidity of migraine and epilepsy was explained by a state of neuronal hyperexcitability that increases the risk of both disorders. Variability in the definitions and subtypes of epilepsy investigated across studies precludes accurate risk estimation based on aggregate findings. Further studies of this association are clearly indicated.

Respiratory Disorders

The association between migraine and allergic conditions, including food allergies, asthma, hay fever, and bronchitis, has been nearly as widely investigated as that with cardiovascular disorders. Irrespective of the specific type of allergic condition assessed in the studies, an association between the allergic conditions and migraine has been found in most clinical studies of both children and adults.

In his classic case-control study, Bille (2) reported that children with migraine had twice the risk of allergies as those without migraine. These findings were confirmed in the epidemiologic studies of Chen et al. (10) and Chen and Leviton (9), who reported relative risks of 1.9 for asthma and 4.1 for allergies, thereby indicating that this relationship cannot be attributed to sampling bias. The average magnitude of the association between allergic conditions and migraine across studies was approximately 2.4.

Gastrointestinal Disorders

Various gastrointestinal conditions also have been linked with migraine. However, it is difficult to discriminate whether these conditions are truly independent or whether they represent manifestations of the gastrointestinal component of migraine. Several studies have examined the association between gastric ulcers and migraine, with the majority reporting significant evidence for this association. Case-control samples from clinical settings yielded relative risks ranging from 1.9 to 2.5 (17). However, Chen et al. (10) reported that ulcers were only associated with migraine among smokers.

Comorbidity between migraine and other gastrointestinal disorders also has been suggested in nonclinical studies. Greater rates of hiatal hernia, colitis, and abdominal pain have been reported among migraineurs than among controls (17), although the occurrence of gastric ulcers and abdominal pain may be a consequence of using migraine drugs.

Depression and Anxiety

Clinicians involved in the treatment of migraine have often described a set of characteristic features of migraineurs, including anxiety, depression, and social fears. Wolff (53) was so convinced of this constellation of attributes that he is often credited as being the initiator of the concept of the purported "migraine personality." However, more careful inspection of his description reveals that the characteristics of "extreme physical fatigue, apathy, and anxious anticipation" are more akin to psychiatric symptoms than personality traits.

Numerous studies of depression in clinical samples of migraine patients and the converse have been conducted. Associations between the two disorders are consistently found, irrespective of the index disorder for which the subjects sought treatment (12,13,16,27,33,39). The results of studies of community samples are summarized in Table 2 (3,4,32,34,36,38,41,42,47). Rates of depression among subjects with migraine in community studies range from 15% to 60%, depending on the definition of depression used. There is remarkable similarity in the magnitude of the association between depression and migraine across the five studies despite the variation in the subjects' characteristics, geographic sites, and specific assessments of migraine and depression. These findings exclude sampling as a source of bias in the cooccurrence of depression and migraine reported in previous clinical samples.

The relationship between migraine and anxiety disorders also has been investigated because of the well-known association between depression and anxiety. When examined alone, anxiety disorders are also associated with migraine in both clinical and community studies, as shown in Table 2 (3,4,23,24,32,34,36,47). However, the simultaneous association with all of these disorders needs to be examined systematically.

Evidence for an association between migraine and the bipolar subtype of depression is particularly strong. Samples of adults (8) and children (54) in treatment for bipolar disorder, as well as epidemiologic studies (3,34,38), support an even stronger association between migraine and bipolar spectrum disorder (major depression with either manic or hypomanic episodes).

Two epidemiologic studies have studied the order of onset of depression, anxiety, and migraine. The results of a prospective longitudinal cohort study of young adults in Zurich, Switzerland, revealed that the onset of anxiety disorders tended to precede that of migraine in about 80% of the cases of migraine with comorbid anxiety/depression, and that the onset of depression followed that of migraine in three fourths of the comorbid cases (34).

Retrospective data from a community survey in Detroit, Michigan, produced strikingly similar findings. The associations between migraine, anxiety, and depression were not only of the same magnitude, but the order of onset of the three conditions also was the same, with anxiety in childhood and adolescence, followed by migraine, and then depression in adulthood (4). More recent evaluation of the prospective data from the Detroit Area Survey supported a bidirectional influence between migraine and major depression, with each disorder increasing the risk for the first onset of the other (5).

Investigation of comorbidity of migraine and depression/anxiety states in family study data revealed that migraine, anxiety, and depression may result from a partially shared diathesis (32,36). Because disturbances in the same neurochemical systems have been implicated in migraine, depression, and anxiety disorders, perturbation of a particular system or systems may produce symptoms of all three conditions, thereby producing one syndrome rather than three discrete entities. These findings underscore the importance of systematic assessment of depression and anxiety in persons with migraine. If there is a subtype of migraine associated with anxiety and depression, it is critical to treat the entire syndrome rather than limiting the treatment goal to headache cessation.

SUMMARY

The results of this review suggest that several disorders are strongly associated with migraine both in clinical samples and in the community. The strongest associations were observed between migraine and allergies, mitral valve prolapse, hypotension, hypertension, stroke, and depression and anxiety (Table 3). Aggregation of the findings of previous studies was partly precluded by methodologic differences across studies, including a lack of standardized diagnostic definitions of both the index and comorbid

TABLE 2. *Association (odds ratio) between migraine with depression and anxiety: community studies*

Authors	N	Depression	Anxiety
Merikangas et al. (34,36)	591	2.2	2.7
Stewart et al. (47)	10,169	—	5.3
Breslau et al. (3,4)	1,007	3.6	1.9
Moldin et al. (38)	914	2.1	2.1
Merikangas et al. (32)	1,218	3.0	2.8

TABLE 3. *Summary of medical disorders most strongly associated with migraine*

System	Disorders	Evidence
Respiratory	Allergies	+++
	Asthma	++
Cardiovascular	Mitral valve prolapse	++
	Hypotension	++
	Myocardial infarction	+
	Hypertension	++
Psychiatric	Depression, anxiety	+++
Gastrointestinal	Colitis, irritable bowel, ulcers	++
Neurologic	Stroke	+++
	Epilepsy	++

disorder; sampling differences with respect to gender, age, and source of the sample; lack of statistical power to detect associations with rare conditions; and wide variability in the inclusion of confounders in the analyses of the associations. Therefore, future studies need to be designed to specifically investigate patterns and causes of comorbidity of migraine and other diseases using standardized diagnostic definitions with reliable methods of assessment of both the index and comorbid conditions. It is particularly critical to formulate the hypotheses regarding the associations in advance in order to avoid the possibility of false-positive errors due to multiple testing, particularly in large samples. Moreover, specific risk factors for each of the conditions need to be identified carefully and their effect on the association investigated systematically. For example, the relationship between heart disease and migraine may be attributed to the greater propensity for smoking among those with tension-type headaches. Indeed, the identification of purported confounding risk factors may be the most important finding with respect to the nature of nonrandom associations between comorbid disorders. Such extrinsic mechanisms can provide targets of prevention for the development of both conditions or for the secondary disorder as a consequence of the index disease, and ultimately yield knowledge regarding the pathogenesis of these disorders.

REFERENCES

1. Berkson J. Limitation of the application of the 4-fold table analysis to hospital data. *Biometrics* 1946;2:47–53.
2. Bille B. Migraine in school children. *Acta Paediatr Scand* 1962;51:3–151.
3. Breslau N, Davis GC. Migraine, physical health and psychiatric disorder: a prospective epidemiologic study in young adults. *J Psychiatr Res* 1993;27:211–221.
4. Breslau N, Davis GC, Andreski P. Migraine, psychiatric disorders, and suicide attempts: an epidemiologic study of young adults. *Psychiatry Res* 1991;37:11–23.
5. Breslau N, Merikangas K, Bowden CL. Comorbidity of migraine and major affective disorders. *Neurology* 1994;44:17–22.
6. Buring JE, Hebert P, Romero J, et al. Migraine and subsequent risk of stroke in the physicians' health study. *Arch Neurol* 1993;52:129–134.
7. Carolei A, Marini C, De Matteis G. History of migraine and risk of cerebral ischaemia in young adults. National Research Council Study Group on Stroke in the Young. *Lancet* 1996;347:1503–1506.
8. Cassidy WL, Flanagan NB. Clinical observations in manic-depressive disease. *JAMA* 1957;164:1535–1546.
9. Chen TC, Leviton A. Asthma and eczema in children born to women with migraine. *Arch Neurol* 1990;47:1227–1230.
10. Chen TC, Leviton A, Edelstein S, Ellenberg JH. Migraine and other diseases in women of reproductive age. *Arch Neurol* 1987;44:1024–1028.
11. Couch JR, Hassanein RS. Headache as a risk factor in atherosclerosis-related diseases. *Headache* 1989;29:49–54.
12. Couch JR, Ziegler DK, Hassanein RS. Evaluation of the relationship between migraine headache and depression. *Headache* 1975;15:41–50.
13. Crisp AH, Kalucy RS, McGuinness B, Ralph PCG, Harris G. Some clinical, social and psychological characteristics of migraine subjects in the general population. *Postgrad Med J* 1977;53:691–697.
14. Dalsgaard-Nielson AT. Migraene og epilepsi. *Ugeskr Laeger* 1964;126:185–191.
15. Depression Guideline Panel. Clinical practice guideline number 5. *Treatment of major depression.* Rockville, MD: U.S. Department of Health and Human Services, Public Health Service, Agency for Health Care Policy and Research, 1993.
16. Diamond S. Depressive headaches. *Headache* 1964;4:255–259.
17. Featherstone HJ. Medical diagnoses and problems in individuals with recurrent idiopathic headaches. *Headache* 1985;25:136–140.
18. Featherstone HJ. Clinical features of stroke in migraine: a review. *Headache* 1986;26:128–133.
19. Feinstein AR. The pre-therapeutic classification of co-morbidity in chronic disease. *J Chronic Dis* 1970;23:455–468.
20. Galiano L, Matias-Guiu J, Vioque J, Falip R, Martin R, Oltra A. A case-control study of the associated factors with migraine. *Cephalalgia* 1993;13:9.
21. Gamberini G, D'Alessandro R, Labriola E, et al. Further evidence on the association of mitral valve prolapse and migraine. *Headache* 1984;24:39–40.
22. Gardner J, Mountain GE, Hinew EA. The relationship of migraine to hypertension and to hypertensive headaches. *Am J Med Sci* 1940;22:50–53.
23. Garvey MJ, Tollefson GD, Schaffer CB. Migraine headaches and depression. *Am J Psychiatry* 1984;141:986–988.
24. Harper M, Roth M. Temporal lobe epilepsy and the phobic anxiety-depersonalization syndrome. Part I: a comparative study. *Compr Psychiatry* 1962;3:129–151.
25. International Headache Society. Classification and diagnostic criteria for headache disorders, cranial neuralgias, and facial pain. *Cephalalgia* 1988;7:1–96.
26. Kaplan MH, Feinstein AR. The importance of classifying initial co-morbidity in evaluating the outcome of diabetes mellitus. *J Chronic Dis* 1974;27:387–404.
27. Kashiwagi T, McClure JN, Wetzel RD. Headache and psychiatric disorders. *Dis Nervous System* 1972;33:659–663.
28. Leviton A, Malvea B, Graham JR. Vascular diseases, mortality, and migraine in the parents of migraine patients. *Neurology* 1974;24:669–672.
29. Lipton RB, Ottman R, Ehrenberg BL, Hauser WA. Comorbidity of migraine: the connection between migraine and epilepsy. *Neurology* 1994;44:28–32.
30. Madans JH, Cox CS, Kleiman JC, et al. 10 years after the NHANES I: Report of initial follow-up. *Public Health Rep* 1986;101:465–473.
31. Markush RE, Karp HR, Heyman A, O'Fallon WM. Epidemiologic study of migraine symptoms in young women. *Neurology* 1975;25:430–435.
32. Merikangas KR. Sources of genetic complexity of migraine. In: Sandler M, Ferrari M, Harnett S, eds. *Migraine: pharmacology and genetics.* New York: Cambridge University Press, 1996:254–281.
33. Merikangas KR, Angst J. Depression and migraine. In: Sandler M, Collins GM, eds. *Migraine: a spectrum of ideas.* Oxford: Oxford University Press, 1990:248–258.
34. Merikangas KR, Angst J, Isler H. Migraine and psychopathology: results of the Zurich cohort study of young adults. *Arch Gen Psychiatry* 1990;47:849–853.
35. Merikangas KR, Fenton B. Comorbidity of migraine and somatic disorders. In: Olesen J, ed. *Headache classification and epidemiology.* New York: Raven, 1994:301–314.
36. Merikangas KR, Merikangas JR, Angst J. Headache syndromes and psychiatric disorders: association and familial transmission. *J Psychiatr Res* 1993;27:197–210.
37. Merikangas K, Fenton B, Cheng SH, Stolar M, Risch N. Association between migraine and stroke in a large-scale epidemic study of the United States. *Arch Neurol* 1997;54:362–368.
38. Moldin SO, Scheftner WA, Rice JP, Nelson E, Knesevich MA, Akisal H. Association between major depressive disorder and physical illness. *Psychol Med* 1993;23:755–761.
39. Morrison DP, Price WH. The prevalence of psychiatric disorder among female new referrals to a migraine clinic. *Psychol Med* 1989;19:919–925.
40. Ottman R, Lipton R. Is the comorbidity of epilepsy and migraine due to a shared genetic susceptibility? *Neurology* 1996;47:918–924.
41. Paulin JM, Waal-Manning HJ, Simpson FO, Knight RG. The prevalence of headache in a small New Zealand town. *Headache* 1985;25:147–151.
42. Philips C, Hunter M. Headache in a psychiatric population. *J Nerv Ment Dis* 1982;1982:34–40.

43. Rasmussen BK, Olesen J. Symptomatic and nonsymptomatic headaches in a general population. *Neurology* 1992;42:1225–1231.

44. Rasmussen BK, Olesen J. Epidemiology of migraine and tension-type headache. *Curr Opin Neurol* 1994;7:264–271.

45. Schele R, Ahlborg B, Ekbom K. Physical characteristics and allergic history in young men with migraine and other headaches. *Headache* 1978;18:80–86.

46. Sternfeld B, Stang P, Sidney S. Relationship of migraine headaches to experience of chest pain and subsequent risk for myocardial infarction. *Neurology* 1995;45:2135–2142.

47. Stewart WF, Linet MS, Celentano DD. Migraine headaches and panic attacks. *Psychosom Med* 1989;51:559–569.

48. Tzourio C, Iglesias S, Hurbert J. Migraine and risk of ischaemic stroke: a case-control study. *BMJ* 1993;307:289–292.

49. Walker CH. Migraine and its relationship to hypertension. *BMJ* 1959;1:1430–1431.

50. Waters WE. Headache and blood pressure in the community. *BMJ* 1971;1:142–143.

51. Weiss NS. Relation of high blood pressure to headache, epistaxis, and selected other symptoms: the United States health examination survey of adults. *N Engl J Med* 1972;287:631–633.

52. Welch KM, Levine SR. Migraine-related stroke in the context of the International Headache Society classification of head pain. *Arch Neurol* 1990;47:458–462.

53. Wolff HG. Personality features and reactions of subjects with migraine. *Arch Neurol Psychiatry* 1937;37:895–921.

54. Younes RP, Delong GR, Neiman G, Rosner B. Comorbidity of migraine and major affective disorders. *J Child Neurol* 1994;1:364–368.

The Headaches, Second Edition,
edited by J. Olesen, P. Tfelt-Hansen, and K.M.A. Welch.
Lippincott Williams & Wilkins, Philadelphia © 2000.

The Migraines

CHAPTER 30

Genetics of Migraine

Michel D. Ferrari and Michael Bjørn Russell

Migraine is a chronic paroxysmal neurovascular disorder, known to often run in families (98). Multiple genetic factors are believed to be involved (95). Anyone can have a migraine attack occasionally, without necessarily being a migraine patient. Attacks appear to involve physiologic mechanisms initiated by migraine-specific triggers. Not the attack but the repeated recurrence of attacks is abnormal. In this respect migraine is similar to other paroxysmal disorders such as epilepsy. Genetic factors seem to set the individual threshold, and both endogenous and exogenous factors modulate this setpoint, making migraine a multifactorial disorder (22,95,98). Unraveling of the genetic basis of migraine will improve the understanding of the pathogenesis of the disease, notably of how, why, and when patients get attacks. This improved insight into the mechanism of the onset of migraine attacks may promote the development of migraine-specific prophylactic drugs and possibly gene-directed therapy. In addition, it may help to establish an objective diagnostic test for the subtypes of migraine (22,112). This chapter reviews the genetic data on migraine without aura, migraine with aura, familial hemiplegic migraine, and related disorders. It discusses the clinical, genetic, and pharmacologic evidence that migraine, at least in part, might be a genetically determined cerebral calcium channelopathy. This chapter also focuses on studies that applied a directed interview of study population by a physician using the criteria of the International Headache Society (IHS), unless otherwise stated (37).

M.D. Ferrari: Department of Neurology, Leiden University Medical Centre, NL-2300 RC Leiden, The Netherlands.

M.B. Russell: Department of Neurology, Glostrup Hospital, University of Copenhagen, DK-2600 Glostrup, Copenhagen, Denmark.

CLINICAL GENETICS

Positive Family History

Transmission of migraine from parents to children was reported as early as the seventeenth century (126). Since then, numerous studies have reported a positive family history of migraine (92). A positive family history is imprecise because it does not specify the number of individuals affected, family size, or relation to the proband. Studies specifying information about parents are more informative. The lifetime prevalence of migraine is 16% to 21% in the general population (88,102). Thus, a positive family history is applicable simply by chance in greater than 80% of probands with six first-degree relatives (parents, siblings and children), and one or both parents are affected in greater than 40% of the families. A positive family history therefore does not prove the presence of a genetic factor. Furthermore, a positive family history does not necessarily mean that the relatives were affected. Migraine assessed by proband report compared with a clinical interview by a physician was not sufficiently sensitive because the probands only identified about half of their affected first-degree relatives (low sensitivity) (94). The misclassification of the specific migraine diagnoses—migraine without aura and migraine with aura—was equally positive and negative. The observed agreement rates were high, whereas kappa values, the chance corrected agreement rates, were low. Kappa values of more than 0.50 to 0.60 are usually considered to represent the minimum acceptable relationship (62,87). Thus, migraine assessed by proband report is not sufficiently precise because the number of affected relatives is highly underestimated and often misclassified. A clinical interview by a physician is indispensable in family studies of migraine. An extensive review of family studies based on proband report has been provided elsewhere (92).

Distinction between Migraine without Aura and Migraine with Aura

Clinical, epidemiologic, pathophysiologic, and genetic differences suggest that migraine without aura and migraine with aura are distinct entities (78,79,89,98,101). An important argument is that the observed number of people with cooccurrence of migraine without aura and migraine with aura is not significantly different from the expected number, that is, the product of the prevalence of migraine without aura and migraine with aura (89,101).

Cooccurrence of migraine without aura and migraine with aura is higher in clinic populations and other selected populations (125). This can be explained by selection bias (4). The authors of this chapter disagree on this issue, but agree that for scientific purposes it seems wise to analyze migraine without aura and migraine with aura separately.

Migraine without Aura

Genetic Epidemiologic Surveys

An increased familial risk can be caused by genetic as well as environmental factors. The risk among spouses can be used to evaluate this relationship because probands and spouses share a common environment but differ in genetic constitution (122). Thus, an increased risk among first-degree relatives and no increased risk among spouses favors the importance of genetic factors, whereas no increased risk among first-degree relatives and spouses favor the importance of environmental factors. Table 1 shows the population relative risk/relative risk (odds ratio) of migraine without aura in different genetic epidemiologic surveys (70,98,107). The Italian study was based on a clinic population. The interviewers of both the Danish and American survey were blind to the diagnostic status of the proband when interviewing the family members (98,107). The probands of the American survey were interviewed and examined by a physician, whereas the first-degree relatives were telephone interviewed by lay interviewers about their most severe type of headache (107). Clinic populations are subject to selection bias, and lay interviews may not be valid. The Danish study found that compared with the general population, first-degree relatives of probands with migraine without aura had a 1.9-fold increased risk of migraine without aura, whereas spouses had 1.5-fold increased risk of migraine without aura (the latter is not shown in Table 2) (98). This cannot be explained by assertive mating because migraineurs are not known to have a specific personality, marital status, education, or employment status (90). Nor can it be explained by environmental factors alone, because the majority of probands and spouses had onset of migraine without aura before age 20 (98). Genetic epidemiologic surveys suggest that migraine without aura is caused by a combination of both genetic and environmental factors.

TABLE 1. *Participants in genetic epidemiological surveys of migraine without aura (MO) and migraine with aura (MA)*

| Disease in probands | Study population | Disease in first-degree relatives | No. of probands | First-degree relatives | | Relative risk[a] | Population relative risk[b] | 95% Confidence intervals |
				No. of affected	No. of total			
Migraine without aura								
Mochie	Clinic	MO	34	64	171	3.62		1.10–6.14
et al. (70)		MO	102				1.86	1.56–2.16
Russell and	General		126		354			
Olesen (98)		MA			42		1.44	1.03–1.85
		MO		30		1.43	0.83–2.47	
Stewart	General		45		156			
et al.[c](107)		MA		10		2.36	0.87–6.38	
Migraine with aura								
Mochie	Clinic	MA	35	13	144	6.95	3.15–10.75	
et al. (70)		MA	111			3.79	3.21–4.38	
Russell and	General		127		359			
Olesen (98)		MO		56		1.02	0.77–1.26	
Kalfakis	Clinic	MA	60	58	328	11.85	7.00–16.70	
et al. (53)		MA		3		1.24	0.28–5.47	
Stewart	General		28		87			
et al.[c](107)		MO		17		1.41	0.71–2.77	

[a]First-degree relatives of probands with migraine compared with first-degree relatives of probands who had never had migraine.

[b]First-degree relatives of probands with migraine compared with the risk of migraine in the general population.

[c]Probands were interviewed by a physician, while first-degree relatives were interviewed by lay interviewers.

TABLE 2. *The numbers of concordant and discordant monozygotic (MZ) and dizygotic (DZ) twin pairs of the same gender*

	Men		Women		Overall	
	MZ	DZ	MZ	DZ	MZ	DZ
Migraine without aura (27)						
Concordant pairs	8	6	30	41	38	47
Discordant pairs	39	69	60	141	99	210
Pairwise concordance rate (%)	17	8	33	23	28	18
Probandwise concordance rate (%)	29	15	50	37	43	31
Migraine with aura (116,117)						
Concordant pairs	12	10	14	6	26	16
Discordant pairs	21	48	30	70	51	118
Pairwise concordance rate (%)	36	17	32	8	34	12
Probandwise concordance rate (%)	53	29	48	15	50	21

Twin Studies

Studies of twin pairs are the classical method of investigating the relative importance of genetic and environmental factors. The majority of twin studies have been case reports or small series; larger samples are limited. Unfortunately, most studies have not discriminated between migraine without aura and migraine with aura. A review of twins studies analyzing unspecified migraine is provided elsewhere (92). A British study included twin pairs from a volunteer-based twin register (66). The twins filled in a self-administered questionnaire. The pairwise concordance rate was 29% (18/18 + 44) among monozygotic and 18% (10/10 + 46) among dizygotic twin pairs. The result suggested that genetic factors play a minor role in migraine without aura. However, the value of nonvalidated questionnaires is doubtful. A self-administered headache questionnaire based on the different diagnostic criteria of the IHS proved invalid for diagnosing migraine (87). A Danish study included 1,013 monozygotic and 1,667 dizygotic twin pairs of the same gender, from a population-based twin register (27). Zygosity was established based on self-reported similarity, which classifies zygosity correctly in 90% to 95% of the twin pairs (67,81). A short screening questionnaire was completed by 87% of the twins. Twin pairs with at least one twin with self-reported migraine or migraine symptoms were interviewed by a physician. The zygosity and questionnaire response was blinded for the interviewer. Self-reported migraine by a single question was previously evaluated and found valid as the chance-corrected agreement rate kappa value was 0.88 (102). Table 2 shows the number of concordant and discordant twin pairs. The pairwise concordance rate was significantly higher among monozygotic than dizygotic twin pairs ($p < 0.05$). Analyzing men and women separately, a similar trend was observed ($p = 0.22$ and $p = 0.08$). Women had slightly higher concordance rates than men, probably reflecting the higher prevalence in women. The significantly higher pairwise concordance rate among monozygotic than dizygotic twin pairs supports the importance of

genetic factors. However, environmental factors also seem to play an important role because the pairwise concordance rate in monozygotic twin pairs never reached 100%. The concordance rate among probands was 31% for dizygotic twin pairs. This risk is comparable with the 30% recurrence risk in Danish siblings (98). Thus, twin studies suggest that migraine without aura is caused by a combination of genetic and environmental factors.

Mode of Inheritance

An Italian study analyzed 34 pedigrees and excluded maternal and X-linked transmission (70). The classic segregation analysis suggested an autosomal-recessive kind of transmission, that is, involvement of a single gene locus. However, a classic segregation analysis only analyzes for autosomal-dominant and -recessive inheritance, whereas a complex segregation analysis also analyzes for multifactorial inheritance, as well as transmissible and nontransmissible environmental factors (59). The Danish study analyzed 127 pedigrees with a complex segregation analysis (95). The complex segregation analysis (Table 3) yielded the sporadic model, no family resemblance, and a poor fit compared with the multifactorial model. There was no evidence of an intergenerational difference for multifactorial inheritance. None of the three models that incorporated a major locus explained the observed segregation pattern better than the multifactorial model. The complex segregation analysis also was performed with transformations of the data, but this did not change the outcome of the segregation analysis. A complex segregation analysis cannot detect genetic heterogeneity. Thus, the results did not exclude that some families may have had a mitochondrial or Mendelian pattern of inheritance. Considering the high prevalence, a single gene is not likely to cause migraine without aura because the gene has to be more common than any known disease-causing gene. A Danish twin study analyzed 85 concordant and 309 discordant twin pairs from a population-based twin register (27). The structural equation modeling was performed with the MX program. The model that combined additive genetic and individual-

TABLE 3. *Results of the complex segregation analyses for migraine without aura and migraine with aura*

Model	Heritability	Z^a	Gene frequency	Displacement between two homozygous means	Degree of dominance	$-2\times lnL$ constant[b]
Migraine without aura (95)						
Sporadic	0^c	—	0^c	—	—	−1239.49
Multifactorial	0.77	1^c	0^c	—	—	−1282.14
Multifactorial with generational difference	0.74	1.31	0^c	—	—	−1283.38
Recessive major locus	0^c	1^c	0.47	1.70	0^c	−1280.32
Additive major locus	0^c	1^c	0.10	2.95	0.5^c	−1281.66
Dominant major locus	0^c	1^c	0.084	1.61	1^c	−1281.33
Migraine with aura (95)						
Sporadic	0^c	—	0^c	—	—	−1236.54
Multifactorial	0.785	1^c	0^c	—	—	−1312.71
Multifactorial with generational difference	0.824	0.754	0^c	—	—	−1313.12
Recessive major locus	0^c	1^c	0.34	1.92	0*	−1310.44
Additive major locus	0^c	1^c	0.064	3.38	0.5*	−1313.23
Dominant major locus	0^c	1^c	0.046	1.87	1*	−1312.52

[a]Takes into account intergenerational differences.
[b]1nL is the natural logarithm of the likelihood.
[c]Fixed parameter.

specific environmental effects gave the best fit. The additive genetic effects accounted for 61% of the total phenotypic variance. This is compatible with multifactorial inheritance. Genetic heterogeneity could not be excluded because structural equation modeling cannot detect it. Family and twin studies suggest that migraine without aura has multifactorial inheritance, and genetic heterogeneity cannot be excluded.

Migraine with Aura

Migraine with aura is subclassified into migraine with typical aura, migraine with prolonged aura, familial hemiplegic migraine, basilar migraine, migraine aura without headache, and migraine with acute onset aura (37). This subclassification may not be useful for separating possible etiologically different types of migraine with aura because of the intraindividual variation of attacks (1,2,35,47,61,63,96,99,100).

Genetic Epidemiologic Surveys

Table 1 shows the population relative risk and the relative risk (odds ratio) of migraine with aura in different genetic epidemiologic surveys (53,70,98,107). All the studies except the American study showed an increased risk of migraine with aura among first-degree relatives. The family members of the American study were only asked about their most severe type of headache. The diagnosis migraine with aura does not require specific headache characteristics (37). However, the American study changed the diagnostic criteria, so that the headache characteristics were similar to those of migraine without aura. This may have caused an underestimation of migraine with aura because the headache in that type is often less severe than it is in migraine without aura (89,101). Furthermore, for an unerring diagnosis, interviews by physicians are preferred. Thus, the American survey seems inconclusive. The Greek and Italian studies were based on clinic populations, which may cause bias (4). The Danish study found that compared with the general population, first-degree relative of probands with migraine with aura had a 3.8-fold increased risk of migraine without aura, whereas spouses of probands had no increased risk of migraine with aura (the latter is not shown in Table 2) (98). Thus, genetic epidemiologic surveys show an increased familial aggregation of migraine with aura, which most likely is attributable to genetic factors.

Twin Studies

Five pairs of monozygotic twins were concordant (19,51,97,108), and one pair of monozygotic twins was discordant for migraine with aura (84). However, case records are subject to selection bias. For example, the discordant twin pair was described in one of a series of articles about discordant monozygotic twins (84). The British study found that the pairwise concordance rate was 29% (4/4 + 20) among monozygotic and 0% (0/0 + 19) among dizygotic twin pairs (66). The result suggested that genetic factors played a minor role in migraine with aura. However, the validity of nonevaluated questionnaires is doubtful (see the section on twin studies of migraine without aura). The results of the Danish population based twin survey are shown in Table 3 (116). The pairwise concordance rate was significantly higher among monozygotic than dizygotic twin pairs ($p < 0.001$). Analyzing each gender separately showed a significant difference in women and a similar trend in men ($p = 0.002$ and $p = 0.07$). The significantly higher pairwise concordance rate among monozygotic than dizygotic twin pairs supports the importance of genetic factors. However, environmental factors also played an important role because the pairwise concordance rate in monozygotic twin pairs was less than 100%. The concordance rate among probands was 21% for dizygotic twin pairs. This risk is comparable with the 27% recurrence risk in Danish siblings (98). Thus, twin studies suggest that migraine with aura is caused by a combination of genetic and environmental factors.

Mode of Inheritance

Five studies have included direct interview by physicians of probands and their relatives (53,70,98,117,118). A detailed description of the study designs is provided in the genetic epidemiologic surveys and twin sections above. The Italian study analyzed 35 pedigrees and excluded maternal and X-linked transmission (70). The classic segregation analysis suggested an autosomal-recessive kind of transmission. The Greek study included 60 families (53). A classic segregation analysis suggested multifactorial inheritance, but the contribution of a major gene could not be excluded. The Danish study analyzed 126 families with a complex segregation analysis (95). The complex segregation analysis (see Table 3) gave the best fit to the multifactorial model without generational differences. The results do not discount the notion that some families have a mitochondrial or mendelian pattern of inheritance. From that point of view it is interesting that another Danish study analyzed the mode of inheritance in high-risk families with migraine with aura (118). The 31 nuclear families consisted of an affected and an unaffected parent and at least one affected and one unaffected child. The nuclear families were expanded with other first-degree relatives, as well as second-degree relatives in case the first-degree relatives were affected. An analysis of the families suggested multifactorial inheritance even in these high-risk families. Until now, only familial hemiplegic migraine, a rare subtype of migraine with aura, seems to have an autosomal-dominant mode of inheritance. The results did not exclude that some families may have a mitochondrial or mendelian pattern of inheritance. Considering the high prevalence, a single gene is not likely to cause migraine with aura because the gene has to be more common than any known disease-causing gene. A Danish twin study analyzed 42 concordant and 169 discordant twin pairs from a population-based twin register (117). Structural equation modeling was performed using the MX program. The model that combined additive genetic and individual-specific environmental effects gave the best fit. The additive genetic effects accounted for 65% of the total phenotypic variance. This is compatible with multifactorial inheritance. Genetic heterogeneity could not be excluded because structural equation modeling is unable to detect it. Migraine with aura most likely has multifactorial inheritance.

Familial Hemiplegic Migraine

Familial hemiplegic migraine was first reported early in the twentieth century (13). It is a rare autosomal-dominantly inherited subtype of migraine with aura (37). Incomplete penetrance has been demonstrated in a pair of monozygotic twin sisters (17). They were discordant for familial hemiplegic migraine, and the unaffected twin sister had a son with familial hemiplegic migraine. Some families are clinically distinct because familial hemiplegic migraine is associated with progressive cerebellar ataxia (12,23,29,41,48,50,72,77,82,83). Patients with familial hemiplegic migraine and their unaffected relatives may have attacks of migraine without aura or nonhemiplegic typical migraine with aura. At present it is unknown whether the risk of the more common types of migraine are increased in these families. An increased risk could suggest that genes involved in familial hemiplegic migraine are candidate genes for migraine without aura and nonhemiplegic typical migraine with aura. Sporadic cases with symptomatology resembling familial hemiplegic migraine exist (5,40), but they are not classified as such because this requires at least one affected first-degree relative with identical attacks (37). At present, familial hemiplegic migraine has been assigned to chromosomes 1 and 19, and at least a third chromosome (see below). Only few clinical differences have been found between chromosome 19–linked and unlinked families. The most striking exception is cerebellar ataxia, which occurs in approximately 50% of the chromosome 19–linked but in none of the unlinked families (21,48, 50,83,109). Most likely, familial hemiplegic migraine and the cerebellar degeneration reflect the similar gene defects (21,34). Other less striking differences are that patients from chromosome 19–linked families are more likely to have attacks which can be triggered by minor head trauma or which are associated with coma (109). A complete list of the early familial hemiplegic migraine literature is provided elsewhere (92).

MOLECULAR GENETICS

Gene-Mapping Approaches

The search for genetic risk factors in paroxysmal diseases such as migraine is complicated by a number of clinical, genetic, and statistical problems. Major clinical issues are how to determine whether or not a person is affected and how to distinguish likely gene carriers from possible phenocopies. Although early onset and severe clinical course are traditionally regarded as indicators for a genetic background, it is unclear how one should address paroxysmal disorders. Are the number of attacks or their severity indicators of the presence of genetic risk factors, or are these merely a consequence of the frequency and intensity of the exposure to environmental triggers? The genetic strategy depends on the available patients, family material, and knowledge of likely candidate genes. When family material is abundant and candidate genes are scarce, a random genome screening for linkage will be the method of choice. The preferred statistical method of analysis is debated, that is, parametric versus nonparametric and the statistical thresholds that provide optimal distinction between linkage and background noise (30,58,60,114). Linkage findings may lead (after independent confirmation) to identification of *positional* candidate genes, as opposed to the *functional* candidates that originate from insights into the biochemical pathways underlying the disease. The involvement of such functional candidates may be evaluated via functional assays, but also by means of linkage tests in multiply affected families. A third, less commonly practiced method of identifying candidate genes for multifactorial disorders is to localize genes that cause rare mendelian variants of that disorder. Such loci can then be evaluated as possible susceptibility loci, assuming that mutations which convey susceptibility to a complex disease are allelic to more serious gene defects leading to mendelian segregation. Tentatively one might call such candidate genes *phenotypic* candidates. Such rare variants usually have a clear inheritance pattern and candidate loci can be identified by using regular LOD score analyses. The advantage of the analysis of functional and phenotypic candidates over a genome search for positional candidates is that the former approach involves fewer statistical tests, and consequently a less stringent statistical correction for multiple testing is required. With respect to functional candidates, one may object that their number is *a priori* not strictly defined and that different investigators may favor different functional candidates. In contrast, for phenotypic candidates the number of alternatives is usually limited. How one should interpret a mildly significant linkage finding for a phenotypic candidate is largely dependent (a) on how plausible a common genetic background is for the common and rare variants of a disease and (b) on independent confirmation. A fourth approach is investigating the *association with genetic markers*. The rationale of such studies is that genetic markers such as DNA polymorphisms may occur in disequilibrium with genes, various alleles of which may lead to differences of the phenotype. Such linkage disequilibrium may have two causes: either the time that elapsed to separate the suspect genes from the tightly linked DNA polymorphism by recombination may not have been sufficient for the disequilibrium to disappear, or the marker allele itself influenced the phenotype to be studied.

Linkage Studies of Familial Hemiplegic Migraine

In 1993, a French group reported the first linkage of familial hemiplegic migraine to chromosome 19p13 (48). Soon after, both the French and a Dutch group found genetic heterogeneity of familial hemiplegic migraine because only about 50% of the families are linked to chromosome 19p13 (50,83). Two groups also have found linkage to chromosome 1 (18,26). The North American group showed, in one large family, an LOD score of 3.04 at $\Theta = 0.09$ with marker D1S249 on chromosome 1q31 (26), whereas the French group showed linkage to chromosome 1q21-q23 in three familial hemiplegic migraine families (18). Further analysis will disclose whether chromosome 1q harbors one or two loci for familial hemiplegic migraine. Some families cannot be linked to either chromosome 1 or 19, indicating that at least a third gene must be involved in familial hemiplegic migraine (18).

CADASIL

Cerebral autosomal-dominant arteriopathy with subcortical infarcts and leukoencephalopathy (CADASIL) is characterized by recurrent subcortical ischemic strokes, extensive white matter signal abnormalities on magnetic resonance imaging, progressive subcortical dementia, and mood disorders with severe depressive episodes (11). Up to one third have cooccurrence of CADASIL and migraine with aura (11,52,120). In one CADASIL family, four of the 10 members affected by magnetic resonance had cooccurrence of familial hemiplegic migraine, whereas one unaffected by magnetic resonance had familial hemiplegic migraine (44). Among another family linked to the CADASIL locus on chromosome 19p12, several individuals had attacks of mainly migraine with aura and white matter lesions on magnetic resonance imaging, segregating with an autosomal-dominant pattern of inheritance (10). However, ischemic stroke, one of the hallmarks of CADASIL, was not present in this family. Initially CADASIL and familial hemiplegic migraine were considered to be allelic (48) because the CADASIL locus was mapped to chromosome 19p12 (115). Further linkage studies revealed that the loci were separate (14,20). The gene responsible for CADASIL has been identified as the *Notch3* gene (49). This suggests that CADASIL and familial hemiplegic migraine are genetically unrelated. The question remains, however, why migraine with aura occurs so frequently in CADASIL.

The *CACNA1A* Gene Mutations

Familial Hemiplegic Migraine

Using exon trapping, a human cDNA highly homologous to a brain-specific rabbit and rat voltage-gated P/Q-type calcium channel α_{1A} subunit gene was identified (71,82,105). The human gene originally designated *CACNL1A4* (15) has subsequently been renamed *CACNA1A* (65). Figure 1 shows four different missense mutations in five unrelated familial hemiplegic migraine families identified by the Dutch group (82). A G-to-A transition at codon 192 resulted in an arginine-to-glutamine substitution (R192Q) within the fourth segment of the first membrane-spanning domain IS4. The highly conserved S4 segment is thought to be part of the voltage sensor. The second mutation occurred within the pore-forming hairpin loop of the second domain, replacing threonine with methionine (T666M). These conserved pore-forming segments, located between each S5 and S6 segment, are involved in the ion selectivity of ion channels and present binding sites for toxins (32). Two other mutations were located in the sixth transmembrane-spanning segment of repeats II and IV. The IIS6 mutation was a T-to-C transition at codon 714, resulting in a valine-to-alanine substitution (V714A). The IVS6 mutation was an A-to-C transversion at codon 1811, resulting in an isoleucine-to-leucine substitution (I1811L). This mutation was found in two independent families both with familial hemiplegic migraine and cerebellar ataxia. The S6 mutations do not change the neutral-polar nature of the amino acid residues, but the original residues are conserved in all calcium channel α_1 subunit genes described (106). Residues in the S6 transmembrane segments may be of influence in the inactivation of the calcium channel (Table 4) (38). The mutations described above were introduced into rabbit α_1 subunits, which show a 94% sequence identity with the human gene (57). The mutant subunits were functionally expressed in *Xenopus laevis* oocytes. The last three of the four familial hemiplegic

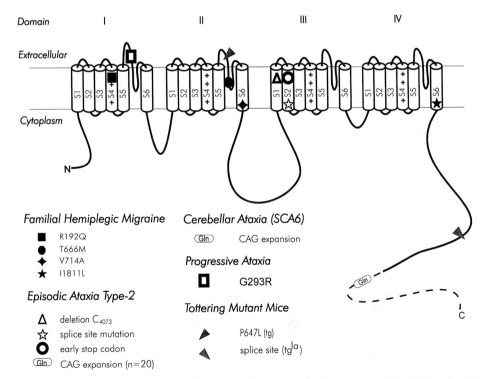

FIG. 1. Membrane topology of α_{1A} subunit of the P/Q-type Ca²⁺ channel, *CACNA1A*. The location and amino acid substitutions are indicated for mutations that cause familial hemiplegic migraine (*FHM*), episodic ataxia type 2 (*EA-2*), tottering mouse (*tg*), leaner mouse (*tgla*), and spinocerebellar ataxia type 6 (*SCA6*).

TABLE 4. *Calcium channel subunits*

Subunit	Nomenclature	Channel type	Pharmacology (blockers)	Location	Distribution	Human disorders	Mouse models
α1A	CACNA1A	P/Q	ω-Agatoxin IVA ω-Conotoxin MVIIC	19p13	Neuronal, endocrine	FHM, EA-2, SCA6	Tottering (*tg*) Leaner (*tg^la*)
α1B	CACNA1B	N	ω-Conotoxin GVIA ω-Conotoxin MVIIA	9q34	Neuronal		
α1C	CACNA1C	L	Dihydropyridines	12p14.3	Cardiac and smooth muscle, neuronal		
α1D	CACNA1D	L	Dihydropyridines	3p14.3	Neuronal, endocrine		
α1E	CACNA1E	R/T	?	1q25–q31	Neuronal		
α1S	CACNA1S	L	Dihydropyridines	1q31–q32	Skeletal muscle	HypoKK, MHS2	
β1	CACNB1			17q11.2–q22	Skeletal muscle, neuronal		
β2	CACNB2			10p12	Heart, aorta, neuronal		
β3	CACNB3			12q13	Neuronal, aorta, trachea, lung, heart, skeletal muscle		
β4	CACNB4			2q22–q23	Neuronal		Lethargic (*lh*)
α2δ	CACNA2			7q21–q22	Skeletal muscle, heart, vascular and intestinal smooth muscle, neuronal		
γ	CACNG			17q24	Skeletal muscle		

FHM, familial hemiplegic migraine; EA-2, episodic ataxia type 2; SCA6, spinocerebellar ataxia type 6; HypoKK, hypokalemic periodic paralysis; MHS2, malignant hyperthermia susceptibility-2.
Data from Ulrich et al. (117,118).

migraine mutations altered the inactivation gating of the calcium channels, increasing or decreasing their functional availability. Similar changes were described when HEK-293 cells containing human α_{1A} and other regulatory subunits were studied (86). Further studies are needed to fully establish the functional consequences of these mutations in human α_1 subunits and calcium channels. The missense mutations in familial hemiplegic migraine suggest a molecular mechanism similar to what is found in other human channelopathies. Both alleles are likely to be expressed with the allele harboring the missense mutation resulting in loss- or gain-of-function variants of the P/Q-type calcium channels. Such mutations have been described in the α subunit of the skeletal muscle sodium channel, resulting in hyperkalemic periodic paralysis, paramyotonia congenita, and the sodium channel myotonias (see Table 2) (9,43). Interestingly, the second familial hemiplegic migraine locus on chromosome 1q is located near *CACNA1E,* a brain-specific R/T calcium channel α_{1E} subunit gene. Mutation analysis will disclose whether this gene is involved in chromosome 1–linked familial hemiplegic migraine families.

Episodic Ataxia Type 2

Episodic ataxia type 2 (EA-2) is also referred to as acetazolamide-responsive paroxysmal cerebellar ataxia,

paroxysmal vestibulocerebellar ataxia, or hereditary paroxysmal cerebellar ataxia (36,56,109,119,123). Onset is usually in childhood or early adulthood (25). Attacks are characterized by generalized ataxia lasting a few hours, usually associated with interictal nystagmus. Patients may experience migrainelike symptoms, during and in between attacks (36,56,109,119,123). Magnetic resonance imaging often shows cerebellar atrophy (33,48,121). Attacks can be precipitated by emotional stress, exercise, or alcohol, whereas acetazolamide often is effective in preventing attacks. After linkage of EA-2 to the same interval on chromosome 19p as familial hemiplegic migraine (36,56,109, 119,123), mutation analysis revealed two different truncating mutations in the *CACNA1A* calcium channel gene in two unrelated EA-2 families shown in Figure 1 (82). One mutation is a nucleotide deletion (deletion C_{4073}), causing a frame shift and a premature stop. The other mutation affects the first invariant G nucleotide of the intron consensus sequence, leading to aberrant splicing. Both mutations result in truncated α_{1A} subunits that are unlikely to form functional calcium channels and may either degrade, resulting in haploinsufficiency, or negatively influence channel assembly in the membrane. A similar mutation, very near to the previously described EA-2 mutations shown in Figure 1, was subsequently described in a patient with nonfamilial episodic vertigo and ataxia responsive to acetazolamide (127).

Spinocerebellar Ataxia Type 6

Spinocerebellar ataxia type 6 (SCA6) is allelic with EA-2, but the two differ clinically because of the presence of progressive, rather than episodic, ataxia in SCA6 (28). Six different cDNA isoforms of the *CACN1A1* gene have been reported, of which three contained a 5-nucleotide insertion prior to the above described stop codon, resulting in a shift of the open reading frame in which the CAG repeat is predicted to encode a polyglutamine stretch (82,128). Small triplet expansions of the intragenic CAG repeat ranging from 21 to 30 repeat units were observed in those with SCA6, whereas normal chromosomes displayed 4 to 20 repeats (45,68,82,91,128). The CAG repeat length is inversely correlated with age at onset (45,68,91). Anticipation of the disease was observed clinically, but intergenerational allele size change was not observed in contrast to other spinocerebellar ataxias and Huntington's chorea, also caused by CAG repeats (68). Two homozygotic cases have been reported. The first patient did not demonstrate an unequivocal gene dosage effect on age at onset (68), whereas the second patient showed an earlier age of onset and more severe clinical manifestations than her sister, a heterozygote carrying an expanded allele with the same repeat length as the homozygote. SCA6 has been estimated to occur in 10% of Germans and 30% of Japanese with spinocerebellar ataxias (68,91). Can the mutations that cause chromosome 19–linked familial hemiplegic migraine or EA-2 cause progressive cerebellar ataxia independent of the number of CAG repeats? The I1811L point mutation that causes familial hemiplegic migraine seems sufficient to cause both familial hemiplegic migraine and cerebellar ataxia because there is no evidence of CAG repeat expansions (113). Two families with small CAG expansions of the *CACNA1A* gene were investigated (46). In one family with a clinical diagnosis of EA-2, a CAG23 repeat allele segregated in patients showed different interictal symptoms, ranging from nystagmus only to severe progressive cerebellar ataxia. No additional mutations in coding and intron-exon junction sequences in disequilibrium with the CAG expansion were found. In the second family, initially classified as having autosomal-dominant cerebellar ataxia of unknown type, an intergenerational allele size change showed that a CAG20 allele was associated with an EA-2 phenotype and a CAG25 alelle with progressive cerebellar ataxia. Thus, it is likely that SCA6 and EA-2 are the same disorder with a high phenotypic variability, at least partly related to the number of repeats.

Tottering and Leaner Mice

Simultaneously with the identification of mutations in familial hemiplegic migraine and EA-2, mutations in the CACNA1A gene were found in the tottering (*tg*) and leaner mouse (*tg^{la}*) phenotypes (Fig. 1) (16,24,39). These recessive tottering mice have been studied extensively as models for human epilepsy (55). The mutation in the tottering mouse is a missense mutation close to the pore-forming P loop of the second transmembrane domain, very similar to one of the familial hemiplegic migraine missense mutations, and most likely affecting the pore function of the P/Q-type calcium channel. The more severe leaner mouse is associated with a splice site mutation producing an aberrant intracellular terminus and resembling the mutations found in two EA-2 families. Mutations at the mouse tottering locus result in intermittent convulsions similar to human absence epilepsy, motor seizures, and mild ataxia. The leaner (*tg^{la}*) mouse suffers from absence seizures, but no motor seizures. The *tg^{la}* mutants are more ataxic and often do not survive past weaning. The profound chronic ataxia is associated with pervasive Purkinje and granule cell loss throughout the anterior cerebellum, as well as reduced cerebellar size. Recent whole-cell and single-channel patch-clamp recordings have shown that the leaner mutant mice have significantly altered P-type calcium channel currents (64). A third mouse strain, the rolling Nagoya (*tg^{rol}*) presents an intermediate phenotype; the ataxia is more severe than in the *tg* mouse, motor seizures do not occur, and they have a normal life span (24). No mutation for the *tg^{rol}* mouse has yet been identified. It has been suggested that tottering mutant mice have a significantly increased threshold for cortical spreading depression, which is a phenomenon thought to be involved in the pathophysiology of the migraine aura. In the tottering mouse a proliferation of noradrenaline axons arising from the locus coeruleus is considered to be one of the neuronal mechanisms underlying the generation of absence seizures (55). Interestingly, positron emission tomography studies in acute migraine attacks suggested that a brainstem area, most likely comprising the locus coeruleus and the dorsal raphe nucleus, might represent the "migraine generator centre" in humans (124). Therefore, the tottering mice may serve not only as a model for epilepsy and ataxia, but also for migraine. The lethargic mouse (*lh*) is another naturally occurring mouse mutant associated with ataxia and seizures (7). Homozygotes of the *lh* mouse are characterized by ataxia, lethargic behavior, motor seizures, and seizures resembling absence seizures of human petit mal epilepsy. It has been shown to be due to a mutation in the calcium channel β4 subunit gene (7).

Linkage and Associations Studies of Migraine

Migraine without aura and migraine with aura have been linked with many disorders; however, caution is necessary due to the high prevalence of both types of migraine, which means that spurious associations frequently occur. Single families with cosegregation of two disorders can supply important knowledge, but the generalizability of the results must subsequently be established in the general population. All linkage and association studies generally should be regarded as preliminary evidence until independently confirmed.

The CACNA1A Gene

A German-Dutch affected sibling pair analysis of 28 families suggests that the *CACNA1A* gene on chromosome 19p13 is involved in migraine without aura and migraine with aura (69). The maximum multipoint LOD score was 1.29 ($p \approx 0.013$), but the major contribution was made by one large family. The results were inconclusive with respect to the relative importance in migraine without aura and migraine with aura, respectively. Subsequently, in a larger second and independent affected sibling pair analysis involving 36 extended Dutch families with migraine with and without aura, significant increased sharing of the marker alleles in siblings with migraine with aura was confirmed (110). No such increased sharing was found for migraine without aura. A combined analysis for both migraine types, including sibling pairs in which one had migraine without aura and the other migraine with aura, resulted in increased allele sharing. The relative risk ratio for a sibling (λ_s) to suffer from migraine with aura, defined as the increase in risk of the trait attributable to the 19p13 locus, was $\lambda_s = 2.4$. When combining migraine with and without aura, λ_s was 1.25. When the results of both studies were combined, the maximum multipoint LOD score increased to 2.27 ($p \approx 0.001$). A Dutch genotype-phenotype relationship study found the I1811L familial hemiplegic migraine mutation in patients with familial hemiplegic migraine and in two unaffected family members with nonhemiplegic migraine (113). This result suggests that the I1811L mutation might be involved in non-hemiplegic migraine. However, it might as well be two unaffected carriers of familial hemiplegic migraine, like one of the monozygotic twin sisters mentioned above in the clinical section on familial hemiplegic migraine (17). Two classical linkage studies have been performed. A Finnish study did not find linkage to chromosome 19 in four multigenerational families with migraine without aura and migraine with aura, but they used the unlikely single gene assumption model (42). An Australian study included several multigenerational families (75). One large tested family showed both cosegregation and significant allele sharing for markers situated within or adjacent to the familial hemiplegic migraine locus. Other tested families showed neither cosegregation nor excess allele sharing to chromosome 19 markers. An American family with dominantly inherited migraine, episodic vertigo, and essential tremor that responded to acetazolamide did not link to chromosome 19p13 (3). Thus, it seems likely that some families with migraine without aura or migraine with aura are caused by mutation in one or more gene(s) on chromosome 19p13. This is in line with family studies of migraine without aura and migraine with aura (53,70, 95,98,107). Future direct mutation analysis of persons with migraine without aura and migraine with aura will establish the precise role of the calcium channel gene in these conditions. Migraine without aura and migraine with aura remarkably has many characteristics in common with established neurologic channelopathies (Table 5). These include a paroxysmal presentation with attacks that can be provoked by both endogenous and exogenous stimuli, which may last from minutes to hours or days, and which may come in a frequency ranging from once in a lifetime to one per day; onset is usually at puberty, amelioration and complete remission may occur after age 40, and pen-

TABLE 5. *Heritable neurologic disorders of ion channels*

Disorder	Ion channel gene	Chromosomal location
Hyperkalemic periodic paralysis	SCNA4 (skeletal muscle sodium channel)	17q23–25
Paramyotonia congenita	SCNA4 (skeletal muscle sodium channel)	17q23–25
Pure myotonias (fluctuans, permanens, acetazolamide-responsive)	SCNA4 (skeletal muscle sodium channel)	17q23–25
Hypokalemic periodic paralysis	CACNA1S (skeletal muscle calcium channel)	1q31–32
Malignant hyperthermia susceptibility-2	CACNA1S (skeletal muscle calcium channel)	1q31–32
Familial hemiplegic migraine	CACNA1A (neuronal calcium channel)	19p13
Episodic ataxia-2	CACNA1A (neuronal calcium channel)	19p13
Spinocerebellar ataxia-6	CACNA1A (neuronal calcium channel)	19p13
Episodic ataxia-1	KCNA-1 (neuronal potassium channel)	12p14
Malignant hyperthermia susceptibility-1	RYR1 (ryanodine calcium channel)	19q13.1
Autosomal dominant nocturnal frontal lobe epilepsy	CHRNA4 (neuronal nicotinic acetylcholine receptor)	20q13.2–q13.3
Hyperekplexia	GLRA1 (neuronal glycine receptor)	
Thomsen's myotonia congenita	CLCN1 (skeletal-muscle chloride channel)	7q35
Becker's myotonia congenita	CLCN1 (skeletal-muscle chloride channel)	
Myotonia levior	CLCN1 (skeletal-muscle chloride channel)	

All disorders have an autosomal dominant inheritance except for Becker's myotonia congenita, which has autosomal recessive inheritance.
Data from Gardner et al. (26), Vahedi et al. (11a), and Verlin et al. (120).

etrance and expression is gender related. Thus, there is also clinical evidence, although still circumstantial, supporting the notion that migraine might be a cerebral ion channelopathy.

The Serotonin System

Serotonin is implicated in migraine pathophysiology (104). An Australian study tested three large multigenerational pedigrees for the Mspl polymorphism in the human 5-hydroxytryptamine 2A (5-HT$_{2A}$) receptor gene (73). In the association analyses, no significant difference was found between the migraine without aura and control population. The subsequent linkage analysis was not informative. A Danish-British association study on allelic variation on codon 23 on the 5-HT$_{2C}$ receptor gene indicated that it did not contribute to the genetic predisposition to migraine without aura and migraine with aura (8). An American study found no evidence of linkage to the 5-HT$_{2A}$ or 5-HT$_{2C}$ receptor genes (6). The mutation analysis indicated that DNA-based mutations in the 5-HT$_{2A}$ and 5-HT$_{2C}$ receptors are not generally involved in the pathogenesis of migraine. A Danish-Scottish association study investigated the role of allelic variation of the human serotonin transporter gene in susceptibility to migraine (76). The results support the notion that susceptibility to migraine without aura and migraine with aura has a genetic component, that these disorders are distinct, and that genetic susceptibility in some cases may be associated with a locus at or near the serotonin transporter gene.

Nitric Oxide Synthase Genes

Nitric oxide has been implicated in the pathophysiology of migraine (80). An Australian study investigated the endothelial nitric oxide synthase polymorphism (31). No evidence of association or linkage was found. No data are available on the importance of the other NOS genes.

Dopamine D2 Receptor Gene

An American study investigated the dopamine D2 receptor gene (85). Individuals with migraine with aura have significantly increased frequency (0.84) of the dopamine D2 Nco 1 C allele compared with controls (0.71) and individuals with migraine without aura (0.70). Migraine with aura was present in 27% of the C/C individuals, 16% of the C/T individuals, and 5% of the T/T individuals. These data suggest that activation of the dopamine D2 receptor plays a modifying role in the pathophysiology of migraine with aura.

Vascular Retinopathy and Raynaud's Phenomenon

A Dutch family with 289 members had occurrence of migraine, autosomal-dominant vascular retinopathy, and Raynaud's phenomenon (111). Retinopathy was found in 20 (7%) family members, migraine in 65 (22%), and Raynaud's phenomenon in 50 (17%). A combination of all three symptoms was found in 11 family members. At the moment, 75% of the genome, including the CACNA1A gene, has been excluded, and further genome search is underway. The family pattern may be caused by a single gene, but might as well be caused by cooccurrence of two or more genes in the same family.

The X Chromosome

The female preponderance of migraine without aura and migraine with aura suggests that genes on the X chromosome might be important in the etiology. An Australian study investigated three large multigenerational migraine pedigrees and found evidence of significant excess allele sharing to chromosome Xq markers in two families (74). Overall analysis of data from all three pedigrees gave significant evidence in support of linkage to chromosome Xq. Confirmation in other families and sporadic cases would be important as well as analyzing migraine without aura and migraine with aura separately.

Mitochondrial Disorders

Mitochondrial function is involved in the oxidative pathways. It is encoded by the mitochondrial and the nuclear genome. Diseases caused by alterations of the mitochondrial genome have a maternal inheritance, because mitochondrial DNA is transmitted from mothers to children. Migraine has been associated with MELAS (mitochondrial myopathy, encephalopathy, lactic acidosis and stroke-like episodes) and less frequently with MERRF (mitochondrial disease, myoclonic epilepsy with ragged-red fibers) (54). MELAS is caused by a point mutation at base pair 3243, and MERRF is caused by a point mutation at base pair 8344. However, neither of the two base pair point mutations nor large scale deletion were found in 23 Germans with migraine with aura (54), excluding a significant role of this mutation in whites. A point mutation in mitochondrial nucleotide pair 11084 was reported in Japanese migraineurs (103). Twenty-five percent (13 of 53) of the Japanese migraineurs had this mutation, whereas none of 39 normal and 60 tension-type headache sufferers did (103). The mutation was not detected in Danes (93). Most likely it represents a common polymorphism in the Japanese population.

THE FUTURE

The other familial hemiplegic migraine genes are likely to be identified in the near future. These genes are suspected to be ion channel genes. Migraine without aura and migraine with aura also have many clinical characteristics in common with established neurologic channelopathies (see Table 4). It is likely, therefore, that these types of migraine also will prove to be channelopathies. The identification of genes for migraine without aura and migraine with aura is expected to be difficult because of the complex mode of inheritance and the relative strong influence of environmental factors.

REFERENCES

1. Airy H. On a distinct form of transient hemiopsia. *Philos Trans R Soc Lond Biol* 1870;160:247–264.
2. Alvarez WC. The migrainous scotoma as studied in 618 persons. *Am J Ophthalmol* 1960;49:489–504.
3. Baloh RW, Foster CA, Yue Q, Nelson SF. Familial migraine with vertigo and essential tremor. *Neurology* 1996;46:458–460.
4. Berkson J. Limitations of the application of fourfold table analysis to hospital data. *Biometrics* 1947;2:47–53.
5. Bradshaw P, Parsons M. Hemiplegic migraine, a clinical study. *Q J Med* 1965;34:65–85.
6. Buchwalder A, Welch S.K, Peroutka S.J. Exclusion of 5-HT$_{2A}$ and 5-HT$_{2C}$ receptor genes as candidate genes for migraine. *Headache* 1996; 36:254–258.
7. Burgess DL, Jones JM, Meister MH, Noebels JL. Mutation of the Ca^{2+} channel beta subunit gene Cchb4 is associated with ataxia and seizures in the lethargic (lh) mouse. *Cell* 1997;88:385–392.
8. Burnet PW, Harrison PJ, Goodwin GM, et al. Allelic variation in the serotonin 5-HT$_{2C}$ receptor gene and migraine. *Neuroreport* 1997;18: 2651–2653.
9. Cannon SC. Ion-channel defects and aberrant excitability in myotonia and periodic paralysis. *Trends Neurosci* 1996;19:3–10.
10. Chabriat H, Tournier Lasserve E, Vahedi K, et al. Autosomal dominant migraine with MRI white-matter abnormalities mapping to the CADASIL locus. *Neurology* 1995;45:1086–1091.
11. Chabriat H, Vahedi K, Iba Zizen MT, et al. Clinical spectrum of CADASIL: a study of 7 families. Cerebral autosomal dominant arteriopathy with subcortical infarcts and leukoencephalopathy [see Comments]. *Lancet* 1995;7:934–939.
12. Chrast B. Migraena cerebellaris. *Lokarsk Listy* 1954;9:271–276.
13. Clarke JM. On recurrent motor paralysis in migraine. *Br Med J* 1910; 1:1534–1538.
14. Dichgans M, Mayer M, Muller Myhsok B, Straube A, Gasser T. Identification of a key recombinant narrows the CADASIL gene region to 8 cM and argues against allelism of CADASIL and familial hemiplegic migraine. *Genomics* 1996;15:151–154.
15. Diriong S, Lory P, Williams ME, Ellis SB, Harpold MM, Taviaux S. Chromosomal localization of the human genes for alfa1A, alfa1B, and alfa1E voltage-dependent Ca^{2+} channel subunits. *Genomics* 1995;30: 605–609.
16. Doyle J, Ren X, Lennon G, Stubbs L. Mutations in the Cacnl1a4 calcium channel gene are associated with seizures, cerebellar degeneration, and ataxia in tottering and leaner mutant mice. *Mamm Genome* 1997;8:113–120.
17. Ducros A, Joutel A, Labauge P, Pages M, Bousser MG, Tournier-Lasserve E. Monozygotic twins discordant for familial hemiplegic migraine. *Neurology* 1995;45:1222.
18. Ducros A, Joutel A, Vahedi K, et al. Mapping of a second locus for familial hemiplegic migraine to 1q21-q23 and evidence of further heterogeneity. *Ann Neurol* 1997;42:885–890.
19. Dupuis MJM, Pierre PH, Gonsette RE. Transient global amnesia and migraine in twin sisters. *J Neurol Neurosurg Psychiatry* 1987;50: 816–817.
20. Duvoisin RC, Parker GW, Kenoyer WL. The cluster headache. *Arch Intern Med* 1961;108:111–116.
21. Elliott MA, Peroutka SJ, Welch S, May EF. Familial hemiplegic migraine, nystagmus, and cerebellar atrophy. *Ann Neurol* 1996;39: 100–106.
22. Ferrari MD. Migraine. *Lancet* 1998;351:1043–1051.
23. Fitzsimons RB, Wolfenden WH. Migraine coma. *Brain* 1985;108: 555–577.
24. Fletcher CF, Lutz CM, O'Sullivan TN, et al. Absence epilepsy in tottering mutant mice is associated with calcium channel defects. *Cell* 1996;87:607–617.
25. Gancher ST, Nutt JG. Autosomal dominant episodic ataxia: a heterogeneous syndrome. *Mov Disord* 1986;1:239–253.
26. Gardner K, Barmada MM, Ptacek LJ, Hoffman EP. A new locus for hemiplegic migraine maps to chromosome 1q31 [see Comments]. *Neurology* 1997;49:1231–1238.
27. Gervil M, Ulrich V, Kaprio J, Olesen J, Russell MB. The relative role of genetic and environmental factors in migraine without aura. *Neurology* 1999 (in press).
28. Geschwind D.H, Perlman S, Figueroa KP, Karrim J, Baloh RW, Pulst SM. Spinocerebellar ataxia type 6. Frequency of the mutation and genotype-phenotype correlations [see Comments]. *Neurology* 1997; 49:1247–1251.
29. Golden GS, French JH. Basilar artery migraine in young children. *Pediatrics* 1975;56:722–726.
30. Greenberg DA, Hodge SE, Vieland VJ, Spence MA. Affecteds-only linkage methods are not a panacea. *Am J Hum Genet* 1996;58: 892–895.
31. Griffiths LR, Nyholt DR, Curtain RP, Goadsby PJ, Brimage PJ. Migraine association and linkage studies of an endothelial nitric oxide synthase (NOS3) gene polymorphism. *Neurology* 1997; 49:614–617.
32. Guy HR, Durell SR. Three-dimensional models of ion channel proteins. In: Narahashi T, ed. *Ion channels*. New York: Plenum Press, 1996.
33. Haan J, Terwindt GM, Bos PL, Ophoff RA, Frants RR, Ferrari MD. Familial hemiplegic migraine in The Netherlands. Dutch Migraine Genetics Research Group. *Clin Neurol Neurosurg* 1994;96:244–249.
34. Haan J, Terwindt GM, Ferrari MD. Genetics of migraine. *Neurol Clin* 1997;15:43–60.
35. Hare EH. Personal observations on the spectral march of migraine. *J Neurol Sci* 1966;3:259–264.
36. Hawkes CH. Familial paroxysmal ataxia: report of a family. *J Neurol Neurosurg Psychiatry* 1992;55:212–213.
37. Headache C, Committee of the International Headache Society. Classification and diagnostic criteria for headache disorders, cranial neuralgias and facial pain. *Cephalalgia* 1988;8:1–96.
38. Hering S, Aczel S, Grabner M, et al. Transfer of high sensitivity for benzothiazepines from L-type to class A (BI) calcium channels. *J Biol Chem* 1996;271:24471–24475.
39. Hess E.J. Migraine in mice? *Cell* 1996;87:1149–1151.
40. Heyck H. Varieties of hemiplegic migraine. *Headache* 1973;12:135–142.
41. Holub V, Chrast B, Saxl O. [Fatal outcome of a migraine attack in children.] *Kinderarztl Prax* 1965;33:539–546.
42. Hovatta I, Kallela M, Farkkila M, Peltonen L. Familial migraine: exclusion of the susceptibility gene from the reported locus of familial hemiplegic migraine on 19p. *Genomics* 1994;23:707–709.
43. Hudson AJ, Ebers GC, Bulman DE. The skeletal muscle sodium and chloride channel diseases. *Brain* 1995;118:547–563.
44. Hutchinson M, O'Riordan J, Javed M, et al. Familial hemiplegic migraine and autosomal dominant arteriopathy with leukoencephalopathy (CADASIL). *Ann Neurol* 1995;38:817–824.
45. Ishikawa K, Tanaka H, Saito M, et al. Japanese families with autosomal dominant pure cerebellar ataxia map to chromosome 19p13.1-p13.2 and are strongly associated with mild CAG expansions in the spinocerebellar ataxia type 6 gene in chromosome 19p13.1. *Am J Hum Genet* 1997;61:336–346.
46. Jodice C, Mantuano E, Veneziano L, et al. Episodic ataxia type 2 (EA2) and spinocerebellar ataxia type 6 (SCA6) due to CAG repeat expansion in the *CACNA1A* gene on chromosome 19p. *Hum Mol Genet* 1997;6:1973–1978.
47. Jolly F. Ueber flimmerskotom und migraine. *Berl Klin Wochenschr* 1902;42:973–976.
48. Joutel A, Bousser MG, Biousse V, et al. A gene for familial hemiplegic migraine maps to chromosome 19. *Nat Genet* 1993;5:40–45.
49. Joutel A, Corpechot C, Ducros A, et al. Notch3 mutations in CADASIL, a hereditary adult-onset condition causing stroke and dementia [see Comments]. *Nature* 1996;24:707–710.
50. Joutel A, Ducros A, Vahedi K, et al. Genetic heterogeneity of familial hemiplegic migraine. *Am J Hum Genet* 1994;55:1166–1172.
51. Juel-Nielsen N. Individual and environmental. A psychiatric investigation of monozygotic twins reared apart. *Acta Psychiatr Scand* 1964; 40:1–292.
52. Jung HH, Bassetti C, Tournier Lasserve E, et al. Cerebral autosomal dominant arteriopathy with subcortical infarcts and leukoen-

cephalopathy: a clinicopathological and genetic study of a Swiss family. *J Neurol Neurosurg Psychiatry* 1995;59:138–143.

53. Kalfakis N, Panas M, Vassilopoulos D, Malliara Loulakaki S. Migraine with aura: segregation analysis and heritability estimation. *Headache* 1996;36:320–322.

54. Klopstock T, May A, Seibel P, Papagiannuli E, Diener HC, Reichmann H. Mitochondrial DNA in migraine with aura. *Neurology* 1996;46:1735–1738.

55. Kostopoulos GK. The tottering mouse: a critical review of its usefulness in the study of the neuronal mechanisms underlying epilepsy. *J Neural Transm Suppl* 1992;35:21–36.

56. Kramer PL, Yue Q, Gancher ST, et al. A locus for the nystagmus-associated form of episodic ataxia maps to an 11-cM region on chromosome 19p. *Am J Hum Genet* 1995;57:182–185.

57. Kraus R.L, Sinnegger MJ, Glossmann H, Hering S, Striessnig J. Familial hemiplegic migraine mutations change alpha1A Ca^{2+} channel kinetics. *J Biol Chem* 1998;6:5586–5590.

58. Kruglyak L. Nonparametric linkage tests are model free. *Am J Hum Genet* 1997;61:254–255.

59. Lalouel JM, Morton NE. Complex segregation analysis with pointers. *Hum Hered* 1981;31:312–321.

60. Lander E, Kruglyak L. Genetic dissection of complex trait: guidelines for interpreting and reporting linkage results. *Nat Genet* 1995;11:241–247.

61. Lashley KS. Patterns of cerebral integration indicated by the scotoma of migraine. *Arch Neurol Psychiatry* 1941;46:331–339.

62. Leone M, Filippini G, D'Amico D, Farinotti M, Bussone G. Assessment of International Headache Society diagnostic criteria: a reliability study. *Cephalalgia* 1994;14:280–284.

63. Lord GDA. A study of premonitory focal neurological symptoms in migraine. In: Clifford Rose F, ed. *Advances in migraine research and therapy.* New York: Raven Press, 1982:45–48.

64. Lorenzon NM, Lutz CM, Frankel WN, Beam KG. Altered calcium channel currents in Purkinje cells of the neurological mutant mouse leaner. *J Neurosci* 1998;15:4482–4489.

65. Lory P, Ophoff RA, Nahmias J. Towards a unified nomenclature describing voltage-gated calcium channel genes. *Hum Genet* 1997;100:149–150.

66. Lucas R.N. Migraine in twins. *J Psychosom Res* 1977;21:147–156.

67. Magnus P, Berg K, Nance WE. Predicting zygosity in Norwegian twin pairs born 1915–1960. *Clin Genet* 1983;24:103–112.

68. Matsuyama Z, Kawakami H, Maruyama H, et al. Molecular features of the CAG repeats of spinocerebellar ataxia 6 (SCA6). *Hum Mol Genet* 1997;6:1283–1287.

69. May A, Ophoff RA, Terwindt GM, et al. Familial hemiplegic migraine locus on 19p13 is involved in the common forms of migraine with and without aura. *Hum Genet* 1995;96:604–608.

70. Mochi M, Sangiorgi S, Cortelli P, et al. Testing models for genetic determination in migraine. *Cephalalgia* 1993;13:389–394.

71. Mori Y, Friedrich T, Kim MS, et al. Primary structure and functional expression from complementary DNA of a brain chacium channel. *Nature* 1991;350:398–402.

72. Münte TF, Müller Vahl H. Familial migraine coma: a case study. *J Neurol* 1990;237:59–61.

73. Nyholt DR, Curtain RP, Gaffney PT, Brimage P, Goadsby PJ, Griffiths LR. Migraine association and linkage analyses of the human 5-hydroxytryptamine (5HT$_{2A}$) receptor gene. *Cephalalgia* 1996;16:463–467.

74. Nyholt DR, Dawkins JL, Brimage PJ, et al. Evidence for an X-linked genetic component in familial typical migraine. *Hum Mol Genet* 1998;7:459–463.

75. Nyholt DR, Lea RA, Goadsby PJ, Brimage PJ, Griffiths LR. Familial typical migraine: linkage to chromosome 19p13 and evidence for genetic heterogeneity. *Neurology* 1998;50:1428–1432.

76. Ogilvie AD, Russell MB, Dhall P, et al. Altered allelic distribution of the serotonin transporter gene in migraine without aura and migraine with aura. *Cephalalgia* 1998;18:23–26.

77. Ohta M, Araki S, Kuroiwa Y. Familial occurrence of migraine with a hemiplegic syndrome and cerebellar manifestations. *Neurology* 1967;17:813–817.

78. Olesen J, Larsen B, Lauritzen M. Focal hyperemia followed by spreading oligemia and impaired activation of rCBF in classic migraine. *Ann Neurol* 1981;9:344–352.

79. Olesen J, Tfelt-Hansen P, Henriksen L, Larsen B. The common migraine attack may not be initiated by cerebral ischaemia. *Lancet* 1981;2:438–440.

80. Olesen J, Thomsen LL, Iversen H. Nitric oxide is a key molecule in migraine and other vascular headaches. *Trends Pharmacol Sci* 1994;15:149–153.

81. Ooki S, Yamaha K, Asaka A, Hayakawa K. Zygosity diagnosis of twins by questionnaire. *Acta Genet Med Gemellol (Roma)* 1990;39:109–115.

82. Ophoff RA, Terwindt GM, Vergouwe MN, et al. Familial hemiplegic migraine and episodic ataxia type-2 are caused by mutations in the Ca^{2+} channel gene CACNL1A4. *Cell* 1996;1:543–552.

83. Ophoff R.A, van Eijk R, Sandkuijl LA, et al. Genetic heterogeneity of familial hemiplegic migraine. *Genomics* 1994;1:21–26.

84. Pembrey ME. Discordant identical twins. VI. Psoriasis and migraine. *Practitioner* 1972;209:846–850.

85. Peroutka SJ, Wilhoit T, Jones K. Clinical susceptibility to migraine with aura is modified by dopamine D2 receptor (DRD2) NcoI alleles. *Neurology* 1997;49:201–206.

86. Pietrobon D, Luvisetto S, Spagnolo M, et al. Effect of mutations linked to familial hemiplegic migraine of the biophysical properties of human alpha1A containingcalcium channels. *Soc Neurosci* 1998;24:21.

87. Rasmussen BK, Jensen R, Olesen J. Questionnaire versus clinical interview in the diagnosis of headache. *Headache* 1991;31:290–295.

88. Rasmussen BK, Jensen R, Schroll M, Olesen J. Epidemiology of headache in a general population—a prevalence study. *J Clin Epidemiol* 1991;44:1147–1157.

89. Rasmussen BK, Olesen J. Migraine with aura and migraine without aura: an epidemiological study. *Cephalalgia* 1992;12:221–228.

90. Rasmussen BK. Migraine and tension-type headache in a general population: psychosocial factors. *Int J Epidemiol* 1992;21:1138–1143.

91. Riess O, Schols L, Bottger H, et al. SCA6 is caused by moderate CAG expansion in the alpha1A-voltage-dependent calcium channel gene. *Hum Mol Genet* 1997;6:1289–1293.

92. Russell MB. Genetic epidemiology of migraine and cluster headache. *Cephalalgia* 1997;17:683–701.

93. Russell MB, Diamant M, Norby S. Genetic heterogeneity of migraine with and without aura in Danes cannot be explained by mutation in mtDNA nucleotide pair 11084. *Acta Neurol Scand* 1997;96:171–173.

94. Russell MB, Fenger K, Olesen J. The family history of migraine. Direct versus indirect information. *Cephalalgia* 1996;16:156–160.

95. Russell MB, Iselius L, Olesen J. Investigation of the inheritance of migraine by complex segregation analysis. *Hum Genet* 1995;96:726–730.

96. Russell MB, Iversen HK, Olesen J. Improved description of the migraine aura by a diagnostic aura diary [see Comments]. *Cephalalgia* 1994;14:107–117.

97. Russell MB, Olesen J. The genetics of migraine without aura and migraine with aura. *Cephalalgia* 1993;13:245–248.

98. Russell MB, Olesen J. Increased familial risk and evidence of genetic factor in migraine. *BMJ* 1995;311:541–544.

99. Russell MB, Olesen J. A nosographic analysis of the migraine aura in a general population. *Brain* 1996;119:355–361.

100. Russell MB, Rasmussen BK, Brennum J, Iversen HK, Jensen RA, Olesen J. Presentation of a new instrument: the diagnostic headache diary. *Cephalalgia* 1992;12:369–374.

101. Russell MB, Rasmussen BK, Fenger K, Olesen J. Migraine without aura and migraine with aura are distinct clinical entities: a study of four hundred and eighty-four male and female migraineurs from the general population [see Comments]. *Cephalalgia* 1996;16:239–245.

102. Russell MB, Rasmussen BK, Thorvaldsen P, Olesen J. Prevalence and sex-ratio of the subtypes of migraine. *Int J Epidemiol* 1995;24:612–618.

103. Shimomura T, Kitano A, Merukawa H, Takahashi K. Mutation in platelet mitochondrial gene in patients with migraine. *Cephalalgia* 1995;15:10.

104. Sicuteri F, Testi A, Anselmi B. Biochemical investigations in headache: increase in the hydroxyindoleacetic acid excretion during migraine attacks. *Int Arch Allergy* 1961;19:55–58.

105. Starr TV, Prystay W, Snutch TP. Primary structure of a calcium channel that is highly expressed in the rat cerebellum. *Proc Natl Acad Sci U S A* 1991;88:5621–5625.

106. Stea A, Soon TW, Snutch TP. Voltage-gated calcium channels. In: North RA, ed. *Handbook of receptors and channels. Ligand- and voltage-gated ion channels.* Boca Raton, FL: CRC Press, 1995:113–153.

107. Stewart WF, Staffa J, Lipton RB, Ottman R. Familial risk of migraine: a population-based study. *Ann Neurol* 1997;41:166–172.

108. Svendsen B.B. Different course of migraine in monozygotic twins. *Acta Psychiatr Scand* 1952;27:165–174.

109. Teh BT, Silburn P, Lindblad K, et al. Familial periodic cerebellar ataxia without myokymia maps to a 19-cM region on chromosome 19p13. *Am J Hum Genet* 1995;56:1443–1449.

110. Terwindt GM. *Clinical genetics of migraine.* Leiden: Terwindt, 1998.

111. Terwindt GM, Haan J, Ophoff RA, et al. Clinical and genetic analysis of a large Dutch family with autosomal dominant vascular retinopathy, migraine and Raynaud's phenomenon. *Brain* 1998;121:303–316.

112. Terwindt GM, Ophoff RA, Haan J, Sandkuijl LA, Frants RR, Ferrari MD. Migraine, ataxia and epilepsy: a challenging spectrum of genetically determined calcium channelopathies. Dutch Migraine Genetics Research Group. *Eur J Hum Genet* 1998;6:297–307.

113. Terwindt GM, Ophoff RA, Haan J, et al. Variable clinical expression of mutations in the P/Q-type calcium channel gene in familial hemiplegic migraine. Dutch Migraine Genetics Research Group. *Neurology* 1998;50:1105–1110.

114. Thomson G. Identifying complex disease genes: progress and paradigms. *Nat Genet* 1994;8:108–110.

115. Tournier Lasserve E, Joutel A, Melki J, et al. Cerebral autosomal dominant arteriopathy with subcortical infarcts and leukoencephalopathy maps to chromosome 19q12. *Nat Genet* 1993;3:256–259.

116. Ulrich V, Gervil M, Kyvik KO, Olesen J, Russell MB. Evidence of a genetic factor in migraine with aura: a population based Danish twin study. *Ann Neurol* 1999;45:242–246.

117. Ulrich V, Gervil M, Kyvik KO, Olesen J, Russell MB. The inheritance of migraine with aura estimated by means of a structural equation modelling. *J Med Genet* 1999;36:225–227.

118. Ulrich V, Russell MB, Østergaard S, Olesen J. Analysis of 31 families with an apparently autosomal dominant transmission of migraine with aura in the nuclear families. *Am J Med Genet* 1997;74:395–397.

119. Vahedi K, Joutel A, Van Bogaert P, et al. A gene for hereditary paroxysmal cerebellar ataxia maps to chromosome 19p [see Comments]. *Ann Neurol* 1995;37:289–293.

120. Verin M, Rolland Y, Landgraf F, et al. New phenotype of the cerebral autosomal dominant arteriopathy mapped to chromosome 19: migraine as the prominent clinical feature. *J Neurol Neurosurg Psychiatry* 1995;59:579–585.

121. Vighetto A, Froment J.C, Trillet M, Aimard G. Magnetic resonance imaging in familial paroxysmal ataxia. *Arch Neurol* 1988;45:547–549.

122. Vogel F, Motulsky AG. *Hum Genet* 1986.

123. von Breederlow B, Hahn AF, Koopman WJ, Ebers GC, Bulman DE. Mapping the gene for acetazolamide responsive hereditary paroxymal cerebellar ataxia to chromosome 19p. *Hum Mol Genet* 1995;4:279–284.

124. Weiller C, May A, Limmroth V, et al. Brain stem activation in spontaneous human migraine attacks. *Nat Med* 1995;1:658–660.

125. Wilkinson M, Blau JN. Are classical and common migraine different entities? *Headache* 1985;25:211–212.

126. Willis T. *Opera Omnia.* Amstelaedami: Henricum Wetstenium, 1682.

127. Yue Q, Jen JC, Thwe MM, Nelson SF, Baloh RW. *De novo* mutation in *CACNA1A* caused acetazolamide-responsive episodic ataxia. *Am J Med Genet* 1998;26:298–301.

128. Zhuchenko O, Bailey J, Bonnen P, et al. Autosomal dominant cerebellar ataxia (SCA6) associated with small polyglutamine expansions in the alpha 1A-voltage-dependent calcium channel. *Nat Genet* 1997;15:62–69.

The Headaches, Second Edition,
edited by J. Olesen, P. Tfelt-Hansen, and K.M.A. Welch.
Lippincott Williams & Wilkins, Philadelphia © 2000.

The Migraines

CHAPTER 31

Biochemistry of Systemic and Jugular Venous Blood

Michel D. Ferrari and Flemming W. Bach

Since the observation by Sicuteri and colleagues (47) that the urinary excretion of 5-hydroxyindoleacetic-acid (5-HIAA), the main metabolite of serotonin (5-hydroxytryptamine; 5-HT), may be increased during migraine attacks, many biochemical studies on migraine have been published (1,10). Most of these addressed the role of platelets and are discussed in Chapter 33. In this chapter, only the most striking and best substantiated observations for plasma and urine are reviewed. Where necessary, the relevant changes in the platelet are discussed as well. Often, several studies measuring the same substances disagree on the results, not the least on differences within clinical subgroups. It should be emphasized that the frequently seen low ratio between estimated differences between groups and intragroup variations implies that results from studies including few subjects may not be meaningful.

SEROTONIN METABOLISM

In blood, most 5-HT is stored in platelets. The changes that are found in migraine in this intracellular and pharmacologically inactive portion of 5-HT in blood are remarkably consistent. There is much confusion, however, regarding the changes in the pharmacologically active extracellular portion of 5-HT in blood (1,10,21, 31). This is largely due to the inconsistent use of designations such as plasma and serum 5-HT. The term

M. D. Ferrari: Department of Neurology, Leiden University Medical Centre, NL-2300 RC Leiden, The Netherlands.
F. W. Bach: Department of Neurology, University of Århus, Århus Kommunehospital, DK-8000 Århus, Denmark.

"plasma 5-HT" should be reserved for the 5-HT content of platelet-free plasma. It should not be used when the 5-HT concentration of platelet-rich plasma is investigated because this reflects predominantly the 5-HT content of platelets (1). Likewise, serum 5-HT refers to the level of 5-HT in the supernatant of clotted blood. During the process of serum preparation, blood is coagulated, causing activation and aggregation of platelets and thus releasing 5-HT. In this chapter, the term "plasma 5-HT" is used to indicate the concentration of 5-HT in platelet-free plasma.

A clear and consistent finding is that platelet 5-HT content decreases by approximately 40% during migraine attacks without aura (1,10,29,21,31). It should be noted, however, that during migraine attacks with aura in 10 subjects, no such decrease could be demonstrated (19). The release of platelet 5-HT during attacks of migraine without aura has been suggested to be due to a serotonin-releasing factor (1). However, methodologic and statistical flaws were pointed out in the studies that have suggested such a releasing factor (18). Thus, although often this is not recognized, there is no conclusive evidence that plasma obtained during a migraine attack induces release of platelet 5-HT.

In contrast to the markedly different behavior of platelet 5-HT, (platelet-free) plasma levels of 5-HT and 5-HIAA show similar changes during migraine attacks with and without aura. Between attacks, migraine patients have significantly lower 5-HT and higher 5-HIAA levels in plasma than do controls (19). During migraine attacks, plasma 5-HT levels are about twice as high as during the attack-free period (19,49), reaching control levels, whereas the 5-HIAA concentration is reduced (19).

The increase of plasma 5-HT during migraine attacks is not due solely to release of platelet 5-HT. More likely, systemic turnover of 5-HT is enhanced in migraine patients between attacks, causing low interictal plasma 5-HT levels. During attacks, turnover of 5-HT is reduced, resulting in transient normalization of plasma 5-HT levels. Because the activities of enzymes involved in 5-HT metabolism are reduced during migraine attacks (1,10,19), the ictal reduction in turnover rate may be due to a transient decrease in enzymatic degradation. Serum 5-HT concentrations were found to be increased between attacks in migraine with aura compared with healthy control subjects and migraine without aura (20). The same study showed twofold increments in 5-HT serum concentrations in the first 3 hours of migraine attacks both with and without aura (20).

It thus appears that migraine occurs in patients with reduced pharmacologically active 5-HT, which in turn may affect the cranial vascular system. The ictal increase in plasma 5-HT may then be regarded as a self-defense mechanism of the body. The observations that intravenously injected 5-HT (31) and 5-HT$_1$ receptor agonists (13,31,44) abort migraine attacks do indeed support this hypothesis.

Urine data on 5-HT metabolism are less consistent. The often cited finding of Sicuteri et al. (47) of increased urinary excretion of 5-HIAA during migraine attacks has been confirmed by two other groups but has been negated by at least three others (1,10,14). This may have been related to wide interindividual variation for 5-HIAA excretion and important methodologic differences between the various studies. These include method of urine sampling, addition of acid to the urine, correction for differences in excretion of creatinine, and differentiation of diurnal and nocturnal urine. In fact, by comparing the same patients outside and during an attack and by accounting for the circadian rhythm, Ferrari and Odink (14) found reduced diurnal urinary excretion of 5-HIAA per mol creatinine during migraine attacks compared with the diurnal excretion during headache-free periods. This finding and Anthony's (1) observation that urine 5-HT was increased during attacks are indeed in keeping with the hypothesis that systemic 5-HT metabolism may be reduced during migraine attacks.

During attack-free periods, Bousser and colleagues have found a marked reduction of urinary 5-HIAA per mol creatinine in female migraine patients compared with sex-matched controls (9). No such difference was found for male migraine patients. From the description of methods, it was not clear whether this reflected 24-hour, diurnal, nocturnal, or mixed urine samples. In the study of Ferrari and Odink (14), diurnal (but not nocturnal) urinary 5-HIAA tended to be lower in (mainly female) migraine patients, without, however, reaching statistical significance. In fact the most important finding in that study was reversal of the circadian rhythm of urinary 5-HIAA excretion in migraine patients compared with controls.

NEUROEXCITATORY AND -INHIBITORY AMINO ACIDS AND MAGNESIUM

Glutamic (Glu) and aspartic (Asp) acids are important neuroexcitatory amino acids in the brain. Their endogenous release and action of N-methyl-D-aspartate (NMDA) receptors play a pivotal role in the initiation, propagation, and duration of spreading depression (SD), which is implicated in the mechanism of the migraine aura (34). Magnesium may modulate the sensitivity of the NMDA receptor to Glu: low magnesium levels potentiate and high levels inhibit (37). Finally, excessive oral intake of Glu may induce migrainelike features in sensitive subjects (45).

We have found that migraine patients have substantially higher Glu and Asp plasma levels during attack-free periods than do controls (15). Patients with migraine attacks with aura have significantly higher levels than do those who suffer from attacks without aura (15). During attacks, Glu (and to a lesser extent Asp) levels are even further increased, the highest levels being reached in patients with migraine with aura (15).

In blood, Glu is stored mainly in the erythrocytes due to an active cellular uptake mechanism, thereby keeping the plasma Glu content low. The function of the Glu carrier system in blood cells seems to reflect the function of the same system at the neuronal-glial cell level. We therefore have hypothesized that the elevated plasma levels of Glu and Asp are caused by a defect of the Glu/Asp

TABLE 1. *Review of mean (x) red blood cell magnesium levels (mM) in migraine patients between attacks.*

	Schoenen (47)		Gallai (22)		Facchinetti (11)		Smeets (48)	
	n	x̄	n	x̄	n	x̄	n	x̄
Migraine without aura	38	1.9*	60	2.1[a]			23	2.1
Migraine with aura	6	2.1	30	2.1[a]			9	2.3
Familial hemiplegic migraine (FHM)							38	2.1
Non-afflicted FHM							11	2.1
Menstrual migraine					20	1.6		
Controls	19	2.1	30	2.4	15	1.7	32	2.1

Measures of variability are omitted for clarity.
[a]Significantly different from control.

uptake mechanism of the erythrocyte, reflecting a similar defect at the neuronal-glial cell level. This may lead to elevated levels of Glu and Asp at the NMDA receptor, predisposing the brains of migraine patients to develop SD. Patients whose migraine attacks were virtually always preceded by an aura (and thus by SD) had much higher plasma levels of Glu and Asp than did patients whose attacks were virtually never preceded by an aura. Interestingly, D'Andrea et al. found elevated platelet levels of Glu and Asp only in migraine patients with aura and not in migraine patients without aura (7,8), whereas plasma glutamic acid concentrations were only increased in migraine without aura and normal in subjects with aura (7). It thus appears that patients who suffer migraine attacks with aura are just more prone to develop SD than are patients who suffer migraine attacks without aura.

This hypothesis is corroborated by the observations that in migraine patients intracellular Mg^{2+} is reduced during attacks in brain (42) and serum (23,43) and between attacks in blood (12,23,43,46), which may potentiate the sensitivity of the NMDA receptor to Glu. Interestingly, Mg^{2+} supplementation did seem to ameliorate menstrual migraine attacks (12). On the other hand, platelet Mg^{2+} levels were similar in patients with or without aura and in control subjects (39), and Smeets et al. (48) found no differences in either plasma or blood cell levels between migraine patients and healthy controls. Importantly, neither were there differences between afflicted and nonafflicted members of families with familial hemiplegic migraine. Based on the accumulated evidence summarized in Tables 1 and 2, we conclude that no consistent pattern can be detected with respect to circulating magnesium levels in migraine patients. Differences between migrainous and nonmigrainous subjects, if any, are small and variable, and they certainly do not parallel presence or absence or severity of aura symptoms. A causal relationship between reduced total blood magnesium levels and migraine pathophysiology therefore seems unlikely. However, a role of magnesium in the brain might be involved in migraine pathophysiology.

TABLE 2. *Review of mean (x) serum magnesium levels (mM) in migraine between attacks.*

	Schoenen (47)		Gallai (22)		Sarchielli (43)	
	n	x	n	x	n	x
Migraine without aura	38	0.92	31	0.71*	41	0.72*
Migraine with aura	6	0.67	15	0.74*	29	0.81*
Control	19	0.94	31	1.03	40	1.02

Measures of variability are omitted for clarity.
[a]Significantly different from control.

Platelet concentrations of the inhibitory amino acid GABA were similar in migraine without aura between attacks and in healthy control subjects (33).

OPIOID PEPTIDES

Data on changes in plasma levels of endogenous opioid peptides are conflicting, most likely due to methodologic differences and difficulties (2,11). Thus far, it has not been convincingly shown that β-endorphin levels are altered in migraine patients (2,11), or that the levels change during attack (3) or following sumatriptan therapy (25). Recently, Leone et al. (35) suggested that peripheral blood mononuclear cell β-endorphin concentrations are reduced in migraine patients with and without aura during attack-free periods. No change in plasma dynorphin was seen during migraine attacks (4). Measurements of plasma and platelet levels of methionine-enkephalin seem to be reasonably consistent despite the methodologic obstacles of large quantities in platelets and much lower levels in plasma (6, 17,40,41). The general picture is that migraine patients have low plasma and high platelet methionine-enkephalin levels during attack-free periods compared with control subjects, and both platelet and plasma methionine-enkephalin levels increase considerably during attacks (6, 17,40,41). So far, no satisfactory pathophysiologic explanation has been provided for these changes.

Before conclusions are made from measurements on circulating opioid peptides, it should be emphasized that the peptides do not cross the blood–brain barrier to a significant extent and do not act directly on central neural pathways. Secondly, it still remains to be shown that circulating opioid peptides may influence peripheral pain mechanisms or vascular headache mechanisms. However, like other substances, the peptides may serve as markers of more or less specific pathophysiologic events during migraine.

VASOACTIVE NEUROPEPTIDES

Moskowitz has presented compelling evidence, although still based only on animal experiments, that vasoactive neuropeptides and the trigeminovascular system are implicated in the pathophysiology of the headache in migraine (see Chapter 17). In support of this theory are the human experiments of Goadsby et al. (26,28). They showed that thermocoagulation of the trigeminal ganglion causes marked ipsilateral elevation in the plasma levels of substance P and calcitonin gene-related peptide (CGRP), coinciding with ipsilateral facial flushing. Furthermore, during migraine attacks, there was a selective increase of plasma levels of the powerful vasodilator CGRP but not of other neuropeptides such as neuropeptide Y (NPY), vasoactive intestinal polypeptide (VIP), and substance P (28). Finally, they demonstrated that the selective 5-HT receptor agonist sumatriptan (44), which is highly effective in the treatment of migraine attacks (13), normalizes

TABLE 3. *Release of vasoactive peptides to plasma during attacks of migraine with or without aura*

Release	No release
• CGRP	• Substance-P
• Neurokinin A	• NPY
• Endothelin-1	• VIP
	• ACTH
	• Vasopressin

CGRP levels during migraine attacks (26). In these studies, changes were observed only in blood withdrawn from the external jugular vein, not in blood withdrawn from the antecubital vein, suggesting localized craniovascular changes during the attack. Friberg et al. presented data from four patients who developed migraine during carotid angiography (22). No systematic differences in CGRP, substance P, NPY, or VIP concentrations were seen between internal jugular vein and carotid artery blood. It may be debated if dilution in the internal jugular vein or the small number of subjects explains the divergence from the data of Goadsby et al. (26,28).

Using measurements of peripheral venous blood, Gallai et al. reported increased concentrations of CGRP and neurokinin A (NKA) (24). As in a previous study (5), they saw no change in substance P levels. Neither did VIP, vasopressin (5), or adrenocorticotrophin (ACTH) (3) change during attacks. Although strictly speaking not a neuropeptide, the strongly vasoactive peptide endothelin-1 should be mentioned here. Peripheral plasma concentrations increase particularly in the early phase of migraine attacks (24,32).

It may be appreciated from Table 3 that studies measuring peptides in the circulation have provided means of testing the clinical relevance in humans of experimental models of pathophysiologic factors in migraine.

CATECHOLAMINES AND PURINES

Plasma levels and urinary excretion patterns of catecholamines and their metabolites generally have been inconclusive (1), possibly due to researchers not accounting for circadian rhythms. The enzyme dopamine-beta-hydroxylase (DBH) was found to be elevated in headache-free migraine patients (29,36), increasing further during the attack (1). This would point to sympathetic overactivity in migraine patients. Available biochemical data are insufficient to confirm this hypothesis (38).

TABLE 4. *Differences between migraine with aura (MA) and migraine without aura (MO) between and during attacks*

Parameter	Period	Diagnosis MA (N = 10)	Diagnosis MO (N = 21)	Difference[a] MA-MO	Effect[b] attack	Diag[c] attack
5-HIAA (plasma)	A-free	143**	105	<0.01		
				<0.005	<0.02	NS
	Attack	113	92			
GLU (plasma)	A-free	173**	129	NS		
				<0.05	<0.001	NS
	Attack	248***	168**	<0.01		
TRP (plasma)	A-free	106	92	NS		
				<0.05	NS	NS
	Attack	105	85	<0.05		
HIS (plasma)	A-free	94	82**	<0.02		
				<0.05	NS	NS
	Attack	94	84**	NS		
MET (platelet)	A-free	268	448**	NS		
				<0.05	<0.001	NS
	Attack	359**	691**	<0.01		
5-HT (platelet)	A-free	110	124	NS		
				NS	<0.005	<0.02
	Attack	115	71	NS		
PST-M (platelet)	A-free	79	97	NS		
				NS	<0.005	<0.05
	Attack	80	83	NS		

Mean values are expressed as percentage of mean control values.

[a] p_1 for difference between attack-free values; p_2 for difference when using both attack and attack-free values; p_3 for difference between attack values.

[b] Difference between attack and attack-free value.

[c] Difference between effect of MA and MO attacks, values for difference from control values: **$p < 0.005$, ***$p < 0.001$.

TRP, tryptophane; HIS, histidine; PST-M, phenol-sylfo-transferase-M.

One study found a 68% increase in circulating levels of the vasodilator adenosine during attacks of migraine without aura (30).

BIOCHEMICAL DIFFERENCES BETWEEN MIGRAINE WITH AND WITHOUT AURA

Ferrari et al. (15–19) have investigated whether, and to what extent, patients who have virtually always (in greater than 80% of their attacks) migraine attacks with aura and patients who have virtually always migraine attacks without aura differ biochemically. All subjects investigated were free of medication for at least 12 days. The most striking differences are summarized in Table 4.

Patients with migraine attacks with aura showed more elevated plasma Glu (15,16) but less elevated platelet methionine-enkaphalin levels (compared with healthy controls) than did patients with attacks without aura (16, 17). Plasma histidine (HIS) concentration was reduced compared with controls in patients who had attacks without aura but not in those who had attacks with aura (15, 16). The biochemical effect of the attack also differed markedly: platelet 5-HT and platelet phenol-sulfo-transferase-M activity clearly decreased during migraine attacks without aura but not during attacks with aura (15, 18).

In conclusion, patients who get migraine attacks with aura are biochemically clearly distinct from patients who get attacks without aura. Although we found primarily quantitative differences between the two patient groups (i.e., in both groups abnormal compared with healthy controls but differing in degree), qualitative differences (abnormal in only one group) also appear to exist. Because the prevailing attack type may change over life, it would be interesting to see if the biochemical variables also change.

BIOCHEMICAL DIFFERENCES BETWEEN MIGRAINE WITHOUT AURA AND TENSION-TYPE HEADACHE

We also investigated whether, and to what extent, patients with migraine without aura and patients with tension-type headache differ biochemically (15–19). The most important differences are summarized in Chapter 78. It appears that there are striking biochemical differences between patients with migraine and patients with tension-type headache, suggesting the feasability of a discriminant diagnosis based on biological markers. This should be confirmed in a validation study.

REFERENCES

1. Anthony M. The biochemistry of migraine. In: Vinken PJ, Bruyn GW, Clifford Rose F, eds. *Handbook of clinical neurology.* Vol. 4 (48). Headache. Amsterdam: Elsevier Science, 1986:85–105.
2. Bach FW. Opioid peptides in primary headaches. In: Olesen J, Edvins-son L, eds. *Frontiers in headache research.* Vol. 7. Headache pathogenesis. Monoamines, neuropeptides, purines, and nitric oxide. Philidelphia: Lippincott-Raven, 1997:193–200.
3. Bach FW, Jensen K, Blegvad N, Fenger M, Jordal R, Olesen J. β-endorphin and ACTH in plasma during attacks of common and classic migraine. *Cephalalgia* 1985;5:177–182.
4. Bach FW, Jensen K, Ekman R, Olesen J. Dynorphin-immunoreactivity in plasma during migraine attacks. *Cephalalgia* 1987;7[suppl 6]: 232–233.
5. Blegvad N, Jensen K, Fahrenkrug J, Schaffalitzky de Muckadell OB, Olesen J. Plasma VIP and substance-P during migraine attack. *Cephalalgia* 1986;5[suppl 5]:352–353.
6. Boiardi A, Picotti GB, Di Giulio AM, et al. Platelet MET-enkephalin immunoreactivity and 5-hydroxytryptamine concentrations in migraine patients: effects of 5-Hydroxy-tryptophan, amitriptyline and chloorimipramine treatment. *Cephalalgia* 1984;4:81–84.
7. Cananzi AR, D'Andrea G, Perini F, Zamberlan F, Welch KMA. Platelet and plasma levels of glutamate and glutamine in migraine with and without aura. *Cephalalgia* 1995;15:132–135.
8. D'Andrea G, Cananzi AR, Joseph R, et al. Platelet glycine, glutamate and aspartate in primary headache. *Cephalalgia* 1991;11:197–200.
9. de Lignieres B, Vincens M, Mauvais-Jarvis P, Mas JL, Touboul PJ, Bousser MG. Prevention of menstrual migraine by percutaneous oestradiol. *Br Med J* 1986;293:1540.
10. Eadie MJ, Tyrer JH. *The biochemistry of migraine.* Lancaster: MTP Press, 1985.
11. Facchinetti F, Genazzani AR. Opioids in cerebrospinal fluid and blood of headache sufferers. In: Olesen J, Edvinsson L, eds. *Basic mechanism of headache.* Amsterdam: Elsevier Science, 1988:261–269.
12. Facchinetti F, Sances G, Borella P, Genazzani AR, Nappi G. Magnesium prophylaxis of menstrual migraine: effects on intracellular magnesium. *Headache* 1991;31:298–301.
13. Ferrari MD, Melamed E, Gawel M, et al. (The Subcutaneous Sumatriptan International Study Group.) Treatment of migraine attacks with sumatriptan. *N Engl J Med* 1991;325:316–321.
14. Ferrari MD, Odink J. Urinary excretion of biogenic amines in migraine and tension headache. In: Clifford Rose F, ed. *New advances in headache research.* London: Smith-Gordon & Co, 1989:85–88.
15. Ferrari MD, Odink J, Bos KD, Malessy MJA, Bruyn GW. Neuro-excitatory plasma aminoacids are elevated in migraine. *Neurology* 1990;40: 1582–1586.
16. Ferrari MD, Odink J, Bruyn GW. Biochemical differences between classic migraine, common migraine and tension headache. In: Ferrari MD, Lataste X, eds. *New trends in clinical neurology: migraine and other headaches.* Carnforth, NJ: Parthenon, 1989:151–160.
17. Ferrari MD, Odink J, Frölich M, Portielje JEA, Bruyn GW. Methionine-enkephalin in migraine and tension headache. Differences between classic migraine, common migraine and tension headache, and changes during attacks. *Headache* 1990;30:160–164.
18. Ferrari MD, Odink J, Frölich M, Tapparelli C, Portielje JEA. Release of platelet MET-enkephalin, but not serotonin, in migraine. *J Neurol Sci* 1989;93:51–60.
19. Ferrari MD, Odink J, Tapparelli C, Van Kempen GMJ, Pennings EJM, Bruyn GW. Serotonin metabolism in migraine. *Neurology* 1989;39: 1239–1242.
20. Fontes Ribeiro CA, Cotrim MD, Morgadinho MT, Ramos MI, Seabra Santos E, Macedo TRA. Migraine, serum serotonin and platelet 5-HT₂ receptors. *Cephalalgia* 1990;10:213–219.
21. Fozard JR. Serotonin, migraine and platelets. *Prog Pharmacol* 1982; 4:135–146.
22. Friberg L, Olesen J, Skyhøj Olsen T, Karle A, Ekman R, Fahrenkrug J. Absence of vasoactive peptide release from brain to cerebral circulation during onset of migraine with aura. *Cephalalgia* 1994;14:47–54.
23. Gallai V, Sarchielli P, Coata G, Firenze C, Morucci P, Abbritti G. Serum and salivary magnesium levels in migraine. Results in a group of juvenile patients. *Headache* 1992;32:132–135.
24. Gallai V, Sarchielli P, Firenze C, et al. Endothelin 1 in migraine and tension-type headache. *Acta Neurol Scand* 1994;89:47–55.
25. Gallai V, Sarchielli P, Floridi A, et al. Vasoactive peptide levels in the plasma of young migraine patients with and without aura assessed both interictally and ictally. *Cephalalgia* 1995;15:384–390.
26. Goadsby PJ, Edvinsson L. The trigeminovascular system and migraine: studies characterizing cerebrovascular and neuropeptide changes seen in humans and cats. *Ann Neurol* 1993;33:48–56.

27. Goadsby PJ, Edvinsson L, Ekman R. Release of vasoactive peptides in the extracerebral circulation of humans and the cat during activation of the trigeminovascular system. *Ann Neurol* 1988;23:193–196.

28. Goadsby PJ, Edvinsson L, Ekman R. Vasoactive peptide release in the extracerebral circulation of humans during migraine headache. *Ann Neurol* 1990;28:183–187.

29. Gotoh F, Kandra T, Sakai F, Yamamoto M, Takeoka T. Serum dopamine-beta-hydroxylase activity in migraine. *Arch Neurol* 1976;33:656–657.

30. Guieu R, Devaux C, Henry H, et al. Adenosine and migraine. *Can J Neurol Sci* 1998;25:55–58.

31. Humphrey PPA. 5-Hydroxytryptamine and the pathophysiology of migraine. *J Neurol* 1991;238[suppl]:38–44.

32. Kallela M, Färkkilä M, Saijonmaa O, Fyhrquist F. Endothelin in migraine patients. *Cephalalgia* 1998;18:329–332.

33. Kowa H, Shimomura, T, Takahashi K. Platelet gamma-aminobutyric acid levels in migraine and tension-type headache. *Headache* 1992;32:229–232.

34. Lauritzen M. Cortical spreading depression as a putative migraine mechanism. *Trends Neurosci* 1987;10:8–13.

35. Leone M, Sacerdote P, D'Amico D, Panerai AE, Bussone G. Beta-endorphin concentrations in the peripheral blood mononuclear cells of migraine and tension-type headache patients. *Cephalalgia* 1992;12:155–157.

36. Magos AL, Brincat M, Zilkha KJ, Studd JWW. Serum dopamine-beta-hydroxylase activity in menstrual migraine. *J Neurol Neurosurg Psychiatry* 1985;48:328–331.

37. Marrannes R, Willems R, De Prins E, Wauquier A. Evidence for a role of the *N*-methyl-*D*-aspartate (NMDA) receptor in cortical spreading depression in the rat. *Brain Res* 1988;457:226–240.

38. Mascia A, Áfra J, Schoenen J. Dopamine and migraine: a review of pharmacological, biochemical, neurophysiological, and therapeutic data. *Cephalalgia* 1998;18:174–182.

39. Mishima K, Takeshima T, Shimomura T, et al. Platelet ionized magnesium, cyclic AMP, and cyclic GMP levels in migraine and tension-type headache. *Headache* 1997;37:561–564.

40. Mosnaim AD, Chevesich J, Wolf ME, Freitag FG, Diamond S. Plasma methionine enkephalin. Increased levels during a migraine episode. *Headache* 1986;26:278–281.

41. Mosnaim AD, Wolf ME, Chevesich J, Callaghan OD, Diamond S. Plasma methionine enkephalin levels. A biological marker for migraine? *Headache* 1985;25:259–261.

42. Ramadan NM, Halvorson H, Vande-Linde A, Levine SR, Helpern JA, Welch KMA. Low brain magnesium in migraine. *Headache* 1989; 29:416–419.

43. Sarchielli P, Coata G, Firenze C, Morucci P, Abbritti G, Gallai V. Serum and salivary magnesium levels in migraine. Results in a group of adult patients. *Cephalalgia* 1992;12:21–27.

44. Saxena PR, Ferrari MD. 5-Hydroxytryptamine$_1$-like receptor agonists and migraine: possible impact on the pathophysiology of migraine. *Trends Pharmacol Sci* 1989;10:200–204.

45. Schaumburg HH, Byck R, Gerstl R, Mashman JH. Monosodium L-glutamate: its pharmacology and role in the Chinese restaurant syndrome. *Science* 1969;163:826–828.

46. Schoenen J, Sianard-Gainko J, Lenaerts M. Blood magnesium levels in migraine. *Cephalalgia* 1991;11:97–99.

47. Sicuteri F, Testi A, Anselmi B. Biochemical investigations in headache: increase in the hydroxyindoleacic acid excretion during migraine attacks. *Int Arch Allerg* 1961;19:55–58.

48. Smeets MC, Vernooy CB, Souverijn JHM, Ferrari MD. Intracellular and plasma magnesium in familial hemiplegic migraine and migraine with and without aura. *Cephalalgia* 1994;14:29–32.

49. Somerville BM. Platelet-bound and free serotonin levels in jugular and forearm venous blood during migraine. *Neurology* 1976;26:41–45.

The Headaches, Second Edition,
edited by J. Olesen, P. Tfelt-Hansen, and K.M.A. Welch.
Lippincott Williams & Wilkins, Philadelphia © 2000.

The Migraines

CHAPTER 32

Influence of Female Hormones on Migraine

Hélène Massiou and Marie-Germaine Bousser

The evidence is plentiful for a link between female hormones and migraine. The female preponderance of migraine appears after puberty; in many patients, migraine occurs at the time of menses and improves during pregnancy; hormonal treatments may modify the course of the migrainous disease.

MENARCHE AND MIGRAINE FEMALE PREPONDERANCE

The female:male ratio of migraine is around 1:1 during childhood, with even a small preponderance in boys. This trend is completely reversed after puberty, and the female:male incidence ratio in adults reaches 2:1 to 4:1. The female preponderance in adults is found for both types of migraine (40) and is related to the peak incidence of migraine in women at menarche, which concerns 10% to 20% of migraineurs. The influence of puberty might be different according to the type of migraine. In two studies (4,31), female preponderance was evident during childhood for migraine with aura, but not for migraine without aura; this difference, however, was not observed by other researchers (23).

MENSTRUAL MIGRAINE

There is no universally accepted definition of menstrual migraine, which is not recognized as such in the International Headache Society (IHS) classification. The peak incidence of migraine during the cycle is situated in a period stretching from 2 days before menstruation to the first few days of menstruation (18,45). More recently

menstrual migraine has been defined as attacks occurring from 2 days prior menses to the second, third, or last day of menstruation. The prevalence figures of menstrual migraine depend on its definition, as well as on the method of recording data. Studies based on patients' self-assessment usually lead to an overestimation. In studies using prospective diary cards, the percentage of migraineurs who suffer from menstrual migraine associated with other attacks during the cycles ranges from 24% to 56% (4,31). Pure menstrual migraine is defined as attacks that occur only at the time of menstruation and at no other time of the cycle. In the study of MacGregor et al. (18), 7.2% of the migraineurs had pure menstrual migraine. In some women, attacks occur at each menstruation, whereas in others they are inconstant, occurring only in some cycles. The link with menstruation is different for migraine without aura and migraine with aura. In the studies of Russell et al. (31) and Johannes et al. (13), migraine without aura but not migraine with aura showed a significant association with menstruation. Cupini et al. (4) found that menstrual migraine and pure menstrual migraine were significantly more frequent in patients with migraine without aura than in patients with migraine with aura. Menstrual migraine without aura is more frequent in women whose onset of this type of migraine takes place at menarche (31). It is still debated whether menstrual migraine is significantly associated with the psychological and physical symptoms of the premenstrual syndrome (8). It is classical to state that menstrual migraine attacks last longer, are more severe, and are more resistant to therapy than other attacks. This current view has not yet been confirmed by any comparative study. The efficacy of sumatriptan and zolmitriptan appears similar in menstrual attacks and in others (5,36). However, a higher rate of recurrence after sumatriptan has been observed in menstrual migraine (43).

H. Massiou: Department of Neurology, Hospital Lariboisière, 75475 Paris Cedex 10, France.

M.-G. Bousser: Department of Neurology, Lariboisière Medical Faculty, Paris VII University, and Department of Neurology, Hospital Lariboisière, 75475 Paris, France.

Attempts to find differences in ovarian hormone levels between women with menstrual migraine and controls have not yielded consistent results. Although some researchers have reported in patients with menstrual migraine higher estrogen and progestin levels, most researchers have not (34). Most found that testosterone, follicle-stimulating hormone, and luteinizing hormone (LH) levels were similar to those in controls. According to the experiments of Somerville (37,38), menstrual migraine appears related to the abrupt decrease in estradiol that occurs immediately before menstruation, after several days of exposure to high levels of estrogens. Estrogens given premenstrually, but not progesterone, can delay the onset of migraine. Why this abrupt decrease in plasma estradiol should precipitate an attack of migraine remains obscure. Serotonin receptors are modulated by estrogen and progesterone. Serotonin may increase prolactin release by inhibiting dopamine and by stimulating thyrotropin-releasing hormone (TRH). In women with menstrual migraine, enhanced prolactin release by dopaminergic antagonists occurs throughout the menstrual cycle, which suggests a central serotonin dysmodulation. Decreased functional hypothalamic opioid activity may explain the loss of LH response to naloxone in the last luteal phase in women with menstrual migraine, and a postsynaptic alpha 2 adrenoceptor hyposensitivity the lack of hormonal response to clonidine during the premenstrual period. Estrogen withdrawal increases the secretion of prostaglandins, which sensitize pain receptors and increase neurogenic inflammation (34).

The treatment of menstrual migraine relies first on the use of acute treatments of attacks with analgesics, nonsteroidal antiinflammatory drugs (NSAIDs), ergot derivatives, and triptans. Prophylactic perimenstrual treatments have been proposed, for a period lasting from 3 to 7 days before menstruation until 1 to 6 days after. Usual prophylactic drugs have been used, as have NSAIDs, ergotamine tartrate, and DHE nasal spray, but few properly controlled studies have been conducted to assess their efficacy in this specific indication. Numerous hormonal manipulations have been tried to prevent menstrual migraine. Progesterone was found ineffective, whereas some success has been observed with the use of synthetic androgen (danazol), antiestrogen (tamoxifen), dopamine agonists (bromocriptine), and LH-releasing hormone (LH-RH) analogues. However, these were mostly open studies or anecdotal reports so that the benefit:risk ratio of these hormonal treatments has not been scientifically established. Because estrogen withdrawal is the trigger of menstrual migraine, estrogen replacement prior to menstruation is the most logical approach and has long been attempted to prevent menstrual attacks. Estradiol implants have a good efficacy but suppress ovulation and all cyclic ovarian activity (19). The best results so far have been obtained with percutaneous estradiol gel, which was found superior to placebo in two double-blind control studies (6,7). Treat-

ment has to be started 48 hours before the anticipated migraine attack and used daily for the next 7 days, at a dose of 1.5 mg estradiol in 2.5 g of gel, which allows attainment of mean estradiol plasma levels of 80 pg/mL. This treatment is especially recommended for pure and regular menstrual migraine in women with regular cycles. In migraineurs suffering from menstrual migraine and from other migraine attacks during the cycle, the efficacy is less convincing. Patches of transcutaneous estradiol also have been studied in the prevention of menstrual migraine. Three dosages are available: Transdermal Therapeutic Express (TTS) 25, which delivers 25 µg of estradiol per 24 hours; TTS 50, which delivers 50 µg of estradiol per 24 hours; and TTS 100, which delivers 100 µg of estradiol per 24 hours. The estradiol serum levels reached with these patches are, respectively, 23 pg/mL, 39 pg/mL, and 74 pg/mL. TTS 50 was not found superior to placebo for the prevention of menstrual migraine in two double-blind trials (28,35), maybe due to too low a serum level. TTS 100 was found superior to TTS 25 in one open trial (29).

OVULATION

Some women establish a link between their migraine attacks and ovulation. This has not been confirmed in any epidemiologic study, where the observed and expected number of attacks associated with ovulation were not significantly different either in migraine without aura or in migraine with aura (18,31,45). This may be so because the peak of estrogen at ovulation is of short duration and the decrease of serum estrogen must be preceded by several days of exposure to high levels of estrogen in order to precipitate the attack. It is nevertheless possible that some women may go through a hypoestrogenic postovulatory phase long enough to trigger an attack.

MIGRAINE AND PREGNANCY

For details and references, the reader is referred to Chapter 131.

Influence of Pregnancy on the Course of Migraine

An improvement or a disappearance of migraine during pregnancy has been observed in 55% to 90% of cases. This beneficial effect of pregnancy is observed more frequently in women whose migraine began at menarche and in those with menstrual attacks. Some researchers have found that this improvement was limited to migraine without aura, was observed mainly in women in the last two trimesters of pregnancy, and tapered off in multiparous mothers, but such was not the case in all studies. Migraine may remain unchanged during pregnancy in 5% to 30% of cases. A worsening or a new onset of migraine also has been observed during this period, especially in migraine with aura.

Postpartum

About 30% to 40% of women suffer from headache during the first postpartum week. These headaches occur most often between day 3 and day 6 postpartum: some are tension-type headaches, sometimes related to the postpartum depression, but others meet the definition of migraine. Women with a prior history of migraine are more likely to develop postpartum migraine. These patients often describe their postpartum headaches as less painful than their usual attacks, but severe and repeated migraine attacks with and without aura also have been reported. Migraine frequently restarts or can begin *de novo* in the postpartum period.

Mechanisms

Sustained high estrogen levels have been proposed as the mechanism of migraine relief that often occurs during pregnancy, and the rapid decrease of these hormones at the time of delivery might then trigger postpartum headaches. It cannot explain, however, the worsening or new appearance of migraine that sometimes occurs. No statistical difference in progesterone levels, measured near term, are found between women who did and women who did not have migraine relief during pregnancy, suggesting that migraine relief does not depend on the absolute blood level of progesterone. Other suggestions concern changes of the serotonin metabolism during pregnancy and increased endorphin levels during the preceding two trimesters.

Consequences of Migraine on Pregnancy

Several researchers have studied the correlation between migraine and pregnancy-induced hypertension. Three of four studies concluded positively (20,22,30), one negatively (44). The two oldest studies (30,44) had important methodologic bias. In the most recent study (20), a positive correlation was found between migraine and preeclampsia [adjusted odds ratio, 2.44; confidence interval (CI), 1.42–4.20], and between migraine and gestational hypertension (adjusted odds ratio, 1.7; CI, 1.02–2.85). However, the IHS criteria for the diagnosis of migraine were not used in this study.

Treatment of Migraine during Pregnancy

Because migraine usually improves during pregnancy, many women can manage their headaches with nonpharmacologic methods, such as relaxation, biofeedback, or local application of ice. Some women, however, continue to have severe attacks, which require drug treatments. Few data are available about the risks of antimigrainous drugs during pregnancy, delivery, and breastfeeding. Whether a drug is present in breast milk and in which amount is often difficult to know because of the variability of the composition of the milk and the frequent lack of specific information. Recommendations about drug use during pregnancy come from sometimes conflicting sources (references in 33). All the details on the birth defect risks from antimigraine drugs exposure are developed in Chapter 131, and we will give here only the main guidelines for the treatment of migraine during pregnancy.

For acute treatment, paracetamol is the first choice drug. In case of inefficacy, aspirin and NSAIDs may be prescribed. Their use should be limited during the third trimester because they inhibit labor, prolong pregnancy, increase maternal and newborn bleeding, and may narrow the ductus arteriosus. Paracetamol and NSAIDs are compatible with breastfeeding, and caution is required with aspirin. Ergot derivatives are classically contraindicated during pregnancy because of their uterotonic effect; their teratogenic effects are uncertain, and they are contraindicated during lactation. There have been no adequate, well-controlled studies in pregnant women with the serotonin agonists (triptans). Metoclopramide may be used in case of nausea or vomiting.

Prophylactic drugs should be discontinued when pregnancy is considered because they are rarely necessary during pregnancy. If needed, beta-blockers may be proposed. There is no evidence of teratogenicity, but fetal and neonatal toxicity may occur, leading to intrauterine growth retardation, hypoglycemia, bradycardia, and respiratory depression. Caution is required in case of migraine with aura because cases of worsening of this type of migraine have been reported with beta-blockers. Their use is compatible with lactation. The data on amitriptyline are conflicting: malformations have been reported, but its teratogenicity has not been confirmed. It may be used, especially in case of status migrainosus. It should be stopped at least 7 weeks prior to delivery to decrease the risk of a neonatal withdrawal syndrome, including respiratory distress and feeding difficulties. Amitriptyline should be avoided during lactation.

MIGRAINE AND ORAL CONTRACEPTION

Prescribing oral contraceptives in migrainous women raises two issues: What is the influence of oral contraception on the course of migraine? What is the risk of stroke in migraineurs who take oral contraceptives?

Influence of Oral Contraception on the Course of Migraine

The influence of oral contraception on the course of migraine is largely variable according to the researchers. A worsening in frequency or severity has been reported in 18% to 50% of the cases, with a net tendency for attacks to occur during the drug-free interval of the cycle

(14,15,32). By contrast, as many as 30% to 40% of women report an improvement or no change of their migraine. A migrainous disease can begin during oral contraceptive use, usually during the first months' cycles, sometimes after prolonged use. Such new-onset migraines occur more often in women with a family history of migraine. However, Kudrow (14) found a family history less frequently in women with a migraine starting with oral contraceptive use (40%) than in those who had migraine before oral contraceptive use (72%). This suggests that the pill may induce attacks in susceptible persons, but in some cases may also play a direct role in the initiation of a migrainous disease. Stopping oral contraceptives when migraine starts with their use may have a variable effect: the relief may occur immediately, or after a delay of 6 to 12 months, and in some patients migraine can continue on a long-term basis. The role of the pills' content remains debated. No large comparative trials are available to determine whether some pills are preferable to others in a migraineur. Empirical strategies are then necessary to determine the best solution in each patient.

Migraine, Oral Contraceptives, and Risk of Stroke

Oral contraceptive use is associated with an increased risk of ischemic stroke. The relative risk depends on the estrogen content of the pill. Recent studies (11,16,26,46) have shown that the adjusted odds ratio for ischemic stroke ranges from 3.5 to 5.3 with pills containing 50 mg or more of ethynil-estradiol, and from 1.5 to 3.2 with pills containing less than 50 mg of ethynil-estradiol (Table 1). In some of these studies (16,46), the ischemic risk was even not significantly increased with pills containing less than 50 mg of ethynil-estradiol or with pure progestative pills. Heinemann (11) found no significant difference for the risk of ischemic stroke between second-generation and third-generation pills, the latter containing gestodene or desogestrel. Because pills currently used contain low doses of ethinyl estradiol, they represent a minimal risk of ischemic stroke.

The association between migraine and ischemic stroke has long raised interest. Among the eight studies concerning the link between migraine and ischemic stroke, six are case-control studies (2,3,12,17,41,42) and two are cohort studies (1,21) (Table 2). One of the main biases of theses studies is the way migraine is diagnosed. Three recent studies using the IHS criteria (2,41,42) found migraine to be strongly associated with ischemic stroke in women under 45 years of age. The adjusted odds ratio ranges from 1.9 to 4.3. The risk of ischemic stroke is about twice as high in women suffering from migraine with aura than it is in those who have migraine without aura (see Table 2). In the study of Tzourio et al. (42), the association of migraine with heavy smoking (more than 20 cigarettes per day) increased the odds ratio for ischemic stroke to 10.2, and the association of migraine with oral contraceptives to 13.9. The absolute risk of ischemic stroke in young women nevertheless remains low: 10 per 100,000 women/year, 6 per 100,000 in non-migrainous women, and 19 per 100,000 in migrainous women. The absolute risk, however, increases with age: it is 10 times as high at 40 years as at 20 years of age. Considering these figures, migraine should not be considered as a contraindication to oral contraception. Nevertheless, special caution is necessary in migrainous women who are on the pill: tobacco should be forbidden, and the use of low-dose estrogen pills is recommended.

Should some migrainous women not take the pill? Most researchers agree on the necessity to contraindicate estroprogestatives in case of severe, prolonged, or frequent attacks, especially with aura. However, the thresholds of migraine severity or frequency that entail the contraindication or discontinuation of oral contraceptives are still to be determined. The risks and benefits of oral contraception should be weighed in each patient. In case of worsening or of a new onset of migraine related to the pill, one should take into account the patient's age, the type of migraine, the frequency and severity of attacks, and the presence of other vascular risk factors. In some

TABLE 1. *Odds ratios of ischemic stroke in relation to OC use by estrogen dose and progestagen type*

Study	Adjusted OR (95% CI) Ethinyl-estradiol ≥50μg	Adjusted OR (95% CI) Ethinyl-estradiol <50μg
Lidegaard (16)	2.9 (1.6–5.4)	1.8 (1.1–2.9)
		PP: 0.9 (0.4–2.4)
WHO (46)		
Europe	5.30 (2.56–11.0)	1.53 (0.71–3.31)
Developing countries	2.71 (1.75–4.19)	3.26 (2.19–4.86)
Petitti (26)		1.18 (0.54–2.59)
Heinemann (11)		
1st generation (≥50 μg EE)	4.4 (2.0–9.9)	
2nd generation[a]		3.4 (2.1–5.5)
3rd generation[b]		3.9 (2.3–6.6)

pp, pure progestagens.
[a]Less than 50μg ethinyl estradiol (EE) and other gestagens than gestodene and desogestrel.
[b]Progestagens: gestodene, desogestrel.

TABLE 2. *Migraine and risk of ischemic stroke*

Study	Design	Patients	IHS criteria	OR or RR (95% CI)
CGSSYW (3)	Case-control	140 women, 15–44	No	
		controls: neighbors		OR: 1.7 (1.2–2.6)
		hospitalized controls		OR: 1.2 (0.8–1.8)
Henrich Horwitz (12)	Case-control	89, 2 sexes, 15–65	No	
		all patients		OR: 1.8 (0.9–3.6)
		"classic migraine"		OR: 2.6 (1.1–6.6)
Lidegaard (17)	Case-control	692 women, 15–44	No	OR: 2.8 (*p* < 0.001)
Buring (1)	Cohort	22,071 males, 40–84	No	RR: 2.0 (1.1–3.6)
Merikangas (21)	Cohort	12,220, 2 sexes, 25–74	No	RR: 2.8 (1.5–5.4) at 40
Tzourio (41)	Case-control	212, 2 sexes, 15–80 all	Yes	OR: 1.3 (0.8–2.3)
		patients women < 45		OR: 4.3 (1.2–16.3)
Tzourio (42)	Case-control	72 women <45	Yes	
		all patients		OR: 3.5 (1.8–6.4)
		MWA		OR: 3.0 (1.5–5.8)
		MA		OR: 6.2 (2.1–18.0)
Carolei (2)	Case-control	308, 2 sexes, 15–44	Yes	
		all patients		OR: 1.9 (1.1–3.1)
		women <35		OR: 3.7 (1.5–9.0)
		MA		OR: 8.6 (1–75)

OR, Odds ratio; RR, relative risk; MWA, migraine without aura; MA, migraine with aura.

cases, it may be decided, before discontinuing oral contraceptives, to try a different pill (e.g., pure progestatives) or to modify the antimigrainous treatment (e.g., to introduce a prophylactic drug). One shall be more restrictive in women with migraine with aura, in smokers, and in elderly women, who are all at increased risk of stroke.

Any unusual headache, with a sudden onset, a long duration, or associated with focal neurologic symptoms different from a typical aura should prompt appropriate neurologic investigations in order to rule out a cerebrovascular complication.

Treatment of Migraine in Women on Oral Contraceptives

The treatment of migraine in women on oral contraceptives does not basically differ from the treatment of other women. No antimigrainous drug is so far contraindicated in these patients. When attacks are purely menstrual, percutaneous estradiol is particularly easy to use because the expected date of the attack is usually precisely known. In most cases, it will be administered during the 7 days off the pill.

MIGRAINE AND MENOPAUSE

The prevalence of migraine decreases with age in both sexes, and the feminine preponderance, although less important, persists after menopause. The female:male incidence ratio of migraine is still 2.5:1 after 70 years of age. Data about menopause and migraine are conflicting. The classical view is that of a worsening just before or during menopause and of an improvement thereafter. However, no change or worsening has been observed in

up to 50% of the patients in some studies. Neri et al. (24) reported an improvement after spontaneous menopause in two thirds of the women. In contrast, a worsening occurred in two thirds of the women after surgical menopause, which should under no circumstances be proposed as a treatment of migraine.

Hormonal replacement therapy (HRT) with estrogens, alone or in combination with progestins, is used to prevent menopausal symptoms and osteoporosis. Various types of estrogens are used: pure estrones, estradiols, and synthetic ethinyl-estradiol. Estrogens are available orally and parenterally in the form of injections, percutaneous gels, transdermal patches, and vaginal creams. Adjunct hormones include progestins and sometimes androgens. Unopposed estrogens and combined regimens can be administered sequentially for 25 days per month, or continuously. The prescribed therapy varies widely from one country to another. The impact on liver function and on the coagulation system is not the same for the different types of estrogens. Parenteral 17-beta-estradiol produces fewer hepatic and metabolic effects.

Hormone replacement therapy is not contraindicated in migrainous women. Migraine no longer appears as a risk factor for stroke after age 45. Whereas hormonal replacement therapy has a protective effect for coronary heart disease, its consequences on the risk of ischemic stroke are still debated. In the studies devoted to the issue, different types, doses, and associations of estrogens and progestins have been used; the definition of HRT exposure varied (current use or ever use); and transient ischemic attacks were sometimes included and sometimes not. This lack of consistency may account for the discrepancy between the results. Four studies out of five did not find a significant association between HRT and the risk of ischemic stroke (9,25,27,39), and one found a slight increase in risk (10).

The influence of hormonal replacement therapy on the course of migraine is variable. It can improve, worsen or leave it unchanged (34). The treatment of postmenopausal migraine is the usual one. Migraine management may be difficult in women in whom hormonal replacement therapy leads to a worsening of migraine. The treatment of migraine should be intensified, and several empirical strategies may be used: reduce the dose of estrogen, change the estrogen type, or convert from interrupted to continuous administration in case of estrogen withdrawal migraine.

In conclusion, these observations point to the strong link between migraine and female hormones. Estrogens seem to play the major role, but there is a large variability in their effects on migraine pattern, which might be explained by the intrinsic estrogen receptor sensitivity of the hypothalamic neurons. In most women, rising or sustained estrogen levels improve migraine, but in some, the same changes could worsen it. There seems to be a difference in hormonal responsiveness between migraine without aura and migraine with aura. Migraine without aura is more likely to appear *de novo* at puberty and to be triggered by declining sex hormone levels at the time of menstruation. Migraine with aura is more likely to begin *de novo* with sustained high sex hormone levels during pregnancy. Although migraine represents a risk factor of ischemic stroke in young women, the absolute risk remains low. Therefore, migraine is not a contraindication to oral contraceptives in most cases. It is nevertheless important to strongly advise migraineurs who take oral contraceptives not to smoke and to choose low-dose estrogen pills.

REFERENCES

1. Buring JE, Hebert P, Romero J, et al. Migraine and subsequent risk of stroke in the physicians health study. *Arch Neurol* 1995;52:129–134.
2. Carolei A, Marini C, De Matteis G, and the Italian National Research Council Study Group on Stroke in the Young. History of migraine and risk of cerebral ischemia in young adults. *Lancet* 1996;347:1503–1506.
3. Collaborative Group for the Study of Stroke in Young Women. Oral contraceptives and stroke in young women. Associated risk factors. *JAMA* 1975;231:718–722.
4. Cupini LM, Matteis M, Troisi E, Calabresi P, Bernardi G, Silvestrini M. Sex-hormone-related events in migrainous females. A clinical comparative study between migraine with aura and migraine without aura. *Cephalalgia* 1995;15:140–144.
5. Dalessio DJ, Brown DL, Solbach P, Adelman JU, Elkind AH, Stark SR. Oral 311C90 is effective in treatment of menstrual migraine. *Cephalalgia* 1996;16:400–401.
6. De Lignières B, Vincens M, Mauvais-Jarvis P, Mas JL, Touboul PJ, Bousser MG. Prevention of menstrual migraine by percutaneous estradiol. *Br Med J* 1986;293:1540.
7. Dennerstein L, Morse C, Burrows G, Oats J, Brown J, Smith M. Menstrual migraine: a double blind trial of percutaneous oestradiol. *Gynecol Endocrinol* 1988;2:113–120.
8. Facchinetti F, Neri I, Martignoni E, Fioroni L, Nappi G, Genazzani AR. The association of menstrual migraine with the premenstrual syndrome. *Cephalalgia* 1993;13:422–425.
9. Falkeborn M, Persson I, Terent A, Adami HO, Lithell H, Bergström R. Hormone replacement therapy and the risk of stroke: follow-up of a population-based cohort in Sweden. *Arch Intern Med* 1993;153:1201–1209.
10. Grodstein F, Stampfer MJ, Manson JE, et al. Postmenopausal estrogen and progestin use and the risk of cardiovascular disease. *N Engl J Med* 1996;335:453–461.
11. Heinemann LAJ, Lewis MA, Thorogood M, Spitzer WO, Guggenmoos-Holzmann I, Bruppacher R, and the Transnational Research Group on Oral Contraceptives and the Health of Young Women. Case-control study of oral contraceptives and risk of thromboembolic stroke: results from international study on oral contraceptives and health of young women. *BMJ* 1997;315:1502–1504.
12. Henrich JB, Horwitz RI. A controlled study of ischaemic stroke risk in migraine patients. *J Clin Epidemiol* 1989;42:773–780.
13. Johannes CB, Linet MS, Stewart WF, Celentano DD, Lipton RB, Szklo M. Relationship of headache to phase of the menstrual cycle among young women: a daily diary study. *Neurology* 1995;45:1076–1082.
14. Kudrow L. The relationship of headache frequency to hormone use in migraine. *Headache* 1975;15:37–40.
15. Larsson-Cohn U, Lundberg PO. Headache and treatment with oral contraceptives. *Acta Neurol Scand* 1970;46:267–278.
16. Lidegaard O. Oral contraception and risk of a cerebral thromboembolic attack: result of a case-control study. *BMJ* 1993;306:956–963.
17. Lidegaard O. Oral contraceptives, pregnancy and the risk of cerebral thromboembolism: the influence of diabetes, hyptertension, migraine and previous thrombotic disease. *Br J Obstet Gynaecol* 1995;102:153–159.
18. MacGregor EA, Chia H, Vohrah RC, Wilkinson M. Migraine and menstruation: a pilot study. *Cephalalgia* 1990;10:305–310.
19. Magos AL, Zilkha KJ, Studd JWW. Treatment of menstrual migraine by oestradiol implants. *J Neurol Neurosurg Psychiatry* 1983;46:1044–1046.
20. Marcoux S, Berube S, Brisson J, Fabia J. History of migraine and risk of pregnancy induced hypertension. *Epidemiology* 1992;3:53–56.
21. Merikangas KR, Fenton BT, Cheng SH, Stolar MJ, Risch N. Association between migraine and stroke in a large-scale epidemiological study of the United States. *Arch Neurol* 1997;54:362–368.
22. Moore MP, Redmann CWG. Case control study of severe preeclampsia of early onset. *BMJ* 1983;287:581–583
23. Mortimer MJ, Kay J, Jaron A. Childhood migraine in general practice: clinical features and characterisics. *Cephalalgia* 1992;12:238–243
24. Neri I, Granella F, Nappi R, Manzoni GC, Facchinetti F, Genazzani AR. Characteristics of headache at menopause: a clinico-epidemiologic study. *Maturitas* 1993;17:31–37.
25. Pedersen AT, Lidegaard O, Kreiner S, Ottesen B. Hormone replacement therapy and risk of non-fatal stroke. *Lancet* 1997;350:1277–1283.
26. Petitti DB, Sidney S, Bernstein A, Wolf D, Quesenberry C, Ziel HK. Stroke in users of low-dose oral contraceptives. *N Engl J Med* 1996;335:8–15.
27. Petitti DB, Sidney S, Quesenberry CH P, Bernstein A. Ischemic stroke and use of estrogen and estrogen/progestogen as hormone replacement therapy. *Stroke* 1998;29:23–28.
28. Pfaffenrath V. Efficacy and safety of percutaneous estradiol versus placebo in menstrual migraine. *Cephalalgia* 1993;13[Suppl 13]:244.
29. Pradalier A, Vincent D, Beaulieu PH, Baudesson G, Launay JM. Correlation between oestradiol plasma level and therapeutic effect on menstrual migraine. In: Clifford-Rose F, ed. *New advances in headache research*. London: Smith-Gordon, 1994:129–132.
30. Rotton WN, Sachtleben MR, Friedman EA. Migraine and eclampsia. *Obstet Gynecol* 1959;14:322–330.
31. Russell MB, Rasmussen BK, Fenger K, Olesen J. Migraine without aura and migraine with aura are distinct clinical entities: a study of four hundred and eighty-four male and female migraineurs from the general population. *Cephalalgia* 1996;16:239–245.
32. Ryan RE. A controlled study of the effect of oral contraceptives on migraine. *Headache* 1978;17:250–252.
33. Silberstein SD. Headaches and women treatment of the pregnant and lactating migraineur. *Headache* 1993;33:533–540.
34. Silberstein SD, Merriam GR. Estrogens, progestins, and headache. *Neurology* 1991;41:786–793.
35. Smits MG, Van Der Meer YG, Pfeil JP, Rijnierse JJ, Vos AJ. Perimenstrual migraine: effect of estraderm TTS and the value of contin-

gent negative variation and exterotemporalis muscle suppression test. *Headache* 1993;34:103–106.

36. Solbach P, Waymer RS. Treatment of menstruation-associated migraine headache with subcutaneous sumatriptan. *Obstet Gynecol* 1993;82: 769–772.

37. Somerville BW. The role of estradiol withdrawal in the etiology of menstrual migraine. *Neurology* 1972;22:355–365.

38. Somerville BW. Estrogen withdrawal migraine. I. Duration of exposure required and attempted prophylaxis by premenstrual estrogen administration. *Neurology* 1975;25:239–244.

39. Stampfer MJ, Colditz GA, Willett WC, et al. Postmenopausal estrogen therapy and cardiovascular disease: ten-year follow-up from the Nurses Health Study. *N Engl J Med* 1991;325:756–762.

40. Stewart WF, Lipton RB, Celentano DD, Reed ML. Prevalence of migraine headache in the United States. Relation to age, income, race, and other sociodemographic factors. *JAMA* 1992;267:64–69.

41. Tzourio C, Iglesias S, Hubert JB, et al. Migraine as a risk of ischemic stroke: a case-control study. *BMJ* 1993;307:289–292.

42. Tzourio C, Tehindrazanarivelo A, Iglesias S, et al. Case-control study of migraine and risk of ischemic stroke in young women. *BMJ* 1995; 310:830–833.

43. Visser WH, Jaspers NMWH, de Vriend RHM, Ferrari MD. Risk factors for headache recurrence after sumatriptan: a study in 366 migraine patients. *Cephalalgia* 1996;16:246–249.

44. Wainscott G, Volans GN. The outcome of pregnancy in women suffering from migraine. *Postgrad Med J* 1978;54:98–102.

45. Waters WE, O'Connor PJ. Prevalence of migraine. *J Neurol Neurosurg Psychiatry* 1975;38:613–616.

46. WHO Collaborative Study of Cardiovascular Disease and Steroid Hormone Contraception. Ischaemic stroke and combined oral contraceptives: results of an international, multicentre, case-control study. *Lancet* 1996;348:498–505.

The Headaches, Second Edition,
edited by J. Olesen, P. Tfelt-Hansen, and K.M.A. Welch.
Lippincott Williams & Wilkins, Philadelphia © 2000.

The Migraines

CHAPTER 33

Platelets and Adaptive Responses in Migraine

Rajiv Joseph, Jacqueline deBelleroche, and Giovanni D'Andrea

Platelets are anuclear cellular components of blood that function primarily to secure hemostasis. They are metabolically adapted to expend large amounts of energy rapidly during aggregation, secretion, and clot formation. Platelets have been likened to a sponge due to their remarkable propensity to absorb various substances from plasma, including serotonin and amino acids (59). The sequence of platelet response to stimulation is called the basic platelet reaction (54). Vascular injury results first in the adhesion of platelets to the vessel wall. The platelets then change shape from their normal discoid appearance into spheres with pseudopodia and adhere to one another in the process of primary aggregation. Simultaneously, a constricting wave of microtubular contraction results in dense bodies and α granules being shifted to the center of the platelet, and the granular contents are secreted into the tubular system for release to the exterior. The dense bodies contain substances such as adenine nucleotides and serotonin, whereas the α granules contain fibrinogen, β-thromboglobulin, and platelet factor-4. Platelet secretory products, together with thromboxane A_2 synthesized within platelets from arachidonic acid, cause irreversible secondary aggregation, leading to thrombus formation and hemostasis.

R. Joseph: Department of Neurology, Baylor Medical Center, Garland, Texas, 75042.

J. deBelleroche: Division of Neuroscience and Psychological Medicine, Department of Neuromuscular Diseases, Imperial College School of Medicine, Charing Cross Hospital, London W6 8RF, United Kingdom.

G. D'Andrea: Neurophysiopathology Service, Headache and Cerebrovascular Diseases Center, San Bortolo Hospital, 36100 Viceza, Italy.

PLATELET STUDIES IN MIGRAINE

Platelet aggregation and secretion has conventionally been studied using the optical principle in platelet-rich plasma, prepared to be free of other blood cells (12). Although this method does not fully reflect the *in vivo* state, increased spontaneous (48), serotonin- (58), adenosine diphosphate- (18), and epinephrine-induced (66) platelet aggregation have been observed in migraine sufferers between attacks. As a result, inhibition of platelet aggregation was postulated to be of therapeutic value in migraine (33). Indeed, drugs such as methysergide (44,70,96) and ergotamine (45), beneficial in treating migraine, also inhibit platelet aggregation (6,19). However, the inhibitory effect of ergotamine on platelet aggregation was found to be unrelated to clinical efficacy (52). The prophylactic efficacy of beta-blockers (102) and naproxen sodium (106), a potent inhibitor of platelet aggregation, was also unrelated to inhibition of platelet aggregation. Furthermore, serial study of platelet aggregation during acute migraine has revealed no correlation with migraine-associated neurologic symptoms (18). Subsequent studies in whole blood using the impedance technique, a better reflection of the *in vivo* state, confirmed normal aggregability in migraine sufferers (64).

Tests of platelet activity have a degree of intrinsic variability, and more than three decades ago it was recommended that limits of variability be ascertained before comparing results in groups of patients (50). Platelet studies in migraine sufferers have not established the normal range of variability for the tests. Frequently, conclusions on the role of platelets in migraine have been drawn on the basis of trends seen in a solitary test of platelet activity. This is hazardous for the following reasons. First, normal platelet function combines several activities including adhesion, aggregation, and secretion, which are not all reflected by any one test. Second, the platelet is susceptible to a wide range of physiologic changes, such as age, gender and stress. The possibility that one of these variables might account for the platelet changes would be higher if only a single test were performed. Finally, because the tests per se have a great deal of intrinsic variability, it will be more reliable if consistent changes are seen in a complete range of platelet investigations.

PLATELET ACTIVITY IN ACUTE MIGRAINE

Platelet activity is altered in acute migraine. After the establishment of an index of variability for each test of platelet activity in migraine sufferers, estimations of changes in aggregation, secretion, plasma thromboxane, and circulating platelet microaggregates during acute migraine attacks were made (59). These measurements of platelet activity were tested in a prospective manner in eight migraineurs carefully selected for their cooperativity. All subjects had readily identifiable migraine attacks occurring two to four times per month. They were administered (single-blind) placebo capsules matched for Inderal (Wyeth-Ayerst) LA 160 mg (propranolol) once per day for up to 8 consecutive weeks. Four patients had no migraine attacks, and each of the other four subjects were studied serially during one of their migraine attacks that occurred during the study period. The duration of individual attacks varied from 24 to 36 hours. Platelet activity tests were performed weekly in these subjects, and three times during an acute migraine attack at the beginning, peak, and end. All platelet measurements were increased in acute migraine, and, except for plasma thromboxane, which was raised above the normal range, the other tests were within the normal range of variability seen in these subjects. A platelet activity index derived by integrating all the tests was maximal shortly after cessa-

tion of the attack and not at the start, as would be predicted if platelets had a causal role in migraine pathogenesis (Fig. 1).

SIGNIFICANCE OF PLATELET ACTIVATION IN MIGRAINE

Although not of causal importance, the reason for platelet activation in migraine is not known. One possibility is that platelet activation is a consequence of stress (61). There is a well-recognized relationship between stress and migraine (86). Stress precipitates migraine, and migraine worsens stress. The manifestations of migraine are easily related to those of excessive circulating catecholamines. Catecholamines and free fatty acids, known platelet-stimulating agents, increase during migraine (55) and after stress (10,16,76). Platelet activity is increased nonspecifically in several apparently unrelated conditions, such as cerebrovascular disease (60,65), multiple sclerosis (82), anorexia nervosa (75), psoriasis (8), alcohol withdrawal (56), and smoking (79). Physiologic stress is also associated with increased platelet activity (50). Whatever be the cause for platelet activation in migraine, it is not without clinical significance. Increased platelet activity may contribute to a prothrombotic state, leading to stroke, a well recognized complication of migraine (13,18,66). Consequently, it would appear safer to avoid the use of drugs that increase platelet activity in migraineurs (61).

PLATELET SEROTONERGIC FUNCTION

The wealth of information contained in studies of platelets in migraine sufferers provides support for a biochemical abnormality in migraine (62). Although, the platelet is not directly involved in migraine causation, it is a biochemical storehouse and contains a number of substances such as serotonin and catecholamines, and is easily available for study. Therefore, platelets have been used as a model to study the function of certain of these substances in migraine (77).

Serotonergic nerve endings and platelets share many morphologic, biochemical, and physiologic characteristics. These similarities are believed to derive from their common ectodermal origin (15). Both tissues accumulate, store, and release serotonin. They possess α_2-, β_2-, 5-hydroxytryptamine 2 (5-HT$_2$-), and specific imipramine-binding sites and use Ca^{2+} and metabolites of the phosphoinositol and prostaglandin pathways as mediators of secretion (37,71,87,88,90). Therefore, the metabolism of serotonin in the platelet dense body may mirror that in the nervous system (77). This has justified studying the platelet, particularly its dense body, as a model of central serotonergic metabolism and function. Almost all of the serotonin present in blood is located in dense bodies and is released upon platelet activation (49). The amount of

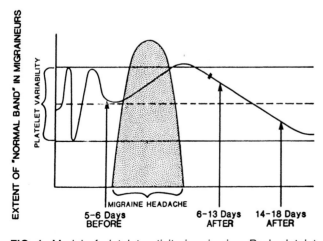

FIG. 1. Model of platelet activity in migraine. Peak platelet activity soon after cessation of headache; normality restored within 2 weeks; migraine causes increased platelet activity.

free serotonin in plasma is extremely low and its estimation difficult (24). A transient increase in plasma serotonin may cause a sterile inflammatory response in vascular walls and increase their permeability (23). Serotonin is mainly converted to 5-hydroxyindole acetic acid (5-HIAA) for renal excretion (22,26). Increase of 5-HIAA in urine and cerebrospinal fluid has been reported in migraine sufferers (65,67). Controversy surrounds the relationship of these observations to platelet serotonin content. Some investigators have noticed an inverse correlation between increased urinary 5-HIAA and decreased platelet serotonin (2,20,92), but others have not (21,92,104). Hannington and colleagues showed that the release of platelet serotonin within 3 days of a migraine attack was reduced compared with migraine-free intervals (48). However, it has not been established whether changes in platelet serotonin are due to a primary platelet abnormality or secondary to a plasma factor (3,39, 99,108).

There are indications that the platelets of migraine sufferers exhibit in the interval between attacks decreased serotonin turnover, increased numbers of dense bodies, decreased dense body secretion, and a defective link between activation of cytoplasmic ionized calcium and platelet activation (63). Taken together, these findings add up to decreased secretion and turnover of platelet serotonin possibly caused by an abnormality in the coupling of cytoplasmic calcium to platelet dense body secretion. Accepting that the platelet dense body is a model for neuronal vesicular function, a similar abnormality in the brain, central serotonergic hypofunction, can be postulated.

PLATELET MONOAMINE OXIDASE AND PHENOLSULFOTRANSFERASE

Monoamine oxidase (MAO) exists in two forms, A and B (57), with platelets containing mainly the latter (81). Tyramine and tryptamine substrates are oxidized by both A and B forms of the enzyme. Hannington noted that foods commonly reported to trigger migraine attacks contain tyramine and that the symptoms of migraine were similar to those caused by ingestion of tyramine-containing foods in patients taking MAO inhibitor drugs. The suggestion that MAO, which inactivates tyramine, might be reduced in migraine sufferers seemed logical (46). Migraine sufferers were subgrouped into those with and without a tyramine-containing food trigger for their attacks (dietary migraineur), and low platelet MAO activity was observed in these patients (43,97). On the other hand, the experience of other investigators has not supported a role for tyramine in migraine, and the theory has received little attention (80,91). Platelet MAO activity may be decreased during headache (39,42), but interpretation of these results is limited because MAO activity is known to fluctuate during menstruation (7). The reason

for changes in MAO activity is unknown but is thought to be due to a plasma factor released during headache (94). However, other studies have not observed a difference in MAO levels between healthy controls and headache-free dietary migraineurs (103). Furthermore, reduction in platelet MAO activity is not specific for migraine because it is also reduced by stress and menstruation and in tension headache sufferers (42).

The P (phenol-inactivating) form of phenolsulfotransferase (PST), for which no endogenous substrate has been identified, is reduced in dietary migraine sufferers (74,100). Alleged triggering factors for migraine, such as cheese, chocolate, and red wine, may contain unidentified phenolic substrates of PST (73). It is unlikely that low platelet PST itself is of primary importance in migraine. However, if the defect is mirrored in the gastrointestinal tract, large amounts of potentially toxic phenolic substances might be absorbed, thus linking diet and migraine (74).

PLATELET ADENINE NUCLEOTIDE, TAURINE, AND ENKEPHALIN

The data are again limited and conflicting. Some studies have shown that the platelet adenine nucleotide content in migraine sufferers was greater than in controls (47,93), whereas others have not observed a difference (53). The finding that adenosine triphosphate release from platelet dense bodies is decreased in migraine sufferers is somewhat consistent with an increased platelet adenine content (64).

Taurine, a sulfur-containing amino acid, is concentrated in platelets and is believed to have smooth muscle–relaxing properties (1,32). Abnormally low platelet taurine levels are seen following a migraine headache (34). This finding may be an epiphenomenon because platelet taurine levels are also reduced during epileptic seizures (4,5). Platelet met-enkephalin is stored in the dense bodies and liberated concomitantly with serotonin during the release reaction (35). Migraineurs may have platelet met-enkephalin immunoreactivity similar to that in healthy controls (11). However, preliminary studies indicate that relative changes in plasma and platelet met-enkephalin levels may be altered in headache subgroups (38).

PLATELET α GRANULE RELEASE AND MEMBRANE COMPOSITION

β-thromboglobulin (βTG), a protein with a molecular weight of 35,800 daltons, is a product of the platelet α granule release reaction and may be a marker of generalized platelet activation. Increased plasma βTG has been observed in some patients during a migraine attack, but this was not associated with changes in thromboxane or prostacyclin as might be expected with generalized platelet activation (25,41,66).

The composition of platelet membranes in migraine sufferers probably does not differ from that in normal subjects. Fatty acid profiles, cholesterol content, and the cholesterol/phospholipid ratio of platelets in migraine sufferers and controls are similar (14). However, some researchers have noticed differences in some aspects of phosphocholines within subgroups of migraine sufferers (84).

CELL SIGNALING IN MIGRAINE AND CLUSTER HEADACHE

No single receptor abnormality has yet been detected that explains why some people are more prone to suffer headache than others. Numerous factors such as stress, hormonal changes, and dietary factors can trigger or predispose to migraine attacks. However, many of the identifiable factors are known to channel into a common pathway of cell signaling.

A ubiquitous mechanism mediating signaling in the nervous system is receptor-mediated transduction (9,83). Neurotransmitters such as noradrenaline, dopamine, serotonin, and neuropeptides, and hormones such as glucagon, use similar mechanisms. The structurally specific interaction of a hormone or neurotransmitter with its receptor in a target tissue leads to the production or suppression of a second messenger, which then mediates the intracellular action of the hormone or transmitter. There are three components that mediate this transduction process: the receptor, a regulatory protein known as a G protein, and an effector system. G proteins are a family of guanine nucleotide-binding proteins encoded by at least 20 genes that transduce the effects of several hundred receptors into a range of specific intracellular responses such as the activation or inhibition of adenyl cyclase, activation of the polyphosphoinositide (PPI) system with the generation of inositol triphosphate (IP_3) and diacylglycerol, modulation of Ca^{2+} and K^+ channels, and the activation of cyclic guanosine monophosphate (cGMP)-phosphodiesterase. G proteins exist as heterotrimers—α, β, and γ—with the α subunit governing specificity of response in most cases. For example, the αs and αi subunits are coupled to the activation and inhibition of adenylate cyclase respectively; the αt subunit, transducin, in the retina regulates cGMP-phosphodiesterase activity in response to light; G_o, which is abundant in the brain, regulates calcium channels; and the Gq/11 family regulates the PPI system. Levels of individual G proteins are subject to regulation by posttranslational modification, by increased degradation or activation of transcription.

ABNORMALITIES IN CELL SIGNALING

Abnormalities in signal transduction in migraine and cluster headache show specificity for the headache phenotype and indicate that an adaptive response has occurred because this difference is present both during and between headache attacks (27–31,69,85,95). In particular, there is a significant decrease in neutrophilic PPI responsiveness in migraineurs following challenge with chemotactic factor, and in the responsiveness of platelets to stimulation with thrombin (31). In each case the generation of radioactively labeled inositol phosphates was followed after preloading with ^{3}H-inositol. Migraine patients with chronic daily headache secondary to analgesic abuse showed a significant improvement in headache following discontinuation of analgesics, and this improvement coincided with changes in PPI responsiveness (51). These and other long-term changes in PPI responsiveness (36,107) indicate that this transduction process can exhibit reversible adaptive changes that persist even after the acute challenge is removed.

Furthermore, abnormalities of the PPI system in migraine and cluster headache are also associated with upstream changes in the expression of G-protein mRNA. The G-protein mRNAs, G_s, G_i, and G_q, represent activation of adenyl cyclase, inhibition of adenyl cyclase, and stimulation of the PPI system, respectively. When studied in lymphocytes, $G_{i\alpha}$ mRNA was reduced by about 50% in migraineurs both during and between attacks compared with normal individuals (40); however, the expression of G_s and G_q was similar in both populations. As in migraineurs, G_i mRNA was also reduced in cluster headache patients, particularly in those who were unmedicated.

DOWNREGULATION OF $G_{I\alpha}$ IN MIGRAINE

A consistent downregulation of $G_{i\alpha}$ mRNA occurs in migraineurs with and without aura, and is apparently unaffected by acute symptoms. This may either reflect an adaptive response to headache, may be due to a precipitating factor causing the headache, or could represent a genetic predisposition. The basis for this may relate to endocrine, neurotransmitter, or glucocorticoid effects, all of which are known to influence the expression of G_i mRNA. G-protein mRNA levels are known to be regulated in response to fluctuations in levels of progesterone and estradiol as shown by changes in $G_{i\alpha}$ mRNA in the myometrium during pregnancy (17,72,78). Both G_i2_α protein and mRNA are increased following estradiol administration and in the final stages of pregnancy, when myometrial concentrations of estradiol are increased. Hence, low levels of $G_{i\alpha}$ mRNA in migraine patients might be associated with deficient estrogen levels. A number of lines of evidence indicate a link between migraine and the female sex hormones estrogen and progesterone: the preponderance of migraine in women and the association of migraine with changes in the menstrual period (98). Migraine typically improves in pregnancy, which may reflect a sustained elevation of estrogen (101), and frequency may worsen at menopause, but consistent correlations between absolute hormone levels and headache frequency are not seen (105).

ADAPTATION MEDIATED BY ALTERATION IN TRANSDUCTION

Although it is well established that receptor upregulation and downregulation can be brought about in response to agonist or antagonist exposure, it is also known that adaptation can occur in postreceptor components of the transduction process. The adenylate cyclase system is sensitive to factors such as age and smoking (68), and the PPI system is upregulated by denervation (89), with alterations occurring at the level of gene expression (36,107). Therefore, measurement of receptor-mediated transduction can provide a basis for studying adaptive responses leading to an improved understanding the pathogenesis of headache and possible novel mechanisms for therapeutic intervention.

ACKNOWLEDGMENT

We are grateful to the Migraine Trust (United Kingdom) for financial support, as well as the National Institutes of Health (United States) and the American Heart Association-National Center.

REFERENCES

1. Ahtee L, Boullin DJ, Passonen MK. Transport of taurine by normal human blood platelets. *Br J Pharmacol* 1974;52:245–251.
2. Anthony M, Hinterberger H, Lance JW. Studies of serotonin metabolism in migraine. *Proc Aust Assoc Neurol* 1968;5:109–112.
3. Anthony M, Hinterberger H, Lance JW. The possible relationship of serotonin to the migraine syndrome. *Res Clin Stud Headache* 1969; 2:29–59.
4. Baskin SI, Dhopish VP, Schraeder PL, Orr PI, Delvitt WS. Relationships of platelet taurine levels to epilepsy. *Clin Res* 1976;24:517a.
5. Baskin SI, Leibman AJ, Con EM. Possible functions of taurine in the central nervous system. In: Costa E, Giaobini E, Paolett R, eds. *Advances in biochemical psychopharmacology*. New York: Raven, 1976:152–164.
6. Baumgartner HR, Born GVR. Effects of 5-hydroxytryptamine on platelet aggregation. *Nature* 1968;218:137–141.
7. Belmaker RH, Murphy DL, Wyatt RJ, Loriaux DL. Human platelet monoamine oxidase changes during the menstrual cycle. *Arch Gen Psychiatry* 1974;31:553–556.
8. Berretini M, Parise P, Costantini V, Grasselli S, Nenci GG. Platelet activation in psoriasis. *Thromb Haemost* 1985;55:195–197.
9. Berridge MJ, Irvine RF. Inositol triphosphate, a novel second messenger in cellular signal transduction. *Nature* 1984;312:315–321.
10. Biggs R, MacFarlane RG, Pilling J. Observations on fibrinolysis. Experimental activity produced by exercise or adrenaline. *Lancet* 1947;1:402–405.
11. Boiardi A, Picoti GB, DiGiulio A, et al. Platelet met-enkephalin immunoactivity and 5-hydroxytryptamine concentrations in migraine patients: effects of 5-hydroxytryptophan, amitriptyline and chlorimipramine treatment. *Cephalalgia* 1984;4:81–84.
12. Born GVR. Quantitative investigations into the aggregation of blood platelets. *J Physiol* 1962;16267–16268.
13. Bosen E. Strokes in migraine: report on seven strokes associated with severe migraine attacks. *Dan Med Bull* 1975;22:100–106.
14. Bottomley JM, Hanington E, Jones RJ, Chapman D. Platelet lipid composition in human migraine. *Headache* 1982;22:256–260.
15. Campbell IC, Marangos PJ, Murphy DL, Pearse AGE. Neuron specific enolase (NSE) in human blood platelets: implications for the neuronal model. *Rec Adv Neuropsychopharmacol* 1981;31:203–211.
16. Castren O. Urinary excretion of noradrenaline and adrenaline in late normal and toxemic pregnancy. *Acta Pharmacol Toxicol* 1963;20 [Suppl 2]:1–98.
17. Cohen-Tannoudji J, Mahouty S, Elwardy-Merezak J, et al. Regulation of myometrial Gi2, Gi3 and Gq during pregnancy. Effects of progesterone and oestradiol. *Biol Reprod* 1995;53:55–64.
18. Couch JR, Hassanein RS. Platelet aggregability in migraine. *Neurology* 1977;27:843–884.
19. Cummings JN, Hilton BP. Effects of methysergide on platelets incubated with reserpine. *Br J Pharmacol* 1971;42:611–619.
20. Curran DA, Hinterberger H, Lance JW. Total plasma serotonin, 5-hydroxyindoleaectic acid and p-hydroxy-methoxymandelic acid excretion in normal and migrainous subjects. *Brain* 1965;88: 997–1010.
21. Curzon G, Barrie M, Wilkinson M. Relationship between headache and amine changes after administration of reserpine to migrainous patients. *J Neurol Neurosurg Psychiatry* 1969;32:555–561.
22. Curzon G, Teaker P, Philipps B. Excretion of 5-hydroxyindole acetic acid (5-HIAA) in migraine. *J Neurol Neurosurg Psychiatry* 1966;29: 85–90.
23. Dalessio DJ. The relationship of vasoactive substances to vascular permeability, and their role in migraine. *Res Clin Stud Headache* 1976; 4:76–84.
24. Dalsgaard-Nielsen J, le Fivre Honore P, Zeeberg IB. Changes in platelet function and blood serotonin level in migraine patients during treatment with femoxetine. *Acta Neurol Scand* 1982;66:191–198.
25. D'Andrea G, Toldo M, Cortelazzo S, Milone FF. Platelet activity in migraine. *Headache* 1982;22:207–212.
26. Deanovic Z, Iskric S, Dupelj M. Fluctuation of 5-hydroxyindole compounds in the urine of migrainous patients. *Biomedicine* 1975;23: 346–349.
27. de Belleroche J. Differential abnormalities in signal transduction in migraine and cluster headache. In: Sandler M, Collins G, eds. *Migraine: a spectrum of ideas*. Oxford, England: Oxford Medical Publications, 1990:269–277.
28. de Belleroche J, Cook GE, Das I, et al. Erythrocyte choline levels in cluster headache. *BMJ* 1984;288:268–270.
29. de Belleroche J, Gardiner IM, Howley P, et al. Membrane transduction in migraine and cluster headache: studies on G-protein activation. In: Clifford Rose F, ed. *New advances in headache research* 2. London: Smith Gordon & Co, 1991:161–163.
30. de Belleroche J, Kilfeather S, Das I, Rose FC. Abnormal membrane composition and membrane dependent transduction mechanisms in cluster headache. *Cephalalgia* 1986;6:147–153.
31. de Belleroche J, Morris R, Davies PT, Clifford Rose F. Differential changes in receptor-mediated transduction in migraine and cluster headache: studies on polymorphonuclear leukocytes. *Headache* 1988; 28:409–413.
32. Dellepiane G. The action of bile and its chief components on the contraction of uterine smooth muscle. *Folia Gynaecol* 1924;19:217–239.
33. Deshmukh SV, Meyer JS. Cyclic changes in platelet dynamics and the pathogenesis and prophylaxis of migraine. *Headache* 1977;17: 101–108.
34. Dhopish VP, Baskin SI. Change in platelet taurine and migraine. *Headache* 1982;22:165–166.
35. Di Giulio AM, Picoti GB, Cesura AM, Pomerai AE, Mantegazze P. Metenkephalin immunoreactivity in blood platelets. *Life Sci* 1982;30: 1605–1614.
36. Essali MA, Das I, de Belleroche J, Hirsch SR. The platelet polyphosphoinositide system in schizophrenia: the effects of neuroleptic treatment. *Biol Psychiatry* 1990;28:475–587.
37. Exton JH. Molecular mechanisms involved in adrenergic responses. *Mol Cell Endocrinol* 1981;23:233–264.
38. Ferrari MD, Odink J, Frolich M, Portielje JEA, Bruyn GW. Methionine-enkephalin in migraine and tension headache, and changes during attacks. *Headache* 1990;30:160–164.
39. Ferrari MD, Odink J, Tapparelli C, Van Kempen GMJ, Pennings EJM, Bruyn GW. Serotonin metabolism in migraine. *Neurology* 1989;39: 1239–1242.
40. Gardiner IM, Ahmed F, Steiner TJ, McBain A, Kennard C, de Belleroche J. A study of adaptive responses in cell signalling in migraine,

and cluster headache: correlations between headache type and changes in gene expression. *Cephalalgia* 1998;18:192–196.

41. Gawel M, Burkitt R, Rose FC. The platelet release reaction during migraine attacks. *Headache* 1979;19:323–327.

42. Glover V, Peatfield R, Zammit-Pace R, Littlewood J, Gawel M, Rose FC, Sandler M. Platelet monoamine oxidase activity and headache. *J Neurol Neurosurg Psychiatry* 1981;44L:676–790.

43. Glover V, Sandler M, Grant E, Rose FC, Orton D, Wilkinson M, Stevens D. Transitory decrease in platelet monoamine oxidase activity during migraine attacks. *Lancet* 1977;1:391–393.

44. Graham JR. Methysergide for prevention of migraine. *N Engl J Med* 1964;270:57–73.

45. Graham JR. Ergot preparations. In: *Treatment of migraine.* Boston: Little, Brown, 1956:43–76.

46. Hanington E. Preliminary report on tyramine headache. *Br Med J* 1967;2:550–551.

47. Hanington E, Jones RJ, Amess JAL. Platelet nucelotides in migraine. *Lancet* 1982;1:437.

48. Hanington E, Jones RJ, Amess JAL, Wachowicz B. Migraine: a platelet disorder. *Lancet* 1981;2:720–723.

49. Hardisty RM, Stacey RS. 5-Hydroxytryptamine in normal human platelets. *J Physiol* 1955;130:711–720.

50. Harrison MJG, Emmons PR, Mitchell JRA. The variability of human platelet aggregation. *J Atheroscler Res* 1967;7:197–205.

51. Hering R, Gardiner I, Catarci T, Whitmarsh T, Steiner T, de Belleroche J. Cellular adaptation in migraineurs with chronic daily headache. *Cephalalgia* 1993;13:261–266

52. Hilton BP, Cummings JN. 5-Hydroxytryptamine levels and platelet aggregation responses in subjects with acute migraine headache. *J Neurol Neurosurg Psychiatry* 1972;35:505–509.

53. Hinterberger H, Anthony M, Vagholkar MK. Platelet 5-hydroxytryptamine and adenine nucleotides, serum arginylesterase and plasma 11-hydroxycorticosteroids in migraine. *Clin Sci* 1968;34:271–276.

54. Holmsen H. Platelet secretion. In: Colman RW, Hirsh J, Marder VJ, Salzman EW, eds. *Hemostasis and thrombosis: basic principles and clinical practice,* 2nd ed. Philadelphia: JB Lippincott, 1987:606–617.

55. Hsu LKG, Crisp AH, Koval J, Chen CN, Carruthers M, Zika KJ. Early morning migraine: nocturnal plasma levels of catecholamines tryptophan, glucose and free fatty acids and sleep encephalographs. *Lancet* 1977;1:447–450.

56. Hutton RA, Fink R, Wilson DT, Marjot DH. Platelet hyperaggregability during alcohol withdrawal. *Clin Lab Haematol* 1981;3:223–229.

57. Johnston JP. Some observations upon a new inhibitor of monoamine oxidase in brain tissue. *Biochem Pharmacol* 1968;17:1285–1297.

58. Jones RJ, Forsythe AM, Amess JAL. Platelet aggregation in migraine patients during the headache-free interval. *Adv Neurol* 1982;33: 275–278.

59. Joseph R. The platelet theory of migraine: a controlled clinical and laboratory evaluation [M.Phil. thesis]. Faculty of Medicine, University of London, 1991.

60. Joseph R, D'Andrea G, Oster SB, Welch KMA. Whole blood platelet function in acute ischemic stroke: importance of dense body secretion and the effects of antithrombotic agents. *Stroke* 1989;20:38–44.

61. Joseph R, Steiner TJ, Schultz LUC, Rose FC. Platelet activity and selective beta blockade in migraine prophylaxis. *Stroke* 1988;19: 704–708.

62. Joseph R, Welch KMA. The platelet and migraine: a nonspecific association. *Headache* 1987;27:3735–3780.

63. Joseph R, Welch KMA, D'Andrea G. Serotonergic hypofunction in migraine: a synthesis of evidence based on platelet dense body dysfunction. *Cephalalgia* 1989;9:293–299.

64. Joseph R, Welch KMA, D'Andrea G, Levine SR. ATP hyposecretion from platelet dense bodies: evidence for the purinergic hypothesis and a marker of migraine. *Headache* 1986;26:403–410.

65. Joseph R, Welch KMA, Oster SB, Grunfeld S, D'Andrea G. A plasmatic factor may cause platelet activation in acute ischemic stroke. *Circ Res* 1989;65:1679–1687.

66. Kalendovsky Z, Austin JH. Complicated migraine: its association with increased platelet aggregability and abnormal plasma coagulation factors. *Headache* 1975;15:18–35.

67. Kangasniemi P, Sonnimen V, Rinne UK. Excretion of free and conjugated 5-HIAA in urine and concentration of 5-HIAA and HVA in CSF during migraine attacks and free intervals. *Headache* 1972;12:62–65.

68. Kilfeather SA, Dawson K, de Belleroche J. Lymphocytes, beta adrenoceptors and multiple prostaglandin receptors: effects of aging and smoking. *Br J Pharmacol* 1986;87:113P.

69. Kilfeather S, Gorgolewska G, Massarella A, Ansell E, Turner P. Beta adrenoceptor and epoprostenol responsiveness of lymphocytes in migraine patients. *Postgrad Med J* 1984;60:391–393.

70. Lance JW, Anthony M, Somerville B. Comparative trial of serotonin antagonists in the management of migraine. *Br Med J* 1970;2: 327–330.

71. Langer SZ, Zarifian E, Briley M, Raisin R, Setter D. High-affinity binding of ^{3}H-impramine in brain and platelets and its relevance to the biochemistry of affective disorders. *Life Sci* 1981;29:211–220.

72. Lest KP, Hugh CJ, Allah CS, et al. Fluoxetine modulates G-protein alpha s, alpha q and alpha 12 subunit mRNA expression in rat brain. *Eur J Pharmacol* 1992;277:233–237.

73. Littlewood J, Gibb C, Glover K, et al. Red wine as a migraine trigger. In: *Proceedings of the 6th International Migraine Symposium.* London, UK. 1986:31–32.

74. Littlewood J, Glover V, Sandler M, Petty R, Pearfield R, Rose FC. Platelet phenolsulphortransferase deficiency in dietary migraine. *Lancet* 1982;11:983–988.

75. Luck P, Mikhailidas DP, Dashwood MR, et al. Platelet hyperaggregability and increased adrenoceptor density in anorexia nervosa. *J Clin Endocrinol Metab* 1983;57:911–914.

76. Macfarlane RG, Biggs R. Observations on fibrinolysis. Spontaneous activity associated with surgical operations, trauma etc. *Lancet* 1946; 2:862–864.

77. Malmgren R, Hasselmark L. The platelet and the neuron: two cells in focus in migraine. *Cephalalgia* 1988;8:7–24.

78. Manji HK, Chen G, Shimon H, Hsiao JK, Potter WZ, Belmaker RH. Guanine nucleotide-binding proteins in bipolar affective disorder. Effects of long-term lithium treatment. *Arch Gen Psychiatry* 1995;52: 135–144.

79. McVerry B, Levine PH. Effect of cigarette smoking on the function of blood platelet. In: Donoso E, Hafm JE, eds. *Thrombosis, platelets, anti-coagulation and acetyl salicylic acid,* Vol. 2. Stuttgart: Thieme, 1976:122–130.

80. Moffett A, Swash M, Scott DF. Effect of tyramine in migraine: a double blind study. *J Neurol Neurosurg Psychiatry* 1972;35:469–499.

81. Murphy DL, Donnelly CH. In: Usdin E, ed. *Neurophyschopharmacology of monoamines and their regulatory enzymes,* New York, 1974:71.

82. Neu IS, Prosegel M, Pfaffenrath V. Platelet aggregation and multiple sclerosis. *Acta Neurol Scand* 1982;66:497–504.

83. Nishizuka Y. Turnover of inositol phospholipids and signal transduction. *Science* 1984;225:1365–1370.

84. Oxman TE, Hitzemann RJ, Smith R. Platelet membrane lipid composition and the frequency of migraine. *Headache* 1982;22:261–267.

85. Peatfield RC, Rose FC. Exacerbation of migraine by treatment with lithium. *Headache* 1981;21:140–142.

86. Perkin GD, Joseph R. Neurological manifestations of the hyperventilation syndrome. *J R Soc Med* 1986;79:448–450.

87. Peters JR, Grahame-Smith DG. Human platelet 5-HT receptors: characterization and functional association. *Eur J Pharmacol* 1980;68: 243–256.

88. Pletscher A, Laubascher A. Blood platelets as a model for neurons: uses and limitations. *J Neural Transm* 1980;7[Suppl 16]:7–16.

89. Reed LJ, de Belleroche J. Increased polyphosphoinositide responsiveness in the cerebral cortex induced by cholinergic denervation. *J Neurochem* 1988;50:1566–1571..

90. Rotman A. Blood platelets in psychopharmacological research. *Prog Neuropsychopharmacol* 1983;7:135–151.

91. Ryan RE. A clinical study of tyramine as an etiological factor in migraine. *Headache* 1974;14:43–48.

92. Rydzevsky W. Serotonin (5-HT) in migraine levels in whole blood in and between attacks. *Headache* 1976;16:16–19.

93. Rydzewski W, Wachowicz B. Adenine nucleotides in platelets in and between migraine attacks. In: Green R, ed. *Current concepts in migraine research.* New York: Raven, 1978:153–158.

94. Sandler M. Transitory platelet monoamine oxidase deficit in migraine: some reflections. *Headache* 1977;17:153–158.

95. Selmaj K, de Belleroche J, Das I, Rose FC. Leukotriene B$_4$ generation by polymorphonuclear leukocytes: possible involvement in the pathogenesis of headache. *Headache* 1986;26:460–464.

96. Sicuteri F. Prophylactic treatment of migraine by means of lysergic acid derivatives. *Triangle* 1963;6:116–125.

97. Sicuteri F, Buffoni F, Anseimi B, Del Bianco PL. An enzyme (MAO) defect on the platelets in migraine. *Res Clin Stud Headache* 1972; 3:245.

98. Silberstein SD, Merriam GR. Estrogens, progestins and headache. *Neurology* 1991;41:786–793.

99. Sjaastad O. The significance of blood serotonin levels in migraine. *Acta Neurol Scand* 1975;51:200–210.

100. Soliman HR, Pradalier A, Launay JM, Dry J, Dreux C. Common migraine platelet phenosulfotransferase activity. In: *Proceedings of the 6th International Migraine Symposium.* 1986:29–30.

101. Somerville BW. A study of migraine in pregnancy. *Neurology* 1972; 22:824–828.

102. Steiner TJ, Joseph R, Rose FC. Migraine is not a platelet disorder. *Headache* 1985;25:434–440.

103. Thomas DV. Platelet monoamine oxidase in migraine. *Adv Neurol* 1982;33:279–281.

104. Tretyakova KA, Fets AN. The general blood serotonin contents in patients with migraine during attacks and in the interparoxysmal period. *Zh Neuropathol Psikhiatr* 1969;69:831–835.

105. Waters WE, O'Connor PJ. Epidemiology of headache and migraine in women. *J Neurol Neurosurg Psychiatry* 1971;34:148–153.

106. Welch KMA, Elis DJ, Keenan PA. Successful migraine prophylaxis with naproxen sodium. *Neurology* 1985;35:1304–1310.

107. Wood H, de Belleroche J. Excitotoxin lesion of nucleus basalis causes a specific decrease in Go mRNA in cerebral cortex sensitivity to MK-801. *FEBS Lett* 1990;273:63–67.

108. Ziegler DK, Hassanein RS, Ward DF. Migraine, tryptamine and blood serotonin. *Headache* 1976;16:53–57.

The Headaches, Second Edition,
edited by J. Olesen, P. Tfelt-Hansen, and K.M.A. Welch.
Lippincott Williams & Wilkins, Philadelphia © 2000.

The Migraines

CHAPTER 34

Immunologic Aspects of Migraine

André Pradalier

In 1927 Vaughan (47) published one of the first observations linking migraine with allergy. He investigated 33 patients suffering from migraine by skin tests and elimination diets and found marked improvement after diet therapy in 10 patients, 5 of whom reported recurrence of migraine after reintroduction of suspected foods. In their article "Migraine is a Food Allergic Disease," Monro et al. (29) relaunched the theory of an allergic mechanism in the physiopathology of migraine.

The concept of a possible involvement of the immune system in migraine may be supported by biochemical abnormalities found in blood cells, plasma, urine, or the cerebrospinal fluid of migraine patients:

Changes in immunoglobulin or complement split product levels during an attack (2,15,18,19)

Local mast cell degranulation during an attack (40,41)

Increase in plasma histamine levels during attack compared with controls and nonmigraine headache patients (11,12,33)

Increased levels of circulating immune complexes and T cells after oral food challenge accompanied by an increase in interleukin 2 release from the cells of some patients (23)

Transferral of migraine from mother to son after bone marrow transplantation (17)

Increased levels of prostaglandins D_2 and F_2 together with increased cerebral blood flow (33,39)

However, blood eosinophilia is a rare feature in migraine, and several of the above findings have not been confirmed by other researchers; for example, the involvement of immune complexes was not confirmed by Rubin and Boyer (36) or by Visintini et al. (48). Furthermore, Selmaj (37) found no change in leukotriene B_4 during an attack. Many migraine patients have circulating specific immunoglobulin G (IgG) antibodies against foods (22), but this phenomenon merely reflects these patients' regular ingestion of this food because no correlation between the presence of IgG antibodies (or their subtypes) and atopy has been convincingly described so far (45). The involvement of basophils or mast cells (40,41) together with the increased levels of plasma histamine (11,12) suggest a type I reaction. Olson et al. (33) found a 5- to 38-fold increase in plasma histamine levels during oral challenge with food items concomitantly eliciting migraine in five patients, whereas placebo challenges produced no increase. Prostaglandin D_2 was elevated both in the acute phase and again 4 to 6 hours after challenge. The present findings need to be confirmed before being interpreted as causal because alternatively they might be a consequence of the attack or a manifestation of the immunologic contact with the food with no causal relationship.

ATOPY AND MIGRAINE

Migraine and allergy are common diseases. Migraine affects at least 10% of the population (up to 25% of all women), whereas allergy affects approximately 15%. By chance, these diseases may be present concomitantly in the single patient, thus being linked together even if no causal relationship exists. Various forms of allergy may be accompanied by headache (anaphylaxis, serum sickness, urticaria, rhinitis complicated by sinusitis), but these forms of headache do not comply with the migraine classification as defined by the Headache Classification Committee of 1988.

A. Pradalier: Xavier Bichat Paris VII University, 75018 Paris, and Service de Médecine Interne, Hôpital Louis Mourier, 92700 Colombes Cedex, France.

Little is known about a possible relationship between inhalant allergy (animal dander, mites, pollen) and migraine. As an estimate, concurrent migraine and atopy are present in 15% to 60% of migraine patients (10,42). In the study conducted by the French Groupe de Recherche et d'Étude de la Migraine, atopy was found in 23.6% of the migraine patients (35). Waters (49) reported an increased incidence of allergic symptoms, particularly rhinitis or urticaria, in patients with migraine as compared with nonmigrainous headache patients or to controls. A case history, however, never suffices to establish a causal relationship between allergy and migraine; a definite relationship requires the detection of a specific allergen and the establishment of its responsibility for precipitating the migraine attack as demonstrated by a double-blind technique, demonstrating cessation of symptoms when the allergen is eliminated and recurrence of symptoms upon challenge. Furthermore, because the natural history of migraine is unpredictable in the single patient, with a varying frequency of attacks and with several additional external and internal factors possibly precipitating an attack, placebo challenges are of mandatory importance (28,34).

Various reports relate ingestion of specific foods to migraine. In many cases of suspected food hypersensitivity, the frequency of reported positive reactions to placebo amounts to more than 35% (4). Such reactions are particularly frequent in patients with subjective symptoms only, in whom no objective signs can he demonstrated. The double-blind, placebo-controlled food challenge (DBPCFC) thus remains the only reliable diagnostic tool for the establishment of a causal link between migraine and food allergy (28,34).

IMMUNOGLOBULIN E

Conflicting reports on the levels of total and specific IgE in migraine patients have been published. In 3 of 10 studies (3,7,13) an increase in total serum IgE was demonstrated in a large proportion (28–39%) of the patients, but in Egger's study (7) half of the patients were described as atopic, as were one third of Bentley's (3) patients. The remaining seven papers (26,27,32,35,36,48) failed to demonstrate any increase in total serum IgE except in patients with established atopy. Thus, measurement of total serum IgE does not seem to be valuable in the diagnosis of migraine.

SPECIFIC IgE

Most studies have found measurement of specific IgE against food to be of little diagnostic value. In only three of eight published papers (3,7,13,27,29,30,32,35) was specific IgE against specific foods detected. In Monro's study (29,30), the positive radio allergosorbent test (RAST) values found in 26 of 33 migraine patients were used to design the subsequent elimination diet on which 23 of the 26 patients responded. However, double-blind challenges with foods in order to confirm the findings were not performed. Idris et al. (13) reported 63% of the patients to be RAST positive but overall for inhalant allergens, whereas Bentley (3) found detectable specific IgE against food in only 4 of 10 children who benefited from dietary manipulation. These four patients also were atopic and had elevated total IgE. In five studies no specific IgE against foods was detected in either nonselected migraine patients (16,35) or dietary migraine patients (7,27,31). In a nonselected adult migraine group of patients in whom specific IgE against at least 10 different foods was measured, only six patients were RAST positive in each study, and all food challenges with the RAST-positive foods were negative. Nattero et al. (32) found no detectable specific IgE against 40 food items in 40 dietary migraine patients, whereas Merrett et al. (27) found some positive values but no significant difference between a group of dietary migraine patients and a control group of nondietary migraine patients. Finally, Egger et al. (7) demonstrated specific IgE against foods in only 8 of 76 patients, whereas total IgE levels were elevated in 28%. This observation led the authors to conclude that IgE might not be important in the mechanism of the presumed allergy.

SKIN PRICK TEST

Like measurement of specific IgE, the value (sensitivity and specificity) of skin prick testing with food allergens is highly variable and dependent on the quality of the extract used. When fresh food items are used, skin prick testing is usually a reliable, inexpensive, and fast diagnostic tool (28).

Skin prick testing in migraine patients has proven useful in two of six studies. Mansfield et al. (21) found that 16 of 43 patients with severe migraine tested positive in the skin to a range of 1 to 29 of 83 food allergens. Five of the seven patients who were subsequently challenged in a double-blind protocol experienced headache when challenged with the skin prick test–positive food item. In contrast, Nattero et al. (32) and Pradalier et al. (35) found no diagnostic value of skin prick test in 105 and 50 adult migraine patients, respectively. Similar results were obtained by Egger et al. (7), whereas Monro et al. (30) found an intradermal but not a skin prick test useful in identifying incriminating foods; in the latter study, challenges were not performed, hampering the value of this finding.

OTHER POSSIBLE IMMUNOALLERGIC MECHANISMS

Although a mechanism mediated by IgE seems unlikely in the mechanism of migraine, other mechanisms are theoretically possible even if proving them is difficult given the present level of our knowledge: direct cytotoxic action of mediators or cytokines, effect of circulating immunocomplexes (type III allergy), and other mediators by a non-IgE mechanism. Lord and Duckworth (18,19) and Jerzmanovski and Klimek (15) proposed a role for IgG or IgA immune complexes or activation of the complement, but their studies were not confirmed (31,36,48). Selmaj et al. (37) did not observe changes in LTB4 during or between attacks. However, for these researchers the increased ionophore-stimulated release of LTB4, in vitro from leukocytes, could reflect a state of activation of these cells during migraine attack. The observation of specific IgG against foods in a lot of patients (22) and the presence of IgE immune complexes (29,37) are today difficult to interpret.

Martelletti et al. (23), studying 21 food-induced migraine patients before and during a food challenge found during the challenge an increased incidence of circulating immune complexes (28.6% compared with 10% in the control group), a significant increase of total T cells at 4 hours after challenge and activated T cells, no changes for IgG4. This increase in activated T cells suggests an involvement of some lymphokines released by the lymphocytes, especially interleukin 2 (IL-2), whereas they observed an increase of IL-2 plasma levels in the juvenile form of food-induced migraine. It would be of great interest to explore more precisely the cytokines in migraine. Cytokines are produced by different cells: lymphocytes, monocytes, macrophages, mast cells, and eosinophils.

Their activities are not limited to the immune system. Their actions are essentially in immunology (IL-2, IL-4, IL-10), in the hematopoiesis (IL-3, IL-5, IL-7), and in the inflammatory reaction (IL-1, IL-6, IL-8). Some of them even have an effect on the central nervous system. For example, IL-1 and tumor necrosis factor (TNF) induce sleep, fever, and anorexia and stimulate the release of adrenocorticotropic hormone. There is increasing argument for the reciprocal modulation of the brain and immune system. For example, this relationship is suggested by evidence of the IL-1 immunoreactive innervation of the hypothalamus (5).

In 1990, Covelli et al. (6) reported an exaggerated spontaneous release of TNF in patients with migraine without aura in comparison with control subjects, but Van Hilten et al. (44), in a different study measuring plasma IL-1 alpha and beta and TNF alpha during and between attacks in 20 migraine patients, found no evidence of an increase in these cytokines during the attack. Martelletti et al. (25) in 1993 investigated IL-4, IL-6, IFN gamma, and granulocyte macrophage colony-stimulating factor (GM-CSF) in plasma from migraine patients during and between challenged migraine attacks. Martelletti et al. observed a decrease after a challenge test for IL-4 and IL-6 and an opposite trend for IFN gamma and GM-CSF, but the implication of this phenomenon in dietary migraine do not seem readily evident. Martelletti et al. have proposed for explanation of their observations an activation of this cytokine network together with the impairment in the neuropeptidergic system if we consider the close links between interleukins and the neuromediators of pain such as histamine and serotonin. Martelletti et al. studied in 1997 the mechanisms involved in the "sterile" inflammation in migraine, by flow cytometry [measurement of the intercellular adhesion molecule type 1 (ICAM 1) and the IL-1 receptor (IL-1R)] and enzyme-linked immunosorbent assay [soluble ICAM 1 (sICAM 1) and IL-4] in patients with migraine during an attack, in those with tension-type headache, and in controls (24). A sharp decrease in the expression of ICAM 1, sICAM 1, and IL-4 was observed during spontaneous or isosorbide dinitrate (nitric oxide donor)-induced migraine but no change in the two other groups tested with isosorbide, suggesting that migraine patients were more susceptible to NO than were controls. Moreover, this decrease of IL-4 and ICAM 1 inhibit the transendothelial migration into the cerebral tissues of activated leukocytes.

In another way, sensory neuropeptides, substance P, neurokinin A (NKA), calcitonin gene–related peptide (CGRP), and vasointestinal peptide (VIP) can modulate the immune function in vitro (8,9,14). For example, substance P modulates lymphocyte proliferation antibody synthesis, activates mast cell degranulation, and stimulates the production of inflammatory cytokines by mononuclear cells; CGRP enhances the mitogenic response to phytohemagglutin; and IL-1 beta enhances in rats axonal transport of opiate receptors in sensory neurons. This suggests that IL-1 beta represents a major mediator to sensitize nociceptors during inflammation. Because activation of the trigeminovascular system is involved in the pathophysiology of migraine attacks and plays an important role in the mediation of nociception in the brain, the relationship between neuropeptides and the immune system could explain, at least in part, the inflammation, duration of pain, and hemodynamic changes of the migraine attack. Gallai et al. (9) studied the monocyte functions (chemotactism, phagocytosis, value of respiratory burst, cytokine production) during and between attacks and in vitro in contact with neuropeptides: substance P, NKA, and CGRP. They concluded to a defect in the monocyte function during headache-free periods. In contrast, monocyte functions increased during attacks, suggesting that one or more mediators of neurogenic inflammation could be implicated in the monocyte changes occurring ictally. Of course, these results must be corroborated by other teams before migraine can be connected to an immunoallergic mechanism, especially because these laboratory techniques are difficult and often made on a very small number of patients.

These modifications may be the causal factor of a migraine attack; they may happen consecutively to the attack; or they may be the manifestation of the immunologic contact with the allergenic food, without the latter having a pathologic role. Further confirmation is needed.

CLINICAL TRIALS

The theory of an allergic etiology of migraine, originally proposed by Vaughan (47), was further substantiated by Unger and Unger in 1952 and 1970, who described complete recovery after an elimination diet in 35 of 55 migraine patients (42,43). Similar results were obtained by Grant (10), who reported complete recovery in 51 of 60 patients placed on a strict elimination diet consisting of pears and lamb. In a 1980 study comprising 36 patients, Monro et al. (29) found 23 patients capable of identifying foods provoking migraine after an elimination diet.

Various other studies have suggested a beneficial effect of food avoidance, but they all suffer from the lack of confirmation by DBPCFC, pointing to the traditional high percentage of false-positive diet results in food hypersensitivity. Egger et al. (7) placed 88 children with migraine on elimination diets for up to two 4-week periods, during which time 78 of the 88 who complied with the regimen recovered completely. Subsequent DBPCFC revealed that 26 of the 40 patients could correctly identify the active challenge (recurrence of migraine) without reaction to the placebo challenge, whereas if positive results of the skin prick test had been used, only three patients would have benefited from diet therapy. Mansfield (21) placed 43 consecutive adult migraine patients on a diet excluding wheat, milk, and eggs and found a substantial effect in 13, of whom 7 underwent DBPCFC, 5 correctly identifying the active challenge. Similar results were demonstrated (20) in 20 of 51 adult patients placed on a diet excluding milk, eggs, corn, and wheat, and positive DBPCFC results were obtained in 11 of 14 patients subsequently challenged. Markedly different results were obtained by Atkins et al. (1), who by medical history and skin prick test found 16 suspected foods in 36 children. The researchers performed 19 DBPCFCs in these 16 children without precipitating an attack of migraine in any of them.

The most recent study (46) investigated 104 adults, 69 of whom reported fewer headaches during elimination diet therapy. Of these, only 8 became headache free. Twenty-three underwent DBPCFC, 15 showing positive results. The foods eliciting attacks of migraine in this study were once again milk, eggs, corn, and wheat.

Pharmacologic agents in foods have been incriminated as inducing migraine. Studies on tyramine, for example, have shown conflicting results ranging from no correlation when performing DBPCFC in 80 patients (50) to positive DBPCFC results in the majority of 45 patients (38). The same applies to nitrites in foods, phenylethylamine, and ethanol.

It may be concluded that some migraine patients may benefit from diet therapy, although only a small percentage (<10%) will become symptom free. The only reliable diagnostic tool is properly performed DBPCFC, whereas skin testing or measurement of specific IgE will only occasionally be valuable. In most cases the offending foods reported have been milk, eggs, corn, and wheat, thus minimizing the need for extensive and elaborate exclusion diets.

REFERENCES

1. Atkins FM, Ball BD, Bock SA. The relationship between the ingestion of specific foods and the development of migraine in children. *J Allergy Clin Immunol* 1988;81:185.
2. Behan W, Behan P, Durward W. Complement studies in migraine. *J Headache* 1981;21:55–57.
3. Bentley D, Katch Burian A, Brostoff J. Abdominal migraine and food sensitivity in children. *Clin Allergy* 1984;14:499–500.
4. Bindsley-Jensen C. Rhinitis and food allergy. In: Mygind N, Naclerio RM, eds. *Allergic rhinitis: clinical aspects.* Copenhagen: Munksgaard, 1992:33–39.
5. Breder CD, Dinarello CA, Saper CB. Interleukin-1 immunoreactive innervation of the human hypothalamus. *Science* 1988;240:321–324.
6. Covelli V, Munno I, Pellegrino NM, Di Venere A, Jirillo E, Buscaino GA. Exaggerated spontaneous release of tumor necrosis factor-alpha/cachectinin patients with migraine without aura. *Acta Neurol* 1990;12: 257–263.
7. Egger J, Carter C, Wilson J, Turner M, Soothill JF. Is migraine food allergy? *Lancet* 1983;2:865–869.
8. Fox FE, Kubin M, Cassin M. Calcitonin gene-related peptide inhibits proliferation and antigen presentation by human peripheral blood mononuclear cells: effects on B7, interleukin 10, and interleukin 12. *J Invest Dermatol* 1997;108:43–48.
9. Gallai V, Sarchielli P, Floridi A, Franceschini M, Trequattrini A, Firenze C. Monocyte function in migraine patients with and without aura. *Headache Q* 1994;5:214–227.
10. Grant E. Food allergies and migraine. *Lancet* 1979;1:966–969.
11. Haimart M, Pradalier A, Launay JM, Dreux C, Dry J. Whole blood and plasma histamine in common migraine. *Cephalalgia* 1987;7:39–42.
12. Heatley R, Denburg J, Bayer N, Bienenstock J. Increased plasma histamine levels in migraine patients. *Clin Allergy* 1982;12:145–149.
13. Idris A, Ishak R, Hassan K. Platelet function and allergic tendency in migraine patients before treatment: a preliminary study. *Cephalalgia* 1989;9:95–96.
14. Jeanjean AP, Maloteaux JM, Laduron PM. IL-1 beta like Freund's adjuvant enhances axonal transport of opiate receptors in sensory neurons. *Neurosci Lett* 1994;177:75–78.
15. Jerzmanowski A, Klimek A. Immunoglobulins and complement in migraine. *Cephalalgia* 1983;3:119–123.
16. Lenarduzzi P, Forget P, Schoenen J. Evaluation of food allergy in migraine with a sensitive RAST. *Cephalalgia* 1987;7:226.
17. Lonnqvist B, Ringden O. Migraine precipitated by red wine after bone-marrow transplantation. *Lancet* 1990;19:364–365.
18. Lord G, Ducworth J, Charlesworth J. Complement activation in migraine. *Lancet* 1977;1:781–782.
19. Lord G, Ducworth J, Charlesworth J. Complement activation in migraine. *J Headache* 1977;17:163–166.
20. Mansfield L, Vaughan TR, Waller S, Haverly R, Ting S. Food allergy and adult migraine: double-blind and mediator confirmation of an allergic etiology. *Ann Allergy* 1985;55:186–189.
21. Mansfield LE. The role of food allergy in migraine: a review. *Ann Allergy* 1987;58:313–317.
22. Marini S, Fois D, Fornara R, Moschetta A, Guidetti V. Allergic aspects in childhood and adolescence headache and migraine [Abstract]. III IHS Int Symposium, Rome, March 6–9, 1991. *Proc Int Juvenile Headache Congress* 1991.
23. Martelletti P, Disabato F, Giacovazzo M. Derangement of IL2 receptor expression associated with growing IL2 plasma levels in juvenile forms

of food induced migraine [Abstract]. III IHS Int Symposium, Rome, March 6–9, 1991. *Proc Int Juvenile Headache Congress* 1991.

24. Martelletti P, Stirparo G, Morrone S, Rinaldi C, Giacovazzo M. Inhibition of intercellular adhesion molecule-1 (ICAM-1), soluble ICAM-1 andinterleukin-4 by nitric oxide expression in migraine patients. *J Mol Med* 1997;75:448–453.

25. Martelletti P, Stirparo G, Rinaldi C, Frati L, Giacovazzo M. Disruption of the immunopeptidergic network in dietary migraine. *Headache* 1993;33:524–527.

26. Median JL, Diamond S. Migraine and atopy. *J Headache* 1976;16:271–274.

27. Merrett J, Peatfield R, Cliffort-Rose F, Merrett TG. Food related antibodies in headache patients. *J Neurol Neurosurg Psychiatry* 1983;46:738–742.

28. Metcalfe D, Sampson HA. Workshop on experimental methodology for clinical studies on adverse reactions to foods and food additives. *J Allergy Clin Immunol* 1990;86:421–442.

29. Monro J, Carini C, Brostoff J. Migraine is a food allergic disease. *Lancet* 1984;2:719–721.

30. Monro J, Carini C, Brostoff J, Zilkha K. Food allergy in migraine. *Lancet* 1980;2:1–4.

31. Nattero G, Savi L, Cadario G, Agliata S, Valenzano C. Relationship between headache and diet in children and adolescents in comparison with adults. III IHS Int Symposium, Rome, March 6–9, 1991. *Proc Int Juvenile Headache Congress* 1991.

32. Nattero G, Savi L, Cadario G, Valenzano C. Dietary migraine as adverse reactions. *Cephalalgia* 1989;9:193–194.

33. Olson CG, Vaughan TR, Ledoux RA. Food induced migraine: search for immunologic mechanisms [Abstract]. *J Allergy Clin Immunol* 1989;83:238.

34. Pearson DJ. Psychologic and somatic interrelationships in allergy and pseudoallergy. *J Allergy Clin Immunol* 1988;81:351–360.

35. Pradalier A, Weinmann S, Launay JM, Baron JF, Dry J. Total IgE, specific IgE and prick tests against food in common migraine. *Cephalalgia* 1984;3:231–234.

36. Rubin L, Boyer J. A correlative study of immunoglobulin isotype expression in common migraine. *J Headache* 1986;26:137–141.

37. Selmaj K, de Belleroche J, Das I. Leukotriene B4 levels in migraine and cluster headache. In: Clifford-Rose F, ed. *Current problems in neurology.* New York: John Libbey, 1987.

38. Smith I, Mullen PE, Hanington E. Dietary migraine and tyramine metabolism. *Nature* 1971;230:246–248.

39. Steinberg M, Page R, Wolfson S, Friday G, Fireman P. Food induced late phase headache [Abstract]. *J Allergy Clin Immunol* 1988;81:185.

40. Thonnard-Neumann E. Some interrelations of vasoactive substances and basophil leukocytes in migraine headaches. *J Headache* 1969;9:130–140.

41. Thonnard-Neumann E, Taylor W. The basophil leukocyte and migraine. *J Headache* 1968;8:98–106.

42. Unger AH, Unger L. Migraine is an allergic disease. *J Allergy* 1952;23:429–440.

43. Unger L, Cristol JL. Allergic migraine. *Ann Allergy* 1970;28:106–109.

44. Van Hilten JJ, Ferrari MD, van der Meer JWM, Gijsman HJ, Looij BJ Jr. Plasma interleukin-1, tumour necrosis factor and hypothalamic-pituitary-adrenal axis responses during migraine attacks. *Cephalalgia* 1991;11:65–67.

45. Van Metre TE Jr. Unproven procedures for diagnosis and treatment of food allergy. *N Engl Reg Allergy Proc* 1987;8:17–21.

46. Vaughan TR, Mansfield LE. Neurologic reactions to foods and food additives. In: Metcalfe DD, Sampson HA, Simon RA, eds. *Food allergy. Adverse reactions to foods and food additives.* Boston: Blackwell Scientific, 1991:355–369.

47. Vaughan WT. Allergic migraine. *JAMA* 1927;88:1383–1386.

48. Visintini D, Trabattoni G, Manzoni G, Lechi A, Bortone L, Behan P. Immunological studies in cluster headache and migraine. *J Headache* 1986;26:398–402.

49. Waters WE. *The epidemiology of migraine.* Bershire: Boehringer Ingelheim, 1979.

50. Ziegler DK, Stewart R. Failure of tyramine to induce migraine. *Neurology* 1977;27:725–726.

The Headaches, Second Edition,
edited by J. Olesen, P. Tfelt-Hansen, and K.M.A. Welch.
Lippincott Williams & Wilkins, Philadelphia © 2000.

The Migraines

CHAPTER 35

Hemodynamics and Neuroimaging of Migraine

Jes Olesen and Hans-Christoph Diener

The study of vascular mechanisms of migraine falls into three epochs: Throughout the nineteenth century and the first half of the twentieth century, studies emphasized the pulsating nature of headache, the existence of vasodilator-induced headaches, and the efficacy of vasoconstrictor agents in the treatments of migraine (43). The group of Harold G. Wolff (59) utilized with ingenuity available primitive techniques to collect evidence for the vascular nature of migraine and formulated what was for decades the textbook concept of migraine mechanisms. The aura symptoms were thought to be secondary to cerebral vaso-constriction-induced ischemia and the headache secondary to reactive hyperemia. The second epoch came with the possibility of measuring regional cerebral blood flow (rCBF) quantitatively and the demonstration of altered rCBF during attacks. The rCBF pattern was shown to be much more complicated than previously thought and incompatible with spasm of major arteries as the initiating event (38). An extensive account of the circulatory mechanisms of migraine and other headaches as of 1991 can be found in Olesen (35). For older literature, the reader is referred to this source and to another extensive review (36). Therefore, only the best of the older studies are cited in the present text. The third and present epoch uses techniques with a high spatial [positron emission tomography (PET) and magnetic resonance (MR)] and temporal [transcranial Doppler (TCD) and MR) resolution. Metabolism, diffusion, and receptor binding can be measured using PET and MR, and brain arteries can be depicted accurately and noninvasively by MR angiography.

J. Olesen: Department of Neurology, Glostrup Hospital, University of Copenhagen, DK-2600 Glostrup, Copenhagen, Denmark.

H.-C. Diener: Department of Neurology, University of Essen, and Department of Neurology, University Hospital Essen, D-45122 Essen, Germany.

BRAIN BLOOD FLOW CHANGES IN MIGRAINE WITH AURA

Interictal Studies

Most (1,27,38,41) but not all (8) studies of rCBF using [133]-xenon (^{133}Xe) inhalation with stationary detectors or single-photon computerized tomography (SPECT) found the interictal absolute flow as well as the flow pattern to be normal. Lauritzen and Olesen (26) found one case with persistent rCBF asymmetry despite normal CT. Also, other studies indicated the existence of asymmetries (29). In juvenile patients, persistent asymmetries were described in 4 of 20 patients (51).

Several of these studies can be criticized for one or more methodologic features, such as the representativity of the case material, the statistical methods, the possibility of mass significance as a result of regions of interest defined *post hoc* or of multiple comparisons, lack of partial pressure of carbon dioxide (PCO_2) control or influence from extracerebral tissues; however, the largest study, which used a brain-dedicated SPECT system, found significant asymmetries (11) that could not be related to the clinical symptoms. On balance, an interictal mild dysregulation of rCBF is possibly present interictally in migraine with aura.

Triggering of Attacks by Angiography

Of 54 patients with "migraine accompagnee," that is, those who have aura symptoms involving the extremities, 16 developed their typical aura symptoms following angiography after a lag phase of 0.5 to 1 hours (22). In four cases, vertebral angiography was performed without any migraine reaction. Induced and spontaneous attacks were similar. We observed the same in our subsequent rCBF series (27,37,38). Mechanisms of migraine induction are uncertain. Disruption of the blood–brain barrier resulting from hypertonic contrast was favored by Janzen et al. (22), who observed spasm of a major cerebral artery in only four patients, two of whom did not develop migraine attacks. Skinhoj (46) and Skinhoj and Paulson (47) studied intracarotid rCBF followed by carotid angiography. At the height of aura symptoms and rCBF reduction, the angiography was normal except for filling of the top of the basilar artery through the circle of Willis, which could be due to increased vascular resistance in the carotid distribution. Spasm is therefore an unlikely mechanism, but there are several other possibilities: an irritating effect of contrast materials on the arterial endothelium, cold temperature of the injectate, the passage of non–oxygen-carrying contrast material, pressure from the injection distending the artery, or the simple mechanical irritation of a puncture or a catheter tip in the artery. We favor the idea that it is the forcible distention of the internal carotid artery caused by injection that induces activity in perivascular nerves and an arterial-arteriolar reflex response, which in return may cause focal flow reduction and thereby trigger a cortical spreading depression (*vide infra*).

rCBF in the Early Phase of the Attack (Induced Attacks)

Studies of rCBF during the aura phase have shown a reduction (14,20,26,27,34,37,38,41,45,48,52). Focal as well as global reductions in rCBF have been reported, but investigations that used equipment with a high spatial resolution all showed a focal start for the reduction in rCBF (Fig. 1).

This finding was first made clear in the study of Olesen et al. (38) and was confirmed by Lauritzen et al. (27) and Skyhoj Olsen et al. (48). Each of the 254 detectors in this camera measures rCBF in an area of approximately 1 cm² of the cortical mantle of the brain. It is possible to measure rCBF in the same patient up to ten times at 5- to 10-min intervals. Until now, measurements have been published from 27 patients who were monitored from the preaura phase, during the aura phase, and in some cases into the headache phase (14,27,37,38,48). In a few cases, the first abnormality observed is a focal hyperperfusion followed by hypoperfusion, which was observed in three of six patients by Olesen et al. (38), in two of three cases by Friberg et al. (14), and not at all by other authors. Its significance is thus uncertain, and further verification and analysis are necessary. In the great majority of cases, the first phenomenon observed has been a reduction of brain blood flow at the posterior pole of the brain (posterior middle cerebral artery territory or posterior border zone) (Fig.1). This low-flow area often manifests before the patient observes any aura symptoms (37,48) and usually enlarges to involve the parietal-occipital-temporal area and occasionally the whole hemisphere (Fig. 1) (27,38).

A focal low-flow area may appear in the central part of the frontal region, perhaps because the posterior hypoperfusion has spread through the insula into the frontal lobe, sparing the primary sensorimotor cortex (27) (Fig.1). The frontal hypoperfusion, again, spreads gradually in all directions, approximately 2 mm per minute, so that occasionally all of the frontal lobe becomes affected. Friberg et al. (14) described three cases in which migraine aura, which did not involve visual symptoms, was associated primarily with frontal lobe hypoperfusion. Gradual enlargement and spread backwards to involve the precentral and post central regions were observed.

The gradual enlargement of the low-flow area was denoted as *spreading oligemia* by Olesen et al. (38). *Spreading hypoperfusion* is, however, a more correct term and will be used in this chapter. It progresses at approximately 2 to 3 mm per minute in the posterior to anterior direction (27) (Fig.1). Because of the convoluted cerebral cortex and the relatively scattered observations, however, this calculation is not accurate.

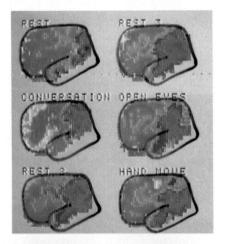

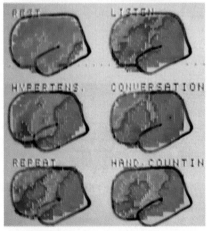

FIG. 1. Original flow results from patients studied before and during the development of a migraine attack with aura. Note the gradual spread of hypoperfusion and the seemingly independent focus in the frontal lobe. There is lack of functional activation in the focal area. [From Lauritzen et al. (27).]

Woods et al. (60) reported changes of rCBF in a woman beginning with the start of an unexpected spontaneous migraine attack. The patient was studied while participating in a visual activation paradigm planned to involve 12 successive measurements of rCBF. After the sixth scan, she developed unilateral headache, nausea, photophobia, and phonophobia. The visual activation paradigm was stopped and rCBF was analyzed while the patient kept her eyes closed during the next six scans. The first decrease in rCBF, noted during the seventh scan, was found bilaterally in the visual association cortex. In each subsequent scan, every 12 minutes, the decrease in rCBF spread forward across the cortical surface toward parietal and occipitotemporal areas at a relatively constant rate, sparing the cerebellum, basal ganglia, and thalamus. The authors estimated the maximal decrease of rCBF (oligemia) to be about 40%, potentially approaching an ischemic level. Most of these changes, however, were of relatively short duration, with substantial recovery by the time of the next measurement 12 to 15 minutes later.

This case report illustrated for the first time, using PET, a bilateral spreading hypoperfusion in a spontaneous migraine attack in a human subject. Even more remarkable is the fact that this patient described only vague visual disturbances that did not fulfill the diagnostic criteria for a visual aura. The result reported by Woods et al. could indicate that "subclinical" spreading oligemia might occur in migraine without aura not reaching the threshold for perceptual deficits. The typical hyperperfusion in the front line of spreading depression known from animal experiments was not detected in this patient. One explanation is the relatively poor spatial and temporal resolution (integration over 90 seconds) of rCBF measurements with PET. The observed changes were relatively short lasting, with substantial recovery in a relatively short time. Investigations later would probably miss them. Despite all the logistic problems, there is a clear need to investigate migraine attacks by using PET or MR as early as possible in the aura phase to confirm these results.

After the slow spread of hypoperfusion, rCBF usually remains relatively unchanged for at least 0.5 to 1 hour. For ethical reasons, it is not possible to continue measurements longer using the intracarotid technique. Spontaneous attacks, on the other hand, usually cannot be studied earlier than 1 hour after onset. At this stage, rCBF has been focally reduced or normal in all published studies (1,20,26,37). rCBF reduction in SPECT studies has virtually always been posterior, involving a smaller or larger part of one hemisphere. With SPECT, typical blood flow abnormalities have been observed mostly in patients who experience both visual and sensory auras, rarely in patients with pure visual auras. This is probably due to technical factors because marked changes were observed with perfusion-weighted MR in pure visual aura (5).

Patients with typical aura symptoms, that is, a slow march of visual and sensory symptoms, virtually always have flow reduction, whereas less typical aura symptoms, such as diffuse hazy vision or spots, usually are associated with normal rCBF (unpublished results). The case of Woods et al. (60) is, however, an exception to this rule.

Completely "out of tune" with others are the findings by Andersson et al. (2) of normal and cerebral metabolic rate (CMR) glucose in induced attacks of migraine with aura. Wrong timing, differences in patient classification, or differences in technical features may be responsible for the lack of positive findings.

Migraine Aura as a Clinical Manifestation of Cortical Spreading Depression (CSD)

The possible relation was already pointed out by Leao and discussed extensively by Lauritzen (25). In Chapter 22 on the basic characteristics of CSD, further data are given. The spread of symptoms and the spread of CSD have the same speed. Also, the spread of hypoperfusion propagates at a similar speed (27). The recent PET study of Woods and colleagues (60) found the same. It remains highly likely but still unproven that CSD is the cortical disturbance resulting in the clinical manifestations of the migraine aura (Table 1).

TABLE 1. *Comparison of migraine with aura and Leao's spreading depression (SD)*

Factor	Migraine	SD
Site of origin	Primary visual cortex	High neuron density
Way of spread	Contiguous, cortical	Contiguous, cortical
Exit/depression	Yes	Yes
Rate of spread	2–6 mm/min	2–6 mm/min
Unilateral	Yes	Yes
Repeated waves	Yes	Yes
Initial hyperemia	(Yes)	Yes
Oligemia lasting	Hours	Hours
Degree of oligemia	Ischemic threshold	Less marked?
Cerebrovascular tone instability	Yes	?
Autoregulation	Preserved?	Preserved
CO_2 reactivity	Abolished?	Impaired
Provocation by arteriography	Yes	?

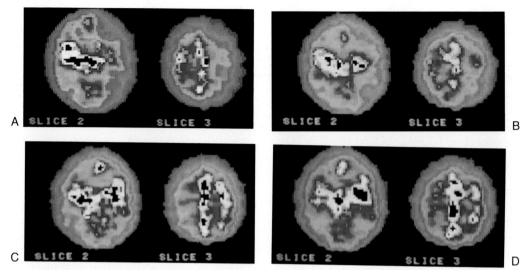

FIG. 2. Regional cerebral blood flow (*rCBF*) during a spontaneous attack of migraine with aura determined by [133]-Xenon inhalation and a brain-dedicated multicrystal single-photon computerized tomography (*SPECT*) system. Two slices 5 and 9 cm above the orbitomeatal line are shown, respectively. **A:** At 30 minutes after onset of migraine aura, a marked reduction of cerebral blood flow in most of the cortex of the right hemisphere is seen (the head is seen from above, low blood flow values are blue, high blood flow values white as seen on the scale to the right). **B:** At 3 hours, the hypoperfusion is still clearly visible but less marked. **C:** At 6 hours, the previously hypoperfused area is now hyperperfused (white, black, and red). This is seen clearly in both slices. **D:** At 24 hours, there is still some increase in blood flow in the right hemisphere, but it is no longer statistically significant. [From Andersen et al. (1).]

rCBF in the Headache Phase

According to Wolff (59), the headache phase of migraine should be due to vasodilatation and hyperperfusion. Several of the early rCBF studies apparently supported this mechanism of pain by demonstrating focal or global hyperperfusion in the headache phase of patients having migraine with aura (34,41,46). The concept was first challenged by Olesen et al. (38) and later by Lauritzen et al. (27). These studies used the intracarotid

method and were extended until 0.5 to 1 hour into the headache phase, at which time rCBF remained depressed. Herold et al. (20) used PET to study a patient who had migraine with aura 2.5 hours after onset of the aura while the patient was experiencing residual neurologic deficits and headache. rCBF was reduced in the temporooccipital region. Woods et al. (60), in their PET study, also found reduced rCBF during headache. A more systematic longitudinal study was performed by Andersen et al. (1) (Fig. 2), who monitored seven patients by using ^{133}Xe inhala-

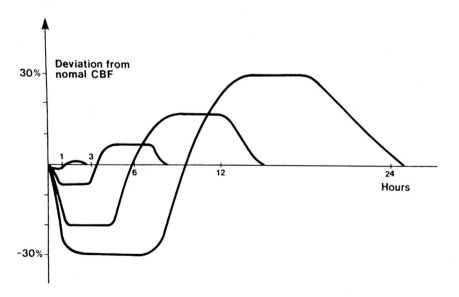

FIG. 3. On the basis of the results of Andersen et al. (1) as well as other experience, the present authors suggest that severity and duration of aura symptoms are related to the severity and duration of blood flow alterations. With short-lasting and mild aura symptoms, such as a typical 20-minute scintillation scotoma, the regional cerebral blood blow (*rCBF*) changes are not marked and may last for only half an hour. With more severe aura symptoms, rCBF changes become more marked and may last several hours before the period of hypoperfusion changes into hyperperfusion. Times and degrees of hypo- and hyperperfusion in the figure are arbitrary.

tion and SPECT from the earliest possible time during the aura (30 minutes to hours after onset) and into the headache phase (after 3–5 hours and 6–8 hours) and in the postheadache phase (after 20–24 hours). Initially, a focal low-flow area was present posterior in the relevant hemisphere. After 3 to 5 hours, three patients had developed hyperemia in the previous low-flow area, and two patients still had a pronounced low-flow area. After 6 to 8 hours, three additional patients had developed hyperperfusion in the previously hypoperfused area. After 20 to 24 hours, CBF had normalized in three patients, whereas two others still showed a slight focal hyperperfusion, and two were not studied at this time. A week after attack, rCBF was normal in all patients. This study clearly showed that timing is crucial to demonstrating hyperperfusion during attacks of migraine with aura. A relationship between the severity of the aura symptoms, the severity of ischemia, and degree as well as duration of hyperemia was indicated (Fig. 3). Similar findings were made in juvenile patients (51). A possible explanation for the hyperperfusion could be previous arteriolar vasoconstriction and oxygen debt, but such a mechanism is likely to be too short lasting. Possibly, liberation of calcitonin gene-related peptide (CGRP) during the aura may be the mechanism (16). At variance with all other previous studies are the findings of normal rCBF during the early headache phase by Andersson et al. (2) using PET.

Temporal and Spatial Relations between Aura Symptoms, rCBF, and Headache

In 63 patients studied serially with either intracarotid flow or SPECT, the sequence of events was described from the early aura to the end of the attack (37). The first observable event was rCBF decrease posterior in one cerebral hemisphere (exempting three frontal cases, a few bilateral cases, and two cases of initial hyperperfusion). Further development of rCBF was accompanied by the aura symptoms. In no case did headache precede the aura symptoms. Thereafter, headache occurred while rCBF remained decreased (Fig.4). During the headache phase, rCBF gradually changed from abnormally low to abnormally high without an apparent change in headache. In some patients, headache disappeared but rCBF remained increased. Thus, headache was dissociated from hyperperfusion at its onset and often also at its termination. It was concluded that headache is associated with the initial cerebral cortical disturbance, which we can observe through its associated rCBF reduction, and that hyperperfusion is probably a secondary phenomenon without direct relationship to headache. In the great majority of patients, aura symptoms were unilateral, as were rCBF changes. The aura symptoms always originated from the hemisphere affected by the low flow (one exception), and the headache was localized over the same hemisphere in

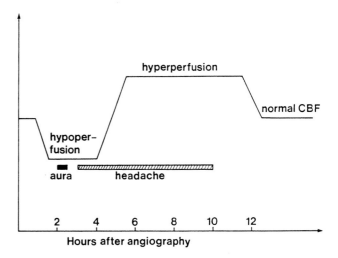

FIG. 4. Schematic drawing illustrating the temporal relation between angiography (time 0 hour), hypoperfusion, aura, headache, hyperperfusion, disappearance of headache, and disappearance of hyperperfusion. The time axis is chosen to illustrate what is typical. The angulation of the flow curve is to show that we do not know details about how fast flow changes. The real course of regional cerebral blood blow (rCBF) changes is smooth. [From Olesen et al. (37).]

35 of 38 cases. The remaining three cases had headache over the presumably unaffected cerebral hemisphere. One third had unilateral aura and rCBF changes but bilateral headache. In conclusion, there is a clear temporal and topographic relation between areas of reduced rCBF, aura symptoms, and headache. The strongly fluctuating course of rCBF changes dictates caution in interpreting point studies of rCBF or metabolism in migraine patients during attacks.

Degree of Blood Flow Reduction

Directly observed rCBF varies from being entirely normal to severely depressed in clinically typical cases. Normal rCBF was observed in 1 of 9 patients (27), 3 of 11 patients (26), and 3 of 12 patients (1). The average blood flow reduction in the study by Olesen et al. (38) was 35%, whereas Lauritzen et al. (27) found a 25% reduction. Using ^{133}Xe inhalation and SPECT, Lauritzen and Olesen (26) found rCBF reductions averaging 17% in eight patients. In each of these studies, one or two cases displayed rCBF in the ischemic range. Skyhoj Olesen et al. (48) attempted to correct measured rCBF for Compton scattered radiation. The estimated true rCBF reduction averaged 50% or more, corresponding to a level of 20 to 25 ml/100g/min. These estimates may not be correct, however. For example, occasional patients have had rCBF reduction in the whole hemisphere, which eliminates the possibility of Compton scatter, but blood flow nevertheless has not always been reduced to ischemic values in such patients (26,27,37,46). The tracer ^{99m}Tc-D,L-hexamethyl-propylene-amine-oxime (^{99}Tc-HMPAO) causes less Compton scatter than ^{133}Xe. Nevertheless, measured values have not approached ischemic levels, except in a few patients, and several patients have had normal rCBF (6,11). A similar picture emerges from studies using PET, when Compton scatter is less important (20,60) and MR where Compton scatter is not involved (5). Thus, Cutrer et al. (5) studied five spontaneous visual auras in four patients. In the gray matter of the occipital cortex contralateral to the affected visual hemifield, rCBF was significantly decreased by 16% to 53%. Regional cerebral blood volume (rCBV) was preserved (6%–33% decrease) and mean transit time (rMTT) was elevated ranging from 10% to 54%. No changes in the apparent diffusion coefficient were observed.

In conclusion, ischemia may occur in a few patients, but ischemia cannot possibly be the cause of the migraine aura. On the other hand, the rCBF reduction is at least partially caused by vasoconstriction which exceeds a possible reduction in brain oxidative metabolism as reflected on increased arterovenous oxygen extraction (13).

RCBF IN MIGRAINE WITHOUT AURA

Interictal Studies

Interictally, most previous studies found a normal flow distribution in patients suffering from migraine without aura (6,26,39,41). In a recent PET study, no interictal abnormalities were found (58). Contrasting with these studies, several previous studies, including a relatively recent and large study using ^{133}Xe inhalation of ^{99}Tc HMPAO and brain-dedicated SPECT showed significant asymmetrics (11). At present, it is difficult to know whether reported inhomogeneities of resting state blood flow outside of migraine attack are real.

rCBF During Attack

The first study that focused exclusively on rCBF during attacks of migraine without aura was done in 1981, with the aim of disclosing a possible early period of hypoperfusion such as that seen in migraine with aura (39). Since the onset of migraine without aura is usually insidious, Olesen et al. selected patients in whom attacks could be provoked within approximately 1 hour by red wine or specific foods. The rCBF measurements were done before provocation, after provocation, and then repeated until a full-blown attack developed. At no point were any focal low-flow areas disclosed in any of the six patients. It was concluded that the migraine attack without aura is not initiated by focal hypoperfusion, similar to what is seen in migraine with aura. Possibly contrasting with these findings is a recent case studied by PET (60). Several studies examined rCBF during the spontaneous attack and then compared the findings with those in the attack-free state. Some early studies described hyperemia, but this is almost certainly an artifact because a large number of subsequent studies using different techniques have all shown normal global as well as focal CBF during attacks (6,9,26). Herold et al. (32) studied one patient by using PET 3 hours after onset of migraine without aura. rCBF was normal and no difference between the two hemispheres was observed.

In a study of 13 patients (three men, ten women; age, 24–57 years), Weiller et al. (58) investigated rCBF during spontaneous migraine attacks without aura and in the headache-free interval with the $C^{15}O_2$ inhalation technique using an ECAT 953-15 PET scanner. Patients with spontaneous, untreated, unilateral migraine headaches during the first 6 hours of the attack were included. Using a region-of-interest analysis and statistical parametric mapping, no differences in rCBF were found between the hemispheres ipsilateral and contralateral to the headache side. Furthermore, no migraine-specific differences in rCBF were found between repeated measurements during the attack and the headache-free interval. This finding is in line with the data of Andersson et al. (2) in ten patients using PET. Weiller and associates (58) found increased activation in the inferior anterocaudal cingulate cortex as well as in the visual and auditory association cortices during the attack. These changes were not detectable after treatment of the attack or in the interval and were considered secondary to pain activation. In an experimental study using painful injections of capsaicin in the frontotemporal region, a similar pattern of activation was seen (31).

In a recent PET study (4) in nine patients experiencing migraine without aura, a small reduction of CBF and CBV with unchanged oxygen metabolism and oxygen extraction was described. The time interval between onset of the attack and the PET measurements varied between 3.8 and 24.5 hours. The results were suggested to indicate an uncoupling of blood flow and metabolism during a migraine attack.

In summary, rCBF in the cerebral hemispheres, apart from unspecific pain activation, is normal in migraine without aura interictally and during attack.

Brainstem Changes

Raskin and colleagues (40) reported in 1987 that patients who underwent implantation of electrodes in the raphe nucleus or periaqueductal gray for the treatment of chronic pain reported migraine-like unilateral headache with nausea, vomiting, photophobia, and phonophobia. This was also the case in patients who did not suffer from migraine. These observations indicate that there might be an anatomic structure in the brainstem or midbrain involved in the "generation" of either headache or the attack as a whole (7). Nine patients (7 women, 2 men; age 29–57 years) suffering from migraine without aura were

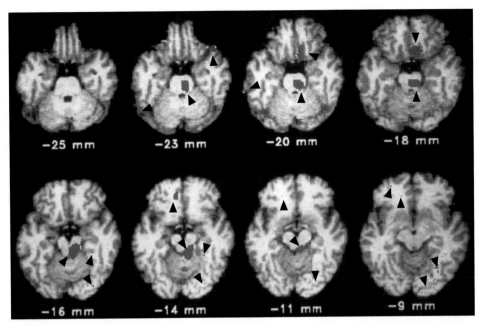

FIG. 5. Regional cerebral blood flow (rCBF) measurements of nine migraine patients. The arrows point to areas of increased blood flow. Data are calculated by subtracting rCBF during the headache-free phase from the migraine attack. rCBF data are superposed on a normalized magnetic resonance image. Note the increase in rCBF in the brainstem and midbrain. The activation of the cingulum is unspecific.

studied during a spontaneous, acute migraine attack with right-sided headache. Headache was classified as migraine without aura according to the Headache Classification Committee of the International Headache Society (19). All nine patients were studied within 6 hours of onset of untreated migraine symptoms. Each patient had three rCBF measurements: (a) during the acute attack, (b) after the relief of headache and other related symptoms by subcutaneous administration of 6 mg of sumatriptan, and (c) during the headache-free interval 3 days to 4 months later.

Significantly higher rCBF values (+11%) were found during the acute attack compared with the headache-free interval in median brainstem structures over several planes, slightly contralateral to the headache side (Fig. 5). The consistent increases in rCBF in the brainstem (covering periaqueductal gray, midbrain reticular formation, and locus coeruleus) persisted, even after sumatriptan induced complete relief from headache, nausea, phonophobia, and photophobia. This increase was not seen outside the attack. Therefore, it is unlikely that the observed activation is due only to pain perception or increased activity of the endogenous antinociceptive system. It does not seem to be a consequence of headache or related to the relief from headache, but it may be inherent to the migraine attack itself, which could explain why sumatriptan, with its short half-life, and other compounds are effective in mitigating the symptoms of migraine but are sometimes unable to terminate the actual attack and why

the headache may recur after the effect of the treatment has "worn off."

It is beyond the resolution of the PET scanner to attribute foci of rCBF increases to distinct brainstem nuclei. The foci of maximum increase coincided, in the Talairach space, with the anatomic location of the dorsal raphe nucleus and the locus coeruleus. Dysfunction of the regulation of these brainstem nuclei involved in antinociception and extracerebral and intracerebral vascular control provides a far-reaching explanation for many of the facets in migraine. It is attractive to consider the observed activation in the brainstem as the first direct visualization of the postulated "migraine center" in humans. Another possibility was proposed by Goadsby and Fields (15): the area of increased activity could reflect neuron projection to the thalamus, modulating pain transmission.

Vascular Reactivity in Migraine With or Without Aura

Functional tests, such as speech, reading, listening, and arm work, elicit increased rCBF in specific areas of the brain. During attacks of migraine with aura, these activation procedures were not accompanied by the usual increase in rCBF in the low-flow areas, whereas a normal, focal rCBF increase was observed in the nonaffected parts of the brain (28,38). The rCBF response to $PaCO_2$ and systemic blood pressure changes in patients investigated with ^{133}Xe inhalation and stationary detectors was impaired (42). Lauritzen et al. (28) concluded from their studies with ^{133}Xe intracarotid injection and 254 stationary detectors that autoregulation was normal during migraine attacks. They recorded an impaired but not abolished reactivity to hyperventilation. Recently, Skyhoj Olesen and Lassen (49) reestimated these reactivity data and concluded that the CO_2 response in the migraine area may reflect Compton scatter from nonaffected areas. With regard to normal autoregulation, they calculated that if flow in the normal area was 40 mL/100 g per minute or more, it would be impossible to measure even large changes of true flow in the low-flow area. On balance, it must be concluded that it is impossible to know whether the $PaCO_2$ reactivity is completely abolished or only impaired. It is most likely but not definitely established that autoregulation is normal.

Friberg et al. (14), in their report of "frontal migraine," observed that the washout curves recorded over the low-flow area were nonlinear in the semilogarithmic plot. Severe ischemia seemed to alternate with hyperemia over periods lasting 20 to 60 seconds. The average flow calculated from the 1-minute slope was always reduced. The suggested explanation was a transient constriction of the arterioles that alternated with short episodes of vasodilatation, a state denoted as "vascular tone instability." The phenomenon needs validation by formal statistical procedures.

Studies of the regulation of rCBF during migraine without aura are sparse. Using ^{133}Xe inhalation and stationary detectors, a decreased response to arterial PCO_2 changes during headache but no side differences were described (42). By 48 hours or longer after the attack, the response to hypercapnia was excessive, whereas the response to hypocapnia was normal. The opposite, a decreased response to 5% CO_2 outside of attacks also has been described as well as normal reactivity (42,44). Using TCD, a normal reactivity to hyperventilation was shown both during and outside of attacks (44,61). Others found an exaggerated response to hypocapnia in migraine with aura outside of attack (10,55). Autoregulation was normal in two patients (42). The response to breathing 100% oxygen was reported by some to be exaggerated (42). An abnormal response to the cold pressor test has been described in migraine with aura (32). Further studies of the regulation of rCBF during attacks of migraine without aura are much needed.

ARTERIOVENOUS SHUNTING

Since the turn of nineteenth century, the hypothesis that migraine could be due to arteriovenous (AV) shunting has lingered. Scrutiny of the evidence for this hypothesis reveals that it is close to nonexistent, and therefore numerous older studies that have not used modern scientific methods are not discussed here. Because this hypothesis is, from time to time, mentioned and because it led to animal experimental models that have proved highly suc-

cessful in predicting the activity of antimigraine drugs (see Chapter 23), the uniformly negative reports from CBF studies in regard to AV shunting must be mentioned. Studies with intraarterial ^{133}Xe are eminently effective in detecting AV shunting. Thus, even small degrees of shunting in intracranial tumors may be seen easily as so-called *shunt peaks*, which are clearly distinguished from so-called *tissue peaks* seen in smaller hyperperfused areas without shunting. Arteriovenous malformations are revealed by enormous shunt peaks. Despite this low detection level, shunting never has been observed in any of the more than 30 migraine patients studied during an attack using the intracarotid injection method and [133]Xe. It may therefore be concluded with absolute certainty that AV shunting in the internal carotid artery territory does not occur during migraine attacks. Most studies in the territory of the external carotid artery have used the local injection of ^{133}Xe, which measures from just a tiny area of injected tissue. Shunting in this territory would normally increase the temperature and cause flushing, however, but this has not been observed in migraine. Furthermore, shunting, which occurs frequently in the fingers, toes, ears, and nose, is not known to be painful. Therefore, it must be concluded that shunting in the internal carotid artery territory is not possible and that shunting in the external carotid artery territory is highly unlikely in migraine.

INTRACRANIAL ARTERIAL RESPONSES

Blood flow studies reflect arteriolar diameter and indicate little or nothing about the arteries. Arteriograms during migraine attacks generally revealed no abnormalities except for abnormal filling of the basilar artery after intracarotid injections, indicating increased cerebral vascular resistance in the carotid territory but not in the basilar artery territory (22,46,47,52). Occasional reports of spasms in migraine have appeared. This literature was reviewed by Solomon et al. (50), who found a total of 14 published cases, two with ophthalmoplegic migraine (MO), nine with aura, and three without aura. Their own case and several cases in the literature involved an unusual, prolonged attack of headaches prompting the angiography. In two cases a stenosis was demonstrated after the patient became asymptomatic, and in four cases the arteriographic changes did not correlate with focal symptoms such as the side of headache. Solomon et al. (50) concluded that arterial narrowing is rare in migraineurs and most likely an epiphenomenon unrelated to headache.

Transcranial Doppler measures linear velocity of blood in large arteries. Measured alterations may, however, reflect changes in flow in the area supplied by the artery (volume flow in the artery) as well as changes in diameter of the artery without change in volume flow and may finally be caused by any combination of the two. The relationship between flow (F), velocity (V), and cross-sectional area (A) of an artery can be described as follows: $A = rCBF/V \times K$, where K is a constant.

When both rCBF and V are known, relative changes in A may be calculated, and when rCBF remains constant, as in MO, TCD changes are inversely related to A. Unfortunately, TCD findings in MO show no uniform picture. Some have described completely normal TCD during and outside of attacks (30,61,62), whereas others described reduced velocity bilaterally (57) or specifically on the side of pain (12,56). In other studies, the TCD response to glyceryl trinitrate has been exaggerated in migraineurs compared with normal subjects (3,54).

EXTRACEREBRAL BLOOD FLOW AND ARTERIAL RESPONSES

Direct measurements using local ^{133}Xe clearance from temporal subcutaneous tissue and temporal muscle have revealed no abnormalities during migraine attacks with or without aura (23,24). Also the regulation of local blood flow was normal in these tissues during as well as outside of attacks in migraineurs compared with normal controls (23,24). The application of various indirect methods has unfortunately confused the picture. Definite statements about blood flow in extracranial tissues cannot be made at present. The superficial temporal artery has been a focus of interest in studies of migraine pathophysiology over several decades. Wolff (59) regarded dilatation and increased pulsations of the superficial temporal artery and other extracranial arteries as the most important mechanism of migraine pain. Several indirect methods used to study this artery will not be reviewed here; however, the application of high-frequency ultrasound equipment has made possible direct measurement of the diameter of this artery (33). Both radial arteries and the superficial temporal artery contralateral to pain constricted during migraine attacks, probably secondary to pain-induced increase in sympathetic outflow (21). The superficial temporal artery on the side of unilateral migraine attacks had significantly larger diameter than on the nonsymptomatic side. These findings were interpreted as the effect of migraine-associated vasodilatation superposed on a systemic vasoconstriction (21). The balance between opposing influences explains why not all migraine patients exhibit a dilated temporal artery. Palpation of the superficial temporal artery did not increase migraine pain. The exact role of this artery in pain mechanisms remains uncertain.

NEUROGENIC CONTROL OF EXTRACEPHALIC ARTERIES AND THE HEART

For older studies, mostly done with less than optimal design and techniques, see Olesen (36). Among the findings suggested were abnormal cardiovascular reflexes, abnormal response to heating, abnormal vasoconstriction caused by a cold stimulus, increased coincidence of Raynaud's syndrome and Prinzmetal's angina, increased heart rate, and increased spontaneous fluctuations of heart rate.

A number of investigators recently analyzed cardiovascular responses in migraineurs during headache-free intervals using one or several of the following procedures: variations of R-R intervals on the electrocardiogram during normal breathing or Valsalva's maneuver, blood pressure measurements during Valsalva's maneuver, body tilting, isometric work tests, and Aschner's test. Detailed studies were performed by Havanka-Kanniainen et al. (17,18) in 49 migraineurs aged 11 to 22 years and in 60 migraineurs aged 23 to 50 years. No significant differences were found between the group of young migraineurs and a control group. In adult migraineurs, however, significant abnormalities were disclosed, suggesting sympathetic hypofunction and mild parasympathetic hypofunction. No differences were found in cardiovascular responses between various clinical subgroups of migraine patients. In ten migraineurs, Havanka-Kanniainen and colleagues (18) found that sympathetic hypofunction was more pronounced during than outside of an attack.

Thomsen and colleagues (53) could not confirm the presence of sympathetic dysfunction but found an abnormal response to Vasalva's maneuver suggesting a mild parasympathetic hypofunction. On balance, the only relatively consistent finding is that of a parasympathetic hypofunction. Large, well-designed prospective studies are needed to confirm or refute the other findings described herein.

REFERENCES

1. Andersen AR, Friberg L, Olsen TS, Olesen J. SPECT demonstration of delayed hyperemia following hypoperfusion in classic migraine. *Arch Neurol* 1988;45:154–159.
2. Andersson JLR, Muhr C, Valind S, Lundberg PO, Langström B. Regional cerebral blood flow and oxygen metabolism during migraine with and without aura. *Cephalalgia* 1997;17:570–579.
3. Bellantonio P, Micieli G, Buzzi MG, et al. Haemodynamic correlates of early and delayed responses to sublingual administration of isosorbide dinitrate in migraine patients: a transcranial Doppler study. *Cephalalgia* 1997;17:183–187.
4. Bednarczyk EM, Remler B, Weikart C, Nelson AD, Reed, RC. Global cerebral blood flow, blood volume, and oxygen metabolism in patients with migraine headache. *Neurology* 1998;50:1736–1740.
5. Cutrer FM, Sorensen AG, Weisskopf RM, et al. Perfusion-weighted imaging defects during spontaneous migrainous aura. *Ann Neurol* 1998;43:25–31.
6. Davies PTG, Steiner TJ, Costa DC, Jones BE, Jewkes RF, Rose FC. Caution in extrapolating from regional cerebral blood flow studies of migraine to hypotheses of pathogenesis. In: Rose FC, ed. *New advances in headache research*. London: Smith-Gordon, 1989:169–174.
7. Diener HC, May A. New aspects of migraine pathophysiology: lessions learned from positron emission tomography: editorial review. *Curr Opin Neurol* 1996;9:199–201.
8. Facco E, Munari M, Baratto F, et al. Regional cerebral blood flow (rCBF) in migraine during the interictal period: different rCBF patterns in patients with and without aura. *Cephalalgia* 1996;16:161–168.
9. Ferrari MD, Haan J, Blokland JA, et al. Cerebral blood flow during migraine attacks without aura and effect of sumatriptan. *Arch Neurol* 1995;52:135–139.

10. Fiermonte G, Pierelli F, Pauri F, Cosentino FI, Soccorsi R, Giacomini P. Cerebrovascular CO_2 reactivity in migraine with aura and without aura: a transcranial Doppler study. *Acta Neurol Scand* 1995;92: 166–169.

11. Friberg L, Olesen J, Iversen HK, et al. Interictal "patshy" regional cerebral blood flow patterns in migraine patients: a single phaton emission comuterized tomographic study. *Eur J Neurol* 1994;1:35–44.

12. Friberg L, Olesen J, Iversen HK, Sperling B. Migraine pain associated with middle cerebral artery dilatation: reversal by sumatriptan. *Lancet* 1991;338:13–17.

13. Friberg L, Olesen J, Lassen NA, Olsen TS, Karle A. Cerebral oxygen extraction, oxygen consumption, and regional cerebral blood flow during the aura phase of migraine. *Stroke* 1994;25:974–979.

14. Friberg L, Skyhoj Olsen T, Roland PE, Lassen NA. Focal ischemia caused by instability of cerebrovascular tone during attacks of hemiplegic migraine. *Brain* 1987;110:917–934.

15. Goadsby PJ, Fields HL. On the functional anatomy of migraine. *Ann Neurol* 1998;43:272–272.

16. Goadsby PJ, Edvinsson L, Ekman R. Vasoactive peptide relese in the extracerebral circulation of humans during migraine headache. *Ann Neurol* 1990;28:183–187.

17. Havanka-Kanniainen H, Tolone U, Myllylaua VV. Cardiovascular reflexes in young migraine patients. *Headache* 1986;26:420–424.

18. Havanka-Kanniainen H, Tolona U, Myllylaura VV. Autonomic dysfunction in adult migraineurs. *Headache* 1986;26:425–430.

19. Headache Classification Committee of the International Headache Society. Classification and diagnostic criteria for headache disorders, cranial neuralgias and facial pain. *Cephalalgia* 1988;8(Suppl 7):1–96.

20. Herold S, Gibbs JM, Jones AKP, Brooks DJ, Frackowiak RSJ, Legg NJ. Oxygen metabolism in migraine. *J Cereb Blood Flow Metab* 1985; 5(Suppl 1):445–446.

21. Iversen HK, Nielsen TH, Olesen J, Tfelt-Hansen P. Arterial responses during migraine headache. *Lancet* 1990;336:837–839.

22. Janzen R, Tanzer A, Zschocke S, Dieckmann H. Postangiographische Spätreaktionen der Hirngefässe bei Migräne-Kranken. *Z Neurol* 1972;201:24–42.

23. Jensen K. Subcutaneous blood flow in the temporal region of migraine patients. *Acta Neurol Scand* 1987;75:310–318.

24. Jensen K, Olesen J. Temporal muscle blood flow in common migraine. *Acta Neurol Scand* 1985;72:561–570.

25. Lauritzen M. Cerebral blood flow in migraine and cortical spreading depression. *Acta Neurol Scand* 1987;76(Suppl 113):1–40.

26. Lauritzen M, Olesen J. Regional cerebral blood flow during migraine attacks by xenon-133 inhalation and emission tomography. *Brain* 1984;107:447–461.

27. Lauritzen M, Skyhoj Olsen T, Lassen NA, Paulson OB. The changes of regional cerebral blood flow during the course of classical migraine attacks. *Ann Neurol* 1983;13:633–641.

28. Lauritzen M, Skyhoj Olsen T, Lassen NA, Paulson OB. The regulation of regional cerebral blood flow during and between migraine attacks. *Ann Neurol* 1983;14:569–572.

29. Levine SR, Welch KMA, Ewing JR, Robertson WM. Asymmetric cerebral blood flow patterns in migraine. *Cephalalgia* 1987;7:245–248.

30. Limmroth V, May A, Auerbach P, Wosnitza G, Eppe T, Diener HC. Changes in cerebral blood flow velocity after treatment with sumatriptan or placebo and implications for the pathophysiology of migraine. *J Neurol Sci* 1996;138:60–66.

31. May A, Kaube H, Buchel C, et al. Experimental cranial pain elicited by capsaicin: a PET study. *Pain* 1998;74:61–66.

32. Micieli G, Tassorelli C, Bosone D, et al. Increased cerebral blood flow velocity indued by cold pressor test in migraine: a possible basis for pathogenesis? *Cephalalgia* 1995;15:494–498.

33. Nielsen TH, Iversen HK, Tfelt-Hansen P. Determination of the luminal diameter of the radial artery in man by high frequency ultrasound: a methodological study. *Ultrasound Med Biol* 1990;16:787–791.

34. Norris JW, Hachinski VC, Cooper PW. Changes in cerebral blood flow during a migraine attack. *BMJ* 1975;3:676–677.

35. Olesen J, ed. *Migraine and other headaches: the vascular mechanisms.* New York: Raven Press, 1991:1–358.

36. Olesen J. Hemodynamics. In: Olesen J, Tfelt-Hansen P, Welch KMA, eds. *The headaches.* New York: Raven Press, 1993:209–222.

37. Olesen J, Friberg L, Olsen TS, et al. Timing and topography of cerebral blood flow, aura and headache during migraine attacks. *Ann Neurol* 1990;28:791–798.

38. Olesen J, Larsen B, Lauritzen M. Focal hyperemia followed by spreading oligemia and impaired activation of rCBF in classic migraine. *Ann Neurol* 1981;9:344–352.

39. Olesen J, Tfelt-Hansen P, Henriksen L, Larsen B. The common migraine attack may not be initiated by cerebral ischemia. *Lancet* 1981;2:438–440.

40. Raskin NH, Hosobuchi Y, Lamb S. Headcache may arise from preturbation of the brain. *Headache* 1987;27:416–420.

41. Sakai F, Meyer JS. Regional cerebral hemodynamics during migraine and cluster headache measured by the 133-Xe inhalation method. *Headache* 1978;18:122–132.

42. Sakai F, Meyer JS. Abnormal cerebrovascular reactivity in patients with migraine and cluster headache. *Headache* 1979;19:257–266.

43. Schiller F. The migraine tradition. *Bull Hist Med* 1975;49:1–19.

44. Silvestrini M, Cupini LM, Troisi E, Matteis M, Bernardi G. Estimation of cerebrovascular reactivity in migraine without aura. *Stroke* 1995;26:81–83.

45. Simard D, Paulson OB. Cerebral vasomotor paralysis during migraine attack. *Arch Neurol* 1973;29:207–209.

46. Skinhoj E. Hemodynamic studies within the brain during migraine. *Arch Neurol* 1973;29:95–98.

47. Skinhhoj E, Paulson OB. Regional cerebral blood flow in internal carotid distribution during migraine attack. *BMJ* 1969;3:569–570.

48. Skyhoj Olsen T, Friberg L, Lassen NA. Ischemia may be the primary cause of the neurological deficits in classic migraine. *Arch Neurol* 1987;44:156–161.

49. Skyhoj Olsen T, Lassen NA. Blood flow and vascular reactivity during attacks of classic migraine: limitations of the Xe-133 intraarterial technique. *Headache* 1988;29:15–20.

50. Solomon S, Lipton RB, Harris PY. Arterial stenosis in migraine: spasm or arteriopathy? *Headache* 1990;30:52–61.

51. Soriani S, Feggi L, Battistella PA, Arnaldi C, De Carlo L, Stipa S. Interictal and ictal phase study with Tc 99m HMPAO brain SPECT in juvenile migraine with aura. *Headache* 1997;37:31–36.

52. Staehelin Jensen T, Voldby B, Olivarius BF, Jensen FT. Cerebral hemodynamics in familial hemiplegic migraine. *Cephalalgia* 1981;1:121–125.

53. Thomsen LL, Iversen HK, Boesen F, Olesen J. Transcranial Doppler and cardiovascular responses during cardiovascular autonomic tests in migrainerus. *Brain* 1995;118:1319–1327.

54. Thomsen LL, Iversen HK, Brinck TA, Olesen J. Arterial supersensitivity to nitric oxide (nitroglycerin) in migraine sufferers. *Cephalalgia* 1993;13:395–399.

55. Thomsen JJ, Iversen HK, Olesen J. Increased cerebrovascular pCO_2 reactivity in migraine with aura: a transcranial Doppler study during hyperventilation. *Cephalalgia* 1995;15:211–215.

56. Thomsen JJ, Iversen HK, Olesen J. Cerebral blood flow velocities are reduced during attacks of unilateral migraine without aura. *Cephalalgia* 1995;15:109–116.

57. Totaro R, De Matteis G, Marini C, Baldassarre M, Carolei A. Sumatriptan and cerebral blood flow velocity changes during migraine attacks. *Headache* 1997;37:635–639.

58. Weiller C, May A, Limmroth V, et al. Brain stem activation in spontaneous human migraine attacks. *Nat Med* 1995;1:658–660.

59. Wolff HG. *Headache and other head pain*, 2nd ed. New York: Oxford University Press, 1963.

60. Woods RP, Iacoboni M, Mazziotta JC. Bilateral spreading cerebral hypoperfusion during spontaneous migraine headache. *N Engl J Med* 1994;331:1689–1692.

61. Zwetsloot CP, Caekebeke JFV, Odink J, Ferrari MD. Vascular reactivity during migraine attacks: a transcranial Doppler study. *Headache* 1991;31:593–595.

62. Zwetsloot CP, Caekebeke JFV, Ferrari MD. Lack of asymmetry of middle cerebral artery blood velocity in unilateral migraine. *Stroke* 1993;24:1335–1338.

The Headaches, Second Edition,
edited by J. Olesen, P. Tfelt-Hansen, and K.M.A. Welch.
Lippincott Williams & Wilkins, Philadelphia © 2000.

The Migraines

CHAPTER 36

Cerebral Metabolic and Cerebrospinal Fluid Studies

K. Michael A. Welch

CEREBROSPINAL FLUID

Routine Diagnostic Findings

The standard diagnostic tests in cerebrospinal fluid (CSF) usually show no abnormality of pressure, protein, or cell count in migraine patients. This finding holds true even when migraine is associated with moderately severe neurologic deficits (11,50). For example, no abnormality was found in two series of patients with hemiplegic migraine or in a series of patients with migraine associated with stupor or coma (34). Nevertheless, CSF protein can be elevated as a result of a disordered blood–brain barrier when migraine is frequent and severe (18,22) or when it is associated with cerebral infarction (39). Elevated CSF protein also was reported in six patients with migraine associated with mitochondrial encephalomyopathy (20). Two of these patients had oligoclonal bonding. The CSF was examined late in the course of the disease, and residual neurologic deficit was present resulting from frequent attacks of migraine and seizures. The CSF changes thus were probably due partly to an altered blood–brain barrier and were reflected in the severity and chronicity of the disorder. Also, migraine most likely was symptomatic in these cases.

The issue of migraine attacks being symptomatic of an underlying process causing CSF pleocytosis or the CSF abnormality simply being a result of migraine underlies most of the cases with CSF abnormality reported in the literature. These cases were accompanied by neurologic deficit; CSF was sampled presumably because of difficulty with differential diagnosis or because of atypical clinical features of migraine. Bartleson et al. (8) held the former opinion of their seven patients who did not have a prior migraine history and suffered a series of migraine-like attacks associated with CSF lymphocytosis, increased protein, and increased CSF pressure. They considered these cases to be symptomatic of a transient inflammatory disorder of the central nervous system (CNS) of uncertain cause. Two other cases resembling these cases were later reported in the literature these cases (31,45). In other reported cases with CSF pleocytosis, angiography or pneumoencephalography may have accounted for a polymorphonuclear leukocytosis (19,57). Many of these cases were reported before contemporary imaging techniques had been developed, however, raising diagnostic uncertainties.

Gomez-Aranda et al. published the largest series in the most recent literature, comprising 50 patients who suffered a total of 164 episodes of what they called *pseudomigraine* (we prefer the term *symptomatic migraine*) with temporary neurologic symptoms and lymphocytic pleocytosis (26). The disorder presented between the ages of 14 and 39 years and was most frequent in male patients (68%). Eight male (24%) and five female (31%) subjects had a prior history of migraine. Twenty-five percent had had a viral-like illness up to 3 weeks before onset of the syndrome. Patients suffered one to 12 episodes of neurologic deficit for a mean duration of 5 hours, accompanied by moderate to severe headache for a mean of 19 hours and occasionally fever. They complained commonly of sensory symptoms, aphasia and motor deficits. Visual symptoms were uncom-

---

K. M. A. Welch: Department of Neurology, University of Kansas School of Medicine, University of Kansas Medical Center, Kansas City, Kansas 66106.

mon. All patients were asymptomatic between episodes and after the symptomatic period that lasted up to 49 days. The CSF lymphocytic pleocytosis ranged from 10 to 760 cells/mm³ CSF. Protein was increased in 96% of patients, immunoglobulin G (IgG) was normal in 80% of cases, and oligoclonal bands were not found. Extensive microbiologic studies were negative. Brain computed tomography (CT) and magnetic resonance imaging (MRI) were always within normal limits, whereas electroencephalograpy (EEG) frequently showed focal slowing. In one patient of 12 in whom the procedure was performed, an abnormal cerebral angiogram suggested localized vascular inflammation coincident with the focal neurologic symptoms. Single-photon emission computed tomography (SPECT), performed in only three patients in the symptomatic period, revealed focal areas of decreased uptake consistent with the clinical symptoms. Similar SPECT findings were reported from a separate center in similar patients (12). Because a number of patients had experienced a prodromal viral-like illness, the authors hypothesized that an aseptic inflammation of the leptomeningeal vasculature possibly accounted for the clinical picture. It seems reasonable to conclude that, even when a secondary illness cannot be confirmed, migraine-like symptoms associated with elevated CSF protein and a pleocytosis most likely reflect a disorder of unidentified cause, of which migraine symptoms are symptomatic.

Biochemical Abnormalities in CSF

A number of studies have examined the biochemistry of CSF with the objective of understanding the mechanisms of the disorder because the CSF acts as a "sink" for compounds produced in the CNS. These studies are of particular value because of the limited number of investigations of cerebral metabolism in migraine patients. This approach has contributed information, albeit indirect, on disturbances of cerebral metabolic and neurotransmitter function in the CNS of migraine sufferers.

Skinhoj (47) documented significant elevation of lactate in the CSF in patients whose cerebral blood flow (CBF) also was measured. This finding was used as evidence to support the concept of cerebral ischemia being the cause of the migraine aura and now should be considered in the light of brain lactate elevation documented by *in vivo* nuclear magnetic resonance (NMR) spectroscopy (see section on metabolism). No other metabolites of the brain energetic system have been examined in CSF. Also, the ionic constituents of CSF have not been studied, with the exception of magnesium (Mg^{2+}), which Jain et al. (28) found to be reduced in CSF sampled between migraine attacks.

The biogenic amines have been studied because of their putative involvement in migraine and chronic pain states. Serotonin (5-HT) was the first neurotransmitter to be studied by means of measuring its metabolite,

5-hydroxyindoleacetic acid (5-HIAA), in CSF. During an attack, 5-HIAA was reported to be low (41), high (29), or unchanged (7) in different series. In another study (30), CSF 5-HIAA was higher than in controls when sampled between and during migraine attacks. The most recent and largest study carried out found no evidence of change in 5-HT or 5-HIAA between attacks (43). Thus, no clear statement can be made about exactly how CNS serotonin metabolism is altered, either between or during attacks.

Catecholamine studies also have been performed in CSF as part of investigations into migraine pathogenesis. Homovanilic acid (HVA), a dopamine metabolite, has been measured less often in CSF, and, although trends toward an increase have been reported both during and between attacks (29,30), no significant differences have been documented. Castillo et al. studied the biochemical parameters related to central dopaminergic neurotransmission in migraine patients during attacks (15). They determined the tyrosine and 3,4-dihydroxyphenylacetic acid (DOPAC) levels in the CSF of 47 patients, 29 suffering migraine without aura and 18 suffering migraine with aura and compared these levels with those of 27 control subjects. Tyrosine levels did not differ significantly between patients and controls. The CSF concentration of DOPAC was 0.73 ± 0.55 ng/mL in the control population, 3.84 ± 2.08 ng/mL in patients with migraine without aura, and 3.30 ± 1.49 ng/mL in patients suffering migraine with aura. The concentration of DOPAC correlated positively with the intensity of headache. In sum, tyrosine levels in CSF during migraine were normal, but DOPAC levels in CSF were significantly higher during migraine than in controls in patients with and without aura. In a previous study, the authors observed lower plasma and CSF levels of noradrenaline and adrenaline in migraine patients during crisis compared with controls (36). Taken together, these findings suggested that the migraine attack is associated with dopaminergic hyperfunction and noradrenergic hypofunction at a central level. The results should be viewed in the light of MRI studies that showed activation of the substantia nigra during an attack (reported in the next section).

Histamine is the final biogenic amine to be studied, although rarely in migraine and more often in cluster headache. Castillo et al. obtained plasma CSF samples during attacks from 29 patients with migraine without aura and 18 with aura (14). Histidine levels were approximately double those of controls in both migraine subtypes. The precise mechanisms whereby this precursor of histamine is involved in migraine remain to be determined.

The opioid system (because of its role in central pain mechanisms) also has been studied. CSF endorphin (E), the main endogenous opioid substance, is consistently low in migraine patients (2,21,25). More recently, a marked increase in CSF *N*-acetyl endorphin (AcE), a posttranslational product of E, has been reported (21). AcE does not bind to opiate receptors and may counter the analgesic activity of E. Thus, AcE could act as a physiological opiate antagonist and induce imbalance of the endogenous nociceptive system in migraine patients.

In a study yet to be replicated (48), somatostatin, neuropeptide Y, and beta-endorphin levels were measured during migraine attacks without aura. Somatostatin levels were decreased between attacks compared with a mixed control group comprising psychiatric patients and decreased further during an attack. Beta-endorphin also was decreased during an attack. Neuropeptide Y was unaltered. This study is the only one to date to implicate somatostatin in the migraine syndromes.

Cerebrospinal fluid cyclic adenosine monophosphate (cAMP) and aminobutyric acid (GABA) also have been studied in migraine patients (53). Both compounds are involved in cerebral energy metabolism and neurotransmission. In 13 patients, CSF cAMP was elevated compared with controls when sampled during or within 48 hours of an attack. GABA was undetectable in normal controls because of low sensitivity of the fluorimetric analysis but was detected in all of eight patients with migraine with and without aura.

Amino acids have been measured in the CSF of migraine subjects. Levels of glutamic and aspartic acid, both CNS-excitatory neurotransmitters, were evaluated in patients during attacks of migraine with and without aura and compared with the results in controls subjected to physical or psychological stress (35). CSF concentrations of glutamic acid were elevated in migraineurs compared with controls. Glutamic acid levels also were higher in migraine with than in migraine without aura. Aspartic acid levels could not be detected in the CSF of controls or migraineurs because of the low sensitivity of the methods used. Rothrock et al (43) measured CSF levels of glycine, taurine, and glutamine between attacks in 38 migraine patients and compared them with the levels in ten headache-free controls. The levels of taurine, glycine, and glutamine were significantly higher in the migraine patients; no significant differences were found among three migraine subgroups (infrequent migraine, frequent migraine, and transformed migraine). In seven patients subsequently treated with divalproex sodium, CSF taurine levels decreased significantly from pretreatment baseline values.

The data from the above two studies support the concept that migraine is at least in part a disorder of central neurotransmission. Glutamine is a precursor of glutamic acid, an excitatory neurotransmitter that may play a role in migraine pathogenesis by promoting neuronal excitability and initiating and propagating spreading cortical depression. Although glycine and taurine may act as inhibitory neurotransmitters whose role in the migraine attack remain to be determined, Rothrock et al. suggested that their increase in CSF may represent a prolonged sec-ondary effect, perhaps caused by spontaneous neuronal depolarization initiated by glutamic acid (43).

In interpreting the CSF results as a whole, it is clear that shifts in CNS energy and neurotransmitter metabolism take place during migraine attacks. There are limitations to the interpretation of the findings, however, because few patients reported in any of the studies were examined both between and during attacks. It is therefore often difficult to judge whether CSF findings are primary or secondary to the migraine attack. In regard to the latter, it is also difficult to distinguish whether ischemia or spreading depression (SD), the two principal mechanisms thought to underlie the migraine attack, can account for the changes. Thus cerebral ischemia potentially can cause elevation of lactate, cAMP, 5-HIAA, GABA, and glutamate in CSF. On the other hand, lactate, cAMP and GABA elevations have been measured in CNS tissue involved in SD. The elevation of CSF glutamate is especially interesting taken in context with the role of glutamate in initiating and propagating SD (40), together with the added documentation of a low CSF Mg^{2+}. Low-tissue Mg^{2+} enhances the potential of CNS tissue to develop SD (40,42).

CEREBRAL METABOLISM

Studies of CNS metabolism in migraine patients are limited, largely because of the inherent difficulties in applying complex methodologies to the study of a short-lasting paroxysmal disorder. In general, three techniques have been employed in the study of CNS metabolism in migraine: positron emission tomography (PET), magnetic resonance spectroscopy (MRS), and most recently functional blood oxygen level dependent MRI (MRI:BOLD). Most investigations have been limited to energy metabolic pathways, but more recent PET studies have focussed on central neurotransmitter receptor function.

Cerebral Oxygenation in Relation to Blood Flow

Bousser et al. (10) described a patient with migrainous cerebral infarction studied by PET 14 days after occurrence. The infarct region (left occipital cortex) showed a decreased CBF and oxygen extraction fraction (OEF), findings typical of cerebral infarction. There was an increased CBF with normal oxygen extraction in contiguous temporal lobe, probably because of a hyperemic zone surrounding the infarct. The opposite occipital cortex revealed decreased flow, with increased oxygen extraction, which occurred despite there being no involvement of this brain region in the migraine symptomatology. Such a profile of measurements can occur with misery perfusion of brain regions. Herold et al. (27) also reported such a metabolic profile in one patient who had migraine with aura who was studied by PET 90 minutes into an attack. No changes occurred in CBF or oxygen extraction in two other cases studied at 3 and 8 hours after onset of an attack. Friberg et al. (23) used intraarterial ^{133}Xe CBF methods and arteriovenous oxygen difference sampling to measure CBF, oxygen consumption, and oxygen extraction in eight patients. Four developed attacks with aura during the procedure and were found to have occipital cortex hypoperfusion. These patients showed a global increase in oxygen extraction (13%). Oxygen consumption was unchanged. These results did not support metabolic suppression secondary to flow decrease. On the other hand, Andersson et al. investigated 11 cases of migraine with and without aura induced by red wine (1). Regional cerebral blood flow (rCBF), oxygen metabolism (rCMRO2) and oxygen extraction (rOER) were measured during baseline (n = 11), aura (n = 6), and headache (n = 10). These studies revealed a region corresponding to the primary visual cortex with significant reductions in CBF (23.1%) and parallel reductions in oxygen consumption (22.5%) but no change in oxygen extraction during the headache phase compared with baseline. These data support metabolic suppression being secondary to flow reduction, but this reduction was attributed to spreading depression rather than cerebral ischemia. Finally, Bednarczyk et al. (9), using PET found reduction in CBF and cerebral blood volume during an attack but no alterations in oxygen metabolism. Overall, the PET studies of oxygen metabolism, at this time, appear conflicting and do not permit confident interpretation of the findings.

To aid in interpreting these studies, a new technique, functional MRI-BOLD, has now been applied to study the early seconds to minutes of visually triggered migraine attacks (13). This new MRI technique measures relative changes in oxygenation of the brain circulation and now is being used extensively in brain activation and functional localization experiments in humans. In brief, when an activating stimulus evokes a neuronal response, local blood flow increases, possibly by a neurogenic reflex that, at least initially, bypasses metabolically mediated increases in flow. This vascular response carries a redundancy of flow to the activated brain regions from which relatively less oxygen is extracted, with the consequence that hemoglobin becomes hyperoxygenated compared with before activation. The relative reduction in deoxyhemoglobin decreases the paramagnetic influence of free iron on T2* relaxation and produces increased signal intensity on a T2*-weighted MR image. Under physiologic conditions, this signal intensity increase reflects an increase in oxygen perfusing the tissue and is an indirect qualitative measure of perfusion that localizes and identifies the brain regions that are activated. The technique is ideal for monitoring neuronal activation and suppression at the same time as measuring, albeit indirectly, the oxygenation state in the immediate circulatory environment of the involved neurons. Further, this can be achieved nearly continuously in a second-to-second time

frame with millimeter resolution, permitting the monitoring of immediate events in triggered migraine attacks.

Visual activation of headache and visual symptoms using repetitive stimulation with a colored grid at 9 Hz occurred in 8 of 15 subjects with a history of migraine and in none of nine normal. Suppression of neuronal activation was observed before and during attacks in the eight activated headache subjects. Neuronal suppression was accompanied by hyperoxygenation of the occipital cortex during the early minutes of the attack. Hyperoxygenation of the occipital cortex was substantiated in a patient with spontaneous visual aura studied using the BOLD technique (56). Hyperoxia was evident throughout regions of both occipital cortices and in mesencephalic structures, despite the patient experiencing only left homonomous quadrantanopia. Hyperoxia occurred only in cortical gray matter, not what would be expected during ischemia. The intensity changes in draining veins confirmed increased occipital tissue hyperoxygenation.

The mechanisms of these observations remain to be determined. Using T2*-weighted MR imaging and inducing SD by direct application of potassium to rat brain cortices, Gardner-Medwin et al. observed localized signal intensity increases that spread along cortical layers at a rate of 3 mm per minute and interpreted this finding as an oxygen increase in blood perfusing brain tissue during the early vasodilator stage of SD (24). In both our visually activated headache and the spontaneous aura subjects, the increases in T2*-weighted image intensity were more widespread in the occipital cortices than might be expected from the localized nature of the visual symptoms. This dissociation between abnormal CBF, metabolism, and neurologic dysfunction in migraine attacks was substantiated by a recent case report and PET study in which bilateral occipital cortex oligemia was observed approximately 45 minutes before any complaint of visual symptoms (59). Finally, ischemia should decrease, not increase, T2*-weighted image intensity in both gray and white matter, arguing in favor of a spreading depression-like event explaining these findings.

Cerebral Glucose Metabolism

Cerebral glucose consumption (CMRGL) was measured by PET using the tracer 2-deoxyglucose in five migraine patients before and after reserpine treatment (44). In most patients given reserpine who experienced headache, CMRGL was globally reduced by between 5% and 30% from baseline, in contrast to control subjects, who did not develop headache after reserpine and who had an increase in CMRGL compared with baseline. From this study, it was evident that glucose hypometabolism occurs during migraine-like headache initiated by reserpine. On the other hand, Mathew et al. found increased CMRGL in patients who suffer status aura (37). The apparent conflict in the results of these studies could be reconciled by increased demand for substrate in brain tissue subjected to repeated depolarization and repolarization during repeated aura in the latter study. The hypometabolism found in the former study could be explained by measurements being made in the late neuronally suppressed phase of spreading depression.

Mullani et al. also studied 27 migraine patients during headache using PET (38). Each patient underwent a blood flow scan using oxygen-15 labeled water followed by a metabolism scan using flourine-18–labeled deoxyglucose (FDG). Statistically significant asymmetries were recorded in blood flow and metabolism in the temporal, mesial temporal, thalamus, and subthalamic brainstem regions of the brain in the migraine headache patients. Four of the patients who underwent rescanning showed a change in the asymmetry with a change in the pain level. The cingulate and the medial occipital regions also showed increased uptake of glucose and blood flow during the pain phase. In these cases, the asymmetric distribution of cortical glucose metabolism and blood flow in migraine headache patients suggested functional involvement of the temporal lobes, thalamus, and brainstem regions, most likely as a result of the pain phase of the headache rather than changes being related to the primary mechanisms of the attack. In addition, the asymmetries were reversible in some patients when head pain lessened.

Cerebral Lactate Metabolism

Proton spectroscopy detects lactate in abnormally metabolizing brain. To date, only one report of lactate detection in migraine subjects has appeared. Watanabe et al. measured lactate in the occipital cortex of five migraine sufferers within 2 months of an attack (52). One of their patients had lactate detected during a headache but had suffered stroke previously (51). It is difficult to interpret the significance of these reports in relation to metabolic changes during an attack. The persistent lactate increases might have been caused by structural damage to brain tissue before the measurements were made. The authors also put forward these findings as supportive of a mitochondrial disorder of brain tissue in migraine.

Phosphate Energy Metabolism

Phosphorous-31RS has documented significant alterations in brain energy metabolism between and during attacks of migraine (54). The decrease in phosphocreatine (PCr) and the increase of inorganic phosphate (Pi) were documented during attacks, particularly in migraine with aura. Also, an increase in Pi was found between attacks. No change in cerebral pH occurred during or between attacks. In another study using ^{31}P-MRS in eight patients studied during attack-free periods (4), PCr was decreased and Pi increased. Of interest, muscle spectroscopy performed in four of these patients showed a decrease in the PCr/Pi ratio at rest and abnormal energy metabolism of the muscle after light exercise. A mitochondrial abnormality in muscle was suggested to explain these findings, which raises the possibility that the disordered cerebral energy metabolism between attacks in migraine patients may be due to a general defect in mitochondrial function. In this study, however, most patients had also suffered strokes attributed to migraine by CT-documented hypodensities in the same occipital regions that were studied by ^{31}P-MRS. Nevertheless, in a further study of 12 attack-free patients who have migraine with aura conducted by the same group (3), ^{31}P-MRS disclosed a low PCr content, a high adenosine diphosphate (ADP), and a low phosphorylation potential in all patients, features suggestive of unstable cerebral metabolism. Abnormal mitochondrial metabolism was also present in 9 of the 12 patients examined.

Finally, by processing ^{31}P-MR spectra, intracellular free Mg^{2+} can be measured and expressed as pMg. The pMg was significantly elevated in migraine patients during a migraine attack, reflecting a decrease in intracellular free Mg^{2+} of 20% of normal control levels (42). No significant abnormality in brain pMg was found in two separate studies in which migraineurs were examined between attacks (3,42). On the other hand, Barker et al. documented low Mg^{2+} values in occipital cortex of a family with hemiplegic migraine (6). This finding was thought either to reflect low Mg^{2+} or, based on abnormal presynaptic P/Q calcium channels, Mg^{2+} bound to NMDA receptors and cell membranes to maintain cellular homeostasis and normal cellular excitability. Also, Barbirolli et al. assessed brain free Mg^{2+} in different types of migraine and compared Mg^{2+} with bioenergetic measurements by in vivo ^{31}P-MRS (5). All patients were in attack-free periods and free from medication. The brain free [Mg^{2+} was reduced significantly in all patients. The lowest content was found in migraine stroke and the highest in patients with migraine without aura. The phosphorylation potential, an index of brain bioenergetics, was proportional to free Mg^{2+}. These results suggested that the extent of free Mg^{2+} reduction was proportional to the degree of impairment of brain bioenergetics. Low brain Mg^{2+} concentration is associated with easily elicited SD and cortical excitability (42). Finally, phosphomonoesters measured by ^{31}P spectroscopic imaging were reduced in the brain between and during a migraine attack (55), suggesting instability of membrane phospholipids and supporting cellular inhomeostasis that might be the basis of hyperexcitability.

In interpreting these cerebral metabolic findings together, it is perhaps pertinent to compare metabolic changes reported in migraine to those of cerebral ischemia and SD. Ischemic infarction is associated with decreased CBF, OEF, and CMRGL as measured by PET and decreased PCr/Pi ratio and pH as measured by MRS.

Cerebral infarction probably accounted for these findings in some of the reported cases of migraine. Transient cerebral ischemia can cause decreased CBF with increased OEF and CMRGLU measured by PET, decreased PCr/Pi and pMg measured by MRS, and decreased pH measured by both techniques. On the other hand, SD causes a short-lived increase in CBF, followed by a prolonged oligemia lasting for hours (33). Hyperoxia seems to accompany the early phase of SD and now has been documented during a migraine attack. CMRGL is either unchanged or increased during the repolarization phase (46). Oxygen consumption also is increased during the repolarization phase, and high-energy phosphates are decreased due to either impaired synthesis or increased consumption (32). Lactate acid levels rise, and pH can be acidotic or unchanged. On balance, either ischemia or SD could explain the metabolic findings in migraine patients studied in the past. More recently developed techniques with improved anatomic and temporal resolution such as functional MRI, however, seem to support the spreading depression hypothesis over ischemia being associated with the migraine aura.

Central Neurotransmitter Metabolism

Considering the longevity of PET and SPECT technology, it is disappointing that so few studies of central neurotransmitter metabolism have been accomplished in recent years. Verhoeff et al. studied two migraine patient by *in vivo* SPECT using the dopamine D2-receptor specific radioligand 1231-3-iodo-6-methoxybenzamide ([123I]IBZM) during ergotamine abuse and after withdrawal (49). No differences were found in striatal uptake of [123I]IBZM between healthy controls and the patients when on or off ergotamine. Wöber et al. studied *in vivo* the influence of flunarizine on dopamine D2 receptors and investigated whether dopamine D2 receptor blockade was involved in its antimigraine action (58). Eleven migraine patients, treated with flunarizine 10 mg per day, underwent SPECT using [[123I]]-labeled iodobenzamide, a ligand with high affinity and high specificity for D2 receptors. There was a reduction of the dopamine D2 receptor binding potential in all patients compared with age-matched controls. The efficacy of flunarizine in migraine prophylaxis failed to correlate with the degree of the dopamine D2 receptor blockade. The first small series would suggest an abnormality of dopamine receptor function in migraine, but the latter study provided no baseline evidence.

Chabriat et al. used PET and 18-F-fluorosetoperone, a 5-HT2 specific radioligand, to investigate migraine patients between attacks (16) They found no evidence of alteration of 5-HT2 receptor function in either migraine with or without aura (16). Chugani et al. performed PET studies using the compound C11-alpha-methyl-tryptophan to measure the whole-brain serotonin synthesis rates

in ten normal volunteers and three patients with migrainous stroke (17). Whole-brain serotonin synthesis rates were increased significantly, by 55%, in the migrainous stroke patients compared with the normal volunteers. In a separate communication to the American Neurological Society in 1997, this laboratory reported similar increased synthesis rates in migraine patients without stroke. Clearly, these observations are important but are difficult to critique at this time, before definitive papers are published.

REFERENCES

1. Andersson JL, Murh C, Lilja A, et al. Regional cerebral blood flow and oxygen metabolism during migraine with and without aura. *Cephalalgia* 1997;17:570–579.
2. Anselmi B, Baldi E, Casacci F, Salmon S. Endogenous opioids in cerebrospinal fluid and blood in idiopathic headache sufferers. *Headache* 1980;21:294–299.
3. Barbirolli B, Montagna P, Cortelli P, et al. Abnormal brain and muscle energy metabolism shown by ^{31}P magnetic resonance spectroscopy in patients affected by migraine with aura. *Neurology* 1992;42:1209–1214.
4. Barbirolli B, Montagna P, Cortelli P, et al. Complicated migraine studied by phosphorous magnetic resonance spectrochscopy. *Cephalalgia* 1990;10:263–272.
5. Barbirolli B, Lodi R, Cortelli P, et al. Low brain free magnesium in migraine and cluster headache: an interictal study by in vivo phosphorus magnetic resonance spectroscopy on 86 patients. Proceedings of the 8th Congress HIS. *Cephalalgia* 1997;
6. Barker PB, Boska MD, Butterworth EJ, et al. Phosphorus and proton MR spectroscopic imaging in migraine. *Proceedings of the Society of Magnetic Research* 1995;1:139.
7. Barrie M, Jowett A. A pharmacological investigation of cerebrospinal fluid from patients with migraine. *Brain* 1967;90:785–794.
8. Bartleson JD, Swanson JW, Whisnant JP. A migrainous syndrome with cerebrospinal fluid pleocytosis. *Neurology* 1981;31:1257–1262.
9. Bednarczyk EM, Remler B, Weikart C, et al. Global cerebral blood flow, blood volume, and oxygen metabolism in patients with migraine headache. *Neurology* 1998;50:1736–1740.
10. Bousser MG, Baron JC, Iba-Zizen MT, Comar D, Caganis E, Castaigne P. Migrainous cerebral infarction: a tomographic study of cerebral blood flow and oxygen extraction fraction with the oxygen-15 inhalation technique. *Stroke* 1980;11:145–148.
11. Bradshaw P, Parsons M. Hemiplegic migraine, a clinical study. *QJM* 1965;34:65–85.
12. Caminero AB, Pareja JA, Arpa J, et al. Migrainous syndrome with CSF pleocytosis. *Headache* 1997;37:511–515.
13. Cao Y, Aurora S, Vikingstad E, Welch KMA. Functional MRI (fMRI) of visually triggered headache: activation, suppression and propagation of the BOLD effect. *J Cereb Blood Flow Metab* 1997;17(Suppl 1):S176.
14. Castillo J, Martinez F, Corredera E, et al. Migraine and histamine: determining histidine in plasma and cerebrospinal fluid during migraine attacks. *Rev Neurol* 1995;23:749–751.
15. Castillo J, Martinez F, Suarez C, et al. Cerebrospinal fluid tyrosine and 3,-dihydroxyophenylacetic acid levels in migraine patients. *Cephalalgia* 1996;16:56–61.
16. Chabriat H, Tehindrazanarivelo A, Vera P et al. 5HT2 receptors in cerebral cortex of migraineurs studied using PET and 18F-fluorosetoperone. *Cephalalgia* 1995;15:104–108.
17. Chugani DC, Chaturvedi S, Niimura K, et al. Whole brain serotonin synthesis in patients with migrainous cerebral infarction: a positron emission tomography study: proceedings of the AAN. *Neurology* 1998:S51:002.
18. Cohen RJ, Taylor JR. Persistent neurologic sequelae of migraine: a case report. *Neurology* 1979;29:1175–1177.
19. Dooling EC, Sweeney VP. Migrainous hemiplegia during breast feeding. *Am J Obstet Gynecol* 1974;118:568–570.
20. Dvorkin GS, Anderman F, Carpenter S, et al. Classical migraine,

intractable epilepsy and multiple strokes: a syndrome related to mitochondrial encephalomyopathy. In: Anderman F, Lugaresi E, eds. *Migraine and epilepsy*. London: Butterworths, 1987:203–232.

21. Facchinetti F, Sances G, Martignoni E, Pagani I, Nappi G, Genazzani AR. Evidence of alpha-N-acetyl β-endorphin in human cerebrospinal fluid. *Brain Res* 1992;586:1–5.

22. Ferguson KS, Robinson SS. Life threatening migraine. *Arch Neurol* 1982;39:374–375.

23. Friberg L, Olesen J, Lassen NA, et al. Cerebral oxygen extraction, oxygen consumption, and regional cerebral blood flow during the aura phase of migraine. *Stroke* 1994;25:974–979.

24. Gardner-Medwin AR, Tepley N, Barkley GL, et al. Welch KMA: magnetic fields associated with spreading depression in anesthetized rabbits. *Brain Res* 1991;562:153–158.

25. Genazzani AR, Nappi G, Facchinetti F, et al. Progress in impairment of CSF B-EP levels in igraine sufferers. *Pain* 1984;127–133.

26. Gomez-Aranda F, Canadillas F, Marti-Massi JF, et al. Pseudomigraine with temporary neurological symptoms and lymphocytic pleocytosis: a report of 50 cases. *Brain* 1997;120:1105–1113.

27. Herold S, Gibbs JM, Jones AKP, et al. Oxygen metabolism in classical migraine. *J Cereb Blood Flow Metab* 1985;5:5445–5446.

28. Jain AC, Sethi NC, Babbar PK. A clinical electroencephalographic and trace element study with special reference to zinc, copper and magnesium in serum and cerebrospinal fluid (CSF) in cases of migraine. *J Neurol* 1985;232(Suppl):161.

29. Kangasniemi P, Sonninen U, Rinne K. Extraction of free and conjugated 5-HIAA and VMA in urine and concentration of 5-HIAA and HVA in CSF during migraine attacks and free intervals. *Headache* 1972;3:62–65.

30. Kovacs K, Bors L, Tothfalusi L, et al. Cerebrospinal fluid (CSF) investigations in migraine. *Cephalalgia* 1989;9:53–57.

31. Kremenitzer M, Golden GS. Hemiplegic migraine: cerebrospinal fluid abnormalities. *J Pediatr* 1974;85:139.

32. Krivanek J. Some metabolic changes accompanying Leao's spreading cortical depression in the rat. *J Neurochem* 1961;6:183–189.

33. Lauritzen M, Diemer NH. Uncoupling of cerebral blood flow and metabolism after single episodes of cortical spreading depression in the rat brain. *Brain Res* 1986;370:405–408.

34. Lee CH, Lance JW. Migraine stupor. *Headache* 1977;17:32–38.

35. Martinez F, Castillo J, Rodriguez JR, Leir R, Noya M. Neuroexcitatory amino acid levels in plasma and cerebrospinal fluid during migraine attacks. *Cephalalgia* 1993;13:89–93.

36. Martinez F, Castillo J, Pardo J, et al. Catecholamine levels in plasma and CSF. *J Neurol Neurosurg Psychiatry* 1993;56:1119–1121.

37. Mathew NT, Mullani NA, Gould KL. Migraine with persistent visual aura-sustained metabolic activation in the medial occipital cortex measured by PET: proceedings of the AAN. *Neurology* 1998;S51:003.

38. Mullani NA, Mathew NT, Gould KL. Asymmetric glucose metabolism and blood flow in the temporal lobes, thalamus, and the brain stem regions in migraine headache patients suggests a functional involvement of these regions: proceedings of the AAN. *Neurology* 1998;S51:005.

39. Murphey JF. Cerebral infarction in migraine. *Neurology* 1955;5:359–361.

40. Nowak L, Bregestovski P, Ascher P, Herbet A, Prochiantz A. Magnesium gates glutamate-activated channels in mouse central neurones. *Nature* 1984;307:462–465.

41. Poloni M, Nappi G, Arrigo A, Savoldi I. Cerebrospinal fluid 5-hydroxyindoleacetic acid levels in migrainous patients during spontaneous attacks, during headache free periods and following treatment with 1-tryptophine. *Experentia* 1974;30:640–641.

42. Ramadan NM, Halvorson H, Vande-Linde AMQ, Levine SR, Helpern JA, Welch KMA. Low brain magnesium in migraine. *Headache* 1989;29:590–593.

43. Rothrock JF, Mar KR, Yaksh TL, et al. Cerebrospinal fluid analysis in migraine patients and controls. *Cephalalgia* 1995;15:489–493.

44. Sachs H, Wolf A, Russell JAG, Christman DR. Effect of reserpine on regional cerebral glucose metabolism in control and migraine subjects. *Arch Neurol* 1986;43:1117–1123.

45. Schraeder PL, Burns RA. Hemiplegic migraine associated with an aseptic meningeal reaction. *Arch Neurol* 1980;37:377–399.

46. Shinohara M, Dollinger B, Brown G, Rapoport S, Sokoloff L. Changes in local cerebral glucose utilization during and following recovery from spreading cortical depression. *Science* 1979;203:188–190.

47. Skinhoj E. Hemodynamic studies within the brain during migraine. *Arch Neurol* 1973;29:95–98.

48. Vecsei L, Widerlov E, Ekman R, et al. Suboccipital cerebrospinal fluid and plasma concentrations of somatostatin, neuropeptide Y and betaendorphin in patients with common migraine. *Neuropeptides* 1992;22:111–116.

49. Verhoeff NPLG, Visser WH, Ferrari MD, Saxena PR, van Royen EA. Dopamine D2-receptor imaging with 123I-iodobenzamide SPECT in migraine patients abusing ergotamine: does ergotamine cross the blood brain barrier? *Cephalalgia* 1993;13:325–329.

50. Verret S, Steel JC. Alternating hemiplegia in childhood: a report of eight patients with complicated migraine beginning in infancy. *Pediatrics* 1971;47:675–680.

51. Watanabe H, Kuwabara T, Ohkubo M, et al. Elevation of cerebral lactate detected by localized 1H-magnetic resonance spectroscopy in migraine during the interictal period. *Neurology* 1996;47:1093–1095.

52. Watanabe H, Kuwabara T, Ohkubo M, et al. Elevation of cerebral lactate detected by localized 1H-magnetic resonance spectroscopy in a patient with migraine. *Rinsho Shinkeigaku* 1994;34:504–507.

53. Welch KMA, Chabi E, Nell JH, et al. Biochemical comparison of migraine and stroke. *Headache* 1976;16:160–167.

54. Welch KMA, Levine SR, D'Andrea G, Schultz LR, Helpern JA. Preliminary observations on brain energy metabolism in migraine by in vivo phosphorous 31 NMR spectroscopy. *Neurology* 1989;39:538–541.

55. Welch KMA, Cao Y, Aurora S, et al. Hyperoxia of the occipital cortex, red nucleus and substantia nigra during visual aura of migraine. *Neurology* 1998;51:1465–1469.

56. Welch KMA, Boska MD, Nelson JA, et al. 31-Phosphorus Spectroscopic Imaging (^{31}P-SI) in migraine: proceedings of the AAN. *Neurology* 1998;S51:004.

57. Whitty CWM. Familial hemiplegic migraine. *J Neurol Neurosurg Psychiatry* 1953;16:172–177.

58. Wöber C, Brücke T, Wöber-Bingöl C, Asenbaum S, Wessely P, Podreka I. Dopamine D2 receptor blockade and antimigraine action of flunarizine. *Cephalalgia* 1994;14:135–140.

59. Woods RP, Iacoboni M, Mazziotta JC: Bilateral spreading cerebral hypoperfusion during spontaneous migraine headache. *N Engl J Med* 1994;331:1689–1692.

The Headaches, Second Edition,
edited by J. Olesen, P. Tfelt-Hansen, and K.M.A. Welch.
Lippincott Williams & Wilkins, Philadelphia © 2000.

The Migraines

CHAPTER 37

Neurophysiology and Autonomic Dysfunction in Migraine

Jean Schoenen and Lars Lykke Thomsen

CLINICAL NEUROPHYSIOLOGY

An impressive number of neurophysiologic studies have been performed in patients with chronic headache, particularly in those with migraine. Some of their results are difficult to interpret due to the lack of normative data or because of insufficient homogeneity of patients groups. Therefore, the objective of the first part of this chapter is not to review in detail all published studies, but merely to underscore major reproducible findings and to examine their potential diagnostic and pathophysiologic interest. In order to avoid tedious enumerations, most of the available data are synoptically presented in tables, in which the reader can also find relevant references.

The neurophysiologic methods that have been used in migraine patients can be subdivided into two major groups: electroencephalography (EEG) and evoked potentials (EPs).

Electroencephalography

It is not surprising that the most numerous studies have been devoted to EEG. Unfortunately, however, the subjective interpretation of recordings and the lack of uniformity in methodology and diagnostic classification preclude any coherent synthesis of the results obtained with routine EEG. Daly and colleagues commented that "reports on EEG in patients with migraine are a mine-

field for uncritical readers, a maze of ill-conceived studies and inadequately reported results" (25). Nonetheless, the more recent methods of EEG quantification have in part reduced subjectivity and produced sets of data that are comparable and, to some extent, similar between different laboratories.

The Interictal EEG

Electroencephalography is traditionally considered to be a useful adjunct to the clinical evaluation of headache, but there is unfortunately little scientific backing for this tradition. Few articles describing EEG findings meet generally accepted criteria for determining the clinical usefulness of a diagnostic test (52). Comprehensive reviews of EEG findings in migraine have been published by Hockaday and Debney (59) and by Sand (111). In subjects with migraine, an incidence of EEG abnormalities as high as 70% has been reported. However, many EEG findings previously considered to be "abnormal," such as posterior slowing, sensitivity to hyperventilation, or 14- and 6-Hz positive spikes, are nearly as prevalent in normal controls as in migraineurs and do not change the probability of the presence of migraine in a clinically significant way.

The only abnormality consistently reported in headache patients, as opposed to controls, in studies of a relatively nonflawed design is a prominent photic driving response at high flash stimulation rates beyond 20 Hz, the well known H response of Golla and Winter (48). This response has been confirmed by spectral analysis (127, 128), but because of its low specificity, it is of little clinical utility in migraine. In conjunction with the results

J. Schoenen: University Department of Neurology, CHR Citadelle, and University of Liège, B-4000 Liège, Belgium.

L. L. Thomsen: Department of Neurology, Glostrup Hospital, University of Copenhagen, DK-2600 Glostrup, Copenhagen, Denmark.

obtained in studies of other visual responses, it nevertheless suggests a permanent dysfunction of visual processing between attacks (see section on evoked responses).

A recent critical review of the literature (52) yielded the following conclusions: (a) EEG is less effective than clinical criteria in distinguishing patients with headache from individuals without headaches or migraine from other headache types, and (b) EEG is not an effective screening method for structural causes of headache, nor an effective means for identifying headache subgroups with different prognoses. In consequence, the Quality Standard Subcommittee of the American Academy of Neurology recommended that EEG is not indicated in the routine evaluation of patients presenting with headache, but that it may be used to evaluate headache patients with associated symptoms suggesting a seizure disorder or with atypical migrainous auras. It also adopted the view of Gronseth and Greenberg (52) that "numerous interesting and potentially fruitful areas of research on the EEG in the setting of chronic headache remain" (107).

The Ictal EEG

During migraine attacks, EEG provides interesting pathophysiologic information. There are anecdotal reports of focal slowing during attacks of migraine with visual or complex neurologic aura, or during hemiplegic migraine (6,19,35). In the study of Lauritzen et al. (76), however, such an abnormality was present in only 20% of patients. During migraine without aura the routine EEG is usually normal (76). Spectral analysis and topographic EEG mapping disclose a unilateral 50% or greater reduction of alpha power accompanied by a less severe reduction of theta power in attacks with a strictly visual aura, but also during attacks of migraine without aura (118, 139). In most cases, the alpha reduction is located on the side of the hemicrania. It can appear up to 12 to 18 hours before the attack, as suggested by the sequential study of women with menstrual migraine, and may outlast the attack by up to 48 hours. When there is a complex neurologic aura or a prolonged aura (3,19), the unilateral reduction of alpha activity may be associated by ipsilateral increase of slow waves. In a small study of four children, attacks of migraine with aura were found to produce a diffuse increase of theta activity (53,127), but it remains to be determined whether such slowing could be due to hyperventilation (62).

The ictal quantitative EEG data are strikingly similar to those observed with spectral analysis of magnetoencephalography (MEG) (11,12). Long-lasting suppressions in spectral power in all frequencies faster than 1 Hz were found in MEG studies during attacks of migraine with aura (8 of 13 patients) or without aura (1 of 2 patients). In addition, prolonged DC shifts lasting 10 to 13 minutes were recorded with MEG during and between attacks.

As stated by Aminoff (5), "the routine EEG is of no interest in the diagnosis of migraine" and, following the recommendations by the Quality Standard Subcommittee of the American Academy of Neurology, one can add "nor is the diagnosis of any other headache." The EEG could be useful as a screening test in a minority of "atypical" headache patients, and more studies are needed on the relationship between sleep (101) or sensitivity to hypocapnia (111) and headache or on the effectiveness of EEG in screening for intracranial pathology compared with imaging techniques taking into account cost and patients' preferences.

From a pathophysiologic point of view, quantified and topographic EEG studies have unraveled two reproducible results. First, a unilateral reduction of alpha activity characterizes attacks of migraine with visual aura as well as attacks of migraine without aura. Because this reduction may precede and outlast the attack by 24 hours or more, it might explain alpha asymmetries reported between attacks, chiefly in migraine with aura and when the recordings were made shortly before or after an attack. Second, attacks of migraine with prolonged or complex neurologic auras are accompanied by a unilateral increase of slow waves over the relevant hemisphere, in addition to the decrease in alpha power. Reported alpha asymmetrics between attacks (65) could be related to the recency of the last attack. Interhemispheric alpha asymmetrics can be found in normal subjects, the alpha power usually being more pronounced over the right hemisphere (34,62,67). Unilateral alpha reduction also may be the sole EEG abnormality in other conditions, for example, extracerebral mass lesions such as meningioma or subdural hematoma (70). In case of a focal ischemic event, however, it is usually accompanied by an increase of slow waves (137), as it is in certain cases of migraine with aura. Interestingly, local depression of electrocortical activity is also the electrophysiologic hallmark of Leão's spreading depression (77,78), which has been postulated to be the primary cause for the blood flow changes during attacks of migraine with aura (74).

The aforementioned data suggest that migraine attack with aura, as that without aura, is accompanied (and even preceded) by a unilateral disturbance of electrocortical activity, which most probably reflects underlying metabolic modifications. Migraine with aura and certain attacks of migraine without aura might thus have similar pathophysiologic mechanisms and differ only by the severity of the cortical dysfunction. Whether these cortical modifications are primarily neuronal (or neuronoglial) or secondary to microcirculatory changes and ischemia remains to be determined (113).

Evoked Responses

Following the seminal observation by Golla and Winter (48) of an increased photic drive of the EEG in patients with migraine, the reactivity of electrocortical activity to visual stimuli has been assessed with a number of different techniques. Event-related potentials have yielded interesting results in relation to a biobehavioral model of migraine (43). More recently, auditory evoked cortical potentials have been studied, and transcranial magnetic stimulation has been used to assess cortical excitability.

Visual Evoked Responses

As mentioned before, enhanced photic driving of the EEG has a prevalence of up to 90% in migraine, but it has also been found in 78% of normal controls (15) (Table 1). There are physiologic similarities between the H response and the abnormalities of the *steady-state response* evoked by a sine wave visual stimulus described by Nyrke et al. (94–97). According to Nyrke et al., this stimulus modality is able to distinguish migraine with aura from migraine without aura, and the abnormalities it discloses are improved after beta-blockers.

Studies of classical visual evoked potentials (VEPs) obtained after flash or checkerboard pattern stimulation have shown increased or normal amplitude of the major cortical component during headache-free intervals (see Table 1). In one study (29), the P100 amplitude was decreased after a treatment with beta-blockers. The same researchers pointed out that none of their migraine patients had P100 latency or amplitude values exceeding the mean of healthy controls by 3 standard deviations (28). Ictal VEP recordings are scarce, but most of them

have shown reduced amplitudes during attacks of migraine with aura (82,108). With hemifield stimulations, prolonged amplitude reduction of P100 and later components of the VEP can be recorded when the affected visual hemifield is stimulated (116).

When the amplitude change of the VEP is sequentially studied during sustained pattern reversal stimulation, migraineurs are characterized by a lack of habituation or a potentiation of the response, whereas healthy controls display habituation (Fig. 1). The deficient habituation of the VEP is found in migraine with and without aura both during short (2 minutes) and long (15 minutes) duration of stimulation (2,123).

Fast EEG activities (20–30 Hz) following flash or checkerboard stimulation were found to be exaggerated in migraine (see Table 1). This was presented as a reliable diagnostic test for migraine in children, but also for childhood periodic syndrome or acephalgic migraine (87,91, 92). Unfortunately, these results have not yet been reproduced in other laboratories, and at least one other group failed to replicate them in adult migraineurs (136).

Auditory Evoked Potentials

Results on brainstem auditory evoked potentials in migraine are inconclusive (114). By contrast, in a recent study (140) the intensity dependence of the cortical auditory evoked potential was significantly different between migraine patients and healthy controls. In migraine, the amplitude of the potential is strongly dependent on the

TABLE 1. *Visual evoked responses in migraine between attacks*

Without aura	With aura

H response: photic driving >20 Hz (48)
  92% (but also 78% of controls) (15)
  Confirmed by spectral analysis (126,127)
	idem

Steady-state visual effect potential to sine wave stimulus
  ↑ Fundamental component 16–22 Hz (94)
  Reduced by propranolol (95)
	↓ 2nd harmonic
	↑ interhemispheric asymmetry (96)

Visual evoked potential
  Transient flash (luminance) stimulus
    ↑ P3 amplitude (79,80)
    ↑ N3 amplitude (9,20,79)
    ↑ P2 amplitude (18)
	idem
	idem
	↑ N3 latency (142)

Pattern (contrast) stimulus
    Normal (18,32,86,105,124,129)
    ↑ Mean P100 latency (68,69)
    ↑ Mean amplitude (4,27,28,69)
    ↓ P100 amplitude after beta-blockers (29)
    P100 potentiation during repetitive stimulation (124)
    Lack of habituation during long duration stimulation (15 min) (1)
	Normal (13,18,105)
	idem
	↑ Mean P100 amplitude (69,125)
	P100 asymmetry with 1/2 field stimulation (24,142)
	idem
	idem

Visual provoked fast activity in migraine
  ↑ to flash (adults) (87)
  ↑↑ Children <13 yr (92)
  ↑ White/red flash ratio (children) (50)
  ↑↑ In childhood "periodic syndrome" (91)
  Normal (5 patients) (136)
	↑ to pattern (87) (adults)
	↑↑ >16 yr (92)
	↓ White/red flash ratio (children) (50)
	↑↑ In adult "acephalgic" migraine (92)
	Normal (3 patients) (136)

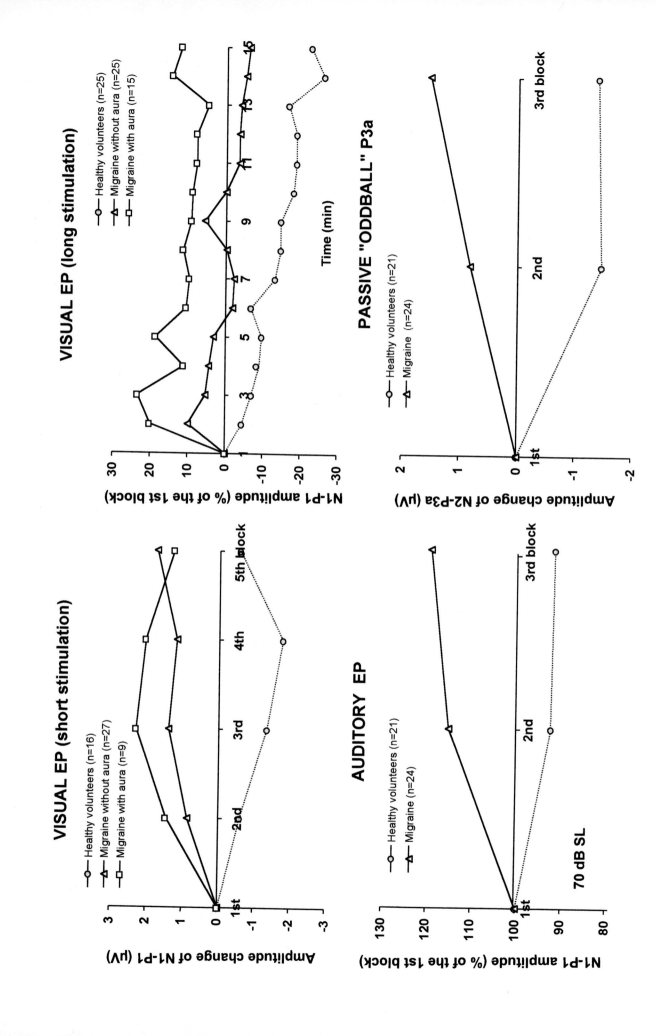

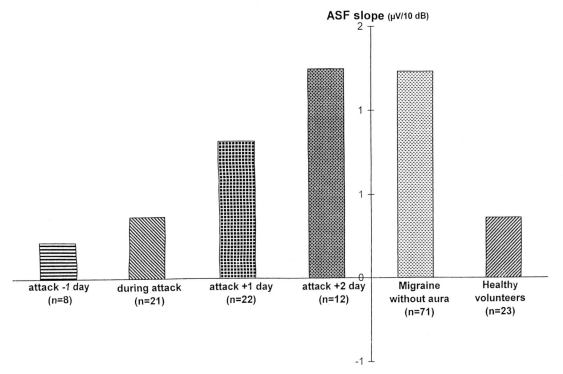

FIG. 2. Mean values of amplitude-stimulus function slopes of auditory evoked cortical potentials in patients with migraine without aura 1 day before, during, and 2 days after an attack compared with results obtained between attacks in groups of migraineurs without aura and healthy volunteers.

intensity of the auditory stimulus, which results in a steep amplitude-stimulus function slope (Fig. 2). The intensity dependence of the auditory evoked potential has little diagnostic usefulness because of its inter- and intraindividual variability. However, it is thought to be inversely related to the levels of central serotonergic activity (58), which makes it an interesting pathophysiologic and pharmacologic tool. Proietti-Cecchini et al. (106) have shown that zolmitriptan, a 5-hydroxytryptamine 1B/1D (5-HT$_{1B/1D}$) agonist with central nervous system penetration, can increase significantly the intensity dependence of auditory evoked cortical potentials in a dose-dependent manner, probably because it decreases central 5-HT release.

Event-Related Potentials

A more posterior scalp distribution of the P3 component with topographic EEG mapping also has been reported (119). Event-related potentials were chiefly studied during headache-free intervals. Results are partly contradictory. For auditory event-related potentials with the oddball paradigm, increased P3 latencies (32,139) and reduced P3 amplitudes (139) were found, but not in every study (31). A recent study suggests that the P3 abnormalities are due to a small subgroup of migraineurs who also have slight cognitive impairment (139). When no task is involved during the auditory oddball paradigm, the P3a component reflects processing of a novel stimulus. Compared with healthy controls, migraine patients between attacks lack habituation of the N2-P3a amplitude during stimulus repetition (138), which is reminiscent of the abnormality found for other evoked- and event-related potentials (see Fig. 1). Deficient habituation also has been found in a study of latency changes of the visual evoked P3 during repeated stimulations (37).

Contingent negative variation (CNV), a slow negative potential appearing during a reaction-time task with a

FIG. 1. Synopsis of results of evoked potential studies designed to assess amplitude changes in successive blocks of averages during continuous stimulation. *Upper left:* PR visual evoked potential during a 2-minute stimulation at 3.1 Hz. *Upper right:* PR visual evoked potential during a 15-minute stimulation. *Lower left:* Auditory evoked cortical potential at a stimulation intensity of 70 dB. *Lower right:* Novel P3 auditory event-related potential. For each modality there is habituation, that is, a decrease in amplitude, in healthy volunteers, but no habituation or even potentiation, that is, an increase in amplitude, in migraine with or without aura.

warning and an imperative stimulus, has on average an increased amplitude in migraine without aura between attacks (17,71,84,121), but not in migraine with aura (81). In a combined electrophysiologic and biochemical study during the menstrual cycle, an inverse relationship was found between CNV amplitude and plasma estradiol or catecholamine levels (93).

The most consistent abnormality of CNV, however, is its lack of habituation during repetition of the trial (17,43, 71,84,117,121). There seems to be a dynamic change of CNV amplitude in relation to the migraine attacks: during attacks, CNV is reduced (72,132), whereas it tends to increase 48 hours before the attack (42). Interictal CNV amplitude may return to normal values in migraineurs treated with beta-blockers (85,122).

Transcranial Magnetic Stimulation

Results obtained with electromagnetic stimulations of the motor cortex are not fully concordant (Table 2). They tend to indicate, nonetheless, that excitability is decreased over the hemisphere that is responsible for the aura symptoms (83,135).

During stimulation of the visual cortex, prevalence of phosphenes in migraine with aura patients was found to be increased in one study (8), but decreased in another (2). These discrepancies may be due to differences in methods, patient selection, and timing of the procedure in relation to attacks.

Evoked or event-related potentials are of little usefulness for the diagnosis of migraine because of their inter- and intraindividual variability. EEG and evoked potentials suggest that the migrainous brain is hypersensitive to visual stimuli during the headache-free period, which is in line with studies showing that migraineurs are hypersensitive to environmental light stimuli (57,133) and that they have modified performances on visual psychophysical tests (19,102,142).

The principal functional abnormality of information processing in migraine may be the lack of habituation (or

TABLE 2. Transcranial magnetic stimulation in migraine

Authors	Patients	Time	Stimulation	Threshold	MEP_{max}/M_{max}	CMCT	Correlation	Interpretation
Bettucci et al. (14)	10 MM 10 HV	Day 2 of menses and mid-cycle	Vertex 2 sides FDI at rest?	↑ in MM Both sides at any time	—	Normal	?	Cortical hypo-excitability
Maertens et al. (85)	12 MA uni-lateral 10 MO uni-lateral 20 HV	≥1 week before/after attack	Vertex 2 sides FDI at rest and 20% contraction	↑ in MA over affected hemisphere	↓ MA affected side	Normal	None with attack duration/frequency	Cortical hypo-excitability or hyper-excitability of inhibitory interneurons
van der Kamp et al. (134)	10 MO 10 MA uni-lateral 10 HV	≥3 days after last attack; before?	Vertex 2 sides ABP at slight contraction	No difference	↑ MO + MA	Normal	+ with attack frequency	Cortical hyper-excitability
van der Kamp et al. (135)	10 FHM 10 MA 10 HV	≥3 days after last attack; before?	Vertex 2 sides ADM at 10% contraction	↑ FHM	↑ MA ↓ affected side in FHM	↑ FHM	+ with attack frequency in MA	Cortical hyper-excitability and hypo-excitability on affected side in FHM
Aurora et al. (8)	11 MA 11 HV	≥1 week after last attack	Occiput	↓ for phosphenes and ↑ prevalence				Cortical hyper-excitability
Afra et al. (2)	25 MA 33 MO 27 HV	≥3 days before and after attack	Occiput Motor cortex Paired stimuli	↓ phosphenes prevalence ↑ threshold in MA	Normal		None None	Cortical hypo-excitability and normal intracortical inhibition

MA, migraine with aura; MO, migraine without aura; MM, menstrual migraine; HV, healthy volunteers; FHM, familial hemiplegic migraine; FDI, first dorsal interosseous muscle; ADM, abductor digiti minimi; CMCT, central motor conduction time.

even potentiation) of cortical responses during repetitive stimulation. It can indeed be demonstrated for various evoked- and event-related potentials (see Fig. 1). One has to keep in mind that this cortical dysfunction undergoes prominent changes in temporal relationship to the attack, during which evoked responses tend to normalize (72, 132) (see Fig. 2). The changes occurring just before an attack could explain why neurophysiologic results may differ in a study where it has not been ascertained that patients did not have an attack during the 3 days following the recordings.

It is at present not clear whether deficient habituation and increased intensity dependence are due to the same underlying neuronal dysfunction in migraine. Both abnormalities have a strong genetic basis and are differentially influenced by prophylactic antimigraine drugs (112). However, they do not necessarily occur together in the same patient. Intensity dependence (i.e., the augmenting-reducing response) is thought to be inversely proportional to central 5-HT transmission (58). Multiple transmitters are involved in habituation/potentiation, including acetylcholine, noradrenaline, dopamine, GABA, and nitric oxide, but 5-HT is thought to play a crucial role (44, 61,66). Cortical information processing may thus be abnormal in migraine because of a dysfunction of sub-cortico-cortical pathways, particularly of the serotonergic raphe-cortical pathway, which tune the state of excitability of the cerebral cortex (117).

Interestingly, the gene on chromosome 19 found abnormal in familial hemiplegic migraine (100) (see Chapter 30) codes for the ionophore of a neuronal voltage-dependent P/Q calcium channel that controls neurotransmitter (e.g., 5-HT) release.

Knowing the role of habituation in preventing lactate accumulation in the cortex during repetitive functional activation and considering the possibility of a reduced mitochondrial energy reserve in the brain of migraineurs (10,90), one may speculate that the lack of habituation might favor biochemical shifts in the cerebral cortex that may lead to a migraine attack (115).

Conclusion

The interest of neurophysiologic studies in migraine is mainly a pathophysiologic one. Taken globally, their results argue in favor of the neurovascular theory of migraine, in which the neuronal dysfunction plays a primary role. Abnormal activity in aminergic brainstem nuclei would on the one hand modify excitability and information processing of sensory cortices, particularly the visual cortex, and favor the occurrence of biochemical and potential shifts, the summation of which would ultimately lead to a cortical phenomenon similar to spreading depression, initiating the migraine aura. The brainstem dysfunction would, on the other hand, be responsible for a reduced descending control of trigemi-

nal nociception, favoring trigeminovascular activation and the migraine headache.

AUTONOMIC DYSFUNCTION

A possible dysfunction of the autonomic nervous system in migraine has long been a subject of considerable interest. Based on cardiovascular tests, vasomotor reactions to temperature changes, and responses to pharmacological tests, as well as changes in biochemical parameters, hypo- as well as hyperfunctioning of both the sympathetic and parasympathetic nervous system have been suggested. In this part of the chapter we review these contradictory results.

Cardiovascular Reflexes

A number of studies have focused on sympathetically mediated cardiovascular reflexes such as the orthostatic test, cold pressor test, and isometric work test (Tables 3 and 4). Havanka-Kanniainen and colleagues (55,56) found no abnormalties in young migraineurs (11–22 years old) outside of an attack, but significant changes suggesting sympathetic hypofunction in older migraineurs (23–50 years of age). Based on decreased R-R variation during normal and deep breathing and a decreased Valsalva ratio, the same researchers concluded that parasympathetic hypofunction was also present in migraine. Gotoh et al. (51) compared responses to a Valsalva maneuver, an orthostatic test, and Achner's test (reflex bradycardia induced by pressure on the eyeballs) interictally in migraine patients suffering from migraine either with or without aura and age-matched healthy controls. In addition, noradrenaline bolus injections and eye instillation tests were evaluated. Sympathetic hypofunction with denervation hypersensitivity and parasympathetic hyperfunction was surmised from these studies.

In contrast, other studies using similar cardiovascular tests have concluded in favor of normal or enhanced sympathetic function (see Table 3). Normal parasympathetic function (23) and more recently parasympathetic hypofunction (131) also have been reported interictally based on an altered heart rate response to a Valsalva maneuver combined with unaltered cardiovascular tests reflecting sympathetic function. Variation in the duration of migraine (54) and differences in age or migraine subtype are not a satisfactory explanation for the discrepancy of results, as indicated by the clinical data in Tables 3 and 4.

Arterial and Arteriolar Vasomotor Reactivity

Reduced vasodilatation in the forehead and hands after heating has been reported in migraineurs (7). In one study, increase of digital blood volume during heating was only absent in male migraineurs (103). By contrast, a peripherally applied cold stimulus failed to induce

TABLE 3. *Interictal studies of cardiovascular reflexes in migraine*

Studies	Mean duration of migraine (yr)	Mean age (yr)	MO/MA/HV (No. of subjects)	Tests
Studies concluding sympathetic hypofunction				Performed sympathetic tests
Gotoh et al. (51)	NA	29	11/10/30	O, adrenal.inj.
Havanka-Kanniainen et al. (56)	15	35	30/30/35	I,O
Mikamo et al. (89)	9	41	12/3/15	I,O
Pogacnik et al. (104)	12	37	41/21/45	I,O
Boccuni et al. (16)	NA	35	32/0/18	O
Studies concluding normal sympathetic function				
Havanka-Kanniainen et al. (55)	6	17	33/16/25	I,O
Havanka-Kanniainen (54)	22	42	4/6/10	I,O
Cortelli et al. (21)	19	39	10/0/10	O
Cortelli et al. (22)	NA	NA	7/0/7	O
Thomsen et al. (131)	22	42	23/27/30	C,O
Micieli et al. (88)	7		15/12/11	C
Studies concluding sympathetic hyperfunction				
Cortelli et al. (23)	NA	34	13/0/18	C,I,O
Studies concluding parasympathetic hypofunction				Performed parasympathetic tests
Havanka-Kanniainen et al (56)	15	35	30/30/35	RR,D,(V)
Thomsen et al. (131)	22	42	23/27/30	RR,D,(V)
Studies concluding parasympathetic hyperfunction				
Gotoh et al. (51)	NA	29	11/10/30	Increased bradycardia to Achners test

RR, RR interval; D, deep breathing; I, isometric handgrip; V, Valsalva; C, cold pressor; O, orthostatic test; MO, migraine without aura; MA, migraine with aura; HV, healthy volunteers.

decreased hand blood flow in migraineurs (30). Finally, normal peripheral vasomotor reactivity in migraineurs also has been described (60).

Local autonomic control regarding the cranial arterial bed is obviously more relevant than studies of systemic vascular reactivity but more difficult to investigate. With transcranial Doppler, decreased blood flow velocity in the middle cerebral artery (MCA), suggestive of dilatation, was found on the painful side during unilateral migraine attacks in some studies (40,130), but not in all (143). No difference in MCA blood velocity responses to tests of cardiovascular sympathetic function was found between migraineurs studied during or outside of an attack and healthy controls (131). This suggests normal MCA reactivity during increased sympathetic drive.

It is likely, though not definitely established, that autoregulation in the cerebral circulation is normal during attacks of migraine with or without aura (75,110). How-

TABLE 4. *Interictal studies of cardiovascular reflexes in migraine*

Studies	Mean patient age (range)	MO/MA/HV (No. of subjects)	Tests
Studies concluding sympathetic hypofunction			
Cortelli et al. (21)	39 (22–53)	10/0/10	O
Havanka-Kanniainen (54)	42 (26–56)	4/6/10	RR,D,V,I,O
Normal sympathetic function			
Thomsen et al. (132)	42 (19–66)	10/0/0 cross over	RR,D,V,C,O
Comparison of parasympathetic function during versus outside			
Havanka-Kanniainen (54)	42 (26–56)[a]	4/6/— cross-over	RR,D,V,I,O
Thomsen et al. (132)	42 (19–66)[a]	10/0/— cross-over	RR,D,V,C,O

[a]In both studies parasympathetic hypofunction was reported outside of attacks compared with controls. No further changes were observed in parasympathetic tests during attack.

RR, RR interval; D, deep breathing; I, isometric handgrip; V, Valsalva; C, cold pressor; O, orthostatic test; MO, migraine without aura; MA, migraine with aura; HV, healthy volunteers.

ever, functional activations such as speech, reading, listening, and arm movement during attacks of migraine with aura provoked by angiography were not accompanied by the usual increase in regional cerebral blood flow in oligemic areas, whereas the response was normal in the nonaffected parts of the brain (75,99).

Dilatation of the superficial temporal artery has been demonstrated on the headache side during attacks (63). This dilatation was relative to a generalized vasoconstriction suggestive of systemic sympathetic activation. The temporal extracranial blood flow response to an orthostatic test was only slightly decreased on the headache side as compared with the nonheadache side during an attack (64).

Pupillometry and Central Sympathetic Function

Autonomic function may be studied by pupillometry. The various studies performed in migraine generally suggest sympathetic hypofunction with denervation supersensitivity. Thus, interictally the mydriatic response to tyramine, phenylephrine, guanethidine, and adrenaline was enhanced in adult migraineurs but not in children (9,39,51), whereas the response to noradrenaline-releasing compounds such as fenfluramine (39) was reduced. Concordantly, a reduced pupillary response to the cold pressor test was reported (109). Studies of the pupillary adaptation to dark light have concluded to sympathetic hyperfunction (88), sympathetic dys- (hypo ?) function, (33) or parasympathetic hypofunction (88). In one study (9) using eye instillations of fenfluramine and phenylephrine, findings were normal.

Involvement of the locus coeruleus in migraine has been suggested but never demonstrated (73). As discussed above, CNV may be modulated be catecholamine afferents to the frontal cortex. Therefore, studies of CNV in migraine may indicate a central sympathetic involvement (84,120).

Other Studies

Other functional tests exploring the autonomic nervous system have led to the following, partly contradictory, conclusions in migraine. A venotest suggested adrenoreceptor supersensitivity (26), sweating studies sympathetic hypofunction (49), a tyramine test increased sensitivity (45), the sympathetic skin response hypofunction (36), and the recording of sympathetic fibers in muscle nerves normal activity (38).

Plasma levels and urinary excretion of catecholamines and their metabolites have been studied often but with contradictory results (120) (see Chapter 31).

NPY and VIP, markers of sympathetic and parasympathetic nerves, respectively, were normal during migraine attacks in external and internal jugular vein blood (41,47). Parasympathetic denervation supersensitivity in migraine has been suggested based on an exaggerated response to cholinergic agents. Thus, a larger increase in the second messenger cyclic GMP after methacholin provocation has been described in peripheral venous blood (98). Evidence points toward a role for the vasoactive amine 5-HT in migraine (see Chapter 31). In this regard it is worth mentioning that there is a close interaction between the central serotonergic and noradrenergic systems (46), but it remains to be determined whether this is relevant to migraine pathogenesis.

Conclusion

A clear dysfunction of the autonomic nervous system in migraine still remains to be proven. If sympathetic dysfunction really exists by itself, then most studies suggest hypofunction. However, considering that several studies, applying different methodologic approaches, have not cleared the ground and that the response of cranial arteries is normal during increased sympathetic activity, it seems unlikely that a sympathetic dysfunction plays any major role in the etiopathogenesis of migraine. There is some evidence suggesting that a mild parasympathetic hypofunction with denervation supersensitivity may be present. The origin and significance of such possible disturbances are unknown.

REFERENCES

1. Áfra J, Mascia A, Gérard P, Maertens de Noordhout A, Schoenen J. Interictal cortical excitability in migraine: a study using transcranial magnetic stimulation of motor and visual cortices. *Ann Neurol* 1998; 44:209–215.
2. Áfra J, Proietti Cecchini A, De Pasqua V, Albert A, Schoenen J. Visual evoked potentials during long-lasting pattern-reversal stimulations in migraine. *Brain* 1998;121:233–241.
3. Agnoli A, Martucci N, Mann V. Complicated and common migraine: EEG mapping and computed telethermography. *Cephalagia* 1985; 5(3):452.
4. Aloisi P, Marrelli A, Porto C, Tozzi E, Cerone G. Visual evoked potentials and serum magnesium levels in juvenile migraine patients. *Headache* 1997;37:383–385.
5. Aminof MJ. *Electrodiagnosis in clinical neurology*, 1st ed. New York: Churchill Livingstone, 1995.
6. Andermann F. Migraine-epilepsy relationships. *Epilepsy Res* 1987;1: 213–227.
7. Appenzeller O. Reflex vasomotor functions: clinical and experimental studies in migraine. *Res Clin Stud Headache* 1978;6:160–166.
8. Aurora SK, Ahmad BK, Welch KMA, Bhardhwaj P, Ramadan NM. Transcranial magnetic stimulation confirms hyperexcitability of occipital cortex in migraine. *Neurology* 1998;50:1111–1114.
9. Balottin V, Arisi D, Frigo GM, Lanzi G. Iris adrenergic sensitivity and migraine in pediatric patients. *Headache* 1983;23:32–33.
10. Barbiroli B, Montagna P, Cortelli P, et al. Abnormal brain and muscle energy metabolism shown by ^{31}P magnetic resonance spectroscopy in patients affected by migraine with aura. *Neurology* 1992;42: 1209–1214.
11. Barkley GL, Tepley N, Nagel-Leiby, et al. Magnetoencephalographic studies of migraine. *Headache* 1990;30:428–434.
12. Barkley GL, Tepley N, Simkins R, et al. Neuromagnetic fields in migraine preliminary findings. *Cephalalgia* 1990;10:171–176.
13. Benna P, Biaco C, Costa P, Piazza D, Bergamasco B. Visual evoked potentials and brainstem auditory evoked potentials in migraine and transient ischemic attack. *Cephalalgia* 1985;2:53–58.

14. Bettucci D, Cantello M, Gianelli M, Naldi P, Mutani R. Menstrual migraine without aura: cortical excitability to magnetic stimulation. *Headache* 1992;32:345–347.

15. Bille B, Koersner PE. Electroencephalographic investigations. In: Bille B, ed. Migraine in school children. *Acta Paediatr* 1962;51[suppl 136]:101–113.

16. Boccuni M, Alessandi M, Fusco BM, Cangi F. The pressor hyperresponsiveness to phenylephrine unmask sympathetic hypofunction in migraine. *Cephalalgia* 1989;9:239–245.

17. Böcker KBE, Timsit-Berthier M, Schoenen J, Brunia CHM. Contingent negative variation in migraine. *Headache* 1990;30:604–609.

18. Brinciotti M, Guidetti V, Matricardi M, et al. Responsiveness of the visual system in childhood migraine studied by means of VEPs. *Cephalalgia* 1986;6:183–185.

19. Camp WA, Wolff HG. Studies on headache. Electroencephalography abnormalities in patients with vascular headache of the migraine type. *Arch Neurol* 1961;4:474–485.

20. Connolly JF, Gawel M, Clifford Rose F. Migraine patients exhibit abnormalities in the visual evoked potential. *J Neurol Neurosurg Psychiatry* 1982;45:464–467.

21. Cortelli P, De Carolis P, Staurani A, et al. Cardiovascular and biochemical assessment in migraine patients submitted to tilt test. *Funct Neurol* 1986;1:285–290.

22. Cortelli P, Lugaresi A, Contin E, Agati R, Tinuper P, Saguegne T. Cardiovascular reflex in migraine patients during and out of migraine attack. *Cephalalgia* 1987;7[suppl 6]:289–290.

23. Cortelli P, Pierangeli G, Parchi P, Contin M, Baruzzi A, Lugaresi E. Autonomic nervous system function in migraine without aura. *Headache* 1991;31:457–462.

24. Dalla Volta G, Anzola GP. Are there objective criteria to follow up migrainous patients? A prospective study with thermography and evoked potentials. *Headache* 1988;28:423–425.

25. Daly DD, Markland OM. Focal brain lesion. In: Daly DD, Pedley TA, eds. *Current practice of clinical electroencephalography.* New York: Raven, 1990.

26. Del Bianco PL, Franchi G, Anselmi B, Sicuteri F. Monoamine sensitivity of smooth muscle *in vivo* in nociceptive disorders. In: Critchley M Friedman AP, Gorini S, Sicuteri F, eds. *Advances in neurology, headache, physiopathological and clinical concepts.* Vol 33. New York: Raven, 1982:391–398.

27. Diener HC. Biological markers in migraine diagnosis. *News Headache* 1991;1:3–5.

28. Diener HC, Ndosi NK, Koletzki E, Langohr HD. Visual evoked potentials in migraine. In: Pfaffenrath V, Lundberg PJ, Sjaastad O, eds. *Updating in headache.* Berlin: Springer-Verlag, 1984:439–465.

29. Diener HC, Scholz E, Dichgans J, Gerber WD. Central effects of drug used in migraine prophylaxis evaluated by visual evoked potentials. *Ann Neurol* 1989;25:125–130.

30. Downey JA, Frewin DB. Vascular responses in the hands of patients suffering from migraine. *J Neurol Neurosurg Psychiatry* 1967;35:258–263.

31. Drake ME, Pakalnis A, Hietter SA, Padamadan H. Visual and auditory evoked potentials in migraine. *Electromyogr Clin Neurophysiol* 1990;30:77–81.

32. Drake ME, Pakalnis A, Padamadan H. Long-latency auditory event-related potentials in migraine. *Headache* 1989;29:238–240.

33. Drummond PD. Disturbances in occular sympathetic function and facial blood flow in unilateral migraine headache. *J Neurol Neurosurg Psychiatry* 1990;53:121–125.

34. Eeg-Olofson O. The development of the electroencephalogram in normal adolescents from the age of 16 through 21 years. *Neuropaediatrie* 1971;3:11–45.

35. Engel GL, Ferris EB, Romano J. Focal electroencephalographic changes during the scotomas of migraine. *Am J Med Sci* 1945;209:650–657.

36. [Deleted in proofs.]

37. Evers S, Bauer B, Suhr B, Husstedt IW, Grotemeyer KH. Cognitive processing in primary headache: a study on event-related potentials. *Neurology* 1997;48:108–113.

38. Fagius J. Muscle nerve sympathetic activity in migraine. Lack of abnormality. *Cephalalgia* 1985;5:197–203.

39. Fanciullaci M. Iris adrenergic impairment of idiopathic headache. *Headache* 1979;19:8–13.

40. Friberg L, Olesen J, Iversen HK, Sperling B. Migraine pain associated with middle cerebral artery dilatation: reversal by sumatriptan. *Lancet* 1991;338:13–17.

41. Friberg L, Olesen J, Olsen TS, Karle A, Ekman R, Fahrenkrug J. Absence of vasoactive peptide release from brain to cerebral circulation during onset of migraine with aura. *Cephalalgia* 1994;14:47–54.

42. Gerber WD, Kropp P. The predictable migraine attack? *News Headache* 1994;4:3.

43. Gerber WD, Schoenen J. Biobehavioral correlates in migraine: the role of hypersensitivity and information-processing dysfunction. *Cephalalgia* 1998;18 Suppl;21;5–11.

44. Geyer MA, Puerto A, Menkes DB, Segal DS, Mandell AJ. Behavioral studies following lesions of the mesolimbic serotoergic pathways. *Brain Res* 1976;106:257–270.

45. Ghose K, Coppen A, Carroll D. Intravenous tyramine response in migraine before and during treatment with indoramin. *Br Med J* 1977;1:1191–1193.

46. Gillespie DD, Manier DH, Sanders-Bush E, Sulser F. The serotonin/norepinephrine-link in brain. II. Role of serotonin in the regulation of beta adrenoceptors in the low agonist affinity conformation. *J Pharmacol Exp Ther* 1988;244:154–159.

47. Goadsby PJ, Edvinsson L, Ekman R. Vasoactive peptide release in the extracerebral circulation of humans during migraine headache. *Ann Neurol* 1990;28:183–187.

48. Golla FL, Winter AL. Analysis of cerebral responses to flicker in patients complaining of episodic headache. *EEG Clin Neurophysiol* 1959;11:539–549.

49. Gomi S, Gotoh F, Komatsumoto S, Ishikawa Y, Araki N, Hamada J. Sweating function and retinal vasomotor reactivity in migraine. *Cephalalgia* 1989;9:179–185.

50. Good PA, Mortimer MJ. A test for migraine in children:differentiation between migraine with and without aura using the VER to white, blue and red light stimuli. *New Advances in Headache Research.* Vol. 2. London: Smith-Gordon, 1991:93–100.

51. Gotoh F, Komatsumota S, Araki N, Gomi S. Noradrenergic nervous activity in migraine. *Arch Neurol* 1984;41:951–955.

52. Gronseth GS, Greenberg MK . The utility of the electroencephalogram in the evaluation of patients presenting with headache:a review of the literature. *Neurology* 1995;45:1263–1267.

53. Guidetti V, Seri S, Cerquiglini A, et al. Computerized EEG topography in childhood headache. *Cephalalgia* 1989;9[suppl 10]:191–192.

54. Havan ka-Kanniainen H. Cardiovascular reflex responses during migraine attack. *Headache* 1986;26:442–446.

55. Havanka-Kanniainen H, Tolonen U, Myllyla VV. Cardiovascular relexes in young migraine patients. *Headache* 1986;26:420–424.

56. Havanka-Kanniainen H, Tolonen U, Myllyla VV. Autonomic dysfunction in adult migraineurs. *Headache* 1986;26:425–430.

57. Hay KM, Mortimer MJ, Barker DC, Debney LM, Good PA. 1044 women with migraine: the effect of environmental stimuli. *Headache* 1994;34:166–168.

58. Hegerl U, Juckel G. Intensity dependence of auditory evoked potentials as an indicator of central serotonergic neurotransmission: a new hypothesis. *Biol Psychiatry* 1993;33:173–187.

59. Hockaday JM, Debney LM. The EEG in migraine. In: Olesen J, Edvinsson L, eds. *Basic Mechanisms of Headache.* Amsterdam: Elsevier Science Publishers BV (Biomedical Division), 1988:365–376.

60. Hockaday JM, Macmillan AL, Whitty CW. Vasomotor-reflex responses in idiopathic and hormone dependent migraine. *Lancet* 1967;1:1023–1026.

61. Hole K, Johnson GE, Berge OG. 5,7-Dihydroxytryptamine lesions of the ascending 5-hydroxytryptamine pathways: habituation, motor activity and agonistic behaviour. *Pharmacol Biochem Behav* 1977;7:205–210.

62. Hughes JR, Robbins LD. Brain mapping in migraine. *Clin Electroencephalogr* 1990;21:14–24.

63. Iversen HK, Nielsen TH, Olesen J, Tfelt-Hansen P. Arterial responses during migraine headache. *Lancet* 1990;336:837–839.

64. Jensen K. Subcutaneous blood flow in the temporal region of migraine patients. *Acta Neurol Scand* 1987;75:310–318.

65. Jonkman EJ, Lelieveld MHJ. EEG computer analysis in patients with migraine. *EEG Clin Neurophysiol* 1981;52:652–655.

66. Kandel ER, Abrams T, Bernier L, Carew TJ, Hawkins RD, Schwartz JH. Classical conditioning and sensitization show aspects of the same molecular cascade in Aplysia. *Cold Spring Harb Symp Quant Biol* 1983;48:821–830.

67. Kellaway P. An orderly approach to visual analysis: parameters of the normal EEG in adults and children. In: Klaas DW, Daly DD, eds. *Current practice of clinical electroencephalography*. New York: Raven, 1979:69–147.

68. Kennard C, Gawel M, Rudolf N, Clifford Rose F. Visual evoked potentials in migraine subjects. *Res Clin Stud Headache* 1978;6:73–80.

69. Khalil NM. Investigations of visual function in migraine using visual evoked potentials and visual psychophysical test [PhD thesis]. London: University of London, 1991.

70. Kiloh LG, McComas AJ, Osselton JW. *Clinical electroencephalography*, 3rd ed. London: Butterworths, 1972:55.

71. Kropp P, Gerber WD. Is increased amplitude of contingent negative variation in migraine due to cortical hyperactivity or to reduced habituation? *Cephalalgia* 1993;13:37–41.

72. Kropp P, Gerber WD. Contingent negative variation during migraine attack and interval: evidence for normalization of slow cortical potentials during the attack. *Cephalalgia* 1995;15:123–128.

73. Lance JW. *Mechanism and management of headache*. Oxford, Butterworth-Heinemann, 1993.

74. Lauritzen M. Cerebral blood flow in migraine and cortical spreading depression. *Acta Neurol Scand* 1987;76:1–40.

75. Lauritzen M, Olsen TS, Lassen NA, Paulson OB. Regulation of regional cerebral blood flow during and between migraine attacks. *Ann Neurol* 1983;14:569–572.

76. Lauritzen M, Trojaborg W, Olesen J. EEG during attacks of common and classical migraine. *Cephalalgia* 1981;1:63–66.

77. Leaõ AA. Spreading depression of activity in cerebral cortex. *J Neurophysiol* 1944;7:359–390.

78. Leaõ AA. Morrisson RS. Propagation of spreading cortical depression. *J Neurophysiol* 1945;8:33–35.

79. Lehtonen JB. Visual evoked potentials for single flashes and flickering light in migraine. *Headache* 1974;14:1–12.

80. Lehtonen JB, Hyyppa MT, Kaihola H-L, Kangasniemi P, Lang AH. Visual evoked potentials in menstrual migraine. *Headache* 1979;19:63–70.

81. Lenarduzzi P, Timsit-Berthier M, Gerard P, Schoenen J. Variation contingente négative (CNV) dans la migraine avec aura (migraine classique) en période intercritique. Société Française d'Etudes des Migraines et Céphalées (réunion du 7.10.1988). Association pour la Neuro-psycho-pharmacologie, 1988:17–18.

82. MacLean C, Appenzeller O, Cordourdo JT, et al. Flash evoked potential in migraine. *Headache* 1975;14:193–198.

83. Maertens de Noordhout A, Pepin JL, Schoenen J, Delwaide PJ. Percutaneous magnetic stimulation of the motor cortex in migraine. *Electroencephalogr Clin Neurophysiol* 1992;85:110–115.

84. Maertens de Noordhout A, Timsit-Berthier M, Schoenen J. Contingent negative variation in headache. *Ann Neurol* 1986;19:78–80.

85. Maertens de Noordhout A, Timsit-Berthier M, Timsit M, Schoenen J. Effects of beta-blockage on contingent negative variation in migraine. *Ann Neurol* 1987;21:111–112.

86. Mariani E, Moschini V, Pastorino G, Rizzi F, Severgnini A, Tiengo M. Pattern-reversal visual evoked potentials and EEG correlations in common migraine patients. *Headache* 1988;28:269–271.

87. Marsters JB, Good PA, Mortimer MJ. A diagnostic test for migraine using the visual evoked potential. *Headache* 1988;28:526–530.

88. Micielli G, Tassorelli C, Magri M, Sandrini G, Cavallini A, Nappi G. Vegetative imbalance in migraine. A dynamic TV pupillometric evaluation. *Funct Neurol* 1989;4:105–111.

89. Mikamo K, Takeshima T, Takahashi K. Cardiovascular sympathetic hypofunction in muscle contraction headache and migraine. *Headache* 1989;29:86–89.

90. Montagna P, Cortelli P, Monari L, et al. ^{31}P-magnetic resonance spectroscopy in migraine without aura. *Neurology* 1994;44:666–668.

91. Mortimer MF, Good PA. The VEP in acephalgic migraine. *Headache* 1990;30:285–288.

92. Mortimer MF, Good PA. The VER as a diagnostic marker of childhood abdominal migraine. *Headache* 1990;30:642–645.

93. Nagel-Leiby S, Welch KMA, D'Andrea G, et al. Event-related slow potentials and associated catecholamine function in migraine. *Cephalalgia* 1990;10:317–329.

94. Nyrke T, Kangasniemi P, Lang AH. Difference of steady-state visual evoked potential in classic and common migraine. *EEG Clin Neurophysiol* 1989;73:284–294.

95. Nyrke T, Kangasniemi P, Lang AH. Transient asymmetries of steady-state visual evoked potentials in classic migraine. *Headache* 1990;30:133–137.

96. Nyrke T, Kangasniemi P, Lang AH, Petersen E. Steady-state visual evoked potentials during migraine prophylaxis by propranolol and femoxetine. *Acta Neurol Scand* 1984;69:9–14.

97. Nyrke T, Lang AH. Spectral analysis of visual potentials evoked by sine wave modulated light in migraine. *EEG Clin Neurophysiol* 1982;53:436–442.

98. Okada F, Miyagishi T, Honma M, Michio U. Plasma cyclic nucleotide responses to methacholine and epinephrine in patients with migraine. *Headache* 1984;24:26–29.

99. Olesen J, Larsen B, Lauritzen M. Focal hyperemia followed by spreading oligemia and impaired activation of rCBF in classic migraine. *Ann Neurol* 1981;9:344–352.

100. Ophoff RA, Terwindt GM, Vergouwe MN, et al. Familial hemiplegic migraine and episodic ataxia type-2 are caused by mutations in the Ca^{2+} channel gene CACNL1A4. *Cell* 1996;87:543–552.

101. Paiva T, Batista A, Martins P, et al. The relationship between headaches and sleep disturbances. *Headache* 1995;35:590–596.

102. Palmer JE, Chronicle EP. Cognitive processing in migraine: a failure to find facilitation in patients with aura. *Cephalalgia* 1998;18:125–132.

103. Passchier J, Van Der Helm-Hylkema H, Orlebeke JF. Psychophysiological characteristics of migraine and tension headache patients. Differential effects of sex and pain state. *Headache* 1984;24:131–139.

104. Pogacnik T, Sega S, Pecnik B, Kiauta T. Autonomic function testing in patients with migraine. *Headache* 1993;33:545–550.

105. Polich J, Ehlers CL, Dalessio DJ. Pattern shift visual evoked responses and EEG in migraine. *Headache* 1986;26:451–456.

106. Proietti Cecchini A, fra J, Schoenen J. Intensity dependence of the cortical auditory evoked potentials as a surrogate marker of CNS serotonin transmission in man: demonstration of a central effect for the 5-HT$_{1B/1D}$ agonist zolmitriptan (311C90, Zomig). *Cephalalgia* 1997;17:849–854.

107. Quality Standards Subcommittee of the American Academy of Neurology. Practice parameter: the electroencephalogram in the evaluation of headache. *Neurology* 1995;45:1411–1413.

108. Regan MD, Heron JR. Simultaneous recording of visual evoked potentials from the left and right hemisphere in migraine. In: Cochrane T, ed. *Background to migraine*. London: Heinemann, 1970:66.

109. Rubin LS, Graham D, Pasker R, Calhaun W. Autonomic nervous system dysfunction in common migraine. *Headache* 1985;25:40–48.

110. Sakai F, Meyer JS. Abnormal cerebrovascular reactivity in patients with migraine and cluster headache. *Headache* 1979;19:257–266.

111. Sand T. EEG in migraine: a review of the literature. *Funct Neurol* 1991;6:7–22.

112. Sandor PS, Mascia A, Áfra J, Schoenen J. Differential effects of prophylactic anti-migraine medication on the intensity dependence of cortical auditory evoked potentials. *Funct Neurol* 1998;13:199–200.

113. Schoenen J. Migraines et céphalées de tension: progrès diagnostiques, physiopathologiques et thérapeutiques. *Med Hyg* 1987;45:3607–3617.

114. Schoenen J. Clinical neurophysiology studies in headache: a review of data and pathophysiological hints. *Funct Neurol* 1992;7:191–204.

115. Schoenen J. Pathogenesis of migraine:the biobehavioural and hypoxia theories reconciled. *Acta Neurol Belg* 1994;94:79–86.

116. Schoenen J. Clinical neurophysiology of headache. In: Mathew NT, ed. *Neurologic clinics. Advances in headache*. Vol. 15. Philadelphia: WB Saunders, 1997:85–105.

117. Schoenen J. Cortical electrophysiology in migraine and possible pathogenetic implications. *Clin Neurosci* 1998;5:10–17.

118. Schoenen J, Jamart B, Delwaide PJ. Topographic EEG mapping in common and classic migraine during and between attacks. In: Clifford Rose F, ed. *Advances in headache research*. London: Smith Gordon, 1987:25–33.

119. Schoenen J, Jamart B, Maertens de Noordhout A, De Pasqua V, Delwaide PJ. Auditory event-related potentials in migraine. *Cephalalgia* 1989;9[suppl 10]:113–114.

120. Schoenen J, Maertens de Noordhout A. The role of the sympathetic nervous system in migraine and cluster headache. In: Olesen J, Edvinsson L, eds. *Basic mechanisms of headache 1983*. Amsterdam: Elsevier Science Publisher, 1983:393–410.

121. Schoenen J, Maertens de Noordhout A, Timsit-Berthier M, Timsit M. Contingent negative variation (CNV) as a diagnostic and physio-

pathologic tool in headache patients. In: Clifford Rose F, ed. *Proceedings of the 5th International Migraine Symposium (London 1984)*. Basel: Karger, 1985:17–25.

122. Schoenen J, Maertens de Noordhout A, Timsit-Berthier M, Timsit M. Contingent negative variation and efficacy of beta-blocking agents in migraine. *Cephalalgia* 1986;6:229–233.

123. Schoenen J, Wang W, Albert A, Delwaide P. Potentiation instead of habituation characterizes visual evoked potentials in migraine patients between attacks. *Eur J Neurol* 1995;2:115–122.

124. Schoenen J, Wang W, Gérard P. Modulation of temporalis muscle exteroceptive suppression by limb stimulation in normal man. *Brain Res* 1994;657:214–220.

125. Shibata K, Osawa M, Iwata M. Simultaneous recording of pattern reversal electroretinograms and visual evoked potentials in migraine. *Cephalagia* 1997;17:742–747.

126. Simon RH, Zimmerman AW, Pasman A, et al. Spectral analysis of photic stimulation in migraine. *EEG Clin Neurophysiol* 1982;53:270–276.

127. Simon RH, Zimmerman AW, Sanderson P, et al. EEG markers of migraine in children and adults. *Headache* 1983;23:201–205.

128. Sturgis Et, Schaefer CA, Ahles TA, et al. Effect of movement and position in the evaluation of tension headache and non-headache controls. *Headache* 1984;24:88–93.

129. Tagliati M, Sabbadini M, Bernardi G, Silvestrini M. Multichannel visual evoked potentials in migraine. *Electroencephalogr Clin Neurophysiol* 1995;96:1–5.

130. Thomsen LL, Iversen HK, Boesen F, Olesen J. Transcranial Doppler and cardiovascular responses during cardiovascular autonomic tests in migraineurs during and outside of attacks. *Brain* 1995;118:1319–1327.

131. Thomsen LL, Iversen HK, Olesen J. Cerebral blood flow velocities are reduced during attacks of unilateral migraine without aura. *Cephalalgia* 1995;15:109–116.

132. Timsit M, Timsit-Berthier M, Schoenen J, Maertens de Noordhout A. Intérêt de l'étude de la VCN dans les migraines et les céphalées de tension. *Rev EEG Neurophysiol Clin* 1987;17:259–270.

133. Vanagaite J, Pareja JA, Storen O, White LR, Sand T, Stovner LJ. Light-induced discomfort and pain in migraine. *Cephalalgia* 1997;17:733–741.

134. Van der Kamp W, Maassen VanDenBrink A, Ferrari D, van Dijk JG. Interictal cortical hyperexcitability in migraine patients demonstrated with transcranial magnetic stimulation. *J Neurol Sci* 1996;139:106–110.

135. Van der Kamp W, Maassen VanDenBrink A, Ferrari MD, van Dijk JG. Interictal cortical excitability to magnetic stimulation in familial hemiplegic migraine. *Neurology* 1997;48:1462–1464.

136. Van Dijk JF, Dorresteijn M, Haan J, Ferrari M. Visual evoked potentials and background EEG activity in migraine. *Headache* 1991;31:392–395.

137. Van Huffelen AC, Poortvliet DCJ, Van Der Wulp CJ, Magnus O. Quantitative EEG in cerebral ischemia. In: Lechner H, Aranibar A, eds. *EEG and clinical neurophysiology*. Amsterdam: Excerpta Medica International Congress Series 526, 1980:115–143.

138. Wang W, Schoenen J. Interictal potentiation of passive "oddball" auditory event-related potentials in migraine. *Cephalalgia* 1998;18:261–265.

139. Wang W, Schoenen J, Timsit-Berthier M. Cognitive functions in migraine without aura between attacks: a psychological approach using the "oddball" paradigm. *Neurophysiol Clin* 1995;25:3–11.

140. Wang W, Timsit-Berthier M, Schoenen J. Intensity dependence of auditory evoked potentials is pronounced in migraine: an indication of cortical potentiation and low serotonergic neurotransmission? *Neurology* 1996;46:1404–1409.

141. Winter AL, Cooper R. Neurophysiological measures of the visual system in classic migraine. In: Clifford Rose F, ed. *Proceecings of the 5th International Migraine Symposium (London 1984)*. Basel: Karger, 1985:11–16.

142. Wray SH, Mijovic-Prelec D, Kosslyn SM. Visual processing in migraineurs. *Brain* 1995;118:25–35.

143. Zwetsloot CP, Caekebeke JVF, Ferrari MD. Lack of asymmetry of middle cerebral artery blood velocity in unilateral migraine. *Stroke* 1993;24:1335–1338.

The Headaches, Second Edition,
edited by J. Olesen, P. Tfelt-Hansen, and K.M.A. Welch.
Lippincott Williams & Wilkins, Philadelphia © 2000.

The Migraines

CHAPTER 38

Psychological Mechanisms of Migraine

Peter D. Drummond

When patients are asked what triggers their episodes of migraine, the majority of them nominate "stress." By itself this is not very informative, because the situational context can range from minor problems or time pressures to major life changes. Nevertheless, it is well established that negative moods and personality traits that increase emotional vulnerability heighten the risk of migraine headaches.

From a conceptual point of view, one of the most convenient ways to define stress is that it develops when demands outweigh resources. Clearly, what is demanding varies enormously from one person to another, because each of us has different strengths and weaknesses and we are each faced with different challenges. However, when demands do outweigh resources, the outcome is likely to be a negative emotional state (e.g., fear, anger, anxiety, or depression) and activation of protective autonomic and neuroendocrine responses. Persistent stress depletes hormonal supplies and energy reserves and, ultimately, may increase susceptibility to inflammatory processes and disease.

In the past 20 years, the link between psychological factors and migraine has become the focus of systematic research. Reviewed in this chapter is evidence that documents an association between stress and migraine, as well as studies that have investigated the role of personality factors and negative emotions in increasing susceptibility to migraine. One of the most stressful aspects of a migraine sufferer's life may be having to endure the pain and disruption of recurrent migraine attacks. Thus, recent contributions to knowledge about the consequences of

having migraine are addressed. Finally, some speculations about how stressful experiences might trigger migraine by activating specific physiologic mechanisms are presented.

PROSPECTIVE STUDIES OF STRESS AND MIGRAINE

The most direct test of association between stress and migraine is to prospectively investigate stressful events and mood changes preceding attacks of migraine. Information from a representative sample of such studies is presented in Table 1.

Studies published before 1992 indicate that the frequency of stressful events was greater than normal 1 day or more preceding attacks of migraine (18,20). However, this effect varied somewhat between studies, possibly because of variation in headache frequency between different samples of subjects or because of variation in the length of data collection. In some, but not all studies, mood changes also preceded headache by a day or more (8,13), the most conspicuous changes being increases in fatigue, time pressures, alertness, and depressed mood. However, similar effects were not detected in all studies, possibly because only a limited set of emotional states were investigated; in addition, the relationship between mood and migraine could not be assessed in some studies because information on headache symptomatology was not collected prospectively.

In the most comprehensive study published since 1992, Sorbi et al. (28) collected mood ratings (alertness, tension, annoyance, irritability, depression, and fatigue), headache symptomatology, ratings of the incidence and stressfulness of daily problems, sleep quality, and stage of the menstrual cycle in 19 female migraine patients for 10 weeks. Data

P. D. Drummond: Department of Psychology, Murdoch University, Perth, Western Australia 6150, Australia.

TABLE 1. *Prospective studies of stress and migraine*

Study	Subjects	Ratings	Findings
Arena et al., 1984 (1)	21 migraine, 32 tension headache, 22 combined	VAS ratings for anger, anxiety, depression and headache intensity (not symptoms) recorded once daily for 28–35 days.	Mood ratings were weakly associated with headache intensity on the day of the attack but not beforehand. Headache type and frequency were not reported.
Dalkvist et al., 1984 (8)	5 migraine, 6 tension headache	VAS ratings for nervous, alert, happy, concentrated, and headache intensity (not symptoms) recorded twice daily for 38–61 days.	Ratings for alertness peaked 2 days before headache and was at a minimum on the day of the attack. Headache type and frequency were not reported.
Harrigan et al., 1984 (13)	17 migraine	Ratings on 9 mood scales and headache intensity (not symptoms) recorded 3 times/day for 21–75 days.	Ratings of negative mood were moderately related to headache intensity on the day of the attack; feelings of fatigue and constraint the day before predicted headache intensity. Headaches were reported on 49% of days (type not specified).
Levor et al., 1986 (20)	24 migraine	Ratings of stressful events, physical activity, mood states, migraine intensity and symptoms recorded 3 times/day for 28 days	Subjects averaged 10.7 days migraine/month. Stressful events were greater over the 4 days before headache than on 4 headache-free days. Physical activity decreased over this period.
Köhler and Haimerl, 1990 (18)	13 migraine	Daily stress questionnaire recorded once/day for 180–192 days.	Subjects reported 2.4 attacks of migraine/month. Attacks were consistently preceded by stressful days for 6 of the 13 subjects.
Sorbi et al., 1996 (28)	19 migraine	Incidence and stressfulness of daily hassles, mood ratings, migraine intensity and symptoms recorded 4 times/day for 10 weeks.	Subjects averaged 3.6 attacks of migraine in 10 weeks. Hassles increased the afternoon before an evening or night-time attack. Morning attacks were preceded by a stressful day, with increased tension and fatigue not relieved by sleep. Afternoon attacks were preceded for several days by a build-up of tension and irritability.
Holm et al., 1997 (17)	20 migraine	Subjects completed questionnaires on daily stress, coping strategies, cognitive appraisal and headache intensity once/day for 8 weeks (migraine symptoms were not recorded).	Headache activity correlated with stress ratings before or after the attack for 14 of the 20 subjects, and with cognitive appraisal for 13 subjects. Headache type and frequency were not reported.

VAS, visual analogue scale.

were analyzed in various ways in relation to the time period before attacks of migraine (28–30). In comparison with headache-free days, the incidence of daily problems was greater during the afternoon preceding an evening or night-time attack of migraine. The timing of evening and night-time attacks is consistent with the notion of migraine developing during a period of relaxation after stress, as opposed to during the stressful experience itself. Attacks that started in the morning or afternoon were preceded by an increase in the incidence or stressfulness of daily problems during the previous few hours or day and were preceded by increases in tenseness, irritability, and fatigue for one or more days. Spierings et al. (30) postulated that several days of tension can produce fatigue and irritability, culminating in extreme emotional tension and ultimately resulting in an afternoon attack of migraine. Morning attacks often began after a particularly stressful period, associated with feelings of tension and fatigue that had developed over the preceding few days. The notion that migraine develops during the period of recovery from stress also might apply to morning attacks because feelings of fatigue were not relieved by sleep. Taken together, the results of this prospective study suggest that relaxation after stress, persistent tension, and fatigue not relieved by sleep each increase the likelihood of migraine.

Holm et al. (17) reported recently on headache activity in 20 female undergraduates who were followed prospectively for 8 weeks. Each subject reported symptoms consistent with the diagnosis of migraine in a preliminary questionnaire and telephone interview, but subjects did not record headache symptomatology prospectively. Thus, the findings discussed here apply to headaches in general but not to migraine in particular. Subjects recorded the occurrence and psychological impact of minor stressful events, their appraisal of the events, and how well they coped with them in a daily diary. They also recorded the intensity of headaches four times daily. In a majority of cases, the timing of migraine attacks was associated with the number and intensity of daily problems, the appraisal of these problems as threatening, and whether resources were available to cope with the problems. This relationship appeared to be reciprocal: stress preceded the headache in some cases but developed after the headache in others. It is tempting to speculate that the development of these reciprocal effects in the same patient would contribute to recurrent attacks of headache. A relationship between phase of the menstrual cycle and ratings of stress was identified in 20% of the subjects (21); thus, hormonal changes may sometimes interact with psychological disturbances to influence the onset of headache.

PERSONALITY, PSYCHOPATHOLOGY, AND MIGRAINE

It has been recognized for some time that patients referred to tertiary treatment centers such as specialized pain or headache clinics often have personality traits that influence the referral decision. This point was investigated recently by Ziegler and Paolo (34), who compared the headache symptoms and psychological profiles of clinic patients with others who had not sought medical treatment for headaches in the past 2 years. Clinic patients had higher scores on the hypochondriasis, depression, hysteria, psychaesthenia, and social introversion scales of the Minnesota Multiphasic Personality Inventory-2 (MMPI-2) than did controls, even when findings were adjusted for differences in the severity of the patients' most intense headaches.

The study outlined above indicates that the clinical stereotype of the perfectionistic, rigid, hostile, and resentful migraine sufferer probably derives as much from referral bias as from a specific involvement of these traits in migraine. Nevertheless, a link between migraine and neuroticism has been detected in several well-controlled, community-based studies; furthermore, the prevalence of anxiety disorders and major depression is higher than normal in community-based migraine samples, as reviewed below.

Psychiatric Disorders

The association between migraine and the appearance of affective disorders in young adults was investigated prospectively in two large community-based samples. The advantage of a prospective design over a conventional cross-sectional design is that it provides some insight into the time sequence of any association that may exist. Breslau et al. (6) used structured interviews, based on current diagnostic criteria for migraine and psychiatric disorders, to measure the lifetime history of these disorders; 3.5 years later the interviews were repeated to identify the new development of the psychiatric symptoms and migraine over this time period. A strong association between migraine and major depression was detected in the lifetime history data. Importantly, depression preceded migraine as often as migraine preceded depression both in the lifetime history data and prospectively, indicating no clear direction of causality. A similar association between migraine and specific anxiety disorders was also detected in the same community-based sample (5).

In a second prospective study, Pine et al. (25) followed an initial cohort of 776 children and adolescents for 9 years. Psychiatric diagnoses were established during detailed standard interviews, whereas headache status was investigated by asking subjects if "they had a history of migraine or chronic headache at any time in their life that prevented them from doing things they would usually do" (p. 156). Adolescents with a diagnosis of major depression reported a history of headache approximately twice as often as those without this diagnosis; furthermore, major depression in adolescence predicted the development of chronic headaches in early adulthood. An association between simple phobias, overanxiousness, and headaches was also identified; however, this association seemed to be due to a link with symptoms of depression. The generality of these findings is limited by the superficial assessment of headache and by the likelihood of unreported episodes of major depression between assessments. Nevertheless, the findings document an association between major depression and the later development of chronic headache.

Recent research has also hinted at a relationship between migraine and a range of anxiety disorders meeting the diagnostic criteria of psychiatric classification systems. For example, in a telephone survey of more than half of the residents of Washington County between 12 and 29 years of age, the risk of having a headache in the previous week was increased for those with a history of panic attacks, particularly when the headache was associated with migrainous features (32). The temporal sequence between migraine and panic disorder was not addressed in this survey; however, in a prospective study by Breslau and Davis (5), panic disorder developed more frequently in subjects with migraine than in controls over a 14-month study period.

Neuroticism

Unlike the clinical diagnoses of major depression and the anxiety disorders, neuroticism is conceptualized as an inherited trait that is part of normal personality; it refers to an emotional instability and autonomic overactivity that increases vulnerability to stress. Breslau and Andreski (3) investigated personality traits, including neuroticism, in a community sample of young adults in Detroit, Michigan. Neuroticism scores were markedly higher in those with a history of migraine, with or without aura, than in others without a history of migraine. The relationship between migraine and neuroticism persisted after controlling for sex, a history of major depression, and a history of anxiety disorders. Neuroticism was greatest in those with migraine and a history of depression and anxiety; nevertheless, neuroticism was greater in those with migraine alone than in others without a history of migraine or psychiatric disorders.

These findings suggest that neuroticism may increase the risk of migraine; alternatively, recurrent episodes of migraine could artificially heighten neuroticism scores because some of the items on the neuroticism scale are related to health and bodily concerns, fatigue, and social withdrawal (2). This point was investigated recently in a 5-year prospective investigation of migraine incidence in relation to neuroticism scores at baseline in young adults (4). In women, the risk of developing migraine during the 5-year follow-up period increased in direct proportion to neuroticism scores at baseline; there were insufficient data to test this relationship in men. The results of this study suggest that neuroticism, or some factor that heightens neuroticism, increases the risk of migraine.

CONSEQUENCES OF MIGRAINE

Migraine sufferers often have to endure intensely painful headaches, frequently associated with nausea, vomiting, and neurologic disturbances. The headaches disrupt normal daily routines, can add to time pressures, and often necessitate withdrawal from pleasurable activities. Not surprisingly, the headache itself can become a major source of stress and anticipatory anxiety.

Most patients who attend specialist pain treatment centers or headache clinics for treatment do not cope well with their headaches (27,35). This depends less on the type of headache (migraine versus tension) than on the belief that chance factors influence headache (27). Disability appears to be greater in clinic patients than in others who rarely seek treatment for their headaches, particularly in terms of how the headache disrupts work activities (35).

One option available to patients with migraine is to take medication to decrease the intensity of pain. However, for various reasons there is often some reluctance to take medication (e.g., fear of side effects, giving in to the headache, financial concerns about the cost of medication, or worry about taking too much medication). Negative emotions (depression, anger, disappointment, fear, and helplessness) often peak before patients decide to take medication (24). Thus, a critical part of medical treatment is to convince the patient to take the medication early on in the course of the attack, when it is most likely to be effective.

MECHANISM OF INTERACTION BETWEEN STRESS AND MIGRAINE

The mechanism that links stress with migraine is unknown. The susceptibility to migraine during periods of recovery from prolonged stress suggests that the mechanism might involve a switch in autonomic balance from sympathetic to parasympathetic dominance. Alternatively, attacks might develop during the exhaustion phase of Selye's general adaptation syndrome, which is characterized by a depleted neuroendocrine response to prolonged stress and an increased susceptibility to inflammatory disease (31). The prospective studies needed to test these ideas have not yet been conducted.

The large body of literature on psychophysiologic responses to laboratory stress in migraine sufferers has yielded only limited insight into the link between stress and migraine. A series of studies by the author (10) indicated that scalp vessels dilated more readily in migraine sufferers than in controls during brief periods of harassment, particularly in subjects who showed signs of extracranial vascular distension during attacks of migraine. Similar findings have been reported by others (14,19,26); however, still other investigators did not detect an effect of migraine on extracranial vascular reactivity (15) or identified signs of more intense vasoconstriction in the scalp vessels of migraine sufferers during stressful activities (23). Clearly, any general statement about extracranial vascular reactivity in migraine cannot be made with confidence at present. However, the variation in results across studies indicates that any link between stress, vascular reactivity, and the predisposition for migraine is tenuous, at best. This is in line with the notion that distension of scalp vessels is a secondary source of pain that develops occasionally during some attacks of migraine (9).

One of the limitations of the psychophysiologic literature on migraine is that responses to brief, artificial sources of stress have been investigated in most studies; the findings of these studies may not be relevant for processes that might only be active during migraine, or that require a stronger or more persistent stimulus than is usually employed. In an attempt to address these issues, Stronks et al. (33) measured cardiovascular responses and changes in serotonin and catecholamine levels during 45 minutes of mental arithmetic in migraine and chronic tension headache sufferers, as well as in nonheadache controls; they also monitored the development of headache during the task. In general, autonomic and hormonal responses to mental stress were similar in all three groups, irrespective of the presence or absence of headache. Thus, the findings do not support the view that some aspect of the acute response to stress contributes to a migraine predisposition.

One of the hypotheses currently being explored in the psychophysiologic literature on migraine is that increases in autonomic activity return more slowly than usual toward baseline during the recovery period after a brief laboratory stress. In a recent investigation of this effect, Holm et al. (16) measured cardiovascular and electromyographic responses while subjects delivered a speech in front of a video camera. Pulse rate increased to the same extent in migraine sufferers, tension headache sufferers, and controls during the speech but remained somewhat elevated in migraine sufferers during the 12-minute recovery period after the speech. Similarly, Kröner-Herwig et al. (19) noted that extracranial vascular responses dissipated more slowly after stressful tests in migraine sufferers than in controls. Because the delay in recovery did not generalize to other autonomic measures in either study, the findings provide only limited support for the idea that susceptibility to migraine may be linked in some way to persistent autonomic arousal after periods of stress (15).

The association between migraine, depression, and anxiety may reflect a common predisposition to these disorders (22), perhaps because of similar neurotransmitter or receptor disturbances in the brain stem or midbrain.

Activation of the hypothalamic-pituitary adrenocortical axis with the serotonin receptor agonist *m*-chlorophenyl-piperazine provokes an initial release of cortisol, followed several hours later by a migrainelike headache whose strength is proportional to the extent of cortisol release (7,12). It is tempting to assume that the endogenous release or depletion of cortisol in response to psychological stress also could set headaches in motion.

CONCLUSIONS

Over the past decade, several well-controlled prospective studies have confirmed a link between psychological factors and migraine. Their findings indicate that tension, fatigue, and irritability often precede headaches by a day or more, consistent with the notion that mood disturbances can trigger attacks. At a more general level, the association between neuroticism and migraine suggests that a vulnerability to stress increases the risk of migraine. The high prevalence of anxiety disorders and depression in migraine sufferers further supports an association with emotional vulnerability. These psychiatric disorders should be diagnosed and treated in their own right, apart from any benefits that might flow on to migraine.

A range of nonpharmacologic approaches are effective in the management of recurrent headaches (11); elements common to most of these approaches include stress reduction, relaxation, and an enhanced sense of control over the demands of life, including headaches. These approaches should be used to supplement pharmacologic treatment of migraine, particularly when the patient shows clear signs of psychological distress.

REFERENCES

1. Arena JG, Blanchard EB, Andrasik F. The role of affect in the etiology of chronic headache. *J Psychosom Res* 1984;28:79–86.
2. Baskin SM. Personality and migraine. *Headache* 1995;35:380–381.
3. Breslau N, Andreski P. Migraine, personality, and psychiatric comorbidity. *Headache* 1995;35:382–386.
4. Breslau N, Chilcoat HD, Andreski P. Further evidence on the link between migraine and neuroticism. *Neurology* 1996;47:663–667.
5. Breslau N, Davis GC. Migraine, physical health and psychiatric disorder: a prospective epidemiologic study in young adults. *J Psychiatr Res* 1993;27:211–221.
6. Breslau N, Davis GC, Schultz LR, Peterson EL. Migraine and major depression: a longitudinal study. *Headache* 1994;34:387–393.
7. Brewerton TD, Murphy DL, Mueller EA, Jimerson DC. Induction of migrainelike headaches by the serotonin agonist *m*-chlorophenylpiperazine. *Clin Pharmacol Ther* 1988;43:605–609.
8. Dalkvist J, Ekbom K, Waldenlind E. Headache and mood: a time-series analysis of self-ratings. *Cephalalgia* 1984;4:45–52.
9. Drummond PD, Lance JW. Facial temperature in migraine, tension-vascular and tension headache. *Cephalalgia* 1984;4:149–158.
10. Drummond PD, Lance JW. Contribution of the extracranial circulation to the pathophysiology of headache. In: Olesen J, Edvinsson L, eds. *Basic mechanisms of headache.* Amsterdam: Elsevier, 1988;321–330.
11. Gauthier JG, Ivers H, Carrier S. Nonpharmacological approaches in the management of recurrent headache disorders and their comparison and combination with pharmacotherapy. *Clin Psychol Rev* 1996; 16:543–571.

12. Gordon ML, Lipton RB, Brown SL, et al. Headache and cortisol responses to *m*-chlorophenylpiperazine are highly correlated. *Cephalalgia* 1993;13:400–405.

13. Harrigan JA, Kues JR, Ricks DF, Smith R. Moods that predict coming migraine headaches. *Pain* 1984;20:385–396.

14. Haynes SN, Gannon LR, Bank J, Shelton D, Goodwin J. Cephalic blood flow correlates of induced headaches. *J Behav Med* 1990;13:467–480.

15. Hermann C, Blanchard EB. Psychophysiological reactivity in pediatric migraine patients and healthy controls. *J Psychosom Res* 1998;44:229–240.

16. Holm JE, Lamberty K, McSherry WC, Davis PA. The stress response in headache sufferers: physiological and psychological reactivity. *Headache* 1997;37:221–227.

17. Holm JE, Lokken C, Myers TC. Migraine and stress: a daily examination of temporal relationships in women migraineurs. *Headache* 1997;37:553–558.

18. Köhler T, Haimerl C. Daily stress as a trigger of migraine attacks: results of thirteen single-subject studies. *J Consult Clin Psychol* 1990;58:870–872.

19. Kröner-Herwig B, Fritsche G, Brauer H. The physiological stress response and the role of cognitive coping in migraine patients and non-headache controls. *J Psychosom Res* 1993;37:467–480.

20. Levor RM, Cohen MJ, Naliboff BD, McArthur D. Psychosocial precursors and correlates of migraine headache. *J Consult Clin Psychol* 1986;54:347–353.

21. Lokken C, Holm JE, Myers TC. The menstrual cycle and migraine: a time-series analysis of 20 women migraineurs. *Headache* 1997;37:235–239.

22. Merikangas KR, Stevens DE. Comorbidity of migraine and psychiatric disorders. *Neurol Clin* 1997;15:115–123.

23. Passchier J, Goudswaard P, Orlebeke JF. Abnormal extracranial vasomotor response in migraine sufferers to real-life stress. *J Psychosom Res* 1993;37:405–414.

24. Passchier J, Mourik J, Brienen JA, Hunfeld JAM. Cognitions, emotions, and behavior of patients with migraine when taking medication during an attack. *Headache* 1998;38:458–464.

25. Pine DS, Cohen P, Brook J. The association between major depression and headache: results of a longitudinal epidemiologic study in youth. *J Child Adolesc Psychopharmacol* 1996;6:153–164.

26. Rojahn J, Gerhards F. Subjective stress sensitivity and physiological responses to an aversive auditory stimulus in migraine and control subjects. *J Behav Med* 1986;9:203–212.

27. Scharff L, Turk DC, Marcus DA. The relationship of locus of control and psychosocial-behavioral response in chronic headache. *Headache* 1995;35:527–533.

28. Sorbi MJ, Maasan GH, Spierings ELH. A time series analysis of daily hassles and mood changes in the 3 days before the migraine attack. *Behav Med* 1996;22:103–113.

29. Spierings ELH, Sorbi M, Haimowitz BR, Tellegen B. Changes in daily hassles, mood and sleep in the 2 days before a migraine headache. *Clin J Pain* 1996;12:38–42.

30. Spierings ELH, Sorbi M, Maassan GH, Honkoop PC. Psychophysical precedents of migraine in relation to the time of onset of the headache: the migraine time line. *Headache* 1997;37:217–220.

31. Sternberg EM, Chrousos GP, Wilder RL, Gold PW. The stress response and the regulation of inflammatory disease. *Ann Intern Med* 1992;117:854–866.

32. Stewart W, Breslau N, Keck PE. Comorbidity of migraine and panic disorder. *Neurology* 1994;44[Suppl 7]:23–27.

33. Stronks DL, Tulen JHM, Verheij R, et al. Serotonergic, catecholaminergic, and cardiovascular reactions to mental stress in female migraine patients: a controlled study. *Headache* 1998;38:270–280.

34. Ziegler DK, Paolo AM. Headache symptoms and psychological profile of headache-prone individuals: a comparison of clinic patients and controls. *Arch Neurol* 1995;52:602–606.

35. Ziegler DK, Paolo AM. Self-reported disability due to headache: a comparison of clinic patients and controls. *Headache* 1996;36:476–480.

The Headaches, Second Edition,
edited by J. Olesen, P. Tfelt-Hansen, and K.M.A. Welch.
Lippincott Williams & Wilkins, Philadelphia © 2000.

The Migraines

CHAPTER 39

5-Hydroxytryptamine Involvement in Migraine

Edith Hamel and Pramod R. Saxena

Migraine is a complex disorder that has been best described as "the manifestation of a hereditary or predisposed sensitivity of neurovascular reactions to certain stimuli or to cyclic changes in the central nervous system" (26). It appears quite clear from its many facets and manifestations that migraine originates in the brain and, in its process and evolution, impacts on the cranial and cerebral blood vessels and leads to the generation and transmission of head pain. It would be simplistic to try to explain the complexity of migraine symptoms based on dysfunctions in a single molecule or neurotransmitter system. As such, individual changes should be seen as part of more complex biochemical abnormalities that together are likely to provide a comprehensive understanding of the pathology. In this regard, there is compelling evidence to suggest that 5-hydroxytryptamine (5-HT or serotonin) might be particularly important to some aspects of migraine pathophysiology. The reported changes in its overall metabolism, the accumulating evidence for abnormal processing in central 5-HT–mediated responses during and between migraine attacks, together with the fact that effective antimigraine drugs target specific populations of 5-HT receptors have all contributed to reinforce its putative pivotal role in migraine pathogenesis (11,13,21,43). Quite convincingly, migraine might be a consequence of a central derangement, most likely involving a chronic hypofunction of serotonergic neurotransmission (11,13,21,37,46).

E. Hamel: Department of Neurology and Neurosurgery, Montréal Neurological Institute, McGill University, Montréal, Québec H3A 2B4, Canada.

P. R. Saxena: Department of Pharmacology, Erasmus University, 3000 DR Rotterdam, The Netherlands.

HISTORICAL BACKGROUND

5-HT, originally discovered as a serum vasoconstrictor agent, was isolated and characterized in 1948 (42) and later identified as an important brain neurotransmitter (51). 5-HT is actively taken up and stored in blood platelets and is synthesized in mast cells and nerve terminals, including those that innervate the cranial and cerebral vasculature (2,6,28,36,51). Shortly after its discovery, 5-HT was implicated in the pathophysiology of migraine based on the original finding by Sicuteri and colleagues (49) of an increased urinary excretion of 5-HT's primary metabolite, 5-hydroxyindoleacetic acid (5-HIAA) during migraine attacks. This observation, however, has proven not to be as reproducible as expected (11), possibly due to individual variations in metabolism between various populations of migraine sufferers (21). In contrast, consistent and indisputable increases in plasma 5-HT content concomitant with decreases in 5-HIAA levels have been found during migraine attacks, whereas the reverse is true between attacks, and this irrespective of migraine with and without aura (11,21,43,46). In keeping with these observations, platelet 5-HT content has been shown to decrease during migraine attacks (11,21), a change that may be absent or much more subtle in migraine without aura (12). The changes in the levels of 5-HT and its metabolite seen in plasma and urine are thought to reflect dysfunctions occurring not only at the level of blood platelets, but primarily so in the brain (21). This is in keeping with the reported increase in cerebrospinal fluid 5-HIAA levels in migraine patients (13), a finding that further suggests that migraine is accompanied by an enhanced turnover of central 5-HT.

Together these observations have supported the hypothesis that a chronically low serotonin disposition forms the biochemical basis of migraine etiology (12,46), and that migraine attacks are triggered by a sudden increase in 5-HT release (21,24,26). However, arguments that do not substantiate this view also have been asserted (37).

MIGRAINE AS A CHRONIC LOW-SEROTONIN SYNDROME

The synthesis of brain serotonin depends on the activity of its rate-limiting enzyme tryptophan hydroxylase and the availability of its precursor, the essential amino acid tryptophan that originates exclusively from dietary intake. Similar to migraine, depression is considered as a disorder of low brain serotonergic activity and, as such, the mechanism of action of most effective antidepressant drugs is to enhance and stabilize 5-HT neurotransmission (1). Epidemiologic studies have shown the comorbidity of migraine with depression and anxiety (34), observations that support a common locus of neurochemical disturbances. Interestingly, pharmacologically controlled depressed patients submitted to a rapid tryptophan depleting diet experienced a depressive relapse together with some symptoms reminiscent of migraine, such as increased nausea or vomiting, drowsiness, and, in some cases, headache (10). A decrease in migraine frequency and intensity with ultimate cessation over a 3-year period was reported in a patient with classic migraine concomitantly with the development of a 5-HT–producing carcinoid tumor, together with recurrence of migraine attacks upon surgery and relative reduction in plasma 5-HT and 5-HIAA levels (20). This anecdotal finding tends to suggest that long-term exposure to 5-HT has a protective role on migraine attacks, possibly through normalization of 5-HT levels and desensitization or downregulation of 5-HT receptors that would otherwise be in a sensitized or hypersensitized state due to a chronic low 5-HT syndrome.

A most convincing piece of evidence, however, in favor of migraine being a low serotonergic syndrome has recently been provided from physiologic studies on the evaluation of auditory evoked potentials. The amplitude of these evoked potentials has been shown to be inversely related to central serotonergic neurotransmission (19). In migraine patients, a marked increase in amplitude was observed between attacks, in support of a low 5-HT transmission and abnormal cortical processing of sensory information (53). The implication of serotonergic pathways in this response has further been confirmed by the observation that 5-HT$_{1B/1D}$ receptor agonists, which can penetrate the brain and activate cortical inhibitory prejunctional 5-HT$_{1B/1D}$ autoreceptors, can increase the amplitude of auditory evoked potentials in normal subjects as well as migraine sufferers (41). Together with previous observations of increased amplitudes of visual evoked potentials in migraine sufferers (7), these observations all converge to support the notion that migraine is

associated with a cortical hypersensitivity to stimulus in the headache-free interval, which is, at least in part, due to low 5-HT transmission (19,53).

HIGH SEROTONIN AS A TRIGGER OF MIGRAINE ATTACKS

Such a scenario of a chronically low availability of 5-HT could result in a sensitization of all or specific populations of 5-HT receptors in migraine sufferers. Interestingly, pharmacologic and molecular evidence seem to support the original hypothesis that migraine is the consequence of an inappropriate increased sensitivity of 5-HT$_{2B}$ receptors (16,24). More specifically, these researchers suggested that activation of cerebrovascular endothelial 5-HT$_{2B}$ receptors, following an increased bioavailability of 5-HT at the onset of a migraine attack, would induce the endothelial production and release of nitric oxide (NO). Nitric oxide can dilate cranial blood vessels and activate trigeminovascular afferents, thus invoking two aspects of the neurogenic inflammatory response thought to be involved in pain generation and transmission (for more details, see Chapters 16 and 17). This mechanism reinforces the view that central dysfunctions in migraine will lead to perturbations of the cranial circulation (26). Indeed, activation of 5-HT$_{1B/1D}$ receptors causing cranial vasoconstriction and inhibition of trigeminovascular activity leads to alleviation of migraine symptoms.

Arguments in favor of the biochemical-triggering event being an increase in 5-HT availability include the observations that several drugs that release 5-HT from neurons and blood platelets (fenfluramine and reserpine) and some 5-HT reuptake inhibitors (zimeldine and femoxetine) are all able to provoke migraine attacks and more frequently so in migraine subjects than in controls (13,21,37). The same may be the case with red wine, which also releases 5-HT from blood platelets, and possibly from neuronal stores (39). However, fenfluramine and reserpine used for extended periods can confer resistance to migraine headache, and 5-HT given during an attack will induce headache relief. It seems therefore that the mobilization of 5-HT from intracellular stores at an early stage will trigger migraine attacks (16,21,24). However, the receptors inducing the migraine attack (possibly the 5-HT$_{2B}$) are different from those (5-HT$_1$ family) that relieve migraine headache (see Chapter 16). The ability of the 5-HT$_{2B/2C}$ receptor agonist m-chlorphenylpiperazine (m-CPP) to induce severe attacks, which were indistinguishable from their spontaneous migraines, in subjects with a personal or family history of migraine (3), together with the 5-HT$_{2B}$ pharmacologic profile of several 5-HT$_2$ receptor antagonists with known prophylactic efficacy in migraine therapy, also provide support to the proposed supersensitivity of 5-HT$_{2B}$ receptors in the predisposition to migraine (16,24,48). On the other hand, one must point out that *m*-CPP is not selective for the 5-HT$_{2B}$ receptor and that several 5-HT$_{2B/2C}$ receptor antagonists, including mianserin and cyproheptadine, are not effective antimigraine agents (45,50,52).

In the event that 5-HT$_{2B}$ receptors are sensitized in migraine sufferers, it would appear interesting to verify whether genetic variations in these receptors would explain the susceptibility to migraine. This does not appear to be the case for the 5-HT$_{2A}$ and 5-HT$_{2C}$ receptors, which have both recently been excluded as candidate genes for migraine susceptibility (4). Similarly, the genetic variants of 5-HT$_{1B}$ (30) and 5-HT$_{1F}$ (29) receptors do not seem to influence the clinical response to sumatriptan in migraine patients.

CENTRAL ORIGIN OF 5-HT DYSFUNCTION

It has been claimed that changes in circulating 5-HT alone can not explain all the facets of a migraine attack (21). However, despite the fact that a low brain serotonergic activity has been evidenced between attacks on the basis of an increase amplitude of auditory action potentials, an increase in central 5-HT neurotransmission at the onset and during an attack has not yet been demonstrated. Thus, whether the pharmacologic manipulations with 5-HT agonists and 5-HT–releasing agents bear any relevance to spontaneous migraine attack is still largely speculative. However, a positron emission tomography study performed in migraine patients during their spontaneous migraine attacks showed increased cerebral blood flow in the brain stem, including in an area corresponding closely in location to the serotonergic dorsal raphe nucleus (54). This fascinating observation may suggest that serotonergic dorsal raphe neurons become activated and release 5-HT during a migraine attack, and as such they have been considered as part of the migraine generator center. These neurons project to many areas of the central nervous system, including the cerebral cortex and the area postrema, where abnormal information processing has been documented during migraine. They are also intricately related to the cranial vasculature, which constitutes the primary locus of pain generation in migraine. These characteristics, together with the known interactions between serotonergic, dopaminergic, and noradrenergic systems in the brain, suggest that dysfunctions of the 5-HT system are likely to have functional repercussions much larger than those expected on the basis of 5-HT neurotransmission alone. This may explain some of the complexity of the neurochemical changes associated with migraine, most specifically those related to other amines (8).

Brain Stem Raphe Neurons as Part of a Possible Migraine Generator Center

Serotonergic neurons located in brain stem raphe nuclei are involved in the regulation of multiple physiologic functions, including stress, pain, appetite, mood, and sleep, to name a few (22), some of these being disturbed during a migraine attack. These neurons also have been shown to change their firing pattern in response to stressful stimuli (2), a behavior compatible with the hypothesis that migraine attacks are triggered by an increased discharge of 5-HT in response to stressful stimuli. A landmark characteristic of raphe 5-HT neurons is the close relationship that exists between their firing pattern and the sleep-wake-arousal cycle. For instance, their firing rate is abolished during rapid eye movement (REM) sleep, but they are at their maximal firing activity during active waking (15). Such an activity pattern with a progressive silence of 5-HT neurotransmission during REM sleep would be accompanied by a concomitant decrease in 5-HT release, and as such could interfere with the evolution of the migraine process. It may explain why the most naturally self-prescribed treatment during a migraine attack is sleep.

Another interesting aspect of brain 5-HT neurons is their intimate association with cortical astroglial cells (5). These cells are important regulators of brain homeostasis, and they have been associated with the development of cortical spreading depression, a suspected mechanism in the initiation of a migraine attack (27). The glycogenolytic activity of astroglial cells, which provides energy not only for the astrocyte itself but also for the activated neurons via the release of lactate and its neuronal uptake, is sensitive to serotonergic stimulation (31). This could represent an additional way via which a disturbed central 5-HT neurotransmission could fail to maintain adequate brain functions. Such a mechanism could possibly explain part of the abnormal processing of cortical sensory information (53).

Dorsal Raphe Neurons as a Possible Link to the Vascular Activation

The endpoint in the migraine process, namely the generation of headache, appears to involve activation of pain-sensitive trigeminovascular fibers releasing vasodilator substances, possibly as a consequence of endothelial 5-HT$_{2B}$ receptor stimulation. Whether the activation of trigeminovascular fibers could be achieved by a change in the firing of dorsal raphe neurons remains an issue still largely speculative, and the mechanisms involved surely are not well described. Although it is quite clear that there is no direct anatomic connections between raphe neurons and the meningeal blood vessels (5,6,33), it is undeniable that these vessels appear to be able to respond to changes in central 5-HT neurotransmission. Of particular interest is the observation that a lesion of the dorsal raphe nucleus induces supersensitivity to serotonin in isolated cerebral arteries (35), a situation that could be compatible with the suggested supersensitivity of cerebrovascular receptors in migraine sufferers due to their chronic low 5-HT disposition. On this basis, the possibility that an abrupt increase in the activity of 5-HT neurons in the raphe nucleus or a platelet discharge of 5-HT following a stressful stimulation activates sensitized $5\text{-}HT_{2B}$ receptors and leads to activation of the pain-generating process cannot be excluded. Another level of interaction is the intra-parenchymal microcirculation, which, at least in the cerebral cortex, has been shown to be intimately regulated by dorsal raphe 5-HT neurons (5). Whether a dysfunctional regulation of local cortical cerebral blood flow by raphe neurons in response to stressful stimuli could contribute or not to the overall abnormal processing of cortical information remains to be demonstrated. However, it is clear that cortical spreading depression, a mechanism postulated to be part of the initial neuronal abnormalities in a migraine attack, is accompanied by changes in local vascular responsiveness (27).

VASCULAR PHARMACOLOGY OF 5-HT

Besides being taken up and stored in sympathetic neurons, 5-HT is synthesized in nerve terminals innervating the cranial and cerebral vasculature (2,6,28,36). The extent of the physiologic importance of 5-HT in the control of vascular smooth muscle tone, either as a co- or neurotransmitter, is not clear. However, cranial blood vessels are particularly sensitive to 5-HT, and they can either contract or relax to 5-HT, acting on $5\text{-}HT_{2A}$, $5\text{-}HT_{1B}$, or $5\text{-}HT_7$ receptors (32,44,52). The affinity of 5-HT for $5\text{-}HT_{1B}$ and $5\text{-}HT_7$ receptors is much higher than for $5\text{-}HT_{2A}$ receptors (32,44,52). Thus, as depicted in Figure 1,

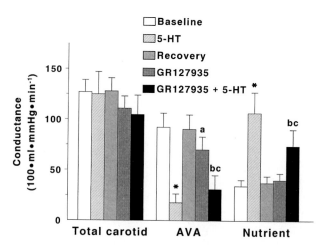

FIG. 2. Effects of two sequential 10-minute intracarotid infusions of 5-HT (2 µg/kg/min) on total carotid, arteriovenous anastomotic (*AVA*), and nutrient vascular conductances in ketanserin-pretreated (0.5 mg/kg) pigs. The initial 5-HT infusion decreased AVA and increased nutrient conductance without changing total carotid conductance. Thirty minutes after stopping the infusion, a full recovery was obtained. In the presence of GR127935 (0.5 mg/kg), the 5-HT–induced AVA constriction and arteriolar dilatation were only slightly inhibited. $*p < 0.05$ versus baseline; $^a p < 0.05$ versus recovery; $^b p < 0.05$ versus state after GR127935; $^c p < 0.05$ versus first response to 5-HT.

5-HT constricts large conducting arteries and arteriovenous anastomoses mainly via the $5\text{-}HT_{1B}$ receptor and dilates arterioles via the $5\text{-}HT_7$ receptor. If either plasma or neuronal 5-HT is involved in the maintenance of vessel wall tone, a decrease in the concentration of 5-HT at the neurovascular junction can lead to constriction of arterioles, but a dilatation of large arteries and arteriovenous anastomoses. There is some evidence of such hemodynamic changes occurring during the headache phase of migraine (44,52).

Whether or not 5-HT plays a pathologic role in migraine at the neurovascular junction, there is no denial that acutely acting antimigraine drugs (ergots and triptans) constrict cranial arteries and arteriovenous anastomoses (9,44,52). It seems clear that the constriction of arteriovenous anastomoses by the triptans and, partly, also the ergot alkaloids involves the $5\text{-}HT_{1B}$ receptor (9). However, it is surprising that the contractile effect of 5-HT itself on porcine carotid arteriovenous anastomoses is not affected much by GR127935, a selective and potent $5\text{-}HT_{1B/1D}$ receptor antagonist (Fig. 2) (9). This unexpected finding suggests that arteriovenous constriction by 5-HT in the pig involves a novel receptor subtype.

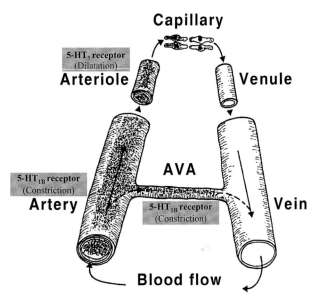

FIG. 1. A schematic representation of the cranial vascular bed, showing dilator and constrictor responses to 5-HT and the main receptor types involved. *AVA,* arteriovenous anastomoses.

PHARMACOLOGIC IMPLICATIONS

Some $5\text{-}HT_{2B}$ receptor antagonists and, in particular, $5\text{-}HT_{1B/1D}$ receptor agonists are effective antimigraine drugs, the former in preventive treatment and the latter in the acute relief of migraine headache (for a review, see Chapter 16). This observation underscores the fact that 5-HT can interact with multiple receptors in the brain and blood vessels, which, depending on their localization, the action they mediate, and time of activation in the migraine process, can either initiate or abort an attack. In this regard, it is interesting to note that the ubiquitous distribution of $5-HT_{2B}$ receptors in human brain and peripheral tissues did raise the possibility of their association with vascular cells which are common to all tissues (25,47). The most recent studies in human brain vessels have supported this contention (5,48) and further confirmed their localization to the endothelium, but also to the myocytes of human cerebral blood vessels (5) (see also Chapter 16). Forbes et al. have recently described some selective $5-HT_{2B}$ receptor antagonists, including SB204741 (14). Clinical effectiveness of such selective drugs in migraine prophylaxis would substantiate the hypothesis of the development of functional hypersensitivity of vascular $5-HT_{2B}$ receptors and therein the initiation of the painful neurogenic inflammatory response (5,16,24,48).

In the acute treatment of migraine symptoms, sumatriptan has been and still is the gold standard. Its clinical efficacy has been associated with its ability to constrict distended cranial vessels or block the release of calcitonin gene–related peptide (CGRP) and substance P from trigeminovascular afferents (see Chapters 16, 17, and 52). The latter action would reverse the vasodilatation and block the initiation of vascular pain. The vascular and neuronal sites of action have been identified as postsynaptic $5-HT_{1B}$ receptors on smooth muscle cells that mediate cerebral constriction and presynaptic $5-HT_{1D}$, and possibly $5-HT_{1F}$ (23,40), receptors on trigeminovascular afferents that block the development of neurogenic inflammation. These receptors in humans also have been found to be present in brain stem centers involved in the transmission of pain centrally, as well as in the cerebral cortex (38). Newer triptan derivatives that selectively target these different $5-HT_1$ receptors have become available (Table 1) and those that penetrate the brain (e.g., naratriptan, rizatriptan, zolmitriptan) may have the possibility to interact with $5-HT_1$ receptors in cortical (41) as well as subcortical brain areas (17,18). The beneficial or detrimental outcome of such interactions is not fully understood at the present time (see Chapter 16). Lastly, the novel 5-HT receptor identified in porcine arteriovenous anastomoses may prove to be another target for identifying antimigraine drugs.

In conclusion, available evidence, albeit indirect and circumstantial, supports the notion that 5-HT exerts a pivotal role in the pathogenesis of a migraine attack. The availability of better tools and technologies to study the level of activity of 5-HT neurotransmission in migraine sufferers and of better pharmacologic compounds to selectively target specific populations of 5-HT receptors,

TABLE 1. *Binding profile of some anti-migraine compounds at $5-HT_1$ receptors*

	$5-HT_{1B}$	$5-HT_{1D}$	$5-HT_{1F}$
Sumatriptan	8.1	8.5	7.6
Naratriptan	8.7	8.3	8.3
Zolmitriptan	8.3	9.2	7.1
Rizatriptan	7.4	7.9	6.7
Frovatritan	8.6	8.4	7.0
Alniditan	8.7	9.0	<6.0
IS-159	8.5	8.8	<5.0
LY 334370	6.9	6.9	8.8

Affinities at the different 5-HT receptor subtypes are expressed as pIC_{50} or pKi values and were taken from various papers in the literature. Although the majority of triptan derivatives are nonselective compounds at these receptors, alniditan and IS-159 are agonists at $5-HT_{1B/1D}$ receptors with no or very low activity at the $5-HT_{1F}$ receptor. In contrast, new compounds, such as LY334370, are being developed to target the $5-HT_{1F}$ receptor. Compounds such as naratriptan, zolmitriptan, and rizatriptan are brain penetrant and could exert effects centrally at the level of the trigeminalis nucleus caudalis.

together with the progress in molecular genetics, may all converge in the near future to provide a much clearer picture of the exact mode of action of 5-HT in the pathogenesis and manifestation of migraine headache.

ACKNOWLEDGEMENTS

Dr. Hamel would like to thank the Medical Research Council of Canada (Grant MA-9967) and the Heart and Stroke Foundation of Québec for supporting the work performed in her laboratory.

REFERENCES

1. Blier P, de Montigny C. Current advances and trends in the treatment of depression. *Trends Pharmacol Sci* 1994;15:220–226.
2. Bonvento G, MacKenzie ER, Edvinsson L. Serotonergic innervation of the cerebral vasculature: relevance to migraine and ischaemia. *Brain Res Rev* 1991;16:257–263.
3. Brewerton TD, Murphy DL, Mueller EA, Jimerson DC. Induction of migraine-like headaches by the serotonin agonist m-chlorophenylpiperazine. *Clin Pharmacol Ther* 1988;43:605–609.
4. Buchwalder A, Welch SK, Peroutka SJ. Exclusion of $5-HT_{2A}$ and $5-HT_{2C}$ receptor genes as candidate genes for migraine. *Headache* 1996; 36:254–258.
5. Cohen Z, Bonvento G, Lacombe P, Hamel E. Serotonin in the regulation of brain microcirculation. *Prog Neurobiol* 1996;50:335–362.
6. Cohen Z, Bonvento G, Lacombe P, MacKenzie ET, Seylaz J, Hamel E. Cerebrovascular nerve fibers immunoreactive for tryptophan-5-hydroxylase in the rat: distribution, putative origin and comparison with sympathetic noradrenergic nerves. *Brain Res* 1992;598:203–214.
7. Connolly JF, Gawel M, Clifford RF. Migraine patients exhibit abnormalities in the visual evoked potential. *J Neurol Neurosurg Psychiatry* 1982;45:464–467.
8. Curzon G, Barrie M, Wilkinson MIP. Relationships between headache and amine changes after administration of reserpine to migrainous patients. *J Neurol Neurosurg Psychiatry* 1969;32:555–561.
9. De Vries P, Villalón CM, Heiligers JP, Saxena PR. Characterization of 5-HT receptors mediating constriction of porcine carotid arteriovenous anastomoses; involvement of $5-HT_{1B/1D}$ and novel receptors. *Br J Pharmacol* 1998;123:1561–1570.

10. Delgado PL, Charney DS, Price LH, Aghajanian GK, Landis H, Heninger GR. Serotonin function and the mechanism of antidepressant action. Reversal of antidepressant-induced remission by rapid depletion of plasma tryptophan. *Arch Gen Psychiatry* 1990;47:411–418.

11. Ferrari MD. Biochemistry of migraine. *Pathol Biol* 1992;40:287–292.

12. Ferrari MD, Odink J, Tapparelli C, Van Kempen GM, Pennings EJ, Bruyn GW. Serotonin metabolism in migraine. *Neurology* 1989;39:1239–1242.

13. Ferrari MD, Saxena PR. On serotonin and migraine: a clinical and pharmacological review. *Cephalalgia* 1993;13:151–165.

14. Forbes IT, Ham P, Booth DH, et al. 5-Methyl-1-(3-pyridylcarbamoyl)-1,2,3,5-tetrahydropyrrolo[2,3-f]indole: a novel $5\text{-}HT_{2C}/5\text{-}HT_{2B}$ receptor antagonist with improved affinity, selectivity, and oral activity. *J Med Chem* 1995;38:2524–2530.

15. Fornal CA, Litto WJ, Metzler CW, Marrosu F, Tada K, Jacobs BL. Single-unit responses of serotonergic dorsal raphe neurons to $5\text{-}HT_{1A}$ agonist and antagonist drug administration in behaving cats. *J Pharmacol Expl Ther* 1994;270:1345–1358.

16. Fozard JR, Kalkman HO. 5-Hydroxytryptamine (5-HT) and the initiation of migraine: new perspectives. *Naunyn Schmiedebergs Arch Pharmacol* 1994;350:225–229.

17. Goadsby PJ, Hoskin KL. Serotonin inhibits trigeminal nucleus activity evoked by craniovascular stimulation through a $5HT_{1B/1D}$ receptor: a central action in migraine? *Ann Neurol* 1998;43:711–718.

18. Goadsby PJ, Knight Y. Inhibition of trigeminal neurones after intravenous administration of naratriptan through an action at 5-hydroxytryptamine $(5\text{-}HT_{1B/1D})$ receptors. *Br J Pharmacol* 1997;122:918–922.

19. Hegerl U, Juckel G. Intensity dependence of auditory evoked potentials as an indicator of central serotonergic neurotransmission. A new hypothesis. *Biol Psychiatry* 1993;33:173–187.

20. Hopf HC, Johnson EA, Gutmann L. Protective effect of serotonin on migraine attacks. *Neurology* 1992;42:1419.

21. Humphrey PPA. 5-Hydroxytryptamine and the pathophysiology of migraine. *J Neurol* 1991;238[Suppl]:38–44.

22. Jacobs BL, Azmitia EC. Structure and function of the brain serotonergic system. *Physiol Rev* 1992;72:165–229.

23. Johnson KW, Schaus JM, Durkin MM, et al. $5\text{-}HT_{1F}$ receptor agonists inhibit neurogenic dural inflammation in guinea pigs. *Neuroreport* 1997;8:2237–2240.

24. Kalkman HO. Is migraine prophylactic activity caused by $5\text{-}HT_{2B}$ or $5\text{-}HT_{2C}$ receptor blockade? *Life Sci* 1994;54:641–644.

25. Kursar JD, Nelson DL, Wainscott DB, Baez M. Molecular cloning, functional expression, and mRNA tissue distribution of the human 5-hydroxytryptamine 2B receptor. *Mol Pharmacol* 1994;46:227–234.

26. Lance JW. Current concepts of migraine pathogenesis. *Neurology* 1993;43[Suppl 3]:11–15.

27. Lauritzen M. Pathophysiology of the migraine aura. The spreading depression theory. *Brain* 1994;117:199–210.

28. Lincoln J. Innervation of cerebral arteries by nerves containing 5-hydroxytryptamine and noradrenaline. *Pharmacol Ther* 1995;68:473–501.

29. MaassenVanDenBrink A, Vergouwe MN, Ophoff RA, et al. Chromosomal localization of the $5\text{-}HT_{1F}$ receptor gene: no evidence for involvement in response to sumatriptan in migraine patients. *Am J Med Genet* 1998;77:415–420.

30. MaassenVanDenBrink A, Vergouwe MN, Ophoff RA, Saxena PR, Ferrari MD, Frants RR. $5\text{-}HT_{1B}$ receptor polymorphism and clinical response to sumatriptan. *Headache* 1998;38:288–291.

31. Magistretti PJ, Sorg O, Martin J-L. Regulation of glycogen metabolism in astrocytes: physiological, pharmacological, and pathological aspects. In: Murphy S, ed. *Astrocytes: pharmacology and function*. London: Academic, 1993:243–265.

32. Martin GR. Vascular receptors for 5-hydroxytryptamine: distribution, function and classification. *Pharmacol Ther* 1994;62:283–324.

33. Mathiau P, Riche D, Behzadi G, Dimitriadou V, Aubineau P. Absence of serotonergic innervation from raphe nuclei in rat cerebral blood vessels—I. Histological evidence. *Neuroscience* 1993;52:645–655.

34. Merikangas KR. Sources of genetic complexity of migraine. In: Sandler M, Ferrari M, Harnett S, eds. *Migraine: pharmacology and genetics*. New York: Chapman & Hall, 1996:254–281.

35. Moreno MJ, Conde MV, De La Fuz Fraile M, Fernandez-Lomana H, Lopez De Pablo AL, Marco EJ. Lesion of the dorsal raphe nucleus induces supersensitivity to serotonin in isolated cat middle cerebral artery. *Brain Res* 1991;538:324–328.

36. Owman C, Chang J-Y, Hardebo JE. Presence of 5-hydroxytryptamine in adrenergic nerves of the brain circulation: its role in sympathetic neurotransmission and regulation of the cerebral vessel wall. In: Saxena PR, Wallis DI, Wouters W, Bevan P, eds. *Cardiovascular pharmacology of 5-hydroxytryptamine*. Dordrecht: Kluwer Academic, 1990: 211–230.

37. Panconesi A, Sicuteri F. Headache induced by serotonergic agonists—a key to the interpretation of migraine pathogenesis? *Cephalalgia* 1997;17:3–14.

38. Pascual J, del Arco C, Romon T, del Olmo E, Castro E, Pazos A. Autoradiographic distribution of [^{3}H]sumatriptan-binding sites in postmortem human brain. *Cephalalgia* 1996;1:317–322.

39. Pattichis K, Louca LL, Jarman J, Sandler M, Glover V. 5-Hydroxytryptamine release from platelets by different red wines: implications for migraine. *Eur J Pharmacol* 1995;292:173–177.

40. Phebus LA, Johnson KW, Zgombick JM, et al. Characterization of LY344864 as a pharmacological tool to study $5\text{-}HT_{1F}$ receptors: binding affinities, brain penetration and activity in the neurogenic dural inflammation model of migraine. *Life Sci* 1997;61:2117–2126.

41. Proietti-Cecchini A, Afra J, Schoenen J. Intensity dependence of the cortical auditory evoked potentials as a surrogate marker of central nervous system serotonin transmission in man: demonstration of a central effect for the $5HT_{1B/1D}$ agonist zolmitriptan (311C90, Zomig). *Cephalalgia* 1997;17:849–854.

42. Rapport MM, Green AA, Page IH. Serum vasoconstrictor (serotonin). IV. Isolation and characterization. *J Biol Chem* 1948;176:1243–1251.

43. Saxena PR. 5-Hydroxytryptamine and migraine. In: Saxena PR, Wallis DI, Wouters W, Bevan P, eds. *Cardiovascular pharmacology of 5-hydroxytryptamine*. Dordrecht: Kluwer Academic, 1990;407–416.

44. Saxena PR. Serotonin receptors: subtypes, functional responses and therapeutic relevance. *Pharmacol Ther* 1995;66:339–368.

45. Saxena PR, Den Boer MO. Pharmacology of antimigraine drugs. *J Neurol* 1991;238[Suppl 1]:28–35.

46. Saxena PR, Ferrari MD. From serotonin receptor classification to the antimigraine drug sumatriptan. *Cephalalgia* 1992;12:187–196.

47. Schmuck K, Ullmer C, Engels P, Lubbert H. Cloning and functional characterization of the human $5\text{-}HT_{2B}$ serotonin receptor. *FEBS Lett* 1994;342:85–90.

48. Schmuck K, Ullmer C, Kalkman HO, Probst A, Lubbert H. Activation of meningeal $5\text{-}HT_{2B}$ receptors: an early step in the generation of migraine headache? *Eur J Neurosci* 1996;8:959–967.

49. Sicuteri F, Testi A, Anselmi B. Biochemical investigations in headache: increase in hydroxyindoleacetic acid excretion during migraine attacks. *Int Arch Allergy Appl Immunol* 1961;19:55–58.

50. Tfelt-Hansen P, Saxena PR. Antiserotonin drugs. In: Olesen J, Tfelt-Hansen P, Welch KMA, eds. *The headaches*. New York: Raven, 1993: 373–382.

51. Twarog BM, Page IH. Serotonin content of some mammalian tissues and urine and a method for its determination. *Am J Physiol* 1953;175:157–161.

52. Villalón CM, de Vries P, Saxena PR. Serotonin receptors as cardiovascular targets. *Drug Dev Today* 1997;2:294–302.

53. Wang W, Timsit-Berthier M, Schoenen J. Intensity dependence of auditory evoked potentials is pronounced in migraine: an indication of cortical potentiation and low serotonergic neurotransmission? *Neurology* 1996;46:1404–1409.

54. Weiller C, May A, Limmroth V, et al. Brain stem activation in spontaneous human migraine attacks. *Nat Med* 1995;1:658–660.

The Headaches, Second Edition,
edited by J. Olesen, P. Tfelt-Hansen, and K.M.A. Welch.
Lippincott Williams & Wilkins, Philadelphia © 2000.

The Migraines

CHAPTER **40**

Nitric Oxide Involvement in Migraine

Lars Lykke Thomsen and Jes Olesen

In 1980 Furchgott and Zawadzki reported that vasodilatation induced by acetylcholine depends on the presence of intact endothelium (10). The mediator of this endothelium-dependent vasodilatation was some years later identified as nitric oxide (NO), which previously was considered to be merely an atmospheric pollutant (44). Since then the biology of this small and short-lived messenger molecule has been increasingly and very intensively investigated (35). NO is generated from the terminal guanidino nitrogen of *L*-arginine. The family of enzymes catalyzing NO synthesis are known as NO synthases (NOS) (26). NO synthase activity has been reported in many tissues, including endothelium, brain, peripheral nerves, vascular smooth muscle, myocardium, macrophages, neutrophils, and microglia of several species (26,35). Purification and cloning of NOS has revealed the existence of at least three isoforms (26). Two of these are constitutive, are Ca^{2+}/calmodulin dependent (cNOS), and release NO from, for example, endothelium (eNOS) and neurons (nNOS). This release is accelerated in response to stimulation of several specific membrane-bound receptors by, for example, glutamate, bradykinin, 5-HT, acetylcholine, histamine, endothelin-1, substance P, and probably calcitonin gene–related peptide (CGRP) (12,14,18,32,57) (Fig. 1). Increased flow velocity and the subsequent increase of shear stress in endothelial cells also may stimulate eNOS (32). Another NO synthase is inducible and Ca^{2+} independent (iNOS). iNOS generates

NO for long periods and in large amounts in response to endotoxins and cytokines (26,35). Most physiologic actions of NO are mediated via activation of soluble guanylate cyclase (sGC) and a consequent increase in cyclic guanosine monophosphate (cGMP), eventually leading to a decrease in intracellular Ca^{2+} in target cells (35). NO has an amazing number of physiologic effects throughout the body, of which several, theoretically, may be implicated in the pathophysiology of migraine (11,35). Thus, endothelium-dependent vasodilatation is of importance in cerebrovascular regulation, and neurogenic vasodilatation may be mediated via perivascular nerves, which operate through NO as discussed in Chapter 11. Furthermore, NO mediates neurotransmission in the central nervous system of importance for pain perception (hyperalgesia). Moreover, NO contributes to the control of platelets and, when produced in large amounts, NO contributes to host defense reactions of importance in nonspecific immunity and neurotoxicity. Finally, NO may release CGRP from perivascular nerve endings and may thus play a role in neurogenic inflammatory reactions (58). An increasing volume of evidence actually suggests that NO plays a pivotal role in migraine pain (43,50). This evidence is in large part based on experiences from experimental human headache-inducing substances that seem to share the same common final molecular pathway, namely activation of the NO pathway. The use of these substances as experimental human headache models is described in detail in Chapter 24. Here we draw on our experiences with these models to focus on NO mechanism in migraine. We also provide evidence supporting the view that inhibition of the NO cascade represents a new principle in the treatment of migraine.

L. L. Thomsen and J. Olesen: Department of Neurology, Glostrup Hospital, University of Copenhagen, DK-2600 Glostrup, Copenhagen, Denmark.

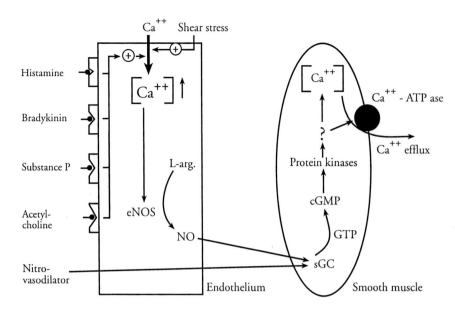

FIG. 1. Molecular events in the nitric oxide pathway illustrated by endothelium-derived synthesis of nitric oxide (*NO*). Endothelium nitric oxide synthase (*eNOS*) is stimulated by an increase in intracellular calcium. NO diffuses from endothelial cells to smooth muscle cells and activates the soluble guanylate cyclase (*cGC*). This in turn leads to an increase in cyclic guanosine monophosphate (*cGMP*) and via activation of protein kinases and subsequent poorly understood intermediary processes stimulates the membrane bound Ca^{2+} ATPase. Ca^{2+} then diffuses out of the cell, eventually leading to smooth muscle relaxation and vasodilatation. Nitrovasodilators act as NO donors and activate the same pathway.

HYPERSENSITIVITY OF MIGRAINEURS TO NO

Glyceryl trinitrate (GTN) is the most suitable substance for experimental studies of NO-induced headache because it is well tolerated and diffuses freely across membranes. GTN itself has no known action in the human body but acts via liberation of NO and is thus generally regarded as an NO donor (7,19,20). Due to its lipid solubility, it may deliver NO to several tissues, including those protected by the blood–brain barrier. Several observations support the notion that GTN induces headache by liberating NO. Thus, GTN-induced headache in healthy controls is very short lived and is therefore unlikely to be caused by metabolites other than NO, because these have a longer half-life (22). Furthermore the long-acting nitrate 5-isosorbide-mononitrate (5-ISMN) induces a dose-dependent headache and arterial dilatation, but its metabolites apart from NO are different from those of GTN (24). Finally, *N*-acetylcysteine, which augments GTN effects in the heart by increasing the formation of NO or by enhancing the effect of NO itself, also augments the headache response to GTN and prolongs GTN-induced arterial dilatation of the superficial temporal artery but not of the radial arteries (21). Previous studies have suggested that migraine patients in some way are particular sensitive to headaches induced by GTN because they more often experience a migrainelike headache in association with nitroglycerin administration than do nonmigraineurs (49). A recent blinded study directly compared headache responses in sufferers of migraine without aura, headache-free individuals, and patients suffering from episodic tension type headache (42). Each person received a staircase intravenous infusion of four increasing doses of GTN, and headache responses were followed prospectively until 1 hour after

termination of the last infusion. Migraineurs reported headaches of stronger intensity and with more migraine characteristics than did the controls (Fig. 2). This difference was most apparent at the higher GTN doses. Most often these immediate headaches were not migraines because the accompanying symptoms characteristic of migraine were lacking. Retrospectively recorded data from 1 to 24 hours after GTN infusions showed that most migraineurs, in addition to the headache experienced in close association with GTN infusions, complained of a delayed

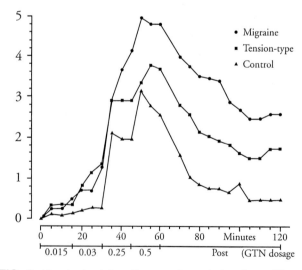

FIG. 2. Headache intensity over time during four different doses of glyceryl trinitrate (GTN). Comparison between responses in migraineurs (n = 17), tension-type headache sufferers (n = 9), and healthy subjects (n = 17). During doses above 0.015 μg/kg/min, migraine patients experienced significantly more headache than controls ($p < 0.05$, Kruskal Wallis and multiple range test). Reproduced from ref. 42.

headache that they labeled as typical migraine. Characteristics of this delayed migraine has been described in detail in Chapter 24. Some of the controls also experienced a delayed headache, which was of milder intensity and only in a single case could be classified as a migraine (42). Thus, migraineurs seem hypersensitive to nitroglycerin-induced headache and most likely therefore to NO in two ways. First, they experience more severe immediate nonmigraine headache than controls; second, most migraineurs in contrast to controls eventually experience a delayed migraine. An increased headache response could reflect a greater general sensitivity to pain, or it could be due to increased physiologic sensitivity to NO. It is well known that nitroglycerin dilates the middle cerebral artery via NO without affecting cerebral blood flow and thereby the arterioles (4,23). Applying the ultrasonographic technique transcranial Doppler (1,53), which provides an indirect measure of large intracranial artery diameters in situations of unchanged blood flow, we examined whether the increased sensitivity to the NO donor GTN was reflected not only in increased headache in migraineurs but also in increased dilatation of the middle cerebral artery. Indeed migraineurs were found to be more sensitive in this aspect as well (55). Furthermore, a decreased platelet aggregability to collagen in combination with increased platelet arginine levels in migraineurs support the notion that migraineurs are supersensitive to the physiologic effects of NO (5). Moreover, migraineurs have been found to be hypersensitive to histamine regarding headache development in controlled trials (6,27,30). The headache induced during histamine infusion (27) as well as a delayed migraine in migraineurs (30) was almost completely blocked by the histamine H_1 blocker mepyramine, whereas the H_2 blocker cimetidine only had a small effect (27). Activation of endothelial H_1 receptors induce the formation of endogenous NO (57). Thus, the increased sensitivity to histamine in migraineurs also may be explained by hypersensitivity to activation of the NO pathway. More direct evidence for the causal relationship between histamine-induced headache and $H1$ receptor–mediated activation of the NO pathway would be provided if inhibition of NOS proved to have any effect on histamine-induced headaches. A recent study, however, did not show any effect of the competitive NOS inhibitor N-monomethyl-L-argenin (L-NMMA) on histamine-induced headaches in healthy subjects (48). One explanation for this may be that the administered doses of L-NMMA were too low to outbalance the administered histamine doses.

Reserpine given intravenously or intramuscularly has been shown to cause headache with some migrainous features in most migraine patients but not in controls (28). Thus, again migraineurs seem particular sensitive. Reserpine depletes not only platelets but also presynaptic nerve terminals of their content of monoamines. Substances released include 5-HT. The 5-HT_{2B} receptor has recently been suggested to play a crucial role in the initiation of migraine attacks (8). The vascular response to 5-HT_{2B} activation, at least in the pig, is primarily a consequence of the release of NO (14). Like reserpine, fenfluramine also causes release of 5-HT, and fenfluramine seems to cause headaches with more migraine features in migraineurs compared with controls (13). Migraineurs also seem particularly sensitive to headache induced by metachlorophenylpiperazine (mCPP) (2,17; see also Chapter 24). mCPP is a direct agonist at the 5-HT_{2Bc} receptor and therefore is likely to cause vascular headache via NO synthesis (8). Infusion of the vasodilator prostacyclin seems to induce bilateral pulsating headaches as well as facial flushing (45). Prostacyclin may act directly on smooth muscle receptors, but in cerebral vessels protected by the blood–brain barrier it is more likely to act via endothelial receptors by liberating NO. We conclude that NO is a likely common denominator for headaches induced by GTN, histamine, reserpine, mCPP, prostacyclin and fenfluramine and that migraineurs show hypersensitivity to activation of the NO cascade.

POSSIBLE MECHANISMS OF SPONTANEOUS MIGRAINE INDUCED BY NO

At present it is not known in further detail where and how activation of the NO pathway may cause experimental migraine headache and how this trigger mechanism may be related to natural migraine triggers. Regarding the latter, natural triggers such as hormones, alcohol, and chocolate may elicit increases in NO directly or via increases in neurotransmitter concentration both in the brain and blood, which in turn may stimulate the formation of NO. This may occur in brain neurons, the arterial endothelium, and in NOS containing nerve terminals (11,32,35). Formation of NO also may be elicited by pathologic reactions such as spreading depression of Leao, which is the proposed mechanism of the migraine aura (16,47). It is therefore interesting that sufferers of migraine with aura also seem particularly sensitive to GTN-induced headache (3). With all the experimental migraine triggers mentioned above, the induced migraine attacks occur up to several hours after infusion. This time lag is not yet understood. The half-life of NO is very short but at least in the anesthetized cat GTN infusion leads to a prolonged (hours) increase in NO concentration (47). Thus, a cascade of physiologic events, which are set up and withheld by the liberation of NO to which migraineurs are hypersensitive, may be implicated. NO seems to be released during spontaneous migraine headache. One study applying electron paramagnetic resonance spectroscopy to estimate systemic nitrosylhemoglobin levels as an index of circulating NO showed slightly increased levels during attacks of migraine without aura compared with the interictal period (37). Furthermore, an NOS inhibitor has shown efficacy treating a full-blown migraine attack as discussed below (29).

In relation to the site where NO-mediated triggering events may be set up, speculation concerning histamine-induced migraines may be more helpful than speculations concerning GTN. Thus, whereas GTN diffuses freely across biologic membranes, histamine does not cross the blood–brain barrier (41) and, when administered systemically, most likely works on endothelial receptors. Moreover, histamine only causes headache when injected into the internal but not into the external carotid artery (39). Due to its short half-life, NO can only diffuse short distances (150–160 μm from a single cell) (31). If histamine-induced migraine headache is set up by H_1-activated liberation of NO, this is therefore likely to involve processes initiated within or just around the intracranial vasculature. Interestingly, human cerebral arteries have long been recognized as pain-sensitive structures (38,46). It is therefore interesting that NO is a powerful vasodilator and that dilatation of the large cranial arteries has been reported during spontaneous migraine headache (9,25,56). A focus on the function of arterial regulatory mechanisms involving NO in migraine has suggested normal endothelial function of NO in peripheral arteries in migraineurs (52). A mild parasympathetic dysfunction may be involved and may, via denervation supersensitivity, be responsible for the observed supersensitivity to NO in cerebral arteries (54). To this end, a larger increase in cGMP after intramuscular injections of a cholinergic agent has been described in peripheral venous blood (40). This may provide a link between parasympathetic hypofunction and arterial NO hypersensitivity in migraine because cholinergic agents seem to liberate NO, at least from the endothelium (10). Direct activation of perivascular sensory nerve fibers (36) by NO may be other possibilities. Thus, increased levels of CGRP, which is present in perivascular sensory nerve endings, has been demonstrated in samples from the external jugular vein during spontaneous migraine attacks (15). Animal studies have suggested that NO may release CGRP from perivascular nerves at least around cerebral arterioles (58). It is tempting to propose an increased sensitivity to such effects of NO in migraineurs. The release of involved peptides may in turn cause prolonged vasodilatation and perhaps sensitization of perivascular nociceptors. Another theoretical possibility is that central pain modulating effects of NO are involved. Animal studies suggest that NO plays a role in central modulation of nociception and produces hyperalgesia (33,34). In humans the role of NO in nociceptive modulation is largely unknown. A recent study examining the influence of intravenous infusion of four increasing doses of the NO donor GTN on the perception of noxious stimulations in humans did not clarify this issue but seemed to have ruled out the idea that central hyperalgesia elicited by NO is involved in GTN-induced headaches (51).

NO AS A TARGET FOR MIGRAINE THERAPY

The molecular mechanisms of action of existing migraine therapy are not known but may involve interaction with the NO pathway. So far the most specific and highly effective acute migraine drugs are the 5-HT$_{1D}$ receptor agonists. These are vasoconstrictors and increase inositol triphosphate (IP$_3$), thus increasing intracellular calcium. Whether they also interact with the NO-cGMP cascade at higher levels is unknown. Regarding drugs with established prophylactic effect in migraine, their mechanism of action has long been an enigma. These drugs include beta-adrenergic blocking drugs without partial agonist activity (i.e., propranolol, metroprolol, atenol, nadolol, and timolol), antiserotonergic drugs (i.e., methysergid, pizotifen) calcium antagonists (i.e., flunarizine and verapamil), and valproate. Many observations suggest that all of these drugs interact with the NO-triggered cascade of reactions. Thus, one calcium antagonist (fenfluramine) blocks the effect of activity in perivascular NANC nerves by inhibiting calcium ion channels and therefore the activation of neuronal NOS (Toda, personal communication at the 7th International Headache Research Seminar, Copenhagen, 1996). Methysergide and pizotifen are 5-HT antagonists that do not discriminate between the 5-HT$_1$ and the 5-HT$_2$ receptors. It has recently been suggested that their effect is via 5-HT$_{2B/2C}$ receptor antagonism. 5-HT$_{2B/2C}$ receptor stimulation liberates NO, as discussed previously. Thus, amine antagonists may well exert their action by reducing NO production. Propranolol blocks isoprenaline-induced relaxation of rat thoracic aortas in an endothelium-dependent fashion. The response is also blocked by the NOS inhibitor L-NOARG. The prophylactic effect of beta-adrenergic blockers in migraine may thus result from blockade of beta-adrenoceptor–induced NO production. Propranolol also antagonizes the 5-HT$_{2B/2c}$ receptor on the endothelium. This is another mechanism whereby it may reduce endothelial NO production. In contrast to propranolol, pindolol, which is ineffective in migraine, lacks affinity to the 5-HT$_{2B}$ receptor (43).

The central role of NO in migraine pain does not only provide possible explanations as to the mechanisms of action of existing antimigraine drugs but is also likely to offer future therapeutic possibilities. Thus, drugs that directly counteract the NO-activated cascade (NOS inhibitors, NO scavengers, guanylate cyclase inhibitors, etc.) may be effective in migraine.

In fact, a recent study suggests that the non-specific NOS inhibitor L-N^G methylarginine hydrochloride (546C88) is effective in the acute treatment of migraine headache (29). In this double-blind placebo-controlled study, patients with migraine without aura randomly received 546C88 (6 mg/kg) or placebo intravenously over 15 minutes for a single migraine attack. Statistically significant efficacy was found 2 hours after dosing regard-

TABLE 1. *Effect of NOS inhibition in acute migraine*

	546C88 (L-N^G methylarginine hydrochloride)	Placebo	p^a
Headache intensity (severe or moderate to mild or absent)	$n=15$	$n=14$	
30 min	5	1	
60 min	8	1	<0.05
120 min	10	2	<0.05
Nausea (present to absent)	$n=13$	$n=10$	
30 min	8	3	
60 min	8	3	
120 min	10	5	
Phonophobia (present to absent)	$n=11$	$n=12$	
30 min	4	1	
60 min	5	1	
120 min	9	2	<0.05
Photophobia (present to absent)	$n=10$	$n=13$	
30 min	4	0	
60 min	6	0	<0.05
120 min	8	1	<0.05

Data from Lassen et al. (29).
^{a}Fisher's exact test.

ing headache relief and the relief of phono- and photophobia (Table 1), and a similar albeit not significant trend for nausea was found. Due to the nonspecific nature of this compound, systemic side effects such as an increase in mean arterial blood pressure of 17% are likely to limit its clinical usefulness. More specific compounds are therefore warranted. Drugs that selectively inhibit the different NOS enzymes or inhibit the NO-cGMP cascade at lower levels are already available today, although not yet in clinical trials. When these tools enter clinical trials, they will no doubt shed further light on our hypothesis and make possible further elucidation of the mechanisms involved in the complex pathophysiology of migraine.

REFERENCES

1. Aaslid R, Markwalder TM, Nornes H. Non-invasive transcranial doppler ultrasound recording of flow velocity in basal cerebral arteries. *J Neurosurg* 1982;57:769–774.
2. Brewerton TD, Murphy DL, Mueller EA, Jimerson DC. Induction of migraine like headaches by the serotonin agonist *m*-chlorophenylpiperazine. *Clin Pharmacol Ther* 1988;43:605–609.
3. Christiansen I, Thomsen LL, Daugaard D, Ulrich V, Olesen J. Glyceryltrinitrate induced headache in migraine with aura. (Submitted for publication).
4. Dahl A, Russell D, Nyberg-Hansen R, Rootwell K. Effect of nitroglycerin on cerebral circulation measured by transcranial Doppler and SPECT. *Stroke* 1989;20:1733–1736.
5. D'Andrea G, Cananzi AR, Perini F, et al. Decreased collagen-induced platelet aggregation and increased arginine levels in migraine: a possible link with the NO pathway. *Cephalalgia* 1994;14:352–357.
6. De-Marinis M, Feliciani M, Janiri L, Cerbo R, Agnoli A. Increased reactivity with a met-enkephalin analog in the control of autonmic responses in migraine patients. *Clin Neurophamacol* 1990;13:507–521.
7. Feelisch M, Noack EA. Correlation between nitric oxide formation during degradation of organic nitrates and activation of guanylate cyclase. *Eur J Pharmacol* 1987;139:19–30.
8. Fozard JR, Kalkman HO. 5-Hydroxytryptamine (5-HT) and the initiation of migraine: new perspectives. *Naunyn Schmiedebergs Arch Pharmacol* 1994;350:225–229.
9. Friberg L, Olesen J, Iversen HK, Sperling B. Migraine pain associated with middle cerebral artery dilatation: reversal by sumatriptan. *Lancet* 1991;338:13–17.
10. Furchgott RF, Zawadzki JV. The obligatory role of endothelial cells in the relaxation of arterial smooth muscle by acetylcholine. *Nature* 1980; 288:373–376.
11. Garthwaite J. Nitric oxide signalling in the nervous system. *Neurosciences* 1993;5:171–180.
12. Garthwaite J, Charles SL, Chess-Williams R. Endothelium-derived relaxing factor release on activation of NMDA receptors suggests a role as intercellular messenger in the brain. *Nature* 1988;336:385–388.
13. Glover V, Ahmed F, Hussein N, Jarman J, Peatfield R. Central 5-hydroxytrptamine supersensitivity in migraine. In: Sandler M, Ferrari M, Harnett S, eds. *Migraine: pharmacology and genetics.* London: Chapman & Hall, 1996:117–126.
14. Glusa E, Richter M. Endothelium-dependent relaxation of porcine pulmonary arteries via 5-HT$_{1c}$-like receptors. *Naunyn Schmiedebergs Arch Pharmacol* 1993;347:471–477.
15. Goadsby PJ, Edvinsson L, Ekman R. Vasoactive peptide release in the extracerebral circulation of humans during migraine headache. *Ann Neurol* 1990;28:183–187.
16. Goadsby PJ, Kaube H, Hoskin KL. Nitric oxide synthesis couples cerebral blood flow and metabolism. *Brain Res* 1992;595:167–170.
17. Gordon ML, Lipton RB, Brown S, et al. Headache and cortisol responses to *m*-chlorophenylpiperazine are highly correlated. *Cephalalgia* 1993;13:400–405
18. Gray DW, Marshall I. Human alpha-calcitonin gene-related peptide stimulates adenylate cyclase and guanylate cyclase and relaxes rat tharacic aorta by releasing nitric oxide. *Br J Pharmacol* 1992;107: 691–696.
19. Gruetter CA, Kadowitz PJ, Ignarro LJ. Methylene blue inhibits coronary arterial relaxation and guanylate cyclase activation by nitroglycerin, sodium nitrate and amyl nitrate. *Can J Physiol Pharmacol* 1981; 59:150–156.
20. Ignarro LJ, Lipton H, Edwards JC, et al. Mechanisms of vascular smooth muscle relaxation by organic nitrates, nitrites, nitroprusside and nitric oxide: evidence for the involvement of S-nitrosothiols as active intermediates. *J Pharmacol Exp Ther* 1981;218:739–749.
21. Iversen HK. N-acetylcysteine enhances nitroglycerin-induced headache and cranial arterial responses. *Clin Pharmacol Ther* 1992;52: 125–133.
22. Iversen HK, Olesen J, Tfelt-Hansen P. Intravenous nitroglycerin as an experimental model of vascular headache. Basic characteristics. *Pain* 1989;38:17–24.
23. Iversen HK, Holm S, Friberg L. Intracranial hemodynamics during intravenous nitroglycerin infusion. *Cephalalgia* 1989;9[Suppl 10]: 84–85.
24. Iversen HK, Nielsen TH, Garre K, Tfelt-Hansen P, Olesen J. Dose-dependent headache response and dilatation of limb and extracranial arteries after three doses of 5-isosorbide-mononitrate. *Eur J Clin Pharmacol* 1992;42:31–35.

25. Iversen HK, Nielsen TH, Olesen J, Tfelt-Hansen P. Arterial responses during migraine headache. *Lancet* 1990;336:837–839.

26. Knowles RG, Moncada S. Nitric oxide synthases in mammals. *Biochem J* 1994;298:249–258.

27. Krabbe AA, Olesen J. Headache provocation by continuous intravenous infusion of histamine. Clinical results and receptor mechanisms. *Pain* 1980;8:253–259.

28. Lance JW. 5-hydroxytrptamine and its role in migraine. *Eur Neurol* 1991;31:279–281.

29. Lassen LH, Ashina M, Christinsen I, Ulrich V, Olesen J. Nitric oxide synthase inhibition in migraine. *Lancet* 1997;349:401–402.

30. Lassen LH, Thomsen LL, Olesen J. Histamine induces migraine via the H1-receptor. Support for the NO-hypothesis of migraine. *Neuroreport* 1995;6:1475–1479.

31. Leone AM, Furst VW, Celleck S, Wiklund NP, Moncada S. Visualizing the cellular release of nitric oxide [Abstract 19]. *Endothelium* 1995; 3[Suppl]:s5.

32. Lüscher TF, Vanhoutte PM. *The endothelium: modulator of cardiovascular functions.* Boca Raton, FL: CRC Press, 1990.

33. McMahon SB, Lewin GR, Wall PD. Central hyperexcitability triggered by noxious inputs. *Curr Opin Neurobiol* 1993;3:602–610.

34. Meller ST, Gebhart GF. Nitric oxide (NO) and nociceptive processing in the spinal cord. *Pain* 1993;52:127–136.

35. Moncada S, Palmer RMJ, Higgs EA. Nitric oxide: physiology, pathophysiology and pharmacology. *Pharmacol Rev* 1191;43:109–142.

36. Moskowitz MA. Neurogenic inflammation in the pathophysiology and treatment of migraine. *Neurology* 1993;43[Suppl 3]:S16–S20.

37. Nattero G, Mengozzi G, Inconis T, Paradisi L. From nitroglycerine induction test to nitric oxide research in migraine [Abstract 05-A36]. *Cephalalgia* 1997;17:349.

38. Nichols FT III, Mawad M, Mohr JP, Stein B, Hilal S, Michelsen J. Focal headache during balloon inflation in the internal carotid and middle cerebral arteries. *Stroke* 1990;21:555–559.

39. Northfield DWC. Some observations on headache. *Brain* 1938;61: 133–162.

40. Okada F, Miyagishi T, Honma M, Michio U. Plasma cyclic nucleotide responses to methacholine and epinephrinc in patients with migraine. *Headache* 1984;24:26–29.

41. Oldendorf WH. Brain uptake of radiolabeled amino acids, amines and hexoses after arterial injection. *Am J Physiol* 1971;221:1629–1639.

42. Olesen J, Iversen HK, Thomsen LL. Nitric oxide supersensitivity. A possible molecular mechanism of migraine pain. *Neuroreport* 1993;4: 1027–1030.

43. Olesen J, Thomsen LL, Lassen LH, Jansen-Olesen I. The nitric oxide hypothesis of migraine and other vascular headaches. *Cephalalgia* 1995;15:94–100.

44. Palmer RMJ, Ferrige AG, Moncada S. Nitric oxide release accounts for the biological activity of endothelium-derived relaxing factor. *Nature* 1987;327:524–526.

45. Peatfield RC, Gawel MJ, Rose FC. The effect of infused prostacyclin in migraine and cluster headache. *Headache* 1981;21:190–195.

46. Ray BS, Wolff HG. Experimental studies on headache. Pain sensitive structures of the head and their significance in headache. *Arch Surg* 1940;41:813–856.

47. Read SJ, Smith MI, Hunter AJ, Parsons AA. Enhanced nitric oxide release during cortical spreading depression following infusion of glyceryl trinitrate in anesthetized cat. *Cephalalgia* 1997;17:159–165.

48. Schmetterer L, Wolzt M, Graselli U, et al. Nitric oxide synthase inhibition in the histamine headache model. *Cephalalgia* 1997;17:175–182.

49. Sicuteri F, Del Bene E, Poggioni M, Bonazzi A. Unmasking latent dysnociception in healthy subjects. *Headache* 1987;27:180–185.

50. Thomsen LL. Investigations into the role of nitric oxide and the large intracranial arteries in migraine headache. *Cephalalgia* 1997;17: 873–895.

51. Thomsen LL, Brennum J, Iversen HK, Olesen J. Effect of a NO donor (glyceryl trinitrate) on nociceptive thresholds in man. *Cephalalgia* 1996;16:169–174.

52. Thomsen LL, Daugaard D, Iversen HK, Olesen J. Normal radial artery dilatation during reactive hyperemia in migraine without aura. *Endothelium* 1996;4:199–206.

53. Thomsen LL, Iversen HK. Experimental and biological variation of three dimensional transcranial Doppler measurements. *J Appl Physiol* 1993;75:2805–2810.

54. Thomsen LL, Iversen HK, Boesen F, Olesen J. Transcranial Doppler and cardiovascular responses during cardiovascular autonomic tests in migraineurs. *Brain* 1995;118:1319–1327.

55. Thomsen LL, Iversen HK, Brinck TA, Olesen J. Arterial supersensitivity to nitric oxide (nitroglycerin) in migraine sufferers. *Cephalalgia* 1993;13:395–399.

56. Thomsen LL, Iversen HK, Olesen J. Cerebral blood flow velocities are reduced during attacks of unilateral migraine without aura. *Cephalalgia* 1995;15:109–116.

57. Toda N. Mechanism underlying responses to histamine of isolated monkey and human cerebral arteries. *Am J Physiol* 1990;258: H311–H317.

58. Wei EP, Moskowitz MA, Baccalini P, Kontos HA. Calcitinon gene related peptide mediates nitroglycerin and sodium nitroprusside induced vasodilation in feline cerebral arterioles. *Circ Res* 1992;70:1313–1319.

The Headaches, Second Edition,
edited by J. Olesen, P. Tfelt-Hansen, and K.M.A. Welch.
Lippincott Williams & Wilkins, Philadelphia © 2000.

The Migraines

CHAPTER 41

Synthesis of Migraine Mechanisms

Jes Olesen and Peter J. Goadsby

Mechanisms of disease are rarely simple. Many years after the introduction of L-DOPA and the description of the nigral pathology of Parkinson's disease there are perhaps as many questions unanswered as answered. A simple explanation for migraine is similarly unlikely. In attempting a synthesis of migraine mechanisms we will try to integrate what we know of the clinical science with what has been observed in the clinic to provide an overview of the systems that are involved. Specifically, we shall consider:

Genetic factors
Environmental predisposition
Interictal physiologic and biochemical traits
Precipitation of attacks
Pathophysiology, both peripheral and central, of the pain
   of the attack

Figure 1 illustrates how some of these factors interact to express migraine as a disease and to initiate the individual attack (Fig. 1).

GENETIC FACTORS

If a person on average has seven first-degree relatives, then, because of the high lifetime prevalence of migraine, there should be an average of one affected first-degree relative just by chance. Because of random unevenness of distribution, many probands by chance will have two, three, or even four affected relatives, and such families would have a high likelihood of being reported as cases of dominant inheritance. Therefore, genetic-epidemio-

logic studies are critical. They have shown a twofold increased risk of migraine without aura among first-degree relatives of probands having migraine without aura and a fourfold increase in migraine with aura (30). Twin studies have recently provided convincing evidence of a genetic component to migraine. Thus, the concordance rate of migraine in monozygous twins was significantly higher than in dizygous twins.

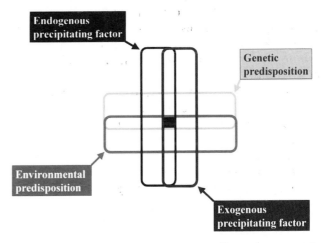

FIG. 1. A genetic predisposition and in many cases an environmental predisposing factor are required for the expression of migraine. By the latter is meant a factor that is present for a long time or permanently. The nature of such environmental factors is unknown, but their existence can be derived from genetic epidemiologic and twin studies. Given the predisposition, there also must be one or more precipitating factors present before the individual attack occurs. These can be endogenous (e.g., menstruation) or exogenous (e.g., drinking red wine). The occurrence of all these factors at the same time is rare, which explains why only a small fraction of an individual's lifetime is spent in attack (dark square in the middle of the figure).

   J. Olesen: Department of Neurology, Glostrup Hospital, University of Copenhagen, DK-2600 Glostrup, Copenhagen, Denmark.
   P. J. Goadsby: The National Hospital for Neurology and Neurosurgery, London WC1N 3BG, United Kingdom.

This comes at a period in research when the description of the first clear mutations to cause a migraine syndrome has been observed, namely mis-sense mutations in the gene on chromosome 19 encoding the α_1 subunit of the voltage-gated P/Q calcium channel in familial hemiplegic migraine (25). However, even this relatively stereotyped condition is genetically heterogeneous, with at least another locus on chromosome 1 (5) and families that do not map to either. Furthermore, as described in Chapter 30, linkage studies in migraine with and without aura are conflicting and indicate that we have only heard the first shots in a long battle.

Genetic work has eliminated some interesting candidate genes, such as the ones coding for the 5-hydroxytryptamine 2A ($5-HT_{2A}$) receptor (19) and for endothelial nitric oxide synthase (eNOS) (8). New candidates have been thrown up by this process, notably those responsible for dopamine receptors (26), although not without causing dissent (17). Perhaps one of the more interesting developments was the attempt to link polymorphisms in the $5-HT_{1B}$ receptor to sumatriptan responses (16). This was not successful, but the principle of being able to link basic disease biology to clinical outcome is very attractive and no doubt will evolve in the next millennium.

ENVIRONMENTAL PREDISPOSITION

The genetic predisposition to migraine does not always express itself. Thus, monozygotic twins with migraine were only concordant in 20% to 50% of cases (30). If this is true, at least 50% of those carrying a genetic disposition to migraine will never manifest attacks because of favorable environmental conditions, or the 50% who do manifest the condition will experience headache because of unfavorable conditions. Furthermore, apparent carriers express migraine only during part of their lifetime because the prevalence of migraine increases up to the age 20 or 30 years and decreases in old age (31). In a meticulous longitudinal cohort study, children with migraine often became migraine free for years or decades, but many of these later had recurrence of attacks (1). Some of the predisposing or triggering factors for the expression of the disease include:

Female sex
Psychosocial stress
Biochemical changes
Certain foods and alcohol

The most important predisposing or priming factor would seem to be the female hormonal environment, although it has not been established beyond question that the male hormonal environment is in some way protective. The sex ratio is approximately equal before puberty, whereas females suffer from migraine three times more frequently than males after puberty (see Chapter 28). What happens after menopause has not been completely defined,

although it seems likely that there is improvement. Psychosocial stress also seems to be an important predisposing factor as discussed in Chapter 38. Patients reporting to a doctor as a consequence of increased attack frequency often do so at times of psychosocial stress, and the attack frequency returns to the usual pattern after removal of, or adaptation to, the stressor. It seems likely that psychosocial stress can also cause the onset of migraine in persons who have not previously expressed it. Similar but less solid evidence indicates that certain foods, alcoholic drinks, and perhaps biochemical and myogenic changes may enhance expression of any genetic predisposition and thereby cause expression or worsening of migraine as discussed in Chapters 24, 30, and 32. Several researchers have discussed the existence of a migraine threshold that may be high or low, depending on genetic as well as environmental predisposing factors. A particularly elegant and penetrating discussion of this concept was given by Welch et al. (35).

One interpretation is that migraine sufferers inherit a lack of ability to adapt to physiologic changes (see Chapter 37), particularly those of a sensory nature. Stimuli or behavior that present no problem to the nonmigraineur may therefore trigger an attack in those disposed to migraine. A migraineur may trigger attacks by sleeping late or getting up too early, by skipping meals or overindulging certain foods, by experiencing too much stress or during periods of relaxation, such as early in a holiday. The migraine sufferer's brain is more sensitive to change, and although there is no fixed trigger, the broad principle of unstable sensory processing, which is probably intimately linked to dysfunction of aminergic control pathways, serves us well when advising patients about life-style changes.

PHYSIOLOGIC AND BIOCHEMICAL ABNORMALITIES OUTSIDE OF ATTACKS

Physiologic and biochemical abnormalities in migraine sufferers outside of attacks may be genetic or environmental, but the former is most likely when changes are present weeks after the last attack and when they persist for years. The interictal abnormal contingent negative variations described in Chapter 37; the interictal biochemical, platelet, and magnesium abnormalities described in Chapter 31; and the interictal inhomogeneity of regional cerebral blood described in Chapter 35 are important examples. Regardless of the genetic or environmental cause of these changes, it is likely that migraine patients have both a biochemical and a physiologic preparedness for developing attacks. This explains why precipitating factors cause attacks in some persons and not in others.

PRECIPITATION OF ATTACKS

Some migraine patients get attacks as rarely as once a year, some as often as once a week, but most do not have it all the time (see Fig. 1). Why does the attack come at a particular time in a particular patient? The answer is sometimes known (red wine, stress, or food), but in most cases it is not. Even in those cases where one or more precipitating factors are thought to explain the migraine attack, relationships are complicated. Not every exposure to the precipitant induces an attack, and it seems most likely that endogenous and exogenous factors must coincide in order to precipitate attacks in most individuals (see Fig. 1). This fact may explain why most patients have rare attacks. How and where do these precipitating factors exert their migraine-triggering effects? More specifically, are these effects generated within or outside of the central nervous system (CNS)? Could both indeed be possible? Some factors such as emotional disturbances, psychosocial stress, and strong light undoubtedly act primarily on the CNS. Other factors are more likely to work systemically, such as fasting and effects of various foods. All of the latter may, however, affect the CNS either by substances crossing the blood–brain barrier or via sensory afferent impulses projecting to the CNS. Most recently the discovery of many different endothelial receptors on the brain and extracerebral arteries (15) has revealed new possibilities for changes in blood chemistry such as changes in plasma 5-HT or glutamate to trigger migraine by affecting cerebral arteries.

HOW AND WHERE PAIN FIBERS (NOCICEPTORS) BECOME EXCITED DURING MIGRAINE ATTACKS

In this section, we discuss the pathophysiology of migraine attacks according to the view that migraine with aura and migraine without aura are identical in terms of the painful phase of the attack but differ at the onset of attack. This view is based on the finding of many similar clinical characteristics of migraine with aura and migraine without aura (27), the frequent cooccurrence of the two conditions (27), a number of pathophysiologic similarities (6), and the identical response of both forms to prophylactic and acute treatment (11).

The Migraine Aura is Probably Caused by Cortical Spreading Depression

A detailed description of the migraine aura is given in Chapter 43. In the present chapter we analyze aspects of the symptomatology that teach us about mechanisms of the aura. Patients without eyes or totally blind have been described to have typical visual auras. This and the clinical characteristics of the aura itself demonstrate that it originates from the cerebral cortex and not from the eyes. The visual disturbance spreads laterally in one hemifield, accelerating and enlarging as it spreads. A disturbance spreading at a steady speed (3–6 mm/min) along the primary visual cortex would have these characteristics

because the cortical representation of the visual field decreases with distance from the center of vision. The edge of the moving visual disturbance is usually flickering at a rate of 10 to 15 Hz, decreasing in the periphery to 3 or 4 Hz, and is followed by a scotoma, indicating an irritative disturbance at the front followed by depressed neuronal function. Sensory auras similarly march at a slow pace, often with tingling at the edge and numbness in its wake. If there is more than one type of aura symptom, such as visual and sensory symptoms, they occur in sequence. The only known disturbance that can explain this slow continuous spread of excitation followed by depression is cortical spreading of Leao, also known as cortical spreading depression (CSD) (12,13).

The association between CSD and migraine was not taken seriously as long as it was based exclusively on clinical observations. In 1981 Olesen et al. (24) provided the first evidence in human patients during migraine attacks of slowly spreading cortical hypoperfusion incompatible with spasm of a major artery but fully compatible with the occurrence of CSD. Several later studies of regional cerebral blood flow discussed in Chapters 22 and 35 and also reviewed by Lauritzen (12) support these observations.

How Cortical Spreading Depression Excites Trigeminovascular Afferents

Migraine pain is not a direct consequence of CBF changes or of the modest changes in arterial diameter described in Chapter 35. However, CSD involves gross disturbances of the brain extracellular environment. The potassium level increases to 60 mmol, the extracellular glutamate level increases considerably, and the extracellular calcium level decreases. Nitric oxide is produced both immediately after CSD and in a second prolonged wave lasting several hours (29). It has been suggested that CSD can excite trigeminovascular afferents directly (18), but these data have recently been questioned (9).

Ray and Wolff (28) observed that convexity pial arteries are insensitive to a variety of noxious stimuli. These are precisely the arteries most likely to be affected by CSD because of their proximity to the cortical mantel. However, Ray and Wolff could not know that temporal and spatial summation may greatly increase pain responses (see Chapters 12 and 13) or that sensory fibers from the trigeminal nerve invest pial arteries throughout their entire length with only a quantitative difference, large proximal arteries having a more dense supply (see Chapter 9). Firing of nerve fibers around a large number of small arteries, particularly if sustained, may result in a pain similar to that which might be elicited from larger arteries. CSD also may directly involve the nerves around the big basal arteries if it spreads to the basal and mesial cortex. We do not know if this happens, because regional cerebral blood flow measurements from those areas are inaccurate with the techniques used in published studies.

In addition to direct firing of nociceptive impulses, perivascular nerve activity results in liberation of a number of transmitter substances, of which the tachykinins (substance P, neurokinin A), calcitonin gene–related peptide (CGRP), and nitric oxide are active in the so-called neurogenic inflammatory response. First described by Lembeck et al. (14), this response involves exudation of fluid and sensitization of peripheral sensory nerve endings. In a series of elegant animal experiments, Moskowitz and associates demonstrated that retrograde activity in the trigeminal nerve is a useful model for selecting candidate antimigraine drugs. This model also has been used to describe a number of pathophysiologic changes that may be relevant to migraine, particularly the well-recognized clinical complaint of sensitivity to movement (3). The neurogenic inflammatory response is discussed more fully in Chapter 17.

Once established, migraine pain may persist for many hours or days. Long-term potentiation of nucleus caudalis neurons secondary to incoming C-fiber impulses, perhaps triggered by long-lasting NO production, is a likely explanation of the long duration of pain. Burstein and Strassman (2,32) have examined mechanisms of sensitization in the trigeminal nucleus that would produce hyperalgesia, allodynia, and enlarged receptive fields that may last many hours. These observations would explain the abnormal sensations that migraineurs report in the head, such as sensitivity to touch, and, if such changes took place in thalamic neurons (36), would explain odd sensory changes reported in other parts of the body (11).

Pial and Extracerebral Arteries are the Source of Pain Both in Migraine With Aura and Migraine Without Aura.

Regional cerebral blood flow, apart from pain activation, remains normal during attacks of migraine without aura, demonstrating that vascular regulation at the level of intraparenchymal arterioles is intact. However, this does not exclude arterial dilatation, as discussed in Chapter 35 (Fig. 2). Thus, dilatation of the middle cerebral artery and the superficial temporal artery on the pain side during migraine attacks has been demonstrated. Intra- and extracranial dilatation has been observed in migraine with and without aura and may be a common denominator for migraine pain. It is thought that the nociception originates from much larger sections of the cephalic arterial tree, including the small convexity arteries, dural arteries, and perhaps extracranial arteries, and is just not possible to measure from smaller arteries.

Arterial dilatations have been observed that were small in magnitude and similar to arterial responses to normal physiologic stimuli, such as changes in arterial blood pressure and pCO_2, which do not cause headache. Pre-

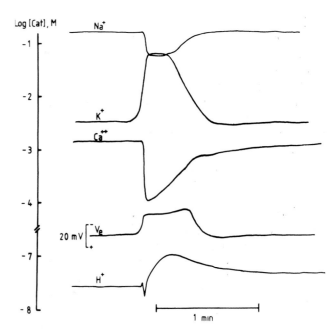

FIG. 2. Ion shifts during cortical spreading depression as recorded by ion-sensitive electrodes. Note the huge increase in extracellular potassium and decrease in extracellular calcium, which together can easily depolarize perivascular nerve fibers. A simultaneous increase in excitatory amino acids occurs that may be chiefly responsible for the propagation of spreading depression and may also stimulate perivascular nerve fibers. Courtesy of Anker Jon Hansen.

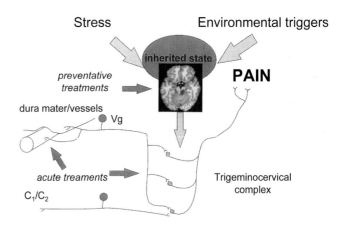

FIG. 3. Migraine is an episodic dysfunction of brainstem or diencephalic sensory modulation systems, as suggested by the finding of activations in the brainstem in positron emission tomography scans during the acute attack (34). These systems control input from pain-producing trigeminal nerves that innervate the large extracerebral intracranial vessels and dura mater and whose cell bodies are found in the trigeminal ganglion (*Vg*). Referral of pain to the back of the neck results from projections from the high cervical nerves (C1/C2) onto neurons of the trigeminal nucleus, which is known to descend to the C2 level of the cervical spinal cord (trigeminocervical complex). It is likely that acute attack treatments, such as triptans, target this trigeminovascular system which is, in essence, responsible for pain expression, whereas preventative medications effect the central control systems involved in the genesis of the attacks (11).

sumably periarterial nociceptors and second- and perhaps third-order neurons are sensitized as discussed in Chapters 12 and 15. The demonstration of increased efflux of CGRP in the external jugular vein during migraine attacks (4) and the demonstration of nitric oxide involvement in migraine (24) suggest that these molecules may be involved in sensitizing peripheral nociceptors and possibly also in central sensitization. Given that there is a disturbance at the hypothalamic level (as indicated by the characteristics of the premonitory symptoms) with the possible consequence of autonomic dysregulation, and evidence from PET studies of changes in brainstem areas (34) implicated in cerebrovascular control (7), it is likely that migraine represents a syndrome of neurovascular dysfunction (Fig. 3).

CENTRAL PROCESSING OF MIGRAINE AFFERENT PAIN IMPULSES (NOCICEPTION)

In most painful disorders there is only a weak relationship between peripheral injury/nociception and the perception of pain. This is because the CNS strongly modulates incoming nociceptive impulses. For example, boxers and soldiers may have severe injury and feel little or no pain. The CNS also may increase gain in the afferent pain pathways, for example, when attention is directed toward the painful stimulus. These mechanisms are described in previous chapters. They have been studied most extensively in the extremities but are probably no less important in the head. They help us understand why the severity of migraine aura and migraine pain are not always well correlated and why it is possible to have migraine auras and no headache. Olesen (21) offered a model of migraine pain perception, including not only the source of pain but also its central modulation. Neurons in the nucleus caudalis are known to integrate nociceptive input from intracranial as well as extracranial tissues and to receive supraspinal facilitatory as well as inhibitory inputs (Fig. 4). They sum all these inputs and project the net results to the thalamus and onto the cortex. Even if the migraine pain is primarily vascular or dural, additional nociceptive input from muscles and other cranial tissues may therefore contribute to migraine pain. The strong vascular input of the migraine attack is usually enough to fire these neurons but causes partial depolarization at other times. Modest additional input from pericranial muscles, then, is sufficient to fire the neurons and cause pain. This explains the increased tenderness of pericranial structures during migraine attacks (10) and the effect of trigger point injections (33). Supraspinal control may enhance or diminish the pain caused by a certain nociceptive input. The aggravating effect of psychosocial stress and other factors, discussed in Chapter 38, and the ameliorating effect of relaxation are most likely effected via supraspinal control of neurons of the trigeminal nucleus caudalis.

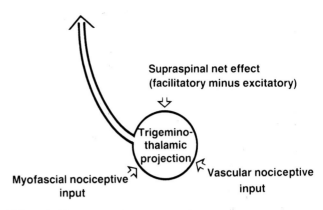

FIG. 4. The vascular-supraspinal-myogenic integration model of migraine. No painful disorder can be understood fully by the mere study of its peripheral noxious mechanisms. There is a marked modulation in the CNS, and neurons in the nucleus caudalis of the tract of the trigeminal nerve probably are of key importance in this respect. They receive input not only from the vasculature but also from many other structures of the head. There are good reasons to believe that myofascial input interacts with vascular input. This marked myofascial input may trigger migraine attacks and worsen migraine. Also, the supraspinal control of these neurons is important, some pathways increasing the sensitivity of these neurons, others decreasing the sensitivity via the so-called endogenous antinociceptive system. Emotional factors play primarily on this supraspinal control system. The net result of these complicated interactions is the final determinant of migraine pain as perceived by the subject.

The vascular-supraspinal-myogenic (VSM) model of migraine pain perception (21) provides a rationale for the different, generally accepted treatment modalities in migraine. Pharmacologic treatment reduces vascular neuronal input. Psychological and behavioral techniques reduce supraspinal facilitation or increase supraspinal inhibition, and physiotherapy, biofeedback, and trigger point injections reduce myofascial input. Although vascular nociception is a dominant factor in migraine, a full understanding of each patient requires an evaluation of factors along each arm of the VSM model. Such an individual evaluation and an explanation of the complex mechanisms of migraine allow a logical choice of treatments and optimize patient satisfaction and compliance.

REFERENCES

1. Bille BA. 40 year follow-up of school children with migraine. *Cephalalgia* 1997;17:488–491.
2. Burstein R, Yamamura H, Malick A, Strassman AM. Chemical stimulation of the intracranial dura induces enhanced responses to facial stimulation in brain stem trigeminal neurons. *J Neurophysiol* 1998;79:964–982.
3. Cutrer FM, Limmroth V, Waeber C, Yu X, Moskowitz MA. New targets for antimigraine drug development. In: Goadsby PJ, Silberstein SD, eds. *Headache.* Philadelphia: Butterworth-Heinemann, 1997:59–72.
4. Edvinsson L, Goadsby PJ. Neuropeptides in headache. *Eur Neurol* 1998;5:329–341.

5. Gardner K, Barmada M, Ptacek LJ, Hoffman EP. A new locus for hemiplegic migraine maps to chromosome 1q31. *Neurology* 1997;49:1231–1238.
6. Goadsby PJ. Animal models of migraine: which model, why and for what? In: Edvinsson L, ed. *Experimental headache models in animals and man.* London: Martin Dunitz, 1999.
7. Goadsby PJ, Lance JW. Brainstem effects on intra- and extracerebral circulations. Relation to migraine and cluster headache. In: Olesen J, Edvinsson L. *Basic mechanisms of headache.* Amsterdam: Elsevier Science Publishers, 1988:413–427.
8. Griffiths LR, Nyholt DR, Curtain RP, Goadsby PJ, Brimage PJ. Migraine association and linkage studies of an endothelial nitric oxide synthase (NOS3) gene polymorphism. *Neurology* 1997;49:614–617.
9. Ingvardsen BK, Laursen H, Olsen UB, Hansen AJ. Possible mechanism of c-fos expression in trigeminal nucleus caudalis following spreading depression. *Pain* 1997;72:407–415.
10. Jensen K, Tuxen C, Olesen J. Pericranial muscle tenderness and pressure—pain threshold in the temporal regions during common migraine. *Pain* 1988;35:279–284.
11. Lance JW, Goadsby PJ. Mechanism and Management of headache. London: Butterworth-Heinemann, 1998.
12. Lauritzen M. Pathophysiology of the migraine aura. The spreading depression theory. *Brain* 1994;117:199–210.
13. Leao AAP. Spreading depression of activity in cerebral cortex. *J Neurophysiol* 1944;7:359–390.
14. Lembeck F, Holzer P. Substance P as a neurogenic mediator of antidromic vasodilatation and neurogenic plasma extravasation. *Naunyn Schmiedebergs Arch Pharmacol* 1979;310:175–183.
15. Luscher TF, Vanhoutte PM. The endothelium: modulator of cardiovascular function. Boca Raton, FL: CRC Press, 1990.
16. Maassen VanDenBrink A, Vergouwe MN, Ophoff RA, Saxena PR, Ferrari MD, Frants RR. 5-HT$_{1B}$ receptor polymorphism and clinical response to sumatriptan. *Headache* 1998;38:288–291.
17. Mascia A, Afra J, Schoenen J. Dopamine and migraine: a review of pharmacological, biochemical, neurophysiological, and therapeutic data. *Cephalalgia* 1998;18:174–182.
18. Moskowitz MA, Nozaki K, Kraig RP. Neocortical spreading depression provokes the expression of C-fos protein–like immunoreactivity within the trigeminal nucleus caudalis via trigeminovascular mechanisms. *J Neurosci* 1993;13:1167–1177.
19. Nyholt DR, Curtain RP, Gaffney PT, Brimage P, Goadsby PJ, Griffiths LR. Migraine association and linkage analyses of the human 5-hydroxytryptamine (5HT$_{2A}$) receptor gene. *Cephalalgia* 1996;16:463–467.
20. Nyholt DR, Dawkins JL, Brimage PJ, Goadsby PJ, Nicholson GA, Griffiths LR. Evidence for an X-linked genetic component in familial typical migraine. *Hum Mol Gen* 1998;7:459–463.
21. Olesen J. Clinical and pathophysiological observations in migraine and tension-type headache explained by integration of vascular, supraspinal and myofascial inputs. *Pain* 1991;46:125–132.
22. Olesen J, Bousser MG. *The genetics of headache disorders.* Philadelphia: Lippincott Williams & Wilkins, 1999 (in press).
23. Olesen J, Larsen B, Lauritzen M. Focal hyperemia followed by spreading oligemia and impaired activation of rCBF in classic migraine. *Ann Neurol* 1981;9:344–352.
24. Olesen J, Thomsen LL, Lassen LH, Jansen Olesen I. The nitric oxide hypothesis of migraine and other vascular headaches. *Cephalalgia* 1995;15:94–100.
25. Ophoff RA, Terwindt GM, Vergouwe MN, et al. Familial hemiplegic migraine and episodic ataxia type-2 are caused by mutations in the Ca^{2+} channel gene CACNLA4. *Cell* 1996;87:543–552.
26. Peroutka SJ. Dopamine and migraine. *Neurology* 1997;49:650–656.
27. Rassmussen BK, Olesen J. Migraine with aura and migraine without aura: an epidemiological study. *Cephalalgia* 1992;12:221–228.
28. Ray BS, Wolff HG. Experimental studies on headache. Pain sensitive structures of the head and their significance in headache. *Arch Surg* 1940;41:813–856.
29. Read SJ, Smith MI, Hunter AJ, Parsons AA. Enhanced nitric oxide release during cortical spreading depression following infusion of glycerol trinitrate in the anaesthetized cat. *Cephalalgia* 1997;17:159–165.
30. Russell MB, Olesen J. Increased familial risk and evidence of a genetic factor in migraine. *Br Med J* 1995;311:541–544.
31. Stewart WF, Lipton RB, Celentano DD, Reed ML. Prevalence of migraine headache in the United States: relation to age, income, race and other sociodemographic factors. JAMA 1992;267:64–69.
32. Strassman AM, Raymond SA, Burstein R. Sensitization of meningeal sensory neurons and the origin of headaches. *Nature* 1996;384:560–563.
33. Tfelt-Hansen P, Lous I, Olesen J. Prevalence and significance of muscle tenderness during common migraine attacks. *Headache* 1981;21:49–54.
34. Weiller C, May A, Limmroth V, et al. Brain stem activation in spontaneous human migraine attacks. *Nature Med* 1995;1:658–660.
35. Welch KMA, D'Andrea G, Tepley N, Barkeley GL, Ramadan NM. The concept of migraine as a state of central neuronal hyperexcitability. *Headache* 1990;8:817–828.
36. Zagami AS, Lambert GA. Craniovascular application of capsaicin activates nociceptive thalamic neurons in the cat. *Neurosci Lett* 1991;121:187–190.

The Headaches, Second Edition,
edited by J. Olesen, P. Tfelt-Hansen, and K.M.A. Welch.
Lippincott Williams & Wilkins, Philadelphia © 2000.

The Migraines

CHAPTER 42

Symptomatology of Migraine without Aura

Alessandro S. Zagami and Birthe Krogh Rasmussen

DEFINITION OF MIGRAINE WITHOUT AURA

IHS code and diagnosis: 1.1 Migraine without aura.
WHO code and diagnosis: G43.0. Migraine without aura.
Short description (Headache Classification Committee, 1988) (22): Idiopathic, recurring headache disorder manifesting in attacks lasting 4 to 72 hours. Typical characteristics of headache are unilateral location, pulsating quality, moderate or severe intensity, aggravation by routine physical activity, and association with nausea, photophobia, and phonophobia.
Other terms: Common migraine, hemicrania simplex.
IHS diagnostic criteria for migraine without aura (Headache Classification Committee 1988):

At least five attacks fulfilling B–D
Headache attacks lasting 4 to 72 hours (untreated or unsuccessfully treated)
Headache has at least two of the following characteristics:
Unilateral location
Pulsating quality
Moderate or severe intensity (inhibits or prohibits daily activities)
Aggravation by walking stairs or similar routine physical activity
During headache at least one of the following:
Nausea and/or vomiting
Photophobia and phonophobia

At least one of the following:
History, physical, and neurologic examinations do not suggest one of the disorders listed in groups 5–11 of the IHS classification.
History, physical, and/or neurologic examinations do suggest such disorder, but it is ruled out by appropriate investigations.
Such disorder is present, but migraine attacks do not occur for the first time in close temporal relation to the disorder.

Migraine without aura may occur almost exclusively at a particular time of the menstrual cycle (so-called menstrual migraine). Generally accepted criteria for this entity are not available. It seems reasonable to demand that 90% of attacks should occur between 2 days before menses and the last day of menses, but further epidemiologic knowledge is needed.

INTRODUCTION

Migraine without aura, previously called common migraine or hemicrania simplex, is the most common form of migraine (9). The diagnostic criteria of migraine without aura are detailed above. They are proposed by the Headache Classification Committee of the International Headache Society (IHS) (22) and are adopted in this chapter. Blau (5) has suggested that the migraine episode be divided into five distinct phases: (a) premonitory symptoms, (b) aura, (c) headache and associated symptoms, (d) resolution, and (e) recovery (Fig. 1). In migraine without aura, headache is an essential part of the diagnosis, and, although not preceded by any identifiable focal symptoms of neurologic disturbance, as is the case in migraine with aura (classic migraine), it may be preceded by premonitory symptoms, sometimes quite

A. S. Zagami: Department of Medicine, University of New South Wales, and Institute of Neurological Sciences, Prince of Wales Hospital, Randwick, Sydney, New South Wales 2031, Australia.
B. K. Rasmussen: Department of Neurology, Hilleroed Hospital, DK-3400 Hilleroed, Denmark.

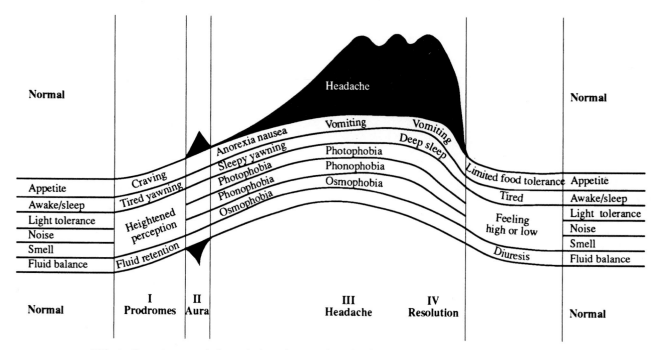

FIG. 1. Symptoms and signs during phases of a migraine attack. Reproduced from Blau (6).

characteristic for the individual patient and clearly identifiable as the warning symptoms of an impending attack.

PREMONITORY SYMPTOMS

The Headache Classification Committee (22) states
that in migraine without aura, such symptoms may precede a migraine attack by hours or up to 1 or 2 days. They
usually consist of physical or mental hyper- or hypoactivity, depression, craving for special foods, repetitive yawning, and similar atypical symptoms. Premonitory symptoms have been known to precede a migraine attack for
centuries (25) and have been classified on clinical
grounds as excitatory or inhibitory (4). *Excitatory premonitory symptoms* include irritability, being "high,"
physical hyperactivity, being obsessional and witty,
yawning, excessive sleepiness, increased sensitivity to
light and sounds, craving for food, increased bowel and
bladder activity, and thirst. Under the heading of
inhibitory symptoms are included being mentally withdrawn, mental slow-down, behavioral sluggishness, feeling tired, difficulty focusing, slurred speech, difficulty
finding the right word, poor concentration, slow thinking,
muscle weakness, and feelings of cold, anorexia, constipation, and abdominal bloatedness. In a study by
Waelkens (60), such premonitory symptoms were classified under the headings of (a) general complaints, (b)
symptoms related to the head, (c) abnormalities of eyes or
sight, (d) sensory intolerance, (e) mood and behavior
variations, and (f) abdominal symptoms. Children tend to
have more abdominal symptoms, particularly pain, as
well as attacks of vertigo preceding their migraine

headache without aura (42). In the various series reported
so far (5,25,48,53,60,61) the incidence of premonitory
symptoms has varied widely from 7% to 88%.

Early studies of premonitory symptoms, however,
lacked scientific rigor. A recent population-based study
found similar vague symptoms preceding tension-type
headache (45). In two recently published, population-
based studies, the frequency of premonitory symptoms in
subjects with tension-type headache (9%) was similar to
that found among migraineurs (48,53). These results
seem to call into question the specificity and importance
of premonitory symptoms. Further investigations looking
prospectively at the incidence of premonitory symptoms
and using adequate controls are therefore needed.

PRECIPITATING FACTORS

Precipitants (also called trigger factors) are factors that
alone or in combination with other exogenous exposures
induce headache attacks in susceptible individuals. The
factors precede the onset of an attack by a relatively short
time interval. Precipitants induce headache attacks in predisposed subjects and are not regarded as causal agents.
Precipitants are not universal because the presence of a
factor does not always trigger an attack in the same individual and only subgroups of headache sufferers are sensitive to any specific factor. This suggests a multifactorial trigger mechanism for individual attacks.

One or more precipitating factors have been described
in 64% to 90% of patients with migraine (44,48,53,58),
and overall they appear to be more common in patients
with migraine without aura than in those with migraine

with aura (48). The nature and frequency of the most common precipitants are listed in Table 1. Previous studies (44,48,50,53,55) have consistently reported that stress and mental tension are the most common provoking factors for migraine. Although this is undoubtedly true, it has to be remembered that in some patients such mental tension may be a prodromal sign (58). Menstruation is a common precipitant cited by women with a frequency of 24% to 62% (44,48,50,55,58) and again appears to be more frequent in migraine without aura (48,53). It needs to be remembered that hormonal factors may act as both predisposing as well as precipitating factors. This is discussed in more detail in Chapter 32.

Many patients identify dietary factors as precipitants for their migraines. Between 20% and 52% of patients report that alcoholic drinks of one sort or another can precipitate their migraines (38,39,44,48,58). Whereas some patients are sensitive to all forms of alcohol, a smaller number report sensitivity only to red wine or, less commonly, beer (38). An association between sensitivity to red wine and to foods such as cheese and chocolate has been described (38) but the metabolic mechanisms responsible remain to be determined.

Certain foods have been implicated as triggers by 10% to 45% of migraineurs (38,39,44,48,50,53,55,58). The most common foods reported are chocolate, dairy food (particularly cheese), citrus fruit, and fried fatty foods. In a study by Peatfield et al. (39), only about 19% of migraineurs claimed to be sensitive to cheese or chocolate or both, and 11% to citrus fruit. Most diet-sensitive patients were sensitive to all three foods. Interestingly, two double-blind, placebo-controlled trials testing whether chocolate was a trigger for migraine came to opposite conclusions (21,32). The mechanism whereby some substances in food trigger migraine in some patients remains unclear, although a role for both a chemical mechanism and food allergy have been suggested. The latter is discussed further in Chapter 34. Other

ingested agents such as chemicals and drugs can precipitate headache, and these are discussed in detail in Chapter 114.

Apart from stress, mental tension, and hormonal changes, other endogenous precipitating factors have been described. Missing a meal has been quoted as precipitating headache in 25% of children (29) and migraine in 40% of adult migraineurs (50). Both oversleeping and undersleeping have been cited as precipitants. Tiredness and fatigue also have been described as trigger factors (53,58).

Various exogenous factors have been described as precipitating attacks of migraine. Between 7% and 43% of patients claim that a change in the weather is a precipitant (44,48,49,58), and they often maintain that they are able to predict such weather changes. Specific studies to test this possibility have given contradictory results, however (12,15,41,63). Between 12% and 47% of patients reported that various sensory stimuli precipitate their migraine (50,53,55,58). Bright lights, glare, and flickering lights have been quoted as precipitants of migraine in several studies (50,55,58) but in a more recent study, bright light was a precipitant for migraine with aura but not for migraine without aura (53). Other less common exogenous trigger factors include angiography, head trauma, exertion, and high altitude. Interestingly, sexual activity does not appear to be a precipitant for migraine (44,48,50).

ONSET OF THE ATTACK

In many instances, the initial phase of the headache cannot be localized to any particular part of the head, nor does it appear to be throbbing. Almost certainly this is the reason why patients are uncertain as to whether they are experiencing an attack and hesitate to take their usual antimigraine treatment at the onset of their attacks (5). Furthermore, headaches that might represent the onset of

TABLE 1. *Frequency of precipitating factors in migraine (%)*

Precipitants (not mutually exclusive)[a]	Selby and Lance (55) (n = 500)	Peatfield et al. (39) (n = 490)	Van den Berg et al. (58) (n = 217)	Rasmussen and Olesen[b] (48) (n = 58)	Rasmussen (44) (n = 119)	Peatfield (38) (n = 490)	Robbins (50) (n = 494)	Russell et al.[b] (53) (n = 222)
Stress/mental tensions	67	—	49	43	44.5	—	62	38
Certain foods	25	19	45	12	10	17	30	34[c]
Wine, beer, spirits	—	29	52	28	20	30	—	11[d]
Weather changes	—	—	7	16	11	—	43	—
Menstruation	62	—	48	29	24	—	50	—
Sensory stimuli	47	—	12	—	—	—	38	12
Fatigue	—	—	16	—	—	—	—	19
One or more precipitants	—	—	85	90	64	—	—	79

[a]Other precipitants at a lower frequency are mentioned but not included in this table.
[b]Migraine without aura patients only in these studies.
[c]Includes red wine.
[d]Beer, spirits only.

a migraine attack often disappear without therapy or with simple analgesics. The pain progresses over a period of 0.5 to 2 hours or more from a mild ache to a pain of moderate or marked severity, localized in about two thirds of patients to one side of the head. Associated symptoms usually follow the onset of severe pain, but occasionally photophobia and nausea occur before pain fully develops.

THE FULLY DEVELOPED ATTACK

Duration and Timing of Onset of Attacks

Most attacks last half a day to a full day, but the duration may vary from 4 hours to 3 days. Patients in whom the headache persists for more than 3 days despite treatment are said to be in status migrainosus (11). In a recent study (53) this occurred in less than 1% of patients. In about two thirds of patients the headache lasts for a day or less, in one sixth it continues for 24 to 48 hours, and in the remainder it persists for more than 48 hours (54). Women more often than men experience attacks of long duration according to one study (53). Headaches can begin in the morning on waking or at the end of a stressful day. Heavy or prolonged sleep on weekends or holidays may provoke a migraine attack (17), but otherwise attacks are not more frequent on weekends (35). More commonly, attacks begin in the afternoon or evening and may be preceded by one or more premonitory symptoms that the patient has come to recognize as a warning of an impending attack.

Quality of Pain

The word "hemicrania" is derived from the Greek, meaning literally "half the head," and the component of pain or headache is implied. The headache commonly begins as an awareness of a discomfort in the head that soon becomes painful, initially being a mild ache and then increasing to be moderate or severe in intensity over a period of 0.5 to 2 hours. In a survey of 750 patients questioned during the attack, 47% said that the pain was pulsating (37), whereas in other more recent population-based studies, patients (outside of an attack) reported that this was so in 78% (46) and 82% (53) of cases. The remaining patients described the pain as pressing or bursting, or used other terms instead. Be that as it may, the words "throbbing" and "pulsating" are frequently misunderstood, most patients taking them to mean severe, whereas an expression such as "throbbing with your heart beat" is plain enough to be fully understood by the patient, as suggested by Campbell (9). Physical activity of any form aggravates the headache: coughing, breath-holding, or rapid rotation of the head from side to side accentuated the headache in 49 of 50 patients (7). In fact, aggravation of the headache by routine physical activity is a sensitive feature of migraine without aura, occurring in over 95% of sufferers (46,53). Severe pain intensity as measured by interference with the ability to perform daily activities is the most sensitive and specific pain characteristic of migraine without aura (26,37,46,48,53).

Location of Pain

In more than 50% of patients the headache is hemicranial (9,28,46,48), whereas the remainder experience a bilateral or generalized headache. Unilateral headache may occur more frequently in women (53). Whether hemicranial or bilateral, the pain tends to be more intense in the frontotemporal and ocular regions, at least initially, before it spreads to the parietal and occipital areas. Sjaastad et al. (56) found that 75% of patients with migraine without aura felt their initial pain in the oculo-fronto-temporal region. In contrast, basilar migraine produces pain that is felt predominantly in the occipital region, although not infrequently it may radiate to the anterior parts of the head, particularly in its later stages. So-called lower half headache, an entity not recognized at present by the IHS, is said to be experienced in the ocular area and radiates downward into the cheek and lower jaw.

Idiopathic stabbing headache with ice-pick pains or jabs and stabs, consisting of momentary sharp, shooting pains in various parts of the head, including the eye, are common in patients with frequent attacks of migraine (49) and tend to occur more frequently on the side habitually affected by headache (20,43) (see also Chapter 100).

Frequency of Attacks

As stated in the definition, the diagnosis of migraine should not be made until or unless the patient has had five attacks fulfilling all the criteria listed. Attacks may vary from once a year to several attacks weekly. Frequent migrainous episodes may be mixed with frequent attacks of tension-type headache and may eventually end up as chronic daily headaches, often as a result of daily use of analgesics (33).

The high frequency of attacks is one of the characteristics that distinguish migraine without aura from other variants of the syndrome. In clinic populations, over 50% of patients suffer from one to four attacks per month, less than 15% experience a few attacks annually, while up to 35% have up to three attacks per week. The headache frequency in the individual patient varies not only from year to year, but also at different times of the year, depending on environmental circumstances (54). In population-based samples the frequency is somewhat lower (36,47,48), which is to be expected, because high headache frequency may be a reason for referral.

Accompanying Symptoms

The nature and frequency of such symptoms are listed in Table 2. The most distressing associated symptoms are those arising from disturbance of the gastrointestinal tract

TABLE 2. *Migraine without aura: prevalence of associated symptoms (%)*

Symptoms[a]	Selby and Lance (55) (n = 500)	Lance and Anthony (28) (n = 500)	Olesen (37) (n = 750)	Solomon et al. (57) (n = 100)	Davies et al. (14) (n = 354)	Rasmussen and Olesen (48) (n = 58)	Russell et al. (53) (n = 342)
Nausea	87	93	86	95	89	95	87
Vomiting	55	55	47	59	60	62	45
Diarrhea	—	19	9	—	—	8	—
Photophobia	82	49	—	91	—	95	92
Phonophobia	—	—	—	61	—	98	82

[a]Other symptoms at lower incidence are mentioned but not recorded in this table.
Em dash denotes that the corresponding symptom is not mentioned in the particular study.

in the form of nausea or vomiting, which can be severe and incapacitating. About 50% of migraineurs vomit during attacks, and nausea occurs in more than 80% (37,46,48,55). Anorexia, food intolerance, and frequent loose motions or even frank diarrhea do occur, but are not as disturbing to the patient. Photophobia and phonophobia also frequently accompany a migraine attack (see Table 2). Several population-based studies have found a positive correlation between pain severity and the occurrence of associated symptoms (2,10,27,40,59). In three previous studies the severity of nausea, photophobia, and phonophobia were graded as mild, moderate, or severe (26,46,52). It was found that these symptoms were not only more prevalent in migraineurs but also more severe than in tension-type headache. It has been suggested that such a grading of accompanying symptoms may improve the differentiation of migraine without aura from tension-type headache (45).

RESOLUTION OF THE ATTACK

In most patients the headache resolves slowly by fading away. A large minority find that sleeping for a few hours even through the course of the day will abolish the headache, whereas others find that vomiting will arrest an attack (3). Children in particular find that sleep or vomiting is highly effective in terminating a migrainous episode (42). Even after the headache has resolved, many patients do not feel entirely back to normal for some time. In one series 47 of 50 patients remained symptomatic after the headache had ended (3). The most frequent symptoms were changes in mood (72%), muscular weakness (54%), physical tiredness (52%), and reduced appetite (32%). Commonly, patients complained of feeling "tired and washed out," reflecting that they felt both physically and mentally below par. The average duration of these symptoms before complete resolution was 23 hours.

SPECIAL TYPES OF MIGRAINE WITHOUT AURA

Menstrual Migraine

As stated in the present definition, this variety of migraine occurs between 2 days before the beginning of

menses and the last day of menses. To be so categorized, 90% of attacks should occur in that particular time frame (22). Menstrual migraine is migraine without aura in the great majority of patients (13,16,31). In a group of 55 women thought to have menstrual migraine, only 4 (7.2%) had migraine conforming to the above criteria, whereas 19 (34.5%) had an increased number of attacks at the time of menstruation in addition to attacks at other times of the cycle (31). The investigators called the headaches in this latter group menstrually related migraine. Otherwise, the prevalence of menstrual migraine reported in various studies has varied from 8% to 70% (14,18,19). As pointed out by Macgregor (30), there are numerous problems with studies of menstrual migraine accounting for such widely divergent findings. Lack of a proper definition of menstrual migraine is the major one. Macgregor has proposed a stricter definition of true menstrual migraine as migraine attacks occurring on or between 2 days prior to menstruation and the first 2 days of menstruation with no attacks at any other time of the cycle. Using this definition, Russell et al. (53) found that menstrual migraine occurred in 25% of women with migraine without aura, but only 8% of those with migraine with aura. Similarly, Cupini et al. (13) found that menstrual migraine occurred almost exclusively in women with migraine without aura. Whether menstrual migraine is a special subtype of migraine without aura will be determined by future studies. Because the topic is addressed more specifically in Chapter 32, it will not be discussed further here.

Status Migrainosus

The term *status migrainosus* refers to a prolonged attack of migraine without aura lasting for more than 72 hours and which is refractory to treatment. It is highly unlikely that throughout the entire attack the patient is suffering from vascular headache (62). Rather, an attack of migraine (vascular headache) is succeeded by a tension (nonvascular) headache, which in turn is followed by recurrence of the vascular component before the tension-type headache has resolved. Thus, there is a repetition of migrainous attacks bridged by intervals of tension-type headache (11).

The mechanism of status migrainosus is not known or understood clearly, although cerebral edema (8) and cerebral hyperemia (34) have been suggested, but they are difficult to prove in practice.

Factors involved in the causation of migraine status are more clearly understood. Psychological disturbances in the form of emotional stress, depression, and anxiety are reported by the majority of patients, followed by medication abuse in about 30%, ergotamine being the substance most widely abused (11). Treatment of this condition is detailed in Chapter 66.

Atypical Migraine

Included in this group are those subjects who fulfill all but one of the criteria for migraine and do not fulfill criteria for tension-type headache as set out by the Headache Classification Committee (code 1.7) (22). In a Danish population-based study using the IHS criteria, 11% of subjects with migraine fulfilled the criteria of migrainous disorder (code 1.7). All these subjects had headache without aura. One subject had experienced fewer than five attacks, six had headache attacks lasting less than 4 hours (but more than 30 minutes), four did not have nausea or vomiting but had photophobia or phonophobia, and criterion C regarding the characteristics of the pain was not met by two others (46). Henry et al. (23) reported on the epidemiology of migraine in a nationwide survey in France. In that study a standardized questionnaire and a diagnostic algorithm applied by lay interviewers were used as the method of data collection. The algorithm was based on IHS diagnostic criteria (22). In the study a group of borderline cases was described encompassing subjects with migraine where either the duration of attacks was between 2 and 4 hours or there was photophobia or phonophobia but not both. In a validation study they found that the borderline cases were all considered by the neurologist involved as definite migraine (24), which is in accordance with the IHS classification of migraine including code 1.7.

Russell and Olesen (51), in a large population-based study of 4,000 patients, found 48 with a migrainous disorder. Forty of these had migrainous disorder without aura. More than half of these failed to achieve the criteria for migraine because of an insufficient number of attacks, whereas in 12 the headaches were of too short a duration. Unilateral location, aggravation by routine physical activity, and the associated features of nausea, vomiting, and photophobia were all significantly less common than in patients with migraine without aura. From their genetic epidemiologic studies they provided evidence that in some cases migrainous disorder without aura is a type of migraine without aura. In contrast, migrainous disorder with aura may be unrelated to migraine with aura (51).

Some patients with migraine may develop a headache of prolonged duration, lasting several days or even weeks at a time. This may be due to excessive use of medications, which is discussed further in Chapter 115. It also has been suggested that some of these patients may have an atypical form of occipital neuralgia (1). Anthony has investigated this condition and found that 60% of 74 such patients had a previous history of migraine before their headache became daily (1).

REFERENCES

1. Anthony M. Unilateral migraine or occipital neuralgia? In: Rose FC, ed. *New advances in headache research.* London: Smith-Gordon, 1989: 39–43.
2. Bakal DA, Kaganow JA. Symptom characteristics of chronic and non-chronic headache sufferers. *Headache* 1979;19:285–289.
3. Blau JN. Resolution of migraine attacks: sleep and the recovery phase. *J Neurol Neurosurg Psychiatry* 1982;45:223–226.
4. Blau JN. Clinical characteristics of premonitory symptoms in migraine. In: Amery WK, Wauquir A, eds. *The prelude to the migraine attack.* London: Baillière Tindall, 1986:39–43.
5. Blau JN. Adult migraine: the patient observed. In: Blau JN, ed. *Migraine: clinical, therapeutic, conceptual and research aspects.* London: Chapman & Hall, 1987:3–30.
6. Blau JN. Migraine: theories of pathogenesis. *Lancet* 1992;339: 1202–1207.
7. Blau JN, Dexter SL. The site of pain origin during migraine attacks. *Cephalalgia* 1981;1:143–147.
8. Blau JN, Solomon F. Migraine and intracranial swelling: an experiment of nature. *Lancet* 1985;2:718.
9. Campbell JK. Manifestations of migraine. *Neurol Clin* 1990;8: 841–855.
10. Celentano DP, Stewart WF, Linet MS. The relationship of headache symptoms with severity and duration of attacks. *J Clin Epidemiol* 1990; 43:983–994.
11. Couch JR, Diamond S. Status migrainosus: causative and therapeutic aspects. *Headache* 1983;23:94–101.
12. Cull RE. Barometric pressure and other factors in migraine. *Headache* 1981;21: 102–104.
13. Cupini LM, Matteis M, Troisi E, Calabresi P, Bernardi G, Silvestrini M. Sex-hormone-related events in migrainous females. A clinical comparative study between migraine with aura and migraine without aura. *Cephalalgia* 1995;15:140–144.
14. Davies PTG, Peatfield RC, Steiner TJ, Bond RA, Rose FC. Some clinical comparisons between common and classical migraine: a questionnaire-based study. *Cephalalgia* 1991;11:223–227.
15. De Matteis G, Vellante M, Marrelli A, Santalucia P, Tuzi P, Prencipe M. Geomagnetic activity, humidity, temperature and headache: is there any correlation? *Headache* 1993;34:41–43.
16. Dennerstein L, Morse C, Burrows G, Oats J, Brown J, Smith M. Menstrual migraine: a double-blind trial of percutaneous oestradiol. *Gynaecol Endocrinol* 1988;2:113–120.
17. Dexter JD, Riley TL. Studies in nocturnal migraine. *Headache* 1975; 15:51–62.
18. Diamond S, Dalessio DJ. *The practising physician's approach to headache.* Baltimore: Williams & Wilkins, 1982.
19. Diegre K, Damasio H. Menstrual migraine: differential diagnosis, evaluation and treatment. *Clin Obstet Gynaecol* 1987;30:417–430.
20. Drummond PD, Lance JW. Neurovascular disturbances in headache patients. *Clin Exp Neurol* 1984;20:93–99.
21. Gibb CM, Davies PTG, Glover V, Steiner TJ, Clifford Rose F, Sandler M. Chocolate is a migraine-provoking agent. *Cephalalgia* 1991;11: 93–95.
22. Headache Classification Committee of the International Headache Society. Classification and diagnostic criteria of headache disorders, cranial neuralgias and facial pain. *Cephalalgia* 1988;8[Suppl 7].
23. Henry P, Michel P, Brochet B, et al. A nationwide survey of migraine in France: prevalence and clinical features in adults. *Cephalalgia* 1992; 12:229–237.

24. Henry P, Michel P, Dartigues JF, et al. Migraine prevalence in France. In: Rose FC, ed. *New advances in headache research.* London: Smith-Gordon, 1991:11–14.

25. Isler H. Frequency and course of premonitory phenomena. In: Amery WK, Waquir A, eds. *The prelude to the migraine attack.* London: Baillière Tindall, 1986:44–53.

26. Iversen HK, Langemark M, Anderson PG, et al. Clinical characteristics of migraine and episodic tension-type headache in relation to old and new diagnostic criteria. *Headache* 1990;30:514–519.

27. Kaganov JA, Bakal DA, Dunn BE. The differential contribution of muscle contraction and migraine symptoms to problem headache in the general population. *Headache* 1981;21:157–163.

28. Lance JW, Anthony M. Some clinical aspects of migraine. *Arch Neurol* 1966;15:356–361.

29. Leviton A, Slack VW, Masek B, Bana D, Graham JR. A computerised behavioural assessment for children with headaches. *Headache* 1984;24:182–185.

30. Macgregor EA. Menstrual migraine: towards a definition. *Cephalalgia* 1996;16:11–21.

31. Macgregor EA, Chia H, Vohrah RC, Wilkinson M. Migraine and menstruation: a pilot study. *Cephalalgia* 1990;10:305–310.

32. Marcus DA, Scharff L, Turk D, Gourley LM. A double-blind provocative study of chocolate as a trigger of headache. *Cephalalgia* 1997;17:855–862.

33. Mathew NT, Stubits E, Nigam MP. Transformation of episodic migraine into daily headache: analysis of factors. *Headache* 1982;22:66–68.

34. Meyer JS, Hata T, Imai A, Zetusky WJ. Migraine and intracranial swelling. *Lancet* 1985;2:1308–1309.

35. Morrison DP. Occupational stress in migraine—is weekend headache a myth or reality? *Cephalalgia* 1990;10:189–193.

36. Nikiforow R. Headache in a random sample of 200 persons: a clinical study of a population in northern Finland. *Cephalalgia* 1981;1:99–107.

37. Olesen J. Some clinical features of the acute migraine attack. An analysis of 750 patients. *Headache* 1978;18:268–271.

38. Peatfield RC. Relationships between food, wine, and beer-precipitated migrainous headaches. *Headache* 1995;35:355–357.

39. Peatfield RC, Glover V, Littlewood JT, Sandler M, Clifford Rose F. The prevalence of diet-induced migraine. *Cephalalgia* 1984;4:179–183.

40. Philips C. Headache in general practice. *Headache* 1977;16:322–329.

41. Piorecky J, Becker WJ, Rose MS. Effect of Chinook winds on the probability of migraine headache occurrence. *Headache* 1997;37:153–158.

42. Prensky AL. Migraine in children. In: Blau JN, ed. *Migraine: clinical, therapeutic and conceptual and research aspects.* London: Chapman & Hall, 1987:31–54.

43. Raskin NH, Schwartz RK. Icepick-like pain. *Neurology* 1980;30:203–205.

44. Rasmussen BK. Migraine and tension-type headache in a general population: precipitating factors, female hormones, sleep pattern and relation to lifestyle. *Pain* 1993;53:65–72.

45. Rasmussen BK. Epidemiology of headache. *Cephalalgia* 1995;15;45–68.

46. Rasmussen BK, Jensen R, Olesen J. A population-based analysis of the diagnostic criteria of the International Headache Society. *Cephalalgia* 1991;11:129–134.

47. Rasmussen BK, Jensen R, Schroll M, Olesen J, Epidemiology of headache in a general population study. *J Clin Epidemiol* 1991;44:1147–1157.

48. Rasmussen BK, Olesen J. Migraine with aura and migraine without aura: an epidemiological study. *Cephalalgia* 1992;12:221–228.

49. Rasmussen BK, Olesen J. Symptomatic and non-symptomatic headaches in a general population. *Neurology* 1992;42:1225–1231.

50. Robbins L. Precipitating factors in migraine: a retrospective review of 494 patients. *Headache* 1994;34:214–216.

51. Russell MB, Olesen J. Migrainous disorder and its relation to migraine without aura and migraine with aura. A genetic epidemiological study. *Cephalalgia* 1996;16:431–435.

52. Russell MB, Rasmussen BK, Brennum J, et al. Presentation of a new instrument: the diagnostic headache diary. *Cephalalgia* 1992;12:369–374.

53. Russell MB, Rasmussen BK, Fenger K, Olesen J. Migraine without aura and migraine with aura are distinct clinical entities: a study of four hundred and eighty-four male and female migraineurs from the general population. *Cephalalgia* 1996;16:239–245.

54. Selby G. Clinical features of migraine and its variants. In: Selby G, ed. *Migraine and its variants.* Sydney: Adis Press, 1983:31–40.

55. Selby G, Lance JW. Observations on 500 cases of migraine and allied vascular headache. *J Neurol Neurosurg Psychiatry* 1960;23:23–32.

56. Sjaastad O, Bovim G, Stovner LJ. Common migraine (migraine without aura): localization of the initial pain of attack. *Funct Neurol* 1993;8:27–32.

57. Solomon S, Cappa KG, Smith CR. Common migraine: criteria for diagnosis. *Headache* 1987;27:124–129.

58. Van den Bergh V, Amery WK, Waelkens J. Trigger factors in migraine: a study conducted by the Belgian Migraine Society. *Headache* 1987;27:191–196.

59. Waters WE. The Pontypridd headache survey. *Headache* 1974;14:81–90.

60. Waelkens J. Warning symptoms in migraine: characteristics and therapeutic implications. *Cephalalgia* 1985;5:223–228.

61. Waelkens J, Caers J, Amery WK. Effects of therapeutic measures taken during the premonitory phase. In: Amery WK, Wauguir A, eds. *The prelude to the migraine attack.* London: Baillière Tindall, 1986:78–83.

62. Wilkinson M. Drug therapy during migraine attacks. In: Blau JN, ed. *Migraine: clinical, therapeutic, conceptual and research aspects.* London: Chapman & Hall, 1987:205–213.

63. Wilkinson M, Woodrow J. Migraine and weather. Headache 1979;19:375–378.

The Headaches, Second Edition,
edited by J. Olesen, P. Tfelt-Hansen, and K.M.A. Welch.
Lippincott Williams & Wilkins, Philadelphia © 2000.

The Migraines

CHAPTER 43

Migraine with Aura and Its Subforms

Jes Olesen and F. Michael Cutrer

DEFINITION OF MIGRAINE WITH AURA

IHS code and diagnosis: 1.2 Migraine with aura
WHO code and diagnosis: G43.1 Migraine with aura
Short description (Headache Classification Committee, 1988) (23): Idiopathic, recurring disorder manifesting with attacks of neurologic symptoms unequivocally localizable to cerebral cortex or brain stem, usually gradually developed over 5 to 20 minutes and usually lasting less than 60 minutes. Headache, nausea, and/or photophobia usually follow neurologic aura symptoms directly or after a free interval of less than 1 hour. The headache usually lasts 4 to 72 hours but may be completely absent.
Other terms: Classic migraine; classical migraine; ophthalmic, hemiparesthetic, hemiplegic, or aphasic migraine; migraine accompagnée; complicated migraine.
IHS diagnostic criteria for migraine with aura
(Headache Classification Committee, 1988) (23):
A. At least two attacks fulfilling B.
B. At least three of the following four characteristics:
　1. One or more fully reversible aura symptoms indicating focal cerebral cortical and/or brain stem dysfunction.
　2. At least one aura symptom develops gradually over more than 4 minutes or two or more symptoms occur in succession.

　3. No aura symptom lasts more than 60 minutes. If more than one aura symptom is present, accepted duration is proportionally increased.
　4. Headache follows aura with a free interval of less than 60 minutes. (It may also begin before or simultaneously with the aura.)
C. At least one of the following:
　1. History, physical, and neurologic examinations do not suggest one of the disorders listed in groups 5–11 of the IHS classification.
　2. History and/or physical and/or neurologic examinations do suggest such disorder, but it is ruled out by appropriate investigations.
　3. Such disorder is present, but migraine attacks do not occur for the first time in close temporal relationship to the disorder.

The transient neurologic symptoms of the aura are among the most striking features of migraine and frequently factors that motivate patients to seek consultation from a physician. The present chapter will concentrate on the migraine aura because the premonitory symptoms (hours before headache), the headache, and the post-headache phases of migraine are similar in attacks both with and without aura and are discussed in Chapter 42 and elsewhere (46). There is ongoing debate as to whether migraine with aura and migraine without aura represent two distinct pathophysiologic processes. Those researchers who consider them to be the same entity point to (a) the similarity in the clinical features of the prodromal, headache, and resolution phases of migraine with and without aura; (b) the fact that many sufferers experience attacks of both migraine with and without aura in the course of their lives; and (c) the apparent similarity of therapeutic response in the two types (8). Arguments that they represent two different processes are bolstered by (a)

　J. Olesen: Department of Neurology, Glostrup Hospital, University of Copenhagen, DK-2600 Glostrup, Copenhagen, Denmark.
　F.M. Cutrer: Department of Neurology, Harvard Medical School, and Partners Headache Center, Massachusetts General Hospital/Brigham and Women's Hospital, Boston, Massachusetts 02114-3117.

genetic epidemiologic studies showing differing familial accumulation of the two types of migraine; (b) other population-based epidemiologic studies indicating that the occurrence of both forms within the same patient might not be more common than is expected from cooccurrence of two relatively common entities; (c) the observation that the headache following aura is often less severe and of shorter duration; (d) the fact that auras are not consistently followed by headache; (e) studies of regional blood flow in migraine that show areas of spreading hypoperfusion in migraine with aura but not in migraine without aura; and (f) biochemical studies indicating differences in the migraineurs with and without aura (45).

GENERAL CHARACTERISTICS OF MIGRAINE AURA

Unfortunately, the description of aura symptoms is not easy. The most detailed and precise descriptions originate from self-observation by doctors and other professionals who had migraine themselves. However, such accounts can be criticized for lack of representativity because they are likely to be biased toward complicated and interesting symptomatology. The other approach has been to collect clinical data, mostly retrospectively, from hospital charts but also using patient questionnaires, interviews, and drawings prospectively (Fig. 1). With this method representativity is good but accuracy varies.

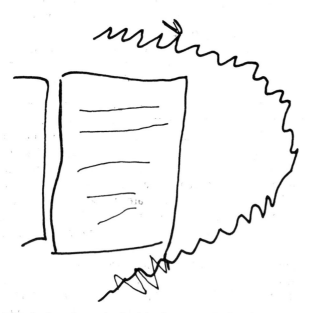

FIG. 1. A patient who had had numerous visual auras was unable to describe them retrospectively. He became interested in his own symptomatology and drew his next visual aura, which is depicted above. In the center of vision, he is looking at a book, and there is a typical zigzag-shaped fortification line in his right hemifield of vision. There is no scotoma.

In 1996, Russell and Olesen published a nosographic analysis of migraine aura in 163 sufferers identified in a sampling of 4,000 Danish citizens (48). Because it was drawn from the general population, it was less likely to be affected by selection bias for more striking cases. In this series, 62 subjects had some migraine auras with headache and some attacks without headache, whereas 7 subjects experienced only auras without headache. In Russell's study population, visual aura was overwhelmingly the most common aura symptom, occurring in 99% of cases, followed by sensory, aphasic, and motor auras. Visual aura occurred without any other aura symptoms in 64% of cases, whereas other aura types usually occurred in combination with another aura type (usually visual). These findings are similar to those seen in a small prospective study published 2 years earlier in which 54 migraine auras in 20 patients were described in detail (47). In this study, visual and sensory aura symptoms developed over 15 to 25 minutes and persisted for 20 to 55 minutes. When visual and sensory symptoms preceded a headache, the headache was typically migrainoid. However, if a headache preceded the aura symptoms, the headache was of the tension type. The various subforms of migraine are often determined by the type, number, and duration of aura symptoms discussed in the following sections.

TYPES OF AURA SYMPTOMS

Visual Aura

According to Schiller (50), the term *fortifications* was first used by Fothergill in his 1778 account of sick headache. He noted that during a migraine aura objects appear surrounded with luminous angles like those of fortifications. Over the next 100 years a number of British scientists described and accurately mapped their visual symptoms. Some of them experienced fortifications, others only hemianopsia. Hubert Airy (1) coined the term *teichopsia* (a translation of "seeing fortifications") and published precise drawings of his own visual symptoms, which were not followed by headache (migraine aura without headache) (Fig. 2). Jolly (29) accurately recorded and drew 24 visual auras. In addition, he reported on his experience with several hundred visual auras over the years. His first symptom was usually a hazy spot close to the center of vision (Fig. 3). The spot was followed after 2 to 15 minutes by a star-shaped figure, which was shining and flickering, and then by a semicircular zigzag line (fortification). The fortification slowly moved away from the center of vision while expanding in size and finally disappeared at the extreme lateral margin of the visual field. Sometimes the disturbance was more pronounced in the upper quadrant, sometimes in the lower quadrant, but it never crossed the midline. In 3 or 4 of about 100 instances, visual symptoms

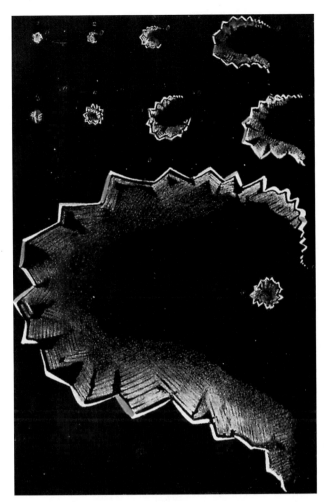

FIG. 2. The visual auras of Hubert Airy (1). The upper line shows the development of fortification lines in the left hemifield of vision. A spot begins close to the center of vision (0), and gradually enlarges and spreads laterally. Another visual aura is shown in the middle line. In this instance, it began below and a few degrees to the left of the center of vision, but otherwise resembled the first. The large figure below demonstrates a fully developed fortification figure and the beginning of a second attack while the first has not yet disappeared. Such attacks never developed fully, unless they arose on the opposite side.

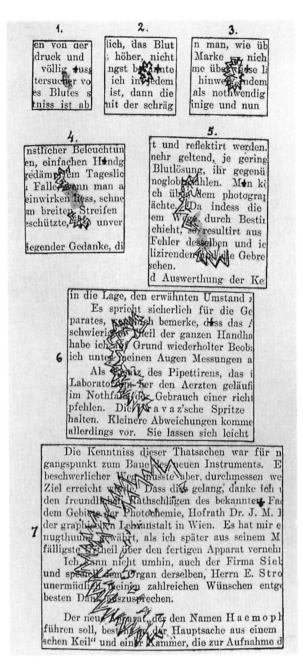

FIG. 3. One of the visual auras experienced by Jolly (29). The typical features are obvious from the illustration. Little or no scotoma was associated with the fortification line.

developed in the reverse order, that is, starting laterally in the visual field. Concerning the location of headache, Jolly observed a few attacks that were ipsilateral to the visual symptoms, but the vast majority of attacks were associated with contralateral or bilateral headache. In his later years, the visual auras were no longer followed by headache. Lashley (31) suffered from visual auras without headache and mapped his auras very accurately. His profound knowledge of the visual system (he was a visual physiologist himself) enabled him to add considerably to existing descriptions of visual auras. There were a number of common features. The auras always started at or near the center of fixation and gradually spread laterally. They were almost symmetrical in both eyes and never

impinged on the midline. Some of the scotomas were exclusively negative, whereas others scintillated at the edge, which appeared zigzag shaped (fortifications). In some instances only part of the scotoma scintillated above or below a certain point. As the scotoma moved laterally it increased in size and the rate of drift increased. In some auras the shape of the scotoma was very well preserved as it drifted, whereas the shape changed during other auras (Fig. 4). Usually the scotoma affected both the upper and lower quadrant of the right or left hemifield of vision (Fig. 4A and B), but occasionally only the lower

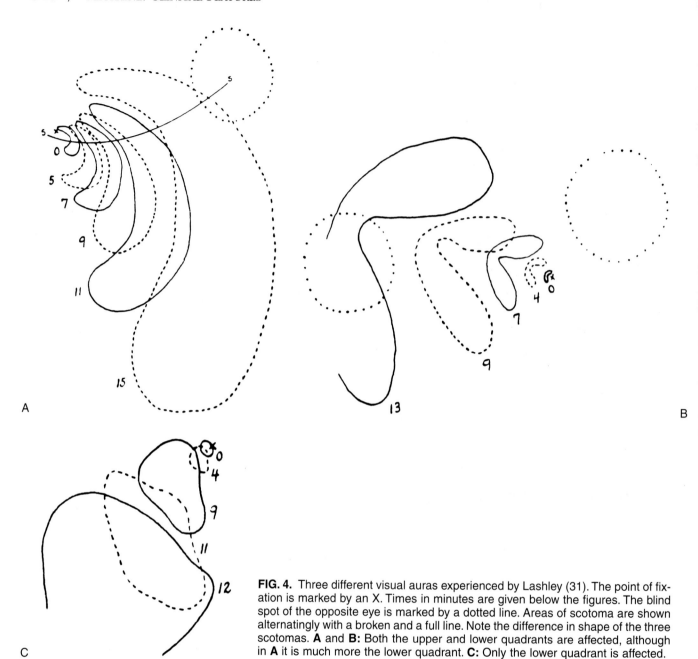

FIG. 4. Three different visual auras experienced by Lashley (31). The point of fixation is marked by an X. Times in minutes are given below the figures. The blind spot of the opposite eye is marked by a dotted line. Areas of scotoma are shown alternatingly with a broken and a full line. Note the difference in shape of the three scotomas. **A** and **B:** Both the upper and lower quadrants are affected, although in **A** it is much more the lower quadrant. **C:** Only the lower quadrant is affected.

or upper quadrant was affected (Fig. 4C). The size and density of scotomas varied, and complete hemianopsia was observed in only one instance from more than 100. Close examination of the scintillations revealed series of parallel zigzag lines. There was a tendency for the pattern of figures in each part of the advancing front to remain relatively constant in both size and shape as the fortification drifted laterally. The period of inhibition after scintillations had passed varied (as indicated by the size of the scotoma) from approximately 5 minutes to approximately half an hour. Only a few auras were completely without scotoma, in contrast to the reports of Jolly (29), who usually had fortifications without scotoma (see Fig. 3). The rate of scintillations was estimated at 10 cycles/s. A neg-

ative scotoma might completely escape observation. Hare (22) confirmed Lashley's findings and added accurate measurements of the vertical diameter of the fortification figure. It was found to increase exponentially with time (Fig. 5). The rate of shimmer of the fortification line diminished during the march. After 3 or 4 minutes, it was on the order of 10 to 15 cycles/s, decreasing to about 3 or 4 cycles/s toward the end. In contrast to the previous findings of Schumacher and Wolff (50), amyl nitrite had only minor and very short-lasting effects on the diameter of the fortification figure.

In studies of larger numbers of patients, Alvarez (2) reported somewhat unsystematic observations in 618 migraine patients. The above pattern generally was con-

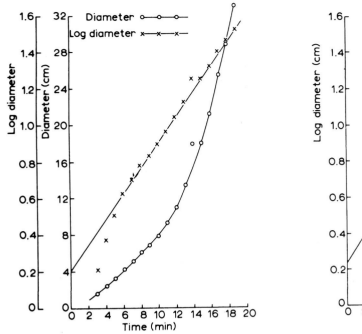
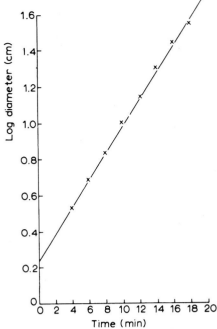

FIG. 5. The vertical diameter of the fortification figure as measured by Hare (22). To the left, a logarithmic and a linear plot of this diameter at various times during a single aura. To the right, the mean of nine attacks plotted logarithmically. Note that the vertical diameter of the figure increases exponentially because it becomes a straight line in a logarithmic plot.

firmed. Most scintillations were uncolored, but sometimes colored lines appeared, usually behind the advancing scintillation. The scintillations varied in intensity from being almost blinding to being almost unnoticeable. The failure to observe negative scotomas was stressed by several patients, and Alvarez himself once noticed left-sided hemianopsia only when he failed to observe a car coming from the left. There was a preference for the hours between 11 a.m. and 1 p.m. in his own case, but this has not been described by others. He occasionally had two scotomas in a day, and in one instance a second scotoma started 10 minutes after another had disappeared. Such repetitive scotomas also had been observed by others (1,31), and occasionally more than one fortification figure has been seen at a time. Twelve percent of men, but only 0.7% of women, suffered from scotomas without headache according to Alvarez (2). Hachinski et al. (21) obtained drawings of visual symptoms from 100 children with migraine. Diffuse blurring, scotomas, distortions, and hallucinations were described, but the drawings were made retrospectively.

Bücking and Baumgartner (10) analyzed the symptomatology of auras in 87 migraine patients with aura, but it is not clear if it was by history alone or by prospective observation, probably the former. Only three did not have visual symptoms in addition to sensory, speech, or motor symptoms. The following numbers are therefore based on 84 patients. Six different types of visual disturbances were described (Table 1). They were mostly uncolored, but in eight cases spectral colors were reported, usually close to a fortification line. Only the fortification lines were clearly lateralized to one visual field, whereas other disturbances affected both sides. The different visual disturbances occurred in a typical order. Initially, unclear vision often changed into diffuse flickering spots that, again, progressed to grouped dysopsias and finally into a scintillating fortification line with scotoma. In 40 patients a gradual development of visual disturbances could clearly be described. Symptoms were reported to vary from attack to attack in the individual patient, but no quantitative data were given to support this observation.

TABLE 1. *Localization of components of the visual aura in 84 patients with classic or hemiplegic migraine*

	First symptom	Diffuse spots	Grouped dysopsias	Scintillating	Scotomas
Whole field	27	22	2	2	0
More in one hemifield	7	18	18	19	2
Only in one hemifield	0	0	1	2	2
Not known	18	8	2	3	0

Translated from Bücking and Baumgartner (10).

In the 161 cases of visual aura studied by Russell and Olesen, 108 patients (69%) reported that symptoms were limited to one hemifield of vision, whereas 49 (31%) reported that symptoms were bilateral. Most commonly, the visual disturbance consisted of an uncolored, flickering zigzag-shaped line that usually appeared near the center of vision (62%) and moved toward the periphery. A scotoma was left in the wake of the expanding visual disturbance about 50% of the time. The progression of the visual symptoms most often lasted less than 30 minutes (82%), and the total duration of the aura was under an hour in 111 patients (69%). When more than one symptom type occurred, the mean duration of the aura was increased (48).

Sensory Aura

Sensory migrainous symptoms are second in frequency to visual symptoms. The following frequencies have been given in patients with migraine with aura: 40% (27), 31% (48), 30% (35), and 41% (10). Of 36 patients in the latter study, 23 reported unilateral occurrence, usually in the upper extremity and periorally. This so-called cheirooral (hand-mouth) distribution was also noted in most of the patients of Manzoni et al. (35). Specifically, the spread of paresthesias to involve the tongue is very typical and rarely seen in cerebrovascular attacks (16). In 10 cases a slow spread was noted, usually starting in the thumb and gradually spreading to the whole hand and to the perioral region. In 6 cases the leg was affected. Paresthesias affected only the hand, the face, or the foot in the rest of the patients. The affected side changed from attack to attack. Quite often paresthesias were the first sensory symptom leaving numbness in their wake. Heyck (24) noted a cheirooral distribution of sensory symptoms in 20 of 40 patients with sensory symptoms, and gradual spread of symptoms in 6 of 7 patients where sufficiently reliable information was available. Russell found that among 51 patients with sensory aura, the hand (96% of cases) and face (67%) were the body parts most often affected, whereas the leg (24%) and trunk (18%) were much less commonly involved. In Russell's series, sensory symptoms tended to progress less than 30 minutes (82%), and the total duration was usually less than 1 hour (80%). When occurring with motor aura, the symptoms tended to last longer. The Australian neurologist Lord (34) was able to describe his sensory symptoms very accurately:

> In attacks commencing with tingling of the hands or face, orderly march was the rule, and attack details were predictable using the sensory homunculus. In some right hemisphere attacks, a gradual progression occurred, beginning with a disturbance of hand sensation with tingling, then numbness followed by loss of awareness of position of the arm, and then visual disturbance with teichopsia moving from the periphery centrally, also conforming to known neuroanatomical boundaries. Typically, a band of tingling marched along a limb or face with the region remaining numb for many minutes thereafter.

In a group of patients selected because they had aura symptoms in the extremities, the duration of limb symptoms varied markedly (9) (Table 2). There are no published self-observations with accurate timing or plotting of sensory disturbances similar to those available for the visual aura. The findings of one of our cases are shown in Figure 6.

Motor Aura

Motor weakness was described by 21% of Bücking and Baumgartner's (10) patients with migraine with aura. They noted that paresis usually developed focally and gradually spread to involve more and more muscles. In 10 patients the paresis was unilateral, whereas eight indicated bilateral weakness in arms or legs. Quite often paresis was associated with impaired coordination, and in one patient severe dyscoordination occurred without paresis. In his excellent article on hemiplegic migraine, Heyck (24) provided accurate information about motor symptoms (Table 3). Jensen et al. (27) found motor weakness in 18% of patients with classic migraine, and Bradshaw and Parson (9) described weakness in 62% of their patients, selected because they had sensory or motor symptoms as part of their aura. Bana and Graham (4) found motor weakness in only 18 of 325 patients in a retrospective study. Similarly, Russell and Olesen found motor weakness in only 6% of their patients (48). In their series, no body part that was affected by the motor aura was unaffected by sensory symptoms. Motor aura symptoms were unilateral and affected the arm and hand. Progression of motor symptoms occurred in under 30 minutes in 56% of patients, but in 22% symptoms continued to progress for over an hour. The duration of motor symptoms was often prolonged beyond 1 hour in 67% of cases. In a population-based retrospective study, 13% of migraines with aura were accompanied by weakness (46). In 164 patients with aura, Manzoni et al. (35) found none with convincing weakness. The presence or absence of paresis and its severity varies from attack to attack. In our experience, sensory ataxia is often misinterpreted as weakness. True paresis is rare and always half-sided (39).

TABLE 2. *Duration of limb symptoms in the average attack (%)*

Duration	Group A	Group B	Combined
<1 hour	56	59	58
1–3 hours	18	9	14
3–24 hours	10	16	12
1–7 days	16	16	16

From Bradshaw and Parsons (9).

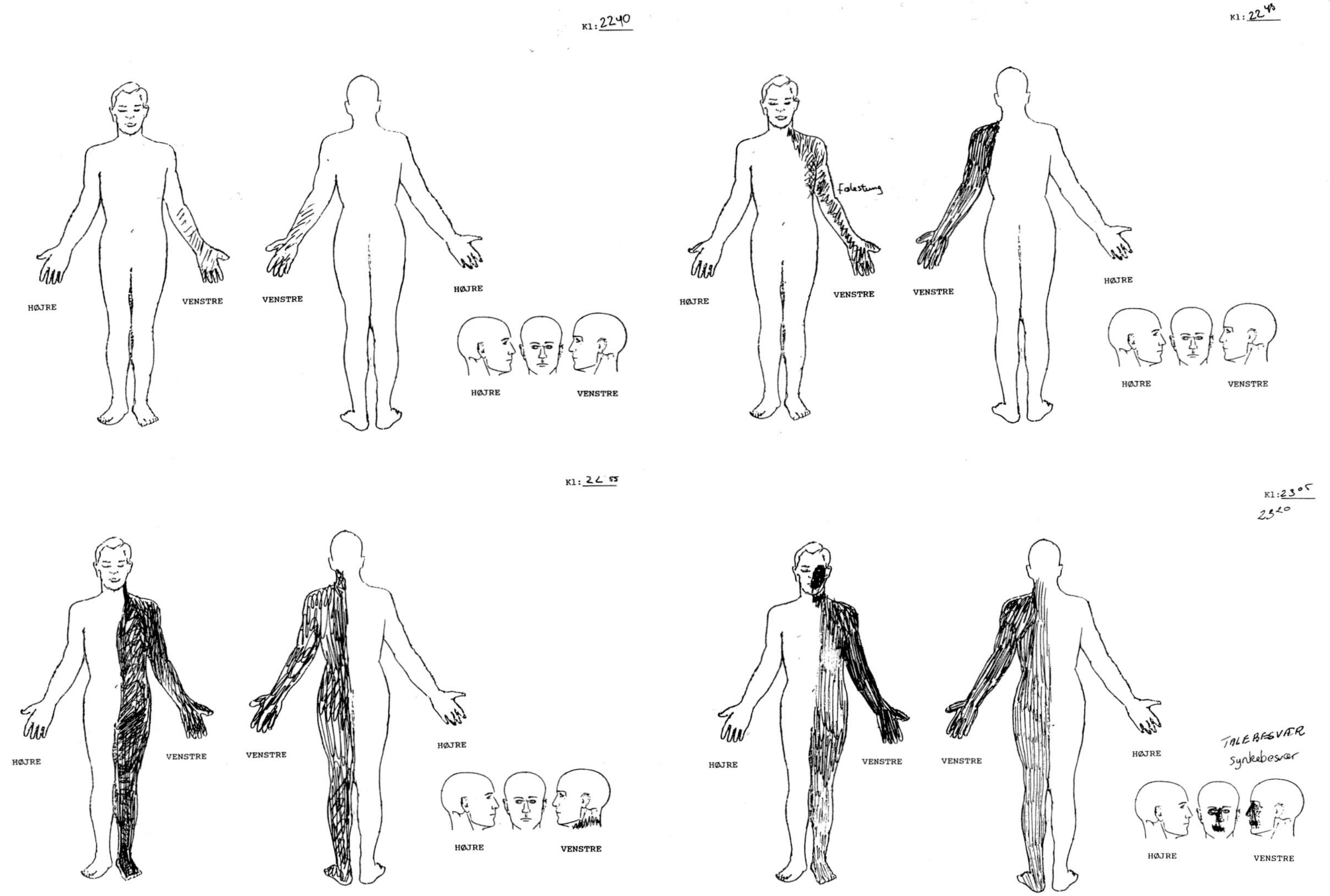

FIG. 6. Sensory aura.

TABLE 3. *Differentiation of motor symptoms*

Motor pareses	
Combined with sensory symptoms	17 cases
Without sensory symptoms	3 cases
Unilateral pareses	
Right side	
Hand or arm only	4 cases
Face only	1 case
Face, arm, and leg	2 cases
Arm and leg	1 case
Left side	
Hand or arm only	4 cases
Arm and leg	3 cases
Face, arm, and leg	3 cases
Bilateral pareses	
Arm only, alternately	1 case
Arm and leg, simultaneously or alternately	1 case
Jacksonian jerks	
Face, right side with aphasia	1 case
Left arm, followed by paresis	2 cases
Feeling of stiffness	
Right hand 1, left arm 1, thumb both sides 1	3 cases

From Heyck (22).

Language Aura

Language or aphasic aura is less common than sensory and visual symptoms but more common than weakness (39). Speech disturbances in migraine patients have been observed with the following frequencies: 22% (10), 20% (27), 18% (48), 17% (35), and 9% (4). In patients with so-called hemiplegic migraine, it was found in 47% (9). In the latter study the disturbance was characterized as aphasia in 44 and as dysarthria in 3 patients. Bücking and Baumgartner (10), on the other hand, felt that it was difficult to decide in many cases whether dysarthria or aphasia was present. In most but not all patients, speech difficulty has been associated with other evidence, indicating involvement of the dominant hemisphere. Heyck (24) described 25 patients with speech disturbance (Table 4). It is interesting that five right-handed patients were aphasic and yet had a left hemiparesis. The author observed several similar cases. Not infrequently, patients report

TABLE 4. *Differentiation of speech disturbances*

Motor and/or amnesic aphasia or dysphasia	21 cases
Sensory symptoms and motor aphasia	2 cases
Together with hemipareses	
Right	11 cases
Left	5 cases
Bilateral, simultaneous or alternating	4 cases
Without other neurological symptoms	2 cases
Dysarthric speech disturbance	4 cases
Together with hemipareses	
Right	2 cases
Left	1 case
Both sides	1 case

From Heyck (24).

that speech disturbance occurs as the spreading paresthesias reach the face or the tongue. Russell and Olesen found that the duration of language aura symptoms was usually under 30 minutes (59%). Paraphasic errors (76%) and other types of impaired language production (72%) were common, and impaired comprehension also occurred (38%).

Less Typical Aura Symptoms

As previously discussed in Chapters 29 and 35, a pathophysiologic disturbance (probably cortical spreading depression or its human analogue) that gradually spreads through the cerebral cortex underlies the aura symptoms. From this it would be expected that virtually any cortical symptom could be encountered during the aura. This is supported by a number of case histories but has not been documented by systematic observations. Other symptoms are less frequent and much more difficult to describe. Neglect has been described by Lord (34). During a cerebral blood flow study, showing much decreased perfusion in the right parietal region, we have observed neglect (unpublished observations). Because the basis of neglect is inattention, it is easily understandable why lay patients do not report this symptom. Spatial and geographic disorientation also has been recorded by Lord (34). Strong emotion, particularly anxiety, has been described in a number of convincing case histories by Sacks (49). Such anxiety was clearly pathologic because it continued to occur with every new attack even if patients knew very well that it was part of the migraine aura. Decreased visual attention during attacks originating from the left hemisphere but not from the right hemisphere without residual symptoms outside of attacks was described by Sinforiani et al. (53). A number of neuropsychological symptoms lasting 10 to 15 minutes and occurring immediately before migraine attack were described by Ardita and Sanchez (3). In addition to symptoms previously discussed, they recorded ataxia, acalculia, depersonalization (alteration in the usual sense of one's own reality), automatic behavior, achromatopsia (disappearance of colors), palinopsia [visual perseveration; which had already been recorded by Selby and Lance (52)], gustatory hallucinations, and transient global amnesia. It has been proposed that the latter syndrome could be caused by a spreading depression in the dominant hippocampus (40). As yet, there is no solid evidence to support this hypothesis and no quantitative documentation of increased incidence of transient global amnesia in patients suffering from migraine with aura. Olfactory hallucinations have been described by a number of researchers (3,18,60). Oscillacusis (fluctuation in the intensity of ambient sounds) also has been described in at least one case (57). Metamorphopsia or distorted vision has been recorded for decades during aura symptoms. This includes macropsia and micropsia, telescopic vision, mosaic vision, deja vu, jamais vu, and a number of other disturbances. The best insight into the complexity of the migraine aura is probably gained by reading Chapter 3 in Sacks's highly interesting book (49).

Symptoms that May or May Not Be Part of a Migrainous Aura

When people are asked to record any symptom occurring just before headache, vertigo/dizziness is often reported (46). In one epidemiologic study, patients having migraine without aura reported vertigo/dizziness less often (46), suggesting that this sensation may actually be part of the migraine aura. In another series, 91 patients were identified from the population of a neurotologic specialty clinic whose recurrent episodes of dizziness had no other identifiable cause than migraine. Forty-five percent of the subjects had migraine with aura, 44% had migraine without aura, and 11% reported recurrent auras without headache (again migraine with aura is disproportionately represented). Vertiginous dizziness (illusion of movement) occurred in 69%, whereas nonvertiginous dizziness (severe imbalance, nausea, and motion sensitivity) was present in 31%. Many of the patients who reported vertigo also experienced episodes of nonvertiginous dizziness. The duration of the episodes of dizziness had a bimodal distribution, with 31% having episodes lasting from minutes to under 2 hours and 57% having attacks lasting from 6 to greater than 24 hours. Most subjects (70%) experienced dizziness both in the context of and independent of migraine attacks. However, 3 patients had dizziness that occurred exclusively in the minutes prior to the onset of a migraine attack (11). The pathophysiologic mechanism of migraine-associated dizziness is not well understood. Dizziness that lasts minutes and tends to occur just before the onset of a migraine attack is suggestive of an auralike phenomenon. Although it is clear that disturbed cortical function may cause a sensation of dizziness, it remains unclear whether true vertigo can occur. When occurring during the headache phase, nausea, malaise, and pain may be misreported as dizziness. In any case, the presence of vertigo/dizziness should never be used to differentiate between migraine with aura and migraine without aura.

Decreased level of consciousness again is a very difficult concept to deal with by history. Blau (7) wrote: "Do patients lose consciousness in migraine? A sleepy patient with slurred or dysphasic speech may seem to relatives to be confused and possibly semiconscious. Furthermore, it is not difficult to visualize a patient lying in bed, vomiting, then rising to go to the bathroom and suffering an attack of syncope." Nausea and vomiting may induce vasovagal attacks resulting in syncope due to bradycardia and decreased blood pressure, but it may also elicit changes in cardiac rhythm (33). It is our opinion that most reports of decreased level of consciousness or syn-

cope are of a secondary nature. On the other hand, a number of reports document that severe migrainous aura, especially of the hemiplegic type in children, may include confusion, psychosis, or decreased consciousness (6,12,13,32). On occasion such severe migraine aura may be life threatening by inducing respiratory arrest. Lethal outcome has been described (14,26,37). The patient in the latter report was febrile, and other patients have had febrile attacks (20,26,36). Such attacks were dominantly inherited, and it seems most likely that somehow the underlying inherited cerebellar/cerebral disturbance may have been associated with a very low migraine threshold. On balance, severe migrainous aura, especially of the hemiplegic type in children, may occasionally be associated with decreased level of consciousness or syncope. In adults this is exceedingly rare and often associated with other signs of neurologic disease or febrile illness.

Combinations of Aura Symptoms

The various combinations of typical aura symptoms (speech symptoms excluded) have been nicely illustrated by Peatfield (44) (Fig. 7). Only visual symptoms frequently occur in isolation, whereas sensory, speech, and motor symptoms are usually associated with visual symptoms or with one or more of the other symptoms (2,4,10,24,27,48). When two or more aura symptoms are present, they virtually always occur in succession and not simultaneously (15,16,34). By far the most common is for the aura to begin with visual symptoms, followed by sensory symptoms, speech difficulty, or hemiparesis. The reverse order is relatively rare (24,34, personal observations). If less typical symptoms are included, combinations of aura symptoms become legion. Meticulous individual case histories demonstrate the complexity best

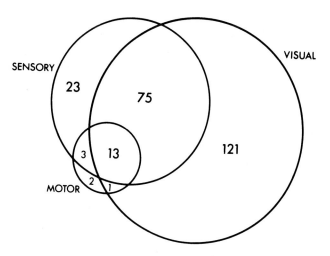

FIG. 7. Frequencies of visual, sensory, and motor aura symptoms and their combinations. From Peatfield (44) with permission.

(49). It is uncertain if aura symptoms can be bilateral. In our prospectively observed series (39) this seemed to be the case, with visual symptoms in a small proportion of cases, whereas sensory and motor symptoms were always unilateral. In a couple of patients an aura affected one side first; a new aura subsequently affected the other side before the first aura symptoms had disappeared. This may be one explanation for bilateral aura symptoms.

The duration of visual auras is usually 20 to 30 minutes, ranging from 5 to 60 minutes. The duration of other aura symptoms has been less well described, and little is known about the duration of combinations of aura symptoms. Duration is clearly longer the more symptoms a patient encounters. Even an aura composed of all the four typical symptoms mentioned above does not usually last more than 2 to 4 hours.

THE HEADACHE PHASE AND ITS RELATIONSHIP TO AURA

Population-based studies are necessary to determine whether the headache phases of migraine with and without aura are similar because apparent differences might reflect referral patterns rather than real differences. One such population-based study by Rasmussen and Olesen (46) examined 38 patients with aura and 58 patients without aura diagnosed among a randomly selected group of 1,000 normal Danes. In this study, the headache phase of migraine with aura was less intense and shorter lasting than attacks of migraine without aura. There was a trend toward fewer attacks in patients with aura. The location, character, and aggravation during physical activity were similar in the two groups. The tendency for nausea, vomiting, and photo- and phonophobia also were identical. In a clinic population, Manzoni et at. (35) found that headache was generally not severe and was short-lived in patients with aura. In all published studies there is a tendency for men to have less pronounced headache than women, and for the headache phase to gradually fade away over the years. Thus, a middle-aged man is much more likely to have migraine aura without headache than is a young woman. Sacks (49) also described the disappearance of the headache phase with persisting aura symptoms during pregnancy. Even if aura symptoms are unilateral, headache often is bilateral (39). Bilateral aura symptoms are usually associated with bilateral headache.

Much confusion has existed regarding the timing of aura symptoms and headache. The International Headache Classification Committee accepted that headache may occur before the aura (23). It is difficult for patients to remember such temporal relationships, and no systematic prospective study has been conducted. In a large series of patients studied with regional cerebral blood flow, the evolution of symptoms was directly observed during the attack (39). In a single case, aura symptoms and headache began simultaneously, and in 58 cases aura symptoms came first. When a headache occasionally is reported before a migraine aura, it may be a tension-type headache, a headache associated with febrile illness, or some other headache. An aura may pass unnoticed during sleep or if symptoms are exclusively negative (e.g., a scotoma). It may then appear that the headache came first if a second aura develops later. Another problem has been the location of aura symptoms and headache. Several reports in the literature have indicated that half-sided aura symptoms may be associated with headache on the same or opposite side quite haphazardly. Patients, however, cannot remember sides, and in a prospectively studied series where symptoms were recorded during the actual attack by the investigator, headache occurred over the hemisphere affected by the aura in 33 of 36 cases (39). A similar picture is brought out when patients prospectively record their aura symptoms and their headache by standardized forms (47).

SUBTYPES OF MIGRAINE WITH AURA

Migraine with Typical Aura

IHS code and diagnosis: 1.2.1 Migraine with typical aura

WHO code and diagnosis: G43.10 Migraine with typical aura

Short description (23): Migraine with an aura consisting of homonymous visual disturbances, hemisensory symptoms, hemipareses, or dysphasia, or combinations thereof. Gradual development, duration under 1 hour, and complete reversibility characterize the aura that is associated with headache.

Other terms (23): Ophthalmic, hemiparesthetic, hemiparetic, hemiplegic, or aphasic migraine; migraine accompagnée.

Diagnostic criteria (23):
  A. Fulfills criteria for 1.2, including all four criteria under B.
  B. One or more aura symptoms of the following types:
    1. Homonymous visual disturbance
    2. Unilateral paresthesias and/or numbness
    3. Unilateral weakness
    4. Aphasia or unclassifiable speech difficulty

This diagnosis depends entirely on the history. Many patients do not necessarily fulfill diagnostic criteria for migraine with typical aura at the first interview, but when they are encouraged to study their symptoms prospectively, they become typical. The symptomatology of migraine with typical aura has been described earlier in this chapter.

Migraine with Prolonged Aura

IHS code and diagnosis: 1.2.2 Migraine with prolonged aura

WHO code and diagnosis: G43.11 Migraine with prolonged aura

Short description (23): Migraine with one or more aura symptoms lasting more than 60 minutes and less than 1 week. Results of neuroimaging are normal.

Other terms (23): Complicated migraine, hemiplegic migraine.

Diagnostic criteria (23): Fulfills criteria for 1.2, but at least one symptom lasts more than 60 minutes and no more than 7 days. If neuroimaging reveals a relevant ischemic lesion, code 1.6.2 migrainous infarction regardless of symptom duration.

This diagnosis is given to patients with long-lasting but otherwise typical aura symptoms. This generally occurs in a few attacks in patients who otherwise have a typical aura and patients who virtually always have hemisensory or hemiparetic symptoms. The distinction of the patients with prolonged motor/sensory aura from familial hemiplegic migraine based on symptomatology is often difficult.

Familial Hemiplegic Migraine

IHS code and diagnosis: 1.2.3 Familial hemiplegic migraine

WHO code and diagnosis: G43.IX5 Familial hemiplegic migraine

Short description (23): Migraine with aura including hemiparesis and where at least one first-degree relative has identical attacks.

Diagnostic criteria (23):
A. Fulfills criteria for 1.2.
B. The aura includes some degree of hemiparesis and may be prolonged.
C. At least one first-degree relative has identical attacks.

The basis of this syndrome is a number of families in which several members have been afflicted by the same type of migraine attacks, which seemed to be dominantly inherited. The aura is usually long lasting and includes weakness (9,20,24,28,43,58). Such cases have been reported since the late nineteenth century. For older references, see the cited literature. The severity of migrainous aura varies in the individual from those with mild sensory symptoms to those with severe hemisensory disturbances and paresis. The duration of aura symptoms varies similarly, but in hemiplegic (strict sense) attacks the duration is often from several hours up to a few days. Complete restitution is the rule, but a few cases with permanent sequelae exist. Most patients experienced onset in childhood or adolescence, and in many patients symptoms disappear before the age of 30 (28). Familial hemiplegic migraine is the first migraine syndrome to be associated with a single gene defect. In several families, familial hemiplegic migraine has been linked to a missense mutation on the short arm of chromosome 19 (30,42). See Chapter 30 for more details. More recently, a different gene defect has been mapped to chromosome 1 in another family with familial hemiplegic migraine (19).

Basilar Migraine

IHS code and diagnosis: 1.2.4 Basilar migraine

WHO code and diagnosis: G43.IX3 Basilar migraine

Short description (23): Migraine with aura symptoms clearly originating from the brain stem or from both occipital lobes.

Other terms (23): Basilar artery migraine, Bickerstaff's migraine, syncopal migraine.

Diagnostic criteria (23):
A. Fulfills criteria for 1.2.
B. Two or more aura symptoms of the following types: visual symptoms in both the temporal and nasal fields of both eyes, dysarthria, vertigo, tinnitus, decreased hearing, double vision, ataxia, bilateral paresthesias, bilateral pareses, decreased level of consciousness.

Bickerstaff (5,6) proposed this term for patients in whom the aura symptoms indicated dysfunction of the basilar artery territory. Virtually all these patients had one or more of the typical aura symptoms described above and, in addition, decreased level of consciousness, vertigo, diplopia, or ataxia. Sturzenegger and Meienberg (54) found 95 patients with "basilar artery migraine" in one department over a 10-year period. Diagnostic uncertainty regarding this syndrome is thus considerable. Basilar migraine may be a reality in children or young adolescents. Hockaday (25) described a large number of children who by history had altered consciousness or vertigo, and a few had diplopia, tinnitus, or dysarthria. It remains uncertain whether the brain stem is really involved. Electroencephalographic tracings during attacks indicate bihemispheric dysfunction (32,55), as does a single regional cerebral blood flow (RCBF) study (41). Absence of evidence for basilar artery spasm during migraine attacks and uncertainty about the origin of symptoms prompted the IHS to remove the word "artery" from the diagnosis. Systematic clinical description and RCBF studies during more attacks are needed to definitively establish or disprove the existence of migraine aura originating in the brain stem. The diagnosis of basilar migraine is sometimes made in a rather facile manner in patients who present with episodes of syncope followed by headache. Given the uncertainty surrounding basilar migraine, the diagnosis should be made only after the other possible causes (especially cardiac causes) of syncope have been eliminated. For further details, see elsewhere in this volume.

Migraine Aura without Headache

IHS code and diagnosis: 1.2.5 Migraine aura without headache

WHO code and diagnosis: G43.IX4 Migraine aura without headache

Short description (23): Migrainous aura unaccompanied by headache.

Other terms (23): Migraine equivalents, acephalic migraine.

Diagnostic criteria (23):
  A. Fulfills criteria for 1.2.
  B. No headache.

The existence of migraine aura without headache has been documented for at least a century (1). Several articles have described a number of cases (15,16,38,59). The symptoms of migraine aura without headache are no different from those of aura followed by a headache phase. General population studies indicate that migraine aura without headache is common, especially in men and especially in those with advancing age (46). Many patients have some attacks with headache and others without headache (48).

Migraine with Acute Onset Aura

IHS code and diagnosis: 1.2.6 Migraine with acute onset aura

WHO code and diagnosis: G43.12 Migraine with acute onset aura

Short description (23): Migraine with aura developing fully in less than 5 minutes.

Diagnostic criteria (23):
  A. Fulfills criteria for 1.2.
  B. Neurologic symptoms develop within 4 minutes.
  C. Headache lasts 4 to 72 hours (untreated or unsuccessfully treated).
  D. Headache has at least two of the following characteristics:
    1. Unilateral location
    2. Pulsating quality
    3. Moderate or severe intensity (inhibits or prohibits daily activities)
    4. Aggravated by walking stairs or similar routine physical activity
  E. During headache at least one of the following:
    1. Nausea and/or vomiting
    2. Photophobia and phonophobia
  F. Thromboembolic transient ischemic attack (TIA) and other intracranial lesion ruled out by appropriate investigations.

Fisher (15,16) described a number of patients in whom the onset of neurologic symptoms was abrupt but whom he nevertheless thought had migraine. This was based on absence of angiographic abnormalities, recurrence of the episodes, and a benign course during long-term follow-up. Occasional cases of abrupt onset also have been noted by others (9, personal observation). Russell and Olesen reported that 4 of 163 patients with migraine with aura

experienced exclusively acute onset aura (48). However, because there are many reasons why a patient might report sudden onset of symptoms even if it were gradual (e.g., expansion of a negative scotoma or initiation of symptoms during sleep), the diagnostic entity is probably quite rare. Because it may be mimicked by embolic episodes, the diagnosis should be given cautiously.

INTERRELATIONSHIPS BETWEEN SUBFORMS OF MIGRAINE WITH AURA

As already indicated above, subforms of migraine with aura are not mutually exclusive. They tend to mix, and one form may shift into another during the years. Other affected family members often have a different subform of migraine with aura. The preceding chapters imply, perhaps incorrectly, that all forms of migraine with aura share a common pathophysiology and that they can all be treated with the same drugs with equal effectiveness. It is to be hoped that future epidemiologic/genetic studies will make it possible to subclassify migraine with aura in a more logical fashion.

REFERENCES

1. Airy H. On a distinct form of transient hemiopsia. *Philos Trans R Soc Lond B Biol Sci* 1870;160:247–264.
2. Alvarez WC. The migrainous scotoma as studied in 618 persons. *Am J Ophthalmol* 1960;49:489–504.
3. Ardila A, Sanchez E. *Neuropsychologic* symptoms in the migraine syndrome. *Cephalalgia* 1988;8:67–70.
4. Bana DS, Graham JR. Observations on prodromes of classic migraine in a headache population. *Headache* 1986;26:216–219.
5. Bickerstaff ER. Basilar artery migraine. In: Rose FC, ed. *Handbook of clinical neurology.* Vol. 4 (48). Amsterdam: Elsevier, 1986:135–140.
6. Bickerstaff ER, Birm MD. Basilar artery migraine. *Lancet* 1961; 1: 15–17.
7. Blau JN. *Migraine: clinical, therapeutic, conceptual and research aspects.* London: Chapman & Hall, 1987.
8. Blau JN. Migraine with aura and migraine without aura are not different entities. *Cephalalgia* 1995;15:186–190.
9. Bradshaw P, Parsons M. Hemiplegic migraine, a clinical study. *Q J Med* 1965;34:65–85.
10. Bücking H, Baumgartner G, Klinik und Pathophysiologie der initialen neurologischen Symptome bei fokalen Migraenen (Migraine ophthalmique, migraine accompagnd). *Arch Psychiatr Nervenkr* 1974;219: 37–52.
11. Cutrer FM, Baloh RW. Migraine-associated dizziness. *Headache* 1992; 32:300–304.
12. Ehyai A, Fenichel GM. The natural history of acute confusional migraine. *Arch Neurol* 1978;35:368–369.
13. Feely MP, O'Hare J, Veale D, Callaghan N. Episodes of acute confusion or psychosis in familial hemiplegic migraine. *Acta Neurol Scand* 1982; 65:369–375.
14. Ferguson KS, Robinson SS. Life-threatening migraine. *Arch Neurol* 1982;39:374–376.
15. Fisher CM. Late-life migraine accompaniments as a cause of unexplained transient ischemic attacks. *Can J Neurol Sci* 1980;7:9–17.
16. Fisher CM. Late-life migraine accompaniments: further experience. *Stroke* 1986;17:1033–1042.
17. Fitzsimons RB, Wolfenden WH. Migraine coma. Meningitic migraine with cerebral oedema associated with a new form of autosomal dominant cerebellar ataxia. *Brain* 1985;108:555–577.
18. Fuller GN, Guiloff RJ. Migrainous olfactory hallucinations. *J Neurol Neurosurg Psychiatry* 1987;50:1688–1690.
19. Gardner K, Barmada MM, Ptacek LJ, Hoffman EP. A new locus for hemplegic migraine maps to Chromosome 1q31. *Neurology* 1997;49: 1231–1238.

20. Glista GG, Mellinger JF, Rooke ED. Familial hemiplegic migraine. *Mayo Clin Proc* 1975;50:307–311.
21. Hachinski VC, Porchawka J, Steele JC. Visual symptoms in the migraine syndrome. *Neurology* 1973;23:570–579.
22. Hare EH. Personal observations on the spectral march of migraine. *J Neurol Sci* 1966;3:259–264.
23. Headache Classification Committee of the International Headache Society. Classification and diagnostic criteria for headache disorders, cranial neuralgias and facial pain. *Cephalalgia* 1988;8[Suppl 7]:1–96.
24. Heyck H. Varieties of hemiplegic migraine. *Headache* 1973;12:135–142.
25. Hockaday JM. Basilar migraine in childhood. *Dev Med Child Neurol* 1979;21:455–463.
26. Holub V, Chrast B, Saxi 0. Toedlicher Ausgang eines kindlichen Migraineanfalles. *Kinderärztl Prax* 1965;33:539–546.
27. Jensen K, Tfelt-Hansen P, Lauritzen M, Olesen J. Classic migraine. A prospective recording of symptoms. *Acta Neurol Scand* 1986;73: 359–362.
28. Jensen TS, Olivarius BF, Kraft M, Hansen HJ. Familial hemiplegic migraine: a reappraisal and a long-term follow-up study. *Cephalalgia* 1981;1:33–39.
29. Jolly F. Über Flimmerskotom und Migraene. *Berlin Klin Wschr* 1902; 42:973–976.
30. Joutel A, Bousser MG, Biousse V, et al. A gene for familial hemiplegic migraine map to chromosome 19. *Nat Genet* 1993;5:40–45.
31. Lashley KS. Patterns of cerebral integration indicated by the scotomas of migraine. *Arch Neurol Psychiatry* 1941;46:259–264.
32. Lee CH, Lance JW. Migraine stupor. *Headache* 1977;17:32–38.
33. Lewis NP, Fraser AG. Syncope while vomiting during migraine attack. *Lancet* 1988;2:400–401.
34. Lord GDA. Clinical characteristics of the migrainous aura. In: Amery WK, Wauquier A, eds. *The prelude to the migraine attack.* London: Baillière Tindall, 1986:87–98.
35. Manzoni GC, Farina S, Lanfranchi M, Solari A. Classic migraine: clinical findings in 164 patients. *Eur Neurol* 1985;24:163–169.
36. Mfinte TF, Mijiler-Vahl H. Familial migraine coma: a case study. *J Neurol* 1990;237:59–61.
37. Neligan P, Harriman DGF, Pearse J. Respiratory arrest in familial hemiplegic migraine: a clinical and neuropathological study. *Br Med J* 1977;2:732–734.
38. O'Connor PS, Tredici TJ. Acephalgic migraine. Fifteen years experience. *Ophthalmology* 1981;88:993–1003.
39. Olesen J, Friberg L, Olsen TS, et al. Timing and topography of cerebral blood flow, aura and headache during migraine attacks. *Ann Neurol* 1990;28:791–798.
40. Olesen J, Jorgensen MB. Leao's spreading depression in the hippocampus explains transient global amnesia. *Acta Neurol Scand* 1986;73: 219–220.
41. Olesen J, Larsen B, Lauritzen M. Focal hyperemia followed by spreading oligemia and impaired activation of RCBF in classic migraine. *Ann Neurol* 1981;9:344–352.
42. Ophoff RA, Terwindt GM, Vergouwe MN, et al. Familial hemiplegic migraine and episodic ataxia type-2 are caused by mutations in the Ca^{2+} channel gene CACNL1A4. *Cell* 1996;87:543–552.
43. Parrish RM, Stevens H. Familial hemiplegia migraine. *Minnesota Med* 1972;60:709–715.
44. Peatfield R. *Headache.* New York: Springer-Veriag, 1986.
45. Rasmussen BK. Migraine with aure and migraine without aura are two different entities. *Cephalalgia* 1995;15:183–186.
46. Rasmussen BK, Olesen J. Migraine with aura and migraine without aura. An epidemiological study. *Cephalalgia* 1992;12:221–228.
47. Russell MB, Iversen HK, Olesen J. Improved description of the migraine aura by a diagnostic aura diary. *Cephalalgia* 1994;14: 107–117.
48. Russell MB, Olesen J. A nosographic analysis of the migraine aura in a general population. *Brain* 1996;119:335–361.
49. Sacks 0. *Migraine.* London: Faber & Faber, 1991.
50. Schiller F. The migraine tradition. *Bull Hist Med* 1975;49:1–19.
51. Schumacher JA, Wolff HJ. Experimental studies on headache. *Arch Neurol Psychiatry* 1941;45:199–214.
52. Selby G, Lance JW. Observations on 500 cases of migraine and allied vascular headache. *J Neurol Neurosurg Psychiatry* 1960;23:2332.
53. Sinforiani E, Zineiii P, Faglia L, et al. Lateralization of visual attention in patients with classic migraine and unilateral prodromes. *Funct Neurol* 1989;4:247–252.
54. Sturzenegger MH, Meienberg 0. Basilar artery migraine: a follow-up study of 82 cases. *Headache* 1985;25:408–415.
55. Swanson JW, Vick NA. Basilar artery migraine. 12 patients, with an attack recorded electroencephalographically. *Neurology* 1978;28: 782–786.
56. Tietjen G. Migraine with aura and migraine without aura: one entity, two or more? *Cephalalgia* 1995;15:182–183.
57. Whitman BW, Lipton RB. Oscillocusis: an unusual auditory aura in migraine. *Headache* 1995;35:428–429.
58. Whitty CWM. Familial hemiplegic migraine. *J Neurol Neurosurg Psychiatry* 1953;16:172–177.
59. Whitty CWM. Migraine without headache. *Lancet* 1967;2:283–285.
60. Wolberg FL, Ziegler DK. Olfactory hallucinations in migraine. *Arch Neurol* 1982;39:382.

The Headaches, Second Edition,
edited by J. Olesen, P. Tfelt-Hansen, and K.M.A. Welch.
Lippincott Williams & Wilkins, Philadelphia © 2000.

The Migraines

CHAPTER 44

Diagnosis and Differential Diagnosis

J. Keith Campbell and Fumihiko Sakai

The diagnosis of migraine is made clinically; there are no blood tests, imaging, or electrophysiologic tests to confirm the diagnosis. Investigations are needed to rule out structural, biochemical, and other causes of headache that can mimic migraine.

Migraine is easy to diagnose when it is episodic, is associated with an aura, or is accompanied by gastrointestinal symptoms and associated symptoms such as photophobia, phonophobia, and pallor (3). Relief with sleep, aggravation of the pain by a Valsalva maneuver or the head-low position, pain involving half of the head, and attacks triggered by such factors as the menstrual cycle, fasting, oversleeping, indulgence in alcohol, or tyramine-containing foods are all helpful in the diagnosis. Recurrent headaches of this type, especially if there is a family history of similar headaches, over a period of years separated by periods of freedom make the diagnosis of migraine so likely that investigations are rarely necessary (2). When the history is less typical, when the subject is seen with or shortly after the initial headache, or when anxiety is such that more than reassurance is needed, neuroimaging may be necessary. Computerized tomography (CT) or, preferably, magnetic resonance imaging (MRI) would be the investigation of choice to exclude structural abnormalities mimicking migraine.

Migraine can simulate or be simulated by most of the primary and secondary headaches; as a consequence, the

J.K. Campbell: Department of Neurology, Mayo Clinic and Mayo Medical School, Rochester, Minnesota 55905.

F. Sakai: Department of Medicine, Kitasato University, 1-15-1 Kitasato, Sagamihara, 228 Kanagawa, Japan.

TABLE 1. *Causes of headache in the differential diagnosis of migraine*

Cerebrovascular disorders
  Transient ischemic attacks
  Cerebral infarction
  Cerebral hemorrhage
  Subarachnoid hemorrhage, especially sentinel leaks
  Intracranial hematoma
  Intracranial aneurysm and AVM
  Arterial dissection, carotid or vertebral
  Venous thrombosis
  Arterial hypertension
  Cranial vasculitis
Nonvascular intracranial disorders
  Benign intracranial hypertension (pseudotumor)
  Low CSF pressure
  Intracranial neoplasm
Chemical, metabolic, endocrine abnormalities
  Nitrites, nitrates, other vasodilators
  Hypoxia, hypoglycemia, dialysis, hypercarbia
Cranium, neck, eyes, and nose
  Arnold-Chiari malformation
  Cervical spine abnormalities
  Purulent sinusitis
  Sinus and base of skull neoplasms
  Glaucoma, refractive errors (children)
  Tolosa-Hunt syndrome
  Raeder's syndrome
Others
  Epilepsy
  Trauma
  Other primary headaches
  Fever, systemic disease

AVM, arteriovenous malformation; CSF, cerebrospinal fluid.

differential diagnosis is essentially that of almost all conditions that can present with headache. Table 1 lists many disorders that must be considered.

HEADACHES ASSOCIATED WITH VASCULAR DISORDERS

Transient Ischemic Attack (TIA)

Headache as a manifestation of transient cerebral ischemia is relatively common (7,11), but the focal neurologic symptoms of the attack need to be differentiated from an aura of migraine. The motor or sensory symptoms contralateral to hemispheric ischemia, like the weakness or subjective sense of heaviness and the paresthesias of a migraine aura, can involve the face, limbs, or trunk. A motor or sensory march of symptoms may occur but tends to be much quicker in a TIA than in migraine. The motor or sensory spread of a TIA is rapid, taking only seconds to a minute to move from the face to the hand, then marching up the arm to the trunk. Progression down the trunk to the lower limb can occur in both conditions. The march of motor and sensory changes in migraine is slow, taking a number of minutes to reach to its maximum distribution. The sensory symptoms in migraine are commonly a positive phenomenon, that is, a tingling sensation rather than a sense of numbness or sensory loss. Whereas the former can occur in a TIA, a sense of numbness or deadness is more often described. In both conditions, the sensory disturbances still can be spreading to new areas of involvement while simultaneously clearing from previously involved areas.

The weakness of a TIA is usually far greater than in a migrainous aura, but in the case of hemiplegic migraine, the difference can be minor and not diagnostic. Recovery can be over a similar period in both TIAs and migraine, but most TIAs are very short-lived, and recovery is within minutes. A long history of similar attacks, onset in youth or early adult life, a personal or family history of migraine, and a normal clinical and noninvasive neurovascular examination all point to a migraine aura as the cause of the transient symptoms. Even in later life, when TIAs are more common, migraine can be the cause of such events (8,10).

A hemianopia is a relatively rare manifestation of a TIA and does not generally have the scintillating and spreading features of the visual aura of migraine. The visual loss of a TIA is usually a negative scotoma (black) rather than the positive scotoma (bright) of migraine. *Amaurosis fugax* is a sudden onset of monocular blindness followed by gradual clearing of vision in 5 to 10 minutes. This pattern of visual disturbance is contrasted with an initial small area of scintillating scotoma that spreads gradually in the visual field in migraine.

Transient ischemic events can result in brainstem and temporo-occipital dysfunction, leading to vertigo, tinnitus, bilateral visual disturbances, weakness of both sides of the body, and such symptoms as dysarthria, dysphagia, and diplopia. A similar constellation of symptoms occurs in basilar artery migraine (1). Headache can occur in both conditions, but in basilar migraine the headache is severe and almost always presents as the neurologic symptoms subside. Basilar migraine is most common in teenagers or in early adult life, whereas vertebrobasilar TIAs usually occur later in life. An overlap does occur; therefore, age alone is not an arbiter. Arteriography (MR or conventional) may be required for clarification.

Thromboembolic Stroke

Cerebral infarction, particularly cerebral embolism, often is associated with headache (7,17) and sometimes with positive visual symptoms, such as phosphenes or other visual hallucinations, when the vertebrobasilar arterial system is involved. It is rarely confused with migraine, because the resulting neurologic deficit generally suggests the presence of the structural lesion. Arteriography or noninvasive vascular studies, echocardiography, and coagulation studies may be required for final diagnosis. The dominantly inherited arteriopathy associated with recurrent subcortical infarction (CADASIL) can, at least early in its course, mimic migraine attacks. The family history, the progressive course, and the characteristic subcortical infarcts shown on MRI make the diagnosis clear.

Intracranial Hematoma

In most instances, an intracranial hematoma, if it gives rise to headache, also produces other neurologic symptoms. Impaired consciousness, focal neurologic deficits, and a progressive course are characteristic. A hematoma in the head of the caudate nucleus or periventricular area may cause severe headache without obvious neurologic symptoms. A subcortical hematoma in a nonsymptomatic area may cause only dull headache, and careful neurological examination of mental and higher cortical function may suggest the diagnosis. Confusion with migraine could occur in a patient with a prior history of the primary headache disorder. The recent and sudden onset of a headache, a history of head trauma, or the development of neurologic signs, especially if progressive, should lead to examination by CT or MRI, which will reveal the hematoma.

Subarachnoid Hemorrhage and Intracranial Aneurysms

Many patients who eventually have a subarachnoid hemorrhage (SAH) report a history of headaches that were not recognized as warnings of an impending catastrophic hemorrhage (14). Such sentinel or warning headaches are due to small, self-limited hemorrhages from the aneurysm or (more rarely), arteriovenous malformation (AVM), which eventually gives rise to the major hemorrhage. Many sentinel headaches are ignored or dismissed as migraine, tension-type headache, or due to other benign causes. Neck stiffness may be absent, and the pain may have subsided by the time the patient is examined. An unenhanced CT scan to look for blood in the basal subarachnoid cisterns should be obtained. If the CT is normal, a cerebrospinal fluid (CSF) examination should be performed. Unfortunately, a normal CT and CSF examination does not completely exclude a small SAH or help to distinguish between a migraine and the potentially far more serious headache. MR angiography or conventional angiography should be obtained when there is any doubt about the nature of the headache.

Day and Raskin (6) described a headache of dramatic suddenness known as the *thunderclap* headache. Investigations sometimes reveal an aneurysm that has not bled but that is associated with diffuse spasm of the surrounding vessels. The sudden onset of the headache is unlikely to be confused with migraine in most instances, although a sudden-onset variety of migraine has been referred to as a *crash* or *blitz* migraine (9). As with other extremely severe headaches of abrupt onset, neuroimaging is a serious consideration.

Unruptured Intracranial Vascular Malformations

A headache indistinguishable from migraine with or without aura can occur ipsilateral to a vascular malformation. The unlikely presence of an AVM is but one of the reasons a CT or MRI scan should be considered in the evaluation of any patient with a migrainous history. The coexistence of migraine and seizures should especially prompt investigation, because an AVM is even more likely to produce epilepsy than headache.

Dural AVMs of the sigmoid or cavernous sinus region can produce episodic headache with the features of migraine. They also can cause raised intracranial pressure and a variety of visual symptoms. Neurovascular imaging is required for definitive diagnosis.

Arteritis

Giant cell arteritis (temporal arteritis) is characteristically a cause of headache in patients aged over 65 years (4). The headache tends to be constant, progressive, and associated with tenderness of the scalp, jaw claudication, and often systemic symptoms such as fatigue, myalgias, and low-grade fever. The headaches are often worse at night and on exposure to cold. The progressive nature of the headache and the associated features help distinguish it from migraine. The elevated sedimentation rate and abnormal temporal artery biopsy confirm the diagnosis.

Carotid or Vertebral Artery Pain

Dissection of one of the great cervical vessels usually results in unilateral pain of sudden onset. Carotid dissec-

tion causes local neck pain and pain behind the ipsilateral eye (16). The pain is persistent for some days to several weeks. An ipsilateral Horner syndrome is commonly noted. Migraine usually is excluded easily by the history, although the pain may wax and wane and may be made worse by coughing, sneezing, and bending. Angiography is the definitive investigation, although MR angiography and carotid ultrasound also may be diagnostic. Vertebral artery dissection produces neck and occipital pain. The abrupt onset and occasional association of brainstem ischemic symptoms should prevent confusion with migraine.

Idiopathic carotidynia can be recurrent and result in neck and ipsilateral head and facial pain. The carotid artery in the neck is exquisitely tender. An initial attack is difficult to distinguish from a carotid dissection. The relationship of this disorder to migraine is uncertain.

Arterial Hypertension

Rapid elevation of blood pressure from any cause can result in headache. Pheochromocytoma or certain vasoactive drugs such as amphetamines, phenylpropanolamine, or a monamine oxidase (MAO) inhibitor in the presence of an amine can produce severe episodic headaches. When headache is a manifestation of sustained severe hypertension, it may be associated with papilledema. The early morning headache of hypertension can mimic migraine. Measurement of the blood pressure leads to the diagnosis. A CT or MRI scan of the head is necessary to rule out an intracranial mass or hydrocephalus causing the papilledema.

HEADACHES ASSOCIATED WITH NONVASCULAR INTRACRANIAL DISORDERS

Elevated Cerebrospinal Fluid Pressure

Pseudotumor cerebri can result in episodic headache and vomiting (5), but it is unlikely to be confused with migraine for long, because the development of visual blurring, visual obscurations, and persistent headache prompts the subject to seek medical help. The association of headache, obesity, menstrual irregularity, and papilledema in a young woman is likely due to benign intracranial hypertension. A CT, or preferably an MRI, to rule out an intracranial mass, particularly in the posterior fossa, is essential.

Low Cerebrospinal Fluid Pressure Headache

This type of headache occurs after a lumbar puncture or may be due to the loss of fluid through the nose, ears, or operative site (13). The headache is characteristic. Standing increases the pain and recumbency gives almost immediate relief. This orthostatic pattern is quite unlike migraine, but demonstration of low CSF pressure (<80 mm H_2O) is needed to confirm the diagnosis of a hypoliquorrheic headache. Traumatic or spontaneous rupture of the thecal sac in the spine is the usual cause of orthostatic headache (13). Unilateral or bilateral subdural hematoma sometimes occurs as a consequence of low CSF pressure and may add a different type of headache. Radionuclide cisternography or CT myelography may be required in the investigation of a spontaneous low CSF pressure headache.

Intracranial Infection, Sarcoidosis, and Other Noninfectious Inflammatory Diseases

Although these conditions can produce episodic headaches of a throbbing type that worsens with coughing, they are usually progressive and may be associated with fever, cranial nerve deficits, and neck stiffness. After noninvasive imaging with CT or MRI, a CSF examination confirms the presence of a meningeal process.

Intracranial Tumors

Headache caused by an intracranial tumor initially may be episodic and quite lateralized, mimicking migraine. With time, the headache may change to that of raised intracranial pressure, wakening the subject during the night and becoming associated with nausea and vomiting. The temporal profile depends on whether the lesion obstructs the CSF pathways early or late in its development. Posterior fossa lesions have a much shorter time course.

Colloid cysts and other ventricular tumors, such as ependymomas, can present with episodic headache, nausea, and vomiting and hence are the most likely of intracranial masses to mimic migraine. Examination by CT or preferably MRI reveals the cause.

HEADACHES ASSOCIATED WITH SUBSTANCES OR THEIR WITHDRAWAL

Many substances responsible for the headache are, ironically, used for relief of headaches. Ergotamine preparations and combination analgesics are the main offenders when taken daily or in excessive amounts. Alcohol, nitrites and nitrates, monosodium glutamate, indomethacin, nifedipine, and many other substances can induce headache resembling migraine or simply trigger migraine. Removal or avoidance of the offending substances with relief of the headache confirms their role as migraine triggers or the cause of the headache.

HEADACHES ASSOCIATED WITH METABOLIC DISORDERS

Hypoxia

High altitude, hypoxia due to pulmonary disease, or sleep apnea can result in a pounding headache resembling migraine without aura. Migrainous subjects are particularly susceptible to the headaches of high altitude.

Carbon dioxide retention secondary to emphysema, often associated with hypoxia, also results in a vascular headache. Hypoglycemia and renal dialysis are both capable of producing a throbbing headache with migrainous features.

In each instance, the history should provide the clue to the cause of the headache. Pulmonary function studies, overnight polysomnography, arterial blood gas analysis, and determination of the plasma glucose may be required. In some instances, CT or MRI examination of the head will be needed to exclude an intracranial cause, especially when severe carbon dioxide retention results in papilledema.

HEADACHES ASSOCIATED WITH DISEASES OF THE NECK, CRANIUM, EYES, EARS, SINUSES, TEETH, AND OTHER STRUCTURES

Cervical Spine

The role of the neck in the pathogenesis of headache is controversial. It has been stated that a cervicogenic headache radiates from the neck, often unilaterally to the orbital or retroorbital region ipsilaterally (19). Associated autonomic features can include ipsilateral overflow of tears and conjunctival injection. More generally accepted is an occipital-cervical pain secondary to cervical muscle tension triggered by bony and postural abnormalities of the cervical spine. The headache is not accompanied by autonomic features and should be readily distinguished from migraine. The history, pain, and limitations of movement of the cervical spine and cervical spine radiographic findings are helpful in the diagnosis.

Eyes

In children, refractive errors can give rise to episodic frontal headaches resembling migraine without aura. This rarely occurs in adults.

Acute glaucoma in adults can result in severe eye and supraorbital pain. Attacks may occur at night and resemble migraine. The affected globe may be hard and the cornea steamy. Ophthalmologic examination confirms the diagnosis.

Sinuses

Contrary to common lay opinion, sinus abnormalities other than acute purulent sinusitis are rarely the cause of headache.

Teeth, Jaws, and Temporomandibular Joint Disease

Referred pain from these structures can cause headache but rarely with the characteristics of migraine. Pain on chewing or pain on exposure of the teeth to hot and cold stimuli should help to pinpoint the source of the pain.

HEADACHES ASSOCIATED WITH HEAD TRAUMA

Acute attacks of migraine, especially migraine with aura, can be triggered by recurrent minor head trauma, for example, footballer's (soccer players) migraine from "heading" the ball (15). Acute posttraumatic headache is not likely to be confused with migraine if the history is ascertained. Chronic posttraumatic headaches, although they tend to be persistent, can be episodic and may be confused with migraine. Neuroimaging is necessary to exclude such conditions as a chronic subdural hematoma.

MISCELLANEOUS HEADACHES OCCASIONALLY CONFUSED WITH MIGRAINE

Benign cough headache, benign exertional headache, and the headaches associated with sexual activity can occur in migraineurs or totally independently. The history of a sudden onset of headache during exertion or during sexual activity or in relation to a cough or sneeze differentiates the headache from that of migraine.

Epilepsy can result in recurrent headaches, but the seizure prior to the headache indicates the nature of the disorder.

Recurrent migrainelike episodes have been described in persons infected with human immunodeficiency virus (HIV) in the absence of intracranial infection. In many patients who have been studied, anticardiolipin antibodies have been detected (18).

Migraine can be a feature of the MELAS (mitochondrial myopathy, encephalopathy, lactic acidosis, and strokelike episodes) syndrome and other mitochondrial disorders. Recurrent strokes in the MELAS syndrome and myoclonic epilepsy in association with a mitochondrial myopathy help distinguish these rare disorders from migraine (12).

REFERENCES

1. Bickerstaff ER. Basilar artery migraine. *Lancet* 1961;1:15–17.
2. Blau JN. Headache: history, examination, differential diagnosis and special investigations. In: Vinken PJ, Bruyn GW, Klawans HL, eds. *Handbook of clinical neurology*, vol 48. New York: Elsevier, 1986:43–58.
3. Campbell JK. Manifestations of migraine. In: Mathew NT, ed. *Neurologic clinics*, vol 8. Philadelphia: WB Saunders, 1990:841–855.
4. Caselli RJ, Hunder GG. Giant cell (temporal) arteritis as a cause of headache in the elderly. In: Goadsby PJ, Silberstein SD, eds. *Headache*. Boston: Butterworth-Heinemann, 1997:299–311.
5. Corbett JJ. Headache due to idiopathic intracranial hypertension. In: Goadsby PJ, Silberstein SD, eds. *Headache*. Boston: Butterworth-Heinemann, 1997:279–283.
6. Day JW, Raskin NH. "Thunderclap" headache: symptom of unruptured cerebral aneurysm. *Lancet* 1986;2:1247–1248.
7. Edmeads J. The headaches of ischemic cerebrovascular disease. *Headache* 1979;19:345–349.
8. Fisher CM. Late-life migraine accompaniments as a cause of unexplained transient ischemic attacks. *Can J Neurol Sci* 1980;7:9–17.
9. Fisher CM. Painful states: a neurological commentary. *Clin Neurosurg* 1984;31:32–53.
10. Fisher CM. Late-life migraine accompaniments—further experience. *Stroke* 1986;17:1033–1042.
11. Gorelick PB, Heir DB, Caplan LR, Langenberg P. Headache in acute cerebrovascular disease. *Neurology* 1986;36:1445–1450.
12. Klopstock T, May A, Seibel P, Papagiannuli E, Diener HC, Reichmann H. Mitochondrial DNA in migraine with aura. *Neurology* 1996;46:1735–1738.
13. Lay CL, Campbell JK. Low cerebrospinal fluid pressure headache. In: Goadsby PJ, Silberstein SD, eds. *Headache*. Boston: Butterworth-Heinemann, 1997:355–367.
14. Leblanc R. The minor leak preceding subarachnoid hemorrhage. *J Neurosurg* 1987;66:35–39.
15. Matthews WB. Footballer's migraine. *BMJ* 1972;2:326–327.
16. Mokri B, Sundt TM Jr, Houser OW, Piepgras DG. Spontaneous dissection of the cervical internal carotid artery. *Ann Neurol* 1986;19:126–138.
17. Portenoy RK, Abissi CJ, Lipton RB, et al. Headache in cerebrovascular disease. *Stroke* 1984;15:1009–1012.
18. Rinaldi R, Manfredi R, Azzimondi G, et al. Recurrent migrainelike episodes in patients with HIV disease. *Headache* 1997;37:443–448.
19. Sjaastad O, Fredriksen TA, Pfaffenrath V. Cervicogenic headache: diagnostic criteria. *Headache* 1998;38:442–445.

The Headaches, Second Edition,
edited by J. Olesen, P. Tfelt-Hansen, and K.M.A. Welch.
Lippincott Williams & Wilkins, Philadelphia © 2000.

The Migraines

CHAPTER 45

Prognosis of Migraine

Birthe Krogh Rasmussen and Richard B. Lipton

Information about the prognosis of migraine is sparse. It is still not clear how often attacks increase or decrease, completely remit, or change in character over the life span. Nor is it clear which genetic or environmental risk factors determine prognosis. Cross-sectional epidemiologic data have provided limited insight into how migraine evolves over time. If migraine sufferers from a representative general population are asked about how their headaches have changed over time, some may have difficulty remembering events of many years ago. Recall errors may vary with the time interval from the first or most recent attack and with the severity of illness. Moreover, possible cohort effects may not be detected.

Longitudinal prospective epidemiologic data with periodic contacts and examinations are necessary to draw valid conclusions about the prognosis and natural history of migraine. To date, few studies of representative migraine populations include follow-up evaluations. Bille (2–6) conducted follow-up studies of 73 children (aged 7–15 at study onset) 6, 16, 22, 30, and 40 years after an initial assessment. In the migraine group, 34% were free of migraine at the 6-year follow-up and 62% were free of migraine for at least 2 years at the 16-year follow-up. By the 22-year follow-up, about one third of this group were having migraine regularly. Thus, only 40% of the migraine children were free of migraine at the age of 30 years (Fig. 1). In the 30-year follow-up, 53% had migraine and 47% were migraine free. The 40-year follow-up showed that 29% of the original 73 migraine children had suffered from migraine the whole time since

childhood. Another 22% still had migraine, although they had experienced one or more migraine-free periods of 2-year duration or longer. Thus, over a 40-year period, more than half the migraineurs continued to report migraine attacks (see Fig. 1). Bille found an unfavorable prognosis in girls compared with boys and also in children with visual aura (3,5).

Sillanpää conducted follow-up of 2,921 Finnish schoolchildren, when they entered school at age 7 years and again at age 14 years. Of the children who had migraine at the age of 7 years, 22% had complete remission and 37% showed some alleviation; so a total of 59% improved. On the other hand, 41% were unchanged or experiencing more severe migraine (14). The prognosis for migraine that had begun before school age was better for boys than for girls, and migraine with onset at age 8 to 14 years had a better prognosis in girls than in boys (14). In another recent Finnish study of the outcome of migraine in early school-aged children (12), boys at age 11 to 12 had a worse prognosis than girls, as measured by attack frequency.

In a cross-sectional study of young adults (21 to 30 years old), the last-year persistence rate of migraine was defined as the proportion of those meeting lifetime criteria for migraine who reported a migraine attack in the preceding year. In men the persistence rate was 48% and in women 79%, suggesting a higher rate of remission in young adulthood among men compared with women (8). In general, men had an earlier average age of onset than females, a finding that was confirmed in another American study using reconstructed cohort methods (16).

Whitty and Hockaday (19) conducted follow-up of 92 migraine patients for periods of 15 to 20 years and found cessation in about one third of patients and improvement in more than two thirds of those with continuing attacks. Some patients showed a long-term picture of migraine in

B. K. Rasmussen, Department of Neurology, Hilleroed Hospital, DK-3400 Hilleroed, Denmark.

R. B. Lipton: Departments of Neurology, Epidemiology, and Social Medicine, Albert Einstein College of Medicine, and Headache Unit, Montefiore Medical Center, Bronx, New York 10467.

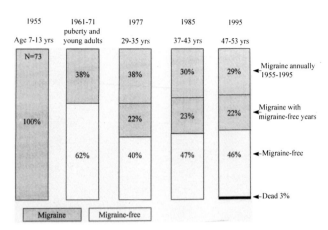

FIG. 1. The prognosis for schoolchildren with pronounced migraine during a 40-year follow-up period. (From ref. 6, with permission.)

which attacks ceased completely in early adult life and recurred later. Even after migraine remits, in many patients, the capacity to have migraine remains, as demonstrated by reactivation of the disorder after a headache-free period (5–7,19). No age factor (age itself, age at onset, time since onset) was of prognostic value (19). Also, Fry (10), by collecting information for 15 years from his general practice, found a tendency for the severity and frequency of migraine attacks to become less over the years and found cessation in 32% of males and 42% of females after 15 years. The condition thus seems to be self-limiting according to several studies.

A number of studies suggest that the prevalence of migraine increases steadily from infancy until approximately the age of 40 years (3,5,9,14,17). A decrease in migraine with increasing age begins in the fifth or sixth decade of life (1,13,17). The lower prevalence in older age groups observed in cross-sectional studies may be due to spontaneous remission, treatment, or increased incidence in younger age cohorts. There is no systematic evidence to suggest increased mortality among older subjects with migraine. Leviton and colleagues (11) reported that the risk for migraine sufferers dying before age 70 years is 1.9 times higher than that of subjects without migraine. On the other hand, Waters and colleagues (18), in a 12-year follow-up of the Pontypridd Survey, found significantly lower mortality in women with one or more migrainous features compared with women with headache only or no headache. This unexpected finding may be due to higher consultation rates with general practi-

tioners among migraineurs, which would increase detection and improve treatment of other diseases. Some evidence for an increased incidence of migraine in younger age cohorts has been observed (15), but further confirmation of such secular trends is required.

In summary, it seems likely that migraine becomes attenuated or disappears with advancing age, although in some subjects recurrence of attacks is seen after a shorter or longer migraine-free period. Additional long-term follow-up studies are needed to evaluate prognosis, mortality, morbidity, and incidence of migraine more precisely.

REFERENCES

1. Abramson JH, Hopp C, Epstein LM. Migraine and non-migrainous headaches: a community survey in Jerusalem. *J Epidemiol Community Health* 1980;34:188–93.
2. Bille B. Migraine in school children. *Acta Paediatr* 1962;51(Suppl 136):1–151.
3. Bille B. The prognosis of migraine in childhood. *Dan Med Bull* 1975; 22:112.
4. Bille B. Migraine in childhood and its prognosis. *Cephalalgia* 1981;1: 71–75.
5. Bille B. Migraine in childhood: a 30 year follow-up. In: Lanzi G, Balottin U, Cernibori A, eds. *Headache in children and adolescents.* Amsterdam: Elsevier Science Publishers B.V., 1989:19–26.
6. Bille B. A 40-year follow-up of school children with migraine. *Cephalalgia* 1997;17:488–491.
7. Blau JN. Loss of migraine: when, why and how. *J R Coll Physicians Lond* 1987;21:140–142.
8. Breslau N, Davis GC, Andreski P. Migraine, psychiatric disorders, and suicide attempts: an epidemiologic study of young adults. *Psychiatry Res* 1991;37:11–23.
9. Dalsgaard-Nielsen T, Engberg-Pedersen H, Holm HE. Clinical and statistical investigations of the epidemiology of migraine. *Dan Med Bull* 1970;17:138–148.
10. Fry J. *Profiles of disease.* Edinburgh: Livingstone, 1966, 142–143.
11. Leviton A, Malvea B, Graham JR. Vascular diseases, mortality, and migraine in the parents of migraine patients. *Neurology* 1974;24: 669–672.
12. Metsähonkala L, Sillanpää M, Tuominen J. Outcome of early school-age migraine. *Cephalalgia* 1997;17:662–665.
13. Nikiforow R. Headache in a random sample of 200 persons: a clinical study of a population in Northern Finland. *Cephalalgia* 1981;1:99–107.
14. Sillanpää M. Changes in the prevalence of migraine and other headaches during the first seven school years. *Headache* 1983;23: 15–19.
15. Sillanpää M, Anttila P. Increasing prevalence of headache in 7-year-old schoolchildren. *Headache* 1996;36:466–470.
16. Stewart WF, Linet MS, Celentano DD, Van Natta M, Ziegler D. Age- and sex-specific incidence rates of migraine with and without visual aura. *Am J Epidemiol* 1991;134:1111–1120.
17. Stewart WF, Lipton R, Celentano DD, Reed ML. Prevalence of migraine headache in the United States. *JAMA* 1992;267:64–69.
18. Waters WE, Campbell MJ, Elwood PC. Migraine, headache, and survival in women. *BMJ* 1983;287:1442–1443.
19. Whitty CWM, Hockaday JM. Migraine: a follow-up study of 92 patients. *BMJ* 1968;1:735–736.

The Headaches, Second Edition,
edited by J. Olesen, P. Tfelt-Hansen, and K.M.A. Welch.
Lippincott Williams & Wilkins, Philadelphia © 2000.

The Migraines

CHAPTER 46

General Approach to Treatment

Peer Tfelt-Hansen and Ninan T. Mathew

The first step in treatment is to establish the diagnosis of migraine. Migraine associated with neurologic signs and symptoms other than typical aura should be investigated via neuroimaging to exclude underlying conditions such as cerebral arteriovenous malformation, encephalomalacia, and, rarely, cerebral neoplasm. Headaches of recent onset without previous history, even if they manifest like migraine, should be investigated. In a patient with an established history of headache, a change in the pattern of headache should elicit concern and might warrant investigation to rule out the development of any new serious pathology.

COMORBIDITIES OF MIGRAINE

The clinician should be able to recognize coexisting conditions with migraine. These include frequent tension-type headache, as well as psychological and behavioral comorbidities such as anxiety, depression, panic episodes, bipolar illness, social phobias, and addictive tendencies. Asthma, allergies, and gastrointestinal disorders such as irritable bowel syndrome and hypertension are not infrequent comorbidities. Less well recognized are the gynecologic comorbidities in women with migraine. As the frequency of migraine and interictal tension-type headache increases, patients tend to take analgesics frequently, which eventually results in drug-induced chronic daily headache. This is often seen in patients who use multiple analgesics, particularly those containing caffeine, barbiturates, and codeine.

P. Tfelt-Hansen: Department of Neurology, Glostrup Hospital, University of Copenhagen, DK-2600 Glostrup, Copenhagen, Denmark.
N. T. Mathew: Houston Headache Clinic, Houston, Texas 77004.

DOCTOR–PATIENT RELATIONSHIP

It is imperative that a good doctor–patient relationship be developed that results in confidence on the part of the patient. Physicians who demonstrate an interest in the patient's symptoms and overall well-being are trusted more by patients. Patients appreciate an explanation of their illness by the physician. Good management of headache results from a partnership between doctor and patient.

HEADACHE DIARY

Patients should be encouraged to keep a headache diary, which should include the frequency, severity, duration, associated symptoms, and medications they are taking. Triggers for each attack, if identifiable, also should be recorded.

REALISTIC EXPECTATIONS

Physicians should encourage the patient to develop realistic expectations of the treatment of chronic migraine. It is important to explain that migraine is a recurrent disorder and that there is no total cure; the best that can be done is to keep the headaches under some control with abortive as well as preventive medications. Unrealistic expectations usually lead to therapeutic failure.

It is natural for the physician to become frustrated when dealing with chronic conditions such as migraine, but it is important that the physician not communicate that frustration to the patient. Expressions of encouragement and hope are important therapeutic strategies. A general practitioner with limited experience with headache patients may have an equal chance of success or failure as the more experienced headache specialist. A great deal depends on the ability of the physician to handle the patient with confidence, sympathy, and interest.

EDUCATION

Education of the patient is extremely important. The clinician may wish to provide the patient with educational materials on headache disorders and the clinical features of migraine, with an emphasis on the biological aspects. Educational materials also should attempt to dispel the myths about headaches. Good educational materials should encourage the patient to seek help, taking advantage of modern treatments available for these conditions. It is easier to treat a well-informed patient over the long term; education leads to cost-effective management of headache, avoiding unnecessary doctor visits, emergency room visits, and unnecessary tests.

BIOLOGICAL NATURE OF MIGRAINE WITH EMPHASIS ON TRIGGERS

Migraine is a disorder of the neurovascular system and is a special response of the human brain to both external and internal triggers. This tendency toward peculiar central nervous system response is probably genetically determined. Migraine patients have a lower threshold for triggering migraine attacks than non-migraneurs. This threshold is influenced by various factors, including female hormones, which account for hormone-related fluctuations in headache, such as in menstrual migraine. Other triggers also must be explained to the patient. Patients should be given a list of common triggers for migraine so that they can avoid headache episodes. Patients should be taught to look for the triggers that initiate their attacks and to record those triggers in their headache diaries. Common triggers are listed in Table 1. Clinicians should teach their patients behavioral modifications to avoid triggers. A simple explanation is all that is necessary in the majority of patients, which can be offered even by the busiest general practitioner. The importance of regular eating and sleeping habits should be emphasized. Too much and too little sleep can induce headaches, as can missing a meal.

Patients should scrutinize their diets carefully. The physician should acquire a detailed history of patients' diets, particularly regarding caffeine intake. Decreasing caffeine intake is extremely important in reducing the frequency of migraine. The myths about allergy to food should be dispelled. The most accurate explanation is that any dietary activators are usually chemicals, which cause a chemical reaction rather than an allergic response, and that the chemical reaction influences neurotransmitter functions, resulting in a migraine attack. This understanding of food triggers may circumvent the need for consultation with allergists and various expensive and extensive allergy tests with no beneficial outcome.

TREATMENT STRATEGIES

The first step in treatment is to recognize and avoid trigger factors. The patient should be asked to begin a headache diary; during subsequent office visits, the diary should be checked so that the patient can be instructed to avoid any triggers, if any can be identified from the diary. Medical and gynecologic comorbidities such as hypertension and ovarian steroid dysfunction should be corrected and controlled.

If stress is identified as a major factor, it is worthwhile to initiate a stress-management program while proceeding with pharmacologic therapy. Pharmacologic therapy alone, without addressing stress factors, may not be adequate treatment. Thus, behavioral and nonpharmacologic treatment should be administered concurrently with pharmacotherapy. For stress management, any form of relaxation exercise, including biofeedback training, is recommended. Physical exercise, relaxing to many patients, also should be encouraged. Exercise improves sleep, reduces weight, and gives the patient an overall sense of well-being. In the majority of patients, simple instructions from the physician about the broad principles of stress management are sufficient; however, in more complex cases, referral to a clinical psychologist or a behavioral therapist is beneficial.

Psychotherapy and psychiatric counseling may become necessary in patients with significant comorbidities such as depression, anxiety, poor coping abilities, and personality disorders. The practitioner will usually have to make an assessment over time concerning the need for psychotherapy. The question of psychotherapy should not be introduced to the patient during the first interview because the patient may get the incorrect impression that

TABLE 1. *Common provocational triggers for migraine*

Triggers for migraine	
Hormonal	Menstruation, ovulation, oral contraceptive, hormonal replacement
Dietary	Alcohol, nitrite-laden meat, monosodium glutamate, aspartame, chocolate, aged cheese, missing a meal
Psychological	Stress, poststress (weekend or vacation), anxiety, worry, depression
Physical-environmental	Glare, flashing lights, visual stimulation, fluorescent lighting, odors, weather changes, high altitude
Sleep-related	Lack of sleep, excessive sleep
Miscellaneous	Head trauma, physical exertion, fatigue
Drugs	Nitroglycerine, histamine, reserpine, hydralazine, ranitidine, estrogen

the physician views the problem as psychological. On the other hand, if the patient suggests the approach, the clinician should follow through.

Nonpharmacologic approaches should be initiated whether or not the patient is ready for pharmacotherapy. Principles that are outlined in the section on general principles of pharmacotherapy should be instituted (see Chapter 49). The difference between abortive and prophylactic treatment must be explained to the patient. The need for taking abortive medications at the onset of headache should be emphasized. Compliance is important in prophylactic therapy. The headache diary should note adverse effects from medications.

Other types of nonpharmacologic treatment may be considered, including physiotherapy, particularly with limited stretching of neck muscles. Massage, short-wave diathermy, and hot packs may be beneficial in those patients who have pericranial tenderness with their migraine attacks, or in those patients with tension-type headache in addition to migraine. If the interictal tension-type headache and muscle spasm can be reduced, it may secondarily reduce the migraine attacks as well.

The patient who fails to respond to conventional treatment may resort to alternative medications. The physician must warn the patient about the lack of information about many of the medications, which are often sold in health food stores. Other techniques such as acupuncture and hypnotherapy have not been evaluated in controlled scientific studies. Therefore, the physician may find it difficult to recommend those to the patient. Although individual patients may benefit from some of these alternative managements, the rationale for use of alternative medicines varies from unknown to, at best, uncertain.

The Headaches, Second Edition,
edited by J. Olesen, P. Tfelt-Hansen, and K.M.A. Welch.
Lippincott Williams & Wilkins, Philadelphia © 2000.

The Migraines

CHAPTER 47

Psychological and Behavioral Treatments of Migraine

Patrick J. McGrath, Kenneth A. Holroyd, and Marjolijn J. Sorbi

Behavioral treatments for migraine have been developed and well validated in carefully designed clinical trials. In contrast, psychotherapists using other techniques may treat patients with migraine with some success, but there has been a dearth of properly designed scientific trials evaluating psychotherapy in migraine. At best, psychotherapy is unproven as a treatment for migraine. As a result, this chapter will focus on behavioral treatments that have been scientifically evaluated.

Behavioral methods include a broad range of techniques. The most commonly investigated behavioral treatments for migraine are finger temperature biofeedback and relaxation, or a combination of these. Electromyographic (EMG) biofeedback and cephalic artery biofeedback have received limited attention as treatment for migraine and will not be reviewed. Operant methods (16) involving extinction of pain behavior and reinforcement of active, healthy behavior have been widely used in the treatment of patients with chronic pain, many of whom may suffer from migraine. However, operant strategies have not often been studied in migraine treatment. Cognitive therapy or stress coping training has been studied and will be reviewed.

The first report of behavioral treatment of migraine was Sargent's (42) serendipitous discovery of finger warming as a treatment for migraine. This has been followed by over 100 studies (excluding case studies) examining the effectiveness of behavioral treatments with migraine-type headaches (24).

In finger temperature warming, patients learn to warm their hands via visual or auditory feedback of changes in their finger temperature as measured by a simple thermistor. For example, a tone may increase or decrease in pitch or loudness as the finger temperature increases. Patients are encouraged to try what works but are often taught to use imagery, suggestions, and various types of relaxation training. Cephalic artery biofeedback uses the same principle, but blood flow in an external cephalic artery is monitored. It is not widely used because it is technically challenging and does not produce superior results. Muscle tension biofeedback uses EMG measurements of tension in the muscles of the head and neck and is commonly used in the treatment of tension headache but less often in the treatment of migraine.

Relaxation training includes progressive muscle relaxation modeled after Jacobson (28), imagery- and suggestion-based relaxation such as that described originally by Schultz and Luthe (43), and relaxation by way of breathing exercises (4). Progressive muscle relaxation involves a set of exercises in which muscles are tensed and then relaxed. The tension phase helps patients identify the difference between tension and relaxation and produces a relaxation rebound when the tension is released. Imagery-based relaxation uses pleasant imagery to induce relaxation. For example, a patient might use the image of lying on a beach and enjoying the warmth of the sun and gentle breezes. Imagery should be tailored to the individual patient because one patient's relaxing imagery may induce distress in another patient. Relaxation via suggestion involves repeated, often hypnotic-like sugges-

P. J. McGrath: Department of Psychology, Dalhouise University, Halifax, Nova Scotia B3H 4J1, Canada.

K. A. Holroyd: Department of Psychology, Ohio University, Athens, Ohio 45701-2979.

M. J. Sorbi: Department of Health Psychology, Utrecht University, 3508 TC Utrecht, The Netherlands.

TABLE 1. *Typical biofeedback/relaxation treatment programs*

Session	Content
1	Explanation of program and rationale. Relaxation training (tension-relaxation) with 16 muscle groups. Instruction in home practice.
2	Problems encountered with relaxation, relaxing imagery.
3	Relaxation training, discrimination training, relaxing imagery.
4	Relaxation training, discrimination training, relaxing imagery.
5	Relaxation with eight muscle groups, relaxing imagery.
6	Relaxation training with four muscle groups, relaxation by recall.
7	Introduce thermal biofeedback training and home biofeedback device. Use autogenic phrases.
8	Check problems with home biofeedback; thermal biofeedback training; cue control relaxation.
9	Thermal biofeedback training, cue controlled relaxation by recall.
10	Thermal biofeedback training.
11	Thermal biofeedback training; relax by recall.
12	Thermal biofeedback training.
13	Thermal biofeedback training; relax by recall.
14	Thermal biofeedback training.
15	Thermal biofeedback training; relax by recall.
16	Thermal biofeedback training; discuss problems, schedule posttreatment follow-up.

Revised from Blanchard and Andrasik (7).

tions to relax, let go, and loosen or smooth specific muscle groups. Suggestions of heaviness, warmth, calmness, and peacefulness are often used. Typically, patients are instructed in the procedure, the method is demonstrated, the patient practices under supervision, and then practices at home. Often an audiotape of the exercise is made for home practice. Hybridized forms of relaxation are often used, and there is little evidence to distinguish their efficacy from each other. However, there may be some advantage of combining relaxation with biofeedback or cognitive therapy (7,25,45).

Stress coping training—which is also called stress management, cognitive coping training, or cognitive therapy—includes identification of stresses and reactions to stress, change of thoughts and images about stressful situations, and learning coping strategies to manage stress. These methods derive from the pioneering work of Beck (3) in depression and Meichenbaum (36) in self-instruction. Typically, therapeutic interactions involve discussion of both cognitive and behavioral reactions to stressful situations and rehearsal of more adaptive coping strategies. Use is made of identifying and changing inner speech (i.e., what the patient is thinking or saying to him or herself). Special attention is directed to identifying and correcting thinking patterns that are causing distress. Catastrophic thinking (47), in which excessively negative and often vague outcomes are anticipated (e.g., "It is terrible that my boss doesn't understand me" or "I can't manage—it is impossible if I get a headache"), is a frequent target of therapy. Patients are taught to become aware of their thinking, to assess the usefulness or truth of their thinking, and to institute more helpful or realistic patterns of thinking. Unrealistic beliefs (e.g., "I must always be liked") and core beliefs that cause stress (e.g.,

"I am not a worthy person") are identified and the patient is taught how to refute them. Patients are often asked to keep a diary of specific situations and how they reacted to them.

Table 1 summarizes the content of typical treatment protocols used in cognitive therapy, and Table 2 presents a typical temperature biofeedback training protocol. These are standardized protocols; in clinical practice, the number and nature of sessions is likely to be tailored to the preferences of the individual patient and therapist, to be modified in response to the perceived effectiveness of the treatment, and to be influenced by the demands of the agency paying the bills.

Behavioral treatments have been used primarily for preventive or prophylactic treatment. They are also used by patients as palliative (to reduce pain during a headache) or abortive interventions (to interrupt headaches)

TABLE 2. *Typical cognitive therapy/relaxation program*

Session	Content
1	Rationale and explanation of stress-migraine model; first coping exercise and relaxation with tension.
2	Cognitive restructuring. Review of relaxation.
3	Examining unrealistic beliefs and their role in creating stress. Changing beliefs. Relaxation without tension.
4	Distraction strategies.
5	Imagery, behavior rehearsal, mental activities, relaxation with imagery.
6	Assertiveness, aggressivity, and passivity.
7	Problem solving.
8	Review of coping strategies.

Revised from McGrath et al. (35).

within a preventive treatment program. However, the efficacy of behavioral treatments in these latter capacities has not been evaluated. Behavioral treatments are unlikely to be used as stand-alone palliative or abortive interventions.

OUTCOME OF PSYCHOLOGICAL AND BEHAVIORAL TREATMENTS

Methodology in Outcome Studies

In evaluating outcome, one good study should be more highly regarded than a dozen poorly designed or poorly executed studies. The International Headache Society's Committee on Clinical Trials in Migraine (26) produced the Guidelines for controlled trials of drugs in migraine. Although intended for drug trials, these guidelines are of use to those designing nonpharmacologic trials. For example, they recommend that the headache index that sums headache ratings across time not be used because it confounds intensity, duration, and frequency. Some of the guidelines are clearly inappropriate for psychological studies, such as crossover designs, which are unlikely to be of use in evaluation of psychological treatments. Others, such as the requirement of a placebo, present significant difficulties in psychological studies because there is no agreement on what a psychological placebo should be. However, designers of clinical trials of psychological treatments would be wise to consult the guidelines for advice. The guidelines are now under revision.

It is common, but incorrect, to assume that a successful treatment can tell us about cause. So, for example, the finding that sufferers find relief with stress management does not mean that their headaches were caused by stress. Nor does finger temperature biofeedback success indicate that migraine is caused by cold fingers.

Short-Term Effects of Behavioral Treatments

Average percentage reductions in headache activity reported with the most commonly used relaxation and biofeedback therapies calculated in recent metanalytic (statistical) reviews are summarized in Table 3. It can be seen that relaxation training combined with thermal biofeedback training has yielded about a 50% reduction in migraine activity, but relaxation training and biofeedback training procedures alone have yielded somewhat smaller improvements. The few studies that have directly compared combined relaxation training and thermal biofeedback to either relaxation training alone or biofeedback alone have not consistently supported the superiority of combined relaxation and thermal biofeedback training (6). The use of different treatment protocols and different patient populations across studies may have obscured differences in treatment efficacy; some studies also appear to have included too few patients to possess adequate statistical power, or to have included a significant number of patients unlikely to benefit from behavioral treatment (e.g., patients with chronic substance-induced headache). Thus, the hypothesis that combined relaxation/thermal biofeedback training is more effective than either relaxation training or biofeedback training alone is tentative. However, improvements reported with relaxation and biofeedback therapies have been at least three times as numerous as improvements with medication placebo control treatments. Considerable evidence is thus available indicating that relaxation/biofeedback therapies produce clinically significant improvements in headache activity.

Even when relaxation and biofeedback therapies produce similar outcomes, it does not imply that these therapies are interchangeable. Some patients who fail to respond to relaxation training will benefit from biofeedback training (11). There is no evidence, however, to indicate there is an advantage for beginning treatment with one, rather than another, of these interventions.

The evidence for the efficacy of stress management or cognitive therapy for migraine is less clear. Several studies have shown that cognitive therapy alone or in combination with relaxation is an effective treatment (30,35,39,40,45,46). However, in a clinical trial, Blanchard (13) found no difference in the effectiveness of thermal biofeedback training and thermal biofeedback plus cognitive therapy. A recent metanalysis of a subset of studies meeting stringent research design and data-reporting criteria reported, on average, that stress-man-

TABLE 3. *Average improvement by type of treatment*

Type of treatment	Average % improvement	Treatment groups (n)	Improvement range (%)
Combined relaxation and biofeedback training	56	35	11 to 93
Relaxation training	37	38	5 to 81
Thermal biofeedback training Cephalic vasomotor	35	14	−8 to 80
Biofeedback training	34	11	2 to 82
Placebo control (medication placebo)	12	20	−23 to 32
Headache monitoring control	3	15	−30 to 33

Data from Holroyd et al. (24).

agement training yielded improvements in migraine activity that were very similar in magnitude to improvements reported with relaxation and thermal biofeedback therapies alone (34). It thus appears that cognitive therapy can be effective in managing migraine but that cognitive and relaxation-based treatments may not be additive in their effect. One limitation of existing studies is that cognitive therapy procedures were adopted largely unchanged from those originally developed for the management of tension-type headache. Somewhat different and more effective interventions might be developed specifically for migraine, where, for example, relationships between daily life stresses and headache onset are typically less obvious than in tension headache. Nonetheless, there is no evidence that currently available stress-management interventions can improve upon results obtained from relaxation/biofeedback therapies alone.

Cognitive therapies have the disadvantage of being more complex than relaxation and biofeedback. On the other hand, cognitive approaches may have the advantage of teaching strategies that are generalizable to a wide range of situations or stressors giving rise to headache (7). Moreover, these skills may be useful in combating depression, anxiety, and other problems that migraine patients may experience. However, the differential impact of cognitive therapy and relaxation/biofeedback therapies on other symptoms has not been evaluated.

Long-Term Effectiveness of Behavioral Treatments

Approximately one half to two thirds of patients successfully treated with psychological treatment for migraine have good maintenance of effects 1 to 5 years later (5,46). The problem in interpreting such long-term follow-up data is that a significant proportion of patients are typically lost during follow-up, and other patients may have initiated medical treatment during the follow-up period. However, even in the subset of studies that has addressed these methodologic problems (17), long-term follow-up results have been quite positive. Thus, it appears that improvements achieved with behavioral treatments are frequently well maintained.

Treatments incorporate strategies to encourage maintenance, the most frequent being booster sessions spaced out over time once the active treatment is over. In controlled studies, booster sessions have not been found to enhance the maintenance of improvements, possibly because good maintenance has frequently been found without booster sessions (1). It is possible, however, that patients at high risk for relapse would benefit from booster sessions.

Effects on Disability and Handicap

Although chronic pain research frequently examines the specific activities interrupted by pain (disability) and the impact of pain on social role functioning (handicap), headache studies have not typically examined these variables. Headache research has almost exclusively relied on measures of headache activity as the only outcome measures. Although many individuals who suffer from migraine have minimal disability and handicap, migraine headache produces a significant level of disability and handicap in many patients. The measurement of disability and handicap should be included in studies and in clinical work.

Effects with Special Populations

The treatment of childhood and adolescent migraine has not been as widely investigated as that of adult migraine. This is probably because severe migraine in children does not appear to be as common as in adults, and children's pain has generally been ignored. The evidence suggests that relaxation treatment, finger temperature biofeedback, and cognitive therapy are all effective (31,35,40). At this time, there is no evidence that one is more effective than another. Although no direct treatment comparisons of adolescents and adults have been conducted, psychological treatment of adolescents appears to be as effective as that of adults.

The behavioral treatment of the elderly with migraine was once thought to be less effective than for younger adults (10). However, work in which the behavioral treatment was modified to be more appropriate to the elderly has been more successful (29).

CLINICAL ISSUES

Although chronic headaches from undetected serious pathology are rare, patients receiving psychological treatment for migraine should have a thorough medical evaluation by a physician experienced in migraine.

Some migraine sufferers may prefer one type of treatment to another. For example, psychologically oriented individuals may prefer cognitive therapy, whereas the less psychologically oriented may prefer more physically based therapies such as biofeedback or relaxation. Clinically the choice of intervention may thus be influenced by the client's preferences.

Patients who are seriously depressed (other than those who are depressed because of their migraine headaches) may have difficulty participating in psychological treatment for migraine. Treatment of the depression, either by means of cognitive therapy or by medical means, may be required prior to headache treatment. Some individuals who are susceptible to panic attacks may find it initially difficult to engage in relaxation training without triggering fear of a panic attack.

Patients suffering from drug-induced migraine may have to substantially reduce their medication usage before or while they are receiving psychological treatment in order to benefit from treatment.

Predicting Who Will Benefit

Effective and efficient treatment of migraine is a pressing issue because migraine is such a common and costly disorder. One way of improving cost efficiency of treatment is to determine who will and will not benefit from psychological treatment. Unfortunately, research on predicting who responds to a particular treatment and who does not has been scarce. Although, the proportion of successes is generally high (30%–80%), a considerable number of patients do not benefit. One can distinguish five sets of predictors of benefit from psychological treatment, although the variables used differ somewhat between studies. Almost all studies quoted pertain to psychophysiologic treatments, and most results are not exclusively specific to migraine but refer also to other types of nonorganic headache.

Several studies have found that psychological treatments are more effective in younger adult patients (7,12), but age seems to have no predictive value within the pediatric age group (44). Adult patients with somatic complaints in addition to headache are less likely to benefit from psychological treatment in adults (7,12), whereas the reverse may be true in adolescents (32). Shorter headache history, especially less than 2 years (8) and appropriate use of medications (14) are also related to good outcome.

The predictive value of headache diagnosis per se (2,44) is inconclusive. Continuous pretreatment headache as opposed to intermittent headache is related to treatment failure (2), whereas a high frequency of intermittent headache at baseline seems to be related to treatment success (32,40). In addition, no distinctive differential profiles of predictors for different types of headache have as yet been identified, despite the effort of a large and well designed study conducted by Blanchard (7).

Low scores on depression scales (7,11,27), high scores on state and trait anxiety (6), low scores on assertiveness (8), and low scores on several Minnesota Multiphasic Personality Inventory scales, particularly the scales for hysteria and hypochondriasis (7), are found to be positively related to treatment success.

Motivation to comply with home practice exercises on the basis of a pretreatment willingness to accept self-responsibility has been shown to be related to the long-term maintenance of effect of treatments (46). Secondary gain from headache is, from a clinical point of view, considered to be a potent determinant of treatment failure. However, research evaluation of secondary gain has proven to be very difficult, if not impossible.

A few studies made use of psychophysiologic measures, such as frontal EMG, skin temperature, skin resistance, and heart rate, for the purpose of effect prediction. Higher baseline levels of frontal EMG and higher physiological reactivity to stress, as well as initial levels of responses more removed from normal, have been shown to be associated with poorer outcome (9). The psychophysiologic variables tended to produce better prediction than did the psychological variables. In addition, slightly better and more consistent prediction was possible when headache diagnosis was taken into account in analyzing the results.

The variance of effect resulting from different sets of predictors range roughly between 30% and 70%. It is clear that, although we have come a long way in studying the effect of psychological treatments, much work remains to be done.

How Can Psychological and Drug Therapies Be Combined?

The effectiveness of behavioral and drug therapies have been compared directly in only a few trials (21). However, the effectiveness of these two treatment modalities has been examined via metanalysis, a methodology that allows findings from clinical trials of each treatment to be combined for analysis. Metanalysis revealed (31) that improvements in migraine reported in 25 prophylactic drug therapy (propranolol HCl) trials and in 35 relaxation/thermal biofeedback trials (over 2,400 patients) were virtually identical. Propranolol and relaxation/thermal biofeedback training have each yielded a 55% reduction in migraine activity in the typical patient. In contrast, patients treated with placebo showed only a 12% reduction in migraine activity. This suggests that prophylactic drug and behavioral therapies may be equally viable treatment options for many patients. However, these two treatment modalities may well have different advantages and disadvantages in particular subgroups of patients, for example, in patients with frequent disabling headaches versus patients with less frequent and severe migraines, or in patients seen in primary care and in patients seen in specialty headache treatment centers.

Combined propranolol and relaxation/thermal biofeedback therapy has proven highly effective in controlling recurrent migraines in two trials yielding more than a 70% reduction in migraine activity on average (23,33). In one trial conducted at a headache specialty center, the combined treatment proved only slightly more effective than propranolol, which in turn was more effective than relaxation/biofeedback training alone (33). This suggests that prophylactic drug therapy may be a necessary component of treatment in this difficult to treat population. The second smaller trial, conducted with patients more similar to those seen in a primary care setting, also found the combined treatment more effective than relaxation/biofeedback training alone (23). However, two thirds of the patients who received propranolol and relaxation/biofeedback training in this study were able to effectively control migraines with only a low dose of propranolol (60 mg/day). This raises the possibility that combined therapy may enable patients with less severe migraines to control their headaches with low-dose prophylactic therapy.

An algorithm to guide the choice of drug and nondrug therapies (24) suggests that, when migraines are frequent or severe, or comorbid anxiety or mood disorders are present, conjoint behavior and preventive drug therapy should be considered. However, when migraines are less frequent and uncomplicated by the presence of a psychological disorder, behavioral and drug therapies may be equally viable treatment alternatives. In the latter case, patient preference, treatment costs, presence of medication contraindications (e.g., possibility of pregnancy, breastfeeding) might then influence the treatment modality chosen.

A recent metanalysis of the pediatric literature found thermal biofeedback training (either when administered alone or when combined with relaxation training) and propranolol yielded similar improvements in pediatric migraine (20). Improvements reported with thermal biofeedback training were more significant than improvements reported with either serotonergic drugs (a heterogeneous grouping that included amitriptyline, trazadone, cyproheptadine, pizotifen, and tryptophan) or calcium channel blockers (flunarizine or nimodipine). Unfortunately, this metanalysis was limited by the small number of available trials of any sort with pediatric migraine. The one study to directly compare behavior therapy and prophylactic drug therapy in children (6–12 years of age) found that combined relaxation and self-hypnosis training (five treatment sessions) yielded significantly better results than did propranolol (3 mg/kg/day), which failed to produce better results than placebo. Additional studies that compare drug and behavioral therapies in pediatric migraine are needed.

The efficacy of 5-hydroxytryptamine type 1 (5-HT$_1$) agonists or triptans has led to the growing role of abortive medications in the management of migraine. Unfortunately, little information is available about how behavioral interventions and these new abortive therapies can best be integrated. The high cost of the triptans will probably encourage the development of interventions to help patients use these medications effectively. However, triptans are potent vasoconstrictors that may block some of the physiologic changes induced by handwarming or relaxation exercises, attenuating the effects of these behavioral interventions, although no hard data on this possibility are available. Nonetheless, in the next decade behavioral interventions may increasingly focus on teaching headache-management skills, rather than on the modification of specific physiologic responses via biofeedback training. Methods for deciding when to use analgesic, abortive, or other medications, as well as psychological and behavioral skills, for managing headaches may therefore play a prominent role in future self-management interventions. In the case of children and adolescents, clinicians have been reluctant to use triptans with children and adolescents because they have not been shown to be effective in this population (19). Thus, behavioral interventions may be particularly useful for children and adolescents.

Poor adherence probably limits the effectiveness of both abortive and prophylactic therapies for migraine. On the basis of 100 patient interviews, Packard and O'Connell (38) concluded that over 50% of headache sufferers fail to properly adhere to drug treatment regimens. Furthermore, when patients were assessed 1 year after initiating drug therapy, only 24% of patients reported they had used headache medications as instructed (15). One third of patients were judged noncompliant with prophylactic medication when an electronic device was used to monitor pill bottle opening (37), although this level was lower (20%) when only once-a-day regimens were considered. Behavioral interventions may thus prove of value in facilitating patients' effective use of prescribed medications.

The one study to focus on improving adherence with abortive medications examined the use of ergotamine (22). Patients who received a brief adherence intervention (a meeting with an allied health professional following the neurologist's prescription of ergotamine, three telephone calls to identify and remedy problems with ergotamine use, and a workbook to help identify and correct adherence problems) attempted to abort 70% of migraine attacks and showed clinically significant reductions in migraine activity (40% reduction). In contrast, patients who received standard ergotamine therapy attempted to abort only about 40% of their migraine attacks and showed smaller reductions in migraine activity (26% reduction). These results suggest that interventions to facilitate the effective use of prescribed medications deserve more attention than they have received to date. For many patients, brief interventions that successfully improve adherence with existing medical regimens might yield greater benefits than will new pharmacologic agents.

Making Behavioral Treatments More Available

Given the prevalence of migraine, it is inconceivable that all migraine patients could or would need to be treated individually by qualified psychologists. Moreover, the cost would be prohibitive. Several strategies for increasing the availability and cost-effectiveness of psychological treatments have been examined. One strategy for cost-effective treatment is the use of groups. Behavioral group treatment of migraine has not been widely reported, but our own experience is positive, with group treatment being as effective as individual treatment. Where patient flow is adequate, it should be feasible to reduce the costs of treatment and to make good use of health professionals' time by administering treatment in small groups rather than individually. However, this requires not only that health professionals be able to administer behavioral treatments, but also that they be adept at handling problems that arise during group treatment.

A second strategy is the use of primarily home-based treatment formats. In a minimal-contact or home-based treatment program, headache management skills are introduced in periodic clinic sessions, but written materials and audiotapes are used to enable patients to acquire skills at home that typically would be taught in clinic sessions. As a result, only three to four (monthly) clinic sessions may be required to complete limited-contact behavioral treatment. This contrasts with the 10 to 20 (often weekly) clinic sessions required for completely therapist-administered clinic-based treatment. In the studies that have directly compared the effectiveness of the same behavioral intervention provided in therapist-administered and minimal-contact treatment formats, these two treatment formats have yielded similar outcomes in adults, but somewhat smaller improvements in children (18,41). Using the following formula for cost effectiveness (percentage improvement in headache activity/clinician contact time), Haddock (18) determined that home-based therapy was five times more cost effective as clinic-based individual therapy. Some proportion of patients will, of course, continue to require more therapist intensive treatment. Individuals who excessively use analgesic medication, are clinically depressed, or suffer from nearly daily headache problems may require more intensive treatment. Other patients simply do not persist in efforts to learn or apply self-regulation skills without regular contact with a health professional. Perhaps the greatest cost savings could be realized with home-based treatment administered by allied health professionals or even by nonprofessional technicians under the supervision of a health professional. The third is to have treatment delivered by allied health professionals such as nurses, social workers, or occupational therapists or by technicians under supervision of a health psychologist. No specific certification designates a health professional competent to treat migraine. It is our opinion that the person be broadly trained in one of the health professions and specifically trained in understanding and administering behavioral treatment of headache. No studies have evaluated this strategy.

In sharp contrast to pharmacologic treatments, which only require that patients take their medicine, psychological treatments require the active participation of patients. Psychological treatments are often referred to as self-regulatory treatments. In psychological treatments, patients must learn to change their physiologic and/or psychological reactions. These treatments emphasize taking control of their treatment. Although this commitment and responsibility are welcomed by many patients, the demands on the patient have been an impediment to treatment for some patients.

FUTURE DIRECTIONS

Psychological treatment has been shown to be an effective and efficient treatment for migraine. However, several issues require more study. Psychological treatments should become more widely available. This will require a variety of strategies, including the addition of psychologists to headache treatment units, the training of other professionals, such as nurses and social workers, to administer treatments, and increasing use of treatments that are largely self-administered.

The mechanisms by which psychological treatments are effective need to be elucidated. Discovery of mechanisms will allow for the refinement of treatments and the better matching of patients to treatments. The matching of patients to treatments also can be discerned from a purely empirical approach. These two approaches can complement each other.

The interaction of pharmacologic and psychological treatments should be more widely investigated. We need to know which patients are most likely to benefit from each strategy. Are combined regimens of use with specific patients?

More attention should be directed to treatment failures. Can second-order treatments be developed for those who do not benefit from standard psychological interventions? In patients with multiple types of headaches, do behavioral interventions affect specific headaches? The use of the International Classification System that focuses on headaches, not on patients, should help clarify this issue.

Cost effectiveness must become a standard feature of all migraine outcome studies. Almost all studies of psychological treatment of headache have been conducted in specialty clinics or universities. The field trials to evaluate these treatments in primary or secondary care have not yet been undertaken.

REFERENCES

1. Andrasik, FA, Blanchard EB, Neff DF, Rodichok LD. Biofeedback and relaxation training for chronic headache: a controlled comparison of booster treatments and regular contacts for long-term maintenance. *J Consult Clin Psychol* 1984;52:609–615.
2. Bakal DA, Demjen S, Kaganov JA. Cognitive behavioral treatment of chronic headaches. *Headache* 1981;21:81–86.
3. Beck AT. *Depression: causes and treatment.* Philadelphia: University of Pennsylvania Press, 1972.
4. Benson H. *Beyond the relaxation response.* New York: Times Books, 1984.
5. Blanchard EB. Long term effects of behavioral treatment of chronic headache. *Behav Ther* 1987;8:375–385
6. Blanchard EB, Andrasik F. Psychological assessment and treatment of headache: recent developments and emerging issues. *J Consult Clin Psychol* 1982;50:859–879.
7. Blanchard EB, Andrasik F, eds. *Management of chronic headaches: a psychological approach.* New York: Pergamon, 1985.
8. Blanchard EB, Andrasik F, Arena JG, et al. Prediction of outcome from the nonpharmacological treatment of chronic headache. *Neurology* 1983;33:1596–1603.
9. Blanchard EB, Andrasik F, Arena JG, et al. Psychophysiological responses as predictors of response to behavioral treatment of chronic headache. *Behav Ther* 1983;14:357–374.

10. Blanchard EB, Andrasik F, Evans DD, Hillhouse J. Biofeedback and relaxation treatments for headache in the elderly: a caution and a challenge. *Biofeedback Self Regul* 1985;10:69–73.
11. Blanchard EB, Andrasik F, Neff DF, et al. Biofeedback and relaxation training with three kinds of headache: treatment effects and their prediction. *J Consult Clin Psychol* 1982;50:562–575.
12. Blanchard EB, Andrasik F, Evans DD, Neff DF, Appelbaum KA, Rodichok LD. Behavioral treatment of 250 chronic headache patients: a clinical replication series. *Behav Ther* 1985;16:308–327.
13. Blanchard EB, Appelbaum KA, Radnitz CL, et al. A controlled evaluation of thermal biofeedback and thermal biofeedback combined with cognitive therapy in the treatment of vascular headache. *J Consult Clin Psychol* 1990;58:216–224.
14. Diener HC, Wilkinson M, eds. *Drug induced headache.* New York: Springer Verlag, 1988.
15. Fitzpatrick RM, Hopkins AP, Harvard-Watts O. Social dimensions of healing: a longitudinal study of outcomes of medical management of headaches. *Soc Sci Med* 1983;8:501–510.
16. Fordyce WE. *Behavioral methods for chronic pain and illness.* St. Louis: CV Mosby, 1976.
17. Gauthier JG, Carrier S. Long-term effects of biofeedback on migraine headache: a prospective follow-up study. *Headache* 1991; 31:605–612.
18. Haddock CK, Rowan AB, Andrasik FA, Wilson PG, Talcott GW, Stein RJ. Home-based behavioral treatments for chronic benign headache—a meta-analysis of controlled trials. *Cephalalgia* 1997; 17:113–118.
19. Hamalainen ML, Hoppu K, Santavuori PR. Sumatriptan for migraine attacks in children: a randomized, placebo-controlled trial (do children with migraine respond differently to oral sumatriptan from adults?). *Neurology* 1997;48:1100–1103.
20. Hermann C, Kim M, Blanchard EB. Behavioral and pharmacological intervention studies of pediatric migraine: an exploratory meta-analysis. *Pain* 1995;60:239–256.
21. Holroyd KA, Cordingley GE, Pingel JD, et al. Enhancing the effectiveness of abortive therapy: a controlled evaluation of self-management training. *Headache* 1989;29:148–153.
22. Holroyd KA, France JL, Cordingley GE, et al. Enhancing the effectiveness of relaxation-thermal biofeedback training with propranolol hydrochloride. *J Consult Clin Psychol* 1995;63:327–330.
23. Holroyd K. Integrating pharmacologic and non-pharmacologic treatments. In: Tolison CD, Kunkel RS, eds. *Headache diagnosis and interdiciplinary treatment.* Baltimore: Williams & Wilkins, 1993:309–320.
24. Holroyd KA, Lipchik GL, Penzien DB. Psychological management of recurrent headache disorders: empirical basis for clinical practice. In: Dobson KS, Craig KD, eds. *Best practice: developing and promoting empirically supported interventions.* Newbury Park, CA: Sage Publications, 1998:187–236.
25. Holroyd KA. Penzien DB. Pharmacological versus non-pharmacological prophylaxis of recurrent migraine headache: a meta-analytic review of clinical trials. *Pain* 1990;42:1–13
26. International Headache Society, Committee on Clinical Trials in Migraine. Guidelines for controlled trials of drugs in migraine. First edition. *Cephalagia* 1991;11:1–12.
27. Jacob RG, Turner SM, Szekely BC, Eidelman BH. Predicting outcome of relaxation therapy in headaches: the role of depression. *Behav Ther* 1983;14;457–465.
28. Jacobson E. *Progressive relaxation.* Chicago: University of Chicago Press, 1938.
29. Kabela E, Blanchard EB, Appelbaum KA, Nicholson N. Self-regulatory treatment of headache in the elderly. *Biofeedback Self Regul* 1989;14:219–228.
30. Knapp TW. Treating migraine by training in temporal artery vasoconstriction and/or cognitive behavioral coping: a one-year follow-up. *J Psychosom Res* 1982;26:551–557.
31. Labbe EE, Williamson DA. Treatment of childhood migraine using autogenic feedback training. *J Consult Clin Psychol* 1984;52: 968–976.
32. Larsson B, Melin L. The psychological treatment of recurrent headache in adolescents: short-term outcome and its prediction. *Headache* 1988;28:187–195.
33. Mathew NT. Prophylaxis of migraine and mixed headache: a randomized controlled study. *Headache* 1981;21:105–109.
34. McCrory DC, Penzien DB, Rains JC, Hasselblad V. Efficacy of behavioral treatments for migraine and tension-type headache: meta-analysis of controlled trials. *Headache* 1996;36:272.
35. McGrath PJ, Humphreys P, Keene D, et al. The efficacy and efficiency of a self-administered treatment for adolescent migraine. *Pain* 1992;49:321–324.
36. Meichenbaum D. *Cognitive behavior modification: an integrative approach.* New York: Plenum Press, 1977.
37. Mulleners WM, Whitmarsh TE, Steiner TJ. Noncompliance may render migraine prophylaxis useless, but once-daily regimens are better. *Cephalalgia* 1998;18:52–56.
38. Packard RC, O'Connell P. Medication compliance among headache patients. *Headache* 1986;26:416–419.
39. Richardson GM, McGrath PJ. Cognitive-behavioral therapy for migraine headaches: a minimal-therapist-contact approach versus a clinic-based approach. *Headache* 1990;29:352–357.
40. Richter I, McGrath PJ, Humphreys PJ, Goodman JT, Firestone P, Keene D. Cognitive and relaxation treatment of pediatric migraine. *Pain* 1986;25:195–203.
41. Rowan AB, Andrasik FA. Efficacy and cost-effectiveness of minimal therapist contact treatments of chronic headache: a review. *Behav Ther* 1996;27:207–234.
42. Sargent JD, Green EE, Walters ED. Preliminary report on the use of autogenic feedback training in the treatment of migraine and tension headaches. *Psychosom Med* 1973;35:129–135.
43. Schultz JH, Luthe W. *Autogenic training: a psychophysiologic approach to psychotherapy.* New York: Grune & Stratton, 1959.
44. Smith MS, Womack WM, Chen AC. Hypnotizability does not predict outcome of behavioral treatment in pediatric headache. *J Clin Hypnosis* 1989;31:237–241.
45. Sorbi M. *Psychological intervention in migraine.* Delft: Eburon, 1988.
46. Sorbi M, Tellegen B, Du Long A. Long-term effects of training in relaxation and stress-coping in patients with migraine: a three-year follow-up. *Headache* 1989;29:111–121.
47. Sullivan MJL, Bishop SR, Pivik J. The Pain Catastrophizing Scale: development and validation. *Psychol Assess* 1995;7:524–532.

The Headaches, Second Edition,
edited by J. Olesen, P. Tfelt-Hansen, and K.M.A. Welch.
Lippincott Williams & Wilkins, Philadelphia © 2000.

The Migraines

CHAPTER 48

Unconventional Treatments for Migraine

John G. Edmeads

It may surprise some readers of this mainstream medical text to learn that more people go to unconventional practitioners than to physicians for health care in general and for the treatment of headaches in particular. Between 34% (14) and 40% (4) of the population of the United States regularly consult alternative practitioners. A Canadian study (13) revealed that, for migraine, 48% of the population surveyed had used unconventional therapies, 44% had taken prescription medications, and 91% had consumed over-the-counter analgesics.

People who use unconventional treatments do so because they find them effective; they are neither ignorant nor prejudiced because of dissatisfaction with mainstream medicine. An American study (4) found that in general people using alternative therapies were more educated than those using traditional treatments alone and that they tended to use alternative treatments in combination with mainstream therapies. Only 4.4 % of those surveyed relied exclusively on alternative medicine, and this small minority were more likely to be dissatisfied with or mistrustful of conventional therapy. In this survey of users of alternative medicine, it was found that 24% of those using these therapies were doing so for the complaint of headache.

Do these unconventional treatments work? We do not know. Some of them are quite old and widely used, but in general they have not been submitted to the rigorous controlled studies of efficacy demanded of conventional medical therapies, and so they remain in intellectual and scientific limbo.

J.G. Edmeads: Department of Medicine, Sunnybrook Health Science Center, University of Toronto, Toronto, Ontario M4N 3M5, Canada.

LOCAL THERAPY TO THE HEAD

Pressure applied to the head during headache is an ancient remedy that only recently has been evaluated systematically. Binding of the head was used in Sumeria and ancient Egypt (12) and was a commonplace treatment long afterward, as evidenced by Shakespeare who had Desdemona say, on hearing from Othello that he had a headache, "Let me but bind it hard, within this hour it will be well." Presumably, pressure works in vascular headache either by compressing painfully distended extracranial vessels or through the effects of "counterirritation." Blau and Dexter (6) found that 28 of 50 migraine sufferers gained some headache relief from occluding the scalp circulation either with fingers or a blood pressure cuff; Drummond and Lance (11) noted that one third of their 66 migraineurs had their headaches eased by pressure on the temporal artery; and Vijayan (49) reported that his 23 migraine patients gained some relief in 87% of their aggregate headaches by using an elastic head band with a Velcro fastener and rubber discs to apply localized pressure.

Application of cold to the head is another historic method of treating migraine headaches. The earliest medical textbook on cryotherapy, published in 1849 (3), advocated putting salt and ice on the aching head. The theoretic basis for the efficacy of local cold is that it both constricts dilated vessels and numbs pain fibers. Recent studies (9,41) report that local application of cold helps 35% to 80% of migraine patients. Sheftell and colleagues (43) found that mild, dull headaches were more likely to respond than severe ones. Lance (30) used an impressive machine that cooled the circumference of the head and neck to 2 °C and warmed the vertex to 41 °C; he reported that 15 of 20 migraine sufferers had less severe headaches from using this Migra-Lief apparatus (Fig. 1). All the studies cited concluded that local appli-

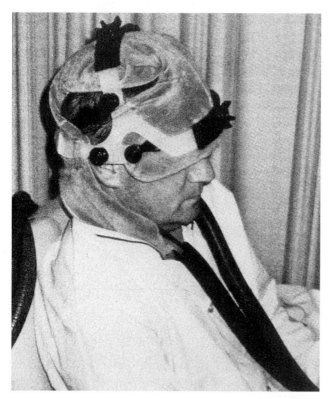

FIG. 1. Lance's Migra-Lief apparatus (see text). Hot and cold water are pumped through the tubes into the cap, warming the vertex and cooling the neck and the periphery of the scalp. (From ref. 30, with permission.)

cation of cold can be a valuable adjunct to other forms of headache therapy.

Electric stimulation of the head and neck as a treatment for pain in that region is not new. In 1888 Gowers commented, in his classic neurology text (20), that for migraine "electricity is not often of service. Faradism usually does harm. The voltaic current passed through the head occasionally gives transient, but rarely permanent relief." In modern times, three studies (25,46,47) reported some success in controlling headache with electric stimulation by transcutaneous electric nerve stimulation (TENS), but two of these studies used patients with mixtures of tension headache and migraine; whereas differences between TENS and placebo were demonstrated in some of the studies, the clinical significance of the changes was dubious. In a variation on this theme, another group of investigators (44) applied pulsed electromagnetic fields to the thighs of migraine sufferers and found significant and sustained reduction in the frequency of headaches. This study appears to have been, however, a small study of an atypical population. In summary, there is no compelling evidence of the worth of cranial electrotherapy in migraine.

Injection of the nerves or soft tissues of the head and neck with local anaesthetic, either alone or in combination with corticosteroid, is a widely and perhaps exces-

sively used therapy for migraine, usually migraine that is refractory to pharmacologic therapy. The rationales cited for this treatment range from the simplistic to the sophisticated. At one extreme is the school of thought that holds that a numb head cannot ache; at the other is that which holds that blockade of any nerve fiber that impinges on the caudal nucleus of the trigeminal nerve may reduce the firing frequency of that nucleus to a level where it can no longer sustain nociceptive transmission, thereby terminating the migraine attack. Given the large volumes of corticosteroid and local anaesthetic that are repeatedly injected into the necks and scalps of some unfortunate migraine sufferers, systemic absorption cannot be discounted as a mechanism of action; certainly this author has seen several cases of Cushing's syndrome resulting from this therapy. Although a number of articles have been published citing the benefits of such therapy for migraine and other headaches (2,8,18,42), there is a dearth of controlled studies and thus no scientific proof of efficacy. This author believes that blocking of the occipital nerves with local anaesthetic in judiciously selected cases, as part of a combination with other types of treatment, may confer some benefit sometimes.

Dental treatment is used by some practitioners to treat migraine. Disorders of the teeth and jaws may produce various head and face pain syndromes (21), but migraine generally is not considered to be one of them. Some dentists, however, believe that structural imbalances generate muscular hyperactivity that can aggravate or even initiate migraine pain (33) and on this basis have treated migraine with splints and other devices (29,32,38). Studies of dental treatment are difficult or impossible to conduct in a controlled fashion; so the results of these studies must be viewed with caution (51). There is no scientific proof that dental therapy, however skilled, helps migraine.

MANIPULATION OF THE NECK

Manipulation of the head and neck for the treatment of migraine encompasses two facets: stretching and massage of muscles and changing the relationships between articulated structures. No studies of muscle massage in migraine have been reported, unlike tension-type headache, for which a few studies have been reported; nor have there been any reports of adverse effects from massage. On the other hand, reports of serious complications, notably stroke, arising from chiropractic manipulation of the neck (17,19) have appeared. Fairness compels the comments that these complications are rare and that physicians probably do more harm with misused medications than chiropractors do with ill-advised manipulations. Nevertheless, given the occurrence of these complications, it seems self-evident that manipulation should not be recommended by physicians unless or until its efficacy has been established.

Numerous studies of manipulation in headache have been done (48), but all have had some methodologic faults, including failure to specify diagnostic criteria, inadequate or no randomization procedures, lack of controls, lack of blinding, lack of objectively verifiable outcome measurements, and inadequate or no statistical evaluations of results. One study was methodologically sound in design, although difficulties occurred in its execution (36). In this study, 85 patients with migraine were randomized into one of three groups: one group had neck manipulation beyond the normal range of motion (but not the appropriate chiropractic maneuvers) by a physician or physiotherapist, another group had chiropractic manipulation by a chiropractor, and the third (control) group had small physiologic mobilization movements by a physician or physiotherapist. Patients were not told which modality they were receiving. Subjects were evaluated during a 2-month pretreatment baseline period, a 2-month treatment period, and a 2-month posttreatment period. The average number of treatments was seven. Overall improvement was the same in all three groups: 28%. The severity of headaches was reduced more in the chiropractic group ($p = 0.01$), but the authors, noting the higher level of enthusiasm in the patients and practitioners within the chiropractic group, cautioned that this reduction in headache intensity might be attributable to placebo response. In a subsequent follow-up study 20 months later (37), these authors found that frequency of migraine attacks had further decreased in all three groups, each by 19%, and attributed this improvement over time to the natural history of the condition.

In assessing these and other studies, Vernon (48), the dean in charge of research at a major chiropractic college, concluded that "Only by evolving to a level of scientific quality will chiropractors really be able to determine if their therapeutic approaches truly offer anything of value to the vast number of headache sufferers awaiting our efforts."

ACUPUNCTURE FOR MIGRAINE

Originally believed to work by redirecting the flow of vital forces along meridians (52), acupuncture is now thought to exert its analgesic effects by increasing endorphins or metenkephalins. It may be that low-frequency electroacupuncture, like classic needle acupuncture, stimulates opioidergic mechanisms, whereas higher-frequency electroacupuncture may activate nonopioidergic gating mechanisms (23,24).

Studies of the efficacy of acupuncture have been beset by methodologic difficulties, including subject self-selection bias (enthusiasts volunteer, skeptics abstain), the impossibility of blinding the therapist when sham procedures are used, the employment of inappropriate control modalities, the risk of breaking the blind when crossover designs are used, protocol violations, high dropout rates, suboptimal outcome evaluations, and inappropriate or no statistical analysis. In 1986 Richardson and Vincent (40)

critically reviewed the evaluative literature on acupuncture and commented on the dearth of acceptable studies. The few methodologically acceptable studies of acupuncture in migraine have shown variable results. Henry et al (26) found no benefit from genuine acupuncture compared with sham acupuncture. Dowson et al (10) showed a modest superiority (about 20%) of acupuncture over placebo, a difference of dubious clinical significance. Vincent (50) demonstrated a 40% reduction in pain scores and medication in the acupuncture group, with improvement sustained at a one year follow-up.

It is difficult to understand how acupuncture could exert prolonged effects. Boivie and Brattberg (7) and Baischer (5) maintained that the benefits of acupuncture are significant and prolonged over months or years, but their studies were uncontrolled, and each had a dropout rate of 16%. Certainly, it was Lance's empirical experience (31) that patients improved with acupuncture but relapsed shortly afterward. In summary, the few sound studies on this subject suggest that the benefits of acupuncture for migraine are, if they exist, modest.

HYPNOSIS

Hypnosis, like acupuncture, has a long tradition and a short list of controlled studies of its efficacy. It is difficult to envisage a sham hypnosis technique, and so the controlled study strategies remaining are hypnosis versus comparators, such as medication or biofeedback, hypnosis versus wait-list controls, or (least satisfactory but widely used) the comparison within subjects of headache status before and after hypnotherapy. Two of the classic studies (1, 22) used this last technique and reported a high degree of efficacy, but their results must be viewed cautiously. Reich's (39) study compared the results of combined hypnotherapy, relaxation, and cognitive therapy with those of biofeedback and of TENS and found that all were beneficial to patients with migraine and tension headaches; biofeedback was most effective, TENS was next, and the hypnotherapy-relaxation-cognitive therapy group showed the least, but still measurable, improvement. A metanalysis (28) of largely uncontrolled studies also suggested that hypnotherapy was beneficial for headache when combined with cognitive–behavioral therapy.

Another study (35) compared self-hypnosis with propranolol and placebo in the treatment of juvenile classic migraine and concluded that hypnosis reduced the frequency of headaches but that propranolol and placebo did not. This study exemplifies how design influences outcome. The children were randomized to propranolol or placebo for 3 months, crossed over to the other modality for 3 months, and finally all the children were taught self-hypnosis. It may well have been that the improvement after 6 months was not due to hypnosis but to the passage of time. Another study (1) found hypnosis more effective than prochlorperazine in a randomized trial, but prochlorperazine by the route used is not generally accepted as a migraine treatment and thus was an invalid comparator. Although many in the field of headache (the author included) believe that hypnosis may be a useful adjunct to migraine therapy, none of the published studies that purport to prove this will survive critical scrutiny.

HERBAL THERAPY

Physicians have been using preparations from plants, vines and trees (botanicals) to treat disease since mankind appeared on earth (Fig. 2). In a Neanderthal grave 60,000 years old in northern Iraq, pollens were found from various plants that still grow in that area and still are used by local inhabitants for medicinal purposes. It is evident from their placement that these pollens did not find their way accidentally into the grave but rather were placed there purposefully, and it is speculated that the occupant was a shaman, or medicine man (45). Among the five varieties of pollen was yarrow (*Achillea millefolia* L.) which was documented by French explorers in 1633 as

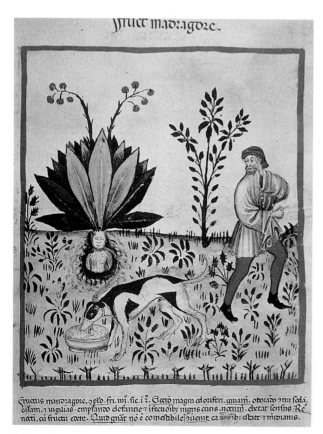

FIG. 2. A fourteenth century herbalist gathers mandrake root, often used as a poultice for headache. Because this root, when pulled from the ground, was believed to emit a piercing scream that could drive those who heard it mad, the herbalist has tied the root to a dog, so that when the dog moves off, it will pull the root, hopefully out of the herbalist's earshot.

being used by North American Indians (who put the pulverized leaves up their noses) for the treatment of "megrim." The Chippewa Indians, as recently as 1926, were described as sniffing the burning leaves of yarrow for their headaches (15). It is symptomatic of the uncoordinated state of the herbal medicine literature that another major work on this subject (16), although it lists yarrow as being used for other conditions, makes no mention of its use for headaches.

Another characteristic of the herbal medicine literature is the paucity of controlled studies of efficacy and the scarcity of reports of adverse effects. Of the three score botanicals listed as useful for headache in two major guides to medicinal plants and trees found in the author's geographic area, only one, feverfew (*Tanacetum parthenium* L.), has been demonstrated through randomized controlled trials to be efficacious for headache (27,34). It may be, given the tendency not to report negative results, that other herbal preparations have been tested, but the data were not published. This is unfortunate, because the long tradition of use of some of these plants for headaches (e.g., valerian has been used for migraine by physicians from Galen to Gowers) and what is known of some of their components (e.g., the balsam poplar contains salicylate) suggest that there is potential for some of these botanicals, or perhaps more likely their derivatives, to be useful in the treatment of headaches.

Clearly, herbal remedies do have some potential to create adverse effects, despite the popular misbelief that, if ineffective, they are at least harmless. The roots of Indian hemp (*Apocynum cannabinum* L.) and of spreading dogbane (*Apocynum androsaemifolium* L.), recommended to be taken internally for headache, can be cardiotoxic; and taken internally instead of applied externally to the head, decoctions of great lobelia (*Lobelia siphilitica* L.) and great rhododendron (*Rhododenron maximum* L.) are lethal. Preparations from the fringetree (*Chionanthus virginum* L.) and from the black locust (*Robinia pseudoacacia* L.), which are taken for liver disease and constipation, respectively, actually may produce headache.

Given the wide use of herbal remedies, the possibility that some of them might be efficacious, and the potential that some can be harmful, there is a clear need for the same kind of randomised controlled trials of safety and efficacy that are demanded of pharmaceuticals. Until this need is met, herbal remedies for headache cannot be recommended.

SUMMARY

The popularity and longevity of some of these unconventional techniques suggest either a strong placebo effect or true efficacy. Some of these techniques merit the effort of well-designed, punctiliously executed, randomized, controlled clinical trials.

REFERENCES

1. Anderson JAD, Bastian MA, Dalton R. Migraine and hynotherapy. *International Journal of Experimental Hypnosis* 1975;23:48–58.
2. Anthony M. Unilateral migraine or occipital neuralgia? In: Rose FC, ed. *New advances in headache research*, London: Smith Gordon, 1989:39–43.
3. Arnott J. *Practical illustrations of the treatment of principal varieties of headache by the local application of benumbing cold (with remarks on the remedial and anaesthetic uses of congelation in diseases of the skin and surgical operations).* London: Churchill, 1849.
4. Astin J. Why patients use alternative medicine: results of a national survey. *JAMA* 1998;279:1548–1553.
5. Baischer W. Acupuncture in migraine: long term outcome and predicting factors. *Headache* 1995;35:472–474.
6. Blau JN, Dexter SL. The site of pain origin during migraine attacks. *Cephalalgia* 1981;1:143–147.
7. Boivie J, Brattberg G. Are there longstanding effects on migraine headaches after one series of acupuncture treatments? *Am J Clin Med* 1987;15:69–75.
8. Caputi CA, Firetto V. Therapeutic blockade of greater occipital and supraorbital nerves in migraine patients. *Headache* 1997;37:174–179.
9. Diamond S, Freitag F. Cold as an adjunctive therapy for headache. *Postgrad Med* 1986;75:305–309.
10. Dowson DI, Lewith GT, Machin D. The effects of acupuncture versus placebo on the treatment of headache. *Pain* 1985;21:35–42.
11. Drummond P, Lance JW. Extracranial vascular changes, and the source of pain in migraine headache. *Ann Neurol* 1983;13:32–37.
12. Edmeads J. The treatment of headache: a historical perspective. In: Gallagher RM, ed. *Drug therapy for headache.* New York: Marcel Dekker, 1991:1–8.
13. Edmeads J, Findlay H, Tugwell P, Pryse-Phillips W, Nelson RF, Murray TJ. Impact of migraine and tension-type headache on life-style, consulting behaviour, and medication use: a Canadian population survey. *Can J Neurol Sci* 1993;20:131–137.
14. Eisenberg DM, Kessler RC, Foster C, Norlock FE, Calkins DR, Delbanco TL. Unconventional medicine in the United States: prevalence, costs, and patterns of use. *N Engl J Med* 1993;328:246–252.
15. Erichsen-Brown C. *Use of plants.* Aurora, Ontario: Breezy Creeks Press, 1979.
16. Foster S, Duke JA. *A field guide to medicinal plants—eastern and central North America. The Peterson field guide series.* Boston: Houghton Mifflin, 1990.
17. Franklin LR, Baloh RW. Wallenberg's syndrome following neck manipulation. *Neurology* 1990;40:611–615.
18. Gawel MJ, Rothbart PJ. Occiptal nerve block in the management of head and cervical pain. *Cephalalgia* 1992;12:9–13.
19. Gotlib A, Thiel H. A selected annotated bibliography of the core biomedical literature pertaining to stroke, cervical spine manipulation, and head-neck movement. *Journal of the Canadian Chiropractic Association* 1985;29:80–89.
20. Gowers W. *A manual of diseases of the nervous system.* Philadelphia: P. Blakiston, Son, 1888:1189.
21. Graff-Radford S. Oromandibular disorders and headache: a critical appraisal. *Neurol Clin* 1990;8:929 945.
22. Graham GW. Hypnotic treatment for migraine headaches. *International Journal of Clinical and Experimental Hypnosis* 1975;23:165–171.
23. Han JS, Terenius L. Neurochemical basis of acupuncture analgesia. *Annu Rev Pharmacol Toxicol* 1982;22:193–220.
24. Hardebo JE, Ekman R, Eriksson M. Low CSF met-enkephalin levels in cluster headache are elevated in acupuncture. *Headache* 1989;29:494–497.
25. Hay KM. Control of head pain in migraine using transcutaneous electrical nerve stimulation. *Practitioner* 1982;226:771–775.
26. Henry P, Baille H, Dartigues J, Jogeix M. Headaches and acupuncture. In: Pfaffenrath V, Lundberg PO, Sjaastad O, eds. *Updating in headache.* Berlin: Springer-Verlag, 1985:208–216.
27. Johnson ES, Kadam SP, Hylands DM. Efficacy of feverfew as prophylactic treatment of migraine. *BMJ* 1985;291:569–573.
28. Kirsch I. Hypnosis as an adjunct to cognitive-behavioral psychotherapy: a meta-analysis. *J Consult Clin Psychol* 1995;63:214–220.
29. Lamey PJ, Barclay SC. Clinical effectiveness of occlusal splint therapy in patients with classical migraine. *Scott Med J* 1987;32:11–12
30. Lance JW. The controlled application of cold and heat by a new device (Migra-lief apparatus) in the treatment of headache. *Headache* 1988;28:458–461.
31. Lance JW. *Mechanism and management of headache.* 4th ed. London: Butterworth Scientific, 1982:181.
32. Lapeer GL. Reduction of the painful sequelae of migraine headache by the use of the occlusal diagnostic splint: an hypothesis. *Cranio* 1988;6:82–86.
33. Moss RA. A structural imbalance/muscular hyperactivity interactional theory of common migraine pain. *Cranio* 1988;6:87–89.
34. Murphy JJ, Hepinstall S, Mitchell JRA. Randomised double-blind placebo-controlled trial of feverfew in migraine prevention. *Lancet* 1988;2:189–192.
35. Olness K, MacDonald JT, Uden DL. Comparison of self-hypnosis and propranolol in the treatment of juvenile classical migraine. *Pediatrics* 1987;79:593–597.
36. Parker GB, Tupling H, Pryor DS. A controlled study of cervical manipulation for migraine. *Aust N Z J Med* 1978;8:589–593.
37. Parker GB, Pryor DS, Tupling H. Why does migraine improve during a clinical trial? Further results from a trial of cervical manipulation for migraine. *Aust N Z J Med* 1980;10:193–194.
38. Quayle AA, Gray RJ, Metcalfe R, Guthrie E, Wastell D. Soft occlusal splint therapy in the treatment of migraine and other headaches. *J Dent* 1990;18:123–129.
39. Reich BA. Non-invasive treatment of migraine and muscle contraction headache: a comparative longitudinal clinical study. *Headache* 1989;29:34–41.
40. Richardson PH, Vincent CA. Acupuncture for the treatment of pain : a review of evaluative research. *Pain* 1986;24:15–40.
41. Robbins L. Cryotherapy for headache. *Headache* 1989;29:598–600.
42. Saadah HA, Taylor FB. Sustained headache syndrome associated with occipital nerve zones. *Headache* 1987;27:201–204.
43. Sheftell F, Rapoport A, Kudrow L. Efficacy of symptomatic treatment of tension and migraine headaches with the suboccipital ice pillow. *Headache* 1989;29:327 (abst).
44. Sherman RA, Robson L, Marden LA. Initial exploration of pulsing electromagnetic fields for treatment of migraine. *Headache* 1998;38:208–213.
45. Solecki RS. Shanidar IV. A Neanderthal flower burial in northern Iraq. *Science* 1975;190:880–881.
46. Solomon S, Elkind A, Freitag F, Gallagher RM, Moore K, Swerdlow B, Malkin S. Safety and efficacy of cranial electrotherapy in the treatment of tension headache. *Headache* 1989;29:445–450.
47. Solomon S, Guglielmo KM. Treatment of headache by transcutaneous electrical stimulation. *Headache* 1985;25:12–15.
48. Vernon HT. The effectiveness of chiropractic manipulation in the treatment of headache: an exploration in the literature. *J Manipulative Physiol Ther* 1995;18:611–617.
49. Vijayan N. Head band for migraine relief. *Headache* 1993;33:40–42.
50. Vincent CA. A controlled trial of the treatment of migraine by acupuncture. *Clin J Pain* 1989;5:305–312.
51. Watts PG, Peet KM, Juniper RP. Migraine and the temporomandibular joint: the final answer? *Br Dent J* 1986;16:170–173.
52. Wong TW, Fung KP. Acupuncture from needle to laser. *Fam Pract* 1991;8:168–170.

The Headaches, Second Edition,
edited by J. Olesen, P. Tfelt-Hansen, and K.M.A. Welch.
Lippincott Williams & Wilkins, Philadelphia © 2000.

The Migraines

CHAPTER 49

General Principles of Pharmacological Treatment of Migraine

Peer Tfelt-Hansen and K. Michael A. Welch

Table 1 is a "problem check list," to be considered in the pharmacologic treatment of migraine. Treating physicians should familiarize themselves with items in the table and may refer to them when discussing options for pharmacotherapy with the patient and their family. In the majority of migraine patients, only acute, abortive treatment of migraine attacks is required. Abortive treatment always should be optimized before prophylaxis is considered. Even in patients treated with prophylactic drugs who continue to suffer from migraine, the main emphasis of pharmacotherapy should be on treating the attack. Attacks vary considerably among and within subjects in terms of severity, associated symptoms, disability, and social impact. The bioavailability of the migraine abortive drugs varies considerably (see Chapters 51 and 52 on drug treatment), so treatment must be tailored to the individual patient. The same principles hold true for prophylactic treatment.

TREATMENT OF ACUTE MIGRAINE ATTACKS

The clinician must first consider the diagnosis. Specific antimigraine drugs such as ergotamine and triptans are only effective against migraine attacks and not useful in the treatment of episodic tension-type headaches. Accordingly, the treating physician must be aware that patients with frequent migraine attacks have interval

P. Tfelt-Hansen: Department of Neurology, Glostrup Hospital, University of Copenhagen, DK-2600 Glostrup, Copenhagen, Denmark.

K. M. A. Welch: Department of Neurology, University of Kansas School of Medicine, University of Kansas Medical Center, Kansas City, Kansas, 66106.

headaches, usually of the tension type. This puts the patient at risk for overuse of antimigraine drugs. Whenever possible the physician must clarify for the patient which headaches are migraine and which are not. A careful history should be supplemented by asking the patient to keep a diagnostic headache diary (see Chapter 6). This should be reviewed carefully with the patient to ascertain if he or she can distinguish migraine attacks from other headache types. The patient should be instructed to use antimigraine drugs only for migraine attacks and treat other headaches as discussed in Chapter 87.

The *choice of drugs* may depend on the characteristics of the migraine attacks; not all attacks in the same patient may require the same drug. Thus, mild and sometimes moderate attacks may be treated with aspirin or nonsteroidal antiinflammatory drugs (NSAIDs), optionally combined with drugs that promote their absorption, such as metoclopramide. When attacks are severe, the 5-hydroxytryptamine 1B and 1D (5-HT$_{1B/1D}$) agonists ergotamine, dihydroergotamine, sumatriptan, zolmitriptan, naratriptan, or rizatriptan should be used. When patients are uncertain if a headache will develop into a migraine attack, they may choose to stage their treatment, first using less specific drugs such as aspirin, paracetamol (acetaminophen), or NSAIDs. Using a specific antimigraine drug is best when there is an aura, when an impending migraine attack is recognized based on experience as potentially severe, or when the attack is already severe. When a short-lasting aura of 30 minutes or less is expected, ergotamine or triptans that are known to penetrate the central nervous system may be used, although the effective use of sumatriptan during the aura phase remains to be established. Again, some patients who

TABLE 1. *Problems to be considered in the pharmacologic treatment of migraine*[a]

Problems	Brief comments (see text for extensive comments)
Treatment of migraine attacks	
Is it migraine?	Have the patient keep a diagnostic headache diary for at least 1 month. Observe for drug over use.
Choice of drug(s)	
Mild or severe attacks?	Use aspirin for mild and specific drugs for severe attacks.
Treatment during aura phase?	If duration of aura is less than 30 min ergotamine can be used. Sumatriptan is not effective given in the aura phase.
Associated symptoms?	Nausea/vomiting can be treated with antiemetic and preferably prokinetic drugs such as metoclopramide
Previous experience with drugs?	Was the drug previously used in optimal doses? Were there prohibitive side effects?
Contraindications?	Risk of ischemic vascular disease for ergotamine and triptans. Pregnancy
Side effects?	Patients should be informed about the most frequent ones.
Dose of drug?	Should be tailored to the individual patients. Start with low doses and have the patient treat two attacks before gradually increasing the dose.
Route of administration?	If vomiting prohibits oral administration, subcutaneous injections, rectal or nasal routes can be used.
Prophylactic treatment	
When to use?	More than two attacks per month, that cannot be treated with optimized abortive treatment. If frequent attacks evaluate drug overuse.
Documentation of problem and effect?	Have the patient keep a headache diary before and during treatment.
Treatment for how long?	Try to withdraw even successful treatment after one year at the most.
Choice of drug	
Contraindications?	Asthma with beta-blockers, depression with flunarizine, obesity with pizotifen, peptic ulcer and bleeding disorders with NSAIDs.
Side effects?	Inform patients.
Previous experience?	Was the drug used in optimal dose and time frame? Was it used during actual drug abuse?
Dose of drugs?	No "standard" dose for all patients. Tailor individual dose. Start with small doses.

[a]For prolonged and severe attacks, possible drug interaction, and pregnancy, see text.

experience aura may choose to stage treatment, using drugs such as aspirin, until establishing for themselves whether their headache is mild.

The *associated symptoms* of a migraine, such as nausea and vomiting, may be as disabling as headache. Absorption of oral medications may be delayed due to gastric stasis. Starting treatment with antiemetic and prokinetic drugs such as metoclopramide may ameliorate the gastrointestinal manifestations of migraine and improve gastric peristalsis with consequent rapid and more complete absorption (see Chapter 54). Most triptans ameliorate nausea and vomiting and, uniquely to the antimigraine drugs, relieve photophobia. Most are now available by parenteral routes of administration, although their effectiveness may prove variable under these circumstances.

Prior experience with efficacy or adverse drug effects is of considerable importance. For example, a previously ineffective drug may not have been used in the optimal dose or by the best route of administration, and therefore may merit a new trial. Experience can dictate whether patients choose to stage their treatment or not. Adverse drug effects—for example, nausea accompanying ergotamine use—may be due to high dosage (see Chapter 51).

Side effects occur with all drugs and should be explained carefully to the patients. Patients should be asked about side effects during follow-up and, when appropriate, the dose adjusted to minimize side effects.

Contraindications

A prior history or risk factors, personal or familial, of ischemic heart or cerebrovascular disease, uncontrolled hypertension, and pregnancy contraindicate ergotamine and triptan use. Although cautionary labeling may vary, some practitioners consider it prudent to regard all the 5-HT$_{1B/1D}$ agonists as sharing the same risk profile in vascular diseases. Enteric ulcers and bleeding disorders contraindicate the use of aspirin and NSAIDs (see chapters on individual drugs).

Drug Dosage

Absorption of antimigraine drugs, especially ergotamine, varies among individuals. When used for the first time, an antimigraine drug should be taken in low doses that may be increased subsequently based on experience gained by treating several attacks. Then, the maximal safe and effective dose of the chosen drug should be given at onset of the attack.

The appropriate route of drug administration may depend on the characteristics of the attack, or the circumstances under which treatment must be taken. If vomiting prohibits oral administration of a drug, then subcutaneous injection, suppository, or intranasal preparations may be used. In attacks where speed of relief is important, the parenteral route of administration is preferable.

Customarily, having received appropriate advice from their physician, patients are able to treat themselves. For severe and prolonged migraine attacks, medical attendance may be essential. The appropriate courses of action under these circumstances are discussed in Chapters 66 and 132.

PROPHYLACTIC TREATMENT

When to Use?

To use preventive pharmacotherapy for migraine attacks is a decision that must not be made without considerable forethought by physician and patient. Migraine is an episodic disorder of an otherwise healthy population, and drug use can be accompanied by adverse effects. Issues of compliance and expense must also be considered. Prophylactic therapy should be considered only under one or more of the following circumstances:

1. Incidence of attacks is more than two or three per month.
2. Attacks are severe and impair normal activity.
3. Patient is psychologically unable to cope with the attacks.
4. Optimal abortive therapies have failed or produced serious side effects.

Migraine prophylaxis should not be used in patients planning pregnancy. Some form of birth control, preferably not steroidal, should be instituted before prophylactic treatment in women of childbearing potential. Monotherapy should be the rule in providing prophylaxis. No rigorous clinical trials have yielded convincing evidence of the additive effects of a second or third preventive drug. Such a therapeutic strategy also increases side effects, and potential interactions among the common preventive drugs are not understood. Nevertheless, it has become common practice to combine prophylactic agents in some countries, often making it impossible to know which is the effective agent.

The patients should keep a diagnostic headache diary (see Chapter 6) for at least 1 month so that the character and amount of the problem is documented before prophylactic treatment is begun. Some patients often suffer frequent migraine attacks and interval headaches, and overuse or abuse of drugs will become apparent when the diary is reviewed. These problems must be addressed before embarking on prophylactic treatment (see Chapters 115 and 127). During prophylactic treatment, patients should keep a simplified headache activity diary (Fig. 1) to help document the effect of treatment. Each medication should be given for an adequate time to judge its effectiveness, ideally 2 to 3 months. This often introduces a compliance problem, however. After the initial visit, patients should be observed at 2- to 3-month intervals or sooner depending on the severity and frequency of the migraine attacks or on the potential for adverse drug effects, for example, methysergide.

Treatment for How Long?

The frequency of migraine attacks varies over time, and there is often uncertainty when benefit occurs whether it is due to the drug or whether the disorder has gone into natural remission. This should be suspected whenever major life situations change that in themselves promote resolution of the attack frequency. Even with successful prophylactic treatment, gradual withdrawal after 6 to 12 months is an important goal to achieve.

Choice of Drug

Contraindications for common migraine preventive drugs include asthma and bradycardia for beta-blockers; peptic ulcer for NSAIDs; morbid obesity for pizotifen, tricyclic antidepressants, and valproic acid; and depression for flunarizine.

Side effects, even relatively minor, often limit the daily use of drugs in migraine. Patients should be warned to expect them and informed in advance about the nature of the most common ones. The importance of involving patients in decisions about their own therapy is never more in evidence than when deciding to take the available preventive medications.

In questioning about previous experiences with prophylactic treatment, the physician should check whether optimal doses were used and for how long. In addition, many patients may have tried prophylactic treatment without success due to overuse of symptomatic medications. Under these circumstances the drug should not be judged ineffective. Unresponsive patients have multiple preventive drug experiences, often making such judgments impossible.

Dose of Drug

The bioavailability of preventive migraine drugs varies; propanolol, for example, can vary by up to 10-fold (see Chapter 56). Accordingly there is no standard dose to be recommended for any migraine preventive medication. Customarily, drug levels are not measured in blood or urine, so the approach of relating levels to effect has never been pursued rigorously. Treatment should be initi-

For your **migraine attacks** indicate the severity as:

1, mild;   2, medium;   3, severe.

1)   A mild attack does not inhibit work or other activities.

2)   A medium attack inhibits but does not prohibit work or other activities.

3)   A severe attack prohibits work and/or other activities.

For your **tension-type headaches** use one or more crosses to indicate severity as defined above:

x, mild;   xx, medium;   xxx, severe.

For attacks of **cluster headache** use letters a, b and c for severity as defined above:

a, mild;   b, medium;   c, severe.

HEADACHE CALENDAR

The year 19____

The headache calender is used to record all episodes of headache during an entire year. This information will greatly assist your doctor in selecting the best treatment, and it may help yourself to identify factors in your life which worsen or improve your headache condition.
Bring this calender to each consultation with your doctor.

Name:

Social security no.:

Address:

Telephone:

The owner of this card is being treated for headache/migraine by Dr.:

(STAMP)

	Jan.	Feb.	Mar.	Apr.	May	June	July	Aug.	Sept.	Oct.	Nov.	Dec.	
1													1
2													2
3													3
4													4
5													5
6													6
7													7
8													8
9													9
10													10
11													11
12													12
13													13
14													14
15													15
16													16
17													17
18													18
19													19
20													20
21													21
22													22
23													23
24													24
25													25
26													26
27													27
28													28
29													29
30													30
31													31

FIG. 1. Suggested simple headache diary used to monitor headache activity during prophylactic treatment of migraine.

ated with low doses that, depending on efficacy and side effects, are increased gradually at 2- to 4-week intervals (see chapters on individual drugs).

POSSIBLE DRUG INTERACTIONS

Simultaneous use of prophylactic and abortive medications has the potential to cause their interaction. For example, NSAIDs used for acute attacks can increase the risk of gastrointestinal distress and hemorrhage when drugs of the same class are given preventively. Although not confirmed, methysergide combined with ergot preparations or a triptan could increase the risk of vasoconstrictive complications. Sumatriptan used for acute treatment of patients receiving selective serotonin reuptake inhibitors for prevention has in a few cases produced a serotonin syndrome that involves excessive agitation, movement disorders, and pyrexia. Clinicians must check drug information sources for drug interactions before prescribing.

PREGNANCY

Few data are available on the risks of most antimigraine drugs during pregnancy. For the treatment of migraine attacks, paracetamol (acetaminophen) with or without metoclopramide can be used. Hospital admission and intravenous fluids may be required for severe intractable migraine that may be judged life threatening. Migraine prevention may be considered for similar reasons. Propranolol in low doses can be used (for detailed guidelines, see Chapter 130). The decision to provide migraine preventive drugs should be taken together with a high-risk obstetric specialist.

The Headaches, Second Edition,
edited by J. Olesen, P. Tfelt-Hansen, and K.M.A. Welch.
Lippincott Williams & Wilkins, Philadelphia © 2000.

The Migraines

CHAPTER 50

Nonsteroidal Antiinflammatory Drugs in the Acute Treatment of Migraine

Peer Tfelt-Hansen and John McEwen

Whereas aspirin has been used for the treatment of migraine and other headaches for many years, the newer nonsteroidal antiinflammatory drugs (NSAIDs) were introduced in migraine therapy based mainly on indirect evidence of the involvement of prostaglandins in the pathophysiology of the migraine process. Thus, infusion of the two vasodilating prostaglandins prostaglandin E_1 (4,9) and prostacyclin (17,48) to either healthy volunteers or migraine sufferers induced flushing and a vascular headache, which, however, resembled migrainous symptoms in only a few patients (51). Another argument for the use of NSAIDs in migraine prophylaxis was based on their effect in opposing the suggested hyperaggregability of platelets in migraine, an effect since thought unlikely to contribute to their efficacy (see Chapter 60). However, subsequent controlled trials have demonstrated the efficacy of the NSAIDs in migraine therapy.

PHARMACOLOGIC BACKGROUND

Nonsteroidal antiinflammatory drugs possess antiinflammatory, analgesic, and antipyretic properties. The principal types of drugs are listed in Table 1. They exert their effect by blocking cyclooxygenase, thereby inhibiting the synthesis of prostaglandins from arachidonic acid (Fig. 1), but they have little or no effect on lipoxygenase and therefore no effect on the formation of leukotrienes.

Both prostaglandins and leukotrienes are involved in the inflammatory process (29).

Prostaglandins are associated with the development of pain that accompanies injury or inflammation. The NSAIDs, which inhibit the synthesis of these prostaglandins, are usually classed as mild peripheral analgesics, and a consideration of the type of pain that they suppress is important. They are particularly effective in settings in which inflammation has caused sensitization of pain receptors to normally pain-free mechanical or chemical stimuli. This sensitization appears to result from a lowering of the threshold of the polymodal nociceptor situated on C fibers (29). Although generally described as peripherally acting analgesics, an additional inhibitory effect on the central nociceptive system also may be responsible for their analgesic effect (6,7,37). The mode of action of the central effect of NSAIDs is unknown, but possible relevant effects include the following (6,10):

1. Inhibition by NSAIDs of prostaglandin synthesis in brain neurons.
2. Prolongation of catecholamine and serotonin turnover in brain neurons.
3. Blockade of the release of serotonin in response to noxious stimuli.

NSAIDs also inhibit platelet cylooxygenase with consequent inhibition of the formation of thromboxane A_2, a potent aggregating agent. The NSAID can either bind reversibly to this enzyme or, as in the case of aspirin, for the life of the platelet due to acetylation (8–11 days) (29). This effect on platelets can sometimes result in a prolonged bleeding time. An exception to this general description of NSAID properties is paracetamol, which

P. Tfelt-Hansen: Department of Neurology, Glostrup Hospital, University of Copenhagen, DK-2600 Glostrup, Copenhagen, Denmark.

J. McEwen: Department of Clinical Pharmacology and Therapeutics, Ninewells Hospital and Medical School, Dundee DD1 9SY, United Kingdom.

TABLE 1. *Nonsteroidal antiinflammatory drugs and their efficacy in migraine*

Carboxylic acids	Enolic acids
Acetic acids	
Indole acetic acids	Pyrazolones
Indomethacin	Phenylbutazone
Phenylacetic acids	Azapropazone
Diclofenac[a]	Oxicams
Fenclofenac	Piroxicam
Other heterocyclic acetic acids	
Sulindac	
Tolmetin	
Ketorolac[b]	
Salicylic acids	
Aspirin[a,c]	
Benorylate	
Propionic acids	
Fenoprofen[d]	
Ibuprofen[a]	
Ketoprofen[c,d]	
Naproxen[a,e]	
Indoprofen[c]	
Flurbiprofen[d]	
Pirprofen[a]	
Anthranilic acids	
Meclofenamic acid	
Mefenamic acid[c]	
Tolfenamic acid[a,e]	

[a] With demonstrated efficacy in the treatment of migraine attacks (at least two trials demonstrating efficacy).

[b] Only compared with other injections without placebo control.

[c] With possible efficacy in migraine prophylaxis (only one "positive" trial); (see Chapter 60).

[d] With possible effect in migraine attacks (only one "positive" trial).

[e] With demonstrated efficacy in the prophylaxis of migraine (at least two trials demonstrating efficacy).

has only weak antiinflammatory activity and does not cause inhibition of cyclooxygenase (29).

Possible Mode of Action in Migraine

The early prostaglandin infusion experiments (4,9,17) lent little support to the involvement of prostaglandins in the pathophysiology of migraine; only in a few cases were true migraine attacks provoked (51). Furthermore, intravenous infusion of prostacyclin to eight migraine patients induced only one migrainelike headache, and in two subjects given the infusion after a migraine attack had started, only a short-lived worsening occurred, suggesting that vasodilating prostaglandins were not the sole mediators of vascular headache in these patients (48). These experiments do not exclude an involvement of prostaglandins in inflammation of neurogenic origin such as the extravasation of plasma in the rat dura mater after trigeminal stimulation, an effect blocked by indomethacin and aspirin (8). The poor efficacy of indomethacin in migraine (51) might be taken as evidence against this possibility. Another possible explanation for the beneficial effects of aspirin and NSAIDs in the treatment of migraine attacks is their analgesic effect or more specific effects on the trigeminal (35) and antinociceptive (19) system in the brainstem.

Pharmacokinetics

In the treatment of migraine attacks the important pharmacokinetic parameter is the speed of absorption, which can of course be improved by appropriate formulation technology. NSAIDs are generally well-absorbed after oral administration with a time-to-peak plasma concentration (t_{max}) of less than 2 hours (29). Aspirin is absorbed very quickly, with a t_{max} of less than half an hour, and is metabolized quickly to salicylic acid (29,53). Naproxen sodium has a t_{max} of 1 hour, whereas naproxen has a t_{max} of 2 hours (29,43). Due to the slower

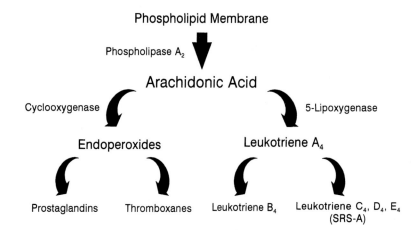

FIG. 1. Principal metabolic pathways of arachidonic acid. NSAIDs block cyclooxygenase, thereby inhibiting the synthesis of prostaglandins from arachidonic acid, but have little or no effect on lipoxygenase and therefore no effect on the formation of leukotrienes (29).

absorption of oral drugs during migraine attacks (50; see Chapter 7), NSAIDs are often combined with the prokinetic antiemetic drug metoclopramide. Ketorolac is given as an intramuscular injection, with a t_{max} of 45 to 60 minutes (18).

RESULTS OF RANDOMIZED CONTROLLED CLINICAL TRIALS

Placebo-Controlled Trials

A summary of 23 placebo-controlled double-blind randomized trials on the efficacy of NSAIDs or their combinations with either metoclopramide or caffeine in the treatment of migraine attacks are given in Table 2. A total of 1,898 migraine patients were administered NSAIDs or their combinations, 1,910 received placebo, and 286 received a comparator drug. The size of the trials varied

from a small crossover trial (25) with only 20 patients to several trials with parallel group design with more than 100 evaluable patients in each treatment group (11,28, 40,58). Except for five trials (28,32,39,41,59), in which only migraine patients without aura were included, the trials included a mixture of patients suffering from migraine both with and without aura. The crossover design, which causes few problems in trials concerning treatment of the acute attacks, was used in 16 of 23 trials. As indicated in Table 1, except for enolic acids, NSAIDs have been found to have some efficacy in the acute therapy of migraine.

Aspirin, 500 to 1000 mg, was superior to placebo in three trials (5,25,59). Aspirin plus metoclopramide was not superior to aspirin in one trial (59). Highly soluble aspirin salts (equivalent to 900 mg aspirin) combined with 10 mg metoclopramide were superior to placebo in three trials (11,28,58) and in one trial were comparable with 100 mg

TABLE 2. *Double-blind randomized, placebo-controlled, trial with NSAIDs or combinations containing NSAIDs in the treatment of migraine attacks*

Trial (ref.)	Drug, dosage Initial (maximum) (mg)	Study design	No. of attacks treated[a]	No. of patients evaluated	Result of trial
(59)	Metocl + ASA 10 + 650 ASA 650 Pl	CO	1	85	Escape medication: Metocl + ASA (63/92) = ASA (51/86) > Pl (75/95) Effect on pain: Metocl + ASA = ASA > Pl
(25)	Tfa 200 Erg 1 ASA 500 Pl	CO	2	20	Mean duration of attacks (h): Tfa (3.2) = Erg (3.8) = ASA (4.2) > Pl (7.1). Preference: all drugs > Pl
(5)	ASA 1,000 Parac 400 + CA 25 Pl	CO	1	198	Success rate[b]: ASA (52%) = Parac +CA (50%) > Pl (30%)
(11)	ASA 900 + Metoc 10 Pl	Pa	2 2	111 114	Success rates[b]: ASA + Metoc (59%) > Pl (29%)
(58)	ASA 900 + Metoc 10 Sum 100 Pl	Pa	2 2 2	133 119 124	Success rates[b]: ASA + Metoc (56%) = Sum (53%) > Pl (24%)
(28)	ASA 900 + Metoc 10 Pl	Pa	1	127 131	Success rates[b]: ASA + Metoc (54%) > Pl (26%)
(40)	ASA 600 + Parac 400 +Ca 200 Pl	Pa	1	602 618	Success rates[b]: ASA + Parac + C (59%) > Pl (33%)
(14)	Parac 1,000 (3,000) Metoc 10 (30) Pl	Pa	>4	42	Duration of attacks and amount of rescue medication: Parac + Metoc >Pl Severity: Parac+Metoc vs Pl NS
(15)	Parac[c] 650 (1,625) Pl	CO	2	56	Relief ranking: Parac = Pl
(60)[d]	Tfa 200 (400) Pl	CO	2	43–48	Duration of attacks (h): Tfa (5.6) > Pl (7.5)
(44)	TfaR 200 (400) Sum 100 Pl	Pa	2	43 42 41	Success rates[b]: TfaR (77%) = Sum (79%) > Pl (29%) for the first attack treated.
(45)	Napx 750 (1,250) Pl	CO	6	32	Headache severity[e]: Napx (2.1) > Pl (2.3) Napx > Pl for overall rating. Escape medication: Napx (24%) > Pl (46%)
(2)	Napx 750 (1,250) Pl	CO	6	32	Headache severity after 2h[e]: Napx (2.0) > Pl (2.2). Headache severity[e] for whole attack: Napx (2.2) vs. Pl (2.2) NS

TABLE 2. *Continued*

Trial (ref.)	Drug, dosage Initial (maximum) (mg)	Study design	No. of attacks treated[a]	No. of patients evaluated	Result of trial
(30)	NapxS 825 (1,375) PI	Pa	10	61	Change in headache severity[f]: NapxS (3.8) > PI (5.0). Escape medication: NapxS (44%) > PI (67%).
(18)	Ibupr 800 (1,200) PI	CO	5	27	Duration of attacks: Ibupr (5 h) > PI (11 h). Mild attacks: Ibupr (33%) > PI (7%)
(37)	Ibupr 1,200 (1,600) PI	CO	3	25	Headache severity[e] Ibupr (1.78) > PI (2.33) Migraine index[g]: Ibupr (25) > PI (46)
(54)	IbuprA 400 PI	CO	1	29	IbuprA > PI for pain reduction.
(13)	Diclo 75 IM PI	CO	3	32	Response to treatment[h]: Diclo (3.4) > PI (1.7). Preference: Diclo (21) > PI (1).
(41)	Diclo 50 (100) PI	CO	2	91	Attack aborted within 2 h: Diclo (27%) > PI (19%). Escape medication: Diclo (54%) > PI (66%).
(36)	Pirp 200 (500) CO	CO	1	55	Escape medication: Pirp (18/58) = Erg (18/59) > PI (32/60).
	Erg[i] 2 (5) PI				Duration of attacks (h): Erg (6.5) > PI (10.5) but vs Pirp NS. For most parameters Pirp vs. Erg Ns
(21)	Pirp 600 rectally PI	CO	2	20	Escape medication: Pirp (58%) > PI (98%)
(3)	Flurbp 100 (300) PI	CO	2	19	Relief score[j]: Flurbp (3.2) > PI (0.7)
(32)	Ketop 100 rectally	CO	6	50	Median change in pain on VAS scale: Ketop (15%) > PI (7%)
	Erg 2 do PI				Ketop = Erg (12%) Working ability: Ketop > Erg = PI

[a]Maximum number of attacks treated with each drug (in some trials the trial was terminated at a fixed date).
[b]A success defined as a decrease in headache from severe or moderate to none or mild.
[c]Only results for paracetamol and placebo given, see (15).
[d]A complicated study comparing Tfa, caffeine, metoclopramide, and their combinations with placebo (60). Only the comparison with placebo is shown here.
[e]Severity on a 4-point verbal scale (0 = none, 1 = mild, 2 = moderate, 3 = severe).
[f]Score: 2 = complete relief, 3 = substantial relief, 4 = slight relief, 5 = no change, 6 = worse.
[g]Severity times duration in hours.
[h]Response scale: 4 (excellent) to 1 (insufficient).
[i]An ergotamine combination with 1 mg ergotamine tatrate, 100 mg caffeine, 50 mg butalbital, and 0.125 mg bellafoline.
[j]Relief score: 4 (very good relief) to 0 (no relief).
ASA, aspirin; CA, caffeine; Diclo, diclofenac; Erg, Ergotamine; Flurb, flurbiprofen; Ibupr, ibuprofen; IGUprA, ibuprofen-arginine; Ketop, ketoprofen; Mefa, mefanamic acid; Metocl, metoclopramide; Napx, naproxen; NapxS, naproxen sodium; Parac, paracetamol (acetaminophen); Pirp, pirprofen; Sum, sumatripan; Tfa, tolfenamic acid; TfaR, rapid release tolfenamic acid; PI, placebo; CO, Crossover; Pa, Parallel group; NS or =, no statistical significant difference; > more effective than; VAS, visual analogue scale; IM, intramascularly.

sumatriptan (58). If one combines the results of these three trials, the therapeutic gain (success rate for active drug minus success rate for placebo) is 29% [95% confidence interval (CI) 23%–35%], a therapeutic gain in the same range as for 100 mg sumatriptan (see Chapter 52). For a combination of 600 mg aspirin plus 400 mg acetaminophen and 200 mg caffeine, a therapeutic gain of 26% (95% CI 21%–31%) was found in three trials (40), but it should be noted that patients with the most severe migraine attacks were excluded from these trials.

Paracetamol combined with metoclopramide was superior to placebo in one trial (14), whereas 650 mg paracetamol alone was no better than placebo (15). A combination of 400 mg paracetamol and 25 mg codeine was found to be superior to placebo (5).

Tolfenamic acid 200 mg was shown in three trials to be more effective than placebo (25,44,60), and in one of these (44), a rapid-release form was comparable with 100 mg sumatriptan. The latter result needs confirmation in larger trials. In one of the other trials (25), tolfenamic acid was comparable with 500 mg aspirin and 1 mg ergotamine, with fewer side effects than ergotamine. In a small crossover trial (n = 10) (23), the addition of caffeine to tolfenamic acid was found to be superior to the addition of pyridoxine to tolfenamic acid, but in a larger double-blind crossover trial (n = 49), the effect of the addition of caffeine to tolfenamic acid was not superior to that of tolfenamic acid alone (60). In contrast, the addition of metoclopramide to tolfenamic acid was significantly, if marginally, better than tolfenamic acid alone (60).

Naproxen was shown to be superior to placebo in one trial (45), whereas in another similar trial the effect of naproxen was only superior to placebo after 2 hours, but not for the whole attack (2). Naproxen sodium, which due to quicker absorption of the naproxen molecule should be more suitable than naproxen per se (see Pharmacokinetics section), was superior to placebo in one trial (30).

Ibuprofen 800 to 1,200 mg or 400 mg as an arginine salt was more effective than placebo in three trials (27,37,54). In one trial in children, ibuprofen and paracetamol were comparable, and both were superior to placebo (26).

In two trials, oral (41) and intramuscular diclofenac (13) were superior to placebo, with the most convincing results following intramuscular diclofenac (13).

Pirprofen was comparable with an ergotamine combination in one trial, and both were superior to placebo (36). In a trial including episodic tension-type headache, the results for migraine treated with rectal pirprofen were superior to those for placebo (21). Flurbiprofen was superior to placebo in one trial (3). Ketoprofen by suppository was superior to placebo and superior to ergotamine for working capacity in one trial (32).

Comparative Trials without Placebo Control

In two trials aspirin taken at the onset of an attack was inferior to ergotamine and a dextropropoxyphene compound in preventing migraine attacks (22,24) (see Table 2 and Chapter 51). In one trial the success rate of the combination of 1,000 mg aspirin and 10 mg metoclopramide (45%) was not significantly different from 100 mg sumatriptan (56%) for the primary efficacy parameter, the effect on head pain in the first attack, but inferior to sumatriptan for all other parameters (46).

Tolfenamic acid was superior to paracetamol in a reasonably large crossover trial with 58 evaluable patients (39), but there was no difference between the efficacy of 200 and 400 mg tolfenamic acid. Thus, no dose-response relationship has been established for tolfenamic acid in migraine or for that matter with any other NSAID.

In one trial, naproxen sodium was found to be superior to an ergotamine combination for some parameters (52), but in other studies naproxen sodium was found to be equally effective as ergotamine (61) or ergotamine plus caffeine (55).

Ibuprofen was superior to paracetamol in one trial (47), and intramuscular diclofenac was superior to intramuscular paracetamol in one trial (33), whereas mefenamic acid was not superior to paracetamol (49).

Ketorolac 30 mg intramuscularly was found to be less effective than 75 mg meperidine (38), whereas a dose of 60 mg ketorolac was as effective as 75 mg meperidine (plus 25 mg promethazine) (12), 100 mg meperidine (plus 50 mg hydroxyzine) (16), and 25 mg chlorpromazine intravenously (57) in rather small (n = 30–47)

randomized trials in emergency departments. In one trial (n = 64), 30 mg intravenous ketorolac was inferior to 10 mg intravenous prochlorperazine (56). There have been no placebo-controlled trials with ketorolac (18). Ketoprofen 100 mg intramuscularly was superior to an injection of 500 mg paracetamol (34). A combination drug Fiorinal with codeine (butalbital 50 mg, caffeine 50 mg, aspirin 325 mg, and codeine phosphate 30 mg) was found to be inferior to intranasal butorphanol 1 mg for treating migraine pain during the first 2 hours (20) (see Chapter 54).

Side effects after NSAIDs in all of the aforementioned trials were minor and mostly referable to the gastrointestinal tract, such as epigastric pain. One major argument for the original introduction of NSAIDs in migraine treatment has been the high incidence of the side effects of the then standard drug ergotamine (25,52). In several trials with NSAIDs (25,32,36,52,55,61), ergotamine has been the reference drug, and generally the NSAIDs were comparable with oral ergotamine with regard to efficacy. The differences have been mainly those of tolerability: on the whole, ergotamine caused more gastrointestinal side effects such as nausea and vomiting, although this was only statistically significant in two trials (25,55). In one trial (58), 100 mg sumatriptan caused more side effects than the combination of aspirin and metoclopramide.

In some randomized controlled clinical trials of NSAIDs (5,11,28,40,44,58), the use of currently accepted trial methodology (see Chapter 7) allows a fair judgment of their efficacy. In contrast, the clinical relevance of the results of older trials is difficult to judge. Even if the NSAIDs are statistically significantly superior to placebo, the beneficial effects often seem marginal in some trials (2,30,32,37,41,45,59). The results of many trials of these drugs may have not yet been published. We suggest that in order to justify the use of an NSAID in acute migraine therapy there should be at least two controlled trials showing a significantly better effect than placebo. So far there is no good reason to choose tolfenamic acid, naproxen sodium, ibuprofen, pirprofen, or diclofenac rather than aspirin, especially aspirin combined with metoclopramide, because no controlled trial has shown a newer NSAID to be superior to aspirin in the treatment of migraine attacks.

THERAPEUTIC USE

Aspirin and paracetamol are the most frequently used drugs for the treatment of migraine, and many patients have already tried them before consulting a physician. For those for whom self-medication has proved ineffective, one can endeavor to optimize aspirin or paracetamol treatment by giving the drugs in effervescent form in combination with metoclopramide 10 mg orally or highly soluble aspirin salts plus metoclopramide, if available. One should also maximize the dose and ensure that med-

TABLE 3. *Recommended dose of NSAIDs in the treatment of migraine attacks*

Drug	Initial dose (mg)	Repeated dose if necessary after 1–2 h[a] (mg)
Aspirin	900 or 1,000	900 or 1,000
Aspirin + metoclopramide	900 + 10	900 + 10
Paracetamol (acetaminophen)	1,000	1,000
Tolfenamic acid	200	200
Naproxen sodium	825	550
Piprofen	200	200
Ibuprofen	1,200	400
Ketoprofen by suppository	100	
Diclofenac intramuscularly	75	

[a]There are no trials demonstrating that repeated dosing increases the effectiveness of NSAIDs.

ication is taken at the onset of the first symptoms. If the patient does not respond to this, then either other NSAIDs plus metoclopramide, triptans, or ergotamine should be tried (see Chapter 55). The relative effectiveness of NSAIDs and triptans remains to be established.

NSAIDs can be used during the drug withdrawal period in patients with a history of ergotamine abuse (1,42) and probably also after triptan abuse. In the emergency room intramuscular diclofenac is often useful.

The recommended doses of the NSAIDs are given in Table 3. Side effects include epigastric pain and diarrhea. Contraindications include hypersensitivity to aspirin or any NSAID, peptic ulcer, and concomitant treatment with anticoagulants.

REFERENCES

1. Ala-Hurula V, Myllylä VV, Hokkanen E, Tokola O. Tolfenamic acid and ergotamine abuse. *Headache* 1981;21:240–242.
2. Andersson PG, Hinge HH, Johansen O, Andersen CU, Lademann A, Götzke PC. Double-blind study of naproxen vs placebo in the treatment of acute migraine attacks. *Cephalalgia* 1989;9:29–32.
3. Awidi AS. Efficacy of flurbiprofen in the treatment of acute migraine attacks: a double blind cross-over study. *Curr Ther Res* 1982;32:492–497.
4. Bergström S, Carlson LA, Erelund LG, Oro L. Cardiovascular and metabolic response to infusion of of prostaglandin E 1 and simultaneous infusion of noradrenaline and PGE 1 in man. *Acta Physiol Scand* 1965;64:332–339.
5. Boureau F, Joubert JM, Lasserre V, Prum B, Delecoeuillerie G. Double-blind comparison of an acetaminophen 400 mg–codeine 25 mg combination versus aspirin 1000 mg and placebo in acute migraine attack. *Cephalalgia* 1994;14:156–161.
6. Bromm B, Forth W, Ricther E, Sharein E. Effects of acetaminophen and antipyrine on non-inflammatory pain and EEG activity. *Pain* 199250:213–221.
7. Brune K, Bek WS, Geislinger G, et al. aspirin-like drugs may block pain independent of prostaglandin synthesis inhibition. *Experientia* 1991;47:257–261.
8. Buzzi MG, Sakas DE, Moskowitz MA. Indomethacin and acetylsalicylic acid block neurogenic plasma protein extravasation in rat dura mater. *Eur J Pharmacol* 1989;165:251–258.
9. Carlson LA, Eklund LG, Oro L. Clinical and metabolic effects of different doses of PGE 1 in man. *Acta Med Scand* 1968;183:423–430.
10. Cashman JN. The mechanisms of action of NSAIDs in analgesia. *Drugs* 1996;52[Suppl 5]:13–23.
11. Chabriat H, Joire JE, Danchot J, Grippon P, Bousser MG. Combined oral lysine acetylsalicylate and metoclopramide in the acute treatment of migraine: a multicentre double-blind placebo-controlled study. *Cephalalgia* 1994;14:297–300.
12. Davis CP, Torre PR, Williams C, et al. Ketorolac versus meperidine-plus-promethazine treatment of migraine headache: evaluations by patients. *Am J Emerg Med* 1995;13:146–150.
13. Del Bene E, Poggioni M, Garagiola U, Maresca V. Intramuscular treatment of migraine attacks using diclofenac sodium: a crossover clinical trial. *J Int Med Res* 1987;15:44–48.
14. Dexter SL, Graham AN, Johnson ES, Ratcliffe DM, Wilkinson MIP, Rose AJ. Double-blind controlled study of Paramax in the acute treatment of common and classical migraine. *Br J Clin Pract* 1985;39:388–392.
15. Diamond S. Treatment of migraine with isometheptene, acetaminophen, and dichlorphenazone combination: a double-blind, crossover trial. *Headache* 1976;16:282–287.
16. Duarte C, Dunaway F, Turner L, Aldag J, Frederick R. Ketorolac versus meperidine and hydroxyzine in the treatment of acute migraine headache: a randomized, prospective, double-blind trial. *Ann Emerg Med* 1992;21:1116–1121.
17. Fitzgerald GA, Friedman LA, Miya M, O'Grady J, Lewis PJ. A double-blind placebo controlled crossover study of prostacyclin in man. *Life Sci* 1979;25:665–672.
18. Gillis JC, Brogden RN. Ketorolac. A reappraisal of its pharmacodynamic and pharmacokinetic properties and therapeutic use in pain management. *Drugs* 1997;53:139–188.
19. Gobel H, Ernst M, Jeschke J, Keil R, Weigle L. Acetylsalicylic acid activates antinociceptive brain-stem reflex activity in headache patients and in healthy subjects. *Pain* 1992;48:187–195.
20. Goldstein J, Gawel MJ, Winner P, et al., on behalf of the Stadol Nasal Spray/Fiorinal C study group. Comparison of butorphanol nasal spray and Fiorinal with codeine in the treatment of migraine. *Headache* 1998;38:516–522.
21. Guidotti M, Zanasi S, Garagiola U. Pirprofen in the treatment of migraine and episodic headache attacks: a placebo-controlled crossover clinical trial. *J Int Med Res* 1989;17:48–54.
22. Hakkarainen H, Gustafsson B, Stockman O. A comparative trial of ergotamine tartrate, acetylsalicylic acid and a dextropropoxyphene compound in acute migraine attacks. *Headache* 1978;18:35–39.
23. Hakkarainen H, Parantainen J, Gothoni G, Vapaatalo H. Tolfenamic acid and caffeine: a useful combination in migraine. *Cephalalgia* 1982;2:173–177.
24. Hakkarainen H, Quiding H, Stockman O. Mild analgesics as an alternative to ergotamine in migraine. A comparative trial with acetyl salicylic acid, ergotamine tartrate and a dextropropoxyphene compound. *J Clin Pharmacol* 1980;20:590–595.
25. Hakkarainen H, Vapaatalo H, Gothoni G, Paratainen J. Tolfenamic acid is as effective as ergotamine during migraine attacks. *Lancet* 1979;2:326–328.
26. Hamalainen ML, Hoppu K, Valkeila E, Santavuori P. Ibuprofen or acetaminophen for the acute treatment of migraine in children: a double-blind, randomized, placebo-controlled, crossover study. *Neurology* 1997;48:103–107.
27. Havanka-Kanniainen H. Treatment of acute migraine attack: ibuprofen and placebo compared. *Headache* 1989;29:507–509.
28. Henry P, Hiesse-Provost O, Dillenschneider A, Ganry H, Insuasty J. Efficacité et tolérance de l association effevescente aspirine-métoclopramide dans le traitement de la crise de migraine sans aura. Essai randomisé en double avuegle contre placebo. *Presse Med* 1995;24:254–258.
29. Insel PA. Analgesic-antipyretics and antiinflammatory agents and drugs employed in the treatment of gout. In: Goodman LS, Limbird LE, Milinoff PB, Gilman AG, Hardman JG, eds. *Goodman and Gilman's the pharmacological basis of therapeutics,* 9th ed. New York: McGraw-Hill, 1996:617–657.
30. Johnson ES, Ratcliffe DM, Wilkinson M. Naproxen sodium in the treatment of migraine. *Cephalalgia* 1985;5:5–10.
31. Jurna I, Brune K. Central effect of the non-steroid anti-inflammatory agents, indomethacin, ibuprofen, and diclofenac, determined in C fibre-evoked activity in single neurones of the rate thalamus. *Pain* 1990;41:71–80.
32. Kangasneimi P, Kaaja R. Ketoprofen and ergotamine in acute migraine. *J Intern Med* 1992;231:551–554.

33. Karachalios GN, Fotiadou A, Chrisikos N, Karabetsos A, Kehagioglou K. Treatment of acute migraine attack with diclofenac sodium:a double-blind study. *Headache* 1992;32:98–100.

34. Karabetsos A, Karachalios G, Bourlinou P, Reppa A, Koutri R, Fotiadou A. Ketoprofen versus paracetamol in the treatment of acute migraine. *Headache* 1997;37:12–14.

35. Kaube H, Hoskin KL, Goadsby PJ. Intravenous acetylsalicylic acid inhibits central trigeminal neurons in the dorsal horn of the upper cervical spinal cord in the cat. *Headache* 1993;33:541–544.

36. Kinnunen E, Erkinjuntti T, Färkkilä M, et al. Placebo-controlled double-blind trial of pirprofen and an ergotamine tartrate compound in migraine attacks. *Cephalalgia* 1988;8:175–179.

37. Kloster R, Nestvold K, Vilming ST. A double-blind study of ibuprofen versus placebo in the treatment of acute migraine attacks. *Cephalalgia* 1992;12:169–171.

38. Larkin GL, Prescott JE. A randomized, double-blind, comparative study of the efficacy of ketorolac tromethamine versus meperidine in the treatment of severe migraine. *Ann Emerg Med* 1992;21:919–924.

39. Larsen BH, Christiansen LV, Andersen B, Olesen J. Randomized double-blind comparison of tolfenamic acid and paracetamol in migraine. *Acta Neurol Scand* 1990;81:464–467.

40. Lipton RB, Stewart WF, Ryan RE Jr, Saper J, Sheftell F. Efficacy and safety of acetaminophen, aspirin, and caffeine in alleviating migraine headache pain: three double-blind, randomized, placebo-controlled trials. *Arch Neurol* 1998;55:210–217.

41. Massiou H, Serrurier D, Lassere O, Bousser M-G. Effectiveness of oral diclofenac in the acute treatment of common migraine attacks: a double-blind study versus placebo. *Cephalalgia* 1991;11:59–63.

42. Mathew NT. Amelioration of ergotamine withdrawal symptoms with naproxen. *Headache* 1987;27:130–133.

43. Moyer S. Pharmacokinetics of naproxen sodium. *Cephalalgia* 1986;6 [Suppl 4]:77–80.

44. Myllylä VV, Havanka H, Herrala L, et al. Tolfenamic acid rapid release versus sumatriptan in the acute treatment of migraine: comparable effect in a double-blind, randomized, controlled, parallel-group study. *Headache* 1998;38:201–207.

45. Nestvold K, Kloster R, Partinen M, Sulkava R. Treatment of acute migraine attack: naproxen and placebo compared. *Cephalalgia* 1985;5:115–119.

46. Oral Sumatriptan and Aspirin Plus Metoclopramide Comparative Study Group. A study to compare oral sumatriptan with oral aspirin plus metoclopramide in the treatment of migraine. *Eur Neurol* 1992;32:177–184.

47. Pearce I, Frank GJ, Pearce JMS. Ibuprofen compared with paracetamol in migraine. *Practioner* 1983;227:465–467.

48. Peatfield RC, Gawel MJ, Clifford Rose F. The effect of infused prostacyclin in migraine and cluster headache. *Headache* 1981;21:190–195.

49. Peatfield RC, Petty RG, Rose FC. Double blind comparison of mefenamic acid and acetaminophen (paracetamol) in migraine. *Cephalalgia* 1983;3:129–134.

50. Pini LA, Bertolotti M, Trenti T, Vitale G. Disposition of naproxen after oral administration during and between migraine attacks. *Headache* 1993;33:191–194.

51. Pradalier A, Clapin A, Dry J. Treatment review: non-steroid anti-inflammatory drugs in the treatment and long-term prevention of migraine attacks. *Headache* 1988;28:550–557.

52. Pradalier A, Rancurel G, Dordain G, Verdure L, Rascol A, Dry J. Acute migraine attack therapy: comparison of naproxen sodium and an ergotamine tartrate compound. *Cephalalgia* 1985;5:107–113.

53. Ross-Lee LM, Eadie MJ, Heazlewood V, Bochner F, Tyrer JH. Aspirin pharmacokinetics in migraine. The effect of metoclopramide. *Eur J Clin Pharmacol* 1983;24:777–785.

54. Sandrini G, Franchini S, Lanfranchi S, Granella F, Manzoni GC, Nappi G. Effectiveness of ibuprofen-arginine in the treatment of acute migraine attacks. *Int J Clin Pharmacol Res* 1998;18:145–150.

55. Sargent JD, Baumel B, Peters K, et al. Aborting a migraine attack: naproxen sodium v ergotamine plus caffeine. *Headache* 1988;28:263–266.

56. Seim MB, March JA, Dunn KA. Intravenous ketorolac vs intravenous prochlorperazine for the treatment of migraine headaches. *Acad Emerg Med* 1998;5:573–576.

57. Shrestha M, Singh R, Moreden J, Hayes JE. Ketorolac vs chlorpromazine in the treatment of acute migraine without aura. A prospective, randomized, double-blind trial. *Arch Intern Med* 1996;156:1725–1728.

58. Tfelt-Hansen P, Henry P, Mulder LJ, Scheldewaert RG, Schoenen J, Chazot G. The effectiveness of combined oral lysine acetylsalicylate and metoclopramide compared with oral sumatriptan for migraine. *Lancet* 1995;346:923–926.

59. Tfelt-Hansen P, Olesen J. Effervescent metoclopramide and aspirin (Migravess) versus effervescent aspirin or placebo for migraine attacks: a double-blind study. *Cephalagia* 1984;4:107–111.

60. Tokola RA, Kangasneimi P, Neuvonen PJ, Tokola O. Tolfenamic acid, metoclopramide, caffeine and their combinations in the treatment of migraine attacks. *Cephalagia* 1984;4:253–263.

61. Treves TA, Streiffler M, Korczyn AD. Naproxen sodium versus ergotamine tartrate in the treatment of acute migraine attacks. Headache 1992;32:280–282.

The Headaches, Second Edition,
edited by J. Olesen, P. Tfelt-Hansen, and K.M.A. Welch.
Lippincott Williams & Wilkins, Philadelphia © 2000.

The Migraines

CHAPTER 51

Ergot Alkaloids in the Acute Treatment of Migraine

Peer Tfelt-Hansen and Pramod R. Saxena

He gently prevails on his patients to try

The magic effects of the ergot of rye.

Lord Alfred Tennyson (1809–1892) (66)

In the Middle Ages, grain contaminated with ergot (*Claviceps purpurea*) caused epidemics of gangrene known as the "Holy Fire" or "St. Anthony's Fire" (7,78,115). Ergotamine (Fig 1), one of the ergot alkaloids mainly responsible for this effect, was isolated from ergot in 1918 (105) and found to have sympatholytic activity. Its introduction for the treatment of migraine in 1926 was based on the belief that migraine was caused by heightened sympathetic activity (75). In 1938 Graham and Wolff concluded that the efficacy of ergotamine was probably due to vasoconstriction of the extracranial vasculature (36). Yet, soon afterward, in 1945, dihydroergotamine was introduced in migraine therapy as a more potent sympatholytic agent than ergotamine (49). The vasoconstrictor activity of these ergot alkaloids is most likely involved in their effect on migraine pain, although other possible mechanisms for the beneficial effect of ergotamine have been suggested, including an action on central serotonergic neurones (50,89) and an effect on neurogenic inflammation (76) (see Chapter 17).

P. Tfelt-Hansen: Department of Neurology, Glostrup Hospital, University of Copenhagen, DK-2600 Glostrup, Copenhagen, Denmark.

P. R. Saxena: Department of Pharmacology, Erasmus University, 3000 DR Rotterdam, The Netherlands.

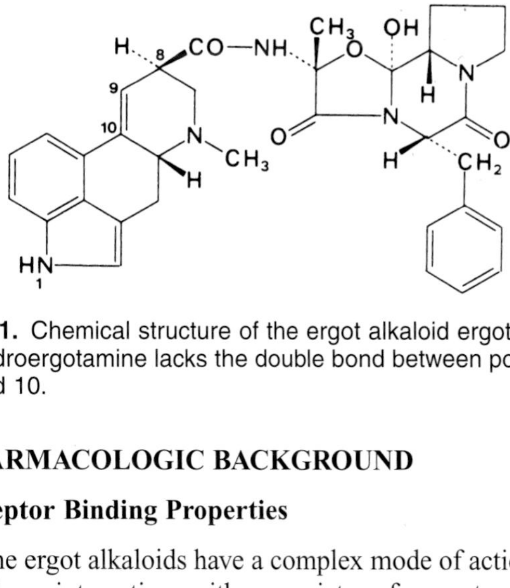

FIG. 1. Chemical structure of the ergot alkaloid ergotamine. Dihydroergotamine lacks the double bond between positions 9 and 10.

PHARMACOLOGIC BACKGROUND

Receptor Binding Properties

The ergot alkaloids have a complex mode of action that involves interaction with a variety of receptors (82). Indeed, as shown in Table 1 (2,32,52,53,68,69), both ergotamine and dihydroergotamine have affinities for 5-hydroxytryptamine (5-HT), dopamine, and noradrenaline receptors. In contrast, sumatriptan is much more selective, showing high affinity for 5-HT$_{1B}$ and 5-HT$_{1D}$ receptors and a moderate affinity for 5-HT$_{1A}$ and 5-ht$_{1F}$ receptors.

The α-adrenoceptor blocking property of ergotamine, first described in 1906 (17), is a textbook knowledge (48); however, this property is often overemphasized, in that it has been observed only with high doses used in some animal models, which bears no relevance to therapeutic use in human (27). In lower therapeutically relevant concentrations, ergotamine acts as an agonist at α-adrenoceptors, 5-HT (particularly 5-HT$_{1B/1D}$), and dopamine D$_2$ receptors (19,81,82,97,121). In addition, there is evidence that both

TABLE 1. *Receptor profile of ergotamine and dihydroergotamine as compared to sumatriptan*

Receptor type	PK$_i$ value on human cloned receptors in radioligand binding assay[a]		
	Ergotamine	Dihydroergotamine	Sumatriptan
5-HT$_{1A}$	7.89[b]	9.30[c]	6.43[c]
5-HT$_{1B}$	7.88[b]	9.22[c]	7.82[c]
5-HT$_{1D}$	8.36[b]	8.60[c]	8.46[c]
5-ht$_{1E}$	6.22[d]	6.22[c]	5.80[c]
5-ht$_{1F}$	6.77[d]	6.96[c]	7.86[c]
5-HT$_{2A}$	7.69$_o$, functional[f]	8.54[c], *functional*	<5.0 (pIC50)[c]
5-HT$_{2B}$	8.17 (pEC$_{50}$, pig)	7.70 (pEC$_{50}$, pig)[f]	ND
5-HT$_{2C}$	7.25 (pig, native)[e]	7.43 (pig)[c]	<5.0 (pIC$_{50}$, pig)[c]
5-HT$_3$	ND	<5.0 (pIC$_{50}$, mouse)[c]	<5.0 (pIC$_{50}$, mouse)[c]
5-HT$_4$	ND	6.52 (guinea-pig)[c]	<5.0 (pIC$_{50}$, guinea-pig)[c]
5-ht$_{5A}$	7.26[b]	7.34[b]	5.50[d]
5-ht$_{5B}$	8.50 (pK$_d$, rat)[g]	ND	ND
5-ht$_6$	ND	6.78[b]	5.31[d]
5-HT$_7$	7.49 (pK$_d$, rat)[g]	7.17[b]	6.51[d]
α$_1$ adrenoceptor	8.00 (?)[h]	8.00 (rat)[c]	<5.0 (pIC$_{50}$, rat)[c]
α$_2$ adrenoceptor	8.20 (?)[h]	8.00 (rat)[c]	<5.0 (pIC$_{50}$, rat)[c]
β$_1$ adrenoceptor	ND	5.27[c]	<5.0 (pIC$_{50}$)[c]
β$_2$ adrenoceptor	ND	<5.0 (pIC$_{50}$)[c]	<5.0 (pIC$_{50}$)[c]
Dopamine D$_1$	ND	5.32 (rat)[c]	<5.0 (pIC$_{50}$, rat)[c]
Dopamine D$_2$	8.50 (?)[h]	8.21[c]	<5.0 (pIC$_{50}$)[c]

?, species and test not specified; ND, not determined.
[a]Unless otherwise stated.
[b]Data from Pauwels PJ, personal communication.
[c]Data from Leysen JE, Gommeren W, Leylen, L, et al. (69).
[d]Data from Adham N, Kao HT, Schecter LE, et al. (2).
[e]Data from Hoyer D (52).
[f]Data from Glusa E, Roos A (32).
[g]Data from Hoyer D, Clarke DE, Fozard JR, et al. (53).
[h]Data from Leysen JE, Gommeren W (68).

ergotamine and dihydroergotamine can activate novel, not yet characterized receptors (19).

Vasoconstrictor Properties

The most important and conspicuous pharmacologic effect of ergot alkaloids is undeniably their vasoconstrictor action (81,82). Extensive studies in animal models have shown that this vasoconstrictor effect is particularly marked within the carotid vascular bed. This selectivity further extends to the arteriovenous anastomotic part of the carotid circulation; blood flow to a number of tissues, including that to the brain, is affected only minimally (19,58). Similar vasoconstrictor effects on cephalic arteriovenous anastomoses also have been observed with the use of sumatriptan as well as other triptans (98).

In humans, ergotamine can constrict several isolated blood vessels, including the pulmonary (14), cerebral (81), temporal (83), and coronary (74) arteries. The drug seems to be more active on large arteries (conducting vessels) than on arterioles (resistance vessels). Dihydroergotamine constricts veins, as demonstrated locally by local infusion into hand veins (3), and its contractile effect on human basilar arteries is equipotent but with a smaller maximal effect than ergotamine (81).

In humans, arterial blood pressure transiently increased moderately after parenteral therapeutic doses of ergota-

mine and dihydroergotamine (6,108,109). For ergotamine, the hypertensive response is due to increased total peripheral resistance (111). Basal cerebral blood flow (CBF) and acetazolamide-stimulated CBF remain unchanged after both ergotamine and dihydroergotamine (6). Basal myocardial blood flow also is unchanged after intravenous ergotamine, but the coronary vasodilator reserve decreases, probably by an effect on the microcirculation (33). In contrast to the short-lasting (about 3 hours) effect on blood pressure, ergotamine causes long-lasting (at least 24 hours) vasoconstriction of leg arteries (108,109). A similar long-lasting venoconstrictor effect (at least 8 hours) has been observed after a single dose of dihydroergotamine (5). For dihydroergotamine, no effect on peripheral arteries was found (6). An important feature of ergotamine and dihydroergotamine, observed *in vitro*, is that their effect on blood vessels is resistant to repeated wash (74,80,83), which appears to be due mainly to slow diffusion from the receptor biophase; therefore, their effects last far longer than can be expected from plasma concentrations (5,113).

Neuronal Properties

Ergotamine and dihydroergotamine have been reported to inhibit dural plasma extravasation after stimulation of the trigeminal ganglion in rat (11,12,76) by a C fiber-dependent mechanism, perhaps coupled to blockade of neuropeptide release from perivascular nerves (see Chapter 17). Furthermore, dihydroergotamine binds to receptors in the trigeminal nucleus caudalis and in the dorsal horn of the first and second cervical segments of the spinal cord in the cat (35), which, in turn, may inhibit activity in the central trigeminal neurons (50) (see Chapter 23). Probably, ergotamine has the same effect. Both the peripheral and central effects on the trigeminovascular system have been suggested to contribute toward the antimigraine effect of ergot alkaloids.

Effect on the Cranial Vasculature and Possible Mode of Action in Migraine

In the now classic study by Graham and Wolff (36), a parallel decrease in pulsation of the temporal artery and headache intensity was observed in 16 of 20 experiments after intravenous ergotamine. When the amplitude of pulsation decreased slowly, headache likewise diminished slowly. If the amplitude dropped precipitously, the headache ended promptly (Fig. 2). Similar decreases in pulsation of the temporal artery was found for dihydroergotamine later (9). No evidence was found of changes in the diameter of intracranial arteries (36). This study apparently demonstrated an extracranial pain source, the dilated temporal artery, during migraine attacks, and also demonstrated that ergotamine acts by its vasoconstrictor effect. As pointed out subsequently by Brazil and Friedman (9), however, pulse-wave contour can vary considerably and depends not only on the tone in the arterial wall but also on the pulse amplitude and the blood flow. Thus, an increase in amplitude does not necessarily imply vasodilatation, nor does diminution of amplitude necessarily imply vasoconstriction. Furthermore, the likelihood of a specific vasoconstrictor effect on the extracranial arteries as being the effect solely responsible for the efficacy of ergot alkaloids has been weakened by the demonstration that in only one third of migraine patients is the pain arguably of extracranial vascular origin (23). In addition, the temporal artery was only relatively dilated to a small extent on the pain side during migraine attacks (57). Thus, the effect of ergot alkaloids may not be entirely due to extracranial vasoconstriction.

The parallel decreases in pulse amplitude and headache still point to a vascular action of ergotamine, but this effect might have been brought about by actions of the drug on other parts of the cranial vascular bed. Thus, in male volunteers, 0.5 mg of ergotamine administered intravenously caused an increase in blood velocity in the middle cerebral artery (116). In another study, however, ergotamine (0.5 mg, administered imtramuscularly) was effective in nine of ten migraine patients, but it did not affect blood velocity in the middle cerebral artery as would have been expected in case this artery dilated during migraine attacks (20). This finding might suggest indirectly that some other action of ergot alkaloids, such as an effect on neurogenic inflammation (76) or central inhibition of trigeminalvascular pathways (34,50), might be responsible for its antimigraine effect. Alternatively, a combination of effects may be necessary for the therapeutic effect.

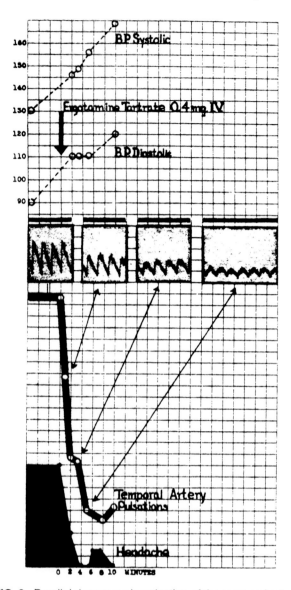

FIG. 2. Parallel decreases in pulsation of the temporal artery and headache in a migraine patient treated with 0.4 mg ergotamine intravenously. [From Grahamm and Wolf (36).]

PHARMACOKINETICS OF ERGOTAMINE AND DIHYDROERGOTAMINE

Ergotamine

With tritium-labeled ergotamine, 66% of the orally administered ergotamine was absorbed (4), but subsequently it was shown that the oral bioavailability of ergotamine was less than 1% (10,55). Thus, even if ergotamine is well absorbed, most of the drug is metabolized during the first pass through the liver.

After intravenous injection, ergotamine is distributed quickly, with a half-life of 2 to 3 minutes and an elimination half-life of 2 hours (54). It is cleared extensively during its passage through the liver, with an extraction fraction of greater than 0.75 (111). The intramuscular bioavailability is about 50%, and the peak plasma concentration is seen after 10 minutes (54). For other routes of administration, it is often impossible to detect ergotamine in plasma. Based on measurements with high-performance liquid chromatography (24) and mass spectrometry (95), the oral and sublingual bioavailability of ergotamine is estimated to be less than 1%, whereas the rectal and inhalational bioavailabilities are estimated to be 1% to 3 % (10,26,54,55,95,114).

Dihydroergotamine

Dihydroergotamine also has a low oral bioavailability (about 1%) as a result of extensive liver first-pass metabolism (72,124). Despite formation of an active metabolite, 8'-hydroxydihydroergotamine, with an area under the curve about seven times greater than the parent dihydroergotamine (77), the "total oral bioavailability" of dihydroergotamine is still quite low.

After intravenous injection, dihydroergotamine is distributed quickly and eliminated, with a mean terminal half-life of 13 to 15 hours (110,124). The peak plasma concentration occurs 30 minutes after intramuscular injection (4) and 45 minutes after subcutaneous administration (70). Nasally administered dihydroergotamine becomes rapidly available to the systemic circulation, with peak plasma levels achieved in 0.75 (110) to 0.9 hour (51) (Fig. 3). The bioavailability of intranasal dihydroergotamine is about 40% (51,110).

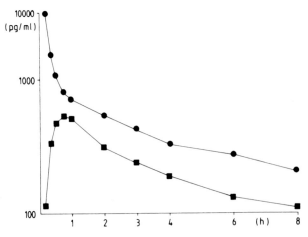

FIG. 3. Mean plasma concentrations of dihydroergotamine (*DHE*) after intravenous and intranasal administration in 12 volunteers: Mean plasma concentrations of DHE after 1 mg DHE intravenously (•) and as a nasal spray (■); log-scale. [From Tfelt-Hansen et al. (110).]

RESULTS OF CLINICAL TRIALS WITH ERGOTAMINE

Because it was an old drug, ergotamine did not undergo the controlled clinical trial program that would be expected of a new drug today. Nevertheless, oral ergotamine has been used over the past 30 years as the standard comparative drug in controlled trials of other medicines. Even so, the number of good clinical trials incorporating so widely a used drug such as ergotamine is not great. In a recent review, it was stated that little evidence exists that it is significantly more effective than placebo (16). Despite information that is generally not up to date (56) (see Chapter 7) from clinical trials with ergotamine, some evidence for the efficacy of ergotamine has been reported in the literature, which is summarized briefly in the following.

Randomized Controlled Clinical Trials with Ergotamine

A summary of 15 controlled double-blind trials of oral ergotamine, or oral ergotamine plus caffeine, is given in Table 2. In seven trials (28,43,62,84,94,96,122), ergotamine was compared with placebo, whereas ergotamine served as the standard comparative drug in eight other trials (1,41,42,67,79,87,120,125) without placebo control. The initial dose of ergotamine varied from 1 to 5 mg, and in several trials repeated intake of test drugs was used (see Table 1). The reported parameters for efficacy varied considerably from benefit based on a clinical interview (122) to use of changes on a verbal headache scale (28,79,125).

Ergotamine (1–5 mg) was superior to placebo for some parameters in six trials (28,43,62,84,94,96) and no better than placebo in one study using a dose of 2 to 3 mg (122). In two comparative trials, ergotamine was superior to aspirin (500 mg) (41,42), and inferior to an isometheptene compound in one trial (125) and superior to it in another trial (1). As shown in Table 1, the new drugs ergocristine, tolfenamic acid, dextropropoxyphene, naproxen sodium, and pirprofen, were generally found to be comparable to ergotamine. Exceptions include sumatriptan (100 mg orally), which was superior to 2 mg of ergotamine plus 200 mg of caffeine (79), and the combination of calcium carbasalate (equivalent to 900 aspirin) plus metoclopramide (10 mg), which was superior to a rather small dose of 1 mg ergotamine plus 100 mg caffeine (67).

These trials of ergotamine, some placebo controlled, demonstrate that oral ergotamine is effective in the treatment of migraine; however, the clinical relevance of the different parameters of efficacy used in the studies (see Table 1) can be questioned, and no uniform picture of the effectiveness of oral ergotamine emerges from these trials. The use of escape medication is a clinically relevant

TABLE 2. *Double-blind randomized trials with pure oral ergotamine (Erg) or an ergotamine compound with caffeine (ErgC) in the treatment of migraine attacks*

Trial	Drug	Dosage Initial (maximum) mg	Study design	Number of attacks treated[a]	Number of patients (number evaluated)	Results of trial
84	Ergotamine Placebo	5	Crossover	1	44	More than 50% headache relief: Erg (70%) > placebo (39%)
122	Ergotamine Placebo	2–3	Crossover	?[b]	88 (79)	Benefited based on clinical interview: Erg (51%) = placebo (58%)
94	ErgC ErgS Placebo	2 (6) 2 (6)	Crossover	1	48	Escape medication: ErgC (22/48) = Ergs (22/46) > placebo (33/46)
1	ErgC Isometheptene compound	2 (6) 130 (130)	Crossover	2	54	Mean headache duration: ErgC > Isometheptene compound.
125	ErgC Isometheptene compound[c]	2 (6) 130 (390)	Crossover	1	38	Headache intensity[d]: Isometheptene compound (2.8) > ErgC (3.3). Nausea[d]: Isometheptene compound (1.1) > ErgC (2.0)
43	Ergotamine Tolfenamic acid Aspirin Placebo	1 200 500	Crossover	2	20	Mean duration of attack in h: Erg (3.8) = tolfenamic acid (3.2) = aspirin (4.2) > placebo (7.1). Preference: all drugs > Placebo
41	Ergotamine DextC[e] Aspirin	1 (3) 65(195) 500 (1500)	Crossover	7	25	Mean of attack prevented: Erg (3.6) = DextC (2.6) > placebo (1.1)
42	Ergotamine DextC[e] Aspirin	1 (2) 100 (200) 500 (1000)	Crossover	7	25	Attack not prevented: Erg (53%) = DextC (59%) > placebo (82%)
87	ErgC[f] Naproxen sodium	2 (4) 825 (1375)	Parallel group	6	114 (95)	For test drug taken within 2 h: Naproxen sodium > ErgC for headache relief. Later intake of test drug, NS.[g]
96	ErgC Naproxen sodium Placebo	2 (3) 825 (1100)	Parallel group	6	169 (122)	Relief of headache at 1 h: Naproxen sodium > placebo, ErgC = placebo. Overall efficacy: ErgC > placebo, naproxen sodium = placebo
62	ErgC[f] Pirprofen Placebo	2 (5) 200 (500)	Crossover	1	67 (61)	Escape medication: ErgC (18/59) = Pirprofen (18/58) > Placebo (32/60). Duration of attacks in h: ErgC (6.5) > Placebo (10.5) but vs. Pirprofen NS. For most parameters ErgC vs. Pirprofen NS.
28	ErgC[f] Placebo	2 (6)	Parallel group	2	? (104)	Mean improvement from baseline on a 5 point headache scale after 2 hours: ErgC (1.0) > Placebo (0).[h]
79	ErgC Sumatriptan	2 100	Parallel group	3	580 (577)	Headache relief[i]: Sumatriptan (66%) > ErgC (48%)
120	Ergotamine Naproxen sodium	2 (4) 750 (1750)	Parallel group	6	79 (71?)	Naproxen sodium > Erg for overall efficacy rating of treatments on a 6 point scale (none to excellent). Improvement of headache: Naproxen sodium = Erg
67	ErgC CASA + M	1 900 + 10	Parallel group	3	268	Headache relief[i]: CASA + M (54%) > ErgC (36%)

[a]Maximum number of attacks treated.

[b]Approximately one quarter of patients did not have migraine (122).

[c]Only dose of isometheptene given (for other components, confer reference).

[d]Verbal scale: 1, very mild; 2, mild; 3, moderate; 4, severe; 5, very severe.

[e]Only doses for dextropropoxyphen (65 mg of the chloride [41] or 100 mg of the napsylate [42]) are indicated (for other components, see references).

[f]Contains other components in addition to caffeine, see references.

[g]Study conclusions weakened by the lack of use of double dummy technique.

[h]Patients refractory to ergot therapy were excluded.

[i]A decrease from severe or moderate headache to none or mild headache.

CASA + M, calcium carbasalate (equivalent to 900 mg ASA) plus metoclopramide; ErgC, ergotamine compound with caffeine (1 mg ergotamine + 100 mg caffeine); Ergs, ergostine (+ caffeine); NS or, no statistical significant difference; > signifies more effective than.

efficacy parameter (56), which was used by 31% (62), 44% (79), and 46% (94) of patients treated with ergotamine.

Other routes of administration of ergotamine, which from a kinetic point of view should be more efficacious, have scarcely been investigated. In one trial, inhaled ergotamine (maximum dose, 1.8 mg) was superior to sublingual ergotamine (maximum dose, 2 mg), and sublingual ergotamine did not produce better results than sublingual placebo (15). In one double-blind, placebo-controlled study, a suppository of ergotamine (2 mg) was no better than placebo, whereas ketoprofen (100 mg administered as a suppository) was superior to placebo (61). In a recent randomized, crossover, double-blind trial including 251 patients (106), ergotamine–caffeine suppositories (2–100 mg) plus one optional suppository after 1 h were superior to 25 mg sumatriptan suppositories with response rates of 73% and 63% after 2 hours, respectively. Because more side effects occurred after ergotamine suppositories, slightly but not significantly more patients preferred sumatriptan suppositories (44%) than ergotamine suppositories (36%).

Randomized Double-Blind Clinical Trials with Dihydroergotamine

Intranasal dihydroergotamine was compared with placebo in nine double-blind trials, but most of these trials were published in abstract form only and therefore are difficult to evaluate, and results varied considerably. For a review of these trials and open trials, see the first edition of this book and the review by Scott (99).

Recently, intranasal dihydroergotamine was compared with placebo in three trials (21,31). In two studies reported in the same paper (21), only the changes in headache incidence from baseline after 1 mg plus 1 mg dihydroergotamine or placebo were reported, making it difficult to judge the clinical relevance of the findings. Dihydroergotamine was superior to placebo after 1 and 3 hours, respectively (21). In another trial (31), doses of 2 mg and 3 mg of dihydroergotamine had superior results to placebo as judged from the response rates (Table 3). Only the 2-mg dose had an effect after 30 minutes; 3 mg of dihydroergotamine was apparently less effective than 2 mg and superior to placebo only after 2 hours. The therapeutic gain (i.e., the success rate minut the active success rate for placebo) for 2 mg of dihydroergotamine was 41% (95% confidence interval: 29%–54%) and is in the same range as found for intranasal sumatriptan (see Chapter 52). In contrast, in one small trial that included only 16 to 19 patients in each treatment group, neither 0.5 mg nor 1 mg (plus optional 1 mg) of intranasal dihydroergotamine was superior to placebo (119). In one study, intranasal dihydroergotamine 1 mg (plus an optional dose of 1 mg after 30 minutes) was clearly inferior to 6 mg of subcutaneous sumatriptan up to 2 hours after intake (118) but recurrences were less (see Table 3).

In the three placebo-controlled trials (21,31), dihydroergotamine caused nasal congestion (21% and 50%) and taste disturbances (9% and 12%) more frequently than placebo. Also, nausea (4% and 17%) occurred more frequently with intranasal dihydroergotamine.

Subcutaneous dihydroergotamine 1 mg was inferior to 6 mg subcutaneous sumatriptan for the first 2 hours but apparently comparable thereafter (123) and with less recurrences (see Table 3). The latter results, however, are equivocal because 30% of the patients in the dihydroergotamine group got a second injection after 2 hours compared with only 15% in the sumatriptan group who got a second injection (of placebo) and because there were more severe headaches in the sumatriptan group. The tendency of the effect of dihydroergotamine being less rapid but more long lasting than the effect of sumatriptan is theoretically interesting. It fits with the time-effect curve

TABLE 3. *Recent double-blind, randomized clinical trials with subcutaneous and intranasal dihydroergotamine*

Trial	Drug	Dose (mg)	Study	Number of	Response[a] at hr				Recurrence rate
					0.5	1	2	4	
123	Dihydroergotamine	1[b]SC	Parallel group	145		57	73	86	18
	Sumatriptan	6 SC		150		78[x]	85[x]	83	45
118	Dihydroergotamine	1 + 1[c]IN	Crossover	266	20	34	53		17
	Sumatriptan	6 SC			48[d]	71[d]	81[d]		31
31	Dihydroergotamine	2 IN	Parallel group	105	28[e]	50[e]	65[e]	70[a]	15
	Dihydroergotamine	3 IN		97	12	30	45[e]	60[a]	
	Placebo			98	9	18	23	28	33

[a]A decrease from severe or moderate headache to none or mild.
[b]43 ptt. received a second dose of 1 mg dihydroergotamine after 2 hours.
[c]1 mg dihydroergotamine plus an optional 1 mg dose after 30 minutes.
[d]Sumatriptan superior to dihydroergotamine (p < 0.01).
[e]Dihydroergotamine superior to placebo (p < 0.01).
SC, subcutaneous; IN, intranasal.

for the vasoconstrictor effect of ergot alkaloids both *in vitro* as well as *in vivo* (113). A slow dissociation from the receptor site, in addition to a long-lasting effect, would result in a slow onset of action (108).

Intravenous dihydroergotamine was compared with placebo in one complicated crossover trial, and the results indicated some superiority of dihydroergotamine (13). In one small double-blind trial (n = 9), the intravenous combination of dihydroergotamine with metoclopramide was superior to placebo (63). In children, oral dihydroergotamine (20–40 μg/kg) was marginally better than placebo (*p* = 0.06) in a crossover trial that evaluated 12 children (44). For trials comparing parenteral dihydroergotamine with other drugs or drug combinations, see Chapter 54.

THERAPEUTIC USE OF ERGOTAMINE AND DIHYDROERGOTAMINE

Ergotamine

Ergotamine still is widely used in some countries for the treatment of severe migraine attacks. It is generally regarded as a safe and useful drug when prescribed in the correct dose and in the absence of contraindications (86,88,102). For information about choosing between ergotamine and the triptans, which in many countries now are the drugs of first choice for severe attacks, if both are available and affordable, see Chapter 55.

Dosages and Routes of Administration

Ergotamine can be given, in ascending order of efficacy and side effects, as sublingual and oral tablets, by inhalation, by suppository, and by injection (not available in all countries). In all but the parenteral route, low bioavailability results in marked interpatient variability with regard to the amounts of the drug reaching the circulation. Thus, there is no "standard dose"; rather, the dose should be tailored to the individual patient. The safer option is to begin with a small dose and to increase it gradually, depending on efficacy and side effects, until the optimal dose for the individual patient has been achieved. Serious side effects, such as angina pectoris and intermittent claudication, should lead to discontinuation of ergotamine, regardless of dose. In clinical practice, however, nausea is encountered in 10% to 20% of patients after oral and rectal administration of ergotamine. The frequent occurrence of this side effect most often limits ergotamine's use. The drug has a direct effect on the chemoreceptor trigger zone in medulla (86).

Patients vary considerably in their sensitivity to this effect of ergotamine. Regardless of the route of administration, it is often useful to have the patient try ergotamine during the headache-free interval to ensure that no nausea occurs. The initial recommended dose of ergotamine (*vide infra*), for example, 1 mg rectally, should be tried first; if this dose does not cause nausea, it can be used in the treatment of an attack. Also, the next increment, if necessary, should be tested and found not to cause nausea-inducing effect before being used in the treatment of migraine. Nausea caused by an effective dose of ergotamine may be prevented by the simultaneous administration of metoclopramide. Ergotamine should be administered in the selected dose as soon as the patient is sure that a migraine attack is developing. The dose of ergotamine should not be divided, as is often recommended.

For oral ergotamine, sublingual tablets, ordinary tablets, and in some countries effervescent tablets are available. The recommended starting dose is 2 mg, the maximum dose 6 mg. In tablets, 1 mg of ergotamine tartrate often is combined with 100 mg of caffeine, which increases the absorption of ergotamine. The recommended starting dose for ergotamine by inhalation is 1.08 mg (three puffs), and the maximum recommended dose is 2.16 mg (six puffs). Inhalation is a convenient mode of administration, but in our experience only a few patients can use the inhalational device effectively. For rectal ergotamine, the recommended starting dose is 1 mg (half a suppository), and the recommended maximum dose is 4 mg (two suppositories). The rectal route is probably the most effective in clinical practice and is useful for attacks associated with severe nausea and or vomiting. Ergotamine can be given by subcutaneous or intramuscular injections with a starting dose of 0.25 mg and a maximum dose of 0.5 mg. The use of injections is hampered by the high frequency of side effects, especially nausea, and they are not in general use.

Frequency of Dosing

A persistent (at least 24 hours) vasoconstrictor effect occurs after a single therapeutic dose of ergotamine (109). Ergotamine thus should not be given daily, as this will lead to chronic vasoconstriction or habituation (see Chapter 115); ideally, patients should not be allowed more than two doses per week (88).

Can ergotamine be used in migraine with aura?

Because of its vasoconstrictor effect, it has long been debated whether ergotamine can be used safely in migraine with aura, where decreased CBF, continuing into the headache phase, occurs (see Chapter 35). Studies in migraine patients during attacks (39,103), in nonmigrainous patients (40), and in normal subjects (6) failed to show any effect of ergotamine on CBF. In large intravenous doses, however, ergotamine can cause a small constriction of cerebral arteries in volunteers (116) and may do so to a greater extent in susceptible persons, causing symptomatic arterial vasospasm, as has been confirmed angiographically (47). Therefore, ergotamine perhaps is best avoided in treating migraine attacks preceded by an aura lasting for more than 30 minutes.

Side Effects

The side effects of ergotamine are listed in Table 4. After a single dose, side effects include nausea [occurring in 10% after oral administration (86)] and vomiting, abdominal discomfort, acroparaesthesia, and leg cramps. After chronic daily intake, unwanted symptoms include those attributable to vasospasm (such as intermittent claudication) and ergotamine-induced headache (see Chapter 115).

Overt ergotism (29,45,78,115) is rare but should be treated early and vigorously with a direct-acting vasodilator for at least 24 hours (e.g., intravenous nitroglycerin in at starting dose of 0.5 µg/kg per minute) (112). Even if pregangrenous symptoms such as cyanosis are not present, treatment should be started if the patient has resting limb pain to avoid ischaemic neuropathy (Tfelt-Hansen, personal observation). If the vasodilator treatment is ineffective and gangrene is imminent, mechanical intraarterial dilatation with a balloon-tipped catheter may be necessary (101). Alternatively, prostaglandin infusion has been suggested (25).

In patients with ischemic heart disease, ergotamine, given in therapeutic doses, has in a few cases caused variant angina, myocardial infarction, and cardiac arrest (30,64,93). Even sudden death in a case without atherosclerosis has been described (8). Also, cerebral vasospasm may be caused by ergotamine (47). Anorectal ulcers, although usually reported after chronic use of ergotamine, also has been reported after a single rectal dose (59,60). A few cases of fibrotic disorders, involving pleura, pericardium, heart valves, and retroperitoneum have been reported (46,92,104,107). Palsy of the peroneal nerve, probably caused by constriction of the vasa vasorum, also can be caused by ergotamine (78,85); and neurophysiological investigations have demonstrated signs of peripheral neuropathy and dorsal column lesion after chronic use of ergotamine (38,73).

Contraindications

As summarized in Table 4, ergotamine is contraindicated in cardiovascular disease, sepsis, liver and kidney disease, pregnancy (because of the prominent uterotonic action (18,37,91), and breastfeeding. Ergotamine should not be used concomitantly with certain drugs, including triacetyloleandomycin and erythromycin, which decrease the metabolism of ergotamine (65).

Precautions

One-half the normally effective dose of ergotamine should be tried in patients on methysergide because of the vasoconstrictor action of methysergide (30). Caution is advocated in patients on β-adrenoceptor antagonists. Triptans have a minor peripheral vasoconstrictory effect (22,100,117) and generally should not be used together with ergotamine.

Dihydroergotamine

Dihydroergotamine Injections

Dihydroergotamine can be given as in a dose of 1 mg as a subcutaneous or intramuscular injections or in doses of 0.5 mg to 1 mg intravenously in the treatment of severe migraine attacks. These doses are based mainly on clinical experience. Parenterally, 3 mg of dihydroergotamine is the recommended maximum daily dose (88,102). Concerning intravenous dihydroergotamine for status migrainosus, see Chapter 66.

TABLE 4. *Side effects of and contraindications for ergotamine (for references, see text)*

	Side effects
Single dose	Nausea/vomiting, abdominal pain, acroparaesthesia, swollen fingers, leg cramps, diarrhea, tremor, syncope, globus feeling.[a] (In patients with ischemic heart disease: angina and myocardial infarction).
Chronic daily intake	Ergotamine-induced chronic headache,[b] ergotamine withdrawal headache,[b] intermittent claudication, acrocyanosis, constant nausea, acroparaesthesia, anorectal ulcers, ischemic neuropathy, dorsal column lesion, fibrotic disorders involving the pleura, pericardium, and retroperitoneum, overt ergotism.
Contraindications	Cardiovascular disease, pregnancy, breast-feeding, liver and kidney disease, sepsis, concomitant use of triacetyloleandomycin, or erythromycin.
Cautions	Concomitant use of methysergide, β-blockers and triptans (see text).

[a]After parenteral use.
[b]See Chapter 115.

Intranasal Dihydroergotamine

The recommended initial dose for intranasal dihydroergotamine is 1 mg (one puff in each nostril). If needed, the patient can repeat the dose of 1 mg after 15 minutes . We would recommend, however, that the patient be instructed to titrate the effective dose of intranasal dihydroergotamine between 1 and 2 mg, which then should be administered as a single dose. Higher doses seem not to be more effective.

Side Effects

With parenteral dihydroergotamine, the most common side effect is nausea, and concomitant administration of an antiemetic is recommended for intravenous use (90). Leg pain, paraesthesia, and a few cases of angina and ergotism have been reported (90). With intranasal dihydroergotamine, the most common side effects are transient nasal congestion, nausea, and throat discomfort (71).

Contraindications

Contraindications include known hypersensitivity to ergot alkaloids, pregnancy, breastfeeding, coronary arterial disease, inadequetly controlled hypertension.

REFERENCES

1. Adams M, Aikman P, Allardyce K, et al. General practioner clinical trials: treatment of migraine. *Practitioner* 1971;206:551–554.
2. Adham N, Kao HT, Schechter LE, et al. Cloning of another human serotonin receptor (5-HT$_{1F}$): a fifth 5-HT$_1$ receptor subtype coupled to the inhibition of adenylate cyclase. *Proc Natl Acad Sci U S A* 1993;90: 408–412.
3. Aellig WH. Venoconstrictor effect of dihydroergotamine in superficial hand veins. *Eur J Clin Pharmacol* 1974;7:137–139.
4. Aellig WH, Nüesch E. Comparative pharmacokinetic investigations with tritium-labelled ergot alkaloids after oral and intravenous administration in man. *Int J Clin Pharmacol* 1977;15:106–112.
5. Aellig WH, Rosenthaler J. Venoconstrictor effect of dihydroergotamine (DHE) after intranasal and i.m. administration. *Eur J Clin Pharmacol* 1986;30:581–584.
6. Andersen AR, Tfelt-Hansen P, Lassen NA. The effect of ergotamine and dihydroergotamine on cerebral blood flow in man. *Stroke* 1987;18:120–123.
7. Barger G. *Ergot and ergotism.* Edinburgh: Gurney & Jackson, 1931.
8. Benedict CR, Robertson D. Angina pectoris and sudden death in the absence of atherosclerosis following ergotamine therapy for migraine. *Am J Med* 1979;67:177–178.
9. Brazil P, Friedman AP. Further observations in craniovascular studies. *Neurology* 1957;7:52–55.
10. Bülow PM, Ibraheem JJ, Paalzow G, Tfelt-Hansen P. Comparison of pharmacodynamic effects and plasma levels of oral and rectal ergotamine. *Cephalalgia* 1986;6:107–111.
11. Buzzi, MG, Moskowitz MA. Evidence for 5-HT$_{1B/1D}$ receptors mediating the antimigraine effect of sumatriptan and dihydroergotamine. *Cephalalgia* 1991;11:165–168.
12. Buzzi MG, Moskowitz MA, Peroutka SJ, Byun B. Further characterization of the putative 5-HT receptor which mediates blockade of neurogenic plasma extravasation in rat dura mater. *Br J Pharmacol* 1991;103:1421–1428.
13. Callaham M, Raskin N. A controlled study of dihydroergotamine in the treatment of acute migraine headache. *Headache* 1986;26: 168–171.
14. Cortijo J, Marti-Cabrera M, Bernabeu E, et al. Characterization of 5-HT receptors on human pulmonary artery and vein: functional and binding studies. *Br J Pharmacol* 1997;122:1455–1463.
15. Crooks J, Stephen SA, Brass W. Clinical trial of inhaled ergotamine tartrate in migraine. *BMJ* 1964;1:221–224.
16. Dahlöf C. Placebo-controlled clinical trials with ergotamine in the acute treatment of migraine. *Cephalalgia* 1993;13:166–171.
17. Dale HH. On some physiological actions of ergot. *J Physiol (Lond)* 1906;34:163–206.
18. de Groot ANJA, van Dongen PWJ, van Roosmalen J, Eskes TKAB. Ergotamine-induced fetal stress: review of side effects of ergot alkaloids during pregnancy. *Eur J Obstet Gynecol Reprod Biol* 1993;51: 71–77.
19. De Vries P, Villalon CM, Heiligers JP, Saxena PR. Characterization of 5-HT receptors mediating constriction of porcine carotid arteriovenous anastomoses; involvement of 5-HT$_{1B/1D}$ and novel receptors. *Br J Pharmacol* 1998;123:1561–1570.
20. Diener H-C, Peters C, Rudzio M, et al. Ergotamine, flunarizine and sumatriptan do not change cerebral blood flow velocity in normal subjects and migraineurs. *J Neurol* 1991;238:245–250.
21. Dihydroergotamine Nasal Spray Multicenter Investigators. Efficacy, safety, and tolerability of dihydroergotamine nasal spray as monotherapy in the treatment of acute migraine. *Headache* 1995;35:177–84.
22. Dixon RM, Meire HB, Evans DH, et al. Peripheral vascular effects and pharmacokinetics of the antimigraine compound, zolmitriptan, in combination with oral ergotamine in healthy volunteers. *Cephalalgia* 1997;17:639–646.
23. Drummond PD, Lance JW. Extracranial vascular changes and the source of pain in migraine headache. *Ann Neurol* 1983;13:32–37.
24. Edlund P-O. Determination of ergot alkaloids in plasma by high performance liquid chromatography and fluorescence detection. *J Chromatogr* 1981;226:107–115.
25. Edwards RJ, Fulde GWO, McGrath. Successful limb salvage with prostaglandin infusion: a review of ergotamine toxicity. *Med J Aust* 1991;155:825–827.
26. Ekbom K, Krabbe AÆ, Paalzow G, Paalzow L, Tfelt-Hansen P, Waldenlind E. Optimal routes of administration of ergotamine tartrate in cluster headache patients: a pharmacokinetic study. *Cephalalgia* 1983;3:15–20.
27. Fozard JR. The animal pharmacology of drugs used in the treatment of migraine. *J Pharm Pharmacol* 1975;27:297–321.
28. Friedman AP, Di Serio FJ, Hwang D-S. Symptomatic relief of migraine: multicenter comparison of Cafergot P-B, Cafergot, and placebo. *Clin Ther* 1989;11:170–182.
29. Fukui S, Coggia M, Goëau-Brissonnière O. Acute upper extremity ischemia during concomitant use of ergotamine tartrate and ampicillin. *Ann Vasc Surg* 1997;11:420–424.
30. Galer BS, Lipton RB, Solomon S, Newman LC, Spierings ELH. Myocardial ischemia related to ergot alkaloids: a case report and literature review. *Headache* 1991;31:446–450.
31. Gallagher RM. Dihydroergotamine Working Group. Acute treatment of migraine with dihydroergotamine nasal spray. *Arch Neurol* 1996;53:1285–1291.
32. Glusa E, Roos A. Endothelial 5-HT receptors mediate relaxation of porcine pulmonary arteries in response to ergotamine and dihydroergotamine. *Br J Pharmacol* 1996;119:330–334.
33. Gnecchi-Ruscone T, Lorenzoni R, Anderson D, et al. Effects of ergotamine on myocardial blood flow in migraineurs without evidence of atherosclerotic coronary artery disease. *Am J Cardiol* 1998;81: 1165–1168.
34. Goadsby PJ, Edvinsson L. The trigeminovascular system and migraine: studies characterizing cerebrovascular and neuropeptide changes seen in humans and cats. *Ann Neurol* 1993;33:48–56.
35. Goadsby PG, Gunlach AL. Localization of ^{3}H-dihydroergotamine-binding sites in the cat central nervous system: relevance to migraine. *Ann Neurol* 1991;29:91–94.
36. Graham JR, Wolff HG. Mechanism of migraine headache and action of ergotamine tartrate. *Arch Neurol Psychiatry* 1938;39:737–763.
37. Graves CR. Agents that cause contraction or relaxation of the uterus. In: Hardman JG, Limbird LE, Molinoff PB, Ruddon RW, Gilman AG, eds. *Goodman & Gilman's the pharmacological basis of therapeutics.* New York: McGraw-Hill, 1996:939–949.
38. Grotemeyer KH, Hussstedt IW, Schalke HP. Die Nervus suralis-Leitgeschwindigkeit und die relative Refraktairperiode bei Patienten unter

einer Ergotalkaloidetherapie. *EEG EMG Z Elektroenzephalogr Verwandte Geb* 1986;17:16–19.

39. Hachinsky V, Norris JW, Cooper PW, et al. Migraine and the cerebral circulation. In: Green R, ed. *Current concepts in migraine research.* New York: Raven Press, 1978:11–15.

40. Hachinski V, Norris JW, Edmeads J, Cooper PW. Ergotamine and cerebral blood flow. *Stroke* 1978;9:594–596.

41. Hakkarainen H, Gustafsson B, Stockman. A comparative trial of ergotamine tartrate, acetyl salicylic acid and dextropropoxyphene compound in acute migraine attacks. *Headache* 1978;18:35–39.

42. Hakkarainen H, Quiding NH, Stockman O. Mild analgesics as an alternative to ergotamine in migraine: a comparative trial with acetylsalicylic acid, ergotamine tartrate, and a dextropropoxyphene compound. *J Clin Pharmacol* 1980;20:590–595.

43. Hakkarainen H, Vapaatalo H, Gothoni G, Parantaine. Tolfenamic acid is as effective as ergotamine during migraine attacks. *Lancet* 1979;2: 326–328.

44. Hämäläinen ML, Hoppu K, Santavuori PR. Oral dihydroergotamine for therapy-resistant migraine attacks in children. *Pediatr Neurol* 1997;16:114–117.

45. Harrison TE. Ergotaminism. *Journal of the American College of Emergency Physicians* 1978;7:162–169.

46. Hendrikx M, van Dorpe J, Flameng W, Daenen W. Aortic and mitral valve disease induced by ergotamine therapy for migraine: a case report and review of the literature. *J Heart Valve Dis* 1996;5:235–237.

47. Henry PY, Larre P, Aupy M, et al. Reversible cerebral arteriopathy associated with the administration of ergot derivatives. *Cephalalgia* 1984;4:171–178.

48. Hoffman BB, Lefkowitz RJ. Catecholamines, sympathomimetic drugs, and adrenergic receptor antagonists. In: Hardman JG, Limbird LE, Molinoff PB, Ruddon RW, Gilman AG, eds. *Goodman & Gilman's the pharmacological basis of therapeutics.* New York: McGraw-Hill, 1996:199–248.

49. Horton BT, Peters GA, Blumenthal LS. A new product in the treatment of migraine: a preliminary report. *Mayo Clin Proc* 1945;20: 241–248.

50. Hoskin KL, Kaube H, Goadsby PG. Central activation of the trigeminovascular pathway in the cat is inhibited by dihydroergotamine. A c-Fos and electrophysiological study. *Brain* 1996;119:249–256.

51. Humbert H, Cabiac M-D, Dubray C, Lavene D. Human pharmacokinetics of dihydroergotamine administered by nasal spray. *Clin Pharmacol Ther* 1996;60:265—275.

52. Hoyer D. Functional correlates of serotonin 5-HT$_1$ recognition sites. *J Rec Res* 1988;8:59–81.

53. Hoyer D, Clarke DE, Fozard JR, et al. International Union of Pharmacology classification of receptors for 5-hydroxytryptamine (Serotonin). *Pharmacol Rev* 1994;46:157–203.

54. Ibraheem JJ, Paalzow L, Tfelt-Hansen P. Kinetics of ergotamine after intravenous and intramuscular administration to migraine sufferers. *Eur J Clin Pharmacol* 1982;23:235–240.

55. Ibraheem JJ, Paalzow L, Tfelt-Hansen P. Low bioavailability of ergotamine tartrate after oral and rectal administration in migraine suffers. *Br J Clin Pharmacol* 1983;16:695–699.

56. International Headache Society Committee on Clinical Trials in Migraine. Guidelines for controlled trials of drugs in migraine. First edition. *Cephalalgia* 1991;11:1–12.

57. Iversen HK, Nielsen TH, Olesen J, Tfelt-Hansen P. Arterial responses during migraine headaches. *Lancet* 1990;336:837–839.

58. Johnston BM, Saxena PR. The effect of ergotamine on tissue blood flow and the arteriovenous shunting of radioactive microspheres in the head. *Br J Pharmacol* 1978;63:541–549.

59. Jost WH, Raulf F, Müller-Lobeck H. Anorectal ergotism. Induced by migraine therapy. *Acta Neurol Scand* 1991;84:73–74.

60. Jost WH, Schimrigk. Ergotamine-induced rectal lesions in asymptomatic patients. *Wien Klin Wochenschr* 1994;106:171–173.

61. Kangasneimi P, Kaaja R. Ketoprofen and ergotamine in acute migraine. *J Intern Med* 1992;231:551–554.

62. Kinnunen E, Erkinjuntti T, Färkkliä, et al. Placebo-controlled double-blind trial of pirprofen and an ergotamine tartate compound in migraine attacks. *Cephalalgia* 1988;8:175–179.

63. Klapper J, Stanton J. The emergency treatment of acute migraine headache; a comparison of intravenous dihydroergotamine, dexamethasone, and placebo. *Cephalgia* 1991;11(Suppl 11):159–160.

64. Koh KK, Roe IH, Lee MM, Cho SK, Kim SS. Variant angina complicating ergot therapy of migraine. *Chest* 1994;105:1259–1260.

65. Krupp P, Haas G. Effects indesirables et interactions medicamenteuse des alcaloides de l'ergot de seigle. *J Pharmacol (Paris)* 1979;10: 401–412.

66. Lawrence DR. *Clinical pharmacology*, 3rd ed. London: Churchill, 1966:514.

67. Le Jeunne C, Gomez JP, Pradalier A, et al. Comparative efficacy and safety of calcium carbasalate plus metoclopramide versus ergotamine tartrate plus caffeine in the treatment of acute migraine attacks. *Eur Neurol* 1999;41:37–43.

68. Leysen JE, Gommeren W. *In vitro* binding profile of drugs used in migraine. In: Amery WK, Van Nueten JM, Wauquier A, eds. *The pharmacological basis of migraine therapy.* London: Pitman Publishing, 1984:255–266.

69. Leysen JE, Gommeren W, Heylen L, et al. Alniditan, a new 5-hydroxytryptamine$_{1D}$ agonist and migraine-abortive agent: ligand-binding properties of human 5-hydroxytryptamine$_{1Da}$, human 5-hydroxytryptamine$_{1D\beta}$, and calf 5-hydroxytryptamine$_{1D}$ receptors investigated with [^{3}H]5-hydroxytryptamine and [^{3}H]alniditan. *Mol Pharmacol* 1996;50:1567–1580.

70. Lindblad B, Abisch E, Bergqvist D. The pharmacokinetics of subcutaneous dihydroergotamine with and without a dextran indfusion. *Eur J Clin Pharmacol* 1983;24:813–818.

71. Lipton RB. Ergotamine tartrate and dihydroergotamine mesylate: safety profiles. *Headache* 1997;37(Suppl 1):S33–S41.

72. Little PJ, Jennings GL, Skews H, Bobik A. Bioavailability of dihydroergotamine in man. *Br J Clin Pharmacol* 1982;13:785–790.

73. Ludolph AC, Husstedt IW, Schalke HP, Grotemeyer KH, Brune GG. Chronic ergotamine abuse: evidence for functional impairment of long ascending spinal tracts. *Eur Neurol* 1988;28:311–316.

74. Maassen VanDenBrink A, Reekers M, Bax WA, Ferrari MD, Saxena PR. Coronary side-effect potential of current and prospective antimigraine drugs. *Circulation* 1998;98:25–30.

75. Maier HW. L'ergotamine inhibitteur du sympathique etudie en clinique, comme moyen d'exploration et comme agent therapeutique. *Rev Neurol* 1926:33:1104–08.

76. Markowitz S, Saito K, Moskowitz MA. Neurogenically mediated plasma extravasation in dura mater: effect of ergot alkaloids. A possible mechanism of action in vascular headache. *Cephalalgia* 1988;8: 83–91.

77. Maurer G, Frick W. Elucidation of the structure and receptor binding studies of the major primary, metabolite of dihydroergotamine in man. *Eur J Clin Pharmacol* 1984;26:4463–470.

78. Merhoff GC, Porter JM. Ergot intoxication: historical review and description of unusual clinical manifestations. *Ann Surg* 1974;180: 773–779.

79. Multinational Oral Sumatriptan and Cafergot Comparative Study Group. A randomized, double-blind comparison of sumatriptan and Cafergot in the acute treatment of migraine. *Eur Neurol* 1991;1: 314–322.

80. Müller-Schweinitzer E. *In vitro* studies on the duration of action of dihydroergotamine. *Int J Clin Pharmacol Ther Toxicol* 1980;18:88–91.

81. Müller-Schweinitzer E. Ergot alkaloids in migraine: is the effect via 5-HT receptors? In: Olesen J, Saxena PR, eds. *5-Hydroxytryptamine mechanisms in primary headaches.* New York: Raven Press, 1992: 297–304.

82. Müller-Schweinitzer E, Weidmann H. Basic pharmacological properties. In: Berde B, Schild HO, eds. *Ergot alkaloids and related compounds.* Berlin: Springer-Verlag, 1978:87–232.

83. Stergaard JR, Mikkelsen E, Voldby B. Effects of 5-hydroxytryptamine and ergotamine on human superficial temporal artery. *Cephalalgia* 1981;1:223–228.

84. Ostfeld AM. A study of migraine pharmacotherapy. *Am J Med Sci* 1961;241:192–198.

85. Perkin GD. Ischaemic lateral popliteal plasy due to ergotamine intoxication. *J Neurol Neurosurg Pscychiatry* 1974;37:1389–1391.

86. Peroutka SJ. Drugs effective in the therapy of migraine. In: HardmanJG, Limbird LE, Molinoff PB, Ruddon RW, Gilman AG, eds. *Goodman and Gilman's the pharmacological Basis of Therapeutics, 9th Ed.* New York: McGraw-Hill, 1996:487–502.

87. Pradalier A, Rancurel G, Dordain G, Verdure L, Rascol A, Dry J. Acute migraine attack therapy: comparison of naproxen sodium and an ergotamine tartrate compound. *Cephalalgia* 1985;5:107–113.

88. Quality Standards Subcommittee of the American Academy of Neu-

rology. Practice parameter: appropiate use of ergotamine tartrate and dihydroergotamine in the treatment of migraine and status migrainosus (summary statement). *Neurology* 1995;45:585–587.

89. Raskin NH. Pharmacology of migraine. *Annu Rev Pharmacol Toxicol* 1981;21:463–478.

90. Raskin NH. *Headache*, 2nd ed. New York: Churchill Livingstone Inc., 195p1.28870

91. Raymond GV. Teratogen update: ergot and ergotamine. *Teratology* 1995;51:344–347.

92. Robert M, Derbaudrenghien J-P, Blampain J-P, et al. Fibrotic processes associated with long-term ergotamine therapy. *N Engl J Med* 1984;311:601–602.

93. Roithinger FX, Punzengruber C, Gremmel F, Hinterreiter M, Holzner F, Pachinger O. Myocardial infarction after chronic ergotamine abuse. *Eur Heart J* 1993;14:1579–1581.

94. Ryan RE. Double-blind evaluation of the efficacy and safety of ergostine-caffeine, ergotamine-caffeine and placebo in migraine headache. *Headache* 1970;9:212–222.

95. Sanders SW, Haering N, Mosberg H, Jaeger. Pharmacokinetics of ergotamine in healthy volunteers following oral and rectal dosing. *Eur J Clin Pharmacol* 1986;30:331–334.

96. Sargent JD, Baumel B, Peters K, et al. Aborting migraine attack: naproxen sodium v ergotamine plus caffeine. *Headache* 1988;28:263–266.

97. Saxena PR, Cairo-Rawlins WI. Presynaptic inhibition by ergotamine of the responses to cardioaccelerator nerve stimulations in the cat. *Eur J Pharmacol* 1979;58:305–312.

98. Saxena PR, Ferrari MD. Pharmacology of antimigraine 5-HT$_{1D}$ receptor agonists. *Exp Opin Invest Drugs* 1996;5:581–593.

99. Scott AK. Dihydroergotamine: a review of its use in the treatment of migraine and other headaches. *Clin Neuropharmacol* 1992;15:289–296.

100. Seidelin KN, Tfelt-Hansen P, Mendel C, Stephanage M. Peripheral haemodynamic study of MK-462, ergotamine and their combination in man. *Cephalalgia* 1995;15(Suppl 14):207.

101. Shifrin E, Perel A, Olschwang D, et al. reversal of ergotamine-induced arteriospasm by intra-arterial dilatation. *Lancet* 1980;2:1278–1279.

102. Silberstein SD, Young WB. Safety and efficacy of ergotamine tartrate and dihydroergotamine in the treatment of migraine and status migrainosus. *Neurology* 1995;45:577–584.

103. Simard D, Paulson OB. Cerebral vasomotor paralysis during migraine attack. *Arch Neurol* 1973;29:207–209.

104. Stecker JF Jr, Rawls HP, Devine CJ Jr, et al. Retroperitoneal fibrosis and ergot derivatives. *J Urol* 1974;112:30–32.

105. Stoll A. Zur Kenntnis der Mutterkornalkaloide. *Verh Naturf Ges (Basel)* 1920;101:190–191.

106. Swedish Medical Product Agency. http://www.mpa.se/sve/mono/imig.sht (Monograph in Swedish on sumatriptan suppositories published on the Internet by Swedish Medical Product Agency).

107. Tall BG, Spierings ELH, Hilvering C. Pleuropulmonary fibrosis associated with chronic and excessive intake of ergotamine. *Thorax* 1983;38:396–398.

108. Tfelt-Hansen P. The effect of ergotamine on the arterial system in man. *Acta Pharmacol Toxicol* 1986;59(Suppl 3):1–30.

109. Tfelt-Hansen P, Eickhoff JH, Olsen J. The effect of single dose ergotamine tartrate on peripheral arteries in migraine patients: methodological aspects and time effect curve. *Acta Pharmacol Toxicol* 1980;47:151–156.

110. Tfelt-Hansen P, Holm JW, Fahr A, Rosenthaler J. Bioavailability of dihydroergotamine as a nasal spray. In: Lance JW, ed. *Recent trends in the management of migraine.* Aulendorf : Editio Cantor, 1987:23–25.

111. Tfelt-Hansen P, Kanstrup I-L, Christensen NJ, Winkler K. General and regional haemodynamic effects of intravenous ergotamine. *Cli Sci* 1983;65:599–604.

112. Tfelt-Hansen P, Østergaard JR, Gøhgen I, Jacobsen E, Rasmussen JP, Husum B. Nitroglycerin for ergotism: experimental studies *in vitro* and in migraine patients and treatment of an overt case. *Eur J Clin Pharmacol* 1982;22:105–109.

113. Tfelt-Hansen P, Paalzow L. Intramuscular ergotamine: plasma levels and dynamic activity. *Clin Pharmacol Therap* 1985;37:29–35.

114. Tfelt-Hansen P, Paalzow L, Ibraheem JJ. Bioavailability of sublingual ergotamine. *Br J Clin Pharmacol* 1982;13:239–240.

115. Tfelt-Hansen P, Saxena PR, Ferrari MD. Ergot alkaloids. In: de Wolf FA, ed. *Handbook of clinical neurology*, vol 21. *Intoxications of the nervous system.* Part II. Amsterdam: Elsevier Science B.V. 1995:61–78.

116. Tfelt-Hansen P, Sperling B, Andersen AR. The effect of ergotamine on human cerebral blood flow and cerebral arteries. In: Olesen J, ed. *Frontiers in headache research:* migraine and other headaches: the vascular mechanisms. New York: Raven Press, 1991:339–343.

117. Tfelt-Hansen P, Sperling B, Winter PDO'B. Transient additional effect of sumatriptan on ergotamine-induced constriction of peripheral arteries in man. *Clin Pharmacol Ther* 1992;51:149.

118. Touchon J, Bertin L, Pilgrim AJ, Ashford E, Bès A. A comparison of subcutaneous sumatriptan and dihydroergotamine in the acute treatment of migraine. *Neurology* 1996;47:361–365.

119. Treves TA, Kuritzky A, Hering R, Korczyn AD. Dihydroergotamine nasal spray in the treatment of acute migraine. *Headache* 1998;38:614–617.

120. Treves TA, Streiffler M, Korczyn AD. Naproxen sodium versus ergotamine tartrate in the treatment of acute migraine attacks. *Headache* 1992;32:280–282.

121. Villalón CM, De Vries P, Rabelo G, Centurión D, Sánchez-López A, Saxena PR. Canine external carotid vasoconstriction to methysergide, ergotamine and dihydroergotamine: role of 5-HT$_{1B/1D}$ receptors and a$_2$-adrenoceptors. *Br J Pharmacol* 1999;126:585–594.

122. Waters WE. Controlled clinical trial of ergotamine tartrate. *BMJ* 1970;2:325–327.

123. Winner P, Ricalde O, Le Force B, Saper J, Margul B. A double-blind study of subcutaneous dihydroergotamine vs subcutaneous sumatriptan in the treatment of acute migraine. *Arch Neurol* 1996;53:180–184.

124. Wyss PA, Rosenthaler J, Nüesch E, Aellig WH. Pharmacokinetic investigation of oral and IV dihydroergotamine in healthy subjects. *Eur J Clin Pharmacol* 1991;41:597–602.

125. Yuill G. A double-blind crossover trial of a isometheptene mucate compound and ergotamine in migraine. *Br J Clin Pract* 1973;26:73–79.

The Headaches, Second Edition,
edited by J. Olesen, P. Tfelt-Hansen, and K.M.A. Welch.
Lippincott Williams & Wilkins, Philadelphia © 2000.

The Migraines

CHAPTER 52

Triptans, 5-HT$_{1B/1D}$ Receptor Agonists in the Acute Treatment of Migraine

Pramod R. Saxena and Peer Tfelt-Hansen

The triptans are a completely new class of compounds known as 5-hydroxytryptamine $_{1B/1D}$ [5-HT$_{1B/1D}$, previously 5-HT$_1$–like/5-HT$_{1D}$ (195)] receptor agonists. The first of this family, sumatriptan, was undoubtedly a significant advance in migraine therapy (44,99,173,217, 237). The idea that compounds mimicking 5-HT at craniovascular receptors should abort migraine attacks stems from the following observations (196):

1. Urinary excretion of 5-hydroxyindole acetic acid increases, whereas platelet 5-HT decreases during migraine attacks
2. Migrainelike symptoms can be precipitated by reserpine and alleviated by 5-HT, which causes carotid vasoconstriction via 5-HT$_1$–like receptors
3. Ergotamine and methysergide elicit a selective carotid vasoconstriction (at least partly via 5-HT$_1$–like receptors), which is confined to cephalic arteriovenous anastomoses that seem to be involved in migraine pathophysiology (194).

Based on the aforementioned, tryptamine derivatives were synthesized to achieve selectivity at the craniovascular 5-HT$_1$–like receptor, and this culminated in the design and development of sumatriptan (100).

Despite its great utility in migraine treatment, sumatriptan has certain limitations; for example, low oral bioavailability, high headache recurrence—possibly due to a short half-life—and contraindication in patients with

coronary artery disease. Therefore, a number of pharmaceutical companies decided to develop newer triptans having agonist activity at 5-HT$_{1B/1D}$ receptors. Several such compounds (zolmitriptan, rizatriptan, and naratriptan) are already on the market, whereas others (eletriptan, almotriptan, and frovatriptan) are in advance stages of clinical development (for chemical structures, see Fig. 1). Although avitriptan (189), BMS181885 (243), and the nontriptan alniditan (83) were found effective in the treatment of migraine, these compounds are no longer in clinical development.

In this chapter we will review the pharmacology of triptans and rationale for their use in migraine, the randomized clinical trials with triptans demonstrating their efficacy and evaluating the optimum dose, randomized clinical trials comparing triptans, randomized clinical trials comparing sumatriptan with other treatments, long-term studies with triptans, tolerability and safety problems with triptans, and finally the therapeutic use of triptans.

PHARMACOLOGY OF TRIPTANS

Receptor-Binding Profile

Sumatriptan as well as the newer triptans display high affinities at 5-HT$_1$ receptor subtypes, mainly the 5-HT$_{1B}$ and 5-HT$_{1D}$ receptors (Table 1) (10,13,28,118,130,152, 236,242). The triptans have high affinity for both 5-HT$_{1B}$ and 5-HT$_{1D}$ receptors, with sumatriptan being the weakest at the 5-HT$_{1B}$ receptor. Moreover, some triptans also show a high affinity at the 5-HT$_{1A}$ and 5-HT$_{1F}$ receptors. At the 5-HT$_{1F}$ receptor, however, rizatriptan is the least potent. Sumatriptan, zolmitriptan, eletriptan, and frovatrip-

P.R. Saxena: Department of Pharmacology, Erasmus University, 3000 DR Rotterdam, The Netherlands.

P. Tfelt-Hansen: Department of Neurology, Glostrup Hospital, University of Copenhagen, DK-2600 Glostrup, Copenhagen, Denmark.

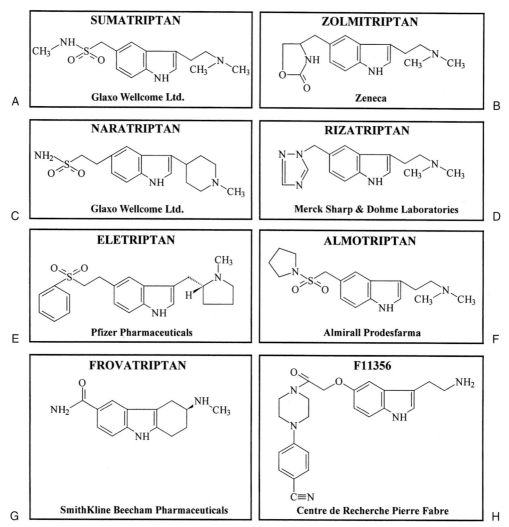

FIG. 1. Chemical structures of sumatriptan and second-generation triptans (for pharmacology of F11356, see Chapter 53 and refs. 107, 108, and 165).

tan display an M affinity at the 5-HT₇ receptor, which mediates smooth muscle relaxation (58,195).

Cardiovascular Effects

Systemic Hemodynamics

Human volunteer studies showed that sumatriptan (126), zolmitriptan (53), and rizatriptan (198) slightly increase arterial blood pressure. This hypertensive response, which has little clinical relevance, is probably related to peripheral vasoconstriction. Interestingly, in anesthetized animals given high intravenous doses, suma-triptan (45,161), eletriptan (238), and rizatriptan (161) decrease blood pressure, which appears to be due to reduction of sympathetic outflow (55,99,161).

Carotid Hemodynamics

Sumatriptan increases internal carotid and middle cerebral artery blood flow velocity in human volunteers

(23). This effect is probably caused by constriction of intracranial arteries, consistent with findings in animal models. Although this is yet to be established, based on similar pharmacologic properties, other triptans are likely to have comparable effects.

As shown in Table 2 (10,28,45,89,108,128,162,202, 238), sumatriptan as well as the other triptans decrease carotid blood flow in anesthetized animals. The apparent rank order of agonist potency (based on intravenous dose needed to decrease canine carotid blood flow by 50%) was: frovatriptan (0.4 μg/kg) (162), greater than zolmitriptan (2.3 μg/kg) (128), greater than eletriptan (12 μg/kg) (89), equal to naratriptan (19 μg/kg) (28), greater than or equal to rizatriptan (30 μg/kg) (202), and equal to sumatriptan (39 μg/kg) (28). Almotriptan also reduces carotid blood flow in the cat (10). Using intracarotid administered radiolabeled microspheres, it also has been shown that the carotid vasoconstriction by sumatriptan (45,48), zolmitriptan (128), and eletriptan (238) is confined to arteriovenous anastomoses, which may dilate during migraine headaches (97,194). Similarly, sumatrip-

TABLE 1. *pK$_i$ values of triptans at 5-HT receptors*

Receptor	Sumatriptan	Zolmitriptan	Naratriptan	Rizatriptan	Eletriptan	Almotriptan	Frovatriptan
5-HT$_{1A}$	6.43 (118) 6.90 (152)	9.20 (130)	7.12[a] 7.10 (rat) (28) 7.58 (152)	6.37[a]	7.35[b]	6.3 (10)	7.3 (13)
5-HT$_{1B}$	7.82 (118)	8.30 (130)	8.12[a] 8.70 (28)	8.14[b] 6.86[a] 7.74 (242)	8.00[a]	8.0 (10)	8.6 (13)
5-HT$_{1D}$	8.46 (118)	9.20 (130)	8.37[a] 8.30 (28)	8.63[b] 7.88[a]	8.94[a]	8.0 (10)	8.4 (13)
5-HT$_{1E}$	5.80 (118)	7.95[b]	7.69[a]	6.77[a]	7.25[a]		<6.0 (13)
5-HT$_{1F}$	7.86 (118) 6.30[c] (236)	7.20 (130) 6.21[c] (236)	8.65 (rat)[a] 7.37[c] (236)	7.08 (rat)[a] 5.27[c] (236)	8.18 (rat)[a]		7.0 (13)
5-HT$_{2A}$	<5.0 (pEC$_{50}$) (118)	<5.5[a]	<5.5[a]	<5.5[a]	<5.5[a]		<5.3 (13)
5-HT$_{2B}$		7.19[a]		6.59[a]			
5-HT$_{2C}$	<5.0 (pEC$_{50}$, pig) (118)	4.10 (gp) (130)	<5.5[a]	<5.5[a]	<5.5[a]		<5.3 (13)
m5-HT$_3$	<5.0 (pEC$_{50}$) (118)	<5.5[a]	<5.5[a]	<5.5[a]	<5.5[a]		<6.0 (13)
gp5-HT$_4$	<5.0 (pEC$_{50}$) (118)	<5.5[a]	<5.5[a]	<5.5[a]	<5.5[a]		
5-HT$_{5A}$	5.50[b] <5.5 (rat)[a]	6.40 (rat)[a]	5.47 (rat)[a]	5.26 (rat)[a]	6.01 (rat)[a]		
5-HT$_{5B}$							
5-HT$_6$	5.31[b]	<5.5[a]	<6.0[a]	<5.5[a]	6.28[a]		
5-HT$_7$	6.51[b]	7.02[a]	<5.5[a]	5.73[a]	6.70[a]	<6.5 (10)	6.70 (13)

[a]P. Gupta, personal communication.
[b]PI Pauwels, personal communication.
[c]pEC$_{50}$, [^{35}S]GTPτS binding to cells expressing the 5-HT$_{1F}$ receptor.
All values refer to the human receptor, except when stated otherwise. References are provided in parentheses.
gp, guinea-pig; m, mouse.

tan (infused into the brachial artery) can decrease human forearm blood flow by a selective vasoconstrictor action on arteriovenous anastomoses (228). The extracerebral blood flow, in contrast, increases in response to 5-HT$_{1B/1D}$ receptor agonists (45,48,238), although a decrease has been reported with zolmitriptan (128). Interestingly, cerebral blood flow does not seem to be affected by triptans, as shown with sumatriptan (46,48) and even with the much more lipophilic, brain-penetrant compounds zolmitriptan (128), eletriptan (238), and rizatriptan (209).

Using SB224289 [selective 5-HT$_{1B}$ receptor antagonist (92,201)] and BRL15572 [selective 5-HT$_{1D}$ receptor antagonist (92,174)], it has been shown that sumatriptan

constricts porcine carotid arteriovenous anastomoses (Fig. 2) as well as canine external carotid vasculature via 5-HT$_{1B}$ receptors and not via 5-HT$_{1D}$ receptors (46,48). Considering their similar receptor-binding profile, it is likely that newer triptans also exert vascular effects via this receptor. The latter is consistent with the low expression of 5-HT$_{1D}$ receptor messenger RNA (mRNA) (11,226,229) or the corresponding protein (123) in blood vessels. Notwithstanding, some lines of evidence suggest that a novel 5-HT receptor, possibly identical to that reported by Castro et al. (24), mediates 5-HT–induced constriction of porcine carotid arteriovenous anastomoses (47). Similarly, ergotamine and dihydroergotamine constrict the carotid vascular bed considerably via non–5-

TABLE 2. *ED$_{50}$ of intravenous triptans producing changes in carotid blood flow*

	Sumatriptan	Zolmitriptan	Naratriptan	Rizatriptan	Eletriptan	Almotriptan	Frovatriptan
Total (↓)	39 (dog) (28) 30–100 (pig) (45)	2.3 (dog) (128) 1.0 (cat) (128)	19 (dog) (28)	30 (dog) (202)	12 (dog) (89) 30–100 (pig) (238)	10 (cat) (10)	0.4 (dog) (162)
AVA (↓)	<30 (pig) (45)	<10 (cat) (128)			30–100 (pig) (238)		
Extracerebral	↑ (pig) (45)	↓ (dog) (128)			↑ (pig) (238)		
Cerebral	= (pig) (45)	= (dog) (128)		= (man) (209)	= (pig) (238)		

AVA, arteriovenous anastomoses; ↓, decrease; ↑, increase; =, no changes.
Values are given in μg/kg.

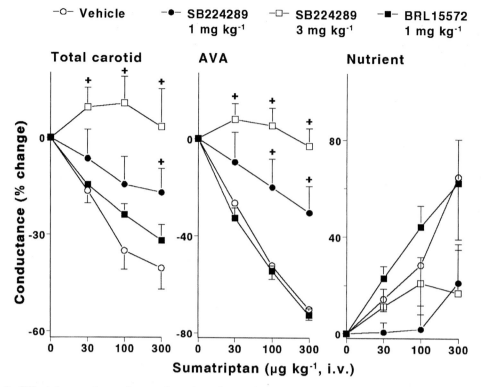

FIG. 2. Effect (percentage change from baseline values) of intravenous sumatriptan (30, 100, and 300 μg/kg) on total carotid, arteriovenous anastomotic (AVA), and nutrient conductances in vagosympathectomized, anesthetized pigs, treated with vehicle (n = 6), 1 mg/kg^{-1} of SB224289 (n = 6), 3 mg/kg^{-1} of SB224289 (n = 3), or 1 mg/kg BRL15572 (n = 6). All values are presented as mean ± SEM. +, $p < 0.05$ versus response by corresponding dose in vehicle-treated animals. Data from De Vries et al. (48).

HT$_{1B/1D}$ receptors (47,230). Significantly, it was recently shown that the ergot-induced carotid vasoconstriction in the anesthetized dog is abolished by a combination of 5-HT$_{1B/1D}$ receptor and α$_2$-adrenoceptor antagonists (230). Possibly, the novel 5-HT receptors and α$_2$-adrenoceptors may be targeted for future antimigraine drugs because constriction of the carotid vasculature and carotid arteriovenous anastomoses is highly predictive for antimigraine potential (194).

Constriction of Isolated Blood Vessels

As shown in Table 3, a number of isolated blood vessels from several species contract in response to triptans (7,10,13,28,90,91,121,122,124,125,129,130,163,227). This effect is more marked in cranial vessels, where, contrary to most peripheral arteries, 5-HT1B rather than 5-HT2 receptors are predominant (6,29). All compounds resemble sumatriptan in their action and potency, but naratriptan appears to be more efficacious (higher maximum contraction) than sumatriptan in the canine basilar artery (28). Moreover, eletriptan seems to behave as a partial agonist in the dog saphenous vein (91), whereas zolmitriptan shows a somewhat lower maximal contraction in the rabbit saphenous vein compared with sumatriptan (130).

In a number of isolated blood vessels [canine basilar (206) and coronary (216) arteries, canine (206) and rabbit (179) saphenous vein, and human middle meningeal artery (180)], the contractile effect of the triptans is antagonized by selective 5-HT$_{1B/1D}$ receptor antagonists, such as GR127935 (164,206). Further studies using selective 5-HT$_{1B}$ and 5-HT$_{1D}$ receptor antagonists will undoubtedly reveal the exact nature of receptors involved. Indeed, it has been shown that sumatriptan constricts the isolated human temporal artery via 5-HT$_{1B}$, but not 5-HT$_{1D}$ receptors (229).

Coronary Vascular Effects

In the human coronary artery, 5-HT$_2$ receptors are more important, but about 20% to 30% of the response is mediated by 5-HT$_1$ receptors (6,29). Accordingly, sumatriptan moderately constricts the human coronary artery, both *in vivo* (126) and *in vitro* (Table 3). Other triptans for which data are available are slightly more potent (except eletriptan), but show similar efficacy (Fig. 3, upper panels) (124,125,163). Figure 3 (lower panel) (124,125) presents the ratio between the unbound maximum plasma concentration (C$_{max}$) after administration of clinically effective doses and the concentration eliciting 50% of maximum contraction (E$_{max}$) of the human iso-

TABLE 3. *pEC$_{50}$ values of triptans in producing contraction of isolated blood vessels*

	Sumatriptan	Zolmitriptan	Naratriptan	Rizatriptan	Eletriptan	Almotriptan	Frovatriptan
Human basilar artery	6.93 (1.11) (163)					5.46 (10)	7.86 (1.25) (163)
Dog basilar artery	6.16 (0.63) (129) 6.80 (0.89) (90)	6.63 (0.61) (129)	6.96 (1.05) (28)		7.20 (0.77) (90)		
Primate basilar artery	6.46 (0.48) (130)	6.92 (0.56) (130)					
Rabbit basilar artery	6.00 (13)						7.20 (13)
Dog middle cerebral artery	7.80 (1.08)[a]		7.15 (1.14) (28)				
Human middle meningeal artery	7.15 (0.66) (122)			7.05 (0.83) (122)	7.30 (0.79) (125)	7.52 (10)	
Human saphenous vein	6.14 (0.54) (227)				5.91 (0.48) (227)		
Dog saphenous vein	6.10 (0.85) (91)				6.30 (0.57) (91)		
Rabbit saphenous vein	6.48 (0.97) (130)	6.79 (0.77) (130)		6.64 (0.90) (7)			
Human coronary artery	6.10 (0.24) (124) 6.70 (0.35) (130) 6.14 (0.21) (28) 6.20 (0.43) (121)	6.32 (0.20) (124) 7.30 (0.37) (130)	6.77 (0.17) (124) 6.77 (0.33) (28)	6.35 (0.17) (124) 5.99 (0.22) (121)	5.37 (0.33) (125)		7.38 (0.42) (163)

[a]F.D. Yocca, personal communication.
If known, the intrinsic activity relative to 5-HT (5-HT = 1) is given in parentheses. References are provided in parentheses on a separate line.

tated conronary artery (EC$_{50}$) of the different compounds. A C$_{max}$/EC$_{50}$ ratio of 1 indicates that the drug [active metabolite excluded, see Maassen Van Den Brink et al. (124)] would elicit 50% of its maximum contraction in a clinical situation. Because in each case the C$_{max}$/EC$_{50}$ ratio is well below 0.4 (zolmitriptan and eletriptan even below 0.05), the triptans are expected to cause only a little coronary constriction upon therapeutic doses in migraine patients without any coronary artery affliction. However, in patients with coronary artery disease (stenosis or hyperreactivity), the second-generation triptans may still cause myocardial ischemia (124).

Trigeminal Inhibitory Effects

As described previously, the vascular effects of triptans are mediated mainly by the 5-HT$_{1B}$ receptor. Given that cranial vasoconstriction is the most important therapeutic mechanism, it implies that agonist action at the 5-HT$_{1D}$ receptor (and 5-HT$_{1F}$ receptor) is not required for the antimigraine action. However, several other mechanisms, which do not seem to be mediated solely by the 5-HT$_{1B}$ receptor, also have been implicated in migraine relief.

These mechanisms include inhibition of the trigeminovascular system either peripherally (145) or centrally (78).

Peripheral Trigeminal Neuronal Inhibition

As depicted in Table 4 (10,28,32,73–76,130,202,203, 239), the triptans (although yet to be established for frovatriptan) inhibit dural plasma protein extravasation following electrical stimulation of the trigeminal nerve (10,28,89,130,239). Because sumatriptan was ineffective in 5-HT$_{1B}$ receptor knockout mice, this effect seems to involve the 5-HT$_{1B}$ receptor (245). Similarly, this receptor mediates the effects of sumatriptan in the guinea pig dura mater (244,245), where the 5-HT$_{1F}$ (109,170) as well as a novel (244,245) receptor also play an important role. In the rat, the inhibition of plasma protein extravasation involves non–5-HT$_{1B}$ receptors, possibly 5-HT$_{1D}$ receptors, and another CP122288-sensitive receptor (203). Importantly, it should be noted that the inhibition of plasma protein extravasation alone is not consistent with antimigraine activity because CP122288 (in doses devoid of vasoconstrictor effect) was ineffective in migraine (185). Moreover, May et al. (137) have ques-

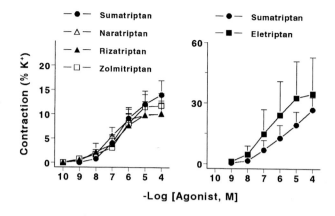

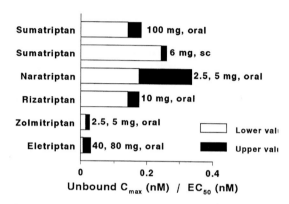

FIG. 3. Coronary effects of triptans. **Upper panels:** Concentration–response (expressed as percentage of response to 100 mM K$^+$) curves in human isolated coronary arteries obtained with sumatriptan, naratriptan, rizatriptan, and zolmitriptan [n = 9, upper left panel; data taken from Maassen Van Den Brink et al. (124)] and sumatriptan and eletriptan [n = 9, upper right panel; data from Maassen Van Den Brink et al. (125)]. **Lower panel:** Relationship between reported C_{max} concentration (corrected for plasma protein binding) in patients and EC_{50} values in the contracting human isolated coronary artery. Frovatriptan, which also constricts the human coronary artery (163), has not been included because the exact therapeutic dose and plasma protein binding level is not known.

tioned the involvement of plasma extravasation in migraine, mainly based on the lack of retinal permeability changes during migraine attacks.

Sumatriptan (73) and zolmitriptan (74) have been shown to inhibit neuropeptide release (mainly calcitonin gene–related peptide) elicited by trigeminal ganglion stimulation. Moreover, sumatriptan and rizatriptan, but not CP122288, inhibit neurogenically induced dural vasodilatation, an effect that, at least in rats, seems to be mediated by the 5-HT$_{1B}$ receptor (203).

Central Trigeminal Neuronal Inhibition

Goadsby and colleagues have shown that intravenous administration of zolmitriptan (75) as well as naratriptan (76) inhibits action potentials generated in the trigeminal nucleus caudalis after superior sagittal sinus stimulation in cats. Similarly, in rats, (intravenous) rizatriptan inhibits such potentials evoked by dural stimulation (32). Thus, these drugs exhibit a central inhibitory effect within the trigeminal system, which may contribute in part to their therapeutic effect in migraine. However, due to its poor central penetration, intravenous sumatriptan did not affect c-*fos* mRNA expression in the trigeminal nucleus caudalis following trigeminal ganglion stimulation in rats (204). This raises the question of whether central trigeminal inhibition is predictive of antimigraine potential. On the other hand, it remains to be clarified whether during migraine headaches the blood–brain barrier is partly disrupted. Indeed, after disruption of the blood–brain barrier by infusion of hyperosmolar mannitol, sumatriptan did inhibit c-*fos* mRNA expression (204).

The central trigeminal inhibitory effects of naratriptan in the cat, being susceptible to blockade by GR127935, are mediated by 5-HT$_{1B/1D}$ receptors (76). Because ketanserin displaced zolmitriptan from its binding sites in the cat brainstem, the involvement of 5-HT$_{1D}$ receptors is

TABLE 4. ED_{50} of intravenous triptans in producing trigeminal neuronal inhibition

	Sumatriptan	Zolmitriptan	Naratriptan	Rizatriptan	Eletriptan	Almotriptan
Inhibition of plasma protein extravasation after trigeminal ganglion stimulation	4 (rat) (28) 31 (rat) (203)	10–30 (guinea-pig) (130)	4.1 (rat) (28)	31 (rat) (239)	30–300 (rat) (89)	200 (guinea-pig) (10)
Inhibition of CGRP Release after cat trigeminal ganglion stimulation	Yes (73)	Yes (74)				
Inhibition of dural vasodilatation after rat trigeminal ganglion stimulation	1,000–10,000 (203)			1,000–3,000 (239)		
Inhibition of activity in trigeminal nucleus caudalis after stimulation[a]	Inactive (rat) (204)	100 (cat) (75) 300–1,000 (rat) (33)	30–100 (cat) (76)	1,000–3,000 (rat) (32)		

[a]Stimulation of the superior sagittal sinus in cats or dural meninges in rats.
CGRP, calcium gene-related peptide.
Values are given in µg/kg.
No data are available for frovatriptan.

likely (141). Also in rats, 5-HT$_{1D}$ receptors, but not 5-HT$_{1B}$ receptors, seem to mediate the central trigeminal anti-nociceptive action by zolmitriptan (33).

Possible Mechanisms of Action of Triptans in Migraine

The theoretically possible mechanisms of actions of triptans in migraine are discussed thoroughly in Chapter 17. In our view, the main action of triptans in migraine is to constrict dilated cranial extracerebral blood vessels (64,101,102) (Fig. 4). In addition, the triptans can reduce neuropeptide release and plasma protein extravasation across dural vessels (145,146) and inhibit impulse transmission centrally within the trigeminovascular system (71,78) (Fig. 4). The possible contribution of the neuronal effect of triptans can first be judged when pure 5-HT$_{1D}$ receptor agonists have been developed and tested for efficacy in migraine.

Pharmacokinetics

The pharmacokinetic characteristics of triptans have been studied in human volunteers and migraine patients (Table 5) (15,18,27,52,54,56,65,66,82,103,111,116,117, 142,143,144,166,175,183,198). Subcutaneous sumatriptan (6 mg) is quickly absorbed with a time to maximum plasma concentration (t_{max}) of approximately 10 minutes and an average bioavailability of 96% (56,65). After oral administration of therapeutic doses (100 mg) of sumatriptan, however, the t_{max} is substantially longer (1.5 hours) and, more importantly, the bioavailability is rather low (~14%) (65,115). Intranasal or rectal administration of sumatriptan does not seem to improve these parameters much (56,116,143). The oral bioavailability of newer triptans, especially naratriptan and almotriptan, is much improved. The latter can be partly attributed to the more lipophilic nature of these drugs. Interestingly, the t_{max} after oral administrations of zolmitriptan (52,54), naratriptan (66,111), almotriptan (18,183), and frovatriptan

(15) is not much better (even worse for some) than that of sumatriptan, whereas rizatriptan (27,198) and eletriptan (103,142,144) seem to reach their peak plasma levels quicker compared with sumatriptan. It may be noted that the unbound C_{max} values (C_{max} corrected for plasma protein binding) of newer triptans are lower than that of sumatriptan. This is apparently due to two main factors: lower therapeutic concentrations are needed because these drugs have a higher affinity at 5-HT$_{1B/1D}$ receptors (see Table 1) and these drugs have been better titrated, thus reducing therapeutic penalty. For the latter reason, low-dose formulations of sumatriptan have been marketed in some countries.

With the exception of rizatriptan, triptans are degraded slower than sumatriptan. Frovatriptan has a plasma half-life of 26 to 30 hours (15), and in view of the putative relationship of this parameter to headache recurrence, the results of clinical trials with frovatriptan are awaited with interest. In contrast to sumatriptan and naratriptan, active metabolites have been reported for zolmitriptan (52), rizatriptan (82), and eletriptan (103). It is not known whether (and if so, to what extent) the metabolites contribute to therapeutic activity. We do not know whether the metabolism of almotriptan and frovatriptan results in the formation of active metabolites.

RANDOMIZED CLINICAL TRIALS WITH TRIPTANS

First, it should be demonstrated in randomized, double-blind, placebo-controlled, clinical trials that a drug is more effective than placebo. Then the dose–response curve should be established, and the optimum dose (taking both efficacy and tolerability into account) and minimum effective dose should be determined. The drug should then in the optimum dose be compared with currently established treatment for efficacy and tolerability.

Other questions that have been addressed in randomized clinical trials, mainly with sumatriptan, the first triptan, are listed as follows:

1. Does a second dose increase efficacy?
2. Can a second dose prevent recurrence of headache?
3. Is a second dose effective in the treatment of recurrences?
4. What is the onset of action compared with placebo/control?
5. Can a triptan, being a vasoconstrictor, be given safely during the aura phase?
6. Can a triptan given in the aura phase prevent the headache?
7. Is the efficacy sustained in multiple attacks?

In current randomized clinical trials, headache relief with triptans is defined as a decrease from an initial moderate or severe headache to none or mild (171) after a certain time (1, 2, or 4 hours). In this section, response rates

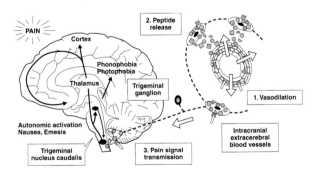

FIG. 4. Triptans could theoretically have three possible mechanisms of actions in migraine: **(1)** Constriction of dilated cranial extracerebral blood vessels; **(2)** reduction of neuropeptide release from peripheral nerve endings around blood vessels; and **(3)** inhibition of impulse transmission centrally in the trigeminal nucleus caudalis.

TABLE 5. *Pharmacokinetic parameters for triptans*

Drug	Route of administration	Dose (mg)	T_{max} (h)	C_{max} (ng/ml)	Bioavailability (%)	$t_{1/2}$ (h)	AUC (ng/h/ml)	Active metabolites	Plasma protein binding (%)	CL_R (ml/min)	Log $D_{pH7.4}$ (175)	References
Sumatriptan	s.c.	6	0.17	72	96	2	90	–	14–21	220	–1.5	(56,65)
	p.o.	100	1.5	54	14	2	158			260		(65,117)
	i.n.	10	1.5	8.5	15.8	2	31			210		(56,143)
	rectal	25	1.5	27	19.2	1.8	78			200 (20 mg)		(56,116)
Zolmitriptan	p.o.	5	1.5	10	46	3.0	42	+	25[a]	193	–1.0	(166)
	p.o.	10	2.5	13.4	46	2.8	87			179		(52,54)
Naratriptan	p.o.	2.5	2	12.6	74	5.5	98	–	20[a]	220	–0.2	(66,111)
Rizatriptan	p.o.	10	1.0	19.8	40	2.0	50	+	14[a]	414	–0.7	(27,82, 198)
Eletriptan	p.o.	40	1.8[a]	82[a]	50[a]			+	85[a]	597[a]	+0.5	(103,142, 144)
	p.o.	80	1.4	246	50	6.3	1,661					
Almotriptan	p.o.	12.5	2.5	49.5	80	3.1	266					(18,183)
Frovatriptan	p.o	2.5	3.0	7.0	29.6	25.7	94					(15)
	p.o.	40	5.0	53.4	17.5	29.7	881					
	i.v.	0.8	—	24.4	100	23.6	104			132		

[a]A. McHarg, personal communication.

AUC, area under curve; PPB, plasma protein binding; CL_R, renal clearance; Log$D_{pH7.4}$, measure of lipophilicity with increasing numbers indicating greater lipid solubility; s.c., subcutaneous; p.o., Oral; i.n., intranasal; i.v., intravenous.

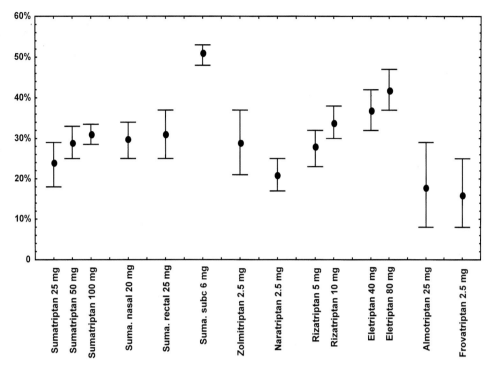

FIG. 5. Mean therapeutic gains (proportion of patients responding to active drug minus proportion of patients reponding to placebo) (•) and 95% CIs (bars) for oral (25, 50, and 100 mg), intranasal (20 mg), rectal (25 mg), and subcutaneous (6 mg) sumatriptan, zolmitriptan (2.5 mg), naratriptan (2.5 mg), rizatriptan (5 and 10 mg), eletriptan (40 and 80 mg), almotriptan (25 mg), and frovatriptan (2.5 mg). For number of patients treated with each dose of drugs and placebo, see text. Note that the therapeutic gain is determined with the most certainty, as shown by the narrow CIs, for 100 mg sumatriptan and 6 mg subcutaneous sumatriptan (approximately 4,000 and 3,000 patients, respectively).

at 1 hour after injection and at 2 hours after other routes of administration will be considered as the primary responses for active drugs and placebo. These response rates vary considerably in different trials, for example, from 56% to 88% after subcutaneous sumatriptan (218), most likely due to a variable placebo response. Therefore, the results of the trials will be given as the therapeutic gain (percentage response for active drug minus percentage response for placebo) with 95% confidence intervals (95% CIs). As will be shown, the mean therapeutic gains for two triptans or two doses of a triptan have, in most cases, overlapping 95% CIs (Fig. 5), and it should be noted that the relative efficacy of two doses or drugs can only be established definitely in comparative trials (Table 6).

Randomized Clinical Trials with Sumatriptan

Subcutaneous Sumatriptan

Subcutaneous sumatriptan has a reasonably well defined dose–response curve, with 1 mg being the minimum effective dose and with 6 mg being the optimum dose with no gain by increasing to 8 mg (217).

Six milligrams subcutaneous sumatriptan has been evaluated against placebo in 13 randomized double-blind placebo-controlled clinical trials (12,20,22,59,86,94,106, 135,148,186,210,211) where headache relief was reported after 1 hour. As shown in Figure 5, 6 mg subcutaneous sumatriptan [based on 1994 patients treated with sumatriptan (headache relief in 69%) and 1,265 patients treated with placebo (headache relief in 19%)] has a mean therapeutic gain of 51% (95% CI 48%–53%) after 1 hour. After 2 hours in 10 of these trials, the therapeutic gain was the same [52% (95% CI 40%–56%)] as after 1 hour (Tfelt-Hansen, personal observation), indicating that the response to subcutaneous sumatriptan should be evaluated after 1 hour. In two trials with subcutaneous sumatriptan in which headache relief was reported after 1½ hours (2,21), the mean therapeutic gain was 45% (95% CI 34%–56%). In 11 of these trials the total number of adverse events were reported: 930 of 1,456 after sumatriptan (64%) versus 290 of 890 after placebo (31%). There were thus 33% (95% CI 29%–37%) more adverse events after subcutaneous sumatriptan than after placebo. Most of these adverse events were, however, mild to moderate and short term.

Subcutaneous sumatriptan also has been shown in one placebo-controlled trial (20) to reduce productivity loss during a migraine attack.

TABLE 6. *Randomized clinical trials comparing a new triptan with sumatriptan*

Trial	Drug and dose (mg)	No. of patients	Success rate[a] (%)	Therapeutic gain[b] (%)	Pain free[c] (%)	Recurrence[d] (%)
Oral administration						
(51)[e]	PL	55	44		13	25
	ZO 5	491	59	15	29	26
	SU 100	498	61	17	30	28
Success rates						
ZO 5 vs. SU 100	−2% (−8% to +4%)					
Pain free						
ZO 5 vs. SU 100	−1% (−7% to +5%)					
(40)	PL	91	31 39[f]			36
	NA 1	85	58 64[f]	27		31
	NA 2.5	87	52 63[f]	21		17
	NA 5	93	54 65[f]	23		32
	NA 7.5	93	68 80[f]	37		30
	NA 10	96	69 80[f]	38		29
	SU 100	98	60 80[f]	29		44
Success rates						
NA 2.5 vs. SU 100	−8% (−23% to +6%)					
Success rates at 4h						
NA 2.5 vs. SU 100	*−16% (−29% to −3%)*					
Recurrence rates						
NA 2.5 vs SU 100	−27% (−42% to −13%)					
(5)	PL	104	22 27[f]			10
	NA 0.1	207	30 36[f]	8		30
	NA 0.25	214	29 36[f]	7		43
	NA 1	208	38 52[f]	18		42
	NA 2.5	199	50 66[f]	28		19
	SU 100	229	59 76[f]	37		36
Success rate						
NA 2.5 vs. SU 100	−9% (−18% to +1%)					
Success rates at 4 hours						
NA 2.5 vs. SU 100	*−9% (−18% to −1%)*					
Recurrence rates						
NA 2.5 vs. SU 100	−17% (−27% to −7%)					
(80)[g]	NA 2.5	215	76[f]			43[h]
	SU 100	216	84[f]			57
Success rates at 4 hours						
NA 2.5 vs. SU 100	*−8% (−15% to 0%)*					
Recurrence rates						
NA 2.5 vs. SU 100	−14% (−24% to −3%)					
(235)	PL	85	18		3	36
	RI 10	89	52	34	26	41
	RI 20	82	56	38	35	53
	RI 40	120	67	49	49	42
	SU 100	72	46	28	22	43
Success rates						
RI 10 vs. SU 100 +6% (−10% to +21%)	RI 40 vs. SU 100 +21% (+7% to +35%)					
Pain free						
RI 10 vs. SU 100 +4% (−10% to +17%)	RI 40 vs. SU 100 +27% (+14% to +40%)					
(119)	PL	80	23		3	33
	RI 5	352	63	40	27	38
	SU 50	356	67	44	32	34
Success rates						
RI 5 vs. SU 50	−4% (−11% to +3%)					
Pain free						
RI 5 vs. SU 50	−6% (−12% to +2%)					
(85)	PL	141	38		9	32
	RI 5	294	68	30	33	33
	RI 10	305	72	34	41	35
	SU 25	297	62	24	27	32
	SU 50	291	68	30	37	31
Success rates						
RI 10 vs. SU 50+ 4% (−3% to +11%)	RI 5 vs. SU 25 +6% (−2% to +14%)					
Pain free						
RI 10 vs. SU 50+ 4% (−4% to +12%)	RI 5 vs. SU 25 +6% (−1% to +13%)					
(223)	PL	159	40		9	20
	RI 5	164	60	20	25	48

TABLE 6. *Continued*

Trial	Drug and dose (mg)	No. of patients	Success rate[a] (%)	Therapeutic gain[b] (%)	Pain free[c] (%)	Recurrence[d] (%)
Oral administration (cont'd)						
(223) *(cont'd)*	RI 10	385	67	27	40	35
	SU 100	387	62	22	33	32
Success rates						
RI 10 vs. SU 100	+5% (−2% to +12%)					
Pain free						
RI 10 vs. SU 100	+7% (+1% to +14%)					
(105,172)	PL	126	24		6	23
	EL 20	129	54	30	19	27
	EL 40	117	65	41	29	33
	EL 80	118	77	53	37	32
	SU 100	115	55	31	23	33
Success rates						
EL 20 vs. SU 100	−1% (−13% to +12%)	EL 40 vs. SU 100	+10% (−2% to +23%)			
EL 80 vs. SU 100	+22% (+11% to +34%)					
Pain free						
EL 20 vs. SU 100	−4% (−14% to +6%)	EL 40 vs. SU 100	+6% (−6% to +17%)			
EL 80 vs. SU 100	+14% (+2% to +25%)					
(172)	PL	80	31		4	25
	EL 40	169	64	33	31	19
	EL 80	160	67	36	37	16
	SU 50	176	50	19	19	26
	SU 100	160	53	22	18	27
Success rates						
EL 40 vs. SU 50	+14% (+4% to +24%)	EL 40 vs. SU 100	+11% (0 to +21%)			
EL 80 vs. SU 50	+17% (+6% to +27%)	EL 80 vs. SU 100	+14% (+3% to +24%)			
Pain free						
EL 40 vs. SU 50	+12% (+3% to +21%)	EL 40 vs. SU 100	+13% (+3% to +22%)			
EL 80 vs. SU 50	+18% (+9% to +28%)	EL 80 vs. SU 100	+19% (+9% to +28%)			
(172)	PL	86	40		9	19
	EL 40	175	62	22	19	6
	EL 80	170	70	30	26	8
	SU 25	171	53	13	17	14
	SU 50	175	56	16	18	6
Success rates						
EL 40 vs. SU 25	+10% (−1% to +20%)	EL 40 vs. SU 50	+6% (−4% to +17%)			
EL 80 vs. SU 25	+17% (+7% to +28%)	EL 80 vs. SU 50	+14% (+4% to +24%)			
Pain free						
EL 40 vs. SU 25	+2% (−6% to +11%)	EL 40 vs. SU 50	+1% (−7% to +10%)			
EL 80 vs. SU 25	+10% (+1% to +18%)	EL 80 vs. SU 50	+8% (−0.5% to +17%)			
(19)	PL	99	42			20
	AL 12.5	184	57	15		18
	AL 25	191	57	15		15
	SU 100	194	64	22		25
Success rates						
AL 12.5 vs. SU 100	−7% (−17% to +3%)	AL 25 vs. SU 100	−7% (−17% to +3%)			
Subcutaneous administration						
(38)	PL	63	41		17	35
	NA 0.5	60	65	24	30	39
	NA 1	55	75	34	44	41
	NA 2.5	42	83	42	60	49
	NA 5	34	94	53	79	22
	NA 10	34	91	50	88	29
	SU 6	47	89	48	55	45
Success rates						
NA 5 vs. SU 6	+5% (−7% to +17%)	NA 10 vs. SU 6	+2% (−11% to +15%)			
Pain free						
NA 5 vs. SU 6	+24% (+4% to +44%)	NA 10 vs. SU 6	+33% (+15% to +51%)			

Percentages in parentheses are 95% CIs.
[a]A decrease in headache from severe or moderate to none or mild at 2 hours.
[b]Percentage success with active drug minus percentage success with placebo.
[c]At 2 hours.
[d]Percentage of patients with an initial success who had an increase in headache to moderate or severe within 24 hours.
[e]Secondary efficacy parameter (51).
[f]Success rate at 4 hours.
[g]Patients selected as having frequent recurrences (≥50% of attacks treated with any medication).
[h]Statistically significant difference at p<0.01.
AL, almotriptan; EL, eletriptan; NA, naratriptan; PL, placebo; RI, rizatriptan; SU, sumatriptan; ZO, zolmitriptan.

Oral Sumatriptan

The lower part of the dose–response curve for oral sumatriptan until recently (169) was not well established (217). The minimum effective dose is 25 mg (85,169) and the optimum dose 50 to 100 mg, with no gain in efficacy, but more adverse events, when the dose is increased to 200 to 300 mg (155,217).

Oral sumatriptan 100 mg has been evaluated against placebo in 20 randomized double-blind placebo-controlled clinical trials (5,19,26,35,40,51,77,105,149,151, 155,156,169,172,182,192,220,223,235). As shown in Figure 5, 100 mg oral sumatriptan (based on 3,090 patients treated with sumatriptan (headache relief in 59%) and 1,741 patients treated with placebo (headache relief in 28%) has a mean therapeutic gain of 31% (95% CI 28%–33.5%) after 2 hours.

In 12 of these trials, the total number of adverse events were reported: 755 of 1,948 after sumatriptan (39%) versus 284 of 1,236 after placebo (23%). There were thus 16% (95% CI 13%–19%) more adverse events after 100 mg oral sumatriptan than after placebo. However, most of these adverse events were mild and short term.

The lower doses of oral sumatriptan, 25 and 50 mg, have been investigated less, in five and seven clinical trials, respectively. For 50 mg sumatriptan (based on 1,599 patients treated with sumatriptan (headache relief in 59%) and 653 patients treated with placebo (headache relief in 30%), the mean therapeutic gain was 29% (95% CI 29%–33%) (35,85,169,172,192,193), a therapeutic gain similar to that of 100 mg sumatriptan (Fig. 5), and in two direct comparative trials the efficacy of the two doses of sumatriptan were comparable (169,190). The total number of adverse events was 357 of 1,034 after 50 mg sumatriptan (35%) versus 164 of 509 after placebo (32%), with no difference between the two (35,85,169, 192,193). In the two comparative trials (169,190), 50 mg sumatriptan caused fewer adverse events than 100 mg sumatriptan. The response rate of 50 mg sumatriptan was superior to that of placebo at 30 minutes (85, 169,193).

The mean therapeutic gain for 25 mg sumatriptan was 24% (95% CI 18%–29%) [based on 1,113 patients treated with sumatriptan (headache relief in 56%) and 428 patients treated with placebo (headache relief in 32%)] (35,85,169,172,192) (Fig. 5). In two direct comparative trials (169,190), 25 mg sumatriptan was found inferior to 50 and 100 mg sumatriptan. After 25 mg sumatriptan, 38% (273 of 714) of patients experienced the same incidence of adverse events as after placebo 37% (132 of 353). In one trial (85), 25 mg sumatriptan was superior to placebo after 30 minutes.

Concerning the oral dose of sumatriptan, one can conclude that 100- and 50-mg doses have the same efficacy, superior to that of the 25-mg dose. Both the 25- and 50-mg doses cause fewer adverse events than 100 mg suma-triptan, both lower doses cause apparently no more adverse events than placebo. Based on these results, 50 mg should be the optimum dose, but even if 100 mg caused more adverse events than 50 mg in one crossover trial (190) almost the same percentage of patients (35% and 31%, respectively) preferred the two doses of suma-triptan, whereas only 21% preferred the 25 mg dose. This could be due to the fact that more patients on 100 than on 50 mg reported complete relief of pain (190). So some patients seem to prefer a more effective dose and will endure the cost of more, transient and often mild, adverse events.

Intranasal Sumatriptan

The minimum effective dose of intranasal sumatriptan is 5 mg; 10 mg is also effective, but less so than 20 mg (168), and 20 mg intranasal sumatriptan is the optimum dose (168), with no gain when the dose is increased to 40 mg (168,191).

Intranasal sumatriptan 20 mg has been evaluated against placebo in seven trials (3,36,49,167,176,187,191). As shown in Figure 5, 20 mg intranasal sumatriptan [based on 1,205 patients treated with sumatriptan (headache relief in 61%) and 701 patients treated with placebo (headache relief in 31%)] had a mean therapeutic gain of 30% (95% CI 25%–34%) after 2 hours.

Intranasal sumatriptan 20 mg caused 21% (95% CI 16%–26%) more adverse effects than placebo (3); the most common adverse event was taste disturbances (36, 49,167,187,191).

In one trial, 73 of 200 patients (37%) treated with intranasal sumatriptan 20 mg had headache relief after 30 minutes (the primary efficacy parameter) compared with 45 of 207 patients (22%) treated with oral sumatriptan 100 mg (131,138). Intranasal sumatriptan thus had a therapeutic gain over oral sumatriptan of 15% (95% CI −6% to +23%) after 30 minutes. Similar therapeutic superiority of intranasal sumatriptan was also found at 15 minutes, as well as at 45 and 60 minutes. After 4 hours, oral sumatriptan was almost superior to intranasal sumatriptan [9% difference in response (95% CI −0.2% to +19%)]. For the second and third attacks treated, no superiority of intranasal over oral sumatriptan could be demonstrated from 15 to 120 minutes, and oral sumatriptan was superior to intranasal sumatriptan after 4 hours ($p < 0.01$).

Rectal Sumatriptan

Two trials comparing the recommended 25-mg rectal dose of sumatriptan have been published (79,215). In addition, two trials have been presented as posters (93,113). For 25 mg given rectally, sumatriptan [based on 426 patients treated with sumatriptan (headache relief in 70%) and 403 patients treated with placebo (headache relief in 39%)] had a mean therapeutic gain of 31% (95% CI 25%–37%) after 2 hours (Fig. 5).

In three of these clinical trials the total number of adverse events are given (79,93,215): 76 of 301 after sumatriptan (25%) versus 24 of 171 after placebo (14%). There were thus 11% (95% CI 4%–18%) more adverse events after 25 mg rectal sumatriptan than after placebo.

Rectal sumatriptan 25 mg was significantly superior to placebo after 30 minutes (215) and 60 minutes (79,93). Higher doses of 50 and 100 mg did not increase the efficacy compared with 25 mg (79), and 12.5 mg can be considered as the minimum effective dose (79,93,113,215).

Does a Second Dose of Sumatriptan Increase Efficacy?

In two trials on subcutaneous sumatriptan 6 mg or placebo given 1 hour after the first dose of sumatriptan to patients without headache relief, there was no difference in headache response at 2 hours between the 6 mg plus 6 mg of sumatriptan and the 6 mg of sumatriptan plus placebo regimens (22,210). In two trials, patients initially took 100 mg oral sumatriptan and all patients then at 2 hours (63) or at 4 hours (199) took either another dose of 100 mg sumatriptan or placebo in a double-blind fashion. Headache relief rates 4 hours (63) and 8 hours (199) after the initial, open-label dose of 100 mg sumatriptan were 80% and 77% (63), and 85% and 84% (199) for the 100 mg plus 100 mg of sumatriptan group and the 100 mg of sumatriptan plus placebo group, respectively. Taken together, these four trials demonstrate that neither a second dose of sumatriptan to patients not responding to the first dose nor the routine use of a second dose increases the efficacy of sumatriptan.

Sumatriptan in the Prevention and Treatment of Recurrences

Headache recurrence, or secondary treatment failure, is a problem with all triptans, as well as with other acute migraine treatments. With sumatriptan it occurs in 20% to 40% of primary successfully treated patients in controlled clinical trials. In clinical pratice it is also a major clinical problem; and about 75% of patients are reported to experience headache recurrence in at least some attacks and up to 40% in most of their attacks (232). Multiple recurrences, in some cases prolonging the migraine attack for several days, also can occur (62). Patients with headache recurrence tend to have longer attacks than patients without recurrences (233), and neither pharmacokinetic (half-life) nor pharmacodynamic differences (effect on carotid arteries) for sumatriptan were observed in recurrence-prone patients compared with other migraine patients (231).

Oral sumatriptan has been evaluated for prevention of recurrence by administering 100 mg 2 hours (63) or 4 hours (199) after 100 mg sumatriptan, or 4 hours after 6 mg subcutaneous sumatriptan (178). In all three trials the patients were first given open-label sumatriptan, and then either 100 mg sumatriptan or placebo. In neither of the studies did 100 mg sumatriptan decrease the incidence of headache recurrences compared with placebo. After subcutaneous sumatriptan plus 100 mg sumatriptan or placebo, the recurrence rate in both groups was 39%, but the 100 mg sumatriptan dose delayed the median time to recurrence from 10.3 hours after placebo to 15.6 after sumatriptan (178). In the study where the second oral dose was given after 2 hours (63), both groups (100 mg plus 100 mg of sumatriptan or 100 mg of sumatriptan plus placebo) had similar incidences of headache recurrence, 22% and 25%, respectively; and the median times to recurrence were approximately 16 hours in both groups. Similarly, administering 100 mg sumatriptan after 4 hours (199) resulted in no decrease in headache recurrence (25% for patients treated with 100 mg plus 100 mg of sumatriptan and 23% for patients treated with 100 mg of sumatriptan plus placebo). Prevention of recurrence with a second dose of sumatriptan is thus not recommended (63,178,199).

The efficacy of sumatriptan in treating recurrent headache has been investigated in four trials (31,63, 169,199). In all four trials sumatriptan was superior to placebo. Oral sumatriptan 100 mg seems to have the same efficacy in the treatment of headache recurrences [mean therapeutic gain after 2 hours of 32% (95% CI: 18%–45%) (63)] as in the treatment of migraine attacks (see above) (Fig. 5). In another trial with oral sumatriptan (199), the therapeutic gain was approximately 37% after 4 hours. In one trial (31), subcutaneous sumatriptan 6 mg had a 84% response rate compared with 50% for placebo for the first attack. The therapeutic gain was thus 34% (95% CI: 15%–52%). In conclusion, a second dose of sumatriptan is effective in the treatment of headache recurrence, as is a second dose of rizatriptan (214) (see below).

Sumatriptan During the Migraine Aura

Subcutaneous sumatriptan was compared with placebo during the aura phase in one trial (4). The purpose was to investigate whether sumatriptan, a cerebral vasoconstrictor, would prolong or modify the aura. Furthermore, the aim was to investigate whether sumatriptan prevented or delayed development of the headache. Eighty-eight patients treated themselves with 6 mg sumatriptan, and 83 patients received placebo during a typical aura. The median duration of aura was 25 minutes after sumatriptan and 30 minutes after placebo ($p = $ NS). The proportion of patients who developed a moderate or severe headache after administration of test drugs were similar in the two groups (68% after sumatriptan and 75% after placebo). In an open fashion, patients could later treat their attacks successfully with sumatriptan 6 mg. The lack of effect of sumatriptan during the aura phase on the subsequent development of headache remains obscure.

Randomized Clinical Trials with Zolmitriptan

Zolmitriptan has a well established dose–response curve, with 1 mg being the minimum effective dose, 2.5 mg zolmitriptan the optimum dose (61,197). Doses of up to 25 mg zolmitriptan have been evaluated (37,51,61, 177,197,208,234), and generally no increase in efficacy was observed above the 2.5- to 5-mg dose range, but an increase in side effects was observed (61). An exception is the high therapeutic gain of 58% (95% CI 47%–68%) for 20 mg zolmitriptan in one trial (37), a result normally only seen after subcutaneous sumatriptan.

The recommended dose of 2.5 mg zolmitriptan has been compared with placebo in two trials (177,208). As shown in Figure 5, 2.5 mg zolmitriptan [based on 438 patients treated with zolmitriptan (headache relief in 64%) and 213 patients treated with placebo (headache relief in 35%)] has a mean therapeutic gain of 29% (95% CI 21%–37%) after 2 hours. After 1 hour, the mean therapeutic gain was 14% (95% CI 6%–21%) (177,208). Based on a metanalysis of all phase II/III studies, a slightly higher therapeutic gain of 34% (95% CI 27%–41%) was reported for 2.5 mg zolmitriptan (72). In these two trials (177,208) adverse events occurred in 223 of 498 patients (45%) treated with zolmitriptan and in 70 of 239 patients (29%) treated with placebo. Zolmitriptan 2.5 mg thus caused 15% (95% CI 8%–23%) more adverse events than placebo. For an overview of adverse events after zolmitriptan, see Table 9.

A recurrence rate of 22% after 2.5 mg zolmitriptan was reported in one trial (208). Overall recurrence rates in dose range-finding studies was 31% with 2.5 or 5 mg zolmitriptan (197).

Randomized Clinical Trials with Naratriptan

Oral naratriptan has been evaluated in a wide dose range from 0.1 to 10 mg (5,40,112,134), with 100 mg sumatriptan used as the control treatment in two trials (5,40) (see Table 6). The minimum effective dose is 1 mg, and 2.5 mg naratriptan was chosen as the dose causing no more adverse events than placebo (88). Higher oral doses of 7.5 mg and 10 mg naratriptan were quite comparable in efficacy to 100 mg sumatriptan in one trial (40).

Oral naratriptan 2.5 mg, the recommended dose, has been evaluated against placebo in four trials (5,40, 112,134). As shown in Figure 5, 2.5 mg naratriptan had [based on 1,009 patients treated with naratriptan (headache relief in 48%) and 912 patients treated with placebo (headache relief in 27%)] a mean therapeutic gain of 21% (95% CI 17%–25%) after 2 hours. Escape medication could first be taken after 4 hours, and at this time the mean therapeutic gain was 33% (95% CI 29%–37%) (5,40,112,134).

Naratriptan 2.5 mg was superior to placebo in producing headache relief after 60 minutes (88). Recurrence rates for 2.5 mg naratriptan were 27% (134), 28% (112), 17% (40), and 19% (5).

In one early relatively small, dose-ranging study, subcutaneous naratriptan in the dose range of 0.5 to 10 mg was compared with placebo and 6 mg sumatriptan (see Table 6) (38). After 2 hours, all doses of naratriptan were superior to placebo, with response rates of 65% (0.5 mg), 75% (1 mg), 83% (2.5 mg), 94% (5 mg), and 91% (10 mg) versus 41% for placebo. For sumatriptan the response rate was 89%. Naratriptan 2.5 mg (and higher doses) was thus quite comparable with 6 mg sumatriptan, but as shown by the wide 95% CI, the trial is too small to demonstrate comparability (see Table 6). The recurrence rates were 45% for sumatriptan and quite comparable with the lower doses of naratriptan [38% (0.5 mg), 41% (1 mg), and 49% (2.5 mg)], whereas the 5- and 10-mg doses resulted in lower, but not significantly so, recurrence rates of 22% and 29%, respectively.

Randomized Clinical Trials with Rizatriptan

For rizatriptan, the minimum effective dose is 5 mg, the optimum dose being 10 mg (39); 2.5 mg rizatriptan is a noneffective dose (70), whereas the high 40-mg dose had a therapeutic gain of 49% (235) but caused too many adverse events.

Ten milligrams rizatriptan has been evaluated in six placebo-controlled trials (70,85,115,214,223,235). As shown in Figure 5, 10 mg rizatriptan [based on 1,961 patients treated with rizatriptan (headache relief in 69%) and 836 patients treated with placebo (headache relief in 34%)] had a mean therapeutic gain of 35% (95% CI 31%–39%) after 2 hours. In four of these trials (85,214,223,235) the total number of adverse events were reported: 545 of 1,196 after rizatriptan (46%) versus 177 of 620 after placebo (29%). There were thus 17% (95% CI 12%–22%) more adverse events after 10 mg rizatriptan than after placebo.

The 5-mg dose of rizatriptan, recommended for use in patients on propranolol has been evaluated in five controlled trials (70,85,119,214,223). As shown in Figure 5, 5 mg rizatriptan [based on 1,397 patients treated with rizatriptan (headache relief in 62%) and 749 patients treated with placebo (headache relief in 34%)] has a mean therapeutic gain of 28% (95% CI 23%–32%) after 2 hours. In four of these trials (85,119,214,223), the total number of adverse events were reported: 448 of 1,268 after rizatriptan (35%) versus 188 of 686 after placebo (27%). There were thus 8% (95% CI 4%–12%) more adverse events after 5 mg rizatriptan than after placebo.

A rapidly dissolving wafer of rizatriptan has been compared with placebo in two trials (1, and Merk Sherpe &

Dohme data on file). The 10 mg dose rizatriptan in wafer form [based on 288 patients treated with rizatriptan (headache relief in 70%) and 265 treated with placebo (headache relief in 34%)] had a mean therapeutic gain of 37% (95% CI 29%–45%); and 5 mg rizatriptan in wafer form (headache relief in 62% of 271 patients) had a mean therapeutic gain of 28% (95% CI 20%–36%). Ten milligrams rizatriptan in wafer form was superior to placebo after 30 minutes and had a small therapeutic gain of 11% (95% CI 3%–18%) (1).

In one trial (214), rizatriptan 10 mg was superior to placebo in the treatment of headache recurrence, with a therapeutic gain of 38% (95% CI 23%–52%) after 2 hours, whereas 5 mg rizatriptan was not significantly superior to placebo in the treatment of recurrences.

Randomized Clinical Trials with Eletriptan

Thus far, no peer-reviewed papers on eletriptan have been published. An early dose-finding study evaluating doses from 5 to 30 mg eletriptan found only minor difference from the placebo response (60). Based on five placebo-controlled trials (96,105,172,181), the mean therapeutic gain for 80 mg eletriptan [based on 1,103 patients treated with eletriptan (response rate 68%) and 624 patients treated with placebo (response rate 25%)] was 43% (95% CI 39%–47%) after 2 hours (Fig. 5). For 40 mg eletriptan the mean therapeutic gain was 36% (95% CI 32%–41%) after 2 hours (96,172,181) (Fig. 5). In the trial program for eletriptan, adverse events were reported to occur in 50%, 42%, and 31% of patients treated with 80 mg eletriptan, 40 mg eletriptan, and placebo, respectively (95). Asthenia was the most common adverse effect and occurred in 5% of patients treated with 40 mg eletriptan and 10% of patients treated with 80 mg eletriptan (95).

Randomized Clinical Trials with Almotriptan

To date, no peer-reviewed papers on almotriptan have been published. The first efficacy trial demonstrated that 6- and 10-mg doses of subcutaneous almotriptan were superior to placebo (17). Based on two placebo-controlled trials (16,19) the mean therapeutic gain for 25 mg almotriptan [based on 226 patients treated with almotriptan (response rate 61%) and 130 patients treated with placebo (response rate 42%)] was 18% (95% CI 8%–29%) after 2 hours (Fig. 5). Higher doses of up to 150 mg almotriptan were not superior to the 25-mg dose (16). A recurrence rate of 15% was reported in one trial after 25 mg almotriptan (19).

Randomized Clinical Trials with Frovatriptan

Based on the abstracts of two placebo-controlled trials (84,188), the mean therapeutic gain for 2.5 mg frovatriptan [based on 225 patients treated with frovatriptan

(response rate 40%) and 214 patients treated with placebo (response rate 24%)] was 16% (95% CI 8%–25%) after 2 hours (Fig. 5). Higher doses of up to 40 mg frovatriptan were not superior to the 2.5-mg dose (188), and lower doses were not superior to placebo (84). Recurrence rates of 11% (188) and 14% (84) were reported for 2.5 mg frovatriptan.

Randomized Trials with Other 5-HT1B/1D Receptor Agonists

Avitriptan (BMS180048) 75 mg had a mean therapeutic gain of 40% (95% CI 27%–51%) in two trials (30,189), but the development program for avitriptan was stopped due to toxicity.

Subcutaneous alniditan, a nontriptan 5-HT$_{1B/1D}$ receptor agonist, in a dose of 1.4 mg had a therapeutic gain of 45% (95% CI 26%–65%) after 1 hour in one trial (83). A decrease in recurrence rate with increasing dose of alniditan was observed (83), but because alniditan did not result in fewer recurrences than sumatriptan in a comparative clinical trial (Jansen, data on file), the development of alniditan was stopped.

Comparative Trials of Triptans

The second-generation triptans—zolmitriptan, naratriptan, rizatriptan, eletriptan, and almotriptan—have been compared with oral sumatriptan in 12 randomized, double-blind clinical trials (see Table 6). Furthermore, one trial compared subcutaneous naratriptan, an administration form not in use for naratriptan, with subcutaneous sumatriptan (see Table 6) (38). As shown in Table 6, 40 mg rizatriptan was superior to 100 mg sumatriptan at 2 hours (235), but this dose was later dropped because of too high an incidence of adverse events. Eletriptan 80 mg was superior to 100 mg (172) and 25 mg and 50 mg sumatriptan (172), in most cases also for the clinically more relevant parameter *pain free* after 2 hours (132). Forty milligrams eletriptan was superior to (172) or comparable with 100 mg sumatriptan (172), whereas this dose of eletriptan was not superior to 25 or 50 mg sumatriptan in one trial, with a rather high placebo response of 40% (172). For 5 mg zolmitriptan (51), 5 mg (85,119) and 10 mg rizatriptan (85,223), 20 mg eletriptan (172), and 12.5 and 25 mg almotriptan (19), the results at 2 hours were similar to the comparative sumatriptan dose (see Table 6). Naratriptan in oral doses of 7.5 mg and 10 mg was quite comparable with 100 mg sumatriptan (40), but the 2.5-mg oral dose of naratriptan [which was chosen for clinical use based on incidence of adverse events, being comparable with placebo (88)] was inferior to 100 mg sumatriptan in three trials for the chosen primary efficacy parameter *headache relief* after 4 hours (5,40,80). Subcutaneous naratriptan in doses of 2.5 to 10 mg was comparable with 6 mg subcutaneous sumatriptan (38).

The recurrence rates for 100 mg sumatriptan varied considerably among trials (see Table 6). In one trial (172) with generally extremely low recurrence rates for all drugs (see Table 6), the recurrence rate was as low as 6%. In recurrence-prone patients, the recurrence rate was expectedly high, 57% (80). In the other eight trials the recurrence rates for 100 mg sumatriptan were between 27% and 44%. This variability in recurrence rates demonstrates that recurrence rates for two drugs can only be compared in comparative trials. As shown in Table 6, there are, apart from naratriptan, no consistent differences in recurrence rates between the new triptans and sumatriptan. Naratriptan 2.5 mg resulted in fewer recurrences than 100 mg sumatriptan in two trials (5,40), and this was also the case in recurrence-prone migraine patients in one trial (80) (see Table 6). Thus, even if there are statistical concerns about comparing recurrence rates in two groups of patients responding to two different drugs (62), these results strongly indicate that the longer half-life for naratriptan than for sumatriptan results in fewer recurrences. That this is not always the case is illustrated by the high recurrence rates after some of the subcutaneous naratriptan doses (38) (see Table 6).

Based on the quicker absorption of rizatriptan versus sumatriptan, two trials (85,223) compared the speed of onset of headache relief between oral rizatriptan and oral sumatriptan, with time to headache relief analysis up to 2 hours. This analysis suggests that approximately 15% more patients are likely to achieve headache relief within 2 hours after 5 and 10 mg rizatriptan than after 25 and 50 mg sumatriptan, respectively (85). In the other trial (223), the sumatriptan-treated group was marginally but significantly older than the rizatriptan group, and older age was correlated with better response. After correction for age imbalance, the results suggest that 21% more patients are likely to achieve headache relief within 2 hours after 10 mg rizatriptan than 100 mg sumatriptan (223). As shown in Table 6, more patients treated with 10 mg rizatriptan (40%) than patients treated with 100 mg sumatriptan (33%) were pain free after 2 hours. A post hoc analysis of the results suggests that 29% more patients are likely to be pain free within 2 hours after 10 mg rizatriptan than after 100 mg sumatriptan.

Comparative Trials with Drugs Other than Triptans

Sumatriptan, the first triptan, is the only triptan that has been compared with several standard treatments for migraine attacks. Eletriptan has been compared with Cafergot in one clinical trial (181). A brief summary of these nine randomized, double-blind, clinical trials is shown in Table 7. Oral sumatriptan 100 mg was superior to Cafergot (2 mg ergotamine tartrate plus 200 mg caffeine), with a quicker onset of action, but with more recurrences (41% versus 30%) within 48 hours (150). Sumatriptan 100 mg was not significantly superior to a combination of 900 mg aspirin and 10 mg metoclopramide for the first treated attack, the primary efficacy parameter, but was superior for the second and third treated attacks, and for other parameters (154). A combination of a highly soluble aspirin salt, lysine acetylsalicylate 1,620 mg (equivalent to 900 mg aspirin), and 10 mg metoclopramide was equivalent to 100 mg sumatriptan (220). Apparently, a rapid soluble form of tolfenamic acid, given in a dose of 200 mg plus 200 mg, was comparable with 100 mg sumatriptan (149), but as demonstrated by the wide 95% CI (Table 7), this finding needs confirmation in a larger trial. Subcutaneous sumatriptan 6 mg was considerably superior to dihydroergotamine (DHE) nasal spray (1 mg plus 1 mg), and at 15 minutes sumatriptan was superior to DHE (225). Recurrence of headache occurred less often after DHE (17%) than after sumatriptan (31%). Compared with subcutaneous DHE (1 mg plus optional 1 mg), subcutaneous sumatriptan was superior for the first 2 hours, but after 3 and 4 hours the effects of both treatments were similar (240). After DHE there were significantly fewer recurrences than after sumatriptan, 18% and 45%, respectively. Intranasal sumatriptan 20 mg was numerically superior to intranasal DHE (1 mg + optional 1 mg) at all time points, with a statistically significant difference from 60 minutes and beyond (131), but there were fewer recurrences after DHE (13%) than after sumatriptan (23%). Rectal sumatriptan 25 mg was inferior to Cafergot suppositories (2 mg ergotamine tartrate plus 100 mg caffeine) taken by two thirds of the patients twice within 30 minutes, and there were fewer recurrences after Cafergot (11%) than after sumatriptan (22%) (139). Due to adverse events, 44% preferred sumatriptan and 37% preferred Cafergot in this crossover study ($p = $ NS). Both 40- and 80-mg doses of eletriptan were superior to Cafergot (2 mg ergotamine tartrate plus 200 mg caffeine) and placebo (181). Patients who took Cafergot tended to have fewer recurrences than those who took eletriptan.

Sumatriptan 100 mg caused more adverse events than aspirin plus metoclopramide (154) and lysine acetylsalicylate plus metoclopramide (220), and subcutaneous sumatriptan 6 mg caused more adverse events than intranasal DHE (1 mg + optional 1 mg) (225). Rectal sumatriptan 25 mg caused less nausea and vomiting than Cafergot suppositories (2 mg ergotamine tartrate plus 100 mg caffeine) (139) (Table 7). In most cases the adverse events were mild to moderate, but one case of atrial fibrillation after 100 mg sumatriptan required hospitalization (220).

An interesting observation (Table 7) is that in all five trials (131,139,150,225,240) comparing sumatriptan with either ergotamine or DHE, the recurrence rate was lower after the ergot alkaloid than after sumatriptan. A similar tendency was observed for ergotamine versus eletriptan (181). This is most likely due to the long duration of the vascular effects of a single dose of an ergot alkaloid, see Chapter 51.

TABLE 7. *Randomized, clinical trials comparing sumatriptan and eletriptan with standard treatments for migraine attacks*

Trial	No. of patients	Drugs and dose (mg)	Success rate (%) At 2 hours	At 4 hours	Adverse events (%)	Recurrence (%)
Oral sumatriptan						
(150)	220	SU100	66[a]		45	41[a]
	246	E2 + C200	48		39	30
Success rates						
SU 100 vs. E2 + C200	+18% (+9% to +27%)					
(154)	133	SU100	56		42[a]	42
	138	A900 + M10	45		29	33
Success rates						
SU100 vs. A900 + M10	+11% (−1% to +23%)					
(220)	119	SU100	53[b]		28[a]	38
	133	LA1620 + M10	57[b]		18	36
	124	PL	24		13	30
Success rates						
SU100 vs. LA 1620 + M10	−4% (−17% to +8%)					
(149)	43	RTA200 + RTA200	77[b]		30	23
	42	SU100	79[b]		41	22
	41	PL	29		19	25
Success rates						
SU100 vs. RTA200 + RTA200	+2% (−17% to +20%)					
Subcutaneous sumatriptan						
(225)	266	SU6	80[a]		43[a]	31[a]
	266	DHEn1 + 1DHEn	50		22	17
Success rates						
SU6 vs. DHEn1 + 1DHEn	+30% (+19% to +41%)					
(240)	150	SU6	85[a]	83	?	45[a]
	145	DHEs1 + DHEs1	73	86	?	18
Success rates (2 h)						
SU6 (134/158) vs. DHEs1 + DHEs1 (111/152)	+12% (+3% to +21%)					
Success rates (4 h)						
SU6 (131/158) vs. DHEs1 + DHEs1 (131/152)	−3% (−11% to +5%)					
Intranasal sumatriptan						
(131)	327	SU20	63[a]			23[c]
	327	DHEn1 + DHEn1	51			13
Success rates						
SU20 vs. DHEn1 + 1DHEn	+12% (+4% to +20%)					
Rectal sumatriptan						
(139)	241	SU25	58		2[d]	22%[c]
	241	E2.5 + C100 +E2.5 + C100	69[c]		14[a,d]	11%
Success rates						
SU25 vs. E2.5 + C100 + E2.5 + C100	−12% (−20% to −3%)					
Oral eletriptan						
(181)	206	EL40	54[a,b]			21
	209	EL80	68[a,b]			22
	197	E2 + C200	33[e]			8
	102	PL	21			44
Success rates						
EL40 vs. E2 + C200	+21% (+11% to +30%)					
EL80 vs. E2 + C200	+35% (+26% to +44%)					

Percentages in parentheses are 95% CIs. Recurrence rate definition differs (see individual trials).
[a]Statistically significant difference at $p < 0.01$.
[b]Statistical significant difference from placebo at $p < 0.01$.
[c]Statistically significant difference at $p < 0.05$.
[d]Only nausea and/or vomiting are given as adverse events.
[e]Statistical significant difference from placebo at $p < 0.05$.
 A, aspirin; C, caffeine; DHEn, intranasal dihydroergotamine; DHEs, subcutaneous dihydroergotamine; E, ergotamine; EL, eletriptan; LA, lysine acetylsalicylate; M, metoclopramide; PL, placebo; RTA, rapid release tolfenamic acid; SU, sumatriptan.

Consistency of Response in Multiple Attacks

In patients treating three attacks with 100 to 300 mg sumatriptan, 47% responded to all three treatments compared with 8% responding to placebo in all three attacks (155). However, this trial was not designed to investigate consistency of response.

Consistency to subcutaneous sumatriptan 6 mg was investigated in 120 patients treating three attacks with sumatriptan and one attack with placebo in a double-blind, randomized, crossover trial (21). Relief rates were 78%, 85%, 84%, and 84% 60 minutes postdose for the first through the fourth attacks, respectively, indicating that the efficacy of sumatriptan did not diminish with repeated use. Seventy-three percent of patients responded to all sumatriptan-treated attacks. In another double-blind crossover trial, consistency of the response to 100 mg sumatriptan was evaluated by letting 154 migraine patients treat up to nine attacks with sumatriptan and up to three attacks with placebo (182). Patients were randomized to receive sumatriptan or placebo in a 3:1 ratio for three four-attack blocks. The response to sumatriptan (49%–50%, mean of three attacks) and placebo (16%–20%) was similar for each of the three four-attack blocks. In a subset of patients who treated nine moderate or severe attacks, 62% experienced headache relief in seven of nine attacks.

The consistency of the effect of 10 mg rizatriptan was investigated in one placebo-controlled trial (115) in which 407 patients treated up to four attacks in a special crossover design. Percentage of patients responding at 2 hours to 10 mg rizatriptan were consistent (75%–80%) over the four attacks, whereas the response to placebo varied somewhat (28%–54%). Of the 315 patients who treated at least three migraine attacks with rizatriptan, 272 (86%) had relief in at least two of the attacks.

Apart from these three trials, consistency of response to a triptan has been claimed but not proven in long-term studies.

Long-Term Studies with Triptans

Long-term studies with a duration of 6 to 12 months have evaluated the tolerability and efficacy of sumatriptan (87,213), zolmitriptan (104), naratriptan (9), and rizatriptan (8). In these long-term studies a considerable number of patients were recruited and a large number of migraine attacks were treated. Thus, 288 patients treated 8,094 attacks with 100 mg sumatriptan; 275 patients treated 8,931 attacks up to three times with 100 mg sumatriptan within 24 hours (213); 366 patients treated 9,448 attacks with up to two doses of 6 mg sumatriptan within 24 hours (87,213); 2,058 patients treated 31,579 attacks with up to two doses of 5 mg zolmitriptan (104); 414 patients treated 7,709 attacks with up to two doses of 2.5 mg naratriptan (9); and 1,767 patients treated 46,773 attacks with either 10 mg rizatriptan, 5 mg rizatriptan (both up to three doses within 24 hours), or standard care

in a study where patients were randomized to these treatment options (8). In total, 4,439 patients thus treated 104,406 migraine attacks with a triptan in these long-term studies.

It has been argued that these studies are needed because the double-blind trials are of short duration and migraine usaually persists for years. Thus, to be of clinical benefit, an acute treatment for migraine must therefore be effective and well tolerated, have an acceptable safety profile, and have no abuse potential in the long term (213). It is dubious whether these studies help in addressing these problems (219). In all but one (9), these studies included patients who previously had participated in randomized, double-blind, clinical trials with the drugs. This selection of patients most likely introduced a bias, probably resulting in increased efficacy because patients not responding in the double-blind trial to active drug are less likely to participate in these extension studies. In fact, in the larger extension studies (8,104,213) with 100 mg sumatriptan, 5 mg zolmitriptan, and 10 mg rizatriptan, the mean response rates for treating moderate and severe attacks were 80% to 85% and thus considerably higher than in the randomized controlled trials. In our view, one should thus regard these reported mean efficacy rates as what one can expect in a selected population of responders. Consistency of response over time has been claimed in all these studies, but the clinical relevance of these results is difficult to judge because of the selection bias.

For tolerability, there is probably also a selection bias because patients with previous adverse events in the controlled trials are less likely to participate, and no new adverse events problems turned up in these studies (8,9,87,104,213). These studies excluded the same patients as in the controlled trials. In contrast to clinical practice, only healthy patients without any risk factors were included, and these studies probably do not help much in evaluating the safety problems of these triptans. Also, abuse-prone patients were excluded. Thus, even with more than 4,000 patients treating more than 100,000 migraine attacks for 6 to 12 months, these studies failed to identify the abuse potential of these triptans.

The general major pitfall in these studies was that they were not population-based long-term studies and thus quite different from clinical practice (219).

Tolerability and Safety of Triptans Based on Randomized Controlled Trials

In randomized controlled trials, and in clinical practice, the triptans cause typical adverse events, so-called triptan symptoms (133). These triptan symptoms are reported somewhat differently for the different triptans but include, among others, tingling, numbness, warm/hot sensation, heaviness, and pressure or tightness in different parts of the body, including the chest and neck. In

TABLE 8. *Percentage incidence of the most common adverse events[a] in controlled trials of 4 to 8 mg subcutaneous sumatriptan[b]*

	Sumatriptan (n = 1,924)	Placebo (n = 868)
Injection site reaction[c]	40	17
Nausea/vomiting	10	10
Tingling	9	3
Warm/hot sensation	9	3
Dizziness/vertigo	8	4
Heaviness	8	1
Pressure sensation	6	1
Flushing	6	2
Burning sensation	5	<1
Chest symptoms (mainly tightness and pressure)	5	1
Neck pain/stiffness	3	<1
Tightness	3	<1
Weakness	2	<1
Headache	2	<1

[a]Adverse events were defined as any untoward medical event occurring during treatment and were not necessarily related to drug treatment.
[b]Adapted from Brown et al. (14)
[c]Mainly mild pain and redness lasting less than 60 min.

addition, symptoms more likely to be of central nervous system (CNS) origin, such as dizziness and sedation, occur. In most cases these adverse events have been reported to be short lived and mild to moderate (14,57,205), but in long-term studies, adverse events led to withdrawal in 6% to less than 10% of patients treated

with 6 and 100 mg sumatriptan (87,213) and 8% of patients treated with 5 mg zolmitriptan (104).

The incidence of adverse events for the different triptans or forms of administration is given above. The incidence varies from 33% more adverse after subcutaneous sumatriptan 6 mg, the highest incidences, to no more adverse events after 2.5 mg naratriptan than after placebo. However, even doses of a drug with apparently no more associated adverse events than placebo in randomized controlled trials (e.g., 25 and 50 mg sumatriptan and 2.5 mg. naratriptan) probably have the potential to induce the typical triptan symptoms in some patients due to individual disposition.

The typical adverse events after a triptan is illustrated with subcutaneous sumatriptan (4–8 mg) in Table 8. The most common adverse events were injection site reactions, generally not a triptan adverse event. Tingling, flushing, burning, and warm/hot sensations occurred more frequently with subcutaneous sumatriptan than with placebo, as did symptoms variously described as heaviness, pressure, or tightness in different parts of the body, including the chest and neck. These adverse events were generally mild and short term and disappeared within 30 minutes in almost all patients.

Zolmitriptan has been evaluated in a wide dose range, from 1 to 25 mg, and as shown in Table 9, the incidence of adverse events increased with increasing doses of zolmitriptan. Based on this dose–response curve for adverse events and the efficacy response, which did not increase in doses of 2.5 and 5 mg zolmitriptan, the 2.5 mg dose was chosen as the optimum dose (61,197). It is

TABLE 9. *Incidence, most common adverse events, and chest-related adverse events in placebo-controlled trials after oral administration of zolmitriptan that has been investigated in a wide dose range*

	Placebo (n = 401)	1 mg zolmitriptan (n = 163)	2.5 mg zolmitriptan (n = 498)	5 mg zolmitriptan (n = 1012)	10 mg zolmitriptan (n = 514)	20 mg zolmitriptan (n = 210)
Patients with at least one adverse event						
	117 (29%)	68 (42%)	227 (46%)	587 (58%)	359 (70%)	158 (75%)
Most common adverse events						
Asthenia	13 (3%)	8 (5%)	16 (3%)	89 (9%)	64 (12%)	45 (21%)
Heaviness other than chest or neck	2 (<1%)	2 (1%)	10 (2%)	51 (5%)	30 (6%)	33 (16%)
Dry mouth	7 (2%)	8 (5%)	16 (3%)	32 (3%)	25 (5%)	12 (6%)
Nausea	15 (4%)	6 (4%)	45 (9%)	63 (6%)	41 (8%)	20 (10%)
Dizziness	16 (4%)	9 (6%)	42 (8%)	96 (9%)	67 (13%)	34 (16%)
Somnolence	12 (3%)	8 (5%)	30 (6%)	78 (8%)	55 (11%)	28 (13%)
Paresthesia	6 (1%)	8 (5%)	29 (6%)	77 (8%)	56 (11%)	28 (18%)
Warm sensation	7 (2%)	5 (3%)	21 (4%)	52 (5%)	36 (7%)	12 (6%)
Chest-related adverse events						
Chest tightness	2 (<1%)		13 (3%)	15 (1%)	21 (4%)	(0%)[a]
Chest pain	1 (<1%)		1 (<1%)	8 (1%)	6 (1%)	(3%)[a]
Chest heaviness	0 (0%)		1 (<1%)	4 (<1%)	3 (<1%)	(1%)[a]
Chest pressure	1 (<1%)		1 (<1%)	8 (1%)	8 (2%)	(1%)[a]

[a]Data from Dahlöf et al. (37).
Modified from Edmeads and Millson (57).

worth noting that although the typical triptan symptoms such as asthenia, heaviness other than chest or neck, dizziness, somnolence, and paresthesia show a strong tendency to be dose dependent, and with an incidence for the highest dose of 20 mg zomitriptan comparable with that of subcutaneous sumatriptan (see Table 8), no such clear tendency for dose dependency is apparent for the relatively seldomly occurring chest-related adverse events (see Table 9). In one trial comparing 100 mg sumatriptan and 5 mg zolmitriptan (51), the incidence of CNS-related adverse events was comparable to that given for 5 mg zolmitriptan (Table 9) (57).

The occurrence in the early clinical evaluation of intravenous sumatriptan of a single case of possible myocardial ischemia (14) combined with the frequently reported tightness or pressure in the chest led to electrocardiographic (ECG) monitoring in more than 1,000 patients. In 120 patients who complained of these chest symptoms, a 12-lead ECG was obtained during the event, without any significant changes being observed except in the above case (205).

Safety Problems with Triptans not Reported in Controlled Clinical Trials

In general clinical use of the triptans, safety problems with triptans are more likely to be revealed than in controlled trials both because patients with possible risk factors are not excluded to the same extent as in trials and because a much larger migraine population is likely to be exposed to the triptans. Because sumatriptan is the triptan used most widely, so far the safety problems mentioned in the following are mainly related to this triptan.

In clinical practice, between 20% (tablets) and 40% (subcutaneous injection) of patients are reported to experience tightness, heaviness, or pressure in the chest, neck, or throat in association with sumatriptan treatment (43). After reports of coronary vasospasm, myocardial infarction, and cardiovascular arrest after sumatriptan (34,43, 120,147,153,157,159) the main concern has been the cardiovascular safety of the triptans. In one report from the Netherlands Centre for Monitoring of Adverse Reactions to Drugs, there were 29 reports of chest pain and 4 reports of myocardial infarction attributed to the use of sumatriptan (160). In a recent review, however, it was remarked that fatal cardiovascular events are remarkably rare (43). Thus, between 1991, the year sumatriptan was introduced, and December 1996, 39 deaths due to cardiovascular causes were spontaneously reported worldwide within 24 hours of administration of sumatriptan tablets or injections for more than 100 million treated migraine attacks (43).

All triptans have some, albeit weak, constrictor effect on human coronary arteries *in vitro*. Based on these results, the triptans are expected to cause little coronary constriction in migraine patients without any coronary artery affliction, but in patients with coronary artery disease they may possibly cause myocardial ischemia (124). *In vivo* it was shown that 6 mg subcutaneous sumatriptan caused a 14% reduction in coronary artery diameter in patients undergoing coronary angiography without any clinical symptoms (126,127). In contrast, 1.5 mg subcutaneous naratriptan failed to induce coronary constriction in 10 patients with known or suspected coronary artery disease in a placebo-controlled study (212).

Although the triptans have the potential for coronary constriction, the vast majority of the frequent chest-related symptoms that occasionally mimic angina pectoris are, however, most likely not due to coronary constriction (43). Thus, as mentioned above, ECGs recorded in 119 patients complaining of chest symptoms after sumatriptan did not show any significant changes; and in 23 migraine patients with these symptoms after an oral dose of 150 mg avitriptan, ECG Holter monitoring and echocardiographic monitoring did not show signs of myocardial ischemia (42). Alternatively, it has been suggested (43) that these chest symptoms after triptans could be due to esophageal spasm (98), intercostal muscle spasm, skeletal muscle mitochondrial impairment, or facilitation of nociceptive neurotransmission.

Other rare adverse events reported after sumatriptan administration include cerebrovasular disorders (140) and ischemic colitis (114), in both cases most likely due to vasospasm, and the serotonin syndrome (136).

Sumatriptan 8 mg subcutaneously (222), rizatriptan 10 mg orally (200), and zolmitriptan 20 mg orally (53) have all been shown to cause a minor short-lived constriction of peripheral leg arteries. Claudication, however, seems not to be an adverse event of the triptans.

THERAPEUTIC USE OF TRIPTANS

The triptans in clinical use for the moment are sumatriptan, zolmitriptan, naratriptan, and rizatriptan. Soon eletriptan, almotriptan, and frovatriptan will probably be introduced, but their recommended doses are yet unknown. Thus, only the first four triptans mentioned previously will be considered for therapeutic use. An overview of therapeutic use of triptans is given in Table 10.

In recent years the tolerability (side effects) and, more important, cardiovascular safety of triptans have received much attention (43,158). In our view the cardiovascular safety problem should not be overemphasized and should be viewed in perspective with the alternative specific antimigraine drugs such as ergotamine with its well known cardiovascular risks (see Chapter 51) (221). For the time being, caution is advised in treating migraine patients with known risk factor for cardiovascular diseases—a small minority of migraine patients—and patients with ischemic heart disease should of course not be treated with triptans. This and the other contraindications to triptans are listed in Table 10.

TABLE 10. *Therapeutic use of marketed triptans (as of April 1, 1999) in currently recommended doses*

Contraindications to triptans	Ischemic heart disease, variant angina, cerebral and peripheral vascular disease, and uncontrolled hypertension; pregnancy; use of ergot alkaloids within 24 h; current use or use of MAO inhibitors within the last 2 weeks; hypersensitivity to the triptan; hemiplegic and basilar migraine.
Cautious use	Patients on SSRIs can be treated with triptans but should be warned about the symptoms of the serotonin syndrome.
Recommended doses of triptans	*Daily dosage* *Maximum* 6 mg subcutaneous sumatriptan — 12 mg 50–100 mg oral sumatriptan — 300 mg (25 mg tablets available in the United States) 20 mg intranasal sumatriptan — 40 mg 25 mg sumatriptan as suppositories — 50 mg 5 mg oral zolmitriptan — 10 mg 2.5 mg oral naratriptan — 5 mg 10 mg oral rizatriptan[a] — 20 mg 10 mg oral rizatriptan wafer[a] — 20 mg
Clinical efficacy in the treatment of migraine attacks	Subcutaneous sumatriptan (6 mg) > oral sumatriptan (50–100 mg) = intranasal sumatriptan (20 mg) = rectal sumatriptan (25 mg) = oral zolmitriptan (2.5–5 mg) = oral rizatriptan (10 mg) > oral sumatriptan (25 mg), oral naratriptan (2.5 mg)
Speed of onset of effect compared with placebo	Subcutaneous sumatriptan (10 min) > intranasal sumatriptan (15 min) > oral sumatriptan = oral rizatriptan (30 min) > rectal sumatriptan (30–60 min) > oral zolmitriptan and oral naratriptan (60 min). It should be noted, however, that these "early responses," apart from subcutaneous sumatriptan, are often of relatively small magnitude (see Fig. 6).
Speed of onset of effect compared directly among two triptans or two administration forms of a triptan	Oral rizatriptan > oral sumatriptan. Intranasal sumatriptan (>) oral sumatriptan.
Adverse events with triptans	So-called "triptan" symptoms: tingling, numbness, warm/hot sensation, pressure or tightness in different part of the body, including chest and neck; rarely regular chest pain; dizziness and sedation.
Choice of form of administration	Tablets generally most convenient. If severe nausea/vomiting is present the patient could alternatively use an injection, nasal spray, or a suppository.
Additional dose if the first dose of a triptan is not effective	There is no evidence that a second dose of a triptan increases the efficacy. Instead, if the chosen dose of a triptan is ineffective, the patient should try another dose or different forms of administration or another triptan.
Recurrence or secondary treatment failure	Most triptans have the same recurrence rate of 20%–40%. In some trials, naratriptan has had a lower recurrence rate than sumatriptan and could be tried in recurrence-prone patients.
Use of a second dose for the treatment of a recurrence when the first dose of a triptan is primarily effective	A second dose of a triptan will probably be effective, but with multiple recurrence for days alternative drugs should probably be tried.
Abuse or inappropriate use of triptans	Triptans should not be used on a daily basis (except in the treatment of chronic cluster headache). Set an upper limit of 10 doses per month. Use triptans with extreme caution in previous drug abusers.
Breastfeeding	Sumatriptan can be used if milk is expressed and discarded for 8 h after the dose. Not recommended with the other triptans.
Possible drug interactions	Except for the interaction between rizatriptan and propranolol, there are no drug interactions of triptans and currently used prophylactic drugs for migraine and some SSRIs.

[a]5 mg rizatriptan in patients on propranolol.
SSRIs, selective serotonin reuptake inhibitors.

Due to the comorbidity of migraine and depression and some anxiety disorders, migraine patients may also require treatment for these psychiatric disorders, most often with selective serotonin reuptake inhibitors [SSRIs]. The combination of sumatriptan and an SSRI has been reported to cause the serotonin syndrome in a few patients (136), but in a recent review, compelling clinical evidence supporting the strict avoidance of suma-triptan in patients receiving other serotonergic agents was not found (69). In 82 migraine patients using SSRIs and treated with 10 and 20 mg intranasal sumatriptan in controlled clinical trials, there were no more adverse events than in patients not using SSRIs (3). Thus, triptans can be used with caution in patients on SSRIs. However, the use of a triptan is still contraindicated in patients treated with monoamine oxidase (MAO) inhibitors (Table 10).

The recommended doses of sumatriptan, zolmitriptan, naratriptan, and rizatriptan are shown in Table 10. There is no doubt that subcutaneous sumatriptan (6 mg) has the highest therapeutic gain (50%) among the currently available forms of triptans (Fig. 5). Oral (50–100 mg), intranasal (20 mg), and rectal (25 mg) sumatriptan have the same therapeutic gain (30%–35%) as oral zolmitriptan (2.5 mg) and rizatriptan (10 mg), as shown in Figure 5. In contrast, the recommended 2.5-mg dose of naratriptan has a lower therapeutic gain of approximately 20% (Fig. 5).

Speed of onset is highly valued by patients (81), and compared with placebo, subcutaneous sumatriptan has an onset of action after 10 minutes (Fig. 6). Intranasal sumatriptan has an onset of action after 15 minutes, whereas 50 to 100 mg sumatriptan (Fig. 6) (193,218) and 10 mg rizatriptan (39) are superior to placebo after 30 minutes. Rectal sumatriptan 25 mg is superior to placebo after 30 to 60 minutes. Zolmitriptan 2.5 mg and naratriptan 2.5 mg are superior to placebo after 60 minutes. It should be noted that, apart from subcutaneous sumatriptan, the very early therapeutic gains for the triptans are relatively small in magnitude, as illustrated for intranasal and oral sumatriptan in Figure 6. Direct comparison of speed of onset between two triptans or a triptan delivered by two different routes has only been done in a few cases. Thus, after oral administration, rizatriptan patients are 15% to 20% more likely to experience a response within 2 hours than after oral sumatriptan (85,223). Intranasal sumatriptan 20 mg was superior (15% higher success rate) to oral sumatriptan 100 mg after 30 minutes for the first treated attack, but this superiority was not sustained over subsequently treated attacks (131).

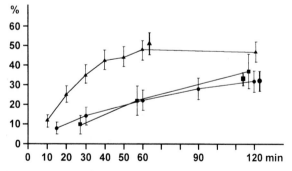

FIG. 6. Therapeutic gain (proportion of patients responding to sumatriptan minus proportion of patients responding to placebo) and 95% CIs for 6 mg subcutaneous sumatriptan (—▲—), 20 mg intranasal sumatriptan (—●—) and 100 mg oral sumatriptan (—■—) up to 2 hours after administration. The combined therapeutic gains for each form of administration are also shown [reproduced from Tfelt-Hansen (218)]. Apart from an early onset of action and greater overall efficacy, subcutaneous sumatriptan has a clinically relevant effect after 20 minutes, whereas this is first the case for intranasal and oral sumatriptan after 1 hour.

The typical so-called triptan symptoms (133) are listed in Table 10. Chest symptoms (mainly tightness and pressure) have been reported to occur in up to 40% of patients treated with sumatriptan at some time (41). Such symptoms can be a frightening experience for the patients, and they should be warned in advance of the risk of these symptoms and should be informed about their generally benign nature. However, if the chest symptoms are severe and persistent, patients should immediately seek medical advice. Sedation (41) also can be a problem, and we warn patients about driving and about performing complicated tasks in the first hour after administration.

Most patients prefer the oral route of administration. However, if severe nausea or vomiting is present, this route of administration may be suboptimal due to slow absorption, which has been described for several drugs (see Chapter 54), including sumatriptan (173) and zolmitriptan (224), and the drug may actually be vomited. Subcutaneous sumatriptan is probably the best alternative in this situation, but it is more expensive and some patients dislike injecting themselves. For these patients intranasal or rectal administration forms, so far only available with sumatriptan, may be good alternatives. We often recommend that the patient have different forms available so that they can choose the most convenient for the actual attack.

If a dose of a triptan is not effective, does a second dose then increase efficacy? This question has been studied for subcutaneous (repeated dose after 1 hour) and oral sumatriptan (repeated dose after 2 hours), and in both cases the repeated dose was not superior to a repeated dose of placebo. If a patient does not experience an effect after a dose of a triptan in, for example, three attacks, either the dose should be increased if possible in future attacks or another form of administration or another triptan should be tried.

Recurrence of headache after a primary successful response within 2 hours occurs in clinical practice in 40% of patients in nearly all attacks treated with sumatriptan (232) and is a major problem with all drugs, including triptans, used for the treatment of migraine attacks. The risk of recurrence is related to long-lasting migraine attacks (233). Naratriptan has in several trials, but not in all, resulted in fewer recurrences than sumatriptan; naratriptan is worth trying in patients with such recurrence problems. The efficacy of a second dose for the treatment of a recurrence has been proven versus placebo for sumatriptan and rizatriptan, and most likely the other triptans are also effective in the treatment of headache recurrences. In clinical practice we have observed patients treating repeated recurrences over several days with a triptan. If multiple recurrences occur, then probably other drugs should be used for the treatment of these recurrences.

Daily intake of sumatriptan, which, apart from patients with chronic cluster headache, must be considered an abuse or inappropriate use of the drug, has been reported

(25,110) (see Chapter 115) and is most often observed in patients who previously had abused such drugs as ergotamine or analgesics. A study using prescription data suggests that sumatriptan abuse is a real problem, with 1% of sumatriptan users taking 60 doses of sumatriptan or more within 30 days (67). This clearly inappropriate use of sumatriptan is often observed in patients treating drug-induced headaches (68). In order to avoid this problem, migraine patients should not be allowed daily use of triptans, and an upper limit of 10 doses of a triptan per month should be instituted. In previous drug abusers it has been recommended to limit the use of triptans to one dose per week (25). In addition, triptans should not be used for the treatment of the rebound/withdrawal headache after ergot abuse (Chapter 115). In one placebo-controlled study it was shown that subcutaneous sumatriptan was temporally very effective in the treatment of the withdrawal headache after ergotamine abuse, but the headache reoccurred within 12 hours (50). To switch patients who have been abusing ergotamine directly to a triptan probably risks making the patient a triptan abuser with intake of a triptan several times a day.

It has been shown that sumatriptan is excreted in small amounts in the milk of breastfeeding women (241), but if the milk is expressed and discarded for 8 hours after the administration of sumatriptan, there should be no risk for the baby. No such data are available for the other triptans, and for the moment they may not be used during breastfeeding.

The possible drug interaction of triptans has mainly been investigated in pharmacokinetic studies concerning drugs used for migraine prophylaxis or drugs likely to be coadministered with a triptan in the treatment of migraine attacks. The pharmacokinetics of sumatriptan was not influenced by concomitant administration of propranolol, pizotifen, flunarizine, dihydroergotamine mesylate, paroxetine, buthorphanol, or naratriptan (168). For zolmitriptan there were no clinically significant changes in pharmacokinetics after dihydroergotamine, propranolol, pizotifen, fluoxetine, metoclopramide, or paracetamol (acetaminophen) (184). The mean plasma level of rizatriptan was increased by 70% after administration of a high dose of propranolol (39), but this interaction appears to be unique to propranolol because nadolol and metoprolol had no such effect on plasma levels of rizatriptan (39). As a safety precaution, 5 mg rizatriptan is recommended for patients taking propranolol (Table 10). Paroxetine did not affect the plasma levels of rizatriptan (39). Rizatriptan did not affect plasma concentrations of ethinyl estradiol and norethindrone (oral contraceptive pills) (39). In contrast, administration of the MAO-A selective inhibitor moclobemide increased the plasma levels of sumatriptan, zolmitriptan, and rizatriptan (39,168,184).

Finally, with several triptans on the market one has the opportunity to try several in the treatment of the migraine patient. So far there are no controlled trials investigating whether nonresponders to one triptan can benefit from another triptan, but it is our clinical experience that if one triptan is not effective one can often have success with another triptan or another mode of administration. Finally, in clinical practice we recommend a trial with subcutaneous sumatriptan before deciding that the patients do not benefit from triptans.

REFERENCES

1. Ahrens SP, Visser WH, Jiang K, Reines SA and the Rizatriptan RPD^{TMr} Study Group. Rizatriptan RPD^{TM} for the acute treatment of acute migraine. *Eur J Neurol* 1998;5(Suppl 3):52.
2. Akpunonu BE, Mutgi AB, Federman DJ, et al. Subcutaneous sumatriptan for treatment of acute migraine in patients admitted to the emergency department: a multicenter study. *Ann Emerg Med* 1995;25: 464–469.
3. Ashford E, Salonen R, Saiers J, Woessner M. Consistency of response to sumatriptan nasal spray across patient subgroups and migraine types. *Cephalalgia* 1998;18:273–277.
4. Bates D, Ashford E, Dawson R, et al. Subcutaneous sumatriptan during migraine aura. *Neurology* 1994;44:1587–1592.
5. Bates D, Winter P. Efficacy and tolerability of naratriptan tablets (0.1–2.5 mg) in the acute treatment of migraine. *Eur J Neurol* 1998; 5(Suppl 3):48–49.
6. Bax WA, Renzenbrink GJ, Van Heuven-Nolsen D, et al. 5-HT receptors mediating contractions of the isolated human coronary artery. *Eur J Pharmacol* 1993;239:203–210.
7. Beer MS, Middlemiss DN, Stanton JA et al. *In vitro* pharmacological profile of the novel 5-HT$_{1D}$ receptor agonist MK-462. *Cephalalgia* 1995;15:203.
8. Block GA, Goldstein J, Polis A, Reines SA, Smith ME, and the Rizatriptan Multicenter Study Group. Efficacy and safety of rizatriptan versus standard care during long-term treatment for migraine. *Headache* 1998;38:764–771.
9. Bomhof MAM, Heywood J, Pradalier A, Enahoro H, Winter P, Hassani H, on behalf of the Naratriptan Long-Term Study Group. The tolerability and efficacy of naratriptan tablets with long-term treatment (6 months). *Cephalalgia* 1998;18:33–37.
10. Bou J, Domenech T, Gras J, et al. Pharmacological profile of almotriptan, a novel antimigraine agent. *Cephalalgia* 1997;17:421.
11. Bouchelet I, Cohen Z, Case B, et al. Differential expression of sumatriptan-sensitive 5-hydroxytryptamine receptors in human trigeminal ganglia and cerebral blood vessels. *Mol Pharmacol* 1996;50:219–223.
12. Bousser MG, d'Allens H, Richard A, and the Early-Morning Migraine Sumatriptan Study Group. Efficacy of subcutaneous sumatriptan in the acute treatment of early-morning migraine: a placebo-controlled study. *J Intern Med* 1993;234:211–216.
13. Brown AM, Parsons AA, Raval P, et al. SB 209509 (VML 251), a potent constrictor of rabbit basilar artery with high affinity and selectivity for human 5-HT$_{1D}$ receptors. *Br J Pharmacol* 1996;119:110P.
14. Brown EG, Endersby CA, Smith RN, Talbot JCC. The safety and tolerability of sumatriptan: an overview. *Eur Neurol* 1991;31:339–344
15. Buchan P, Keywood C, Ward C. The pharmacokinetics of frovatriptan (VML 251/SB 209509), a potent, selective 5-HT$_{1B/1D}$ agonist, following single dose administration by oral and intravenous routes to healthy male and female volunteers. Presented at the Annual meeting of the American Association for the study of Headache, San Fransisco, 1998.
16. Cabarrocas X, on behalf of the Almotriptan Oral Study Group. Efficacy data on oral almotriptan, a novel 5HT$_{1B/1D}$ agonist. *Headache* 1998;38:377.
17. Cabarrocas X, on behalf of the Almotriptan Subcutaneous Study Group. First efficacy data on subcutaneous almotriptan, a novel 5HT$_{1D}$ agonist. *Cephalalgia* 1997;17:420–421.
18. Cabaroccas X, Salva M. Pharmacokinetic and metabolic data on almotriptan, a new antimigraine drug. *Cephalalgia* 1997;17:421.
19. Cabarrocas X, Zayas JM, Suris M, for and on behalf of the Almotriptan Comparative Study Group. Equivalent efficacy of oral almotriptan, a new 5-HT$_{1B/1D}$ agonist, compared with sumatriptan 100 mg. *Headache* 1998;38:377–378.

20. Cady RC, Ryan R, Jhingran P, O'Quinn S, Pait G. Sumatriptan injection reduces productivity loss during a migraine attack. Results of a double-blind, placebo-controlled trial. *Arch Intern Med* 1998;158: 1013–1018.

21. Cady RK, Dexter J, Sargent JD, Markley H, Osterhaus JT, Webster CJ. Efficacy of subcutaneous sumatriptan in repeated episodes of migraine. *Neurology* 1993;43:1363–1368.

22. Cady RK, Wendt JK, Kirchner JR, Sargent JD, Rothrock JF, Skaggs H. Treatment of acute migraine with subcutaneous sumatriptan. *JAMA* 1991;265:2831–2835.

23. Caekebeke JF, Ferrari MD, Zwetsloot CP, et al. Antimigraine drug sumatriptan increases blood flow velocity in large cerebral arteries during migraine attacks. *Neurology* 1992;42:1522–1526.

24. Castro ME, Romon T, Castillo MJ, et al. Identification and characterization of a new serotonergic recognition site with high affinity for 5-carboxamidotryptamine in mammalian brain. *J Neurochem* 1997;69: 2123–2131.

25. Catarci T, Lenzi GL, Cerbo R, Fieschi C. Sumatriptan and daily headache. *J Neurol Neurosurg Psychiatry* 1995;58:508.

26. Centonze V, Polito MB, Di Bari M, et al. Evaluation of the efficacy of oral sumatriptan in the therapy of acute migraine [in Italian]. *Clin Ter* 1995;146:721–728.

27. Cheng H, Polvino WJ, Sciberras D, et al. Pharmacokinetics and food interaction of MK-462 in healthy males. *Biopharm Drug Dispos* 1996;17:17–24.

28. Connor HE, Feniuk W, Beattie DT, et al. Naratriptan: biological profile in animal models relevant to migraine. *Cephalalgia* 1997;17: 145–152.

29. Connor HE, Feniuk W, Humphrey PP. 5-Hydroxytryptamine contracts human coronary arteries predominantly via 5-HT$_2$ receptor activation. *Eur J Pharmacol* 1989;161:91–94.

30. Couch JR Jr, Saper J, Meloche JP. Treatment of migraine with BMS180048: response at 2 hours. North American BMS180048 Study Group. *Headache* 1996;36:523–530.

31. Cull RE, Price WH, Dunbar A. The efficacy of subcutaneous sumatriptan in the treatment of recurrence of migraine headache. *J Neurol Neurosurg Psychiatry* 1997;62:490–495.

32. Cumberbatch MJ, Hill RG, Hargreaves RJ. Rizatriptan has central antinociceptive effects against durally evoked responses. *Eur J Pharmacol* 1997;328:37–40.

33. Cumberbatch MJ, Hill RG, Hargreaves RJ. The effects of 5-HT$_{1A}$, 5-HT$_{1B}$ and 5-HT$_{1D}$ receptor agonists on trigeminal nociceptive neurotransmission in anaesthetized rats. *Eur J Pharmacol* 1998;362:43–46.

34. Curtin T, Brooks AP, Roberts JA. Cardiorespiratory distress after sumatriptan given by injection. *Br Med J* 1992;305:713–714.

35. Cutler N, Mushet GR, Davis R, Clements MS, Whitcher L. Oral sumatriptan for the acute treatment of migraine: evaluation of three dosage strengths. *Neurology* 1995;45(Suppl 7):5–9.

36. Dahlöf C. Sumatriptan nasal spray: a review of data from multinational clinical trials. *Funct Neurol* 1996;11:150.

37. Dahlöf C, Diener H-C, Goadsby PJ, et al. Zolmitriptan, a 5-HT receptor agonist for the acute oral treatment of migraine: a multicentre, dose-range finding study. *Eur J Neurol* 1998;5:535–543.

38. Dahlöf C, Hogenhuis L, Olesen J, et al. Early clinical experience with subcutaneous naratriptan in the acute treatment of migraine: a dose-ranging study. *Eur J Neurol* 1998;5:469–477.

39. Dahlöf C, Lines C. Rizatriptan: a new 5-HT$_{1B/1D}$ receptor agonist for the treatment of migraine. *Exp Opin Invest Drugs* 1999;8:671–686.

40. Dahlöf C, Winter P, Whitehouse H, Hassani H. Randomized, double-blind, placebo-controlled comparison of oral naratriptan and oral sumatriptan in the acute treatment of migraine. *Neurology* 1997; 48(Suppl 3):A85–A86.

41. Dahlöf CGH. How does sumatriptan perform in clinical practice? *Cephalalgia* 1995;15(Suppl 15):21–28.

42. Dahlöf CGH, Falk L, Risenfors M, Lewis CP. Safety trial with the 5HT$_{1B/1D}$ agonist avitriptan (BMS-180048) in patients with migraine who has experienced pressure, tightness, and/or pain in the chest, neck, and/or throat following sumatriptan. *Cephalalgia* 1998;18: 546–551.

43. Dahlöf CGH, Mathew N. Cardiovascular safety of 5HT$_{1B/1D}$ agonists—is there a cause for concern? *Cephalalgia* 1998;18:539–545.

44. Dechant KL, Clissod SP. Sumatriptan. A review of its pharmacodynamic and pharmacokinetic properties, and therapeutic efficacy in the acute treatment of migraine and cluster headache. *Drugs* 1992;43: 776–798.

45. De Vries P, Heiligers JPC, Villalón CM, Saxena PR. Blockade of porcine carotid vascular response to sumatriptan by GR127935, a selective 5-HT$_{1D}$ receptor antagonist. *Br J Pharmacol* 1996;118: 85–92.

46. De Vries P, Sánchez-López A, Centurión D, et al. The canine external carotid vasoconstrictor 5-HT$_1$ receptor: blockade by 5-HT$_{1B}$ (SB224289), but not by 5-HT$_{1D}$ (BRL15572) receptor antagonists. *Eur J Pharmacol* 1998;362:69–72.

47. De Vries P, Villalón CM, Heiligers JPC, Saxena PR. Characterisation of 5-HT receptors mediating constriction of porcine carotid arteriovenous anastomoses; involvement of 5-HT$_{1B/1D}$ and novel receptors. *Br J Pharmacol* 1998;123:1561–1570.

48. De Vries P, Willems EW, Heiligers JPC, Villalón CM, Saxena PR. Investigation of the role of 5-HT$_{1B}$ and 5-HT$_{1D}$ receptors in the sumatriptan-induced constriction of porcine carotid arteriovenous anastomoses. *Br J Pharmacol* 1999;127:405–412.

49. Diamond S, Elkind A, Jackson T, Ryan R, DeBussey S, Asgharnejad M. Multiple-attack efficacy and tolerability of sumatriptan nasal spray in the treatment of migraine. *Arch Fam Med* 1998;7:234–240.

50. Diener HC, Haab J, Peters C, Ried S, Dichgans J, Pilgrim A. Subcutaneous sumatriptan in the treatment of headache during withdrawal from drug-induced headache. *Headache* 1991;31:205–209.

51. Diener HC, Klein K, for the Multinational Oral 311C90 and Sumatriptan Comparative Study Group. The first comparison of the efficacy and safety of 311C90 and sumatriptan in the treatment of migraine. *Funct Neurol* 1996;11:152.

52. Dixon R, Gillotin C, Gibbens M, et al. The pharmacokinetics and effects on blood pressure of multiple doses of the novel anti-migraine drug zolmitriptan (311C90) in healthy volunteers. *Br J Clin Pharmacol* 1997;43:273–281.

53. Dixon RM, Meire HB, Evans DH, Watt H, On N, Posner, Rolan P. Peripheral vascular effects and pharmacokinetics of the antimigraine compound, zolmitriptan, in combination with oral ergotamine in healthy volunteers. *Cephalalgia* 1997;17:639–646.

54. Dixon R, On N, Posner J. High oral bioavailability of the novel 5-HT$_{1D}$ agonist 311C90. *Cephalalgia* 1995;15:218.

55. Dreteler GH, Wouters W, Saxena PR. Comparison of the cardiovascular effects of the 5-HT$_{1A}$ receptor agonist flesinoxan with that of 8-OH-DPAT in the rat. *Eur J Pharmacol* 1990;180:339–349.

56. Duquesnoy C, Mamet JP, Sumner D, Fuseau E. Comparative clinical pharmacokinetics of single doses of sumatriptan following subcutaneous, oral, rectal and intranasal administration. *Eur J Pharm Sci* 1998;6:99–104.

57. Edmeads JG, Millson DS. Tolerability profile of zolmitriptan (ZomigTM, 311C90), a novel dual central and peripherally acting 5HT$_{1B/1D}$ agonist. International experience based on >3000 subjects treated with zolmitriptan. *Cephalalgia* 1997;17(Suppl 18):41–52.

58. Eglen RM, Jasper JR, Chang DA, Martin GR. The 5-HT$_7$ receptor: orphan found. *Trends Pharmacol Sci* 1997;18:104–107.

59. Facchinetti F, Bonellie G, Kangasneimi P, Pascual J, Shuaib A, for the Sumatriptan Menstrual Migraine Study Group. The efficacy and safety of sumatriptan in the acute treatment of menstrual migraine. *Obstet Gynecol* 1995;86:911–916.

60. Färkkilä M, Diener H-C, Dahlöf C, Steiner TJ, on behalf of the Eletriptan Steering Committee. A dose-finding study of eletriptan (UK-116,044) (5–30 mg) for the acute treatment of migraine. *Cephalalgia* 1996;16:387.

61. Ferrari MD. 311C90: increasing the options for therapy with effective acute antimigraine 5HT$_{1B/1D}$ receptor agonists. *Neurology* 1997; 48(Suppl 3):21–24.

62. Ferrari M. How to assess and compare drugs in the management of migraine: success rates in term of response and recurrence. *Cephalalgia* 1999;19(Suppl 23):2–8.

63. Ferrari MD, James MH, Bates D, et al. Oral sumatriptan: effect of a second dose, and treatment of headache recurrence. *Cephalalgia* 1994;14:330–338.

64. Ferrari MD, Saxena PR. Clinical and experimental effects of sumatriptan in humans. *Trends Pharmacol Sci* 1993;14:129–133.

65. Fowler PA, Lacey LF, Thomas M, et al. The clinical pharmacology, pharmacokinetics and metabolism of sumatriptan. *Eur Neurol* 1991; 31:291–294.

66. Fuseau E, Baille P, Kempsford RD. A study to determine the absolute oral bioavailability of naratriptan. *Cephalalgia* 1997;17:417.

67. Gaist D, Andersen M, Aarup AL, Hallas J, Gram LF. Use of sumatrip-

tan in Denmark in 1994–5: an epidemiological analysis of nationwide prescription data. *Br J Clin Pharmacol* 1997;43:429–433.

68. Gaist D, Tsiropoulos I, Sindrup SH, et al. Inappropriate use of sumatriptan: population-based register and interview study. *BMJ* 1998;316: 1352–1353.

69. Gardner DM, Lynd LD. Sumatriptan contraindications and the serotonin syndrome. *Ann Pharmacother* 1998;32:33–38.

70. Gijsman H, Kramer MS, Sargent J, et al. Double-blind, placebo-controlled, dose-finding study of rizatriptan (MK-462) in the acute treatment of migraine. *Cephalalgia* 1997;17:547–651.

71. Goadsby PJ. Current concepts of the pathophysiology of migraine. *Neurol Clin* 1997;15:27–42.

72. Goadsby PJ. A triptan too far? *J Neurol Neurosurg Psychiatry* 1998; 64:143–147.

73. Goadsby PJ, Edvinsson L. The trigeminovascular system and migraine: studies characterizing cerebrovascular and neuropeptide changes seen in humans and cats. *Ann Neurol* 1993;33:48–56.

74. Goadsby PJ, Edvinsson L. Peripheral and central trigeminovascular activation in cat is blocked by the serotonin (5HT)-$_{1D}$ receptor agonist 311C90. *Headache* 1994;34:394–399.

75. Goadsby PJ, Hoskin KL. Inhibition of trigeminal neurons by intravenous administration of the serotonin (5HT)$_{1B/D}$ receptor agonist zolmitriptan (311C90): are brain stem sites therapeutic target in migraine? *Pain* 1996;67:355–359.

76. Goadsby PJ, Knight Y. Inhibition of trigeminal neurones after intravenous administration of naratriptan through an action at 5-hydroxytryptamine (5-HT$_{1B/1D}$) receptors. *Br J Pharmacol* 1997;122: 918–922.

77. Goadsby PJ, Zagami AS, Donnan GA, et al. Oral sumatriptan in acute migraine. *Lancet* 1991;338:782–783.

78. Goadsby PJ, Zagami AS, Lambert GA. Neural processing of craniovascular pain: a synthesis of the central structures involved in migraine. *Headache* 1991;31:365–371.

79. Göbel H. A placebo-controlled, dose-defining study of sumatriptan suppositories in the acute treatment of migraine. *Front Headache Res* 1997;6:203–206.

80. Göbel H, Boswell D, Winter P, Crisp A. A comparison of the efficacy, safety and tolerability of naratriptan and sumatriptan. *Cephalalgia* 1997;17:426.

81. Göbel H, Petersen-Braun M, Heinze A. Which properties do patients expect of new and improved drugs in the treatment of primary headache disorders? In: Olesen J, Tfelt-Hansen P, eds. *Headache treatment:* trial methodology and new drugs. New York: Lippincott-Raven, 1997;93–97.

82. Goldberg MR, Lee Y, Ermlich S, et al. Single and multiple-dose pharmacokinetics and tolerability of rizatriptan, a novel 5-HT$_{1B/1D}$ agonist for migraine. Presented at the American Association for the Study of Headache, New York, 1997.

83. Goldstein J, Dahlöf CG, Diener H-C, et al. on behalf of the Subcutaneous Alniditan Study Group. Alniditan in the acute treatment of migraine attacks: a subcutaneous dose-finding study. *Cephalalgia* 1996;16:497–502.

84. Goldstein J, Keywood C. A low dose range finding study of frovatriptan, a potent selective 5-HT$_{1B/1D}$ agonist for the treatment of migraine. *Funct Neurol* 1998;13:178.

85. Goldstein J, Ryan R, Jiang K, et al. and the Rizatriptan Protocol 046 Study Group. Crossover comparison of rizatriptan 5 mg and 10 mg versus sumatriptan 25 mg and 50 mg in migraine. *Headache* 1998; 38:737–747.

86. Gross MLP, Kay J, Turner AM, Hallett K, Cleal AL, Hassani H, on behalf of the United Kingdom Study Group. Sumatriptan in acute migraine using a novel cartridge system self-injector. *Headache* 1994;34:559–563.

87. Gross MLP, Kay J, Turner AM, Jewsbury J, Cleal AL. Long-term efficacy of subcutaneous sumatriptan using a novel self-injector. *Headache* 1995;35:601–606.

88. Gunasekara NS, Wiseman LR. Naratriptan. *CNS Drugs* 1997;8: 402–408.

89. Gupta P, Brown D, Butler P, et al. Pre-clinical *in vivo* pharmacology of eletriptan (UK-116,044): a potent and selective partial agonist at "5-HT$_{1D}$–like" receptors. *Cephalalgia* 1996;16:386.

90. Gupta P, Napier CM, Shepperson NB, Wallis R. Further characterization of the *in vitro* pharmacology of eletriptan. *Cephalalgia* 1997; 17:413.

91. Gupta P, Scatchard J, Shepperson N, et al. *In vitro* pharmacology of

92. Hagan JJ, Slade PD, Gaster L, et al. Stimulation of 5-HT$_{1B}$ receptors causes hypothermia in the guinea pig. *Eur J Pharmacol* 1997; 331:169–174.

93. Henriksson A. Safety and efficacy of sumatriptan suppositories in the acute treatment of migraine attacks. *Cephalalgia* 1995;15(Suppl 14):235.

94. Henry P, d'Allens H, and the French Migraine Network Bordeaux-Lyon-Grenoble. Subcutaneous sumatriptan in the acute treatment of migraine in patients using dihydroergotamine as prophylaxis. *Headache* 1993;33:432–435.

95. Hettiarachichi J. Adverse event profile of oral eletriptan: review of clinical trial experience. *Cephalalgia* 1999;19:355.

96. Hettiarachichi J, on behalf of the Eletriptan Steering Group. Efficacy, safety and tolerability of oral eletriptan versus placebo in the acute treatment of migraine:a phase III randomised trial [Abstract]. *Headache* 1999;89:358–359.

97. Heyck H. Pathogenesis of migraine. *Res Clin Stud Headache* 1969; 2:1–28.

98. Houghton LA, Foster JM, Whorwell PJ, Morris J, Fowler P. Is chest pain after sumatriptan oesophageal in origin? *Lancet* 1994;344: 985–986.

99. Humphrey PP, Feniuk W, Perren MJ, et al. The pharmacology of the novel 5-HT$_1$–like receptor agonist, GR43175. *Cephalalgia* 1989;9: 23–33

100. Humphrey PPA, Apperley E, Feniuk W, Perren MJ. A rational approach to identifying a fundamentally new drug for the treatment of migraine. In: Saxena PR, Wallis DI, Wouters W, Bevan P, eds. *Cardiovascular pharmacology of 5-hydroxytryptamine: prospective therapeutic applications.* Dordrecht: Kluwer Academic, 1990:416–431.

101. Humphrey PPA, Feniuk W. Mode of action of the anti-migraine drug sumatriptan. *Trends Pharmacol Sci* 1991;12:444–446.

102. Humphrey PPA, Goadsby PJ. The mode of action of sumatriptan is vascular? A debate. *Cephalalgia* 1994;14:401–410.

103. Hyland R, Jones BC, McCleverty P, et al. *In vitro* metabolism of eletriptan in human liver microsomes. *Cephalalgia* 1998;18:404.

104. The International 311C90 Long-term Study Group. The long-term tolerability and efficacy of oral zolmitriptan (Zomig, 311C90) in the acute treatment of migraine. An international study. *Headache* 1998; 38:173–183.

105. Jackson NC on behalf of the Eletriptan Steering Committee. Clinical measures of efficacy, safety and tolerability for the acute treatment of migraine: a comparison of eletriptan (20–80 mg), sumatriptan (100 mg) and placebo [Abstract]. *Neurology* 1998;50(Suppl 4):376.

106. Jensen K, Tfelt-Hansen P, Hansen EW, Krris EH, Pedersen OS. Introduction of a novel self-injector for sumatriptan. A controlled clinical trial in general practice. *Cephalalgia* 1995;15:423–429.

107. John GW, Valentin JP, LeGrand B, et al. *In vitro* vascular and neuronal actions of F11356, a novel high efficacy 5-HT$_{1B/D}$ receptor agonist, in models relevant to migraine. *Naunyn Schmiedebergs Arch Pharmacol* 1998;358:R523.

108. John GW, Verscheure Y, Infanti F, et al. *In vivo* pharmacological actions of F11356, a novel high efficacy 5-HT$_{1B/D}$ receptor agonist. *Naunyn Schmiedebergs Arch Pharmacol* 1998;358:R523.

109. Johnson KW, Schaus JM, Durkin MM, et al. 5-HT$_{1F}$ receptor agonists inhibit neurogenic dural inflammation in guinea pigs. *Neuroreport* 1997;8:2237–2240.

110. Kaube H, May A, Diener HC, Pfaffenrath V. Sumatriptan. *BMJ* 1994; 308:1573–1574.

111. Kempsford RD, Baille P, Fuseau E. Oral naratriptan (2.5–10 mg) exhibit dose-proportional pharmacokinetics. *Cephalalgia* 1997;17: 408.

112. Klassen A, Elkind A, Asgharnejad M, Webster C, Laurenza A, on behalf of the Naratriptan S2WA3001 Study Group. Naratriptan is effective and well-tolerated in the acute treatment of migraine. Results of a double-blind, placebo-controlled, parallel-group study. *Headache* 1997;37:640–645.

113. Klassen AC, Gabriel H, Hobbs S, Woessner M, on behalf of the Study Group. Safety and efficacy of sumatriptan suppositories in the acute treatment of migraine attacks. *Cephalalgia* 1995;15(Suppl 14):234.

114. Knudsen JF, Friedman B, Chen M, Goldwasser JE. Ischemic colitis and sumatriptan use. *Arch Intern Med* 1998;158:1946–1948.

115. Kramer MS, Matzura-Wolfe D, Polis A, et al. and the Rizatriptan Multiple Attack Study Group. A placebo-controlled crossover study of

eletriptan (UK-116,044) at the "5-HT$_{1D}$–like" receptor in the dog saphenous vein. *Cephalalgia* 1996;16:386.

rizatriptan in the treatment of multiple attacks. *Neurology* 1998; 51:773–781.

116. Kunka RL, Hussey EK, Shaw S, et al. Safety, tolerability, and pharmacokinetics of sumatriptan suppositories following single and multiple doses in healthy volunteers. *Cephalalgia* 1997;17:532–540.

117. Lacey LF, Hussey EK, Fowler PA. Single dose pharmacokinetics of sumatriptan in healthy volunteers. *Eur J Clin Pharmacol* 1995;47:543–548.

118. Leysen JE, Gommeren W, Heylen L, et al. Alniditan, a new 5-hydroxytryptamine$_{1D}$ agonist and migraine-abortive agent: ligand-binding properties of human 5-hydroxytryptamine$_{1Da}$, human 5-hydroxytryptamine$_{1Dβ}$, and calf 5-hydroxytryptamine$_{1D}$ receptors investigated with [^{3}H]5-hydroxytryptamine and [^{3}H]alniditan. *Mol Pharmacol* 1996;50:1567–1580.

119. Lines C, Visser WH, Vandormael K, Reines SA. Rizatriptan 5 mg versus sumatriptan 50 mg in the acute treatment of migraine. *Headache* 1997;37:319–320.

120. Liston H, Bennett L, Usher B, Nappi J. The association of the combination of sumatriptan and methysergide in myocardial infarction in a premenopausal woman. *Arch Intern Med* 1999;159:511–513.

121. Longmore J, Boulanger CM, Desta B, et al. 5-HT$_{1D}$ receptor agonists and human coronary artery reactivity *in vitro*: crossover comparisons of 5-HT and sumatriptan with rizatriptan and l-741,519. *Br J Clin Pharmacol* 1996;42:431–441.

122. Longmore J, Razzaque Z, Hargreaves RJ, et al. Rizatriptan selectively contracts human middle meningeal over coronary artery: comparison with sumatriptan. *Cephalalgia* 1997;17:388–389.

123. Longmore J, Shaw D, Smith D, et al. Differential distribution of 5-HT$_{1D}$- and 5-HT$_{1B}$-immunoreactivity within the human trigeminocerebrovascular system: implications for the discovery of new antimigraine drugs. *Cephalalgia* 1997;17:833–842.

124. Maassen Van Den Brink A, Reekers M, Bax WA, et al. Coronary side-effect potential of current and prospective antimigraine drugs. *Circulation* 1998;98:25–30.

125. Maassen Van Den Brink A, Van Den Broek RWM, De Vries R, Saxena PR. Human middle meningeal and coronary artery contraction to eletriptan and sumatriptan. *Cephalalgia* 1999;19:398.

126. MacIntyre PD, Bhargava B, Hogg KJ, et al. Effect of subcutaneous sumatriptan, a selective 5HT$_1$ agonist, on the systemic, pulmonary, and coronary circulation. *Circulation* 1993;87:401–405.

127. MacIntyre P, Gemmill J, Hogg K, Bhargava B. The effect of subcutaneous sumatriptan on central haemodynamics and the coronary circulation. *Clin Pharmacol Ther* 1992;51:152.

128. MacLennan SJ, Cambridge D, Whiting MV, et al. Cranial vascular effects of zolmitriptan, a centrally active 5-HT$_{1B/1D}$ receptor partial agonist for the acute treatment of migraine. *Eur J Pharmacol* 1998;361:191–197.

129. Martin GR. Inhibition of the trigemino-vascular system with 5-HT$_{1D}$ agonist drugs: selectively targeting additional sites of action. *Eur Neurol* 1996;36:13–18.

130. Martin GR, Robertson AD, MacLennan SJ, et al. Receptor specificity and trigemino-vascular inhibitory actions of a novel 5-$_{1B/1D}$ receptor partial agonist, 311C90 (zolmitriptan). *Br J Pharmacol* 1997;121:157–164.

131. Massiou H. Sumatriptan nasal spray—comparator clinical trials. Presented at the 3rd European Headache Federation Conference, Sardinia, June 1996.

132. Massiou H, Tzourio C, El Amrani M, Bousser MG. Verbal scales in the acute treatment of migraine: semantic categories and clinical relevance. *Cephalalgia* 1997;17:37–39.

133. Mathew NT. Serotonin 1$_D$ (5-HT$_{1D}$) agonists and other agents in acute migraine. *Neurol Clin* 1997;15:61–83.

134. Mathew NT, Asgharnejad M, Peykamian M, Laurenza A, on behalf on the Naratriptan S2Wa3003 Study Group. Naratriptan is effective and well tolerated in the acute treatment of migraine. Results of a double-blind, placebo-controlled crossover study. *Neurology* 1997;49:1485–1490.

135. Mathew NT, Dexter J, Couch J, et al. Dose ranging efficacy and safety of subcutaneous sumatriptan in the acute treatment of migraine. *Arch Neurol* 1992;49:1271–1276.

136. Mathew NT, Tietjen GE, Lucker C. Serotonin syndrome complicating migraine pharmacotherapy. *Headache* 1996;35:488–489.

137. May A, Shepheard SL, Knorr M, et al. Retinal plasma extravasation in animals but not in humans: implications for the pathophysiology of migraine. *Brain* 1998;121:1231–1237.

138. Medical Products Agency, Sweden. Monograph on sumatriptan nasal spray. 1997-08-15. http://www.mpa.se/sve/mono/imig.sht. (Monograph in Swedish on sumatriptan nasal spray published on the Internet by the Swedish Medical Products Agency).

139. Medical Products Agency, Sweden. Monograph on sumatriptan suppositories. 1997-08-15. http://www.mpa.se/sve/mono/imig.sht. (Monograph in Swedish on sumatriptan suppositories published on the Internet by the Swedish Medical Products Agency).

140. Meschia JF, Mallkoff MD, Biller J. Reversible segmental cerebral arterial vasospasm and cerebral infarction. Possible association with excessive use of sumatriptan and Midrin. *Arch Neurol* 1998;55:712–714.

141. Mills A, Rhodes P, Martin GR. [^{3}H]311C90 binding sites in cat brain stem: implications for migraine treatment. *Cephalalgia* 1995;15:116.

142. Milton KA, Buchanan TJ, Haug-Pihale G, Molz KH. The pharmacokinetics, safety and tolerability of oral eletriptan in subjects with impaired hepatic function. *Cephalalgia* 1998;18:411–412.

143. Moore KHP, Hussey EK, Shaw S, Fuseau E, Duquesnoy C, Pakes GE. Safety, tolerability, and pharmacokinetics of sumatriptan in healthy subjects following ascending single intranasal doses and multiple intranasal doses. *Cephalalgia* 1997;17:541–550.

144. Morgan P, Rance D, James G, et al. Comparative absorption and elimination of eletriptan in rat, dog and human. *Cephalalgia* 1997;17:414.

145. Moskowitz MA. Neurogenic versus vascular mechanisms of sumatriptan and ergot alkaloids in migraine. *Trends Pharmacol Sci* 1992;13:307–311.

146. Moskowitz MA. Neurogenic inflammation in the pathophysiology and treatment of migraine. *Neurology* 1993;43(Suppl 3):16–20.

147. Mueller L, Gallagher M, Ciervo CA. Vasospasm-induced myocardial infarction with sumatriptan. *Headache* 1996;36:329–331.

148. Mushet GR, Cady RK, Baker CC, Clements B, Gutterman DL, Davis R. Efficacy and tolerability of of subcutaneous sumatriptan administered using the IMITREXR STATdose™ system. *Clin Ther* 1996;18:687–699.

149. Myllylä VV, Havanka H, Herrala L, et al. Tolfenamic acid rapid release versus sumatriptan in the acute treatment of migraine: comparable effect in a double-blind, randomized, controlled, parallel-group study. *Headache* 1998;38:201–207.

150. Multinational Oral Sumatriptan and Cafergot Comparative Study Group. A randomized, double-blind comparison of sumatriptan in the acute treatment of migraine. *Eur Neurol* 1991;31:314–322.

151. Nappi G, Sicuteri F, Byrne M, Roncolaro M, Zerbini O. Oral sumatriptan compared with placebo in the acute treatment of migraine. *J Neurol* 1994;41:138–144.

152. Newman-Tancredi A, Conte C, Chaput C, et al. Agonist activity of antimigraine drugs at recombinant human 5-HT$_{1A}$ receptors: potential implications for prophylactic and acute therapy. *Naunyn Schmiedebergs Arch Pharmacol* 1997:355:682–688.

153. O'Connor P, Gladstone P. Oral sumatriptan-associated transmural myocardial infraction. *Neurology* 1995;45:2274–2276.

154. Oral Sumatriptan and Aspirin plus Metoclopramide Comparative Study Group. A study to compare oral sumatriptan with oral aspirin plus oral metoclopramide in the acute treatment of migraine. *Eur Neurol* 1992;32:177–184.

155. Oral Sumatriptan Dose-Defining Study Group. Sumatriptan—an oral dose-defining study. *Eur Neurol* 1991;31:300–305.

156. Oral Sumatriptan International Multiple-Dose Study Group. Evaluation of a multiple-dose regimen of oral sumatriptan for the acute treatment of migraine. *Eur Neurol* 1991;31:306–313.

157. Ottervanger JP, Paalman HJA, Boxma GL, Stricker BHC. Transmural myocardial infarction with sumatriptan. *Lancet* 1993;341:861–862.

158. Ottervanger JP, Stricker BHC. Cardiovascular adverse reactions to sumatriptan: cause for concern? *CNS Drugs* 1995;3:90–98.

159. Ottervanger JP, Valkenburg HA, Grobbee DE, Stricker BH. Characteristics and determinants of sumatriptan-associated chest pain. *Arch Neurol* 1997;54:1387–1392.

160. Ottervanger JP, Wilson JHP, Stricker BHC. Drug-induced chest pain and myocardial infrarction. Reports to a national centre and review of the literature. *Eur J Clin Pharmacol* 1997;53:105–110.

161. Pagniez F, Valentin JP, Vieu S, et al. Pharmacological analysis of the haemodynamic effects of 5-HT$_{1B/D}$ receptor agonists in the normotensive rat. *Br J Pharmacol* 1998;123:205–214.

162. Parsons AA, Parker SG, Raval P, et al. Comparison of the cardiovascular effects of the novel 5-HT(1B/1D) receptor agonist, SB 209509

(VML251), and sumatriptan in dogs. *J Cardiovasc Pharmacol* 1997; 30:136–141.

163. Parsons AA, Raval P, Smith S, et al. Effects of the novel high-affinity 5-HT$_{(1B/1D)}$-receptor ligand frovatriptan in human isolated basilar and coronary arteries. *J Cardiovasc Pharmacol* 1998;32:220–224.

164. Pauwels PJ. Pharmacological properties of a putative 5-HT$_{1B/D}$ receptor antagonist GR127935. *CNS Drug Rev* 1996;2:415–428.

165. Pauwels PJ, Palmier C, Tardif S, et al. F11356, a new 5-HT derivative, with selective, potent and highly efficacious agonist properties at 5-HT$_{1B/1D}$ receptors. *Naunyn Schmiedebergs Arch Pharmacol* 1998; 358:R523.

166. Peck RW, Seaber EJ, Dixon RM, et al. The pharmacodynamics and pharmacokinetics of the 5HT$_{1B/1D}$-agonist zolmitriptan in healthy young and elderly men and women. *Clin Pharmacol Ther* 1998;63: 342–353.

167. Peikert A, Becker WJ, Ashford EA, Dahlof C, Hassani H, Salonen RJ. Sumatriptan nasal spray: a dose-ranging study in the acute treatment of migraine. *Eur J Neurol* 1999;6:43–49.

168. Perry CN, Markham A. Sumatriptan. An updated review of its use in migraine. *Drugs* 1998;55:889–922.

169. Pfaffenrath V, Cunin G, Sjonell G, Prendergast S. Efficacy and safety of sumatriptan tablets (25 mg, 50 mg, 100 mg) in the acute treatment of migraine: defining the optimum doses of oral sumatriptan. *Headache* 1998;38:184–190.

170. Phebus LA, Johnson KW, Zgombick JM, et al. Characterization of LY344864 as a pharmacological tool to study 5-HT$_{1F}$ receptors: binding affinities, brain penetration and activity in the neurogenic dural inflammation model of migraine. *Life Sci* 1997;61:2117–2126.

171. Pilgrim AJ. Methodology of clinical trials of sumatriptan in migraine and cluster headache. *Eur Neurol* 1991;31:295–299.

172. Pitman V, Forster E, Jackson N. Comparison of the efficacy of oral eletriptan and oral sumatriptan for the acute treatment of migraine: combined analysis across three clinical trials [Abstract]. *Headache* 1999;39:374.

173. Plosker GL, McTavish D. Sumatriptan. A reappraisal of its pharmacology and therapeutic efficacy in the acute treatment of migraine and cluster headache. *Drugs* 1994;47:622–651.

174. Price GW, Burton MJ, Collin LJ, et al. SB-216641 and BRL-15572-compounds to pharmacologically discriminate h5-HT$_{1B}$ and h5-HT$_{1D}$ receptors. *Naunyn Schmiedebergs Arch Pharmacol* 1997;356: 312–320.

175. Rance D, Clear N, Dallman L. Physicochemical comparison of eletriptan and other 5-HT$_{1D}$–like agonists as a predictor of oral absoption potential. *Headache* 1997;37:328.

176. Rapoport AM. Sumatriptan nasal spray: a review of randomised, double-blind, placebo-controlled clinical trials conducted in the USA. *Funct Neurol* 1996;11:150.

177. Rapoport AM, Ramadan NM, Adelman JU, et al. on behalf of The 017 Clinical Trial Study Group. Optimizing the dose of zolmitriptan (ZomigTM, 311C90) for the acute treatment of migraine. A multicenter, double-blind, placebo-controlled, dose range-finding study. *Neurology* 1997;49:1210–1218.

178. Rapoport AM, Visser WH, Cutler NR, et al. Oral sumatriptan in preventing headache recurrence after treatment of migraine attacks with subcutaneous sumatriptan. *Neurology* 1995;45:1505–1509.

179. Razzaque Z, Longmore J, Hill RG. Differences in the effects of ketanserin and GR127935 on 5-HT-receptor mediated responses in rabbit saphenous vein and guinea-pig jugular vein. *Eur J Pharmacol* 1995;283:199–206.

180. Razzaque Z, Shaw D, Smith D, et al. Pharmacological analysis of 5-HT-receptor mediated vasoconstriction of human isolated middle meningeal arteries: determining the contribution of 5-HT$_{1D\beta}$- and 5-HT$_{1F}$-receptor activation. *Br J Pharmacol* 1997;120:211P.

181. Reches A on behalf of the Eletriptan Steering Committee. Comparison of the efficacy, safety and tolerability of oral eletriptan and Cafergot^R for the acute treatment of migraine [Abstract]. *Cephalalgia* 1999;19:355.

182. Rederich G, Rapoport A, Cutler N, Hazelrigg R, Jamerson B. Oral sumatriptan for the long-term treatment of migraine: clinical findings. *Neurology* 1995;45(Suppl 7):15–20.

183. Robert M, Warrington SJ, Zayas JM, et al. Electrocardiographic effects and pharmacokinetics of oral almotriptan in healthy subjects. *Cephalalgia* 1998;18:406.

184. Rolan PE, Martin GR. Zolmitriptan: a new acute treatment for migraine. *Exp Opin Invest Drugs* 1998;7:633–652.

185. Roon K, Diener HC, Ellis P, et al. CP-122,287 blocks neurogenic inflammation, but is not effective in aborting migraine attacks: results of two controlled clinical trials. *Cephalalgia* 1997;17:245.

186. Russel MB, Holm-Thomsen OE, Nielsen MR, Cleal A, Pilgrim AJ, Olesen J. A randomized, double-blind, placebo-controlled crossover study of subcutaneous sumatriptan in general practice. *Cephalalgia* 1994;14:291–296.

187. Ryan R, Elkind A, Baker CC, Mullican W, DeBussey S, Asgharnejad M. Sumatriptan nasal spray for the acute treatment of migraine. Results of two clinical studies. *Neurology* 1997;49:1225–1230.

188. Ryan R, Keywood C on behalf of the US multi-centre study of VML251. A preliminary study of VML251 (SB209509) a novel 5HT1B/1D agonist for the treatment of migraine attacks. *Cephalalgia* 1997;17:418.

189. Ryan RE Jr, Elkind A, Goldstein J. Twenty-four-hour effectiveness of BMS 180048 in the acute treatment of migraine headaches. *Headache* 1997;37:245–248.

190. The S2BM11 Study Group. Patients preference between 25, 50 and 100 mg oral doses of sumatriptan. *Eur J Neurol* 1996;3(Suppl 3):86.

191. Salonen R, Asford E. Dahlöf C, et al. for the International Intranasal Sumatriptan Study Group. Intranasal sumatriptan for the acute treatment of migraine. *J Neurol* 1994;241:463–469.

192. Sargent J, Kirchner JR, Davis R, Kirkhart B. Oral sumatriptan is effective and well tolerated for the acute treatment of migraine: results of a multicenter study. *Neurology* 1995;45(Suppl 7):10–14.

193. Savani N, Brautaset NJ, Reunanen M, et al. A double-blind placebo-controlled study assessing the efficacy and tolerability of sumatriptan 50-mg tablets in the acute treatment of migraine. *Int J Clin Pract* (in press).

194. Saxena PR. Cranial arteriovenous shunting, an *in vivo* animal model for migraine. In: Olesen J, Moskowitz MA, eds. *Experimental headache models*. Philadelphia: Lippincott-Raven, 1995:189–198.

195. Saxena PR, De Vries P, Villalón CM. 5-HT$_1$-like receptors: a time to bid goodbye. *Trends Pharmacol Sci* 1998;19:311–316.

196. Saxena PR, Ferrari MD. From serotonin receptor classification to the antimigraine drug sumatriptan. *Cephalalgia* 1992;12:187–196.

197. Schoenen J, Sawyer J. Zolmitriptan (Zomig™, 311C90), a novel dual central and peripheral 5HT1B/1D agonist: an overview of efficacy. *Cephalalgia* 1997;17(Suppl 18):28–40.

198. Sciberras DG, Polvino WJ, Gertz BJ, et al. Initial human experience with MK-462 (rizatriptan): a novel 5-HT$_{1D}$ agonist. *Br J Clin Pharmacol* 1997;43:49–54.

199. Scott RJ, Aitchison WRC, Barker PR, McLaren GI. Oral sumatriptan in the acute treatment of migraine and migraine recurrence in general practice. *Q J Med* 1996;89:613–622.

200. Seidelin KN, Tfelt-Hansen P, Mendel C, Stephanage M. Peripheral haemodynamic study of MK-462, ergotamine and their combination in man. *Cephalalgia* 1995;15(Suppl 14):207.

201. Selkirk JV, Scott C, Ho M, et al. SB-224289—a novel selective (human) 5-HT$_{1B}$ receptor antagonist with negative intrinsic activity. *Br J Pharmacol* 1998;125:202–208.

202. Shepheard SL, Williamson DJ, Baker R, et al. *In vivo* pharmacology of the novel 5-HT$_{1D}$ receptor agonist MK-462. *Cephalalgia* 1995;15: 204.

203. Shepheard SL, Williamson DJ, Beer MS, et al. Differential effects of 5-HT$_{1B/1D}$ receptor agonists on neurogenic dural plasma extravasation and vasodilation in anaesthetized rats. *Neuropharmacology* 1997;36: 525–533.

204. Shepheard SL, Williamson DJ, Williams J, et al. Comparison of the effects of sumatriptan and the NK1 antagonist CP-99,994 on plasma extravasation in dura mater and c-*fos* mRNA expression in trigeminal nucleus caudalis of rats. *Neuropharmacology* 1995;34:255–261.

205. Simmons VE, Blakeborough P. The safety profile of sumatriptan. *Rev Contemp Pharmacother* 1994;5:319–328.

206. Skingle M, Beattie DT, Scopes DIT, et al. GR127935: a potent and selective 5-HT$_{1D}$ receptor antagonist. *Behav Brain Res* 1996;73: 157–161.

207. Smith MI, James MF, Bockhorst KH, et al. Cortical spreading depression (CSD) in the cat visualized with magnetic resonance imaging (MRI). *Cephalalgia* 1998;18:400.

208. Solomon GD, Cady RK, Klapper JA, Earl NL, Saper JR, Ramadan N, on behalf of the 042 Clinical Study Group. The clinical efficacy and tolerability of 2.5 mg zolmitriptan for the acute treatment of migraine. *Neurology* 1997;49:1219–1225.

209. Sperling B, Tfelt-Hansen P, Lines C. Lack of effect of MK-462 on cerebral blood flow in humans. *Cephalalgia* 1995;15(Suppl 14):206.

210. Subcutaneous Sumatriptan International Study Group. Treatment of migraine attacks with sumatriptan. *N Engl J Med* 1991;325:316–321.

211. Sumatriptan Auto-Injector Study Group. Self-treatment of acute migraine with subcutaneous sumatriptan using an auto-injector device. *Eur Neurol* 1991;31:323–331.

212. Swan L, Birnie DH, Hood S, et al. The effect of subcutaneous naratriptan 1.5 mg on the systemic, pulmonary, and coronary circulation in patients with suspected coronary disease. *Cephalagia* 1988;17:428.

213. Tansey MJB, Pilgrim AJ, Martin PM. Long-term experience with sumatriptan in the treatment of migraine. *Eur Neurol* 1993;33:310–310.

214. Teall J, Tuchman M, Cutler N, et al. and the Rizatriptan 022 Study Group. Rizatriptan (MAXALT) for the acute treatment of migraine and migraine recurrence. *Headache* 1998;38:281–287.

215. Tepper SJ, Cochran A, Hobbs S, Woessner M, on behalf of the S2B351 Study Group. Sumatriptan suppositories for the acute treatment of migraine. *Int J Clin Pract* 1998;52:31–35.

216. Terrón JA. GR127935 is a potent antagonist of the 5-HT$_1$–like receptor mediating contraction in the canine coronary artery. *Eur J Pharmacol* 1996;300:109–112.

217. Tfelt-Hansen P. Sumatriptan for the treatment of migraine attacks—a review of controlled clinical trials. *Cephalalgia* 1993;13:238–244.

218. Tfelt-Hansen P. Efficacy and adverse events of subcutaneous, oral, and intranasal sumatriptan used for migraine treatment: a systematic review based on number needed to treat. *Cephalalgia* 1998;18:532–538.

219. Tfelt-Hansen P. Pitfalls in long-term studies assessing acute migraine therapy. *Cephalalgia* (in press).

220. Tfelt-Hansen P, Henry P, Mulder K, Scheldewaert RG, Schoenen J, Chazot G. The effectiveness of combined oral lysine acetylsalicylate and metoclopramide compared with oral sumatriptan for migraine. *Lancet* 1995;346:923–926.

221. Tfelt-Hansen P, Saxena PR, Ferrari MD. Ergot alkaloids. In: de Wolf FA, ed. *Handbook of clinical neurology*. Vol. 21 (65): Intoxications of the nervous system. Part II. Amsterdam: Elsevier Science, 1995:61–78.

222. Tfelt-Hansen P, Sperling B, Winter PDO. Transient additional effect of sumatriptan on ergotamine-induced constriction of peripheral arteries in man. *Clin Pharmacol Ther* 1992;51:149.

223. Tfelt-Hansen P, Teall J, Rodriguez F, et al. and Rizatriptan 030 Study Group. Oral rizatriptan versus oral sumatriptan: a direct comparative study in the acute treatment of migraine. *Headache* 1998;38:748–755.

224. Thomsen LL, Dixon R, Lassen LH, et al. 311C90 (zolmitriptan), a novel centrally and peripherally acting oral 5-hydroxytrypyamine-1D agonist: a comparison of its absorption during a migraine attack and in a migraine-free period. *Cephalalgia* 1996;16:270–275.

225. Touchon J, Bertin L, Pilgrim AJ, Ashford E, Bes A. A comparison of subcutaneous sumatriptan and dihydroergotamine nasal spray in the acute treatment of migraine. *Neurology* 1996;47:361–365.

226. Ullmer C, Schmuck K, Kalkman HO, Lubbert H. Expression of serotonin receptor mRNAs in blood vessels. *FEBS Lett* 1995;370:215–221.

227. Van Den Broek RWM, Maassen Van Den Brink A, de Vries R, et al. Pharmacological analysis of contraction to eletriptan and sumatriptan in human isolated coronary artery and saphenous vein. *Cephalalgia* 1999;19:399.

228. Van Es NM, Bruning TA, Camps J, et al. Assessment of peripheral vascular effects of antimigraine drugs in humans. *Cephalalgia* 1995;15:288–291.

229. Verheggen R, Hundeshagen AG, Brown AM, et al. 5-HT$_{1B}$ receptor-mediated contractions in human temporal artery: evidence from selective antagonists and 5-HT receptor mRNA expression. *Br J Pharmacol* 1998;124:1345–1354.

230. Villalón CM, De Vries P, Rabelo G, et al. Canine external carotid vasoconstriction to methysergide, ergotamine and dihydroergotamine: role of 5-HT$_{1B/1D}$ receptors and α_2-adrenoceptors. *Br J Pharmacol* 1999;126:585–594.

231. Visser WH, Burggraaf J, Muller LM, et al. Pharmacokinetic and pharmacodynamic profiles of sumatriptan in migraine patients with headache recurrence or no response. *Clin Pharmacol Ther* 1996;60:452–460.

232. Visser WH, de Vriend RH, Jaspers MW, Ferrari MD. Sumatriptan in clinical practice: a 2-year review of 453 migraine patients. *Neurology* 1996;47:46–51.

233. Visser WH, Jaspers NM, de Vriend RH, Ferrari MD. Risk factors for headache recurrence after sumatriptan: a study in 366 migraine patients. *Cephalalgia* 1996;16:264–269.

234. Visser WH, Klein KB, Cox RC, Jones D, Ferrari MD. 311C90, a new central and peripherally acting 5-HT1D receptor agonist in the acute oral treatment of migraine: a double-blind, placebo-controlled, dose-range finding study. *Neurology* 1996;46:522–526.

235. Visser WH, Terwindt GM, Reines SA, Jiang K, Lines CR, Ferrari MD, for the Dutch/US Rizatriptan Study Group. Rizatriptan vs sumatriptan in the acute treatment of migraine. A placebo-controlled, dose-ranging study. *Arch Neurol* 1996;53:1132–1137.

236. Wainscott DB, Johnson KW, Phebus LA, et al. Human 5-HT$_{1F}$ receptor-stimulated [^{35}S]GTPgammaS binding: correlation with inhibition of guinea pig dural plasma protein extravasation. *Eur J Pharmacol* 1998;352:117–124.

237. Wilkinson M, Pfaffenrath V, Schoenen J, Diener H-C, Steiner T. Migraine and cluster headache—their management with sumatriptan: a critical review of the current clinical experience. *Cephalalgia* 1995;15:337–357.

238. Willems E, De Vries P, Heiligers JP, Saxena PR. Porcine carotid vascular effects of eletriptan (UK-116,044): a new 5-HT$_{1B/1D}$ receptor agonist with anti-migraine activity. *Naunyn Schmiedebergs Arch Pharmacol* 1998;358:212–219.

239. Williamson DJ, Shepheard SL, Hill RG, Hargreaves RJ. The novel anti-migraine agent rizatriptan inhibits neurogenic dural vasodilation and extravasation. *Eur J Pharmacol* 1997;328:61–64.

240. Winner P, Ricalde O, Le Force B, Saper J, Margul B. A double-blind study of subcutaneous dihydroergotamine vs subcutaneous sumatriptan in the treatment of acute migraine. *Arch Neurol* 1996;53:180–184.

241. Wojnar-Horton RE, Hackett LP, Yapp P, Dusci LJ, Paech M, Ilett KF. Distribution and excretion of sumatriptan in human milk. *Br J Clin Pharmacol* 1996;41:217–221.

242. Wurch T, Palmier C, Colpaert FC, Pauwels PJ. Recombinant saphenous vein 5-HT$_{1B}$ receptors of the rabbit: comparative pharmacology with human 5-HT$_{1B}$ receptors. *Br J Pharmacol* 1997;120:153–159.

243. Yocca FD, Gylys JA, Smith DW et al. BMS-181885: a clinically effective migraine abortive with periperovascular and neuronal 5-HT$_{1D}$ agonist properties. *Cephalalgia* 1997;17:404.

244. Yu XJ, Cutrer FM, Moskowitz MA, Waeber C. The 5-HT$_{1D}$ receptor antagonist GR-127,935 prevents inhibitory effects of sumatriptan but not CP-122,288 and 5-CT on neurogenic plasma extravasation within guinea pig dura mater. *Neuropharmacology* 1997;36:83–91.

245. Yu XJ, Waeber C, Castanon N, et al. 5-Carboxamido-tryptamine, CP-122,288 and dihydroergotamine but not sumatriptan, CP-93,129, and serotonin-5-O-carboxymethyl-glycyl-tyrosinamide block dural plasma protein extravasation in knockout mice that lack 5-hydroxytryptamine$_{1B}$ receptors. *Mol Pharmacol* 1996;49:761–765.

The Headaches, Second Edition,
edited by J. Olesen, P. Tfelt-Hansen, and K.M.A. Welch.
Lippincott Williams & Wilkins, Philadelphia © 2000.

The Migraines

CHAPTER 53

Novel Compounds in Development for Acute Treatment of Migraine

Carl G. H. Dahlöf and Pramod R. Saxena

In the last decade of the twentieth century, tremendous progress was made in the acute therapy of migraine. Sumatriptan, a member of the new class of drugs known as 5-hydroxytryptamine$_{1B/1D}$ (5-HT$_{1B/1D}$) receptor agonists, has provided the lead (19,20,53). This seminal discovery by Humphrey and colleagues (19,20) was based on the findings that a novel 5-HT (now 5-HT$_{1B}$) receptor mediates selective carotid vasoconstriction, which is also observed following small doses of the well-known antimigraine drug ergotamine (44,45). The success of sumatriptan in migraine therapy undoubtedly resulted in heightened research interest in the field of migraine, which in turn led to a better understanding of the pathophysiologic processes involved in migraine as well as the development of new triptans (8,11) and other prospective drugs. This chapter reviews the compounds that are in an early phase of development:

1. 5-HT$_1$ receptor agonists
2. Calcitonin gene-related peptide (CGRP) receptor antagonists
3. Neurokinin NK$_1$ receptor antagonists
4. Spreading depression antagonists
5. Drugs affecting nitric oxide biosynthesis

5-HT$_1$ RECEPTOR AGONISTS

The main mechanism of the therapeutic action of triptans undoubtedly involves constriction of dilated cranial

C. G. H. Dahlöf: Department of Clinical Pharmacology, Sahlgrenska University Hospital, and Gothenburg Migraine Clinic, S-41117 Göteborg, Sweden.

P. R. Saxena: Department of Pharmacology, Erasmus University, 3000 DR Rotterdam, The Netherlands.

extracerebral blood vessels mediated by the 5-HT$_{1B}$ receptor (8,12,18,46). In addition, these drugs may inhibit the release of proinflammatory neuropeptides and plasma protein extravasation across dural vessels through 5-HT$_{1D/1F}$ receptors (23,34,35) and central nociceptive transmission within the trigeminovascular system, probably involving 5-HT$_{1B/1D}$ receptors (15).

Attempts are being made to identify compounds that might be effective against migraine but lack vasoconstrictor action, particularly on the coronary arteries (2,32,33); however, there is still vigorous debate over whether compounds that solely inhibit neuropeptide release and plasma protein extravasation will have significant antimigraine activity (12,18,34). In any case, the headache relief may be relatively slow by decreasing perivascular edema (47).

Among the 5-HT$_1$ receptor ligands, three types of drugs are in development:

1. 5-HT$_{1B/1D}$ receptor agonists
2. Selective 5-HT$_{1D}$ receptor agonists
3. Selective 5-HT$_{1F}$ receptor agonists

5-HT$_{1B/1D}$ Receptor Agonists

The most important compound of this type in preclinical development is F11356 (Pierre Fabre, Castres, France) (Table 1) (22). Among the triptans, F11356 has the highest affinity at 5-HT$_{1B/1D}$ receptors. It selectively and potently decreases carotid blood flow in both anesthetised pigs and conscious dogs and increases outward hyperpolarizing Ca^{2+}-dependent K$^+$ current in the guinea pig trigeminal ganglion. Based on preclinical data, F11356 has an excellent potential for antimigraine efficacy.

TABLE 1. *Receptor binding profile of some 5-HT$_1$ receptor agonists in development at human 5-HT$_1$ receptor subtypes*

Drug	5-HT$_{1A}$	5-HT$_{1B}$	5-HT$_{1D}$	5-HT$_{1E}$	5-HT$_{1F}$
Sumatriptan[a]	6.4	8.3	8.5	5.6	7.6
F11356[b]	7.6	9.4–10.1	9.3–10.2	5.9	5.5
L775606[c]	7.3	7.1	9.2	<5.0	5.4
PNU109291[d]	6.0	5.2	9.0	—	—
LY344864[e]	6.3	6.3	—	6.2	8.2
LY334370[f]	—	6.9	6.9	—	8.8

F11356 (4-[4-(2-[3-(2-aminoethyl)-1H-indol-5-yloxy]-acetyl]-piperazin-1-yl)-benzonitrile hydrochloride; L775606 (1-(3-[5-(1,2,4-triazol-4-yl)-1H-indol-3-yl]propyl)-4-(2-(3-fluorophenyl)ethyl) piperazine); PNU109291 (S(-)-1-(1-ethyl-4-methoxyphenyl piperazin)-6-methyl-carboxamido-isochromane); LY344864 (N-[3-(dimethylamino)-2,3,4,9-tetrahydro-1H-carbazol-6-yl]-4-fluorobenzamide); LY334370 (4-fluoro-N-[3-(1-methyl-4-piperidinyl)-1H-indol-5-yl]-benzamide). Except otherwise indicated, all data are given as pK$_i$ at human receptors. Data from[a] (1, 3, 29);[b] (22);[c] pIC$_{50}$ (5);[d] (10);[e] (40);[f] (23).

Selective 5-HT$_{1D}$ Receptor Agonists

PNU-109291 (10) and L775606 (5) have been described as highly selective 5-HT$_{1D}$ receptor agonists (see Table 1). These compounds inhibit protein plasma extravasation in response to trigeminal nerve stimulation but lack potent vasoconstrictor activity. Although inhibition of dural plasma extravasation by itself is not predictive of antimigraine activity (42), the 5-HT$_{1D}$ receptor seems to mediate inhibition of the central component of the trigeminovascular system (8). Therefore, selective 5-HT$_{1D}$ receptor agonists are valuable for probing migraine mechanisms (10).

5-HT$_{1F}$ Receptor Agonists

Two potent 5-HT$_{1F}$ agonists, LY344864 (40) and LY334370 (23), have been described (see Table 1). Both compounds inhibit dural plasma protein extravasation without significant vasoconstrictor activity. Because SB224289, which displays little affinity at the 5-HT$_{1F}$ receptor (17), completely antagonizes sumatriptan-induced carotid vasoconstrictor effects (8), the 5-HT$_{1F}$ receptor is apparently not involved in the vascular effects of triptans. This finding implies that, if LY334370 (which has undergone clinical evaluation but may not be further developed as a result of animal toxicology data) turns out to be effective in migraine at doses devoid of 5-HT$_{1B/1D}$ receptor interaction, the mechanism of action will not be through cranial vasoconstriction. In the absence of the importance of dural plasma protein extravasation, further experiments will be needed to explain the efficacy of LY334370 (8,42). It should be noted that the efficacy of LY334370 would have no bearing on the importance of 5-HT$_{1B}$ receptor-mediated cranial vasoconstriction in view of poor affinity displayed by the potent antimigraine drug alniditan at the 5-HT$_{1F}$ receptor (29).

CGRP RECEPTOR ANTAGONISTS

Another strategy currently under evaluation is the use of selective antagonists of sensory vasoactive neuropeptides that are released during a migraine attack. Compared with inhibition of peptide release through a prejunctional effect (60), this strategy has the disadvantage of targeting only one of the neuropeptides. Its success will depend on the importance of that particular peptide in migraine pathogenesis. The enriched localization of CGRP in trigeminal sensory ganglia (57) indicates a role in the neurogenic inflammation associated with migraine. Thus, CGRP antagonists may represent a novel therapeutic approach to the treatment of migraine. To our knowledge, however, no CGRP antagonist has been evaluated in migraine as yet. We believe that a proof-of-concept study using even a peptide antagonist (41) will be worthwhile.

NEUROKININ NK$_1$ RECEPTOR AGONISTS

Substance P is distributed throughout the cranial vasculature and in the trigeminal sensory afferent nerve fibers, and its release can be demonstrated following activation of the trigeminovascular system in animals and humans (57). The recently developed selective neurokinin NK$_1$ receptor antagonists inhibit substance P-mediated dilatation and plasma protein extravasation in the cranial circulation (39,48,59), suggesting that they may provide an effective and novel acute treatment for migraine. Initial clinical results from migraine patients show that NK$_1$ receptor antagonists (RPR 100,893 and LY 303,870) do not differ from placebo in providing headache relief in acute migraine attacks at 2 hours after dosing (9,16). These findings question the role of substance P in migraine pathogenesis.

Preclinical studies with NK$_1$ receptor antagonists have demonstrated inhibition of c-*fos* mRNA and FOS protein expression in trigeminal nucleus caudalis following electric stimulation of the trigeminal ganglion (49) or noxious chemical stimulation of the brain meninges (7). This inhibition of trigeminal c-*fos* responses was maximally around 60%, suggesting that even brain-penetrant NK_1 receptor antagonists will be inactive against migraine if the threshold for inhibition of central nociceptive transmission that gives clinical pain relief is greater. After opening the blood–brain barrier, sumatriptan markedly decreases neuronal firing in trigeminal nucleus caudalis in response to sagittal sinus stimulation (24) and reduces the c-*fos* expression in response to trigeminal ganglion stimulation to a greater extent than the NK_1 receptor antagonist CP 99,994 (49). These observations are consistent with a general prejunctional inhibition of neuropeptide transmitter release from central trigeminal sensory nerve fibers rather than inhibition of a single neuropeptide.

Acute antimigraine strategies based on preventing neurogenic extravasation appear to be misdirected because once headache has manifested, this process already may have occurred. It is therefore worth exploring the utility of NK_1 receptor antagonists in migraine prophylaxis. NK_1 receptor antagonists lack general analgesics properties (43), but they are effective against facilitated nociceptive responses evoked centrally in the spinal and medullary dorsal horn by prolonged noxious sensory input (26,31). Thus, although the clinical findings to date suggest that NK_1 receptor antagonists cannot reverse intense trigeminal nociceptive processes that are under way once a migraine attack has become established, it remains possible that they may be able to prevent or ameliorate migraine headaches if given prophylactically.

In preclinical assays, NK_1 receptor antagonists showed antiemetic property, acting centrally in the vicinity of the vomiting center in the brainstem (4,13,52,58) against a wide range of peripheral and central emetogenic stimuli (30). The clinical antiemetic effectiveness of NK_1 receptor antagonists was demonstrated in chemotherapy-induced emesis when used in combination with other antiemetic agents (25). It is not yet known whether these drugs would be useful against nausea and vomiting associated with migraine.

SPREADING DEPRESSION ANTAGONISTS

Cortical spreading depression is characterized by a transient, reversible depression of electroencephalographic activity, which advances across the cortical surface at a velocity of 2 to 5 mm per min^{-1}. Cortical spreading depression originally was linked to the aura phase of migraine and later to the headache phase on the basis that it may activate meningeal trigeminal C-fibers causing neurogenic inflammation and pain (36,38). It also was suggested that C-fiber activation is caused by hyperosmolar KCl/NaCl, not by cortical spreading depression

(21). Morphine, but not sumatriptan, reduced c-*fos* expression in both the ipsilateral and contralateral trigeminal nucleus caudalis, confirming that nociceptors were activated. No positive correlation was seen between the number of cortical spreading depressions and the extent of c-*fos* expression in trigeminal nucleus caudalis, but a positive linear correlation between the number of KCl injections and the extent of c-*fos* expression was demonstrated (21).

The role of cortical spreading depression in migraine remains controversial because of difficulty in demonstrating it clinically; however, a promising technique using magnetic resonance imaging has been developed (38), which seems to offer new opportunities for investigating cortical spreading depression in humans. Meanwhile, animal studies show that cortical spreading depression leads to cranial vasodilatation (38). Inhibition of this vasodilator response appears to be a novel avenue for developing antimigraine drugs without vasoconstrictor action per se. Indeed, Chan et al. (6) reported a series of compounds, in particular SB220453, which block cortical spreading depression by an unknown, probably a channel, mechanism. Some other compounds, such as the calcium channel blocker KB-2796 (51) and a glutamate antagonist blocking voltage-sensitive sodium channels, lamotrigine (27), also have been described. SB220453 is in clinical trials in acute migraine; lamotrigine was found to be effective in a pilot trial of migraine prophylaxis (27).

DRUGS AFFECTING NITRIC OXIDE BIOSYNTHESIS

It is well known that nitroglycerin, a nitric oxide donor effective in angina pectoris, causes headaches as a side effect and can precipitate migraine and cluster attacks. Nitroglycerin increases (55) and inhibition of nitric oxide biosynthesis decreases (56) carotid arteriovenous anastomotic blood flow in the pigs. Olesen and co-workers suggested that nitric oxide released from blood vessels, perivascular nerve endings, or brain tissue is a molecule trigger mechanism for migraine pain (37,54). The blood concentration of cyclic guanosin 3,5'-monophosphate (cGMP) increases during migraine attack (50). Furthermore, the propensity of migraine to occur in women may be due to the capacity of estrogen to alter myogenic tone by increasing cerebrovascular nitric oxide production and its action (14). These observations dictate that drugs that block the synthesis of nitric oxide may abort migraine attacks. Indeed, the nitric oxide-synthase (NOS) inhibitor L-N^G-methylarginine hydrochloride (546C88) was reported to be effective in acute migraine (28), but this trial might have a bias as a result of the inclusion of historical controls. Nevertheless, this approach using preferably selective nNOS or iNOS inhibitors is worth exploring.

REFERENCES

1. Adham N, Kao HT, Schechter LE, et al. Cloning of another human serotonin receptor (5-HT$_{1F}$): a fifth 5-HT$_1$ receptor subtype coupled to the inhibition of adenylate cyclase. *Proc Natl Acad Sci U S A* 1993;90: 408–412.
2. Bax WA, Saxena PR. Sumatriptan and ischaemic heart disease [Letter; Comment]. *Lancet* 1993;341:1420.
3. Beer MS, Heald MA, McAllister G, Stanton JA. Pharmacological characterisation of a cloned dog 5-HT$_{1B}$ receptor cell line. *Eur J Pharmacol* 1998;360:117–121.
4. Bountra C, Bunce K, Dale T, et al. Anti-emetic profile of a non-peptide neurokinin NK$_1$ receptor antagonist, CP-99,994, in ferrets. *Eur J Pharmacol* 1993;249:R3–R4.
5. Chambers MS, Street LJ, Goodacre S, et al. 3-(Piperazinylpropyl)indoles: selective, orally bioavailable h5-HT$_{1D}$ receptor agonists as potential antimigraine agents. *J Med Chem* 1999;42:691–705.
6. Chan WN, Evans JN, Hadley MS, et al. Identification of (-)-*cis*-6-acetyl-4S-(3-chloro-4-fluoro-benzoylamino)3,4-dihydro-2,2-dimethyl-2H-benzo[b]pyran-3S-ol as a potential antimigraine agent. *Bioorg Med Chem Lett* 1999;9:285–290.
7. Cutrer FM, Moussaoui S, Garret C, Moskowitz MA. The non-peptide neurokinin-1 antagonist, RPR 100893, decreases c-fos expression in trigeminal nucleus caudalis following noxious chemical meningeal stimulation. *Neuroscience* 1995;64:741–750.
8. De Vries P, Villalón CM, Saxena PR. Pharmacology of triptans. *Emerg Drug Rev* 1999;4:In Press.
9. Diener HC, Group for the RPR100893-201 Migraine Study Group. Substance–P antagonist RPR100893 is not effective in human migraine attacks. Abstract. 6th International Headache Research Seminar-Headache Treatment Trial Methodology and New Drugs, November 17-19, 1995. Copenhagen, Denmark 1995:63.
10. Ennis MD, Ghazal NB, Hoffman RL, et al. Isochroman-6-carboxamides as highly selective 5-HT$_{1D}$ agonists: potential new treatment for migraine without cardiovascular side effects. *J Med Chem* 1998;41: 2180–2183.
11. Ferrari MD. Migraine. *Lancet* 1998;351:1043–1051.
12. Ferrari MD, Saxena PR. Clinical and experimental effects of sumatriptan in humans. *Trends Pharmacol Sci* 1993;14:129–133.
13. Gardner CJ, Twissell DJ, Dale TJ, et al. The broad spectrum anti-emetic activity of the novel non-peptide tachykinin NK$_1$ receptor antagonists GR203040. *Br J Pharmacol* 1995;116:3158–3163.
14. Geary GG, Krause DN, Duckles SP. Estrogen reduces myogenic tone through a nitric oxide-dependent mechanism in rat cerebral arteries. *Am J Physiol* 1998;275:H292–300.
15. Goadsby PJ. How do the currently used prophylactic agents work in migraine? . *Cephalalgia* 1997;17:85–92.
16. Goldstein DJ, Wang O, Saper JR, Stoltz R, Silberstein SD, Mathew NT. Ineffectiveness of neurokinin-1 antagonist in acute migraine: a crossover study. *Cephalalgia* 1997;17:785–790.
17. Hagan JJ, Slade PD, Gaster L, Jeffrey P, Hatcher JP, Middlemiss DN. Stimulation of 5-HT$_{1B}$ receptors causes hypothermia in the guinea pig. *Eur J Pharmacol* 1997;331:169–174.
18. Humphrey PP, Feniuk W. Mode of action of the anti-migraine drug sumatriptan. *Trends Pharmacol Sci* 1991;12:444-446.
19. Humphrey PP, Feniuk W, Perren MJ, et al. GR43175, a selective agonist for the 5-HT$_1$-like receptor in dog isolated saphenous vein. Br *J Pharmacol* 1988;94:1123–1132.
20. Humphrey PPA, Apperley E, Feniuk W, Perren MJ. A rational approach to identifying a fundamentally new drug for the treatment of migraine. In: Saxena PR, Wallis DI, Wouters W, Bevan P, eds. *Cardiovascular pharmacology of 5-hydroxytryptamine:* prospective therapeutic applications. Dordrecht: Kluwer academic publishers, 1990: 416–431.
21. Ingvardsen BK, Laursen H, Olsen UB, Hansen AJ. Possible mechanism of c-*fos* expression in trigeminal nucleus caudalis following cortical spreading depression. *Pain* 1997;72:407–415.
22. John GW, Pauwels PJ, Perez M, et al. F11356, a novel 5-HT derivative with potent, selective and unique intrinsic activity at 5-HT$_{1B/D}$ receptors in models relevant to migraine. *J Pharmacol Exp Ther* 1999;290:83–95.
23. Johnson KW, Schaus JM, Durkin MM, et al. 5-HT$_{1F}$ receptor agonists inhibit neurogenic dural inflammation in guinea pigs. *Neuroreport* 1997;8:2237–2240.
24. Kaube H, Keay KA, Hoskin KL, Bandler R, Goadsby PJ. Expression of c-*fos*-like immunoreactivity in the caudal medulla and upper cervical spinal cord following stimulation of the superior sagittal sinus in the cat. *Brain Res* 1993;629:95–102.
25. Kris MG, Radford JE, Pizzo BA, Inabinet R, Hesketh A, Hesketh PJ. Use of an NK$_1$ receptor antagonist to prevent delade emesis after cisplatin. *J Natl Cancer Inst* 1997;89:817–818.
26. Laird JMA, Hargreaves RJ, Hill RG. Effect of RP67580, a non-peptide neurokinin-1 receptor antagonist, on facilitation of a nociceptive spinal flexion reflex in the rat. *Br J Pharmacol* 1993;109:713–718.
27. Lampl C, Buzath A, Klinger D, Neumann K. Lamotrigine in the prophylactic treatment of migraine aura—a pilot study. *Cephalalgia* 1999;19:58–63.
28. Lassen LH, Ashina M, Christiansen I, et al. Nitric oxide synthase inhibition: a new principle in the treatment of migraine attacks. *Cephalalgia* 1998;18:27–32.
29. Leysen JE, Gommeren W, Heylen L, et al. Alniditan, a new 5-hydroxytryptamine$_{1D}$ agonist and migraine-abortive agent: ligand-binding properties of human 5-hydroxytryptamine$_{1D\alpha}$, human 5-hydroxytryptamine$_{1D\beta}$, and calf 5-hydroxytryptamine$_{1D}$ receptors investigated with [^{3}H]5-hydroxytryptamine and [^{3}H]alniditan. *Mol Pharmacol* 1996;50: 1567–1580.
30. Longmore J, Hill RG, Hargreaves RJ. Neurokinin-receptor antagonists: pharmacological tools and therapeutic drugs. Can J *Physiol Pharmacol* 1997;75:612–621.
31. Ma QP, Woolf CJLeaR. Tachykinin NK$_1$ receptor antagonist RP67580 attenuates progressive hypersensitivity of flexor reflex during experimental inflammation in rats. *Eur J Pharmacol* 1997;322:165–171.
32. MaassenVanDenBrink A, Reekers M, Bax WA, Ferrari MD, Saxena PR. Coronary side-effect potential of current and prospective antimigraine drugs. *Circulation* 1998;98:25–30.
33. MacIntyre PD, Bhargava B, Hogg KJ, Gemmill JD, Hillis WS. Effect of subcutaneous sumatriptan, a selective 5HT$_1$ agonist, on the systemic, pulmonary, and coronary circulation. *Circulation* 1993;87:401–405.
34. Moskowitz MA. Neurogenic versus vascular mechanisms of sumatriptan and ergot alkaloids in migraine. *Trends Pharmacol Sci* 1992;13: 307–311.
35. Moskowitz MA. Neurogenic inflammation in the pathophysiology and treatment of migraine. *Neurology* 1993;43:S16–S20.
36. Moskowitz MA, Macfarlane R. Neurovascular and molecular mechanisms in migraine headaches. *Cerebrovasc Brain Metab Rev* 1993;5: 159–177.
37. Olesen J, Thomsen LL, Lassen LH, Olesen IJ. The nitric oxide hypothesis of migraine and other vascular headaches. *Cephalalgia* 1995;15: 94–100.
38. Parsons AA. Recent advances in mechanisms of spreading depression. *Curr Opin Neurol* 1998;11:227–231.
39. Phebus LA, Johnson KW, Stengel PW, Lobb KL, Nixon JA, Hipskind PA. The non-peptide NK-1 receptor antagonist LY303870 inhibits neurogenic dural inflammation in guinea pigs. *Life Sci* 1997;60: 1553–1561.
40. Phebus LA, Johnson KW, Zgombick JM, et al. Characterization of LY344864 as a pharmacological tool to study 5-HT$_{1F}$ receptors: binding affinities, brain penetration and activity in the neurogenic dural inflammation model of migraine. *Life Sci* 1997;61:2117–2126.
41. Rist B, Lacroix JS, Entzeroth M, Doods HN, Beck-Sickinger AG. CGRP 27-37 analogues with high affinity to the CGRP$_1$ receptor show antagonistic properties in a rat blood flow assay. *Regul Pept* 1999;79: 153–158.
42. Roon K, Diener HC, Elllis Pea. CP122,288 blocks neurogenic inflammation but is not effective in aborting migraine attacks: Results of two clinical trials. *Cephalalgia* 1997;17:245.
43. Rupniak NM, Boyce S, Williams AR, et al. Antinociceptive activity of NK$_1$ receptor antagonists: non-specific effects of racemic RP67580. *Br J Pharmacol* 1993;110:1607–1613.
44. Saxena PR. The effects of antimigraine drugs on the vascular responses by 5-hydroxytryptamine and related biogenic substances on the external carotid bed of dogs: possible pharmacological implications to their antimigraine action. *Headache* 1972;12:44–54.
45. Saxena PR, De Vlaam-Schluter GM. Role of some biogenic substances in migraine and relevant mechanism in antimigraine action of ergotamine-studies in an experimental model for migraine. *Headache* 1974; 13:142–163.
46. Saxena PR, Ferrari MD. 5-HT$_1$-like receptor agonists and the pathophysiology of migraine. *Trends Pharmacol Sci* 1989;10:200–204.

47. Shepheard SL, Williamson DJ, Beer MS, Hill RG, Hargreaves RJ. Differential effects of 5-HT$_{1B/1D}$ receptor agonists on neurogenic dural plasma extravasation and vasodilation in anaesthetized rats. *Neuropharmacology* 1997;36:525–533.

48. Shepheard SL, Williamson DJ, Hill RG, Hargreaves RJ. The non-peptide neurokinin$_1$ receptor antagonist RP67580 blocks neurogenic plasma extravasation in the dura mater of rats. *Br J Pharmacol* 1993;108:11–12.

49. Shepheard SL, Williamson DJ, Williams J, Hill RG, Hargreaves RJ. Comparison of the effects of sumatriptan and the NK$_1$ antagonist CP-99,994 on plasma extravasation in dura mater and c-*fos* mRNA expression in trigeminal nucleus caudalis of rats. *Neuropharmacology* 1995;34:255–261.

50. Stepien A, Chalimoniuk M. Level of nitric oxide-dependent cGMP in patients with migraine. *Cephalalgia* 1998;18:631–634.

51. Takagi H, Takashima M, Liou SY. Effect of KB-2796, a novel calcium channel blocker, on spreading depression in rat hippocampal slices. *Nippon Yakurigaku Zasshi* 1998;115:309–316.

52. Tattersall FD, Rycroft W, Francis B, et al. Tachykinin NK$_1$ receptor antagonists act centrally to inhibit emesis induced by the chemotherapeutic agent cisplatin in ferrets. *Neuropharmacology* 1996;35:1121–1129.

53. The Subcutaneous Sumatriptan International Study Group. Treatment of migraine attacks with sumatriptan. *N Engl J Med* 1991;325:316–321.

54. Thomsen LL, Olesen J. Nitric oxide theory of migraine. *Clin Neurosci* 1998;5:28–33.

55. van Gelderen EM, De Bruijne EL, Agteresch HJ, Saxena PR. The effect of nitric oxide donors on haemodynamics and blood flow distribution in the porcine carotid circulation. *Br J Pharmacol* 1995;114:1303–1309.

56. Van Gelderen EM, Saxena PR. Inhibition of nitric oxide biosynthesis and carotid arteriovenous anastomotic shunting in the pig. *Br J Pharmacol* 1994;111:961–967.

57. van Rossum D, Hanisch UK, Quirion R. Neuroanatomical localization, pharmacological characterization and functions of CGRP, related peptides and their receptors. *Neurosci Biobehav Rev* 1997;21:649–678.

58. Watson JW, Gonsalves SF, Fossa AA, et al. The anti-emetic effects of CP-99,994 in the ferret and the dog: role of the NK$_1$ receptor. *Br J Pharmacol* 1995;115:84–89.

59. Williamson DJ, Hargreaves RJ, Hill RG, Shepheard SL. Intravital microscope studies on the effects of neurokinin agonists and calcitonin gene-related peptide on dural vessel diameter in the anaesthetized rat. *Cephalalgia* 1997;17:518–524.

60. Williamson DJ, Hargreaves RJ, Hill RG, Shepheard SL. Sumatriptan inhibits neurogenic vasodilation of dural blood vessels in the anaesthetized rat—intravital microscope studies. *Cephalalgia* 1997;17:525–531.

The Headaches, Second Edition,
edited by J. Olesen, P. Tfelt-Hansen, and K.M.A. Welch.
Lippincott Williams & Wilkins, Philadelphia © 2000.

The Migraines

CHAPTER 54

Antiemetic, Prokinetic, Neuroleptic, and Miscellaneous Drugs in the Acute Treatment of Migraine

Peer Tfelt-Hansen

Nausea and vomiting are common symptoms of migraine (48) and are often as distressing as the headache. Thus, in addition to analgesics or more specific antimigraine drugs, antinauseant agents are often used. For possible future use of antiemetics in migraine, the reader is referred to Dahlöf and Hargreaves (15).

During a migraine attack the absorption of orally administered drugs may be delayed (50,51,53,63,64,66, 68,69). This is possibly due to gastric stasis, which contribute to the failure of some patients to respond to treatment (68). These pharmacokinetic observations led to the use of metoclopramide in migraine by virtue of its antiemetic property and its ability to promote gastric emptying, the so-called gastric prokinetic effect (9,47).

Neuroleptics have been used in the acute treatment of migraine, as analgesics, and as antiemetics. Neuroleptics are also frequently used in the treatment of status migrainous (14). Probably their most important role today is as an alternative to narcotics in emergency departments.

Several miscellaneous, alternative drugs for the treatment of migraine attacks deserve mention. These include drugs in common use despite limited evidence of efficacy in controlled double-blind trials (isometheptene combinations, dextropropoxyphen combinations, analgesic combination with antihistamines, morphinomimetics, and lidocaine).

ANTIEMETIC AND PROKINETIC DRUGS

Metoclopramide

Pharmacologic Background

Metoclopramide is a benzamide derivative and, although related to the neuroleptics, has no significant antipsychotic or sedative properties. Metoclopramide is a dopamine and 5-hydroxytryptamine 3 (5-HT$_3$) receptor antagonist (25,47) and also possesses some 5-HT$_4$ agonist activity (10,47). The actions of metoclopramide include antagonism of emesis induced by apomorphine or ergotamine (9); it also induces hyperprolactinemia, a characteristic of dopaminergic blockade (9,31,49). It can cause serious extrapyramidal dysfunction, especially after high intravenous dosage (9,31,49).

In the gastrointestinal tract, metoclopramide enhances the motility of smooth muscle from the esophagus through to the proximal small bowel. It thereby accelerates gastric emptying and the transit of intestinal contents from the duodenum to the ileocecal valve (9,47). The mechanism of this prokinetic effect has not been fully elucidated, but an agonistic effect on 5-HT$_4$ receptors on the enteric nerve plexus has been postulated (10,47).

Pharmacokinetics

Metoclopramide is rapidly and completely absorbed after oral administration, but due to hepatic first-pass metabolism its bioavailability is reduced to about 75%. Metoclopramide is distributed rapidly to most tissues and

P. Tfelt-Hansen: Department of Neurology, Glostrup Hospital, University of Copenhagen, DK-2600 Copenhagen, Denmark.

readily crosses the blood–brain barrier and placenta. The half-life of the drug in plasma is 4 to 6 hours (9).

Pharmacokinetic Investigations of Oral Absorption during Migraine Attacks

In the first classical study by Volans on aspirin absorption during migraine attacks (68), it was shown that during established migraine attacks salicylate concentrations determined 30 and 60 minutes after administration of 900 mg effervescent aspirin were significantly lower than those in the control subjects, but between migraine attacks the same patients demonstrated normal aspirin absorption. The impairment of aspirin absorption was ascribed to delayed gastric emptying because radiologic investigations had shown gastric stasis during migraine (37,39). In the next studies two antinauseant agents, metoclopramide and thiethylperazine (the latter lacking the prokinetic activity), were tested for their possible effect on aspirin absorption during a migraine attack (69,71). Both drugs were given in a dose of 10 mg intramuscularly followed 10 minutes later by 900 mg effervescent aspirin. As was previously found, aspirin absorption was impaired during migraine, but metoclopramide normalized it. In those who had received thiethylperazine, aspirin absorption remained impaired. In a later study in which both aspirin and salicylate concentrations were measured following effervescent aspirin administration to patients during migraine attacks (53), the delay observed for aspirin reaching its absorption sites was not seen after 10 mg metoclopramide, given orally or intramuscularly. The oral absorption of the nonsteroidal antiinflammatory drug (NSAID) tolfenamic acid was found to be impaired during migraine attacks, but the decreased absorption was reversed after 20 mg metoclopramide rectally (66). The absorption of paracetamol (64), naproxen (50), sumatriptan (51), and zolmitriptan (63) also was found to be slightly delayed during migraine attacks.

Clinical Trials with Metoclopramide

For controlled clinical trials concerning the combination of NSAIDs plus metoclopramide, the reader is referred to Chapter 50.

Metoclopramide alone was not better than placebo in treating nausea (65), whereas the combinations of metoclopramide and tolfenamic acid (65), metoclopramide and paracetamol and diazepam (62), and metoclopramide and aspirin (61) were better than placebo. This might be interpreted paradoxically as indicating that metoclopramide itself was not an effective migraine antinauseant in the absence of an analgesic.

The possible enhancing effect of metoclopramide on the efficacy of analgesics in migraine has been difficult to demonstrate formally. Thus, metoclopramide just failed to enhance analgesia in one study (62) ($p = 0.06$), and increased the efficacy of tolfenamic acid only for some parameters, such as intensity of attack as a whole (65), whereas it failed to enhance the analgesic effect of effervescent aspirin (61). The efficacy of combinations of highly soluble aspirin salt and metoclopramide (see Chapter 50) indicate, however, that metoclopramide enhances the analgesic effect of analgesics. In controlled trials there was no convincing evidence for the usefulness of the combination of metoclopramide and ergotamine (28,55).

Metoclopramide (10 mg intravenously) was found to be better than placebo in patients with severe migraine presenting at an emergency department (60), indicating that metoclopramide per se might have an effect on the migraine attack, apparently confirming an earlier anecdotal observation (33). In contrast, intramuscular metoclopramide was without any effect on migraine pain (62). In one study, intravenous metoclopramide (0.1 mg/kg) was as successful as intravenous chlorpromazine (0.1 mg/kg) both given in repeated doses up to three times every 15 minutes (11), but the lack of a placebo control precludes firm conclusions. In another trial in emergency departments, 10 mg metoclopramide intravenously was inferior to 10 mg prochloperazine intravenously and not different from placebo (13). In controlled trials there is thus no convincing evidence for the effect of metoclopramide per se on migraine attacks.

Therapeutic Use

Metoclopramide is combined with orally administered drugs in the treatment of migraine attacks based on a twofold rationale: it is an antiemetic, and it can normalize the delayed absorption of orally administered drugs, thereby optimizing their use. For the use of metoclopramide in combination with NSAIDs, the reader is referred to Chapter 50. Based on clinical experience, metoclopramide can probably also be used to increase the efficacy of oral triptans in some patients.

The dose of metoclopramide is 10 to 20 mg orally, 20 mg by suppository, or 10 mg intramuscularly. If there is a risk of vomiting, we recommend that patients wait 10 to 20 minutes after taking or receiving the metoclopramide before taking the analgesic drugs by mouth in order to allow sufficient time for the prokinetic effect to develop.

The side effect of metoclopramide 10 mg intravenously, akathisia, normally precludes its use in the treatment of migraine attacks. Metoclopramide (5 mg intravenously) is sometimes used as an antiemetic when intravenous dihydroergotamine is given (see Chapter 66).

Other side effects include sedation and dystonic reactions such as torticollis, trismus, facial spasm, and oculogyric crisis (the extrapyramidal side effects are usually seen after single parenteral doses of metoclopramide).

Contraindications include pheochromocytoma, breastfeeding, and treatment with neuroleptics. Use in children under 12 years of age is also contraindicated.

Domperidone

Domperidone is a derivative of benzimidazole that possesses both antiemetic and prokinetic properties. It is a dopaminergic antagonist and produces marked hyperprolactinemia (8,9). The effects of domperidone on gastrointestinal motility closely resemble those of metoclopramide. Domperidone, however, crosses the blood–brain barrier poorly and therefore rarely causes extrapyramidal side effects.

Domperidone is rapidly absorbed after oral administration [time to peak plasma concentration (t_{max}) = 30 minutes)], whereas rectal absorption is slower (t_{max} = 60 minutes). Its oral and rectal bioavailability is only about 15%. The half-time for its elimination from plasma is about 7.5 hours (8).

In one double-blind crossover controlled trial, domperidone 20 mg and 30 mg orally plus 1 g paracetamol in repeated doses was found to decrease the duration of migraine attacks compared with placebo plus paracetamol, whereas there was no statistically significant effect on headache and nausea (44).

In addition, in two placebo-controlled trials, domperidone 30 mg given orally at the start of premonitory symptoms of migraine was better than placebo for the prevention of impending attacks of migraine (3,70). The mechanism for this effect of domperidone remains unclear but has been ascribed to hypersensitivity of dopamine receptors in migraine patients (70).

Therapeutically, domperidone is an alternative for patients who have previously experienced side effects to metoclopramide. It also can be recommended for children below the age of 12, a group especially at risk of developing extrapyramidal side effects after metoclopramide. The dose in children is 0.2 mg/kg. For adults the oral dose is 10 to 20 mg and 30 to 60 mg by suppository. Our personal experience with the use of domperidone during premonitory symptoms have been rather disappointing.

Side effects include sedation, acute dystonia (rarely), hyperprolactinemia, and galactorrhea. Contraindications include pheochromocytoma and concomitant treatment with neuroleptics.

Other Antiemetics

Despite the fact that neuroleptics such as chlorpromazine and prochlorperazine have, for many years, been given either by injection or suppository to combat the nausea of migraine, there is little evidence from controlled clinical trials to substantiate their usefulness. In one small study (36), prochlorperazine 10 mg intravenously was superior to placebo in treating nausea and vomiting, with success rates of 10 of 10 and 2 of 7, respectively. In another trial, chlorpromazine 1 mg/kg intramuscularly was superior to placebo for relief of nausea (46).

Therapeutically, neuroleptics and neuroleptic-type antiemetics can be used in the treatment of severe nausea and vomiting accompanying migraine attacks. The doses of chlorpromazine are 25 mg orally, 50 to 100 mg by suppository, and 25 mg intramuscularly. For prochlorperazine the doses are 10 mg orally, 25 mg by suppository, and 10 mg intramuscular. Thiethylperazine can be given as 10 mg orally, by suppository, and intramuscularly (9). Some of these drugs may have an effect per se on the migraine attack, as discussed later in this chapter.

Several histamine H_1-receptor antagonists (e.g., diphenhydramine, cyclizine, and promethazine) are muscarinic receptor antagonists, a property that may add to their antiemetic effect (4,47). The major disadvantage in the use of these drugs is drowsiness. In some countries these drugs (e.g., buclizine) are used as antiemetics in fixed combinations with analgesics.

Therapeutically, for the treatment of nausea and vomiting the dose of diphenhydramine is 25 to 50 mg by all routes of administration. For cyclizine the dose is 50 mg orally or intramuscularly. The dose of promethazine is 12.5 to 25 mg by all routes (9).

Side effects include drowsiness, dizziness, and dry mouth. Contraindications include hypersensitivity, glaucoma, and prostatic hypertrophy.

Neuroleptics

Pharmacologic Background

The phenothiazines are dopamine antagonists with a broad spectrum of pharmacologic activity. They also have varying degrees of activity on the serotonergic, histaminic, adrenergic, and cholinergic neurotransmitter systems, giving them differing efficacy and toxicity profiles (5,24,43). The diverse actions with an effect on so many neurotransmitters makes the mode of action in acute migraine therapy highly speculative.

Regarding other actions of phenothiazines, the neuroleptics are believed to exert their powerful antiemetic effects by blocking dopamine receptors in the chemoreceptor trigger zone on the floor of the fourth ventricle. The phenothiazine methotrimeprazine has an analgesic effect (42). The phenothiazines are often strong α-adrenergic antagonists and can induce postural hypotension. This is less prominent with the piperazine phenotiazine prochlorperazine, which is mainly used as an antiemetic. Chlorpromazine as well as methotrimeprazine have sedative effects, whereas this is less prominent with prochlorperazine. The risk for acute extrapyramidal reactions is greatest with prochlorperazine (5).

Results of Clinical Trials with Neuroleptics

A summary of four placebo-controlled randomized clinical trials (13,35,36,46) with parenteral neuroleptics in

TABLE 1. *Placebo-controlled, double-blind randomized trials of neuroleptics for the treatment of migraine attacks in emergency departments*

Trial (ref.)	Drug	Drug dosage (mg)	Study design	No. of patients evaluated	Result of trials
(46)	CPZ PL	1/kg (IM)	Pa	36	Treatment success[a] CPZ (9/19) versus PI (4/17), NS Relief of nausea: CPZ (15/17) > PI (4/14)
(36)[b]	PCPZ PI	10 (IV)	Pa	82	Complete headache relief: PCPZ (31/42) > PI (5/40)
(13)	PCPZ Metoc PI	10 (IV) 10 (IV)	Pa	70	Clinical success[c]: PCPZ (82%) > Metoc (46%) = PI (29%)
(35)	PCPZ Metoc PI	10 (IM) 10 (IM)	Pa	86	Changes in median pain score (10 cm VAS scale): PCPZ (67%) > Metoc (34%) = PI (16%)

[a]Enough improvement to perform everyday activities and complete relief.

[b]Plus 5 mg dimenhydrinate IV; the trial included both migraine attacks (n = 41), tension-type headaches (n = 18), and combined migraine-tension headaches (n = 23); only 10 of 23 migraine patients had nausea and vomiting.

[c]Patients satisfied and a decrease of more than 50% in pain score on a VAS scale after 30 minutes.

CPZ, chlorpromazine; Metoc, metoclopramide; PCPZ, prochlorperazine; Pa, parallel group; PI, placebo; VAS, visual analogue scale; NS, no significant difference; >, significantly better; IM, intramuscularly; IV, intravenously.

the treatment of migraine attacks in emergency departments is given in Table 1. In one trial (36) investigating prochloperazine, both patients with severe migraine and tension-type headaches were included, and the pure migraine attacks accounted only for 50% of 82 attacks treated. In this trial prochloperazine (10 mg intravenously) was superior to placebo. The efficacy of prochlorperazine (10 mg intravenously) was, however, confirmed in a trial (13) demonstrating its superiority compared with both metoclopramide (10 mg intravenously) and placebo. Intramuscular prochlorperazine (10 mg) was found superior to metoclopramide (10 mg intramuscularly) and placebo (35) regarding decrease in perceived pain, but rescue medication was necessary in the majority of patients treated with both prochloperazine (16 of 28) and metoclopramide (23 of 29), suggesting that neither drug is effective as single-agent therapy. In contrast, chlorpromazine (1 mg/kg intramuscularly) was not superior to placebo for headache relief, but better for relief of nausea (46). The efficacy parameters used varied considerably among trials (see Table 1), making it difficult to compare the results and judge their clinical relevance.

In two trials comparing the efficacy of repeated intravenous chlorpromazine [0.1 mg/kg (40) and 12.5 mg (7) with meperidine (0.4 mg/kg) (40), and dihydroergotamine (1 mg) and lidocaine (50 mg) (7)], chlorpromazine was superior to the comparative drugs. Use of escape medication, a clinically relevant parameter, was only needed in 8% (40) and 21% (7) of patients after chlorpromazine. The use of the single-blind design (7) weakens the conclusions to some extent, but the two trials taken together indicate some efficacy of intravenous chlorpromazine for the treatment of migraine attacks.

In one trial comparing methotrimeprazine intramuscularly (37.5 mg) with mepiridine (75 mg) in combination with dimenhydrinate (50 mg), the results were quite similar in the two treatment groups (59). The lack of a placebo control weakens the conclusion that can be drawn.

In one double-blind trial in an emergency department, prochlorperazine (25 mg rectally) was superior to placebo in the treatment of migraine attacks (34).

The side effects of neuroleptics are a major concern when given parenterally. Intramuscular chlorpromazine caused more drowsiness (79%) and asymptomatic blood pressure decrease than did placebo (18%) (46), whereas intravenous chlorpromazine in patients pretreated with normal intravenous saline induced either the same incidence of side effects as mepiridine (7) or less than dihydroergotamine (40). Methotrimeprazine intramuscularly caused more prolonged drowsiness (52%) than did mepiridine (17%) (59). In contrast, intravenous prochlorperazine caused no more side effects than placebo (36), and intramuscular prochloperazine caused no more side effects than metoclopramide (35).

In conclusion, there is evidence for prochlorperazine being effective in the treatment of migraine attacks. Based on its being more effective than mepiridine, intravenous chlorpromazine probably have some efficacy in migraine attacks.

Therapeutic Use

The phenothiazine neuroleptics have been studied primarily in emergency departments as an alternative to narcotics, and to triptans because of their costs (38).

Prochlorperazine 10 mg intravenously can be given without the need for administering saline, and repeated after 30 minutes. The patient should rest for 1 hour. Methotriperazine can be given intramuscularly in doses of 12.5 to 25 mg. Again, there should be at least 1 hour of rest and the patient should be accompanied and advised to remain in bed for 6 hours (59). This scheme limits the use of methotriperazine. Given the risk of hypotension, an intravenous line should be established and 500 ml normal saline should be administered before chlorpromazine. We recommend an initial dose of 10 mg chlorpromazine intravenously, to be repeated if necessary after 30 to 60 minutes. At least 1 hour of bed rest is required after chlorpromazine administration. Concerning the use of neuroleptics as antiemetics, the reader is referred to the preceding section. The most common side effects after parenteral neuroleptics are sedation and postural hypotension (both less with prochlorperazine), and extrapyramidal symptoms such as a feeling of restlessness (probably akathisia). Acute dystonic reactions are in our experience rare.

Contraindications include hypersensitivity to the drugs, pregnancy, treatment with neuroleptics, patients with a history of seizures, low blood pressure, postural hypotension, treatment with antihypertensive drugs, and cardiac disease.

MISCELLANEOUS DRUGS

Isometheptene

Isometheptene, a sympathomimetic amine, is used in combination medications together with dichloralphenazone (in the United States) and paracetamol (acetaminophen). The rationale for this combination is the supposed combined action of a vasoconstrictor, isometheptene, a mild sedative, dichloralphenazone, and a mild analgesic, paracetamol. However, as described below, there is no evidence from controlled trials that the combination is more effective than isometheptene alone (54).

Pharmacologic Background

Isometheptene is an indirectly acting sympathomimetic that causes vasoconstriction and stimulation of the heart (57). Isometheptene is believed to exert its efficacy in migraine by a vasoconstriction in the head. In cats isometheptene caused a decrease in carotid blood flow and vigorously reduced the fraction of carotid blood flow shunted through the arteriovenous anastomoses, similar to the effect reported with ergotamine and dihydroergotamine (57). There have been no further investigations into the possible mechanisms of isometheptene in migraine. The pharmacokinetics of isometheptene mucate are not well established.

Results of Controlled Double-Blind Trials with Isometheptene

In two trials the isometheptene combination (65 mg isometheptene mucate 100 mg, dichloralphenazone 100 mg, and mg paracetamol 325; two tablets at onset and up to five to six tablets at 1-hour intervals, if necessary) was found to be superior (54) or marginally superior (17) to placebo. Isometheptene 130 mg (maximum three tablets) was found to be superior to placebo (19) and comparable with the isometheptene combination (54). In one trial the isopmethepene combination was not superior to paracetamol alone (17). In these studies there were similar side effects with the different treatment. In two trials, the isometheptene combination was either found marginally inferior (2) or superior (72) to a combination of ergotamine and caffeine. Side effects, mainly nausea and vomiting, occurred less frequently with the isometheptene combination than with ergotamine in both studies (2,72). In conclusion, these controlled trials demonstrate some efficacy of the isometheptene combination in the treatment of migraine attacks, but the combination has not been shown to be better than isometheptene alone.

Therapeutic Use

Two capsules can be given at onset of attack, followed by 1 capsule every hour if necessary (maximum five capsules in 12 hours). Caution is advised in patients with frequent headaches; anecdotal evidence suggests that this medication may cause rebound headache.

Side effects include dizziness and circulatory disturbances. Contraindications include glaucoma, concomitant treatment with monoamine-oxidase inhibitors or within 2 weeks of this treatment, porphyria, severe cases of renal disease, hypertension, organic heart disease, and hepatic disease.

Combinations of Analgesics and Antihistamines

The combination of an analgesic and an antihistamine with antiemetic effects in one tablet is motivated by the desire to simultaneously treat two symptoms of a migraine attack: head pain and nausea and vomiting. The analgesics used have been paracetamol and small doses of codeine (8–15 mg) with probably only minor analgesic effects. The histamine H_1-receptor antagonists used are buclizine and doxylamine. For pharmacology of these antiemetics, the reader is referred to preceding sections.

Results of Controlled Trials

Three double-blind, placebo-controlled randomized trials (1,56,67) with the combination of analgesics and antihistamines have been conducted.

In one trial the combination with doxylamine (Mersyndol; paracetamol 450 mg, codeine phosphate 9.75 mg, caffeine 30 mg, and doxylamine 5 mg) was found to be superior to placebo (56). The only side effect was drowsiness, which occurred more frequently with Mersyndol (57%) than with placebo (18%).

Two studies (1,67) compared the buclizine combination [Migraleve; paracetamol 500 mg, buclizine 6.25 mg, and codeine 8 mg (1) or 15 mg (67)] with placebo, and in our opinion even the study (1) claiming superiority for

Migraleve is questionable given the choice of endpoint variable. In this study the mean duration of attacks was quite similar after Migraleve (8.6 hours) and placebo (9.9 hours) (1). In the other study there was no evidence of a benefit compared with placebo (67).

In conclusion, there is no convincing evidence from these trials demonstrating that Migraleve is superior to placebo, and the comparability with other drugs remains to be elucidated.

Therapeutic Use

The combination of buclizine and analgesics can be given as two tablets containing 12.5 mg buclizine at the onset of a migraine attack, followed by two tablets without buclizine but the other components every 4 hours if necessary, to a maximum of six extra tablets.

Side effects include drowsiness, fatigue, and dry mouth. Contraindications include hypersensitivity to drugs, glaucoma, and driving a car or operating dangerous instruments.

Dextropropoxyphen Combinations

Dextropropoxyphene has been evaluated in the acute treatment of migraine with drug combinations consisting of dextropropoxyphene chloride (65 mg), acetyl salicylic acid (350 mg), and phenazone (150 mg) (30) or these drugs plus phentiazin caboxyl chloride (5 mg) and caffeine (50 mg) (29). Dextropropoxyphene produces analgesic and other central nervous system effects by binding primarily to μ-opioid receptors (52). Combinations of dextropropoxyphen and aspirin afford a higher level of analgesia than does either agent alone (6).

In two randomized, double-blind crossover trials (29,30), 25 female migraine patients treated seven attacks with each treatment. The drugs were taken at the onset of attacks, and the main efficacy parameter was prevention of an attack. The dextropropoxyphen combination prevented 37% to 41% of attacks and was comparable with ergotamine, which prevented 47% to 51% of attacks; both were superior to aspirin, which prevented only 16% to 18% of attacks (29,30).

These two trials demonstrate a moderate efficacy of the dextropropoxyphen combination with aspirin and phenazone in the treatment of migraine attacks [for contraindications and side effects, see e.g., ref. (52)].

Morphinomimetics

Despite evidence of poor efficacy and a high addiction potential, meperidine and other opioid analgesics remain in common use as abortive migraine drugs, particularly in the emergency room. Butorphanol nasal spray has been introduced for self-treatment of migraine attacks.

In a double-blind trial, meperidine with dimenhydrinate given intravenously was found inferior to chlorpromazine intravenously (40), and in another double-blind trial where this combination was given intramuscularly, it was comparable with methotrimeperazine (59). The NSAID ketorolac 30 mg intramuscularly was found to be less effective than meperidine 75 mg (41), whereas a dose of 60 mg ketorolac intramuscularly was as effective as 75 mg meperidine (plus 25 mg promethazine) (16), and 100 mg meperidine (plus 50 mg hydroxyzine) (20). In one double-blind trial, 1 mg dihydroergotamine intramuscularly was found to have similar effect as meperidine (1.5 mg/kg intramuscularly), both combined with the antinauseant hydroxyzine (12). All these trials with meperidine lacked placebo controls, precluding a real judgment of the effect of meperidine in migraine attacks.

The available clinical studies fail to support firmly the usefulness of parenteral morphinomimetics in the treatment of migraine headache, and with the current alternatives we find no support for their use.

Transnasal butorphanol, a synthetic opioid agonist (κ-opioid receptor) antagonist (μ-opioid receptor) analgesic, has been introduced as a noninvasive presentation of an analgesic for moderate to severe pain (26). It also has been registered for use for migraine in the United States, where its ease of administration has been used as a selling point. There is no pharmacokinetic interaction between intranasal butorphanol and sumatriptan (58). In a double-blind trial in migraine and a few cluster headache patients in an emergency department, 2 mg and 3 mg butorphanol intramuscularly produced more pain relief than 1 mg butorphanol (22).

Transnasal butorphanol 1 mg in repeated doses has been compared with placebo in two double-blind trials. In the first trial, butorphanol 1 mg followed by 1 mg 1 hour later, given to 32 patients, was more effective than placebo (n = 31) in relieving moderate to severe pain over the 6-hour study period (18). Butorphanol was also superior to methadone 10 mg intramuscularly given to 32 patients at some but not all time points (18). In another trial, migraine patients with moderate or severe headache could use up to 12 sprays of either butorphanol (n = 107) or placebo (n = 50) over 24 hours (32). From half an hour up to 40 hours, butorphanol was significantly better than placebo ($p < 0.01$), with a therapeutic gain (success rates for active minus success rates for placebo) of from 28% [95% confidence interval (CI) 18%–39%] at half an hour to 41% (95% CI 26%–56%) at 6 hours. The adverse events drowsiness (29% versus 0%) and dizziness (58% versus 4%) were often intense; and 26% of butorphanol-treated patients chose not to repeat use of the drug for the remainder of the headache due to side effects. In addition, 7% of butorphanol-treated patients experienced euphoria versus none on placebo; and a few patients described strong psychotropic effects such as an out-of-body sensation. Fifty-seven percent of patients rated the drug as poor.

In a comparative double-blind trial, the combination of the oral drug Fiorinal with codeine (butalbital 50 mg, caffeine 50 mg, aspirin 325 mg, and codeine phosphate 30 mg; n = 139) was found inferior to intranasal butorphanol 1 mg plus an optional 1 mg (n = 136) for treating migraine pain during the first 2 hours as measured by pain intensity difference and time to response (27). At 2 hours, more patients treated with butorphanol (60%) than patients treated with Fiorinal with codeine (47%) had responded. In contrast, more patients rated Fiorinal with codeine (46%) than butorphanol (27%) as good to excellent, most likely due to more adverse events with butorphanol (78%) than with Fiorinal with codeine (31%). In conclusion, these trials with transnasal butorphanol demonstrated a rapid onset of action, but its use is hampered by many adverse events, probably leading to the low rating of the drug by the patients in the controlled trials (27,32). Furthermore, the addiction potential of the drug is not sufficiently elucidated (23) and may be a problem according to the unpublished experiences of many headache experts. The use of transnasal buthorphanol in migraine must therefore be regarded as controversial. Transnasal butorphanol should only be used as a last resort in patients failing to respond to several other acute migraine treatments. Its use should probably be restricted to a maximum of eight doses per month.

Other Drugs

Intranasal lidocaine administered as a 4% solution was found superior to placebo in the treatment of migraine attacks in one double-blind controlled trial (45). Within 15 minutes, 29 of 53 lidocaine-treated patients had a more than 50% reduction in headache, whereas this was only the case in 6 of 28 placebo-treated patients. Relapse of headache occurred in 42% of patients responding to lidocaine, usually within the first hour after treatment. Intranasal lidocaine can thus be tried when a quick effect is needed, but probably only in a minority of attacks will a sustained effect result. Repeated dosing may be needed.

In open clinical studies, corticosteroids have mainly been used in the treatment of status migrainosus, a migraine attack lasting more than 72 hours (see Chapter 66). Based on the anecdotal evidence, corticosteroids, particularly dexamethasone 12 to 20 mg intravenously, can be used in the treatment of status migrainosus. A repeated parenteral dose, or its oral equivalent, may be necessary in 8 to 12 hours, but treatment beyond 24 hours is not generally recommended (21). If corticosteroids have not terminated status migrainosus within 24 hours, they are unlikely to do so later (21).

REFERENCES

1. Adam EI. A treatment for the acute migraine attack. *J Intern Med Res* 1987;15:71–75.
2. Adams M, Aikman P, Allardyce K, Baird H, et al. General practitioner clinical trials:treatment of migraine. *Practitioner* 1971;206:551–554.
3. Amery WK, Waelkens J. Prevention of the last chance: an alternative pharmacological treatment of migraine. *Headache* 1983;23:37–38.
4. Babe KS Jr, Serafin WE. Histamine, bradykinin, and their antagonists. In: Hardman JG, Limbird LE, Molinoff PB, Ruddon RW, Gilman AG, eds. *Goodman and Gilman's: the pharmacological basis of therapeutics,* 9th ed. New York: McGraw-Hill, 1996:581–600.
5. Baldessarini RJ. Drugs and the treatment of psychiatric disorders: psychosis and anxiety. In: Hardman JG, Limbird LE, Molinoff PB, Ruddon RW, Gilman AG, eds. *Goodman and Gilman's: the pharmacological basis of therapeutics,* 9th ed. New York: McGraw-Hill, 1996:399–430.
6. Beaver WT. Impact of non-narcotic oral analgesics on pain management. *Am J Med* 1988;84[Suppl 5A]:3–15.
7. Bell R, Montoya D, Shuaib A, Lee M. Comparative trial of three agents in the treatment of acute migraine. *Ann Emerg Med* 1990;19:1079–1082.
8. Brogden RN, Carmine AA, Heel RC, Speight TM, Avery GS. Domperidone. A review of its pharmacological activity, pharmacokinetics and therapeutic efficacy in the symptomatic treatment of chronic dyspepsia and as an antiemetic. *Drugs* 1982;24:360–400.
9. Brunton LL. Agents affecting gastrointestinal water flux and motility; emesis and antiemetics; bile acids and pancreatic enzymes. In: Hardman JG, Limbird LE, Molinoff PB, Ruddon RW, Gilman AG, eds.. *Goodman and Gilman's: the pharmacological basis of therapeutics,* 9th ed. New York: McGraw-Hill, 1996:917–936.
10. Buchheit K-H, Buhl T. Prokinetic benzamides stimulate peristaltic activity in the isolated guinea pig ileum by nactivation of 5-HT$_4$ receptors. *Eur J Pharmacol* 1991;205:203–208.
11. Cameron JD, Lane PL, Speechley M. Intravenous chlorpromazine vs intravenous metoclopramide in acute migraine headache. *Acad Emerg Med* 1995;2:597–602.
12. Carleton SC, Shesser RF, Pietrzak MP, et al. Double-blind, multicenter trial to compare the efficacy of intramuscular dihydroergotamine plus hydroxyzine versus intramuscular meperidine plus hydroxyzine for the emergency department treatment of acute migraine headache. *Ann Emerg Med* 1998;32:129–138.
13. Coppola M, Yealy DM, Leibold RA. Randomized, placebo-controlled evaluation of prochlorperazine versus metoclopramide for emergency department treatment of migraine headache. *Ann Emerg Med* 1995;26:541–546.
14. Couch JR, Diamond S. Status migrainous, causative and therapeutic aspects. *Headache* 1983;23:94–101.
15. Dahlöf CGH, Hargreaves RJ. Pathophysiology and pharmacology of migraine. Is there a place for antiemetics in future treatment strategies? *Cephalalgia* 1998;18:593–604.
16. Davis CP, Torre PR, Williams C, et al. Ketorolac versus meperidine-plus-promethazine treatment of migraine headache: evaluations by patients. *Am J Emerg Med* 1995;13:146–150.
17. Diamond S. Treatment of migraine with isometheptene, acetaminophen, and dichloralphenazone combination: a double-blind, crossover trial. *Headache* 1976;15:282–287.
18. Diamond S, Freitag FF, Diamond ML, et al. Transnasal butorphanol in the treatment of migraine headache pain. *Headache Q* 1992;3:164–171.
19. Diamond S, Medina J. Isometheptene—a non-ergot drug in the treatment of migraine. *Headache* 1975:15:212–213.
20. Duarte C, Dunaway F, Turner L, Aldag J, Frederick R. Ketorolac versus meperidine and hydroxyzine in the treatment of acute migraine headache: a randomized, prospective, double-blind trial. *Ann Emerg Med* 1992;21:1116–1121.
21. Edmeads J. Emergency management of headache. *Headache* 1988;28:675–679.
22. Elenbaas RM, Iacono CU, Koellner KJ, et al. Dose effectiveness and

safety of butorphanol in acute migraine headache. *Pharmacotherapy* 1991;11:56–63.

23. Fisher MA, Glass S. Butorphanol (Stadol): a study in problems of current drug information and control. *Neurology* 1997;48:1156–1160.

24. Fozard J. Basic mechanisms of antimigraine drugs. *Adv Neurol* 1982;33:295–307.

25. Fozard JR, Morabarok Ali ATM. Blockade of neuronal tryptamine receptors by metoclopramide. *Eur J Pharmacol* 1978;49:109–112.

26. Gillis JC, Benfield P, Goa KL. Transnasal butorphanol. A review of its pharmacodynamic and pharmacokinetic properties, and therapeutic potential in acute pain management. *Drugs* 1995;50:157–175.

27. Goldstein J, Gawel MJ, Winner P, et al., on behalf of the Stadol Nasal Spray/Fiorinal C study group. Comparison of butorphanol nasal spray and Fiorinal with codeine in the treatment of migraine. *Headache* 1998;38:516–522.

28. Hakkarainen H, Allonen H. Ergotamine vs. metoclopramide vs. their combination in acute migraine attacks. *Headache* 1982;22:10–12.

29. Hakkarainen H, Gustafsson B, Stockman O. A comparative trial of ergotamine tartrate, acetyl salicylic acid and a dextropropoxyphene compound in acute migraine attacks. *Headache* 1978;18:35–39.

30. Hakkarainen H, Quiding H, Stockman O. Mild analgesics as an alternative to ergotamine in migraine. A comparative trial with acetylsalicylic acid, ergotamine tartrate, and a dextropropoxyphene compound. *J Clin Pharmacol* 1980;20:590–595.

31. Harrington RA, Hamilton CW, Brogden RN, Linkewich JA, Romankiewicz JA, Heel RC. Metoclopramide. A updated review of its pharmacological properties and clinical use. *Drugs* 1983;25:451–494.

32. Hoffert MJ, Couch JR, Diamond S, et al. Transnasal butorphanol in the treatment of acute migraine. *Headache* 1995;35:65–69.

33. Hughes JB. Metoclopramide in migraine. *Med J Aust* 1977;2:580.

34. Jones EB, Gonzalez ER, Boggs JG, Grillo JA, Elswick RK Jr. Safety and efficacy of rectal prochlorperazine for the treatment of migraine in the emergency department. *Ann Emerg Med* 1994;24:237–241.

35. Jones J, Pack S, Chun E. Intramuscular prochloperazine versus metoclopramide as a single-agent therapy for the treatment of acute migraine headache. *Am J Emerg Med* 1996;14:262–265.

36. Jones J, Sklar D, Dougherty J, White W. Randomized double-blind trial of intravenous prochorperazine for the treatment of acute headache. *JAMA* 1989;261:1174–1176.

37. Kaufman J, Levine I. Acute gastric dilatation of stomach during attack of migraine. *Radiology* 1936;27:301–302.

38. Kelly A-M, Ardagh M, Curry C, D'Antonio J, Zebic S. Intravenous chlorpromazine versus intramuscular sumatriptan for acute acute migraine. *J Accid Emerg Med* 1997;14:209–211.

39. Kreel L. The use of metoclopramide in radiology. *Postgrad Med J* 1973;49[Suppl 4]:42–46.

40. Lane P, McLellan B, Baggoley C. Comparative efficacy of chlorpromazine and meperidine with dimenhydrinate in migraine headache. *Ann Emerg Med* 1989;18:360–365.

41. Larkin GL, Prescott JE. A randomized, double-blind, comparative study of the efficacy of ketorolac tromethamine versus meperidine in the treatment of severe migraine. *Ann Emerg Med* 1992;21:919–924.

42. Lasagna L, Dekornfeld J. Methotrimeprazine: a new phenothiazine derivative with analgesic properties. *JAMA* 1961;178:887–890.

43. Leysen J, Niemegeers C, Tollenaere J, Laduron P. Serotoninergic component of neuroleptic receptors. *Nature* 1978;272:169–171.

44. MacGregor EA, Wilkinson M, Bancroft K. Domperidone plus paracetamol in the treatment of migraine. *Cephalalgia* 1993;13:124–127.

45. Maizels M, Scott B, Cohen W, Chen W. Intranasal lidocaine for treatment of migraine: a randomized, double-blind, controlled trial. *JAMA* 1996;276:319–321.

46. McEwen J, O'Connor H, Dinsdale H. Treatment of migraine with intramuscular chlorpromazine. *Ann Emerg Med* 1987;16:758–763.

47. Mitchelson F. Pharmacological agents affecting emesis. A review (part I). *Drugs* 1992;43:295–315.

48. Olesen J. Some clinical features of the acute migraine attack. An analysis of 750 patients. *Headache* 1978;18:268–271.

49. Pinder RM, Brogden LN, Sawyer PR, Speight TM, Avery GS. Metoclopramide: a review of its pharmacological properties and clinical use. *Drugs* 1976;12:81–131.

50. Pini LA, Bertolotti M, Trenti T, Vitale G. Disposition of naproxen after oral administration during and between migraine attacks. *Headache* 1993;33:191–194.

51. Plosker GL, McTavish D. Sumatriptan. A reappraisal of its pharmacology and therapeutic efficacy in the acute treatment of migraine and cluster headache. *Drugs* 1994;47:622–651.

52. Reisine T, Pasternak G. Opioid analgesics and antagonists. In: Hardman JG, Limbird LE, Molinoff PB, Ruddon RW, Gilman AG, eds. *Goodman and Gilman's: the pharmacological basis of therapeutics,* 9th ed. New York: McGraw-Hill, 1996:521–555.

53. Ross-Lee LM, Eadie MJ, Heazlewood V, Bochner F, Tyrer JH. Aspirin pharmacokinetics in migraine. The effect of metoclopramide. *Eur J Clin Pharmacol* 1983;24:277–785.

54. Ryan R. A study of midrin in the symptomatic relief of migraine headache. *Headache* 1974;14:33–42.

55. Slettness O, Sjaastad O. Metoclopramide during attacks of migraine. In: Sicuteri F, ed. *Headache: new vistas.* Florence: Biomedical Press, 1977:201–204.

56. Somerville B. Treatment of migraine attacks with an analgesic combination (mersyndol). *Med J Aust* 1976;1:865–866.

57. Spierings ELH, Saxena PR. Effect of isometheptene on the distribution and shumting of 15 microM microspheres throughout the cephalic circulation of the cat. *Headache* 1980;20:103–106.

58. Srinivas NR, Shyu WC, Upmalis D, Lee JS, Barbhaiya RH. Lack of pharmacokinetic interaction between butorphanol tartrate nasal spray and sumatriptan succinate. *J Clin Pharmacol* 1995;35:432–437.

59. Stiell I, Dufour D, Moher D, et al. Methotrimeprazine versus meperidine and dimenhydrinate in the treatment of severe migraine: a randomized, controlled trial. *Ann Emerg Med* 1991;20:1201–1205.

60. Tek DS, McClellan DS, Olshaker JS, Allen CL, Arthur DC. A prospective, double-blind study of metoclopramide hydrochloride for the control of migraine in the emergency department. *Ann Emerg Med* 1990;19:1083–1087.

61. Tfelt-Hansen P, Olesen J. Effervescent metoclopramide and aspirin (Migravess) versus effervescent aspirin or placebo for migraine attacks: a double-blind study. *Cephalalgia* 1984;4:107–111.

62. Tfelt-Hansen P, Olesen J, Aebelholt-Krabbe A, Melgaard B, Veilis B. A double-blind study of metoclopramide in the treatment of migraine attacks. *J Neurol Neurosurg Psychiatry* 1980;43:369–371.

63. Thomsen LL, Dixon R, Lassen LH, et al. 311C90 (zolmitriptan), a novel centrally and peripherally acting oral 5-hydroxytrypyamine-1D agonist: a comparison of its absorption during a migraine attack and in a migraine-free period. *Cephalalgia* 1996;16:270–275.

64. Tokola RA. The effect of metoclopramide and prochlorperazine on the absorption of effervescent paracetamol in migraine. *Cephalagia* 1988;8:139–147.

65. Tokola RA, Kangasneimi P, Neuvonen PJ, Tokola O. Tolfenamic acid, metoclopramide, caffeine and their combinations in the treatment of migraine attacks. *Cephalalgia* 1984;4:253–263.

66. Tokola RA, Neuvonen PJ. Effects of migraine attacks and metoclopramide on the absorption of tolfenamic acid. *Br J Clin Pharmacol* 1984;17:67–85.

67. Uzogara E, Sheehan DV, Manschreck TC, Jones KJ. A combination drug for acute common migraine. *Headache* 1986;26:1986.

68. Volans GN. Absorption of effervescent aspirin during migraine. *BMJ* 1974;4:265–269.

69. Volans GN. The effect of metoclopramide on the absorption of effervescent aspirin in migraine. *Br J Clin Pharmacol* 1975;2:57–63.

70. Waelkens J. Dopamine blockade with domperidone: bridge between prophylactic and abortive treatment of migraine? A dose-finding study. *Cephalalgia* 1984;4:85–90.

71. Wainscott G, Kaspi T, Volans GN. The influence of thiethylperazine on the absorption of effervescent aspirin in migraine. *Br J Clin Pharmacol* 1976;3:1015–1021.

72. Yuill G. A double-blind crossover trial of isometheptene cucate compound and ergotamine in migraine. *Br J Clin Pract* 1973;26:73–79.

The Headaches, Second Edition,
edited by J. Olesen, P. Tfelt-Hansen, and K.M.A. Welch.
Lippincott Williams & Wilkins, Philadelphia © 2000.

The Migraines

CHAPTER 55

Prioritizing Acute Pharmacotherapy of Migraine

Peer Tfelt-Hansen

Treatment should be prioritized as a joint venture between doctor and patient. The vast majority of migraine attacks are and should be treated by the patients at home or at work. The following discussion focuses on information necessary to the physician in helping patients choose the best treatment for their migraine attacks (for treatment in a surgery setting or in an emergency department, see Chapter 132).

As mentioned in the discussion of general principles of pharmacologic treatment (see Chapter 49), acute treatment should be tailored to the individual patient, taking into account available drugs, efficacy versus side effects, contraindications, suitability, convenience, acceptability of route of administration, and costs. An overview of some of these factors is given in Table 1. In addition, treatment should be selected based on the overall severity of the patient's disease. The patient with occasional mild migraine has different treatment needs than the patient with frequent disabling migraine. Finally, treatment also should be tailored to the individual attack, taking into account severity, duration, and whether treatment is taken at the beginning of an attack or whether a full-blown attack is to be treated as when an attack is fully developed upon awakening.

As shown in Table 1, the availability of drugs differs considerably. Whereas aspirin is available worldwide, this is not the case for the triptans. The author's opinions on efficacy and occurrence of side effects for the current drugs for treatment of migraine attacks are indicated in Table 1. The variability of reporting results in different controlled clinical trials for older drugs such as ergotamine and nonsteroidal antiinflammatory drugs (see Chapters 50 and 51) makes it impossible to compare

these results with the results reported for the triptans in recent years in controlled clinical trials (see Chapter 52). Relatively few controlled clinical trials, eight with sumatriptan and one with eletriptan (see Chapter 52), have compared standard treatment with a triptan, and we will probably never have a definite scientific foundation for the rating of efficacy and side effects as given in Table 1.

Sumatriptan given as a subcutaneous injection has therapeutic gain (proportion of patients responding to active drug minus proportion of patients responding to placebo) of 50% after 1 hour in controlled clinical trials (for results with the triptans, see Chapter 52) and is rated as the most efficacious. Oral, intranasal, and rectal sumatriptan are less effective than subcutaneous sumatriptan, with therapeutic gains of approximately 30% after 2 hours, and similar results are reported for oral zolmitriptan and oral rizatriptan. Oral naratriptan in the low dose chosen for clinical use has a therapeutic gain of approximately 20% after 2 hours. Oral sumatriptan was found to be superior to oral ergotamine and somewhat more effective than aspirin plus metoclopramide in one trial and comparable with this combination in another trial. Intranasal and subcutaneous sumatriptan were both superior to intranasal dihydroergotamine, whereas rectal sumatriptan was inferior to rectal ergotamine plus caffeine in one trial. Subcutaneous sumatriptan was superior to subcutaneous dihydroergotamine for the first 2 hours, but the two drugs were comparable at later time points.

Speed of onset is highly valued by patients (2), and subcutaneous sumatriptan has an onset of action after 10 minutes, intranasal sumatriptan after 15 minutes, and 50 to 100 mg sumatriptan and 10 mg rizatriptan after 30 minutes. Oral rizatriptan has demonstrated a quicker onset of action than oral sumatriptan in comparative clinical trials. It should be noted that, apart from subcutaneous sumatriptan, this early effect of the triptans is of

P. Tfelt-Hansen: Department of Neurology, Glostrup Hospital, University of Copenhagen, DK-2600 Glostrup, Copenhagen, Denmark.

TABLE 1. *Availability, efficacy, side effects, convenience/acceptability of route of administrations, and costs for currently used medication for migraine attacks rated from + to ++++*

Drug	Availability worldwide	Efficacy	Side effects	Convenient/ acceptable[a]	Costs
Aspirin	++++	+ to ++	+	++++	+
Paracetamol	++++	+	+	++++	+
Triptans					
Sumatriptan					
Tablets	++	+++	+ to ++	++++	++++
Intranasal	++	+++	+ to ++	+++	++++
Suppositories	++	+++	+ to ++	++	
Subcutaneous injection[b]	++	++++	++	+ to ++	++++
Zolmitriptan tablets	++	+++	+ to ++	++++	++++
Naratriptan tablets	++	++	+[c]	++++	++++
Rizatriptan tablets	++	+++	+ to ++	++++	++++
Rizatriptan wafer[d]	++	+++	+ to ++	++++	++++
Ergot alkaloids					
Ergotamine					
Tablets	+++	+ to ++	++	++++	++
Suppositories	++	+++	+++	++	++
Injections[e]	+	+++[f]	++++	+	++
Inhalator[g]	+	+	+	++	++
Dihydroergotamine					
Injections	++	+++[h]	++	+	++
Intranasal	+	++	+ to ++	+++	++
NSAIDs	+++	++	+	++++	++
NSAIDS + metoclopramide	++	++ to +++	+	++++	++

The ranking is based on a combination of my judgment of the literature and my personal experience and may be different in the experience of others.

[a]Convenience/acceptability depends heavily on cultural factors (see text).

[b]An autoinjector device is used.

[c]In controlled clinical trials, the low 2.5-mg dose of naratriptan caused no more side effects than placebo.

[d]A rapidly dissolving oral wafer.

[e]Not generally suitable for self-medication because of the side effects.

[f]Based on old uncontrolled trials (4) and my personal experience.

[g]In my experience it is only a minority of patients that can use this device effectively.

[h]Subcutaneous dihydroergotamine has a slower onset of action than subcutaneous sumatriptan (see text).

relatively small magnitude (see Fig. 6 in Chapter 52). Thus, if a quick and clinically significant effect is needed, subcutaneous sumatriptan is probably the best alternative. Due to their pharmacodynamic properties, ergot alkaloids are generally more slowly acting drugs than the triptans (see Chapter 51).

The classic drug ergotamine, which has effects on many receptors (see Chapter 51), undoubtedly also has the most side effects, and increased nausea may limit oral use of the drug. Using routes of administration with higher bioavailability such as suppositories or injections may increase side effects such as nausea and vomiting. A subnauseating dose of ergotamine suppositories should be determined (see Chapter 51). Injections with ergotamine are not generally suitable for self-medication because of the side effects, but subcutaneous dihydroergotamine causes fewer side effects than parenteral ergotamine. Nonsteroidal antiinflammatory drugs (NSAIDs) have been comparable with oral ergotamine and generally have fewer side effects (see Chapter 50). Subcutaneous sumatriptan 6 mg causes more transient side effects than

100 mg oral sumatriptan, which causes generally the same side effects as oral zolmitriptan and oral rizatriptan. The lower 25- and 50-mg doses of sumatriptan and the 2.5-mg dose of naratriptan cause in controlled clinical trials no more side effects than placebo. Sumatriptan 100 mg causes more side effects than the combination of aspirin plus metoclopramide, whereas rectal sumatriptan causes fewer side effects than rectal sumatriptan.

Contraindications can determine the choice of drugs. Whereas NSAIDs are contraindicated in patients with a peptic ulcer, they can be the drug of first choice for migraine patients with cardiovascular diseases, in whom ergot alkaloids and triptans are contraindicated.

The choice between routes of administration depends on convenience, suitability, and acceptability by patients. The most convenient way to administer drugs is normally by the oral route, but this may not be suitable in a migraine attack with severe nausea and vomiting. In this situation one can either treat the nausea with an antiemetic and prokinetic drug such as metoclopramide (see Chapter 54) or try alternative routes of administration to circumvent the problems. The alternatives routes of administration are subcutaneous injection, rectal administration, sublingual administration, inhalation, and intranasal administration; but only a few of the drugs for acute migraine treatment—sumatriptan and the ergot alkaloids ergotamine and dihyergotamine—are available in these forms. Even if a route of administration is convenient and suitable, it may not be acceptable for the patient; for example, some patients detest injecting themselves. Furthermore, there are considerable cultural differences in the acceptability of routes of administration, as exemplified by the following citation from a British textbook on clinical pharmacology (3) on the use of ergotamine: "Suppositories are more effective than oral administration, though less effective than injection, but they are unpopular with all except a perverse minority." This statement would, of course, be unlikely in a French textbook.

If a migraine patient has, for example, one attack per month, then the abuse potential is not important, but in patients with frequent migraine attacks or a mixture of migraine attacks and frequent or daily tension-type headaches, the abuse potential should be a primary factor in drug selection (see Chapter 115). Thus, any instant-relief drug for headache, when taken daily or almost daily, seems to induce more migraine or headache, leading to a vicious circle. The risk is greatest with opioids, which in my opinion are never indicated for migraine. Ergotamine is also easily abused and should not be taken more than twice a week (see Chapter 51). Abuse of triptans, most often in previous drug abusers, also has been reported (see Chapter 52).

The costs of migraine drugs should be taken into account. Depending on the country and the availability of health insurance, cost may be an issue for the health-care system, the government, or the patient. In some countries, patients do not pay for their medication. The drugs used for treatment of migraine attacks vary, from inexpensive drugs such as aspirin and paracetamol (acetaminophen), the drugs used for most migraine attacks worldwide, to relatively inexpensive drugs such as ergotamine and NSAIDs, to expensive drugs such as the triptans. It can be argued that a very expensive but effective drug such as sumatriptan is not that expensive when the cost and benefits for the patients and the society are taken into account (see Chapter 5). In one placebo-controlled clinical trial, subcutaneous sumatriptan was found to reduce productivity loss during migraine attacks (1). Even if there is a general benefit to society, the price of triptans may still limit their use in many patients. Currently, many of our patients are aware of the price differences, especially between ergot alkaloids, NSAIDs combined with metoclopramide, and triptans, and ask advice on which of the these drugs to use, because they envisage the use of drugs for migraine for years. We advise patients to treat three attacks with each of these alternatives. Patients can then decide whether there is a difference in effectiveness and side effects that justifies the price difference. Similar single-case experiments also can be undertaken for other drugs or forms of administration of a drug.

REFERENCES

1. Cady RC, Ryan R, Jhingran P, O'Quinn S, Pait G. Sumatriptan injection reduces productivity loss during a migraine attack. Results of a double-blind, placebo-controlled trial. *Arch Intern Med* 1998;158: 1013–1018.
2. Göbel H, Petersen-Braun M, Heinze A. Which properties do patients expect of new and improved drugs in the treatment of primary headache disorders? In: Olesen J, Tfelt-Hansen P, eds. *Headache treatment: trial methodology and new drugs.* New York: Lippincott-Raven, 1997:93–97.
3. Laurence DR. *Clinical pharmacology,* 4th ed. Edinburgh: Churchill Livingstone, 1973:12.7.
4. Lennox WG. Ergonovine versus ergotamine as a terminator of migraine headaches. Am J Med Sci 1938;195:458–468.

The Headaches, Second Edition,
edited by J. Olesen, P. Tfelt-Hansen, and K.M.A. Welch.
Lippincott Williams & Wilkins, Philadelphia © 2000.

The Migraines

CHAPTER 56

β-Adrenoceptor Blocking Drugs in Migraine Prophylaxis

Peer Tfelt-Hansen and Robin G. Shanks

Beta-blockers (β-adrenoceptor antagonists) were introduced into medicine for the treatment of angina pectoris and cardiac arrhythmias, but they have subsequently proved valuable in many other conditions, including hypertension and migraine. The hypotensive action of these drugs was not predicted from their pharmacologic properties and was observed initially in patients receiving treatment for angina (39). Similarly, the value of propranolol in migraine was discovered in 1966 by Rabkin (41), who reported that migraine improved in a patient receiving propranolol for angina pectoris. Many controlled trials have since confirmed that propranolol is effective in the prophylaxis of migraine, and other beta-blocking drugs—namely nadolol, metoprolol, atenolol, and timolol—also have been demonstrated to be effective in the prophylaxis of migraine. In contrast, several beta-blocking drugs with partial agonist activity—alprenolol, oxprenolol, pindolol, and acebutolol—have not been demonstrated to be effective in migraine prophylaxis. Several reviews of the prophylactic use of beta-blocking drugs in the treatment of migraine have been published (3,46,53,55,57).

The mode of action of beta-blocking drugs in migraine remains to be elucidated, but the effective drugs are at present the drugs of first choice in migraine prophylaxis.

PHARMACOLOGIC BACKGROUND

The adrenergic receptors on which noradrenaline, the principal neurotransmitter at the peripheral sympathetic synapses, evokes responses have been classified as α and β types (1). α-receptors are abundant in the resistance vessels of the skin, mucosa, and kidney and result in vasoconstriction when stimulated. β-receptors have been subdivided into β_1-receptors, which predominate in the heart subserving myocardial excitation, and β_2-receptors in the arteries of the skeletal muscle and bronchi, subserving vasodilatation and bronchodilatation (28).

A beta-blocking drug, for example, propranolol, which has equal affinity for β_1- and β_2-receptors, is described as being a nonselective drug, whereas agents such as metoprolol and atenolol have greater affinity for β_1- than for β_2-receptors and are examples of β_1-selective blocking drugs, even though the selectivity is not absolute. Propranolol is a pure antagonist and has no capacity to activate β-adrenoceptors. Several beta-blocking drugs, for example, pindolol and acebutolol, activate β-receptors, but the intrinsic activities of these drugs are less than the full agonist, such as isoprenaline. These partial agonists are said to have intrinsic sympathomimetic activity (31). Some beta-blocking drugs possess properties in addition to their effect in blocking β-receptors. Membrane-stabilizing activity has a direct effect on nervous tissue in the heart and is similar to the effect of local anesthetics. Membrane-stabilizing activity is present for some of these agents (Table 1).

There are considerable differences in the pharmacokinetics of the beta-blocking drugs. The difference that could be important in the treatment of migraine might be expected to relate to the penetration of the drugs into the central nervous system. The entry of beta-blocking drugs into the central nervous system depends on protein binding, ionization and lipid solubility. Of these, the most important factor determining entry into the brain is lipid

P. Tfelt-Hansen: Department of Neurology, Glostrup Hospital, University of Copenhagen, DK-2600 Glostrup, Copenhagen, Denmark.

R. Shanks: Department of Therapeutics and Pharmacology, Queen's University of Belfast, Belfast BT9 7BL, United Kingdom.

TABLE 1. *Efficacy of β-adrenoreceptor blockers in migraine prophylaxis and their properties*

	Efficacy in migraine	Penetration into CNS	MSA	Cardioselective	PAA	Affinity for 5-HT in CNS[a]
Alprenolol	no	yes	yes	no	yes	high
Oxprenolol	no	yes	yes	no	yes	high
Propranolol	yes	yes	yes	no	no	high
Pindololol	no	yes	yes	no	yes	high
Nadolol	yes	—	no	no	no	—
Timolol	yes	yes	no	no	no	—
Acebutol	no	yes	yes	yes	yes	—
Atenolol	yes	poorly	no	yes	no	low
Metoprolol	yes	yes	no	yes	no	—
Practolol	?[b]	poorly	no	yes	yes	—

[a]As judged from inhibition of specific ^{3}H–5-HT binding to crude synaptic membrane from rats (35).
[b]Only an open trial reported efficacy of practolol before it was withdrawn due to side effects.
MSA, membrane-stabilizing activity; PAA, partial agonist activity.

solubility, for which there are great differences in beta-blocking drugs. Propranolol, alprenolol, oxprenolol, and metoprolol are extremely lipophilic and readily pass into the central nervous system. In contrast, atenolol is much more hydrophilic and passes into the central nervous system poorly (11).

For many years it has been suggested that 5-hydroxytryptamine (5-HT) may be involved in the development of a migraine attack, and several beta-blocking drugs have substantial affinity for the 5-HT binding site in the brain (see Table 1). Thus, alprenolol, oxprenolol, propranolol and pindolol, have high affinity for these binding sites, whereas atenolol has low affinity.

As clearly illustrated in Table 1 the fact that a beta-blocking drug is effective in migraine prophylaxis does not depend on whether it penetrates easily into the central nervous system, whether it is cardioselective, or has membrane-stabilizing activity or binds to 5-HT sites in the brain. The only common property that the active beta-blocking drugs have in common is the lack of partial agonist activity. It does seem that partial agonist activity prevents beta-blocking drugs from exerting a beneficial effect in migraine prophylaxis, but the mechanism behind this remains obscure.

On the basis of one trial, it has even been questioned whether the efficacy of beta-blocking drugs in migraine is related to blockade of β-adrenoceptors (50). It was reported that propranolol, in the clinically used racemic form *d,l*-propranolol, and *d*-propranolol, which has only a slight beta-blocking effect, were significantly superior to placebo with no differences between the two forms of propranolol, indicating that an effect not related to beta-blockade was an important factor in the action of propranolol in the prophylaxis of migraine (50). However, when the results were reanalyzed using conventional statistical methods, there was a significant effect for *d,l*-propranolol on the headache index, but no significant effect for *d*-propranolol compared with placebo (53). For headache days there were no difference between the three treatments.

The trial thus did indicate that the beta-blocking effect per se is important in migraine prophylaxis.

WHAT IS THE MODE OF ACTION OF BETA-BLOCKING DRUGS IN MIGRAINE?

It was originally hypothesized that beta-blocking drugs were effective in migraine prophylaxis by inhibiting the vasodilatory phase of migraine. How this should be reconciled with the effectiveness of beta-blocking drugs in migraine with aura, where a decrease in cerebral blood flow is present, is not clear. In a study on migraine with aura there was no increase in aura without headache (26), and one might presume that the preventive effect of beta-blocking drugs must occur on the first phase of the attack, which clearly is perpetuating in the central nervous system.

There are some indications that beta-blocking drugs exert their effect on the central catecholaminergic system. The contingent negative variation (CNV)—an event-related, slow, negative cerebral potential recorded over the scalp in simple reaction time tasks with warning stimulants—is significantly increased and its habituation reduced in untreated migraine patients in comparison with controls and tension-type headache sufferers. The CNV returned to normal values after migraine prophylaxis with beta-blocking drugs (45). Furthermore, after 3 months' treatment with metoprolol or propranolol, it was shown that there was a significant correlation between CNV before treatment and the clinical response of beta-blocking drugs: patients with higher CNVs tended to respond better to therapy. This would indicate that in patients with central catecholaminergic hyperactivity, the chance of a positive response to beta-blocking drugs in migraine prophylaxis is better and indirectly points to an effect in the central nervous system being responsible for the migraine prophylactic effect. However, one cannot rule out that what is observed in this study is an epiphenomenon, and the mode of action of beta-blocking drugs still remains an enigma.

PHARMACOKINETICS OF BETA-BLOCKING DRUGS EFFECTIVE IN MIGRAINE

Propranolol is highly lipophilic and is well absorbed. Much of the drug is metabolized by the liver during its first passage through the portal circulation, resulting in 25% bioavailability. There is great interindividual variation in the presystemic clearance of propranolol, resulting in enormous variability in plasma concentration after oral administration of the drug (approximately 20-fold). Propranolol is extensively metabolized, and one of the products of hepatic metabolism is 4-hydroxypropranolol, which possess some beta-blocking effect. The half-life in plasma is about 4 hours but, as in hypertension, the drug is effective when administered twice daily. A sustained-release formulation of propranolol has been developed to maintain the concentration of propranolol in plasma over a 24-hour period (21).

Nadolol is hydrophilic and is incompletely absorbed. The bioavailability is 35%, and interindividual variability in bioavailability is less than with propranolol. Nadolol is not extensively metabolized and is largely excreted intact in the urine. The half-life of nadolol in plasma is in the range of 12 to 20 hours, and it can consequently be administered once daily. Nadolol may accumulate in patients with renal failure.

Timolol is well absorbed and is subject to moderate first-pass metabolism, resulting in a bioavailability of 50%. It is metabolized by the liver, and the half-life in plasma is about 4 hours. It can be administered twice daily.

Metoprolol is well absorbed, but there is considerable first-pass metabolism, resulting in about 40% bioavailability. Plasma concentrations of the drug vary widely (up to 17-fold), and the plasma half-life of metoprolol is 3 to 4 hours. It can be given twice daily. A sustained-released formulation of metoprolol has been developed to maintain the concentration in plasma over a 24-hour period; this formulation can be given once daily.

Atenolol is incompletely absorbed, but most of the absorbed drug reaches the systemic circulation, resulting in a bioavailability of 50%. There is relatively little variation in the plasma concentration of atenolol, with a four-fold range between patients. The drug is excreted largely unchanged in the urine, and the half-life in plasma is 5 to 8 hours. It can be given once daily and may accumulate in patients with renal failure.

RESULTS OF CLINICAL TRIALS WITH BETA-BLOCKING DRUGS IN MIGRAINE

On the basis of controlled clinical trials in which a beta-blocking drug was compared with a placebo, it can be concluded that propranolol, metoprolol, timolol, nadolol, and atenolol have documented efficacy in migraine prophylaxis (3).

The main effect has been to reduce the frequency of attacks in patients with migraine with aura and without aura. In most trials a mixed population of patients with migraine with aura and without aura have been included, but some trials (26,38,54) have studied these two forms of migraine separately and found similar results, as in the mixed patient populations. There is thus no reason to believe that the two forms of migraine respond differently to prophylaxis with beta-blocking drugs.

In this chapter, only trials in which beta-blocking drugs have been compared with placebo or in which two beta-blocking drugs have been compared with each other will be reviewed. In addition, for many years, propranolol has been the standard comparative drug for migraine prophylaxis and has been compared with several agents that are not beta-blocking drugs. These trials will be mentioned in the chapters concerning these agents, but generally the results have shown similar efficacy for the new drug and propranolol.

The crossover design comparing active drug against placebo has been used in most trials (Table 2). The

TABLE 2. *Controlled double-blind clinical trials comparing beta-blocking drugs with placebo in the prophylaxis of migraine*

Trial (ref)	Drug, dosage (mg)	Study design	No. of patients (no. evaluated), type of migraine	Run-in	Duration of treatment	Factors evaluated	Investigators' conclusion
(56)	Prop 20 qid	CO	25 (19) MO, MA		3 mo × 2	"Symptomatic response"	Prop > P1
(32)	Prop ? mg	CO	31 (29) MO	30 days open	6 wk × 2	Preference, headache units per day, relief medication	Prop very effective in some patients
(59)	Prop 40 qid	CO	45 (30) MO, MA (responders in pilot)	Open pilot study of Prop for 2–11 mo	3 mo × 2	Attack rate, preference	Prop > P1
(7)	Prop 40 qid	CO	45 (30) MO, MA	4 wk no drug	12 wk × 2	Frequency, preference	Prop > P1

TABLE 2. *Continued*

Trial (ref)	Drug, dosage (mg)	Study design	No. of patients (no. evaluated), type of migraine	Run-in	Duration of treatment	Factors evaluated	Investigators' conclusion
(30)	Prop 20/40 tid	CO	32 (28) children MO, MA		13 wk × 2	Frequency	Prop > Pl
(16)	Prop 80 tid	CO	40 (32) MO, MA	10 wk no drug	12 wk × 2	Attack rate, headache days, "integrated head-headache," relief medication	Prop > Pl
(12)	Prop 80–160/day	CO	83 (62) MO, MA		4–8 wk × 2	Preference, head-ache index, relief medication index	Pro > Pl
(22)	Prop 40 bid–tid	Pa	53 (36) MO, MA		12 wk	Migraine index, subjective rating	Pro = Pl
(34)	Prop 20–80 qid	CO	64 (41) MO, MA	6 wk dose-finding	12 wk × 2	Headache unit index, relief medication index	Prop > Pl
(31)	Prop LA	CO	38 (31) MO, MA		8 wk × 2	Frequency, severity, duration	PropLA > Pl
(40)	Prop LA 160	Pa	55 (41) MO	4 wk P1	12 wk	Frequency	Prop LA > Pl
(2)	Pro LA 80 Prop LA 160	CO	45 (30)	4 wk P1	8 wk (1 wk wash-out)	Frequency, duration, severity	Prop La 80 and Prop LA 160 vs. Pl NS
(47)	Pind 7.5–15 per day	CO	28 (24) MO, MA	3 wk no drug	4 wk × 2 (3 wk wash-out)	Headache index, headache days	Pind vs. Pl NS
(13)	Alpren 200 bid	CO	33 (28) MO, MA		6 wk × 2 (1 wk wash-out)	Frequency, preference, headache index	Alpren vs. Pl NS
(15)	Oxpren 80 tid	CO	34 (30) MO, MA		8 wk × 2 (1 wk wash-out)	Frequency, preference	Oxpren vs. Pl, NS
(35)	Acebut 400 bid	CO	43 (33) "migraine"	4 wk no drug	12 wk × 2 (4 wk washout)	Frequency	Acebut vs. Pl NS
(8)	Tim 10 bid	CO	14 MO, MA	4 wk no drug	6 wk × 4[a]	Frequency, preference	Tim > Pl
(49)	Tim 10 bid	CO	107 (94) MO, MA	4 wk P1	8 wk × 2	Frequency, global preference	Tim > Pl
(43)	Nad 80 od Nad 80 bid Nad 80 tid	Pa	80 (79) MO, MA	2 mo P1	3 mo	Frequency, severity	Nad in all groups > Pl
(4)	Met LA 200 od	Pa	71 (62) MO, MA	4 wk no drug	8 wk	Frequency migraine days, severity score, relief medication.	Met LA > Pl
(26)	Met LA 200 od	CO	77 (74) MA	4 wk no drug	8 wk × 2 (4 wk wash-out)	Frequency, migraine days, global dura-ion, relief medication	Met LA > Pl
(48)	Met 50–100 bid	Pa	59 (54) MO, MA	4 wk P1	8 wk	Frequency severity score, relief medication	Met vs. Pl NS[b]
(17)	Aten 100 od	CO	24 (20) MO, MA	60 days no drug	90 days × 2 (2 wk wash-out)	Frequency, integrated headache, relief medication	Aten > Pl
(25)	Aten 100 od	CO	72 (63) MO, MA	8 wk	12 wk × 2 (2 wk wash-out)	Integrated headache, migraine days	Aten > Pl

[a]Patients crossed over twice, receiving timolol during two periods and placebo during two.

[b]In the initial double-blind 12-week treatment there was no difference between metoprolol and placebo; but in a further follow-up of 12 weeks, nonresponders to placebo or metoprolol switching to metoprolol 50 bid or metoprolol 100 mg bid, respectively, resulted in significant improvement. *Acebut,* acebutol; *Alpren,* alprenolol; *Aten,* atenolol; *Met,* metoprolol; *Nad,* nadolol; *Oxpren,* oxprenolol; *Pind,* pindolol; *Prop,* propranolol; *Tim,* timolol; *LA,* long-acting, slow-release formulation; *Pl,* placebo; *od,* once daily; *bid,* twice daily; tid, three times daily; qid, four times daily; *CO,* crossover; *Pa,* parallel groups; *MO,* migraine without aura; *MA,* migraine with aura; *NS,* no statistically significant difference; >, more effective than.

Modified and extended from Andersson and Vinge (3).

blinding of the patients in these trials may be open to question because patients can often determine that they are on a beta-blocking drug because of the pulse-slowing effect, particularly during effort. There are also negative trials with beta-blocking drugs, however, suggesting that the blinding problem is not that great. In addition, it is reassuring that beta-blocking drugs also have been found effective in the parallel group design, where the problem with blinding is less important.

Beta-Blocking Drugs
Compared with Placebo

A number of double-blind controlled clinical trials comparing one beta-blocking drug against placebo are summarized in Table 2. A total of 1,184 patients were recruited for the trials, and 82% of the patients completing the treatments were evaluable. By modern standards, many of the early studies can be criticized from a methodologic point of view. In many studies there are too few patients and the treatment periods are short (e.g., 4 to 6 weeks). However, the conclusion that propranolol is effective in migraine prophylaxis has been confirmed in more recent trials with better methodology. In addition, nadolol, timolol, metoprolol, and atenolol have shown better efficacy than placebo in double-blind controlled clinical trials (see Table 2). However, in some trials propranolol failed to show a significant difference from placebo (2,22,51). It is most likely that the apparent lack of effect in these trials may be a statistical type 2 error (i.e., lack of power to detect the difference).

Beta-blocking drugs possessing partial agonist activity, pindolol, alprenolol, oxprenolol, and acebutolol showed no significant difference from placebo in several early trials (see Table 2). It was suggested by an open study with practolol that partial agonist activity does not exclude efficacy in migraine prophylaxis because good results were obtained in 39 and 43 patients treated (44), but this result has never been confirmed in a double-blind trial. The fact that the beta-blocking drugs with partial agonist activity were only studied in relatively small trials some time ago has led reviewers to state that the beneficial effect may have escaped detection (3). Since propranolol was found to be effective in similar small trials, the beta-blocking drugs with partial agonist activity probably are not effective in migraine.

In contrast to the demonstration of the prophylactic effect of beta-blocking drugs in migraine, two double-blind placebo-controlled trials (6,18) have not shown any effect of propranolol in the acute treatment of the migraine attack.

Clinical Trials Comparing
Two Beta-Blocking Drugs or Two Doses
of the Same Beta-Blocking Drug

Controlled double-blind clinical trials comparing the effect of two different beta-blocking drugs or two doses of one drug are summarized in Table 3.

The general results are that when two beta-blocking drugs are used in equipotent doses, determined by their effect on heart rate and blood pressure, they will be equally effective in migraine prophylaxis. The exception is one study in which nadolol 160 mg per day was significantly more effective than propranolol 160 mg per day (52).

These comparative clinical trials are in most cases probably too small to demonstrate any differences between two active treatments. Comparability should be evidenced by giving narrow confidence intervals. As illustrated in Figure 1, even when metoprolol and propranolol resulted in similar responses (27), wide confidence intervals showed that considerable differences in efficacy between the two drugs could have remained undetected. In a much larger crossover study (N = 80) (54), no difference between timolol and propranolol was found, although the study had a power of 0.88 to detect a difference of less than 25% between the two treatments. Thus, in this clinical trial, the two drugs were equipotent in their clinical effects. Another problem with most of the comparative trials is the lack of inclusion of placebo. Strictly speaking, a placebo also should be included in comparative trials to demonstrate that the active drugs had a significant effect (24). If two beta-blocking drugs are given, and there is a decrease compared with run-in, it could be due to the time effect (a decrease in frequency with time regardless of treatment) (24).

Generally, attempts to correlate plasma concentrations of beta-blocking drugs and their effect in migraine prophylaxis have failed (5,10,60), even when active metabolites of propranolol were taken into account (10). This does not excluded a dose-response relationship in the individual patients, and in some studies (9,48) higher doses seem to be more effective than the lower doses of a beta-blocker investigated.

The Efficacy of Beta-Blocking Drugs
in Clinical Trials

As demonstrated in Tables 2 and 3, the different designs and ways of reporting the results, sometimes with complicated headache indices, make it difficult to judge the percentage of patients benefiting from beta-blocker treatment in these trials. In a metanalysis (25) of results of both controlled trials and published open studies, with 2,403 patients treated with a modal dose of 160 mg pro-

TABLE 3. *Controlled double-blind clinical trials comparing 2 beta-blocking drugs or 2 doses of a beta-blocking drug in migraine prophylaxis*

Trial (ref)	Drug, dosage (mg)	Study design	No. of patients (no. evaluated), type of migraine	Run-in	Duration of treatment	Factors evaluated	Investigators' conclusion
(14)	Pind 2.5 tid Pind 5 tid	Pa	30 (26) MO, MA	4 wk no drug	4 wk	Frequency headache index, duration	Pind vs. PI, NS[a]
(50)	d,l-Prop 40 qid d-Prop	CO	20 (19) MO, MA		4 wk × 3 (1 wk washout)	Headache days, headache index	d,l-Prop > PI d-Prop vs. PI, NS[b]
(51)	Aten 50 bid Prop 80 bid	CO?	35 (28) MO, MA		6 wk × 2	Headache index, migraine days	Aten vs. Prop NS, Aten > PI, Prop vs. PI NS
(54)	Tim 10 bid Prop 80 bid	CO MO	96 (80)	4 wk no drug	12 wk × 3	Frequency, headache indices	Tim vs. Prop NS Tim > PI Prop > PI
(42)	Nad 80/day Nad 160/day Prop 160/day	Pa	48 (45) MO, MA	4 wk PI	12 wk	Frequency, headache index	"Suggest that both Nad and Prop reduce frequency and severity"
(37)	Nad 80–160/day Prop 80–160/day	Pa	28 (27) MO, MA	4 wk	24 wk 120 days PI?	Frequency, relief medication, duration	Nad vs. Prop NS[a]
(52)	Nad 80/day Nad 160/day Prop 160/day	Pa	140 (98) MO, MA	4–8 wk	12 wk	Several headache indices	Nad 160 > Prop 160 Nad 160 vs. Nad 80 NS
(27)	MetLA 200 od Prop 80 bid	CO	36 (35) MO, MA	4 wk PI (4 wk washout)	8 wk × 2	Frequency, severity, migraine days, relief medication	MetLA vs. Prop NS both > PI run-in
(38)	Met 50 bid Prop 80 bid	CO	56 (56) MO, MA	4 wk PI (4 wk washout)	8 wk × 2	Frequency, migraine days, severity, relief medication	Met vs. Prop NS, both > PI run-in
(20)	Prop LA 80 od Prop LA 160 od	CO	48 (42) MO, MA	4 wk PI (4 wk washout)	12 wk × 2	Frequency, migraine days, severity	Pro LA 80 vs. Prop LA 160 NS
(9)	Prop LA 80 od Prop LA 160 od Prop LA 80	CO	51 (37) MO, MA	4 wk PI (2 wk washout)	12 wk × 2	Frequency, duration, severity	Prop LA 160 >

[a]Too small a parallel trial to demonstrate a difference in our opinion.
[b]Not the author conclusion, but the conclusion after reanalysis with conventional statistical methods (56).
For abbreviations, see footnote to Table 2.
Modified and extended from Andersson and Vinge (3).

pranolol, it was reported that based on a headache index, the improvements were 44% compared with pretreatment and 33% compared with placebo. However, the composite nature of the headache index, taking both severity and duration of attacks into account, makes it difficult to extrapolate these results to clinical practice.

Side Effects in Clincal Trials of Beta-Blocking Drugs in Migraine Prophylaxis

The tolerability of beta-blocking drugs in migraine prophylaxis is an important issue because clinical expe-

rience has shown that some patients stop treatment because of the side effects produced by the drugs. In many of the above-mentioned controlled clinical trials there were not significantly more side effects with active drug than with placebo. This may be due to the trials including too few patients, to an inadequate side effects reporting system, or to an actual effect in which the drug did not produce side effects. In one relatively large crossover trial (54), two beta-blocking drugs, timolol and propranolol, resulted in significantly more side effects than placebo (Table 4). Timolol and propranolol induced side effects in 46% and 42%, respectively,

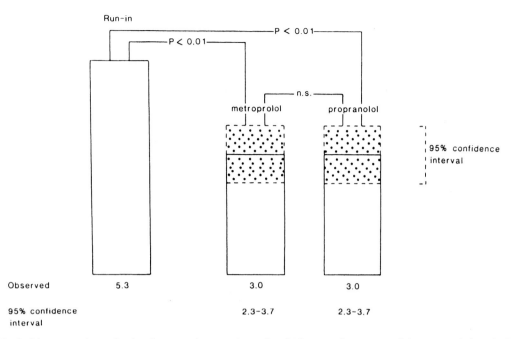

FIG. 1. Mean number of migraine attacks per 4 weeks during run-in, metoprolol, propanolol periods (*bars with unbroken lines*) (27). The dotted areas represent the 95% confidence intervals for the difference between the two drugs. Note that for both beta-blocking drugs the real mean frequency of attacks could be in the range of 2.3 to 3.7 per 4 weeks instead of the measured 3.0. The trial is thus too small to demonstrate comparability. From Tfelt-Hansen (53).

whereas 28% experienced side effects from placebo, and 11 of 96 patients withdrew from the trial because of side effects (9 patients on beta-blockers and 2 patients on placebo). Thus, in a well-designed trial there are more side effects on active drug than on placebo.

TABLE 4. *Side effects in 83 migraine patients in a double-blind three-way crossover trial comparing timolol (10 mg twice daily) and propranolol (80 mg twice daily) with placebo*

	Timolol	Propranolol	Placebo
With side effects	38	35	23
Without side effects	45	48	60
Most commonly reported side effects			
Fatigue/tiredness	18 (22%)	11 (13%)	15 (18%)
Dizziness	5 (6%)	4 (2%)	2 (2%)
Nausea	2 (2%)	5 (6%)	2 (2%)
Sleep disturbances	4 (5%)	3 (4%)	2 (2%)
Depression	2 (2%)	3 (4%)	0
Abnormal dreaming	2 (2%)	0	0

From Tfelt-Hansen et al. (54).

THERAPEUTIC USE OF BETA-BLOCKING DRUGS IN MIGRAINE PROPHYLAXIS

The doses and pharmacokinetic properties of beta-blocking drugs effective in migraine are summarized in Table 5. The effective therapeutic dosage range is wide, probably due to the large variability in bioavailability, which occurs with most beta-blocking drugs. Consequently, the dose of a beta-blocking drug should be titrated for each individual patient. The patients should start with the lowest dose indicated in Table 5; then, depending on efficacy and side effects, the dose can be increased gradually with 4 to 8 weeks between increases in doses. Until the patient has reached the final dose, the pulse and blood pressure should be controlled at each visit. The patients should try the highest dose they can tolerate without side effects for 2 months before the beta-blocking drug is deemed to be ineffective, and if there is no effect, another avenue of therapy should be explored.

To ensure a high level of compliance, it is recommended that patients take beta-blocking drugs twice a day, a frequency of dosing that has been found to be effective in controlled trials. With very low doses of propranolol the patient should probably take the dose three times a day. Nadolol and atenolol, which haves long half-lives, can be administered once a day. The same is the

TABLE 5. *Doses and pharmacokinetic properties of beta-blocking drugs effective in migraine*

	Tablets sizes (mg)	Daily dosage, range (mg)	Dosing (frequency per day)	Bioavailability	Half-life (h)	Primary metabolic route
Propranolol						
Regular	10,20,40,80,90	40–320	twice	25%	3–5	Hepatic
Long-acting	60,80,120,160	60–320	once			
Metoprolol						
Regular	50,100	50–200	twice	40%	3–4	Hepatic
Long-acting	50,100,200	50–200	once			
Nadolol	40,80,120,160	40–240	once	35%	12–20	Renal
Atenolol	50,100	50–200	once	50%	5–8	Renal
Timolol	10,20	10–20	twice	50%	3–5	Hepatic

case for the long-acting preparations of propranolol and metoprolol, which can be substituted for the short-acting forms in the same dosage once the effective dosage has been found.

Withdrawal symptoms can occur occasionally after a sudden cessation of propranolol therapy, but this is rare among migrainous patients. However, to avoid this potential but rare hazard, treatment with a beta-blocking drug should not be stopped abruptly, but the dose reduced gradually over a period of about 2 weeks. A few patients may note a worsening of their migraine when propranolol is begun. If this occurs, the dosage should be reduced. Patients should be warned in advance about this problem.

Which Beta-Blocking Drug Should Be Used in the Prophylactic Treatment of Migraine?

In our opinion, there is no evidence for one drug being more effective in migraine prophylaxis than another among those with proven efficacy. One should choose one of the effective beta-blocking drugs and make oneself familiar with that drug. However, if adverse effects of a central nervous system origin occur with, for example, propranolol, a change to atenolol could be made. The failure to respond to one beta-blocking drug does not generally predict the failure to respond to another; if available, several beta-blocking drugs could be used consecutively in the same patient.

Side Effects

Side effects to beta-blocking drugs generally occur in 10% to 15% of patients. The most common side effects are fatigue, cold extremities, gastrointestinal symptoms (flatulence, diarrhea, constipation), and dizziness. Side effects of central nervous system origin (19,21) include vivid dreams, nightmares, insomnia, depression, and memory disturbances. Impotence is a relatively rare side effect.

Contraindications

Contraindications to the use of beta-blocking drugs include asthma and chronic obstructive lung disease, congestive heart failure, partial or complete arterioventricular conduction defects, Raynaud's disease, peripheral vascular disease, and brittle diabetes.

Cautions

Beta-blocking drugs should not be used during actual abuse of ergotamine because it may precipitate overt ergotism (58).

REFERENCES

1. Ahlquist, RP. A study of the adrenotropic receptors. *Am J Physiol* 1948; 153:586–600.
2. Al-Qassab HK, Findley LJ. Comparison of propranolol LA 80 mg and propranolol LA 160 mg in migraine prophylaxis: a placebo controlled study. *Cephalalgia* 1993;13:128–131.
3. Andersson K-E, Vinge E. β-Adrenoceptor blockers and calcium antagonists in the prophylaxis and treatment of migraine. *Drugs* 1990;39: 355–373.
4. Andersson P-G, Dahl S, Hansen JH, et al. Prophylactic treatment of classical and non-classical migraine with metoprolol—a comparison with placebo. *Cephalalgia* 1983;3:207–212.
5. Baldrati A, Cortelli P, Procaccianti G, et al. Propranolol and acetylsalicylic acid in migraine propphylaxis. Double-blind crossover study. *Acta Neurol Scand* 1983;67:181–186.
6. Banerjee M. Findley L. Propranolol in the treatment of acute migraine attacks. *Cephalalgia* 1991;11:193–196.
7. Børgesen SE, Lang Nielsen J, Møller CE. Prophylactic treatment of migraine with propranolol. *Acta Neurol Scand* 1974;50:651–656.
8. Briggs RS, Millac PA. Timolol in migraine prophylaxis. *Headache* 1979;19:379–381.
9. Carroll JD, Reidy M, Savundra PA, Cleave N, McAinsh. Long-acting propranolol in the prophylaxis of migraine:a comparative study of two doses. *Cephalalgia* 1990;10:101–105.
10. Cortelli P, Sacquegna T, Albani F, et al. Propranolol plasma levels and relief of migraine:relationship between plasma propranolol and 4-hydroxypropranolol concentrations and clinical effects. *Arch Neurol* 1985;42:46–48.
11. Cruichshank JM, Prichard BNC. *Beta-blockers in clinical practice.* London: Churchill Livingstone, 1988:177–274.
12. Diamond S, Medina JL. Double blind study of propranolol for migraine prophylaxis. *Headache* 1982;22:268–271.
13. Ekbom K. Alprenolol for migraine prophylaxis. *Headache* 1975;15: 129–132.
14. Ekbom K, Lundberg PO. Clinical trial of LB-46 (d,1-4 (2-hydroxy-3-

isopropylaminopropoxy)indol). An adrenergic beta-receptor blocking agent in migraine prophylaxis. *Headache* 1972;12:15–17.

15. Ekbom K, Zetterman M. Oxprenolol in the treatment of migraine. *Acta Neurol Scand* 1977;56:181–184.

16. Forssman B, Henriksson KG, Johansson V, Lindvall L, Lundin H. Propranolol for migraine prophylaxis. *Headache* 1976;16:238–245.

17. Forssman B, Lindblad CJ, Zbornikova V. Atenolol for migraine prophylaxis. *Headache* 1983;23:188–190.

18. Fuller GN, Guiloff RJ. Propranolol in acute migraine: a controlled study. *Cephalalgia* 1990;10:229–233.

19. Gleiter CH, Deckert J. Adverse CNS-effects of beta-adrenoceptor blockers. *Pharmacopsychiatry* 1996;19:201–211.

20. Havanka-Kannianinen H, Hokkanen E, Myllylä VV. Long acting propranolol in the prophylaxis of migraine. Comparison of daily doses of 80 mg and 160 mg. *Headache* 1988;28:607–611.

21. Hoffman BB, Lefkowitz RJ. Catecholamines, sympathomimetic drugs, and adrenergic receptor anatagonists. In: Hardman JG, Limbird LE, Molinoff PB, Ruddon RW, Gilman AG, eds. *Goodman and Gilman's. The pharmacological basis of therapeutics*, 9th ed. New York: McGraw-Hill, 1996:199–248.

22. Holdorff B, Sinn M, Roth G. Propranolol in der Migräneprophylaxe. *Med Klin* 1977;72:1115–1118.

23. Holroyd KA, Penzien DB, Cordingley GE. Propranolol in the management of recurrent migraine: a meta-analytic review. *Headache* 1991;31:33–340.

24. International Headache Society committee on clinical trials in migraine. Guidelines for controlled trials in migraine. *Cephalalgia* 1991;11:1–12.

25. Johannson V, Nilsson LR, Widelius T, et al. Atenolol in migraine prophylaxis: a double-blind cross-over multicenter study. *Headache* 1987;27:372–374.

26. Kangasniemi P, Andersen AR, Andersson PG, et al. Classic migraine: effective prophylaxis with metoprolol. *Cephalalgia* 1987;7:231–238.

27. Kangasniemi P, Hedman C. Metoprolol and propranolol in the prophylactic treatment of classical and common migraine: a double-blind study. *Cephalalgia* 1984;4:91–96.

28. Lands AM, Arnold A, McAuliff JP, Ludena FP, Brown TG. Differentiation of receptor systems activated by sympathomimetic amines. *Nature* 1967;214:597–598.

29. Kuritzky A, Hering R. Prophylactic treatment of migraine with long acting propranolol—a comparison with placebo. *Cephalalgia* 1987;7:457–458.

30. Ludvigsson J. Propranolol used in prophylaxis of migraine in children. *Acta Neurol Scand* 1974;50:109–115.

31. McDevitt DG. The assessment of beta-adrenoceptor blocking drugs in man. *Br J Clin Pharmacol* 1977;4:413–425.

32. Malvea BP, Gwon N, Graham JR. Propranolol prophylaxis of migraine. *Headache* 1973;13:163–167.

33. Middlemiss DN, Blakeborough L, Leather SR. Direct evidence for an interaction of beta-adrenergic blockers with the 5-HT receptor. *Nature* 1977;267:289–290.

34. Nadelmann JW, Phil M, Stevens J, Saper JR. Propranolol in the prophylaxis of migraine. *Headache* 1986;26:175–182.

35. Nanda RN, Johnson RH, Gray J, Keogh HJ, Melville ID. A double blind trial of acebutol for migraine prophylaxis. *Headache* 1978;18:20–22.

36. Nies AS, Shand DG. Clinical pharmacology of propranolol. *Circulation* 1975;52:6–15.

37. Olerud B, Gustavsson C-L, Furberg B. Nadolol and propranolol in migraine management. *Headache* 1986;26:490–493.

38. Olsson J-E, Behring HC, Forssman, et al. Metoprolol and propranolol in migraine prophylaxis: a double blind multicentre study. *Acta Neurol Scand* 1984;70:160–168.

39. Prichard BNC. Hypotensive action of of pronethalol. *Br Med J* 1964;1:1227–1228.

40. Pradalier A, Serratrice G, Collard M, et al. Long-acting propranolol in migraine prophylaxis:results of a double-blind, placebo-controlled study. *Cephalalgia* 1989;9:247–253.

41. Rabkin R, Stables DP, Levin NW, Suzman MM. Propranolol and prophylaxis of angina pectoris. *Am J Cardiol* 1966;18:370–380.

42. Ryan RE. Comparative study of nadolol and propranolol in prophylactic treatment of migraine. *Am Heart J* 1984;108:1156–1159.

43. Ryan Sr RE, Ryan RE Jr, Sudilovsky A. Nadolol: its use in the prophylactic treatment of migraine. *Headache* 1983;23:26–31.

44. Sales F, Bada JL. Practolol and migraine. *Lancet* 1975;1:742.

45. Schoenen J, Maertens de Noordhout A, Timsit-Berthier M, Timsit M. Contingent negative variation and efficacy of beta-blocking agents in migraine. *Cephalalgia* 1986;6:229–233.

46. Shank RG. Mechanism of of action of beta-adrenoceptor antagonists in migraine. In: Carrol JD, Pfaffenrath V, Sjaastad O, eds. *Migraine and beta-blockade*. Uddevalla: AB Hässle, 1985:45–53.

47. Sjaastad O, Stenrud P. Clinical trial of a beta-receptor blocking agent (LB 46) in migraine prophylaxis. *Acta Neurol Scand* 1972;48:124–128.

48. Steiner TJ, Joseph R, Hedman C, Rose FC. Metoprolol in the prophylaxis of migraine: parallel-groups comparison with placebo and dose-ranging follow-up. *Headache* 1988;28:15–23.

49. Stellar S, Ahrens SP, Meibohm AR, Reines SA. Migraine prevention with timolol. *JAMA* 1984;252:2576–2579.

50. Stensrud P, Sjaastad O. Short-term clinical trial of propranolol in racemic form (Inderal), D-propranolol and placebo in migraine. *Acta Neurol scand* 1976;53:229–232.

51. Stensrud P, Sjaastad O. Comparative trial of Ternormin (atenolol) and Inderal (propranolol) in migraine. *Headache* 1980;20:204–207.

52. Sudilovsky A, Elkind AH, Ryan RE Sr, Saper JR, Stern MA, Meyer JH. Comparative efficacy of nadolol and propranolol in the management of migraine. *Headache* 1987;27:421–426.

53. Tfelt-Hansen P. Efficacy of beta-blocking drugs in migraine: a critical review. *Cephalalgia* 1986;6[Suppl 5];15–24.

54. Tfelt-Hansen P, Standnes B, Kangasniemi P, Hakkarainen H, Olesen J. Timolol vs propranolol vs placebo in common migraine prophylaxis: a double blind multicenter study. *Acta Neurol Scand* 1984;69:1–8.

55. Turner P. Beta-blocking drugs in migraine. *Postgrad Med J* 1984;60[Suppl 2]:51–55.

56. Weber RB, Reinmuth OM. The treatment of migraine with propranolol. *Neurology* 1972;22:366–369.

57. Weerasuriya K, Patel L, Turner P. β-Adrenoceptor blockade and migraine. *Cephalalgia* 1982;2:33–45.

58. Venter CP, Joubert PH, Buys AC. Severe peripheral ischaemia during concommitant use of beta blockers and ergot alkaloids. *Br Med J* 1984;289:288–289.

59. Widerœ T-E, Vigander T. Propranolol in the treatment of migraine. *BMJ* 1974;2:699–701.

60. Ziegler DK, Hurwitz A, Preskorn S, Hassanein R, Seim J. Propranolol and amitriptyline in the prophylaxis of migraine. Pharmacokinetic and therapeutic effects. *Arch Neurol* 1993;50;825–830.

The Headaches, Second Edition,
edited by J. Olesen, P. Tfelt-Hansen, and K.M.A. Welch.
Lippincott Williams & Wilkins, Philadelphia © 2000.

The Migraines

CHAPTER 57

Antiserotonin Drugs in Migraine Prophylaxis

Peer Tfelt-Hansen and Pramod R. Saxena

Antiserotonin drugs were the first group of effective agents available for migraine prophylaxis. Originally, these drugs were thought to act via antagonism at serotonin (5-hydroxytryptamine; 5-HT) D receptors (39), which are now classified as 5-HT$_2$ receptors (46,88). This view, however, does not seem tenable for several reasons. First, several selective and potent 5-HT$_2$ receptor antagonists, including ketanserin, ICI 169,369, sergolexole, and mianserin, are either ineffective or only weakly effective in migraine (83). Second, the antimigraine potency of these drugs does not correlate with their affinity at the 5-HT$_{2A}$, 5-HT$_{2B}$, or 5-HT$_{2C}$ receptors (91). Furthermore, the antimigraine drugs ergotamine and dihydroergotamine have an agonist (not antagonist) action at the 5-HT$_{2C}$ receptor (11). Thus, while conceding that the title of this chapter may be a misnomer, from the outset we wish to emphasize that the prophylactic effect of antiserotonin drugs in all likelihood does not depend on their antiserotonin property. For further discussion of mechanisms, see the discussions of the individual drugs.

METHYSERGIDE

Methysergide is a semisynthetic compound derived from the ergot alkaloid methylergometrine by adding a methyl group at the indole nitrogen (Fig. 1). It was introduced in pharmacotherapy as a specific 5-HT receptor antagonist (29,89). Methysergide has been considered the most potent 5-HT receptor antagonist for human use and has been used as an experimental tool to investigate the role of 5-HT in, for example, endocrinologic regulation

and certain central nervous system (CNS) functions (30,33,68).

Pharmacokinetics

Pharmacokinetic studies in humans have indicated that methysergide is probably only a prodrug; its main metabolite is methylergometrine (10). After oral administration, the bioavailability of methysergide was about 13%, most likely due to a high degree of first-pass metabolic conversion to methylergometrine (see Fig. 1) (10). Whereas the area under the plasma concentration curve (AUC) for methysergide and methylergometrine after intravenous administration of methysergide was in the same range, oral administration of methysergide resulted in an AUC that was 10 times greater for methylergometrine than for the parent drug (Fig. 2). The elimination half-lives of methysergide and methylergometrine were 60 and 220 minutes, respectively.

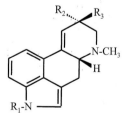

	Methysergide	Methylergonovine	Lisuride
R$_1$	-CH$_3$	-H	-H
R$_2$	-CO-NH-CH-CH$_2$-CH$_3$ ⌐CH$_2$OH	-CO-NH-CH-CH$_2$-CH$_3$ ⌐CH$_2$OH	-H
R$_3$	-H	-H	-NH-CO-N(CH$_2$CH$_3$)$_2$

FIG. 1. Chemical structure of methysergide, its metabolite methylergometrine, and lisuride.

P. Tfelt-Hansen: Department of Neurology, Glostrup Hospital, University of Copenhagen, DK-2600 Glostrup, Copenhagen, Denmark.

P. R. Saxena: Department of Pharmacology, Erasmus University, 3000 DR Rotterdam, The Netherlands.

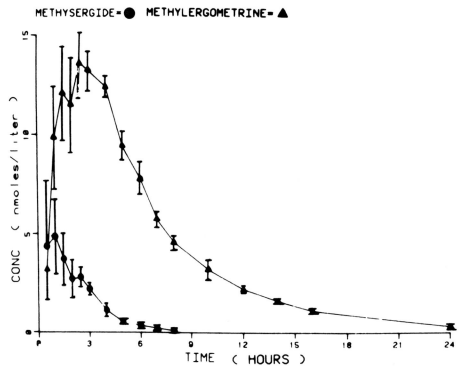

FIG. 2. Plasma concentration profiles of methysergide and methylergometrine after an oral dose of 2.0 mg methysergide (values are means ± SD, n = 5). From Bredberg et al. (10).

In contrast to methysergide, methylergometrine has dopaminergic activity (8). The metabolism of methysergide to methylergometrine probably explains why methysergide has little dopaminergic activity upon parenteral administration (8), but its oral administration can result in a significant decrease in the plasma prolactin level (30,33,68). Thus, when the "pure" 5-HT ligand methysergide is used orally in humans, there are serotonergic effects due both to the parent drug and the metabolite methylergometrine, as well as some dopaminergic effects due to the metabolite methylergometrine.

Pharmacologic Background

It is well known that methysergide is a potent a 5-HT$_2$ receptor antagonist, but it does not distinguish between the 5-HT$_{2A}$, 5-HT$_{2B}$, and 5-HT$_{2C}$ subtypes (91). Thus, methysergide antagonizes the contractile effects of 5-HT on vascular and nonvascular smooth muscles with a pA$_2$ of more than 8 (66). Indeed, in the human isolated temporal artery, which contains predominantly 5-HT$_2$ receptors (27), both methysergide and its active metabolite methylergometrine are potent antagonists; the latter compound is some 40 times more active than the parent drug (98). In the early 1970s, Saxena and co-workers reported that the vasoconstrictor effect of 5-HT within the canine carotid vascular bed was not much modified by methysergide or by two other potent 5-HT$_2$ receptor antago-

nists, mianserin and cyproheptadine (Fig. 3) (79,81,85). Therefore, the receptors for 5-HT in the external carotid vascular bed appeared to be of a novel type, which were later named 5-HT$_1$–like receptor (84). Interestingly, methysergide proved to be an agonist at these receptors

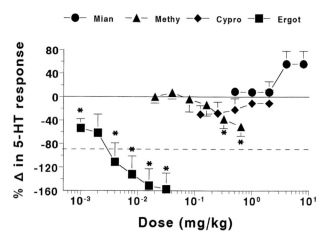

FIG. 3. Dog external carotid vascular bed. Effect of mianserin (*Mian*), methysergide (*Methy*), cyproheptadine (*Cypro*), and ergotamine (*Ergot*) on the vasoconstrictor response to serotonin. Values below the interrupted line (i.e., change more than -100%) mean that serotonin caused vasodilatation instead of vasoconstriction. *Significant ($p < 0.05$) change compared with parallel administration of saline. Data from Saxena et al. (85) and Saxena (79).

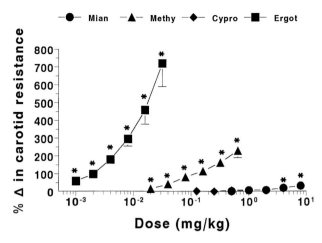

FIG. 4. Dog external carotid vascular bed. Effect of mianserin (*Mian*), methysergide (*Methy*), cyproheptadine (*Cypro*), and ergotamine (*Ergot*) on the carotid vascular resistance. *Significant (p < 0.05) change compared with the respective baseline value. Data from Saxena et al. (85) and Saxena (79).

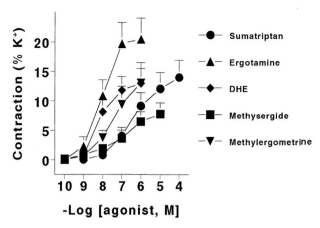

FIG. 5. Concentration response (expressed as a percentage of the response to 100 mM K^+) curves in human isolated coronary arteries (n = 9) obtained with ergotamine, dihydroergotamine (*DHE*), sumatriptan, methysergide, and its metabolite methylergometrine. Data, displayed as means ± SEM, are from MaassenVanDenBrink et al. (58).

and selectively decreased carotid blood flow (46,81,87) by constricting arteriovenous anastomoses (Fig. 4) (87). Although this effect of methysergide is much less marked than that of ergotamine or sumatriptan (23–25), its mediation by novel 5-HT$_1$–like receptors undeniably provided incentive for the development of sumatriptan, which at the time of its introduction was regarded as a selective 5-HT$_1$–like receptor agonist (49).

As recently argued (82), the term 5-HT$_1$–like receptor is now redundant because the composition of this heterogeneous group has been delineated. This group comprises the sumatriptan-insensitive 5-HT$_7$ receptor, which mediates tachycardia in cats and vasorelaxation (21,28,100), as well as sumatriptan-sensitive 5-HT$_{1B}$, 5-HT$_{1D}$, and, in some tissues, even 5-HT$_{1F}$ receptors. Methysergide is a potent antagonist at the 5-HT$_7$ (and 5-HT$_2$) receptor and an agonist at 5-HT$_{1B}$ and, possibly, also 5-HT$_{1D}$ receptors. *In vitro* functional and radioligand studies confirm that methysergide acts on 5-HT$_{1B}$ receptors. Thus, methysergide contracts canine, bovine, and human cerebral arteries (63–65), and the methysergide-induced contraction of the dog isolated saphenous vein is antagonized by the nonselective 5-HT$_1$ and 5-HT$_2$ receptor antagonist methiothepin, but not by the 5-HT$_2$ receptor antagonist ketanserin (49,63).

The pharmacology of the metabolite methylergometrine has been investigated less thoroughly. However, it is a more potent vasoconstrictor than methysergide both *in vivo* (59) and *in vitro* on, for example, canine saphenous veins and human basilar (65) and coronary (58) arteries (Fig. 5). The last two effects may bestow efficacy in migraine (62) and coronary side effect potential (67) to methylergometrine.

Lastly, chronic but not acute treatment with methysergide has been reported to attenuate dural plasma

extravasation following electric stimulation of the trigeminal ganglion in the rat (78). The discrepancy between the effect of acute and chronic treatment with methysergide in this model is most likely due to the presence of methylergometrine during chronic administration of methysergide. Although Saito and colleagues have implied a presynaptic inhibition of the release of calcitonin gene-related peptide (CGRP) from perivascular sensory nerves, functional antagonism (via vasoconstriction) of the vasodilator effects of CGRP cannot be ruled out. Indeed, such a functional antagonism between methysergide and CGRP has recently been described in the rabbit eye (52) and should be investigated further with the use of methylergometrine.

Possible Mechanism of Antimigraine Action

The mechanism of action of methysergide in migraine is not well understood. The efficacy of methysergide has been ascribed to its 5-HT$_2$ receptor antagonist property, but this is unlikely because potent 5-HT$_2$ receptor antagonists such as mianserin, sergolexole, ketanserin, and ICI 169,369 seem to have no prophylactic effect in migraine, and for cyproheptadine the claimed efficacy (66) has never been confirmed in controlled clinical trials. Therefore, it is highly improbable that 5-HT$_2$ receptor antagonism plays any role in migraine prophylaxis (83,99). It should be noted that, in essence, these same arguments also apply against the advocated role of 5-HT$_{2C}$ receptor antagonism [methysergide is a potent 5-HT$_{2C}$ receptor antagonist (66)] in migraine (36,37).

We believe that the vasoconstrictor action of methysergide within the carotid vascular bed (80,87), which is mediated by 5-HT$_{1B}$ receptors (100), is most likely involved in the therapeutic activity. The carotid vaso-constrictor effect of methysergide is weaker, both in potency and efficacy, than that of ergotamine (see Fig. 4) (24) or sumatriptan (23,25), which have the ability to abort migraine attacks (for more details, see Chapter 52). Thus, it is possible that methysergide owes its therapeutic effect in migraine to its metabolic product methylergometrine. Indeed, methylergometrine has a more potent vasoconstrictor action than methysergide (58,65).

Apart from 5-HT$_{1B}$ receptors, the craniovascular effects of methysergide (or methylergometrine) also may involve 5-HT$_7$ receptor blockade (21,28,100). Also worth investigating is the involvement of dopamine receptors because Bell (6,7) has presented evidence that dilatation of arteriovenous anastomoses can be mediated by a neural release of dopamine.

Inhibition of peptide release from perivascular sensory nerve endings as well as neurogenic inflammation by methysergide, as demonstrated in the rat, also has been invoked as a mechanism of action in migraine (78). As argued elsewhere (22), however, there is considerable doubt whether inhibition of neurogenic inflammation in experimental animals is connected with antimigraine efficacy because several such compounds were found clinically ineffective in migraine.

Results of Clinical Trials

Open Trials

In open studies including approximately 1,400 migraine patients (18,38,40,55), methysergide was found to decrease migraine attack frequency in the majority of patients. However, about 10% (18,55) to 20% (38,40) of the patients had to stop the drug because of side effects. The most common side effects, occurring in more than 5% of patients (38,40), were dizziness, nausea and vomiting, weight gain, epigastric pain, psychic reactions, peripheral arterial insufficiency, and peripheral edema. One case of ergotism was observed, and in one case angina pectoris was precipitated (38). Thus, the open trials with methysergide indicated not only a useful prophylactic effect, but also side effect problems.

During the first years of clinical use of methysergide it became evident that continuous use of the drug for longer periods can induce retroperitoneal fibrosis, as well as pleural and heart valve fibrosis, with an estimated incidence of 1 in 5,000 treated patients (41,42). In most cases the fibrotic process regressed after discontinuation of methysergide (41). The metabolism of methysergide was unchanged in patients who had developed this side effect (9), and its mechanisms remain elusive. This side effect of methysergide limits its clinical use.

Controlled Clinical Trials

Methysergide has been compared with placebo or another drug in nine double-blind randomized clinical trials (2,5,34,43,71,75,76,93,97). The daily dosage of methysergide varied from 3 to 6 mg, and in most trials a mixed migraine population (with or without aura) was studied. In two trials methysergide was superior to placebo for either severe headaches (93) or frequency of attacks (71), but in one trial methysergide was not superior to placebo (76). In four trials (2,34,71,76), methysergide was found comparable with pizotifen (Table 1). Methysergide was also found comparable with lisuride (25 µg three times daily) (44), propranolol (40 mg tid) (5), and flunarizine (10 mg daily) (97).

The side effects reported in these trials were similar to those observed in the open studies (see above). Although in some trials only a few patients stopped treatment with methysergide because of side effects (5,34,75,76,97), in others discontinuation of therapy was more frequent: 5% (2), 7% (71), 20% (44), and 26% (93). The higher drop-out rates of 20% (44) and 26% (93) occurred with a daily dosage of 6 mg methysergide, but apparently this dosage was tolerated in other studies (34,97). There was thus no dose-response relationship for the side effects of methysergide.

Being the first drug introduced for migraine prophylaxis, methysergide has not been evaluated in randomized trials with current methodology (see Chapter 7). However, taken together, the controlled trials with methysergide show that the drug is efficacious in migraine prophylaxis. The problems with side effects also have been demonstrated for this potent drug.

Therapeutic Use

Due to potentially grave side effects, methysergide should be reserved for severe cases for which other attempts of migraine prophylaxis have not produced optimal results. The daily dosage of methysergide in migraine prophylaxis is 3 to 6 mg given in three divided doses. In order to minimize the acute side effect, the dosage should be increased gradually, starting with 1 mg per day and increasing with 1 mg every third day. Methysergide should not be taken continuously for long periods, which can result in retroperitoneal fibrosis (4,41,42). Instead, the drug should be given for 6 months, with a 2-month interruption before starting the drug again. When methysergide is stopped it should be weaned off gradually over 1 week in order to avoid rebound headache.

The side effects of methysergide are nausea and vomiting, dyspepsia, edema, dizziness, sedation, and depression. Long-term use may lead to retroperitoneal fibrosis, as well as heart valve and pleural fibrosis. The starting symptoms of retroperitoneal fibrosis, in which the ureters are constricted, are low back pain, leg pain, and urologi-

TABLE 1. *Controlled double-blind trials comparing pizotifen with placebo or another drug for migraine prophylaxis*

Trial	Drug dosage (mg)	Study design	No. of patients (no. evaluated) and type of migraine	Run-in and duration of treatment	Factors evaluated	Investigators' conclusion(s)
Lance and Anthony (53)	Pizotifen 1 tid	Parallel groups	50	4 wk	Improvement	Pizotifen = placebo
	Placebo tid		?			
Hughes and Foster (48)	Pizotifen 1 tid	Crossover	26	2 mo × 2	Frequency, severity and preference	Pizotifen = placebo, Pizotifen > placebo
	Placebo		?			
Ryan (77)	Pizotifen 1 tid	Parallel groups	60 (51) MO, MA	4 wk, 12 wk	Frequency, headache index[a]	Placebo > pizotifen, Placebo = pizotifen[b,c]
	Placebo					
Arthur and Hornabrook (3)	Pizotifen 1 tid Placebo tid	Crossover	52 (41) MO, MA, CH	4 wk, 4 wk × 2	Frequency	Pizotifen > placebo
Carrol and Maclay (13)	Pizotifen 1 tid Placebo tid	Crossover	27 (14) MO, MA	4 wk[d] 2 mo × 2	Headache index[a]	Pizotifen = placebo[e]
Lawrence et al. (56)	Pizotifen 1 tid Placebo	Parallel group	36 (28) ?	12 wk	Headache index[a]	Pizotifen > placebo
Cleland et al. (16)	Pizotifen 1.5 mg nightly Placebo nightly	Crossover	88 MO, MA	12 weeks x 2 4 weeks washout	Frequency of attacks	Pizotifen > placebo (Median attacks per month: 3.5 vs 3.9)
Ryan (76)	Pizotifen 2 bid Methysergide 2 bid	Crossover	62 MO, MA	4 wk × 3	Frequency, Headache index[a]	Pizotifen > methysergide = placebo[f]
Presthus (75)	Pizotifen 0.5 tid Methysergide 1 tid	Crossover	21 (19) MO, MA	1 wk, 5 wk × 2 1 week washout	Freqeuncy, severity, duration	Pizotifen = methysergide
Forssman (34)	Pizotifen 1 tid Methysergide 2 tid	Crossover	22 (17) MO, MA	6 wk, 10 wk × 2	Frequency headache index[a]	Pizotifen = methysergide
Andersson (2)	Pizotifen 0.5 qid Methysergide 1 qid	Crossover	73 (49) MO, MA	1 mo, 3 mo × 2	Frequency, headache index[a]	Pizotifen = methysergide, both better than run-in
Hübbe (47)	Pizotifen 1 tid Perchlorperazine 5 tid	Crossover	43 (40) ?	8 wk × 2	Frequency	Pizotifen = perchlorperazine
Osterman (69)	Pizotifen 1 tid 1-Iso 5 tid Placebo tid	Crossover	30 (28) MO, MA	8 wk × 3	Frequency, headache index[a] preference	Pizotifen > 1-Iso = placebo
Kangasneimi (50)	Pizotifen 0.5 tid 1-Iso 5 tid	Crossover	50 (34) MO, MA	14 wk × 2 4 wk washout	Frequency headache index[a]	Pizotifen = 1-Iso = placebo[c]
Capildeo and Clifford Rose (12)	Pizotifen 0.5 tid Pizotifen 1.5 nightly	Crossover	17 MO, MA	2 mo × 2	Headache index[a]	Pizotifen tid = pizotifen 1.5 nightly

For comparison with calcium blockers, see Chapter 58.

[a] Frequency times severity.
[b] In pretreatment period, more attacks in pizotifen group (12 / 4 weeks) than in placebo group (7 / 4 weeks).
[c] The opinion of the present reviewers.
[d] Pizotifen during run-in to determine optimal dosage (in most cases 3 mg per day).
[e] No statistics given, but Wilcoxon's test on raw data gives $p > 0.2$.
[f] No statistical evaluation.

1-Iso, 1-isopropyl-3-hydroxy-5-semicarbazono-6-oxo-2.3.5.6-tetrahydroindol; bid, twice daily; tid, thrice daily; qid, four times daily; MO, migraine without aura; MA, migraine with aura; CH, cluster headache; = , no statistical significant difference; >, signifies more effective than.

cal disturbances (4,41,42). The drug should be discontinued immediately even on suspicion of retroperitoneal fibrosis.

Contraindications include cardiovascular diseases, severe hypertension, a history of thrombophlebitis, peptic ulcers, pregnancy, familial fibrotic disorders such as Dupuytren's disease, lung diseases, collagenoses, and liver and kidney diseases.

As a cautionary note, one should try to half the dose of ergotamine normally effective in aborting an acute attack of migraine because of the additional vasoconstrictor effect of methysergide.

PIZOTIFEN

Pizotifen was introduced in migraine prophylaxis as an antiaminic drug based on the idea that not only 5-HT but also other biogenic amines might be involved in migraine (90). In open studies, improvement during pizotifen therapy has been reported in 42% to 68% of patients (95), and in controlled trials the drug has been more effective than placebo. Its general use is hampered by its main side effects, weight gain and sedation.

Pharmacologic Background

Pizotifen is a potent 5-HT$_2$ receptor antagonist with a pA$_2$ value of around 9.2 (66,72). Pizotifen also has antihistaminic and weak anticholinergic actions and, in some animals, sedative and antidepressant properties (95). The antidepressant property has been confirmed in humans (96). Furthermore, in both dogs (63) and humans (1), a modest venoconstrictor activity of pizotifen has been demonstrated. It has been suggested that pizotifen acts as a calcium channel blocker (74), but this is unlikely in the concentrations in plasma reached with therapeutic doses in humans (63). In our opinion, the diversity of pharmacologic properties of pizotifen precludes a meaningful hypothesis concerning its efficacy in migraine (70).

Pharmacokinetics

The pharmacokinetics of pizotifen has only been studied with [^{3}H]-labeled drug (60). Thus, measured concentrations in plasma (total radioactivity) include both parent drug and metabolites. The study indicated a maximal therapeutic plasma level of pizotifen of 9 ng/mL and an extensive metabolism of the drug, with less than 1% being excreted unchanged in the urine (60). Due to the method used, the study allows no conclusion about how often pizotifen should be administered.

Results of Clinical Trials

A summary of 15 randomized double-blind controlled clinical trials comparing pizotifen with placebo (3,13,16,48,53,56,77) or other drugs (2,12,34,47,50,69, 75,76) is given in Table 1. In most trials mixed populations of migraine patients with and without aura were studied. The daily dosage of pizotifen was 1.5 to 3 mg. In addition, pizotifen reportedly has been equally effective as the calcium blockers flunarizine (four trials) and nimodipine (two trials) (see Chapter 58).

Pizotifen was superior to placebo for frequency of attacks or headache index in several studies (3,16,56,69) and comparable with placebo for frequency but superior to placebo for severity of headaches in one study (48). In two trials with low power to detect a difference, no significant difference was found between pizotifen and placebo (13,53), and another trial (77) indicated that pizotifen was inferior to placebo, probably due to unsuccessful randomization (see Table 1). In one of these trials (16) investigating whether pizotifen prophylaxis improved migraine beyond the benefit offered by acute sumatriptan therapy alone, the effect must be judged as clinically insignificant.

In the comparative trials with methysergide, pizotifen was found to be as efficacious as methysergide (2,34,75), and in one trial without any statistics pizotifen was reported to be superior to methysergide (76). Pizotifen was found comparable with prochlorperazine in one trial (47) and better than (69) or comparable with (50) 1-isopropyl-noradrenochrome-5-monosemicarbazono. In addition, one study indicated that pizotifen 1.5 mg at night was as effective as 0.5 mg three times daily (12). However, apart from one trial (76), these comparative trials with pizotifen lack a placebo control, and it is thus difficult to judge the significance of these results.

The side effects in these controlled trials included drowsiness, increased appetite, and weight gain. Thus, in one placebo-controlled trial with pizotifen 3 mg per day in 30 patients, the drug induced drowsiness in 15, increased appetite in 12, and caused weight gain in 24 (>1.5 kg in 21 and >4 kg in 3) patients; the numbers of patients with these side effects with placebo were 4, 3, and 2, respectively (69). Drowsiness, however, often diminished with time (69).

In conclusion, the controlled clinical trials demonstrated efficacy of pizotifen in migraine prophylaxis, but side-effects, especially weight gain, were frequent and limit the use of the drug.

Therapeutic Use

Pizotifen is normally used in migraine prophylaxis in a daily dosage of 1.5 mg, which can either be taken as 0.5 mg three times daily or as one dose in the evening (12) in order to increase compliance and cause less sedation. The dosage should be increased gradually, starting with 0.5 mg once a day, increasing with 0.5 mg every third day to 0.5 mg three times daily or 1.5 mg at night. In refractory cases, dosage up to 3 to 4.5 mg daily, taken in three divided doses, can be used.

Side-effects include increase in appetite and weight gain, as well as sedation. Contraindications include obesity. Patients should refrain from driving at the start of the treatment.

LISURIDE

After its synthesis in 1959, the ergot alkaloid derivative lisuride (see Fig. 1) was first developed as a peripheral 5-HT receptor antagonist, and its similarity to methysergide led to its clinical use in migraine prophylaxis (45). Later, lisuride's dopaminergic effect was established, and it is now also used in higher doses in the treatment of Parkinson's disease.

Pharmacologic Background

Lisuride is a dopamine (D_2) receptor agonist (72), but also has a potent antagonist at 5-HT_2 (66) as well as at 5-HT_7 (21). In addition, lisuride may act as an agonist on CNS 5-HT receptors (45). The mode of action of lisuride in migraine prophylaxis remains elusive, but the doses used in migraine are probably without any dopaminergic effect (45).

Results of Clinical Trials

In open studies, success rates (more than 50% reduction in frequency of attacks) from 34% (54) to 61% (94) have been reported after lisuride (0.025 mg three times daily). In two double-blind placebo-controlled trials with parallel group design, lisuride (0.025 mg three times daily) was reported to be superior to placebo (44,92). In these trials a total of 390 patients were recruited, and 83% completed the trials. In both trials (44,92), patients with up to 21 to 30 attacks per month were included, making the diagnosis of migraine, which is only defined in one of the trials (92), dubious, at least in some patients. In a double-blind trial, lisuride (0.025 mg three times daily) was found comparable with methysergide (2 mg three times daily) in 253 patients (43). In this study, 11 patients with cluster headache were included, and 40% of patients had more than 10 attacks per month, making it unlikely that only migraine attacks were treated. In one trial, there was no difference between lisuride in dosages of 0.025 and 0.05 mg three times daily (101).

The most common side effects of lisuride reported were nausea, gastrointestinal complaints, and dizziness. A case of visual hallucinations during lisuride treatment also was reported (92).

In conclusion, the controlled clinical trials suggest that lisuride has some efficacy in migraine prophylaxis, but the selection of patients with uncertain diagnosis of migraine for these trials prevents a definitive statement.

Therapeutic Use

Lisuride can be tried in migraine prophylaxis in a dosage of 0.025 mg three times daily. Side effects include nausea, gastrointestinal complaints, and dizziness. Contraindications include peripheral vascular diseases, coronary artery disease, and psychosis.

CYPROHEPTADINE

Cyproheptadine is mainly used as an antihistaminic drug, but it also has been used in the past in migraine prophylaxis. The drug is a potent antagonist at 5-HT_2 receptors (pA_2 of around 8.8), but it also antagonizes responses mediated by histamine H_1 and muscarinic cholinergic receptors (66). In addition, cyproheptadine acts as a calcium channel blocker in the canine basilar artery (73). The drug does not seem to act on 5-HT_1 receptors and is unable to block the 5-HT–induced vasoconstriction in the carotid vascular bed (see Figs. 2 and 3) (79,86).

In open studies success rates (headache free or considerably improved) for cyproheptadine in migraine prophylaxis of 43% (54), 46% (18), and 65% (51) were reported. In one study cyproheptadine was found inferior to methysergide (18). Furthermore, the effect of cyproheptadine was not significantly different from that of placebo in another study (53). There are no double-blind randomized placebo-controlled trials with cyproheptadine, and the proof of its efficacy as a migraine prophylactic drug is virtually nonexistent.

Therapeutic Use

Cyproheptadine is sometimes used in migraine prophylaxis in a dosage of 8 to 32 mg daily, taken in three to four divided doses. The initial dose is 2 mg, increased by 2 mg every third day until beneficial effect is observed or side effects occur.

Side effects include drowsiness, dizziness, dry mouth, increased appetite, and weight gain. Contraindications include glaucoma.

OTHER 5-HT_2 RECEPTOR ANTAGONISTS

Mianserin

The antidepressant drug mianserin is a potent 5-HT_2 receptor antagonist with a pA_2 of 9.3 (66). Mianserin neither blocks the vasoconstrictor effects of 5-HT nor elicits vasoconstriction within the canine external carotid vascular bed (see Figs. 2 and 3) (85). It has been claimed to be effective in migraine prophylaxis (26,61). However, this claim is based on two controlled studies that, even if they were double-blind and placebo-controlled, were full of methodologic faults (99). There were thus no clear indications for mianserin being better than placebo (99).

Sergolexole

Sergolexole is a 5-HT$_2$ receptor antagonist with a pA$_2$ value of approximately 9 (17). The drug also can act as an antagonist at the 5-HT$_7$ receptor (19). Based on the possible involvement of 5-HT in migraine, it was investigated in one prophylactic migraine trial (14) and found no better than placebo. In small open pilot studies, the selective 5-HT$_2$ antagonists ketanserin (102) and ICI 169,369 (20) were without convincing prophylactic effect in migraine. Overall, these 5-HT$_2$ antagonists seem to have only minor or no prophylactic effect in migraine.

5-HT$_3$ RECEPTOR ANTAGONISTS

It has been hypothesized that 5-HT, released at perivascular nerve endings, causes migraine pain via activation of neuronal 5-HT$_3$ receptors on pain afferents present in cranial microvasculature (35). Initially, a small trial conducted with the 5-HT$_3$ receptor antagonist MDL 72222 in acute migraine attacks seemed to support the above hypothesis (57). This trial has been criticized on several grounds (31).

The potent 5-HT$_3$ receptor antagonist tropisetron has been evaluated in migraine prophylaxis in two double-blind placebo-controlled trials (32). In both trials, the parallel group design was used; 204 patients were recruited and 182 were evaluated. The results with none of the doses of tropisetron (15 mg, n = 38; 25 mg, n = 47; 50 mg, n = 50) were different from those with placebo (n = 79) during a 3 months treatment. The main side effect was constipation, which occurred in 42% to 55% of patients treated with tropisetron. Due to wide confidence intervals, an effect of tropisetron could not be excluded (32). As reviewed by Ferrari (31), the efficacy of 5-HT$_3$ receptor antagonists in migraine therapy remains hypothetical. Another 5-HT$_3$ receptor antagonist, zatosetron, also has been found ineffective in the treatment of migraine attacks (15).

REFERENCES

1. Aellig WH. Influence of pizotifen and ergotamine on the vasoconstrictor effect of 5-hydroxytryptamine and noradrenaline in man. *Eur J Clin Pharmacol* 1983;25:759–762.
2. Andersson PG. BC-105 and deseril in migraine porphylaxis: a double-blind study. *Headache* 1973;13:68–73.
3. Arthur GP, Hornabrook RW. The treatment of migraine with BC 105 (pizotifen): a double blind trial. *N Z Med J* 1971;73:5–9.
4. Bana DS, MacNeal PS, LeCompte PM, Shah Y, Graham JR. Cardiac murmurs and endocardial fibrosis associated with methysergide therapy. *Am Heart J* 1974;88:640–655.
5. Behan PO, Reid M. Propranolol in the treatment of migraine. *Practitioner* 1980;224:201–204.
6. Bell C. Benztropine-induced prolongation of responses to vasodilator nerve stimulation in the canine paw pad. *Br J Pharmacol* 1982;76:231–233.
7. Bell C, Lang WJ. Evidence for dopaminergic vasodilator innervation of the canine paw pad. *Br J Pharmacol* 1979;67:337–343.
8. Berde B, Stürmer E. Introduction to the pharmacology of ergot alkaloids and related compounds as a basis of their therapeutic application. In: Berde B, Schild HO, eds. *Ergot alkaloids and related compounds. Handbook of experimental pharmacology.* Vol. 49. Berlin: Springer-Verlag, 1978:1–28.
9. Bianchine JR, Friedman AP. Metabolism of methysergide and retroperitonal fibrosis. *Arch Intern Med* 1970;126:252–254.
10. Bredberg U, Eyjolfdottir GS, Paalzow L, Tfelt-Hansen P, Tfelt-Hansen V. Pharmacokinetics of methysergide and its metabolite methylergometrine in man. *Eur J Clin Pharmacol* 1986;30:75–77.
11. Brown AM, Patch TL, Kaumann AJ. The antimigraine drugs ergotamine and dihydroergotamine are potent 5-HT$_{1C}$ receptor agonists in piglet choroid plexus. *Br J Pharmacol* 1991;104:45–48.
12. Capildeo R, Clifford Rose F. Single-dose pizotifen, 1.5 mg nocte: a new approach in the prophylaxis of migraine. *Headache* 1982;22:272–275.
13. Carrol JD, Maclay WP. Pizotifen (BC-105) in migraine prophylaxis. *Curr Med Res Opin* 1975;3:68–71.
14. Chappell AS, Bay JM, Botzum GD. Sergolexole maleate and placebo for migraine prophylaxis. *Cephalalgia* 1991;11[Suppl 11]:170–171.
15. Chappell AS, Bay JM, Botzum GD, Cohen ML. Zatosetron, a 5-HT$_3$ receptor antagonist in a multicenter trial for acute migraine. *Neuropharmacology* 1994;33:509–513.
16. Cleland PG, Barnes D, Elrington GM, Loizou LA, Rawes GD. Studies to assess if pizotifen prophylaxis improves migraine beyond the benefit offered by acute sumatriptan therapy alone. *Eur Neurol* 1997;38:31–38.
17. Cohen ML, Robertson DW, Bloomquist WE, Wilson HC. LY215840, a potent 5-hydroxytryptamine (5-HT)$_2$ receptor antagonist, blocks vascular and platelet 5-HT$_2$ receptors and delays occlusion in a rabbit model of thrombosis. *J Pharmacol Exp Ther* 1992;261:202–228.
18. Curran DA, Lance JW. Clinical trial of methysergide and other preparations in the management of migraine. *J Neurol Neurosurg Psychiatry* 1964;27:463–469.
19. Cushing DJ, Zgombick JM, Nelson DL, Cohen ML. LY215840, a high-affinity 5-HT$_7$ receptor ligand, blocks serotonin-induced relaxation in canine coronary artery. *J Pharmacol Exp Ther* 1996;277:1560–1566.
20. Davies PTG, Steiner TJ. Serotonin S$_2$ receptors and migraine: a study with the selective receptor antagonist ICI 169,369. *Headache* 1990;30:340–343.
21. De Vries P, Villalón CM, Heiligers JP, Saxena PR. Nature of 5-HT$_1$-like receptors mediating depressor responses in vagosympathectomized rats; close resemblance to the cloned 5-HT$_7$ receptor. *Naunyn Schmiedebergs Arch Pharmacol* 1997;356:90–99.
22. De Vries P, Villalón CM, Saxena PR. Pharmacological aspects of experimental headache models in relation to acute antimigraine therapy. *Eur J Pharmacol* 1999 (in press).
23. De Vries P, Willems EW, Heiligers JPC, Villalón CM, Saxena PR. Constriction of porcine carotid arteriovenous anastomoses as indicator of antimigraine activity: the role of 5-HT$_{1B/1D}$, as well as unidentified receptors. In: Edvinsson L, ed. *Migraine & headache pathophysiology.* London: Martin Dunitz, 1999:119–132.
24. Den Boer MO, Villalón CM, Heiligers JPC, Humphrey PPA, Saxena PR. Carotid vascular effects of ergotamine and dihydroergotamine in the pig: no exclusive mediation via 5-HT$_1$–like receptors. *Br J Pharmacol* 1991;104:183–189.
25. Den Boer MO, Villalón CM, Heiligers JPC, Humphrey PPA, Saxena PR. The role of 5-HT$_1$–like receptors in the reduction of porcine cranial arteriovenous anastomotic shunting by sumatriptan. *Br J Pharmacol* 1991;102:323–330.
26. Denaro A, Martucci N, Ruggieri S, Manna V, Agnoli A. Headache and noradrenergic involvement: the effects of α$_2$-stimulants and α$_2$-antagonists. *Acta Psychiatr Scand* 1985;72[Suppl 320]:20–25.
27. Edvinsson L, Jansen IJO. Characterization of human craniovascular 5-hydroxytryptamine receptors. In: Olesen J, Saxena PR, eds. *5-Hydroxytryptamine mechanisms in primary headaches.* New York: Raven, 1992:129–136.
28. Eglen RM, Jasper JR, Chang DA, Martin GR. The 5-HT$_7$ receptor: orphan found. *Trends Pharmacol Sci* 1997;18:104–107.
29. Fanchamps A, Doepfner W, Weidman H, Cerletti A. Pharmakologische Charakterisierung von Deseril, einem Serotonin-Antagonisten. *Schweiz Med Wochenschr* 1960;51:1040–1046.
30. Ferrari C, Caldera R, Rampini P, et al. Inhibition of prolactin release by serotonin receptor antagonists in hyperprolactinemic subjects. *Metabolism* 1978;27:1499–1504.

31. Ferrari MD. 5-HT$_3$ receptor antagonists and migraine therapy. *J Neurol* 1991;238[Suppl 1]:53–56.

32. Ferrari MD, Wilkinson M, Hirt D, Lataste X, Notter M. Efficacy of ICS 205-930, a novel 5-hydroxytryptamine$_3$ (5-HT$_3$) receptor antagonist, in the prevention of migraine attacks. A complex answer to a simple question. *Pain* 1991;45:283–291.

33. Flückiger E, del Pozo E. Influence on the endocrine system. In: Berde B, Schild HO, eds. *Ergot alkaloids and related compound. Handbook of experimental pharmacology.* Vol. 49. Berlin: Springer-Verlag, 1978:615–690.

34. Forssman B, Henriksson K-G, Kihlstrand S. A comparison between BC 105 and methysergide in the prophylaxis of migraine. *Acta Neurol Scand* 1972;48:204–212.

35. Fozard JR. Basic mechanisms of antimigraine drugs. *Adv Neurol* 1982;33:295–307.

36. Fozard JR. 5-HT$_{1C}$ receptor agonism as an initiating event in migraine. In: Olesen J, Saxena PR, eds. *5-Hydroxytryptamine mechanisms in primary headaches.* New York: Ravens, 1992:200–212.

37. Fozard JR, Gray J. 5-HT$_{1C}$ receptor activation: a key step in the initiation of migraine? *Trends Pharmacol Sci* 1989;8:307–309.

38. Friedman AP, Elkind AH. Appraisal of methysergide in treatment of vascular headaches of migraine type. *JAMA* 1963;184:125–128.

39. Gaddum JH, Picarelli ZP. Two kinds of tryptamine receptors. *Br J Pharmacol* 1957;12:323–328.

40. Graham JR. Methysergide for prevention of migraine. *N Engl J Med* 1964;270:67–72.

41. Graham JR. Cardiac and pulmonary fibrosis during methysergide therapy for headache. *Am J Med Sci* 1967;254:1–12.

42. Graham JR, Suby HI, LeCompte PR, Sadowsky NL. Fibrotic disorders associated with methysergide therapy for headache. *N Engl J Med* 1966;274:360–368.

43. Herrmann WM, Horowski R, Dannehl K, Kramer U, Lurati K. Clinical effectiveness of lisuride hydrogen maleate: a double-blind trial versus methysergide. *Headache* 1977;17:54–60.

44. Herrmann WM, Kristof M, Sastre y Hernandez M. Preventive treatment of migraine headache with a new isoergonyl derivative. *J Intern Med Res* 1978;6:476–482.

45. Horowski R. Some aspects of the dopaminergic action of ergot derivatives and their role in the treatment of migraine. *Adv Neurol* 1982;33: 325–334.

46. Hoyer D, Clarke DE, Fozard JR, et al. International Union of Pharmacology classification of receptors for 5-hydroxytryptamine (serotonin). *Pharmacol Rev* 1994;46:157–203.

47. Hübbe P. The prophylactic treatment of migraine with an antiserotonin pizotifen (BC 105). *Acta Neurol Scand* 1973;49:108–114.

48. Hughes RC, Foster JB. BC 105 in the prophylaxis of migraine. *Curr Ther Res* 1971;13:63–68.

49. Humphrey PPA, Apperley E, Feniuk W, Perren MJ. A rational approach to identifying a fundamentally new drug for the treatment of migraine. In: Saxena PR, Wallis DI, Wouters W, Bevan P, eds. *Cardiovascular pharmacology of 5-hydroxytryptamine: prospective therapeutic applications.* Dordrecht: Kluwer Academic, 1990: 416–431.

50. Kangasneimi P. Placebo, l-isopropylnoradrenochrome-5-monosemicarbazono and pizotifen in migraine prophylaxis. *Headache* 1979;19: 219–222.

51. Klimek A. Cyproheptadine (Peritol) in the treatment of migraine and related headache. *Ther Hung* 1979;27:93–94.

52. Krootila K, Oksala O, Zschauer A, Palkama A, Uusitalo H. Inhibitory effect of methysergide on calcium gene-related peptide–induced vasodilatation and ocular irritative changes in the rabbit. *Br J Pharmacol* 1992;106:404–408.

53. Lance JW, Anthony M. Clinical trial of a new serotonin receptor antagonist, BC 105, in the prevention of migraine. *Med J Aust* 1968;1:54–55.

54. Lance JW, Anthony M, Sommerville B. Comparative trial of serotonin receptor antagonists in the management of migraine. *Br Med J* 1970;2:327–329.

55. Lance JW, Fine RD, Curran DA. An evaluation of methysergide in the prevention of migraine and other vascular headaches. *Med J Aust* 1963;1:814–818.

56. Lawrence ER, Hossain M, Littlestone W. Sandomigran for migraine prophylaxis: controlled multicenter trial in general practice. *Headache* 1977;17:112.

57. Loisy C, Beorchia S, Centzone V, Fozard JR, Schechter PJ, Tell GP. Effects on migraine headache of MDL 7222, an antagonist at neuronal 5-HT receptors. Double-blind, placebo-controlled study. *Cephalalgia* 1985;5:79–82.

58. MaassenVanDenBrink A, Reekers M, Bax WA, Ferrari MD, Saxena PR. Coronary side-effect potential of current and prospective antimigraine drugs. *Circulation* 1998;98:25–30.

59. MacLennan SJ, Martin GR. Comparison of the effects of methysergide and methylergometrine with GR43175 on feline carotid blood flow distribution. *Br J Pharmacol* 1990;99:221P.

60. Meier J, Schreier E. Human levels of some anti-migraine drugs. *Headache* 1976;16:96–104.

61. Monro P, Swade C, Coppen A. Mianserin in the prophylaxis of migraine: a double-blind study. *Acta Psychiatr Scand* 1985;72[Suppl 320]:98–103.

62. Mueller L, Gallagher RM, Ciervo CA. Methylergonovine maleate as a cluster headache prophylactic: a study and review. *Headache* 1997; 37:437–442.

63. Müller-Schweinitzer E. Pizotifen, an antimigraine drug with venoconstrictor activity *in vivo. J Cardiovasc Pharmacol* 1986;8: 805–810.

64. Müller-Schweinitzer E. Serotonergic receptors in brain vessels. In: Owman C, Hardebo JE, eds. *Neural regulation of brain circulation.* Amsterdam: Elsevier, 1986:219–234.

65. Müller-Schweinitzer E. Ergot alkaloids in migraine: is the effect via 5-HT receptors. In: Olesen J, Saxena PR, eds. *5-Hydroxytryptamine mechanisms in primary headaches.* New York: Raven, 1992:297–304.

66. Mylechrane EJ. 5-HT$_2$ receptor antagonists and migraine therapy. *J Neurol* 1991;238[Suppl 1]:45–52.

67. Oneglia C, Marchetti A, Rusconi C. Methylergometrine-induced myocardial ischemia in a previously asymptomatic premenopausal woman. *Cardiovasc Drugs Ther* 1995;9:631–632.

68. Oppizzi G, Verde G, De Stefano L, et al. Evidence for a dopaminergic activity of methysergide in humans. *Clin Endocrinol* 1977;7:267–272.

69. Osterman PO. A comparison between placebo, pizotifen and 1-isopropyl-3-hydroxy-5-semicarbazono-6-oxo-2.3.5.6-tetrahydroindol (Divascan) in migraine prophylaxis. *Acta Neurol Scand* 1977;56: 17–28.

70. Peatfield RC, Fozard JR, Clifford Rose F. Drug treatment of migraine, handbook of clinical neurology. In: Clifford Rose F, ed. *Headache.* Vol. 48. Amsterdam: Elsevier Science, 1986:173–216.

71. Pedersen E, Møller CE. Methysergide in migraine prophylaxis. *Clin Pharmacol Ther* 1966;7:520–526.

72. Peroutka SJ. Drugs effective in the therapy of migraine. In: Hardman JG, Limbird LE, Molinott PB, Ruddon RW, Gilman AG, eds. *Goodman and Gilman's: the pharmacological basis of therapeutics,* 9th ed. New York: Macmillan, 1996:487–502.

73. Peroutka SJ, Allen GS. The calcium receptor antagonist properties of cyproheptadine: implications for antimigraine action. *Neurology* 1984;34:304–309.

74. Peroutka SJ, Banghart SB, Allen GS. Calcium channel antagonism of pizotifen. *J Neurol Neurosurg Psychiatry* 1985;48:381–383.

75. Presthus J. BC 105 and methysergide (Deseril) in migraine prophylaxis. *Acta Neurol Scand* 1971;47:514–518.

76. Ryan RE. Double-blind crossover comparison of BC-105 methysergide and placebo in the prophylaxis of migraine. *Headache* 1968;8: 118–126.

77. Ryan RE. BC-105 a new preparation for the interval treatment of migraine—a double-blind evaluation compared with placebo. *Headache* 1971;11:6–18.

78. Saito K, Markowitz S, Moskowitz MA. Ergot alkaloids block neurogenic extravasation in dura mater: proposed action in vascular headaches. *Ann Neurol* 1988;27:732–737.

79. Saxena PR. The effects of antimigraine drugs on the vascular responses by 5-hydroxytryptamine and related biogenic substances on the external carotid bed of dogs: possible pharmacological implications to their antimigraine action. *Headache* 1972;12:44–54.

80. Saxena PR. Selective carotid vasoconstriction in carotid vascular bed by methysergide: possible relevance to its antimigraine effect. *Eur J Pharmacol* 1974;27:99–105.

81. Saxena PR, De Vlaam-Schluter GM. Role of some biogenic substances in migraine and relevant mechanism in antimigraine action of ergotamine—studies in an experimental model for migraine. *Headache* 1974;13:142–163.

82. Saxena PR, De Vries P, Villalón CM. 5-HT$_1$-like receptors: a time to bid goodbye. *Trends Pharmacol Sci* 1998;19:311–316.

83. Saxena PR, Den Boer MO. Drug therapy of migraine. *J Neurol* 1991;238[Suppl 1]:28–35.

84. Saxena PR, Duncker DJ, Bom AH, Heiligers J, Verdouw PD. Effects of MDL 72222 and methiothepin on carotid vascular responses to 5-hydroxytryptamine in the pig: evidence for the presence of "5-hydroxytryptamine$_1$-like" receptors. *Naunyn Schmiedebergs Arch Pharmacol* 1986;333:198–204.

85. Saxena PR, Van Houwelingen P, Bonta IL. The effect of mianserin hydrochloride on the vascular responses to 5-hydroxytryptamine and related substances. *Eur J Pharmacol* 1971;13:295–305.

86. Saxena PR, Verdouw PD. Redistribution by 5-hydroxytryptamine of carotid arterial blood at the expense of arteriovenous anastomotic blood flow. *J Physiol (Lond)* 1982;332:501–520.

87. Saxena PR, Verdouw PD. Effects of methysergide and 5-hydroxytryptamine on carotid blood flow distribution in pigs: further evidence for the presence of atypical 5-HT receptors. *Br J Pharmacol* 1984;82:817–826.

88. Saxena PR, Villalón CM. Cardiovascular effects of serotonin agonists and antagonists. *J Cardiovasc Pharmacol* 1990;15[Suppl 7]:17–34.

89. Sicuteri F. Prophylactic and therapeutic properties of 1-methyllysergic acid butanolamide in migraine. *Int Arch Allergy* 1959;15:300–307.

90. Sicuteri F, Franchi G, del Bianco PL. An antiaminic drug, BC 105, in the prophylaxis of migraine. *Int Arch Allergy* 1967;31:78–93.

91. Silberstein SD. Methysergide. *Cephalalgia* 1998;18:421–435.

92. Sommerville BW, Herrmann WM. Migraine prophylaxis with lisuride hydrogen maleate—a double-blind study of lisuride versus placebo. *Headache* 1978;18:75–79.

93. Southwell N, Williams JD, Mackenzie I. Methysergide in the prophylaxis of migraine. *Lancet* 1964;1:523–524.

94. Soyka D, Frieling B. Lisurid in der Migräneprophylaxe. *Fortschr Med* 1989;107:763–766.

95. Speight TM, Avery GS. Pizotifen (BC-105): a review of its pharmacological properties and its therapeutic efficacy in vascular headaches. *Drugs* 1972;3:159–203.

96. Standal JE. Pizotifen as an antidepressant. *Acta Psychiatr Scand* 1977;56:276–279.

97. Steardo L, Marano E, Barone P, Denman DW, Monteleone P, Cardone G. Prophylaxis of migraine attacks with a calcium-channel blocker: flunarizine versus methysergide. *J Clin Pharmacol* 1986;26:524–528.

98. Tfelt-Hansen P, Jansen I, Edvinsson L. Methylergometrine antagonizes 5-HT in the temporal artery. *Eur J Clin Pharmacol* 1987;33:77–79.

99. Tfelt-Hansen P, Pedersen HR. Migraine prophylaxis with 5-HT$_2$ partial agonists and receptor antagonists. In: Olesen J, Saxena PR, eds. *5-Hydroxytryptamine mechanisms in primary headaches.* New York: Ravens, 1992:305–310.

100. Villalón CM, De Vries P, Rabelo G, Centurión D, Sánchez-López A, Saxena PR. Canine external carotid vasoconstriction to methysergide, ergotamine and dihydroergotamine: role of 5-HT$_{1B/1D}$ receptors and α_2-adrenoceptors. *Br J Pharmacol* 1999;126:585–594.

101. Wilkinson M, Agnoli A, Gerber WD, Grotemeyer KH, Langor HD, Runge I. Multicentre migraine study. Cuyalit (lisuride 0.025 mg) vs. lisuride 0.05 mg tds. *Cephalalgia* 1989;9[Suppl 10]:353–354.

102. Winther K. Ketanserin a selective serotonin receptor antagonist, in relation to platelet aggregation and migraine attack rate. *Cephalalgia* 1985;5[Suppl 3]:402–403.

The Headaches, Second Edition,
edited by J. Olesen, P. Tfelt-Hansen, and K.M.A. Welch.
Lippincott Williams & Wilkins, Philadelphia © 2000.

The Migraines

CHAPTER 58

Calcium Antagonists in Migraine Prophylaxis

Noboru Toda and Peer Tfelt-Hansen

Calcium antagonists have been introduced in migraine prophylaxis because of two effects considered to be of potential benefit (3):

1. Their vasodilatory effect on cerebral vessels (e.g., nimodipine and verapamil), which inhibits vasospasm of the cerebral arteries (19,59)
2. Their protective action (e.g., flunarizine) against cerebral hypoxia, which is thought to be present during migraine attacks (2).

Cerebral blood flow and transcranial Doppler studies have made it unlikely, however, that either of these phenomena occur during a migraine attack (see Chapter 35). Thus, as with many other drugs used in migraine therapy, the original rationale is equivocal. Herein two calcium antagonists, verapamil with possible efficacy and flunarizine with proven efficacy in migraine prophylaxis, are reviewed and their therapeutic use described briefly. The results of 11 trials of the use of nimodipine, which is not registered for migraine prophylaxis, and the results of using other calcium antagonists are reviewed briefly.

PHARMACOLOGIC BACKGROUND

A common feature of Ca^{2+} antagonists is to block the transmembrane influx of Ca^{2+} across cell membranes through slow, voltage-dependent channels of which several types exist in cardiac muscle and vascular smooth muscle (18,30,71). Therefore, the antagonists are also called *slow channel inhibitors*, or Ca^{2+} *entry blockers*,

which are more accurate terms because they characterize the nature of the drug. For historical reasons, however, *calcium antagonist* is still the preferred term (71). Most of the antagonists in concentrations sufficient to inhibit the vascular and cardiac functions do not impair the Ca^{2+} influx in peripheral neural and vascular endothelial cells (18,68), but flunarizine and cildipine act prejunctionally to inhibit the release of neurotransmittors from nitroxidergic and adrenergic nerves (5,25). The calcium antagonists are a heterogenous group of drugs (Fig. 1) with several subtypes blocking different types of Ca^{2+} channels (71).

The calcium antagonists have relatively selective effect on cerebral arteries compared with that on peripheral arteries (7,49,54,70). One reason may be that they are highly dependent on extracellular calcium for their activation; however, results from *in vitro* studies of this selectivity vary considerably among species. Thus, for nimodipine, the difference in potency for inhibiting the contraction of cerebral and peripheral arteries in animal studies was of the order of several thousandfold (49,70), whereas in humans this difference was recently reported to be only about tenfold (27).

The other pharmacologic property of calcium antagonists considered possibly beneficial in migraine is the cytoprotective effect, that is, protection against excessive Ca^{2+} influx/release during cerebral ischemia. This cytoprotective effect has been demonstrated convincingly in animal studies for both flunarizine and nimodipine (31). It has also been suggested that calcium antagonists may be effective in migraine prophylaxis by inhibiting cortical spreading depression (CSD) (see Chapter 22). In one study in rats using a high dose of flunarizine (40 mg/kg intraperitoneally), flunarizine increased the threshold for CSD (72). A later study with the same dose but a modified technique failed to reproduce this result (39). In

N. Toda: Department of Pharmacology, School of Medicine, Shiga University of Medical Sciences, Seta, Ohtsu 520-2192, Japan.

P. Tfelt-Hansen: Department of Neurology, Glostrup Hospital, University of Copenhagen, DK-2600 Glostrup, Copenhagen, Denmark.

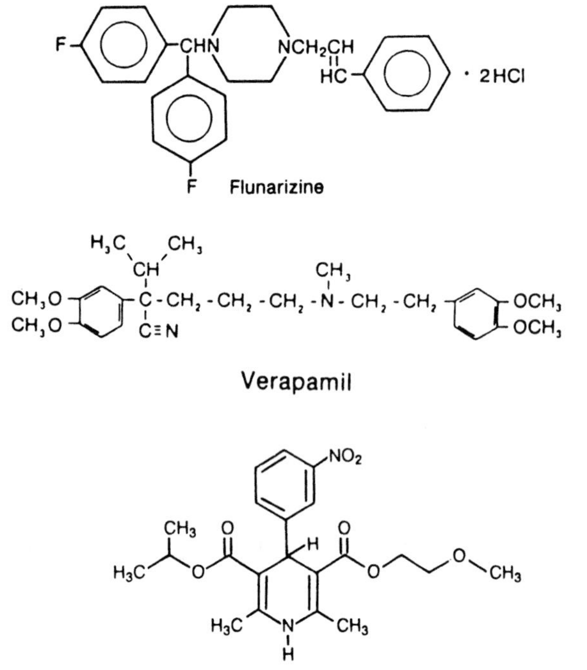

FIG 1. Chemical structures of flunarizine (*Flun*), a difluorinated piperazine derivative, verapamil (*Ver*), a synthetic papaverine derivative, and nimodipine (*Nim*), a 1,4-dihyropyridine derivative, with proven (*Flun*) or possible (*Ver, Nim*) efficacy in migraine prophylaxis.

another study, using an oral doses of 20 mg/kg flunarizine had no any effect on CSD (21).

The brain contains a high density of binding sites for calcium antagonists (19), and the drugs have central nervous system (CNS) effects that could be relevant for their effect in migraine. In humans, experimental evidence has been found that nimodipine can affect neurotransmission (26), and flunarizine has proven efficacy as an add-on drug for epilepsy (48,69). In addition, the side effects of flunarizine, such as sedation, weight gain, parkinsonism, and depression, strongly suggest interaction with CNS neurotransmittors. In addition, flunarizine has antihistaminic effects (69).

POSSIBLE MODE OF ACTION IN MIGRAINE

Cerebral arterial vasospasm is unlikely to occur in migraine, and flunarizine, the best proven calcium antagonist for migraine, exerts minimal calcium antagonistic effect on cerebral vessels in therapeutic doses (27). This drug does, however, appear to impair the synthesis and release of nitric oxide (NO), a substance possibly responsible for migraine pain (see Chapter 40), from perivascular nerves (5) and possibly endothelium in cerebral vasculatures. On the other hand, nimodipine in doses used in migraine prophylaxis can exert an effect on cerebral vessels (27), but it has only minor or no pro-

phylactic effect (*vide infra*). The cytoprotective effect of calcium antagonists is probably irrelevant, because the most convincing effect of calcium antagonists is in migraine without aura (64), in which cerebral blood flow is normal during attacks (see Chapter 35). The mechanism of action of calcium antagonists in migraine prophylaxis is most likely through their interaction with CNS neurotransmission.

PHARMACOKINETICS

The half-life of verapamil is 3 to 7 hours (24), and the drug is given in three daily doses. Sustained-release preparations of verapamil can be given once or twice daily. Flunarizine has a terminal elimination half-life of 18 days (69) and is given once daily.

RESULTS OF CONTROLLED CLINICAL TRIALS WITH VERAPAMIL

The three small double-blind crossover trials (38,58, 59) with verapamil for migraine prophylaxis are summarized in Table 1. In two of the trials, high dropout rates of 48% (59) and 30% (38) were reported, leaving only 12 (59) and 14 (38) evaluable patients. In total, only 41 patients were evaluable in these trials; therefore, the results cannot be applied directly to the general migraine population.

In two trials, verapamil (240 and 320 mg daily) was better than placebo (38,59), and in one study verapamil (320 mg) had an effect that was similar to that of long-acting propranolol (120 mg daily) but also similar to that of placebo (58) (see Table 1). In two double-blind trials, probably performed simultaneously, 320 mg daily verapamil had better results than 240 mg daily compared with placebo control (57), but the lack of randomization precludes drawing any conclusions.

In conclusion, the scientific proof for a prophylactic effect of verapamil in migraine is almost nonexistent, and its use in migraine prophylaxis in some countries is based on open clinical studies that indicated some efficacy of the drug (56).

Therapeutic Use

Verapamil can be tried in migraine prophylaxis when other well-established drugs have not been effective (see Chapters 56, 57, and 59–61). The optimal daily dose is probably 240 to 320 mg given in divided doses of 80 mg or when avaliable as sustained-release preparations.

- Side effects: constipation, hypotension, artrioventricular block, edema, headache, and nausea
- Contraindications: bradycardia, second- and third-degree heart block, sick sinus syndrome, and beta-blockers

TABLE 1. *Controlled double-blind randomized trials of verapamil (Ver) in migraine prophylaxis*

Trial	Drug, dosage (mg)	Study design	No. of patients (no. evaluated), type of migraine	Run-in	Duration of treatment	Factors evaluated	Investigators' conclusions
(59)	Ver 80 qid	CO	23 (12) MO,MA	3 mo 5 days washout		Frequency of headache unit index[a]	Ver > Pl
(38)	Ver 80 tid	CO	20 (14) MO,MA	4 wk, no drug	8 wk	Weekly headache score,[b] frequency	Ver > Pl
(58)[c]	Ver 80 tid	CO	? (15) MO,MA		2 mo × 3	Frequency, intensity duration	Ver = PropLA 120 od PropLA. PropLA > Pl Ver = Pl[d]

Ver, verapamil; CO, crossover; Pl, placebo; MA, migraine with aura; MO, migraine without aura; PropLA, longacting propranolol; od, once daily; tid, three times daily; qid, four times daily; >, more effective than.
[a]Total score of headache severity divided by the total number of days observed.
[b]Severity times duration, then summing scores for each week.
[c]Only reported as an abstract.
[d]Verapamil was only better than placebo for intensity.

RESULTS OF CONTROLLED CLINICAL TRIALS WITH FLUNARIZINE

For previous reviews of controlled trials with flunarizine, see the reports by Andersson and Vinge, Tfelt-Hansen and co-workers, and Todd and Benfield (3,66,69). A summary of seven placebo-controlled, double-blind, randomized trials that used flunarizine for migraine prophylaxis in both adults and children is presented in Table 2. In two trials, patients with migraine aura (41) or without aura (64) were studied. Both the parallel group (14,34,41,61) and the crossover (60,64,67) designs were used. A total of 299 patients were recruited for these trials, and 87% of the patients completing the trials were evaluable. The dropout rate of 13% is similar to the dropout rates found in other trials investigating migraine prophylaxis (see Chapters 56 and 57).

Flunarizine (10 mg daily in adults and 5 mg in children) produced better results than placebo in six studies (14,34,41,60,61,64) using both kinds of study designs, whereas there was only a trend in favor of the drug in one small trial (67). In one trial studying only migraine without aura, the efficacy of flunarizine in this form of migraine was confirmed (64) (Fig. 2), and one study indicated an effect in migraine with aura (41).

Based on the pooled raw data for frequency of attacks reported in six trials (14,34,41,60,61,64), one can—although with due acknowledgment to the pitfalls of doing so—calculate the mean frequency of attacks to be 1.9 during flunarizine treatment and 3.2 during placebo

TABLE 2. *Controlled double-blind, placebo-controlled trials of flunarizine (Flun) in the prophylaxis of migraine*

Trial	Drug, dosage (mg)	Study design	No. of patients (no. evaluated), type of migraine	Run-in (wk)	Duration of treatment (mo)	Factors evaluated	Investigators' conclusions
(34)	Flun 10	Pa	58 MA,MO		3	Frequency, duration, severity	Flun > Pl (frequency)
(14)	Flun 10	Pa	35 MA,MO		3	Overall efficacy	Flun > Pl
(41)	Flun 10	Pa	30 (20) MA	4	3	Frequency, duration, severity	Flun > Pl
(61)[a]	Flun 5	Pa	48 (42) MA,MO		3	Frequency duration	Flun > Pl
(64)	Flun 10	CO	29 (27) MO	4	4 × 2	Frequency, duration, intensity	Flun > Pl (frequency)
(60)[a]	Flun 5	CO	70 (63)	4 (4 wk washout)	3 × 2	Frequency duration	Flun > Pl
(67)	Flun 10	CO	29 (15) MO		3 × 2	Headache index	A trend in favor of Flun

From Andersson and Vinge (3).
[a]Children.
Flun, flunarizine; for other abbreviations, see Table 1.

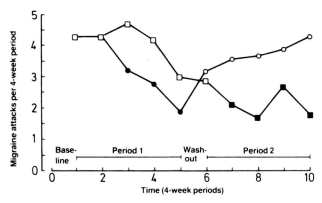

FIG 2. The effect of flunarizine on the frequency of attacks in a placebo-controlled crossover study in 27 patients with migraine without aura. [From Sørensen et al. (64).]

treatment. The calculated mean reduction of frequency during flunarizine treatment compared with placebo is thus 42%, a figure comparable to the effect of propranolol (see Chapter 56).

The comparablity of flunarizine (10 mg daily) with propranolol (120 mg daily) was also indicated by three comparative multicenter trials (36,37) that had a parallel group design and included a total of 464 evaluable migraine patients in whom similar decreases in the frequency of attacks were observed. In one trial, fluarizine 10 mg was found to be comparable to 160 mg propranolol (15). Definite proof of comparability, however, cannot be deduced from these trials because they were not placebo controlled.

Flunarizine also was found to produce comparable results to metoprolol (200 mg daily) in two trials (20,65), pizotifen (1.5 to 3 mg daily) in four trials (11,35,51,73), cinnarizine (225 mg daily) in one trial (13), and methysergide (2 mg daily) in one trial (62). None of these trials was placebo controlled, however.

Side Effects

In most of the placebo-controlled trials, significantly more side effects were not found with flunarizine than with placebo, probably because of the small sizes of the trials (see Chapter 7). Taken together, the trials indicate that sedation is associated with flunarizine treatment: Sedation was reported to occur in 0% (41) to 53% (67) of patients, with a mean of 13% for all flunarizine-treated patients compared with 2% for patients on placebo (14,34,41, 60,61,64,67). In addition, weight gain was reported in some trials, that is, in 22% (60) to 53% (67) of patients on flunarizine, whereas in another trial body weight was unchanged (41). One case of galactorrhea was reported (67). In comparative trials, flunarizine seemd to induce sedation (mean 19%) and weight gain (mean, 21%) with the same frequency as pizotifen (mean, 17% and 27%, respectively) (11,35,51) and sedation in the same range as propranolol (mean, 11% and 8%, respectively) (36,37).

One study reported two cases of depression during or after flunarizine therapy (51). After reports of extrapyramidal symptoms and depression occurring during flunarizine treatment (for literature, see 43), attention has been drawn to depression during flunarizine used for migraine prophylaxis. In one comparative trial, depression occurred in 6 of 72 [8%, 95% confidence intervals (CI) 3–17%] treated with flunarizine and in 2 of 75 (3%, 95% CI 0–9%) treated with metoprolol (200 mg daily) (65). Depression during flunarizine therapy occurred with some latency (after 3 to 5 months of treatment)(65). An open crossover trial comparing 5 and 10 mg of flunarizine daily reported depression to occur more frequently with the higher dose of flunarizine (in 5 of 40 patients) (10). Long-term open trials of flunarizine for migraine prophylaxis (8,32), on the other hand, indicate an incidence below 1% per year.

In conclusion, flunarizine has proven efficacy for migraine prophylaxis in both adults and children, and it seems comparable to other currently used drugs for migraine prophylaxis. Side effects, such as sedation, weight gain, and depression, can limit the use of flunarizine.

Therapeutic Use

Flunarizine can be used for migraine prophylaxis if the drugs of first choice, that is beta-blockers, are either ineffective or contraindicated. The standard dose is 10 mg once daily, but 5 mg can be tried if side effects occur. Flunarizine probably should be tried for 2 months before deemed ineffective. The dose in children is 5 mg daily.

- Side effects: Sedation, weight gain, depression, extrapyramidal symptoms (parkinsonism)
- Contraindications: Pregnancy, parkinsonism, previous depresssion or excessive mood changes, first-degree relatives with a history of depression.

RESULTS OF CONTROLLED CLINICAL TRIALS WITH NIMODIPINE

The possible prophylactic effect of nimodipine (120 mg daily) was investigated in six placebo-controlled, double-blind, randomized trials, including a total of 491 migraine patients (4,16,22,45,46,63). In all but two trials (45,46), both patients with and without migraine aura were included.

Nimodipine (120 mg daily) had superior results to placebo in the two first published trials (16,22). One trial (63) indicated some efficacy of nimodipine, but three later trials (4,45,46) found no significant difference between nimodipine and placebo. Because of the marked placebo effect and the use of the parallel group design, even the largest trial (45), in which 161 patients who had migraine without aura were evaluable, was not powerful and could not rule out that nimodipine could have up to 30% effect on a single main outcome parameter; however, the uniform lack of response in all tested parameters made this unlikely (45). The authors concluded that 'nimodipine probably has only a small or no effect in migraine without aura (45).

In one placebo-controlled trial (6) in children, the efficacy of nimodipine was not demonstrated. Two doses of nimodipine, 60 mg and 120 mg daily, were compared in a crossover trial (42), and the higher dose seemed to reduce headache frequency more than the lower; but both migraine and chronic cluster headache patients were investigated. In two comparative crossover trials, nimodipine (120 mg daily) was found to have results comparable to those of pizotifen (1.5 mg daily); these trials included 43 (23) and 20 evaluable patients (44). Nimodipine also showed results comparable to those of flunarizine (20 mg daily) in one small (n = 25) parallel group trial (9). All these trials lack power and a placebo control and therefore contribute little. In conclusion, some effect in migraine with aura cannot be excluded, but more than a minor effect in migraine without aura is unlikely. As a consequence, nimodipine has not been registered for migraine prophylaxis in any country.

OTHER CALCIUM ANTAGONISTS

Diltiazem (90 mg daily) was given to 15 patients who experienced frequent attacks of migraine; it significantly decreased the number of attacks and the severity of attacks (52). In a pilot study, patients who did not respond to nadolol had significant benefit from diltiazem therapy (55). No double-blind, controlled trials have been performed using diltiazem.

In a double-blind, crossover trial that included eight patients with migraine associated with idiopathic Raynaud's phenomenon, nifedipine (30 mg daily) showed better results than placebo (29). In an open study, about 70% of patients who had migraines, both with aura or without aura, reported benefit from nifedipine (28). In a randomized, open-label study, nifedipine (60 mg daily) had inferior results compared with propranolol (120 mg daily), and 9 of 20 patients treated with nifedipine withdrew from the study because of side effects (1). In a double-blind trial including 24 patients with migraine with aura, nifedipine (60–90 mg daily) achieved no better results than placebo and induced significantly more side effects, such as dizziness and edema (40). Thus, the limited trials do not support the use of nifedipine for migraine prophylaxis.

The atypical calcium antagonist cyclandelate (50) has been compared with propranolol and placebo. In one trial with parallel group design, cyclandelate (1,200–1,600 mg) was found to be comparable to propranolol (120–160 mg) in 62 evaluable patients (17), but the trial lacks placebo control, and the observed effects could be due to the so-called time effect (47). In another trial, also with parallel group design, neither cylandelate (1,200 mg) nor propranolol (120 mg) was statistically significantly superior to placebo in 214 patients (12). In contrast, cyclan-

delate (1,200–1,600 mg) was found to be superior to placebo in a small double-blind trial that included 15 and 10 patients in the two treatment groups, respectively (53). Thus, the scientific evidence for the use of cyclandelate in migraine prophylaxis remains to be established.

Finally, in a double-blind crossover trial that included 30 patients suffering from migraine without aura, nicardipine (40 mg daily) had better results than placebo in decreasing the frequency, intensity, and duration of attacks (33). Based on only one published trial, however, nicardipine cannot be recommended for migraine prophylaxis.

REFERENCES

1. Albers GW, Simon LT, Hamik A, Peroutka SJ. Nifedipine versus propranolol for the initial prophylaxis of migraine. *Headache* 1989;29:214–217.
2. Amery WK. Brain hypoxia: the turning-point in the genesis of the migraine attack? *Cephalalgia* 1982;2:83–109.
3. Andersson K-E, Vinge E. β-adrenoceptor and calcium antagonists in the prophylaxis and treatment of migraine. *Drugs* 1990;39:355–373.
4. Ansell E, Fazzone T, Festenstein R, Johnson ES, Thavapalan M, Wilkinson M. Nimodipine in migraine prophylaxis. *Cephalalgia* 1988;8:269–272.
5. Ayajiki K, Okamura T, Toda N. Flunarizine, an anti-migraine agent, impairs nitroxidergic nerve function in cerebral arteries. *Eur J Pharmacol* 1997;329:49–53.
6. Battistella PA, Ruffilli R, Moro R, et al. A placebo-controlled crossover trial of nimodipine in pediatric migraine. *Headache* 1990;30:264–268.
7. Bian K, Toda N. Vasodilator actions of flunarizine in isolated dog cerebral and extracerebral arteries. *Jpn J Pharmacol* 1989;49:83–94.
8. Bono G, Manzoni GC, Martucci N, et al. Flunarizine in common migraine: Italian cooperative trial II. Long-term follow-up. *Cephalalgia* 1985;5(Suppl 2):155–158.
9. Bussone G, Baldini S, D'Andrea G, et al. Nimodipine versus flunarizine in common migraine: a controlled pilot study. *Headache* 1987;27:76–79.
10. Centonze V, Magrone D, Vino M, et al. Flunarizine in migraine prophylaxis: efficacy and tolerability of 5 mg and 10 mg dose levels. *Cephalalgia* 1990;10:17–24.
11. Cerbo R, Casacchia M, Formisano R, et al. Flunarizine-pizotifen single-dose double-blind cross-over trial in migraine prophylaxis. *Cephalalgia* 1986;6:15–18.
12. Diener HC, Foh M, Iaccarino C, et al. on behalf of the study group. Cyclandelate in the prophylaxis of migraine: a randomized, parallel, double-blind study in comparison with placebo and propranolol. *Cephalalgia* 1996;16:441–447.
13. Drillisch C, Girke W. Ergebnisse der Behandlung von Migräne Patienten mit Cinnarizin und Flunarizin. *Medizinische Welt* 1980;31:1870–1872.
14. Frenken CWGM, Nuijten STM. Flunarizine, a new preventive approach to migraine. *Clin Neurol Neurosurg* 1984;86:17–20.
15. Gawel MJ, Kreeft J, Nelson RF, Simard D, Arnott WS. Comparison of te efficacy and safety of flunarizine to propranolol in the prophylaxis of migraine. *Can J Neurol Sci* 1992;19:340–345.
16. Gelmers HJ. Nimodipine, a new calcium antagonist, in the prophylactic treatment of migraine. *Headache* 1983;23:106–109.
17. Gerber WD, Schellenberg R, Thom M, et al. Cyclandelate versus propranolol in the prophylaxis of migraine—a double-blind placebo-controlled study. *Funct Neurol* 1995;10:27–35.
18. Godfraind T, Miller R, Wibo M. Calcium antagonism and calcium entry blockade. *Pharmacol Rev* 1986;38:321–416.
19. Greenberg DA. Calcium channel antagonists and the treatment of migraine. *Clin Neuropharmacol* 1986;9:311–328.
20. Grotemeyer K-H, Schlake H-P, Husstedt IW, Rolf LH. Metoprolol versus flunarizine: a double blind cross-over study. *Cephalalgia* 1987;7(Suppl 6):465–466.
21. Hansen AJ, Lauritzen M, Tfelt-Hansen P. Spreading cortical depression and antimigraine drugs. In: Amery WK, van Nueten JM, Wauquier A, eds. *The pharmacological basis of migraine therapy*. London: Pitman, 1984:161–170.
22. Havanka-Kannianinen H, Hokkanen E, Myllylä VV. Efficacy of nimodipine in the prophylaxis of migraine. *Cephalalgia* 1985;5:39–43.

23. Havanka-Kanniainen H, Hokkanen E, Myllylä VV. Efficacy of nimodipine in comparison with pizotifen in the prophylaxis of migraine. *Cephalalgia* 1987;7:7–13.

24. Henry PD. Comparative pharmacology of calcium antagonists: nifedipine, verapamil and diltiazem. *Am J Cardiol* 1980;46:1047–1058.

25. Hosono M, Fujii S, Himura T, et al. Inhibitory effect of cilnidipine on vascular sympathetic neurotransmission and subsequent vasoconstriction in spontaneously hypertensive rats. *Jpn J Pharmacol* 1995;69: 127–134.

26. Itil TM, Itil KZ, The comparative CNS pharmacology of nimodipine in man. In: Betz E, Deck K, Hoffmeister F, eds. *Nimodipine: pharmacological and clinical properties.* Stuttgart: Schattauer Verlag, 1985:1 85–202.

27. Jansen I, Tfelt-Hansen P, Edvinsson L. Comparison of the calcium entry blockers nimodipine and flunarizine on human cerebral and temporal arteries: role in cerebrovascular disorders. *Eur J Clin Pharmacol* 1991;40:7–15.

28. Jonsdottir BA, Meyer JS, Rogers Rl. Efficacy, side effects and tolerance compared during headache treatment with three different calcium blockers. *Headache* 1987;27:364–369.

29. Kahan A, Weber S, Amor B, Guerin F, Degeorges M. Nifedipine in the treatment of migraine in patients with Raynaud's phenomenon. *N Engl J Med* 1983;308:1102–1103.

30. Khalil R, Lodge N, Saida K, van Breemen C. Mechanism of calcium activation in vascular smooth muscle. *J Hypertens* 1987;5:S5–S15.

31. Lazarewicz JW, Pluta R, Salinska E, Puka M. Beneficial effect of nimodipine on on metabolic and functional disturbances in rabbit hippocampus following complete cerebral ischemia. *Stroke* 1989;20: 70–77.

32. Leandri M, Parodi C, Bacigalupo F, Farinini D. Long-term study on effectiveness of flunarizine i headache prophylaxis. *Cephalalgia* 1985; 5(Suppl 3):556–557.

33. Leandri M, Rigardo S, Schizzi R, Parodi CI. Migraine treatment with nicardine. *Cephalalgia* 1990;10:11–116.

34. Louis P. A double-blind placebo-controlled prophylactic study of flunarizine in migraine. *Headache* 1981;21:235–239.

35. Louis P, Spierings ELH. Comparison of flunarizine and pizotifen in migraine treatment: a double-blind study. *Cephalalgia* 1982;2: 197–203.

36. Ludin HP. Flunarizine and propranolol in the treatment of migraine. *Headache* 1989;29:219–223.

37. Lücking CH, Oestreich W, Schmidt R, Soyka D. Flunarizine vs. propranolol in the prophylaxis of migraine: two double-blind comparative studies in more than 400 patients. *Cephalagia* 1988;8:(Suppl 8):21–26.

38. Markley H, Cheronis J, Piepho R. Verapamil prophylactic therapy of migraine. *Neurology* 1984;34:973–976.

39. Marranes R, Wauquier A, Reid K, De Prins E. Effects of drugs on cortical spreading depression. In: Amery WK, Wauquier A, eds. *The prelude to the migraine attack.* London: Bailliere Tindall, 1986:158–173.

40. McArthur JC, Marek K, Pestronk A, McArthur J, Peroutka SJ. Nifedipine in the prophylaxis of classic migraine: A crossover, double-masked, placebo-controlled study of headache frquency and side effects. *Neurology* 1989;39:284–286.

41. Mendenopoulos G, Manafi T, Logothesis I, Bostantjopoulou S. Flunarizine in the prevention of classical migraine: a placebo-controlled evaluation. *Cephalalgia* 1985;5:31–37.

42. Meyer JS, Hardenberg J. Clinical effectiveness of calcium entry blockers in prophylactic treatment of migraine and cluster headache. *Headache* 1983;23:266–277.

43. Micheli FE, Pardal MMF, Giannaula R, et al. Movement disorders and depression due to flunarizine and cinnarizine. *Mov Disord* 1989;4: 139–146.

44. Micieli G, Trucco M, Agostinis C, Mancuso A, Papalia F, Sinforiani E. Nimodipine vs pizotifen in common migraine: results of a double-blind cross-over trial. *Cephalalgia* 1985;5(Suppl 3):532–533.

45. Migraine–Nimodipine European study Group (MINES). European multicenter trial of nimodipine in the prophylaxis of common migraine (migraine without aura). *Headache* 1989;29:633–638.

46. Migraine–Nimodipine European study Group (MINES). European multicenter trial of nimodipine in the prophylaxis of classic migraine (migraine with aura). *Headache* 1989;29:639–642.

47. Olesen J, Krabbe AÆ, Tfelt-Hansen P. Methodological aspects of prophylactic drug trials in migraine. *Cephalalgia* 1981;1:127–141.

48. Overweg J, Binnie CD, Meijer JWA, et al. Double-blind placebo-controlled trial of flunarizine as add-on therapy in epilepsy. *Epilepsia* 1984;25:217–222.

49. Peroutka SJ, Banghart SB, Allen GS. Relative potency and selectivity of calcium antagonists used in the treatments of migraine. *Headache* 1984;25:55–58.

50. Perrier ML, Scatton B, Benavides J. Dihydropyridine- and omega-conotoxin resistant, neomycin-sensitive calcium channels mediate the depolarization-induced increase in internal calcium levels in cortical slices from immature rat brain. *J Pharmacol Exp Ther* 1992;261: 324–330.

51. Rascol A, Montastruc J-L, Rascol O. Flunarizine versus pizotifen: a double-blind study in the prophylaxis of migraine. *Headache* 1986;26: 83–85.

52. Riopelle RJ, McCans JL. A pilot study of the calcium antagonist diltiazem in migraine syndrome prophylaxis. *J Can Sci Neurol* 1982;9: 269.

53. Siniatchkin M, Gerber W-D, Vein A. Clinical efficacy and central mechanisms of cyclandelate in migraine: a double-blind placebo-controlled study. *Funct Neurol* 1998;13:47–56.

54. Shimizu K, Ohta T, Toda N. Evidence for greater susceptibility of isolated dog cerebral arteries to Ca antagonists than peripheral arteries. *Stroke* 1980:11:261–266.

55. Smith R, Schwartz A. Diltiazem prophylaxis in refractory migraine. *N Engl J Med* 1984;310:1327–1328.

56. Solomon GD. The actions and uses of calcium channel blockers in migraine and cluster headache. *Headache Quarterly* 1990;1:152–159.

57. Solomon GD, Diamond S, Freitag FG. Verapamil in migraine prophylaxis; comparison of dosages. *Clin Pharmacol Ther* 1987;41:202.

58. Solomon GD, Scott AFB. Verapamil and propranolol in migraine prophylaxis: a double-blind, crossover study. *Headache* 1986;26:325.

59. Solomon GD, Steel JG, Spaccavento LJ. Verapamil prophylaxis of migraine: a double-blind, placebo-controlled trial. *JAMA* 1983;250: 2500–2502.

60. Sorge F, De Simone R, Marano E, Nolano M, Orefice G, Carrieri P. Flunarizine in prophylaxis of childhood migraine. A double-blind, placebo-controlled, cross-over study. *Cephalalgia* 1988;8:1–6.

61. Sorge F, Marano E. Flunarizine v. placebo in childhood migraine: a double-blind study. *Cephalalgia* 1985;5(suppl 2):145–148.

62. Steardo L, Marano E, Barone P, Denman DW, Moteleone P, Cardone G. Prophylaxis of migraine attacks with a calcium-channel blocker: flunarizine versus methysergide. *J Clin Pharmacol* 1986;26:524–528.

63. Stewart DJ, Gelston A, Hakim A. Effect of prophylactic administration of nimodipine in patients with migraine. *Headache* 1988;28:260–262.

64. Sørensen PS, Hansen H, Olesen J. A placebo-controlled, double-blind, cross-over trial of flunarizine in common migraine. *Cephalalgia* 1986; 6:7–14.

65. Sørensen PS, Larsen BH, Rasmussen MJK, et al. Flunarizine versus metoprolol in migraine prophylaxis: a double-blind, randomized parallel group study of efficacy and tolerability. *Headache* 1991;31: 650–657.

66. Tfelt-Hansen P, Edvinsson L, Olesen J. Treatment of migraine with calcium entry blockers. *Progress in Basic Clinical Pharmacology* 1989;2: 143–154.

67. Thomas M, Behari M, Ahuja GK. Flunarizine in migraine prophylaxis: an Indian trial. *Headache* 1991;31:613–615.

68. Toda N, Okamura T. Different susceptibility of vasodilator nerve, endothelium and smooth muscle functions to Ca++ antagonists in cerebral arteries. *J Pharmacol Exp Ther* 1992;261:234–239.

69. Todd PA, Benfield P. Flunarizine—a reappraisal of its pharmacological properties and therapeutic use in neurological disorders. *Drugs* 1989;38:481–499.

70. Towart R. The selective inhibition of serotonin induced contraction of rabbit cerebral vasculatur smooth muscle by calcium-antagonistic dihyropyridines. *Circ Res* 1981;48:650–657.

71. Vanhoutte PM, Paoletti R. The WHO classification of calcium antagonists. *Trends in Pharmacological Sciences* 1987;8:4–5.

72. Wauquier A, Ashton D, Marranas R. The effects of flunarizine in experimental models related to the pathogenesis of migraine. *Cephalalgia* 1985;5(Suppl 2):119–123.

73. Wörz R, Drillisch C. Migräne-Prophylaxe durch einen Kalziumeintrittsblocker: Ergebnisse einer Doppelblindstudie Flunarizin vs. Pizotifen. *MMW Munich Med Wochenschr* 1983;125:711–714.

rior to placebo (see Table 1), but the trial failed to show a clear dose–response relationship across this range. Unfortunately, although the same principal measure of efficacy (mean attack frequency) was adopted in the dose-ranging study, outcome on this measure was not actually reported; together with a substantial baseline difference between the placebo (6.1 per 4 weeks) and all active treatment groups (4.5 to 4.7 per 4 weeks), this lack of outcome data makes comparison with other studies difficult. Responder rates (attack frequency reduced by ≥50% compared with run-in) on divalproex (44%), however, were compatible with those in the earlier trial (48%) (31).

The most common adverse events in one trial (31), which recorded considerably more frequent events than others, were nausea (46% of patients), asthenia (31%), drowsiness (30%), vomiting (19%), tremor (13%), and alopecia (13%). Discontinuations from divalproex (13%) were nevertheless not significantly higher than from placebo (5%).

Comparative Trials

No randomized double-blind, placebo-controlled trials have compared valproate or divalproex with other antimigraine drugs. In open or single-blind trials, valproate had similar efficacy to propranolol (23) and flunarizine (36) and divalproex to propranolol (21).

Therapeutic Use

Valproate may be used in migraine prophylaxis when the first-choice drugs, beta-blockers, are contraindicated or ineffective. Because no clear dose–response curve for the prophylactic effect of valproate in migraine has been established, doses lower than those used in epilepsy, for example 500 mg daily, may be used to initiate therapy. Depending on the efficacy and side effects, this dose may be increased. Valproate probably should not be deemed ineffective before it is demonstrated that doses resulting in antiepileptic plasma concentrations lack efficacy.

A sizeable minority of patients taking valproate will experience side effects (32,41), principally but not entirely gastrointestinal, and these can be reduced by enteric coating (43). Other side effects are weight gain, hair loss, and tremor. Fulminant hepatitis, not consistently preceded by abnormal tests of liver function, occurs rarely with valproate monotherapy in epilepsy (32). In most countries, routine hematologic screening and biochemical tests of liver function are considered necessary before starting and during valproate or divalproex treatment.

Contraindications

Persons with thrombocytopenia and liver disease should not take valproate. These drugs are associated with an increased incidence of neural tube defects (19) and other fetal abnormalities and, in the treatment of migraine, should not be used at any time during pregnancy.

NEWER ANTIEPILEPTIC DRUGS

Gabapentin

The possible mode of action of gabapentin in migraine is unclear (52). It penetrates the blood–brain barrier but does not interact with GABA receptors (14). Gabapentin was evaluated in one double-blind parallel-group comparison with placebo (51). In 14 patients taking gabapentin, 900 mg daily, the mean attack frequency was reduced from 6.5 to 4.1 per month. In an open study of 34 patients, doses of 600 to 1,800 mg daily resulted in decreases in attack frequency of 50% or more in 59% of patients (30).

Vigabatrin

Vigabatrin has some pharmacological similarities to valproate (32). It is a selective irreversible inhibitor of GABA transaminase. In a double-blind study (13), 23 patients with migraine with or without aura refractory to other treatments were randomly allocated to vigabatrin titrated to 1,000 to 2,000 mg daily over 6 weeks or placebo. Treatment was maintained for an additional 6 weeks before crossover, with 4 weeks of washout between treatments. Attack frequency was reduced by 40% or more in 10 of 16 (63%) patients who completed the study, but the level of statistical significance was not reported.

Lamotrigine

Lamotrigine blocks voltage-sensitive sodium channels, leading to inhibition of neuronal release of glutamate (24,27,34), which is essential to the propagation of spreading depression (42). In an open study, ten patients with migraine with aura responded favorably to lamotrigine (9). In a double-blind trial (45), 77 patients with migraine with or without aura were randomly allocated to lamotrigine, 200 mg daily, or placebo. Treatment in parallel groups was continued for up to 3 months. Mean attack frequency was reduced from 4.4 to 3.0 per 4 weeks on placebo and from 3.6 to 3.2 on active medication. These differences were not statistically significant but indicated that lamotrigine was ineffective in attack prevention.

CONCLUSIONS

Among the several antiepileptic drugs, old and new, that have been evaluated for migraine prophylaxis, only valproate/valproic acid is of proven efficacy. Defining its place in migraine prophylaxis awaits comparative trials, but it may be among the most effective prophylactic drugs available. Nevertheless, its use in women of child-bearing potential is not without problems. No other drug has been sufficiently investigated to disprove useful effect; whereas gabapentin and vigabatrin may have some promise, lamotrigine does not.

REFERENCES

1. Andermann F. Migraine and epilepsy: an overview. In: Andermann F, Lugaresi E, eds: *Migraine and epilepsy*. Boston: Butterworths, 1987: 405–422.
2. Anthony M, Lance JW, Somerville B. A comparative trial of prindolol, clonidine and carbamazepine in the interval therapy of migraine. *Med J Austr* 1972;1:1343–1346.
3. Basser LS. The relation of migraine and epilepsy. *Brain* 1969;92: 285–300
4. Bloom FE. Neurotransmission and the central nervous system. In: Hardman JG, Limbird LE, Molinoff PB, Ruddon RW, Gilman AG, eds. *Goodman and Gilman's The pharmacological basis of therapeutics*, 9th ed. New York: McGraw-Hill, 1996:267–293.
5. Coria F, Sempere AP, Duarte J, et al. Low-dose sodium valproate in the prophylaxis of migraine. *Clin Neuropharmacol* 1994;17:569–573.
6. Cotariu D, Zaidman JL, Evans S. Neurophysiological and biochemical changes evoked by valproic acid in the central nervous system. *Progr Neurobiol* 1990;34:343–354.
7. Cutrer FM, Limmroth V, Ayata C, Moskowitz MA. Attenuation by valproate of c-*fos* immunoreactivity in trigeminal nucleus caudalis induced by intracisternal capsaicin. *Br J Pharmacol* 1995;116: 3199–3204.
8. Cutrer FM, Moskowitz MA. The actions of valproate and neurosteroids in a model of trigeminal pain. *Headache* 1996;36:265.
9. D'Andrea G, Granella F. Effectiveness of lamotrigine in the prophylaxis of migraine with aura. An open pilot study. *Cephalalgia* 1997; 17:4138.
10. Derman H, Hasson S. Low dose Depakote in migraine prophylaxis. *Headache* 1996;36:265.
11. Donnet A, Bartolomei F. Migraine with visual aura and photosensitive epileptic seizures. *Epilepsia* 1997;38:1032–1034.
12. Ferrari MD, Odnik J, Bos KD, Malessy MJA, Bruyn GW. Neuroexcitatory plasma amino acids are elevated in migraine. *Neurology* 1990; 40:1582–1586.
13. Ghose K, Niven B, McLeod A, Berry B. Vigabatrin in the prophylaxis of drug resistant migraine: a double blind crossover comparison with placebo. *Cephalalgia* 1996;16:367.
14. Gidal BE, Wagner ML, Privitera MD, et al. Current developments in neurology, part I: advances in the pharmacotherapy of headache, epilepsy and multiple sclerosis. *Ann Pharmacother* 1996;30:1272–1276.
15. Goldstein J. The emergence of an anticonvulsant drug in the management of migraine. *Headache Quart* 1996;7(Suppl 1):13–15.
16. Graham JR. The migraine connection. *Headache* 1981;21:243–250.
17. Headache Classification Committee of the International Headache Society. Classification and diagnostic criteria for headache disorders, cranial neuralgias and facial pain. *Cephalalgia* 1988;8(Suppl 7):1–96.
18. Hering R, Kuritzky A. Sodium valproate in the prophylactic treatment of migraine: a double-blind study versus placebo. *Cephalalgia* 1992; 12:81–84.
19. Jeavons PM. Sodium valproate and neural tube defects. *Lancet* 1982; 2:1282–1283.
20. Jensen R, Brinck T, Olesen J. Sodium valproate has a prophylactic effect in migraine without aura: a triple-blind, placebo-controlled crossover study. *Neurology* 1994;44:647–651.
21. Kaniecki RG. A comparison of divalproex with propranolol and placebo for the prophylaxis of migraine without aura. *Arch Neurol* 1997;54:1141–1145.
22. Klapper J, on behalf of the Divalproex Sodium in Migraine Prophylaxis Study Group. Divalproex sodium in migraine prophylaxis: a dose-controlled study. *Cephalalgia* 1997;17:103–108.
23. Kozubski W, Prusinski A. Sodium valproate versus propranolol in the prophylactic treatment of migraine. *Neurol Neurochir Polska* 1995; 29:937–947.
24. Lamb RJ, Leach MJ, Miller AA, Wheatley PL. Anticonvulsant profile in mice of lamotrigine, a novel anticonvulsant. *Br J Pharmacol* 1985; 85(Suppl):235.
25. Lauritzen M. Spreading cortical depression as a mechanism of the aura in classic migraine. In: Amery WK, Wauquier A, eds: *The prelude to the migraine attack*. London: Bailliere Tindall 1986:134–141.
26. Leao AAP. Spreading depression of activity in the cerebral cortex. *J Neurophysiol* 1944;7:359–390.
27. Leach MJ, Marden CM, Miller AA. Pharmacological studies on lamotrigine, a novel potential antiepileptic drug. II. Neurochemical studies on the mechanism of action. *Epilepsia* 1986;27:490–497
28. Lee WS, Limmroth V, Ayata C, et al. Peripheral GABA$_A$ receptor-mediated effects of sodium valproate on dural plasma protein extravasation to substance P and trigeminal stimulation. *Br J Pharmacol* 1995; 116:1661–1667.
29. Marks DA, Ehrenberg BR. Migraine-related seizures in adults with epilepsy, with EEG correlation. *Neurology* 1993;43:2476–2483.
30. Mathew N. Gabapentin in migraine prophylaxis. *Cephalalgia* 1996; 16:367.
31. Mathew NT, Saper JR, Silberstein SD, et al. Migraine prophylaxis with divalproex. *Arch Neurol* 1995;52:281–286.
32. McNamara JO. Drugs effective in the therapy of the epilepsies. In: Hardman JG, Limbird LE, Molinoff PB, Ruddon RW, Gilman AG, eds. *Goodman and Gilman's The pharmacological basis of therapeutics*, 9th ed. New York: McGraw-Hill, 1996:461–486.
33. McQuay H, Carroll D, Jadad AR, Wiffen P, Moore A. Anticonvulsant drugs for management of pain: a systematic review. *BMJ* 1995;311: 1047–1052.
34. Millar AA, Wheatley P, Sawyer DA, et al. Pharmacological studies on lamotrigine, a novel potential antiepileptic drug. I. Anticonvulsant profile in mice and rats. *Epilepsia* 1986;27:483–489.
35. Mitsikostas DD. The valproate mechanisms of action in migraine [Letter]. *Cephalalgia* 1994;14:465.
36. Mitsikostas DD, Polychronidis I. Valproate versus flunarizine in migraine prophylaxis: a randomized, double-open, clinical trial. *Funct Neurol* 1997;12:267–276.
37. Nishikawa T, Scatton B. Inhibitory influence of GABA on central serotonergic transmission: raphe nuclei as the neuroanatomical site of the GABAergic inhibition of cerebral serotonergic neurons. *Brain Res* 1985;331:91–103.
38. Panayiotopoulos CP, Sharoqi IA, Agathonikou A. Occipital seizures imitating migraine aura. *J R Soc Med* 1997;90:255–257.
39. Ramadan NM, Schultz LL, Gilkey SJ. Migraine prophylactic drugs: proof of efficacy, utilization and cost. *Cephalalgia* 1997;17:73–80.
40. Rompel H, Bauermeister PW. Aetiology of migraine and prevention with carbamazepine (Tegretol): results of a double-blind cross-over study. *S Afr Med J* 1970;44:75–80.
41. Rothrock JF. Clinical studies of valproate for migraine prophylaxis. *Cephalalgia* 1997;17:81–83.
42. Scheller D, Heister U, Dengler K, Tegtmeier F. Extracellular changes of aspartate and glutamate during generation and during propagation of cortical spreading depression in rats. In: Olesen J, ed. *Migraine and other headaches:* the vascular mechanisms. New York: Raven Press 1991:161–165.
43. Silberstein SD. Divalproex sodium in headache: literature review and clinical guidelines. *Headache* 1996;36:547–555.
44. Sorensen KV. Valproate: a new drug in migraine prophylaxis. *Acta Neurol Scand* 1988; 78:346–348.
45. Steiner TJ, Findley LJ, Yuen AWC. Lamotrigine versus placebo in the prophylaxis of migraine with and without aura. *Cephalalgia* 1997;17: 109–112.
46. Stensrud P, Sjaastad O. Clonazepam (Rivotril) in migraine prophylaxis. *Headache* 1979;19:333–334.
47. Taylor K. High-dose versus low-dose valproic acid as a prophylactic medication. *Headache* 1996;36:514–515.
48. Tran BN, Vivian VS, Burch KJ. Can valproate prevent migraine headaches? *J Pharm Technol* 1997;13:163–168.
49. Weiller C, May A, limmroth V, Juptner M, Kaube H, Schayck RV, Coenen HH, Diener HC. Brain stem activation in spontaneous human migraine attacks. *Nat Med* 1995;1:658–660.

50. Welch KMA, D Andrea G, Tepley N, Barkly G, Ramadan NM. The concept of migraine as a state of central neuronal hyperexcitability. *Neurol Clin* 1989;8:817–828.

51. Wessely P, Baumgartner C, Klingler D, Kreczi J, Meyerson N, Sailer L, Saltuari L, Schütt P. Preliminary results of a double blind study with the new migraine prophylactic drug gabapentin. *Cephalalgia* 1987;7(Suppl 6):476–477.

52. Wetzel CH, Connelly JF. Use of gabapentin in pain management. *Ann Pharmacother* 1997;31:1082–1083.

53. Wong SL, Cavanaugh J, Shi H, Awni, WM, Granneman GR. Effects of divalproex sodium on amitriptyline and nortriptyline pharmacokinetics. *Clin Pharmacol Ther* 1996;60:48–53.

54. Zaccara G, Messori A, Moroni F. Clinical pharmacokinetics of valproic acid. *Clin Pharmacokinet* 1988;15:367–389.

The Headaches, Second Edition,
edited by J. Olesen, P. Tfelt-Hansen, and K.M.A. Welch.
Lippincott Williams & Wilkins, Philadelphia © 2000.

The Migraines

CHAPTER 60

Nonsteroidal Antiinflammatory and Miscellaneous Drugs in Migraine Prophylaxis

Ewan J. Mylecharane and Peer Tfelt-Hansen

The rationale for using nonsteroidal antiinflammatory drugs (NSAIDs) in the prophylaxis of migraine is based on the possible general involvement of prostaglandins in the inflammatory/algesic pathophysiologic components of the migraine process (see Chapter 50) as well as the proposal that migraine is a primary platelet disorder (84) with aggregation releasing vasoactive products, including 5-hydroxytryptamine (5-HT, serotonin) and prostaglandins, a hypothesis that has been effectively challenged (74). Furthermore, NSAIDs may relieve the abdominal pain associated with menstruation and, because about 15% of women migraineurs suffer migraine only during menstruation (22), it has been suggested that NSAIDs might be effective for menstrual-related migraine (see Chapter 32).

Many other miscellaneous drugs have been tested for migraine prophylaxis, but this chapter is confined to drugs that have been assessed seriously over the last 30 years: some ergot alkaloids (e.g., dihydroergotamine); some antihypertensive agents with affinity for α-adrenoceptors (e.g., clonidine and indoramin); some antidepressants (e.g., amitriptyline, monoamine oxidase inhibitors, and some selective 5-HT uptake inhibitors); and nonorthodox drugs such as magnesium, riboflavin, and feverfew. For drugs with established efficacy in migraine prophylaxis, details of their therapeutic use are mentioned briefly.

E. J. Mylecharane: Department of Pharmacology, University of Sydney, Sydney, New South Wales 2006, Australia.

P. Tfelt-Hansen: Department of Neurology, Glostrup Hospital, University of Copenhagen, DK-2600 Glostrup, Copenhagen, Denmark.

NONSTEROIDAL ANTIINFLAMMATORY DRUGS (NSAIDS)

Pharmacologic Background

The pharmacologic actions of the NSAIDs relevant to migraine prophylaxis are described in Chapter 50. Briefly, NSAIDs, including aspirin, possess antiinflammatory, analgesic, and antipyretic properties (33). The principal types of drugs are listed in Table 1 in Chapter 50. They exert their effect by inhibiting the ubiquitous cyclooxygenase-1 (*constitutive*) and cyclooxygenase-2 (*inducible*) enzymes, thereby preventing the synthesis of prostaglandins and thromboxanes from arachidonic acid. The inhibition by aspirin, but not other NSAIDs, is irreversible because aspirin acetylates cyclooxygenase. In platelets, which cannot resynthesize cyclooxygenase, the effects of low doses of aspirin are substantial and long lasting, in contrast to the negligible activity of these doses in other tissues where cyclooxygenase can be resynthesized. Inhibition of platelet cyclooxygenase reduces the thromboxane A_2-mediated ability of the platelet to aggregate in response to some endogenous aggregants (33). The NSAIDs usually are classified as peripheral analgesics, although they have central effects as well (see Chapter 50).

Possible Mode of Action in Migraine Prophylaxis

The mode of action of NSAIDs in migraine therapy and whether this mode of action involves prostaglandins in the migraine process are discussed in Chapter 50. One of the major obstacles to inhibition of cyclooxygenase being responsible for the prophylactic efficacy of these

TABLE 1. *Double-blind randomized clinical trials comparing NSAIDs with placebo and other drugs in the prophylaxis of migraine*

Trial	Drug and dosage (mg)	Study design	No. of patients (no. evaluated), type of migraine	Run-in	Duration of treatment	Factors evaluated	Investigators' conclusions
(55)	ASA 650 bid PI bid	CO	12 MO, MA	Nil	3 mo × 2	Frequency	ASA > PI
(7)	ASA 4.5/kg tid Prop 0.6/kg tid	CO	18 (12) MO	30 days open	3 mo × 2 (2 wk washout)	Frequency Headache index[a]	ASA vs Prop, NS [a]Both > run-in
(32)	ASA 160 od PI od	CO	38 (27) MO, MA		3 mo × 2	Frequency, severity	ASA vs PI, NS
(62)	ASA 100–200 od Flun 5–10 od	Pa	30 (29)[b] MO, MA	4 wk open	3 mo	Frequency	ASA vs Flun, NS; both > run-in
(29)	Metop 200 od ASA 1,500 od	CO	28 (21) MO	8 wk	12 wk × 2	Frequency, 50% decrease in frequency	Metop > ASA; both > run-in
(43)	Napx 250 bid PI bid	CO	28 MO, MA	2 mo (no drug)	6 wk × 2 (1 wk washout)	Frequency, duration, headache index,[e] preference	Napx > PI for preference other parameters dubious[d]
(84)	NapxS 550 bid PI bid	CO	34 (28) MO, MA	2 wk PI	8 wk × 2 (2 wk washout)	Rating of efficacy,[e] headache index,[c] duration, medication	NapxS > PI for all parameters
(81)	NapxS 550 bid PI bid	CO	51 (33) MO, MA	2 wk PI	8 wk × 2 (2 wk washout)	Rating of efficacy,[e] headache index,[c] days with severe headache	NapxS > PI for all parameters
(71)	NapxS 550 bid Prop 40 tid PI	Pa	170 (129) MO, MA	2 wk PI	14 wk	Headache days, severity, overall evaluation	NapxS vs. Prop vs PI NS for headache days and severity; Napxs = Prop > PI for patients' evaluation
(10)	NapxS 550 bid Pizo 0.5 tid PI tid	Pa	176 (151) MO, MA	8 wk	12 wk	Headache unit index	NapxS = Pizo > PI
(49)	Tfa 100 tid PI tid	CO	38 (31) MO, MA	Nil	10 wk × 2 (2 wk washout)	Frequency, severity, duration, preference	Tfa > PI for PI all parameters
(50)	Tfa 100 tid Prop 40 tid PI tid	CO	39 (31) MO, MA	Nil	12 wk × 3	Frequency, duration, severity, medication	Tfa = Prop > PI for frequency and medication; Tfa > Prop = PI for severity
(67)	Tfa 100 tid Prop 40 tid	CO	76 (56) MO, MA	4 wk (no drug)	12 wk × 2 (4 wk washout)	Migraine days, duration, severity	Both > run-in Tfa = Prop for all parameters.
(76)	Ketop 50 tid PI tid	CO	26 (24) MO, MA	Nil	6 wk × 2 (1 wk washout)	Headache index[c] headache days	Ketopr > PI for both parameters
(35)	Mefena 500 tid Prop 80 tid PI tid	CO	29 (17) MO, MA	1 mo open	3 mo × 3	Frequency, duration, severity	Frequency: Mefena = Prop > PI severity and duration, NS
(20)	Fenop 200 tid Fenop 600 tid PI tid	Pa	118 (110) MO, MA	4 wk PI	12 wk	Frequency, headache index, medication	Fenop 600 > PI for all parameters; parameters; Fenop 200 vs. PI, NS

TABLE 1. *Continued*

Trial	Drug and dosage (mg)	Study design	No. of patients (no. evaluated), type of migraine	Run-in	Duration of treatment	Factors evaluated	Investigators' conclusions
(17)	Indob 200 bid Pl bid	Pa	42 (35) MO, MA	4 wk (no drug)	3 mo	Frequency, duration headache index,[c] evaluation of treatment	Indob > Pl for all parameters

ASA, aspirin; Fenop, fenoprofen; Flun, flunarizine; Indob, indobufen; Ketop, ketoprofen; Mefena, mefenamic acid; Metop, metoprolol; Napx, naproxen; NapxS, naproxen sodium; NSAIDs, nonsteroidal antiinflammatory drugs; Pizo, pizotifen; Prop, propranolol; Tfa, tolfenamic acid; Pl, placebo; od, once daily; bid, twice daily; tid, three times daily; CO, crossover; Pa, parallel-groups comparison; MO, migraine without aura; MA, migraine with aura; wk, week(s); mo, month(s); NS (or =), no statistical significant difference; >, more effective than.

[a] Frequency × severity × duration.
[b] Children, 7 to 17 years old.
[c] Frequency × severity.

agents is the lack of effect of the potent NSAID indomethacin in a double-blind, placebo-controlled trial in migraine patients (5).

It has been suggested that the prophylactic usefulness of NSAIDs in migraine could be through the inhibition of platelet aggregation, thereby correcting an underlying hyperaggregability (46,84). Moderately high oral doses of aspirin (650–1,300 mg daily) in combination with 75 to 300 mg dipyramidole daily were marginally superior to placebo in one trial (68) and superior to placebo in another (46), but these effects were not correlated with whether the patients had hyperaggregable platelets. Aspirin in doses as low as 40 mg inhibits platelet aggregation (33), but in one placebo-controlled crossover trial in which a low dose of aspirin (160 mg) was evaluated for migraine prophylaxis (see below), the "active" medication was of no benefit despite inhibition of platelet function (32). In the Physicians' Health Study (15) of aspirin (325 mg on alternate days), however, a 20% reduction in the incidence of migraine was suggested compared with placebo (see below). No correlation was observed between the degree of platelet inhibition and the efficacy as a migraine prophylactic of naproxen (81); thus, the concept of migraine as a primary platelet disorder has been challenged (74). Our view is that it is most unlikely that an action on platelets is responsible for the beneficial prophylactic effect of NSAIDs.

Pharmacokinetics of NSAIDs

Absorption after oral aspirin (acetylsalicylic acid), as with other NSAIDs, is high, in excess of 80% (14,21,33). Aspirin is metabolized rapidly by plasma and tissue esterases to salicylic acid before it reaches the systemic circulation; thus, it is likely that low doses of aspirin act on platelets in the portal venous blood. The peak plasma concentration of aspirin is achieved 15 minutes after oral administration, whereas the peak concentration of salicylate is reached after 30 to 60 minutes. The irreversible action of aspirin means that platelet responsiveness is inhibited long after aspirin has been excreted from the body. In contrast, high doses are needed for analgesia, an effect that is reversible within a few hours as new cyclooxygenase is synthesized within the tissues. Salicylic acid is a relatively weak analgesic. The plasma half-life of aspirin is 15 to 30 minutes. Salicylic acid exhibits dose-dependent kinetics; thus, its half-life after 250 mg of aspirin is about 3 hours and after 1 g about 6 hours (42). Naproxen/naproxen sodium, fenoprofen, and mefenamic acid all have high bioavailabilities (>90%), whereas tolfenamic acid has a bioavailability of 60% (60) to 85% (S.B. Pedersen, personal communication). The plasma half-lives of these NSAIDs are in the range of 2 to 4 hours, with the exception of naproxen, which has a half-life of 12 to 15 hours (14,21,33,60).

Results of Controlled Clinical Trials

A summary of 17 controlled double-blind randomized trials on the efficacy of oral NSAIDs in migraine prophylaxis is given in Table 1. All but two trials (7,29) included migraine patients both with and without aura.

Medium doses of aspirin (1,300 mg and 900 mg daily, respectively) showed superior efficacy compared with placebo (55) and were apparently comparable in efficacy to propranolol (7) in two small trials (12 patients in each), although the latter trial was too small to demonstrate comparability. In another trial, however, aspirin (1,500 mg daily) was less effective than metoprolol (29). Trials of low doses of aspirin have not provided convincing evidence of efficacy. Aspirin (160 mg daily) did not achieve better results than placebo (32), and no correlation was found between the number of attacks and inhibition of adenosine diphosphate (ADP)-induced platelet aggregation. In children aged 7 to 17 years, aspirin's effect (100–200 mg daily) was comparable to that of flunarizine

(62); however, because no placebo was used in this trial, conclusions concerning the efficacy of aspirin cannot be made (see Chapter 7). The Physicians' Health Study (15) was not a specific trial on migraine prophylaxis, but it indicated some effect of low-dose aspirin (325 mg every other day for the prevention of cardiovascular disease) with the finding that 6% of subjects reported migraine compared with 7.4% of subjects taking placebo during a 60-month period. The rate of self-reported ordinary headaches was similar in the two groups. The question of whether low-dose aspirin with resulting inhibition of platelet aggregation has a minor effect in migraine prophylaxis thus remains open.

In the first trial of naproxen (500 mg daily), this drug proved only questionably better than placebo (43). Naproxen sodium (1,100 mg daily), however, was demonstrated to have better efficacy than placebo in three trials (10,81,84), and in one of these trials (10) it was comparable to pizotifen. In another trial (71), naproxen sodium (1,100 mg daily) was comparable to propranolol, but the superiority of both drugs over placebo was restricted to patients' evaluations. Comparability in each of these trials was not substantiated by narrow confidence intervals.

Tolfenamic acid had significantly better results than placebo (49,50), and comparability to propranolol was indicated in one of the trials (50) by rather narrow confidence intervals. In another trial (67), tolfenamic acid was comparable to propranolol, but no placebo control was included. Ketoprofen showed marginally superior results compared with placebo in a group of severely afflicted migraine patients (75). In one small trial (17 patients), mefenamic acid had superior efficacy compared with placebo (35), but the claimed comparability to propranolol cannot be substantiated from a trial that included so few patients. Fenoprofen (1,800 mg daily but not 600 mg daily) was superior to placebo (20). Indobufen also had greater effects than placebo in one trial (17). In our opinion, only naproxen sodium and tolfenamic acid have been demonstrated convincingly to be superior to placebo.

Gastrointestinal problems were the most common side effects during NSAID treatment, including dyspepsia and diarrhea, but their frequencies of occurrence were generally not greater than those encountered in subjects who took placebo, probably because of the relatively small size of the trials. In only one trial (naproxen sodium) was it necessary for a patient to withdraw because of peptic ulceration (10).

Menstrual Migraine

Naproxen sodium (550 mg twice daily) has been shown to reduce "pain" (including headache) in the premenstrual syndrome (23). Its specific effects on "menstrual migraine" (550 mg twice daily) have also been evaluated (69,71,79). In one trial (71), a subset of 30 of 129 patients taking naproxen sodium or placebo continuously was analyzed for headache activity occurring before and after the onset of menstruation; patients treated with naproxen sodium reported fewer and less severe headaches during the week before menstruation than patients treated with placebo, but only severity was significantly reduced. In the other two placebo-controlled trials, naproxen sodium, given during 1 week before and 1 week after the start of menstruation, resulted in fewer perimenstrual headaches; in one study (79), severity was not reduced (79), but in the other both severity and analgesic requirements were decreased (69).

Therapeutic Use

When first-line migraine prophylactics (i.e., β-adrenoceptor blockers and antiserotonin drugs) are ineffective, contraindicated, or inappropriate, NSAIDs may be tried. The recommended doses of the two NSAIDs with proven efficacy in migraine prophylaxis are naproxen sodium (or equivalent naproxen), 550 mg twice daily, and tolfenamic acid, 100 mg three times daily. The regimens for other NSAIDs are mefenamic acid, 500 mg three times daily; fenoprofen, 600 mg three times daily; indobufen, 200 mg twice daily; and aspirin, 300 to 600 mg three times daily. For migraine occurring at the time of menstruation, which often does not respond to prophylactic treatment, naproxen sodium, 550 mg twice daily (or equivalent dose of naproxen), can be tried for 1 week before and 1 week after menstruation.

Side effects include dyspepsia, erosive gastritis, peptic ulceration, diarrhea (especially tolfenamic and mefenamic acids), hematologic complications, and hypersensitivity reactions. Contraindications include hypersensitivity to aspirin or any NSAID, active peptic ulceration, liver or kidney disease, coagulation disorders or treatment with other anticoagulants, and age below 12 years.

ERGOT ALKALOIDS

Dihydroergotamine

Among the ergot alkaloids, dihydroergotamine (for pharmacology of dihydroergotamine, see Chapter 51) was traditionally used orally in the prophylaxis of migraine, despite the lack of controlled clinical trials demonstrating its efficacy (for review, see 73). Dihydroergotamine, in a long-acting oral form, has been subjected to six controlled double-blind clinical trials of its efficacy in migraine prophylaxis. In three trials (31,45,53) with treatment periods from 30 to 45 days, dihydroergotamine (10 mg daily) was superior to placebo in reducing the frequency of attacks. In one study (31), however, most patients probably did not suffer from migraine, and one study (45) was reported only briefly, making it difficult to judge, although this trial suggested that dihydroergotamine was most effective in "night" migraine. Three other trials showed that drugs like flunarizine (10 mg once daily) (41), indoramin (25 mg twice daily) (64), and dihydroergocryptine (20 mg twice daily) (26) are better than run-in and no different from dihydroergotamine (5 mg twice daily); all these comparative studies, however, suffer from a lack of placebo control, and the results may be merely a "time effect" (see Chapter 7).

In one double-blind crossover trial, the combination of long-acting dihydroergotamine (10 mg) plus aspirin (80 mg) daily reduced attack frequency compared with placebo (11), but the use of two drugs concurrently in this trial makes it impossible to draw definitive conclusions as to the efficacy of either. In another double-blind trial in children, dihydroergotamine (3–6 mg daily, administered as drops 2 or 3 times per day) did not produce better results than placebo during 3 months treatment (63). Overall, the trials reviewed herein indicate some efficacy of dihydroergotamine in migraine prophylaxis, but definitive scientific proof for efficacy remains weak.

In migraine prophylaxis, dihydroergotamine is used in a dose of 10 mg daily. The main side effects reported during dihydroergotamine trials include nausea, vomiting, diarrhea, and abdominal pain (73). Contraindications include known hypersensitivity to ergot alkaloids, pregnancy, breastfeeding, coronary artery and other vascular disease, and concomitant use of erythromycin and triacetyloleandomycin, which may inhibit the metabolism of dihydroergotamine (39). It should be used with caution in patients with hepatic or renal disease.

Dihydroergocryptine

Dihydroergocryptine is a hydrogenated ergot alkaloid that possesses dopamine D_1 and D_2 receptor agonist activity. In a double-blind crossover trial (16), oral dihydroergocryptine (20 mg daily) was compared with placebo as a prophylactic agent in patients who have migraine without aura. A considerable "time effect" is apparent; dihydroergocryptine was probably superior to placebo, but appropriate statistical evaluation was not presented. As mentioned, dihydroergocryptine was comparable to dihydroergotamine in a subsequent controlled trial and showed a considerable "time effect" (26). Dihydroergocryptine (20 mg daily) was comparable to flunarizine (5 mg daily) in migraine without aura (2), but no placebo control was included. Thus, no conclusion regarding the efficacy of this compound can be drawn.

Ergometrine

Based on a retrospective study (66) and extensive clinical experience (65), ergometrine (also known as ergonovine) in an oral dose of 0.6 to 1.2 mg daily has been recommended for migraine prophylaxis. The known pharmacologic properties of ergometrine are similar to those of methylergometrine, which may explain the possible efficacy of ergometrine, because methylergometrine is most likely the active metabolite of methysergide, which has proven efficacy in migraine prophylaxis (see Chapter 57).

DRUGS WITH AFFINITY FOR α-ADRENOCEPTORS

The antihypertensive agent clonidine is a centrally acting selective α_2-adrenoceptor agonist. It has some vasoconstrictor activity, mediated through a partial agonist action at α_2-adrenoceptors in some vascular smooth muscle. It was introduced as a potential migraine prophylactic agent, however, on the basis of studies in cats; these studies purported to show that low (nonhypotensive) doses of clonidine had a direct inhibitory effect on vasoconstrictor and vasodilator responses to noradrenaline, adrenaline, isoprenaline, and angiotensin (82). Subsequent studies on the monkey cranial vasculature using mediators implicated in migraine could not reproduce these findings, however, and therefore have refuted the pharmacologic basis shown in animal models for an action of clonidine in migraine (52).

Three early double-blind, placebo-controlled trials apparently demonstrated the efficacy of clonidine in migraine prophylaxis, but the methodology used in these trials has been questioned (58). Ten other such trials failed to show superiority of clonidine compared with placebo (12,19,58), whereas in one trial clonidine showed superior effects compared with placebo (36). In crossover comparative trials with β-adrenoceptor antagonists, clonidine had better efficacy than practolol (36), it had equal efficacy to propranolol (38), and it was inferior to metoprolol (44). In most cases, clonidine is clearly ineffective.

Indoramin is a selective, competitive α_1-adrenoceptor antagonist that was introduced as an antihypertensive agent; in addition, competitive antagonism of histamine H_1 and 5-HT receptors is also evident (3). In an initial double-blind, controlled study, indoramin had better efficacy than placebo in migraine prophylaxis (57). In an unpublished trial (cited in 58), indoramin did not have better efficacy than placebo. In another study (64), indoramin was comparable to dihydroergotamine in the prophylaxis of migraine, but the lack of placebo precludes a definitive conclusion.

ANTIDEPRESSANT DRUGS

Monoamine Uptake Inhibitors

The only antidepressant drug with established efficacy in the prophylaxis of migraine is the tricyclic agent amitriptyline. In the clinical trials summarized in the following section, a consistent finding is that its antimigraine effect is unrelated to its antidepressant action. Amitriptyline inhibits both noradrenaline and 5-HT uptake to a similar extent (for pharmacology of amitriptyline, see Chapter 88), but inhibition of uptake does not appear to correlate with efficacy in migraine. Another tricyclic antidepressant, imipramine, which is a relatively selective noradrenaline uptake inhibitor, has little effect in migraine prophylaxis (65), although no controlled trials have been reported. Clomipramine, a tricyclic antidepressant with a selective inhibitory effect on 5-HT uptake, is also inactive in controlled migraine trials (40,54).

Of the nontricyclic antidepressants that selectively inhibit 5-HT uptake, femoxetine had no significant effect in placebo-controlled migraine prophylaxis trials (56,83), and it was inferior to propranolol with regard to headache index (4,37) and attack frequency (37). Zimelidine was reported to be better than placebo (78), but this was a single-blind trial with an unusual design (placebo after zimelidine), and a difference was found for only one parameter. The efficacy of fluoxetine in migraine prophylaxis is uncertain. In a small double-blind, placebo-controlled trial with parallel group design (but 14 of 32 were dropouts), fluoxetine (10–40 mg daily) was superior to placebo (1). In a larger trial of similar design (no dropouts), however, fluoxetine (20–40 mg daily) did not show better efficacy than placebo on any measure (70). A recent study with S-fluoxetine, the longer-acting enantiomer of racemic fluoxetine and equieffective with the R-enantiomer as an uptake inhibitor, showed that 40 mg daily for 3 months was superior to placebo, with attack frequency reduced 52% by S-fluoxetine and 27% by placebo, although attack severity was unaltered (75). The longer half-life of S-fluoxetine (7 days, compared with 8 hours for R-fluoxetine) may have resulted in higher blood levels than those achieved in the previous trials. The only other selective 5-HT uptake inhibitor evaluated for migraine prophylaxis in a controlled trial is fluvoxamine (8), which was compared with amitriptyline; both drugs significantly reduced attack frequency and headache index values to a similar extent, but the relatively low dose of amitriptyline used (25 mg daily) and the lack of placebo make it difficult to gauge efficacy.

Overall, amine uptake inhibition does not seem to be responsible for the prophylactic effect of some antidepressants in migraine. The possibility that 5-HT$_2$ receptor blockade might explain the efficacy of amitriptyline in migraine has been raised (25,58), but 5-HT$_2$ receptor blockade is probably not responsible for the effect of antiserotonin drugs in migraine (see Chapter 57). Many antidepressants (including amitriptyline, imipramine, and fluoxetine) induce a gradual downregulation in central 5-HT$_2$ receptors and β-adrenoceptors, although the data are not always consistent (30). The possible role of such more subtle and localized regulatory effects on receptor

TABLE 2. *Double-blind randomized clinical trials comparing amitriptyline with placebo and other drugs in the prophylaxis of migraine*

Trial	Drug and dosage (mg/day)	Study design	No. of patients (no. evaluated), type of migraine	Run-in	Duration of treatment	Factors evaluated	Investigators' conclusions
(27)	Amitr 10–60[a] Pl	CO	26 (20) MO, MA	Nil	6 mo × 2	Frequency, duration	Amitr > Pl for frequency
(18)	Amitr 50–100 Pl	Pa	162 (100)[b] MO, MA	4 wk Pl	8 wk	Migraine score, depression scores[c]	Amitr > Pl for migraine score; unrelated to depression
(85)	Amitr 50–150 Prop 80–240 Pl	CO	54 (30) MA	4 wk Pl	10 wk × 3 (2 wk washout)	Headache score, depression scores[c]	Amitr = Prop > Pl for headache score; unrelated to depression
(86)	Amitr 40–150 Prop 25–240 Pl	CO	30 MO, MA	4 wk Pl	10 wk × 3 (2 wk washout)	Frequency, severity, headache score	Amitr > Pl for all parameters; Prop > Pl for severity, headache score
(8)	Amitr 25 Fluvox 50	Pa	70 (49) MO, MA	4 wk Pl	12 wk	Frequency, headache index	Amitr > run-in for both parameters Fluvox > run-in for both parameters

Amitr, amitriptyline; Fluvox, fluvoxamine; Prop, propranolol; Pl, placebo; MA, migraine with aura; MO, migraine without aura; CO, crossover; Pa, parallel-groups comparison; wk, week(s); mo, month(s); =, no significant difference; >, more effective than.
[a]Average dose 30–40 mg.
[b]Forty-six patients dropped out during placebo run-in.
[c]Hamilton depression scale and Zung self-rating depression scale.

NONSTEROIDAL ANTIINFLAMMATORY AND MISCELLANEOUS DRUGS / 495

densities and monoaminergic transmission remains to be investigated.

A summary of the five double-blind controlled clinical trials with oral amitriptyline is given in Table 2. The doses of amitriptyline used varied considerably, from 10 to 150 mg daily. Amitriptyline had better efficacy than placebo in all four placebo-controlled trials (18,27,85,86), and it was equieffective to propranolol (85) and fluvoxamine (8) in two of the comparative trials. No clear correlation was found between antidepressant activity and migraine prophylactic effect of amitriptyline in the trials in which depression was assessed objectively (18,85). In two of the placebo-controlled trials (18,85), the results were given only as a composite headache score, and no estimates of the variability in the mean data were provided, which makes it difficult to judge the clinical nature of the results (see Chapter 7), but in the other placebo-controlled trials, amitriptyline reduced attack frequency by 42% (27) and by up to 51% (86) compared with placebo. As noted, the lack of placebo in the comparative trial of amitriptyline and fluvoxamine (8) makes conclusions about efficacy difficult.

In migraine prophylaxis, the effective dosage of amitriptyline varies considerably among subjects, probably reflecting the wide variation in its bioavailability (see Chapter 88). The recommended starting dose is 10 mg taken at night; depending on efficacy and side effects, this dose may be increased by 10 mg every 2 weeks to a daily dose normally between 20 and 50 mg. Migraine patients are often sensitive to the unpleasant side effects of the drug, which in most cases means limiting the dose to 50 mg (27). Others (18,65,85,86) have used doses of the order of 150 to 175 mg daily.

Side effects of amitriptyline include drowsiness (the most common side effect), dry mouth, weight gain, skin reactions, orthostatic hypotension, nausea, and constipation. Contraindications include narrow-angle glaucoma, urinary retention, pregnancy, breastfeeding, and concomitant use of monoamine oxidase inhibitors. It should be used with caution in patients with kidney, liver, cardiovascular, and thyroid disease.

Monoamine Oxidase Inhibitors

These antidepressants were introduced in migraine prophylaxis based on the hypothesis that migraine is a "low 5-HT syndrome" with resulting vasodilation and that the drug would increase plasma 5-HT levels; the only evidence of efficacy, however, comes from two open trials of phenelzine (6,48) and a retrospective analysis of the effects of moclobemide alone or in combination with other migraine prophylactic drugs (47). Modulation of central nervous system monoaminergic neurotransmission is more likely to be responsible for any effects of phenelzine or moclobemide in migraine. Like other antidepressants, monoamine oxidase inhibitors produce a

gradual downregulation in central 5-HT$_2$ and β-adrenergic receptors (30). Because of the serious side effects of monoamine oxidase inhibitors and the caution required regarding serious interactions with foods and drugs (less likely with moclobemide, which is reversible and monoamine oxidase A-selective but still an important risk), their use should be reserved for patients who have frequent attacks and who have failed to respond to other forms of prophylactic or acute treatments.

Other Antidepressants

The atypical antidepressant mianserin appears to have no prophylactic effect in migraine, despite its high affinity for 5-HT$_{2A/2C}$ receptors (see Chapter 57). A placebo-controlled crossover trial of trazodone in paediatric migraine prophylaxis (9) demonstrated significant superiority over placebo, despite a substantial initial improvement with placebo. The most prominent pharmacologic action of trazodone is 5-HT$_{2A/2C}$ receptor antagonism; it also has some α-adrenoceptor antagonist and weak 5-HT uptake inhibitory activity. Paradoxically, its major metabolite, m-chlorophenylpiperazine, can induce a migrainelike headache (13), although no such adverse events were reported in this paediatric migraine trial (9).

NONORTHODOX DRUGS

In recent years, some agents that have not been regarded as orthodox drug therapy for migraine have been subjected to clinical trials. Those considered here are magnesium, riboflavin, and feverfew.

Magnesium has been tested in three double-blind, placebo-controlled trials using a parallel-group comparison design, on the basis of reductions in Mg^{2+} levels in blood, saliva, cerebrospinal fluid, and cortex cells in association with migraine. The first trial (24) included patients with menstrual migraine in whom magnesium was found to be effective in reducing the total index of pain and days with migraine when administered in a total daily oral dose of 360 mg of Mg^{2+} (from day 15 to onset of menses for two menstrual cycles). A larger trial (59) also showed some efficacy in migraine (with or without aura) patients who took a total daily oral dose of 600 mg of Mg^{2+} for 12 weeks. Attack frequency was reduced by 42% compared with 16% in the placebo group; comparable reductions in days with migraine also were reported. The number of responders (> 50% reduction in attack frequency), however, was not significantly higher after magnesium (39%) than after placebo (21%). Another trial, however, concluded that magnesium at a total daily oral dose of 243 mg of Mg^{2+} for 12 weeks had no significant effect on intensity or total duration of migraine attacks in patients who had migraine without aura (61). Only 29% of each group achieved the study's primary endpoint of a 50% or better reduction in attack intensity or total duration. The lower dose used in this trial might account for the apparent lack of efficacy of magnesium, but given the very low absorption of magnesium following oral administration, the range of oral doses used might not be a critical factor in producing increases in extracellular and intracellular Mg^{2+} levels. In one trial (24), blood levels in the migraine patients at the commencement of the trial were lower in lymphocytes and polymorphonucleated cells but were not lower in erythrocytes or plasma, compared with nonmigrainous controls. The magnesium treatment produced generally greater increases in lymphocyte and polymorphonucleated cell Mg^{2+} levels compared with those in the placebo group, but erythrocyte and plasma levels remained unchanged. Diarrhea and gastric irritation were the most commonly reported adverse effects of magnesium in these trials; the only other adverse effect was palpitations (in three patients). The results of these trials suggest that magnesium may prove to be of benefit, but further controlled trials are needed because of the relatively small number of patients recruited into trials thus far.

Riboflavin for migraine prophylaxis has been studied in only one placebo-controlled trial (72). The stimulus for this trial was the identification of impaired oxygen metabolism resulting from mitochondrial dysfunction as a possible pathogenic factor in migraine, the beneficial effect of riboflavin in some other rare mitochondriopathies, and encouraging results from a small open pilot study. The trial was a double-blind, parallel-group comparison design, with results from migraine (with or without aura) patients treated for 3 months with riboflavin (400 mg/day) or placebo. Riboflavin was superior to placebo in reducing attack frequency, intensity, and duration, as well as days with migraine and a migraine index. A 50% or greater reduction in attack frequency, days with migraine, and migraine index was achieved by 56%, 59%, and 41% of the riboflavin group, respectively, compared with 19%, 15%, and 8% of the placebo group. The high dose of riboflavin used resulted in only two minor adverse events (diarrhea, polyuria). These findings justify further controlled trials to define a possible role for riboflavin in migraine prophylaxis.

The first clinical trial of feverfew (*Tanacetum parthenium*) in migraine prophylaxis (34) was initiated after a marked increase in self-medication with this herb when the health food industry responded to demand and marketed a variety of formulations containing dried feverfew; previously, its use had been confined largely to the ingestion of fresh leaves. The active ingredient is thought to be in the sesquiterpene lactone content of the leaves, the principal one being parthenolide. This double-blind, placebo-controlled pilot trial was completed in 17 patients in a parallel-group comparison design. All patients had a history of migraine with or without aura, for which they had been using fresh feverfew leaves daily for at least 3 months before commencement of the trial,

at which point they changed to daily treatment for 24 weeks with capsules containing a standard equivalent dose of freeze-dried feverfew leaves or placebo. The conclusion reached, that feverfew is of benefit in migraine, relied on the indirect finding that migraine frequency and intensity remained unchanged in the feverfew group but increased significantly in the placebo group. The investigators noted, however, that the initial degree of efficacy of the prior self-medication with feverfew is difficult to assess, as it was based solely on recollections of a group of self-selected feverfew users; in addition, in some cases, other drugs with potential migraine prophylactic activity had been used in conjunction with the prior fresh feverfew self-treatment and in the trial period. A larger and more valid double-blind, placebo-controlled trial confirmed that feverfew reduced the attack frequency of migraine with or without aura (51). The duration and severity of attacks were not changed by feverfew, but accompanying nausea and vomiting were reduced. This trial design was a crossover study of treatment with feverfew and placebo (4 months in each case) following a 1-month run-in with placebo, completed in 59 patients. Capsules containing dried feverfew leaves, standardized for parthenolide content, were used at a daily dose rate equivalent to the "average" self-medication dose of feverfew leaves. Only 23% of the trial subjects had previously used feverfew, and all migraine-related treatments were stopped at the beginning of the run-in period. Although feverfew was clearly superior to placebo in some respects, the overall 24% reduction in the frequency of attacks with feverfew use relative to the frequency in the placebo group appears to be a modest improvement. Subsequent investigations have focused on inhibition of platelet aggregation and 5-HT secretion as a possible mechanism for an antimigraine action of feverfew, by means of inhibitory effects on a variety of intracellular pathways that include protein kinase C, phospholipase A_2, cyclooxygenase, and lipoxygenase (28,77). Unfortunately, no further reliable controlled trials have investigated the efficacy of feverfew in migraine prophylaxis. A recent review (80) was critical of two other double-blind, placebo-controlled trials (one in 1994 claiming no benefit, one in 1997 claiming efficacy) on grounds of a lack of important detail, methodology, and small sample size. A third well-conducted trial in 1996 showed no benefit, but in this trial an extract of feverfew with a standardized concentration of parthelonide lactones was used, which may mean that the sesquiterpene lactones in feverfew are not the active ingredients.

REFERENCES

1. Adly C, Straumanis J, Chesson A. Fluoxetine prophylaxis of migraine. *Headache* 1992;32:101–104.
2. Agnoli A, Bussone G, Mailland F, Manzoni GC, Martucci N, Nappi G. Dihydroergokryptine vs flunarizine in the basic treatment of migraine without aura. *Cephalalgia* 1991;11(Suppl 11):216–217.

3. Alps BJ, Hill M, Johnson ES, Wilson AB. Quantitative analysis on isolated organs of the autonomic blocking properties of indoramin hydrochloride (Wy 21901). *Br J Pharmacol* 1972;44:52–62.
4. Andersson PG, Petersen EN. Propranolol and femoxetine, a 5-HT uptake inhibitor, in migraine prophylaxis: a double-blind crossover study. *Acta Neurol Scand* 1981;64:280–288.
5. Anthony M, Lance JW. Indomethacin in migraine. *Med J Aust* 1968;1:56–57.
6. Anthony M, Lance JW. Monoamine oxidase inhibition in the treatment of migraine. *Arch Neurol* 1969;21:263–268.
7. Baldrati A, Cortelli P, Procaccianti G, et al. Propranolol and acetylsalicylic acid in migraine prophylaxis: double-blind crossover study. *Acta Neurol Scand* 1983;67:181–186.
8. Bánk J. A comparative study of amitriptyline and fluvoxamine in migraine prophylaxis. *Headache* 1994;34:476–478.
9. Battistella PA, Ruffilli R, Cernetti R, et al. A placebo-controlled crossover trial using trazodone in pediatric migraine. *Headache* 1993;33: 36–39.
10. Bellavance AJ, Meloche JP. A comparative study of naproxen sodium, pizotyline and placebo in migraine prophylaxis. *Headache* 1990;30: 710–715.
11. Bousser MG, Chick J, Fuseau E, Soisson T, Thevenet R. Combined low-dose acetylsalicylic acid and dihydroergotamine in migraine prophylaxis: a double-blind, placebo-controlled crossover study. *Cephalalgia* 1988;8:187–192.
12. Bredfeldt RC, Sutherland JE, Kruse JE. Efficacy of transdermal clonidine for headache prophylaxis and reduction of narcotic use in migraine patients: a randomized crossover trial. *J Fam Pract* 1989;29: 153–158.
13. Brewerton TD, Murphy DL, Mueller EA, Jimerson DC. Induction of migrainelike headaches by the serotonin agonist m-chlorophenylpiperazine. *Clin Pharmacol Ther* 1988;43:605–609.
14. Brogden RN, Heel RC, Speight TM, Avery GS. Naproxen up to date: a review of its pharmacological properties and therapeutic efficacy and use in rheumatic diseases and pain states. *Drugs* 1979;18:241–277.
15. Buring JE, Peto R, Hennekens CH. Low-dose aspirin for migraine prophylaxis. *JAMA* 1990;264:1711–1713.
16. Canonico PL, Scapagnini U, Genazzani E, Zanotti A. Dihydroergokryptine (DEK) in the prophylaxis of common migraine: double-blind clinical study vs placebo. *Cephalalgia* 1989; 9(Suppl 10):446–447.
17. Carrieri PB, Orefice G, Sorge F. A double-blind placebo-controlled trial of indobufen. *Acta Neurol Scand* 1988;77:433–436.
18. Couch JR, Hassanein RS. Amitriptyline in migraine prophylaxis. *Arch Neurol* 1979;36:695–699.
19. Das SM, Ahuja GK, Narainaswamy AS. Clonidine in prophylaxis of migraine. *Acta Neurol Scand* 1979;60:214–217.
20. Diamond S, Solomon GD, Freitag FG, Mehta ND. Fenoprofen in the prophylaxis of migraine: a double-blind, placebo controlled study. *Headache* 1987;27:246–249.
21. Dollery CT. NSAID monographs. In: Dollery CT, ed. *Therapeutic drugs.* Edinburgh: Churchill Livingstone, 1991;A146–A150,F20–F23, M31–M34,N30–N33.
22. Epstein MT, Hockaday JM, Hockaday TDR. Migraine and reproductive hormones throughout the menstrual cycle. *Lancet* 1975;1:543–548.
23. Facchinetti F, Fioroni L, Sances G, Romano G, Nappi G, Genazzani AR. Naproxen sodium in the treatment of premenstrual symptoms: a placebo-controlled study. *Gynecol Obstet Invest* 1989;28:205–208.
24. Facchinetti F, Sances G, Borella P, Genazzani AR, Nappi G. Magnesium prophylaxis of menstrual migraine: effects on intracellular magnesium. *Headache* 1991;31:298–301.
25. Fozard JR. Basic mechanisms of antimigraine drugs. *Adv Neurol* 1982; 33:295–307.
26. Frediani F, Grazzi L, Zanotti A, Mailland F, Zappacosta BM, Bussone G. Dihydroergokryptine versus dihydroergotamine in migraine prophylaxis: a double-blind clinical trial. *Cephalalgia* 1991;11:117–121.
27. Gomersall JD, Stuart A. Amitriptyline in migraine prophylaxis: changes in pattern of attacks during a controlled clinical trial. *J Neurol Neurosurg Psychiatry* 1973;36:684–690.
28. Groenewegen WA, Heptinstall S. A comparison of the effects of an extract of feverfew and parthenolide, a component of feverfew, on human platelet activity in-vitro. *J Pharm Pharmacol* 1990;42:553–557.
29. Grotemeyer K-H, Scharafinski H-W, Schlake H-P, Husstedt IW. Acetylsalicylic acid vs. metoprolol in migraine prophylaxis a double-blind cross-over study. *Headache* 1990;30:639–641.
30. Heninger GR, Charney DS. Mechanism of action of antidepressant treatments: implications for the etiology and treatment of depressive disorders. In: Meltzer HY, ed. *Psychopharmacology: the third generation of progress.* New York: Raven Press, 1987;535–544.
31. Heuser B, Middendorf E. Migräneprophylaxe mit Dihydroergotamin. *Fortschr Med* 1985;103:966–970.
32. Hosman-Benjaminse SL, Bolhuis PA. Migraine and platelet aggregation in patients treated with low dose acetylsalicylic acid. *Headache* 1986;26:282–284.
33. Insel PA. Analgesic-antipyretic and antiinflammatory agents and drugs employed in the treatment of gout. In: Hardman JG, Limbird LE, Molinoff PB, Ruddon RW, Gilman AG, eds. *Goodman and Gilman's the pharmacological basis of therapeutics,* 9th ed. New York: McGraw-Hill, 1996;617–657.
34. Johnson ES, Kadam NP, Hylands DM, Hylands PJ. Efficacy of feverfew as prophylactic treatment of migraine. *BMJ* 1985;291:569–573.
35. Johnson RH, Hornabrook RW, Lambie DG. Comparison of mefenamic acid and propranolol with placebo in migraine prophylaxis. *Acta Neurol Scand* 1986;73:490–492.
36. Kallanranta T, Hakkarainen H, Hokkanen E, Tuovinen T. Clonidine in migraine prophylaxis. *Headache* 1977;17:169–172.
37. Kangasniemi PJ, Nyrke T, Lang AH, Petersen E. Femoxetine a new 5-HT uptake inhibitor and propranolol in the prophylactic treatment of migraine. *Acta Neurol Scand* 1983;68:262–267.
38. Kåss B, Nestvold K. Propranolol (Inderal) and clonidine (Catapressan) in the prophylactic treatment of migraine: a comparative trial. *Acta Neurol Scand* 1980;61:351–356.
39. Krupp P, Haas G. Effects indésirables et interactions medicamenteuse des alcaloides d l'ergot de seigle. *J Pharmacol* 1979;10:401–402.
40. Langohr HD, Gerber WD, Koletzki E, Mayer K, Schroth G. Clomipramine and metoprolol in migraine prophylaxis a double-blind crossover study. *Headache* 1985;25:107–113.
41. Langohr HD, Reinicke M, Gerber WD, Mangold R. Dihydroergotamin und Flunarizin in der Migräne-Prophylaxe: Eine vergleichende Doppelblind-Studie. *Forstschr Med* 1988;106:39–42.
42. Levy G. Pharmacokinetics of salicylate elimination in man. *J Pharmaceut Sci* 1965;54:959–967.
43. Lindegaard K-F, Övrelid L, Sjaastad O. Naproxen in the prevention of migraine attacks: a double-blind placebo-controlled cross-over study. *Headache* 1980;20:96–98.
44. Louis P, Schoenen J, Hedman C. Metoprolol v. clonidine in the prophylactic treatment of migraine. *Cephalalgia* 1985;5:159–165.
45. Martucci N, Manna V, Mattesi P, et al. Ergot derivatives in the prophylaxis of migraine: a multicentric study with a timed-release dihydroergotamine formulation. *Cephalalgia* 1983;3(Suppl 1):151–155.
46. Masel BE, Chesson AL, Peters BH, Levin HS, Alperin JB. Platelet antagonists in migraine prophylaxis: a clinical trial using aspirin and dipyridamole. *Headache* 1980;20:13–18.
47. Meienberg O, Amsler F. Moclobemide in the prophylactic treatment of migraine: a retrospective analysis of 44 cases. *Eur Neurol* 1996;36: 109–110.
48. Merikangas KR, Merikangas JR. Combination monoamine oxidase inhibitor and -blocker treatment of migraine, with anxiety and depression. *Biol Psychiatry* 1995;38:603–610.
49. Mikkelsen BM, Falk JV. Prophylactic treatment of migraine with tolfenamic acid: a comparative double-blind crossover study between tolfenamic acid and placebo. *Acta Neurol Scand* 1982;66:105–111.
50. Mikkelsen B, Pedersen KK, Christiansen LV. Prophylactic treatment of migraine with tolfenamic acid, propranolol and placebo. *Acta Neurol Scand* 1986;73:423–427.
51. Murphy JJ, Heptinstall, S, Mitchell JRA. Randomised double-blind placebo-controlled trial of feverfew in migraine prevention. *Lancet* 1988;2:189–192.
52. Mylecharane EJ, Duckworth JW, Lord GDA, Lance JW. Effects of low doses of clonidine in the monkey circulation. *Eur J Pharmacol* 1980; 68:163–173.
53. Neuman M, Demaraz JP, Harmey JL, Le Bastard B, Cauquil J. Prevention of migraine attacks through the use of dihydroergotamine. *Int J Clin Pharmacol Res* 1986;6:11–13.
54. Noone JF. Clomipramine in the prevention of migraine. *J Int Med Res* 1980;8(Suppl 3):49–52.
55. O'Neill BP, Mann JD. Aspirin prophylaxis in migraine. *Lancet* 1978;2: 1179–1181.
56. Orholm M, Honoré PF, Zeeberg I. A randomized general practice

group-comparative study of femoxetine and placebo in the prophylaxis of migraine. *Acta Neurol Scand* 1986;74:235–239.

57. Pearce J, Pearce I, Faux GA. α-Adrenergic activity and blockade in migraine. In: Greene R, ed. *Current concepts in migraine research.* New York: Raven Press, 1978;49–52.

58. Peatfield RC, Fozard JR, Clifford Rose F. Drug treatment of migraine. In: Clifford Rose F, ed. *Handbook of clinical neurology,* Vol 4, *Headache.* Amsterdam: Elsevier, 1986;173–216.

59. Peikert A, Wilimzig C, Köhne-Volland R. Prophylaxis of migraine with oral magnesium: results from a prospective, multi-center, placebo-controlled and double-blind randomized study. *Cephalalgia* 1996;16:257–263.

60. Pentikäinen PJ, Neuvonen PJ, Backman C. Human pharmacokinetics of tolfenamic acid, a new anti-inflammatory agent. *Eur J Clin Pharmacol* 1981;19:359–365.

61. Pfaffenrath V, Wessely P, Meyer C et al. Magnesium in the prophylaxis of migraine a double-blind, placebo-controlled study. *Cephalalgia* 1996;16:436–440.

62. Pothmann R. Migräneprophylaxe mit Flunarizin und Azetylsalizylsäure. *Monatsschr Kinderheilkd* 1987;135:646–649.

63. Pothmann R, Winter K. Migraine prophylaxis with dihydroergotamine a double-blind placebo-controlled study. *Cephalalgia* 1989;9(Suppl 10):428–429.

64. Pradalier A, Dry J, Loisy B, et al. Etude comparative indoramine versus dihydroergotamine dans le traitement préventif de la migraine. *Therapie* 1988;43:293–297.

65. Raskin NH. *Headache,* 2nd ed. New York: Churchill Livingstone, 1988;135–213.

66. Raskin NH, Schwartz RK. Interval therapy of migraine: long-term results. *Headache* 1980;20:336–340.

67. Rasmussen M-J K, Larsen BH, Borg L, Sørensen PS, Hansen PE. Tolfenamic acid versus propranolol in the prophylactic treatment of migraine. *Acta Neurol Scand* 1994;89:446–450.

68. Ryan RE Sr, Ryan RE Jr. The use of platelet inhibitors in migraine. *Adv Neurol* 1982;33:247–252.

69. Sances G, Martignoni E, Fioroni L, Blandini F, Facchinetti F, Nappi G. Naproxen sodium in menstrual migraine prophylaxis: a double-blind placebo controlled study. *Headache* 1990;30:705–709.

70. Saper JR, Silberstein SD, Lake AE, Winters ME. Double-blind trial of fluoxetine: chronic daily headache and migraine. *Headache* 1994;34:497–502.

71. Sargent J, Solbach P, Damasio H, et al. A comparison of naproxen sodium to propranolol hydrochloride and a placebo control for the prophylaxis of migraine headache. *Headache* 1985;25:320–324.

72. Schoenen J, Jacquy J, Lenaerts M. Effectiveness of high-dose riboflavin in migraine prophylaxis: a randomized controlled trial. *Neurology* 1998;50:466–470.

73. Scott AK. Dihydroergotamine: a review of its use in the treatment of migraine and other headaches. *Clin Neuropharmacol* 1992;15:289–296.

74. Steiner TJ, Joseph R, Clifford Rose F. Migraine is not a platelet disorder. *Headache* 1985;25:434–440.

75. Steiner TJ, Ahmed F, Findley LJ, MacGregor EA, Wilkinson M. S-fluoxetine in the prophylaxis of migraine: a phase II double-blind randomized placebo-controlled study. *Cephalalgia* 1998;18:283–6.

76. Stensrud P, Sjaastad O. Clinical trial of a new anti-bradykinin, anti-inflammatory drug, ketoprofen (19.583 R.P.) in migraine prophylaxis. *Headache* 1974;14:96–100.

77. Sumner H, Salan U, Knight DW, Hoult JRS. Inhibition of 5-lipoxygenase and cyclo-oxygenase in leukocytes by feverfew: involvement of sesquiterpene lactones and other components. *Biochem Pharmacol* 1992;43:2313–2320.

78. Syvälahti E, Kangasniemi P, Ross SB. Migraine headache and blood serotonin levels after administration of zimelidine, a selective inhibitor of serotonin uptake. *Curr Ther Res* 1979;25:299–310.

79. Szekely B, Merryman S, Croft H, Post G. Prophylactic effects of naproxen sodium on perimenstrual headache: a double-blind, placebo-controlled study. *Cephalalgia* 1989;9(Suppl 10):452–453.

80. Vogler BK, Pittler MH, Ernst E. Feverfew as a preventive treatment for migraine: a systematic review. *Cephalalgia* 1998;18:704–708.

81. Welch KMA, Ellis DJ, Keenan PA. Successful migraine prophylaxis with naproxen sodium. *Neurology* 1985;35:1304–1310.

82. Zaimis E, Hanington E. A possible pharmacological approach to migraine. *Lancet* 1969;2:298–300.

83. Zeeberg I, Orholm M, Nielsen JD, Honore PLF, Larsen JJV. Femoxetine in the prophylaxis of migraine a randomised comparison with placebo. *Acta Neurol Scand* 1981;64:452–459.

84. Ziegler DK, Ellis DJ. Naproxen in prophylaxis of migraine. *Arch Neurol* 1985;42:582–584.

85. Ziegler DK, Hurwitz A, Hassanein RS, Kodanaz HA, Preskorn SH, Mason J. Migraine prophylaxis: a comparison of propranolol and amitriptyline. *Arch Neurol* 1987;44:486–489.

86. Ziegler DK, Hurwitz A, Preskorn S, Hassanein R, Seim J. Propranolol and amitriptyline in prophylaxis of migraine: pharmacokinetic and therapeutic effects. *Arch Neurol* 1993;50:825–830.

The Headaches, Second Edition,
edited by J. Olesen, P. Tfelt-Hansen, and K.M.A. Welch.
Lippincott Williams & Wilkins, Philadelphia © 2000.

The Migraines

CHAPTER 61

Prioritizing Prophylactic Treatment of Migraine

Peer Tfelt-Hansen and K. Michael A. Welch

Prioritizing prophylactic treatment of migraine is a complex task that should be regarded as a joint venture between the doctor and the patient who is participating in a single-case scientific experiment. For general recommendations on when to use prophylactic treatment, on the use of headache diaries, and on tailoring the dose to the individual patient, consult Chapter 49 on general principles of pharmacotherapy in migraine. This chapter focuses on general information necessary for the physician to advise patients about the choice of prophylactic drugs.

The first priority is to use the drug that has the highest risk-to-benefit ratio. At first glance, this task might seem easy based on numerous publications about pharmacologic prophylaxis of migraine. Review of these studies and clinical trials, however, will confirm that most prophylactic drugs have an approximate 40% advantage over placebo in reducing attack frequency (see Chapters 56–58). In part, this may be artifactual, as a result of publication bias occasioned by authors, industrial companies, and editors having a preference for positive results. If a trial of active drug does not produce better results than placebo, or if the new drug has inferior benefits compared with those of an established drug, the trial often remains unpublished. In addition, comparability is seldom substantiated by narrow confidence intervals; even in small trials with grossly inadequate power, the lack of significance is often confused with lack of difference (see Chapter 7). Side effects often are reported as infrequently for active drugs as for placebo in controlled clinical trials,

probably because of either the inclusion of too few patients in the trial or an inadequate system for reporting adverse events (see Chapter 7). In clinical practice, side effects occur with the use of antimigraine drugs, which may limit their use.

In addition to the above-mentioned limitations in transferring results from controlled trials to clinical practice, it should be kept in mind that migraine patients recruited for controlled trials are often hard-core patients from specialized clinics who have participated in multiple trials. Controlled trials probably are not a true reflection of general practice.

Our ranking of prophylactic drugs (summarized in Table 1) is based on a combination of our judgment of the publications and our personal experience and may differ from the experience of others. The table gives a ranking, from + to ++++ (see Table 1), for clinical efficacy, scientific validity of the drug trials, and potential for side effects. The table also includes side effects and contraindications. For a more extensive review of side effects and contraindications, the reader should consult the individual chapters. Drug contraindications should be known before a drug is considered for use. The potential for side effects is an important factor in the choice of prophylactic drug, because use may be prolonged over months to years. Side effects may cause noncompliance with a drug that is otherwise effective. The potential side for effects ranges from verapamil (+ and clonidine (+), which have few side effects, to methysergide (++++), which have potentially serious fibrotic complications after long-term treatment. Accordingly, methysergide can never be the drug of first choice despite its effectiveness.

Physicians also should consider the scientific proof for efficacy when choosing a drug; the contemporary patient is often inquisitive, too. The literature is extremely varied with regard to the scientific support of drugs used in

P. Tfelt-Hansen: Department of Neurology, Glostrup Hospital, University of Copenhagen, DK-2600 Glostrup, Copenhagen, Denmark.

K. M. A. Welch: Department of Neurology, University of Kansas School of Medicine, University of Kansas Medical Center, Kansas City, Kansas, 66106.

TABLE 1. *Clinical efficacy,[a] scientific proof of efficacy[b] and potential for side effects[a] rated on a scale from + to ++++ for some drugs used in migraine prophylaxis*

Drug	Clinical efficacy	Scientific proof for efficacy	Side effect potential	Examples of side effects (Examples of contraindications)
β-blockers (Propranolol, metoprolol, atenolol, nadolol, timolol)	++++	++++	++	Tiredness, cold extremities, vivid dreams, depression (Asthma, brittle diabetes, A–V conduction defects)
Antiepileptics				
Sodium valproate/ divalproex	++	+++	+++	Weight gain, tremor, hair loss (Thrombocytopenia, liver disease,[c] pregnancy)
Antiserotonin drugs				
Methysergide	++++	++	++++	Chronic use: fibrotic disorders (Cardiovascular diseases)
Pizotifen	+++	++	+++	Weight gain, sedation (Obesity)
Calcium antagonists				
Flunarizine	+++	++++	+++	Sedation, weight gain, depression (Depression, Parkinson)
Verapamil	+	+	+	Constipation (Bradycardia, A–V conduction defects)
NSAIDs				Dyspepsia, peptic ulcers
Naproxen	++	+++	++	(Active peptic ulcers)
Tolfenamic acid	++	+++	++	Miscellaneous
Amitriptyline	++	++	++	Sedation, dry mouth, weight gain (Glaucoma)
Clonidine	+	+	+	Dry mouth
Dihydroergotamine	++	+	++	Nausea, diarrhea (Ischemic heart disease)

[a]The rating is based on a combination of the published literature and our personal experience.

[b]As judged by the authors (apparently conflicting with the overwhelming majority of comparative trials claiming equipotency of 2 drugs. This claim of comparability is probably due to small trials, see text).

[c]In most countries, routine haematological screening and biochemical tests of liver function are considered necessary prior to starting and during valproate or divalproex treatment.

DHE, dihydroergotamine; NSAID, non-steroidal antiinflammatory drugs.

migraine prophylaxis (Table 1). Some old, well-established drugs (e.g., methysergide, ranked ++) have not been evaluated using contemporary methods (see Chapter 57); for verapamil (+), results for only 41 patients in three controlled trials have been published (see Chapter 58). In contrast, the beta-blockers, especially propranolol (++++), the calcium antagonist flunarizine (++++), and recently sodium valproate/divalproex (+++) were evaluated extensively in controlled clinical trials and found superior to placebo (see Chapters 56, 58, and 59). Although a recently introduced drug for the phophylaxis of migraine, sodium valproate/divalproex has had an amazing lack of placebo-controlled, double-blind comparative, randomized trials.

Concerning clinical efficacy, the drugs are ranked from the less efficaceous drugs (+), such as verapamil and clonidine, to the most effective drugs (++++), such as β-blockers and methysergide, whereas other drugs, such as flunarizine (+++), pizotifen (+++), sodium valproate/divalproex (++), naproxen (++), tolfenamic acid (++), amitriptyline (++), and dihydroergotamine (++), are judged to be intermediate in their effectiveness (Table 1). This ranking of clinical efficacy should be considered along with the ranking for potential for side effects (Table 1). The options, documented outcomes, relative efficacy, and side effects always should be discussed with the patient.

In general, the drugs of first choice are the beta-blockers, which are in practice the most frequently used agents. No trials have been done to show the superiority of one of the effective beta-blockers over another (see Chapter 56). When beta-blockers are not effective or are contraindicated, the choice of a prophylactic drug depends to some extent on local availability (e.g., pizotifen and flunarizine are not available in United States); based on the ratios for efficacy/side effects, however, all of which should be discussed with the patient, the choice can be either pizotifen, flunarizine, sodium valproate/divalproex, one of the nonsteroidal antiinflammatory drugs listed, or amitriptyline. Verapamil, clonidine, dihydroergotamine, and methysergide (in a specialist's hands) probably should be used only as last resort. Finally, the physician should check the patient at 2- to 3-month intervals, the patients should keep a simple headache diary for monitoring migraine attack frequency (see Fig. 1 of Chapter 49), and the efficacy/safety ratioo should be discussed with the patient, who is ultimately the judge of the prophylactic treatment.

The Headaches, Second Edition,
edited by J. Olesen, P. Tfelt-Hansen, and K.M.A. Welch.
Lippincott Williams & Wilkins, Philadelphia © 2000.

The Migraines

CHAPTER 62

Familial Hemiplegic Migraine

Anne Ducros and J. Keith Campbell

DEFINITION OF FAMILIAL HEMIPLEGIC MIGRAINE

IHS code and diagnosis: 1.2.3 Familial hemiplegic migraine.

WHO code and diagnosis: G43.1x5 Familial hemiplegic migraine.

Short description (Headache Classification Committee, 1988): Migraine with aura including hemiparesis and where at least one first-degree relative has identical attacks.

GENETICS

Like other autosomal-dominant conditions, familial hemiplegic migraine (FHM) affects males and females equally and is transmitted by fathers as well as mothers to 50% of their offspring. Penetrance of the condition is incomplete: not all mutated gene carriers have FHM (9–11). The incomplete penetrance of FHM has several implications for clinicians as well as for geneticists. First, an affected individual may have no first- or even second-degree affected relative, making it difficult to diagnose FHM. Second, an asymptomatic family member may have affected children. Third, in the mapping of FHM genes, only affected recombinants should be considered. Finally, the incomplete penetrance suggests that modifying genetic or environmental factors plays a role in the expression of the FHM phenotype.

Familial hemiplegic migraine is genetically heterogeneous: the existence of at least three different genes has been demonstrated (1,10,26,36) (Fig. 1). The first respon-

sible gene, mapped on chromosome 19 (25), is involved in approximately 50% to 60% of unselected families (10,11,26,36) (Fig. 2). This gene was recently shown to be the alpha 1A subunit of a P/Q type voltage-dependent calcium channel, *CACNA1A* (35). A second FHM gene, mapped on the long arm of chromosome 1 by two independent teams (10,15), is involved in about 20% of families with FHM (10). This gene has not been identified yet. Finally, 20% of families with FHM are unlinked to chromosome 19 and to chromosome 1, suggesting the existence of at least a third locus (10). One recent study compared clinical and genetic data between three family groups: 10 chromosome 19–linked families including 94 patients, 3 chromosome 1–linked families including 24

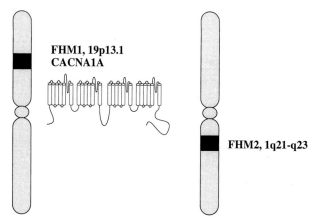

FIG. 1. Genetic heterogeneity of FHM. The two known loci, FHM1 and FHM2, are indicated. The gene located on chromosome 19 has been identified as being *CACNA1A*, coding for the alpha 1A subunit of a voltage-gated calcium channel. The gene located on 1q21-q23 has not been identified yet. A third FHM gene (at least) is still to be localized.

A. Ducros: Laboratoire de Pathologie de l'Immunité, Faculté de Médecine Necker-Enfants Malades, 75730 Paris Cedex 15, France.

J. K. Campbell: Department of Neurology, Mayo Clinic and Mayo Medical School, Rochester, Minnesota, 55905.

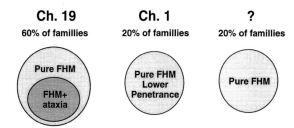

FIG. 2. Genotype-phenotype correlations in FHM. Proportion of families linked to the various FHM loci are indicated.

patients, and 4 unlinked families including 24 patients (11). No significant difference was observed between the three family groups with regard to the characteristics of hemiplegic migraine (HM) attacks, the occurrence of severe attacks, the existence of other migraine subtypes, and the disease course. Two major genotype-phenotype correlations were observed: first, penetrance seems to be much lower in chromosome 1 families; second, associated permanent cerebellar symptoms are observed in 50% of chromosome 19–linked families and in those families only. Moreover, linkage analysis or *CACNA1A* mutation screening demonstrated involvement of the alpha 1A calcium channel subunit in all 13 families with FHM and cerebellar ataxia analyzed so far (11,12,26,35,36).

DIAGNOSIS

The diagnosis of FHM is entirely dependent on obtaining a family history of similar attacks. Due to the incomplete penetrance of FHM, the familial investigation should concern not only first-degree but also second-degree relatives. In the absence of such a history, evaluation of a patient with a transient hemiparesis and a headache requires clinical judgment in the selection of tests, both invasive and noninvasive, as well as a period of observation and follow-up.

The IHS diagnostic criteria for FHM as described by the Headache Classification Committee of the IHS are as follows:

A. Fulfills criteria for migraine with aura 1.2.
B. The aura includes some degree of hemiparesis and may be prolonged.
C. At least one first-degree relative has identical attacks.

Genetic testing for FHM is now theoretically available. However, this condition, which may of course be incapacitating, has a generally good prognosis. Consequently, presymptomatic and prenatal genetic testing should be avoided.

CLINICAL FEATURES

Familial hemiplegic migraine is a hereditary form of migraine with aura characterized by the presence of a

motor weakness during the aura (4,20). It is the only migraine subtype for which a monogenic mode of inheritance, autosomal dominant, has been clearly established. Since the first description by Clarke in 1910 (6) and subsequently by Whitty (45) and by Blau and Whitty (3), more than 50 families have been reported in the literature.

Migraine Attacks

Triggering factors are reported by about two thirds of the patients, the most frequent being stress and minor head trauma (11,40). Less than 10% of patients with FHM identify triggers usually incriminated in other forms of migraine such as dietary factors, visual or auditory stimulations, climatic factors (temperature, wind), and menstrual periods (11). In several cases, a severe HM episode was precipitated by injection of contrast enhancement media during cerebral or extracerebral angiography (2,3).

During the HM aura, motor weakness is always associated with at least one other aura symptom: sensory disturbances (paresthesias, numbness), speech disturbances (dysarthria, reduced speech fluency, paraphasias), or visual symptoms (hemianopia, scintillating scotoma, blurred vision) (11). The degree of motor deficit is highly variable, ranging from mild clumsiness to total hemiplegia. Attacks may alternately be right or left sided or always involve the same side (40%) (11). Bilateral symptoms occur in about 25% of patients, one side after the other or both sides simultaneously (11,19). Other aura symptoms may occur: lack of balance, diplopia, tinnitus, partial hearing loss, drop attacks, confusion, or loss of consciousness (19). The average duration of the aura is 1 to 2 hours, but may range from 10 minutes to several days (11).

Headache generally follows resolution of the aura and lasts a few hours to a few days. The pain may be unilateral or bilateral. If one sided, it may be ipsilateral or contralateral to the weak limbs. Not infrequently, the pain will switch sides or become bilateral during the attack. All degrees may be observed from moderate discomfort to excruciating pain. Moreover, up to 11% of the patients have no headache at all (11). Associated autonomic signs and symptoms are indistinguishable from those accompanying any form of migraine and include nausea and vomiting, photophobia and phonophobia, and pallor.

In addition to usual episodes, up to 40% of the patients will have one or more atypical attacks (11,13–15,30,31). Those atypical episodes may consist of HM with prolonged aura, lasting up to several days. More dramatic episodes are characterized by impaired consciousness ranging from confusion or somnolence to coma with respiratory failure, with or without the usual aura symptoms. Fever or meningismus or both may occur. In rare instances, an epileptic manifestation has been reported during such an episode. Persistent confusion and associated visual and auditory delusions following an HM attack have been reported (13). More than 50% of those severe attacks occur before 20 years of age. They represent the first FHM-related neurologic episode in up to 20% of the cases and are often triggered by minor head trauma (11). Whatever the severity of the various symptoms, they usually entirely resolve within a few days, weeks, or sometimes months.

Other forms of migraine may occur: about 15% of the patients have migraine with nonhemiplegic aura alternating with HM attacks, and 34% have migraine without aura (11,13,14,18,19,22,30,31,33,43).

All the HM features are highly variable (11). Order of onset, progression, topography, intensity, and duration of the various aura symptoms may vary from one attack to another within a given patient as may vary the various headache features. Moreover, those features may be highly variable among patients from a given family (11) and quite similar in affected members from other families (17).

Associated Neurologic Symptoms

Permanent cerebellar symptoms are found in about 20% of families with FHM (7,11,12,14,18,25,26,33,36, 40,43,44). Within those families, cerebellar symptoms cosegregate with FHM but have a lower penetrance: nystagmus (gaze-evoked horizontal, vertical, or multidirectional) is found in about 75% of patients with FHM, and slowly progressive mild to moderate statokinetic ataxia occurs in about 40% of the patients (11). Nystagmus and other abnormal ocular motility findings are most likely the first symptoms of the progressive cerebellar syndrome (12). Some subjects will later develop ataxia. Autonomous gait remains possible even after years of evolution. Age of onset of these cerebellar symptoms is difficult to determine precisely. Nystagmus and ataxia may begin prior to the first HM attack (11,43). Their progression is not correlated to the frequency and severity of HM attacks. Computerized tomographic (CT) or magnetic resonance imaging (MRI) scans in some of those patients reveal cerebellar atrophy mainly affecting the anterior part of the vermis (12,14,18,25).

Other associated neurologic symptoms have been reported in a few families with FHM, including essential tremor (11,45), Usher syndrome and cataracts (43), cognitive impairment (30), and mental retardation (14,44).

Neurologic Investigations

The cerebrospinal fluid (CSF) was examined during 32 attacks of HM in 20 patients. Almost 90% of the HM attacks were severe with impairment of consciousness. An elevated CSF white cell count (12–290 cells) was found in 28% of the cases. Protein and glucose levels were always normal.

During attacks, the electroencephalogram is always abnormal, showing diffuse slow-wave activity predominantly over the hemisphere contralateral to the limb weakness (28). Other abnormalities have been reported rarely, including periodic sharp waves (16) or dysrhythmia (17,31). These abnormalities may persist for several days or weeks after the attack.

Isolated case studies using transcranial Doppler have been reported. During one attack (right hemiplegia and aphasia) in a single patient, Doppler evaluation suggested a diffuse vasoconstriction of the vessels at the base of skull and of small arteries within the hemisphere contralateral to the limb weakness (37).

The few CT scans performed during or just following an HM attack have all been normal, except in one patient in whom the scan showed hemispheric edema during a severe attack with coma and fever (14). The majority of CT scans performed in interictal periods have been normal; but 25% showed cerebellar atrophy, and 10% a focal abnormality of uncertain etiology. Cerebellar atrophy has been found only in patients having FHM associated with cerebellar ataxia. Cerebral MRI was normal in a patient having permanent cognitive dysfunction (30) and disclosed cerebellar atrophy in several patients having FHM with nystagmus and ataxia (12,14,18,25).

Cerebral angiography performed during or after an attack was normal, except for two reports of arterial diameter changes during one HM attack [basilar artery spasm (23) and narrowing of the middle cerebral artery contralateral to the hemiplegic side (44)]. Angiography does not provide any evidence that neurologic symptoms may be due to spasm or arterial occlusion. In addition, angiography is dangerous in patients with FHM, in 60% of cases leading to the onset or aggravation of an attack, always with fever, prolonged aura, and coma (2,3,11).

A single patient was shown on an ictal single photon emission computerized tomography (SPECT) scan to have decreased perfusion in the parietooccipital region and the opposite cerebellar hemisphere, consistent with crossed cerebellar diaschisis (8). Finally, Uncini et al. (42) found spectroscopic magnetic resonance abnormalities of muscle and brain in several patients from the same FHM family, suggesting a mitochondrial dysfunction.

COURSE AND PROGNOSIS

Age of onset is usually between 10 and 15 years. However, onset before 5 years of age is not infrequent, and the initial attack of HM in a 75-year-old patient has been reported (38). The frequency of attacks varies from several per week to only a few in a lifetime, with an average of three or four per year. In some patients, this frequency may range from daily attacks, usually in the first years of evolution, to free intervals lasting for years (11). In general, the attack frequency decreases after 20 to 25 years of age. This is not always the case, and in some, the hemiplegic episodes continue for life.

Despite the recurrent episodes of hemiparetic aura, full recovery between attacks is the rule. In a few patients, speech disturbances and moderate concentration and memory impairment may persist several weeks after an attack before complete recovery. In many individuals, the degree of weakness becomes less severe as they reach late adolescence or early adult life.

MANAGEMENT

Despite the identification of the first FHM gene, the precise mechanisms of this condition are still unknown. Thus, management of FHM is empirically based on what is known about treatment of other forms of migraine with aura. Treatment can be preventive or symptomatic. In most patients, the HM attacks are so infrequent that prophylactic therapy is not considered solely to prevent those rare HM episodes, but it is used when other associated forms of migraine attacks are so frequent as to cause significant disruption of activities or so severe as to justify preventive treatment. In younger subjects, the HM episodes may be sufficiently frequent to warrant such prophylactic measures. However, the relative rarity of FHM has precluded detailed reporting of a large series of patients. Most of those reported have been isolated cases or have been included in larger series of migraine subjects with various nonhemiplegic manifestations.

Rare reports suggest that the beta-blocking agents, specifically propranolol, may be harmful in patients with FHM (32), whereas others have reported apparent benefit (27,28). Therefore, the use of propranolol in FHM must be carefully monitored, although Olesen et al. (34) reported that this beta-blocking agent does not alter regional blood flow in the awake human and is unlikely to affect cerebral metabolism adversely. There are a few experiential reports of the use of calcium-blocking agents (flunarizine, verapamil, and nimodipine) seemingly reducing the frequency and the severity of HM (5,24,28). No meaningful data are available about the use of methysergide for prophylaxis of FHM. On the basis of its vasoconstrictor action, it is probably an unwise choice. Phenytoin was reported by Ross (39) to prevent further HM episodes in one patient. Papaverine and phenobarbital also have been used.

As full recovery from HM is the usual outcome, the use of any symptomatic treatment other than that which provides relief from pain, nausea, and vomiting is debatable. If pharmacologic intervention is undertaken, it is usually to shorten the episode of disability or to relieve the treating physician's anxiety that migrainous infarction will follow. This sequence of events is rare.

There are anecdotal reports of the use of calcium-blocking drugs being given acutely in HM. Intravenous administration of verapamil and sublingual administration of nifedipine have been followed by rapid reversal of the focal neurologic deficit, but the cause-and-effect rela-tionship is hard to prove. The role of ergotamine and dihydroergotamine in migraine with hemiparetic aura is controversial. Although Heyck (21) reported that the intravenous administration of dihydroergotamine on multiple occasions apparently shortened the episodes of hemiparesis in one patient and did not result in any permanent deficit, Tfelt-Hansen and colleagues (41) showed that ergotamine caused a minor degree of constriction of cerebral arteries in young healthy male volunteers, so that most would feel it prudent to avoid ergotamine and dihydroergotamine in migraine with a prolonged or a motor aura. The role of sumatriptan and other triptans in FHM is not known, but because it is not recommended for basilar artery migraine, which has many features in common with FHM (19), its use in the latter cannot be recommended.

REFERENCES

1. Ahmed MA, Reid E, Cooke A, Arngrimsson R, Tolmie JL, Stephenson JB. Familial hemiplegic migraine in the west of Scotland: a clinical and genetic study of seven families. *J Neurol Neurosurg Psychiatry* 1996; 61:616–620.
2. Bergouignan FX, Ferrer X, Julien J. Familial hemiplegic migraine: a new case. *Headache* 1986;26:498–499.
3. Blau JN, Whitty CWM. Familial hemiplegic migraine. *Lancet* 1955;2: 1115–1116.
4. Bradshaw P, Parsons M. Hemiplegic migraine, a clinical study. *Q J Med* 1965;34:65–85.
5. Caers LI, De Beukelaar F, Amery WK. Flunarizine, a calcium-entry blocker, in childhood migraine, epilepsy, and alternating hemiplegia. *Clin Neuropharmacol* 1987;10:162–168.
6. Clarke JM. On recurrent motor paralysis in migraine. With report of a family in which recurrent hemiplegia accompanied the attacks. *Br Med J* 1910;1:1534–1538.
7. Codina A, Acarin PN, Miguel F, Noguera M. Familial hemiplegic migraine associated with nystagmus [in French]. *Rev Neurol* 1971;124: 526–530.
8. Crawford JS, Konkol RJ. Familial hemiplegic migraine with crossed cerebellar diaschisis and unilateral meningeal enhancement. *Headache* 1997;37:590–593.
9. Ducros A, Joutel A, Labauge P, Pagès M, Bousser MG, Tournier-Lasserve E. Monozygotic twins discordant for familial hemiplegic migraine. *Neurology* 1995;45:1222.
10. Ducros A, Joutel A, Vahedi K, et al. Mapping of a second locus for familial hemiplegic migraine to 1q21-q23 and evidence of further heterogeneity. *Ann Neurol* 1997;42:885–890.
11. Ducros A, Joutel A, Vahedi K, Bousser MG, Tournier-Lasserve E. Genotype-phenotype correlations in familial hemiplegic migraine [Abstract]. *Neurology* 1998; 50(Suppl 4):A352.
12. Elliott MA, Peroutka SJ, Welch S, May EF. Familial hemiplegic migraine, nystagmus, and cerebellar atrophy. *Ann Neurol* 1996;39: 100–106.
13. Feely MP, O'Hare J, Veale D, Callaghan N. Episodes of acute confusion or psychosis in familial hemiplegic migraine. *Acta Neurol Scand* 1982; 65:369–375.
14. Fitzsimons RB, Wolfenden WH. Migraine coma. Meningitic migraine with cerebral oedema associated with a new form of autosomal dominant cerebellar ataxia. *Brain* 1985;108:555–577.
15. Gardner K, Barmada MM, Ptacek LJ, Hoffman EP. A new locus for hemiplegic migraine maps to chromosome 1q31. *Neurology* 1997;49: 1231–1238.
16. Gastaut JL, Yermenos E, Bonnefoy M, Cros D. Familial hemiplegic migraine: EEG and CT scan study of two cases. *Ann Neurol* 1981;10: 392–395.
17. Glista GG, Mellinger JF, Rooke ED. Familial hemiplegic migraine. *Mayo Clin Proc* 1975;50:307–311.
18. Haan J, Terwindt GM, Bos PL, Ophoff RA, Frants RR, Ferrari MD.

Familial hemiplegic migraine in The Netherlands. *Clin Neurol Neurosurg* 1994;96:244–249.

19. Haan J, Terwindt GM, Ophoff RA, et al. Is familial hemiplegic migraine a hereditary form of basilar migraine? *Cephalalgia* 1995; 15:477–481.

20. Headache Classification Committee of the International Headache Society. Classification and diagnostic criteria for headache disorders, cranial neuralgias and facial pain. *Cephalalgia* 1988;8(Suppl 7):19–28.

21. Heyck H. Varieties of hemiplegic migraine. *Headache* 1973;12:135–142.

22. Jensen TS, de Fine Olivarius B, Kraft M, Hansen HJ. Familial hemiplegic migraine—a reappraisal and long-term follow-up study. *Cephalalgia* 1981;1:33–39.

23. Jensen TS, Voldby B, de Fine Olivarius B, Jensen FT. Cerebral hemodynamics in familial hemiplegic migraine. *Cephalalgia* 1981;1:121–125.

24. Jonsdottir M, Meyer JS, Rogers RL. Efficacy, side effects and tolerance compared during headache treatment with three different calcium blockers. *Headache* 1987;27:364–369.

25. Joutel A, Bousser MG, Biousse V, et al. A gene for familial hemiplegic migraine maps to chromosome 19. *Nat Genet* 1993;5:40–45.

26. Joutel A, Ducros A, Vahedi K, et al. Genetic heterogeneity of familial hemiplegic migraine. *Am J Hum Genet* 1994;55:1166–1172.

27. Kangasniemi P, Andersen AR, Andersson PG, et al. Classic migraine: effective prophylaxis with metoprolol. *Cephalalgia* 1987;7:231–238.

28. Lai CW, Ziegler DK, Lansky LL, Torres F. Hemiplegic migraine in childhood: diagnostic and therapeutic aspects. *J Pediatr* 1982;101:696–699.

29. Leone M, Frediani F, Patruno G, Valentini S, Bussone G. Is nimodipine useful in migraine prophylaxis? Further considerations. *Headache* 1990;30:363–365.

30. Marchioni E, Galimberti CA, Soragna D, et al. Familial hemiplegic migraine versus migraine with prolonged aura: an uncertain diagnosis in a family report. *Neurology* 1995;45:33–37.

31. Münte TF, Müller-Vahl H. Familial migraine coma: a case study. *J Neurol* 1990;237:59–61.

32. O'Hare JA, Feely MJ, Callaghan N. Clinical aspects of familial hemiplegic migraine in two families. *Irish Med J* 1981;74:291–295.

33. Ohta M, Araki S, Kuroiwa Y. Familial occurence of migraine with a hemiplegic syndrome and cerebellar manifestations. *Neurology* 1967; 17:813–817.

34. Olesen J, Hougard K, Hertz M. Isoproterenol and propranolol: ability to cross the blood-brain barrier and effects on cerebral circulation in man. *Stroke* 1978;9:344–349.

35. Ophoff RA, Terwindt GM, Vergouwe MN, et al. Familial hemiplegic migraine and episodic ataxia type-2 are caused by mutations in the Ca(2+) channel gene *CACNL1A4*. *Cell* 1996;87:543–552.

36. Ophoff RA, van Eijk R, Sandkuijl LA, et al. Genetic heterogeneity of familial hemiplegic migraine. *Genomics* 1994;22:21–26.

37. Pierelli F, Pauri F, Cupini LM, Fiermonte G, Rizzo PA. Transcranial Doppler sonography in familial hemiplegic migraine. *Cephalagia* 1991;11:29–31.

38. Rajput V, Kramer ED. Adult onset familial hemiplegic migraine. *Headache* 1995;35:423–427.

39. Ross RT. Hemiplegic migraine. *Can Med Assoc J* 1958;78:10–16.

40. Terwindt GM, Ophoff RA, Haan J, Frants RR, Ferrari MD. Familial hemiplegic migraine: a clinical comparison of families linked and unlinked to chromosome 19. *Cephalalgia* 1996;16:153–155.

41. Tfelt-Hansen P, Sperling B, Andersen AR. The effect of ergotamine on human cerebral blood flow and cerebral arteries. In: Olesen J, ed. *Migraine and other headaches. The vascular mechanisms.* New York: Raven, 1991:339–343.

42. Uncini A, Di Muzio A, Servidei B, et al. Abnormal brain and muscle mitochondrial function in familial hemiplegic migraine. *J Neurol* 1994; 241(suppl 1):35.

43. Young GF, Leon-Barth CA, Green J. Familial hemiplegic migraine, retinal degeneration, deafness, and nystagmus. *Arch Neurol* 1970;23: 201–209.

44. Zifkin B, Andermann E, Andermann F, Kirkham T. An autosomal dominant syndrome of hemiplegic migraine, nystagmus, and tremor. *Ann Neurol* 1980;8:329–332.

45. Whitty CWM. Familial hemiplegic migraine. *J Neurol Neurosurg Psychiatry* 1953;16:172–177.

The Headaches, Second Edition,
edited by J. Olesen, P. Tfelt-Hansen, and K.M.A. Welch.
Lippincott Williams & Wilkins, Philadelphia © 2000.

The Migraines

CHAPTER 63

Basilar Artery Migraine

Richard C. Peatfield and K. Michael A. Welch

HIS code and diagnosis: 1.2.4 Basilar migraine
WHO code and diagnosis: G43.1X3 Basilar migraine
Short description: Migraine symptoms originating from the brainstem or from both occipital lobes
Other terms: Basilar artery migraine, Bickerstaff's migraine, syncopa migraine
Diagnostic criteria:

Fulfills criteria for 1.2

Two or more aura symptoms of the following types: visual symptoms in both the temporal and nasal fields of both eyes, dysarthria, vertigo, tinnitus, decreased hearing, double vision, ataxia, bilateral paresthesias, bilateral paresis, decreased level of consciousness.

The concept of basilar artery migraine was first proposed by Bickerstaff (2), who later wrote about his attention being drawn to the syndrome when he saw, within a short period, two patients with identical symptoms explicable only on the basis of an abnormality of basilar artery circulation (5). One of these cases was a boy aged 14 years whose symptoms lasted a few hours and were repeated on numerous occasions. The other was an elderly man whose symptoms progressed rapidly to coma and death and in whom infarction of the brainstem and occipital cortex was caused by thrombotic occlusion of the basilar artery demonstrated at autopsy. So it was by clinical analogy with the structural lesion in the basilar artery and the symptoms of basilar artery territory ischemia that the syndrome basilar artery migraine first was described.

R.C. Peatfield: Charing Cross Hospital, London W6 8RF, United Kingdom.

K. M. A. Welch: Department of Neurology, University of Kansas School of Medicine, University of Kansas Medical Center, Kansas City, Kansas 66106.

Bickerstaff (5) attributed the earliest recorded description of basilar artery migraine to Aretaeus, who gave the following description in the first century A.D.:

> If darkness possess the eye, and if the head be whirled round with dizziness, and the ears ring as from the sound of rivers rolling along with a great noise, or like the wind when it roars among the sails, or like the clang of pipes or reeds, or like the rattling of a carriage, we call the affection scotoma (or vertigo). The mode of vertigo is heaviness of the head, sparkles of light in the eyes along with much darkness, ignorance of themselves and those around, and if the disease go on increasing, the limbs sink below them and they crawl on the ground; there is nausea and vomiting of phlegm or of yellow or black bilious matter . . .

There is no specific information on the prevalence of basilar migraine except that it is rare. Longitudinal studies of the natural history of these serious migraine subtypes are needed.

CLASSIFICATION

The International Headache Society (IHS)(14) classified this disorder as basilar migraine (IHS 1.2.4). The Classification Committee suggested that this term replace *basilar artery migraine* and other terms such as *Bickerstaff's migraine* and *syncopal migraine*. The diagnostic criteria include those for migraine with aura (IHS 1.2) plus two or more aura symptoms of the following types: visual symptoms in both the temporal and nasal fields of both eyes, dysarthria, vertigo, tinnitus, decreased hearing, double vision, ataxia, bilateral paresthesias, bilateral paresis, and decreased level of consciousness. The absence of consistent evidence for basilar artery spasm during migraine attacks and uncertainty about the origin of the mechanisms of the symptoms prompted the IHS Classification Committee to remove the word *artery* from the terminology. Further investigative studies were called for to establish definitively or disprove the existence of migraine aura originating in the brainstem.

PATHOGENESIS

Few studies have been done specifically of basilar migraine. It must be assumed that the pathogenetic mechanisms are the same as those of more clearly lateralized migrainous auras and headaches. Frequin et al. (12) described a patient who experienced recurrent, prolonged coma in whom angiography showed profound narrowing of the basilar artery. They attributed this condition to vasospasm, although it remains possible that this appearance actually was produced by an inflammatory swelling of the vessel wall. In a recent transcranial Doppler study, La Spina and colleagues showed an increase in mean flow velocity in both posterior cerebral arteries, again consistent with narrowing of these vessels (18). It remains to be determined whether these changes are the cause, the consequence, or entirely unrelated to the aura symptoms.

CLINICAL FEATURES

Of the 34 cases in Bickerstaff's original series, all were aged younger than 35 years, and 32 were under the age of 23 years (2). Twenty-six of the 34 were female subjects, and 28 reported a family history of migraine. A definite association was found with the menarche, and attacks often were linked to menstruation. The attacks were infrequent but often interspersed with more typical migrainous attacks with aura. In Bickerstaff's series, the headache was bilateral, occipital, and preceded by visual disturbances affecting both sides of the visual field, diplopia, bilateral circumoral or limb paresthesiae, dysarthria, bilateral ataxia, vertigo, and tinnitus, often lasting 20 to 30 minutes and clearly resembling intoxication. The attacks were relieved by sleep. Bickerstaff noted that the attacks tended to become more typically migrainous as the patients grew older.

Several large series of such patients have been published more recently, and these give a breakdown of the proportion of patients with each type of aura symptom. Two of the largest series are presented in Table 1 (15,24). More than a third of subjects have their first attack in the second decade of life, and two-thirds have the first attack in their second or third decade of life (24). The condition also occurs frequently in children (15). A few cases, however, present for the first time in persons over the age of 50. The condition may occur in combination with other forms of migraine, although basilar migraine remains the dominant problem in more than 75% (24).

At first, Bickerstaff noted a predominance of teenage girls in his basilar artery migraine population, but subsequent experience revealed a female incidence that is similar to other forms of migraine (2). The highest sex ratio, approximately 3:1, is found when basilar migraine presents for the first time in the second decade of life (24). Commonly, when basilar artery migraine starts in the teens, the frequency of attacks diminishes, to be replaced in adult life by other forms of migraine (2,5).

Patients who suffer from basilar migraine identify trigger factors that are similar to those for other forms of migraine. Precipitating factors were identified by as many as 71% of subjects (24). Emotion, stress, menstruation, and weather change were the predominant triggers, but head injury, food stuffs, and contraceptive drugs were also common. Of note, vascular risk factors were present in 41% of sufferers, including smoking, oral contraceptives, and diabetes mellitus.

In most cases, the aura lasts between 5 to 60 minutes, but it may extend to up to 3 days. Visual symptoms commonly occur first, predominantly in the temporal and nasal fields of vision. The visual disturbance may consist of blurred vision, teichopsia, scintillating scotoma, graying of vision or total loss of vision. The features may start in one visual field and then spread to become bilateral. Bickerstaff (5) pointed out that, when vision is not completely obscured, diplopia may occur, usually sixth-nerve weakness. Some form of diplopia occurs in up to 16% of cases (24).

TABLE 1. *Symptoms of basilar artery migraine*

	Hockaday (1979) (15)		Sturzenegger and Meienberg (1985) (24)	
n	29		49	
Female	17	65%	32	65%
Alteration of consciousness	13	45%	38	77%
Mood disturbances	8	28%	34	69%
Bilateral sensory changes	4	14%	30	61%
Bilateral visual disturbances	14	48%	42	86%
Vertigo	12	41%	31	63%
Ataxia	5	17%	31	63%
Seizures	Unclear		4	8%

Vertigo and gait ataxia are the next most common symptoms, each occurring in 63% of one series (24). Fenichel described a series of patients who experienced isolated benign recurrent vertigo, which later evolved into migraine (10). This entity, first described by Basser (1), usually starts in preschoolers and progresses into the teens. Abrupt attacks of rotational sensation occur, lasting seconds to minutes, accompanied by loss of balance, pallor, and vomiting. The disorder is self-limiting but may be a precursor to migraine or a migraine equivalent because many sufferers subsequently develop migraine with and without aura (7).

Ataxia sometimes occurs independently of vertigo, and tinnitus may accompany vertigo. Dysarthria is as common as ataxia and vertigo. Tingling and numbness, in the typical cheiro-oral spreading pattern seen in migraine with aura, occurs in more than 60% of cases. These usually are bilateral and symmetric but may alternate sides with a hemidistribution. Occasionally, dysesthesiae extend to the trunk. Bilateral motor weakness occurs in more than 50% of cases.

Impairment of consciousness in some form is common (3,24). Bickerstaff noted in his early work that patients enter a state of impaired consciousness that resembles sleep, from which they may be easily aroused by stimulation, only to return to the same state (3). Rarely, this condition progresses to stupor and prolonged coma (11,19). Other forms of altered consciousness include amnesia and syncope. Drop attacks with very transient loss of consciousness may occur as part of the full clinical syndrome, but this is rare.

Headache occurs in almost all patients. It has an occipital location in most patients, with a throbbing, pounding quality, and is accompanied by severe nausea and vomiting. It is unusual for the headache to be unilateral or localized to the more anterior parts of the cranium. Photophobia and phonophobia occur in a third to half of the patients. As with other forms of migraine, symptoms may occur without headache, but this is usually in no more than 4% of cases (24).

Seizures have been observed in association with basilar migraine (1,4). Of the patients in the study by Sturzenegger and Meinberg, 8% had overt seizure (24). Electroencephalographic (EEG) changes without seizures occurring with attacks of typical basilar artery migraine also have been described (20). These cases are reported to have a good response to anticonvulsants (6,20–22,25). Camfield and colleagues described a syndrome of basilar migraine and unilateral or bilateral temporal occipital EEG abnormality suppressed by opening the eyes. The epileptic seizures were either focal or generalized following the migraine aura (6). In all, EEG abnormalities are detected in fewer than one-fifth of cases with basilar migraine and are mostly independent of any clinical manifestation of the disorder (16). The EEG findings between attacks are usually spike-wave or spike-slow wave complexes. During an attack, diffuse high-voltage slow waves and associated spikes with sharp waves and diffuse beta activity occur. In a recently published long-term follow-up (8 to 16 years) of seven children affected by basilar migraine (7) who had EEG findings of occipital spike and wave complexes, basilar migraine resolved and the EEG became normal in all subjects. In one patient, basilar migraine ceased and tonic clonic seizures occurred 5 years later; these seizures also resolved. Four patients in this series later developed migraine with typical aura, two of whom had migraine aura associated with seizures that were partial with secondary generalization.

TREATMENT

None of the published series of basilar migraine suggests that it should be managed in any significantly different way from more typical migrainous attacks in patients of the same age. Trigger factors are often common in adolescent patients, and appropriate lifestyle changes, including rest and relaxation, are often helpful. Many authorities recommend that potential vasoconstrictor drugs, including ergotamine, sumatriptan, and other triptans, should be avoided in these patients. Some authorities urge caution with prophylactic agents such as propranolol, which may limit any compensatory vasodilator capacitance. Sodium valproate, which has neither vasoconstrictor nor proconvulsant activity, may be more appropriate in the rare patient in whom prophylaxis seems justified. Alternatively, calcium channel blockers have been used.

DIFFERENTIAL DIAGNOSIS

Bickerstaff (5), writing on the ideal approach to differential diagnosis, stated: "Because the clinical picture produced by basilar artery disturbance can be so varied, it is perhaps a little too easy to include under the diagnosis of basilar artery migraine puzzling transient syndromes within this territory. Basilar artery migraine is a diagnosis which is unprovable and great care is required in labeling a patient with such a diagnosis, which, having been made, might be perpetuated without adequate attempts to further elucidate the cause."

A few cases present for the first time in persons over the age of 50. Clearly, in older subjects, vascular pathologies in the basilar artery circulation causing transient ischaemic attacks will need to be considered, and full investigation may be necessary. Possible mechanisms include dissections of the vertebral or basilar circulation, thrombotic or embolic disease, and even basilar tip aneurysms and brainstem arteriovenous malformations. It is probably prudent to arrange a magnetic resonance imaging scan in most patients who have atypical symptoms, but adolescent patients with a strong family history and recurrent stereotyped posterior fossa symptoms followed by headache will seldom require further study.

When episodic vertigo occurs during an attack of basilar migraine, the diagnosis is straightforward if other symptoms of visual and brainstem dysfunction are time locked with headache. When vertigo alone occurs with headache, the diagnosis may be more difficult. Careful history taking is required because other symptoms of brainstem disorder may be understated as a result of the severity of vertigo. A history of repeated stereotypic spells may be helpful in the differential diagnosis of vertigo. Peripheral causes of vertigo, such as Meniere's disease, may be excluded by caloric studies. A response to trials of antimigraine drugs also may enhance the diagnostic probabilities. As noted previously, Basser's syndrome is self-limiting but may be a precursor to migraine or a migraine equivalent (1).

Episodic seizures, particularly of temporal lobe origin, must be considered in the differential diagnosis because symptoms may resemble those of basilar migraine, for example, vertigo, imbalance, confusion, memory disturbance, and disorders of consciousness, and because headache is common as a postictal symptom. Occipital lobe epilepsy, a disorder of children, often is accompanied by headache (13). These children also may suffer from migraine, of which there is frequently a family history. Certain familial disorders present with neurologic deficit in which attacks of hemiplegic or basilar migraine may be part of the symptom complex. This group includes cerebral autosomal dominant arteriopathy with subcortical infarcts and leukoen cephalopathy (CADASIL) (17), mitochondrial encephalomyopathylactic acrosis and strokelike episodes (MELAS) and variants of MELAS, which are associated with seizures, particularly occipital in origin (8). Alternating hemiplegia (9), most frequently seen in children and once thought to be due to migraine (26), also may present with ataxia.

PROGNOSIS

The prognosis of basilar migraine is generally good. The disorder declines in frequency as patients enter their twenties and thirties. Rarely, basilar migraine is complicated by stroke, which most often involves the posterior cerebral artery (5,27), although other terminal arteries may be involved (23).

REFERENCES

1. Basser LS. The relation of migraine and epilepsy. *Brain* 1969;92:285–300.
2. Bickerstaff ER. Basilar artery migraine. *Lancet* 1961:15–17.
3. Bickerstaff ER. Impairment of consciousness in migraine. *Lancet* 1961:2:1057–1959.
4. Bickerstaff ER. The basilar artery and migraine-epilepsy syndrome. *Proc R Soc Med* 1962;55:167–169.
5. Bickerstaff ER. Basilar artery migraine. In: Clifford Rose R, ed. *Handbook of clinical neurology*. New York: Elsevier Science, 1986:135–140.
6. Camfield PR, Metrakos K, Andermann F. Basilar migraine, seizures, and severe epileptiform EEG abnormalities. *Neurology* 1978;28:584–588.
7. De Romanis F, Buzzi MG, Assenza S, Brusa L, Cerbo R. Basilar migraine with electroencephalographic findings of occipital spike-wave complexes: a long-term study in seven children. *Cephalalgia* 1993;13:192–196.
8. Dvorkin GS, Andermann F, Carpenter S. Classical migraine, intractable epilepsy, and multiple strokes: a syndrome related to mitochondrial encephalomyopathy. In: Andermann F, Lugaresi E, eds. *Migraine and epilepsy*. Stoneham, MA: Butterworth-Heineman, 1987;203–232.
9. Dynes JB. Alternating hemiparetic migraine syndrome. *BMJ* 1939;2:446–447.
10. Fenichel GM. Migraine as a cause of benign paroxysmal vertigo in childhood. *J Pediatr* 1967;71:114–115.
11. Ferguson KS, Robinson SS. Life-threatening migraine. *Arch Neurol* 1982;39:374–376.
12. Frequin ST, Linssen WH, Pasman JW, Hommes OR, Merx HL. Recurrent prolonged coma due to basilar artery migraine: a case report. *Headache* 1991;31:75–81.
13. Gastaut H, Zifkin BG. Classification of the epilepsy. *J Clin Neurophysiol* 1985;2:313–326.
14. Headache Classification Committee of the International Headache Society. Classification and diagnostic criteria for headache disorders, cranial neuralgias and facial pain. *Cephalalgia* 1988;8(Suppl 7):1–96.
15. Hockaday JM. Basilar migraine in childhood. *Dev Med Child Neurol* 1979;21:455–463.
16. Jacome DE. EEG features in basilar artery migraine. *Headache* 1987;27:80–83.
17. Joutel A, Bousser M-G, Biousse V, et al. A gene for familial hemiplegic migraine maps to chromosome 19. *Nat Genet* 1993;5:40–45.
18. La Spina I, Vignati A, Porazzi D. Basilar artery migraine: transcranial Doppler, EEG and SPECT from the aura phase to the end. *Headache* 1997;31:43–47.
19. Lawall JS, Oommen JK. Basilar artery migraine presenting as conversion hysteria. *J Nerv Ment Dis* 1978;166:809–811.
20. Lapkin ML, French JH, Golden GS. The EEG in childhood basilar artery migraine. *Neurology* 1977;27:580–583.
21. Lapkin ML, Golden GS. Basilar artery migraine. *Am J Dis Child* 1978;132:276–281.
22. Panayiotopoulos CP. Basilar migraine (?), seizures, and severe epileptic EEG abnormalities. *Neurology* 1980;30:1122–1125.
23. Solomon GD, Spaccavento LJ. Lateral medullary syndrome after basilar migraine. *Headache* 1982;22:171–172.
24. Sturzenegger MH, Meienberg O. Basilar artery migraine: a follow-up study of 82 cases. *Headache* 1985;25:408–415.
25. Swanson JW, Vick NA. Basilar artery migraine. *Neurology* 1978;28:782–786.
26. Verret S, Steele JC. Alternating hemiplegia in childhood: a report of eight patients with complicated migraine beginning in infancy. *Pediatrics* 1971;47:675–680.
27. Welch KMA, Levine SR. Migraine-related stroke in the context of the International Headache Society classification of head pain. *Arch Neurol* 1990;47:458–462.

The Headaches, Second Edition,
edited by J. Olesen, P. Tfelt-Hansen, and K.M.A. Welch.
Lippincott Williams & Wilkins, Philadelphia © 2000.

The Migraines

CHAPTER 64

Ophthalmoplegic Migraine and Retinal Migraine

B. Todd Troost and Alessandro S. Zagami

DEFINITION OF OPHTHALMOPLEGIC MIGRAINE

International Headache Society (IHS) code and diagnosis: 1.3 ophthalmoplegic migraine.

World Health Organization (WHO) code and diagnosis: G43.80 Ophthalmoplegic migraine.

Short description (Headache Classification Committee, 1988): Repeated attacks of headache associated with paresis of one or more ocular cranial nerves in the absence of demonstrable intracranial lesion.

Other terms: Ocular migraine or ophthalmic migraine has been used to describe this condition, but usually those terms describe situations in which the visual complaints are prominent, such as in migraine with aura.

Epidemiology

In a review of 5,000 migraine patients, Friedman and colleagues (16) found eight patients with ophthalmoplegic migraine, thus attesting to its rarity. All eight patients (five men and three women) had periodic migraine headaches and unilateral ophthalmoplegia. Three patients had persistent ophthalmoplegia after several years, and one had a definite family history of migraine. It is now believed that most attacks begin before age the age of 10 years, with a significantly greater incidence in males. Woody and Blaw (45) reported two cases of ophthalmoplegic migraine occurring in infants aged 5 and 7 months. The infants had

recurrent attacks with almost complete clearing between episodes. Both children were treated with prednisone during subsequent attacks, which seemed to shorten the duration of the episodes. Rarely, ophthalmoplegic migraine occurs without headache. Hupp and colleagues (23) believed that ophthalmoplegic migraine occurs in 2% to 17% of patients with migraine. In a survey to attempt to define the incidence and characteristics of ophthalmoplegic migraine, charts from patients admitted over a 10-year period to the departments of neurology, neurosurgery, ophthalmology, and pediatrics serving a population of more than 600,000 inhabitants in Copenhagen County, Denmark, were surveyed (21). An initial four cases of ophthalmoplegic migraine were found (for an annual incidence of 0.7 per 1 million inhabitants), but another four cases were added during the review. Durkan and colleagues (11) described two children with isolated recurrent, painless, oculomotor palsies in whom the results of neurodiagnostic investigations were all normal. The recurrent attacks were believed to be due to ophthalmoplegic migraine.

Genetics

No clear genetic pattern is present in the vast majority of patients. Most patients with ophthalmoplegic migraine do not have a history of familial occurrence. In Nigeria, ophthalmoplegic migraine has been associated with abnormal hemoglobin (35). Whether this represents a genetic predisposition or a chance occurrence is undetermined.

Anatomy and Pathology

No pathologic reports were found of isolated peripheral cranial nerve palsy. Ocular motor deficits occurring

B. T. Troost: Department of Neurology, Wake Forest University School of Medicine, Winston-Salem, North Carolina 27157-1078.

A. S. Zagami: Department of Medicine, University of New South Wales, and Institute of Neurological Sciences, Prince of Wales Hospital, Randwick, Sydney, New South Wales 2031, Australia.

in association with fatal brainstem infarction caused by basilar migraine (1.2.4) are not included in this review.

Pathophysiology

Recent reports have shown abnormalities of the oculomotor nerve using magnetic resonance imaging (MRI) in children with recurrent painful ophthalmoplegia fulfilling the criteria for ophthalmoplegic migraine (34, 43). Ostergaard and colleagues described two patients aged 7 and 18 months when they first developed ophthalmoplegia. Headache was reported a few years later in association with recurrent episodes of ophthalmoplegia. In one patient, the oculomotor nerve was abnormally thickened and showed enchancement with gadolinium in its course from the brainstem, into the prepontine cistern, to the cavernous sinus. In the second case, a swollen oculomotor nerve was demonstrated on MRI after the patient had repeated attacks of painful ophthalmoplegia. Wong and Wong (43) also showed abnormal enhancement of the oculomotor nerve on MRI in a 6-year-old boy whose attacks fulfilled the criteria for opthalmoplegic migraine.

Straube and colleagues (38) described a 23-year old woman with a history of migraine without aura who had two episodes of ophthalmoplegia involving the oculomotor nerve in association with migrainous headaches. MRI showed an enlarged oculomotor nerve in the prepontine cistern extending into the cavernous sinus. These authors suggested that this patient, although apparently fulfilling the criteria for ophthalmoplegic migraine, had instead the "Tolosa-Hunt syndrome."

The pathophysiology of ophthalmoplegic migraine remains obscure. Theories (34) include swelling of the posterior cerebral artery (13), pituitary swelling (14), vascular anomaly with compression of the third nerve (2), and unilateral brain swelling (22). None of these theories has been documented, and cerebral angiography is unrevealing. Walsh and O'Doherty (41) suggested that a swollen intracavernous carotid artery compressed adjacent cranial nerves within the cavernous sinus. Such swelling also would narrow the vessel, which the authors attempted to document angiographically; however, subsequent negative arteriograms during attacks do not support this theory (15). Microvascular constriction with peripheral cranial nerve ischemia would seem to be the most likely cause. As many attacks leave some residual effects and the ophthalmoplegia tends to worsen after repeated attacks, it seems likely that repeated episodes produce progressive microinfarction.

Clinical Features

IHS diagnostic criteria for ophthalmoplegic migraine (Headache Classification Committee, 1988):

A. At least 2 attacks fulfilling B.
B. Headache overlapping with paresis of one or more of cranial nerves III, IV, and VI.
C. Parasellar lesion ruled out by appropriate investigations.

The headaches usually proceed the ophthalmoplegia by 3 to 4 days. The headache is usually unilateral and may be throbbing or constant but is occasionally bilateral or alternating. It is often of the crescendo type, lasting hours to days. The ophthalmoplegia usually follows, affecting one or more nerves and possibly alternating sides in subsequent attacks. Extraocular muscle paralysis may occur with the first attack of headache or, rarely, may precede it; however, the paralysis usually appears subsequent to an established migraine pattern. The pupillomotor fibers are usually involved, producing a mydriatic and poorly responsive pupil. Other third-nerve dysfunction subsequently occurs, including ptosis and limitation of medial upward and downward gaze. Recently, Leone and colleagues (29) described a young woman who had experienced two episodes of internal ophthalmoplegia, without ptosis or external ophthalmoplegia, associated with headache. With sixth-nerve ophthalmoplegic migraine, paralysis of abduction occurs, and, with trochlear nerve involvement, limitation of downward and inward gaze is present. The headache usually resolves, leaving the ophthalmoplegia to recover over a period of as long as 1 month, but usually the ophthalmoplegia resolves within 1 week. Some residual third-nerve dysfunction may persist, such as a slight anisocoria. Only rarely does oculomotor nerve synkinesis develop (*aberrant regeneration*) (32). One of the authors (B.T.T.) examined a patient who had more than 100 attacks of abducens cranial nerve ophthalmoplegic migraine who still had completely normal ocular motility.

A typical clinical syndrome emerges: A child or young adult with periodic headache has ophthalmoplegia involving all functions of the third nerve, beginning at the height of an attack of cephalgia. The pain is primarily unilateral and in the orbital region. The ocular motor dysfunction lasts for days to weeks after cessation of headaches; recovery is gradual and tends to be less complete after repeated attacks.

Reports of transient, otherwise unexplained, unilateral pupillary mydriasis have been attributed tentatively to migraine in young patients (12,20,44). One should be careful to exclude intermittent angle-closure glaucoma with mydriasis, as pointed out by Sarkies and colleagues (37).

Until the 1930s and 1940s, when angiography was introduced in practice, it was impossible in many cases to rule out aneurysms or other lesions in the vicinity of the cavernous sinus. Multiple etiologies were cited as underlying causes of ophthalmoplegic migraine, including aneurysm, basilar arachnoiditis, and tumors. It was believed, in fact, that no separate clinical syndrome of ophthalmoplegic migraine existed but that all patients had a specific underlying organic lesion. Now, however, this is a diagnosis of exclusion, and noninvasive imaging tests such as MRI or magnetic resonance angiography (MRA) should be performed in all cases to exclude the possibility of aneurysm (36). The finding of an entirely normal MRI in a child with a third cranial-nerve palsy following a 4-day history of headache, but otherwise is well, should complete the workup. Aneurysmal third-nerve palsies are extremely rare in children aged under 14 years (17); however, in any adult with sudden onset of headache with a third-nerve palsy involving pupillomotor function, serious consideration should be given to angiography. The usual cause will be a posterior communicating artery aneurysm, which is best excluded by conventional angiography. Newer techniques, however, such as MRA or spiral contrast-enhanced computed tomographic scanning, soon may provide sufficient resolution to exclude aneurysm as a cause (40).

Myasthenia is ruled out if the pupil is involved (and actually should not be considered in the presence of pain) and with a positive response to edrophonium chloride (Tensilon). In the differential diagnosis, suspicion of another cause would be raised by the absence of a migraine history, severe persistent headache with total ophthalmoplegia, onset after age 20 years, and symptoms and signs of subarachnoid hemorrhage. In general, however, angiography is not warranted in a young patient strictly fulfilling the clinical criteria.

Prognosis

The prognosis for complete recovery following initial attacks is excellent. With recurrent attacks, however, progressive limitation of extraocular muscle function may persist as a residual effect. The usual recovery period is 1 to 4 weeks. In a review by Friedman and colleagues (15), four patients had 20 or more attacks, two patients had five to ten attacks, two patients had fewer than five attacks, and only a single patient had one attack. Therefore, after the diagnosis of ophthalmoplegic migraine is made, one may expect further attacks within an interval of 6 to 10 months.

In the differential diagnosis, consideration also should be given to aneurysm, tumor, diabetes, and sphenoid mucocele. The age of onset, negative glucose tolerance tests, and neuroimaging studies usually will rule out these possibilities. Other clinical entities confused with ophthalmoplegic migraine have included myasthenia gravis and the Tolosa-Hunt syndrome, which usually refers to a progressive painful ophthalmoplegia resulting from inflammatory disease in and around the cavernous sinus. Imaging studies may reveal inflammatory changes in the cavernous sinus not seen in ophthalmoplegic migraine (38). The diagnosis of Tolosa-Hunt syndrome is one of exclusion. Particular care should be taken to rule out neo-

plasm. Unlike ophthalmoplegic migraine, in which there may be a background history of migrainous attacks, there is an isolated involvement of cranial nerves III, IV, or VI in the Tolosa-Hunt syndrome; the pain persists, and multiple cranial nerves may be involved over a longer duration. Regarding both ophthalmoplegic migraine and the Tolosa-Hunt syndrome, care should be taken to rule out specific etiologies. Corticosteroid therapy has not been used regularly for ophthalmoplegic migraine. Given the rarity of attacks and the usual good prognosis for recovery in 10 days to 2 weeks, there is currently no evidence that drug therapy would be efficacious in ophthalmoplegic migraine.

Management

With recurrent attacks, standard migraine prophylactic therapy, including -blockers or calcium channel blockers, are recommended. Given the rarity of this condition and the infrequent attacks, prophylactic therapy has not been documented to provide benefit.

DEFINITION OF RETINAL MIGRAINE

IHS code and diagnosis: 1.4 retinal migraine.
WHO code and diagnosis: G43.81 retinal migraine.
Short description (Headache Classification Committee, 1988): Repeated attacks of monocular scotoma or blindness lasting less than one hour and associated with headache. Ocular or structural vascular disorder must be ruled out.
Other terms: ocular migraine, anterior visual pathway migraine, ophthalmic migraine.

Epidemiology

Retinal migraine occurs more frequently than ophthalmoplegic migraine. We estimate the frequency of strictly monocular visual phenomena occurring in conjunction with migraine to be 1 in 200 migraine sufferers. Frequently, however, homonymous visual-field phenomena in migraineurs is incorrectly attributed to a single eye. For example, a patient with transient right homonymous hemianopia might think the right eye is affected, because normally the right temporal hemifield is 30 to 40 degrees larger than the left nasal hemifield (1).

Genetics

The exact genetic predisposition to this subtype of migraine headache is unknown. The familial occurrence is similar to that expected in all patients with migraine preceded by visual aura, with an estimated 25% positive familial history. Retinal migraine is expected to be more common in women than men, which is true of migraine headaches in general, but this also has not been documented.

Anatomy and Pathology

The phrase *anterior visual pathway migraine* (AVPM) may be preferable to the term *retinal migraine*, because on rare occasion other structures are affected (see later). There are two forms of AVPM: (a) transient monocular blindness (TMB) and (b) permanent unilateral visual loss, a much less common occurrence.

The transient form has a relatively stereotyped presentation, consistent with retinal or optic nerve hypoperfusion from spasm of the central retinal or ophthalmic artery. For example, 10 of 24 patients reported by Tomsak and Jergens (39) described concentric contraction of vision, and only five of their patients had an altitudinal or quadratic visual change consistent with spasm of retinal artery branch. Kline and Kelley (25) studied a patient with a history of cluster headache and documented a reduction in central retinal artery blood flow during an attack of ocular migraine by intravenous fluorescein angiography. They noted no change in choroidal perfusion, also suggesting selective spasm of the central retinal artery. Others noted retinal artery constriction during episodes of migrainous transient monocular blindness (6,20) (Figs. 1 and 2) or normal arterial caliber (38). It is of interest to note that, in the case report by Wolter and Burchfield (42), a review of the fundus photographs depicts venous vasoconstriction as well as retinal opacification during an episode. Recently, Burger and co-workers (4) reported amaurosis fugax episodes resulting from documented vascular constriction in the retina. Their patients did not have retinal migraine, but the report showed the ability of retinal vascular constriction to produce monocular episodes of amaurosis in the absence of embolic phenomena. In some cases, retinal migraine may be due to a primary neuronal event, such as retina spreading depression, which has been induced in chick retina and has been blocked reversibly in a concentration-dependent manner by the serotonin (5-HT)$_{1D}$ agonist sumatriptan (31).

Permanent unilateral visual loss from AVPM is well-documented but uncommon. In addition to arterial or venous retinal vascular occlusions (6,17–19,26), central serous retinopathy, vitreous hemorrhage, retinal hemorrhage, and ischemic optic neuropathy have been noted (9,23,24). Newman and colleagues (33) reported bilateral central retinal artery occlusions, disk drusen, and migraine; and other descriptions of AVPM and vascular retinopathy have been reported (7,8). A recent unconfirmed report suggests that up to one third of migraineurs have retinal or optic-nerve visual-field defects found on testing with automated perimetry (30).

Clinical Features

IHS diagnostic criteria for retinal migraine (Headache Classification Committee, 1988):

A. At least 2 attacks fulfilling B and C.
B. Fully reversible monocular scotoma or blindness lasting less than 60 minutes and confirmed by examination during attack or (after proper instruction) by patient's drawing of monocular field defect during an attack.
C. Headache follows visual symptoms with a free interval of less than 60 minutes, but it may precede them.
D. Normal ophthalmoplegic examination outside of attack. Embolism is ruled out by appropriate investigations.

A typical history is that of a young adult with a pattern of common or classic migraine who has recurrent episodes of monocular visual loss or monocular scintillating scotomas. The visual loss is often one-sided and stereotyped in nature and tends to affect the entire monocular visual field (39), although any of the visual patterns described in migraine with aura may occur on a monocular basis in retinal migraine. Carrol (5) suggested that such transient episodes never have a preceding fortification spectra, that the absence of accompanying headache was invariable, and that the visual disturbance never lasted more than 10 minutes. Permanent visual loss is the exception rather than the rule. Transient AVPM is not associated with other neurologic symptoms but may be precipitated by postural change or exercise. Approximately one third of patients have a prior history of migraine (39).

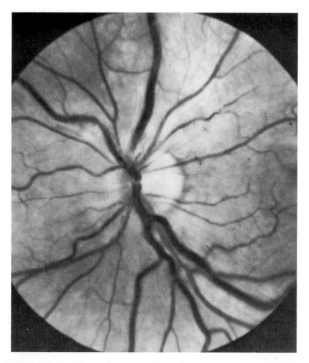

FIG. 1. Early disc edema and moderate venous congestion 4 hours after the start of a retinal migraine attack. Right eye, visual acuity: counting fingers. (From ref. 6, with permission.)

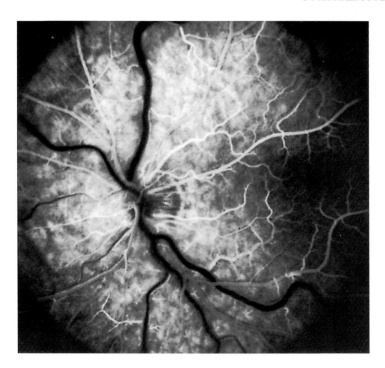

FIG. 2. Intravenous fluorescein angiogram of same eye as in Fig. 1 showing delayed intraretinal circulation. The first evidence of venous filling occurred 68 seconds after the early arterial phase (normal, 6–8 seconds). Poor filling of the optic-nerve capillaries also was noted. From ref. 6, with permission.

Ocular migraine as a cause of transient monocular blindness should be a diagnosis of exclusion, as highlighted by a recent case (10) in which a young medical student had episodes of amaurosis fugax, occasionally accompanied by headache, and was considered to have retinal migraine. He turned out to have a large pituitary tumor!

Prognosis

In general, the prognosis for retinal migraine is similar to that of migraine headache with typical aura. Recurrent attacks are expected, with a variable interval. In that the true incidence of retinal migraine is unknown, it is uncertain whether there is a higher incidence of permanent neuroretinal injury. The visual field data presented previously (30) suggest that there is a higher incidence of end-arteriolar distribution infarction and a higher incidence of permanent visual-field defects in retinal migraine than in clinically manifest cerebral infarctions in migraine with aura; however, there may be a higher than expected incidence of cerebral infarctions in migraineurs with visual aura who are studied with MRI. These would be, in effect, silent strokes revealed by neuroimaging, that were clinically unsuspected. An infarction in the retina, however, is usually apparent to the patient.

A recent study of transient ischemic attacks in young patients, including a large proportion of migraineurs, suggests a benign prognosis for stroke and myocardial infarction as long as other cardiovascular risk factors are not present (28). Another study of retinal strokes in people aged under 30 years found that 8 of 27 had migraine. Only two patients, however, had migraine as the only

association, the others having other systemic and/or ocular risk factor as well (3).

Management

We believe that all patients with retinal migraine should be placed on prophylactic antimigrainous therapy, such as calcium channel-blocking or beta-blocking agents. There is a report of the salutary effects of isoproterenol inhalation on AVPM and other migrainous visual phenomena (27), but we have not had personal experience with this treatment.

REFERENCES

1. Anderson DR. *Perimetry: with and without automation,* 2nd ed. St. Louis: CV Mosby, 1987.
2. Bramwell E. Etiology of ophthalmoplegic migraine. *Trans Ophthalmol Soc UK* 1934;54:204.
3. Brown GC, Margargal LE, Shields JA, Goldberg RE, Walsh PN. Retinal arterial obstruction in children and young adults. *Ophthalmology* 1981;88:18–25.
4. Burger SK, Saul RF, Selhorst JB, Thurston SE. Transient monocular blindness caused by vasospasm. *N Engl J Med* 1991;325:870–873.
5. Carroll D. Retinal migraine. *Headache* 1970;10:9.
6. Cassen JH, Tomsak RL, DeLuise VP. Mixed arteriovenous occlusive disease of the fundus. *J Clin Neuro-ophthalmol* 1985;5:164–168.
7. Coppeto JR, Lessell S, Sciarra R, Bear L. Vascular retinopathy in migraine. *Neurology* 1986;36:267–270.
8. Corbett JJ. Neuro-ophthalmic complications of migraine and cluster headaches. In: Smith CH, Beck RW, eds. *Neurologic clinics.* Symposium on neuro-ophthalmology. Philadelphia: WB Saunders, 1983:973–995.
9. Dalessio DJ, Silberstein SD. *Wolff's headache and other head pain.* 6th ed. New York: Oxford University Press, 1993.
10. Dirr LY, Janton FJ, Troost BT. Non-benign amaurosis fugax in a medical student. *Neurology* 1990;40:349.
11. Durkan GP, Troost BT, Slamovits TL, Kennderdale J. Recurrent painless oculomotor palsy in children: a variant of ophthalmoplegic migraine. *Headache* 1981;21:58.

12. Edelson RN, Levy DE. Transient benign unilateral pupillary dilatation in young adults. *Arch Neurol* 1974;31:12.

13. Ehlers H. On the pathogenesis of ophthalmoplegic migraine. *Acta Psychiatr Neurol Scand* 1928;3:219.

14. Elliot AJ. Ophthalmoplegic migraine: with report of a case. *Can Med Assoc J* 1940;43:242.

15. Friedman AP, Harter DH, Merritt HH. Ophthalmoplegic migraine. *Arch Neurol* 1962;7:320.

16. Friedman MW. Occlusion of central retinal vein in migraine. *Arch Ophthalmol* 1951;45:678.

17. Gabianelli EB, Klingele TG, Burde RM. Acute oculomotor nerve palsy in childhood: is arteriography necessary? *J Clin Neuro-ophthalmol* 1989;9:33–36.

18. Graveson GS. Retinal arterial occlusion in migraine. *BMJ* 1949;2:838.

19. Gronvall A. On changes in the fundus oculi and persisting injuries to the eye in migraine. *Acta Ophthalmol* 1938;16:602.

20. Hallet M, Cogan DG. Episodic unilateral mydriasis in otherwise normal patients. *Arch Ophthalmol* 1970;84:130.

21. Hansen SL, Borelli-Moller L, Strange P. Ophthalmoplegic migraine: diagnostic criteria, incidence of hospitalization and possible etiology. *Acta Neurol Scand* 1990;81:54–60.

22. Harrington DO, Flocks M. Ophthalmoplegic migraine pathogenesis: Report of pathological findings in case of recurrent oculomotor paralysis. *Arch Ophthalmol* 1953;49:643.

23. Hupp SL, Kline LB, Corbett JJ. Visual disturbance of migraine. *Surv Ophthalmol* 1989;33:221–236.

24. Inan LE, Uysal H, Ergun U. Yurdakal M, Karagoz, H. Complicated retinal migraine. *Headache* 1994;34:50–52.

25. Kline LB, Kelley CL. Ocular migraine in a patient with cluster headache. *Headache* 1980;20:253–257.

26. Krapin D. Occlusion of the central retinal artery in migraine. *N Engl J Med* 1964;270:359.

27. Kupersmith MJ, Hass WK, Chase NE. Isoproterenol treatment of visual symptoms in migraine. *Stroke* 1979;10:299–305.

28. Larsen BH, Sorensen PS, Marquardsen J. Transient ischaemic attacks in young patients: a thromboembolic or migrainous manifestation? A ten year follow up of 46 patients. *J Neurol Neurosurg Psychiatr* 1990; 53:1029–1033.

29. Leone, M., Grazzi, L., Moschiano, F., and Bussone, G. Internal ophthalmoplegia associated with migraine attacks. *Cephalalgia* 1994;14: 461–462.

30. Lewis RA, Vijayan N, Watson C, Keltner J, Johnson CA. Visual field loss in migraine. *Ophthalmology* 1989;96:321–326.

31. Maranhao-Filho PA, Martins-Ferreira H, Vincent MB, Ribeiro LJC, and Novis, S.A. P. Summatriptan blocks spreading depression in isolated chick retina. *Cephalalgia* 1997;17:822–825.

32. Miller NR, Newman NJ. *Walsh & Hoyt's clinical neuro-ophthalmology,* 5th ed., vol. 1. Baltimore: Williams & Wilkins, 1998:1220–1225.

33. Newman NJ, Lessell S, Brandt M. Bilateral central retinal artery occlusions, disk drusen, and migraine. *Am J Ophthalmol* 1989;107:236–240.

34. Ostergaard JR, Moller HU, Christensen T. Recurrent opthalmoplegia in childhood: diagnostic and otiologic considerations. *Cephalalgia* 1996; 16:27–69.

35. Osuntoken O, Osuntoken BO. Ophthalmoplegic migraine and hemoglobinopathy in *Nigerians. Am J Ophthalmol* 1972;74:451.

36. Ross JS, Masaryk MD, Modic MT, Harik SI, Wiznitzer M, Selman WR. Magnetic resonance angiography of the extracranial carotid arteries and intracranial vessels: a review. *Neurology* 1989;39:1369–1376.

37. Sarkies NJC, Sanders MD, Gautier-Smith PC. Episodic unilateral mydriasis and migraine (letter). *Am J Ophthalmol* 1985;99:217–218.

38. Straube A, Bandmann O, Buittner U, Schmidt H. A contrast enhanced lesion of the III nerve on MR of a patient with ophthalmoplegic migraine as evidence for a Tolosa-Hynt syndrome. *Headache* 1993;33: 446–448.

39. Tomsak RL, Jergens PB. Benign recurrent transient monocular blindness: a possible variant of acephalgia migraine. *Headache* 1987;27: 66–69.

40. Tomsak RL, Masaryk TJ, Bates JH. Magnetic resonance angiography (MRA) of isolated aneurysmal third nerve palsy. *J Clin Neuro-ophthalmol* 1991;11:16–18.

41. Walsh JP, O'Doherty DS. A possible explanation of the mechanism of ophthalmoplegic migraine. *Neurology* 1960;10:1079.

42. Wolter JR, Burchfield WJ. Ocular migraine in a young man resulting in unilateral transient blindness and retinal edema. *J Pediatr Ophthalmol* 1971;8:173.

43. Wong V, Wong WC. Enhancement of oculomotor nerve-a diagnostic criterion for ophthalmoplegic migraine. *Pediatr Neurol* 1997;17:70–73.

44. Woods D, O'Connor PS, Fleming R. Episodic unilateral mydriasis and migraine. *Am J Ophthalmol* 1984;98:229–234.

45. Woody RC, Blaw ME. Ophthalmoplegic migraine in infancy. *Clin Pediatr* 1986;25:82–84.

The Headaches, Second Edition,
edited by J. Olesen, P. Tfelt-Hansen, and K.M.A. Welch.
Lippincott Williams & Wilkins, Philadelphia © 2000.

The Migraines

CHAPTER 65

Childhood Syndromes Related to Migraine

Ishaq Abu-Arafeh and Mirja Hämäläinen

Common childhood disorders, such as abdominal migraine, cyclic vomiting, and paroxysmal vertigo, have been noted to occur in close association with migraine or in children with a family history of migraine. Because of their close relationship with migraine, they were called *variants of migraine* or *migraine equivalents*. The underlying pathologic process of all these conditions is not clear; however, it is likely to be centrally mediated through a release of neuroactive substances or as a result of autonomic nervous system disturbances. Pathophysiologic investigations into these disorders have not been possible because of the absence of objective biochemical or physiologic markers for the diagnosis of migraine. Therefore, the common epidemiologic, demographic and clinical characteristics were investigated to establish the relationship between all these disorders. Epidemiologic data showed higher rates than expected of the coexistence of these conditions in the same patient or in a single family. Common demographic features included similar patterns for the mean age of onset, peak age of onset, sex distribution, and family history of migraine. All these conditions were shown to share common trigger factors, associated symptoms during attacks, and relieving factors. These disorders are yet to find their places among the migraine syndromes, however, and into the classification and definition of migraine.

Future research is needed into the genetics, the molecular pathology, and the long-term follow-up of patients who have these disorders. Such research is now possible because of the availability of acceptable criteria for the diagnosis of migraine in children [International Headache Society (IHS), 1988] and criteria for the diagnoses of abdominal migraine, cyclic vomiting syndrome, and benign paroxysmal vertigo. Also, the relatively high prevalence rates of migraine and such disorders in schoolchildren would make research feasible.

DEFINITION OF ABDOMINAL MIGRAINE

International Headache Society (IHS) code and diagnosis: 1.5 (no diagnostic criteria were proposed)

World Health Organization (WHO) code and diagnosis: G43.820

Short description: Abdominal migraine is a disorder characterised by recurrent attacks of dull periumbilical abdominal pain associated with anorexia, nausea, vomiting, pallor, and misery. Between attacks, the patient is completely well. No abnormalities can be elicited on physical examination or other investigations.

Other terms: Functional abdominal pain, nonorganic abdominal pain, psychogenic abdominal pain, and recurrent abdominal pain of childhood, periodic syndrome.

Epidemiology

Between 8% and 12% of all schoolchildren may suffer from attacks of recurrent abdominal pain (5,10,37,38). Approximately half of these children may fulfill the criteria for the diagnosis of abdominal migraine (5). A population-based study of abdominal migraine as defined here estimated the prevalence rate at 4.1% among a random sample of more than 2,000 healthy 5- to 15-year-old schoolchildren in Scotland (5). The prevalence of abdominal migraine in children between 3 and 11 years of age was 2.4% in a population of one general practice in England

I. Abu-Arafeh: Department of Paediatrics, Stirling Royal Infirmary, Stirling FK8 2AU, United Kingdom.

M. Hämäläinen: Department of Pediatric Neurology, University of Helsinki, and Department of Pediatric Neurology, Hospital for Children and Adolescents, FIN-00029 HYKS Helsinki, Finland.

(35). Abdominal migraine is well recognized in the adult population (11), but its prevalence rate is not known.

One in four children with abdominal migraine also suffer from migraine headache as defined by the IHS, compared with the prevalence of one in ten in the general childhood population (5). Abdominal migraine affects girls more often than boys at a ratio of 3:2, and it is associated with an increased family history of migraine in first-degree relatives at one in three, compared with one in five in the general population. Symptoms of abdominal migraine may start at any age from the first year of life. The mean age of onset is around 7 years, with two peaks at 5 and 10 years of age (Fig. 1) in a similar pattern to that of childhood migraine (Abu-Arafeh, M.D. thesis, University of Aberdeen, 1996).

Pathophysiology

Studies of children with nonorganic, nonspecific recurrent abdominal pain showed evidence of a reduced plasma level of oxytocin (7) and an increased level of cholecystokinin (CCK) (8). These observations may suggest an association with the vagal modulating mechanisms and gut motility. Similar studies of children with abdominal migraine as a separate entity are not available yet. Studies are needed on the biochemical and physiologic changes during attacks of abdominal migraine compared with those during attacks of migraine headache and with controls.

The relationship between abdominal migraine and childhood migraine has been established on epidemiologic and clinical grounds only. The symptoms during attacks of abdominal migraine are related to systemic disturbances, vasomotor changes, gastrointestinal upset, and sensory impairment. These disturbances are highly suggestive of disease mechanisms similar to those of migraine.

Clinical Features

Abdominal migraine is an episodic disorder characterized by sudden onset of brief attacks of abdominal pain followed by complete remission of symptoms and return to normal health. The frequency of attacks may vary considerably. Population-based studies suggest an average of one attack per month (5,35), but higher frequency has been noted in hospital-based studies (40). The duration of each attack may also vary from 1 to 48 hours. The typical episode is 1 to 2 days.

The attacks of abdominal migraine may be provoked by trigger factors similar to migraine headache, including stress, fatigue, travel, poor sleep, and missing a meal. No specific aura symptoms have been described, but some children have reported prodromal nonspecific symptoms, such as behavioural changes, mood swings, headache, and anorexia during the day preceding onset of the abdominal pain.

The abdominal pain is commonly dull and severe enough to interfere with normal daily activities. The site of maximal intensity of the pain is around the umbilicus, but it may be ill defined. Most attacks are associated with anorexia, nausea, and repeated vomiting. The child looks pale and ill and prefers to be left alone or may go to bed. Some relief of symptoms may follow rest, sleep, and vomiting. The recovery is usually gradual, and the first sign of improvement is the return of appetite. The resolution of symptoms is always complete, and between attacks the child is well.

Physical examination during or between attacks does not reveal any abnormal findings to suggest anemia, jaundice, weight loss, food intolerance, allergy, impaired growth and development, constipation, or organ enlargement. The diagnosis of abdominal migraine should be based on as selective clinical criteria as possible (Table 1) to avoid the

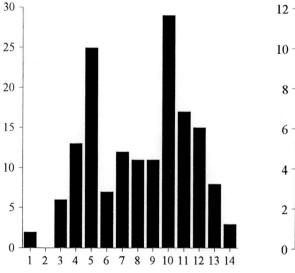
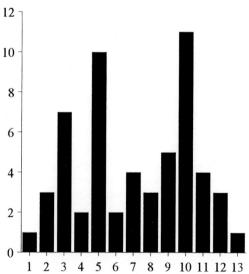

FIG. 1. Age of onset (in years) in children with migraine (*left*) and abdominal migraine (*right*).

TABLE 1. *Criteria for the diagnosis of abdominal migraine*

Attack lasting between 1 to 48 h
Pain severe enough to interfere with normal daily activities
Abdominal pain dull in nature
Periumbilical or poorly localized abdominal pain
Associated with any two of the following:
    Anorexia
    Nausea
    Vomiting
    Pallor
Complete resolution between attacks
Other possible causes excluded on clinical assessment and
    investigations

From ref. 5.

inclusion of doubtful cases (5). Family and personal history of migraine should not be a factor in the definition of abdominal migraine to avoid any diagnosis bias.

Clinical presentation and special investigations may be needed to exclude other conditions such as gastroesophageal reflux, gastritis, peptic ulceration, inflammatory bowel disease, food intolerance, malabsorption syndromes, and renal or menstrual disorders. Celiac disease and lactose intolerance (12) may present without impairment of growth and also should be considered in the differential diagnosis. Most children present to general practitioners after several episodes of abdominal pain, and few patients are brought to the hospital general pediatric or gastroenterology departments. Children presenting during acute attacks may be admitted to pediatric surgery wards and discharged with no spesific diagnosis for acute abdominal pain after excluding acute appendicitis and intestinal obstruction.

Other children may be referred to hospital departments after several pain episodes because of parental concerns about a possible underlying sinister cause. After a negative physical examination, it is worthwhile to run screening tests, including full blood count, erythrocyte sedimentation rate, serum urea and electrolytes, liver function tests, urinanalysis, and culture and abdominal ultrasound scan.

Prognosis

Long-term follow-up studies of children with abdominal migraine are not yet available because the condition only recently has become recognized as a separate entity. Long-term (10–20 years) follow-up of children with recurrent abdominal pain, however, has shown that abdominal pain ceases in about half of these children, continues in one quarter, and is replaced with migraine headache in about one quarter (32).

Management

Reassurance of the patient and the parents about the benign nature of the disorder and the lack of long-term

complications should be based on the exclusion of other possible causes by full physical examination and the necessary investigations. Acknowledgment of the distressing nature of the attacks to both the child and the family would improve compliance and cooperation with future advice and treatment. Children and their families should be encouraged to record diaries of future episodes to help in understanding the condition; assessing prospectively the frequency, duration, and severity of attacks; and also to obtain a baseline for future reference in relation to prognosis and treatment. During attacks, the child should be allowed to rest. Oral fluids should be encouraged in small, frequent volumes as tolerated. Antiemetic drugs, such as metoclopromide, may be used with caution. The efficacy of simple analgesics, such as paracetamol and diclofenac or even codeine, is unclear because no controlled trials on their use in this context have been reported. Also of importance is the presumed association between gastritis and migraine, as has been described in some children (33), which may discourage the use of nonsteroidal antiinflammatory drugs as analgesics.

Nonpharmacologic prophylactic treatment of abdominal migraine may be useful in some patients by identifying and avoiding trigger factors. High dietary fiber intake also may reduce the number of attacks of abdominal pain, possibly by reducing the intestinal transit time, in a fashion similar to that shown in patients with irritable bowel disease (19).

Prophylactic drug treatment with the antimigraine agent pizotifen has been shown to be effective in reducing the number of days of abdominal pain and also the indices of severity and misery in a small number of patients (41). Experience with other drugs is limited to anecdotal reports.

DEFINITION OF CYCLIC VOMITING SYNDROME

IHS code and diagnosis: 1.5 (no diagnostic criteria were proposed)
WHO code and diagnosis: not available
Short description: Cyclic vomiting syndrome (CVS) is a disorder characterized by recurrent episodes of unexplained nausea, vomiting, pallor, intense feeling of ill health, misery, and lethargy. The attacks last between few hours and few days and almost always are followed by complete recovery.
Other terms: Acephalalgic migraine, bilious headache, fitful vomiting, and periodic syndrome.

Epidemiology

Episodes of unexplained vomiting were reported to affect 2.3% of schoolchildren in Western Australia (17). A recent study of the epidemiology of CVS as a specific clinical entity defined by strict clinical diagnostic criteria reported a prevalence rate of 1.9% among 5- to 15-year-old schoolchildren (4). CVS may occur at any age, but it is more common in children than in adults. The mean age of onset is between 5 and 7 years, with more than 70% of cases starting in early childhood before the age of 7 years. Both girls and boys are equally affected, but more boys are affected before the age of 8 years.

Pathophysiology

Although the underlying etiology of CVS is not known, migraine (24,25,27), psychogenic problems (23,29), epilepsy (34), central nervous system disease, and metabolic disorders all have been suggested as possible underlying causes. Both CVS and migraine have similar clinical features (4,25,42), comparable patterns of electroencephalographic (EEG) changes (27), and similar disturbances in gastric motility and autonomic dysfunction (1,43,44). The metabolic changes noted during attacks of CVS are more likely to be the effects rather than the causes of the attacks.

Clinical Features

The frequency of CVS attacks is variable, but on average they occur about eight times per year. Attacks occurring more than ten times per year are rare (10% of patients). Each attack may last from 4 hours to several days, but the average duration of the attack is about 24 hours. Approximately two thirds of children with CVS have episodes of vomiting as the only recurrent problem (4), and around 15% also may suffer from migraine as defined by the IHS (1988). One third of these children may also suffer from travel sickness, and one third may suffer from atopic diseases. Like migraine, the precipitating factors may include travel, stress, excitement, tiredness, and lack of sleep, but these factors are reported only in a minority of children who can identify a trigger factor. Prodromal symptoms, such as nonspecific changes in mood and behavior or even sensory aura symptoms, may precede the attacks.

During the episodes of vomiting, the child is commonly pale, feels unwell, and has anorexia. The child may become so ill and dehydrated that hospital admission and parenteral administration of fluids is the only method of maintaining adequate hydration. Some children may find relief simply from resting or sleeping.

The diagnosis of CVS should be made only on fulfillment of the clinical criteria (Table 2) and by the exclusion of other disorders that may require specific investigations and treatment (26). Children should be reviewed on several occasions during and between attacks before the diagnosis can be safely made.

Children with typical clinical features and normal physical examination, including neurologic assessment and normal blood pressure, may need only minimal investigations, including full blood count, erythrocyte sedimentation rate (ESR), serum urea, electrolytes, creatinine, amy-

TABLE 2. *Criteria for the diagnosis of cyclic vomiting syndrome*

Essential criteria
  Recurrent, severe, discrete episodes of vomiting
  Various intervals of normal health between episodes
  Duration of vomiting episodes from hours to days
  No apparent cause of vomiting
Supportive criteria
  Stereotypical: each episode similar within individuals as to time of onset, intensity, duration, frequency, associated symptoms and signs
  Self-limited: episodes resolve spontaneously if left untreated
Other associated features
  Nausea
  Diarrhoea
  Abdominal pain
  Headache
  Motion sickness
  Photophobia
  Fever
  Pallor
  Dehydration
  Excess salivation
  Social withdrawal

lase, liver function tests, blood glucose, urinalysis, and urine culture. In atypical cases or in the presence of abnormal findings on physical examination or neurological evaluation, full investigations may be needed and may include neuroimaging, metabolic assessment (serum ammonia, plasma amino acids, urinary amino acids, organic acids), gastrointestinal contrast imaging or endoscopy or both, abdominal ultrasonography, and electroencephalography. The investigations aim to exclude a wide variety of conditions as outlined in Table 3.

Prognosis

The disorder runs a protracted, long course of relapses and remissions. Older children and young adults may experience complete cessation or significant reduction in the frequency of attacks. In other children, more typical episodes of migraine with the characteristic headache may replace episodes of CVS. Unfortunately, long-term follow-up studies of children with CVS are not available.

Management

The management of acute attacks aims at the prevention of dehydration, replacement of fluid loss, and relief of pain and misery. Most children can be treated safely at home with small, frequent amounts of oral fluids and rest. In prolonged severe episodes, hospital admission may be necessary for intravenous infusions and the diagnosis and treatment of other possible concurrent infections. Antiemetic treatment with metoclopramide or domperidone may help in reducing nausea and vomiting or even aborting the attack.

TABLE 3. *Differential diagnosis of clinical vomiting syndrome*

Gastrointestinal disorders	Peptic ulcers, gastroesophageal reflux, inflammatory bowel diseases, malabsorption, and food intolerance
Renal disorders	Urinary tract infections, renal calculi, and obstructive lesions
Neurological disorders	Brain tumors, vascular malformations, hydrocephalus, and epilepsy
Metabolic and endocrine disorders	Ornithine transcarbamylase deficiency, medium chain acyl coenzyme-A dehydrogenase deficiency, propionic acidaemia, isovaleric acidaemia, phaeochromocytoma, porphyria, adrenal insufficiency, and diabetes mellitus
Infectious diseases	Chronic sinusitis

Prophylactic treatment may include measures to avoid precipitating factors, when possible, and administration of pharmacological agents. Pizotifen (5-hydroxytryptamine antagonist), the agent used successfully in the prophylaxis of migraine, also has been used with some success in reducing the frequency and severity of attacks of CVS (21). Recent publications suggest response to treatment with erythromycin as a prokinetic agent in an open study (44) and amitriptyline and cyproheptadine in a retrospective review (9). Other antimigraine agents, such as propranolol, have not been investigated.

DEFINITION OF BENIGN PAROXYSMAL VERTIGO

IHS code and diagnosis: 1.5.1
WHO code and diagnosis: G43.821
Short description: Benign paroxysmal vertigo (BPV) is a disorder characterized by transient episodes of unreal sensation of rotation of the patient or the surroundings in the absence of a neurologic or an auditory disorder. The attacks may be associated with nausea, pallor, and nystagmus, but no loss of consciousness occurs. Complete recovery between attacks is always expected.
Other terms: dizziness, giddiness.

Epidemiology

In a population-based study of dizziness in schoolchildren, about 20% of those between 5 and 15 years of age reported suffering from episodes of vertigo over a period of 1 year (3). Most episodes occurred during the course of self-limiting illnesses or trauma. The prevalence rate of BPV, as defined herein (Table 4), in the same population was 2.6%. No other similar population-based studies on BPV in children are available, but the condition was previously regarded as uncommon (13,14). The clinical features of BPV have been described from reports of children attending pediatric neurology (45) and otolaryngology clinics (22). No studies of children attending primary health care services are available.

Etiology and Pathophysiology

Episodes of vertigo occur at all ages and commonly in adults (31), particularly in the elderly (36). In children,

episodes of vertigo may be the result of vascular, neurologic, or auditory underlying disorders or as a side effect to medications such as antiepileptic treatment (6).BPV is commonly idiopathic (15,16) and may represent an early manifestation of migraine (20). It is often called a variant of migraine or a migraine equivalent. The clinical and epidemiologic relationship between BPV and migraine might suggest a shared pathogenesis (3). Migraine has been reported in at least one first-degree relative of 42% of children with BPV, compared with 18% of the general childhood population (3). The prevalence of BPV among children with migraine (8.8%) is three times the prevalence of BPV in the general childhood population (2.6%) (3).

About one third of children with migraine (45) reported vertigo attacks either just before the onset of migraine headache attacks or during the headache phase. Also, vertigo is a characteristic feature of basilar artery migraine (30) in children (basilar artery migraine; see WHO diagnosis G43.1x3).

Clinical Features

The syndrome of BPV of childhood may take one of two forms, depending on the age at first presentation. Early childhood BPV is a specific disorder characterized by severe, sudden, and brief episodes of unsteadiness, nystagmus, and pallor, with no headache or loss of consciousness. Young children between 1 and 4 years of age (18,28) are most commonly affected. In infants under the age of 1 year, benign paroxysmal torticollis has been closely related to vertigo (18). The attacks may last for few hours to few days and are associated with vomiting and tilting of the neck to one side. A relationship to migraine has been suggested for both paroxysmal vertigo and paroxysmal torticollis (45).

TABLE 4. *Criteria for the diagnosis of benign paroxysmal vertigo in children*

Brief attacks of unreal sensation of rotation in otherwise healthy children
Multiple, brief, sporadic episodes of equilibrium, anxiety, and often nystagmus or vomiting
Normal neurological examination
Normal electroencephalogram

In school-age children, idiopathic BPV occurs commonly in association with migraine. It is slightly more common in girls than boys, at a ratio of 5:4 between the ages of 5 and 15 years. About one in four children also suffer from migraine, and 40% also suffer from motion sickness. The attacks vary considerably in frequency between 3 to 100 per year, on average, once per month. Most attacks last 5 to 10 minutes, but in few patients the attacks may be as long as 2 hours. No specific trigger factors are recognized. Pallor and nausea are commonly associated with the attacks of vertigo, occurring in 56% and 44% of children, respectively. Most children find relief from rest.

The diagnosis of BPV is based on the IHS clinical criteria (see Table 4) of at least three transient episodes of unreal sensations of rotation either of the child or the surrounding environment. The attacks are severe enough to interfere with normal activities and are not associated with loss of consciousness or any neurologic or auditory abnormality (3). In atypical attacks, investigations may be necessary to exclude possible underlying pathology (Table 5).

Prognosis

Benign paroxysmal vertigo is a benign disorder with relapses and remissions. The frequency of attacks could be influenced by emotional and environmental factors. BPV of early onset is a self-limiting disorder that improves with time and may remit completely in late childhood. Long-term follow-up (2.6–15.7 years; mean, 8.9 years) of seven children with early onset BPV showed that five patients became free from vertigo, four had migraine-type headache, and two had nonspecific headaches (45).

Late onset BPV may run a longer course and persist into adult life. Patients learn how to deal with attacks, and the impact of the condition on daily activities become less evident.

Management

No specific treatment is necessary. The condition is self-limiting. Most patients require reassurance about the lack of sinister underlying cause. Rest during attacks will help in resolving the symptoms. No trials have been done to assess medications, such as pizotifen or propranolol, in the treatment of BPV as a separate entity.

TABLE 5. *Causes of dizziness in children*

Central nervous disorders
  Cortical lesion (tumor or trauma)
  Posterior fossa lesion
  Brainstem lesion (tumor or trauma)
  Migraine or epilepsy
  Demyelinating disease
  Postmeningitis
Peripheral lesions
  Benign paroxysmal vertigo of childhood
  Paroxysmal torticollis in infancy
  Vestibular neuronitis
  Meniere's disease
  Drug induced ototoxicity
  Paroxysmal positional vertigo
  Posttraumatic labyrinthine dysfunction
  Middle-ear disease
  Labyrinthintis and labyrinthine fistula
Cardiovascular
  Orthostatic hypotension
  Cardiac arrhythmia
Medications
  Antihypertensive drugs
  Antiepileptic drugs
Psychogenic miscellaneous conditions
  Psychosomatic
  Genetic familial disturbances

Modified from ref. 22.

REFERENCES

1. Abell TL, Chung HK, Malagelada JR. Idiopathic cyclic nausea and vomiting—a disorder of gastrointestinal motility? *Mayo Clin Proc* 1988;31:1169–1175.
2. Abu-Arafeh I, Russell G. Prevalence of headache and migraine in schoolchildren. *BMJ* 1994;309:765–769.
3. Abu-Arafeh I, Russell G. Paroxysmal vertigo as a migraine equivalent in children: a population-based study. *Cephalalgia* 1995;15:22–25.
4. Abu-Arafeh I, Russell G. Cyclical vomiting syndrome in children: A population-based study. *J Pediatr Gastroenterol Nutr* 1995;21:454–458.
5. Abu-Arafeh I, Russell G. Prevalence and clinical features of abdominal migraine compared with those of migraine headache. *Arch Dis Child* 1995;72:413–417.
6. Abu-Arafeh IA, Wallace SJ. Unwanted effects of anti-epileptic treatment. *Dev Med Child Neurol* 1988;30:117–121.
7. Alfven G, de la Torre B, Uvnas-Moberg K. Depressed concentrations of oxytocin and cortisol in childrenwith recurrent abdominal pain of non-organic origin. *Acta Paediatr* 1994;83:1076–1080.
8. Alfven G, Uvnas-Moberg K. Elevated cholecystokinin concentrations in plasma in children with recurrent abdominal pain. *Acta Paediatr* 1993;82:967–970.
9. Andersen JM, Sugerman KS, Lockhart JR, Weinberg WA. Effective prophylactic therapy for cyclic vomiting syndrome in children using amitriptyline or cyproheptadine. *Pediatr* 1997;100:977–981.
10. Apley J, Naish N. Recurrent abdominal pains: a field survey of 1000 schoolchildren. *Arch Dis Child* 1958;33:165–170.
11. Axon ATR, Long DE, Jones SC. Abdominal migraine: Does it exist? [Editorial] *J Clin Gastroenterol* 1991;13:615–616.
12. Barr RG, Levine MD, Watkins JB. Recurrent abdominal pain of childhood due to lactose intolerance. *N Engl J Med* 1979;300:1449–1452.
13. Blayney AW, Colman BH. Dizziness in children. *Clin Otolaryngol* 1984;9:77–85.
14. Busis SN. Dizziness in children. *Pediatr Ann* 1988;17:648.
15. Cawthorne T. Vertigo: president's address. *Proc R Soc Med* 1958;52:529–536.
16. Corbin KB, Williams HL. Dizziness. *Med Clin North Am* 1960;44:941–951.
17. Cullen KJ, MacDonald WB. The periodic syndrome: its nature and prevalence. *Med J Aust* 1963;II:167–172.
18. Dunn DW, Snyder CH. Benign paroxysmal vertigo of childhood. *Am J Dis Child* 1976;130:1099–1100.
19. Feldman W, McGrath P, Hodgson C, Ritter H, Shipman RT. The use of

dietary fiber in the management of simple, childhood, idiopathic, recurrent, abdominal pain: results in a prospective, double-blind, randomized, controlled trial. *Am J Dis Child* 1985;139:1216–1218.

20. Fenichel GM. Migraine as a cause of benign paroxysmal vertigo of childhood. *J Pediatr* 1967;71:114–115.

21. Forbes D, Withers G. Prophylactic therapy in cyclic vomiting syndrome. *J Pediatr Gastroenterol Nutr* 1995;21(Suppl):S57–S59.

22. Fried MP. The evaluation of dizziness in children. *Laryngoscope* 1980;90:1548–1560.

23. Gonzalez-Heydrich J, Kerner J, Steiner H. Testing the psychogenic vomiting diagnosis. *Am J Dis Child* 1991;145:913–916.

24. Hockaday J. Migraine and its equivalents in childhood. *Dev Med Child Neurol* 1987;29:258–270.

25. Hoyt CS, Stickler GB. A study of 44 children with the syndrome of recurrent (cyclic) vomiting. *Pediatrics* 1960;25:775–780.

26. International Symposium on Cyclic Vomiting Syndrome. Diagnostic criteria for Cyclic Vomiting Syndrome. *J Pediatr Gastroenterol Nutr* 1995;21(Suppl):vi.

27. Jernigan S, Ware L. Reversible quantitative EEG changes in a case of cyclic vomiting: evidence for a migraine equivalent. *Dev Med Child Neurol* 1991;33:808–815.

28. Koenigsberger MR, Chutorian AM, Gold AP, Schvey MS. Benign paroxysmal vertigo of childhood. *Neurology* 1970;20:1108–1113.

29. Lanzi G, Balottin U, Fazzi E, Tagliasacchi M, Manfrin M, Mira E. Benign paroxysmal vertigo of childhood: a long-term follow-up. *Cephalalgia* 1994;14:458–460.

30. Lapkin M. Golden G. Basilar artery migraine: a review of 30 cases. *Am J Dis Child* 1978;132:278–281.

31. Luxon LM. "A bit dizzy." *Br J Hosp Med* 1984;32:315–321

32. Magni G, Pierri M, Donzelli F. Recurrent abdominal pain in children: a long term follow up. *Eur J Pediatr* 1987;146:72–74.

33. Mavromichalis I, Zaramboukas T, Giala MM. Migraine of gastrointestinal origin. *Eur J Pediatr* 1995;154:406–410.

34. Mitchell W, Greenwood R, Messenheimer J. Abdominal epilepsy. Cyclical vomiting as a major symptom of simple partial seizure. *Arch Neurol* 1983;40:251–252.

35. Mortimer MJ, Kay J, Jaron A. Clinical epidemiology of childhood abdominal migraine in an urban general practice. *Dev Med Child Neurol* 1993;35:243–248.

36. Orma EJ, Koskenoja M. Postural dizziness in the aged. *Geriatrics* 1957;12:49–59.

37. Oster J. Recurrent abdominal pain, headache and limb pains in children and adolescents. *Pediatrics* 1972;50:429–436.

38. Pringle MLK, Butler NR, Davie R. *11,000 seven-year-olds*. London: Longman 1966:184.

39. Reinhart JB, Evans SL, McFadden DL. Cyclic vomiting in children: seen through the psychiatrist's eye. *Pediatrics* 1977;59:371–377.

40. Symon DNK, Russell G. Abdominal migraine: a syndrome defined. *Cephalalgia* 1986;6:223–228.

41. Symon DNK, Russell G. Double blind placebo controlled trial of pizotifen syrup in the treatment of abdominal migraine. *Arch Dis Child* 1995;72:48–50.

42. Symon DNK, Russell G. The relationship between cyclic vomiting syndrome and abdominal migraine. *J Pediatr Gastroenterol Nutr* 1995;21 (Suppl 1):S42–S43.

43. Thompson W, Heaton K. Functional bowel disorders in apparently healthy people. *Gastroenterology* 1980;79:283–288.

44. Vanderhoof JA, Young R, Kaufman SS, Ernst L. Treatment of cyclic vomiting in childhood with erythromycin. *J Pediatr Gastroenterol Nutr* 1993;17:387–91.

45. Watson P, Steele J. Paroxysmal disequilibrium in the migraine syndrome of childhood. *Arch Otolaryngol* 1974;99:177–179.

The Headaches, Second Edition,
edited by J. Olesen, P. Tfelt-Hansen, and K.M.A. Welch.
Lippincott Williams & Wilkins, Philadelphia © 2000.

The Migraines

CHAPTER 66

Status Migrainosus

J. Keith Campbell and Alessandro S. Zagami

DEFINITION

IHS code and diagnosis: 1.6.1 Status migrainosus.
WHO code and diagnosis: G43.2 Status migrainosus.
Short description (Headache Classification Committee, 1988): Attack of migraine with headache phase lasting more than 72 hours despite treatment. Headache-free intervals of less than 4 hours (sleep not included) may occur.

IHS diagnostic criteria for status migrainosus (Headache Classification Committee, 1988) is provided as follows (3):

A. The patient fulfills criteria for 1.1 or 1.2.
B. The present attack fulfills criteria for one form of migraine except that headache lasts more than 72 hours whether treated or not.
C. Headache is continuous throughout the attack or interrupted by headache-free intervals lasting less than 4 hours. Interruption during sleep is disregarded.

Although the IHS definition states that the headache phase must exceed 72 hours, a headache somewhat shorter in duration may be just as severe and refractory to treatment as an episode of status migraine and require the specialized treatment to be described.

CLINICAL FEATURES OF STATUS MIGRAINOSUS

Most episodes that by definition become status migrainosus start as an unremarkable attack of migraine

J.K. Campbell: Department of Neurology, Mayo Clinic and Mayo Medical School, Rochester, Minnesota 55905.

A.S. Zagami: Department of Medicine, University of New South Wales, and Institute of Neurological Sciences, Prince of Wales Hospital, Randwick, Sydney, New South Wales 2031, Australia.

with or without aura. Initially, the attack resembles the individual's typical migraine. It is rare for a status attack to be the first migraine experienced. Although a migraine destined to develop into a status migrainosus may be more severe than usual, it is the persistence and refractory nature of the attack that are characteristic. Almost all attacks are accompanied by nausea and prolonged vomiting to the point of dehydration. Shock, electrolyte imbalance, hypotension, severe pain, and fatigue may ensue.

The severity and recurrence rate of attacks are quite variable. Some individuals will have a single episode in their entire migraine experience; others will suffer recurrent bouts, especially when acute episodes of migraine are not promptly and effectively treated. The incidence and prevalence of status migrainosus are unknown, but it is by no means a rare occurrence in specialized headache clinics.

PRECIPITATING FACTORS

Couch and Diamond reviewed the causative and therapeutic aspects of status migrainosus (1). Based on a questionnaire completed by members of the American Association for the Study of Headache, those factors felt to be the main triggers of status included emotional stress, depression, abuse of medication, anxiety, diet, hormones, and other nonspecific factors.

Since this study in 1983, more and more emphasis has been placed on medication overuse as a cause of status migrainosus (9), which under these circumstances can be considered as a prolonged rebound headache. Avoidance of medication abuse and management of the other trigger factors are considered important in the prevention of status migrainosus.

MANAGEMENT

By the time most patients are seen in status migrainosus, they have already tried several remedies, both over-the-counter and prescription preparations, including the currently available migraine-specific agents, with minimal benefit. Hospital admission is often appropriate, although parenteral sumatriptan is an option for the patient who has not yet tried it, especially if combined with an antiemetic such as metoclopramide 10 mg intramuscularly. If dehydration is not severe and if vomiting subsides, further treatment at home with self-administered subcutaneous, intranasal, or oral sumatriptan may be considered.

Treatment in hospital, an urgent care center, or emergency department includes correction of dehydration with intravenous fluids and provision of a quiet, dark, restful environment. The specific additional treatment options to be described are not mutually exclusive. Many subjects respond better to one regimen than another. The therapeutic choices depend on the preferences of the physician, the past treatment experiences of the patient, and the presence or absence of medical contraindications to various techniques (Fig. 1).

Sumatriptan

There are no significant controlled trial results on the use of sumatriptan in status migrainosus, but in the experience of many headache specialists subcutaneous sumatriptan 6 mg (4) will at least temporarily relieve the persistent headache and associated symptoms of photophobia and phonophobia. Nausea also may be decreased. Recurrence of the headache may require one or two further injections in the next 24 hours.

A dose of sumatriptan theoretically precludes the subsequent use of dihydroergotamine (DHE) for 8 to 12 hours; therefore, some will choose to use DHE first because it has a proven efficacy in status migrainosus (8,9,11).

Dihydroergotamine Mesylate

The intravenous DHE protocol of Raskin (8) or some modification of it (11) has been extensively used in the hospital management of prolonged attacks of migraine with reports of up to 91% of patients becoming headache free within 1 to 2 days.

Metoclopramide (intravenously) is extensively used in the Raskin protocol to overcome the nausea and vomiting induced or aggravated by DHE. Chlorpromazine may be added to provide sedation and further reduce nausea. The dose of DHE must be carefully adjusted for the individual patient based on the presence or absence of vomiting and the response of the headache. Many who have used this protocol have found it logistically troublesome because the DHE has to be injected as a bolus every 8 hours.

Recently, however, Ford and Ford (2) have shown that DHE can be given successfully by continuous intravenous infusion (3 mg in 100 mL normal saline). The infusion rate was adjusted as necessary if side effects developed and, in any case, was gradually reduced as headache diminished. When combined with metoclopramide 10 mg intravenously every 8 hours, the continuous infusion of DHE in saline was as beneficial as the older intermittent intravenous injection technique. Ford and Ford (2) treated 96 patients with prolonged intractable migraine with DHE by infusion; 89 became headache-free, 64.5% of them within 3 days. The most common side effects—nausea, diarrhea, and vomiting—occurred with a similar frequency as in patients treated with repetitive DHE. Until recently, it was believed that DHE was insoluble in water and unstable when exposed to light. However, experiments performed by the manufacturer of DHE have recently confirmed that the drug is soluble in saline and is stable when exposed to light and to plastic tubing.

Phenothiazines

Chlorpromazine given intravenously in doses of 5 mg to 50 mg was reported by Lane and colleagues (6,7) to be effective in breaking medically intractable attacks of migraine. This modality has become widely used in emergency departments. Hypotension is avoided by giving a bolus of 500 mL normal saline intravenously with the chlorpromazine being injected slowly through the intravenous tubing.

Intravenous prochlorperazine 10 mg also has been reported effective in status migrainosus (5). Dystonic reactions to this and to chlorpromazine are most troublesome in young patients and can be minimized by the addition of diphenhydramine 25 mg intravenously. The phenothiazine chosen can be repeated along with the diphenhydramine every 4 to 6 hours until the headache resolves.

Other Treatments

Parenterally administered corticosteroids, intravenous lidocaine (10), intramuscular ketorolac, and, more recently, intravenous droperidol (12) have each been advocated for status migrainosus, but no large or controlled series have been published.

The use of opioids in the management of refractory migraine is controversial, and although there may be a role in providing temporary pain relief if one of the treatments described above is initiated, in the opinion of many researchers, the benefits of opioids are outweighed

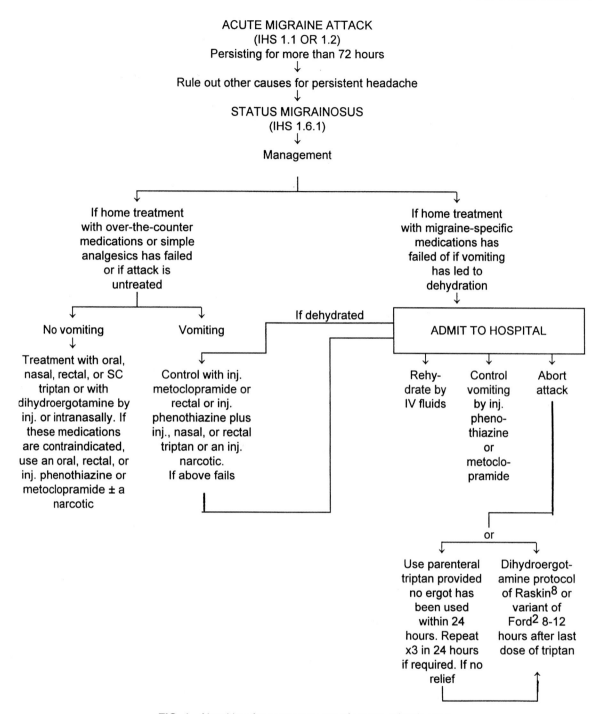

FIG. 1. Algorithm for management of status migrainosus.

by their tendency to induce vomiting, their transient pain-relieving action, and the perpetuation of the analgesic rebound phenomenon.

REFERENCES

1. Couch JR Jr, Diamond S. Status migrainosus: causative and therapeutic aspects. *Headache* 1983;23:94–101.
2. Ford RG, Ford KT. Continuous intravenous dihydroergotamine in the treatment of intractable headache. *Headache* 1997;37:129–136.
3. Headache Classification Committee of the International Headache Society. Classification and diagnostic criteria for headache disorders, cranial neuralgias and facial pain. *Cephalalgia* 1988;8(suppl 7): 26–27.
4. Jauslin P, Goadsby PJ, Lance JW. The hospital management of severe migrainous headache. *Headache* 1991;31:658–660.
5. Jones J, Sklar D, Dougherty J, White W. Randomized double-blind trial of intravenous prochlorperazine for the treatment of acute headache. *JAMA* 1989;261:1174–1176.
6. Lane PL, McLellan BA, Baggoley CJ. Comparative efficacy of chlorpromazine and meperidine with dimenhydrinate in migraine headache. *Ann Emerg Med* 1989;18:360–365.

7. Lane PL, Ross R. Intravenous chlorpromazine—preliminary results in acute migraine. *Headache* 1985;25:302–304.

8. Raskin NH. Repetitive intravenous dihydroergotamine as therapy for intractable migraine. *Neurology* 1986;36:995–997.

9. Raskin NH. Treatment of status migrainosus: the American experience. *Headache* 1990;30(suppl 2):550–553.

10. Reutens DC, Fatovich DM, Stewart-Wynne EG, Prentice DA. Is intravenous lidocaine clinically effective in acute migraine? *Cephalalgia* 1991;11:245–247.

11. Silberstein SD, Schulman EA, Hopkins MM. Repetitive intravenous DHE in the treatment of refractory headache. *Headache* 1990;30: 334–339.

12. Wang S-J, Silberstein SD, Young WB. Droperidol treatment of status migrainosus and refractory migraine. *Headache* 1997;37:377–382.

The Headaches, Second Edition,
edited by J. Olesen, P. Tfelt-Hansen, and K.M.A. Welch.
Lippincott Williams & Wilkins, Philadelphia © 2000.

The Migraines

CHAPTER 67

Migraine and Stroke

K. Michael A. Welch and Marie-Germaine Bousser

Migraine is associated with an increased risk of strokes between and during attacks (27,111). Various forms of migraine are recognized, and they are generally classified according to the transient, though sometimes persistent, neurologic deficits that may precede, accompany, or outlast the headache phase. A number of these clinical syndromes may mimic cerebrovascular syndromes, including migraine with aura of different types, retinal or ocular migraine, ophthalmoplegic migraine, hemiplegic migraine, and basilar artery migraine (BAM) (27,60, 111,147). If the deficit of a migraine attack remains, *migraine-induced stroke* should be suspected.

The clinical features of migraine can occasionally mimic stroke. Visual disturbances account for well over half the transient neurologic manifestations. Most frequently, these consist of positive phenomena such as stars, spark photopsia, complex geometric patterns, and fortification spectra. These positive phenomena may leave in their wake negative phenomena such as scotoma or hemianopia. The symptoms are characteristically slow in onset and slow in progression, although the onset is more abrupt and may be confused with amaurosis fugax. Visual symptoms sometimes progress to visual distortion or misperception, such as micropsia or dysmetropsia. The patterns of symptoms indicate the spread of neurologic dysfunction from the occipital cortex into the contiguous regions of the temporal or parietal lobes. It is critical in making the differential diagnosis from stroke to establish that the neurologic deficit crosses arterial territories. The next most com-

mon symptoms are somatosensory, which characteristically involve the hand and lower face (cheirooral). Less frequently, the symptoms include aphasia, hemiparesis, or clumsiness of the limb. A slow, marchlike progression is characteristic, further distinguishing migraine from stroke.

EPIDEMIOLOGY

A review of mostly uncontrolled hospital-based studies conducted before 1989 of patients under the age of 50 years with a diagnosis of stroke showed that the strokes were attributed to migraine 1% to 17% of the time; in two thirds of these patients, stroke was attributed to migraine 1% to 8% of the time; in one third, stroke was attributed to migraine 11% to 17% of the time (3). A compilation of studies up to the same time showed that of 448 total stroke cases, 4% were attributed to migraine, and 31% had an unknown cause. In clinical studies, stroke is reported as more common in patients with migraine with aura (10,137) and in patients with posterior cerebral artery (PCA) strokes (13). No differences in stroke risk factors were found in migraine sufferers compared with controls without stroke, although those with migraine were more likely to have recurrent stroke, supporting the notion that migraine is an independent stroke risk factor (137). Another study of migraine with aura showed that 91% of patients who had stroke during a migraine attack had no arterial lesions; in contrast, lesions were absent in only 9% of patients with migraine with aura who suffered stroke remote from a migraine attack and in 18% of patients with stroke without a migraine history (11). In some instances, however, stroke risk factors increased stroke risk in migraine with aura.

The overall incidence of "migraine infarction" has been estimated at 3.36 per 100,000 population per year [95% confidence interval (CI) 0.87–4.8], but in the absence of other stroke risk factors becomes 1.44 per

K.M.A. Welch: Department of Neurology, University of Kansas School of Medicine, University of Kansas Medical Center, Kansas City, Kansas 66106.

M.-G. Bousser: Department of Neurology, Lariboisiére Medical Faculty, Paris VII University, and Department of Neurology, Hôpital Lariboisière, 75475 Paris, France.

100,000 population per year (95% CI 0.00–0.07) (82). This rate is similar to that reported later in subjects under 50 (13); migrainous infarction accounted for 25% of cerebral infarcts. To place these data in context, the overall incidence of ischemic stroke under age 50 ranges from 6.5 per 100,000 (98) to 22.8 per 100,000 (94,103).

Epidemiologic studies that have addressed an association between migraine and stroke have been scarce. In a retrospective study of parents of migraine sufferers, no increased risk of stroke was found, but the frequency of hypertension was 1.7 times greater in persons with migraine than in those without (99). In an inconclusive study, the Collaborative Group for the Study of Stroke in Young Women found that the relative risk of thrombotic stroke was twofold higher for women with migraine compared with neighborhood centers but not with hospital controls (72). A hospital-based controlled study of 89 cases found that ischemic stroke was increased more than twofold in patients with migraine with aura (81), but when stroke risk factors were excluded in this group, there was no longer a statistically significant association.

A systematic examination in a large-scale prospective epidemiologic study of men and women showed that, after controlling for established risk factors for stroke, both migraine and severe nonspecific headache were associated with a significantly increased risk for stroke (111). The risk for stroke associated with migraine decreased as the age at stroke increased. In a case-controlled study, there was no overall association between migraine and ischemic stroke, but among women less than 45 years of age, migraine and stroke were significantly associated; there was approximately a fourfold increased risk, more so in women who smoked (148). When this study was extended to a larger population, the results were confirmed and strengthened (25). The risk of stroke among women under 45 years of age was three times that of controls for those with migraine without aura and six times the risk of controls for women with migraine with aura. Furthermore, young women with migraine who smoked increased their stroke risk to approximately 10 times that of controls, more than three times greater than that of young women without migraine who smoked. For young women with migraine on oral contraceptives, the risk of stroke was 14 times that of controls; for those on estrogen, the risk of stroke was four times that of controls (the odds ratio was 4.8 for women taking doses of 50 μg of estrogen, 2.7 for 30–40 μg, 1.7 both for 20 μg and 1 μg for progesterone). In none of these cases was the stroke induced by the migraine attack.

In a more recent published case-controlled study of 308 patients with either transient ischemic attacks or stroke, a history of migraine was more common among these women than among controls (14.9% versus 9.1%) (25). Migraine was the only significant risk factor (odds ratio 3.7) in women under 35 years of age. Although these risk figures appear startlingly high in both studies, the absolute

risk of stroke for this patient population translates to around 19 per 100,000 per year, which is a low rate.

Most recently, a hospital-based case-control study involving five European centers studied 291 women 20 to 44 years of age with ischemic, hemorrhagic, or unclassified arterial stroke compared with 736 age- and hospital-matched controls (27). Adjusted odds ratios associated with a personal history of migraine were 1.78 (95% CI 1.14–2.77), 3.54 (95% CI 1.30–9.61), and 1.10 (95% CI 0.63–1.94) for all strokes, ischemic strokes, and hemorrhagic strokes, respectively. Odds ratios for ischemic stroke were similar to those for migraine with aura (3.81; 95% CI 1.26–11.5) and migraine without aura (2.97; 95% CI 0.66–13.5). A family history of migraine, irrespective of personal history also was associated with increased odds ratios, not only for ischemic stroke, but also for hemorrhagic stroke. Use of oral contraceptives or a history of high blood pressure or smoking had greater than multiplicative effects on the odds ratios for ischemic stroke associated with migraine alone, although only smoking was statistically significant. A change in the frequency or type of migraine associated with oral contraceptive use did not predict subsequent stroke. Between 20% and 40% of strokes may have been induced by a migraine attack.

This study should be interpreted with particular caution on the basis of the methods, working criteria for the classification, and questionnaire used. Concerns are raised by the higher numbers of migraine with as compared to without aura, and the difficulty in diagnosing migraine by questionnaire in family members. Also clinical experience would not support the high incidence of true migraine-induced stroke.

In summation, based especially on case-controlled studies, an association between migraine and stroke appears confirmed. Common risk factors for stroke in general increase this risk. Only one study suggested that a family history of migraine provides increased risk for stroke, independent of those at risk who also had migraine.

PAST CONCEPTS

In 1881, Fere (51), working with Charcot at the Salpetrière Hospital, provided one of the earliest comprehensive descriptions of the problem. He reviewed 12 patients suffering from classic migraine who also experienced language and sensorimotor symptoms. Fere later reported Charcot's fatal case of a 53-year-old man with classic migraine since adolescence who developed permanent aphasia and right faciobranchial paralysis, offering an explanation (52) of vasospasm as the cause. Charcot again emphasized this notion of cerebral ischemia as a result of vasospasm in his discussion of a case of ophthalmoplegic migraine (28).

Among the fatal cases of migrainous cerebral infarction that have been studied at autopsy, characteristic pathologic changes have not been consistently identified (115).

Buckle et al. reported the case of a 16-year-old in whom an angiogram just prior to death showed widespread narrowing (18). Other clinical pathologic studies extended the concept of vasospasm (87,119,122). These reports offered the possibility that repeated attacks of severe migraine presumably accompanied by vasospasm lead to focal arterial injury, whether an endarteritis or intimal proliferation and media myonecrosis, comparable with that observed as a result of spasm induced by subarachnoid hemorrhage (33,50,85). These arterial changes, in turn, presumably predispose the patient to thrombosis or distal embolization. An autopsy of one patient with familial hemiplegic migraine (FHM) was exceptional for its demonstration of small deep infarcts, a distinctly uncommon site of migrainous cerebral infarction, indicating that lenticulostriate arteropathy may be one mechanism, a hypothesis favored by Bruyn (15–17). The clinical-pathologic features of the patients with migraine reported by Guest and Wolf (73) and Polyak (128) are more compatible with cerebral embolism. The hypothesis of local vascular alterations in the course of a migraine attack, particularly the vasodilatory phase (145), contributed to the concept of arterial dissection as a cause of migrainous stroke.

Scattered clinical studies with accompanying laboratory investigations were reported prior to the 1950s, describing serious neurologic consequences of migraine, usually permanent visual field defects (21,76,87,123, 133,135,143,154) prior to the 1990s. Not only was thrombosis related to vasoconstriction considered a sequela of migraine, but so was intracerebral and subarachnoid hemorrhage (2,9,23,39,44,67,126). In 1962, Connor (32) reported on a series of 18 complicated migraine cases, observing a predilection for occipital cortex involvement. The largest series of cases was reported in 1965 by Pearce and Foster (124). Only two vascular malformations were detected among 29 angiograms performed, but these cases had unusual features, including seizures and loss of consciousness. This established the rarity of vascular anomalies in patients with persisting deficits, suggesting that such sequelae are likely due to infarction.

CLINICAL INVESTIGATION

Clinical reports in the past 50 years have provided more convincing evidence for an association between migraine and cerebral infarction, especially those cases documented using angiography, computed tomography (CT) scanning, positron emission tomography (PET), and, most recently, magnetic resonance imaging (MRI). There is little to support any of the possible mechanisms raised by older studies.

Angiography

Kaul et al. (93) reported angiographic findings of four patients with migraine. One had an occlusion of the main trunk of the PCA, presenting with right hemianopia, hemianesthesia, spontaneous pain, transient amnesia, and dysphasia. All four of these patients had branch occlusions of the calcarine artery. Each patient suffered from transient visual disturbances, and the deficits occurred during a severe migraine. Vasospasm attributed to migraine has been documented by arteriography, the first in 1964 by Dukes and Vieth (43). A 44-year-old man suffered from left hemianopia with numbness of the left side of the body, followed by a throbbing right hemicranial headache. The patient underwent arteriography. A first and second set of films demonstrated increasingly poor filling of the intracranial internal carotid system at a time when focal deficit was maximal. During the headache phase, good intracranial filling of the internal carotid was observed. Other cases reported in subsequent years confirm arterial occlusion (65,104).

CT Scanning

The use of CT scanning beginning in the mid-1970s permitted documentation of lesions compatible with cerebral infarction in many cases (4,20,22,37,86,105). In each instance, CT showed a low-density lesion in the cortex, most commonly in the occipital lobe. Review of CT series of selected migrainous patients with or without local focal neurologic deficits showed that the prevalence of abnormalities ranged from 34% to 71%. Cala and Mastaglia (22) reported on 94 patients with a history of "recurrent migrainous headaches," of whom 6 showed evidence of cerebral infarction. Four had fixed visual field defects with mesial occipital low densities. Cerebral edema, particularly in the periventricular white matter, was evident in another six patients. Baker (4) described diffuse low-density zones during a migraine attack, which disappeared on subsequent CT examination. Hungerford et al. (86) studied 53 patients who had "exceptionally severe" migraine or serious clinical complications including hemiplegia. The most frequently encountered abnormalities were cerebral atrophy (30%) and infarction (10%). Similar findings were reported by Mathew and co-workers (105). Rascol and colleagues (130,131) reported CT-confirmed cerebral infarction occurring in the course of a migrainous attack. These researchers required that three conditions be fulfilled before making a diagnosis of complicated migraine or migrainous cerebral infarction:

1. Previous history of migraine attacks conforming to the Ad Hoc Committee's definition.
2. Close chronologic relationship between the migraine attack and the persisting neurologic disorder.
3. Other vascular diseases or predisposing disorders must be excluded.

Ten patients had syndromes referable to the middle cerebral artery, whereas the remaining four had hemianopic defects due to PCA territory infarctions. Arteriography, performed in each patient 2 days to 6 months after stroke onset, gave an abnormal result in nine, showing internal carotid artery occlusion in one, middle or posterior cerebral artery stem occlusion in four, and branch occlusions in the remaining four patients.

Magnetic Resonance Imaging

The diagnosis of migraine-induced stroke, both infarction and neuronal necrosis, has been greatly enhanced by the use of MRI. The greatest value of MRI, however, is in the differential diagnosis of stroke due to migraine from other causes in cases that present as migraine mimics. From the research viewpoint, great interest stemmed from observations of increased white matter lesions in approximately 30% of routinely studied migraine patients compared with healthy controls (12%) (88). Lesions were found in the centrum semiovale and frontal white matter, in some cases extending to deeper structures in the region of the basal ganglia. In some series such findings were more prevalent in migraine subtypes associated with neurologic aura (49). Not all case series found a greater incidence than controls, however (34). Another series found a higher incidence of white matter lesions in patients with migraine, as well as in patients with tension-type headache (41). The mechanisms of these changes remain to be determined. If relevant, they may represent small foci of ischemic infarction of obscure origin, or gliosis.

HEADACHE OF VASCULAR DISEASE

Head pain occurs in various forms of acute cerebrovascular disease, including ischemic stroke. Study of the headache syndromes due to ischemic cerebrovascular disease showed that most patients complained of the symptom at the onset of a persisting neurologic deficit, although in some cases headache was premonitory or accompanied transient ischemic attacks (54,56,57), findings also noted by others (46,70,108,118,153). The headache was usually not throbbing, was often localized, and was frequently lateralized ipsilateral to the presumed arterial occlusion. There was a high frequency of headache in PCA territory infarctions compared with that seen in carotid or basilar disease. Headache was the exception in lacunar strokes with pure motor or pure sensory syndromes, and none occurred in any of 58 patients with transient monocular blindness. Overall, the frequency of headache was 31% in carotid and 42% in vertebrobasilar disease. Headache frequency is higher in ischemia affecting posterior compared with anterior circulations (112). Mitsias and Ramadan have extensively reviewed the literature on this topic up to 1997 (112).

The possible mechanisms of headache due to thromboembolism remain to be determined. Prevailing views include dilatation of collaterals, focal distension of the artery, local ischemia of the arterial muscle, and irritation of the pain-sensitive arterial wall by atheroma (113,153). Serotonin and other vasoactive peptides released from the junctional elements of the trigeminovascular system also may play a role (118). Mitsias and Ramadan reviewed contemporary concepts of the mechanisms of pain in cerebrovascular disorders (113).

CLINICAL SUBTYPES OF MIGRAINE-RELATED STROKE

One drawback in understanding the dilemma that faces the diagnostician has been a lack of consistency in the definition of migraine-related stroke. Three major issues must be considered. Stroke occurs in the course of the migraine attack, causing true migraine-induced cerebral infarction. Migraine may cause stroke because other risk factors for stroke are present to interact with the migraine-induced pathogenesis. Stroke may present as a migraine syndrome, either symptomatic migraine or as a migraine mimic. The International Headache Society (IHS) classification (79) and new techniques of brain imaging have served to clarify the association between migraine and stroke.

Coexisting Stroke and Migraine

Definition: A clearly defined clinical stroke syndrome must occur remotely in time from a typical attack of migraine.

Stroke in the young is rare and migraine is common. Clearly, the two conditions can coexist without migraine being a contributive factor to stroke. When the two conditions coexist in the young, the true pathogenesis of stroke may be difficult to elucidate. A comorbidity of stroke risk in migraine sufferers seems apparent from the case-controlled series reviewed above, where none of the strokes were induced by the migraine attack (148). This increases the clinical significance of coincident stroke and should serve to raise clinical consciousness to the need for stroke risk factor awareness in all migraine sufferers.

Stroke with Clinical Features of Migraine

Definition: A structural lesion unrelated to migraine pathogenesis that presents with clinical features typical of migraine.

Symptomatic Migraine

Established structural lesions of the central nervous system or cerebral vessels episodically cause symptoms typical of migraine with neurologic aura. Such cases should be termed "symptomatic migraine." Cerebral arteriovenous malformations frequently masquerade as migraine with aura. Migraine attacks associated with cerebral autosomal dominant arteriopathy with subcortical infarcts and leukoencephalopathy (CADASIL) also may be symptomatic of the membrane dysfunction associated with this disorder.

Migraine Mimic

In this category, stroke due to acute and progressing structural disease is accompanied by headache and a constellation of progressive neurologic signs and symptoms indistinguishable from those of migraine. This might best be termed a "migraine mimic." The diagnostic discrimination of a migraine mimic can be most difficult to define in patients with established migraine. Many of the cases described in the above section of the conceptual evolution of migraine-related stroke were likely migraine mimics, the diagnosis being hampered by limitation in investigative tools and uncertainty in the knowledge of migraine pathogenesis.

The issue of spontaneous carotid artery dissection is especially relevant because patients with migraine are at increased risk of dissection (38), and the occurrence of dissection as a typical migraine mimic has been reported (129). Although the mechanism of pain production is not clearly understood, the occurrence of headache is an expected finding, present in 60% of patients (77) and probably more prevalent in vertebral dissection. When accompanied by ischemic complications, dissection may mimic migraine, for example, basilar migraine. Fisher (61) analyzed 21 selected cases of angiographically documented cervical carotid dissection, observing that almost all patients (19 of 21) had ipsilateral pain in one or more regions of the head, including the forehead, orbit, temple, retroorbit, side of the head, and the frontal region. In addition, 12 patients had neck pain, usually in the upper neck and localized to a region including the mastoid, upper carotid, behind or below the angle of the jaw, and along the sternocleidomastoid muscle. The pain was usually severe, often sudden in onset, described equally as steady or throbbing, and occasionally by alterations in ipsilateral scalp sensation. The duration ranged from several hours to 2 years, with most lasting no longer than 3 to 4 weeks. About three fourths of Fisher's patients experienced ischemic complications, and in half the headache preceded the ischemic attack by a few hours to 4 days. Other common diagnostic findings were Horner syndrome, subjective bruit, dysgeusia, and visual scintillations. Given this clinical picture, it is difficult to avoid considering the possibility that cases formerly diagnosed as carotidynia (132), paratrigeminal syndrome (59), or migraine cluster with miosis of transient focal deficits (50,95) may have been instances of carotid dissection. The topic of dissection and migraine has been reviewed elsewhere (114).

Migraine-Induced Stroke

Definition

Migrainous cerebral infarction (IHS 1.6.2) is described in the IHS classification as follows: one or more migrainous aura symptoms not fully reversible within 7 days and/or associated with neuroimaging confirmation of ischemic infarction: (a) patient has previously fulfilled criteria for migraine with neurologic aura; (b) the present attack is typical of previous attacks, but neurologic deficits are not completely reversible within 7 days and/or neuroimaging demonstrates ischemic infarction in the relevant area; (c) other causes of infarction must be ruled out by appropriate investigations.

According to this definition, migraine-induced stroke must meet the following criteria:

1. The neurologic deficit must exactly mimic the migrainous symptoms of previous attacks.
2. Stroke must occur during the course of a typical migraine attack.
3. All other causes of stroke must be excluded. Stroke risk factors often must be taken into account.

Another problem is that the IHS classification does not permit the diagnosis of migraine-induced stroke in patients with migraine without aura (see definition). Migraine without aura may begin in "silent" brain areas and may have the same pathogenesis as migraine with aura. There is clearly a need for rigorous analysis of patients with migraine-related stroke without aura and more pathophysiologic information on the latter to refine the IHS classification of this subtype.

True Migraine-Induced Stroke without Stroke Risk Factors

The following satisfies the preceding criteria without identifiable stroke risk.

A 34-year-old woman had suffered a complex of twice yearly episodes of right homonymous hemianopia, right cheirooral numbness, and confusion followed by left hemicranial head pain typical of migraine with aura. In one episode, the neurologic deficit persisted throughout and after the headache. Examination revealed a right homoymous hemianopia, and hemiparesis with Babinski's sign were noted. Only the right hemianesthesia persisted 6 weeks later. An electroencephalogram revealed slow activity in the left occipital and posterior temporal regions. Cerebral blood flow was in the oligemic range in the temporooccipital and parietooccipital cortex. MRI revealed a left thalamic infarct. Cerebral angiography showed fusiform dilatation of the left PCA with narrowing of arterial caliber proximal and distal to the dilatation. No penetrating branches of the PCA were visualized. Repeated angiography 6 weeks later was normal. No stroke risk factors could be elicited.

The arterial lesion in this case clearly involved the PCA and its branches, although the precise arterial pathologic location was not known. No unequivocal radiographic evidence of dissection, fibromuscular disease, or premature atherosclerosis was present, and the subsequent radiographic appearance of the artery was normal. Similar arteriographic findings have been reported, for example, migraine with an in situ thrombus positioned in the fusiform dilatation (2). The impaired filling of small penetrating branches supports the notion of intravascular thrombus formation. Any large thrombus, if present, might have undergone dissolution by the time of arteriography 48 hours after the event. The transient left-sided neurologic deficit could be explained by compressive edema, occlusion of the top of the basilar penetrating branch, or diaschisis. Study of this case and others like it has produced insight into the pathogenesis of both migraine and the process leading to stroke.

True Migraine-Induced Stroke with Stroke Risk Factors

Most reviews that address criteria for true migrainous stroke do not include the modifying statement of risk factors in the definition. This subclassification may be important to understanding mechanisms. For example, oral contraceptives are recognized to increase stroke risk in migraine sufferers and may cause coexisting stroke and migraine. In some instances, however, stroke occurs during the migraine attack, and the medication may have increased the risk of coagulopathy but may not have induced stroke in the absence of the migrainous process. The following intriguing question arises: does migraine cause stroke only because risk factors, as yet unknown, are present to interact with the pathophysiologic mechanisms of the migraine attack? Oral contraceptive use may not only exacerbate preexisting migraine (42,127,157), but also may contribute to the stroke risk in young women with migraine (27). The Collaborative Study Group in Young Women used a case-control method to evaluate the risk of cerebrovascular disease in users of oral contraceptives (31) and later reported the effect of other risk factors, including hypertension, smoking, and migraine. The risk of cerebral thrombosis among women using oral contraceptives was 9.5 times greater than among nonusers. The role of migraine was assessed in both users and nonusers of contraceptives. Among migraineurs not exposed to birth control pills, the risk of stroke was equivocal, depending on the control group used for the comparison. The use of oral contraceptives in combination with migraine, however, increased the relative risk for thrombotic stroke from 2.0 to 5.9. More recent studies reviewed in the epidemiologic section extend the risk to 13 or greater times that of subjects not on oral contraceptives (27,148). Of particular interest in relation to the interactive role of migraine is the pathologic finding of intimal hyperplasia associated with thrombosis in three fatal cases of stroke in young women exposed to oral contraceptives (117).

Uncertain Classification

Complex or Multiple Factors

Many migraine-related strokes cannot be categorized with certainty. The following case provides examples of all the above subtypes.

A 27-year-old woman presented with stuttering, onset of left hemiparesis and left homonymous hemianopia not accompanied by headaches. She had an established history of migraine with visual aura. Three years previously she sustained the sudden onset of left-sided weakness 15 minutes after taking a second, 2-mg dose of ergotamine 30 to 60 minutes into a typical migraine headache. Opercular branches of the middle cerebral artery were occluded on angiography, and the CT scan showed a right frontal infarct. She was using oral contraceptives and smoked 20 cigarettes daily for 20 years. Investigation at the time also revealed false-positive results from a VDRL test and positive test results for rheumatoid factor. Investigation of the most recent stroke revealed positive anticardiolipin antibody test results with high immunoglobulin G titers.

Drug-Induced Migraine-Related Stroke

It is often impossible to confidently exclude an interaction of the drug with migrainous process to induce stroke. The mechanism of action of 5-hydroxytryptamine 1D (5-HT_{1D}) agonists such as ergotamine or sumatriptan may be neurogenic or vasoconstrictive. Recorded cases have been associated with excessive dosage of these drugs, presumably causing vasospasm (12), although in therapeutic doses ergotamine usually has no effect on cerebral blood flow (48,74). Scattered reports have appeared, linking ergotamine use to focal disturbances in the opthalmic and cerebral circulations, manifested by transient monocular blindness, bilateral papillitis, and sensorimotor deficits (14,36,109,134,138). Since the introduction of sumatriptan there have also been scattered reports of strokelike events, but like ergotamine, so far none have been convincing of primary involvement of the drug or can exclude its use in an event that mimics migraine.

Angiography

The precipitation of migrainelike signs and symptoms during cerebral angiography is not uncommon and can potentially progress to stroke, although not all observers agree (139). Angiography performed during migraine carries risk because of potential interaction with the migraine mechanism. Nevertheless, because arteriography can be complicated by stroke in all patients, the true pathogenesis of stroke cannot be attributed with certainty to migraine.

Transient Focal Neurologic Events and Late-Onset Migraine Accompaniments

Headache is not an invariable occurrence in migraine. Adding to the potential for diagnostic confusion is the occurrence of migraine attacks consisting of visual disturbances or focal deficits not accompanied by typical headache, often termed "migraine sine hemicrania." Charcot (28) identified an incomplete form of opthalmic migraine as "migraines opthalmiques frustes" consisting only of "les troubles oculaires." More controversial has been the entity of accompanied migraine without headache, originally described by Whitty (156). Fisher (58,60) emphasized that the migrainous syndrome, despite the absence of headache, could be diagnosed on the basis of characteristic clinical features. Since then, painless transient and persistent migraine accompaniments have become more widely recognized. The cause of late-onset migraine accompaniments has not been established (58). As the name of the syndrome suggests, the clinical features are essentially indistinguishable from migraine without headache. Brain imaging and cerebral arteriography do not reveal accountable structural lesions.

Transient focal neurologic events have recently been extensively analyzed by Teijen et al. (144). Many of these events have features of migraine with aura, especially visual features. The study by Tzourio and his group reviewed in the Epidemiology section found an association with such events and an increased risk for stroke (148). These studies emphasize the wisdom of thorough evaluation for stroke risk of patients suffering from such symptoms.

Encephalopathy

There are rare reports of migrainelike syndromes associated with other manifestations of neurologic disease that are of uncertain pathogenesis and that make the subtyping of these curiosities impossible. Cases involving migrainelike symptoms and persistent neurologic deficit associated with high cerebrospinal fluid (CSF) protein values and pleocytosis are to be found in the literature, and are reviewed in Chapter 36. Cerebral vasculitis or focal encephalitis were proposed as possible causes. Cases of well-documented migraine with aura will show evidence of similar CSF abnormality. Other rare syndromes associated with migraine-related stroke include migraine associated with mitochondrial encephalopathies (45) and "migraine coma" (62).

Hemorrhage

Cases of intracerebral hemorrhage attributable to migraine have been reported only rarely and have been reviewed elsewhere (24). In our view, investigations have failed to establish true migraine-induced hemorrhage, most cases likely being symptomatic migraine or migraine mimics. From the viewpoint of pathogenesis, however, it is not unreasonable that ischemic softening of tissue during true migraine-induced cerebral infarction might become hemorrhagic, so dogmatism must be avoided. Experience with this entity in the context of the current IHS classification is awaited.

Retinal or Ocular Migraine

This group of disorders is designated as uncertain in classification because of limited information, most clinical case reports or series having been communicated prior to the development of contemporary advanced neurologic investigatory techniques. Although transient homonymous scintillations or fortification scotoma are well-recognized cortical migrainous phenomena, monocular visual loss due to retinal involvement is less often a manifestation of migraine (35), although still a differential diagnostic point in the patient presenting with amaurosis fugax (66). Because both retinal and ciliary circulations may be affected, the term "ocular migraine" is preferred (35) and should be distinguished from the term "opthalmic migraine," which refers to any migrainous disturbance of vision, whether ocular or cortical. To include instances of optic nerve dysfunction that may occur as well, Troost (147) has suggested the broader term "anterior visual pathway migraine."

Retinal migraine is an uncommon disorder (26,75), usually occurring in a young adult who experiences recurrent and unaccompanied episodes of visual loss or dimness in one or both eyes almost never exceeding 10 minutes in duration, but rarely persisting for 1 hour or more. Usually there is no preceding fortification spectra or headache, and normal visual function invariably returns, although with repeated attacks a permanent visual defect may develop. Although typical attacks of classic or common migraine occasionally occur at other times, the visual disturbance without headache may be the predominant or sole manifestation of the migrainous disorder migraine sine hemicrania. As a cautionary note, although migrainous transient monocular blindness may occur for the first time late in life, carotid atherosclerosis is the more likely cause (1,55,80).

The pathophysiology of transient monocular visual loss occurring in the setting of migraine is poorly understood (149). Some researchers have interpreted the retinal venous narrowing seen in some cases as venous spasm, although collapse secondary to reduced arterial flow is an alternative explanation (10,147,159). Other reports of funduscopic examination during an attack have confirmed the observation of arteriolar spasm (55,71,136,149,150,158), despite one negative report of five patients, most having binocular visual symptoms (91).

Of the cases in the literature prior to the new IHS classification in 1988, defects in vision included central or centrocecal scotomas, altitudinal defects, monocular constriction, and complete blindness. The mean age of patients was 37 years, with four times as many women as men. The presence of a family history of migraine was variable. The mean duration of migraine was 13 years, with diverse migraine subtypes, the most frequent being classic migraine (11 cases), followed by retinal migraine unaccompanied by headache (10 cases). Other headache types included retinal migraine with headache (3 cases), retinal and classic migraine (1 case), and cluster headache (1 case). The visual loss almost always occurred abruptly, usually in the setting of a headache that appeared as often being or following the onset of the visual disturbance. In a few cases local eye pain was a prominent symptom. A variety of funduscopic abnormalities were reported, as reviewed below. In the four instances where carotid angiography was performed, no abnormalities were evident. Only a small number of cases were fully investigated to exclude alternative causes of abrupt visual loss, although most cases appeared to fulfill the requirements of a prior history of migraine and abrupt visual loss occurring in the context of a migrainous headache.

Many of the cases cited here were reported before modern diagnostic techniques were available, particularly to pursue an embolic etiology, and before the recognition of prothrombotic disorders such as antiphospholipid antibody syndromes that often affect the eye. These are probably the causes most likely to confound a diagnosis of permanent visual loss resulting from retinal migraine. Transient or permanent monocular visual obscurations of migrainous origin, even when accompanied by specific funduscopic abnormalities, are not clinically distinguishable from amaurosis fugax or retinal infarction due to embolism (35,47,68,78).

Central retinal artery occlusion has been reported in association with migraine attacks (32,37,47,78,117). A number of examples of branch retinal arterial occlusions also have been reported (40,64,69,71,125,151). Central retinal vein occlusion has been less frequently encountered (63,69,102). Ischemic optic neuropathy is a rare complication of migraine (107,152). Cases present with abrupt visual loss in the form of a central scotoma or arcuate defect occurring during the course of a typical headache. The mechanisms remain to be determined. Ischemic susceptibility of the prelaminar portion of the optic nerve is a reflection of its watershed position between the retinal and choroidal systems (78,100).

Migraine that Mimics Stroke

Hemiplegic Migraine

Living (101), in 1973, first described transient hemiparesis associated with a migraine attack. In 1910, Clark (29) published the first report of hemiplegic migraine occurring in a family. Whitty (155) classified the disorder into hemiplegic migraine with a family history of migraine with or without aura and familial hemiplegic migraine, in which attacks occur with stereotypic features in family members, often with severe and long-lasting hemiparesis or other persistent aura symptoms, and an autosomal-dominant inheritance pattern. Heyck's monograph in 1956 (83), Bradshaw and Parson's clinical study (12), and Bruyn's review (15) are milestone clinical references. Hemiplegic migraine also has been described in children (19,84,89), including FHM (29).

The IHS (79) classifies hemiplegic migraine under migraine with typical aura (IHS 1.2.1) or prolonged aura (IHS 1.2.2). FHM is classified as a subgroup of migraine with aura (IHS 1.2.3). The working definition includes the criteria for migraine with aura (1.2.1, 1.2.2) with hemiplegic features that may be prolonged and at least one first-degree relative with identical attacks. As noted above, the overall prevalence of migraine with aura is around 4%; this figure includes hemiplegic migraine. There is no specific information associated with a migraine attack.

Hemiplegic migraine attacks are characterized by hemiparesis or hemiplegia (15,31,83). The arm and leg are involved in the majority of attacks, often combined with face and hand paresis. Less frequently, isolated facial and arm paresis occurs. The progression of motor deficit is slow, with a spreading or marching quality. In most cases, symptoms are accompanied by homolateral sensory disturbance, particularly cheirooral in distribution, again with a slowly spreading or marching quality. Infrequently, the hemiparesis may alternate from side to side, even during an attack. Myoclonic jerks have been reported but are rare. They have been described as jacksonian, although there is some resemblance to the limb jerking associated with carotid or basilar artery ischemia. Visual disturbance, which takes the form of hemianopic loss or typical visual aura, is common. Homolateral or contralateral localization of the visual disturbance is often obscure. When dysphasia occurs, it is more often expressive than receptive. The neurologic symptoms last 30 to 60 minutes and are followed by severe pulsating headache, hemicranial or whole head in distribution. Nausea, vomiting, photophobia, and phonophobia are associated features. In severe cases, the aura can persist throughout the headache phase.

Manifestations of severe hemiplegic migraine attacks include fever, drowsiness, confusion, and coma, all of which can be prolonged from days to weeks (116). Severe hemiplegic migraine may lead rarely to persistent minor neurologic deficits; the cumulative effect of repeated attacks progresses to profound multifocal neurologic deficits, even dementia (142).

Familial hemiplegic migraine is characterized by the neurologic deficit described above that is identical in at least one other first-degree relative (79). The disorder has an autosomal-dominant inheritance pattern. Other neurologic deficits have been described in association with FHM. Most frequent is a syndrome of progressive cerebellar disturbance dysarthria, nystagmus, and ataxia (30,120). Retinitis pigmentosa, sensory neural deafness, tremor, dizziness, and oculomotor disturbances with nystagmus also have been described (160,161). These neurologic deficits are present between attacks and are not part of the aura. Hemiplegic migraine attacks also may be part of other familial disorders affecting other systems, for example, MELAS and CADASIL. Attacks of hemiplegic migraine are less likely to be stereotyped in family members with these conditions because the migraine attacks are probably symptomatic of the underlying brain disorder.

A breakthrough in establishing the cause of FHM was achieved during the clinical investigation of a disease condition termed CADASIL (6,146). This is characterized by recurring small deep infarcts, dementia, and leukoencephalopathy. Some patients also experience recurrent attacks of severe migrainelike headache with aura symptoms that include transient headache and hemiparesis. Joutel and colleagues (92) studied two large family pedigrees satisfying the IHS criteria for FHM, one with cerebellar signs and the other without. Linkage analysis was performed with a set of DNA markers spanning the most probable location for CADASIL, which was mapped recently to chromosome 19. FHM did indeed map to chromosome 19, the most likely location for the gene being a 30-cM interval between *D19S216* and *D19S215,* which encompasses the probable position of the history of stroke and dementia, younger age of onset, only rarely a history of stroke and dementia, no white matter abnormalities on MRI, and a good prognosis. Most recently, Ophoff and colleagues (121) isolated, on chromosome 19p13.1, a gene encoding the alpha-1 subunit of a brain-specific voltage-gated P/Q type neuronal calcium channel (*CACNL1A4*) from patients with FHM.

Four different missense mutations were identified in five unrelated FHM families. The investigators also detected premature stops mutations predicted to disrupt the reading frame of *CACNL1A4* in two unrelated patients with episodic ataxia type-2 (EA-2). Thus FHM and EA-2 can be considered as allelic channelopathies but of differing molecular mechanism, the former involving a gain of function variant of the Ca^{2+} channel subunit and the latter a decrease in channel density. The results also indicate that different mutations in a single gene may cause phenotypic heterogeneity.

Since this report the same French group identified 10 different missense mutations in the Notch 3 genes of 14 unrelated families with CADASIL. The Notch genes are intimately involved in intercellular signaling during development. Proteins belonging to the Notch family are transmembrane receptors. Nine of the 10 mutations either added or mutated a cysteine residue in one of the epidermal growth factor (EGF)-like repeats; EGF-like motifs are to be found in the extracellular domain. It is likely that this mutation strongly affects protein conformation, although how this leads to CADASIL remains to be established. Membrane instability and abnormality of cell signaling could be the underlying basis of the migraine attacks in this disorder. The generalizability of the genetic findings in FHM, one of the rarest subtypes of migraine, to the more prevalent migraine subtypes remains to be established. It must be noted that cases of nonfamilial hemiplegic migraine studied by Ophoff et al. (121) failed to show mutations. Also, the same group has suggested that chromosome 19 is the focus for migraine with and without aura (106), but review of other studies suggests that this may be controversial (110). Furthermore, the distribution of the abnormal calcium channel identified is densely cerebellar (140), a structure not obviously involved in the initiation of a migraine attack. This is nevertheless a point of interest, in view of the occurrence of cerebellar atrophy in a small number of FHM families (120). It is tempting to speculate that cerebellar atrophy might be explained by abnormal release of excitatory amino acids such as glutamate, which has cytotoxic consequences.

Basilar Migraine

The concept of BAM was first proposed by Bickerstaff (7,8) (IHS 1.2.4). The diagnostic criteria include those for migraine with aura plus two or more aura symptoms of the following types:

1. Visual symptoms in both the temporal and nasal fields of both eyes
2. Dysarthria
3. Vertigo
4. Tinnitus
5. Decreased hearing
6. Double vision
7. Ataxia
8. Bilateral paresthesias
9. Bilateral paresis
10. Decreased level of consciousness

Bickerstaff noticed 34 patients whose attacks were usually headed by visual disturbances: either complete visual loss or positive phenomena such as teichopsia so dazzling as to obscure the entire field of vision. Other basilar symptoms followed, including dizziness or vertigo, gait ataxia, dysarthria, tinnitus, bilateral acral, perioral, and lingual numbness, or paresthesias. These symptoms persisted for 2 to 60 minutes, ending abruptly, although the visual loss generally recovered more gradually. After the premonitory phase subsided, a severe throbbing occipital headache supervened and was accompanied by vomiting. The patients recovered completely, and between such attacks many had episodes of classic migraine.

Typically affected were adolescent girls. Attacks were usually infrequent and strongly related to menstruation. In Bickerstaff's series, all but two patients were under 23 years of age and 26 of 34 were girls. A clear-cut family history of migraine in close relatives was obtained in 82% of cases. Lapkin et al. (96) encountered this entity in a younger population, reporting on a group of 30 children with a mean age at onset of 7 years (range 7 months to 14 years). The duration of episodes ranged from minutes to many hours; one patient was symptomatic for nearly 3 days. Unlike the adolescent cases, the most common complaint was vertigo (73%), whereas visual disturbances occurred in 43% of cases. In children more severely affected, pyramidal tract dysfunction was observed, as were cranial nerve abnormalities, including internuclear ophthalmoplegia and facial nerve paresis. A family history of migraine was obtained in 86% patients. During the follow-up period of 6 months to 3 years, none of the patients showed signs of progressive neurologic dysfunction, although one child was mentioned as having developed a permanent oculomotor nerve paralysis. In the majority of cases, the aura lasts between 5 and 60 minutes but can extend up to 3 days. Visual symptoms commonly occur first, predominantly in the temporal and nasal fields of vision. The visual disturbance may consist of blurred vision, teichopsia, scintillating scotoma, graying of vision, or total loss of vision. The features may start in one visual field and then spread to become bilateral. Bickerstaff pointed out that when vision is not completely obscured, diplopia may occur, usually as a sixth nerve weakness. Some form of diplopia may occur in up to 16% of cases (141). Vertigo and gait ataxia are the next most common symptoms, each occurring in 63% of one series (141). Ataxia can occur independent of vertigo. Tinnitus may accompany vertigo. Dysarthria is as common as ataxia and vertigo. Tingling and numbness, in a typical cheirooral spreading pattern seen in migraine with aura, occurs in over 60% of cases. This is usually bilateral and symmetric but may alternate sides with a hemidistribution. Occasionally dysesthesias extend to the truck. Bilateral motor weakness occurs in more than 50% of cases.

The syndrome of BAM was later expanded to include alteration in consciousness. Bickerstaff cited four cases in detail and recorded a total of 8 among 32 patients with previously diagnosed BAM. The onset of impaired consciousness occurred in the context of other basilar symptoms with a leisurely onset, not causing the patient to fall or incur self-injury, and was sometimes preceded by a dreamlike state. Ranging from drowsiness to stupor, the altered consciousness was akinetic and usually brief, lasting up to several minutes and not accompanied by rigidity, posturing, tongue biting, urinary incontinence, or changes in the respiratory pattern. Like the usual BAM, a throbbing headache occurred on recovery. Laboratory investigations were generally unrevealing, with normal CSF and electroencephalographic (EEG) results. Although impairment of consciousness in some form is common (141), rarely does this progress to stupor or prolonged coma (53,97). Other forms of altered consciousness include amnesia and syncope.

Headache occurs in almost all patients. It has an occipital location in the majority of patients and a throbbing, pounding quality, and is accompanied by severe nausea and vomiting. It is unusual for the headache to be unilateral or localized to the more anterior parts of the cranium. Photophobia and phonophobia occur in one third to one half of patients. As with other forms of migraine, the symptoms may occur without headache, but this usually occurs in no more than 4% of cases (141).

Seizures have been observed in association with basilar migraine (5). Changes in EEG unaccompanied by seizures also have been described with attacks of typical BAM. In all, EEG abnormalities are detected in fewer than one fifth of patients with basilar migraine (90) and are mostly independent of any clinical manifestation of the disorder. The EEG findings between attacks are usually spike-and-wave or spike-and-slow wave complexes. During an attack, there are diffuse high-voltage slow waves and associated spikes with sharp waves and diffuse beta activity. There is controversy as to whether the association between seizures and basilar migraine are primarily migraine syndromes with secondary epileptic features resulting from functional or ischemic change caused by repeated migraine auras or whether these cases are primarily basilar migraine that evokes epileptogenic features on the EEG and clinical seizures.

Permanent brainstem deficits occurring as a result of BAM have been reported only rarely. None of Bickerstaff's patients had persisting neurologic disturbances; indeed, he stressed return to complete normality as a criterion for the diagnosis. Among the cases of migraine-associated stroke uncovered in the literature, only four of the five have occurred in the vertebrobasilar territory, excluding the PCA. In Connor's presentation (32) of 18 patients with complicated migraine, three were considered to have lesions in the brainstem. In no instance did the transient episodes clearly resemble BAM as defined above.

Cerebrovascular disease is the most serious differential diagnosis of basilar migraine. Ischemic stroke in the brainstem and the posterior cortical regions, either due to cerebral embolism or thrombosis, presents with a constellation of neurologic symptoms and signs of brainstem and posterior circulation defects accompanied in approximately one third of cases by headache. Basilar artery occlusive disease can therefore mimic basilar migraine. Another basilar migraine mimic for which migraine patients are at increased risk is vertebral artery dissection.

The clinical features of embolic and thrombotic infarction in the PCA syndrome have been elegantly described by Fisher (60). The warning features of PCA ischemia include photopsia with single and formed visual hallucinations, hemianopic visual loss, transient numbness, episodic light-headedness, confusional spells, tinnitus, and headache. When stroke becomes established, however, visual complaints are the most dominant. Of importance in the differential diagnosis of basilar migraine, scintillations or shimmering brightness in the visual fields did not occur during transient ischemia but did occur after occipital lobe infarction was established. Thus, PCA ischemia alone can mimic basilar migraine.

Transient ischemic attacks involving any part of the vertebrobasilar territory must figure largely in the differential diagnosis, particularly if basilar migraine presents for the first time in the later years of life. Certain familial disorders present with neurologic deficit in which attacks of hemiplegic or basilar migraine may be part of the symptom complex. This group includes CADASIL, MELAS, and variants of MELAS that are associated with seizures, particularly those occipital in origin (45).

Mechanisms of Migraine-Induced Stroke

It remains to be determined how a migraine attack can induce permanent neurologic deficit and brain damage. Perhaps even more intriguing, what constitutes the comorbid increased risk for stroke between attacks? The latter is the most difficult question because although comorbid factors may be present (such as increased platelet aggregation or mitral valve prolapse), many are uncertain risk factors for stroke. Indeed, when definite risk factors for stroke are present in migraine sufferers, then stroke is attributed to this cause and not to migraine. On the basis of the epidemiologic data described, however, there must be stroke risk factors yet to be identified that are comorbid with migraine. With regard to the mechanisms whereby stroke is induced during a migraine attack, there is information that provides some limited understanding. Spreading cortical depression (SCD) of Leao may induce short-lived increases in cerebrospinal blood flow (CBF) followed by a more profound oligemia. Ischemic foci, however, may occasionally occur during attacks of migraine with aura. SCD may be associated with depolarization of intrinsic neurons that also supply intraparenchymal resistance microvessels, leading to constriction and a consequent flow reduction below the threshold for K^+ release from the neuron. Increased extracellular K^+ then might precipitate depolarization of contiguous cortical neurons. Alternatively, the decreased

extracellular space and brain swelling that accompanies spreading cortical depression and possibly migraine could increase microvascular resistance by mechanical compression. Thus, low flow in major intracerebral vessels may be due to increased downstream resistance, not major intracranial arterial vasospasm. Essentially, a low cerebral blood flow and sluggish flow in large intracerebral vessels during the aura of migraine when combined with factors predisposing to coagulopathy could lead, although rarely, to intravascular thrombosis and, thus, migraine-induced cerebral infarction. Release of vasoactive peptides, endothelin, activation of cytokines, and upregulation of adhesion molecules during the neurogenically mediated inflammatory response that may be responsible for headache also may induce intravascular thrombosis. This could explain why migraine-induced stroke usually respects intracranial arterial territories, although the aura involves more widespread brain regions. In addition, frequent aura, if due to spreading depression, could induce cytotoxic cell damage and gliosis based on glutamate release or excess intracellular calcium accumulation. Persistent neurologic deficit could in this way be due to selective neuronal necrosis without evidence of ischemic infarction. Why stroke occurs during episodes of migraine aura probably relates to variability in the coagulation status, degree of neuronal and hemodynamic changes, and interaction of each during the course of the migraine attack.

REFERENCES

1. Adams HP, Putnam SF, Corbett JJ, et al. Amaurosis fugax: the results of arteriography in 59 patients. *Stroke* 1983;5:742.
2. Adie WJ. Permanent hemianopia in migraine and subarachnoid hemorrhage. *Lancet* 1930;2:237.
3. Alvarez J, Matias-Guiu J, Sumalla J, et al. Ischemic stroke in young adults 1. Analysis of the etiological subgroups. *Acta Neurol Scand* 1989;80:28–34.
4. Baker HL. Computerized transaxial tomography (EMI scan) in the diagnosis of cerebral vascular disease. Experience at the Mayo Clinic. In: Whisnant JP, ed. *Cerebral vascular diseases. Ninth Conference.* Orlando, FL: Grune & Stratton, 1975:195.
5. Basser LS. The relation of migraine and epilepsy. *Brain* 1969;92:285–300.
6. Baudrimont M, Dubas F, Joutel A, et al. Autosomal dominant leukoencephalopathy and subcortical ischemic stroke: a clinicopathological study. *Stroke* 1993;24:122–125.
7. Bickerstaff ER. Basilar artery migraine. *Lancet* 1961:15–17.
8. Bickerstaff ER. The basilar artery and migraine-epilepsy syndrome. *Proc R Soc Med* 1962;55:167–169
9. Blend R, Bull JWD. The radiological investigation of migraine. In: Smith, ed. *Background to migraine. First Migraine Symposium.* London: Heinemann, 1967:1.
10. Bougousslavsky J, Regli F. Ischemic stroke in adults younger than 30 years of age. Cause and prognosis. *Arch Neurol* 1987;44:479–482.
11. Bougousslavsky J, Regli F, Van Melle G, et al. Migraine stroke. *Neurology* 1988;38:223–227.
12. Bradshaw P, Parsons M. Hemiplegic migraine: a clinical study. *Q J Med* 1965;34:65–85.
13. Broderick JP, Swanson JW. Migraine-related strokes: clinical profile and prognosis in 20 patients. *Arch Neurol* 1987;44:868–871.
14. Brohult J, Forsberg O, Hellstrom R. Multiple arterial thrombosis after oral contraceptives and ergotamine. *Acta Med Scand* 1967;181:453.
15. Bruyn GW. Complicated migraine. In: Vinken PJ, Bruyn GW, eds.

Handbook of clinical neurology, vol 5. Amsterdam: North Holland Publishing, 1968:59.

16. Bruyn GW. Cerebral cortex and migraine. *Adv Neurol* 1982;33:151.
17. Bruyn GW, Weenink HR. Migraine accompagnée. A critical evaluation. *Headache* 1966;6:1.
18. Buckle RM, Du Boulay G, Smith B. Death due to vasospasm. *J Neurol Neurosurg Psychiatry* 1964;27:440.
19. Burke EC, Peters GA. Migraine in childhood: a preliminary report. *Am J Dis Child* 1956;92:330–336.
20. Burns RJ, Blumbergs PC, Sage MR. Brain infarction in young men. *Clin Exp Neurol* 1979;16:69.
21. Butler TH. Scotoma in migrainous subjects. *Br J Ophthalmol* 1933; 17:83.
22. Cala LA, Mastaglia FL. Computerized axial tomography findings in patients with migrainous headaches. *BMJ* 1976;2:149.
23. Caldwell A, Kennedy R. Migraine headaches with preheadache retinal and visual disturbances in a case of congenital vascular anomaly and subarachnoid hemorrhage. *Arch Neurol Psychiatry* 1953;61:397.
24. Caplan L. Intracerebral hemorrhage revisited. *Neurology* 1988;38: 624–627.
25. Carolei A, Marini C, De Matteis G. History of migraine and risk of cerebral ischemia in young adults. *Lancet* 1996;347:1503–1506.
26. Carroll D. Retinal migraine. *Headache* 1970;10:9.
27. Chang CL, Donaghy M, Poulter N: Migraine and stroke in young women: case control study. *BMJ* 1999;318:13–18
28. Charcot JM. Sur un cas de migraine ophtalmologique (paralysie oculomotrice periodique). *Prog Med* 1890;18:83.
29. Clarke JM. On recurrent motor paralysis in migraine, with a report in which recurrent hemiplegia accompanied the attacks. *BMJ* 1910;2:1534.
30. Codina A, Acarini PN, Miguel F. Migraine hemiplegique associée à un nystagmus. *Rev Neurol* 1971;124:526–530.
31. Collaborative Group for the Study of Stroke in Young Women. Oral contraception and increased risk of cerebral ischemia or thrombosis. *N Engl J Med* 1973;288:871.
32. Connor RCR. Complicated migraine. A study of permanent neurological and visual defects caused by migraine. *Lancet* 1962;2:1072.
33. Conway LW, McDonald LW. Structural changes of the intradural arteries following subarachnoid hemorrhage. *J Neurosurg* 1972;37:715.
34. Cooney BS, Grossman RI, Farber RE, et al. Frequency of magnetic resonance imaging abnormalities in patients with migraine. *Headache* 1996;36:616–621.
35. Corbett JJ. Neuro-ophthalmic complications of migraine and cluster headaches. *Neurol Clin* 1983;1:973.
36. Cowan CL, Knox DL. Migraine optic neuropathy. *Ann Ophthalmol* 1982;14:164.
37. Cromwell GF, Carlin L, Biller J. Neurologic complications of migraine. *Am Fam Physician* 1982;26:139.
38. D'Anglejan Chatillon J, Ribeiro V, Mas JL, Youl BD, Bousser MG. Migraine—a risk factor for dissection of cervical arteries. *Headache* 1989;29:560–561.
39. Dassen R. Jacqueca oftalmoplejica con paralisis recidivante del III par craneano: muerte en el segundo ataque: necropsia. *Semana Med* 1931; 1:1049.
40. Davis-Jones A, Gregory MC, Whitty CWM. Permanent sequelae in the migraine attack. In: Cummings JN, ed. *Background to migraine, 5th Symposium.* New York: Springer-Verlag, 1972:25.
41. De Benedittis G, Lorenzetti A, Sina C, et al. Magnetic resonance imaging in migraine and tension-type headache. *Headache* 1995;35:264–268.
42. Desrossiers JJ. Headaches related to contraceptive therapy and their control. *Headache* 1973;13:117.
43. Dukes HT, Vieth RG. Cerebral arteriography during migraine prodrome and headache. *Neurology* 1964;14:636.
44. Dunning HS. Intracranial and extracranial vascular accidents in migraine. *Arch Neurol Psychiatry* 1942;48:392.
45. Dvorkin GS, Andermann F, Carpenter S, et al. Classical migraine, intractable epilepsy, and multiple strokes: a syndrome related to mitochondrial encephalomyopathy. In: Andermann F, Lugaresi E, eds. *Migraine and epilepsy.* Stoneham, MA: Butterworth, 1987:203–232.
46. Edmeads J. The headaches of ischemic cerebrovascular disease. *Headache* 1979;19:127.
47. Edmeads J. Complicated migraine and headache in cerebrovascular disease. *Neurol Clin* 1983;1:385.
48. Edmeads JG, Hachinski VC, Norris JW. Ergotamine and the cerebral circulation. *Hemicrania* 1976;7:6.

49. Fazekas F, Koch M, Schmidt R, et al. The prevalence of cerebral damage varies with migraine type: a MRI study. *Headache* 1992;32:287–291.
50. Fein JM, Flor WJ, Cohan SL, Parkhurst J. Sequential changes of vascular unltastructure in experimental cerebral vasospasm. *J Neurosurg* 1974;41:49.
51. Fere C. Contribution a l'étude de la migraine ophthalmique. *Rev Med Paris* 1881;1:40.
52. Fere C. Note sur un cas de migraine ophthalmique à access répétés suivis de mort. *Rev Med Paris* 1883;3:194.
53. Ferguson KS, Robinson SS. Life-threatening migraine. *Arch Neurol* 1982;39:374–376.
54. Fisher CM. Occlusion of the internal carotid artery. *Arch Neurol Psychiatry* 1957;65:346.
55. Fisher CM. Observations of the fundus oculi transient monocular blindness. *Neurology* 1951;65:346–377.
56. Fisher CM. Clinical syndromes in cerebral arterial occlusion. In: Fields WS, ed. *Pathogenesis and treatment of cerebrovascular disease.* Springfield, IL: Charles C Thomas, 1961:126.
57. Fisher CM. Headache in cerebrovascular disease. In: Vinken PJ, Bruyn GW, eds. *Handbook of clinical neurology,* vol 5. Amsterdam: North-Holland, 1968:124.
58. Fisher CM. Migraine accompaniments versus arteriosclerotic ischemia. *Trans Am Neurol Assoc* 1968;93:211.
59. Fisher CM. Reader's benign paratrigeminal syndrome with dysgeusia. *Trans Am Neurol Assoc* 1972;96:234.
60. Fisher CM. Late-life migraine accompaniments as a cause of unexplained transient ischemic attacks. *Can J Med Sci* 1980;7:9.
61. Fisher CM. The headache and pain of spontaneous carotid dissection. *Headache* 1982;22:60.
62. Fitzsimons R, Wolfenden WH. Migraine coma: meningetic migraine with cerebral edema associated with a new form of autosomal dominant cerebellar ataxia. *Brain* 1985;108:555–577.
63. Friedman MW. Occlusion of the central retinal vein in migraine. *Arch Ophthalmol* 1951;45:678.
64. Galezowski X. Ophthalmic megrim. *Lancet* 1882;1:176.
65. Garnic JD, Schellinger D. Arterial spasm as a finding intimately associated with onset of vascular headache. *Neuroradiology* 1983;24:273.
66. Glaser JS. *Neuro-ophthalmology,* vol 2. New York: Harper & Row, 1978.
67. Goldflamm S. Beitrag zur Aetiologie und Symptomatologie der spontanen subarachnoidealen Blutungen. *Disch Z Neervenheilk* 1923;76:158.
68. Goodwin JA, Gorelick P, Helgason C. Transient monocular visual loss: amaurosis fugax or migraine, abstracted. *Neurology* 34[Suppl 1]:246.
69. Graveson GS. Retinal arterial occlusion in migraine. *BMJ* 1949;2:838.
70. Grindal A, Toole J. Headache and transient ischemic attacks. *Stroke* 1975;5:603.
71. Gronvall H. On changes in the fundus oculi and persisting injuries to the eye in migraine. *Acta Ophthalmol* 1938;16[Suppl 14–16]:602.
72. Group for the Study of Stroke in Young Women. Oral contraceptives and stroke in young women. *JAMA* 1975;231:718–722.
73. Guest IA, Wolf AL. Fatal infarction of the brain. *BMJ* 1964;1:225.
74. Hachinski VC, Norris JW, Cooper PW, Edmeads JG. Ergotamine tartrate and cerebral blood flow. *Can J Neurol Sci* 1975;2:333.
75. Hachinski VC, Porchawka J, Steele JC. Visual symptoms in the migraine syndrome. *Neurology* 1973;23:570.
76. Harrington DO. Ophthalmoplegic migraine. A discussion of its pathogenesis: report of the pathological findings in a case of recurrent oculomotor palsy. *Arch Ophthalmol* 1953;49:643.
77. Hart RG, Easton JD. Dissection of cervical and cerebral arteries. *Neurol Clin* 1983;1:155.
78. Hayreh SS. Pathogenesis of visual field defects: role of ciliary circulation. *Br J Ophthalmol* 1970;54:289.
79. Headache Classification Committee of the International Headache Society. Classification and diagnostic criteria for headache disorders, cranial neuralgias, and facial pain. *Cephalagia* 1988;8:27.
80. Hedges TR. An ophthalmologist's view of headache. *Headache* 1979;19:151.
81. Henrich JB, Horowitz RI. A controlled study of ischemic stroke risk in migraine patients. *J Clin Epidemiol* 1989;42:773–780.
82. Henrich JB, Sandercock PAG, Warlow CP, Jones LN. Stroke and migraine in the Oxfordshire Community Stroke Project. *J Neurol* 1986;233:257–262.
83. Heyck H. Neue Beitrage zur Klinik und Pathogenese der Migraine. Stuttgart: G Thieme Verlag, 1956.
84. Holguin J, Fenichel G. Migraine. *J Pediatr* 1967;70:290–297.

85. Hughes JT, Schianchi M. Cerebral artery spasm. A histological study at necropsy of the blood vessels in cases of subarachnoid hemorrhage. *J Neurosurg* 1978;48:515.

86. Hungerford GD, Du Boulay GH, Zilkha KJ. Computerized axial tomography in patients with severe migraine: a preliminary report. *J Neurol Neurosurg Psychiatry* 1976;39:990.

87. Hunt JR. A contribution to the paralytic and other persistent sequelae of migraine. *Am J Med Sci* 1915;150:313.

88. Igarashi H, Sakai F, Kan S, et al. Magnetic resonance imaging of the brain in patients with migraine. *Cephalalgia* 1991;11:69–74.

89. Isler W. Acute hemiplegia and hemisyndromes in childhood. In: *Clinics in development medicine.* London: Heinemann, 1971:41–42.

90. Jacome DE. EEG features in basilar artery migraine. *Headache* 1987;27:80–83.

91. Joffe SN. Retinal blood vessel diameter during migraine. *Eye Ear Nose Throat Mnthly* 1973;52:338.

92. Joutel A, Bousser M-G, Biousse V, et al. A gene for familial hemiplegic migraine maps to chromosome 19. *Nat Genet* 1993;5:40–45.

93. Kaul SN, Du Boulay GH, Kendall BE, Russel WR. Relationship between visual field defect and arterial occlusion in the posterior cerebral circulation. *J Neurol Neurosurg Psychiatry* 1974;37:1022.

94. Kittner SJ, McCarer RJ, Sherwin RW, et al. Black-white differences, in stroke risk among young adults. *Stroke* 1993;24[Suppl 1]:113–115.

95. Kline LB, Lindsley KC. Ocular migraine in a patient with cluster headaches. *Headache* 1980;20:253.

96. Lapkin ML, French JH, Golden GS. The EEG in childhood basilar artery migraine. *Neurology* 1977;27:580–583.

97. Lawall JS, Oommen JK. Basilar artery migraine presenting as conversion hysteria. *J Nerv Ment Dis* 1978;166:809–811.

98. Leno C, Berciano J, Combarros O, et al. A prospective study of stroke in young adults in Cantabria, Spain. *Stroke* 1993;24:792–795.

99. Leviton A, Malvea B, Graham JR. Vascular disease, morality, and migraine in the parents of migraine patients. *Neurology* 1975;24:669–672.

100. Lieberman MF, Maumenee AE, Green RW. Histologic studies of the vasculature of the anterior optic nerve. *Am J Ophthalmol* 1968;82:405.

101. Liveing E. *On megrim, sick headache, and some allied disorders: a contribution to the pathology of nerve storms.* London: J & A Churchill, 1873.

102. Lohlein W. Erblindung durch Migrane. *Dtsch Med Wochenschr* 1922;48:1408.

103. Marini C, Carolei A, Roberts RS, et al. Focal cerebral ischemia in young adults: a collaborative case-control study. *Neuroepidemiology* 1993;12:70–81.

104. Masuzawa T, Shinoda S, Furuse M, et al. Cerebral angiographic changes on serial examination of a patient with migraine. *Neuroradiology* 1983;24:277.

105. Mathew NT. Complicated migraine and differential diagnosis of migraine. In: Mathew RJ, ed. *Treatment of migraine. Pharmacological and biofeedback considerations.* New York: Spectrum, 1981:9.

106. May A, Ophoff RA, Terwindt GM, et al. Familial hemiplegic migraine locus on 19p13 is involved in the common forms of migraine with and without aura. *Hum Genet* 1995;96:604–608.

107. McDonald WI, Sanders MD. Migraine complicated by ischemic papillopathy. *Lancet* 1971;1:521.

108. Medina J, Diamond S, Rubino S. Headaches in patients with transient ischemic attacks. *Headache* 1975;15:194.

109. Merhoff GC, Porter JM. Ergot intoxication: historical review and description. *Ann Surg* 1974;180:773.

110. Merikangas KR. Genetics of migraine and other headache. *Curr Opin Neurol* 1996;9:202–205.

111. Merikangas KR, Fenton BT, Cheng SH, et al. Association between migraine and stroke in a large-scale epidemiological study of the United States. *Arch Neurol* 1997;54:362–368

112. Mitsias P, Ramadan NM. Headache in ischemic cerebrovascular disease. Part I: Clinical features. *Cephalalgia* 1992;12:269–274.

113. Mitsias P, Ramadan NM. Headache in ischemic cerebrovascular disease. Part II: Mechanisms and predictive value. *Cephalalgia* 1992;12:341–344.

114. Mokri B. Spontaneous dissections of cervicocephalic arteries. In: Welch KMA, Caplan LR, Peis DJ, et al., eds. *Primer on cerebrovascular disease.* San Diego, CA: Academic, 1997:390–396.

115. Morenas L, Dechaume J. Migraine aphasique et monoplegique. Etude anatomo-clinique. Les rapports de las migraine avec l' epilepsie. *J Med Lyon* 1929;10:259.

116. Munte TJ, Muller-Vahl H. Familial migraine coma: a case study. *J Neurol* 1990;237:59–61.

117. Murphy JP. Cerebral infarction in migraine. *Neurology* 1955;5:359.

118. Nappi G, Bono G. Headaches and transient cerebral ischemia: comments on Welch's report. *Adv Neurol* 1982;33:41.

119. Neligan P, Harriman DGF, Pearce J. Respiratory arrest in familial hemiplegic migraine: a clinical and neuropathological study. *BMJ* 1977;2:732.

120. Ohta M, Araki S, Kuroiwa Y. Familial occurrence of migraine with a hemiplegic syndrome and cerebeller manifestations. *Neurology* 1967;17:813–817.

121. Ophoff RA, Terwindt GM, Vergouwe MN, et al. Familial hemiplegic migraine and episodic ataxia type-2 are caused by mutations in the Ca^{+2} channel gene CACNL1A4. *Cell* 1996;87:543–552.

122. Oppenheim H. Casuistischer Beitrag zur Prognose der Hemikranie. *Charite-Annalen* 1890;15:298.

123. Ormond AW. Two cases of permanent hemianopsia following severe attacks of migraine. *Ophthalmol Rev* 1913;32:192.

124. Pearce JMS, Foster JB. An investigation of complicated migraine. *Neurology* 1965;15:323.

125. Pessin MS, Duncan GW, Mohr JP, Poskanzer DC. Clinical and angiographic features of carotid transient ischemic attacks. *N Engl J Med* 1977;296:358.

126. Peters R. Todliche gehirnblutung bei menstrueller migraine. *Beitr Pathol* 1934;93:209.

127. Phillips BM. Oral contraceptives and migraine. *BMJ* 1968;2:99.

128. Polyak S. *The vertebrate visual system.* Chicago: University of Chicago Press, 1957.

129. Ramadan NM, Tiejen GE, Levine SR, Welch KMA. Scintillating scotoma associated with internal carotid artery dissection. *Neurology* 1991;41:1084–1087.

130. Rascol A, Cambier J, Guiraud B, et al. Accidents ischemiques cerebraux ax cours de crises migraineuses. A propos des migraines compliquees. *Rev Neurol (Paris)* 1979;135:867.

131. Rascol A, Clanet M, Rascol O. Cerebrovascular accidents complicating migraine attacks. In: Rose FC, Amory WK, eds. *Cerebral hypoxia in the pathogenesis of migraine.* London: Pitman Books, 1982:110.

132. Raskin NE, Prusiner S. Carotidynia. *Neurology* 1977;27:43.

133. Rich WM. Permanent quadrantanopsia after migraine. *BMJ* 1948;116:592.

134. Richter AM, Banker VP. Carotid ergotism. *Radiology* 1973;106:339.

135. Robinson BE. Permanent homonymous migrainous scotomata. *Arch Ophthalmol* 1955;53:566.

136. Rosenstein AM. Beitrag ZU den beiderseitigen Verdunkelungen des Sehvermogens mit vorübergehenden ophthalmoskopischen Befund dei Herzklappenfehler. *Klin Monatsbl Augenheilkd* 1925;75:357.

137. Rothrock J, North J, Madden K, et al. Migraine and migrainous stroke; risk factors and prognosis. *Neurology* 1993;43:2473–2476.

138. Senter HJ, Lieberman AN, Pinto R. Cerebral manifestations of ergotism. Report of a case and review of the literature. *Stroke* 1976;7:88.

139. Shuaib A, Hachinski VC. Migraine and the risks from angiography. *Arch Neurol* 1988;45:911–912.

140. Starr TVB, Prystay W, Snutch TP. Primary structure of a calcium channel that is highly expressed in the rat cerebellum. *Proc Natl Acad Sci U S A* 1991;88:5623–5625.

141. Sturzenegger MH, Meienberg O. Basilar artery migraine: a follow-up study of 82 cases. *Headache* 1985;25:408–415.

142. Symonds C. Migrainous variants. *Trans Med Soc Lond* 1952;67:237.

143. Thomas JJ. Migraine and hemianopsia. *J Nerv Ment Dis* 1907;34:153.

144. Tietjen GE, Levine SR, Brown E, et al. Factors that predict antiphospholipid immunoreactivity in young people with transient focal neurological events. *Arch Neurol* 1993;50:833–836.

145. Torda C, Wolff HG. Experimental studies on headache: transient thickening of walls of cranial arteries in relation to certain phenomena of migraine headache and action of ergotamine tartrate on thickened walls. *Arch Neurol Psychiatry* 1945;53:329.

146. Tournier-Lasserve E, Iba-Zizen MT, Romero N, Bousser MG. Autosomal dominant syndrome with stroke-like episodes and leukoencephalopathy. *Stroke* 1991;22:1297–1302.

147. Troost BT: Migraine. In: Glaser JS, ed. *Neuro-ophthalmology,* vol 2. New York: Harper & Row, 1978.

148. Tzourio C, Tehindrazanarivelo A, Iglesias S, et al. Case-control study of migraine and risk of ischaemic stroke in young women. *BMJ* 1995;310:830–833.
149. Walsh WB, Hoyt WF. *Clinical neuro-ophthalmology,* vol 2. Baltimore: Williams & Wilkins, 1969.
150. Weber LW, Runge W. Storungen und Verandewnger des Sehappartas bei Pychosen und Neurosen. In: Schieck R, Bruckner A, eds. *Kurzes Handbuch der Ophthalmologie,* vol 6. Berlin: Julius Springer, 1931:800.
151. Wegner W. Augenspiegelbefunde bei Migrane. *Klin Monatsbl Augenheilkd* 1926;76:194.
152. Weinstein JM, Feman SS. Ischemic optic neuropathy in migraine. *Arch Ophthalmol* 1982;100:1097.
153. Wells C. Premonitory symptoms in cerebral embolism. *Arch Neurol* 1961;5:490.
154. Wener A. A case of permanent homonymous hemianopia following an attack of migraine. *Med Rec* 1921;99:849.
155. Whitty CWM. Familial hemiplegic migraine. *J Neurol Neurosurg Psychiatry* 1953;16:172.
156. Whitty CWM. Migraine without headache. *Lancet* 1967;2:283.
157. Whitty CWM, Hockaday JM, Whitty MM. The effect of oral contraceptives in migraine. *Lancet* 1967;2:283.
158. Wilbrand H, Saenger A. *Neurologic des auges,* vol 3. Munich: JF Bergmann, 1906.
159. Wolter JR, Burchfield WJ. Ocular migraine in a young man resulting in unilateral transient blindness and retinal edema. *J Pediatr Ophthalmol* 1971;8:173.
160. Young GF, Leon-Barth CA, Green J. Familial hemiplegic migraine, retinal degeneration, deafness, and nystagmus. *Arch Neurol* 1970;23:201–109.
161. Zifkin B, Andermann F, Kirkham T. An autosomal dominant syndrome and hemiplegic migraine, nystagmus, and tremor. *Ann Neurol* 1980;8:329–332.

The Headaches, Second Edition,
edited by J. Olesen, P. Tfelt-Hansen, and K.M.A. Welch.
Lippincott Williams & Wilkins, Philadelphia © 2000.

Tension-Type Headache, Cluster Headache,
and Miscellaneous Primary Headaches

CHAPTER 68

Tension-Type Headache: Introduction

Jes Olesen

Tension-type headache is so prevalent that one could say, with some truth, that it is more normal to have it than not to have it (5). Can tension-type headache then be called a disease? Instinctively, the answer is no, but some conditions that we do not hesitate to regard as abnormal are even more prevalent. Caries of the teeth is one example, the common cold another. Tension-type headache is perhaps more comparable to other prevalent pain disorders, such as low back pain, or to emotional disturbances, such as anxiety. These disorders are extremely prevalent in their milder or infrequent forms; however, they also occur in frequent or severe forms and then constitute major health problems. The high prevalence of tension-type headache and the relation of the milder forms to psychosocial and behavioral disturbances have biased our view of the more severe and frequent forms. The latter cause a great deal of suffering, adversely affect the functional capacity of the individual, and seem to be largely unaffected by psychosocial factors. There are no readily available laboratory parameters or other test results that are abnormal in those suffering from tension-type headache. The disease definition therefore relies exclusively on the symptoms, which, however, are not so distinct as in migraine. The classification of tension-type headache according to the International Headache Society (IHS) (1) is given in Table 1.

RELATIONSHIP BETWEEN EPISODIC AND CHRONIC TENSION-TYPE HEADACHE

Although the classification divides tension-type headache into a number of subforms, all these subforms

really are believed to be varieties of the same disorder. The symptoms of the individual attack in episodic and chronic tension-type headache is largely the same (6), although the general clinical picture varies significantly (3). The chronic and the episodic forms are formally distinguished by a different frequency of days with headache. The reason for this subdivision was originally purely practical: Patients with chronic tension-type headache constitute a large group seen in headache clinics and in specialist practice, whereas patients with episodic tension-type headache are not seen by specialists and rarely consult their general practitioner. The chronic form requires prophylactic treatment, is difficult to treat, and often is associated with the development of drug overuse. A number of other special management problems are common in the chronic group. Adding to these practical reasons for a subdivision is now a growing number of studies showing important pathophysiologic and genetic–epidemiologic differences (see Chapters 71 and 73).

The symptomatology of tension-type headache is not distinct: simply pain in the head without associated symptoms. Many different disturbances can cause pain in the head, fulfilling the criteria for tension-type headache. Therefore, the etiology of tension-type headache is often thought to be mixed. Similar ideas about migraine recently were revealed to be less likely by the fact that the great majority of migraineurs respond to highly specific serotonin 5-HT$_1$ receptor agonists. This finding suggests that migraine mechanisms are rather homogeneous (see Chapter 52). It cannot be excluded that most patients with tension-type headache may respond similarly to a future specific pharmacotherapy because they share pathophysiological mechanisms.

J. Olesen: Department of Neurology, Glostrup Hospital, University of Copenhagen, DK-2600 Glostrup, Copenhagen, Denmark.

TABLE 1. *Classification of tension-type headache*

2.1 Episodic tension-type headache
    2.1.1 Episodic tension-type headache associated with disorder or pericranial muscles
    2.1.2 Episodic tension-type headache unassociated with disorder of pericranial muscles
2.2 Chronic tension-type headache
    2.2.1 Chronic tension-type headache associated with disorder of pericranial muscles
    2.2.2 Chronic tension-type headache unassociated with disorder of pericranial muscles
2.3 Headache of the tension type not fulfilling above criteria

From ref. 1, with permission.

SUBDIVISION OF TENSION-TYPE HEADACHE TO THE THIRD AND FOURTH DIGITS

The International Headache Classification Committee decided to subdivide tension-type headache into a form with and a form without disorder of the pericranial muscles. This was done in the absence of any actual evidence indicating that such a subdivision was accurate or indeed natural. The committee simply hoped that introduction of this subdivision would prompt scientists to study the impact of pericranial muscle tenderness in a more systematic way, and this has also happened (2). The old dispute about muscular and central factors in the pathogenesis of tension-type headache is not yet settled, but parts of the puzzle now can be clearly seen, as discussed in subsequent chapters of this book.

The IHS classification finally subdivides tension-type headache to the fourth digit (Table 2). In listing these causative factors, the committee again realized that it classified ahead of solid scientific evidence in many instances. The subclassification, therefore, was a call for good scientific studies to elucidate the importance of the disorders listed under each individual digit. Unfortunately, only few studies have specifically examined these issues, but subsequent chapters in this book

discuss a wealth of data pertaining to the subclassification in a more indirect fashion.

FOCUS ON TENSION-TYPE HEADACHE

Despite the high prevalence of tension-type headache and its enormous socioeconomic impact (4), research into the mechanisms of this disorder has been limited. Worldwide, only a few students have been trained scientifically to deal with this disorder. The condition remains low on the priority list of public and private foundations that support medical sciences. The enormous amount of money earned by pharmaceutical companies, which legally advertise their over-the-counter compounds for tension-type headache, has not stimulated such companies to support research. Despite problems, significant progress has been made in the understanding of the mechanisms of tension-type headache as described in relevant chapters in this book. Progress has been made by a few pioneering groups but just now seems to be appreciated by a wider circle of clinical and basic scientists. Furthermore, the research-oriented pharmaceutical companies, which so successfully have developed new treatments for migraine, now seem to also extend their interest to tension-type headache. While waiting for further insight into the basic mechanisms of tension-type headache and for new and more effective treatments, patients must still be managed as well as possible. Fortunately, slim scientific knowledge does not make it impossible to manage patients with success. The sum of knowledge available to doctors resulting from accumulated experience is often much greater than that which can be found in scientific studies. Building on the opinion of a number of experts, for a time, can be a useful substitute for p values. As it is, doctors dedicated to headache treatment can help most patients with tension-type headache. Chronic tension-type headache, however, remains one of the largest indications for which a specific pharmacotherapy is not yet available.

TABLE 2. *Subdivision of tension-type headache according to the most likely causative factor(s)*

0	No identifiable causative factor
1	More than one of the factors 2–9
2	Oromandibular dysfunction
3	Psychosocial stress
4	Anxiety
5	Depression
6	Headache as a delusion or an idea (psychogenic headache)
7	Muscular stress
8	Drug overuse for tension-type headache
9	One of the disorders causing secondary headaches (groups 5–11 in the classification)

From ref. 1, with permission.

REFERENCES

1. Headache Classification Committee of the International Headache Society. Classification and diagnostic criteria for headache disorders, cranial neuralgias and facial pain. *Cephalalgia* 1988;8(Suppl 7):1–96.
2. Jensen R, Rasmussen BK. Muscular disorders in tension-type headache. *Cephalalgia* 1996;16:97–103.
3. Langemark M, Olesen J, Loldrup D, Bech P. Clinical characterization of patients with chronic tension headache. *Headache* 1988;28:590–596.
4. Rasmussen BK, Jensen R, Olesen J. Impact of headache on sickness absence and utilization of medical services. A Danish population study. *J Epidemiol Community Health* 1992;46:443–446.
5. Rasmussen BK, Jensen R, Schroll M, Olesen J. Epidemiology of headache in a general population a prevalence study. *J Clin Epidemiol* 1991;44:1147–1157.
6. Rasmussen BK, Jensen R, Schroll M, Olesen J. Interrelations between migraine and tension-type headache in the general population. *Arch Neurol* 1992;914–918.

The Headaches, Second Edition,
edited by J. Olesen, P. Tfelt-Hansen, and K.M.A. Welch.
Lippincott Williams & Wilkins, Philadelphia © 2000.

Tension-Type Headache, Cluster Headache,
and Miscellaneous Primary Headaches

CHAPTER 69

Epidemiology of Tension-Type Headache

Birthe Krogh Rasmussen and Richard B. Lipton

Despite the fact that tension-type headache is by far the most common form of headache, its epidemiology has received relatively little attention, probably because these headaches are viewed as mild and of almost trivial impact. We view tension-type headache as an important disorder because it afflicts so many people and afflicts 2% to 3% of the general population on a daily or almost daily basis (15,21,44,51). Epidemiologic studies of tension-type headache provide estimates of the morbidity in the community and provide policy makers and clinicians with data on the scope, distribution, and treatment needs for this condition.

Until recently, tension-type headache was an ill-defined syndrome. The terms *muscle contraction headache, tension headache, psychogenic headache, psychomyogenic headache, stress headache, essential headache,* and *non-migrainous headache* had been used interchangeably without operational definitions. The classification of the International Headache Society (IHS)(19) provided operational diagnostic criteria for three major subtypes: *episodic* tension-type headache, *chronic* tension-type headache, and *tension-type–like* headache (see Chapter 68). The introduction of these criteria has facilitated epidemiological studies in the general population.

PREVALENCE AND FREQUENCY OF TENSION-TYPE HEADACHE

In surveys of the general population in North America and Western Europe, the 1-year prevalence of tension-type headache ranges from about 30% to about 80% (Table 1). Differences in definitions and methodology may be largely responsible for this variation. Few prevalence studies from other parts of the world have been conducted. In a study from Jerusalem covering Jewish immigrants, the prevalence of nonmigrainous headaches was 65% in men and 66% in women (1). A prevalence study of headache among Nigerian university students showed a prevalence of muscle-contraction headache of 42% (34). A study of an urban population in Zimbabwe reported a prevalence at 10%, but subjects with infrequent attacks were not included (28). Tension-type headache has been estimated to affect 2% of the people in Hong Kong (63). An American study reports a race effect with reduced prevalence in blacks relative to whites (51). Lower rates in Asian and African populations may reflect differences in genetic or environmental risk factors or cultural differences in reporting and behavior regarding pain.

Tension-type headache varies widely in both frequency and severity among individuals, from rare, short-lasting episodes with mild discomfort to frequent, long-lasting, or even continuously disabling headaches. Pooling these extremes in an overall prevalence may be somewhat misleading. When interpreting prevalence data, it is therefore important also to consider disability, severity, and frequency of the disorder. Few studies, however, have dealt with these aspects. In a population-based study of a random general Danish population, 41% of subjects with tension-type headache (according to the IHS criteria) did

B. K. Rasmussen: Department of Neurology, Hilleroed Hospital, Hilleroed Hospital, DK-3400 Hilleroed, Denmark.

R. B. Lipton: Departments of Neurology Epidemiology, and Social Medicine, Albert Einstein College of Medicine, and Headache Unit, Montefiore Medical Center, Bronx, New York 10467.

TABLE 1. *Some prevalence studies of tension-type headache in industrialized countries*

Study and country	Sample-source	Study method	Respondents (No.)	Age (yr)	Time period prevalence	Tension-type headache		
						Males (%)	Females (%)	All (%)
Crisp et al., 1977 (8), UK[a]	General population	Questionnaire	727	Adults	Lifetime	29	35	
Göbel et al. 1994 (15) Germany	General population	Questionnaire	4,061	>18	Lifetime	36	39	38
Nikiforow, 1981 (33), Finland[a]	General population	Clinical interview	200	>15	1	37	42	40
Philips, 1977 (38), UK[a]	General practice	Questionnaire	597	16–60	6	65	68	
Pryse-Philips et al., 1992 (39), Canada	Random sample	Telephone interview	2,737	>15	Lifetime	21	37	29
Rasmussen et al., 1991 (44), Denmark	General population	Clinical interview and examination	740	25–64	Lifetime 1-yr Point	69 63 9	88 86 16	78 74 12
Schwartz et al., 1997 (51), USA	General population	Telephone interview	13,345	18–65	1 yr	36	42	38
						(episodic tension-type headache)		
Waters, 1972 (57), UK[a]	General practitioners	Questionnaire	882	35–54	1 yr	42	61	
Ziegler et al., 1977 (63), US[a]	Church congregations	Questionnaire	1,809	>15	Lifetime	42	34	
						(mild headache)		

[a]Non-International Headache Society based.

not have their daily activities inhibited because of the headache, whereas 59% had moderate or severe impairment of their daily activities because of the headache (43). Among subjects experiencing tension-type headache in the previous year, 59% had it 1 day per month or less often and 37% had it several times a month (Fig. 1). In the total population, 3% had chronic tension-type headache (i.e., headache ≥180 days a year), which is in agreement with other reports (15,21,51). Population-based studies, including data on the frequency of tension-type headache, have agreed with the Danish study in

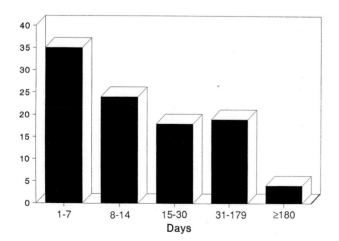

FIG. 1. Number of days with tension-type headache in the previous year. Data are from a Danish population study. (From ref. 44, with permission.)

finding a rather large proportion of subjects with mild and infrequent (once a month or less often) tension-type headache and the 1-year-period prevalence of frequent tension-type headache (more than once a month) seems to be about 20% to 30% (1,13,21,33,39,41,44,51).

SEX AND AGE DISTRIBUTION

Most previous studies confirmed that tension-type headache is slightly more prevalent in women than in men (male-to-female ratio about 1:1.3) (see Table 1); in both sexes, the prevalence seems to peak between the ages of 30 and 39 years and then to decline with age (1,38,39,44,51,57–59). Because most of these studies are cross sectional, they do not support rigorous conclusions about how tension-type headache evolves over time. The lower prevalence in the older groups compared with the younger age groups observed in cross-sectional studies may be a function of remission of the headache with advancing age or an increased incidence in the younger age groups (i.e., cohort effect) or perhaps a combination of the two explanations. Headache remissions with advancing age are most likely spontaneous but could reflect treatment induced remissions. Data on age of onset contribute to the explanation of the observed lower prevalence with advancing age, showing that onset of tension-type headache is low after middle age, adding few new cases to the headache pool (42). Whether the incidence differs in different age cohorts as a result of exposure to different risk factors cannot be assessed from these studies. Distinguishing a real effect of aging from cohort or period effects requires longitudinal follow-up studies. Nonetheless, any comparison of prevalence between populations must take these age and sex differences into account.

Several possible explanations of the sex difference of headache disorders have been explored. Differing perceptions of symptoms and bodily sensations, differing socially defined roles and behavior, differing personality and psychologic traits, and finally the differing influence of hormonal factors were discussed in a recent article (6). Whether underlying physiologic differences rather than sociocultural or psychological processes are responsible for the gender-related headache differences remains unknown. Hormonal factors may contribute to the gender difference. The influence of female hormones has been studied intensively, and some influence, precipitating or predisposing, is likely, although the mechanism is not understood (12,14,17,27,42). In a study of 148 patients with chronic tension-type headache, relief during pregnancy was more common among patients with a history of migraine as well than among patients with exclusively tension-type headache (26). No differences were found between these groups with regard to menstrually associated headache. In a Danish population-based study, 39% of women with tension-type headache (for more than 14 days a year and never migraine) reported menstruation as a precipitating factor; 67% stated that headache was unchanged during pregnancy, 28% reported disappearance or substantial improvement, and 5% reported that headache worsened (42). Corresponding figures for migraine showed that 24% of female migraineurs described menstruation as a precipitating factor; improvement during pregnancy was experienced in about half of the migraineurs (42). Thus, menstruation was more frequently a precipitating factor in tension-type headache, a finding also reported by Waters and O'Connor (62). On the other hand, migraine was more strongly influenced by other clinical factors related to female hormones, such as pregnancy, menarche, menopause, and the use of oral contraceptives. Figures on age at onset of tension-type headache showed that the most common onset was in the second decade for both male and female patients (42). The association between tension-type headache and psychological factors also has received significant attention with the purpose of explaining the gender difference in the occurrence of headache. Several studies using psychometric assessment techniques have supported the existence of a psychosomatic personality in tension-type headache sufferers (2,3,5,18,25,37,41,54), but other studies have not reported this finding (4,20,36). Studies in headache-prone populations, however, should be interpreted with care, because personality traits of patients from headache clinics may be characteristic of persons likely to seek medical care rather than of those with tension-type headache. In one study of a representative general population, gender differences related to tension-type headache were consistent even when controlling for the influence of the psychometric scores (41). Thus, according to these results, the sex difference of tension-type headache cannot be explained solely by differing sex-specific personality traits. Determining whether personality deviations in headache sufferers are causal or rather an effect of recurrent pain requires longitudinal epidemiologic investigations. Probably the sex difference in tension-type headache is a result of a complex of multiple biopsychosocial factors.

EPISODIC AND CHRONIC TENSION-TYPE HEADACHE

The sex distribution of infrequent and mild episodic tension-type headache is controversial. Some studies show a modest female preponderance and others equal prevalence in the two sexes. Some studies show a trend in the direction of increased prevalence in men (1,15,33, 38,55,64). Frequent or chronic tension-type headache consistently shows female predominance (1,21,45,51). In a large U.S. study, the sex ratio for episodic tension-type headache was 1.16, reflecting a modest female preponderance, whereas the corresponding ratio for chronic tension-type headache was 2.0 (51). In a community survey in Jerusalem, the prevalence of frequent tension-type headache (more than once a month) was 21% in men and 30% in women (1). Corresponding figures from a Danish population study were 17% in men and 28% in women (41). In the Danish study, the prevalence of chronic tension-type headache was 2% in men and 5% in women (45), again demonstrating a twofold increased prevalence in women. Remarkably coherent figures for the prevalence and sex distribution of chronic tension-type headache have been reported in recent population-based studies using IHS criteria (15,40,45,51).

The prevalence of frequent or chronic tension-type headache seems to increase with age (15), whereas episodic tension-type headache decreases with increasing age (1,44,51). Thus, the mean age for subjects with chronic tension-type headache is somewhat higher than that of episodic tension-type headache (45). More descriptive and analytical data on episodic and chronic tension-type headache analyzed separately are needed.

SOCIODEMOGRAPHIC FACTORS

Few epidemiologic studies have dealt with possible associations between tension-type headache and marital status, social class, employment status, category of industry, education, or other sociodemographic variables. Several population-based studies have analyzed these factors in relation to headache in general but have not been specific regarding tension-type headache. Impressions based on the experience with clinic patients cannot produce

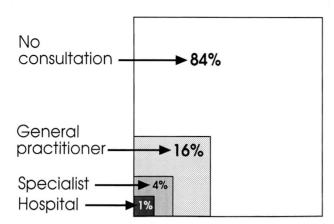

FIG. 2. Consultation rates due to tension-type headache. Among subjects who ever have had tension-type headache. (From ref. 43, with permission.)

information about real associations, because they are based on highly selected subgroups of subjects with tension-type headache. Only 16% of subjects with tension-type headache had consulted a general practitioner at some time because of the headache, and a specialist had been consulted by no more than 4% of subjects with tension-type headache (43) (Fig. 2). Thus, the selection in clinical series is considerable, resulting in limited generalizability. Epidemiologic studies of general populations have shown a fairly uniform prevalence of tension-type headache in various social groups (1,15,33,39,41,56). The methodologies in these studies vary considerably in regard to diagnostic criteria, delineation of socioeconomic status, and sample sizes. In a U.S. study, higher prevalences with increasing educational levels were observed among subjects with episodic tension-type headache, whereas the prevalence of chronic tension-type headache appeared to decline with increasing education (51). This inverse relationship is also reported for migraine (53). Two plausible reasons for a possible link between chronic tension-type headache and low socioeconomic status could be suggested. On the one hand, poor living conditions, stress, or poor access to health care could lead to an increased prevalence. Alternatively, chronic tension-type headache may lead to difficulties with work or in career advancement. In the long term, this would lead to a downward drift in socioeconomic status. Whether these effects are important remains to be determined.

COEXISTING MIGRAINE AND TENSION-TYPE HEADACHE

The terms *tension vascular headache*, *combined headache*, *combination headache*, *mixed headache*, or *vascular* and *muscle-contraction headache* have been used when migraine and tension-type headache coexist in the same person. Thus far, useful criteria have not been developed for mixed headache disorders. Headache suf-

ferers vary from those having pure migraine to those with pure tension-type headache, and some have migraine in combination with greater or lesser amounts of tension-type headache. Clinical observations indicate that rather large proportions of patients with migraine have tension-type headache between their attacks (23,24,26,35,52). Corresponding high percentages of subjects with coexisting migraine and tension-type headache also are found in random populations (13,32,33,44,45,51).

When migraine and tension-type headache coexist, the IHS criteria recommend assigning two independent diagnoses and describing the frequency and impact of each disorder. In persons who clearly experience two independent types of headache, this approach is well accepted; however, there is another group of patients commonly seen in specialized headache clinics whose disorder begins as migraine. Patients report that their headaches increase in frequency over months or years. Often, these persons gradually develop a picture of daily or near-daily headaches. Sometimes the more frequent headaches retain migrainous features, such as nausea, photophobia, or phonophobia. Some authors consider this type of headache a kind of mild migraine, so-called *transformed migraine* (30,31,48). Many such patients use medication excessively, which at least may be partly responsible for some of the headaches, because medication abuse and withdrawal are known to be major causes of headache chronicity (7,29,47). The existence and usefulness of transformed migraine as a clinical construct remains controversial.

The frequent coexistence of migraine and tension-type headache within the same person complicates the clinical practice as well as epidemiologic studies of these disorders. One approach is to study exclusively subjects with pure migraine and pure tension-type headache. Such an approach, however, may result in nonrepresentative results as a result of "diagnostic purity" bias (46). It is therefore important to analyze tension-type headache and migraine separately by means of diaries in patients with both disorders. Such an analysis would provide valuable information about the coexistence and relative importance of the two headache disorders.

PROGNOSIS

Long-term epidemiologic follow-up studies that include large numbers of community-based cases are required to assess prognosis among tension-type headache sufferers. Such studies have never been performed. Waters (60) gave some attention to the prognosis of headache (all headaches combined) using cross-sectional epidemiologic data and assuming that no period or cohort effect was present. From data collected in his Pontypridd study, he concluded that prevalence declines with age and that the severity of headaches does not change with age in men but decreases in women. Headaches, among those who continue to have headaches, become more frequent with age in women but not in men. These conclusions, however, may be somewhat uncertain given the important and unverified assumption noted in the preceding. In a 12-year follow-up study, Waters and co-workers studied the mortality rate from headache; rather surprisingly, the mortality rate was higher in women without headaches than in headache sufferers (61). Women with headaches had a relative risk of dying of 0.72 compared with those without headaches. One possible explanation of this unexpected finding is that subjects with headache are more likely to consult a physician and thereby increase their chances for detection and treatment of other diseases that may influence the mortality rates. Finally, headache sufferers who use aspirin or other analgesics may experience reduced rates of cardiovascular and cerebrovascular diseases.

Some relationship between episodic tension-type headache and chronic tension-type headache and some interrelation between migraine and tension-type headache may exist and influence the prognosis of tension-type headache. Probably subjects with frequent episodic tension-type headache are at increased risk for developing chronic tension-type headache over a period of many years (26), and in subjects with coexisting migraine, the severity and frequency of tension-type headache may be increased (45). Various factors can influence headache frequency and transform episodic tension-type (or migrainous) headache into a chronic form of headache. Among these, the aggravating role of overconsumption of ergotamine or analgesics is well documented. Several studies have clearly demonstrated that chronic abuse of these substances is the most frequent cause of patients evolving from an episodic pattern of headache to a chronic, ultimately daily pattern (16,30,49,50). Unless withdrawal of analgesics can be attained, the prognosis in these patients is worsened with the clinical observation that they are resistant to any prophylactic therapy.

Another factor important at the onset of primary headaches and in their persistence is psychosocial stress. Convincing evidence has been found that chronic headache is associated with the report of a higher frequency as well as severity of minor life events and so-called "daily hassles" (9–11,22). In contrast, major life events do not occur more often in headache patients than in controls. A higher incidence and density of daily hassles have been reported in tension-type headache compared with migraine sufferers (9,11). These studies suggest that the ability to cope with minor daily life events might be a relevant prognostic parameter in tension-type headache.

REFERENCES

1. Abramson JH, Hopp C, Epstein LM. Migraine and non-migrainous headaches. A community survey in Jerusalem. *J Epidemiol Community Health* 1980;34:188–193.
2. Anderson CD, Franks RD. Migraine and tension headache: is there a physiological difference? *Headache* 1981;21:63–71.
3. Andrasik F, Blanchard EB, Arena JG, Teders SJ, Teevan RC, Rodichok LD. Psychological functioning in headache sufferers. *Psychosom Med* 1982;44:171–182.
4. Blanchard EB, Andrasik F, Arena JG, et al. A bio-psycho-social investigation of headache activity in a chronic headache population. *Headache* 1984;24:79–87.
5. Blaszczynski AP. Personality factors in classical migraine and tension headache. *Headache* 1984;24:238–244.
6. Celentano DD, Linet MS, Stewart WF. Gender differences in the experience of headache. *Soc Sci Med* 1990;30:1289–1295.
7. Couch JR, Diamond S. Status migrainosus: causative and therapeutic aspects. *Headache* 1983;23:94–101.
8. Crisp AH, Kalucy RS, McGuinness B, Ralph PC, Harris G. Some clinical, social and psychological characteristics of migraine subjects in the general population. *Postgrad Med J* 1977;53:691–697.
9. Dawans A, Schoenen J, Timsit M, Timsit-Meyer M. Correlative study of psychopathological features and temporalis second exteroceptive silent period in chronic tension-type headache. *Cephalalgia* 1991;11 (Suppl 11):310–311.
10. De Benedittis G, Lorenzetti A, Pieri A. The role of stressful life events in the onset of chronic primary headache. *Pain* 1990;40:65–75.
11. De Benedittis G, Lorenzetti A. The role of stressful life events in the persistence of primary headache: major events vs daily hassles. *Pain* 1992;51:35–42.
12. Dennerstein L, Laby B, Burrows GD, Hyman GJ. Headache and sex hormone therapy. *Headache* 1978;18:146–153.
13. Edmeads J, Findlay H, Tugwell P, Pryse-Philips W, Nelson RF, Murray TJ. Impact of migraine and tension-type headache on life-style, consulting behaviour, and medication use: a Canadian population survey. *Can J Neurol Sci* 1993;20:131–137.
14. Epstein MT, Hockaday JM, Hockaday TDR. Migraine and reproductive hormones throughout the menstrual cycle. *Lancet* 1975;1:543–548.
15. Göbel H, Petersen-Braun M, Soyka D. The epidemiology of headache in Germany: a nationwide survey of a representative sample on the basis of the headache classification of the International Headache Society. *Cephalalgia* 1994;14:97–106.
16. Granella F, Farina S, Malferrari G, Manzoni GC. Drug abuse in chronic headache a clinico-epidemiologic study. *Cephalalgia* 1987;7:15–19.
17. Greenblatt RB, Bruneteau DW. Menopausal headaches- psychogenic or metabolic? *J Am Geriatr Soc* 1974;22:186–90.
18. Harrison RH. Psychological testing in headache: a review. *Headache* 1975;14:177–185.
19. Headache Classification Committee of the International Headache Society. Classification and diagnostic criteria for headache disorders, cranial neuralgias and facial pain. *Cephalalgia* 1988;8(Suppl 7):1–96.
20. Henryk-Gutt R, Rees WL. Psychological aspects of migraine. *J Psychosom Res* 1973;17:141–53.
21. Hollnagel H, Nørrelund N. Headache among 40 year-olds in Glostrup. *Ugeskr Laeger* 1980;142:3071–3077.
22. Holm JE, Holroyd KA, Hursey KG, Penzien DB. The role of stress in recurrent tension headache. *Headache* 1986;26:160–167.
23. Iversen HK, Langemark M, Andersson PG, Hansen PE, Olesen J. Clinical characteristics of migraine and episodic tension-type headache in relation to old and new diagnostic criteria. *Headache* 1990;30:514–519.
24. Johannes CB, Linet MS, Stewart WF, Celentano DD, Lipton RB, Szklo M. Relationship of headache to phase of the menstrual cycle among young women: A daily diary study. *Neurology* 1995;45:1076–1082.
25. Kudrow L, Sutkus BJ. MMPI pattern specificity in primary headache disorders. *Headache* 1979;19:18–24.
26. Langemark M, Olesen J, Poulsen DL, Bech P. Clinical characterization of patients with chronic tension headache. *Headache* 1988;28:590–596.
27. Larsson-Cohn U, Lundberg PO. Headache and treatment with oral contraceptives. *Acta Neurol Scand* 1970;46:267–278.
28. Levy LM. An epidemiological study of headache in an urban population in Zimbabwe. *Headache* 1983;23:2–9.
29. Lippman CW. Characteristic headache resulting from prolonged use of ergot derivatives. *J Nerv Ment Dis* 1955;121:270–273.
30. Mathew NT, Stubits E, Nigam MP. Transformation of episodic migraine into daily headache: analysis of factors. *Headache* 1982;22:66–68.
31. Mathew NT, Reuveni U, Perez F. Transformed or evolutive migraine. *Headache* 1987;27:102–106.
32. Newland CA, Illis LS, Robinson PK, Batchelor BG, Waters WE. A survey of headache in an English City. *Res Clin Stud Headache* 1978;5:1–20.

33. Nikiforow R. Headache in a random sample of 200 persons: a clinical study of a population in Northern Finland. *Cephalalgia* 1981;1:99–107.
34. Ogunyemi AO. Prevalence of headache among Nigerian university students. *Headache* 1984;24:127–30.
35. Olesen J. The clinical features of the acute migraine attack. An analysis of 750 patients. *Headache* 1978;18:268–267.
36. Passchier J, van der Helm-Hylkema H, Orlebeke JF. Personality and headache type: a controlled study. *Headache* 1984;24:140–146.
37. Philips C. Headache and personality. *J Psychosom Res* 1976;20:535–542.
38. Philips C. Headache in general practice. *Headache* 1977;16:322–329.
39. Pryse-Phillips W, Findlay H, Tugwell P, Edmeads J, Murray TJ, Nelson RF. A Canadian population survey on the clinical, epidemiologic and societal impact of migraine and tension-type headache. *Can J Neurol Sci* 1992;19:333–339.
40. Rasmussen, Birthe Krogh. Epidemiology of headache [Thesis]. *Cephalalgia* 1995;15:48–68.
41. Rasmussen BK. Migraine and tension-type headache in a general population: psychosocial factors. *Int J Epidemiol* 1992;21:1138–43.
42. Rasmussen BK. Migraine and tension-type headache in a general population: precipitating factors, female hormones, sleep pattern and relation to lifestyle. *Pain* 1993;53:65–72.
43. Rasmussen BK, Jensen R, Olesen J. Impact of headache on sickness absence and utilisation of medical services: a Danish population study. *J Epidemiol Community Health* 1992;46:443–446.
44. Rasmussen BK, Jensen R, Schroll M, Olesen J. Epidemiology of headache in a general population—a prevalence study. *J Clin Epidemiol* 1991;44:1147–1157.
45. Rasmussen BK, Jensen R, Schroll M, Olesen J. Interrelations between migraine and tension-type headache in the general population. *Arch Neurol* 1992;49:914–918.
46. Sackett DL. Bias in analytic research. *J Chron Dis* 1979; 32: 51–63.
47. Saper JR. Migraine. II. Treatment. *JAMA* 1978;239:2480–2483.
48. Saper JR. The mixed headache syndrome: a new perspective. *Headache* 1982;22:284–286.
49. Saper JR. Ergotamine dependency a review. *Headache* 1987;27:435–438.
50. Schoenen J, Lenarduzzi P, Sianard-Gainko J. Chronic headaches associated with analgesics and/or ergotamine abuse: a clinical survey of 434 consecutive out patients. In: Clifford Rose F, ed. *New advances in headache research.* London: Smith-Gordon, 1989;255–259.
51. Schwartz BS, Stewart WF, Simon D, Lipton RB. Epidemiology of tension-type headache. *JAMA* 1998;279:381–383.
52. Selby G. *Migraine and its variants.* Sydney: Adis Health Science Press, 1983.
53. Stewart WF, Lipton R, Celentano DD, Reed ML. Prevalence of migraine headache in the United States. *JAMA* 1992;267:64–69.
54. Sternbach RA. Survey of pain in the United States: the Nuprin pain report. *Clin J Pain* 1986;2:49–53.
55. Waters WE. Community studies of the prevalence of headache. *Headache* 1970;9:178–186.
56. Waters WE. Migraine: Intelligence, Social Class, and Familial Prevalence. *BMJ* 1971;2:77–81.
57. Waters WE. Headache and migraine in general practitioners. In: *The migraine headache and Dixarit:* proceedings of a symposium held at Churchill College, *Cambridge.* Bracknell, Berkshire: Boehringer Ingelheim, 1972:31–44.
58. Waters WE. The Pontypridd headache survey. *Headache* 1974;14:81–90.
59. Waters WE. Migraine in general practitioners. *British Journal of Preventive and Social Medicine* 1975;29:48–52.
60. Waters WE. Epidemiological data relevant to prognosis in migraine in adults. *Dan Med Bull* 1975;22:89–91.
61. Waters WE, Campbell MJ, Elwood PC. Migraine, headache, and survival in women. *BMJ* 1983;287:1442–1443.
62. Waters WE, O'Connor PJ. Epidemiology of headache and migraine in women. *J Neurol Neurosurg Psychiatry* 1971;34:148–153.
63. Wong TW, Wong KS, Yu TS, Kay R. Prevalence of migraine and other headaches in Hong Kong. *Neuroepidemiology* 1995;14:82–91.
64. Ziegler DK, Hassanein RS, Couch JR. Characteristics of life headache histories in a nonclinic population. *Neurology* 1977;27:265–269.

The Headaches, Second Edition,
edited by J. Olesen, P. Tfelt-Hansen, and K.M.A. Welch.
Lippincott Williams & Wilkins, Philadelphia © 2000.

*Tension-Type Headache, Cluster Headache, and Miscellaneous
Primary Headaches*

CHAPTER 70

Anatomy and Pathology of Tension-Type Headache

Nikolai Bogduk and Rigmor Jensen

The pain of tension-type headache is classically described as bandlike, surrounding the frontal, parietal, and occipital regions of the head. Its physiology is not completely understood and remains under investigation (see Chapters 72–79). Although some models infer that the pain of tension-type headache is central in origin (46), traditional interpretations have maintained that the pain could arise from local structures, such as the muscles of the scalp. Additionally, there are concerns that some forms of tension-type headache might, in fact, constitute referred pain from structures in the upper cervical spine or the temporomandibular apparatus (see Chap. 118 and 121).

A consideration of the anatomy of these structures becomes pertinent as the basis for any consideration of the propriety of these various models of tension-type headache and its treatment. For convenience, the musculoskeletal structures of the head can be considered on a regional basis in three groups: the epicranial scalp muscles, the temporomandibular apparatus, and the upper cervical spine and suboccipital regions.

EPICRANIAL MUSCLES

The scalp muscles are designed to operate on the skin of the head. The occipitofrontalis is a muscle of facial expression that creases the skin of the forehead and raises the eyebrows. Various auricular muscles, designed to operate on the auricle, are almost vestigial in humans in that few persons are accustomed to using these muscles to move their ears.

The occipitofrontalis is a paired muscle consisting of two bellies. The occipital belly stems from the superior nuchal line and covers the occipital bone; it ends in an aponeurosis that glides over the vertex of the skull (Fig. 1). The frontal belly stems from the anterior edge of the epicranial aponeurosis, covers the frontal bone, and inserts into the skin of the forehead (see Fig. 1). The occipital belly receives its motor supply from the posterior auricular branch of the facial nerve (see Fig. 1). The frontal belly is innervated by the temporal branch of the facial nerve. The sensory innervation of these two muscles has not been explicitly demonstrated, but presumably the occipital belly is supplied by the greater and lesser occipital nerves which run over this muscle (see Fig. 1), whereas the frontal belly is supplied by the supraorbital nerve (see Fig. 1).

TEMPOROMANDIBULAR APPARATUS

The temporomandibular apparatus consists of the temporomandibular joint and the muscles that act on it. The joint is an ellipsoid joint containing an articular disc that

N. Bogduk: Department of Anatomy and Musculoskeletal Medicine, University of Newcastle, and Newcastle Bone and Joint Institute, Royal Newcastle Hospital, Newcastle, New South Wales 2300, Australia.

R. Jensen: Department of Neurology, Glostrup Hospital, University of Copenhagen, DK-2600 Glostrup, Copenhagen, Denmark.

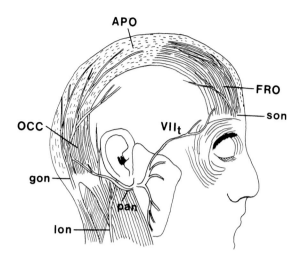

FIG. 1. The muscles of the scalp and their nerves. *OCC*, occipital belly of occipitofrontalis; *FRO*, frontal belly of occipitofrontalis; *APO*, epicranial aponeurosis; *gon*, greater occipital nerve; *lon*, lesser occipital nerve; *pan*, posterior auricular nerve; *VIIt*, temporal branch of facial nerve; *son*, supraorbital nerve.

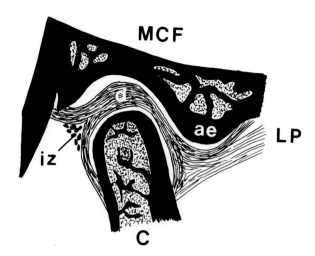

FIG. 2. Internal structure of the temporomandibular joint. *d*, articular disc; *ae*, articular eminence; *iz*, interlaminar zone; *C*, mandibular condyle; *MCF*, middle cranial fossa; *LP*, lateral pterygoid.

divides the joint into an upper and a lower cavity. Its movements consist of sagittal rotation and translation that underlie opening and closing of the jaw and quasi-circular gliding movements that underlie chewing and the grinding movements of the teeth.

Temporomandibular Joint

The zygomatic process of the squamous temporal bone presents a deeply concave, articular fossa that faces downward to receive the convex condyle of the mandible. Interposed between these two bones is the fibrous articular disc, which adapts the shape of the articular surfaces of the temporal bone and mandible. Its presence allows the mandible to undertake gliding movements and translations instead of being locked in the deep recess of the articular fossa, where its movements would be restricted to sagittal rotation.

The joint is enclosed by a fibrous capsule that attaches superiorly to the margins of the articular fossa of the temporal bone and its articular eminence and inferiorly to the neck of the mandibular condyle. Setting astride the condyle like a cap, the articular disc is attached laterally and medially to the neck of the mandible and lies deep to but separate from the joint capsule (27). Anteriorly, the disc is attached to the articular eminence of the temporal bone and to the neck of the mandible; it blends with the anterior capsule of the joint and receives part of the tendon of the lateral pterygoid (Fig. 2). Posteriorly, the disc divides into laminae that blend with the posterior capsule: an inferior lamina that leads to the mandible and a superior lamina that leads to the temporal bone and squamotemporal fissure (27) (see Fig. 2). The space

between the diverging laminae is filled by a plexus of small veins and is pressure sensitive (27). The upper surface of the disc is convex to fit the articular fossa of the temporal bone, whereas the lower surface is slightly concave to receive the condyle of the mandible, but the concavity of the disc is shallower than that of the articular fossa.

In the early phase of jaw opening, the mandibular condyle rolls on the inferior surface of the articular disc. Further opening of the jaw involves anterior translation of both the disc and the condyle, and this requires a muscle to pull both structures forward. The disc translates forward with respect to the temporal bone, carrying with it the mandibular condyle, which rolls and glides on the inferior surface of the disc.

Temporomandibular Muscles

In the upright posture, the jaw can open under gravity. Otherwise, the mandible can be rotated downward by the mylohyoid muscle; the digastric can be recruited if the movement is resisted, but this muscle is involved largely in elevating the hyoid bone rather than opening the jaw.

Anterior translation of the mandible and articular disc is produced by the lateral pterygoid. This muscle arises by two heads, one from the lateral surface of the lateral pterygoid plate, the other from the infratemporal surface of the greater wing of the sphenoid. The two heads converge on the anterior capsule of the temporomandibular joint and insert into the anterior surface of the articular disc and the anterior surface of the neck of the mandible (Fig. 3A). Together, they draw these structures collectively forward to produce anterior translation of the mandible. Moreover, the lateral pterygoid produces a force coupled with the sphenomandibular ligament to

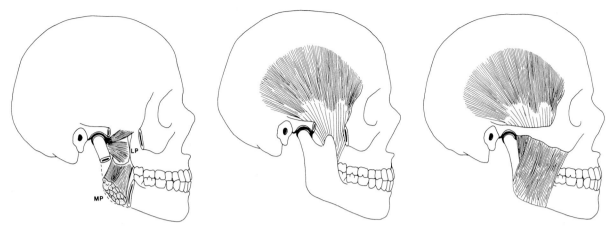

FIG. 3. Muscles of the temporomandibular joint. **A**: Medial pterygoid (MP) and lateral pterygoid (*LP*). **B**: Temporalis. **C**: Masseter.

rotate the mandible about an axis running transversely through its neck.

The other temporomandibular muscles are designed primarily to close the jaw. The medial pterygoid passes downward and slightly backward and laterally from the medial surface of the lateral pterygoid plate to insert into the medial aspect of the angle of the mandible (see Fig. 3A). Its downward inclination allows it to raise the mandible to close the jaw, and its backward and lateral orientations allow it move the mandible forward and medially for grinding movements of the teeth.

The temporalis is a large fan-shaped muscle that arises from the lateral surface of the parietal bone and squamous temporal bone and from the fascia overlying the muscle (Fig. 3B). Its posterior fibers pass downward and forward, and its middle and anterior fibers pass downward, all converging on the coronoid process of the mandible. Collectively, all fibers can elevate the mandible to close the mouth, but the posterior fibers can act independently to retract the mandible, respectively.

The masseter stems from the zygomatic arch and inserts into the lateral aspect of the angle of the mandible (Fig. 3C). Within the muscle, two or three laminae can be recognized. The deepest layer arises more posteriorly and consists of fibers with a mainly downward orientation. Anterior fibers overlap the latter but also are displaced further forward along the zygomatic arch; they pass downward but also backward to reach the mandible. Between these two major layers, a third, intermediate layer can be identified on close dissection.

Innervation

The temporomandibular muscles are innervated by the mandibular division of the trigeminal nerve. Two or three deep temporal nerves innervate the temporalis from its deep surface. The pterygoid muscles each receive a separate nerve. The nerve to masseter passes through the mandibular notch to reach the deep surface of masseter; within the muscle, it runs in the plane between the two major layers of that muscle. The temporomandibular joint receives its innervation anteriorly from the nerve to masseter and posteromedially from the auriculotemporal nerve.

UPPER CERVICAL SPINE

Joints

The skull is supported by the atlas; the occipital condyles nestle into the sockets of the superior articular processes of the atlas, forming the atlantooccipital joints (Fig. 4). These joints are enclosed by a fibrous capsule and allow nodding movements of the head and a small degree of axial rotation.

The atlas, which bears the head, is supported by the axis at the lateral atlantoaxial joints (see Fig. 4). These joiints are essentially planar, synovial joints that allow a large range of gliding movement for rotation of the head and atlas. During rotation, the anterior arch of the atlas slides around the anterior surface of the odontoid process; this movement is accommodated by the median atlantoaxial joint.

Backward movement of the atlas is prevented by impaction of the anterior arch of the atlas against the odontoid process. The reverse movement is prevented by the transverse ligament of the atlas, which constitutes a strong belt passing behind the odontoid process and connecting the left and right lateral masses of the atlas (see Fig. 4). A synovial joint occurs between the ligament and the back of the odontoid process.

The transverse ligament of the atlas is the most important structure stabilizing the atlantoaxial joint. The next most major ligaments in this region are the alar ligaments, which pass laterally and slightly upward from the posterolateral surface of each side of the odontoid

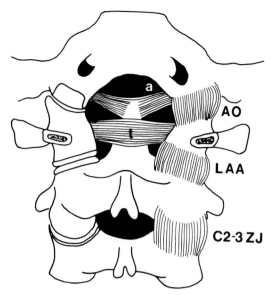

FIG. 4. The upper cervical joints and ligaments viewed from behind. On the right, the joints are enclosed by their capsules; on the left, they are exposed. *AO*, atlantooccipital joint; *LAA11*, lateral atlantoaxial joint; *C2-3 ZJ*, C2-3 zygapophysial joint; *a*, alar ligaments; *t*, transverse ligament.

process to the lateral margin of the foramen magnum (see Fig. 4). Because of their orientation, the alar ligaments prevent distraction of the head from the axis, ipsilateral gliding of the head and atlas on the axis, and excessive contralateral axial rotation of the head (16). The alar ligaments are also sufficiently strong that, if the transverse ligament of the atlas is disabled, they can limit forward sliding of the skull with respect to the axis (21). Complete forward dislocation of the skull and atlas therefore requires destruction of both the transverse ligament and the alar ligaments.

Other ligaments in the craniocervical region, such as the apical ligament of the dens, the longitudinal band of the cruciate ligament, and the accessory atlantoaxial ligaments are not of any major mechanical significance. The anterior and posterior atlantooccipital and atlantoaxial membranes constitute fascial septa separating the vertebral canal from the exterior regions of the vertebral column and are not structures of any mechanical importance.

Below C2 lie the typical joints of the cervical spine. The C2 vertebra rests on an intervertebral disc anteriorly and is connected to the C3 vertebra posteriorly by the C2-3 zygapophysial joints. These are planar, synovial joints that allow gliding movements between the C2 and C3 vertebrae during flexion and rotation of the neck. They are inclined upward and forward and are weight-bearing joints that allow movement.

The anterior longitudinal ligament of the neck terminates largely on the body of C2, but a median extension of it passes to the anterior tubercle of the atlas (51). The posterior longitudinal ligament of the lower cervical spine expands behind the C2 vertebral body to become the membrana tectoria, which covers the atlantoaxial ligaments and attaches to the anterior margin of the foramen magnum. It forms a smooth "carpet" that separates the dural sac and fragile spinal cord from the odontoid process and its joints.

Interspinous ligaments are conspicuously lacking in the cervical spine (48). The interspinous spaces are simply filled with fascia, constituting a feeble midline septum between the deep neck muscles that is continuous with the deep fascia of semispinalis capitis. The ligamen-

FIG. 5. The anatomy of the suboccipital region, by layers. **A:** On the left, the most superficial muscle layer is shown, in which the sternocleidomastoid (*sm*) and trapezius (*T*) attach to the superior nuchal line by way of an aponeurosis (*a*), which connects the two muscles. The greater occipital nerve (*gon*) emerges through an aperture above the aponeurotic sling between these two muscles to become cutaneous. The lesser occipital nerve (*lon*) ascends parallel to sternocleidomastoid to reach the occiput. The third occipital nerve (*ton*) penetrates the trapezius to become cutaneous. On the right, the trapezius and sternocleidomastoid have been resected, leaving their aponeuroses (*a'*) attached to the superior nuchal line to reveal the splenius (*SP*) and the semispinalis capitis (*SS*), through which the greater occipital nerve passes. **B:** On the left, the splenius has been resected to reveal the longissimus capitis (*LG*) and the extent of semispinalis capitis. On the right, the semispinalis capitis (*SS*) has been resected to reveal the course of the greater occipital nerve across the suboccipital muscles: rectus capitis posterior minor (*R*), rectus capitis posterior major (*RM*), obliquus inferior (*OI*), and obliquus superior (*OS*). The attachments of sternocleidomastoid (*SM*), splenius (*SP*), and longissimus capitis (*LG*) to the mastoid process remain in situ. **C:** All posterior muscles have been resected, leaving only their occipital attachments, to show the entire course of the greater occipital nerve and the course of the third occipital nerve (*ton*) across the C2-3 zygapophysial joint. The ganglion of the C2 spinal nerve (*g*) lies behind the lateral atlantoaxial joint. Articular branches (*a*) arise from the C1 ventral ramus to the atlantooccipital joint from the C2 ventral ramus to the lateral atlantoaxial joint and from the third occipital nerve to the C2-3 zygapophysial joint. The C1-3 ventral rami enter the cervical plexus. **D:** Removal of the posterior elements of the occiput and the C1-3 vertebra reveals the C1-3 sinuvertebral nerves, which supply the transverse (*t*) and alar (*a*) ligaments before passing through the foramen magnum to innervate the dura mater over the clivus. The meningeal branches of the vagus (*X*) nerve and hypoglossal nerve (*XII*) are found emerging from the jugular foramen and hypoglossal canal, respectively.

tum nuchae is not a large, sagittal sheet of elastic tissue. Although it has this structure in some quadrupeds, this is not the case in humans. The only substantive structure in the posterior midline of the neck is a cord of tissue known as the *funicular portion* of the ligamentum nuchae (22). It is a raphe, only a few millimetres thick, formed by the interlacing, tendinous fibers of trapezius, splenius, and upper rhomboids. Deep to this cord, what is portrayed as the ligamentum nuchae is only the deep fascia of semispinalis capitis passing along the midline to the interspinous spaces.

Muscles

The intrinsic posterior neck muscles are covered by the trapezius and sternocleidomastoid (Fig. 5A). The trapezius drapes around the upper neck from the medial third of the superior nuchal line and the upper ligamentum nuchae. The sternocleidomastoid encroaches into the suboccipital region by inserting into the mastoid process and the lateral end of the superior nuchal line. These two muscles cover the splenius capitis, the most superficial of the intrinsic posterior neck muscles.

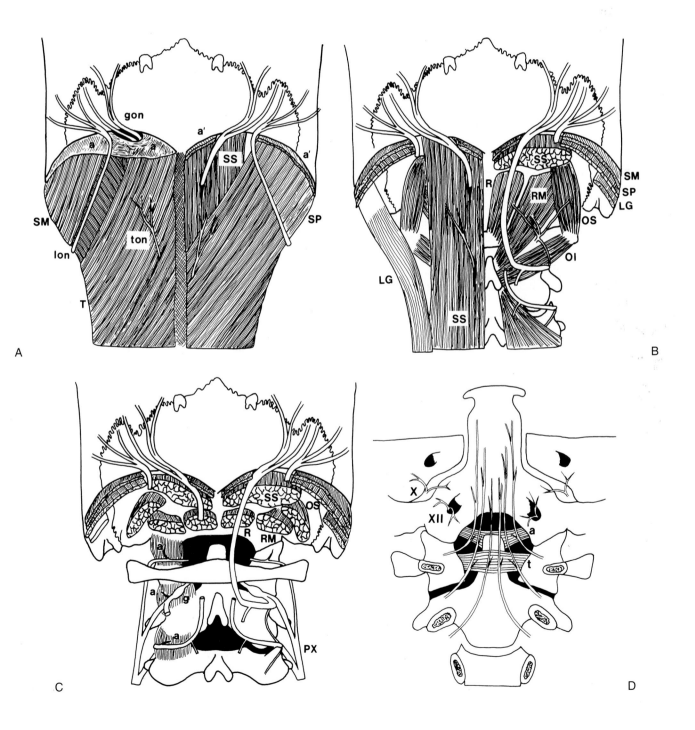

The splenius capitis is a flat muscle whose fibers stem from the funicular portion of the ligamentum nuchae lower in the neck and that pass upward and laterally to assume a linear insertion into the mastoid process and the lateral two thirds or so of the superior nuchal line (Fig. 5A).

Deep to the splenius lies the semispinalis capitis, the largest and most prominent of the posterior neck muscles (Fig. 5B; see Fig. 5A). It arises from the transverse processes of the upper thoracic and the cervical vertebra and forms a large, thick belly that inserts into the occiput below the superior nuchal line. It is flanked in the upper neck by the slender longissimus capitis, which inserts into the mastoid process (see Fig. 5B). Both muscles cover the suboccipital triangle, which is formed by an array of muscles that connect the skull, atlas, and axis (see Fig. 5B). The rectus capitis posterior minor joins the posterior tubercle of the atlas to the skull; the rectus capitis posterior major joins the spinous process of C2 to the skull; the obliquus inferior runs between the spinous process of C2 and the transverse process of C1; and the obliquus superior runs from the transverse process of the atlas to the skull.

At the same depth as the suboccipital muscles, the fascicles of the cervical multifidus radiate caudally from the C2 spinous process and are blended at their origin with the uppermost fibers of the semispinalis cervicis.

The insertions of the posterior neck muscles into the head are largely fleshy, although those inserting about the mastoid process exhibit a mixture of fleshy and tendinous fibers. The origin of trapezius is largely aponeurotic; its more lateral fibers arise from an aponeurotic sling that bridges the tendinous fibers of sternocleidomastoid and the medial third of the superior nuchal line (see Fig. 5A).

Innervation

The C1 and C2 spinal nerves are distinctive in that they do not emerge through intervertebral foramina. The C1 spinal nerve passes across the posterior arch of the atlas behind its superior articular process (Fig. 5C). The C2 spinal nerve crosses the posterior aspect of the lateral atlantoaxial joint (see Fig. 5C), with its ganglion lying opposite the radiologic midpoint of that joint (6,28). Although the C1 spinal nerve lacks a cutaneous branch, it is nonetheless sensory to the suboccipital muscles. Its dorsal root ganglion, however, may be ectopic. When missing from the dorsal root of C1, it is typically found among the rootlets of the spinal accessory nerve (47). The C3 spinal nerve, the first of the typical cervical spinal nerves, lies in the C2-3 intervertebral foramen.

The C1-3 spinal nerves divide into ventral and dorsal rami. Their ventral rami join with that of C4 to form the cervical plexus. From this plexus, muscular branches are distributed to the prevertebral muscles—the longus capitis and cervicis, the rectus capitis anterior and lateralis—

and to the sternocleidomastoid and trapezius. At their origin, the C1-3 spinal nerves form recurrent meningeal branches: the sinuvertebral nerves. These nerves supply the ventral surface of the dura mater of the upper cervical spinal cord before entering the skull through the foramen magnum to supply the dura mater over the clivus (Fig. 5D). En route, they furnish branches to the median atlantoaxial joint, the transverse ligament of the atlas, and the alar ligaments (36). In the posterior cranial fossa, C1-3 sinuvertebral nerves are joined by meningeal branches of the X and XII cranial nerves. Although they arise from cranial nerves, these branches are cervical in origin, having gained the cranial nerves outside the skull, where they communicate with the cervical plexus (36). Other branches of the C1-3 ventral rami join the vertebral nerve, the plexus accompanying the vertebral artery, and furnish sensory branches to the fourth part of the artery (8,35).

The dorsal ramus of C1 innervates the muscles of the suboccipital triangle (see Fig. 5B). The C2 dorsal ramus has lateral branches directed to the longissimus capitis and splenius, but its large medial branch becomes the greater occipital nerve (7), which winds around the inferior border of the obliquus inferior; turns upward and backward through the semispinalis capitis, which it supplies; and enters the scalp through an aperture bound by the superior nuchal line and the aponeurosis of trapezius (5,7,57) (see Fig. 5). Over the occiput, it is joined by the lesser occipital nerve, which is a cutaneous branch of the cervical plexus that reaches the scalp by passing along the posterior border of sternocleidomastoid (see Fig. 5A) (5,7,57).

The C3 dorsal ramus furnishes lateral branches to the longissimus capitis and splenius. It forms two medial branches (7). The deep medial branch crosses the waist of the C3 articular pillar to enter the multifidus muscle. The superficial medial branch constitutes the third occipital nerve, which winds around the lateral and posterior aspect of the C2-3 zygapophysial joint (see Fig. 5B,C). Over the joint, this nerve communicates with the C2 dorsal ramus and furnishes articular branches to the joint. Distally, the third occipital nerve penetrates the semispinalis capitis and trapezius to become cutaneous over the suboccipital region. En route, it furnishes branches to the semispinalis capitis, which joins those from the greater occipital nerves to supply this muscle.

PATHOLOGY

Muscles

Apart from having a similar, segmental innervation, many of the muscles innervated by C1-3 share the feature that they attach to the skull and, therefore, underlie sites that are commonly tender in various forms of headache. Most superficially, the sternocleidomastoid and trapezius attach along the superior nuchal line from the mastoid process to the external occipital protuberance (see Fig. 5). Deep to these, the splenius capitis attaches to the mastoid process and outer half or so of the superior nuchal line (see Fig. 5). In the next deeper layer, the bulky semispinalis capitis is anchored to the occiput below the medial half of the superior nuchal line, and the slender longissimus capitis reaches the mastoid process. Between them, the obliquus superior attaches to the occiput; deep to semispinalis capitis, the rectus capitis posterior major and rectus capitis posterior minor attach to the occiput (see Fig. 5).

These details are pertinent to the description and interpretation of tenderness in this region. There is a proclivity among some physicians to ascribe tenderness in the suboccipital region to entrapment or irritation of the greater occipital nerve or the lesser occipital nerve (30,40,42); however, the attachment sites of these various occipital muscles, notably semispinalis capitis and sternocleidomastoid, are tender even in normal, asymptomatic persons (32). Their tenderness in patients with headaches needs to be distinguished from normal tenderness or decreased perceptual threshold in the course of headache before being arbitrarily ascribed to nerve entrapment (37,39,45).

The basis for tenderness in these regions is that the density of innervation of skeletal muscles is greatest toward their attachment sites. Clinical studies have shown that periosteum and tendons are far more sensitive to stimulation than muscle bellies (31), which correlates with their density of innervation (23). Palpation constitutes a mechanical stimulus that can activate myotendinous nociceptors, and the degree of tenderness is a function of the magnitude of pressure applied, the density of innervation, and the threshold of activation of the nociceptors.

The issue is why patients with headache exhibit greater than normal tenderness. One interpretation is that decreased threshold implies some form of local pathology such as inflammation. A competing paradigm is that the threshold is lowered centrally and that the increased sensitivity to palpation is only an amplification of otherwise normal tenderness and does not imply any local pathology.

There is no firm evidence as to whether and how posterior neck muscles might be a source of pain. Clinical studies have shown that experimental stimulation of muscles innervated by C1-3 can cause headache in normal volunteers (12,15,24), but the nature of pathological conditions that might affect these muscles to cause headache in patients remains elusive. Theoretically, acute tears near their myotendinous junctions could be a cause of acute headache after injury, but such tears attract an inflammatory repair response (25,26,44) and should heal rapidly. Muscular tears, therefore, cannot be entertained as a cause of chronic headache.

Spasm of the posterior neck muscles and of the epicranial muscles is believed by some to be a source of pain, but the evidence is mixed at best (see Chapter 74); nor is it clear how spasm, if it does occur, actually results in pain.

At the attachment site of a muscle, its fleshy fibers become tendinous, and these tendons insert into bone. As they approach bone, the fibers are embedded in a matrix of cartilage and are relatively avascular. This region of transition is called an *enthesis*, and entheses in the appendicular skeleton have attracted attention as putative sources of pain, notably in the rheumatology literature (43). It is believed that entheses can be injured by relatively minor, let alone major, insults that tear the structure, resulting in an enthesopathy. It is believed that enthesopathies can become a source of chronic pain if healing is prolonged or if the region continues to be subjected to repeated trauma. No evidence has been established, however, that any of the suboccipital muscles suffer from enthesopathy. This constitutes only a plausible model that could be investigated by proponents of local causes of muscular pain as the basis for tension-type headaches.

Some investigators believe that headaches can arise as a result of injury and laxity of upper cervical interspinous ligaments and have advocated sclerosis of the ligament as a form of treatment (29,34); this notion still attracts adherents. In the face of the anatomic fact that cervical interspinous ligaments do not exist, this model of headache is nonsense.

The trigger-point theory is fashionable among some medical and paramedical circles, and a variety of trigger-point syndromes affecting the neck muscles are reportedly associated with headache. These are the syndromes of semispinalis capitis, splenius capitis, splenius cervicis, trapezius, and sternocleidomastoid (56). Conspicuously, all these muscles are innervated by C1-3, which is consonant with their capacity to activate the trigeminocervical nucleus. Notably, in contrast, trigger-point syndromes of muscles innervated by lower cervical nerves are not associated with headache but cause referred pain to the shoulder girdle.

The pathology of trigger points is unclear. Biopsy studies have yielded conflicting and inconclusive results (53). The leading current conjecture is that they represent areas of contracted muscle resulting from failure of the sarcoplasmic reticulum to sequestrate calcium; minor trauma, such as sudden, focal stretch, is believed to be the etiology. There is, however, no evidence of this purported pathology or its etiology; trigger-point theory remains essentially a clinically based, empirical interpretation of muscle pain.

An important consideration, however, is the validity of certain upper cervical trigger-point syndromes. Several of the tender sites ascribed to trigger points overlie cervical zygapophysial joints. Consequently, trigger-point syndromes need to be distinguished from painful, tender cervical zygapophysial joints lest the source of pain be ascribed mistakenly to muscles rather than to a cervical joint (10).

Joints

The upper cervical synovial joints can be affected by overt arthritides like rheumatoid arthritis and thereby become a source of neck pain and headache (4,11,49,52, 55). Osteoarthrosis of the atlantoodontoid joint, as seen by computed tomography (CT), is associated with suboccipital headache (60). The lateral atlantoaxial joints also can be affected by osteoarthritis, and anaesthetising these joints relieves a form of headache that can be mistaken for greater occipital neuralgia (20,41). Headaches also can arise from the C2-3 zygapophysial joints in patients who have suffered neck injuries. Blocking these joints or their nerve supply relieves the headache, indicating that the joint is the source of pain (9,38). Radiographically, however, the joints exhibit no obvious arthritic changes, and the actual cause of pain in such cases remains a mystery. The leading contention, however, is that zygapophysial joints can sustain injuries that are not visible on conventional imaging such as plain radiography and CT.

Postmortem studies have shown that injuries to the capsules and meniscoids of cervical zygapophysial joints and small fractures of their articular processes are common in victims of motor-vehicle accidents; but none of these were evident in radiographs of affected spines (33). Injuries to the capsules and meniscoids would not be evident on plain radiography or CT, although early studies using magnetic resonance imagine (MRI) are encouraging (59); however, bony injuries can be demonstrated using contemporary but special procedures.

Otherwise, occult fractures of the cervical zygapophysial joints have been demonstrated using conventional lateral tomography (3,13,58), pillar views (1,2,54), and high-resolution CT scanning (3,13). Between 50% and 100% of the lesions detected by these means were not evident in plain films and were reported as normal.

In a systematic series of studies, Dvorak and colleagues (16,17,18) examined the functional anatomy of the alar ligaments and found that patients with seemingly obscure complaints of upper cervical pain and headache could be identified as having damage to an alar ligament following whiplash injury. The diagnosis became evident when functional CT scanning revealed a unilateral range of rotation of the head and atlas that was significantly greater than normal, implying rupture of the contralateral alar ligament, which normally limits this motion.

Temporomandibular Joint

Models of temporomandibular joint pain fall into two main clusters: internal derangement and myofascial pain dysfunction. It is not clear whether these ultimately represent two distinct entities or constitute different expressions of a common etiology.

In internal derangement, some degree of abnormality is evident in the joint. The condition involves various phases of increasing severity, characterized by displacement of the articular disc and joint clicking progressing to deformation and dislocation of the disc with joint locking and repeated episodes of inflammation, leading eventually to remodelling of the joint and degenerative changes (50). Throughout this evolution, the joint becomes increasingly painful, and pain can be referred to the ear and to the head. Although difficult to demonstrate by plain radiography, the pathology of internal derangement is strikingly revealed by MRI and enhanced by adjunct investigations such as two-compartment arthrography and tomography (50). The aetiology of internal derangement, however, is a contentious issue. Its relationship to abnormalities of occlusion is uncertain (19); direct injuries to the joint are an accepted cause but not a common cause (19). A further contention is that it is secondary to muscle hyperactivity (19).

Myofascial theories of temporomandibular joint pain arose to explain pain unassociated with avert articular changes and to provide a physiologic link between suspected etiologies and the genesis of pain. Malocclusion, malalignment of the jaws, and mandibular parafunction are believed to result in abnormal and excessive activity of the temporomandibular muscles. Pain is believed to occur as a result of muscle fatigue and ischemia or the development of trigger points in them (14,19).

Psychological factors are believed to play a significant role in both internal derangement and myofascial pain dysfunction (19). Psychological stress is said to produce tension in the jaw muscles as a result of anxious jaw clenching, bruxism, or other jaw parafunction.

It is fascinating how the theories concerning temporomandibular joint pain resemble those that have been applied to the cervical spine. In both instances, there is apparent competition between articular, muscular, and behavioral paradigms; but for any particular paradigm, definitive evidence is conspicuously and frustratingly lacking. The link between psychological disturbances and myofascial pain is tenuous and circumstantial; although joint changes are evident in internal derangement, a satisfactory comprehensive explanation of its etiology is still lacking. In this respect, it could be concluded that whoever finally defines the cause of temporomandibular pain will pave the way for an analogous breakthrough for cervical pain or vice versa.

REFERENCES

1. Abel MS. Occult traumatic lesions of the cervical vertebrae. *CRC Critical Reviews in Clinical Radiology and Nuclear Medicine* 1975;6: 469–553.
2. Abel MS. The radiology of chronic neck pain: sequelae of occult traumatic lesions. *Crit Rev Diagn Imaging* 1982;20:27–78.
3. Binet EF, Moro JJ, Marangola JP, Hodge CJ. Cervical tomography in trauma. *Spine* 1977;2:163–172.

4. Bland JH, Davis PH, London MG, et al. Rheumatoid arthritis of the cervical spine. *Arch Intern Med* 1963;112:892–898.
5. Bogduk N. The anatomy of occipital neuralgia. *Clin Exp Neurol* 1980; 17:167–184.
6. Bogduk N. Local anaesthetic blocks of the second cervical ganglion: a technique with application in occipital headache. *Cephalalgia* 1981;1: 41–50.
7. Bogduk N. The clinical anatomy of the cervical dorsal rami. *Spine* 1982;7:319–330.
8. Bogduk N, Lambert G, Duckworth JW. The anatomy and physiology of the vertebral nerve in relation to cervical migraine. *Cephalalgia* 1981; 1:1–14.
9. Bogduk N, Marsland A. On the concept of third occipital headache. *J Neurol Neurosurg Psychiatry* 1986;49:775–780.
10. Bogduk N, Simons DG. Neck pain: joint pain or trigger points? In: Vaeroy H, Merskey H, eds. *Progress in fibromyalgia and myofascial pain.* Amsterdam: Elsevier 1993:267–273.
11. Cabot A, Becker A. The cervical spine in rheumatoid arthritis. *Clin Orthop* 1978;131:130–140.
12. Campbell DG, Parsons CM. 1944 Referred head pain and its concomitants. *J Nerv Ment Dis* 1944;99:544–551.
13. Clark CR, Igram CM, El Khoury GY, Ehra S. Radiographic evaluation of cervical spine injuries. *Spine* 1988;13:742–747.
14. Clark GT, Sakai S. Masticatory muscle hyperactivity and muscle pain. In: Fricton JR, Awad E, eds. *Advances in pain research and therapy,* vol 17. New York: Raven Press, 1990:201–212.
15. Cyriax J. Rheumatic headache. *BMJ* 1938;2:1367–1368.
16. Dvorak J, Panjabi MM. Functional anatomy of the alar ligaments. *Spine* 1987;12:183–189.
17. Dvorak J, Panjabi MM, Greber M, Wichman W. CT-functional diagnostics of the rotatory instability of upper cervical spine. 1: an experimental study on cadavers. *Spine* 1987;12:197–205.
18. Dvorak J, Hayek J, Zehnder R. CT-functional diagnostics of the rotatory instability of the upper cervical spine. Part 2: an evaluation on healthy adults and patients with suspected instability. *Spine* 1987;12:726–731.
19. Dworkin SF, Truelove EL, Bonica JJ, Sola A. Facial and head pain caused by myofascial and temporomandibular disorders. In: Bonica JJ, ed. *The management of pain,* 2nd ed. Philadelphia: Lea & Febiger, 1990:727–745.
20. Ehni G, Benner B. Occipital neuralgia and the C1-2 arthrosis syndrome. *J Neurosurg* 1984;61:961–965.
21. Fielding JW, Cochran G van B, Lawsing JF, Hohl M. Tears of the transverse ligmanet of the atlas. *J Bone Joint Surg* 1974;56A:1683–1691.
22. Fielding JW, Burstein AH, Frankel VH. The nuchal ligament. *Spine* 1976;1:3–14.
23. Feindell WH, Weddell G, Sinclair DC. Pain sensibility in deep somatic structures. *J Neurol Neurosurg Psychiatry* 1948;11:113–116.
24. Feinstein B, Langton JBK, Jameson RM, Schiller F. Experiments on referred pain from deep somatic tissues. *J Bone Joint Surg* 1954;36A: 981–997.
25. Garrett WE, Saffrean MR, Seaber AV, et al. Biomechanical comparison of stimulated and non-stimulated muscle pulled to failure. *Am J Sports Med* 1987;15:448–454.
26. Garrett WE, Nikolau PK, Ribbeck BM, et al. The effect of muscle architecture on the biomechanical failure properties of skeletal muscle under passive tension. *Am J Sports Med* 1988;16:7–12.
27. Griffin CJ, Hawthorn R, Harris R. Anatomy and histology of the human temporomandibular joint. *Monogr Oral Sci* 1975;4:1–26.
28. Guerrier Y, Colin R. Le deuxieme nerf cervical. *Comptes Rendues de l'Association des Anatomistes* 1954;41:813–816.
29. Hackett GS, Huang TC, Raftery A. Prolotherapy for headache. *Headache* 1962;2:20–28.
30. Hammond SR, Danta G. Occipital neuralgia. *Clin Exp Neurol* 1978;15: 258–270.
31. Inman VT, Saunders JB de CM. Referred pain from skeletal structures. *J Nerv Ment Dis* 1944;99:660–667.
32. Jensen R, Rasmussen BK, Pedersen B, Lous I, Olesen J. Cephalic muscle tenderness and pressure pain threshold in a general population. *Pain* 1992;48:197–203.
33. Jonsson H, Bring G, Rauschning W, Sahlstedt B. Hidden cervical spine injuries in traffic accident victims with skull fractures. *J Spinal Dis* 1991;4:251–263.
34. Kayfetz DO, Blumenthal LS, Hackett GS, Hemwall GA, Neff FE. Whiplash injury and other ligamentous headache—its management with prolotherapy. *Headache* 1963;3:24–28.
35. Kimmel DL. The cervical sympathetic rami and the vertebral plexus in the human foetus. *J Comp Neurol* 1959;112:141–161.
36. Kimmel DL. Innervation of the spinal dura mater and dura mater of the posterior cranial fossa. *Neurology* 1960;10:800–809.
37. Langemark M, Olesen J. Pericranial tenderness in tension headache. *Cephalalgia* 1987;7:249–255.
38. Lord SM, Barnsley L, Wallis BJ, Bogduk N. Third occipital nerve headache: a prevalence study. *J Neurol Neurosurg Psychiatry* 1994;57: 1187–1196.
39. Lous I, Olesen J. Evaluation of pericranial tenderness and oral function in patients with common migraine, muscle contraction headache and combination headache. *Pain* 1982;12:385–393.
40. Martin BC, Fagan PJ. The surgical therapy of certain occipital headaches. *Plast Reconstr Surg* 1964;33:266–268.
41. McCormick, CC. Arthrography of the atlanto-axial (C1-C2) joints: technique and results. *J Intervent Radiol* 1987;2:9–13.
42. Murphy JP. Occipital neurectomy in the treatment of headache. *Md Med J* 1969;18:62–66.
43. Niepel GA, Sit'aj S. Enthesopathy. *Clin Rheum Dis* 1979;5:857–872.
44. Nikolau PK, MacDonald BL, Glisson RR, et al. Biomechanical and histological evaluation of muscle after controlled strain injury. *Am J Sports Med* 1987;15:9–14.
45. Oleson J. Some clinical features of the acute migraine attack. An analysis of 750 patients. *Headache* 1978;18:268–271.
46. Olesen J, Langemark M. Mechanisms of tension headache: a speculative hypothesis. In: Olesen J, Edvinsson L, eds. *Basic mechanisms of headache.* Amsterdam: Elsevier, 1988:457–461.
47. Ouaknine G, Nathan H. Anastomotic connections between the eleventh nerve and the posterior root of the first cervical nerve in humans. *J Neurosurg* 1973;38:189–197.
48. Panjabi MM, Oxland TR, Parks EH. Quantitative anatomy of cervical spine ligaments. Part II. Middle and lower cervical spine. *J Spinal Dis* 1991;4:277–285.
49. Robinson HS. Rheumatoid arthritis: atlanto-axial subluxation and its clinical presentation. *Can Med Assoc J* 1966;94:470–477
50. Schellhas KP. Internal derangement of the temporomandibular joint: radiologic staging with clinical, surgical and pathologic correlation. *Magn Reson Imaging* 1989;7:495–515.
51. Schweitzer ME, Hodler J, Cervilla V, Resnick D. Craniovertebral junction: normal anatomy with MR correlation. *AJR Am J Roentgenol* 1992; 158:1087–1090.
52. Sharp J, Purser DW. Spontaneous atlanto-axial dislocation in ankylosing spondylitis and rheumatoid arthritis. *Ann Rheum Dis* 1961;20:47–77.
53. Simons DG. Myofascial pain syndromes: where are we? where are we going? *Arch Phys Med Rehabil* 1988;69:207–212.
54. Smith GR, Beckly DE, Abel MS. Articular mass fracture: a neglected cause of post traumatic neck pain? *Clin Radiol* 1976;27:335–340.
55. Stevens JS, Cartlidge NEF, Saunders M, Appleby A, Hall M, Shaw DA. Atlanto-axial subluxation and cervical myelopathy in rheumatoid arthritis. *QJM* 1971;159:391–408.
56. Travell JG, Simons DG. *Myofascial pain and dysfunction:* the trigger point manual. Baltimore: Williams & Wilkins, 1983.
57. Vital JM, Grenier F, Dautheribes M, Baspeyre H, Lavignolle B, Senegas J. An anatomic and dynamic study of the greater occipital nerve (n. of Arnold). *Surg Radiol Anat* 1989;11:205–210.
58. Woodring JH, Goldstein SJ. Fractures of the articular processes of the cervical spine. *AJR Am J Roentgenol* 1982;139:341–344.
59. Yu S, Sether L, Haughton VM. Facet joint menisci of the cervical spine: correlative MR imaging and cryomicrotomy study. *Radiology* 1987;164: 79–82.
60. Zapletal J, Hekster REM, Straver JS, Wilmink JT, Hermans J. Relationship between atlanto-odontoid osteoarthritis and idiopathic suboccipital nec pain. *Neuroradiology* 1996;38:62–65

The Headaches, Second Edition,
edited by J. Olesen, P. Tfelt-Hansen, and K.M.A. Welch.
Lippincott Williams & Wilkins, Philadelphia © 2000.

*Tension-Type Headache, Cluster Headache, and Miscellaneous
Primary Headaches*

CHAPTER 71

Genetics of Tension-Type Headache

Michael Bjørn Russell and Jes Olesen

Several environmental factors were listed in the International Headache Society (IHS) classification as the most frequent causative mechanisms (1). Until recently, a genetic factor has not been suspected.

EPISODIC TENSION-TYPE HEADACHE

The overall lifetime prevalence of episodic tension-type headache in the general population is 75%, 83% among women and 67% among men (5). The high prevalence causes a positive family history simply by chance in more than 99% of probands with four first-degree relatives (i.e., parents, siblings, and children) and one or both parents are affected by chance in more than 94% of families. Thus, a positive family history does not suggest the presence of a genetic factor. A genetic epidemiologic survey of probands with and without episodic tension-type headache using blind interviews of the relatives is more informative but cannot elucidate the importance of genetic factor as a result of its extremely high prevalence. Episodic tension-type headache is most likely a heterogeneous disorder. The uniform symptomatology makes it likely that nociceptive mechanisms are shared but can be activated by different mechanisms. Each mechanism may be caused by mutation in a single gene inherited in a mendelian fashion. Alternatively, episodic tension-type headache may be caused by multiple genes in a concerted action with environmental factors, or it may be non-genetic. Pathophysiological studies may be a key to discovering different mechanisms that can cause episodic tension-type headache.

CHRONIC TENSION-TYPE HEADACHE

Familial Aggregation

Only a single genetic epidemiologic study has investigated the familial aggregation of chronic tension-type headache (3). It included 122 probands from a headache clinic meeting the criteria of the IHS for chronic tension-type headache (1). The proband's first-degree relatives and spouses aged 18 years or older also were interviewed by a neurologic resident. Table 1 shows chronic tension-type headache assessed by proband report compared with the clinical interview by the neurologic resident. The observed agreement rate was 82%, and kappa, the agreement rate corrected for chance agreement, was 48% (8). The sensitivity was 68%. Thus, direct interviews of probands, first-degree relatives, and spouses are necessary in genetic studies of chronic tension-type headache. The risk of familial occurrence was assessed by estimating the population relative risk (9).

$$\frac{Prob \text{ (relative is affected | proband is affected)}}{Prob \text{ (random member of the population is affected)}}$$

A family aggregation is implied when this risk ratio significantly exceeds 1. The 1-year prevalence of chronic tension-type headache is 3%: 5% among women and 2% among men (6). The lifetime prevalence has been estimated to be twice the 1-year prevalence (8). Because the prevalence of chronic tension-type headache depends on age and gender, the value of the denominator was

M. B. Russell and J. Olesen: Department of Neurology, Glostrup Hospital, University of Copenhagen, DK-2600 Glostrup, Copenhagen, Denmark.

TABLE 1. *Sensitivity, specificity, and predictive values of chronic tension-type headache assessed by proband report compared to the clinical interview*

		Interview			
		Yes n (%)	No n (%)	Total n (%)	Kappa 95% confidence limits
Proband	Yes	48 (13)	43 (11)	91 (24)	0.48 (0.37; 0.60)
	No	23 (6)	263 (70)	286 (77)	
	Total	71 (19)	306 (81)	377 (100)	

Sensitivity: 68% (48/71).
Specificity: 86% (263/306).
PVpos: 53% (48/91).
PVneg: 92% (263/286).
From ref. 8.

adjusted according to the distribution of age and gender in the group of relatives studied.

Figure 1 shows the population relative risk of chronic tension-type headache among first-degree relatives and spouses. Compared with the general population, first-degree relatives had a 3.1-fold significantly increased risk of chronic tension-type headache, whereas spouses had no increased risk of chronic tension-type headache (3). An increased familial risk can be caused by both genetic and environmental factors; however, the results support the importance of genetic factors because first-degree relatives on average share half their genes with the proband, and spouses and probands have different genetic backgrounds, whereas probands, first-degree relatives, and spouses in part share a common environment. The probands in the genetic epidemiologic survey were recruited from a headache clinic, and not from the general population (3). This selection is most likely of minor importance because most Danish patients with chronic tension-type headache consult a specialist or a hospital (4). All interviews were performed by the same inter-

viewer as multiple interviewers invariably increase diagnostic variability (2). The definition of chronic tension-type headache by the International Headache Society makes genetic studies complicated because it is separated from episodic tension-type headache primarily by the attack frequency (1). The Headache Classification Committee chose 180 days per year as the cutoff point in the absence of good scientific evidence. This point is important to take into consideration in future studies.

Mode of Inheritance

A complex segregation analysis of 122 families mentioned above gave the sporadic model (no family resemblance) a poor fit compared with the multifactorial model (7). None of the three models that incorporated a major locus (i.e., recessive, additive, and dominant major locus) explained the observed segregation pattern better than the multifactorial model. Thus, the complex segregation analysis supported that chronic tension-type headache has a genetic cause because the multifactorial model had a significantly better fit than the sporadic model. A complex segregation analysis cannot detect a phenotype caused by different genotypes, that is, genetic heterogeneity. Thus, multifactorial inheritance may alternatively reflect genetic heterogeneity of chronic tension-type headache. To date, it has not been possible to discriminate different subgroups of chronic tension-type by clinical characteristics (7).

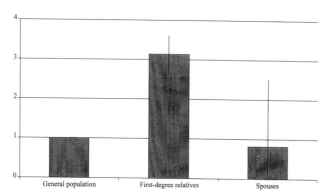

FIG. 1. Age and gender standardized lifetime risk of chronic tension-type headache among first-degree relatives and spouses of probands with chronic tension-type headache. The vertical lines denote 95% confidence intervals.

REFERENCES

1. Headache Classification Committee of the International Headache Society. Classification and diagnostic criteria for headache disorders, cranial neuralgias and facial pain. *Cephalalgia* 1988;8:1–96.
2. Leone M, Filippini G, D'Amico D, Farinotti M, Bussone G. Assessment of International Headache Society diagnostic criteria: a reliability study. *Cephalalgia* 1994;14:280–284.
3. Østergaard S, Russell MB, Bendtsen L, Olesen J. Comparison of first degree relatives and spouses of people with chronic tension-type headache. *BMJ* 1997;314:1092–1093.
4. Rasmussen BK, Jensen R, Olesen J. Impact of headache on sickness

absence and utilisation of medical services: a Danish population study. *J Epidemiol Community Health* 1992;46:443–446.

5. Rasmussen BK, Jensen R, Schroll M, Olesen J. Epidemiology of headache in a general population-a prevalence study. *J Clin Epidemiol* 1991;44:1147–1157.

6. Rasmussen BK, Jensen R, Schroll M, Olesen J. Interrelations between migraine and tension-type headache in the general population. *Arch Neurol* 1992;49:914–918.

7. Russell MB, Iselius L, Østergaard S, Olesen J. Inheritance of chronic tension-type headache investigated by complex segregation analysis. *Hum Genet* 1998;102:138–140.

8. Russell MB, Østergaard S, Bendtsen L, Olesen J. Familial occurrence of chronic tension-type headache. *Cephalalgia* 1999;19:207–210.

9. Weiss KM, Chakraborty R, Majumder PP, Smouse PE. Problems in the assessment of relative risk of chronic disease among biological relatives of affected individuals. *J Chronic Dis* 1982;35:539–551.

The Headaches, Second Edition,
edited by J. Olesen, P. Tfelt-Hansen, and K.M.A. Welch.
Lippincott Williams & Wilkins, Philadelphia © 2000.

Tension-Type Headache, Cluster Headache, and Miscellaneous Primary Headaches

CHAPTER 72

Human Studies of Experimental Pain from Muscle

Peter Svensson and Kai Jensen

Experimental pain studies in healthy subjects represent one of many approaches to gaining more insight into the pathophysiologic mechanisms involved in headache (see Chapter 24) as well as in other clinical pain conditions (1). In research on tension-type headache, special emphasis has been given to the function of the epicranial, temporomandibular, and neck muscles (see Chap. 73–75). This chapter describes human experimental models developed specifically to investigate pain originating from muscle tissue.

In general, experimental pain research involves a standardized induction of pain and the appropriate assessment of the responses (Fig. 1). The evoked pain responses can be recorded by a wide variety of techniques ranging from simple measures of perceived intensity to sophisticated imaging equipment and high-technology measures of motor and autonomic function. The particular assessment technique always depends on the specific aim of the experimental study; the reader is referred to recent comprehensive reviews for more detailed descriptions (1,5). This chapter focuses mainly on the models available to induce pain in the cervicotrigeminal system, including chemical, mechanical, and electric stimulation and exercise-induced activation of human-muscle nociceptors (see Fig. 1).

P. Svensson: Center for Sensory-Motor Interaction, Aalborg University, DK-9220 Aalborg E, and Royal Dental College, University of Århus, DK-8000 Århus C, Denmark.

K. Jensen: Department of Neurology, Hilleroed Hospital, DK-3400 Hilleroed, Denmark.

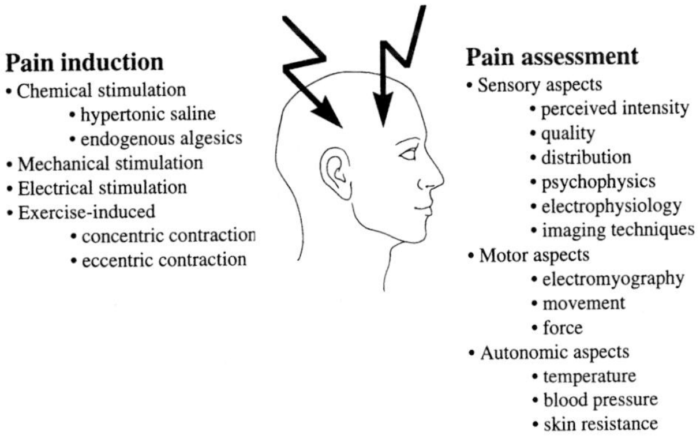

Pain induction
- Chemical stimulation
  - hypertonic saline
  - endogenous algesics
- Mechanical stimulation
- Electrical stimulation
- Exercise-induced
  - concentric contraction
  - eccentric contraction

Pain assessment
- Sensory aspects
  - perceived intensity
  - quality
  - distribution
  - psychophysics
  - electrophysiology
  - imaging techniques
- Motor aspects
  - electromyography
  - movement
  - force
- Autonomic aspects
  - temperature
  - blood pressure
  - skin resistance

FIG. 1. Overview of experimental techniques to induce human muscle pain and to assess pain responses.

CHEMICAL STIMULATION

Hypertonic Saline

Intramuscular injection of hypertonic saline (4%–6%) has been by far the most frequently used chemical stimulus in human experimental muscle-pain research and therefore is described in detail, although potassium chloride and hypotonic saline solutions also can induce pain (11). A major reason for the popularity of hypertonic saline is the safety of this technique; no side effects after numerous intramuscular injections have been reported (30). Unfortunately, this stimulus is a nonspecific painful stimulus in that nonnociceptive afferents may be activated concomitantly with the activation of nociceptive group III and IV afferents (20). In addition, tissue trauma from the injection needle may be a confounding factor. Nevertheless, intramuscular injections of hypertonic saline clearly evoke neuronal activity in convergent spinal dorsal horn neurons and in neurons encoding nociceptive information in the nucleus submedius in the thalamus, and the dominant sensation in conscious humans is a deep aching pain (6,11,14,30,33,40). This evidence indicates that hypertonic saline is indeed a potent chemical stimulus for activation of muscle nociceptors.

Kellgren (14) was the first to describe the quality and intensity of saline-induced pain in the temporomandibular and suboccipital muscles. He noted a rapid increase in pain intensity shortly after a bolus injection of 0.1 mL of 6% saline into the masseter muscle associated with a spread of pain to adjacent regions of the face, including the teeth. The pain peaked after 1 to 2 minutes and faded over a period of 3 to 5 minutes. This preliminary description of one subject was later verified in larger study populations both with bolus injections into the temporalis muscle (11,30) and into the masseter muscle (30,33,34, 36). It is a consistent finding that pain after intramuscular bolus injection of saline starts after a short delay of 10 to 15 seconds, suggesting that a gradual buildup of the osmotic pressure is a prerequisite for activation of the nociceptors. The available data do not suggest major differences in the quality or intensity of the pain from hypertonic saline injections into the temporalis or masseter muscles, and the localization of pain is partly overlapping (Fig. 2). Thus, both sites of experimental muscle pain are represented in regions where patients with tension-type headache often report their symptoms (9). Recently, the bolus injection technique was refined so that a computer-controlled syringe pump can maintain a continuous slow infusion of hypertonic saline up to 15 to 20 minutes with relatively constant pain in the temporomandibular muscles (42) and in the leg and arm muscles (6) (Fig. 3). This type of tonic experimental pain seems to have similar qualities to clinical pain conditions (30) and allows suffi-

cient time for detailed studies of sensory and motor effects of pain (6,36).

An interesting sensory feature of intramuscular saline injection is the spread and referral of pain to adjacent regions. Pain induced in the suboccipital muscles of one subject was perceived as a headache (14), and repeated injections into the temporalis muscle of another single subject caused pain in the neck muscles (28). More recent studies in larger populations showed that pain from the temporalis muscle can be referred to both the upper and lower jaw, ear, and eye region (11) and that pain from the masseter muscle is described as being located above the temporomandibular joint, posterior teeth in the upper and lower jaw, and temple region (30,33,34,36) (see Fig. 2). Generally, the spread and referral patterns from saline-induced pain and from activation of clinical trigger points show strong resemblance (39). The neurophysiologic mechanisms responsible for the spread and referral of muscle pain are not entirely clear but are likely to involve central convergence of peripheral afferents onto wide dynamic-range neurons in the dorsal horn and subnucleus caudalis (26). Another likely mechanism is actually central divergence, because a painful input may open up new spinal/trigeminal connections that formerly were ineffective; the nociceptive input of a single fiber then may become suprathreshold for a greater number of neurons (19). The pathophysiology of trigger points and the associated spread of pain are still discussed. In human experimental subjects, it can be shown that the occurrence of referred pain is correlated to the perceived pain intensity (11) and that the perceived area of masseter pain increases as a function of time with muscle pain (36), in accordance with studies in animal models that have shown increases of receptive fields after noxious stimulation of deep tissues in the trigeminal area (26).

Intramuscular injection of hypertonic saline into the temporomandibular muscles also causes significant increases in the superficial somatosensory sensibility as measured by Von Frey hair stimuli (36) and in deep sensibility as measured by pressure-pain thresholds (11,34). These experimental findings of superficial and deep hyperresponsiveness are consistent with the results from studies in animal models of deep trigeminal pain (26). Thus, there is good evidence to suggest both a qualitative and quantitative change in the processing of somatosensory information during ongoing muscle pain.

In addition to standardized descriptions of somatosensory changes induced by experimental muscle pain, the model with hypertonic saline also can be used to examine the effects of pain on motor function. Muscle dysfunction has long been thought to be an important etiologic factor for the development and maintenance of myogenous symptoms. Thus, induction of pain in healthy subjects may provide insight into the cause-and-effect relationship between pain and muscle function, which is difficult to

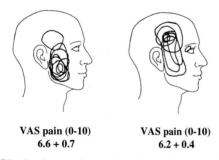

VAS pain (0-10)
6.6 + 0.7

VAS pain (0-10)
6.2 + 0.4

FIG. 2. Distribution and perceived intensity of pain during standardized injection (0.2 mL) of hypertonic saline into the masseter (*left*) and temporalis (*right*) muscle of healthy subjects. Bolus infusion of 5% saline (n = 7). Note the overlap between the two injections and the spread of pain from the injection site.

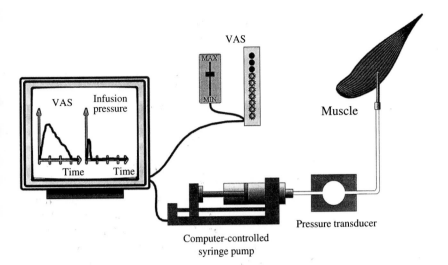

FIG. 3. Experimental setup developed for continuous infusion of small amounts of, for example, hypertonic saline into the muscles. The computer program controls the syringe pump and samples the perceived pain intensity as indicated on the VAS and the infusion pressure.

establish from clinical studies of patients with tension-type headache or temporomandibular disorders.

Experimental pain from the masseter muscle has a profound effect on dynamic repetitive movements such as chewing; that is, the amplitude of the jaw movements are smaller, and there is less electromyographic (EMG) activity in the jaw-closing phase and more EMG activity in the jaw-opening phase, suggesting a guarding and protective effect (33). These experimental results are in strict accordance with the pain-adaptation model presented by Lund and co-workers (17). This model suggests an inhibitory influence of nociceptive activity on the alpha-motoneuron pool through a central pattern generator and brainstem interneurons during agonist function and excitatory influence during antagonist function. Studies in animal models and direct recordings from interneurons in the brainstem support this hypothesis (41). The model with hypertonic saline also shed light on the classic, still controversial problem of increased or nonincreased postural EMG activity in patients with tension-type headache and temporomandibular disorders. Stohler and colleagues (31) showed a small increase (1–2 μV) in the temporalis and masseter muscles during a period of saline-induced pain from the masseter muscle in 20 healthy subjects; however, these authors attributed the small EMG activity recorded by using surface electrodes to contamination from mimic muscles, because similar changes were observed in control experiments in which pain was "imagined." Svensson and colleagues (37) used intramuscular electrodes but could not show any relation between pain intensity and EMG changes. Thus, no experimental evidence has been found to suggest a long-lasting muscle hyperactivity induced by pain in temporomandibular muscles.

A final possibility is to use hypertonic saline as a pain-provoking stimulus in patients with pain. Thus, 12 patients with widespread muscle pain and a clinical diagnosis of fibromyalgia reported significantly more pain

and larger spread of pain induced by hypertonic saline into the anterior tibialis muscle than did healthy control subjects (29). Preliminary results from patients with whiplash syndrome also showed this facilitation of pain responses, probably suggesting a state of hyperexcitability in the central nervous system. As yet, no such studies have been performed in patients with tension-type headache.

In conclusion, injection of hypertonic saline into temporomandibular muscles is a valuable model to study basic sensory and motor effects of pain and has contributed to the recent understanding of pathophysiologic mechanisms in tension-type headache and temporomandibular disorders. Obviously, no experimental pain model in healthy subjects can encompass the entire neurobiologic or psychologic complexity of clinical pain conditions lasting many days, weeks, or longer; however, at present the hypertonic saline model may be the best model for mimicking clinical pain conditions, because pain can be maintained for up to 15 to 20 minutes without damage or side effects.

Endogenous Algogenic Substances

Intramuscular injections of numerous endogenous algogenic substances and neuropeptides also have been tested for chemical activation of human-muscle nociceptors (Table 1). Substantial evidence has been found from studies in animal models that bradykinin (BK) and 5-hydroxytryptamine (5-HT) can trigger action potentials in nociceptive group III and IV fibers (20). When injected into the human temporalis muscle, 5-HT does not induce significant levels of pain, and BK induces only relatively low levels of pain (12). Injections of combinations of 5-HT and BK cause significantly more pain than injections of isotonic saline and a significant reduction of pressure–pain thresholds, a finding that supports the importance of presensitization with 5-HT for BK-

TABLE 1. *Chemical substances used for activation of human-muscle nociceptors*

Hypertonic saline (4%–20%/0.2–1.0 mL)
Hypotonic saline
Potassium chloride (100 mM/0.2 mL)
Bradykinin (10 μM/0.2 mL)
Serotonin (10 μM/0.2 mL)
Substance P (1 μM/0.2 mL)
Calcitonin-gen-related-peptide (1 μM/0.2 mL)
Neurokinin A (1 μM/0.2 mL)
Capsaicin (0.01%, 1 mL)
Nerve growth factor (0.03–1.9 μg/kg)

induced neural activity. E-type prostaglandins also can sensitize muscle afferents to BK, which will release prostaglandin E_2 (PGE_2) from tissue cells, thereby potentiating its own action (20). Other neuropeptides were recently implicated in the modulation of muscle nociceptors, especially glutamate, and the NMDA receptors may play an important role in deep pain (19). Substance P (SP) has been studied extensively in cutaneous pain, but it does not appear to sensitize muscle nociceptors to mechanical stimuli (20). In itself, SP does not produce pain when injected into the human temporalis muscle (13); however, in combination with calcitonin gene-related peptide (CGRP) and BK, it does induce muscle pain and a significant reduction of pressure-pain thresholds in the temporal muscle (SP-BK) (13,23). It should be emphasized that peripheral and central sensitization and direct excitation may be discrete and separate neurobiologic processes. Thus, it is currently speculated that neurokinin-1 and NMDA receptors are involved in hyperexcitability of dorsal horn neurons, causing hyperalgesia; nitric oxid synthesis, on the other hand, seems to be related to spontaneous pain (19).

Apparently, only one study in humans has used intramuscular injection of capsaicin (chili-pepper extract), although this substance has been used extensively in cutaneous pain research. The pain was cramplike, severe, and associated with significant increases in neural activity of group III and IV muscle afferents (18). This stimulus may prove to be useful in future studies of human muscle pain.

Finally, an intriguing finding is that systemic administration of human nerve growth factor (NGF) in 45 healthy subjects induced pain, particularly in the temporomandibular muscles. The pain was more pronounced in women than in men and tended to worsen during function (24). Evidence now exists that estrogen and NGF may interact in the regulation of nociceptive processes; this finding could be important to explaining the female preponderance in tension-type headache and temporomandibular disorders (32).

In conclusion, injection of endogenous algogenic substances and neuropeptides can be helpful in characterizing the neurobiologic basis of human muscle pain, which in turn may be of clinical importance in headache conditions if intracranial changes can trigger the release of critical neuroactive substances by antidromic mechanisms influencing the peripheral conditions for myogenous nociception (9). Furthermore, this experimental approach will give insight into possible pharmacologic interventions and allow the testing of specific antagonists.

MECHANICAL STIMULATION

Few studies have applied mechanical stimuli to the temporomandibular muscles to induce pain. In contrast, mechanical stimuli delivered with pressure algometers have been used to assess the sensitivity of deep tissues (see Chapter 25), despite the fact that mechanical and chemical stimulation can be considered the most relevant stimuli for activating human-muscle nociceptors. Intense mechanical stimuli activate nociceptors in the muscle but, unfortunately, also in the skin. Thus, the evoked pain sensation may have a component from both types of tissue. Anesthetizing the skin will cause a significant elevation of the pressure-pain thresholds on temporomandibular muscles (25). The suggestion has been made that the interrelationship between afferent input from cutaneous and muscle tissues should be evaluated in patients who have muscle pain.

Only a few studies have used mechanical stimulation of the epicranial muscles and tissues to evoke pain. An original, old study applied a head-screw device in which the rubber-coated tips barely touched the scalp (28). Nevertheless, after 15 minutes, all the three of the tested subjects reported excruciating pain coming from the neck and scalp, which was associated with an increase in EMG activity of the neck muscles. Thus, the authors suggested that sustained painful mechanical stimulation of the epicranial muscles would lead to muscle hyperactivity of the neck muscles and that this was the cause of the developing neck pain. Many subsequent controlled EMG studies in headache patients, however, have been unable to demonstrate this muscle hyperactivity (see Chapter 74), and interpretation of the results should be viewed with caution. Clearly, more elaborate studies on longer-lasting mechanical stimulation of epicranial muscles are needed to determine the suitability of this model in experimental headache research.

ELECTRIC STIMULATION

Direct stimulation of muscle afferents can be accomplished by using intramuscular electrodes (40). Thus, the elicited sensation is described as a cramplike pain, often in combination with a visible muscle contraction. One disadvantage of this technique is activation of nonnociceptive afferents, and it cannot be regarded a specific pain stimulus. Furthermore, the peripheral receptors are bypassed and the axons stimulated directly. Nevertheless, this model is able to elicit referred pain areas in a reliable fashion (16) and, in contrast to chemical stimuli, can start and terminate the pain immediately.

Intraneural microstimulation (INMS) is an advanced and powerful but invasive technique for selective stimulation of single human-muscle afferents. The projected pain area increases as a function of stimulus duration (*temporal summation*) and as a function of a number of stimulated afferents (*spatial summation*) (18,27,38). So far, intramuscular electric stimulation of temporomandibular muscles or INMS of trigeminal nerves have not been attempted but might be an interesting technique in headache research because of the easy control of the stimulus parameters and the possibility of eliciting referred pain areas.

EXERCISE-INDUCED STIMULATION

It is a common experience that heavy and unaccustomed physical exercise can lead to significant levels of muscle soreness and pain. Thus, many experimental studies have used various muscle exercises to test the development of head pain. Generally, two different approaches can be used. One technique is based on repeated or sustained concentric contractions of the temporomandibular, epicranial, or suboccipital muscles. The other method involves repeated eccentric contractions that cause forced lengthening of the muscle fibers.

Concentric Contraction Models

In conditions with overloading and insufficient resting periods, concentric dynamic and isometric contractions will elicit muscle pain thought to share the same pathophysiologic mechanisms as ischemic pain (22). Ischemia alone is not sufficient to produce pain, but if it is combined with contractions, strong pain can develop. Accumulation of metabolites, such as lactate, potassium, or the lack of oxidation of metabolic products, in addition to mechanical determinants like the number of contractions, duration and force may play a significant role (20,22). Furthermore, hypoxia and the release of BK, PGE_2, and CGRP, in association with a reduced pH, can cause sensitization of muscle nociceptors, leading to pain evoked by mechanical stimulation during contractions (20).

In the cervicotrigeminal system, many studies have tried to establish an experimental model to induce head pain. A combination of dynamic concentric contractions (chewing) and ischemic block of the superficial temporal artery in healthy subjects causes a continuously increasing, bilateral dull frontal headache (7) with significantly more head pain and significantly shorter onset of pain than chewing without an ischemic block (21). In these models, the ischemia is achieved using scalp shygmomanometers wrapped around the head, which not only reduce blood circulation but also cause activity in cutaneous and deep mechanorecpetors like the head-screw device of Simons and colleagues (28).

Sustained or repeated static tooth-clenching procedures have long been known to cause intense pain with a rapid onset (2,4). The pain quickly disappears, however, and most studies have failed to show any significant pain in the temporomandibular muscles the following days after exercise. Jensen and associates (10) used a sustained tooth-clenching task to provoke pain attacks in migraine patients, but they were unable to show any effect on pericranial tenderness, although patients reported pain in the temporomandibular muscles immediately after the exercise. A recent study showed that even with 5 days of repeated submaximal tooth clenching, it is difficult to elicit longer-lasting muscle pain and soreness in healthy subjects (35). Also, studies with sustained submaximal contraction of the frontalis muscles have failed to produce significant levels of head pain (15).

Thus, it can be concluded that pain in the temporomandibular muscles cannot be readily induced in healthy subjects using the concentric contraction models. The contraction levels and duration have generally been in excess of what is found in clinical populations, which seems to suggest that simple concentric contraction of muscles may be inadequate to explain the pathophysiology of tension-type headache and temporomandibular disorders.

Eccentric Contraction Models

In contrast to the immediate and short-lasting muscle pain evoked by concentric contractions, eccentric contractions are more effective to induce a delayed onset of muscle pain or soreness. The mechanisms underlying this kind of muscle pain seem to be different from that of ischemic muscle pain. Muscle injuries at the ultrastructural level or damages in the connective tissue have been implicated because histologic studies have shown disorganization of myofilaments and extensive disruption of muscle structures localized particularly in the regions of the Z-discs (22). An increased level of intracellular calcium may damage muscle tissues, probably by activating phospholipase A, which acts on membrane phospholipid components and increases the availability of arachidonic acid. Forced lengthening of tetanic-stimulated masticatory muscles in mice demonstrated decreased contractile tension and elevated levels of plasma creatine kinase as indices of muscle injury (8). Experimental tooth grinding for 30 minutes, presumably involving eccentric contractions, originally was reported to cause significant levels of facial pain lasting for several days in nine healthy subjects (3); however, no information on pain intensity was provided for the following days. A later study reproduced the short-term results from Christensen (3) but unfortunately did not provide any data for the following days (2). In a recent study, 45 minutes of strong tooth grinding in 12 subjects caused only moderate levels of pain and tenderness during the following 3 days (Fig. 4). The distribution of pain was quite similar to the experimental mod-

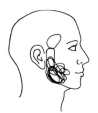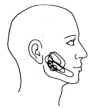

VAS pain (0-10)	VAS pain (0-10)
4.2 + 0.8	1.3 + 0.5

FIG. 4. Distribution and perceived intensity of pain immediately after (*left*) and 1 day after (*right*) a period with toothgrinding for 45 minutes (n = 12). Note the moderate pain intensity the day after the exercise and localization of pain in the masseter region.

els with hypertonic saline infusion, and it was notable that the temporal region was involved less often than the masseter region (see Fig. 4).

These results from exercise-induced activation of human-muscle nociceptors show that excessive and strong contractions of the muscles can cause pain in the head, but the pain is usually of rather short duration. No experimental evidence has been established showing that a self-perpetuating, vicious cycle can be initiated by muscle hyperactivity, leading to pain that again should lead to more muscle hyperactivity.

CONCLUSIONS

The experimental muscle-pain models must be chosen after careful consideration of the aim of the planned study, because each has a number of distinct advantages and also some potential disadvantages. It is important that some of the hypothesized etiologic factors for tension-type headache and temporomandibular disorders can be tested by using the experimental approach. Thus, muscle pain can be induced, and the sensory, motor, and autonomic effects can be described in standardized settings; it is also possible to induce putative painful motor tasks and then analyze the sensory outcome, which allows assumptions about the cause-and-effect relationship between pain and muscle (dys)function that are difficult to derive from basic animal studies and cross-sectional clinical studies. At present, no perfect model is available for tension-type headache, but by combining different experimental pain models in addition to the development of new models, it may be possible to elucidate the pathophysiologic mechanisms in tension-type headache.

ACKNOWLEDGMENT

Center for Sensory-Motor Interaction (SMI) is supported by the Danish National Research Foundation. Thomas Graven-Nielsen and Lars Arendt-Nielsen are greatly thanked for their comments on this manuscript.

REFERENCES

1. Arendt-Nielsen L. Induction and assessment of experimental pain from human skin, muscle, and viscera. In: Jensen TS, Turner JA, Wiesenfeld-Hallin Z, eds. *Proceedings of the 8th World Congress on Pain:* progress in pain research and management, Vol 8. Seattle: IASP Press, 1997: 393–425.
2. Bowley JF, Gale EN. Experimental masticatory muscle pain. *J Dent Res* 1987;66:1765–1769.
3. Christensen LV. Facial pain and internal pressure of masseter muscle in experimental bruxism in man. *Arch Oral Biol* 1971;16:1021–1031.
4. Clark GT, Adler RC, Lee JJ. Jaw pain and tenderness levels during and after repeated sustained maximum voluntary protrusion. *Pain* 1991;45: 17–22.
5. Gracely RH. Studies of pain in normal man. In: Wall PD, Melzack R, eds. *Textbook of pain.* Edinburgh: Churchill Livingstone, 1994: 315–336.
6. Graven-Nielsen T, Arendt-Nielsen L, Svensson P, Staehelin Jensen T. Quantification of local and referred muscle pain in humans after sequential i.m. injections of hypertonic saline. *Pain* 1997;69:111–117.
7. Göbel H, Cordes P. Circadian variation of pain sensitivity in pericranial musculature. *Headache* 1990;30:418–422.
8. Hutchins MO, Skjonsby HS, Brazeau GA, Parikh UK, Jenkins RM. Weakness in mouse masticatory muscles by repetitive contractions with forced lengthening. *J Dent Res* 1995;74:642–648.
9. Jaeger B. Tension-type headache and myofascial pain. In: Fricton JR, Dubner R, eds. *Orofacial pain and temporomandibular disorders.* New York: Raven Press, 1995:205–213.
10. Jensen K, Bülow P, Hansen H. Experimental toothclenching in common migraine. *Cephalalgia* 1985;5:245–251.
11. Jensen K, Norup M. Experimental pain in human temporal muscle induced by hypertonic saline, potassium and acidity. *Cephalalgia* 1992; 12:101–106.
12. Jensen K, Tuxen C, Pedersen-Bjergaard U, Jansen I, Edvinsson L, Olesen J. Pain and tenderness in human temporal muscle induced by bradykinin and 5-hydroxytryptamine. *Peptides* 1990;11:1127–1132.
13. Jensen K, Tuxen C, Pedersen-Bjergaard U, Jansen I. Pain, tenderness, wheal and flare induced by substance-P, bradykinin and 5-hydroxytryptamine in humans. *Cephalalgia* 1991;11:175–182.
14. Kellgren JH. Observations on referred pain arising from muscle. *Clin Sci* 1938;3:175–190.
15. Lacroix JM, Corbett L. An experimental test of the muscle tension hypothesis of tension-type headache. *Int J Psychophysiol* 1990;10: 47–51.
16. Laursen RJ, Graven-Nielsen T, Jensen TS, Arendt-Nielsen L. Quantification of local and referred pain in humans by intramuscular electrical stimulation. *Eur J Pain* 1997;1:105–113.
17. Lund JP, Donga R, Widmer CG, Stohler CS. The pain-adaptation model: a discussion of the relationship between chronic musculoskeletal pain and motor activity. *Can J Physiol Pharmacol* 1991;69: 683–694.
18. Marchettini P, Simone DA, Caputi G, Ochoa JL. Pain from excitation of identified muscle nociceptors in humans. *Brain Res* 1996;740: 109–116.
19. Mense S, Hoheisel U, Kaske A, Reinert A. Muscle pain: basic mechanisms and clinical correlates. In: Jensen TS, Turner JA, Wiesenfeld-Hallin Z, eds. *Proceedings of the 8th World Congress on Pain:* progress in pain research and management, vol 8. Seattle: IASP Press, 1997: 479–496.
20. Mense S. Nociception from skeletal muscle in relation to clinical muscle pain. *Pain* 1993;54:241–289.
21. Meyers DE, McCall WD. Head pain as a result of experimental ischemic exercise of the temporalis muscle. *Headache* 1983;23: 113–116.
22. Newham DJ, Edwards RHT, Mills KR. Skeletal muscle pain. In: Wall PD, Melzack R, eds. *Textbook of pain.* Edinburgh: Churchill Livingstone, 1994:423–440.
23. Pedersen-Bjergaard U, Nielsen LB, Jensen K, Edvinsson L, Jansen I, Olesen J. Calcitonin gene-related peptide, neurokinin A and substance P: effects on nociception and neurogenic inflammation in human skin and temporal muscle. *Peptides* 1991;12:333–337.
24. Petty BG, Cornblath DR, Adornato BT, et al. The effects of systematically administered recombinant human nerve growth factor in healthy human subjects. *Ann Neurol* 1994;36:244–246.

25. Reid KI, Carlson C, Rayens MK, Gracely RH. The influence of cutaneous tissue afferents on masticatory pain-pressure thresholds. *J Orofacial Pain* 1996;10:324–329.

26. Sessle BJ. Masticatory muscle disorders: basic science perspectives. In: Sessle BJ, Bryant PS, Dionne RA, eds. *Temporomandibular disorders and related pain conditions.* Seattle: IASP Press, 1995:47–61.

27. Simone A, Marchettini P, Caputi G, Ochoa JL. Identification of muscle afferents subserving sensation of deep pain in humans. *J Neurophysiol* 1994;72:883–889.

28. Simons DJ, Day E, Goodell H, Wolff HG. Experimental studies on headache: muscles of the scalp and neck as sources of pain. *Assoc Res Nerv Ment Dis* 1943;23:228–244.

29. Sörensen J, Graven-Nielsen T, Henriksson KG, Bengtsson M, Arendt-Nielsen L. Hyperexcitability in fibromyalgia. *J Rheumatol* 1998;25:152–155.

30. Stohler CS, Lund JP. Effects of noxious stimulation of the jaw muscles on the sensory experience of volunteer human subjects. In: Stohler CS, Carlson DS, eds. *Biological and psychological aspects of orofacial pain:* craniofacial growth series 29. Center for Human Growth and Development. Ann Arbor: University of Michigan, 1994:55–73.

31. Stohler CS, Zhang X, Lund JP. The effect of experimental jaw muscle pain on postural muscle activity. *Pain* 1996;66:215–221.

32. Stohler CS. Masticatory myalgias: emphasis on the nerve growth factor-estrogen link. *Pain Forum* 1997;6:176–180.

33. Svensson P, Arendt-Nielsen L, Houe L. Sensory-motor interactions of human experimental unilateral jaw muscle pain: a quantitative analysis. *Pain* 1996;64:241–249.

34. Svensson P, Arendt-Nielsen L, Nielsen H, Larsen JK. Effect of chronic and experimental jaw-muscle pain on pain-pressure thresholds and stimulus-response curves. *J Orofacial Pain* 1995;9:347–356.

35. Svensson P, Arendt-Nielsen L. Effects of 5 days repeated submaximal clenching on masticatory muscle pain and tenderness: an experimental study. *J Orofacial Pain* 1996;10:330–338.

36. Svensson P, Graven-Nielsen T, Arendt-Nielsen L. Mechanical hyperesthesia of human facial skin induced by tonic painful stimulation of jaw-muscles. *Pain* 1998;74:93–100.

37. Svensson P, Graven-Nielsen T, Matre D, Arendt-Nielsen L. Experimental muscle pain does not cause long-lasting increase in resting EMG activity. *Muscle Nerve* 1998;21:1382–1389.

38. Torebjörk HE, Ochoa JL, Schady W. Referred pain from intraneural stimulation of muscle fascicles in the median nerve. *Pain* 1984;18:145–156.

39. Travell JG, Simons DG. *Myofascial pain and dysfunction:* the trigger point manual. Baltimore: Williams & Wilkins, 1983, 219–248.

40. Vecchiet L, Dragani L, Bigontina P, Obletter G, Giamberardino MA. Experimental referred pain and hyperalgesia from muscles in humans. In: Vecchiet L, Albe-Fessard D, Lindblom U, eds. *New trends in referred pain and hyperalgesia.* Amsterdam: Elsevier, 1993:239–249.

41. Westberg K-G, Clavelou P, Schwartz G, Lund JP. Effects of chemical stimulation of masseter muscle nociceptors on trigeminal motoneuron and interneuron activities during fictive mastication in the rabbit. *Pain* 1997;73:295–308.

42. Zhang X, Ashton-Miller JA, Stohler CS. A closed-loop system for maintaining constant experimental muscle pain in man. *IEEE Trans Biomed Eng* 1993;40:344–352.

The Headaches, Second Edition,
edited by J. Olesen, P. Tfelt-Hansen, and K.M.A. Welch.
Lippincott Williams & Wilkins, Philadelphia © 2000.

Tension-Type Headache, Cluster Headache, and Miscellaneous
Primary Headaches

CHAPTER 73

Sensitization of Myofascial Pain Pathways in Tension-Type Headache

Lars Bendtsen and Messoud Ashina

It has been accepted for decades that pericranial myofascial tissues are considerably more tender in patients with tension-type headache than in healthy subjects. Moreover, it has been assumed that the nociceptive impulses from the pericranial myofascial tissues are referred to the head and perceived as headache and that myofascial pain therefore plays an important role in tension-type headache (19). Previously, headache research focused mainly on peripheral factors as the source of muscle pain, because it was believed that muscle pain implied muscle pathology. Basic pain research, however, has revealed that the nervous system is highly plastic, that is, that the response generated by the somatosensory system to a defined input is not fixed or static (30). Of particular importance is the fact that the pain pathways from myofascial tissues to the thalamus/sensory cortex may become sensitized; that is, the excitability of the nociceptive neurons may become increased under certain circumstances (29). In agreement with this fact, recent studies demonstrated that sensitization plays an important role in tension-type headache. The evidence for and possible mechanisms leading to sensitization of myofascial pain pathways in tension-type headache are discussed.

L. Bendtsen and M. Ashina: Department of Neurology, Glostrup Hospital, University of Copenhagen, DK-2600 Glostrup, Copenhagen, Denmark.

PAIN SENSITIVITY IN TENSION-TYPE HEADACHE

Tenderness to Manual Palpation

Manual palpation is by far the most widely used method for the evaluation of myofascial pain sensitivity in patients with tension-type headache both in the clinic and in the laboratory. During manual palpation, the observer evaluates the degree of tenderness (i.e., the pressure-induced pain) elicited by moderate finger pressure (see Chapter 80). As mentioned, it has been accepted for decades that the pericranial myofascial tissues are considerably more tender in patients with tension-type headache than in healthy subjects. This abnormality was documented for the first time in a blinded study in 1987 (23) and was later confirmed in a few blinded (17,18,24) and in numerous open studies (1,4,11). The pericranial tenderness was increased both in patients with episodic and in patients with chronic tension-type headache (16,18). The tenderness seems to be uniformly increased throughout the pericranial region, and both muscles and tendon insertions have been found to be excessively tender (4,18,23) (Fig. 1). In addition, pericranial tenderness is positively associated with both the intensity and the frequency of tension-type headache (18).

Pain Thresholds

Possible mechanisms leading to the increased myofascial pain sensitivity in tension-type headache include (a)

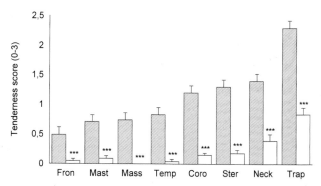

FIG. 1. Local tenderness scores (mean ± SE) at eight pericranial locations in 40 patients with chronic tension-type headache (*hatched bars*) and in 40 healthy controls (*open bars*). The patients had significantly more tenderness than the controls at all locations, *** denotes $p \leq 0.0002$. *Fron*, frontal muscle; *Mast*, mastoid process; *Mass*, masseter muscle; *Temp*, temporal muscle; *Coro*, coronoid process; *Ster*, sternocleidomastoid muscle; *Neck*, neck-muscle insertions; *Trap*, trapezius muscle. (Reproduced from ref. 4, with permission.)

activation or sensitization of peripheral myofascial nociceptors, (b) sensitization of second-order neurons at the level of the spinal dorsal horn/trigeminal nucleus, (c) sensitization of supraspinal neurons, and (d) decreased antinociceptive activity from supraspinal structures. The measurement of pain sensitivity to various types of stimuli applied to various parts of the body provided important information about the nociceptive system in tension-type headache. Thus, the pressure pain detection threshold, that is, the lowest pressure stimulus that is perceived as painful, has been found to be normal in patients with episodic tension-type headache (9,18) and in groups of mixed episodic and chronic tension-type headache patients (7,15) (Table 1). In contrast, pressure pain detection thresholds were decreased in patients with chronic tension-type headache in two studies (4,28) (Fig.

2, see Table 1). The same result was found indirectly in an earlier study that compared patients with chronic tension-type headache with historical controls (22). One population study found normal pressure pain detection thresholds in 14 subjects with chronic tension-type headache (18). This study is, however, difficult to compare with the aforementioned studies because of the low number of subjects examined and, more importantly, because the subjects in the population study probably clinically were affected less than the patients in the three other studies, who were recruited from specialized headache centers. The pressure pain tolerance threshold, that is, the maximal pressure stimulus that is tolerated, has been compared only between chronic tension-type headache patients and healthy controls in one study (4), although pain tolerance is generally considered a better and more reproducible correlate to clinical pain than pain detection (28). In this study (4), pressure pain tolerance thresholds in the finger were significantly lower in chronic tension-type headache patients than in healthy controls (see Fig. 2). The lower pressure pain detection and tolerance thresholds indicate the presence of both allodynia, that is, pain elicited by stimuli that normally are not perceived as painful, and hyperalgesia, that is, increased sensitivity to painful stimuli, in patients with chronic tension-type headache.

Patients with chronic tension-type headache are also hypersensitive to stimuli other than pressure (see Table 1). Langemark and colleagues (22) found significantly decreased pain detection thresholds to thermal stimuli in patients with chronic tension-type headache. Furthermore, both the pain-detection threshold (4) (see Fig. 2) and the pain-tolerance threshold (21) to electric stimuli were decreased in these patients. Sensitivity to the various stimulus modalities (pressure, thermal, electric) is increased at both cephalic and extracephalic locations (4, 21,22,28). The fact that chronic tension-type headache patients are hypersensitive to several types of stimuli

TABLE 1. *Pain threshold studies in tension-type headache*

Population	Pain threshold	Abnormal	Reference
Episodic TH	Pressure-pain detection	No	Göbel et al., 1992 (9)
	Pressure-pain detection	No	Jensen et al., 1993 (18)
Mixed TH	Pressure-pain detection	No	Bovim et al., 1992 (7)
	Pressure-pain detection	No	Jensen et al., 1996 (15)
Chronic TH	Thermal-pain detection	Yes	Langemark et al., 1989 (22)
	Pressure-pain detection	Yes	Schoenen et al., 1991 (28)
	Pressure-pain detection	No	Jensen et al., 1993 (18)
	Electric-pain tolerance	Yes	Langemark et al., 1993 (21)
	Pressure-pain detection	Yes	Bendtsen et al., 1996 (4)
	Pressure-pain tolerance	Yes	Bendtsen et al., 1996 (4)
	Electric-pain detection	Yes	Bendtsen et al., 1996 (4)

TH, tension-type headache.
Overview of studies comparing pain thresholds in tension-type headache patients and in healthy controls. *Mixed* indicates that the population consisted of both patients with episodic and patients with chronic tension-type headache. *Abnormal* indicates increased pain sensitivity in the headache patients.

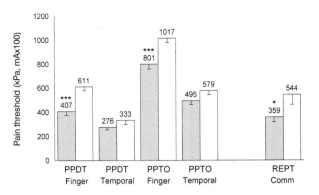

FIG. 2. Pain thresholds to mechanical and electric stimuli in 40 patients with chronic tension-type headache (*hatched bars*) and in 40 healthy controls (*open bars*) (mean ± SE). *PPDT*, pressure pain detection threshold; *PPTO*, pressure pain tolerance threshold; *REPT*, relative electric pain threshold; *Finger*, index finger; *Temporal*, temporal muscle; *Comm*, labial commissure; *** denotes $p \leq 0.0009$; * denotes $p = 0.02$. (From ref. 4, with permission).

applied both at cephalic and at extracephalic, nonsymptomatic locations strongly indicates that the pain sensitivity in the central nervous system is increased in these patients. The widespread and unspecific nature of the hypersensitivity indicates that the general pain sensitivity is affected at the supraspinal level. Thus, it can be concluded that the general pain sensitivity in the central nervous system is increased in patients with chronic tension-type headache, whereas the central pain processing seems to be normal in patients with episodic tension-type headache.

The Stimulus–Response Function for Pressure Versus Pain

The increase in myofascial tenderness is more pronounced than the increase in general pain sensitivity, as can be seen by comparing Figures 1 and 2. Moreover, a significant but not high correlation between general pain hypersensitivity and pericranial tenderness was demonstrated (4,16). Thus, general hypersensitivity can explain only a minor part of the increased pericranial tenderness in patients with chronic tension-type headache. Other factors, therefore, contribute to the increased tenderness. In 1990 Jensen (14) suggested that myofascial tenderness may be the result of a lowered pressure pain threshold, a stronger response to pressures in the noxious range (as illustrated by a steeper stimulus–response function), or a combination of both. It was not possible to study the relation between palpation pressure and pain, however, until the development of a device that allows palpation with a defined pressure, a so-called palpometer (3). By using this instrument, the stimulus–response function for pressure versus pain was investigated in 40 patients with chronic tension-type headache and in 40 healthy controls

(5). The stimulus–response function recorded from normal muscle was well described by a power function. From highly tender muscle, the stimulus–response function was displaced toward lower pressures and, more importantly, it was approximately linear, that is, qualitatively different from that of normal muscle (Fig. 3). This result was confirmed in a study examining tender muscles in patients with fibromyalgia (6). The question is whether these changes are located to peripheral nerve endings, to the spinal cord, or to higher-order neurons.

Spinal dorsal-horn neurons that receive input from deep myofascial tissues can be classified as high-threshold mechanosensitive neurons requiring noxious intensities of stimulation for activation and as low-threshold mechanosensitive neurons, which are activated by innocuous stimuli (26). Yu and Mense (31) showed that high-threshold mechanosensitive dorsal-horn neurons have a positively accelerating stimulus–response function, whereas the stimulus–response function of low-threshold mechanosensitive neurons is approximately linear. This finding suggests that the linear stimulus–response function in tender human muscle may be caused by activity in low-threshold mechanosensitive afferents. At first, this seems unlikely, because low-threshold mechanosensitive afferents normally mediate innocuous sensations. Woolf (30), however, demonstrated that a prolonged noxious input from the periphery is capable of sensitizing spinal dorsal horn neurons, such that low-threshold mechanosensitive afferents can mediate pain. The original finding by Woolf on spinal dorsal-horn sensitization was later confirmed by numerous independent laboratories (12), and a similar sensitization of trigeminal brainstem nociceptive neurons following stimulation of craniofacial muscle afferents has been reported (13). It therefore seems likely that the abnormal stimulus–response function in tender muscle can be explained by changes in neuronal behavior at the spinal/trigeminal level. A decrease in the supraspinal descending inhibition probably does not explain the finding, because it has been reported that the descending inhibition acts through a parallel shift or a decreased slope of the stimulus–response curve (31), whereas it does not change the shape of the stimulus–response curve. Sensitization or increased stimulation of normally active peripheral nociceptors probably would induce a quantitative rather than a qualitative change of the stimulus–response curve (20). Thus, the finding of qualitatively altered nociception from tender muscles indicates that the central nervous system is sensitized at the level of the spinal dorsal horn/trigeminal nucleus in patients with chronic tension-type headache.

Analgesic Effect of Nitric Oxide Synthase Inhibition

Various neurotransmitters, including the freely diffusible gas nitric oxide (NO), have been suggested as playing an important role in central sensitization (8, 25).

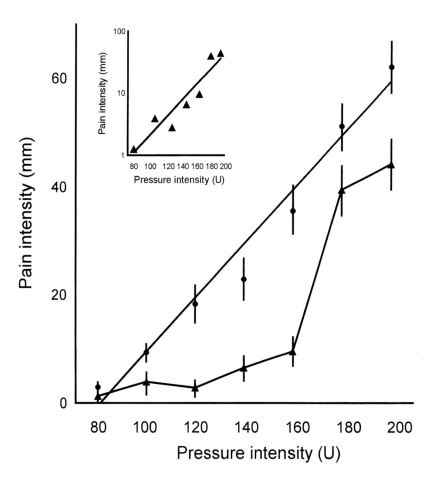

FIG. 3. Stimulus–response functions for pressure versus pain in the trapezius muscle in 40 patients with chronic tension-type headache (*dots*) and in 40 healthy controls (*triangles*)(mean ± SE). Patients had significantly more tenderness than controls, $P = 0.002$. In patients, the stimulus–response function was approximately linear with a slope (β) = 0.50 ± 0.04 mm/U, $p = 0.00004$. In contrast, pain intensities increased in a positively accelerating fashion with increasing pressure intensities in controls, a relation that was well described by a power function. This was demonstrated by obtaining an approximately linear relation between pressure and pain in a double logarithmic plot, B = 3.8 ± 0.61 log*mm*/log*U*, $p = 0.002$ (**inset**). Reproduced from Pain (5) with permission.

The analgesic effect of the nitric oxide synthase (NOS) inhibitor L-N^G methyl arginine hydrochloride (L-NMMA) was investigated in 16 patients with chronic tension-type headache (2). The trial was designed as a double-blind crossover study in which L-NMMA or placebo were administered intravenously over 15 minutes. L-NMMA reduced headache significantly more than placebo. Compared with baseline, the effect was significant already at the end of the infusion period and continued to be significant until the recording of pain intensity was terminated at 120 minutes after start of the infusion (Fig. 4). Acute dosing with a drug with a short half-life, such as L-NMMA, is clearly not ideal for a chronic disorder. The aforementioned study (2) is nevertheless important because it demonstrates, for the first time, that NOS inhibition has an analgesic effect in human chronic pain. With the development of more selective NOS inhibitors that have a longer half-life, chronic dosing with NOS inhibitors may represent a novel principle in the treatment of chronic pain. Furthermore, the study provides information about the pathophysiology of chronic tension-type headache. It is now well established that persistent activity in peripheral nociceptors may lead to sensitization of spinal dorsal horn neurons partly via activation of *N*-methyl-D-aspar-

tate (NMDA) receptors (8). Because many of the effects of NMDA receptor activation are mediated through production of NO (25) and because NOS-like immunoreactivity has been identified in the spinal dorsal horn (27), it is likely that NO plays an important role in hyperalge-

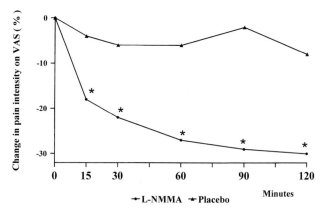

FIG. 4. Change in pain intensity following treatment with the nitric oxide synthase inhibitor L-N^G methyl arginine hydrochloride (L-NMMA) or placebo in 16 patients with chronic tension-type headache. L-NMMA reduced headache significantly more than placebo, $p = 0.01$. * denotes $p < 0.05$ compared with baseline (time = 0). *VAS,* visual analogue scale. (Redrawn from ref. 2, with permission.)

sia in the spinal cord. Supporting this hypothesis are studies in animal models of persistent pain that have shown NOS inhibitors to reduce spinal dorsal-horn sensitization induced by continuous painful input from the periphery (10). Because continuous painful input from the pericranial myofascial tissues probably plays a major role for the development of central sensitization in chronic tension-type headache (see later), it is most likely that the analgesic effect of L-NMMA in tension-type headache is due to reduction of central sensitization (2).

POSSIBLE MECHANISMS LEADING TO SENSITIZATION IN TENSION-TYPE HEADACHE

As mentioned, central sensitization can be generated by prolonged nociceptive input from the periphery (30). Input from muscle nociceptors is more effective in inducing sensitization of spinal dorsal-horn neurons than input from cutaneous nociceptors (29). Comparing pain thresholds in tension-type headache patients with and without abnormal pericranial tenderness recently supported (5) the significance of such mechanisms in tension-type headache. Chronic tension-type headache patients with abnormal tenderness had significantly lower pressure pain detection and tolerance thresholds than chronic tension-type headache patients without abnormal tenderness (16). No such difference was detected in patients with episodic tension-type headache. In addition, chronic tension-type headache patients with abnormal tenderness tended to have lower mechanical pain thresholds than healthy controls, whereas patients without abnormal tenderness had significantly higher pain thresholds than controls (16). Thus, the central nervous system is sensitized only in chronic tension-type headache patients who have increased pericranial tenderness. Experimentally induced tenderness precedes the induced headache in patients with tension-type headache (17), indicating that continuous painful input from pericranial myofascial tissues plays an important role in the development of sensitization at the level of the spinal dorsal horn/trigeminal nucleus in chronic tension-type headache. In turn, the increased nociceptive input to supraspinal structures may result in sensitization at the supraspinal level.

REFERENCES

1. Ashina M, Bendtsen L, Jensen R, Sakai F, Olesen J. Muscle hardness in patients with chronic tension-type headache: relation to actual headache state. *Pain* 1999;79:201–205.
2. Ashina M, Lassen LH, Bendtsen L, Jensen R, Olesen J. Effect of inhibition of nitric oxide synthase on chronic tension-type headache: a randomized crossover trial. *Lancet* 1999;353:287–289.
3. Bendtsen L, Jensen R, Jensen NK, Olesen J. Muscle palpation with controlled finger pressure: new equipment for the study of tender myofascial tissues. *Pain* 1994;59:235–239.
4. Bendtsen L, Jensen R, Olesen J. Decreased pain detection and tolerance thresholds in chronic tension-type headache. *Arch Neurol* 1996;53: 373–376.
5. Bendtsen L, Jensen R, Olesen J. Qualitatively altered nociception in chronic myofascial pain. *Pain* 1996;65:259–264.
6. Bendtsen L, Nørregaard J, Jensen R, Olesen J. Evidence of a qualitatively altered nociception in patients with fibromyalgia. *Arthritis Rheum* 1997;40:98–102.
7. Bovim G. Cervicogenic headache, migraine, and tension-type headache. Pressure-pain threshold measurements. *Pain* 1992;51:169–173.
8. Coderre TJ, Katz J, Vaccarino AL, Melzack R. Contribution of central neuroplasticity to pathological pain: review of clinical and experimental evidence. *Pain* 1993;52:259–285.
9. Göbel H, Weigle L, Kropp P, Soyka D. Pain sensitivity and pain reactivity of pericranial muscles in migraine and tension-type headache. *Cephalalgia* 1992;12:142–151.
10. Hao J-X, Xu X-J. Treatment of chronic allodynia-like response in spinally injured rats: effects of systemically administered nitric oxide synthase inhibitors. *Pain* 1996;66:313–319.
11. Hatch JP, Moore PJ, Cyr Provost M, Boutros NN, Seleshi E, Borcherding S. The use of electromyography and muscle palpation in the diagnosis of tension-type headache with and without pericranial muscle involvement. *Pain* 1992;49:175–178.
12. Hoheisel U, Sander B, Mense S. Myositis-induced functional reorganisation of the rat dorsal horn: effects of spinal superfusion with antagonists to neurokinin and glutamate receptors. *Pain* 1997;69: 219–230.
13. Hu JW, Sessle BJ, Raboisson P, Dallel R, Woda A. Stimulation of craniofacial muscle afferents induces prolonged facilitatory effects in trigeminal nociceptive brain-stem neurones. *Pain* 1992;48:53–60.
14. Jensen K. Quantification of tenderness by palpation and use of pressure algometers. In: Fricton JR, Awad E, eds. *Advances in pain research and therapy*. New York: Raven Press 1990:17;165–181.
15. Jensen R. Mechanisms of spontaneous tension-type headaches: an analysis of tenderness, pain thresholds and EMG. *Pain* 1996;64: 251–256.
16. Jensen R, Bendtsen L, Olesen J. Muscular factors are of importance in tension-type headache. *Headache* 1998;38:10–17.
17. Jensen R, Olesen J. Initiating mechanisms of experimentally induced tension-type headache. *Cephalalgia* 1996;16:175–182.
18. Jensen R, Rasmussen BK, Pedersen B, Olesen J. Muscle tenderness and pressure pain thresholds in headache: a population study. *Pain* 1993;52: 193–199.
19. Kellgren JH. Observations on referred pain arising from muscle. *Clin Sci* 1938;3:175–190.
20. Koltzenburg M, Kress M, Reeh PW. The nociceptor sensitization by bradykinin does not depend on sympathetic neurons. *Neuroscience* 1992;46:465–473.
21. Langemark M, Bach FW, Jensen TS, Olesen J. Decreased nociceptive flexion reflex threshold in chronic tension-type headache. *Arch Neurol* 1993;50:1061–1064.
22. Langemark M, Jensen K, Jensen TS, Olesen J. Pressure pain thresholds and thermal nociceptive thresholds in chronic tension-type headache. *Pain* 1989;38:203–210.
23. Langemark M, Olesen J. Pericranial tenderness in tension headache. A blind, controlled study. *Cephalalgia* 1987;7:249–255.
24. Lipchik GL, Holroyd KA, Talbot F, Greer M. Pericranial muscle tenderness and exteroceptive suppression of temporalis muscle activity: a blind study of chronic tension-type headache. *Headache* 1997;37:368–376.
25. Meller ST, Gebhart GF. Nitric oxide (NO) and nociceptive processing in the spinal cord. *Pain* 1993;52:127–136.
26. Mense S. Nociception from skeletal muscle in relation to clinical muscle pain. *Pain* 1993;54:241–289.
27. Morris R, Southam E, Gittins SR, de Vente J, Garthwaite J. The NO-cGMP pathway in neonatal rat dorsal horn. *Eur J Neurosci* 1994;1: 876–879.
28. Schoenen J, Bottin D, Hardy F, Gerard P. Cephalic and extracephalic pressure pain thresholds in chronic tension-type headache. *Pain* 1991; 47:145–149.
29. Wall PD, Woolf CJ. Muscle but not cutaneous C-afferent input produces prolonged increases in the excitability of the flexion reflex in the rat. *J Physiol (Lond)* 1984;356:443–458.
30. Woolf CJ. Evidence for a central component of post-injury pain hypersensitivity. *Nature* 1983;15:686–688.
31. Yu XM, Mense S. Response properties and descending control of rat dorsal horn neurons with deep receptive fields. *Neuroscience* 1990;39: 823–831.

The Headaches, Second Edition,
edited by J. Olesen, P. Tfelt-Hansen, and K.M.A. Welch.
Lippincott Williams & Wilkins, Philadelphia © 2000.

*Tension-Type Headache, Cluster Headache, and Miscellaneous
Primary Headaches*

CHAPTER 74

Neurophysiology of Tension-Type Headache

Jean Schoenen and Lars Bendtsen

Various neurophysiologic methods have been used in patients with tension-type headache. By far, the most frequent reports have dealt with electromyographic (EMG) recordings of pericranial muscle activity. This situation is explained easily by the fact that in the former Headache Classification of the Ad Hoc Committee (1), *tension headache* was used as a synonym for *muscle-contraction headache* and was considered to be "associated with sustained contraction of the skeletal muscles in the absence of permanent structural change, usually as part of the individual's reaction to life's stress." Recently, attention has focused on the inhibitory reflexes of the jaw-closing muscles (79). Other neurophysiologic methods, in particular those exploring the activity of the brain, such as electroencephalography (EEG), have not disclosed any clear-cut abnormality in tension-type headache (72), as is also the case for contingent negative variation (CNV), an event-related potential, which is abnormal in migraine between attacks but normal in tension-type headache (71,77).

ELECTROMYOGRAPHY

Contraction of head and neck muscles has been thought to play a pathogenetic role in some patients with tension-type headache. This belief is still reflected in the new classification of the International Headache Society (IHS) (31) by the proposal of two subtypes of tension-type headache, of which one is "associated with disorder

of pericranial muscles" (codes 2.1.1. and 2.2.1.), that is, associated with "increased tenderness of pericranial muscles and/or increased EMG level of pericranial muscles at rest or during physiological tests."

Contradictory results have been reported by recording pericranial muscular activity in tension-type headache or, as previously termed, muscle-contraction headache. Relevant data obtained with surface EMG recordings are summarized in Table 1, in which positive data are those that favor a role of increased muscular activity in the pathogenesis of tension-type headache, and negative data represent those that do not. Most of the EMG studies published up to 1983 were critically reviewed by Pikoff (60): About half of the studies appeared to be normal, and in the other half, it was concluded that pericranial EMG levels were increased. Most subsequent studies, however, tend to indicate concordantly that EMG levels are abnormal compared with controls, despite wide variations in experimental conditions. For instance, EMG levels were found to be increased in tension-headache sufferers during postural changes (84), during mental stress (22), and during the headache phase compared with the headache-free interval (61) by analyzing the increment of EMG between rest and maximal contraction (90) or by comparing different electrode placements (35). In a recent study (30) of episodic tension-type headache sufferers recorded in the headache-free phase, higher levels of average temporal EMG levels were found in the patient group compared with controls. Because only 11% of headache subjects had elevated (> mean of controls + 2 SD), EMG activity in at least one muscle, it was believed that EMG data were of little use in assigning individual subjects to diagnostic groups.

We recorded EMG activity in 32 female patients suffering from chronic tension-type headache (code 2.2)

J. Schoenen: University Department of Neurology, CHR Citadelle, and University of Liège, B-4000 Liège, Belgium.

L. Bendtsen: Department of Neurology, Glostrup Hospital, University of Copenhagen, DK-2600 Glostrup, Copenhagen, Denmark.

TABLE 1. *Pericranial surface EMG activity*

"Positive" data	"Negative" data
Increased in 50% of studies (60)	Normal in 50% of studies (60)
Increased on average in CTTH (69,77)	Significantly increased in less than 34% of CTTH patients (69,76)
Increased on average in ETTH (26)	Significantly increased in only 11% of ETTH patients (30)
	Not correlated with headache intensity (14,38,65,69)
Superior stress-induced increase (30,63,64,72,83,88)	Stress-induced increase similar in controls (65)
Increase in frontalis during headache in population-based study (41)	No increase during headache in patients (14,38)
Experimental tooth-clenching produces headache (39)	Headache appears after delay of several hours when EMG is decreased (39); also in migraine (40)
Increased in subgroup 2.2.1 (42)	No difference between 2.2.1 and 2.2.2 (79)

CTTH, chronic tension-type headache; EMG, electromyographic; ETTH, episodic tension-type headache.

over the frontalis, temporalis, and trapezius muscles in supine and standing positions as well as during a mental task (79). On average, EMG activity was significantly higher in patients compared with healthy female volunteers of comparable ages, and this was the case in all three muscles studied and under any condition (Fig. 1). Of the patients, 62.5% had at least one EMG level exceeding the mean control values by 2 SD. Among these patients, five had one abnormal value (of a maximum of six), and only two patients had six abnormal values. If one muscle and one condition were considered, for example, the frontalis in the supine position, 11 patients (34%) would have been considered abnormal. No correlation was found between EMG levels and headache severity or the score on an anxiety scale or pressure pain thresholds. After ten sessions of muscular biofeedback therapy, EMG levels tended to decrease in all muscles, but this modification was significant only in some muscles and under certain recording conditions (43). After biofeedback therapy, a slight but significant positive correlation was

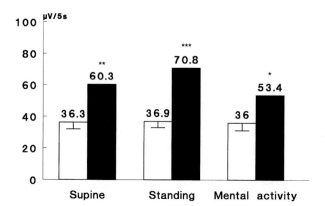

FIG. 1. Electromyographic (*EMG*) levels (mean in μV/5 s-SD) of frontalis, temporalis, and trapezius muscles recorded with the patient in a supine position, in a standing position, and during an arithmetic task. Thirty-two female patients with chronic tension-type headache (*open bars*) and 20 healthy female controls (*tippled bars*) were included. *$p < 0.05$; **$p < 0.002$; ***$p < 0.001$

found between improvement in the headache severity index and maximal reduction of EMG levels, that is, the EMG level that decreased the most considering the three recording sites and the three conditions. Another study found no significant clinical difference between patients with abnormal EMG values and those in whom all EMG recordings were normal (78).

Studies of the possible relation between pericranial EMG activity and stressful situations have produced conflicting results. Increased EMG activity during laboratory stressors have been reported in tension headache patients (15,23,59,88,89). Conversely, a large group of investigations did not find a reliable difference between the EMG activity of tension-type headache patients and headache-free controls in their response to laboratory stressors (2,3,4,6,22,24,50,79,85,91). In a recent study using ambulatory EMG recordings, higher levels of EMG activity were found on "high-stress days" both in headache-free students and in students with episodic tension-type headache; no statistically significant difference was found between the two groups (30,65).

Evidence has been found that pericranial and neck-muscle activity is neither quantitatively nor chronologically related to head pain. The EMG levels are not higher in more severely affected patients (38,69,78,79,80); during prolonged ambulatory EMG recordings, muscle activity varies with daily activities and stress but not with pain levels (14,65). During an actual headache, EMG levels increased over the frontalis muscle in only one population-based study (41) but not in patients (38,14). No difference in EMG levels was found between chronic tension-type headache associated (code 2.2.1) or unassociated (code 2.2.2) with a muscular disorder in one study (78); on the other hand, levels were higher than those in healthy controls in only the 2.2.1 subgroup in another study in which normal EMG levels were found in both subgroups of episodic tension-type headache (42). Two subgroups of episodic tension-type headache sufferers were distinguished on the basis of their pericranial EMG response to experimental pressure-induced pain over the temples, one group with an exaggerated EMG activity and the other with an abnormally low EMG response (26).

Ischemic pain induced in the arm by a tourniquet was not accompanied by higher EMG levels in tension-type headache sufferers compared with controls, although the headache patients rated the tourniquet as more painful (45). Tooth clenching may induce headache in tension-type headache sufferers and has been used as a model to study pathogenetic mechanisms (39). The headache, however, increases gradually over several hours and is associated with pericranial EMG levels that are somewhat lower than the initial ones (39); these levels also can be produced in 54% of migraine patients (40).

It has been argued that myofascial pain syndromes could be related to changes in the viscoelastic properties of muscles, that is, so-called *thixotropy* (82). The recent finding (using a new device, the muscle hardnessmeter) of increased muscle stiffness in tension-type headache sufferers, irrespective of the presence of headache (67), would favor such a mechanism, but this finding needs to be reproduced. Within the same concept, the pain in tension-type headache might be due to muscle contracture, which is electrically silent; in this case, increased electric activity would be localized at the level of trigger points (82). With monopolar needle EMG recordings, increased activity was found at trigger points in patients with chronic tension-type headache (34,62), more often during experimental stress (54). It is not clear whether the EMG activity was recorded from muscle spindles or from the motor endplate zone, and some investigators did not find any abnormality when placing needle electrodes in trigger points (100).

To summarize, EMG recordings have no diagnostic usefulness in tension-type headache, although they may help in understanding its pathogenesis. Contradictory results have been reported for EMG levels of pericranial and neck muscles. Some of these contradictions may be attributable to the different recording conditions. Taken together, however, the published results indicate that there is no causal relationship between the headache and surface EMG activity, although some patients may have EMG levels over certain muscles that exceed those of control subjects. In this respect, the findings may be comparable to those reported in chronic low back pain, where muscle activity is considered a normal protective adaptation and not the cause of pain (5,48). It remains to be determined whether muscular contracture and muscle hardness or localized muscle-fiber contraction under trigger or tender points play a role in the initiation or the boosting of pain in tension-type headache.

BRAINSTEM REFLEXES

The measurement of brainstem reflexes constitutes a noninvasive method for investigating the central processing of sensory information from the cephalic region.

Brainstem reflexes, therefore, have been studied in several neurologic disorders. In tension-type headache, exteroceptive suppression of jaw-closing muscle activity was investigated extensively, and the blink reflex was examined in a single study.

Exteroceptive Suppression

Electric stimulation of the trigeminal nerve fibers normally elicits suppression of voluntary contraction in the masseter and temporal muscles (21). This suppression is mediated by an inhibitory brainstem reflex, which has been called *exteroceptive suppression, cutaneous silent period*, or *inhibitory period*. Traditionally, the term exteroceptive suppression has been used in headache studies (79) to avoid confusion with the proprioceptive silent period of peripheral limb muscles. Exteroceptive suppression is divided into two periods, an early period (ES_1), mediated by an oligosynaptic pathway, and a late period (ES_2), mediated by a polysynaptic pathway (21). Because ES_1 has not been reported to be abnormal in tension-type headache, only ES_2 is considered here. The interneurons responsible for ES_2 probably belong to the bulbar reticular formation (33). This area receives afferents from the periphery but also from limbic structures, the orbitofrontal cortex, the nucleus raphe magnus, and the periaqueductal gray matter (73) (Fig. 2). Studies on ES_2, therefore, may provide information about the excitability control of these brainstem interneurons.

Exteroceptive suppression of jaw-closing muscle activity has been used extensively in investigations of pain mechanisms (52), motor control (21), trigeminal nerve function (18), dysfunction of the temporomandibular joints (37), lesions within the brainstem (34), Parkinson's disease (19), and, more recently, tension-type headache (9,8,27,28,46,55,79,95,96,100). This section briefly discusses the methodology and the results obtained from studies of tension-type headache as well as some data on physiologic or pharmacologic modulation of exteroceptive suppression.

Methodology

Exteroceptive suppression of jaw-closing muscle activity can be measured using a conventional EMG apparatus. The results obtained are, however, heavily influenced by the method used (9,44,73); therefore, standardized, reliable, blinded methods for recording and analyzing ES_2 should be used. The method described briefly here has proved reliable (7,29). While the subject is voluntary clenching his teeth, a slightly painful electric stimulus (e.g., 20 mA) is applied to the labial commissure. The level of voluntary contraction should exceed 50% of maximum (29,73), and the electric stimuli should be applied at intervals of at least 10 seconds to avoid habituation (73). Recording of jaw-closing muscle activity can

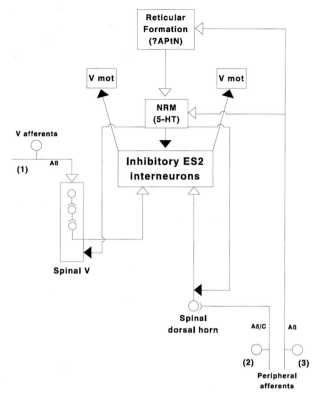

FIG. 2. Diagram illustrating some of the neural pathways and their transmitters involved in the modulation of jaw-closing muscles late exteroceptive suppression.

be performed by using surface electrodes, because this method gives results that are comparable to those obtained with needle electrodes (29). In each recording series, at least ten electric stimuli should be delivered, and the resulting EMG activity should be rectified and averaged to ensure a fairly smooth EMG signal (Fig. 3A). Because suppression periods start and finish gradually, a cutoff point for taking measurements must be defined. From the averaged EMG signal, the duration of ES_2, for example, may be defined as the duration in which there is at least 50% suppression compared with the prestimulus baseline EMG activity (Fig. 3B). The analysis should be performed by a blinded observer.

Temporalis ES_2 is inhibited by a conditioning stimulus applied over the index finger. This peripheral inhibition appears with low-intensity nonpainful stimuli and increases thereafter in proportion to the stimulus intensity (75) (see Fig. 2). High-intensity electric stimuli of the fingers can induce directly a suppression of voluntary EMG activity in jaw-closing muscles, but the prevalence of this response is low (97).

Findings in Headache Patients

In 1987 Schoenen and colleagues (79) reported that the duration of temporalis ES_2 is reduced in chronic tension-

type headache. The 25 patients included in the study all suffered from daily headache and had approximately a 50% reduction of ES_2 compared with 22 healthy controls (Table 2). This original finding was confirmed by Göbel (25), by Nakashima and Takahashi (55) in a study including 17 patients, and by Wallasch and associates (95) in a study including 29 patients with chronic tension-type headache. More recent studies, however, which have used a blinded design, have not confirmed these findings (Table 2). Zwart and Sand (100) found normal ES_2 values in a small blinded study including 11 patients with chronic tension-type headache, and the same result was found by Bendtsen and colleagues (9) in a blinded study comparing 55 patients and 55 healthy controls. Lipchik and colleagues reported normal ES_2 values in a blinded study (46) including 22 young women and in an open study (47) including 27 young women with chronic tension-type headache. The discrepancy between the three earlier and the four later studies cannot be explained easily. As previously discussed (9), it is possible that differences in the methods used for analyzing ES_2 played a role, because the analysis is the most critical part of the methodology (7). Patient characteristics also may have played a role. Thus, at present, it is unclear whether ES_2 per se is abnormal in chronic tension-type headache or only in a subgroup of patients, for example, those suffering from daily headache. In contrast, it has been reported consistently that the duration of ES_2 is not correlated significantly to clinical characteristics, for example, headache frequency, or to various pain parameters, for example, pain thresholds, in patients with tension-type headache (9,46,78).

In patients with episodic tension-type headache and in patients with migraine, ES_2 is normal (27,55,79,95). In postlumbar puncture headache, ES_2 duration is within normal limits (58,93), as it is in cluster headache (70), meningitis, and other symptomatic headaches (58).

Physiological and Pharmacological Modulations of Exteroceptive Suppression

In addition to baseline measurements of ES_2, it is of interest to examine whether ES_2 can be modulated by physiologic or pharmacologic interventions and, if so, whether the effect of such interventions differs between headache patients and healthy controls. In healthy controls, ES_2 is reduced during experimental pain (7,75) and is reduced on the first day compared with the second day of examination (7). The latter tends to be more pronounced in patients with chronic tension-type headache than in healthy controls (9). The finding that ES_2 can be reduced by attentional factors (12) suggests that headache patients are more aroused in the experimental situation than are healthy controls (9). Furthermore, ES_2 duration is reduced by a preceding electric stimulus applied at the periphery (75), and this reduction is more pronounced in

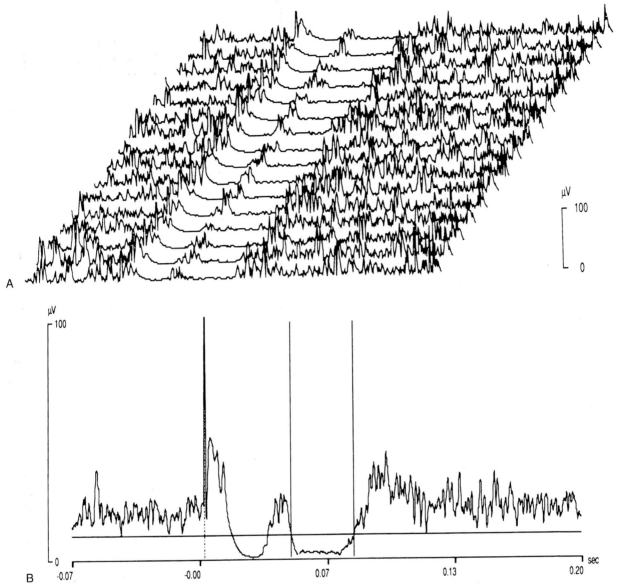

FIG. 3. Exteroceptive suppression of temporalis muscle activity in a healthy volunteer. **A**: Sixteen single signals were recorded and rectified. **B**: Average of the 16 rectified signals. The electric stimulus was delivered at *t* = 0 seconds. A horizontal cursor, placed automatically, indicated 50% of the prestimulus mean electromyographic (*EMG*) amplitude. Vertical cursors, placed manually, indicated the beginning and the end of the ES$_2$ period. Amplitude values must be multiplied by 10. (From ref. 1, with permission.)

patients with tension-type headache than in healthy controls (96) (Fig 4). This last finding may be due to hyperexcitability of brainstem relays interposed between the afferent peripheral input and the medullary interneurons in patients with tension-type headache (96).

In a preliminary study, Schoenen and collagues (74) investigated the modulation of ES$_2$ in healthy volunteers following administration of various serotonergic drugs. The results showed that methysergide, a serotonin antagonist, prolonged ES$_2$; that fluoxetine, a selective serotonin reuptake inhibitor, reduced ES$_2$; and that sumatriptan, a serotonin-agonist that does not penetrate the blood–brain barrier, had no significant effect on ES$_2$.

These data indicate that drugs that increase serotonin levels tend to decrease ES$_2$, whereas drugs that block serotonin receptors tend to increase ES$_2$. This finding was supported by a recent study (8) demonstrating that amitriptyline, a combined serotonin and noradrenaline reuptake blocker, reduced ES$_2$ in patients with chronic tension-type headache. In contrast, Göbel and colleagues (28) could not detect any difference in ES$_2$ before and after treatment with amitriptyline in patients with chronic tension-type headache. The finding by Göbel and associates (26) that acetylsalicylic acid prolongs ES$_2$ in both tension-type headache patients and healthy controls was not confirmed in another study (73). Further pharmaco-

TABLE 2. *Studies of the late exteroceptive suppression period, ES₂, in patients with chronic tension-type headache and healthy controls*

Significant study	Method	Patients' control		difference
		ES₂ duration (n)	ES₂ duration (n)	
Schoenen et al., 1987 (78)	Averaging 10 responses Threshold 80% suppression	25 msec (25)	47 msec (22)	Yes
Göbel, 1990 (25)	Mean of 4 responses at 2Hz Threshold 95% suppression	3.6 msec (15)	12.1 msec (20)	Yes
Nakashima and Takahashi, 1991 (55)	Averaging 32 responses Threshold baseline	21 msec (17)	43 msec (18)	Yes
Wallasch et al., 1991 (95)	Mean of 3 responses Threshold 80% suppression	21 msec (29)	41 msec (19)	Yes
Zwart and Sand, 1995 (100)	Mean of 10 responses (blinded) Threshold 80% suppression	36 msec (11)	34 msec (9)	No
Bendtsen et al., 1996 (9)	Averaging 16 responses (blinded) Threshold 50% suppression	33 msec (55)	35 msec (55)	No
Lipchik et al., 1996 (47)	Averaging 10 responses Threshold baseline	31 msec (27)	34 msec (21)	No
Lipchik et al., 1997 (46)	Averaging 10 responses (blinded) Threshold 50% suppression	11 msec (22)	19 msec (23)	No

ES₂ late exteroceptive suppression period.

logic studies may help to identify the neurotransmitters involved in the regulation of ES₂ and clarify the possible central actions of drugs of interest to headache treatment.

To summarize, temporalis ES₂ has no practical utility for the diagnosis of tension-type headache (73). Measures of its duration may depend on tricky methodologic variables, arousal, and anxiety as well as pharmacologic interventions. Despite these uncertainties, however, there is a possibility that temporalis ES₂ is reduced in a clinical subgroup of severely affected chronic tension-type headache patients who have long-standing daily headache. The decreased excitability of inhibitory brainstem interneu-

rons this abnormality reflects in such patients could be due to hyperactive descending pathways from limbic structures (see Fig. 2).

BLINK REFLEX

Sensory stimulation of the ophthalmic territory evokes reflex responses of the orbicularis oculi muscle, the so-called *blink reflex*. The blink reflex is a protective brainstem reflex that consists of two separate responses, an early ipsilateral (R1) and a late bilateral (R2) component (16). The early component is transmitted through at least

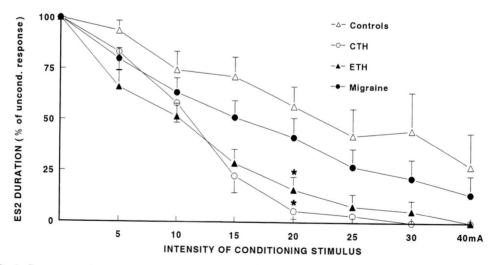

FIG. 4. Decrease of temporalis ES2 duration (expressed as percentage of unconditioned response) with increasing intensities of a conditioning stimulus applied at the index finger 60 ms before the labial commissure stimulation in healthy controls, chronic tension-type headache, episodic tension-type headache and migraine without aura.

one interneuron in the pons, whereas the late component relays in the spinal trigeminal nucleus and then ascends along a bilateral polysynaptic pathway, possibly through the lateral bulbar reticular formation (16). By analogy with the exteroceptive suppression of jaw-closing muscles, the blink reflex may provide information about central mechanisms in tension-type headache. Sand and Zwart (68) compared the blink reflex in 11 patients with chronic tension-type headache and nine healthy controls and found no significant difference in the latencies of the R1 or the R2 component of the two groups. In addition, the latency of R1 was positively correlated to the number of years the patients had suffered from tension-type headache. The importance of the latter finding remains to be determined. In conclusion, this study indicates that the blink reflex is largely normal in patients with tension-type headache.

CONTINGENT NEGATIVE VARIATION

Contingent negative variation (CNV) is an event-related cerebral potential recorded over the frontal cortex in a reaction-time paradigm (see Chap. 37). In patients with the episodic or chronic form of tension-type headache, CNV is on average within normal limits (10,49,71,86), in contrast to the finding of an increased CNV with reduced habituation in migraine without aura (see Chap. 2.1.2.3.4). In patients presenting both migraine and tension-type headache, CNV may be abnormal when migraine is the predominating type of headache (71). When overt depression is associated with tension-type headache, CNV is usually of decreased amplitude, as has been described in depression without headache (87).

REFERENCES

1. Ad Hoc Committee on the Classification of Headache: classification of headache. JAMA 1962;179:717–718.
2. Anderson CD, Franks RD. Migraine and tension headache: is there a physiological difference? Headache 1981;21:63–71.
3. Andrasik F, Holroyd KA. Physiologic and self-report comparisons between tension headache sufferers and non-headache controls. Journal of Behavioral Assessment 1980;2:135–141.
4. Andrasik F, Blanchard EB, Arena JG, Saunders NL, Barron KD. Psychophysiology of recurrent headache: methodological issues and new empirical findings. Behavioral Therapy 1982;13:407–429.
5. Arena JG, Sherman RA, Bruno GM, Young TR. Electromyographic recordings of low back pain subjects and non-pain controls in six different positions: effect of pain levels. Pain 1991;45:23–28.
6. Bakal D, Kaganov JA. Muscle contraction and migraine headache: psychophysiologic comparison. Headache 1977;17:208–214.
7. Bendtsen L, Jensen R, Brennum J, Arendt-Nielsen L, Olesen J. Exteroceptive suppression periods in jaw-closing muscles. Variability and relation to experimental pain and sustained muscle contraction. Cephalalgia 1993;13:184–191.
8. Bendtsen L, Jensen R, Olesen J. Amitriptyline, a combined serotonin and noradrenaline re-uptake inhibitor, reduces exteroceptive suppression of temporal muscle activity in patients with chronic tension-type headache. Electroencephalogr Clin Neurophysiol 1996;101:418–422.
9. Bendtsen L, Jensen R, Brennum J, Arendt-Nielsen L, Olesen J. Exteroceptive suppression of temporal muscle activity is normal in patients with chronic tension-type headache and not related to actual headache state. Cephalalgia 1996;16:251–256.
10. Böcker KBE, Timsit-Berthier M, Schoenen J, Brunia CHM. Contingent negative variation in migraine. Headache 1990;30:604–609.
11. Bratzlavsky M, De Boever J, Van der Eecken H. Tooth pulpal reflexes in jaw musculature in man. Arch Oral Biol 1976;21:491–493.
12. Cadden SW, Newton JP. The effects of attentional factors on an inhibitory jaw reflex in man. Exp Physiol 1995;80:299–305.
13. Cardot H, Laugier H. Le réflexe linguo-maxillaire. C R Soc Biol (Paris) 1922;86:529–530.
14. Clark GT, Sakai S, Merrill R, et al. Cross-correlation between stress, pain, physical activity and temporalis muscle EMG in tension-type headache. Cephalalgia 1995;15:511.
15. Cram JR. EMG biofeedback and the treatment of tension headaches: a systematic analysis of treatment components. Behavioral Therapy 1980;11:699–710.
16. Cruccu G, Bowsher D. Intracranial stimulation of the trigeminal nerve in man. II. Reflex responses. J Neurol Neurosurg Psychiatry 1986;49:419–427.
17. Cruccu G, Agostino R, Fornarelli M, Inghilleri M, Manfredi M. Recovery cycle of the masseter inhibitory reflex in man. Neurosci Lett 1984;49:63–68.
18. Cruccu G, Inghilleri M, Fraioli B, Guidetti B, Manfredi M. Neurophysiologic assessment of trigeminal function after surgery for trigeminal neuralgia. Neurology 1987;37:631–638.
19. Cruccu G, Pauletti G, Agostino R, Berardelli A, Manfredi M. Masseter inhibitory reflex in movement disorders. Huntington's chorea, Parkinson's disease, dystonia, and unilateral masticatory spasm. Electroencephalogr Clin Neurophysiol 1991;81:24–30.
20. Dawans A, Schoenen J, Timsit M, Timsit-Meyer M. Correlative study of psychopathological features and temporalis second exteroceptive silent period in chronic tension-type headache. Cephalalgia 1991;11(Suppl 11):310–311.
21. Desmedt JE, Godaux E. Habituation of exteroceptive suppression and of exteroceptive reflexes in man as influenced by voluntary contraction. Brain Res 1976;106:21–29.
22. Feuerstein M, Bush C, Corpisiero P. Stress and chronic headache: a psychophysiological analysis of mechanisms. J Psychosom Res 1982;26:167–182.
23. Formisano R, Buzzi MG, Cerbo R, et al. Idiopathic headaches : a neuropsychological and computerized electromyographic study. Headache 1988;28:426–429.
24. Gannon LR, Haynes SN, Safranek R, Hamilton J. A psychophysiological investigation of muscle-contraction and migraine headache. J Psychosom Res 1981;25:271–280.
25. Göbel H. Schmerzmessung. Theorie Methodik-Anwenslung bei Kopfschmerz. Stuttgart: Gustav Fischer, 1992:304.
26. Göbel H, Weigle L, Soyka D. Pain sensitivity and pain reactivity of pericranial musculature in migraine and tension-type headache. Cephalalgia 1992;12:142–151.
27. Göbel H, Ernst M, Jeschke J, Keil R, Weigle L. Acetylsalicylic acid activates antinociceptive brain-stem reflex activity in headache patients and in healthy subjects. Pain 1992;48:187–195.
28. Göbel H, Hamouz V, Hansen C, et al. Chronic tension-type headache: amitriptyline reduces clinical headache-duration and experimental pain sensitivity but does not alter pericranial muscle activity readings. Pain 1994;59:241–249.
29. Hansen PO, Svensson P, Nielsen J, Arendt-Nielsen L, Jensen TS. Exteroceptive suppression of masseter muscle: assessment of two methods for quantitating suppression periods. Acta Neurol Scand 1998;97:204–213.
30. Hatch JP, Prihoda TJ, Moore PJ, et al. A naturalistic study of the relationships among electromyographic activity, psychological stress and pain in ambulatory tension-type headache patients and headache-free controls. Psychosom Med 1991;53:576–584.
31. Headache Classification Committee of the International Headache Society. Classification and diagnostic criteria for headache disorders, cranial neuralgias and facial pain. Cephalalgia 1988;8(Suppl 7):1–96.
32. Hoffmann P, Tönnies JF. Nachweis des völlig konstanten Vorkommens des Zungen-Kieferreflexes beim Menschen. Arch Ges Physiol 1948;250:103–108.
33. Hopf HC. Topodiagnostic value of brain stem reflexes. Muscle Nerve 1994;17:475–484.

34. Hubbard DR, Berkoff GM. Myofascial trigger points show spontaneous needle EMG activity. *Spine* 1993;18:1803–1807.

35. Hudzinski LG, Lawrence GS. Significance of EMG surface electrode placement models and headache findings. *Headache* 1988;28:30–35.

36. Hugelin A, Dumont S. Intégrations motrices et vigilance chez l'encéphale isolé. I. Inhibition réticulaire du réflexe d'ouverture de la gueule. *Arch Ital Biol* 1961;99:219–243.

37. Hussein SM, McCall Jr WD. Masseteric silent periods electrically evoked in normal subjects and patients with temporomandibular joint dysfunction. *Exp Neurol* 1983;81:64–76.

38. Jensen R. Mechanisms of spontaneous tension-type headache: an analysis of tenderness, pain thresholds and EMG. *Pain* 1995;64:251.

39. Jensen R, Olesen J. Initiating mechanisms of experimentally induced tension-type headache. *Cephalalgia* 1996;16:175.

40. Jensen K, Büllow P, Hansen H. Experimental tooth clenching in common migraine. *Cephalalgia* 1985;5:245–251.

41. Jensen R, Fuglsang-Frederikseb A, Olesen J. Quantitative surface EMG in headache: a population study. *Electroencephalogr Clin Neurophysiol* 1994;93:335–344.

42. Jensen R, Bendtsen L, Olesen J. Muscular factors are of importance in Tension-type Headache. *Headache* 1998;38:10–17.

43. Juprelle M, Schoenen J. Relaxation avec biofeedback musculaire dans les céphalées de type tension: analyse multifactorielle d'un groupe de 31 patients. *Rev Med Liège* 1990;XLV:630–637.

44. Lavigne G, Frysinger R, Lund JP. Human factors in the measurement of the masseteric silent period. *J Dent Res* 1983;62:985–988.

45. Lehrer PM, Murphy AI. Stress reactivity and perception of pain among tension headache sufferers. *Behav Res Ther* 1991;29:61–69.

46. Lipchik GL, Holroyd KA, Talbot F, Greer M. Pericranial muscle tenderness and exteroceptive suppression of temporalis muscle activity: A blind study of chronic tension-type headache. *Headache* 1997;37:368–376.

47. Lipchik GL, Holroyd KA, France CR, et al. Central and peripheral mechanisms in chronic tension-type headache. *Pain* 1996;64:467–475.

48. Lund JP, Donga R, Widmer CG, Stohler CS. The pain-adaptation model: a discussion of the relationship between chronic musculoskeletal pain and motor activity. *Can J Physiol Pharmacol* 1991;69:683–694.

49. Maertens de Noordhout A, Pepin JL, Schoenen J, Delwaide PJ. Percutaneous magnetic stimulation of the motor cortex in migraine. *Electroencephalogr Clin Neurophysiol* 1992;85:110–115

50. Martin PR, Mathews AM. Tension headache: psychophysiological investigation and treatment. *J Psychosom Res* 1978;22:389–399.

51. Mason P, Strassman A, Maciewicz R. Is the jaw-opening reflex a valid model of pain? *Brain Research Reviews* 1985;10:137–146.

52. Mason P, Strassman A, Maciewicz R. Intracellular responses of raphe magnus neurons during the jaw-opening reflex evoked by tooth pulp stimulation. *Brain Res* 1986;379:232–241.

53. McGrath PA, Sharav Y, Dubner R, Gracely RH. Masseter inhibitory period and sensations evoked by electrical tooth pulp stimulation. *Pain* 1981;10:1–17.

54. McNulty WH, Gerwitz RN, Hubbard DR, Berkoff GM. Needle electromyographic evaluation of trigger point response to a psychosocial stressor. *Psychophysiology* 1994;31:313–316.

55. Nakahima K, Takahashi K. Exteroceptive suppression of the masseter, temporalis and trapezius muscles produced by mental nerve stimulation in patients with chronic headaches. *Cephalalgia* 1991;11:23–28.

56. Olesen J. Clinical and pathophysiological observations in migraine and tension-type headache explained by integration of vascular, supraspinal and myofascial inputs. *Pain* 1991;46:125–132.

57. Ongerboer de Visser BW, Goor C. Cutaneous silent period in masseter muscle : a clinical and electrodiagnostic evaluation. *J Neurol Neurosurg Psychiatry* 1976;39:674–679.

58. Paulus W, Raubüchl O, Strabue A, Schoenen J. Exteroceptive suppression of temporalis muscle activity in various types of headache. *Headache* 1992;32:41–44.

59. Philips C. A psychological analysis of tension headache. In Rachman S, ed. *Contributions to medical psychology*. Oxford: Pergamon, 1977: 91–113.

60. Pikoff H. Is the muscular model of headache will viable? A review of conflicting data. *Headache* 1984;24:186–198.

61. Pritchard DW. EMG cranial muscle levels in headache sufferers before and during headache. *Headache* 1989;29:103–108

62. Proietti Cecchini A, Afra J, Maertens de Noordhout A, Schoenen J. Modulation of pain thresholds showing isometric contraction in patients with chronic tension-type headache and/or generalized myofascial pain compared to healthy volunteers. *Neurology* 1997;48: A258,P04.118.

63. Rasmussen BK, Jensen R, Schroll M, Olesen J. Interrelations between migraine and tension-type headache in the general population. *Arch Neurol* 1992;49:914–918.

64. Reinecke M, Konen T, Langohr HD. Autonomic cerebrovascular reactivity and exteroceptive suppression of temporalis muscle activity in migraine and tension-type headaches. In: Clifford-Rose F, ed., *New advances in headache research*. London: Smith-Gordon, 1991;115.

65. Rugh JD, Hatch JP, Moore PJ. The effects of psychological stress on electromyographic activity and negative affect in ambulatory tension-type headache patients. *Headache* 1990;30:216–219.

66. Sakai S, Mervill R, Clark GT, McCreavy CP. Waking and sleeping EMG levels in chronic daily temporalis region headache patients. *Headache* 1990;30:314.

67. Sakai F, Ebihara S, Akiyama M, Horikawa M. Pericranial muscle hardness in tension-type headache: a non-invasive measurement method and its clinical application. *Brain* 1995;2:523–531.

68. Sand T, Zwart JA. The blink reflex in chronic tension-type headache, migraine, and cervicogenic headache. *Cephalalgia* 1994;14:447–450.

69. Sandrini G, Antonaci F, Pucci E, et al. Comparative study with EMG, pressure algometry and manual palpation in tension-type headache and migraine. *Cephalalgia* 1994;14:451–457.

70. Schoenen J. Exteroceptive silent periods of temporalis muscle in headache. In Van Steenberghe D, De Laat A, eds. *Electromyography of jaw reflexes in man*. Leuven; Belgium: University Press, 1989; 357–368.

71. Schoenen J. Two useful neurophysiological tests in chronic headache. *News in Headache* 1991;1:3–5.

72. Schoenen J. Clinical neurophysiology studies in headache: a review of data and pathophysiological hints. *Funct Neurol* 1992;7:191–204.

73. Schoenen J. Exteroceptive suppression of temporalis muscle activity: methodological and physiological aspects. *Cephalalgia* 1993;13:3–10.

74. Schoenen J, Raubuchl O, Sianard J. Pharmacological modulation of temporalis exteroceptive silent periods in ealthy volunteers. *Cephalalgia* 1991;11(Suppl 11):16–17.

75. Schoenen J, Wang W, Gerard P. Research report: modulation of temporalis muscle exteroceptive suppression by limb stimuli in normal man. *Brain Res* 1994;657:214–220.

76. Schoenen J, Gérard P, De Pasqua V, Juprelle M. EMG activity in pericranial muscles during postural variation and mental activity in healtly volunteers and patients with chronic tension-type headache. *Headache* 1991;31:321–324.

77. Schoenen J, Maertens A, Timsit-Berthier A, Timsit M. Contingent negative variation (CNV) as a diagnostic and physiopathologic tool in headache patients. Rose C, ed. *Migraine Proceedings of the 5th International Migraine Symposium*. London, 1984, Basel: Karger, 1985: 17–25.

78. Schoenen J, Jamart B, Gérard P, Lenarduzzi P, Delwaide PJ. Exteroceptive suppression of temporalis muscle activity in chronic headache. *Neurology* 1987;37:1834–1836.

79. Schoenen J, Gerard P, De Pasqua V, Sianard Gainko J. Multiple clinical and paraclinical analyses of chronic tension-type headache associated or unassociated with disorder of pericranial muscles. *Cephalalgia* 1991;11:135–139.

80. Schoenen J, Bottin D, Juprelle M. De Pasqua V, Gérard P. Chronic tension-type headache: a multifactorial analysis suggesting disturbance of "limbic pathways" to the brainstem. In: Rose C, ed. *New advances in headache research*. London: Smith-Gordon, 1991: 363–368.

81. Sherrington CS. Reflexes excitable in the cat from pinna, vigrissae and jaws. *J Physiol (London)* 1917;51:404–431.

82. Simons DG, Mense S. Understanding and measurement of muscle tone as related to clinical muscle pain. *Pain* 1998;75:1–17.

83. Solomon S, Lipton RB, Newman LO. Evaluation of chronic daily headache: comparison to criteria for chronic tension-type headache. *Cephalalgia* 1992;12:365.

84. Sturgis ET, Schaefer CA, Ahles TA, Sikora TL. Effect of movement and position in the evaluation of tension headache and non-headache controls. *Headache* 1984;24:88–93.

85. Sutton EP, Belar CD. Tension headache patients versus controls: a study of EMG parameters. *Headache* 1982;22:133–136.

86. Timsit M, Timsit-Berthier M, Schoenen J, Maertens de Noordhout A.

Intérêt de l'étude de la VCN dans les migraine et les céphalées de tension. *Rev EEG Neurophysiol Clin* 1987;17:259–270.

87. Timsit-Berthier M, Ansseau M, Mantanus H, Schoenen J, Legros JJ. Contingent negative variation in psychopharmacology. *Event related brain research. EEG Journal* (Suppl 2):1990:31–45.

88. Traue HC, Bischoff C, Zeng H. Sozialer Stress. Muskelspannung und Spaerasgakopfachmerz. *ZF Klin Psychol* 1986;15:57.

89. Van Boxtel A, Van Derven JR. Differential EMG activity in subjects with muscle contraction headaches related to mental effort. *Headache* 1978;17:233–237.

90. Van Boxtel A, Goudswaard P. Absolute and proportional resting EMG levels in chronic headache patients in relation to the state of headache. *Headache* 1984;24:259–265.

91. Vaughn R, Pall ML, Haynes SN. Frontalis EMG response to stress in subjects with frequent muscle-contraction headaches. *Headache* 1977;16:313–317.

92. Wallasch TM. *Use of temporalis inhibitory reflex in the evaluation of chronic headache sufferers. Paneuropean Society of Neurology*, 2nd Congress, 1991;200(abst PO-B1-07).

93. Wallasch TM, Reinecke R. Migräne und Kopfschmerz vom Spannungstyp. Neue Aspekte in der apparativen Diagnostik. *Münch Med Wschr* 1991;113:26–31.

94. Wallasch TM, Reinecke R, Langohr HD. Exterozeptive Suppression der temporalis Muskelaktivität bei Kopfschmerzen. *Nervenheilkunde* 1990;9:58–60.

95. Wallasch TM, Reinecke M, Langohr HD. EMG analysis of the late exteroceptive suppression period of temporal muscle activity in episodic and chronic tension-type headaches. *Cephalalgia* 1991;11: 109–112.

96. Wang W, Schoenen J. Reduction of temporalis exteroceptive suppression by peripheral electrical stimulation in migraine and tension-type headaches. *Pain* 1994;59:327–334.

97. Wang W, Schoenen J. Suppression of voluntary temporalis muscle activity by peripheral limb stimulations in healthy volunteers, migraineurs and tension-type headache sufferers. *Funct Neurol* 1996; 11:307–315

98. Yemm R. The response of the masseter and temporal muscles following electrical stimulation of oral mucous membrane in man. *Arch Oral Biol* 1972;17:23–33.

99. Yemm R. A neurophysiological approach to the pathology and aetiology of temporomandibular dysfunction. *J Oral Rehab* 1985;12:343–353.

100. Zwart JA, Sand T. Exteroceptive suppression of temporalis muscle activity: a blind study of tension-type headache, migraine, and cervicogenic headache. *Headache* 1995;35:338–343.

The Headaches, Second Edition,
edited by J. Olesen, P. Tfelt-Hansen, and K.M.A. Welch.
Lippincott Williams & Wilkins, Philadelphia © 2000.

Tension-Type Headache, Cluster Headache, and Miscellaneous Primary Headaches

CHAPTER 75

Hemodynamics and Muscle Metabolism of Tension-Type Headache

Jes Olesen and Michael Langemark

REGIONAL CEREBRAL BLOOD FLOW

Only one study has focused specifically on regional cerebral blood flow (rCBF) in patients with tension-type headache (1). In several other studies, patients with tension-type headache have been used as controls for comparison with patients suffering from migraine and other neurologic diseases. The article by Andersen and colleagues (1), available only as a short communication, describes their study of 41 patients with chronic tension-type headache, 14 of whom also had rare migraine attacks (i.e., fewer attacks than one per month). Twenty-seven patients had exclusively chronic tension-type headache and never had any migraine symptoms. The study included 19 men and 22 women aged 42.6 ± 14 years. The mean frequency of headache was 28.8 days per month, and the duration of the headache disorder was 8.0 years. The patients were on a standardized medication of paracetamol, 1 to 2 g daily. In 11 patients, the headache was unilateral: five right-sided and six left-sided. Thirty had bilateral headache. The patients were screened carefully both clinically and using computed tomography (CT) scans to exclude organic changes. The patients were studied during headache, and it was not possible to restudy them outside of headache because headache-free days were so rare. rCBF was measured by [133]xenon (^{133}Xe)-inhalation single positron emission computed tomography (SPECT) using brain-dedicated three-slice

J. Olesen: Department of Neurology, Glostrup Hospital, University of Copenhagen, DK-2600 Glostrup, Copenhagen, Denmark.

M. Langemark: Department of Neurology, Hilleroed Hospital, DK-3400 Hilleroed, Denmark.

equipment (Tomomatic 64). The patients also were studied using [99]M-technetium hexa-methyl-propylene-amine-oximine (HMPAO). Side-to-side asymmetry was within normal limits, and no focal areas of hyperperfusion or hypoperfusion were seen by visual inspection. In patients with unilateral headache, no correspondence was noted between laterality of headache and laterality of rCBF, but the numbers of such patients were small. It was concluded that rCBF is normal in chronic tension-type headache.

INTRACRANIAL ARTERIES

In a pilot study, ultrasonically determined CBF velocities were reported to be increased in episodic tension-type headache (24), but in a subsequent study of chronic tension-type headache, no disturbance was found (23).

EXTRACRANIAL BLOOD FLOW

The measurement of extracranial blood flow is difficult (6). Tissues outside the brain are nonhomogeneous and have a variable and largely unknown partition coefficient for diffusible tracers. Therefore, an average extracranial blood flow cannot be measured. Flow must be measured in each homogeneous tissue by local injection of a diffusible tracer. Such measurements are important because pain in chronic tension-type headache (previously called *muscle-contraction headache*) has been hypothesized to be of ischemic origin (22). This conclusion was based on early reports of headache alleviation by vasodilators and lack of effect or worsening by vasoconstrictors in this disorder (15). Support for the ischemic theory also comes from the fact that experimental ischemic exercise of temporal muscle may cause head pain (13).

The finding of a statistically (although not clinically) significant effect of sumatriptan in chronic tension-type headache may indicate involvement of vascular mechanisms (4), because sumatriptan is believed to exert its effect on vascular nociceptors or their projections. It was suggested that the effect of sumatriptan could be explained by convergence of myofascial and vascular input to the same neurons in the brainstem.

Flow in Pericranial Muscles

Blood flow in the splenius capitis muscle was measured by the sodium-24 clearance method in patients with muscle-contraction headache (14). Five patients showed a 56% increase in blood flow during headache compared with outside of headache. In 16 patients studied only during headache, mean blood flow was 33% above the mean blood flow observed in the 44 patients studied only during headache-free intervals. The tracer used in this study is not freely diffusible, which introduces an important source of error. Furthermore, the electromyography (EMG) level was not controlled. A sustained increase in tone may be responsible, through increased muscle metabolism, for these results.

Langemark and colleagues (10) injected ^{133}Xe into the temporal muscle and recorded the washout curve (Fig. 1). This method was used previously to measure temporal muscle blood flow in migraine patients (7,8). Forty patients, 17 men and 23 women, entered the study. They all suffered from chronic tension-type headache of at least 6 months' duration. Patients with migraine headache lasting more than 1 day per month were excluded. Of the 40 patients, 35 had daily headaches, and five reported headache 15 to 25 days per month. None of the patients received opioid, neuroleptic, or vasoactive drugs. Thirteen healthy controls, five men and eight women, were studied similarly. Median age in the control group was 45 years. Temporal muscle flow was determined simultaneously in the two sides. Patients were examined in the supine position after 15 minutes of rest. EMG activity was recorded by surface electrodes on a two-channel amplifier. The subjects were required to rest during the first 8 to 10 minutes while injection trauma subsided. At a given signal, they clenched their jaws, maintaining 30% of maximal EMG signal for 2 minutes. A resting period of at least 2 minutes followed the isometric work. If enough tracer remained to evaluate further exercise, subjects were asked to chew at 20 contractions per minute with approximately half of their maximum EMG. Thirty-six patients reported headache to be present on the day of flow investigation. The resting temporal muscle blood flow was calculated to 3.7

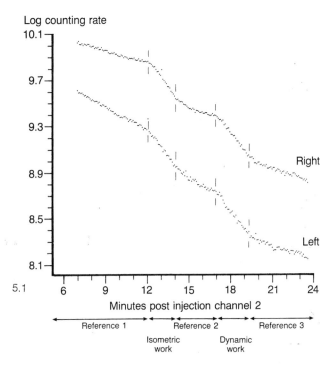

FIG. 1. Logarithmically displayed xenon-133 clearance curves from right and left temporal muscles in a patient with chronic tension-type headache. Note the immediately increased steepness of the curves during isometric and dynamic work, which occurs in parallel on the two sides. (From ref. 10, with permission.)

mL/100 g per minute in the patients and 5.0 mL/100 g per minute in controls; the difference was not statistically significant. Resting blood flows on the two sides were highly correlated, and no right–left differences could be demonstrated. During isometric work, blood flow increased approximately fivefold in both patients and controls (Fig. 2). The increase on the two sides was positively correlated, and no right–left difference could be demonstrated. Reactive hyperperfusion immediately after the 2-minute bite period was observed in eight patients and in one control subject. The hyperperfusion in these cases lasted 20 to 40 seconds, and blood flow values increased up to 60-fold of the resting values or 11-fold of the flow during isometric work. Subjects with and without hyperperfusion did not differ with respect to resting blood flow or relative flow increase during isometric work. The phenomenon, although quite interesting and possibly important, remained unexplained. No trend toward correlation was found between the reported severity of headache and the main flow parameters (resting flow and relative flow increase during exercise). In nine patients with predominantly unilateral headache complaints, no tendency toward relative hypoperfusion or hyperperfusion on the affected side was found during rest or exercise. No correlation was found between pressure pain threshold of the temporal muscle, tenderness

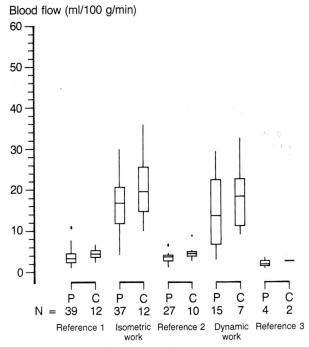

Blood flow (ml/100 g/min)

P	C	P	C	P	C	P	C	P	C
N = 39	12	37	12	27	10	15	7	4	2
Reference 1		Isometric work		Reference 2		Dynamic work		Reference 3	

FIG. 2. Temporal muscle blood flow in patients with chronic tension-type headache (*P*) and headache-free subjects (*C*). Note the lack of difference during rest as well as during isometric and dynamic work. (From ref. 10, with permission).

by manual palpation, and resting flow values or between the tenderness parameters and blood flow during isometric work. Chronic tension-type headache or its related muscle tenderness was therefore not caused by ischemia of the temporal muscle.

Tension-type headache has some characteristics in common with myofascial pain and fibromyalgia (fibromyositis). No evidence of ischemia in these disorders has been found (9,18). Using the method of Langemark and colleagues (10), temporal muscle ischemia might have been overlooked if the phenomenon was intermittent, which is unlikely in light of the relative constancy of pain in this group of patients. The method measures flow in only a small volume of muscle, which might be unaffected. The tracer, however, was injected into the anterior temporal muscle, an area that is tender in most patients with chronic tension-type headache (11).

Conjunctival Blood Flow

In four patients suffering from muscle-contraction headache, constriction of arterioles and venules with blanching of capillary beds was noted (16) and confirmed in a later systematic study of frontally located muscle-contraction headache in 11 patients (15). These studies were unblinded and uncontrolled, however, and the findings require confirmation.

Blood Flow in the Skin

Specific thermographic patterns were not reported in the 27 patients with tension-type headache studied by Drummond and Lance (5). In another study, 11 of 13 patients with muscle-contraction headache showed a symmetric facial thermogram (12). In accordance with these studies, Swerdlow and Dieter (21) found the thermographic pattern of patients with muscle contraction headache to be similar to that of controls. Thus, there is no reason to believe that skin blood flow is altered in tension-type headache.

EXTRACRANIAL ARTERIES

The amplitude of temporal artery pulsations decreased during tension-type headache and was diminished both during and between episodes of headache compared with control values (22). This finding, however, was not confirmed by Brazil and Friedman (3), who pointed out the difficulty of obtaining reproducible pulse-wave contours. Compressing neck and scalp arteries generally has no effect on pain in tension-type headache (2,4). High-frequency ultrasound imaging of extracranial arteries, which has shown relative dilatation on the side of migraine pain (6), has not been applied to the study of tension-type headache. On balance, abnormalities of extracranial arteries during tension-type headache have not been demonstrated convincingly.

MUSCLE METABOLISM

Blood flow in muscle usually reflects the metabolism, and the findings of normal blood flow in the temporal muscle and a normal increase in blood flow during contraction of the temporal muscle strongly indicate that muscle metabolism also is normal. Determination of energy-rich phosphates and calculation of local pH are now possible in temporal muscle using volume-selective magnetic resonance spectroscopy (17).

Investigations in fibromyalgia, a condition that shares several similarities with tension-type headache, found no disturbance in muscle energy metabolism using ^{31}P magnetic resonance spectroscopy at rest and following exercise (19). Using a polarographic oxygen probe, Strobel and colleagues, however, found increased [sic] oxygen tension in tense muscles. This finding was interpreted as being the result of an oversupply of oxygen demanded by the muscle (20). These methods show great promise in increasing the understanding of muscular disturbances, but they have not yet been applied to the study of tension-type headache.

REFERENCES

1. Andersen AR, Langemark M, Olesen J. Regional cerebral blood flow in chronic tension-type headache. In: Olesen J, ed. *Migraine and other*

headaches: the vascular *mechanisms.* New York: Raven Press, 1991: 319–321.

2. Blau JN, Dexter SL. The site of pain origin during migraine headaches. In: Clifford RF, Zilkha KJ, eds. *Progress in migraine research*, vol 1. London: Pitman Medical, 1981:13–14.

3. Brazil P, Friedman AP. Craniovascular studies in headache: a report and analysis of pulse volume tracings. *Neurology* 1956;6:96–102.

4. Brennum J, Kjeldsen M, Olesen J. The 5-HT1-like agonist sumatriptan has a significant effect in chronic tension-type headache. *Cephalalgia* 1992;12:375–379.

5. Drummond PD, Lance JO. Facial temperature in migraine, tension-vascular and tension headache. *Cephalalgia* 1984;4:149–158.

6. Iversen HK, Nielsen TH, Olesen J, Tfelt-Hansen P. Arterial responses during migraine headache. *Lancet* 1990;336:837–839.

7. Jensen K. Headache and extracerebral flow. In: Olesen J, Edvinsson L, eds. *Basic mechanism of headache.* Amsterdam: Elsevier, 1988; 313–320.

8. Jensen K, Olesen J. Temporal muscle blood flow in common migraine. *Acta Neurol Scand* 1985;72:561–570.

9. Klemp P, Nielsen V, Korsgard J, Crone P. Blood flow in fibromyotic muscles. *Scand J Rehabil Med* 1982;14:81–82.

10. Langemark M, Jensen K, Olesen J. Temporal muscle blood flow in chronic tension-type headache. *Arch Neurol* 1990;47:654–658.

11. Langemark M, Olesen J. Pericranial tenderness in tension headache. A blind, controlled study. *Cephalalgia* 1987;7:249–255.

12. Mathew NT, Alvarez L. The usefulness of thermography in headache. In: Clifford RF, ed. *Progress in migraine research,* vol 2. London: Pitman Medical, 1984:232–245.

13. Myers DE, McCall WD Jr. Head pain as a result of experimental ischemic exercise of the temporalis muscle. *Headache* 1983;23:113–116.

14. Onel Y, Friedman AP, Grossman J. Muscle blood flow studies in muscle-contraction headache. *Neurology* 1961;11:935–939.

15. Ostfeld AM, Reis DJ, Wolff HG. Studies in headache. *Arch Neurol Psychiatry* 1957;77:113–119.

16. Ostfeldt AM, Wolff HG. Observations on the behavior of the conjunctival vessels in vascular headache. *Trans Assoc Am Phys* 1955;80:216–217.

17. Sappey-Marinier D, Dheyriat A, Lissac M, Frutoso J, Mallet JJ, Bonmartin A. A metabolism study of human masseter muscle by ^{31}P magnetic resonance spectroscopy during long periods of exercise and recovery. *Eur J Oral Sci* 1998;106:552–558.

18. Schledermann H. Investigations of muscular fibrositis by radioactive sodium injected into the muscle. In: *Proceedings of the Second International Congress of Physical Medicine.* Copenhagen: Munksgaard, 1957: 204–209.

19. Simms RW, Roy SH, Hrovat M, et al. Lack of association between fibromyalgia syndrome and abnormalities in muscle energy metabolism. *Arthritis Rheum* 1994;37:794–800.

20. Strobel ES, Krapf M, Suckfull M, Bruckle W, Fleckenstein W, Muller W. Tissue oxygen measurement and 31P magnetic resonance spectroscopy in patients with muscle tension and fibromyalgia. *Rheumatol Int* 1997; 16:175–180.

21. Swerdlow B, Dieter JN. The validity of the vascular "cold patch" in the diagnosis of chronic headache. *Headache* 1986;26:22–26.

22. Tunis MM, Wolff HG. Studies on headache: cranial artery vasoconstriction and muscle contraction headache. *Arch Neurol Psychiatr* 1954;71: 425–434.

23. Wallasch TM. Transcranial Doppler ultrasonic features in chronic tension-type headache. *Cephalalgia* 1992;12:385–386.

24. Wallasch TM. Transcranial Doppler ultrasonic features in episodic tension-type headache. *Cephalalgia* 1992;12:293–296.

The Headaches, Second Edition,
edited by J. Olesen, P. Tfelt-Hansen, and K.M.A. Welch.
Lippincott Williams & Wilkins, Philadelphia © 2000.

Tension-Type Headache, Cluster Headache, and Miscellaneous Primary Headaches

CHAPTER 76

Oromandibular Dysfunction and Tension-Type Headache

Rigmor Jensen and Steven B. Graff-Radford

Can headache originate from the masticatory system? According to the dental literature, this is often the case (5,7,18,19,23,24). Although temporomandibular disorders and headache occur together frequently, it could be simply by chance, because both disorders are extremely prevalent (2,12,20,21). Guidelines for the evaluation, diagnosis, and management of temporomandibular disorders (TMD) have been presented (3,17) but as yet cannot be regarded as internationally accepted. Of the variables included, only masticatory muscles painful to palpation have been found consistently to have a distinct relationship to headache (5,8,16). Because tenderness may be a part of a generalized myofascial syndrome, the real question of whether occlusal and mandibular abnormalities may be the cause or the effect of tenderness and pain remains largely unanswered. The headache classification committee of the International Headache Society (IHS) tried to obviate such problems by creating a new term, *oromandibular dysfunction* (OMD) (8) as a fourth-digit code number, one of several most likely causative factors to tension-type headache, in the hierachical classification system. These operational diagnostic criteria of OMD include some signs and symptoms of morphologic abnormalities and dysfunctions as well as parafunction of the jaw, tongue, and mouth. It does not include pericranial or jaw-muscle tenderness

(Table 1). Since the introduction of the IHS classification in 1988 (8), only a few studies have dealt with this term, and the terminology and diagnostic criteria in this field are still intensely debated. In the IHS classification (8), diagnostic criteria for the temporomandibular joint (TMJ) disease are also listed as a secondary specific headache form; however, scientific evidence for the exact relation of TMJ disease to headache and orofacial pain is rather limited, and hopefully further research and exchange between the dental and medical specialities can be encouraged (for further discussion, see Chapter 121).

In the following discussion, OMD refers to the fulfillment of the IHS criteria. Some results from population-based investigations are presented. Normative data from healthy subjects are compared with findings in subjects with tension-type headache and related to the clinical literature.

TABLE 1. *Criteria of oromandibular dysfunction (OMD criteria)[a]*

Three or more of the following:
Temporomandibular joint noise on jaw movements
Limited or jerky jaw movements
Pain on jaw function
Locking of jaw on opening
Clenching of teeth
Gnashing (grinding) of teeth
Other oral parafunction (tongue, lips or cheek biting or pressing).

[a]Fourth digit code for group 2 indicates most likely causative factor to tension-type headache.

R. Jensen: Department of Neurology, Glostrup Hospital, University of Copenhagen, DK-2600 Glostrup, Copenhagen, Denmark.

S.B. Graff-Radford: Department of Diagnostic Sciences, U.C.L.A., and The Pain Center, Cedars-Sinai Medical Center, Los Angeles, California 90048.

TABLE 2. *Suggested oromandibular dysfunction (OMD) screening questionnaire*

	Never	Often	Daily
Do you hear noises from jaw joints?			
Do you have pain with jaw function?			
Do you clench your teeth?			
Do you grind your teeth?			
Does your jaw get locked so you can't open or close it?			
Do you bite your tongue, lips or cheek?			
Do you press your tongue against your cheek or teeth?			
Do you have pain in or about the ears, temples, or cheeks?			

DENTAL EXAMINATION

A brief dental interview and examination is easy to perform during examination of a headache patient and will reveal most of the dental dysfunction that may be associated with headache. The items of oromandibular dysfunction 2.1.X.2 in the IHS classification are included in the suggested questionnaire (Table 2) and examination (Table 3). The use of such diagnostic tools is, however, controversial; Gerstner and colleagues reported that a brief questionnaire was valuable to distinguish between patients with temporomandibular disorders and healthy controls but unable to separate these TMD patients from patients with tension-type headache (6).

Because many patients relate their pain to previous trauma, infections, extractions, and joint problems, a short history of these factors also may be included, although the relation between trauma and OMD is quite uncertain. In addition to the present IHS criteria of oromandibular dysfunction, a brief evaluation of the bite function may be recommended as well. A significant loss of molars, impaired chewing ability, or malfunctioning dentures should be noted during the examination, because any of these factors may be a perpetuating factor to the pain (4,22,24). For research purposes, blinded designs must be used because of the subjectivity of the examination and because 13% of a general population had three or more symptoms or signs of OMD, thus fulfilling the IHS criteria (12).

TABLE 3. *Suggested oromandibular dysfunction (OMD) screening examination*

Listen for sounds and clicking of the TMJ
Palpate for jerking of TMJ
Measure interincisal mouth opening (>40 mm)
Palpate the lateral and dorsal TMJ capsules for tenderness
Determine tooth contacts in molar, premolar, and incisor areas, including loss of molars and malfunctioning dentures

TMJ, temporomandibular joint.

PREVALENCE

Disorders affecting the oromandibular system may be occlusal (e.g., lack of molars, occlusal disorders), parafunctional (e.g., bruxism, clenching, tongue pressure), or articular factors (arthritis, arthrosis, clicking at function). Some of these disorders are purely organic, whereas some may have a psychological background. Various terms, such as the *temporomandibular joint pain dysfunction syndrome*, the *myofascial pain dysfunction syndrome*, *craniomandibular disorders*, and *temporomandibular dysfunction*, including jaw-muscle tenderness, have been used. Therefore, the prevalence of a specific disorder is difficult to determine because of this lack of a universally accepted classification system. The complexity of the field is also reflected by the fact that objective signs often show a distribution of age and sex that is different from the distribution of symptoms (12, 19,23,24), and because the correlation between signs and symptoms generally is poor (2). In various series, the proportion of subjects with TMD in need of dental treatment is 3.5% to 9.7%, depending on the definition used (1,20).

NORMATIVE DATA

The prevalence of OMD, headache, and muscle tenderness was studied in a random sample of 735 adults representative of the total Danish population (9,11–13). The investigation was performed in a standardized way, with the observer of OMD and tenderness blinded to the previous history of OMD and headache and any other information about the subjects (9,11–13). The most common symptoms of OMD were clenching (22%) and grinding of teeth (15%), and the most common sign was irregular jaw movements on opening and closing (29%). In total, 13% of the subjects had three or more symptoms or signs of OMD as required by the IHS definition of OMD (12). Female subjects were affected more often than male subjects, but no significant relation to age was noted (12). Similar data were obtained in a Canadian epidemiologic study in which 12.9% reported functional pain or pain at rest, with women and younger age groups more likely than men and older age groups to report one or more symptoms (15). Significant associations between symptoms and potential risk factors as parafunctional behaviors were also reported (15).

RELATION TO HEADACHE TYPE

The prevalence of OMD did not differ between subjects with frequent tension-type headache, migraineurs, and headache-free persons in the Danish population study (13). Subjects with frequent tension-type headache (more than 14 days in the previous year) had the same frequency of three or more symptoms and signs of OMD as the rest of the general population (13). Any causal relationship between OMD and tension-type headache seems therefore to be absent or weak. Nevertheless, a minor positive relation between OMD and increasing frequency of tension-type headache was noted, but no such relation was found with increasing frequency of migraine (13). The lack of relationship between OMD and migraine indicates that dental treatment directed toward the chewing apparatus is inappropriate in migraine patients but may be of use in patients with frequent tension-type headache.

FINDINGS IN TENSION-TYPE HEADACHE

Clinical studies of the association between the former term *craniomandibular disorders* and headache have shown conflicting results (4,5,18,24). Most studies report a positive correlation, but in none of the studies were oromandibular or headache disorders sufficiently classified. Despite the high prevalence of oromandibular disorders and headache in the general population, many clinical studies did not include controls. In one study, headache, facial pain, and pericranial muscle tenderness were included in the definition of these disorders (24). It is not surprising, therefore, that a close relationship was found between headache and craniomandibular disorders, because a highly significant positive association between the frequency of tension-type headache and tenderness in pericranial muscles, quite independent of oromandibular dysfunction, has been reported (9).

Magnusson and Carlsson (16) studied 80 patients referred because of TMJ pain–dysfunction syndrome and 80 patients seeking dental treatment for other reasons. They noted, in correspondence with several others (9,13,24), that the frequency and severity of headache varied with the severity of the tenderness in pericranial muscles, but no other significant correlation was found between headache and TMJ signs or symptoms. In the Danish population study, no relation between OMD and

the intensity of tension-type headache was found, in agreement with Forssell and Kangasniemi (4) but not with others (24).

Solberg studied 735 young subjects from a dental clinic, and headache subjects reported tenderness of their TMJ and muscles in the jaw and head more frequently than nonsufferers of headache, but no other significant differences were reported (23). A significant positive correlation between tenderness and several other TMJ symptoms and signs has been described (5,24), but the use of unprecise classification of headache and TMJ symptoms as well as the use of uncontrolled and unblinded designs explain most of these discrepancies.

In conclusion, pericranial tenderness is increased in patients with frequent tension-type headache (see Chapters 80 and 81), whereas morphologic and articular disorders have no or, at most, an uncertain relation to headache.

Wänmann and Agerberg (24) examined a random group of 285 adolescents aged 17 years for the frequency and intensity of headache and dysfunction of the masticatory system. Tooth grinding and clenching were related to frequency of headache (24). Significant associations between bruxism, limited opening, muscular tenderness, and headache have been presented in other studies (14,18,19). When each sex was analyzed separately in a large sample of the general population, clenching and parafunctions were more frequent in subjects with frequent tension-type headache than in subjects without headache (13) (Fig. 1). In female subjects, but not in male subjects, TMJ noises and irregular movements were also more frequent among headache sufferers. Furthermore, both male and female subjects with clenching and female subjects with grinding had more tenderness than subjects with the identical frequency of headache but without parafunctional complaints (13). Recently, it was demonstrated that sustained tooth clenching provoked headache in 69% of patients with frequent tension-type headache but in only 17% of healthy controls, and this headache development was preceded by increased tenderness. These data indicate that tenderness may be a causative factor to headache (10,11). On balance, an association between parafunction, tenderness, and headache is likely. Tenderness resulting from excessive strain of masticatory muscles may contribute to tension-type headache, or these two disorders may be caused by a common, yet unknown, etiology.

RELATION TO HEADACHE FREQUENCY

Frequent, but not further specified headache, was reported by 48% of heavily affected persons with bruxism (14) compared with only 15% from a general population (12). In the Danish population study (12), OMD was pos-

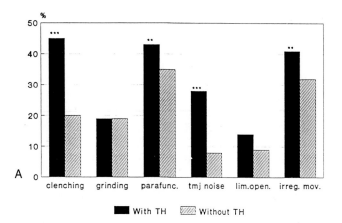

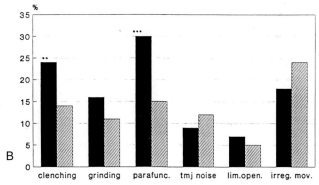

FIG. 1. Distribution of individual symptoms and signs of oromandibular dysfunctions in subjects with frequent tension-type headache (>14 days with tension headache per year) compared with headache-free subjects. **A:** Female subjects. **B:** Male subjects. **Statistical significance with $p < 0.01$. ***$p < 0.001$. (From ref. 13, with permission.)

OCCLUSION

The role of functional occlusal relationships in TMD disorders and headache has been studied intensively but, as is the case with the other hypotheses, none has been scientifically validated. By reviewing the literature, Seligman and Pullinger found no significant association between malocclusion and TMD (22), in line with the Danish population study (10), in which no association between occlusive disorders and headache could be noted (12). Overall, it seems that changes in occlusion do not have a primary role in headache, and complex occlusal therapy in headache patients should therefore be avoided.

CONCLUSION

When tenderness is analyzed separately from other disorders of the masticatory apparatus, as indicated by the IHS criteria, only parafunctional complaints, such as clenching, grinding of teeth, and pain by jaw function, are more prevalent in patients with frequent tension-type headache compared with headache-free subjects. These functional disturbances may be secondary to psychosocial stress or even may be a consequence of headache rather than its cause. Furthermore, the significant relation between parafunctional disorders and headache may represent a common underlying mechanism rather than a causal relationship, and a specific treatment directed toward these parafunctions, therefore, cannot be recommended. It seems clear that headache is not caused by morphologic abnormalities in the great majority of patients.

itively associated with increasing frequency of tension-type headache but not with the frequency of migraine. In correspondence, the few studies (4,24) in which a clinical index to the frequency of headache was calculated also reported increasing values with increasing frequency of headache. Forssell and Kangasniemi found a positive but not a strong ($p = 0.045$) correlation between a clinical index of mandibular dysfunction and the frequency of headache, but the reported symptoms did not correlate with the frequency of headache ($p = 0.78$) (4). Recently, significant correlations between frequent tooth clenching, headache, sleep disorders, and high scores of clinical dysfunction index were reported, but the study was uncontrolled and based on highly selected subjects (14).

A positive association of OMD with the frequency of tension-type headache indicates that OMD may be an aggravating factor for headache, or it may be another denominator of the same underlying pathophysiologic mechanism (5,7,13).

REFERENCES

1. Bakke M, Möller E. Craniomandibular disorders and masticatory muscle function. *Scandinavian Journal of Dental Research* 1992;100: 32–38.
2. De Kanter RJAM, Truin GJ, Burgersdiik RCW, et al. Prevalence in the Dutch adult population and a meta-analysis of signs and symptoms of temporomandibular disorders. *J Dent Res* 1993;72:1509–18.
3. Dworkin SF, Le Resche L. Research diagnostic criteria for temporomandibular disorders: review, criteria, examination and specification critique. *Journal of Craniomandibular Disordorders and Facial Oral Pain* 1992;4:301–355.
4. Forssell H, Kangasniemi P. Mandibular dysfunction in patients with muscle contraction headache. *Proceedings of the Finnish Dental Society* 1984;80:211–216.
5. Gelb H, Tarte J. A two year clinical dental evaluation of 200 cases of chronic headache: the craniocervical-mandibular syndrome. *JADA* 1975; 91:1230–1236.
6. Gerstner GE, Clark GT, Goulet JP. Validity of a brief questionaire in screening asymptomatic subjects from subjects with tension-type headache or temporomandibular disorders. *Community Dent Oral Epidemiol* 1994;22:235–242.
7. Graff-Radford SB. Headache and the temporomandibular joint. In: Goadsby PJ, Silberstein SD, eds. *Blue books of practical neurology.* New York: Butterworth-Heinemann, 1997:383–391.
8. Headache Classification Committee of the International Headache Society. Classification and diagnostic criteria for headache disorders, cranial neuralgias and facial pain. *Cephalalgia* 1988;8(Suppl 7):1–96.

9. Jensen R, Rasmussen BK, Olesen J. Cephalic muscle tenderness and pressure pain threshold in headache. *Pain* 1993;52:193–99.

10. Jensen R, Olesen J. Initiating mechanisms of experimentally induced tension-type headache. *Cephalalgia* 1996;16:175–82.

11. Jensen R, Bendtsen L, Olesen J. Muscular factors are of importance in tension-type headache. *Headache* 1998;38:10–17.

12. Jensen R, Rasmussen BK, Pedersen B, Lous I, Olesen J. Oromandibular disorders in a general population. *J Orofacial Pain* 1993;7:175–182.

13. Jensen R, Rasmussen BK, Lous I, Olesen J. Oromandibular dysfunctions and provocation of headache. In: Olesen J, Schoenen J. *Tension-type headache: classification, mechanisms and treatment.* New York: Raven Press, 1993:219–223.

14. Kampe T, Tagdae T, Bader G, Edman G, Karlsson S. Reported symptoms and clinical findings in a group of subjects with longstanding bruxing behaviour. *J Oral Rehabil* 1997;24:581–587.

15. Locker D, Slade G. Prevalence of symptoms associated with temporomandibular disorders in a Canadian population. *Community Dent Oral Epidemiol* 1988;16:310–313.

16. Magnusson T, Carlsson GE. Comparison between two groups of patients in respect of headache and mandibular dysfunction. *Swed Dent J* 1978;2:85–92.

17. McNeill C, ed. *Temporomandibular disorders: guidelines for classification, assessment and management.* Chicago: AACD Quintessence, 1993, 7–54.

18. Molin C, Carlsson GE, Friling B, Hedegaard B. Frequency of symptoms of mandibular dysfunction in young Swedish men. *J Oral Rehabil* 1976;3:9–18.

19. Nilner M. Epidemiology of functional disturbances and diseases in the stomatognathic system. *Swed Dent J* 1983;(Suppl 17):1–44.

20. Pilley JR, Mohlin B, Shaw WC, Kingdom A. A survey of craniomandibular disorders in 500 19-year olds. *Eur J Orthod* 1997;19:57–70.

21. Rasmussen BK, Jensen R, Schroll M, Olesen J. Epidemiology of headache in a general population—A prevalence study. *J Clin Epidemiol* 1991;44:1147–57.

22. Seligman DA, Pullinger AG. The role of functional occlusal relationships in temporomandibular disorders: a review. *J Craniomandibular Dis* 1991;5:96–106.

23. Solberg WK. Prevalence of mandibular dysfunction in young adults. *J Am Dent Ass* 1979;98:25–34.

24. Wänmann A, Agerberg G. Headache and dysfunction of the masticatory system in adolescents. *Cephalalgia* 1986;6:247–255.

The Headaches, Second Edition,
edited by J. Olesen, P. Tfelt-Hansen, and K.M.A. Welch.
Lippincott Williams & Wilkins, Philadelphia © 2000.

*Tension-Type Headache, Cluster Headache, and Miscellaneous
Primary Headaches*

CHAPTER 77

Psychological Mechanisms of Tension-Type Headache

Frank Andrasik and Jan Passchier

Tension-type headache has variously been labeled muscle contraction headache, psychogenic headache, depression headache, stress headache, conversion headache, psychomyogenic headache, and the like, which reflects the varied views and confusion about its etiology. The Headache Classification Committee of the International Headache Society (10) proposed a creative four-group scheme to help investigators and clinicians sort out the role of various causative factors. The diagnostic groups are sorted on the basis of chronicity (episodic versus chronic) and the presence of identifiable muscle involvement (evidence of pericranial muscle tenderness or elevated electromyographic readings versus the absence of this evidence), resulting in a 2×2 classification table. This more expanded coding format also allows diagnosticians to identify the most likely causative factors with increased precision by specifying whether one or more of the following factors are present: oromandibular dysfunction, psychosocial stress, anxiety, depression, delusion, muscular stress, drug overuse, or other headache condition. This basic approach has been reaffirmed by the World Health Organization (34). Unfortunately, researchers have rarely used the above level of precision when conducting investigations of pathophysiology of tension-type headache. Thus, progress has been slow at partialing out the role of the numerous suspected causes. The present review focuses chiefly on aspects that have been addressed most extensively: stress and muscle

F. Andrasik: Behavioral Medicine Laboratory, University of West Florida, Pensacola, Florida 32514-5751.

J. Passchier: Department of Medical Psychology and Psychotherapy, Erasmus University, 3000 DR Rotterdam, The Netherlands.

involvement. Other suspected etiologic factors are addressed in briefer fashion.

STRESS AS A FACTOR IN TENSION-TYPE HEADACHE

The relationship between stress and tension-type headache has been explored for over four decades, and the volume of available research is extensive. Wittrock and Myers (32) recently conducted a systematic examination of the empirical literature comparing individuals with recurrent tension-type headache and headache-free controls with respect to stress appraisal and coping and to psychophysiologic responses. Studies were numerous and included data collected in laboratory analogues and in the natural environment. Wittrock and Myers (32) developed a model to guide their review, which incorporates the transactional model of stress (15) and adds to it the role that pain itself plays in the experience of headache, especially when it is of a chronic, unremitting nature (Fig. 1). In brief, the model begins with occurrence of an event that is potentially stressful. Emphasis is on *potential* because stress is experienced in an idiosyncratic manner; stress rests within an individual's cognitive interpretive framework. That is, what determines whether any given event is stressful is more a function of how the patient appraises the event. Lazarus and Folkman (15) distinguish two types of appraisal: primary, whether a given event is judged to be significant to the person's well-being, and secondary, whether the person has the resources or options available to respond successfully to the event. If an event is judged to be both relevant and a

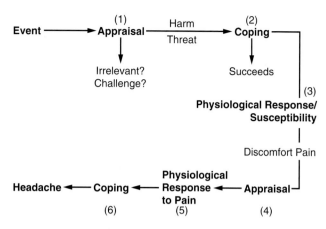

FIG. 1. A model for the appraisal and coping process in tension-type headache. Reproduced with permission from Wittrock and Myers (32).

threat (step 1 in the model), then a coping response is required (step 2). Unsuccessful attempts at coping lead to physiologic arousal (which may involve muscle tension) and pain (step 3). Onset of pain can lead to further negative appraisals (step 4), which then intensify attendant pain (step 5), promote further, perhaps more desperate, efforts to cope (step 6), and ultimately exacerbate headache.

Wittrock and Myers (32) theorize that individuals with tension-type headache may differ from nontension headache sufferers in one or more of five different ways. These hypotheses can be stated in a clear and testable manner and are provided in Table 1. The brief literature review to follow will discuss how studies have examined these aspects and summarize evidence relating to each hypothesis. The present review draws heavily upon the observations and conclusions of Wittrock and Myers (30).

Exposure to Stress

Studies of exposure to stress use scales that focus on distal and/or proximal events. Distal scales typically inquire about major events (positive as well as negative)

TABLE 1. *Possible roles that stress might play with respect to tension-type headache*

1. People with tension-type headache may be exposed more frequently to stressful events.
2. People with tension-type headache may be more likely to appraise situations as stressful.
3. People with tension-type headache may show increased physiologic reactivity to stress.
4. People with tension-type headache may have an increased sensitivity to pain and/or a decreased threshold for pain.
5. People with tension-type headache may cope with stress in a way that increases its impact.

that have occurred over an extended time period (6 months of more) and that have been assigned a weight indicative of the stress demand. Proximal measures, on the other hand, assess everyday stressors over much briefer time frames. A particularly useful instrument is the Daily Stress Inventory (7). This 58-item inventory yields three measures of stress:

1. Event score, the frequency of occurrence of stressful events
2. Impact score, summation of the ratings assigned to each event using a 7-point scale completed by the subject
3. Impact: event ratio, which provides an overall mean stress rating

Available studies reveal a fairly consistent picture (32). Tension-type headache patients typically do not experience a greater number of major stressful events over extended time periods; however, tension-type headache sufferers typically do experience a greater number of everyday life stresses (minor ups and downs or hassles) and judge them to have more impact (9,18,20).

Appraisal of Stress

This aspect has been investigated most commonly by presenting various groups of subjects with taxing laboratory tasks (e.g., mental arithmetic, vigilance, items from intelligence tests, and stressful mental imagery). With few exceptions, available research studies have not found headache subjects to report increased stress in response to these stimuli. A few studies have found that tension-type headache subjects reveal higher baseline levels of stress, but any increases are proportional to those exhibited by the nonheadache comparison groups (32). Exposure to identical stressors in controlled laboratory settings leads to similar increases in stress by tension-type headache subjects. However, the salience of the laboratory stressors used may be questioned.

Physiologic Reactivity to Stress

Although research investigations abound in this area [Wittrock and Myers (32) reported nearly 40 such studies], methodologic complexities have hampered progress. The ideal investigation would examine physiologic responding during adaptation, baseline, stress, and recovery conditions; would include multiple physiologic measures, multiple stress stimuli that simulate real-life circumstances, multiple comparison groups (carefully matched nonheadache controls and carefully matched other headache types), to permit tests of specificity; would conduct assessments when patients were free from headache, when headache was present, and during headache induction; would require subjects to abstain from using substances that are known to affect physiology for a set period prior to study entry (e.g., nicotine, caffeine, and medication); and would use appropriate measurement and analysis procedures that take gender into account (2). Few studies have distinguished between episodic and chronic tension-type headache, and this may be a critical shortcoming (32). No single study has been able to meet all or even most of these criteria. (Most of these rigorous criteria need consideration when evaluating laboratory investigations of stress appraisal and pain sensitivity and thresholds as well.)

In the face of this complexity, it should not be surprising that few findings have been unequivocal or consistently replicated. In the nonheadache state, tension-type headache sufferers reveal no consistent differences in resting levels or in response to stress (31). However, when headache is present, EMG levels do appear to be more elevated (32). Few studies have realized the importance of tracking headache status at the time that assessments are conducted. Greater attention to this aspect in the future may help to clarify matters.

Sensitivity and Threshold Effects

Investigators have used various stimuli to induce mild pain or discomfort in the controlled laboratory setting: thermal (cold pressor and direct application of ice), pressure (pressure algometer and blood pressure cuff), and other (shock and light). These stimuli have been applied to the head, arm, and finger while various psychophysiologic measures, including assessments of muscle tenderness and subjective or self-report measures (pain intensity, threshold, and tolerance) have been collected (32). Findings here are complicated and difficult to interpret. With respect to subjective reports, when differences emerge, they are typically of the nature of tension-type headache sufferers reporting greater sensitivity and a reduced threshold. Analysis of responding in the presence of headache reveals greater pain sensitivity. Researchers have recently begun to examine muscle tenderness, and available findings are fairly consistent in showing increased tenderness for tension-type headache patients versus controls (nonheadache and other headache types; 16–18). Jensen et al. (14) showed that the presence of a muscle disorder significantly affected the pain sensitivity of patients with chronic but not episodic tension-type headache. They speculated that muscular factors may be pivotal for episodic headaches to become chronic.

Wittrock and Myers (32) reported that investigations of psychophysiologic responding to pain stressors have consistently revealed no major differences with respect to EMG measures. However, differences have emerged with respect to cardiovascular parameters, in the direction of revealing heightened sympathetic arousal, to neurochemical measures (β-endorphins, serotonin, and substance P in platelets), and to the later exteroceptive suppression period (ES2) (27), although more recent findings have failed to replicate these ES2 differences (17).

Ukestad and Wittrock (30) exposed tension-type headache subjects and controls to two different cold stressors and then had subjects complete a coping strategies inventory. Headache subjects reported greater catastrophizing about the pain and rated the pain as greater.

Coping Styles

The literature addressing this parameter is limited and inconsistent. Studies assessing coping responses to laboratory stressors have found no differences between tension-type headache patients and controls. Studies quantifying how people cope with life events that disrupted or caused major schedule changes suggest that tension-type headache sufferers tend to report greater use of nonoptimal strategies (e.g., withdrawal, avoidance, self-criticism; 8,11). In response to pain stimuli, individuals with tension-type headache show more tendencies to catastrophize (30).

PSYCHOLOGICAL THEORIES ON TENSION-TYPE HEADACHE

Theories on mental processes can be subdivided into those that emphasize the role of emotional processes and those that focus on cognitive processes. These views can be used to explain many symptoms in addition to those of tension-type headache, and not only physical symptoms but psychological disturbances as well.

Emotional Theories

The psychological theory with the longest history, and both strongly favored and disputed, is that of psychoanalysis. According to this view, psychogenic pain can be considered a solution for an unconscious conflict within the individual. By the presentation of complaints of pain, a person might satisfy both his or her aggressive impulses against other people and his or her own conscience, which forbids its overt expression. Instead of being expressed as an outward reaction, the aggression is directed toward oneself (1,26). Although several empirical researchers have found that tension headache patients are consciously troubled by hostile feelings and anxiety (3,5,25), the unconscious conflicts have seldom been empirically investigated to date. One study (23) did not find an abnormal pattern of defense mechanisms in these patients.

Penzien et al. (25) reviewed nearly 200 headache studies reporting psychological data for headache patients. Of those studies that included headache-free subjects for comparison, 71% found increased maladaptive behavior/psychological test scores for the headache patients. Most studies find the most heightened psychological test scores for tension-type headache patients. The remaining 29% found no significant differences between patients and normative or control samples. Although significantly different (statistically), the levels of psychological symptoms rarely fell into the clinically significant range. In studies reporting clinical significance, only 5% to 15% of headache patients typically fall into the psychopathology category. These conclusions parallel the findings of Merikangas et al. (19), who found no major differences between tension-type headache sufferers and controls subjects 27 to 28 years of age selected from the general population, but they are at odds with a recent study of psychiatric comorbidity conducted with headache clinical patients. Members of the Italian Collaborative Group (13) carefully assessed 217 tension-type headache sufferers from 10 different Italian headache centers and found a high percentage of the cases to meet diagnostic criteria for anxiety, depression, and somatoform disorders. Prevalence rates for anxiety disorder were similar for episodic and chronic cases; chronic cases revealed higher prevalence rates for depression and somatoform disorders. Thus, findings varied significantly as a function of the sample studied. Finally, preliminary findings suggest that tension-type headache patients may suppress and hold in anger (4). It is still unclear if the psychological distress often reported by tension-type headache patients results more from a pain-filled history or serves as an independent source to form an eliciting factor for the headaches. Blanchard et al. (6) offered evidence suggesting that psychopathology may contribute directly to headache for a certain proportion of tension-type patients.

Cognitive Theories

An influential theory that emphasizes the role of attentional processes in the report of symptoms is that of Pennebaker (24). According to Pennebaker, sensations of an internal bodily source compete with those from the environment for gaining the attention of the person. Under conditions of low environmental stimulation (such as stimulus deprivation) or high physiologic activation (such as stress), physical sensations have a higher probability of being perceived. These perceptions can be interpreted as bodily symptoms when the individual structures these perceptions by a cognitive scheme focused on the idea of having a disease. Although this theory has been supported for the perception of symptoms of nasal congestion and pain in general, so far it has not been tested with regard to headache complaints.

Another theory that emphasizes the role of attentional processes in the development of psychosomatic complaints is that of physiologic disregulation of Schwartz (28). Schwartz (28) stated that, when attention is diverted from one's physiologic state and corrective action to return to normal functioning does not occur, physical

dysfunction may be the outcome. Teaching the patient to attend to the afflicted organ by biofeedback can restore proper functioning. So far, some evidence has been collected supporting the theory regarding its usefulness for tension-type headache (12).

CONSEQUENCES OF TENSION-TYPE HEADACHE

Although the intensity of migraine headaches may lead to relatively short but intense interruptions of the daily activities, tension-type headache, with its longer duration, greater frequency, and moderate intensity, tends more to envelop the person's life in a nebula of fatigue and depressive moods. Although absence from school and work as a consequence of these headaches might be found as well, clinical observations indicate that its negative effects are more apparent in the emotional life of the person.

Results from a preliminary investigation of functional impairments in social, behavioral, cognitive, and recreational domains found tension-type headache patients to be less disabled on one measure (composite functional impairment index, which represented the average level of impairment during a day when either a typical or a worst headache occurred) than either migraineurs or those with migraine combined with tension-type headache (33). However, scores for the total functional impairment index (which represented the overall average level of impairment regardless of headache severity) revealed no differences between the three headache groupings. The authors speculated that the three headache groups may differ in the amount of impairment experienced during particular headache episodes but that they may not differ in overall level of impairment endured (due to the more frequent occurrence of tension-type headache). More recent studies have found that tension-type headache patients are as impaired in their lives as are migraine patients (22,29).

SUMMARY

Accumulating evidence suggests that individuals with tension-type headache report experiencing more everyday mild stressors, judge these daily stressors to have high impact, and may use less successful strategies for coping with daily stressors. Furthermore, when experiencing pain or discomfort, individuals with tension-type headache reveal greater pain sensitivity, reduced pain threshold, increased muscle tenderness, and increased overall arousal. When compared with nonheadache controls, individuals with tension-type headache reveal higher elevations on various psychological dimensions, and these differences are most pronounced for samples drawn from clinic settings. However, direction of causality is uncertain.

ACKNOWLEDGMENTS

Preparation of this manuscript was supported in part by Grant NS29855 from the National Institutes of Health–National Institute of Neurologic Disorders and Stroke (NIH-NINDS).

REFERENCES

1. Adler CS, Adler SM. Psychodynamics of head pain: an introduction. In: Adler CS, Adler SM, Packard RC, eds. *Psychiatric aspects of headache.* Baltimore: Williams & Wilkins, 1987:41–55.
2. Andrasik F, Blanchard EB, Arena JG, Saunders NL, Barron KD. Psychophysiology of recurrent headache: methodological issues and new empirical findings. *Behav Ther* 1982;13:407–429.
3. Andrasik F, Blanchard EB, Arena JG, Teders SJ, Teevan RC, Rodichok LD. Psychological functioning in headache sufferers. *Psychosom Med* 1982;44:171–182.
4. Arena JG, Bruno GM, Rozantine GS, Meador KJ. A comparison of tension headache sufferers and nonpain controls on the State-Trait Anger Expression Inventory: an exploratory study with implications for applied psychophysiologists. *Appl Psychophysiol Biofeedback* 1997;22:209–214.
5. Blanchard EB, Andrasik F, Arena JG. Personality and chronic headache. In: Maher BA, Maher WB, eds. *Progress in experimental personality research: normal personality processes*, Vol 13. New York: Academic, 1984:303–364.
6. Blanchard EB, Kirsch CA, Appelbaum KA, Jaccard J. Role of psychopathology in chronic headache: cause or effect? *Headache* 1989;29:295–301.
7. Brantley PJ, Jones GN. *Daily Stress Inventory professional manual.* Odessa, FL: Psychological Assessment Resources, 1989.
8. Ehde DM, Holm JE. Stress and headache: comparisons of migraine, tension, and headache-free subjects. *Headache Q* 1992;3:54–60.
9. Ficek SK, Wittrock DA. Subjective stress and coping in recurrent tension headache. *Headache* 1995;35:455–460.
10. Headache Classification Committee of the International Headache Society. Classification and diagnostic criteria for headache disorders, cranial neuralgias and facial pain. *Cephalalgia* 1988;8(Suppl 7):1–96.
11. Holm JE, Holroyd KA, Hursey KG, Penzien DB. The role of stress in recurrent tension headache. *Headache* 1986;26:160–167.
12. Hovanitz CA, Wander MR. Tension headache: disregulation at some levels of stress. *J Behav Med* 1990;13:539–560.
13. Puca F, Genco S, Prudenzano MP, et al. for the Italian Collaborative Group for the Study of Psychopathological Factors in Primary Headaches. Psychiatric comorbidity and psychosocial stress in patients with tension-type headache from headache centers in Italy. *Cephalalgia* 1999;19:159–164.
14. Jensen R, Bendtsen L, Olesen J. Muscular factors are of importance in tension-type headache. *Headache* 1998;38:10–17.
15. Lazarus RS, Folkman S. Coping and adaptation. In: Gentry WD, ed. *The handbook of behavioral medicine.* New York: Guilford, 1984:282–325.
16. Lipchik GL, Holroyd KA, France CR, et al. Central and peripheral mechanisms in chronic tension-type headache. *Pain* 1996;64:467–475.
17. Lipchik GL, Holroyd KA, Talbot F, Greer M. Pericranial muscle tenderness and exteroceptive suppression of temporalis muscle activity: a blind study of chronic tension-type headache. *Headache* 1997;37:368–376.
18. Lous I, Olesen J. Evaluation of pericranial tenderness and oral function in patients with common migraine, muscle contraction headache, and muscle contraction headache and "combination headache." *Pain* 1982;12:385–393.
19. Merikangas KR, Merikangas JR, Angst J. Headache syndromes and psychiatric disorders: association and familial transmission. *J Psychiatr Res* 1993;27:197–210.
20. Myers TC, Wittrock DA, Foreman G. Appraisal of subjective stress in individuals with tension-type headache: the influence of baseline measures. *J Behav Med* 1998;21:469–484.
21. Mosley TH, Penzien DB, Johnson CA, et al. Time-series analysis of stress and headache. *Cephalalgia* 1991;11(Suppl 11):306–307.
22. Passchier J, de Boo M, Quaak HZA, Brienen JA. Health-related quality of life of chronic headache patients is predicted by the emotional component of their pain. *Headache* 1996;36:556–560.
23. Passchier J, van der Helm-Hylkema H, Orlebeke JF. Personality and headache type: a controlled study. *Headache* 1984;24:140–146.
24. Pennebaker JW. *The psychology of physical symptoms.* New York: Springer-Verlag, 1982.
25. Penzien DB, Rains JC, Holroyd KA. In: Tollison CD, Kunkel RS, eds. *Headache: diagnosis and treatment.* Baltimore: Williams & Wilkins, 1993.
26. Pilowsky I. Psychodynamic aspects of the pain experience. In: Sternbach RA, ed. *The psychology of pain.* New York: Raven, 1978:203–217.
27. Schoenen J. Exteroceptive suppression of temporalis muscle activity in patients with chronic headache and in normal volunteers: methodology, clinical, and pathophysiological relevance. *Headache* 1993;33:3–17.
28. Schwartz GE. Psychosomatic disorders and biofeedback: a psychobiological model of disregulation. In: Maser JD, Seligman MEP, eds. *Psychopathology: experimental models.* San Francisco: WH Freeman, 1977.
29. Solomon JD, Skobieranda FG, Gragg LA. Does quality of life differ among headache diagnoses? Analysis using the medical outcomes study treatment. *Headache* 1994;34:143–147.
30. Ukestad LK, Wittrock DA. Pain perception and coping in female tension headache sufferers and headache-free controls. *Health Psychol* 1996;15:65–68.
31. Wittrock DA. The comparison of individuals with tension-type headache and headache-free controls on frontal EMG levels: a meta-analysis. *Headache* 1997;37:424–432.
32. Wittrock DA, Myers TC. The comparison of individuals with recurrent tension-type headache and headache-free controls in physiological response, appraisal, and coping with stressors: a review of the literature. *Ann Behav Med* 1998;20:118–134.
33. Wittrock DA, Penzien DB, Mosley TH, Johnson CA. The Recurrent Illness Impairment Profile: preliminary results using the headache version. *Headache Q* 1991;2:138–139.
34. World Health Organization. ICD-10 guide for headaches: guide to the classification, diagnosis and assessment of headaches in accordance with the tenth revision of the international classification of diseases and related health problems and its application to neurology. *Cephalalgia* 1997;17(Suppl 19):1–82.

The Headaches, Second Edition,
edited by J. Olesen, P. Tfelt-Hansen, and K.M.A. Welch.
Lippincott Williams & Wilkins, Philadelphia © 2000.

Tension-Type Headache, Cluster Headache, and Miscellaneous Primary Headaches

CHAPTER 78

Biochemistry of Blood and Cerebrospinal Fluid in Tension-Type Headache

Flemming W. Bach and Michel D. Ferrari

The literature on biochemistry in tension-type headache (TTH) is characterized by the pursuit of a large variety of ideas about pathophysiology, and it may therefore appear somewhat dispersed and confusing. Indeed, in many cases similar studies have been performed that yielded contradictory results, and there may be many reasons for this.

First, many different designations, including chronic daily headache, (chronic) muscle contraction headache, tension headache, and chronic migraine; definitions; and criteria have been used in the past to describe clinically patients suffering from unspecified headaches. This severely hampers straightforward comparison of the results. Only in recent years have most investigators used the 1988 criteria (38). Second, exclusion criteria also vary markedly, the most important being the use of medication at the time of biochemical investigation and the coexistence of migraine or depression. Third, timing of the investigation (during headache or during headache-free periods) also varies and, most confusingly, is not always defined.

Our aim is to present the reader with the available data in a systematic fashion and relate to some of the data with a critical eye. However, because of the assorted pattern of studies and multitude of techniques used, it will not for every substance studied be possible to reach a final conclusion on a pathophysiologic or diagnostic role in TTH.

F. W. Bach: Department of Neurology, University of Århus, Århus Kommunehospital, DK-8000 Århus, Denmark.
M. D. Ferrari: Department of Neurology, Leiden University Medical Centre, NL-2300 RC Leiden, The Netherlands.

The subject will be handled in sections on blood chemistry, platelets, immune cells, and cerebrospinal fluid. Data on serotonin in the blood circulation are presented in the platelet section because of the intimate relationship between platelet stores of serotonin and free serotonin in plasma.

BLOOD CHEMISTRY

Magnesium concentrations, which measured in serum may reflect brain level and, thereby, level of inhibition of N-methyl-D-aspartate (NMDA)-type glutamate receptors, were reported to be reduced in patients with TTH in headache-free periods and further lowered during headache in analogy with what was seen in migraine (59). Schoenen et al., on the other hand, found similar magnesium concentrations in chronic TTH and control subjects (60). Lactic and pyruvic acid levels are normal in TTH (55).

Peptides

Several peptides have been studied in TTH, and the endogenous opioid peptides β-endorphin and methionine-enkephalin (met-enkephalin) received much attention for a period. The idea was that headache was a hypoendorphin-syndrome (66). It appears from Table 1 that the data are inconsistent with regard to this idea. Furthermore, because circulating endogenous opioid peptides are not vasoactive or have access to the central nervous system, the role of circulating opioid peptides in relation to headache is obscure (4). Plasma neuropeptide Y (NPY)

TABLE 1. *Plasma levels of opioid peptides*

Peptide	n	Diagnosis	Result	Ref.
β-endorphin	8	DCH	Reduced	(9)
β-endorphin	11	DCH	Reduced	(24)
β-endorphin	47	DCH	Normal	(30)
β-endorphin	41	CTTH	Normal	(7)
β-endorphin	7	ETH	Reduced	(10)
Met-enkephalin	9	TH	Elevated	(28)

DCH, daily chronic headache; CTTH, chronic tension-type headache; ETH, episodic tension-type headache; TH, tension-type headache.

concentrations were normal in patients suffering from episodic TTH and did not differ between headache episodes and pain-free periods (33). Endothelin-1 concentrations in plasma were normal in episodic and chronic TTH (32).

Neuroendocrine Parameters

Adrenocorticotrophic hormone (ACTH) and cortisol were normal in daily chronic headache (24) and chronic TTH (43). Melatonin is synthesized in the pineal gland from serotonin, but possesses negligible serotonin-like activity. Nocturnal levels are high, whereas diurnal concentrations are low or undetectable. Nocturnal plasma melatonin levels have been found to be reduced in a group of female tension headache patients (16). It was not clear from the patient description whether this group also included depressed patients. The pathophysiologic interpretation of these preliminary findings is not simple, but they were suggested to reflect global sympathetic hypofunction.

Amino Acids

Ferrari et al. (26) studied plasma amino acids in migraine patients and used TTH patients and healthy normal individuals as controls. Whereas the neuroexcitatory amino acids glutamic and aspartic acid were clearly elevated in migraine patients, no abnormalities could be demonstrated in TTH patients. Also, homocysteine levels were normal in a study examining 20 patients with episodic TTH (23).

Monoamines

Shimomura et al. (62) found that plasma levels of 3-methoxy-4-hydroxyphenylglycol (MHPG), which seem to reflect central noradrenergic metabolism, predict the clinical response of TTH patients to tizanide hydrochloride. Those patients who showed the best clinical response after 4 weeks of treatment had the highest pretreatment MHPG plasma levels and presumably the highest central noradrenergic activity. Several methodologic

reservations, however, apply to this interesting observation, most importantly the way the clinical response was measured (undefined criteria, open uncontrolled evaluation), how clinical outcome groups were formed and related to the MHGP levels (open or blinded), and lack of clinical information on the patients (use of medication, diet, and depression). Furthermore, those patients who improved most also had by far the shortest duration of the illness, suggesting that other factors were involved. Nevertheless, this approach is most promising and should be confirmed in a prospective, placebo-controlled, double-blind design.

Dopamine β-hydroxylase catalyzes the conversion of dopamine to norepinephrine, and serum levels of this enzyme were found to be reduced in 10 patients with TTH compared with control subjects (31). The same reduction was also seen in migraine patients. Gallai et al. (31) consider serum activity of dopamine β-hydroxylase a useful indicator of sympathetic activity, considering the instability of serum norepinephrine concentrations. Suggesting a reduced noradrenergic tonus in TTH (and migraine), this study should be reproduced on larger groups of patients, and the status of headache at the time of sampling made clear.

Castillo et al. measured plasma concentrations of epinephrine, norepinephrine, and dopamine under standardized conditions in 30 patients with episodic TTH in headache phase. Pain and depression were rated on separate scales. Plasma concentrations of all three catecholamines were lower than in control persons, supporting the idea of reduced sympathetic activity in TTH (15). There was no association between depression scores and catecholamine concentrations. Reduced plasma norepinephrine concentrations also were found in 15 patients with muscle contraction headache (69).

Urinary excretion of 5-hydroxytryptamine (5-HT), noradrenaline, adrenaline, and dopamine and their acidic metabolites have been studied in female, chronic daily headache patients (28). Preliminary data suggested that in these patients the 24-hour excretion of dopamine was reduced and the circadian rhythmicity of the excretion of the metabolites was disturbed. Thus, the normally existing difference between diurnal and nocturnal excretion (diurnal > nocturnal) was absent in the headache patients. Chronic daily headache patients were similar to migraine patients in this respect. More studies are needed.

Martignoni et al. (47) found that baseline β-endorphin plasma levels and the β-endorphin plasma response to clonidine were significantly lower in patients with combined migraine without aura and tension headache than in healthy controls. This was interpreted as evidence for failure of central noradrenergic activity. It is not clear whether similar results could be obtained in patients with pure tension headache without associated migraine.

IMMUNOLOGIC CHANGES

Link and colleagues (45) have investigated several immunologic parameters in cerebrospinal fluid (CSF) and plasma of patients with chronic headache (of unspecified and undefined type). However, in these studies the headache patients were used as controls for patients with multiple sclerosis, and no healthy, normal controls were included. Accordingly, no qualitative conclusions regarding these observations can be drawn.

Nagasawa et al. (51) found slightly higher serum levels of complement C3 and C4 in patients with muscle contraction headache compared with normal individuals. However, the patient group was a mean of 10 years older than the control group, and both C3 and C4 levels increased with age. Accordingly, the conclusion of Nasagawa et al. that inflammatory aspects are involved in muscle contraction headache is interesting but should be confirmed in a study with a matched control group.

Diaz-Mitoma et al. (20) reported that significantly more patients with so-called new daily persistent headaches had evidence of active Epstein-Barr infection (84% versus 25% in controls). It is unknown how frequent this headache syndrome is and how it relates to TTH. We are unaware of similar studies conducted with TTH patients.

Interleukin-2 is a cytokine activating T-lymphocytes. Shimomura et al. found reduced serum levels of interleukin-2 in 46 patients with TTH and similarly reduced levels in migraine (61).

The importance of connections between the immune and nervous systems is becoming increasingly clear, not the least in the field of pain. In a series of experiments, Christoph Stein et al. have provided evidence that β-endorphin may be synthesized in immunocytes and, following stimulation by inflammatory mediators such as corticotropin-releasing hormone and interleukin-1, released into inflamed tissue. Here, β-endorphin may bind to opioid receptors on nociceptive fibers and reduce nociception (14). Three independent groups have measured decreased β-endorphin concentrations in peripheral blood mononuclear cells in patients with episodic TTH during a headache-free period (10,44,48). Although the results are premature in the sense that β-endorphin was not characterized on the molecular level, these data are interesting in the light of development within the field. However, speculations about β-endorphin concentrations in peripheral blood mononuclear cells reflecting central nervous system concentrations of the same substance (44) have no support in scientific data (3).

SEROTONIN (5-HT) METABOLISM AND PLATELET FUNCTION

Many groups have investigated platelet function and platelet-related biochemical factors in relation to TTH, but with often contradictory results. The data are discussed as follows. Relevant data on serotonin are summarized in Table 2.

TABLE 2. *Serotonin metabolism and platelet function in tension headache*

Variable	CDH	N	CMCH-P+	N	CMCHP−	N	THE-P+	N	THE-P−	N	CTTH-P+	N	Ref.
5-HT														
Platelets	↔	9												(29)
Platelets	↓	95												(1)
Platelets			↓	23										(58)
Platelets					↔	14								(65)
Platelets									↑	28				(19)
Platelets							↑	30						(42)
Platelets											↓	31		(52)
Platelets											↓	13		(64)
Platelets											↔	40		(12)
Platelets							↑	13	↔	13				(39)
Plasma											↔	9		(29)
Plasma											↔	40		(12)
Plasma									↑	28				(19)
Plasma					↑	23								(68)
Serum							↔	10						(57)
5-HIAA														
Platelets									↑	28				(19)
Plasma									↑	28				(19)
Plasma	↔	9												(29)
Serum							↔	7						(57)
Urine											↔	39		(12)
5-Hydroxytryptophan														
Plasma	↔	9												(29)
5-HT Uptake platelets											↓	21		(37)
5-HT Uptake platelets									↑	20				(65)

CDH, chronic daily headache; CMCH, chronic muscle contraction headache; P+, during pain; P−, during pain-free period; THE, tension headache episodic type; CTTH, chronic tension-type headache; ↑, increased level; ↔, normal level; ↓, decreased level.

General Methodologic Considerations

Most importantly, when investigating blood levels of 5-HT, it is necessary to discriminate between the two distinct compartments of 5-HT in blood: the 5-HT in platelets with concentrations in the micromolar range and representing a pharmacologically inactive, slow-turnover, reserve pool, and the 5-HT in (platelet-free) plasma with concentrations in the nanomolar range, which shows rapid turnover and is pharmacologically potentially active (2,56). Several researchers have incorrectly used the designation "plasma 5-HT" while indicating the 5-HT concentration in platelet-rich plasma and thus of platelets. In this chapter we reserve the designation "plasma 5-HT" for measurements made in platelet-poor or platelet-free plasma.

Other factors may explain inconsistency between studies. Mean ages of the study populations vary between 29 and 46. Mean duration of illness was between 9 and 12 years. The female to male ratio was at least 3 to 1, except in the studies of Anthony and Lance (1) and Nakano (52), which included more males than females. Freedom from medication was not required in the study of Hannah et al. (37). Patients were free from medication for at least 3 days in the study of Rolf et al. (58) and at least 7 days in the other studies. The use of a diet and coexistence of depression varied by study or are not reported.

Platelet 5-HT

Four groups have found significantly reduced levels of platelet 5-HT in TTH (1,52,58,64), whereas three studies reported normal levels (12,28,65), and two studies increased levels (19,42). The study of Anthony and Lance (1) differs by substantially lower absolute levels of platelet 5-HT in the control and patient groups, compared with those measured by other investigators. It was not stated whether their patients were on a particular diet or were also suffering from depression. The Shukla et al. (65) and D'Andrea et al. (19) studies investigated TTH patients during headache-free periods.

In summary, these studies are seemingly conflicting but in fact are not comparable. The very large study of Anthony and Lance (1) suggests reduced platelet 5-HT in chronic daily headache patients, but this may be restricted to male patients only. Remarkably, Glover et al. (35) also found reduced activity of platelet monoamine oxidase (MAO) in male TTH patients only. Thus, the data of Anthony and Lance should be reanalyzed separately for males and females and should be confirmed by others, taking into account potential sex (and age) differences. It is hard to conclude from so different data, but if only studies using the International Headache Society (IHS) criteria for TTH and with patient materials cleaned of concomitant disorders are included, a picture of normal or reduced platelet 5-HT appears (12,28,64).

Platelet 5-HT Uptake

Shukla et al. (65) found evidence for increased uptake of 5-HT in platelets of TTH patients. However, Hannah et al. (37) found that the 5-HT uptake sites in platelets of TTH patients have reduced affinity for 5-HT, independent of coexisting depression, age, or sex. Binding of serotonin reuptake–inhibiting drugs to platelets may reflect the number of 5-HT transporters and thereby the uptake ability. The number of imipramine binding sites were reduced (46), but studied by paroxetine binding, the number of 5-HT transporters were estimated to be normal (13).

5-HT Binding to Lymphocytes and Monocytes

Giacovazzo et al. (34) found that lymphocytes and monocytes of TTH patients show a complete loss of high-affinity binding sites for 5-HT during the headache but a normal *in vitro* 5-HT binding curve during headache-free periods. No information, however, was given regarding whether the patient and control groups were age matched. In addition, compared with the control group, the patient group contained proportionally more females, who were also using medication. Accordingly, no firm conclusions can be drawn on the validity of these findings.

Platelet Enzymes

No differences have been found for phenolsulphotransferase (PST)-P or -M isoenzyme activity in TTH patients (28), but platelet MAO activity has been found to be reduced during headache in female patients (28) and during headache-free periods in males only (35). Superoxide dismutase activity was normal in TTH and migraine without aura as opposed to reduced activity in migraine without aura (63).

5-HT and 5-HT Precursors and Metabolites in Plasma and Serum

Plasma levels of 5-HT, its precursor 5-hydroxytryptophan (5-HTP), and the 5-HT metabolite 5-hydroxyindole acetic acid (5-HIAA) were found to be normal by Ferrari et al. (28) in female TTH patients during headache. Bendtsen et al. also found normal plasma 5-HT and urine 5-HIAA levels during pain (12), whereas two other studies showed increased levels in headache-free period (19,68). Finally, a study on episodic TTH showed normal plasma 5-HT levels in headache-free periods and increased levels during headache (39).

Ribeiro et al. (57) found normal serum levels of 5-HT and 5-HIAA during headache in TTH patients who were on a phenylethylamine- and tyramine-restricted diet. Serum concentrations are difficult to relate to plasma and platelet levels because during the process of serum preparation, blood is coagulated and platelets are activated, causing release of platelet 5-HT. Indeed, their control values for serum 5-HT were about 50 times higher than values generally considered normal for plasma 5-HT.

Methionine-Enkephalin

Methionine-enkephalin is colocalized with 5-HT in the dense granules of platelets (21) and seems to possess neutralizing activity with respect to the endothelial damaging effects of 5-HT (36). Platelet met-enkephalin levels have been found to be normal in TTH patients, but plasma met-enkephalin levels proved to be markedly increased compared with both normal individuals and migraine patients, during as well as outside of acks (27). Thus, determination of plasma and platelet met-enkephalin levels may prove to be a useful marker to distinguish between TTH and migraine without aura. This should be confirmed in a larger study, especially because in the study of Ferrari et al. (27) patient and control groups were not age matched.

Release of Platelet Methionine-Enkephalin and 5-HT

Plasma collected from migraine patients during an attack has been shown to release met-enkephalin *in vitro* from platelets collected from the same migraine patients during attack-free periods (Fig. 1). No such release could be measured from platelets from TTH patients or healthy control persons (28). This suggests another biochemical difference between migraine and TTH patients. No release of platelet 5-HT was observed by Ferrari et al. (28), either when platelets from migraine patients were used or when platelets from TTH patients or healthy controls were incubated.

Other Platelet Constituents

Gamma-aminobutyric acid (GABA) concentrations in platelets from 27 TTH patients were higher than in 21 healthy control persons (40). Glycine, glutamate, and aspartate concentrations, on the other hand, were normal (18). Substance P concentrations in platelets from patients with TTH during pain were similar to migraine patients and higher than in healthy control persons (52). Ionized magnesium was reduced in platelets from 20 patients with TTH, whereas concentrations of cyclic AMP and cyclic GMP were normal (50).

Conclusions from Platelet Studies

Because the fundamental idea in studying platelet biochemistry in TTH is the concept of platelets being a model of serotonergic neurons, the work of obtaining consistent data between groups of researchers should at this time be redirected toward efforts in validate this concept further.

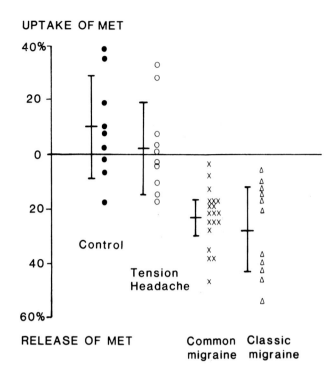

FIG. 1. Change in platelet met-enkephalin content induced by incubation with plasma collected during migraine attacks. Each symbol indicates, per individual, the proportional increase (uptake) or decrease (release) of platelet met-enkephalin content induced by incubation with migraine-attack plasma compared with the met-enkephalin content of the platelets that were only resuspended in water. Vertical lines represent 99% confidence intervals and group means.

CEREBROSPINAL FLUID

Quantitative analysis of the biochemical constituents of CSF are performed on the assumption that CSF concentrations reflect brain or spinal cord tissue concentrations, and perhaps synaptic activity, because CSF is in constant exchange with extracellular fluid of the central nervous system (CNS). Evidence in support of this assumption is available for monoamines (72) and neuropeptides (11). However, some common issues related to biochemical measurements in CSF have to be addressed to validate the results:

1. Most substances of interest exist in both CNS and blood and can be regarded as markers of CNS activity only if the blood–CSF barrier is relatively complete for a given substance and patient group. The evidence to date suggests that CSF monoamines and neuropeptides originate mainly in the CNS and do not leak in from the circulation in patients without CNS lesions (11,73). Exceptions are prolactin, gonadotropins, and cortisol (74).

2. It may be difficult to identify which CNS regions contribute to the CSF pool of a given substance. It is likely that superficial regions located close to the

subarachnoidal space and near the sampling site contribute more than deeper regions at the opposite end of the neuroaxis. Methionine-enkephalin and dynorphin are examples of neuropeptides that are abundant in, and can be released from, the spinal cord (49). CSF obtained by lumbar puncture may therefore be suitable to evaluate processes in the spinal cord, although both peptides are also abundant supraspinally. β-endorphin, on the other hand, is almost entirely supraspinally located (67), and the relevance of lumbar sampling of CSF thus relies on the positive correlation found between central and lumbar CSF β-endorphin concentrations (8).

3. If effects of age, sex, menstrual phase, and diurnal variation on CSF peptide levels are not ruled out, materials and sampling procedures have to be standardized accordingly.

4. Centrally acting drugs may influence neuropeptide production, processing, and secretion. Such drugs should be avoided for weeks before CSF sampling.

5. Neuropeptides such as opioid peptides and tachykinins are processed from precursors in one or more steps, and the products may be further derivatized (54). As a result, radioimmunoassays will rarely be specific for a single neuropeptide. For example, some antisera recognize several β-endorphin–related peptides in CSF (5). Because derivatization usually changes the biological activity of a peptide, ideally it should be examined if the degree of derivatization differs between groups investigated.

With these precautions in mind, CSF examinations may be a valuable tool for the study of nociceptive and antinociceptive mechanisms in headache.

NEUROPEPTIDES

Opioid Peptides

Endogenous opioid peptides are derived from three distinctive gene products—the precursor molecules proopiomelanocortin, proenkephalin A, and proenkephalin B—and are commonly classified as the endorphins, the enkephalins, and the dynorphins, respectively (49). Several forms of derivatization of the peptides with or without preservation of the biological activity exist within each opioid family. β-endorphin may be C-terminally truncated or N-acetylated and loses its opioid activity in the latter case.

β-Endorphin

Lumbar CSF from eight patients suffering from migraine with interparoxysmal headache for 1 to 10 years revealed a mean β-endorphin concentration that was only 20% of the mean of the control subjects. All individual concentrations were below the defined normal range (53). Similar levels of β-endorphin were found in patients with migraine without aura, whereas patients with symptomatic headaches (posttraumatic and postischemic) had normal CSF β-endorphin levels (53). On the other hand, a study including 47 patients with chronic TTH according to the criteria of the IHS showed almost identical CSF β-endorphin levels in the patient group and the control group (7). In contrast to the former study, patients with migraine attacks more than once per month were excluded. Nineteen of the patients included had migraine attacks 1 to 12 days per year. Although migraine was not associated with low β-endorphin concentrations in our study (7), it may be that the low concentrations found by Nappi et al. (53) are related more to migraine than to tension headache. On the other hand, an inverse relationship between chronic pain factors and CSF β-endorphin also has been reported in patients with low back pain (17). Demographic characteristics of the patients and control group were matched in both studies, and both radioimmunoassays applied distinguish between β-endorphin and β-lipotropin. Patients with fibromyalgia, a disorder with many similarities to chronic tension-type headache, have a normal β-endorphin level in CSF (70).

N-Acetylated b-Endorphin

Cerebrospinal fluid concentrations of N-acetylated β-endorphin (Ac-β-EP) in 15 patients with migraine and associated chronic TTH was significantly higher than in 22 controls ($p < 0.01$) (25). β-endorphin concentrations in the same samples, however, were lower in the headache group ($p > 0.05$) (Fig. 2). As a consequence, the β-endorphin:Ac-β-EP ratio was much lower in patients than in controls (25) (see Fig. 2). In this study, there was also a negative relationship between CSF β-endorphin and a headache pain index.

Methionine-Enkephalin

Cerebrospinal fluid from 48 patients of the same group with chronic tension-type headache examined for β-endorphin by Bach et al. (7) revealed a higher mean level of met-enkephalin immunoreactivity (41). Studies on patients suffering from other types of pain have shown that patients with neurogenic pain syndromes had higher met-enkephalin levels than controls, whereas patients with idiopathic pain syndromes had normal levels (71). Increased CSF levels of met-enkephalin-Arg[6]-Phe[7] were found in patients with fibromyalgia, although the control samples were not concurrently obtained (70).

Dynorphin

Dynorphin immunoreactivity was lower in 38 patients from the group with chronic TTH described above than in

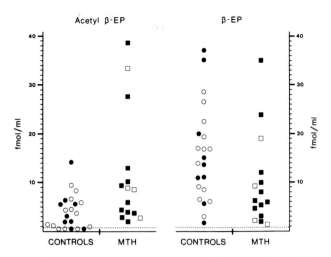

FIG. 2. Individual CSF concentrations of β-endorphin and Ac-β-EP in control subjects (*circles*) and patients with migraine with tension-type headache (MTH) (*squares*). The concentration of peptides in each sample was calculated by adding the peak values to the values for the two adjacent fractions. Open symbols refer to males; solid symbols refer to females.

10 healthy controls (6). Patients with idiopathic pain syndromes revealed lower CSF dynorphin levels than controls (71), whereas fibromyalgia patients had higher levels than a nonconcurrent control group (70).

Other Neuropeptides

Calcitonin gene-related peptide (CGRP) is present in C-fiber afferents colocalized with substance P, and is depleted from the trigeminal nucleus after electrical stimulation. Thus, CSF CGRP levels may reflect the level of activity in C-fiber afferents. Cholecystokinin may on the spinal level act as an analgesic in high doses, but act as an inhibitor of opioid-induced antinociception in lower doses. Somatostatin is thought to exert an inhibitory effect on nociceptive afferents. We determined CSF concentrations of these three neuropeptides in patients with chronic TTH and found normal levels (6).

OTHER SUBSTANCES

CSF levels of prolactin, follicle-stimulating hormone (FSH), and luteinizing hormone (LH) were detectable in 20 patients with chronic tension-type headache but were undetectable in control persons (22). CSF cortisol was lower in the headache patients than in controls (22). However, these differences seem to reflect similar differences in serum (22), which agrees with the view that CSF levels of all these substances correlate with serum or plasma levels (74). Thus, the significance of these findings is unclear.

CONCLUSIONS

Analysis of neuropeptides in CSF from patients with chronic TTH clearly indicates changes in the CNS that may be either adaptive or pathophysiologic (Table 3). The finding of a decreased CSF β-endorphin:Ac-β-EP ratio in patients with migraine and TTH is particularly intriguing, indicating the existence of a disease due to biological inactivation of β-endorphin (25). However, another study, using a radioimmunoassay that does not detect Ac-β-EP to a significant degree, failed to find decreased β-endorphin levels in a patient group who were similar except that they were suffering from fewer migraine attacks (7). Future studies will be needed to show if such an inactivation of β-endorphin occurs in other idiopathic pain syndromes. The finding of decreased dynorphin levels might likewise indicate opioid hypoactivity. Increased CSF met-enkephalin levels in patients with chronic TTH may be the result of an increased input from the nociceptive afferents, followed by increased activity in descending or segmental antinociceptive systems mediated by met-enkephalin. Alternatively, met-enkephalin release is increased compensatorily to insufficiency of other central pain-inhibitory systems acting presynaptically on the primary afferent. The findings outlined here do not easily fit into a simple pathophysiologic model for chronic TTH but provide evidence of disturbances in the endogenous opioid system.

COMPARISON WITH MIGRAINE

Distinguishing between migraine without aura and TTH is not always easy to do on purely clinical grounds. Ferrari and co-workers studied biochemical differences between these two entities (see Chapter 31). Their data show that patients with tension headache and patients with migraine differ biochemically. In addition to these data, Anthony and Lance (1) showed in a large study that platelet 5-HT levels are markedly reduced in TTH patients compared with both

TABLE 3. *CSF findings in chronic tension-type headache*

Substance	Level in CSF	Reference
Opioid Peptides		
β-endorphin	Decreased	(53)
β-endorphin	Normal	(7)
N-acetylated β-endorphin	Increased	(25)
Met-enkephalin	Increased	(41)
Dynorphin	Decreased	(6)
Calcitonin gene-related peptide	Normal	(6)
Cholecystokinin	Normal	(6)
Somatostatin	Normal	(6)
Hormones		
FSH	Normal	(22)
LH	Normal	(22)
Prolactin	Normal	(22)
Cortisol	Normal	(22)

controls and migraine patients (but see above for comments), but Shukla et al. (65) found the opposite. The reviewed studies of neuropeptides in plasma or CSF do not consistently point at parameters that distinguish TTH and migraine. Although some studies reveal biochemical differences that might be of relevance for diagnostic purposes, much more work is needed to validate these options.

REFERENCES

1. Anthony, M, Lance JW. Plasma serotonin in patients with chronic tension headaches [see Comments]. *J Neurol Neurosurg Psychiatry* 1989; 52:182–4.
2. Artigas, F, Sarrias MJ, Martinez E, Gelpi E, Alverez E, Udina C. Increased plasma free serotonin but unchanged platelet serotonin in bipolar patient treated chronically with lithium. *Psychopharmacology* 1989;99:382–392.
3. Bach FW. β-endorphin and migraine. *Cephalalgia* 1992;12:390.
4. Bach FW. Opioid peptides in primary headaches. In: Olesen J, Edvinsson L, eds. *Headache pathogenesis. Monoamines, neuropeptides, purines, and nitric oxide.* Philadelphia: Lippincott-Raven, 1997:193–200.
5. Bach FW, Ekman R, Jensen FM. β-endorphin-immunoreactive components in human cerebrospinal fluid. *Regul Pept* 1986;16:189–198.
6. Bach FW, Langemark M, Ekman R, Rehfeld JF, Schifter S, Olesen J. Effect of sulpiride or paroxetine on cerebrospinal fluid neuropeptide concentrations in patients with chronic tension-type headache. *Neuropeptides* 1994;27:129–136.
7. Bach FW, Langemark M, Secher NH, Olesen J. Plasma and cerebrospinal fluid β-endorphin during chronic tension-type headache. *Pain* 1992;51:163–168.
8. Bach FW, Schmidt JF, Faber T. Radioimmunoassay of β-endorphin in ventricular and lumbar cerebrospinal fluid. *Clin Chem* 1992;38:847–852.
9. Baldi E, Salmon S, Anselmi B, et al. Intermittent hypoendorphinaemia in migraine attack. *Cephalalgia* 1982;2:77–81.
10. Battistella PA, Bordin A, Cernetti R, et al. Beta-endorphin in plasma and monocytes in juvenile headache. *Headache* 1996;36:91–4.
11. Beal MF, Martin JB. Neuropeptides in neurological disease. *Ann Neurol* 1986;20:547–565.
12. Bendtsen L, Jensen R, Hindberg I, Gammeltoft S, Olesen J. Serotonin metabolism in chronic tension-type headache. *Cephalalgia* 1997;17:843–848.
13. Bendtsen L, Mellerup ET. The platelet serotonin transporter in primary headaches. *Eur J Neurol* 1998;5:277-282.
14. Capot PJ, Carter L, Gaiddon C, et al. Immune cell-derived β-endorphin. Production, release, and control of inflammatory pain in rats. *J Clin Invest* 1997;100:142–148.
15. Castillo J, Martinez F, Leira R, Lema M, Noya M. Plasma monoamines in tension-type headache. *Headache* 1994;34:531–535.
16. Claustrat B, Loisy C, Brun J, Beorchia S, Arnaud JL, Chazot G. Nocturnal plasma melatonin levels in migraine:a preliminary report. *Headache* 1989;29:241–244.
17. Cleeland CS, Shacham S, Dahl JL, Orrison W. CSF β-endorphin and the severity of pain. *Neurology* 1984;34:378–380.
18. D'Andrea G, Cananzi AR, Joseph R, et al. Platelet glycine, glutamate and aspartate in primary headache. *Cephalalgia* 1991;11:197–200.
19. D'Andrea G, Hasselmark L, Cananzi AR, et al. Metabolism and menstrual cycle rhythmicity of serotonin in primary headaches. *Headache* 1995;35:216–221.
20. Diaz-Mitoma F, Vanast VJ, Tyrell DL. Increased frequency of Epstein-Barr virus excretion new daily persistent headaches. *Lancet* 1987;1:411–414.
21. DiGiulio AM, Picotti GB, Cesura AM, et al. Met-enkephalin immunoreactivity in blood platelets. *Life Sci* 1982;30:1605–1614.
22. Elwan O, Abdella M, Bayad ABE, Hamdy S. Hormonal changes in headache patients. *J Neurol Sci* 1991;106:75–81.
23. Evers S, Koch HG, Husstedt I. Plasma homocysteine levels in primary headache. In: Olesen J, Edvinsson L, eds. *Headache pathogenesis. Monoamines, neuropeptides, purines, and nitric oxide. Headache pathogenesis.* Philadelphia: Lippincott-Raven, 1997:215–218.
24. Facchinetti F, Nappi G, Savoldi F, Genazzani AR. Primary headaches: reduced circulating β-lipotropin and β-endorphin levels with impaired reactivity to acupuncture. *Cephalalgia* 1981;1:195–201.
25. Facchinetti F, Sances G, Martignoni E, Pagani I, Nappi G, Genazzani AR. Evidence of alpha, N-acetyl β-endorphin in human cerebrospinal fluid. *Brain Res* 1992;586:1–5.
26. Ferrari MD, Odink J, Bos KD, Malessy MJA, Bruyn GW. Neuro-exitatory plasma aminoacids are elevated in migraine. *Neurology* 1990;40:1582–1586.
27. Ferrari MD, Odink J, Frölich M, Portielje JEA, Bruyn GW. Methionine-enkephalin in migraine and tension headache. Differences between classic migraine, common migraine and tension headache, and changes during attacks. *Headache* 1990;30:160–164.
28. Ferrari MD, Odink J, Frolich M, Tapparelli C, Portielje JE. Release of platelet met-enkephalin, but not serotonin, in migraine. A platelet response unique to migraine patients? *J Neurol Sci* 1989;93:51–60.
29. Ferrari MD, Odink J, Tapparelli C, VanKempen GMJ, Pennings EJM, Bruyn GW. Serotonin metabolism in migraine. *Neurology* 1989;39:1239–1242.
30. Fettes I, Gawel M, Kuzniak S, Edmeads J. Endorphin levels in headache syndromes. *Headache* 1985;25:37–39.
31. Gallai V, Gaiti A, Sarchielli P, Coata G, Trequattrini A, Paciaroni M. Evidence for an altered dopamine beta-hydroxylase activity in migraine and tension-type headache. *Acta Neurol Scand* 1992;86:403–406.
32. Gallai, V, Sarchielli P, Firenze C, et al. Endothelin 1 in migraine and tension-type headache. *Acta Neurol Scand* 1994;89:47–55.
33. Gallai V, Sarchielli P, Trequattrini A, Paciaroni M, Usai F, Palumbo R. Neuropeptide Y in juvenile migraine and tension-type headache. *Headache* 1994;34:35–40.
34. Giacovazzo M, Bernoni RM, Di Sabato F, Martelletti P. Impairment of 5HT binding to lymphocytes and monocytes from tension-type headache patients. *Headache* 1990;30:220–223.
35. Glover V, Littlewood JT, Sandler M, Peatfield R, Petty R, Rose FC. Platelet monoamine oxidase activity and headache: relationship to personality and smoking. *Psychopharmacol Bull* 1984;20:536–538.
36. Grossman A, Clement-Jones V. Opiate receptors: enkephalins and endorphins. *Clin Endocrinol Metab* 1983;12:31–56.
37. Hannah P, Jarman J, Glover V, Sandler M, Davies PT, Clifford Rose F. Kinetics of platelet 5-hydroxytryptamine uptake in headache patients. *Cephalalgia* 1991;11:141–145.
38. Headache Classification Commitee of the International Headache Society. Classification and diagnostic criteria for headache disorders, cranial neuralgias and facial pain. *Cephalalgia* 1988;8:1–96.
39. Jensen R, Hindberg I. Plasma serotonin increase during episodes of tension-type headache. *Cephalalgia* 1994;14:219–222.
40. Kowa H, Shimomura T, Takahashi K. Platelet gamma-aminobutyric acid levels in migraine and tension-type headache. *Headache* 1992;32:229–232.
41. Langemark M, Bach FW, Ekman R, Olesen J. Increased cerebrospinal fluid met-enkephalin immunoreactivity in patients with chronic tension-type headache. *Pain* 1995;63:103–107.
42. Leira, R, Castillo J, Martinez F, Prieto JM, Noya M. Platelet-rich plasma serotonin levels in tension-type headache and depression. *Cephalalgia* 1993;13:346–348.
43. Leone M, Biffi M, Leoni F, Bussone G. Leukocyte subsets and cortisol serum levels in patients with migraine without aura and chronic tension-type headache. *Cephalalgia* 1994;14:139–142.
44. Leone M, Sacerdote P, D'Amico D, Panerai AE, Bussone G. Beta-endorphin concentrations in the peripheral blood mononuclear cells of migraine and tension-type headache patients [see Comments]. *Cephalalgia* 1992;12:154–157.
45. Link H, Baig S, Kostulas V, Olsson O, Olsson T. Immunoglobulin-secreting cells in the cerebrospinal fluid from patients with muscle tension headache. *J Neuroimmunol* 1989;25:1–6.
46. Marazziti D, Bonuccelli U, Nuti A, et al. Platelet 3H-imipramine binding and sulphotransferase activity in primary headache. *Cephalalgia* 1994;14:210–214.
47. Martignoni E, Facchinetti F, Rossi R, Sances G, Gennazani AR, Nappi G. Neuroendocrine evidence of deranged noradrenergic activity in chronic migraine. *Psychoneuroendocrinology* 1989;14:357–363.
48. Mazzotta G, Sarchielli P, Gaggioli A, Gallai V. Study of pressure pain and cellular concentration of neurotransmitters related to nociception in episodic tension-type headache patients. *Headache* 1997;37:565–571.
49. Millan MJ. Multible opioid systems and chronic pain. In: Hertz A, ed.

Handbook of experimental pharmacology. Berlin: Springer-Verlag, 1993:127–162.

50. Mishima K, Takeshima T, Shimomura T, et al. Platelet ionized magnesium, cyclic AMP, and cyclic GMP levels in migraine and tension-type headache. *Headache* 1997;37:561–564.

51. Nagasawa A, Teramoto J, Naitou K, Takahashi A. Inflammatory alterations in muscle contraction headache. *Headache* 1991;31:543–545.

52. Nakano T, Shimomura T, Takahashi K, Ikawa S. Platelet substance P and 5-hydroxytryptamine in migraine and tension-type headache. *Headache* 1993;33:528–532.

53. Nappi G, Facchinetti F, Martignoni E, et al. Plasma and CSF endorphin levels in primary and symptomatic headaches. *Headache* 1985;25: 141–144.

54. Nyberg F, Vaeröy H, Terenius L. Opioid peptides and substance P in the cerebrospinal fluid. Regulation and the relation to pain. In: Olesen J, Edvinsson L, eds. *Basic mechanisms of headache 2.* Amsterdam: Elsevier, 1988:241–258.

55. Okada H, Araga S, Takeshima T, Nakashima K. Plasma lactic acid and pyruvic acid levels in migraine and tension-type headache. *Headache* 1998;38:39–42.

56. Ortiz J, Artigas F, Gelpi E. Serotonergic status in human blood. *Life Sci* 1988;43:983–990.

57. Ribeiro CA, Cotrim MD, Morgadinho MT, Ramos MI, Santos ES, de Macedo TdR. Migraine, serum serotonin and platelet 5-HT2 receptors. *Cephalalgia* 1990;10:213–219.

58. Rolf LH, Wiele G, Brune GG. 5-hydroxytryptamine in platelets of patients with muscle contraction headache. *Headache* 1981;21:10–11.

59. Sarchielli P, Coata G, Firenze C, Morucci P, Abbritti G, Gallai V. Serum and salivary magnesium levels in migraine and tension-type headache. Results in a group of adult patients. *Cephalalgia* 1992;12:21–27.

60. Schoenen J, Sianard Gainko J, Lenaerts M. Blood magnesium levels in migraine. *Cephalalgia* 1991;11:97–99.

61. Shimomura T, Araga S, Esumi E, Takahashi K. Decreased serum interleukin-2 level in patients with chronic headache. *Headache* 1991;31: 310–313.

62. Shimomura T, Awaki E, Kowa H, Takahashi K. Treatment of tension-type headache with tizanidine hydrochloride: its efficacy and relationship to the plasma MHPG concentration. *Headache* 1991;31:601–604.

63. Shimomura T, Kowa H, Nakano T, et al. Platelet superoxide dismutase in migraine and tension-type headache. *Cephalalgia* 1994;14:215–218.

64. Shimomura T, Takahashi K. Alteration of platelet serotonin in patients with chronic tension-type headache during cold pressor test. *Headache* 1990;30:581–583.

65. Shukla R, Shanker K, Nag D, Verma M, Bhargava KP. Serotonin in tension headache. *J Neurol Neurosurg Psychiatry* 1987;50:1682–1684.

66. Sicuteri F. Natural opioids in migraine. In: Critchley M, Friedman A, Gorini S, Sicuteri F, eds. *Headache: physiopathological and clinical concepts 33.* New York: Raven, 1982:65–74.

67. Stengaard-Pedersen K, Larsson L-I. Comparative immunocytochemical localization of putative opioid ligands in the central nervous system. *Histochemistry* 1981;73:89–114.

68. Takeshima T, Shimomura T, Takahashi K. Platelet activation in muscle contraction headache and migraine. *Cephalalgia* 1987;7:239–243.

69. Takeshima T, Takao Y, Urakami K, Nishikawa S, Takahashi K. Muscle contraction headache and migraine. Platelet activation and plasma norepinephrine during the cold pressor test. *Cephalalgia* 1989;9:7–13.

70. Vaerøy, H, Nyberg F, Terenius L. No evidence for endorphin deficiency in fibromyalgia following investigation of cerebrospinal fluid (CSF) dynorphin A and met-enkephalin-Arg⁶-Phe⁷. *Pain* 1991;46:139–143.

71. Von Knorring L, Almay BLG, Ekman R, Widerlöv E. Biological markers in chronic pain syndromes. *Nord Psykiatr Tidsskr* 1988;42: 139–145.

72. Wester P, Bergström U, Eriksson A, Gezelius C, Hardy J, Winblad B. Ventricular cerebrospinal fluid monoamine transmitter and metabolite concentrations reflect human brain neurochemistry in autopsy cases. *J Neurochem* 1990;54:1148–1156.

73. Wood JH. Neurochemical analysis of cerebrospinal fluid. *Neurology* 1980;30:645–651.

74. Wood JH. Neuroendocrinology of cerebrospinal fluid: peptides, steroids, and other hormones. *Neurosurgery* 1982;11:293–305.

The Headaches, Second Edition,
edited by J. Olesen, P. Tfelt-Hansen, and K.M.A. Welch.
Lippincott Williams & Wilkins, Philadelphia © 2000.

Tension-Type Headache, Cluster Headache, and Miscellaneous Primary Headaches

CHAPTER 79

Synthesis of Tension-Type Headache Mechanisms

Jes Olesen and Jean Schoenen

One simple etiology and one simple pathophysiologic mechanism cannot be expected in tension-type headache, which, on the contrary, is likely to be multifactorial (4). A few good studies now have comprehensively elucidated the various aspects of the mechanisms of tension-type headache. They have yielded novel but partly conflicting results. Pathogenic models, therefore, cannot yet be entirely specific. Nevertheless, models are necessary for our understanding and for future research strategies. This chapter largely follows the scheme used in the chapter on the synthesis of migraine mechanisms (Chapter 41).

BACKGROUND

Muscle pains are the most frequent of any pains in the body (2,3), and tension-type headaches are more common than myofascial pains in other parts of the body. Myofascial tissues are constructed to move; muscles need exercise, whereas change of position is necessary for joints and fasciae. Long-term immobilization or static posture affects these tissues and causes them to hurt. During normal functioning, there is a constant cross-talk between myofascial tissues and the central nervous system, eliciting the necessary changes in position and the necessary rest. In this way, the normal person is kept free of myofascial pain.

Every time slight discomfort is felt from myofascial tissues, and probably even earlier, there are afferent impulses in small-diameter myelinated Aδ and unmyelinated C fibers (*nociception*). This physiologically important afferent input, however, may be a latent source of pain, depending on the central modulation of nociception, which may explain why myofascial pain is so common. For instance, descending inhibition is stronger on input to dorsal horn neurons from muscle nociceptors than from cutaneous nociceptors (8).

Why, then, is tension-type headache more common than myofascial pain from other areas in the body? One reason may be that pain thresholds to pressure are lower in the cranium than in the extremities (11). A general lowering of pain thresholds (*increased sensitivity*) could result in head pain without pain in the rest of the body. The head also occupies a primary role in body awareness, as evidenced by the rostrocaudal deterioration in patients with decreased levels of consciousness (12), and the head and face have a particularly large cortical representation. Chewing muscles and neck muscles are directly involved in emotional motor behavior, such as facial expression, aggression, defense, sucking, feeding, and gnashing of teeth. Excessive inhibition of motor behaviors, such as facial expressiveness (17), as well as of emotional mechanisms (16) have been described in headache patients, although motor patterns of jaw muscles also may be suppressed as a consequence of the pain (13). Nevertheless, the result could be increased strain, tenderness, and pain. There is increasing evidence that pain perception is not a simple reflection of simultaneous afferent noxious input

J. Olesen: Department of Neurology, Glostrup Hospital, University of Copenhagen, DK-2600 Glostrup, Copenhagen, Denmark.

J. Schoenen: University Department of Neurology, CHR Citadelle, and University of Liège, B-4000 Liège, Belgium.

but a dynamic process that is highly influenced by the effects of past experience. Peripheral and central sensitization of nociceptors plays a pivotal role in these processes, involving striking biochemical and physiologic changes of primary and second-order nociceptive neurons (18) (see Chapter 15). Such considerations do not prove that muscle strain or sensitization plays a primary pathogenetic role, but they provide a background for the understanding of tension-type headache.

GENETIC PREDISPOSITION

If the genetics of migraine are poorly worked out, the situation is clearly worse in tension-type headache. Because of the enormous prevalence and variability in frequency and severity of tension-type headache, any inheritance is almost certain to be polygenic. Sufferers of tension-type headache must by chance have many affected first-degree relatives. The population relative risk in relatives compared with normal controls has been calculated in only a single recent study. In chronic tension-type headache, the risk was increased threefold, indicating a genetic predisposition. The transmission suggested complex inheritance (10). At present, we adopt the view that the great majority of the population, perhaps all, have the potential to develop tension-type headache if exposed to sufficiently strong environmental factors.

ENVIRONMENTAL PREDISPOSITION

We know of only a few environmental factors that increase the likelihood of attacks over a prolonged period. The role of female hormones is clearly less pronounced compared with that in migraines, with a male-to-female ratio of 4:5 (14). No definite changes at menarche or during pregnancy have been described. Oromandibular dysfunction, particularly pressure and grinding of teeth, seem to be associated with an increased prevalence of tension-type headache and especially with increased frequency and severity of tension-type headache as discussed in Chapter 76. An association between tension-type headache and a state of anxiety or depression also is indicated (see Chapter 77). Classic and operant conditioning of behavior might play a role (17). The relationship between short-lasting (weeks or months) aggravation and environmental factors is better known. Thus, psychological stress, daily hassles, oromandibular dysfunction, nonphysiologic working position and other muscle strain, anxiety, and depression are found frequently in patients visiting their doctor because of aggravation of headache.

PHYSIOLOGIC AND BIOCHEMICAL ABNORMALITIES OUTSIDE OF ATTACKS

Most of the changes found outside of attacks are of somewhat uncertain validity, partly because most abnor-

malities have been shown in only one center and partly because it has often not been clearly described whether studies were done on headache-free days or on headache days. Mostly, it is also uncertain whether these abnormalities can be found in the individual patient over a prolonged period. However, recently some of the most important questions have been clarified.

After a dispute of some years, it was finally shown in a double-blind, controlled study that patients with tension-type headache had more tenderness in the pericranial myofascial tissue than did a control group. The same result was found in a blinded population-based study, which also showed that muscle tenderness increased with increasing frequency of tension-type headaches (see Chapter 73). No increase in surface electromyogram (EMG) over the frontal and temporal muscles was found in subjects with episodic tension-type headache, but a modest increase in subjects with chronic tension-type headache was noted (6,15) (see Chapter 74). Recently, a qualitatively changed response to mechanical stimuli in human tender muscle was demonstrated in patients with chronic tension-type headache (1). This response was most pronounced in patients who felt the most tenderness and suggests mediation of pain by low-threshold mechanosensitive afferents projecting to sensitized second-order trigeminal neurons. As discussed in Chapter 74, temporalis exteroceptive suppression is not consistently abnormal in chronic tension-type headache. It could be reduced or abolished in a subgroup of patients with long-standing daily headache in whom it might reflect increased cortical serotoninergic activity.

PRECIPITATION OF ATTACKS

Little scientific evidence can be found about possible precipitating factors, but psychogenic factors and myofascial strain are the primary suspects. Specifically designed experiments have shown that experimental stress in the laboratory can induce headaches in some subjects (see Chapter 74). Experimental change of bite function (7) and experimental clenching of teeth also cause headache (see Chaps. 73 and 76). After tooth clenching, muscle tenderness increased in patients, who subsequently developed headache, and the mechanical pain threshold increased in those who did not develop headache, suggesting a role both for peripheral and central sensitization and central antinociceptive systems (5). The relation to the menstrual period is less clear than for migraine, although some increase in tension-type headache premenstrually and menstrually has been described. There are no good pharmacologic tools to induce tension-type headache.

PHYSIOLOGIC AND BIOCHEMICAL ABNORMALITIES DURING ATTACKS

Few previous studies have compared patients during and outside of tension-type headaches. Changes in cerebrospinal fluid composition have not been consistently reported. Interest has focused on the endogenous opioids, but more evidence is needed, as discussed in Chapter 78. The same conclusion has been drawn in this chapter regarding changes in blood platelets, hormones, and immunologic parameters. Pericranial muscle tenderness is increased during headache compared with outside of headache (see Chapter 73). Thus, hyperalgesia appears initially to be linked reversely to the actual headache episode. Headache and tenderness vary in parallel, and it is difficult to know which causes which. The same was true for increased EMG levels in patients with chronic tension-type headache. The increase in EMG levels was, however, modest, significant only in the frontal muscle and far too small to explain muscle pain on the basis of ischemia resulting from muscle contraction. Correspondingly, Langemark and Olesen showed that local temporal blood flow was normal in patients with chronic tension-type headache (Chapter 75). This finding pertained to those with headache on the day of examination as well as those without headache. The increased tenderness during an actual headache also was not due to an increase in general pain threshold in subjects with tension-type headache on the day of examination compared with matched subjects without actual headache.

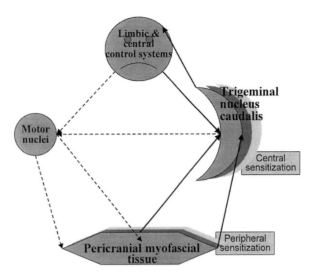

FIG. 1. Illustration of the concept that tension-type headache is the result of a dynamic interaction between peripheral nociceptive and mechanoceptive second-order brainstem neurons and their descending control systems. Peripheral mechanisms might predominate in occasional episodic tension-type headache, whereas central changes play an increasingly important role with more frequent headaches and may become the predominant pathogenetic mechanism in chronic tension-type headache.

A MODEL OF TENSION-TYPE HEADACHE

Individual Episode

An acute episode of tension-type headache usually occurs in a perfectly normal person. Thus, the attack may be viewed as a deflection of the normal mechanisms of nociception and central modulation of nociception from myofascial tissues or increased afferent nociceptive input from the tissues (Fig. 1). Headache may be brought on by physical stress, such as riding a racing bicycle for the first time, or an nonphysiologic working position. In such cases, increased nociception from strained muscle seems to be the primary cause of the attack. Lack of rest and sleep may cause headache by similar mechanisms. Increased input in C fibers and in sensitized mechanoceptive Aδ fibers (pain impulses) may cause an increased sensitivity of neurons of the trigeminal tract, and pain then may propagate itself to some extent (9). Under normal circumstances, such increased nociceptive activation is counteracted by descending antinociceptive systems (Fig. 1). The tension-type headache is favored by an inadequate activation of the pain-controlling pathways, possibly because of stress, anxiety, and emotional disturbances (see Chap, 77). The latter may increase muscle tension through the limbic system of muscle control and input from nociceptive muscle afferents. Possibly, these mechanisms also can activate the so-called *on cells*, which facilitate nociception in the brainstem (Chapter 10).

How Chronicity May Develop

Chronic tension-type headache usually evolves from the episodic form. Prolonged painful input from the periphery may cause central sensitization in the trigeminal system. Such mechanisms have been demonstrated in animal models; irritative stimuli from myofascial deep tissues are much more effective for induction of central sensitization than cutaneous stimuli (see Chapter 15). Myofascial factors are thus likely to contribute to the chronification of pain. When the central sensitization becomes sufficiently strong and widespread, the pain becomes chronic as a result of self-perpetuating disturbances in pain perception. A vicious circle may be initiated, and incoming peripheral stimuli may produce an abnormal reaction and probably maintain it long after the primary causative stimulus or stressor has stopped.

Initiating and chronifying mechanisms are less clear in tension-type headache unassociated with muscular disorder (2.1.2 and 2.2.2). In these rare patients, the central dysfunction might be the only abnormality (Fig. 2).

The cellular and molecular mechanisms involved in peripheral and central sensitization of nociception are increasingly better understood, which has already led to novel strategies for the treatment of pain (see Chapters 12 and 15). With regard to tension-type headache, preventing the evolution from the episodic to the chronic form is without any doubt a major challenge for future therapies.

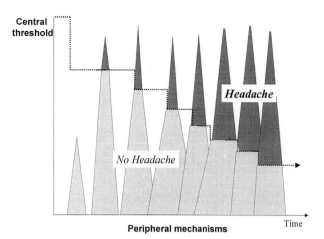

FIG. 2. Diagram illustrating how the interaction of peripheral and central mechanisms may lead to the progressive transformation of episodic tension-type headache into chronic tension-type headache.

REFERENCES

1. Bendtsen L, Jensen R, Olesen J. Qualitatively altered nociception in chronic myofascial pain. *Pain* 1996;65:259–264.
2. Brattberg G, Thorslund M, Wikman A. The prevalence of pain in a general population. *Pain* 1989;37:215–222.
3. Fround F, Fround C. Pain in general practice. *Scand J Prim Health Care* 1986;4:97–10.
4. Headache Classification Committee of the International Headache Society (Jes Olesen, Chairman). Classification and diagnostic criteria for headache disorders, cranial neuralgias and facial pain. *Cephalalgia* 1988;8(Suppl 7):1–96.
5. Jensen R, Olesen J. Initiating mechanisms of experimentally induced tension-type headache. *Cephalalgia* 1996;16:175–182.
6. Jensen R, Fuglsang-Frederiksen A, Olesen J. Quantitative surface EMG of pericranial muscles in headache: a population study. *Electroencephalogr Clin Neurophysiol* 1994;93:335–344.
7. Magnusson T, Enbom L. Signs and symptoms of mandibular dysfunction after introduction of experimental balancing side interferences. *Acta Odontol Scand* 1984;42:129–135.
8. Mense S. Nociception from skeletal muscle in relation to clinical muscle pain. *Pain* 1993;54:241–289.
9. Olesen J. Clinical and pathophysiological observations in migraine and tension-type headache explained by integration of vascular, supraspinal, and myofacial inputs. *Pain* 1991;46:125–132.
10. Stergaard S, Russell MB, Bendtsen L, Olesen J. Increased familial risk of chronic tension-type headache. *BMJ* 1997;314:1092–1093.
11. Petersen KL, Brennum J, Olesen J. Evaluation of pericranial myofascial nociception by pressure algometry: reproducibility and factors of variation. *Cephalalgia* 1992;12:33–37.
12. Plum F, Posner JB. *Diagnosis of stupor and coma.* Philadelphia: FA Davis, 1992, vol 3.
13. Svensson P, Arendt-Nielsen L, Houe L. Sensory-motor interactions of human experimental unilateral jaw muscle pain: a quantitative analysis. *Pain* 1996;64:241–249.
14. Rasmussen BK, Jensen R, Schroll M, Olesen J. Epidemiology of headache in a general population—a prevalence study. *J Clin Epidemiol* 1991;44:1147–1157.
15. Schoenen J, Gérard P, De Pasqua V, Juprelle M. EMG activity in pericranial muscle during postural variation and mental activity in healthy volunteers and patients with chronic tension-type headache. *Headache* 1991;31:321–324.
16. Timsit M. Rorschach movement responses distorsions and chronic headache. *Cephalalgia* 1985;5(Suppl 3):240–241.
17. Traue HC. Behavioral inhibition in stress disorders and myogenic pain. In: Bischoff C, Traue HC, Zenz H, eds. *Clinical perspectives in headache and low back pain.* Toronto: Hogrefe & Huber, 1989;29–45.
18. Woolf CJ. Windup and central sentization are not equivalent. *Pain* 1996;66:105–108.

The Headaches, Second Edition,
edited by J. Olesen, P. Tfelt-Hansen, and K.M.A. Welch.
Lippincott Williams & Wilkins, Philadelphia © 2000.

*Tension-Type Headache, Cluster Headache, and Miscellaneous
Primary Headaches*

CHAPTER 80

Symptomatology of Episodic Tension-Type Headache

Rigmor Jensen and Teresa Paiva

In its milder and infrequent forms, episodic tension-type headache is a nuisance, not a disease; but in its frequent forms, it becomes distressing and socially disturbing, although it rarely incapacitates those affected to the same degree as chronic tension-type headache or migraine. Characteristics of tension-type headache have been described by several authors (10,16,23,24), but a clear-cut classification of tension-type headache and a differentiation between the chronic and the episodic form were not available until the introduction of the International Headache Society (IHS) classification in 1988 (14) (Table 1). Most previous studies in tension-type headache have been performed in specialized headache clinics and dealt with the chronic form, whereas patients with the episodic form rarely consult a specialist. The pattern of tension-type headache seen in general practice clearly differs, although most sufferers have not even consulted a general practitioner (9,34). In recent years, more data from the general population were provided (9,12,28,32,33,42,43) (see also Chapter 69 on epidemiology). The large individual variations in those with episodic tension-type headache have therefore become apparent, and the clinical manifestations will be summarized in the following sections.

CLINICAL PICTURE OF EPISODIC TENSION-TYPE HEADACHE

The reason most patients with episodic tension-type headache do not seek medical assistance is that their

R. Jensen: Department of Neurology, Glostrup Hospital, University of Copenhagen, DK-2600 Glostrup, Copenhagen, Denmark.

T. Paiva: Laboratory EEG/SLEEP, Centro de Estudos Egas Moniz, Hospital Santa Maria, 1600 Lisbon, Portugal.

headache usually is mild in intensity, of relatively short duration, lacks the migraine-associated incapacitating symptoms such as nausea and vomiting, and, most of all, is responsive to most simple analgesics. The clinical picture is therefore not so well described as it is in most other headache disorders. Furthermore, the diagnosis of episodic tension-type headache is also frequently overlooked, because most patients in headache clinics focus on their

TABLE 1. *Diagnostic criteria for episodic tension-type headache*

A. At least ten previous headache episodes fulfilling criteria B–D listed below. Number of days with such headache <180/yr (<15/mo).
B. Headache lasting from 30 min to 7 days.
C. At least two of the following pain characteristics:
  1. Pressing/tightening (non-pulsating quality)
  2. Mild or moderate severity
  3. Bilateral location
  4. No aggravation by walking stairs or similar routine physical activity
D. Both of the following:
  1. No nausea or vomiting (anorexia may occur)
  2. Photophobia and phonophobia are absent, one but not the other is present
E. At least one of the following:
  1. History, physical- and neurologic examinations do not suggest one of the disorders listed in group 5–11 (symptomatic disorders).
  2. History, physical and neurologic examinations do suggest such disorder, but it is ruled out by appropriate investigations.
  3. Such disorder is present, but tension-type does not occur for the first time in close temporal relation to the disorder.

most severe and recent headaches. In the comparative study by Russell and colleagues, headache diagnosis made from a clinical interview was compared with the diagnosis from a diagnostic prospective headache diary. The results showed that fewer than 50% of patients who actually had episodic tension-type headache during the prospective diary recording reported such episodes at the clinical interview, whereas the vast majority of migraineurs were identified initially (39). Because most patients in such specialized headache clinics have several coexisting headache disorders, it is necessary also to focus on these mild headaches, which are important in the differential diagnosis of migraine. In addition, these headaches are probably the main reason for inappropriate drug consumption as well as acceleration of drug consumption, with many patients treating these headaches as mild migraine attacks and thus use antimigraine medications to treat them.

The mean lifetime duration of episodic tension-type headache was reported to be 10.3 years in a German population study (12) and 19.9 years in a clinical study (22) illustrating that tension-type headache is a life-long pain disorder, that subjects suffer several years before seeking medical help, and that there is a considerable referral bias in the relatively few patients who have episodic tension-type headache and are examined in specialized headache centers.

In a clinical study using the IHS criteria, the median frequency of episodes was 6 days per month, ranging from 2 to 12 days per month (17) compared with a median frequency of 2.2 days per month in the general population (12). Because episodic tension-type headache is so widespread and variable in frequency, it is recommended that subjects be defined according to a lower limit of headache days below which subjects may be regarded as headache free, at least from a practical point of view. Previously, we suggested that this lower limit should be at a frequency of 14 days per year (20). The duration of each headache episode also varies widely, with mean values between 4 and 13 hours and extreme values at 30 minutes to 72 hours (16,17,22), rates similar to those reported from older studies that used less strict criteria. The male-to-female ratio at 4:5 and the highly variable temporal profile within and between patients are the main features distinguishing tension-type headache from migraine (38,43).

CHARACTER OF PAIN

Patients usually describe their pain as being "dull" and "nonpulsating," often using descriptions such as "a sensation of tightness," "pressure," or "soreness." Some patients refer to a "band" or a "cap" compressing their head, and some patients mention a great "weight" over the head or the shoulders (10,23,24,26). Several studies confirm this pain quality; in a series of 402 patients, a dull head pain was found in 85% and a tight heaviness in

83% (7). The high incidence of this pressing quality was confirmed in more recent studies by applying the IHS criteria; it was present in 78% of 488 subjects with episodic tension-type headache from the general population (32) but only in 52% of 50 patients with episodic tension-type headache from a prospective diary study (16).

The pulsating character occurs seldom or never in 80% to 86% of the patients from clinical populations (16,17). The most frequent pain quality in tension-type headache is thus nonpulsating and pressing, although it may be experienced as periodically pulsating during severe pain episodes in a minority of subjects (32).

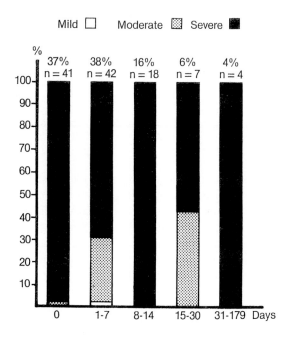

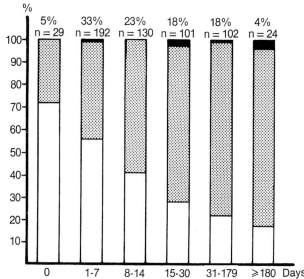

FIG. 1. Pain severity as a function of frequency of migraine (top) and tension-type headache (bottom). *Open bars* indicate mild pain; *shaded bars*, moderate pain; *closed bars*, severe pain. [From Rasmussen (45), with permission.]

SEVERITY OF PAIN

According to IHS criteria, the pain in episodic tension-type headache is typically of mild or moderate intensity (14). In population-based studies, it was mild or moderate in 87% to 99% of subjects with this type of headache (12,32), findings similar to those of Iversen and associates (17). These data correspond with a prospective headache diary study that analyzed the intensity of pain across several headache episodes (16,39).

The severity of tension-type headache increases markedly with increasing frequency; 76% of subjects with more than 30 days of headache per year report moderate or severe intensity compared with 50% of those with less frequent headache (35). These data illustrate the clinical impression that tension-type headache is a graded phenomenon in which intensity increases with greater frequency, in contrast to migraine, which is an "all or nothing" phenomenon that runs its course when started (Fig. 1).

LOCATION

Typically, the pain is considered to be located bilaterally, as reported by 90% of subjects in the population study (32). Nevertheless, pain does not always occur in the same location; a varying site associated with varying intensity has been reported in clinical studies (10), and in the study by Iversen and colleagues, 21% of patients with episodic tension-type headache reported varying location (17). Strictly unilateral pain accounted for 4% to 12.5 % in the episodic form (1,17,27,32). If the location remains unaltered through all of the episodes a patient experiences, an associated localized abnormality, such as triggerpoints, oromandibular dysfunction, or intracranial disorder should be searched. In order of frequency, the location of tension-type headache is occipital, parietal, temporal, or frontal (10,17,23). A bandlike topography, including frontal and occipital areas, is rather typical (10,17).

Lack of aggravation of pain by physical activity is typical of tension-type headache (14,17) and was shown to be one of the best criteria for distinguishing tension-type headache from migraine: 74% of 488 subjects had the episodic form in one population study (35), 83% in another large population study (43), and 84% in a prospective diary study (16) reported no aggravation by routine physical activity, in contrast to only 4% of migraineurs (35).

ACCOMPANYING SYMPTOMS

Nausea and vomiting are not part of the criteria for diagnosing episodic tension-type headache, and their presence actually rules out this diagnosis. Nevertheless, 18% of subjects with tension-type headache have reported mild or moderate anorexia during the headache episode (32). It is therefore important to distinguish between nausea and anorexia during the interview. Photophobia or phonophobia may be present, but the pres-

ence of both symptoms is not allowed in the IHS criteria. The pain criteria are usually graded, but the accompanying symptoms are listed only as present or absent. Accompanying symptoms, however, were graded into mild, moderate, and severe to study the sensitivity and specificity of the criteria. Mild photophobia was present in 10% and mild phonophobia in 7%, although in most subjects their appearance was occasional (17,32). Grading these accompanying symptoms may improve the separation of migraine and tension-type headache, and suggestions for revising the IHS criteria were recently presented (32). Nevertheless, the presence of these accompanying symptoms had no influence on the pain characteristics; not only two, but more frequently three or all four, pain characteristics were fulfilled in episodic tension-type headache (32) (Fig. 2). Clinical characteris-

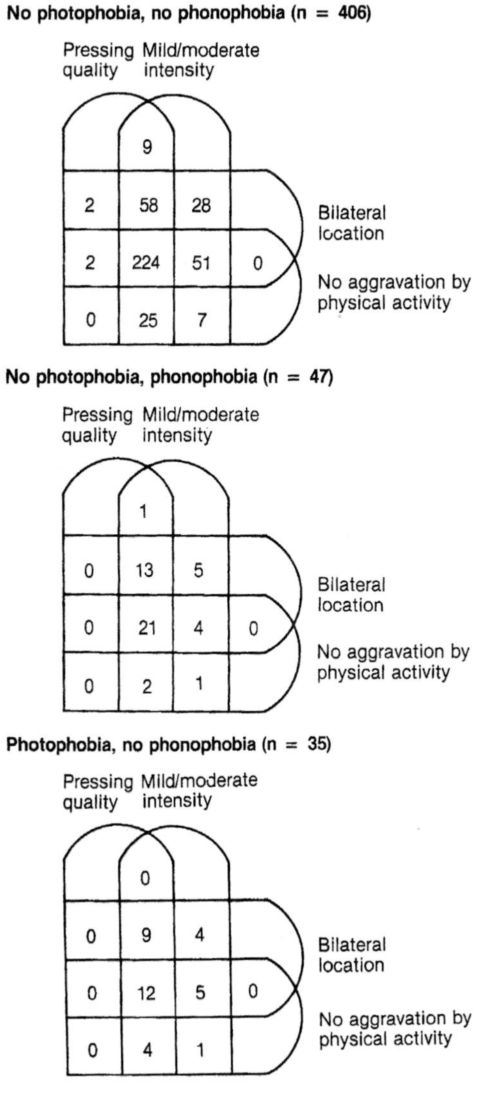

FIG. 2. Venn diagram showing the distribution of subjects with episodic tension-type headache with different combinations of symptoms according to the International Headache Society classification. From Rasmussen et al. (32), with permission.

tics of tension-type headache in migraineurs and in non-migraineurs were compared in a large epidemiologic study of 4,000 subjects (43). The 1-year-prevalence of tension-type headache and the male-to-female ratio were similar in migraineurs and in nonmigraineurs, whereas the frequency of tension-type headache was higher and the episodes lasted significantly longer in migraineurs compared with those who never had migraine. The pain characteristics and the accompanying symptoms of the episodes of tension-type headache were similar; therefore, it was concluded that tension-type headache and migraine are separate disorders, not part of a continuum, although they may coexist in many patients (35,38,43). Migraine may aggravate or even precipitate tension-type headache, confirming the impressions from highly specialized headache clinics, where the vast majority of migraine patients have coexisting frequent tension-type headache (10,23,24).

Patients with tension-type headaches may also complain of other symptoms. In a series of 402 patients, associated symptoms included fatigue (81%), poor sleep (53%), and light headedness (51%) (7).

RELATION TO SLEEP

Whereas many chronic headache sufferers complain of insufficient sleep, lack of restoration after sleep, tender or stiff muscles in their jaw muscles, severe snoring, and similar problems (25–27), there have been no formal studies or even clinical reports of the relations between sleep disorders and episodic tension-type headache. The few studies of a possible relationship between sleep and tension-type headache have not distinguished between the episodic and the chronic forms; so the following discussion refers to tension-type headache in general.

In the Danish population, study subjects with tension-type headache had a higher prevalence of sleeping problems compared with migraineurs (36), whereas a case–control study of children and adolescents reported an equal number of sleeping disturbances between migraine and tension-type headache (6). Complaints of a lack of restoration also have been reported to be positively associated with headache disorders (7,36,43). These associations may indicate a common causal disorder, but because the main precipitating factors in tension-type headache are stress and mental tension (36,43), sleep also may be an indirect measure of such underlying risk factors. In addition, because of the high prevalence of sleep disorders and tension-type headache, it is difficult to ascertain whether their coexistence is spurious or causal. On the other hand, because morning or nocturnal headaches are frequent indicators of a sleep disturbance (29), the relation is complex, and further controlled studies are needed.

Lack of sleep is frequently reported as a precipitating factor for headache (36); headache of tension-type

occurred in 39% of healthy volunteers after sleep deprivation (5). The possible mechanism of sleep-related headache is also discussed in the chapter on headache and sleep (Chapter 129) and chronic tension-type headache (chapter 81).

DIURNAL AND SEASONAL VARIATIONS

Tension-type headache often is reported to start sometime during the day and to increase slowly, in contrast to migraine, but no exact studies of properly classified patients have confirmed this assumption. In the most severe and frequent forms, patients often awaken with headache or notice it shortly after awakening. The headache then remains throughout the day, often unaltered during widely varying activities. In such patients, a disturbed sleep pattern or analgesic overuse should be suspected.

No conclusive studies or clinical reports of seasonal variation in the frequency or intensity of episodic tension-type headache have been reported. Because one of the significant precipitating factors in tension-type headache is weather changes (36), seasonal variations would be likely, and more research is clearly needed.

PHYSICAL EXAMINATION

A diagnosis of tension-type headache requires exclusion of *other* organic disorders; such exclusion is mandatory and is made possible by taking an extensive history of the evolution of the pain and other symptoms and by performing an intensive physical and neurological examination. The physical examination should include manual palpation of the pericranial muscles to identify tender areas and triggerpoints (4,19,25). *Tenderpoints* are areas where manual pressure induces a local pain, and *triggerpoints* are areas of localized deep tenderness where sustained pressure also induces a referred pain in another area in the region. They probably represent different intensities of the same pathogenic mechanism, with local tenderness as a common feature.

As a minimum, pericranial tenderness should be assessed by manual palpation of the temporal, lateral pterygoid, masseter, sternocleidomastoid, and trapezius muscles. The muscle-insertion areas, such as the mastoid process and the neck-muscle insertions also should be palpated (19,25).

Palpation should be done symmetrically and systematically using small rotating movements with the second and third fingers, followed by unilateral examination for a better side-to-side estimation. In each area, a semiquantitative tenderness score from 0 to 3 can be estimated based on the mimic and verbal reaction of the patient (25), and a total sum of the individual scores can be calculated, called the *total tenderness score* (TTS). This method has shown intraobserver reliability, whereas comparisons between observers may vary according to the applied pressure (4). When it is part of a research project, the palpation procedure should be blinded and standardized, and the pressure intensity should be controlled (4). In routine practice, a standardized procedure is also recommended so that the physician can better develop his or her ability to distinguish normal and abnormal conditions.

The texture of pericranial, shoulder, and chewing muscles often is altered in tension-type headache, with tight tender bands or generalized increased consistency (40). Such findings previously were detected only by manual palpation, but a newly invented and validated instrument, a hardness meter, confirmed the observation (2,40). In controlled series, patients with episodic tension-type headache have increased muscle consistency, and no significant difference was found between those with the episodic and those with chronic subform (40). The pathophysiological background and significance of these findings are not yet clarified.

Pain sensitivity as assessed by a pressure algometer is widely used in research, but it plays no role in routine practice. Some methodological precautions should be taken into consideration (19,30).

Findings in Headache Patients

When pericranial muscle tenderness is examined by manual palpation and pressure algometer in a general population, pain sensitivity is lower in women than in men, and pain sensitivity decreases with increasing age (18). Increased tenderness in pericranial muscles is the most consistent abnormal finding and increases with the frequency and intensity of tension-type headache (19). Subjects with the episodic form have increased TTS score compared with migraineurs and healthy controls (11,13,20,22), but they have less tenderness than subjects who have chronic tension-type headache (19,22).

In 1982 Lous and Olesen reported a specific relationship between the location of the headache and muscle tenderness (27), a finding confirmed in the subsequent study of Drummond (8), who found increased tenderness on the usual headache site compared with the other side of the scalp. In addition, pericranial muscle tenderness can persist several days after the headache subsides (8,19). Subjects with frequent headaches are more likely to have had one or several headache episodes within the last few days than subjects with more infrequent headaches. In clinical studies, it is therefore fundamental to control for the usual frequency of headache, location, age, and sex differences. It is also important to emphasize whether the muscle examination is performed during an actual headache episode or during a headache-free period, because tenderness increases 24% during an actual headache episode (21). Concerning pain thresholds recorded by pressure algometry, most studies report normal pain thresholds in patients with episodic tension-type headache at both

cephalic and extracephalic locations (11,19,22). During a spontaneous headache episode, cephalic and extracephalic pain thresholds and tolerances were unaltered by ongoing pain, indicating a widely normal, central pain processing in these patients (21).

The cervical spine should be examined for restricted and painful movements, and the paravertebral muscles should be examined for tender points (45). Cervical radiologic examination cannot be recommended unless a local pathology is suspected clinically, because the prevalence of organic cervical spine lesions in tension-type headache is equivalent to other headache disorders (44). (See Chapter 82 for a discussion of laboratory investigations in headache.)

SUBDIVISIONS OF EPISODIC TENSION-TYPE HEADACHE

The definition of a possible muscular factor in tension-type headache as defined in the IHS classification [i.e., muscle tenderness recorded by manual palpation or by pressure algometer or abnormal electromyelographic (EMG) levels] (14) depends on the assumption that, compared with controls, most tension-type headache sufferers reveal marked tenderness by manual palpation. Only a minority of frequent headache sufferers are completely free of tenderness but otherwise have identical headache symptoms (22–26). In the Danish population study, 65% of subjects with episodic tension-type headache had a muscular factor according to the IHS classification (14,20). Only a few clinical studies have studied these relations in patients with the episodic form of headache. In a recent controlled study, clinical and paraclinical features were studied with respect to muscular disorders in two subgroups of patients with episodic or chronic tension-type headache and compared with healthy controls (22). No significant variations were detected with respect to the clinical features. The study furthermore confirmed that pericranial tenderness recorded by manual palpation was by far the most sensitive and specific test compared with pressure pain thresholds (PPT) and EMG, which were of limited diagnostic value (20,22). Although there are large variations between subjects, moderate tenderness in at least 50% of the palpated pericranial muscles and tendon insertions (see above) indicates a muscular disorder. EMG and pressure pain threshold provide no useful diagnostic information and therefore cannot be recommended for clinical use. Until further research in this area is available, the present criteria should be regarded as complementary (41).

POSSIBLE CAUSATIVE AND PRECIPITATING FACTORS

The most likely causative factors for tension-type headache are listed as the fourth-digit codes in the IHS classification (14) (Table 2). They represent a wide variety of potential causes, but clear evidence for these items is not yet available. This subgrouping was created mainly for research purposes but also can be used as a guideline in the daily clinical approach to headache patients.

The relationship between oromandibular dysfunction and tension-type headache is described in Chapter 76. Other possible causative factors are medication overuse and organic factors listed under "The Secondary Headaches." The possible psychological and psychiatric causative factors (items 3–6) are defined according to the Diagnostic and Statistical Manual of Mental Disorders (DSM)-III-R criteria. Tension-type headaches generally are reported to occur in relation to emotional conflict and psychosocial stress, but the cause–effect relation is not clear. In population studies (36,43), stress and mental tension were the most frequently reported precipitating factors, but they occurred with similar frequency in tension-type headache and migraine. These results are in correspondence with the findings of largely normal personality profiles in subjects with episodic tension-type headache in population studies (28,37) and a large clinical study (31). In conclusion, some of the suspected psychosocial and personality factors may be results of specific coping strategies for recurrent pain rather than being the primary cause of headache. In a controlled study, Holroyd and colleagues reported that a number of personality factors, such as depression, anxiety, and somatization, which were highly abnormal during ongoing pain, normalized again when patients were retested outside the pain period (15). In general, psychological abnormalities in episodic tension-type headache may be viewed rather as secondary to the organic disorder, although they are closely related in most subjects (3). How psychiatric comorbidity otherwise affects tension-type headache is described in Chapter 77.

In conclusion, episodic tension-type headache occurs with a wide variety of frequency and intensity, not only between subjects but also within an individual subject over time. As most cases of chronic tension-type headache evolved from the episodic form and a disturbance in the complex interaction between peripheral and central pain mechanisms is suggested to be of major importance for the conversion of episodic into chronic tension-type headache (22), it is therefore likely that an early identification and treatment of the episodic tension-type headache may prevent development of the chronic pain condition. Furthermore, identification of the episodic tension-type headache is also important in the more complex headache patient because a specific diagnosis is mandatory so that a specific treatment can be prescribed and numerous cases of drug-induced headache thereby be prevented. It is therefore extremely important to study the clinical characteristics and the evolution of episodic tension-type headache in future studies. A better understanding of tension-type headache will lead to better treatment as well as prevention.

TABLE 2. *Possible causative factors for tension-type headache*

0. No identifiable causative factor
1. More than one of the factors 2–9 (list in order of importance)
2. Oromandibular dysfunction
3. Psychosocial stress
4. Anxiety
5. Depression
6. Headache as a delusion or an idea
7. Muscular stress
8. Drug overuse for tension-type headaches
9. One of the disorders listed in groups 5–11 of the IHS classification

IHS, International Headache Society.

REFERENCES

1. Amico D, Leone M, Bussone G. Side-locked unilaterality and pain localization in long-lasting headaches: migraine, tension-type headache, and cervicogenic headache. *Headache* 1994;34:526–530.
2. Ashina M, Bendtsen L, Jensen R, Sakai F, Olesen J. Measurement of muscle hardness: a methodological study. *Cephalalgia* 1998;18:106–111.
3. Bech P, Rasmussen BK, Olesen J. Psychiatric aspects of tension-type headache. In: Olesen J, Schoenen J, eds. *Tension-type headache: classification, mechanisms and treatment.* New York: Raven Press, 1993;143–146.
4. Bendtsen L, Jensen R, Jensen NK, Olesen J. Pressure-controlled palpation: a new technique which increases the reliability of manual palpation. *Cephalalgia* 1995;15:205–210.
5. Blau JN. Sleep deprivation headache. *Cephalalgia* 1990;10:157–160.
6. Bruni O, Fabrizi P, Ottaviano S, Cortesi F, Giannotti F, Guidetti V. Prevalence of sleep disorders in childhood and adolescence with headache: a case–control study. *Cephalalgia* 1997;17:492–498.
7. Chun WX. An approach to the nature of tension headache. *Headache* 1985;25:188–189.
8. Drummond PD. Scalp tenderness and sensitivity to pain in migraine and tension headache. *Headache* 1987;27:45–50.
9. Edmeads J, Findlay H, Tugwell P, Pryse-Philips W, Nelson RF, Murray TJ. Impact of migraine and tension-type headache on life style, consulting behavior , and medication use: a Canadian population survey. *Can J Neurol Sci* 1993;20:131–137.
10. Friedman AP. Characteristics of tension headache: a profile of 1,420 cases. *Psychosomatics* 1979;20:418–422.
11. Goebel H, Weigle L, Kropp P, Soyka D. Pain sensitivity and pain reactivity of pericranial muscles in migraine and tension-type headache. *Cephalalgia* 1992;12:142–151.
12. Goebel H, Petersen-Braun M, Soyka D. The epidemiology of headache in Germany: a nationwide survey of a representatative sample on the basis of the headache classification of the International Headache Society. *Cephalalgia* 1994;14:97–106.
13. Hatch JP, Moore PJ, Cyr-Provost M, Boutros NN, Seleshi E, Borcherding S. The use of electromyography and muscle palpation in the diagnosis of tension-type headache with and without pericranial muscle involvement. *Pain* 1992;49:175–178.
14. Headache Classification Committee of the International Society. Classification and diagnostic criteria for headache disorders, cranial neuralgias and facial pain. *Cephalalgia* 1988;8:1–96.
15. Holroyd KA, France JL, Nash JM, Hursey KG. Pain state as artifact in the psychological assessment of recurrent headache sufferers. *Pain* 1993;53:229–235.
16. Inan LE, Cankalt Tulunay F, Guvener A, Tokgoz G, Inan N. Characteristics of headache in migraine without aura and episodic tension-type headache in the Turkish population according to the IHS classification. *Cephalalgia* 1994:14:171–173.
17. Iversen HK, Langemark M, Andersson PG, Hansen PE, Olesen J. Clinical characteristics of migraine and tension-type headache in

relation to new and old diagnostic criteria. *Headache* 1990; 30:514–519.

18. Jensen R, Rasmussen BK, Olesen J. Cephalic muscle tenderness and pressure pain threshold in a general population. *Pain* 1992;48:197–203.

19. Jensen R, Rasmussen BK, Olesen J. Cephalic muscle tenderness and pressure pain threshold in headache: a population study. *Pain* 1993; 52:193–199.

20. Jensen R, Rasmussen BK. Muscular disorders in tension-type headache. *Cephalalgia* 1996;16:97–103.

21. Jensen R. Mechanisms of spontaneous tension-type headaches: an analysis of tenderness, pain thresholds and EMG. *Pain* 1996;64:251–256.

22. Jensen R, Bendtsen L, Olesen J. Muscular factors are of importance in tension-type headache. *Headache* 1998;38:10–17.

23. Kudrow L. Muscle contraction headaches. In: Rose CF, ed. *Handbook of clinical neurology*. New York: Elsevier Science Publishers BV, 1986;4(48):343–352.

24. Lance JW. Tension headache. In: *Mechanism and management of headache*, 4th ed. London/Boston: Butterworth, 1982:100–120.

25. Langemark M, Olesen J. Pericranial tenderness in chronic tension-type headache: a blind controlled study. *Cephalalgia* 1987;7:249–255.

26. Langemark M, Olesen J, Poulsen DL, Bech P. Clinical characterization of patients with chronic tension headache. *Headache* 1988;28: 590–596.

27. Lous I, Olesen J. Evaluation of pericranial tenderness and oral function in patients with common migraine, muscle contraction headache and combination headache. *Pain* 1982;12:385–393.

28. Merinkangas KR. Psychopathology and headache syndromes in the community. *Headache* 1994;34:17–26.

29. Pavia T, Batista A, Martins P, Martins A. The relationship between headaches and sleep. *Headache* 1995;35:590–596.

30. Petersen KL, Brennum J, Olesen J. Evaluation of pericranial myofascial nociception by pressure algometry: reproducibility and factors of variation. *Cephalalgia* 1992;12:33–37.

31. Pfaffenrath V, Hummelsberger J, Pöllmann W, Kaube H, Rath M. MMPI personality profiles in patients with primary headache syndromes. *Cephalalgia* 1991;11:263–268.

32. Rasmussen BK, Jensen R, Olesen J. A population-based analysis of the criteria of the International Headache Society. *Cephalalgia* 1991;11: 129–134.

33. Rasmussen BK, Jensen R, Schroll M, Olesen J. Epidemiology of headache in a general population: a prevalence study. *J Clin Epidemiol* 1991;44:1147–1157.

34. Rasmussen BK, Jensen R, Olesen J. Impact of headache on sickness absence and utilisation of medical services: a Danish population study. *J Epidemiol Health* 1992;46:443–447.

35. Rasmussen BK, Jensen R, Olesen J. Interrelations between migraine and tension-type headache in the general population. *Arch Neurol* 1992;49:914–918.

36. Rasmussen BK. Migraine and tension-type headache in a general population: Precipitating factors, female hormones, sleep pattern and relation to lifestyle. *Pain* 1993;53:65–72.

37. Rasmussen BK. Migraine and tension-type headache in a general population: Psychosocial factors. *Int J Epidemiol* 1992;21:1138–1143.

38. Rasmussen BK. Migraine and tension-type headache are separate disorders. *Cephalalgia* 1996;16:217–220.

39. Russell M, Rasmussen BK, Brennum J, Iversen H, Jensen R, Olesen J. Presentation of a new instrument: the diagnostic headache diary. *Cephalalgia* 1992;12:369–374.

40. Sakai F, Ebihara S, Akiyama M, Horikawa M. Pericranial muscle hardness in tension-type headache: a non-invasive measurement method and its clinical application. *Brain* 1995;118:523–531.

41. Schoenen J, Gerard P, De Pasqua V, Sianard-Gainko. Multiple clinical and paraclinical analyses of chronic tension-type headache associated or unassociated with disorder of pericranial muscles. *Cephalalgia* 1991;11:135–139.

42. Schwartz BS, Stewart WF, Simon D, Lipton RB. Epidemiology of tension-type headache. *JAMA* 1998;279:381–383.

43. Ulrich V, Russell MB, Jensen R, Olesen J. A comparison of tension-type headache in migraineurs and in non-migraineurs: a population-based study. *Pain* 1996;67:501–506.

44. Wöber-Bingöl C, Wöber C, Zeiler K, et al. Tension headache and the cervical spine: plain x-ray findings. *Cephalalgia* 1992;12:152–154.

45. Zwart JA. Neck mobility in different headache disorders. *Headache* 1997;37:6–11.

The Headaches, Second Edition,
edited by J. Olesen, P. Tfelt-Hansen, and K.M.A. Welch.
Lippincott Williams & Wilkins, Philadelphia © 2000.

Tension-Type Headache, Cluster Headache, and Miscellaneous Primary Headaches

CHAPTER 81

Symptomatology of Chronic Tension-Type Headache

Rigmor Jensen and Giorgio Sandrini

Except for its frequency, chronic tension-type headache is similar to episodic tension-type headache in most of its clinical features (Table 1). The main reason, why the Headache Classification Committee of the International Headache Society (11) distinguished these forms was because of the differences in management rather than in the clinical picture. However, the chronic type is often associated with more severe pain, with more accompanying symptoms, is often combined with medication overuse and is less influenced by daily hassles and stress. In addition, most of the former studies have been carried out in clinical populations of patients with chronic daily headache including patients in whom migraine, and/or analgesic abuse coexisted with chronic tension-type headache. The relationship between migraine and chronic tension-type headache remains controversial (23,34). The problem of the evolution of tension-type headache is very complex, since the data in the literature are exclusively based on retrospective studies. It has been suggested that chronic tension-type headache evolves from migraine in the majority of cases (25,43), and thereby represents the end of a severity spectrum. However, in other series (21) the majority of the chronic patients have evolved from the episodic form of tension-type headache. These different results suggests that the considerable referral bias in studies from specialised headache clinics may play an important role. Data from the general population (31,34,44)

have demonstrated that migraine and tension-type headache have different male:female ratio, age distribution and clinical presentation and that migraine and tension-type headache represent 2 different clinical entities (31,34,44). The so-called continuum severity model, therefore, remains unsubstantiated, and the former term chronic daily headache seems merely to be a diagnostic artefact and should be avoided. At the initial consultation, it can be very difficult to identify whether the patient has

TABLE 1. *Diagnostic criteria for chronic tension-type headache*

A. Average headache frequency ≥15 days/mo (≥180 days/yr) for 6 mo fulfilling criteria B–D listed below.
B. At least two of the following pain characteristics:
   1. Pressing/tightening (nonpulsating quality)
   2. Mild or moderate severity
   3. Bilateral location
   4. No aggravation by walking stairs or similar routine physical activity
C. Both of the following:
   1. No vomiting
   2. No more than one of the following:
      Nausea, photophobia, or phonophobia
D. At least one of the following:
   1. History, physical and neurologic examinations do not suggest one of the disorders listed in groups 5–11 (symptomatic disorders).
   2. History, physical and neurologic examinations do suggest such disorder, but it is ruled out by appropriate investigations.
   3. Such disorder is present, but tension-type does not occur for the first time in close temporal relation to the disorder.

R. Jensen: Department of Neurology, Glostrup Hospital, University of Copenhagen, DK-2600 Glostrup, Copenhagen, Denmark.

G. Sandrini: Department of Neurological Sciences, University of Pavia, and Department of Neurological Rehabilitation, IRCC C. Mondino Foundation, 27100 Pavia, Italy.

only one or several types of headache (see Chapter 132). A specific diagnosis can therefore only seldom be applied and the use of a diagnostic headache diary for one or two months is highly recommended.

Most recently, a report of genetic predisposition for chronic tension-type headache has been published (45), but the transmission seems to be complex. Tension-type headache is in all likelihood a disease where the individual genetic constitution represents only one of several concurrent factors. These factors are complex in chronic tension-type headache and only poorly elucidated. In the following the clinical characteristics, precipitating factors, and clinical findings will be reviewed.

CLINICAL PICTURE OF CHRONIC TENSION-TYPE HEADACHE

The typical patient with chronic tension-type headache is a middle-aged patient, male or female, with a headache history for 10 to 20 years (5,10,13,18,27) and with a more or less continuous daily headache (8-27) which is almost refractory to numerous treatment strategies and quite independent of daily activities (Fig. 1). In most cases there is a history of a coexisting migraine without aura and quite often also a family history of migraine or chronic tension-type headache. The majority of patients have started with an episodic headache disorder in their adolescence, either a migraine or an episodic tension-type headache or both, and then gradually the headache frequency have accelerated over several years without any obvious explanations and have been chronic for several years. No specific associations to other diseases or

relations to other chronic pain conditions can be detected. Most of these patients have adapted to their chronic pain condition, have even lost any hope of new therapeutic strategies and are primarily seeking the specialist because of a change in their migraine pattern or because of other neurological complaints. It is therefore a great clinical and therapeutic challenge to treat these patients.

A minimum headache frequency of at least 15 days per month during at least 6 months is required in the IHS-classification (11) (see Table 1) but the duration of significant headache symptoms is usually much higher when patients seek a specialist. The frequency of days with headache in the chronic form is also very high as the mean frequency in prospective diary studies was between 23-25 days with headache per 4 weeks period (5,18) to a median value at 30 days per month (20,21). These studies support the clinical observation that if the headache frequency is above 15 days per month it very often becomes a daily or almost daily pain. On the other hand, is it important to emphasize that patients may overreport the frequency of their tension-type headache during an initial, clinical interview compared to the frequency in a prospective headache diary (35). It is therefore recommended to use a diagnostic headache diary in the diagnosis of both the episodic and the chronic tension-type headache.

The reported median age at onset is in the second decade (20,42) with a declining prevalence with increasing age in one study (29,31) and increasing prevalence with increasing age in other more recent studies (10,42). The presumed evolution of chronic tension-type headache from the episodic form is indirectly demonstrated by an older mean age in chronic tension-type

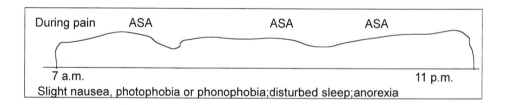

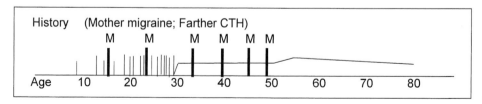

menarche pregnancy I - II   menopause   hypertension

FIG. 1. Illustration of the clinical characteristics of chronic tension-type headache (*CTH*). The *upper box* illustrates the individual headache episode with more or less continuous pain during the day almost refractory to analgesics and daily activities. *ASA*, acetylic salicylic acid. The *lower box* indicates a lifetime history and evolution of pain in the individual patient. *M*, coexisting migraine attacks.

headache (>50 years) than in episodic tension-type headache (42) (see Fig. 1). For further details see Chapter 69.

CHARACTER OF PAIN

Kudrow (19) described the pain of tension headache as dull, aching, pressure-like, constricting, or giving a sense of fullness. Throbbing was considered an uncommon quality. Patients often describe their pain as "wearing a tight hat, wearing a tight band around the head or bearing a heavy burden on the head" (26). Recently, this "pressing" pain quality was confirmed by 83% of chronic tension-type headache sufferers in a general population (30) and varied from 72% to 95% of patients with daily or almost daily tension-type headache from specialized headache clinics (24,27,42).

LOCATION OF PAIN

The bilateral location of the pain is considered a frequent characteristic of tension-type headache and has been included in the IHS diagnostic criteria (see Table 1). The location of pain may vary considerably within and between patients (21,43), however. Rasmussen and colleagues (30) reported that bilateral location was present in 88% of patients with chronic tension-type headache, whereas unilateral location is considered more typical of migraine. In a study from a specialized headache clinic, 98% of 100 consecutive patients reported bilateral location (43), whereas it was only reported by 79% to 85% of patients with chronic tension-type headache in two more recent European studies (24,27). The statement once made by the National Institutes of Heatlth (NIH) Ad Hoc Committee (1962) (1) that headache is usually occipital has been disproven. Thus, the distribution of the pain was frontal, temporal, or frontotemporal in 66% and only occipital in 25% of the patients in a large clinical study done by Langemark and colleagues (21) and similar to the large series of 1,420 patients studied by Friedman in 1979 (8).

SEVERITY OF PAIN

According to the IHS criteria, the pain is usually mild or moderate in severity. The pain may thus inhibit but does not prohibit daily activities (11). In a Danish population study, Rasmussen and colleagues (30) found that 16% of patients with chronic tension headache patients had mild, 78% moderate, and only 4% severe intensity of pain; on the other hand, Goebel and associates reported that 42% of subjects from a German population study had severe and 44% had moderate pain intensity (10). In the clinical study by Langemark and colleagues (21), 51% of the patients reported that the pain did not interfere with daily activities, 42% reported inhibition, and in 7% the

pain was incompatible with normal activity. In the clinical study from Italy, only 7% of patients reported a severe pain intensity, 78% moderate intensity, and 15% mild intensity (24). In the most recent American population-based study, tension-type headache accounted for a considerable part of the reduced effectiveness in the workplace (41). In the Danish population study, tension-type headache accounted for 75% of lost workdays attributable to primary headache disorders (32). Lack of aggravation from walking stairs or similar routine physical activity is a typical feature considered to be a specific characteristic of tension-type headache and is one of the characteristics used in the diagnostic criteria of the IHS (11). Manzoni and colleagues reported that routine physical activity provoked worsening of the pain in 33% of patients, whereas physical activity had no effect or even improved in 67% (24). These data are quite similar to the former study by Langemark and co-workers (21) and to the Danish population study (30), in which 71% of patients reported that physical activity was without any influence on headache intensity, in contrast to only 2% of migraineurs. Aggravation of pain from routine physical activity is one of the best criteria for distinguishing between migraine and tension-type headache, better than unilaterality or throbbing pain quality (13,30).

It can be concluded that although most subjects with chronic tension-type headache have little or moderate interference with daily activities, the social impact on quality of life and effectiveness at work are considerable as a result of the chronicity and daily occurrence of a life-long pain disorder.

ACCOMPANYING SYMPTOMS

From a diagnostic viewpoint, the presence of accompanying symptoms is crucial. According to the IHS classification (11), no vomiting and no more than one of the symptoms (nausea, photophobia, phonophobia) can occur. Although the pain criteria are graded, the accompanying symptoms are listed only as *present* or *absent*. In a study by Langemark and colleagues (21), 32% of patients reported either photophobia or phonophobia, whereas 68% never experienced such symptoms. In the general population, 58% of patients with chronic tension-type headache or tension-type–like headache had none of the associated symptoms; 17% had photophobia or phonophobia, and 25% had nausea but not photophobia or phonophobia (30). Different combinations of these symptoms excluding the IHS diagnosis of chronic tension-type headache appear quite often (43), and coexistence of both photophobia and phonophobia was the main reason for exclusion of 63% of patients from the IHS diagnosis of chronic tension-type headache in the large Italian study of patients with chronic headaches (24). Combinations of nausea, photophobia, and phonophobia were responsible for only 14.8% of the exclusions, whereas most of the pain characteristics were fulfilled (24). To evaluate the sensitivity and specificity of these symptoms, they have been categorized as mild, moderate, or severe (30). Because accompanying symptoms are not only more frequent but also more severe in migraine patients than in tension-type headache, some investigators have suggested that a grading of nausea, photophobia, and phonophobia might improve the distinction between migraine and tension-type headache (13,30).

Furthermore, in some the old studies, it is unclear whether migraine attacks or drug-induced headaches could be responsible for some of the reported accompanying symptoms, as patients were classified as having only one headache diagnosis. In the IHS classification, patients are allowed to have different headache diagnoses although not at the same time (11). In highly specialized headache clinics, patients frequently have two, three, or more different headaches. Because a specific diagnosis is crucial for a specific treatment, identification of these headache disorders is therefore necessary.

RELATION TO SLEEP

Several patients with chronic headache complain of insufficient sleep; lack of rejuvenation in the morning; tender, stiff jaw muscles; severe snoring, and other problems (36). In the general population, subjects with tension-type headache (both the episodic and the chronic forms) had a significantly greater number of sleeping problems compared with migraineurs (33). Sleeping problems were reported by 41% of women and by 24% of men with tension-type headache, in contrast to 18% and 7% of migraineurs, respectively (33). The major specific problems were lack of refreshment on wakening in both sexes and snoring in females (33).

Chronic tension-type headache has sometimes been suggested to be a localized part of the fibromyalgia syndrome because impaired sleep, widespread chronic pain, and recurrent headaches are among the most frequent complaints in fibromyalgia patients. Alternatively, a common biochemical mechanism may be involved in these complex disorders: Sleep disorders, mental depression, fibromyalgia, and chronic tension-type headache may have some clinical features in common. The serotonergic systems are thought to be implicated in the regulation of pain, in mental depression, as well as in sleep; however, the relation is not simple. The highly selective, quite effective serotonergic reuptake inhibitor (SSRI) drugs have a significant effect on depression and sleep disorders but only a modest or no effect on chronic tension-type headache (5). No conclusive sleep studies of properly classified patients have been published, and the cause–effect relationship between chronic pain and sleep disturbances remain to be solved. The possible mechanism of sleep-related headache is also discussed in Chapter 80 and certainly merits further studies.

OTHER DIURNAL VARIATIONS

Tension-type headache often is reported to start sometime during the day and to increase slowly, in contrast to migraine. Most patients with chronic headache, however, awake with the headache or notice it shortly after rising. It usually lasts the whole day, often unaltered during widely varying activities. Langemark and colleagues found that headache worsened in 25% of the patients in the morning and in 14% in the afternoon, whereas 54% reported absence of any diurnal pattern (21). These figures correspond to other large series (43) and allow us to conclude that no specific diurnal variation occurs in the chronic form.

SEASONAL VARIATIONS

These aspects never have been specifically investigated in tension-type headache. Seasonal variations in the *frequency* of headache, according to our experience, are unlikely to be prominent in chronic tension-type headache. Most patients report weather changes, extreme temperatures, or humid environment as aggravating factors (35,44). Seasonal variations in the *intensity* of the headache may therefore be present. Relief during vacation has been described as pronounced in 7% of 148 patients with chronic tension headache and as light in 26%, and 67% reported no changes during vacation (21).

PHYSICAL EXAMINATION

A diagnosis of chronic tension-type headache requires exclusion of other organic disorders. Therefore, a general physical examination including an eye, ear, nose and throat examination, and in particular, a neurologic evaluation is mandatory. If any abnormalities in the history or in the examination are noted, subsequent evaluation should be made by appropriate investigations and specialists. The physical examination also should include manual palpation of the pericranial muscles to identify tender areas (3,14–18,20). For further details, see Chapter 80.

FINDINGS IN HEADACHE PATIENTS

Tenderness of pericranial muscles is the most common abnormal finding in chronic tension-type headache sufferers (3,14–18,20). Langemark and associates (20) found a significantly higher number of tender pericranial muscles in 40 patients with chronic tension-type headache compared with 40 matched controls in a blinded study. Similar findings have been noted in 735 randomly selected subjects from a general population (14) and in several subsequent clinical studies using the same methodology with a semiquantitative score system (3,9,16,38). Subjects with chronic tension-type headache were significantly more tender than subjects without any experience of headache, migraineurs, and subjects with episodic tension-type headache (14) (Fig. 2). Pericranial tenderness increased significantly with increasing frequency and intensity of tension-type headache (14). Is the increased tenderness a cause or an effect of the headache? To elucidate this relationship, 28 patients with frequent episodic or chronic tension-type headache were investigated during and outside an episode of headache, and the tenderness was increased by 24% during ongoing pain compared with the pain-free state (16). Even in the latter state, pericranial tenderness was markedly higher compared with healthy controls; so the tenderness is not a simple effect of ongoing pain.

In the past, experimental tooth clenching has been reported to induce mild headaches; therefore, an attempt was made to study the cause–effect relationship between such sustained muscle contraction and tension-type headache. Fifty-eight patients with frequent episodic or chronic tension-type headache and 30 healthy controls were encouraged to clench their molar teeth slightly for 30 minutes (17). Forty patients (69%) and only 5 (17%) healthy controls developed headache within the following 24 hours after the clenching procedure. Those patients who later developed headache reported increased tenderness at the recording 90 minutes after clenching, whereas those patients who did not develop headache reported unchanged tenderness in their pericranial muscles (17). This study indicates that tenderness may precede the headache and may be an initiating factor. These observations therefore led to the hypothesis of central sensitization as an underlying patophysiologic mechanism of chronic tension-type headache (17,18). Recently, a qualitatively changed response to mechanical stimuli in human tender muscle was demonstrated for the first time in patients with chronic tension-type headache (5). These findings suggested mediation of pain by low-threshold mechanosensitive afferents projecting to sensitized dorsal horn neurons (4) (see also Chap. 73). Thus, perception of pain is not a simple reflection of simultaneous afferent noxious input but a dynamic process that is highly influenced by the effects of past experiences.

Cephalic and extracephalic pressure pain thresholds are decreased in most clinical but not in epidemiologic studies of the chronic form (3,14,16,22,40), in contrast to the episodic form in which normal mechanical pain sensitivity is found (9,14). The mechanical pain thresholds are only slightly affected, however, and large series of patients are needed to detect any statistical difference between groups. The use of pressure algometry and recording of pain thresholds plays no role in daily clinical practice and should be applied only for research purposes.

The texture of pericranial, shoulder and chewing muscles is often altered in tension-type headache, with tight tender bands or increased consistency. Such findings previously were detected only by manual palpation, but a newly invented and validated instrument, a hardness meter, confirmed this observation (2,37). A close correlation between increased tenderness recorded by manual palpation and hardness was reported, whereas no relationship to the presence or absence of actual pain was found (2,37). The pathophysiologic background and significance of these findings are not yet clarified.

SUBDIVISIONS OF CHRONIC TENSION-TYPE HEADACHE

The definition of a possible muscular factor in tension-type headache in the IHS classification [muscle tenderness recorded by manual palpation or by pressure algometer or abnormal electromyelographic EMG (EMG) levels] (11) depended mainly on studies in the chronic form, in which most patients revealed marked tenderness by manual palpation compared with healthy controls. In addition, a small minority of sufferers of chronic tension-type headache were reported to be free of muscle tenderness but revealed otherwise identical symptomatology of the headache (18). The importance of these differences were not clarified at the time the IHS classification (11) was created, and the subdivision was made to encourage to further research in this area. Most EMG studies of these patients have reported slightly increased EMG levels, whereas other, mainly smaller, studies reported normal levels (15–18,38). Application of EMG in these patients is technically complicated and provides only limited information (15). Therefore, and as a result of large interindividual variations, it has been suggested that EMG criteria should be omitted from the diagnostic IHS criteria and restricted to paired experimental studies (15). The relationship between these diagnostic tests is complex, if it exists, and further studies are warranted.

In the past, several terms, for example, *psychogenic headache* and *conversion headache* (1), were used to

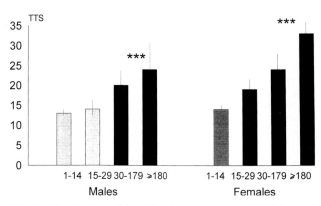

FIG. 2. Distribution of total tenderness score (*TTS*) in pericranial muscles in the general population; subjects without any experience of headache (*Never*), migraineurs (*Migr*), episodic tension-type headache (>14 days per year) (*ETH*), and chronic tension-type headache (*CTH*). Mean values with standard errors of mean for men and women are shown. *Asterisks* indicate significant differences (***p < 0.001) [From Jensen et al. (14)].

define patients in whom abnormal psychological features were prominent. The absence of pericranial muscular tenderness has often been considered typical of these patients (19). A recent comparative study of patients with and without increased pericranial muscle tenderness reported similar clinical characteristics in both groups but marked differences in pain thresholds and EMG levels in patients with chronic but not episodic tension-type headache (19). It was therefore concluded that muscular factors may be of major importance in the conversion of episodic into chronic tension-type headache in most patients, namely, those associated with a muscular disorder, whereas other mechanisms must be considered in those fairly rare patients unassociated with a disorder of pericranial muscles (18). Further investigations in properly classified patients are needed.

CAUSATIVE FACTORS

In the IHS classification, a fourth-digit code indicating the most likely causative factors has been proposed (11). These factors can partly modify and identify some of the clinical and psychological features as well as the therapeutic approach in patients with chronic tension-type headache. In addition, one or several likely etiologic factors capable of inducing the onset or worsening of headache may be identified, but the scientific basis for the evolutive nature and possible causative factors in chronic tension-type headache is still limited.

Because the possible causative factors 2–9 were thoroughly presented in Chapter 80, this chapter discusses only the factors probably involved in turning headache from episodic into chronic. Analgesic abuse is the most important and is involved in more than 50% of cases from highly specialized clinics (7,25,28,39). These chronic patients who abuse drugs may, in some cases, be completely headache free or revert to a pattern of episodic headache if drugs are discontinued (7,25,28,39). Rapaport and co-workers reported highly encouraging data after drug discontinuation in a mixed group of headache patients, with 30% headache free 1 month after discontinuation, but as many as 82% were pain free after 4 months (28). A favorable long-term prognosis also has been reported by Schnider and associates, who reported a 5-year follow-up study of 38 patients with migraine, tension-type headache, or mixed headaches combined with drug abuse according to the IHS classification (39). A tendency toward a better prognosis was found in migraineurs compared with subjects with tension-type headache. (For further details, see Chapter 115.)

Stressful situations may be involved, but the cause–effect relationship has only been sparsely studied. Stress and mental tension are the most frequently reported precipitating factors to tension-type headache, but whether they are causative to the chronic subform is unclear (6,8,33,44). It is likely that mental stress may pre-cipitate an episode of headache, but the chronic subform is widely independent of daily hassles and stress, and a completely different underlying mechanism must be sought. The role of psychological factors, anxiety and depression in particular, remains difficult to clarify, because some of these disturbances may be secondary to the chronic pain condition. These relations were studied by Holroyd and colleagues, who investigated two large groups of patients with migraine or tension-type headache during and outside a period of pain and compared them to healthy controls (12). Anxiety, depression, and somatization was pronounced during the pain episode but similar to healthy controls when patients were examined free of pain, indicating that the pain is an important artifact to these psychological instruments (12) and therefore nearly impossible to eliminate in a chronic pain condition. Whether primary or secondary, psychological factors must be considered in all patients with chronic tension-type headache. Further details about the psychological manifestations are described in Chapter 77 and Chapter 80.

In summary, chronic tension-type headache is a clinical entity different from migraine and is probably a multifactorial disorder with several concurrent pathophysiological mechanisms. It is important to identify and understand the clinical evolution of chronic tension-type headache and thereby, it is hoped, lead us to a better prevention and treatment of the most costly and treatment resistent form of headache.

REFERENCES

1. Ad Hoc Committee on Classification of NIH. *JAMA* 1962;179: 717–718.
2. Ashina M, Bendtsen L, Jensen R, Sakai F, Olesen J. Muscle hardness in patients with chronic tension-type headache: relation to actual headache state. *Pain* 1999;79:201–205.
3. Bendtsen L, Jensen R, Olesen J. Decreased pain detection and tolerance thresholds in chronic tension-type headache. *Arch Neurol* 1996;53: 373–376.
4. Bendtsen L, Jensen R, Olesen J. Qualitatively altered nociception in chronic myofascial pain. *Pain* 1996;65:259–264.
5. Bendtsen, Jensen R, Olesen J. A nonselective (amitriptyline), but not a selective (citalopram), serotonin reuptake inhibitor is effective in the prophylactic treatment of chronic tension-type headache. *J Neurol Neurosurg Psychiatry* 1996;61:285–290.
6. De Benedittis G, Lorenzetti A, Pieri A. The role of stressful life events in the onset of chronic primary headache. *Pain* 1990;40:65–75.
7. Edmeads J, Findlay H, Tugwell P, Pryse-Philips W, Nelson RF, Murray TJ. Impact of migraine and tension-type headache on life style, consulting behavior, and medication use: a Canadian population survey. *Can J Neurol Sci* 1993;20:131–137.
8. Friedman AP. Characteristics of tension headache: a profile of 1420 cases. *Psychosomatics* 1979;20:418-422.
9. Goebel H, Weigle L, Kropp P, Soyka D. Pain sensitivity and pain reactivity of pericranial muscles in migraine and tension-type headache. *Cephalalgia* 1992;12:142–151.
10. Goebel H, Petersen-Braun M, Soyka D. The epidemiology of headache in Germany: a nationwide survey of a representatative sample on the basis of the headache classification of the International Headache Society. *Cephalalgia* 1994;14:97–106.
11. Headache Classification Committee of the International Society. Classification and Diagnostic criteria for headache disorders, cranial neuralgias and facial pain. *Cephalalgia* 1988;8:1–96.

12. Holroyd KA, France JL, Nash JM, Hursey KG. Pain state as artifact in the psychological assessment of recurrent headache sufferers. *Pain* 1993;53:229–235.

13. Iversen HK, Langemark M, Andersson PG, Hansen PE, Olesen J. Clinical characteristic of migraine and episodic tension-type headache in relation to old and new diagnostic criteria. *Headache* 1990;30: 514–519.

14. Jensen R, Rasmussen BK, Pedersen B, Olesen J. Cephalic muscle tenderness and pressure pain threshold in headache: a population study. *Pain* 1993;52:193–199.

15. Jensen R, Rasmussen BK. Muscular disorders in tension-type headache. *Cephalalgia* 1996;16:97–103.

16. Jensen R. Mechanisms of spontaneous tension-type headaches: an analysis of tenderness, pain thresholds and EMG. *Pain* 1996;64:251–256.

17. Jensen R, Olesen J. Initiating mechanisms of experimentally induced tension-type headache. *Cephalalgia* 1996;16:175–182.

18. Jensen R, Bendtsen L, Olesen J. Muscular factors are of importance in tension-type headache. *Headache* 1998;38:10–17.

19. Kudrow L. Muscle contraction headaches. In: Rose C, ed.: *Handbook of clinical neurology. Headache*, vol 48, Amsterdam: Elsevier, 1986:343–352.

20. Langemark M, Olesen J. Pericranial tenderness in chronic tension-type headache: a blind controlled study. *Cephalalgia* 1987;7:249–255.

21. Langemark M, Olesen J, Poulsen DL, Bech P. Clinical characterization of patients with chronic tension headache. *Headache* 1988;28:590–596.

22. Langemark M, Jensen K, Jensen TS, Olesen J. Pressure pain thresholds and thermal nociceptive thresholds in chronic tension-type headache. *Pain* 1989;38:203–210.

23. Leston JA. Migraine and tension-type headache are not separate disorders. *Cephalalgia* 1996;16:220–223.

24. Manzoni GC, Granella F, Sandrini G, Cavallini A, Zanferrari C, Nappi G. Classification of chronic dailay headache by International Headache Society criteria: limit and new propsals. *Cephalalgia* 1995;15:37–43.

25. Mathew NT, Reuveni U, Perez F. Transformed or evolutive migraine. *Headache* 1987;27:102–106.

26. Olesen J. Clinical characterization of tension headache. In: Olesen J, Edvinsson L, eds. *Basic mechanisms of headache.* Amsterdam: Elsevier Science Publishers, 1988:9–14.

27. Pfaffenrath V, Isler H. Evaluation of the nosology of chronic tension-type headache. *Cephalalgia* 1993(suppl 12):60–62.

28. Rapaport A, Weeks R, Sheftell F. Analgesic rebound headache: theoretical and practical implications. *Cephalalgia* 1985;5:448–449.

29. Rasmussen BK, Jensen R, Schroll M, Olesen J. Epidemiology of headache in a general population: a prevalence study. *J Clin Epidemiol* 1991;44:1147–1157.

30. Rasmussen BK, Jensen R, Olesen J. A population-based analysis of the diagnostic criteria of the International Headache Society. *Cephalalgia* 1991;11:130–134.

31. Rasmussen BK, Jensen R, Schroll M, Olesen J. Interrelations between migraine and tension-type headache in the general population. *Arch Neurol* 1992;49:914–918.

32. Rasmussen BK, Jensen R, Olesen J. Impact of headache on sickness absence and utilization of medical services: a Danish population study. *J Epidemiol Health* 1992;46:443–446.

33. Rasmussen BK. Migraine and tension-type headache in a general population: Precipitating factors, female hormones, sleep pattern and relation to lifestyle. *Pain* 1993;53:65–72.

34. Rasmussen BK. Migraine and tension-type headache are separate disorders. *Cephalalgia* 1996;16:217–20.

35. Russel M, Rasmussen BK, Brennum J, Iversen H, Jensen R, Olesen J. Presentation of a new instrument: the diagnostic headache diary. *Cephalalgia* 1992;12:369–374.

36. Sahota PK, Dexter JD. Sleep and the headache syndromes: a clinical review. *Headache* 1990;30:80–84.

37. Sakai F, Ebihara S, Akiyama M, Horikawa M. Pericranial muscle hardness in tension-type headache: a non-invasive measurement method and its clinical application. *Brain* 1995;118:523–531.

38. Sandrini G, Antonaci F, Pucci E, Bono G, Nappi G. Comparative study with EMG, pressure algometry and manual palpation in tension-type headache and migraine. *Cephalalgia* 1994;14:451–457.

39. Schnider P, Auli S, Baumgartner C, et al. Long term outcome of patients with headache and drug abuse after inpatient withdrawal: five-year follow-up. *Cephalalgia* 1996:16;481–485.

40. Schoenen J, Bottin D, Hardy F, Gerard P. Cephalic and extracephalic pressure pain thresholds in chronic tension-type headache. *Pain* 1991; 47:145–149.

41. Schwartz BS, Stewart WF, Simon D, Lipton RB. Lost workdays and decreased work effectiveness associated with headache in the workplace. *J Occup Environ Med* 1997;30:320–327.

42. Schwartz BS, Stewart WF, Simon D, Lipton RB. Epidemiology of tension-type headache. *JAMA* 1998;279:381–3.

43. Solomon S, Lipton RB, Newman LC: Evaluation of chronic daily headache- comparison to criteria for chronic tension-type headache. *Cephalalgia* 1992;12:365–368.

44. Ulrich V, Russell MB, Jensen R, Olesen J. A comparison of tension-type headache in migraineurs and in non-migraineurs: a population-based study. *Pain* 1996;67:501–6.

45. stergaard S, Russell MB, Bendtsen L, Olesen J. Increased familial risk of chronic tension-type headache. *BMJ* 1997;314:1092–1093.

The Headaches, Second Edition,
edited by J. Olesen, P. Tfelt-Hansen, and K.M.A. Welch.
Lippincott Williams & Wilkins, Philadelphia © 2000.

Tension-Type Headache, Cluster Headache, and Miscellaneous Primary Headaches

CHAPTER 82

Differential Diagnosis and Prognosis of Tension-Type Headache

Jean Schoenen and Rigmor Jensen

DIFFERENTIAL DIAGNOSIS

According to the International Headache Society (IHS) Classification of Headaches (codes 2.1 and 2.2), tension-type headache is usually bilateral, of a pressing quality, of mild or moderate intensity, not aggravated by physical activity, and rarely accompanied by mild symptoms such as nausea, photophobia, or phonophobia. Although these characteristics are encountered in the vast majority of patients, it must be kept in mind, as demonstrated by a recent population-based analysis (18), that 18% of patients may have a pulsating headache, 10% unilateral pain, 28% aggravation on routine physical activity, 18% anorexia, 4% nausea, and 11% photophobia (Table 1). Two problems arise, therefore, in diagnosing tension-type headache. On the one hand, tension-type headache, although it is the most frequent [present in up to 78% in the population-based study by Rasmussen and colleagues (18)], is also the least distinct of all headache types; its clinical diagnosis is based chiefly on negative features, that is, on the absence of symptoms that characterize other idiopathic or symptomatic headaches (the absence of unilaterality, pulsatility, aggravation by physical activity, associated symptoms, and so on). On the other hand, a minority of patients may present with symptoms that are found in other headache types. The lack of specificity as well as the uncommon features may make the clini-

cian, and thus the patient, hesitate about the correct diagnosis and explains why paraclinical investigations to exclude organic disease are (and probably should be) performed more frequently in tension-type headache than in other headaches (e.g., migraine). In particular, an atypical history or an abnormality on clinical examination indicates the need for further investigations, for example, for a computed tomography (CT) scan. Several studies confirm that brain imaging studies have a low likelihood of discovering significant intracranial disease in adult or pediatric patients with normal physical and neurologic exams, typical headache patterns, and no change in preexisting headache (20,15,31,5). Many of the various headache types listed under the major headings of the IHS Classification may mimic tension-type headache at some stage of their clinical course. Here we examine only the most frequent among them (Table 2).

Usually, there is little difficulty in distinguishing symptomatic headache caused by sinus or eye disease from tension-type headache. Chronic sinusitis cannot be accepted as a cause of headache on the basis of a simple radiologic thickening of sinus mucosae. At least intermittent radiologic or clinical signs of ongoing sinus disease must be present. Similarly, radiologic evidence of cervical spondylosis is rarely a satisfactory explanation for a headache, because it can be found with equal prevalence in age-matched headache-free subjects (30).

The relation between oromandibular dysfunction and tension-type headache remains controversial (see Chapter 121). Oromandibular dysfunction is listed in the IHS Classification as a possible causative factor at the fourth

J. Schoenen: University Department of Neurology, CHR Citadelle, and University of Liège, B-4000 Liège, Belgium.

R. Jensen: Department of Neurology, Glostrup Hospital, University of Copenhagen, DK-2600 Glostrup, Copenhagen, Denmark.

TABLE 1. *Atypical features of tension-type headache and their incidence*

Feature	Percent
Aggravation by routine physical activity	28
Pulsating headache	18
Anorexia	18
Photophobia	11
Unilateral headache	10
Nausea	4

From ref. 18, with permission.

digit code level. Because of its high prevalence, however, its occurrence with tension-type headache in the same subject could be fortuitous. The similar prevalence of oromandibular dysfunction in subjects from the general population suffering from tension-type headache or migraine or devoid of headache suggests that a causal relationship with tension-type headache is rare (10).

Changes in intracranial pressure are well-known causes of headache. Whereas spontaneous or symptomatic intracranial hypotension is most often distinguishable from other headache types by its clear-cut accentuation when the patient is in the erect position (*orthostatic headache*), intracranial hypertension may produce a headache that can mimic migraine or tension-type headache. Although brain tumors represent only a small minority of the causes of headache, they obviously are a major concern to patients and clinicians. Headache occurs at presentation in approximately 36% to 50% of patients with brain tumors and develops in the course of the disease in 60% (26). Headaches are a more common symptom of brain tumor in children (i.e., in more than 90%). Elevation of intracranial pressure is not necessary for its production. The headache is usually generalized, but in 30% to 80% of patients, it overlies the tumor. Headache awakening the patient from sleep or present on awakening and associated with vomiting is a frequent characteristic of brain tumor but also may occur in some migraineurs.

The syndrome of idiopathic intracranial hypertension, also known as *pseudotumor cerebri or benign intracranial hypertension*, may mimic chronic tension-type headache. The following characteristic features should guide the diagnosis: predominant occurrence in young, obese women (93%); the "most severe headache ever" (93%); pulsatile character (83%); nausea (57%); vomiting (30%); orbital pain (43%); transient visual obscuration (71%);

TABLE 2. *Headache disorders that sometimes mimic chronic tension-type headache*

Analgesic/ergotamine/triptan-abuse headache
Sinus/eye disease
Idiopathic intracranial hypertension
Oromandibular dysfunction
Cervical spondylosis
Brain tumor

diplopia (38%); and visual loss (31%) (28). Papilledema without neuroradiologic abnormalities (except for a possible "empty sella") is pathognomic for this condition (26). Idiopathic intracranial hypertension may occur without papilledema (14). In such patients, who may be indistinguishable from others with intractable chronic daily headache, increased cerebrospinal fluid (CSF) pressure, obesity, and pulsatile tinnitus suggest the diagnosis (29).

In clinical practice, the most frequent cause of chronic daily headache is chronic analgesic or ergotamine or triptan abuse (IHS code 8.2), to which patients may evolve after having presented initially with migraine or with episodic or chronic tension-type headache (23,16,6). (For further details see Chapter. 115.) Recognizing this condition is of crucial importance because any kind of therapy for the initial headache type can be effective only after the patient has been withdrawn from analgesic or specific antimigraine compounds.

Episodic tension-type headache (code 2.1) can be difficult to distinguish from migraine without aura (code 1.1) in patients with atypical, but not necessarily uncommon, clinical features. Primarily for this reason, some authors have hypothesized that migraine and tension-type headache might represent a continuum rather than two distinct entities. Recent epidemiologic studies based on the operational diagnostic criteria of the new IHS Classification do not confirm this hypothesis (17,27). To improve the clinical distinction between these two headache types, a slight modification of the IHS criteria by setting mandatory demands on pain intensity and including graded severity of accompanying symptoms has been proposed. It must be kept in mind that tension-type headache and migraine often coexist in the same patient and that the individual episode of tension-type headache is more severe and more frequent in migraineurs compared with nonmigraineurs (19).

Finally, within the category of tension-type headaches, the validity and clinical usefulness of the subdivision into subgroups "associated or not associated with disorder of pericranial muscles" (code 2.2.2 and 2.2.1) remain to be proven. Pericranial tenderness, a frequent finding in patients with tension-type headache, is by no means pathognomic for this disorder. It can be found in other primary headaches as well as in symptomatic headaches, for instance, in the case of intracerebral lesions, such as tumor or hemorrhage. In the latter case, however, the tenderness tends to be lateralized. Pericranial electromyographic (EMG) levels may be within normal range in most patients with tension-type headache, when recordings are performed at rest in one muscle. The proportion of abnormal findings increases with multiple recording sites, under stress conditions (25), and with the disorder becoming chronic (11). No correlation exists between pericranial tenderness and EMG levels, and patients with increased tenderness do not differ clinically from those without such abnormalities (24,11).

In conclusion, significant overlap exists between the headache of organic brain disease and the tension-type headache. Any headache of recent onset, with fixed localization, that has changed in character, and, obviously, any headache accompanied by a neurologic sign or symptom requires a thorough evaluation. Although a normal electroencephalogram (EEG) may reassure the patient, the doctor must be aware that it does not exclude organic brain disease and plays no role in the workup of headache patients (8). If an intracranial lesion is suspected on the basis of clinical history or examination, a CT or a magnetic resonance imaging (MRI) scan should be performed. The distinction between episodic tension-type headache and migraine without aura may be difficult in some patients. At present, there are no reliable paraclinical tests that are useful in the differential diagnosis. Therefore, a careful history and examination as well a prospective follow-up using diagnostic headache diaries (21) probably constitute the most effective strategy.

PROGNOSIS

The prognosis and clinical course of tension-type headache are variable. Subjects with frequent episodic tension-type headache are probably at increased risk of developing chronic tension-type headache over a period of many years (12). Whether subjects with more severe tension-type headache are at increased risk for developing migraine is still controversial, because patients with coexisting migraine, tension-type headache, and drug-induced headaches represent the vast majority of clinical populations. Recent studies from the general population suggest, however, that migraineurs have the same lifetime prevalence of tension-type headache as nonmigraineurs, but the migraineurs have significantly more frequent and more severe episodes of tension-type headache, indicating that migraine may be one of numerous precipitating factors to tension-type headache (19,27). Various factors can influence headache frequency and transform the episodic into the chronic form; among these, the most frequent is overuse of combined analgesics, ergotamine, or triptans (13,7,22,23,1,6).

Another factor important to the onset of primary headaches, especially for their persistence, is psychosocial stress. Some evidence has been found, particularly in tension-type headache, that chronic recurrent headache is associated with the report of high frequency as well as severity of minor life events and so-called daily hassles (9,3,2,4). These studies suggest that the ability to cope with minor daily life events might be a relevant prognostic parameter in tension-type headache. As a corollary, they offer a rational basis for behavioral therapies designed to improve coping strategies.

The role of sex hormones in primary headaches becoming chronic is a controversial topic, although the role is probably minor. Nonetheless, because menstruation is a frequent precipitating factor of migraine (see Chapter 1) as well as of tension-type headache (17,24), it seems likely that fluctuations of hormonal plasma level, such as those associated with premenopause or inadequate hormonal therapy, can aggravate any primary headache.

In conclusion, it is of major prognostic importance to identify and distuingish episodic tension-type from migraine to initiate an early and specific treatment and to prevent inapropriate and excessive drug consumption.

REFERENCES

1. Celentano DD, Steward WF, Linet MS. The relationship of headache symptoms with severity and duration of attacks. *J Clin Epidemiol* 1990;43:983–994.
2. Dawans A, Schoenen J, Timsit M, Timsit-Berthier M. Comparative study of psychopathological features and temporalis second exteroceptive silent period in chronic tension-type headache: is 5-HT the common denominator? In: Olesen J, Saxena PR, eds. *5-Hydroxytryptamine mechanisms in primary headaches*, vol 2. New York: Raven Press, 1992:220–225.
3. De Benedittis G, Lorenzetti A, Pieri A. The role of stressful life events in the onset of chronic primary headache. *Pain* 1990;40:65–75.
4. De Benedittis G, Lorenzetti A. Minor stressful life events (daily hassles) in chronic primary headache: relationship with MMPI personality patterns. *Headache* 1992;22:140–146.
5. Demaerel P, Boelaert I, Wilms G, Baert AL. The role of cranial computed tomography in the diagnostic work-up headache. *Headache* 1996;36:347–348.
6. Gaist D, Tsiropopulos I, Sindrup S, et al. Inappropriate use of sumatriptan: a population-based register and interview study. *BMJ* 1998;316:1352–1353.
7. Granella F, Farina S, Malferrari G, Manzoni GC. Drug abuse in chronic headache a clinico-epidemiologic study. *Cephalalgia* 7:15–19.
8. Gronseth GS, Greenberg MK. The utility of the electroencephalogram in the evaluation of patients presenting with headache : a review of the literature. *Neurology* 1995;45:1263–1267.
9. Holm JE, Holroyd KA, Hursey KG, Penzien DB. The role of stress in recurrent tension headache. *Headache* 1986;26:160–167.
10. Jensen R, Rasmussen BK, Pedersen B, et al. Oromandibular disorders in a general population. *J Craniomandibular Disorders and Facial Oral Pain* 1993;7:135.
11. Jensen R, Bendtsen L, Olesen J. Muscular factors of importance in tension-type headache. *Headache* 1998;38:10–17.
12. Langemark M, Olesen J, Poulsen DL, Bech P. Clinical characterization of patients with chronic tension headache. *Headache* 1988;28:590–596.
13. Mathew NT, Stubits E, Nigam MP. Transformation of episodic migraine into daily headache: analysis of factors. *Headache* 1982;22:66–68.
14. Mathew NT, Ravishankar K, Sanin LC. Coexistence of migraine and idiopathic intracranial hypertension without papilledema. *Neurology* 1996;46:1226–1230.
15. Maytal J, Bienkowski RS, Patel M, Eviatar L. The value of brain imaging in children with headaches. *Pediatrics* 1995;96:413–416.
16. Olesen J. Analgesic headache. *BMJ* 1995;310:479–480.
17. Rasmussen BK. Migraine and tension-type headache in a general population: precipitating factors, female hormones, sleep patterns and relation to lifestyle. *Pain* 1993;53:65–72.
18. Rasmussen BK, Jensen R, Olesen J. A population-based analysis of the diagnostic criteria of the International Headache Society. *Cephalalgia* 1991;11:129–134.
19. Rasmussen BK, Jensen R, Schroll M, Olesen J. Interrelations between migraine and tension-type headache in general population. *Arch Neurol* 1992;49:914–918.
20. Report of the Quality Standards Subcommittee of the American Academy of Neurology. Practice parameter: the utility of neuroimag-

ing in the evaluation of headache in patients with normal neurologic examinations (summary statement). *Neurology* 1994;44:1353–1354.

21. Russell M, Rasmussen BK, Brennum J, Iversen H, Jensen R, Olesen J. Presentation of a new instrument: the diagnostic headache diary. *Cephalalgia* 1992;12:369–374.

22. Saper JR. Ergotamine dependency: a review. *Headache* 1987;27:435–438.

23. Schoenen J, Lenarduzzi P, Sianard-Gainko J. Chronic headaches associated with analgesics and/or ergotamine abuse: a clinical survey of 434 consecutive out-patients. In: Clifford RF, ed. *New advances in headache research*. London: Smith-Gordon, 1989:255–259.

24. Schoenen J, Gérard P, De Pasqua V, Sianard-Gainko J. Multiple clinical and paraclinical analyses of chronic tension-type headache associated or unassociated with disorder of pericranial muscles. *Cephalalgia* 1991;11:135–139

25. Schoenen J, Gérard P, De Pasqua V, Juprelle M. EMG activity in pericranial muscles during postural variation and mental activity in healthy volunteers and patients with chronic tension-type headache. *Headache* 1991;31:321–324.

26. Silberstein SD, Marcelis J. Headache associated with changes in intracranial pressure. *Headache* 1992;32:84–94.

27. Ulrich V, Russell MB, Jensen R, Olesen J. A comparison of tension-type headache in migraineurs and in non-migraineurs: a population-based study. *Pain* 1996;67:501–506.

28. Wall M. The headache profile of idiopathic intracranial hypertension. *Cephalalgia* 1990;10:331–335.

29. Wang S-J, Silberstein SD, Patterson S, Young WB. Idiopathic intracranial hypertension without papilledema: a case–control study in a headache center. *Neurology* 1998;51:245–249.

30. Wöber-Bingöl C, Wöber C, Zeiler K, et al. Tension headache and the cervial spine-plain X-ray findings. *Cephalalgia* 1992;12:152–154.

31. Wöber-Bingol C, Wöber C, Prayer D, et al. Magnetic resonance imaging for recurrent headache in childhood and adolesence. *Headache* 1996;36:83–90.

The Headaches, Second Edition,
edited by J. Olesen, P. Tfelt-Hansen, and K.M.A. Welch.
Lippincott Williams & Wilkins, Philadelphia © 2000.

Tension-Type Headache, Cluster Headache, and Miscellaneous Primary Headaches

CHAPTER 83

General Approach to Treatment of Tension-Type Headache

Richard C. Peatfield and John G. Edmeads

Tension-type headache is extremely common; Rasmussen (6), for example, using International Headache Society (IHS) criteria, found in suburban Copenhagen that 78% of the population had experienced episodic tension headache during their lifetime, and 3% had chronic headache, defined as suffering for more than 15 days each month. Few tension-type headache sufferers sought medical advice. The large survey undertaken by Lipton and colleagues (4) established that even among patients with unequivocal migraine a considerable majority had not had migraine confirmed by a physician; 8.5% of this population had severe nonmigrainous headaches, and even fewer of these had sought medical advice or prescription medication for their headache. Another Canadian survey (2) demonstrated that only 45% of people with tension-type headaches had ever consulted a physician, as opposed to 64% of people with migraine. Of people with tension-type headache, 34% had consulted nonmedical practitioners, 90% were taking over-the-counter analgesics, and only 24% had received prescription medication. It is clear, therefore, that over-the-counter medication, such as paracetamol (acetaminophen), aspirin, or ibuprofen, remains effective for most patients who see the need to take treatment at all and that patients presenting themselves for med-

ical advice are likely to be among the most distressed or severely affected.

APPROACH TO THE PATIENT

The importance of a thorough history and examination of any patient complaining of headache cannot be overestimated. It is essential that alternative diagnoses have been excluded, including in particular cervical spondylosis, depression, and temporal arteritis, which also gives an opportunity to inquire about aggravating factors and, in particular, to consider the question of abuse of medication. In most cases, and in particular in patients who have a long history of headache who have no physical symptoms or signs, the diagnosis can be considered established without special investigations, but such investigations should be undertaken whenever necessary.

In general, the fact that the physician is taking an interest in the patient's problems will have a therapeutic effect in its own right, particularly if the patient's understandable concern about potentially serious disease, especially brain tumors, can be allayed. It is often helpful to explain the condition as a disturbance of the central pain-modulating system in such a way that normally innocuous stimuli are perceived as painful, with the secondary development of increased muscle tension, anxiety, and depression. It is usually better not to attribute the disease to a single mechanism such as "muscle spasm" or to "a psychosomatic disorder." The patient should be told that cure is rare but that control and symptom suppression are more easily attainable.

R.C. Peatfield: Charing Cross Hospital, London W6 8RF, United Kingdom.

J.G. Edmeads: Department of Medicine, Sunnybrook Health Science Center, University of Toronto, Toronto, Ontario M4N 3M5, Canada.

SELECTING TREATMENTS

Few systematic trials of medication have been done in patients with tension headache. Most studies that are available are small and of nonpharmacologic treatment rather than of the drugs most commonly used; most of these have been on the market for many years, and there is little to motivate drug companies to test them specifically or to develop new remedies specifically for tension-type headache. Unfortunately, many of the earlier trials were undertaken in patients without consistent diagnoses, and many may unwittingly have been abusing analgesics (7). In most available studies, the response rates are similar, and in many cases they are difficult to distinguish from the placebo effect attributable to a caring therapist (Table 1).

Some authorities recommend that patients should keep a written record of their attacks and the likely trigger mechanisms before starting treatment. Others argue that it is better to proceed with treatment at once if only to retain the confidence of the patient and to minimize the use of clinical resources.

It is important to consider and, if possible, to eliminate aggravating factors, especially analgesic abuse. The chronic effects of ergotamine have been recognized for many years, but many more patients are now using opioid analgesics, such as codeine, dihydrocodeine, or dextropropoxyphene (as found in coproxamol). The evidence that simple analgesics, such as aspirin or paracetamol, or antiinflammatory drugs, such as ibuprofen, can be abused is less clear, but more and more patients who seem to perpetuate their headaches by the repeated use of sumatriptan are attending specialist clinics.

Female sex hormones also can perpetuate headache, not only the contraceptive pill, particularly the combined type, but also the progesterone-only pill and hormonal preparations used for perimenopausal and postmenopausal replacement therapy. If patients actually have taken the trouble to seek medical advice about their headaches, and it is considered even remotely likely that the contraceptive pill has made a contribution, it is realistic to suggest that the patient discontinue it, probably for a minimum of 3 months. If the patient is taking hormone replacement therapy for distressing menopausal symptoms, the decision may be more difficult.

Depression and tension-type headache often coexist, and under these circumstances, it is often more straightforward and more successful to treat the patient with a conventional tricyclic antidepressant rather than an analgesic of any kind. There is increasing evidence that tricyclic antidepressants are also effective in patients with chronic headache without overt depression and also that newer antidepressants, especially selective serotonin reuptake inhibitors, may be less effective than tricyclic antidepressants in these patients, possibly because of the beneficial effect of some of the other pharmacologic effects of the tricyclics.

Stress is a more difficult concept, often less easy to influence. It is certainly prudent to identify patients who seem excessively stressed and who, therefore, may respond to stress management or relaxation therapy (7). Holroyd (3) suggests that cognitive-behavioral therapy may be at least as effective. It is certainly reasonable to ensure that patients receive adequate sleep and rest and to identify those in whom a complaint of headache is a cry for help relating to intolerable stresses at work.

Many patients have strong preconceived ideas about treatment and may, for example, strongly dislike daily prophylactic medication. Others reject psychological treatment. Many antipathies are due to previous experience in which treatments may have been used in a less than optimal way, especially by giving too low a dose. Patients with marked pericranial tenderness, young patients, and psychologically intact persons benefit most from biofeedback and physiotherapy. Patients with stress disorders and patients without a significant muscular factor are likely to benefit more from prophylactic medication. Episodic tension-type headache patients may benefit from reduction of psychosocial stress, whereas chronic tension-type headache often is unaffected even by major life events.

TABLE 1. *Summary of treatment options in tension-type headache*

Type of treatment	Examples
Episodic tension-type headache	
Pharmacologic	Acetylsalicylic acid, paracetamol (acetaminophen), ibuprofen, naproxen, muscle relaxants
Nonpharmacologic	Relaxation, heat to the neck
Prevention	Relaxation, muscle biofeedback
Effect questionable	Acupuncture, massage, manipulation, codeine, barbiturates
Contraindicated or ineffective	Opiates, ergotamine, tranquilizers, caffeine
Chronic tension-type headache	
Pharmacologic	Amitriptyline, dozepine, imipramine
Nonpharmacologic	Physical therapy, relaxation, muscle biofeedback, heat, massage
Prevention	*See nonpharmacologic
Effect questionable	Psychotherapy, muscle relaxants, acupuncture, manipulation
Contraindicated or ineffective	Analgesics, ergot alkaloids, opiates, tranquilizers, codeine, barbiturates, beta blockers, neuroleptics

Unfortunately, little scientific evidence has been found to guide the selection of treatment modalities and virtually no large-scale double-blind trials have been done. Often one simply must find the best treatment by trial and error. Therefore, the availability of different treatments is of major importance, and it must be admitted that the personal views of the physician may have a greater effect on the choice of treatment than any proven rational considerations. This situation is likely to be amended only when large-scale comparative trials have been undertaken.

WHO SHOULD BE TREATED WITH WHAT?

Most patients with episodic tension headache already will have tried a variety of over-the-counter analgesics but many may need to be encouraged to persist using aspirin, paracetamol, or ibuprofen. Others will require more potent longer-acting nonsteroidal antiinflammatory drugs, such as naproxen or diclofenac. Usually, the attacks are not disabling enough to justify more potent analgesics; in any case, the evidence, which relates largely to sumatriptan, suggests that this class of drugs is not as efficacious in tension-type headaches as they are in migraine (1). In general, opiates are best avoided; the more potent ones have a well-established potential for addiction, and there is a risk of analgesic abuse in patients who are allowed codeine or dextropropoxyphene on a daily basis.

If the headaches are frequent, tricyclic antidepressants such as amitriptyline, prothiaden, or nortriptyline should be considered. The evidence that selective serotonin reuptake inhibitors are effective is less sound.

For chronic tension-type headache, the first step is to consider risk factors such as the abuse of analgesics, sex hormone treatment, or overt depression. Some patients will benefit from forceful advice about the hazards of chronic analgesic administration without the need for inpatient detoxification, but in others the habit of "pill popping" is so ingrained that admission to the hospital is the only way to enable patients to stop taking medication.

A number of patients will be entirely headache free once detoxified, but in others the original headache pattern (which may be more overtly migrainous) may reemerge and justify treatment in its own right.

In the long term, it is paramount to avoid causing headaches by allowing the patients excessive quantities of codeine, caffeine, or tranquilizers or any kind. Antidepressants remain the mainstay of treatment, and studies suggest that clinical response is independent of the prior psychiatric state of the patient. In many patients, of course, a vicious circle occurs in which depression exacerbates headache and vice versa, and it is now well established that this is much more easily treated by concentrating on antidepressants rather than analgesics. Nevertheless, some centers in the United States have had success with repetitive intravenous dihydroergotamine, but this treatment is by no means available in all countries.

The large number of published studies of small trials of alternative treatments, such as relaxation therapy and biofeedback, suggest that they can be helpful. It is difficult to recommend such treatments, however, particularly at public expense, without much more satisfactory double-blind trials.

REFERENCES

1. Brennum J, Kjeldsen M, Brinck T, et al. Sumatriptan in the treatment of tension-type headache. In: Olesen J, Tfelt-Hansen P, eds. *Headache treatment: trial methodology and new drugs.* Philadelphia: Lippincott-Raven Publishers, 1997:219–222.
2. Edmeads J, Findlay H, Tugwell P, Pryse-Phillips W, Nelson RF, Murray TJ. Impact of migraine and tension-type headache on lifestyle, consulting behaviour, and medication use. *Can J Neurol Sci* 1993;20:131–137.
3. Holroyd KA. Behavioural treatment strategies. In: Olesen J, Schoenen, eds. *Tension-type headache: classification, mechanisms, and treatment.* New York: Raven Press, 1993:245–254.
4. Lipton RB, Stewart WF, Celentano DD, Reed ML. Undiagnosed migraine headaches. *Arch Intern Med* 1992;152:1273–1278.
5. Rasmussen BK, Jensen R, Schroll M, Olesen J. Epidemiology of headaches in a general population—a prevalence study. *J Clin Epidemiol* 1991;44:1147–1157.
6. Rasmussen BK. Epidemiology of headache. *Cephalalgia* 1995;15:45–68.
7. Zagami AS. Chronic tension-type headache. *CNS Drugs* 1995;4:90–98.

The Headaches, Second Edition,
edited by J. Olesen, P. Tfelt-Hansen, and K.M.A. Welch.
Lippincott Williams & Wilkins, Philadelphia © 2000.

Tension-Type Headache, Cluster Headache, and Miscellaneous
Primary Headaches

CHAPTER 84

Psychological Treatments of Tension-Type Headache

Kenneth A. Holroyd and Paul R. Martin

In this chapter we will address the following seven questions:

1. What is psychological treatment?
2. How effective are psychological treatments?
3. Who can benefit from these treatments?
4. How long do improvements achieved with psychological treatments last?
5. Can psychological treatments be administered cost effectively?
6. How do psychological treatments improve tension headache activity?
7. How should psychological and drug therapies be combined?

WHAT IS PSYCHOLOGICAL TREATMENT?

A number of psychological treatments for tension-type headache have been described in the literature, including electromyographic (EMG) biofeedback training, relaxation training, cognitive-behavior therapy, feedback of temporal artery diameter, digital temperature biofeedback training, hypnotic analgesia, transcendental meditation, and covert positive reinforcement. The research evidence is very limited, however, on the latter five approaches, so only the first three approaches will be discussed.

EMG Biofeedback Training

EMG biofeedback provides patients with continuous information pertaining to the state of tension of one or more muscles with a view to helping them learn to control the tension. The most common site used is the frontalis (active electrodes placed one inch above center of each eye), but some researchers have used the temporalis, trapezius, or multiple sites. Some researchers have advocated providing feedback from the site of highest EMG or the most painful region of the head. Figure 1 illustrates a simplified schematic of biofeedback when the frontal area and trapezius muscles are monitored. Feedback can be given in the auditory modality (e.g., clicks varying in rate) or visual modality (e.g., bar varying in length), although the former is more popular and has the appeal of allowing patients to close their eyes. Some researchers advocate giving patients a choice. Sessions usually last about 1 hour and include an adaptation phase, baseline phase, training phase and self-control phase. Researchers typically use 8 to 16 sessions and clinicians 5 to 25 sessions. In addition to biofeedback training, patients are given a rationale for treatment and advice about strategies that they can adopt. Biofeedback training is usually accompanied by instructions for practicing relaxation at home for about 30 minutes daily. EMG biofeedback training has been combined with relaxation training, administered either concurrently or sequentially.

Relaxation Training

The most commonly used forms of relaxation training are progressive relaxation training (PRT) and autogenic training, particularly the former. The research literature

_____

K. A. Holroyd: Department of Psychology, Ohio University, Athens, Ohio 45201-2979.

P. R. Martin: Department of Psychology, University of New England, Armidale, New South Wales 2351, Australia.

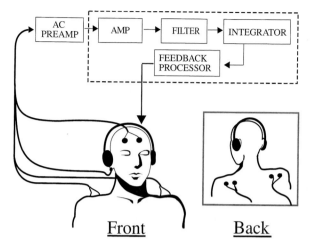

FIG. 1. Schematic of EMG biofeedback training. Frontal area and trapezius muscles are being monitored with the ground on the ear lobe.

provides few guidelines as to which is more effective. Edmund Jacobson originally developed PRT in the 1930s, but most applications to headache are based on an abbreviated version of Jacobson's original procedure. The goal of PRT is to help individuals learn to recognize tension and relaxation as they occur in everyday life. This is accomplished by patients learning to sequentially tense and then release or relax various groups of muscles all through the body. PRT begins with 16 muscle groups, then combines some of these groups to form 7 groups, finally combining more groups to form 4 groups. Latter stages of training involve relaxation by recall (tense stage eliminated from tense-release exercises), cue-controlled relaxation (association of relaxation with a cue word such as "calm"), and differential relaxation (maintaining relaxation in muscles not needed for current activities). Bernstein and Borkovec describe a 10-session program, and most headache researchers use this number or fewer.

Autogenic training was developed by Schultz and Luthe (50). It is based on autosuggestion and seeks to regulate mental and somatic functions simultaneously by passive concentration on formulas such as "my forehead is cool." Schultz and Luthe describe six standard formulas and suggest that it takes 13 to 30 sessions to learn to use them successfully, but most headache researchers use fewer sessions.

Relaxation training is normally accompanied by instructions to practice daily at home, and audiotapes are usually provided for assistance. In fact, relaxation training is sufficiently straightforward that self-administered forms have been advocated.

Cognitive-Behavioral Therapy

A number of researchers have developed treatment packages for tension headache that focus on the mediating role of cognitions and the relationship between stress, coping, and headaches. A diversity of names have been used for this broad-spectrum approach, including cognitive therapy, cognitive-behavioral treatment, stress-coping training, and cognitive skills training, but all will be referred to here as cognitive-behavioral therapy.

Two main variations of cognitive-behavioral therapy have been developed. In the original formulation, Holroyd and colleagues (25,26) focused on altering maladaptive cognitive responses that were assumed to mediate the occurrence of headaches. These researchers offered a rationale in terms of headaches resulting from psychological stress with stress responses determined by cognitions about an event or situation. In contrast, Bakal and colleagues (5) developed a treatment approach that emphasized modifying stress reactions associated with headaches (feelings of helplessness, anxiety, and fear) rather than modifying stress reactions to environmental and interpersonal events. They argued that this shift in emphasis from stress coping skills to headache coping skills was necessary because chronic headache sufferers sometimes experienced attacks in the absence of identifiable external or internal precipitants. More recently, Martin (35) developed a treatment model that includes both a stress coping and headache coping perspective, and emphasizes the importance of behavioral and life-style factors that go beyond the domain of stress. Hence, the model considers the whole range of headache trigger factors and maladaptive reactions of headache sufferers and significant others, as well as the developmental and psychosocial context in which headaches occur.

The most distinctive feature of cognitive-behavioral therapy is cognitive therapy based on the work of theorists such as Donald Meichenbaum (40) and Aaron Beck (7). The goal of cognitive therapy is to teach patients to identify and challenge dysfunctional thoughts, and subsequently the underlying maladaptive assumptions and beliefs. Other elements in cognitive-behavioral therapy include the following. An educational component provides a rationale for the approach. Relaxation training is usually incorporated. Pain management strategies such as imagery training and attention-diversion training are often included. Other techniques may be used depending on the specific features of the case, such as dietary interventions, life-style modification, and contingency management.

Detailed descriptions of psychological treatment techniques as well as discussions of clinical issues that arise in administering psychological treatment and exemplary case studies can be found elsewhere (3,4,11,21,29,33, 35,51).

HOW EFFECTIVE ARE PSYCHOLOGICAL TREATMENTS?

Available studies have been conducted primarily in headache clinics or in specialized university or medical school settings, and generally have been small, averaging about 20 patients per treatment group (15). Information about the results that can be expected when relaxation/biofeedback therapies are integrated into primary care or general neurology settings or when these thera-

TABLE 1. *Mean percentage improvement by type of treatment*

	EMG BF	Relaxation training	BF+ Relaxation training	CBT	Placebo	HA REC
Mean Improvement (%)	48	36	59	53	16	1
No. of treatment groups	28	37	9	15	21	16
Improvement range (%)	−18–96	4–99	37–89	27–76	−70–74	−33–26

EMG BF, EMG biofeedback training; BF+ relaxation training, combined relaxation training and EMG biofeedback; CBT, cognitive-behavior therapy; placebo, placebo and pseudotherapy control conditions; HA REC, headache-recording control.
Data from Borgaards & ter Kuile (15).

pies are administered conjointly with drug therapies thus remains limited.

Metanalytic and narrative reviews have consistently concluded that EMG biofeedback training, relaxation training, and cognitive-behavior therapy effectively reduce tension-type headaches. Table 1 summarizes results from 89 active treatment groups and 37 control groups where daily headache recordings were used to assess treatment outcome.* When results are averaged across studies, EMG biofeedback training, either when administered alone or with relaxation training, and cognitive-behavioral therapy each yield at least a 50% reduction in tension headache activity. Improvements reported with these three treatments as well as with relaxation training alone also are significantly more pronounced than improvements reported with placebo control treatments, or observed in untreated patients. However, these four treatments did not differ significantly among themselves in effectiveness.

Cognitive-behavioral therapy may be particularly helpful where psychological or environmental problems (e.g., chronic work stress, affective distress, other adjustment problems) not effectively addressed by relaxation/biofeedback therapies aggravate headaches or prevent patients from effectively using self-regulation skills. Thus, in one study, patients exhibiting high levels of daily life stress [as assessed by the Hassles Scale (18)] were unlikely to improve with relaxation training alone, but were likely to improve when cognitive-behavioral therapy was added to relaxation training (53). In another study, pretreatment depression was a significant predictor of response to self-management training replicating a common finding, but pretreatment depression was not a significant predictor of response to cognitive therapy, suggesting that a cognitive approach was particularly suited to headache sufferers experiencing depressed mood (38). Cognitive-behavioral therapy may thus enhance the effectiveness of relaxation or EMG biofeedback training for a significant number of patients (10,27).

WHO CAN BENEFIT FROM PSYCHOLOGICAL TREATMENT?

Common clinical problems that arise in administering psychological treatments are discussed here. For the most part, the patients who require special attention in psychological treatment also require special attention when administering drug therapy.

Analgesic Use

Excessive analgesic use limits the benefits likely to be obtained from either psychological treatment or from prophylactic pharmacotherapy. In one retrospective review of patient records (42), less than one third of "high-medication users" showed a 50% or greater reduction in headache activity following psychological treatment, whereas more than half of low-medication users showed this level of improvement. High-medication users in this study were defined by a score of 40 or greater on a frequently used weighted medication index—a score that is obtained by the consumption of at least six aspirins or three Fiorinals (Sandoz) per day, or equivalent medication.

If a patient's headaches are complicated by excessive medication use, withdrawal from the offending medications is probably essential to effective treatment. However, evidence that analgesic withdrawal has therapeutic effects is currently available only for patients who use relatively high levels of medication (6,19). The benefits of analgesic withdrawal are currently unclear for patients who consume marginally problematic levels of analgesics. Psychological treatments appear to help some patients control pain and distress during analgesic withdrawal and to maintain control over their headaches without excessive reliance on analgesics, but these benefits have yet to be evaluated in controlled trials.

Near-Continuous Headaches

Few studies report outcomes specifically for chronic tension-type headache as defined by the International Headache Society (IHS) Classification System, although reported headache frequency data suggest that patient samples in studies evaluating psychological treatments have included a substantial number of patients with the

---

*Daily headache recordings yield relatively conservative estimates of treatment outcome.

chronic form of this disorder. Patients with near-continuous headaches appear less responsive to brief relaxation or biofeedback therapies than are patients with delimited headache episodes. For example, only 13% of patients who recorded near-continuous headaches (6 or more days per week) showed a 50% or greater reduction in headache activity with relaxation/biofeedback treatments in one study (14), whereas more than half of patients who reported at least occasional (1 to 2 days per week) headache-free periods showed this level of improvement. On the other hand, results from a large randomized prospective comparison of nondrug therapies (45,46) suggest that when more than 15 biofeedback/relaxation training sessions are administered, clinically significant reductions in headache activity may be obtained in this population. In this study, patients (N = 522) were randomly assigned to multisite EMG biofeedback training (from trapezius, paracervical, and frontalis muscles), relaxation training, transcutaneous electrical nerve stimulation (TENS), or combinations of these treatments. Combined relaxation/EMG biofeedback training proved highly effective in reducing tension headache activity and in maintaining improvements through 2-, 3-, and 5-year follow-up evaluations, particularly in patients who received more than 15 training sessions. Patients who completed follow-up evaluations (n = 311) had recorded more than 31 hours of headache activity per week before treatment, but showed a 96% reduction in headache hours following relaxation/biofeedback training. Unfortunately, complete data appear to have been collected through 3-year follow-up for only 60% of the patients who began treatment, so reported results probably overestimate the effectiveness of treatment. Nonetheless, these results raise the possibility that near-continuous headaches can be effectively treated by relaxation/biofeedback training, but suggest that effective therapy may require more than 15 training sessions.

Comorbid Psychiatric Disorders

Epidemiologic studies have provided no support for the clinical observation that mood or anxiety disorders are common in individuals with tension-type headache (41). However, the prevalence of psychiatric disorders has not been addressed specifically in chronic tension-type headache sufferers, where psychiatric disorders are most likely to be seen. In clinical samples, chronic tension-type headache appears to be frequently associated with anxiety and mood disorders. In one carefully diagnosed sample, for example, over 40% of individuals with chronic tension-type headaches received a DSM IVR (*Diagnostic and Statistical Manual of Mental Disorders*, 4th ed revised) mood or anxiety disorder diagnosis. More importantly, psychiatric diagnosis was one of the best predictors of headache-related impairments in functioning, suggesting that impairments in functioning associated with pain and with comorbid psychiatric disorders may be difficult to distinguish.

Clinical impressions suggest that patients with comorbid psychiatric disorders are less likely to respond to first-line drug or nondrug therapies than are patients without a comorbid diagnosis, although controlled studies evaluating this possibility are unavailable. The large proportion of patients with comorbid psychiatric disorders typically seen at headache centers that specialize in treating patients who have been refractory to previous treatments is at least consistent with this possibility (39). Treatment outcomes would thus likely be improved if patients in primary care or general neurology settings were routinely screened for the most common anxiety and mood disorders, and if problems identified were appropriately addressed. The Primary Care Evaluation of Mental Disorders [Prime MD (52)], a brief measure designed to screen for the most commonly occurring psychiatric disorders seen in medical settings, is useful for this purpose. Treatment protocols that incorporate elements of cognitive-behavioral therapy or antidepressant medications of demonstrated effectiveness in the treatment of anxiety or mood disorders, also deserve evaluation in this population. Psychological interventions, particularly biofeedback training, may also provide a nonthreatening way to introduce the patient to the process of psychological treatment, and thus to encourage the patient to acknowledge psychological difficulties and accept treatment for psychological disorders.

Children and Adolescents

Despite the fact that approximately 15% of juveniles experience headaches suggestive of tension-type headaches by 15 years of age (9), psychological treatments have rarely been evaluated in young children. Nonetheless, some information supporting the effectiveness of psychological interventions for adolescents is available. Bussone et al. (17) reported that combined EMG biofeedback/relaxation training was more effective than relaxation placebo in reducing episodic tension-type headaches in children (11–15 years of age); notably, the relative benefits of biofeedback training were most evident at 6- and 12-month follow-up evaluations. In a reanalysis of data from three controlled studies, Larsson and colleagues (34) also reported that therapist-administered relaxation training produced larger improvements (63% reduction in what appear to have been episodic tension-type headaches) in adolescents (16–18 years of age) than did group discussion or information-only treatments designed to control for therapist contact and other nonspecific aspects of therapy. No studies have evaluated psychological treatment for pediatric chronic tension-type headache, although this disorder is occasionally seen in children as young as 8 years of age. Clinical observation suggests that headaches in children and adolescents are particularly responsive to self-regulatory therapies, so controlled evaluations of these therapies in children and adolescents with chronic tension-type headache sufferers are needed.

Older Adults

It was first noted in the mid-1980s that relaxation and EMG biofeedback therapies, at least as administered in trials being conducted at that time, were ineffective for tension headache sufferers over the age of about 50 (12,31). Investigators quickly generated complex explanations for this apparent age effect. However, in subsequent studies where relatively simple adjustments were made in treatment protocols, quite positive outcomes were reported, particularly with cognitive-behavioral therapy that included relaxation training (43,44). For example, treating patients who ranged in age from 60 to 78 years (mean 68 years), Moseley found cognitive-behavioral therapy including relaxation training to be more effective than relaxation training alone, with 64% of patients who received 12 sessions of cognitive-behavioral therapy showing clinically significant (greater than 50%) improvements in tension-type headache activity. In this study, audiotapes and written materials designed specifically to assist the acquisition of self-regulatory skills were provided to patients, and weekly phone contacts followed each session to answer questions and identify problems. More recent findings suggest that the provision of more detailed verbal and written explanations of treatment procedures, the review of the material covered, and allowing more time to practice elementary skills before more advanced skills are introduced eliminates the age effect observed in earlier studies.

HOW LONG DO IMPROVEMENTS LAST?

Improvements achieved with psychological treatments have generally been maintained, at least for the 3- to 9-month follow-up periods that have most frequently been assessed. For example, in 22 patient samples included in one metanalytic review, improvements reported at such short-term follow-up evaluation (54% reduction in headache activity) were larger than improvements (45% reduction) reported at immediate posttreatment evaluation (31).

Positive, but much less definitive statements can be made about the long-term (greater than 1 year) maintenance of improvements. In five of six studies that used daily headache recordings, reductions in tension headache activity of 50% or greater were still observed 1 to 3 years following relaxation, EMG biofeedback, or cognitive-behavioral therapy, and in one study, improvements of this magnitude were still observed 5 years following treatment. On the other hand, one study reported poor maintenance 1 year following combined relaxation/EMG biofeedback training (10,27). However, a significant proportion of patients are typically lost to follow-up in these studies, and patients who do complete the follow-up evaluation may have received other treatment during the follow-up period, so these findings must be interpreted cautiously. Booster sessions have not been found to enhance the maintenance of improvements, possibly because good maintenance has frequently been found without booster sessions (1,13). It is possible, however, that patients at high risk for relapse would benefit from booster sessions. Patients discussed in the previous section might thus be reasonable candidates for booster sessions.

CAN PSYCHOLOGICAL TREATMENTS BE ADMINISTERED COST EFFECTIVELY?

For many patients, treatment procedures can be effectively administered in limited-contact or group treatment formats. In a limited-contact or home-based treatment format, headache management skills are introduced in periodic clinic sessions, but written materials and audiotapes are used to enable patients to acquire skills at home that would be typically taught in clinic sessions. As a result, only 3 to 4 (monthly) clinic sessions may be required to complete limited-contact psychological treatment. This contrasts with the 10 to 20 (often weekly) clinic sessions required for completely therapist-administered clinic-based treatment. Across studies, therapist-administered and minimal-contact treatment formats have yielded similar outcomes in adults and children, with the minimal-contact treatment format proving to be significantly more cost effective (20,22,48). To our knowledge, the effectiveness of group and individual administration of psychological treatments for tension-type headache have never been compared; however, relaxation and cognitive-behavioral therapy have been successfully administered in small group treatment formats in a number of studies (24). Limited-contact and small group treatments thus appear to be cost-effective treatment methods. Some proportion of patients require more therapist intensive treatment. Individuals who use excessive amounts of analgesic medication, who are clinically depressed, or who suffer from near daily headache problems are likely to require more intensive treatment. Also, some patients do not persist in efforts to learn or apply self-regulation skills without regular contact with a health professional.

HOW DO PSYCHOLOGICAL TREATMENTS IMPROVE TENSION-TYPE HEADACHES?

Efforts to understand how psychological treatments produce reductions in tension headache activity have focused primarily on EMG biofeedback training. Current models of therapeutic change that emphasize peripheral or central change mechanisms are illustrated in Figure 2. The model that guided the original development of EMG biofeedback training postulated that feedback from pericranial muscles enables the individual undergoing biofeedback training to acquire control of muscle activity associated with tension-type headaches and, thereby, to reduce tension headache activity (Figure 2a). Unfortunately, studies that have

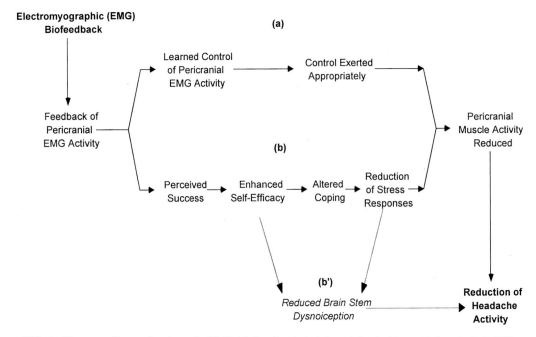

FIG. 2. Therapeutic mechanisms in EMG biofeedback training. Adapted from Holroyd et al. (32).

examined relationships between the self-regulation of pericranial EMG activity and improvement following training have provided little support for this model (2,32,37,47). Especially problematic for this model has been the finding that feedback for increasing (or maintaining constant) pericranial muscle activity can be as therapeutic as feedback for reducing pericranial muscle activity under some conditions (2,32).

The second model postulates that reductions in tension headache activity are consequences of cognitive and behavioral changes set in motion by biofeedback training (Fig. 2b). Studies finding that hypothesized cognitive changes better predict improvement following biofeedback training than do EMG changes provide some support for this model. Improvements in tension-type headache activity following biofeedback training also may reflect the ability of biofeedback training to remedy deficits in central pain modulation contributing to chronic tension-type headache (Fig. 2b) (49). However, attempts to test this modified model using the second exteroceptive suppression period (ES2) of jaw-closing muscles as an index of the integrity of supraspinal pain modulation systems involved in chronic tension-type headache have yielded conflicting results (47,49).

It appears likely that different combinations of peripheral and central factors maintain tension-type headaches in different individuals. This implies that different change mechanisms may be operating in improvements shown by different individuals. Change mechanisms thus need to be evaluated separately in episodic and chronic tension-type headache sufferers, and possibly in more homogenous subgroups of patients within these two broad diagnostic categories.

HOW CAN PSYCHOLOGICAL AND DRUG THERAPIES BE COMBINED?

Surprisingly little attention has been devoted to evaluating strategies to integrate drug and nondrug treatments. In an early study (16), chronic tension headache sufferers (N = 28) were randomized to 16 EMG biofeedback training sessions, or to an individualized medical management program that included drug therapy (antidepressant medication, analgesics, muscle relaxants, sedatives), physical therapy, or combined drug/physical therapy, depending on the clinician's assessment of the patient's needs. Biofeedback training, but not medical management, yielded significant reductions in headache activity, with 54% of patients in the biofeedback training group but only 10% of patients in the medical management group showing at least a 50% reduction in headache activity. Improvements with biofeedback training also were maintained at a 6 month follow-up. Individualized medical management may have had a poor showing in this study because patients had previously been unresponsive to medical therapies and to have been rather severely disabled, with all patients "frequently absent from work, often for long periods, because of headaches" (p. 34). The researchers suggest that in this population, "Drug therapy and physical therapy reinforce a tendency to dependent behavior in many headache patients, but biofeedback educates the patient to control his own well being" (p. 36).

In the only study (30) to directly compare the effectiveness of psychological therapy and prophylactic medication, patients (N = 41) with frequent (either episodic or chronic) tension-type headaches (mean 5 headache days/week) received either cognitive-behavioral therapy (administered in a limited-therapist contact treatment format) or amitriptyline HCl (individualized dose of 25 to 75 mg/day). Cognitive-behavioral therapy and amitriptyline each yielded significant improvements in headache activity, both when improvement was assessed with patient daily recordings (56% and 27% reduction, respectively) and when improvement was assessed by neurologist ratings (94% and 69% of patients rated as at least moderately improved, respectively). Where differences in treatment effectiveness were observed, cognitive-behavioral therapy yielded somewhat more positive outcomes than did amitriptyline. It is unclear if limited-contact cognitive-behavioral therapy would yield equally positive results if only patients with near daily pain were treated because patients who are rarely headache free often do not have an opportunity to make use of the skills for preventing headaches that are an important component of this treatment.

One study (N = 50) has examined the benefits of adding amitriptyline (dose adjustment to 75 mg/day) to EMG biofeedback training from multiple muscle sites (suboccipital, cervical, trapezius, sternocleidomastoid, masseter) over 30 training sessions. Amitriptyline initially enhanced the effectiveness of biofeedback training; however, beginning at month 8 and continuing through the 24-month observation period, the combined treatment showed no advantage over biofeedback training alone. In fact at the 20- and 24-month observation periods, patients who received biofeedback training alone recorded significantly fewer hours of headache activity than patients who received combined amitriptyline/biofeedback training. The relatively poor results obtained with combined treatment at these two follow-up assessments probably reflects the fact that patients were weaned from amitriptyline at month 16. The authors suggest that "the patient's dependence on or expectation of taking medication may actually undermine the intensity or effort applied to learning physiologic control via the biofeedback training" (p. 175), thus reducing the long-term gains that can be achieved with psychological treatment.

Holroyd and colleagues (29) have proposed algorithms to guide the integration of drug and nondrug therapies. For tension-type headache, it is suggested that combined antidepressant medication and psychological therapy be considered if tension-type headaches are unremitting, or a comorbid mood or anxiety disorder is present; if neither condition is present, it is suggested that psychological therapy may be the intervention of choice. However, more intensive psychological treatment including EMG biofeedback training also deserves consideration when headaches are unremitting, and cognitive-behavioral interventions with proven effectiveness in managing mood and anxiety disorders deserve attention when anxiety or mood disorders are present.

It is likely that pharmacologic and nonpharmacologic treatments have different effect profiles, and these differences are likely to go undetected when clinical trials assess treatment outcome narrowly (23). For example, psychological treatments have been observed to produce improvement more slowly than pharmacologic treatment, to yield fewer side effects than pharmacologic treatment (but to require more time and effort to complete), and to produce psychological benefits not observed with pharmacologic treatment in some studies. In order to detect such differences, future clinical trials will need to assess quality of life and the time course of treatment effects as well as simple reductions in headache activity.

CONCLUSION

It is now reasonably well established that psychological therapy can be of value in managing recurrent tension-type headaches. Unfortunately, psychological therapy is more likely to be available at specialized headache treatment centers than at family medicine or general neurology clinics where patients who have not yet developed chronic or intractable headache problems are seen. Psychological therapy may well prove more effective in preventing the development of chronic headaches than in controlling headaches once they have become chronic. Attention thus needs to be devoted to the integration of psychological therapies into general medical practice. See Martin (36) for a general discussion on the relationship between medicine and psychology in the headache field. In this regard, future clinical trials might be conducted in general neurology settings (as well as in psychology clinics and specialized headache treatment centers), and nurses and other health professionals (rather than psychologists) might be trained to administer psychological interventions. Future trials also need to clearly distinguish between episodic and chronic tension-type headaches when evaluating psychological treatments because the intensity of intervention required to manage headaches in these two instances is likely to differ. The effectiveness of psychological treatments that incorporate interventions to manage mood and anxiety disorders also needs to be evaluated in patients who exhibit high levels of affective distress because headaches in these patients may often be ineffectively managed with standard drug therapies.

ACKNOWLEDGMENT

Preparation for this chapter supported in part by a grant from the National Institutes of Health (NINDS #NS 322374).

REFERENCES

1. Andrasik F, Blanchard EB, Neff DF, Rodichok LD. Biofeedback and relaxation training for chronic headache: a controlled comparison of booster treatments and regular contacts for long-term maintenance. *J Consult Clin Psychol* 1984;52:609–615.
2. Andrasik F, Holroyd KA. A test of specific and nonspecific effects in the biofeedback treatment of tension headache. *J Consult Clin Psychol* 1980;48:575–586.

3. Arena JG, Blanchard EB. Biofeedback and relaxation therapy for chronic pain disorders. In: Gatchel RJ, Turk DC, eds. *Psychological approaches to pain management: a practitioner's handbook.* New York: Guilford, 1996.

4. Bakal DA. *The psychobiology of chronic headache.* New York: Springer, 1982.

5. Bakal DA, Demjen S, Kaganov JA. Cognitive behavioral treatment of chronic headache. *Headache* 1981;21:81–86.

6. Baumgartner C, Wesseley P, Bingol C, Maly J, Holzner F. Long-term prognosis of analgesic withdrawal in patients with drug-induced headaches. *Headache* 1989;29:510–514.

7. Beck AT. *Cognitive therapy and the emotional disorders.* New York: International Universities Press, 1976.

8. Bernstein DA, Borkovec TD. *Progressive relaxation training: a manual for the helping professions.* Champaign, IL: Research Press, 1973.

9. Bille B. Migraine in school children. *Acta Paediatr Scand* 1962;51: 1–151.

10. Blanchard EB. Psychological treatment of benign headache disorders. *J Consult Clin Psychol* 1992;60:537–551.

11. Blanchard EB, Andrasik F. *Management of chronic headaches: a psychological approach.* Elmsford, NY: Pergamon, 1985.

12. Blanchard EB, Andrasik F, Evans DD, Hillhouse J. Biofeedback and relaxation treatments for headache in the elderly: a caution and a challenge. *Biofeedback Self Regul* 1985;10:69–73.

13. Blanchard EB, Appelbaum KA, Guarnieri P, et al. Two studies of the long-term follow-up of minimal-therapist contact treatments of vascular and tension headache. *J Consult Clin Psychol* 1988;56:427–432.

14. Blanchard EB, Appelbaum KA, Radnitz CL, Jaccard J, Dentinger MP. The refractory headache patient: I. Chronic, daily, high-intensity headache. *Behav Res Ther* 1989;27:403–410.

15. Bogaards MC, ter Kuile MM. Treatment of recurrent tension headache: a meta-analytic review. *Clin J Pain* 1994;10:174–190.

16. Bruhn P, Olesen J, Melgaard B. Controlled trial of EMG feedback in muscle contraction headache. *Ann Neurol* 1979;6:34–36.

17. Bussone G, Grazzi L, D'Amico D, Leone M, Andrasik F. Biofeedback-assisted relaxation training for pediatric tension-type headache: a controlled study. *Cephalalgia* 1998;18:463–467.

18. DeLongis A, Coyne JC, Dakof G, Folkman S, Lazarus RS. Relationship of daily hassles, uplifts, and major life events to health status. *Health Psychol* 1982;1:119–136.

19. Diener HC, Dichgans J, Scholz E, Geiselhart S, Gerber WD, Bille A. Analgesic-induced chronic headache: long-term results of withdrawal therapy. *J Neurol* 1989;236:9–14.

20. Haddock CK, Rowan AB, Andrasik F, Wilson PG, Talcott GW, Stein RJ. Home-based behavioral treatments for chronic benign headache: a meta-analysis of controlled trials. *Cephalalgia* 1997;17:113–118.

21. Hatch JP. Headache. In: Gatchel RJ, Blanchard EB, eds. Psychophysiological disorders: research and clinical applications. Washington, DC: American Psychological Association, 1993:111–150.

22. Hermann C, Kim M, Blanchard EB. Behavioral and pharmacological intervention studies of pediatric migraine: an exploratory meta-analysis. *Pain* 1995;60:239–256.

23. Holroyd K. Integrating pharmacologic and non-pharmacologic treatments. In: Tolison CD, Kunkel RS, eds. *Headache diagnosis and interdiciplinary treatment.* Baltimore: Williams & Wilkins, 1993:309–320.

24. Holroyd KA, Andrasik F. Coping and the self-control of chronic tension headache. *J Consult Clin Psychol* 1978;46:1036–1045.

25. Holroyd KA, Andrasik F. A cognitive-behavioral approach to recurrent tension and migraine headache. In: Kendall PE, ed. *Advances in cognitive-behavioral research and therapy.* New York: Academic, 1982: 275–320.

26. Holroyd KA, Andrasik F, Westbrook T. Cognitive control of tension headache. *Cogn Ther Res* 1977;1:121–133.

27. Holroyd KA, French D. Recent advances in the assessment and treatment of recurrent headaches. In: Goreczny AJ, ed. *Handbook of health and rehabilitation psychology.* New York: Plenum, 1995:3–30.

28. Holroyd KA, Lipchik GL. Psychological management of recurrent headache disorders: progress and prospects. In: Gatchel RJ, Turk DC, eds. *Psychosocial factors in pain.* New York: Guilford, 1999.

29. Holroyd KA, Lipchik GL, Penzien DB. Psychological management of recurrent headache disorders: empirical basis for clinical practice. In:

Dobson KS, Craig KD, eds. *Best practice: developing and promoting empirically supported interventions.* Newbury Park, CA: Sage, 1998.

30. Holroyd KA, Nash JM, Pingel JD, Cordingley GE, Jerome A. A comparison of pharmacological (amitriptyline HCl) and nonpharmacological (cognitive-behavioral) therapies for chronic tension headaches. *J Consult Clin Psychol* 1991;59:387–393.

31. Holroyd KA, Penzien DB. Client variables in the behavioral treatment of recurrent tension headache: a meta-analytic review. *J Behav Med* 1986;9:515–536.

32. Holroyd KA, Penzien DB, Hursey KG, et al. Change mechanisms in EMG biofeedback training: cognitive changes underlying improvements in tension headache. *J Consult Clin Psychol* 1984;52:1039–1053.

33. Holroyd KA, Penzien DB, Holm JE. Clinical issues in the treatment of recurrent headache disorders. In: Keller PA, Ritt LG, eds. *Innovations in clinical practice: a source book.* Sarasota, FL: Professional Resource Exchange, 1988:433–458.

34. Larsson B, Melin L. The psychological treatment of recurrent headache in adolescents—short-term outcome and its prediction. *Headache* 1988;28:187–195.

35. Martin PR. *Psychological management of chronic headaches.* New York: Guilford, 1993.

36. Martin PR. Headache. In: Bollack AS, Herson M, eds. *Comprehensive clinical psychology,* vol. 2. Oxford: Pergamon;1998:209–220.

37. Martin PR, Mathews AM. Tension headaches: psychophysiological investigation and treatment. *J Psychosom Res* 1978;22:389–399.

38. Martin PR, Nathan PR, Milech D, van Keppel M. Cognitive therapy vs self-management in the treatment of chronic headache. *Br J Clin Psychol* 1989;28:347–361.

39. Mathew NT, Reuveni V, Perez F. Intractable chronic daily headache. A persistant neurobehavioral disorder. *Cephalalgia* 1989;9[Suppl 1a]: 180–181.

40. Meichenbaum DA. *Cognitive behavior modification: an integrative approach.* New York: Plenum, 1977.

41. Merikangas KR, Merikangas JR, Angst J. Headache syndromes and psychiatric disorders: association and family transmission. *J Psychosom Res* 1993;27:197–210.

42. Michultka DM, Blanchard EB, Appelbaum KA, Jaccard J, Dentinger MP. The refractory headache patient: II. High medication consumption (analgesic rebound) headache. *Behav Res Ther* 1989;27:411–420.

43. Mosley TH, Grotheus CA, Meeks WM. Treatment of tension headache in the elderly: a controlled evaluation of relaxation training and relaxation combined with cognitive-behavior therapy. *J Clin Geropsychol* 1995;1:175–188.

44. Nicholson NL, Blanchard EB. A controlled evaluation of behavioral treatment of chronic headache in the elderly. *Behav Ther* 1993;24:67–76.

45. Reich BA. Non-invasive treatment of vascular and muscle contraction headache: a comparitive longitudinal study. *Headache* 1989;29:34–41.

46. Reich BA, Gottesman M. Biofeedback and psychotherapy in the treatment of muscle contraction/tension-type headache. In: Tollison CD, Kunkel RS, eds. *Headache diagnosis and interdisciplinary treatment.* New York: Urban & Schwartzenberg, 1993:167–180.

47. Rokicki LA, Holroyd KA, France CR, Lipchik GL, France JL, Kvaal SA. Change mechanisms associated with combined relaxation/EMG biofeedback training for chronic tension headache. *Appl Psychophysiol Biofeedback* 1997;22:21–41.

48. Rowan AB, Andrasik F. Efficacy and cost-effectiveness of minimal therapist contact treatments of chronic headache: a review. *Behav Ther* 1996;27:207–234.

49. Schoenen J. Exteroceptive silent periods of temporalis muscle in headache. In: van Steenberghe D, DeLaat A, eds. *EMG of jaw reflexes in man.* Leuven, Belgium: Leuven University Press, 1989.

50. Schultz J, Luthe W. *Autogenic training: a psychophysiologic approach in psychotherapy.* New York: Grune & Stratton, 1959.

51. Schwartz MS. Biofeedback: a practitioner's guide. New York: Guilford, 1987.

52. Spitzer AL, Williams JBW, Kroenke K, et al. Utility of a new procedure for diagnosing mental disorders in primary care: The PRIME MD 1000 study. *JAMA* 1994;272:1749–1756.

53. Tobin DL, Holroyd KA, Baker A, Reynolds RVC, Holm JE. Development and clinical trial of a minimal contact, cognitive-behavioral treatment for tension headache. *Cognitive Ther Res* 1988;12:325–339.

The Headaches, Second Edition,
edited by J. Olesen, P. Tfelt-Hansen, and K.M.A. Welch.
Lippincott Williams & Wilkins, Philadelphia © 2000.

Tension-Type Headache, Cluster Headache, and Miscellaneous Primary Headaches

CHAPTER 85

Physiotherapy of Tension-Type Headache

Jane Y. Carlsson and Rigmor Jensen

For decades, physiotherapy has been widely used in the treatment of headache, but the scientific evidence for a positive effect is surprisingly limited. Most of the previous series have been conducted in mixed, not properly classified headache groups. Furthermore, it is difficult to apply a placebo-controlled design in nonpharmacologic treatment studies. Most of the reported studies have therefore consisted of case reports, uncontrolled or comparative with another treatment modality. In tension-type headache as well as in other pain disorders, it is extremely important to consider the placebo effect. It can therefore be recommended that future treatment studies include a randomized and placebo-controlled design. The underlying rationale for physiotherapy, the applied methods, and the available research results will be discussed in the following sections.

PRETREATMENT ASSESSMENT

The patient history should include possible etiologic factors in the home background, work, and leisure activities. The inspection of the patient includes observation of his facial expression (whether he wrinkles his forehead, narrows his eyes, or clenches his jaw) and how he stands, sits, and moves, especially the positioning of the head and shoulders. The mobility of the neck and shoulders is examined with the intention of identification of tense and shortened or impaired neck mobility muscles (16). Neck

mobility can be registered by different methods. The Cybex equipment gives neck mobility in degrees. It is simple and reliable (24).

Increased tenderness of pericranial muscles demonstrated by manual palpation is one of the most consistent abnormal findings in patients with tension-type headache, and to get a more precise quantification of tenderness a palpometer could be used. With a palpometer the investigator can perform palpation with the usual small finger movements and yet keep control over the palpation pressure (1). Alternatively, palpation may be supplemented by means of pressure algometry (12), but although pressure algometry is widely used in research, it plays no practical role in routine clinical work.

The relationship between tension-type headache, muscle contraction, and tenderness is unclear. Muscle tenderness may be found in areas remote from the head pain (22), and electromyographic (EMG) studies indicate only a slightly increased muscle activity, if any. Furthermore, the correlation between EMG amplitudes and tenderness is only slight and is only reported in the chronic, not the episodic, subform of tension-type headache (3). Although this suggests that headache is not directly linked to muscle contraction, the abnormal tenderness is closely related to the frequency and intensity of tension-type headache (14). Although the origin of tension-type headache probably is multifactorial, the muscular factors are considered to be very important in the development and evolution of pain from the episodic to the chronic form (see also Chapter 73). The therapeutic efforts in physiotherapy are primarily designed to produce muscle relaxation and may thereby prevent or minimize the nociceptive input from the periphery to the central nervous system. The physiotherapist must also consider other plausible mechanisms

J. Y. Carlsson: Department of Rehabilitation, College of Health and Caring Sciences, Göteborg University, S-405 30, Göteborg, Sweden.

R. Jensen: Department of Neurology, Glostrup Hospital, University of Copenhagen, DK-2600 Glostrup, Copenhagen, Denmark.

for the development of the tension-type headache in order to give the patients individually adapted treatment programs. Increased tone of cervical muscles (due to poor posture or anxiety) may promote cranial muscle tension because of functional continuity between shoulder, neck, and scalp musculature (5).

Several studies have reported an association between tension-type headache and dysfunction of the masticatory system (see also Chapter 76). In both, muscle tenderness is a predominant feature. Bruxism and other muscular hyperactivity of pericranial and masticatory muscles have been considered as causes of tenderness and pain. Jaw clenching is often combined with a protrusive posture of the head that gives rise to increased tone in the neck muscles.

TREATMENT

Nonpharmacologic Pain Control

Many patients with tension-type headache tend to increase their intake of analgesics, which paradoxically can increase the pain (see also Chapter 115), and nonpharmacologic methods are often a preferable approach. The first step is to wean the patient from analgesic medication gradually or abruptly, substituting with such treatments as transcutaneous electrical nerve stimulation (TENS), heat or cold application, massage, and relaxation. The patient is instructed to use these techniques daily at home in an individually adapted combination.

Relaxation Techniques

It is not known whether pericranial muscle spasm is a cause or an effect of tension-type headache or whether spasm reduction is a cause or an effect of pain relief. Nonetheless, techniques designed to produce muscle relaxation have become conventional therapy for tension-type headache (3).

Relaxation of the whole body can be performed according to a technique described by Jacobson (11). There are currently many abbreviated versions of the original technique, and it is not possible to demonstrate the superiority of one technique over another. The aim of all relaxation techniques is to make the patients aware of the difference between tense and relaxed muscles. The patient is instructed to start the training in a comfortable, recumbent position in a darkened environment, eventually performing the training while sitting in a substantially less peaceful environment. Finally, the tension-type headache sufferer must learn to practice relaxation in everyday life. The patient must be aware of the way he or she stands, sits, and walks and how he or she lies when sleeping. The patient must adopt a new and more economical pattern of muscle use, checking that all muscles that are not essential for the task of the moment are in a state of relaxation. This applies to working situations such as writing, typing, or speaking on the telephone as well as to leisure activities such as watching television or sports. A simple method of helping the patient to notice any warning sensation of muscle tension is to place a piece of tape on the skin over the area of unwanted muscle contraction. When the muscle starts to contract, the patient feels the movement of the tape and can voluntarily stop the contraction and relax the muscle. The importance of short breaks during a day's work, irrespective of what kind of work, cannot be stressed enough. The autogenic relaxation program listed in Table 1 can be recommended.

The biofeedback technique can be used in relaxation training. EMG surface electrodes are placed over the musculature. The electrodes are connected to a small EMG recorder, which transforms the incoming EMG signals into sound and light signals, the strength of which is proportional to the recorded muscle activity. The patient hears and/or sees the signal and can learn to reduce the strength of the signal voluntarily by relaxing the muscle. Relaxation training alone or combined with EMG biofeedback are shown to be superior to no treatment or placebo treatment (3). However, it is probably impossible to predict the treatment outcome by pretreatment demography, medical, and psychological variables (21).

Home Exercise

Several home-based, self-regulatory programs involving relaxation training and strategies for cognitive stress coping have been developed. Such a program can consist of audiotapes supplemented with a manual, containing the same types of instructions as the therapist-assisted regimens. The program has to be easy to accept and to apply. It may start thus: "I want you to concentrate on the muscles of your arm and hand. Good. Now, clench your

TABLE 1. *Autogenic relaxation program during a short break (30 seconds)*

Sit down on a chair with firm support for your back, put your hands on your knees and your feet on the floor:
Lean your head against the wall.
Lower your shoulder.
Relax your jaw so that there is a small gap between the molar teeth.
Close your eyes and breathe calmly and rhythmically.
Feel how your whole body becomes relaxed from your toes up to your forehead.
Use an individually chosen cue word (e.g., "relax") and subvocalize at each inhalation (induces a deeper state of relaxation).
After 30 seconds:
Open your eyes.
Take a deep breath and end with a big yawn and stretch.

hand hard . . . harder." The word "now" is important. It serves as a starting signal for a tension or a relaxation period. "Feel the tension in your whole arm. Hold it (for 5–7 seconds). *Now,* relax. Feel how your fingers, hand, and arm are completely slack. Notice the difference between tense and relaxed muscles. You become more and more relaxed." The last sentence is a pure suggestion. In contrast to Jacobson (10), his pupils Bernstein and Borkovec (2) emphasized the importance of suggestion in relaxation training. The exercise then continues with tension and relaxation (progressive relaxation) of other muscles groups (shoulder, neck, jaw) (Fig. 1). Several controlled studies and a metanalysis (8) have shown that self-regulatory treatments adapted to minimal therapist contact produce comparable or even superior results to clinic-based treatments (8).

When the patient has learned how to prevent the headache from beginning and to eliminate or reduce the headache once it has begun, it is time to build up the patients physical condition, including muscle strength, coordination, litheness, and fitness. The training must be planned according to an individually adapted program, which can be managed by the patient.

Body Awareness

There are various methods, which are based on the body awareness concept. Two well-known programs are presented by Mensendieck (17) and Feldenkreis (7). Mensendieck's training system intends to recreate muscular control in hypo- and hypertonic musculature and thereby reduce a muscular pain state. Feldenkreis suggested that many painful conditions are caused by incorrect movement patterns, which can be adjusted by different physical exercises, and he has described hundreds. However, no scientific evaluations of the Mensendieck and Feldenkreis methods concerning treatments of tension-type headache have ever been published.

Ergonomy and Antistress Training

An ergonomic analysis of the individual's work-related posture and movements is often helpful. Many working positions produce a static load on the neck and shoulder muscles. In several such positions, the cervical spine is not only flexed but rotated, which increases the load (19). A hyperextended position of the neck with an upward turning of the face often coexist with a forward-flexed position of the shoulders in a person who sits working at a desk. During the course of the day's stress, this may progressively give rise to cramping and excessive tone in the neck and shoulder muscles. The symptoms can have many different expressions: headache, dizziness, and pain in the neck with or without decreased range of movement. An important part of the physical therapy program is to make the patient aware of positions that may lead to or aggravate pain and spasm, and that variations between static and dynamic activity is very important.

Although an unfavorable physical load is an essential factor, psychosocial factors at work or at home might contribute to the development of tension-type headache. To that end, the physical therapist may help the patient by describing the relationship between muscle tension and emotional stress.

Massage, Heat/Cold Application, and TENS

Massage is a traditional therapy that has been widely prescribed in diverse cultures for centuries. Although its precise mechanism of action has not been defined, massage is known to relieve spasm and to decrease pain, perhaps through spindle receptor stimulation and reflex muscle relaxation. An increase in plasma β-endorphins has been demonstrated after connective tissue massage (15). Massage incudes stroking (which soothes and relaxes deep muscles) and compression (in which kneading relaxes muscles, decrease edema, and mobilizes tissue adhesions). Therapeutic heat or cold modalities can be useful adjuncts to massage. Superficial heating methods include electric heating pads, moist compresses, and hydrocollator packs. Superficial heat raises the skin and subcutaneous temperature to a depth of 2 to 3 cm. The reflectory increase in superficial blood flow produces cooling in underlying joints and may contribute to pain relief. Superficial cooling produced by ice packs empirically reduces pain and decreases muscle spasm, but there is no scientific evidence for this observation.

Most TENS devices use two frequency areas: high-frequency TENS at 50 to 100 Hz and low-frequency TENS at 1 to 4 Hz. A third type of stimulation gives high-frequency sequences repeated at a low frequency, subcutaneous train stimulation. The pain-reducing effect of TENS is based on the gate-control theory (high-frequency TENS) and the endorphin release theory (low-frequency TENS). Patients with headache are most suitably treated with high-frequency or train stimulation on the pericranial and neck musculature because a pure low-frequency stimulation requires high intensity to be effective, which in turn causes unpleasant muscle contractions. A recommended stimulation time is 20 to 30 minutes, which can be repeated three times per day or as required. A contraindication is present if the patient has a cardiac pacemaker. There are no scientific evaluations of the efficacy of massage, heat/cold application, and TENS in the treatment of tension-type headache.

Manipulation

Manipulation is a technique in which joints are moved a few degrees beyond the physiologic range, in theory to free the joint from restrictive elements. The therapist

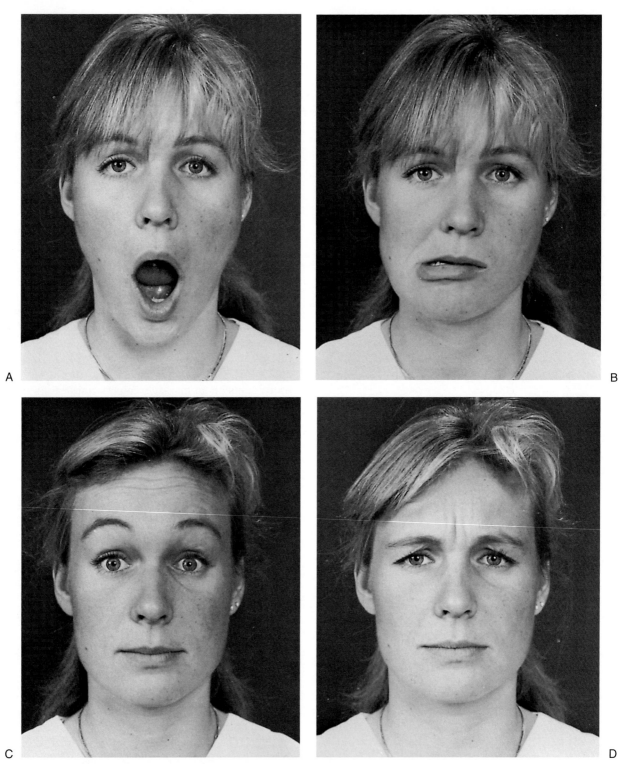

FIG. 1. Progressive relaxing exercises for the jaws, eyes, forehead and shoulders. **A:** Open your mouth and clench your teeth alternately. Relax. **B:** Move your jaw sideways five times in each direction. **C:** Raise your eyebrow as high as you can, then lower them and relax. **D:** Wrinkle your eyebrows, then relax. **E:** Close your eyes tightly, then relax. **F:** Raise your shoulders as high as you can, then let them fall and relax.

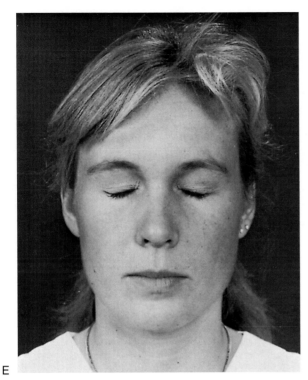
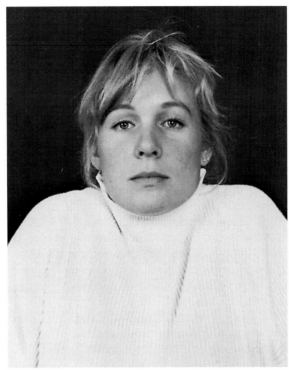

E   F

FIG. 1. (*Continued.*)

positions the joints at the end of normal range, then imparts a rapid, low-amplitude thrust. It is a treatment that is contraindicated in patients with underlying arthritis or vertebral artery disease: cerebrovascular events and death have been reported following manipulation (20). According to two review articles (10,23) there are four randomized clinical studies on manipulation for tension-type headache. Manipulation seems to be better than no treatment, some types of mobilization, and/or ice treatment (4). The effect of cervical manipulation seemed to be equivalent to amitriptyline but had a greater durability and fewer side effects (4).

BALANCE DISORDERS AND OCULOMOTOR DISTURBANCES

Patients with tension-type headache often describe a feeling of unsteadiness when they move in crowded places (5). There might be an association between disequilibrium and the disturbances of oculomotor function observed in patients with tension-type headache consisting of reduction in saccadic velocity and decreases in the smooth pursuit velocity gain (6). It has been argued that the oculomotor abnormalities are caused by pathologic proprioceptive signals from the tense scalp and neck muscles (6). The neck proprioceptors are important for balancing the head and for regulating head movements (18), and connection may exist between neck receptors and the eyes. This connection may be responsible for the

dysregulation of the eye movements. Reported improvements of oculomotor disturbances and dizziness following physiotherapy may be related to a reduction in the abnormal muscle tension (6).

Treatment of the balance disorder associated with tension-type headache therefore includes physiotherapy techniques aimed at decreasing neck and cranial muscle spasm. The patient should be trained to focus his gaze on a stationary object when experiencing the symptoms of disequilibrium.

COMBINATION THERAPY

The form of physical therapy chosen depends on the presumed underlying etiology of the headache to be treated. A combination of active treatments such as relaxation and ergonomic instruction, and passive treatments such as massage, and TENS is often applied.

A standardized, combined treatment program has been evaluated in a randomized, controlled study comprising 58 patients with frequent episodic or chronic tension-type headache (13). The patients were randomized to either 8 weeks of standardized physiotherapy or to a similar observation period without treatment. The treatment group had a significant reduction in the number of days with headache from 17.7 days to 13 days during a 4-week period as well as a reduction of the pericranial tenderness compared with the control group. The effect varied considerably among the treated patients in correspondence with an uncontrolled study of 20 patients by Hammill et al. (9). The positive effect on frequency and intensity of the headache was maintained at a 12-month follow-up examination in the latter study.

CONCLUSION

Most of the described treatments used in patients with tension-type headache are not properly evaluated scientifically. It is apparent that it is very difficult to apply a placebo-controlled design methodology in nonpharmacologic treatment as physiotherapy. Most studies have only found a moderate effect on pain intensity and frequency, and as long as the underlying pathophysiology of tension-type headache is unknown, no specific treatment can yet be offered. However, it has been documented that relaxation training alone or combined with EMG biofeedback are effective and recommendable. Home-based exercise programs produce results that are comparable with or even superior to those of clinic-based treatments, and such therapy can therefore be a valuable part of a combined treatment program. Randomized, controlled studies of the therapeutic effects of various treatment modalities are therefore warranted.

REFERENCES

1. Bendtsen L, Jensen R, Jensen NK, Olesen J. Pressure-controlled palpation; a new technique which increases the reliability of manual palpation. *Cephalalgia* 1995;15:205–101.
2. Bernstein DA, Borkovec TD. *Progressive relaxation training.* Champaign, IL: Research Press, 1973.
3. Bogaards MC, Kuile MM. Treatment of current tension headache. A meta-analytic review. *Clin J Pain* 1994;10:174–190.
4. Boline PD, Kassak K, Bronfort G, Nelsen C, Andersen AV. Spinal manipulation vs. amitriptyline for the treatment of chronic tension-type headache. A randomized clincal trial. *J Manipulative Physiol Ther* 1995;18:148–154.
5. Carlsson J, Fahlcrantz A, Augustinsson L-E. Muscle tenderness in tension headache treated with acupuncture or physiotherapy. *Cephalalgia* 1990;10:131–141.
6. Carlsson J, Rosenhall J. Oculomotor disturbances in patients with tension headache treated with acupuncture or physiotherapy. *Cephalalgia* 1990;10:123–129.
7. Feldenkreis M. *Awareness through movement.* New York: Penguin Books, 1984.
8. Haddock CK, Rowan AB, Andrasik F, Wilson PG, Talcott GW, Stein RJ. Home-based behavioural treatments for chronic benign headache. A meta-analysis of controlled trials. *Cephalalgia* 1997;17:113–118.
9. Hammill JM, Cook TM, Rosecrance JC. Effectiveness of a physical therapy regimen in the treatment of tension-type headache. *Headache* 1996;36:149–153.
10. Hurwitz EL, Aker PD, Adams AH, Meeker WC, Shekelle PG. Manipulation and mobilazation of the cervical spine. A systematic review of the literature. *Spine* 1996;21:1746–1760.
11. Jacobson E. *Progressive relaxation,* 2nd ed. Chicago: University of Chicago Press, 1938:418–419.
12. Jensen K. Quantification of tenderness by palpation and use of a pressure algometer. *Adv Pain Res Ther* 1990;17:165–181.
13. Jensen R, Olesen J. Is there an effect of physiotherapy in tension-type headache? *Cephalalgia* 1996;158[Suppl 14]:152.
14. Jensen R, Rasmussen BK. Muscular disorders in tension-type headache. *Cephalalgia* 1996;16:97–103.
15. Kaada B, Torsteinbo O. Increase of plasma beta-endorphins in connective massage. *Gen Pharmacol* 1989;20:487–489.
16. Kidd RF, Nelson R. Musculoskeletal dysfunction of the neck in migraine and tension headache. *Headache* 1993;33:566–569.
17. Mensendieck BM. *The Mensendieck system of functional exercises.* Portland, ME: The Soutwork Anthoenssen, 1937.
18. Rosenhall U, Tjell C, Carlsson J. The effect of neck torsion on smooth pursuit eye movement in tension-type headache. *J Audiol Med* 1996;5: 130–140.
19. Rundcrantz B-L. Pain and discomfort in the musculoskeletel system among dentist [dissertation]. Lund: University of Lund, 1991.
20. Schellhas KP, Latchaw RE, Wendling LR, Gold LHA. Vertebrobasilar injuries following cervical manipulation. *JAMA* 1980;244:1450–1453.
21. ter Kuile MM, Spinhoven PH, Linssen AC. Responders and no responders to autogenic training and cognitive self-hypnosis: prediction of short- and long-term success in tension-type headache patients. *Headache* 1995;35:630–636.
22. Travell JG, Simons DG. *Myofascial pain and dysfunction. The trigger point manual.* Baltimore: Williams & Wilkins, 1983.
23. Vernon HT. The effectiveness of chiropractic manipulation in the treatment of headache: An exploration in the literature. *J Manipulative Physiol Ther* 1995;18:611–617.
24. Zwart JH. Neck mobility in different headache disorders. Headache 1997;37:6–11.

The Headaches, Second Edition,
edited by J. Olesen, P. Tfelt-Hansen, and K.M.A. Welch.
Lippincott Williams & Wilkins, Philadelphia © 2000.

Tension-Type Headache, Cluster Headache, and Miscellaneous Primary Headaches

CHAPTER 86

Oromandibular Treatment of Tension-Type Headache

Steven B. Graff-Radford and Heli Forssell

Much interest has been focused on the association between oromandibular dysfunction (OMD) and headache. Headache frequency has been shown to be about twice as high among patients with OMD as among the general population (11,14). Correlations between headache and signs and symptoms of OMD have been found both in children and adolescents (3,31) and in adults (4,15,23). Furthermore, correlations between headache and oral parafunctional habits such as tooth grinding and clenching have been described in many studies (2,15,30). Successful treatment of headache with OMD treatments further enhances the association between OMD and headache. This chapter describes oromandibular treatment methods and discusses their role in the treatment of tension-type headache.

MANAGEMENT OF OMD

Oromandibular dysfunction is a collective term embracing a number of clinical problems that involve the masticatory musculature, the temporomandibular joint and related structures. The most frequent presenting symptom is pain, usually localized in the muscles of mastication, the preauricular area, or the temporomandibular joint. The pain is characteristically aggravated by chewing or other jaw functions. Additional characteristics are

limited or asymmetric jaw movements as well as joint noise on movement or locking of jaw on opening.

A number of hypotheses about the prime cause of OMD have been suggested, but scientific evidence is lacking to support any specifically. Muscle hyperactivity, trauma, emotional stress, and malocclusion dominate the literature, but a host of predisposing, initiating, and perpetuating factors have been proposed. No consensus has been reached on the degree to which any of these factors plays a part, but there is general acceptance that multiple factors influence the evolution and progression of these disorders.

Because there are thought to be several etiologic factors involved in OMD, it is to be expected that there are several different therapeutic approaches (Table 1). Unfortunately, most of the literature concerning the treatment methods of OMD consists of uncontrolled observations, and less than 5% of treatment studies have been controlled clinical trials (1). Even these are sometimes compromised by weaknesses in their design. Thus, only general conclusions can be drawn regarding treatment effectiveness. When the effects of different treatments are compared, the results seldom reveal major advantages of one method over another. Elimination of the cause would be the most effective treatment. However, if the cause cannot be identified, symptomatic treatment has to be provided. The goals of treatment are to decrease pain, to decrease adverse loading, and to restore normal function. Because the signs and symptoms of OMD can be transient and self-limiting, simple and reversible treatments have to be preferred over complicated and irreversible procedures.

S. B. Graff-Radford: Department of Diagnostic Sciences, U.C.L.A., and The Pain Center, Cedars-Sinai Medical Center, Los Angeles, California 90048.

H. Forssell: Department of Oral Surgery, Turku University, and Department of Oral Diseases, Turku University Central Hospital, SF-20520 Turku, Finland.

TABLE 1. *Different treatment methods of oromandibular dysfunction*

Patient education
Behavior modification
Physical therapy
Biofeedback/relaxation therapy
Acupuncture
Drug therapy
Occlusal appliances
Occlusal therapy
Temporomandibular joint surgery

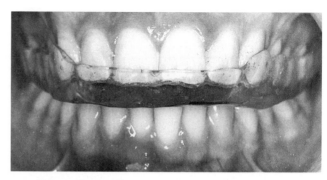

FIG. 1. Full-coverage maxillary stabilization splint.

Patient education and home care constitute the backbone of treatment for OMD. The home care program includes instruction on what can be chewed and behavior modification addressing unconscious postural, clenching, or grinding habits. In an uncontrolled study by Graff-Radford et al. (9) of 25 myofascial headache patients, success was described as 90% reduction of pain at the end of treatment and at 12 months posttreatment. This study suggested that altering perpetuating factors such as posture, body mechanics, and stress was the reason for relief. Different types of physical therapy might also benefit OMD patients, although few data are available to document these. Some evidence is available about the effectiveness of biofeedback/relaxation therapy and acupuncture for OMD symptoms.

Pharmacologic intervention for OMD also may be useful. Antiinflammatories are the most common drugs used and are very helpful in managing symptoms of inflammation associated with myositis and joint synovitis. Tricyclic antidepressants have shown potential in the treatment of nocturnal bruxism and in the treatment of chronic pain problems in general.

Occlusal splint therapy is a physical medicine technique routinely used in management of OMD. Stabilization appliances are flat splints that cover all of the mandibular or maxillary teeth. The occlusal surface of the splint is adjusted to provide a stable mandibular posture by creating even posterior contacts and anterior guidance of lateral and protrusive excursions of the mandible (Fig. 1). It has been proposed that the effects seen with this technique are due to alteration of occlusal disharmony, through an indirect effect on the muscles, or are related to affecting bruxism. Although there is much clinical evidence supporting the effects of appliance treatment, the real reason it may be working is unknown.

Occlusal therapy in the treatment of OMD is controversial. This can include occlusal adjustment to create stable occlusion, restorative dental treatment, including treatment with partial or complete removable dentures, as well as orthodontic therapy. There is some consensus that occlusal therapy should be considered when the existing occlusal support is not adequate or the occlusion is not stable and when these factors directly relate to symptom formation (18). On the individual level, however, it is difficult to determine the causal relationship of occlusion and pain; therefore, treatment aimed at occlusal restoration must be considered with care.

Temporomandibular joint surgery is considered to be a useful treatment for articular disorders in cases when nonsurgical treatment methods have failed or in other specifically indicated situations. The need for surgical treatment is, however, not great.

OROMANDIBULAR TREATMENT FOR HEADACHE

Nonsurgical Treatment

In an uncontrolled study, 33 OMD patients were treated with occlusal splint therapy (11). Following 4 weeks of therapy, 64% of patients reported a decrease in the number of weekly headaches, 30% showing a complete remission of headache. Patients with a high frequency of headaches (four or more per week) seemed to respond more favorably to occlusal splint therapy.

In another uncontrolled study with OMD patients, changes in headache were followed 1 year after the start of OMD treatment (16). The treatment consisted of occlusal splints, therapeutic exercises for masticatory muscles, or occlusal adjustment, most often combinations of these measures. Seventy percent of these patients reported less frequent headaches than 1 year earlier. Forty percent reported less severe head pain. The results achieved seemed to be lasting at a 2.5-year follow-up examination (17). These studies, however, did not control for the placebo effect, and the definition for the type of headache being treated was not clearly stated. Furthermore, one cannot know what part of the treatment was actually necessary.

Vallon and co-workers (27–29) assessed the effects of occlusal adjustment on headache in OMD patients. Fifty patients were randomly assigned to a treatment group and a control group receiving only counseling. The treatment outcome was evaluated after 1, 3, and 6 months and 2 years by a blinded examiner. No significant differences were found at follow-ups regarding changes in frequency of headache. The problem with the study was the great dropout rate of patients from the original treatment groups, ranging from 20% at the 3-month follow-up to 66% at 2 years.

Because OMD is believed to have a multifactorial etiology, it is assumed that the best treatment results are achieved by using several different treatment methods to eliminate as many predisposing and perpetuating factors as possible. This assumption was addressed in a randomized controlled study comparing the effects of occlusal equilibration and other forms of OMD therapy in patients with signs and symptoms of OMD, including headache (32). The OMD therapy consisted of occlusal splints as well as muscle exercises and minor occlusal adjustment in some cases, whereas the comparison group received only occlusal equilibration therapy. The reduction in the symptoms of OMD and in the frequency and intensity of headache was significantly greater in the combined therapy group versus the comparison group.

Some studies focusing on signs and symptoms attributable to OMD have been performed on general headache patients. In a series of studies, 100 recurrent headache patients, referred for neurologic examination, were invited for a functional examination of the stomatognathic system (23). In total, 55 patients displayed pain caused by OMD. In 51 patients the pain was determined to be of myogenous and in four of arthrogenous origin. The 55 patients were divided at random into two groups (24). One group was treated by the neurologist according to conventional headache treatment regimens, and the other group was treated with stabilization splints for 6 weeks and in some cases with physical therapy. In the OMD treatment group, headache frequency decreased in 56% of patients compared with 32% in the neurologic treatment group. There is also a reported significant difference in the reduction of headache intensity as well as in the symptomatic medication taken to control headache. Thus, the clinical result of OMD therapy exceeded the results of the neurologic treatment in patients in whom headache was assumed to be related to OMD. The confounding factor is that the OMD group had a much greater exposure to the treating clinician, which could in part account for the difference.

A randomized controlled trial by Forssell et al. (5) evaluated the effect of occlusal adjustment versus a mock adjustment on tension-type headache using a double-blind study design. The patient population was composed of 56 tension headache patients (20 of whom also had migraine, i.e. combination headache) from a neurologic clinic. Most of them reported subjective symptoms of OMD, and in all patients signs of OMD were registered. Patients were randomly assigned to active and placebo groups, and after a 4- to 8-month follow-up period a neurologist evaluated the treatment outcome. The headache frequency was reduced in 73% and the intensity in 50% of patients in the active treatment group and in 50% and

13% in the placebo group, respectively. Some of the patients from the placebo group having moderate to severe OMD symptoms were afterward treated with occlusal therapy (7). A significant reduction in headache frequency also was observed in these patients. Except for the possible confounder that the same clinician performed both treatments (active and placebo) unblinded, this study again supports the value of OMD treatment for tension-type headache associated with OMD signs and symptoms.

Contradictory results were reported by Quayle and co-workers (20) in an uncontrolled study of headache patients who were treated with soft occlusal splints for 6 weeks. Many patients with migraine type headache improved, but most patients suffering from tension headache failed to benefit from splint therapy. The small number of patients (n = 9) in the tension headache group may reduce the significance of the result.

In the double-blind trial by Karppinen et al. (10), 40 patients seeking treatment for chronic headache, neck, and shoulder pain received a routine battery of physical therapy. In addition, the patients were randomly allocated to the occlusal adjustment group and to a mock adjustment group. Patients were followed up at 6 weeks, 12 months, and 60 months. The short-term response to physical therapy was good in both groups. At 12 months, the effects of treatment began to subside in the mock adjustment group, but further improvement was evident in the real adjustment group. A statistically significant decrease in the occurrence of headache was observed in the real adjustment group compared with the mock adjustment group at 12 and 60 months.

Because several controlled clinical trials seem to suggest that OMD treatment can be effective for headache, the question arises whether there are some special features that could in practice help to single out patients whose headache is related to OMD from other headache patients. Reik and Hale (22) suggested that patients with continuous unilateral headache were patients with OMD. This was not supported by Schokker et al. (25), who found that headaches responsive to OMD treatment were mainly bilateral and showed only a tendency to be present permanently. In that study, patients with headaches linked to OMD showed a greater difference between passive and active mouth opening recorded before treatment. This is considered to be a sign of myogenous origin of OMD. Another study showed that patients who had reported pain while chewing responded more favorably in terms of headache reduction following OMD therapy (6). Pain while chewing is one of the most common subjective symptoms of OMD.

Surgical Treatment

Temporomandibular joint surgery is considered to be useful treatment for certain OMDs. Few studies have examined surgery and response to headache. Vallerand and Hall (26) reported on 50 patients diagnosed with internal temporomandibular joint derangements, myalgia, and headaches who had not responded to nonsurgical management. The surgical procedures they underwent included disc repositioning, repair of disc perforation, disc recontouring, lysis of adhesions, and discectomy. In the retrospective evaluation, the majority of patients reported decreases in headache in addition to decreases in joint pain and noise. The surgeons offer the explanation that the change in head pain is a secondary result of decreasing joint pain, which allowed the patients to cope better with other pains. In another study, Montgomery et al. (19) reported significant changes in temporomandibular joint, ear, neck, and shoulder pains, whereas headaches were less consistently changed following arthroscopy of the temporomandibular joint.

CONCLUSIONS

Treatment of OMD can often help the headache patients, and there is significant evidence that pain can be greatly reduced through nonpharmacologic means. History taking and physical examination of the masticatory system should be parts of the comprehensive evaluation of the headache problem. When OMD is diagnosed, especially with muscular involvement (8,12,13), the patient should receive appropriate OMD treatment for the headache symptom. Due to the large number of nonpatients who display signs and symptoms of OMD but have no pain, the actual role in headache pathogenesis must be carefully reviewed (21). Caution should be taken not to overtreat patients, especially with irreversible treatments, for example, occlusal equilibration or orthodontics. At this time the relationship between occlusion and headache is unclear. Patients are best served by selecting a treatment plan that is tailored toward their presentation rather than presuming that one factor is responsible for the pain.

REFERENCES

1. Antczak-Bouckoms A. Epidemiology of research for temporomandibular disorders. *J Orofacial Pain* 1995;9:226–234.
2. Berlin R, Dessner L. Bruxism and chronic headache. *Lancet* 1960;2:289–291.
3. Egermark-Eriksson I. Mandibular dysfunction in children and individuals with dual bite. *Swed Dent J* 1982;74:118,1121.
4. Forssell H, Kangasniemi P. Correlation of the frequency and intensity of headache to mandibular dysfunction in headache patients. *Proc Finn Dent Soc* 1984;80:223–236.
5. Forssell H, Kirveskari P, Kangasniemi P. Changes in headache after treatment of mandibular dysfunction. *Cephalalgia* 1985;5:229–236.
6. Forssell H, Kirveskari P, Kangasniemi P. Distinguishing between headaches responsive and irresponsive to treatment of mandibular dysfunction. *Proc Finn Dent Soc* 1986;82:219–222.
7. Forssell H, Kirveskari P, Kangasniemi P. Response to occlusal treatment in headache patients previously treated by mock occlusal adjustment. *Acta Odontol Scand* 1987;45:77–80.
8. Graff-Radford SB. Oromandibular disorders and headache. A critical appraisal. *Neurol Clin* 1990;8:929–945.
9. Graff-Radford SB, Reeves JL, Jaeger B. Management of head and neck pain: the effectiveness of altering perpetuating factors in myofascial pain. *Headache* 1987;27:186–190.
10. Karppinen K, Eklund S, Suoninen E, Eskelin M, Kirveskari P. Adjustment of dental occlusion in treatment of chronic cervicobrachial pain and headache. *J Oral Rehabil* (in press)
11. Kemper JT, Okeson JP. Craniomandibular disorders and headaches. *J Prosthet Dent* 1998;49:702–705.
12. Kreisberg MK. Headache as a symptom of craniomandibular disorders II: management. *J Craniomand Pract* 1986;4:219–228.
13. Lous I, Olesen J. Evaluation of pericranial tenderness and oral function in patients with common migraine, muscle contraction headache and combination headache. *Pain* 1982;12:385–393.
14. Magnusson T, Carlsson GE. Comparison between two groups of patients in respect of headache and mandibular dysfunction. *Swed Dent J* 1978;2:85–92.
15. Magnusson T, Carlsson GE. Recurrent headaches in relation to temporomandibular joint pain-dysfunction. *Acta Odontol Scand* 1978;36:333–338.
16. Magnusson T, Carlsson GE. Changes in recurrent headache and mandibular dysfunction after various types of dental treatment. *Acta Odontol Scand* 1980;38:311–320.
17. Magnusson T, Carlsson GE. A 2½-year follow-up of changes in headache and mandibular dysfunction after stomatognathic treatment. *J Prosthet Dent* 1983;49:398–402.
18. McNeill C, ed. Craniomandibular disorders. *Guidelines for evaluation, diagnosis, and management.* Chicago: Quintessence Publishers, 1990.
19. Montgomery MT, Van Sickels JE, Harms SE, Thrash WJ. Arthroscopic TMJ surgery: effects on signs, symptoms, and disc position. *J Oral Maxillofac Surg* 1989;47:1263–1271.
20. Quayle AA, Gray RJM, Metcalfe RJ, Guthrie E, Wastell D. Soft occlusal splint therapy in the treatment of migraine and other headaches. *J Dent* 1990;18:123–129.
21. Reik L Jr. Unnecessary dental treatment of headache patients for temporomandibular joint disorders. *Headache* 1985;25:246–248.
22. Reik L Jr, Hale M. The temporomandibular joint pain-dysfunction syndrome: a frequent cause of headache. *Headache* 1981;21:111–116.
23. Schokker RP, Hansson TL, Ansink BJJ. Craniomandibular disorders in headache patients. *J Craniomandib Disord Facial Oral Pain* 1989;3:71–74.
24. Schokker RP, Hansson TL, Ansink BJJ. The results of treatment of the masticatory system of chronic headache patients. *J Craniomandib Disord Facial Oral Pain* 1990;4:126–130.
25. Schokker RP, Hansson TL, Ansink BJJ. Differences in headache patients regarding their response to treatment of the masticatory system. *J Craniomandib Disord Facial Oral Pain* 1990;4:228–232.
26. Vallerand WP, Hall MB. Improvement in myofascial pain and headaches following TMJ surgery. *J Craniomandib Disord Facial Oral Pain* 1991;5:197–204.
27. Vallon D, Ekberg EC, Nilner M, Kopp S. Short-term effect of occlusal adjustment on craniomandibular disorders including headaches. *Acta Odontol Scand* 1991;49:89–96.
28. Vallon D, Ekberg EC, Nilner M, Kopp S. Occlusal adjustment in patients with craniomandibular disorders including headaches. A 3- and 6-month follow-up. *Acta Odontol Scand* 1995;53:55–9.
29. Vallon D, Nilner M. A longitudinal follow-up of the effects of occlusal adjustment in patients with craniomandibular disorders. *Swed Dent J* 1997;21:85–91.
30. Villarosa GA, Moss RA. Oral behavioral patterns as factors contributing to the development of head and facial pain. *J Prosthet Dent* 1985;54:427–430.
31. Wänman A, Agerberg G. Headache and dysfunction of the masticatory system in adolescent. *Cephalalgia* 1986;6:247–255.
32. Wenneberg B, Nyström T, Carlsson G. Occlusal equilibration and other stomatognathic treatment in patients with mandibular dysfunction and headache. *J Prosthet Dent* 1988;59:478–483.

The Headaches, Second Edition,
edited by J. Olesen, P. Tfelt-Hansen, and K.M.A. Welch.
Lippincott Williams & Wilkins, Philadelphia © 2000.

Tension-Type Headache, Cluster Headache, and Miscellaneous Primary Headaches

CHAPTER 87

Acute Pharmacotherapy of Tension-Type Headache

Ninan T. Mathew and Jean Schoenen

This chapter discusses the treatment of individual attacks of headache in patients with episodic and chronic tension-type headache (TTH). Most headache episodes in these patients are mild to moderate. Patients with mild TTH rarely consult the physician and can manage by using simple analgesics. These patients may consult the physician when the frequency, severity, and duration of the headache increase. Often, such worsening of headache is associated with stress, anxiety, and depression and may be accompanied by pericranial muscle tenderness and spasm. These factors operate in a vicious cycle, and the physician's task is to break this cycle.

METHODOLOGIC CONSIDERATIONS IN CLINICAL STUDIES IN THE ACUTE TREATMENT OF TENSION-TYPE HEADACHE

Several parameters, including visual analog scales (VAS), verbal rating scales (VRS), and global ratings, have been studied to assess the pain relief effected by analgesics (8,17,20,38,39). Global rating was reported to be a sensitive parameter, and this finding was confirmed (7,22). Global rating takes into account overall patient acceptability, including taste, ease of use, side effects, and similar factors, in addition to assessing pain relief. Patient's preference after the intake of two or more different drugs has been a less satisfactory method, because the results depend on the patient's memory of the degree

of effectiveness of a previous medication as well as personal biases about taste and color (18). A strong correlation was found between visual analog pain scales, a verbal pain scale, and verbal pain relief scale (24). A combination of scales that includes global rating gives more reliable assessment of pain relief.

Guidelines for trials of drug treatments for TTH published by the International Headache Society (IHS) Committee on clinical trials (19) recommends VRS or VAS combined with a simple verbal scale for global evaluation efficacy measures.

Patient compliance may become a problem in studies using simple analgesics for the treatment in TTH for the following reasons: (a) Most TTHs are mild and patients therefore may not consider it worthwhile to spend the necessary time and effort for the study. (b) Most patients would have already taken analgesics such as aspirin and may not have confidence in test medications that are not known to be far superior to aspirin. (c) Patients chosen from headache clinics and specialty treatment centers may be more resistant to simple analgesics. Population-based studies are recommended for TTH.

Many controlled studies of *simple analgesics* and *non-steroidal anti-inflammatory drugs* (NSAIDs) have been performed in TTH, using the headache attack as a model for acute pain. Several studies done in recent years fulfill the standards recommended for drug trials in TTH by the IHS (19). From these studies, one may conclude that NSAIDs are the drugs of first choice. The following is a review of some of the previous studies and recent randomized, controlled trials comparing various NSAIDs and simple analgesics. Although differences between

N. T. Mathew: Houston Headache Clinic, Houston, Texas 77004.
J. Schoenen: University Department of Neurology, CHR, Citadelle, and University of Liège, B-4000 Liège, Belgium.

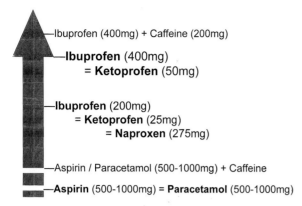

—Ibuprofen (400mg) + Caffeine (200mg)

—Ibuprofen (400mg) = Ketoprofen (50mg)

—Ibuprofen (200mg) = Ketoprofen (25mg) = Naproxen (275mg)

—Aspirin / Paracetamol (500-1000mg) + Caffeine

—Aspirin (500-1000mg) = Paracetamol (500-1000mg)

FIG. 1. Tension-type headache: Acute pharmacotherapy.

drugs may be small or variable, a hierarchical classification of compounds emerges when efficacy data are considered (Fig. 1).

SIMPLE ANALGESICS

Aspirin

Aspirin is the most commonly used analgesic for the acute treatment of TTH. Self-medication with aspirin is universally practiced. The number of studies concerning aspirin in the treatment of TTH is small; one study (28) reported no relief from doses smaller than 650 mg of aspirin, and another (30) found 650 and 1,600 mg of aspirin superior to placebo.

Dose–response curves for aspirin have been established for headache (14,35). These studies indicated 1,000 mg aspirin to be superior to 650 mg. Most studies done on the analgesic effect of aspirin, however, used 650 mg as a standard dose in clinical research. A comparison of the time courses of pain relief after taking 648 mg of solid aspirin and 648 mg of effervescent aspirin was done by using a modified double-dummy technique with solid and effervescent placebo (22). Aspirin had significantly better efficacy than placebo; however, no statistically significant difference was found between solid and effervescent aspirin. Despite high statistical significance in pain scales, the effect was reported as "poor" on the global scale.

Acetaminophen

Compared with placebo, 650 mg and 1,000 mg of acetaminophen were reported to have superior efficacy but were indistinguishable from the effects of similar doses of aspirin (30). Based on this study and the fact that the gastric side-effect profile of acetaminophen is much better, acetaminophen may be a better drug than aspirin for mild to moderate TTH. In most trials, however, the simple analgesics were found to have inferior results compared with the classic antirheumatic NSAIDs.

NONSTEROIDAL ANTIINFLAMMATORY DRUGS (NSAIDS)

Ibuprofen

In a controlled double-blind, crossover trial of ibuprofen (Motrin), aspirin, and placebo that included 50 outpatients with TTH, ibuprofen was repoorted to be as effective as aspirin in the relief of pain (31). Neither aspirin nor ibuprofen produced severe or incapacitating side effects. Curiously, no statistical data were reported, nor was there any mention of the details of the scoring system for headache. Therefore, this study cannot be considered adequately performed.

Two fairly well-documented trials are reviewed here. One trial (11) reported that 108 patients with muscle-contraction headache (done before the IHS classification) completed a double-blind, randomized, parallel trial in which they took either ibuprofen 400 mg, ibuprofen 800 mg, aspirin 650 mg, or placebo for four successive headaches. Acetaminophen was allowed as a rescue analgesic. The intensity of headache pain was recorded pretreatment and again 3 hours posttreatment. A pain intensity difference (PID) score was calculated from the difference. Patients on ibuprofen (both doses) and aspirin had significantly lower pain scores and higher PID scores at 3-hour follow-up than did patients on placebo. Physician's global assessment indicated that both doses of ibuprofen were significantly superior to placebo; aspirin was not. The highest number of side effects occurred with aspirin (26 complaints), followed by placebo (15), ibuprofen 400 mg (4), and ibuprofen 800 mg (3); all were minor. These results suggest that for the treatment of TTH ibuprofen is significantly more effective than placebo and at least as effective as aspirin.

Another double-blind, randomized, placebo-controlled trial (33) determined the onset of action of ibuprofen 400 mg in the treatment of TTH. Headache pain intensity was evaluated on a VAS, and pain relief was measured on a categoric scale 15, 30, 45, 60, 90, and 120 minutes after a single 400-mg dose of ibuprofen or placebo. Efficacy was detected within 15 min on the pain intensity rating scale ($p < .05$) and within 30 minutes and at all subsequent time points on both the pain intensity and pain relief rating scales ($p < .001$). These results indicate an early onset of action of ibuprofen 400 mg in the treatment of tension-type headache.

Recent two studies using the IHS guidelines showed ibuprofen 400 (or 800) mg to be significantly more effective than placebo or paracetamol 1,000 mg (32). Even at a low dose of 200 mg, ibuprofen was superior to aspirin 500 mg (29).

Naproxen Sodium

Naproxen sodium is the sodium salt of naproxen, a phenylalkanoic acid with potent analgesic, anti-inflammatory, and antipyretic properties. Naproxen sodium is more rapidly absorbed and has a more rapid onset of pain relief than naproxen. Rapid absorption and peak plasma levels within 1 hour are desirable qualities for fast relief of headache.

A multicenter, randomized, double-blind, three-way parallel study of naproxen sodium was reported in 1987 (27). The purpose of the study was to compare the efficacy and safety of naproxen sodium (550 mg), acetaminophen (650 mg), and placebo in the treatment of TTH. It included 149 patients, each of whom was treated for one episode of moderate to severe headache with the test medication. The intensity of the headache pain was recorded on 10-cm VAS by patients for up to 12 hours after treatment with the study medication. In addition, the degree of pain relief was recorded in a similar manner. Mean pain intensities, percentage of changes in mean pain intensities, PIDs, and the sum of these differences (SPIDs) were calculated. From the data collected in 124 patients eligible for efficacy analysis, naproxen sodium was shown to provide a significantly greater percentage change in mean pain intensity compared with acetaminophen ($p < 0.01$) or placebo ($p < 0.001$). Mean PID and SPID scores also showed naproxen sodium to be significantly more effective in relieving pain than acetaminophen ($p < 0.02$) or placebo ($p < 0.001$). Mean pain relief scores and calculated total pain relief scores correlated well with the reduction in pain intensity. During the trial, 13 patients reported side effects that included nausea, dizziness, and drowsiness. None of the side effects was considered clinically significant. The results of this study demonstrated naproxen sodium to be a well-tolerated analgesic that provided statistically significantly superior analgesia compared to acetaminophen or placebo in the treatment of tension-type headaches.

Naproxen sodium provided earlier and better pain relief than aspirin in various pain states, including headache, and its effect was consistent over time (35). In the randomized double-blind studies, naproxen sodium was shown to produce a highly significant ($p < 0.001$) greater PID and SPID than aspirin and placebo in patients with musculoskeletal pain, miscellaneous pain (toothache, muscle cramp, etc.), and TTH.

COMPARATIVE CLINICAL TRIALS OF NSAIDS

Table 1 shows recently conducted randomized, controlled trials. Five comparative trials of ketoprofen have been published in recent years (9,21,25,36,37). These studies indicate that ketoprofen 50 mg is more effective than ibuprofen 200 mg or paracetamol 1,000 mg, whereas ketoprofen 25 mg is not clearly superior to the latter. The efficacy of ketoprofen 12.5 mg did not significantly exceed that of placebo in one study, nor did Extra-Strength Tylenol. Naproxen 550 mg provided superior analgesia compared with paracetamol or placebo,

whereas the 220-mg dose was equally effective as ibuprofen 200 mg (2). Other NSAIDs such as ketoralac (16), diclofenac, or indomethacin are also effective but less well studied.

The therapeutic efficacy of NSAIDs in TTH, though undisputable, has to be put in perspective. For instance, the low proportion of patients becoming pain-free 2 hours after dosing in most trials underscores the relative insufficiency of these drugs: 32% for ketoprofen 50 mg, 28% for the 25 mg dose; 17–22% for paracetamol 1000 mg; 17% for placebo. There is thus clearly room for better acute treatments of TTH and a need for prophylactic therapy for frequent TTH attacks.

THERAPEUTIC USE

Aspirin, acetaminophen, ibuprofen, naproxen and ketoprofen are usually bought without a physician's prescription. Many patients do not take an adequate dosage and hence do not get the expected benefit. The recommended doses for the commonly used analgesics for the acute treatment of tension-type headache are given in Table 2.

At present time, ibuprofen (800 mg) can probably be considered the first choice for acute TTH, followed by naproxen sodium (825 mg) because of the all-over better gastrointestinal tolerability (Fig. 1). Several surveys indeed have shown that ibuprofen is associated with the lowest risk of gastrointestinal bleeding or perforation [odds ratio (OR) 2.9], whereas ketoprofen carries a much higher risk (OR 23.7), with naproxen occupying an intermediate position (OR 9.1) (12,23). It remains to be determined whether the newer COX-2 inhibitors, which are assumed to have a lower gastrointestinal toxicity, are also effective as analgesics in TTH.

COMBINATION ANALGESICS AND SEDATIVE ANALGESIC COMBINATIONS

Combination analgesics and sedatives and tranquilizers/analgesic combinations may have a place in the acute treatment of TTH. Just as adding caffeine to an analgesic can enhance its effect, the same can occur when two analgesics with different mechanisms of action are combined. The use of a combination also may reduce the risk of side effects, because lower doses of each medication can be used. The patient's anxiety may be alleviated by the addition of a barbiturate or a benzodiazepine to the regimen, and nausea decreased by the addition of an antiemetic. Compliance with therapy may be encouraged when the patient no longer needs to take several different drugs (3).

Tranquilizers with muscle-relaxant or sedative qualities alone rarely control the discomfort of severe or persistent headache. The important fact is that we are treating not only the perception of pain but also the reaction

TABLE 1. *Recent trials of acute pharmacotherapy in episodic TTH*

Study of objective	Design	Results	Authors (reference no.)
Ibuprofen vs paracetamol	RCT, parallel Ibuprofen 400 mg Paracetamol 1000 mg Placebo	Ibu>para>placebo	Schachtel et al, 1996 (32)
Ketoprofen vs ibuprofen vs naproxen	RCT, parallel Ketoprofen 25 mg Ketoprofen 12.5 mg Ibuprofen 200 mg Naproxen 275 mg	Equal efficacy	Lange and Lentz, 1995 (21)
Ketoprofen vs ibuprofen	RCT, parallel, home-monitored (electr. diary) Ketoprofen 50 mg Ketoprofen 25 mg Ibuprofen 200 mg Placebo	Keto50 = keto25> Ibu200>placebo	Vangerven et al, 1996 (37)
Ketoprofen vs paracetamol	RCT, cross-over Ketoprofen 50 mg Ketoprofen 25 mg Paracetamol 500 mg Paracetamol 1000 mg placebo Placebo	Keto50>placebo Keto50>para Plac< keto25 = Para<keto50	Dahlöf and Jacobs, 1996 (9)
Ketoprofen vs paracetamol	RCT, parallel Ketoprofen 25 mg Paracetamol 1,000 mg Placebo	Keto25 = para>placebo	Steiner and Lange, 1998 (36)
Ketoprofen vs ES Tylenol	RCT, parallel Ketoprofen 25 mg Ketoprofen 12.5 mg ES Tylenol 1,000 mg placebo	Keto25>keto12.5 ES Tylenol = placebo	Mehlisch et al., 1997 (25)
Naproxen sodium vs ibuprofen	RCT, parallel Naproxen 220 mg Ibuprofen 200 mg	Napro = ibu	Autret et al., 1997 (2)
Caffeine as adjuvant	RCT, crossover (6 studies) Para 1,000 + cafl 30 Para + asp500 + cafl 30 Paracetamol 1,000 mg Placebo	1 = 2>3>4	Migliardi et al., 1994 (26)
Caffeine as adjuvant	RCT, parallel Ibu 400 + caf 200 Ibu 400 Caf 200 Placebo	1>2>3 = 4	Diamond et al., 1997 (10)

TTH, tension-type headache; Asp, aspirin; caf, caffeine; ibu, ibuprofen; para, paracetamol; RCT, randomized controlled trial

to pain. Usually, the combination of an analgesic and a tranquilizer with muscle-relaxant or sedative properties provides effective symptomatic treatment of TTH. Many such drug combinations are on the market (Table 3).

The main drawbacks of the combination analgesics are (a) drug dependency and (b) analgesic rebound headache. Therefore, strict monitoring of the intake of these drugs is essential. The number of tablets or capsules taken in a month can be limited by prescribing relatively low doses with only one refill. Table 3 indicates the limits and the number of tablets that can be used.

Controlled Trials

Few published reports are available that use combination analgesics in acute TTH. A single-dose, placebo-controlled study to assess the effectiveness of adding a muscle relaxant to a compound analgesic in the treatment of TTH concluded that such a combination is complementary, with an analgesic for pain relief and an antianxiety agent to relieve the psychic tension (1). A comparison of a combination of meprobamate and aspirin with a butalbital-aspirin-phenacetin combination in 214 patients with TTH found the combinations to be equally effective,

TABLE 2. *Recommended dose of analgesics and NSAIDS in the acute treatment of tension-type headache*

Medication	Initial dose (mg)	Repeat dose in 1–2 h (mg)
Aspirin (325 tablets)	975	975
Acetaminophen	1,000	1,000
Ibuprofen	800	400
Naproxen sodium	825	275
Ketoprofen	75	50
Ketorolac oral	20	10
Ketorolac intermuscular	60	
Indomethacin suppository	50	

NSAIDs, nonsteroidal antinflammatory drugs.

but the latter had significantly more side effects, particularly of the central nervous system (13).

A multicenter double-blind, randomized clinical study comparing the efficacy of Micrainin (meprobamate-acetylsalicylic acid) and aspirin (acetylsalicylic acid) in the treatment of tension-type headache was conducted (14). Each patient treated one episode of moderate to severe TTH and scored the effects for head pain, activity impairment, tension (tense/uptight feeling), muscle stiffness, and overall relief using a VRS and a visual analogue (linear) scale (VAS). In general, overall agreements occurred between the two rating scales. Patient and physician global evaluations also concurred and supported the conclusion that Micrainin was significantly more effective than aspirin in relieving the symptom complex of TTH. Treatment emergent signs and symptoms occurred infrequently in each treatment group; these effects were not serious, however, and were of short duration without sequelae.

In some patients, the combination of analgesics with caffeine, sedatives, or tranquilizers may be more effective than simple analgesics or NSAIDs, but in many cases this impression comes from too low a dosage of the latter. It has been proven, nonetheless, in controlled trials that the adjunction of caffeine (130 or 200 mg) significantly increases the efficacy of simple analgesics (26) and of ibuprofen (10) (see Table 2). Whenever possible, combination analgesics for TTH should be avoided because of the risk of dependency, abuse, and chronification of the headache (see chapter 115).

Muscle Relaxants

A peripherally acting muscle relaxant by itself has not been shown to have any significant effect in acute TTH; however, centrally acting agents like tizanidine may have some benefit as a prophylactic agent in chronic tension-type headache (CTH). This class of drugs is discussed in detail in the next chapter.

OTHER AGENTS

Topical applications on the forehead of Tiger balm (33) and peppermint oil (15) also were superior to placebo in TTH treatment and they were not significantly different from paracetamol.

5-HT₁ Agonists

Brennum and associates (4) showed that sumatriptan has a significant effect in the symptomatic treatment of CTH, whereas it has no clinically relevant effect in the treatment of episodic TTH (5). It also has been shown that migraineurs with TTH respond significantly to sumatriptan, the response being almost equal to that of the response in migraine (6). So it appears that symptomatically CTH and TTH in migraineurs respond to sumatriptan differently from those who have episodic TTH. Further studies are warranted.

CONCLUSION

In conclusion, the mainstay in the acute treatment of tension-type headache is simple analgesics and NSAIDs.

TABLE 3. *Combination analgesics for acute tension-type headache*

Combination	Individual attack	Monthly limit
Aspirin 325 mg Caffeine 40 mg Butalbital 50 mg	1 or 2 tablets or capsules immediately; maximum 6 per attack	10 events, or 24 tablets or capsules
Acetaminophen 325 mg Caffeine 40 mg Butalbital 50 mg	1 or 2 tablets or capsules immediately; maximum 6 per attack	10 events, or 24 tablets or capsules
Aspirin 325 mg Caffeine 40 mg Butalbital 50 mg Codeine 30 mg	1 or 2 capsules immediately; maximum 6 per attack	8 events, or 16 capsules
Acetaminophen 325 g Isometheptene 65 mg Dichloralphenazone 100 mg	2 capsules immediately; maximum 6 per attack	12 events, or 40 capsules

Centrally and peripherally acting muscle relaxants have little place in the acute treatment of TTH, although they may have some prophylactic effect. Combination medications of analgesics and tranquilizers or sedatives are effective for symptomatic relief but are plagued with the potential of habituation and subsequent analgesic rebound headache phenomenon.

REFERENCES

1. Atkinson D. A single dose placebo-controlled study to assess the effectiveness of adding a muscle relaxant to a compound analgesic in the treatment of tension headaches. *J Intern Med* 1979;7:560–565.
2. Autret A, Unger PH, EURAXI group, Lesaichot JL. Naproxen sodium versus ibuprofen in episodic tension headache. *Cephalalgia* 1997;17:446.
3. Beaver WT. Combination analgesics. *Am J Med* 1984;77:38–53.
4. Brennum JK, Kjeldesen M, Olesen J. The 5-HT$_1$-like agonist sumatriptan has a significant effect on chronic tension-type headache. *Cephalalgia* 1992;12:375–379.
5. Brennum J, Brinck T, Schriver L, et al. Sumatriptan has no clinical relevant effect in the treatment of episodic tension-type headache. *Eur J Neurol* 1996;3:223–228.
6. Cady RK, Gutterman D, Saiers JA, Beach ME. Responsiveness of non-IHS migraine and tension-type headache to sumatriptan. *Cephalalgia* 1997;17:588–590.
7. Calimlim JF, Wardell WM, Davis HT, Lasagna L, Gilles AJ. Analgesic efficacy of an orally administered combination of pentazocine and aspirin. *Clin Pharmacol Ther* 1977;21:34–43.
8. Carisson AM. Assessment of chronic pain. 1. Aspects of the reliability and validity of the visual analogue scale. *Pain* 1983;16:97–101.
9. Dahlöf CGH, Jacobs LD. Ketoprofen, paracetamol and placebo in the treatment of episodic tension-type headache. *Cephalalgia* 1996;16:117–123.
10. Diamond S, Freitag FG, Balm TK, Berry DA. The use of a combination agent of ibuprofen and caffeine in the treatment of episodic tension-type headache. *Cephalalgia* 1997;17:446.
11. Diamond S. Ibuprofen versus aspirin and placebo in the treatment of muscle contraction headache. *Headache* 1983;23:206–210.
12. Garcia Rodriguez LA, Jack H. Risk of upper gastrointestinal bleeding and perforation associated with individual non-steroidal anti-inflammatory drugs. *Lancet* 1994;343:769–772.
13. Glassman JM, Soyka JP. Muscle contraction (tension) headache; a double blind study comparing the efficacy and safety of meprobamate-aspirin with butalbital-aspirin-phenacetin-caffeine. *Current Therapeutic Research* 1980;28:904–909.
14. Glassman JM, Soyka JP, Pullack M. Treatment of muscle contraction headache Micrainin vs aspirin. *Headache* 1982;22:101–109.
15. Göbel H, Heinze A, Dworschak M, Stolze H, Lurch A. Oleum menthae piperitae significantly reduces the symptoms of tension-type headache and its efficacy does not differ from that of acetaminophen. *Cephalalgia* 1997;17:446.
16. Harden NR, Carter TD, Gilman CS, Gross AJ, Peter JR. Ketorolac in acute headache management. *Headache* 1991;31:463–464.
17. Houde RW, Wallenstein SL, Beaver W. *Analgesics*. New York: Academic Press, 1963.
18. Huskisson EC. Simple analgesics for arthritis. *BMJ* 1974;4:196–200.
19. International Headache Society—Committee on Clinical Trials: Guidelines for trials of drug treatments in tension-type headache. *Cephalalgia* 1995;15:165–179.
20. Joyce CRB, Zutahl DW, Hrubes V, Mason RM. Comparison of fixed interval and visual analogue scales for rating chronic pain. *Eur J Clin Pharmacol* 1975;8:415–420.
21. Lange R, Lentz R. Comparison ketoprofen, ibuprofen and naproxen sodium in the treatment of tension-type headache. *Drugs Exp Clin Res* 1995;21:89–96.
22. Langemark M, Oleson J. Effervescent ASA versus solid ASA in the treatment of tension headache: a double blind, placebo controlled study: *Headache* 1987;27:90–95.
23. Langman MJS, Weil J, Wainwright P, et al. Risks of bleeding peptic ulcer associated with individual non-steroidal anti-inflammatory drugs. *Lancet* 1994;343:1075–1078.
24. Littman GS, Walker BR, Scheider BE. Reassessment of verbal and visual analog ratings in analgesic studies. *Clin Pharmacol Ther* 1985;38:16–23.
25. Mehlisch DR, Weaver M, Fladung B. Ketoprofen 12.5 and 25 mg, extra strength Tylenol 1000 mg and placebo for the treatment of patients with episodic tension-type headache. *Cephalalgia* 1997;17:274.
26. Migliardi JR, Armellino JJ, Friedman M, Gillings DB, Beaver WT. Caffeine as an analgesic adjuvant in tension headache. *Clin Pharmacol Ther* 1994;56:576–586.
27. Miller DS, Talbot CA, Simpson W, Korey A. A comparison of naproxen sodium, acetaminophen and placebo in the treatment of muscle contraction headache. *Headache* 1987;27:392–396.
28. Murray WJ. Evaluation of aspirin in treatment of headache: *Clin Pharmacol Ther* 1964;5:21–25.
29. Nebe J, Heier M, Diener HC. Low-dose ibuprofen in self-medication of mild to moderate headache: a comparison with acetylsalicylic acid and placebo. *Cephalalgia* 1995;15:531–535.
30. Peters BH, Fraim CJ, Masel BE. Comparison of 650 mg aspirin and 1,000 mg acetaminophen with each other, and with placebo in moderately severe headache. *Am J Med* 1983;74:36–42.
31. Ryan RE. Motrin—a new agent for symptomatic treatment of muscle contraction headache. *Headache* 1977;16:280–283.
32. Schachtel BP, Furey SA, Thoden WR. Nonprescription ibuprofen and acetaminophen in the treatment of tension-type headache. *J Clin Pharmacol 36* 1996;36:1120–1125.
33. Schachtel BP, Thoden WR. Onset of action of ibuprofen in the treatment of muscle contraction headache. *Headache* 1988;28:471–474.
34. Schattner P, Randerson D. Tiger balm as a treatment of tension-headache. A clinical trial in general practice. *Aust Fam Physician* 1996;25:216, 218, 220 passim.
35. Sevelius H, Segre M, Bursick R. Comparative analgesic effects of naproxen sodium, aspirin, placebo. *J Clin Pharm* 1980;20:480–488.
36. Steiner TJ, Lange R. Ketoprofen (25 mg) in the symptomatic treatment of episodic tension-type headache: double-blind placebo-controlled comparison with acetaminophen (1000 mg). *Cephalalgia* 1998;18:38–43.
37. Vangerven JMA, Schoemaker RC, Jacobs LD, et al. Self-medication of a single headache episode with ketoprofen, ibuprofen or placebo, home-monitored with an electronic patient diary. *Br J Clin Pharmacol* 1996;42:475–481.
38. Von Graffenried BV, Hill RC, Nuesch E. Headache as a model for assessing mild analgesic drugs. *J Clin Pharm* 1980;20:131–144.
39. Wallenstein SL, Heidrich III G, Kaiko R, Houde RW. Clinical evaluation of mild analgesics: the measurement of clinical pain. *Br J Clin Pharmacol* 1980;10:319s–327s.

The Headaches, Second Edition,
edited by J. Olesen, P. Tfelt-Hansen, and K.M.A. Welch.
Lippincott Williams & Wilkins, Philadelphia © 2000.

Tension-Type Headache, Cluster Headache, and Miscellaneous Primary Headaches

CHAPTER 88

Prophylactic Pharmacotherapy of Tension-Type Headache

Ninan T. Mathew and Lars Bendtsen

Chronic tension-type headache (CTH) is defined as occurring more than 180 days a year; CTH therefore has a great impact on the quality of life and productivity of the person who experiences it. Other factors that complicate this disorder are analgesic overuse and comorbidities, such as depression, anxiety, and neuroticism. Analgesic overuse makes chronic headaches resistant to prophylactic therapy.

Most patients with CTH require prophylactic approaches, usually a combination of pharmacotherapy, behavioral modalities, and some physical medicine. Stress management, including relaxation therapy, physical exercise, and proper time-management strategies should go hand in hand with prophylactic pharmacotherapy. Analgesic overuse must be recognized and treated before long-term prophylactic pharmacotherapy is prescribed. Significant comorbidities should be treated concomitantly. In this respect, for example, a single medicine, such as tricyclic antidepressants to treat CTH and cormorbid depression, might be chosen. Medications that have been used for prophylaxis of CTH include tricyclic antidepressants, other antidepressants, muscle relaxants, nonsteroidal antiinflammatory agents (NSAIDs), and miscellaneous agents.

MEDICATIONS FOR PROPHYLAXIS OF CHRONIC TENSION-TYPE HEADACHE

ANTIDEPRESSANTS

Pharmacology of Antidepressants

More than three decades ago, the tricyclic antidepressant amitriptyline was reported to be effective in the prophylactic treatment of CTH (18), and amitriptyline is still the only drug with proven prophylactic efficacy in this disorder; however, other tricyclic antidepressants probably are also effective in tension-type headache, especially because several drugs of this group (e.g., clomipramine, imipramine, desipramine) have proved to be effective in the treatment of other chronic pain conditions, such as diabetic neuropathy (25). It is generally agreed that the analgesic effect of the tricyclic antidepressants is independent of their antidepressant effect, but the exact mechanism of action has not been clarified (4).

The tricyclic antidepressants all inhibit the presynaptic reuptake of serotonin and noradrenaline in the central nervous system (CNS), thus potentiating the activity of these neurotransmitters (3). Amitriptyline and doxepin mainly inhibit the reuptake of serotonin, whereas desipramine has its greatest effect on the inhibition of noradrenaline reuptake. Both actions are considered important in the analgesic effect of the tricyclic antidepressants, but the relative importance of these actions is not known. The tricyclic antidepressants have numerous actions besides inhibition of serotonin and noradrenaline reuptake (3). Thus, amitriptyline has potent antimuscarinic and antihistaminergic properties (6), it interacts

N. T. Mathew: Houston Headache Clinic, Houston, Texas 77004.

L. Bendtsen: Department of Neurology, Glostrup Hospital, University of Copenhagen, DK-2600 Glostrup, Copenhagen, Denmark.

with several serotonin receptors subtypes, and it has antagonist effects at α-adrenoceptors (6). Of these effects, the actions on various serotonin receptor subtypes have been considered especially important in the analgesic effect (12). Moreover, it was recently suggested that amitriptyline may act as a N-methyl-^{D}-aspartate (NMDA) receptor antagonist (37) and that the analgesic effect of amitriptyline in chronic pain may be due primarily to this action (8). This suggestion is interesting because the NMDA receptor is known to be involved in the development of central sensitization, which is considered to be of major importance in CTH (see Chapter 73).

Amitriptyline is rapidly absorbed after oral administration, but its bioavailability is only 25% to 50% because of a large first-pass effect. Amitriptyline is metabolized mainly in the liver; the major metabolite, nortriptyline, is pharmacologically active. The half-life of amitriptyline ranges from 13 to 36 hours (6). The pharmacokinetics of amitriptyline, as well as of the other tricyclic antidepressants, are characterized by large interpatient variability, and no clear relationship has been found between plasma concentrations and analgesic effect (6).

Within the last decade, a new generation of antidepressants, the selective serotonin reuptake inhibitors (SSRIs), including fluoxetine, fluvoxamine, and paroxetine, have become the most frequently prescribed antidepressant medications in the United States because of their favorable side-effect profile. Controlled clinical trials suggest, however, that SSRIs have no or only a limited analgesic effect (for review, see reference 16). Other nontricyclic antidepressants include the serotonin receptor (5-HT$_2$) antagonists mianserin and ritanserin and the novel antidepressants mirtazapine and venlafaxine, which potentiate serotonin and noradrenaline neurotransmission with little affinity for receptors mediating tricyclic-like side effects.

The efficacy of the latter medications in the treatment of chronic pain remains to be determined.

Review of Clinical Trials of Antidepressants in Tension-type Headache

The placebo effect must be taken into account in any study of treatment for headache. Therefore, only placebo-controlled trials (Table 1) and trials comparing a well-documented treatment with a new treatment allow definitive statements about efficacy in tension-type headache. Because of the limited number of placebo-controlled trials, however, controlled trials comparing two potentially active treatments are included. It should be kept in mind, however, that the predictable result of such studies, that is, that both treatments are effective and no difference between studies can be detected, is difficult to interpret.

Placebo-controlled Trials

In 1964 Lance and Curran (18) conducted a placebo-controlled, crossover trial of amitriptyline 10 to 25 mg three times daily in 27 patients with CTH. Twelve patients had no improvement during treatment with either amitriptyline or placebo, 12 patients reported a response only to amitriptyline, and three patients responded to both treatments. These results were significantly in favor of amitriptyline.

Diamond and Baltes (7) tested two different dosage ranges of amitriptyline versus placebo, a lower one of 10 to 60 mg daily and a higher one between 25 and 150 mg daily. The results suggested that the lower dose range was more effective than placebo, but no significant effect of the higher dose range was found.

Göbel and colleagues (13) evaluated amitriptyline 75 mg daily. Compared with placebo, headache duration was

TABLE 1. *Summary of randomized, double-blind, placebo-controlled studies of antidepressants in chronic tension-type headache*

Study (reference no.)	Drugs tested design	No. of patients	Results
Lance and Curran (18)	Amitriptyline/Crossover	27	Significantly more responders on A (15/27) than on P (3/27)
Diamond and Baltes (7)	Amitriptyline/Parallel	85	Significant effect of A 10–60 mg/day but not of A 25–150 mg/day
Göbel et al. (13)	Amitriptyline/Parallel	53	Significant effect of A in the last week of the 6-week study
Pfaffenrath et al. (29)	Amitriptyline and AO/Parallel	197	No significant effect of A, no difference in side effects between A and P
Bendtsen et al. (4)	Amitriptyline and CI/Crossover	34	Significant effect of A (headache reduced by 30%), no significant effect of CI
Fogelholm and Murros (10)	Maprotiline/crossover	30	Significant effect of maprotiline
Langemark et al. (19)	Mianserin and CL/parallel	82	Significant effect of mianserin and clomipramine
Ansink et al. (1)	Ritanserin/crossover	44	No effect of ritanserin

A, amitriptyline; P, placebo; AO, amitriptylinoxide; CI: citalopram; CL, clomipramine.

reduced significantly only in the last week of the 6-week study, whereas the intake of analgesics was unaltered. The study did not include a run-in period, and neither headache frequency nor headache intensity was presented. Nevertheless, because headache duration decreased consistently throughout all 6 weeks of active treatment but not throughout placebo treatment, the study favors an effect of amitriptyline.

A large multicenter, parallel-group trial by Pfaffenrath and colleagues (30) compared amitriptyline 50 to 75 mg daily, amitriptyline oxide 60 to 90 mg daily, and placebo. No significant difference was found between the active treatments and placebo for either the primary study endpoint (a reduction of at least 50% of the product of headache duration and frequency *and* a reduction of at least 50% in headache intensity) or for any of the mentioned secondary efficacy parameters. The frequency of side effects was similar with amitriptyline and placebo use. Usually, amitriptyline has marked side effects, and the inability to detect known side effects suggests insensitivity of the trial for reasons that remain obscure.

In a three-way crossover study, Bendsten and associates (4) compared amitriptyline 75 mg daily, citalopram (a highly selective reuptake inhibitor) 20 mg daily, and placebo. The patients had been resistant to numerous previous treatments and were not suffering from depression. Amitriptyline reduced the area under the headache curve (calculated as headache duration times headache intensity) by 30% compared with placebo, which was highly significant, whereas citalopram had only a slight (12%) and insignificant effect (Fig. 1). Amitriptyline also significantly reduced the secondary efficacy parameters: headache duration, headache frequency and intake of analgesics.

Together, these placebo-controlled studies indicate that amitriptyline has a statistically significant and a clinically relevant effect in the prophylactic treatment of CTH. Nonetheless, amitriptyline does not eliminate the headache, and more effective treatment modalities are therefore greatly needed.

Other Antidepressants

A few other antidepressants have been tested in placebo-controlled studies. The tetracyclic antidepressant maprotiline 75 mg daily was found to be effective by Fogelholm and Murros (10), and Langemark and colleagues (20) reported that both clomipramine 75 to 150 mg daily and mianserin 30 to 60 mg daily had superior efficacy to placebo. Ritanserin was reported to be effective in a study that did not include placebo (28), but this promising result was not confirmed in a subsequent placebo-controlled trial (2).

Controlled Trials Comparing Two Potentially Active Treatments without Inclusion of Placebo

Langemark and Olesen (21) compared paroxetine 20 to 30 mg daily with sulpiride, a dopamine antagonist used as a neuroleptic. Patients improved with both treatments, although a tendency to better efficacy was found for sulpiride. Manna and colleagues (22) compared fluvoxamine 50 to 100 mg daily with mianserin 30 to 60 mg daily and found a significant effect of both treatments. Holroyd and associates (14) compared amitriptyline 25 to 75 mg daily with cognitive-behavioral therapy. They found a significant effect of both treatments with a tendency to more positive outcomes of cognitive-behavioral therapy.

Controlled Trials in Patients Suffering from Both Tension-type Headache and Migraine

In patients with mixed migraine and tension-type headache, Mathew (23) found amitriptyline 50 to 75 mg daily to be superior to propranolol, and Morland and colleagues (26) found doxepin 100 mg daily to have significantly better results than placebo. In patients with chronic daily headache, Saper and colleagues (31) found fluoxetine 20 to 40 mg daily to be significantly more effective than placebo in the last month of a 3-month study.

MUSCLE RELAXANTS

About 50% to 60% of patients with tension-type headache have associated pericranial muscle disorder, including muscle spasm and tenderness, and a low pressure-pain threshold (8,19,34). No convincing correlation has been found, however, between these factors and the degree or timing of head pain (38). Moreover, patients

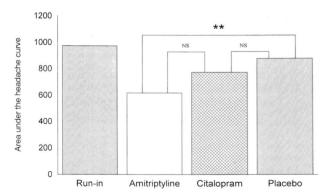

FIG. 1. The prophylactic effect of amitriptyline and of citalopram (a selective serotonin reuptake inhibitor) was compared in a 32-week, double-blind, placebo-controlled, three-way crossover study including 40 patients with chronic tension-type headache. Thirty-four patients completed the study. The bars represent the area under the headache curve (duration times intensity) during a 4-week run-in period and during the last 4 weeks of treatment with amitriptyline, citalopram, and placebo. **$p = 0.002$; *NS,* not significant. [From Bendtsen et al. (2)].

with tension-type headache without the pericranial muscle disorder exhibit clinically identical types of head pain (1). From the exteroceptive silent-period studies, some evidence has accumulated to indicate that a lack of central inhibition (dysfunction of the polysynaptic brainstem inhibitory interneurons) may be involved in the pathophysiology of tension-type headache (26,32).

Pharmacology of Muscle Relaxants

Theoretically, agents that relax skeletal muscles or correct the dysfunction of polysynaptic CNS interneurons should help the pain of tension-type headache. In practice, however, the results of such treatment have been disappointing. The commonly used oral muscle relaxants are listed in Table 2 (5).

Mephenesin-like compounds inhibit the synapses of internuncial neurons in the spinal cord and brainstem, resulting in muscle relaxation. The mechanism of the action of these compounds is unexplained at the neurochemical level. Carisoprodol exhibits a mild atropine-like effect as well as a muscle relaxant effect. Most of these compounds show central muscle-relaxant effects of other sedatives. Mephenesin-like compounds are absorbed well when taken orally. Little is known about the metabolic rate, but the rapid metabolism of the mephenesin group limits its effectiveness. Side effects include sleepiness, weakness, vertigo, and lassitude. Hemolysis and hemoglobinuria have been noted after intervenous administration.

GABA-like Compounds

Baclofen

Baclofen is capable of inhibiting both monosynaptic and polysynaptic rebound at the spinal cord as well as at the supraspinal level. Baclofen is an analogue of the inhibitory neurotransmitter τ-aminobutyric acid (GABA). No conclusive evidence has been found, however, that the actions of GABA systems are involved in the production of its clinical effects. It has CNS depressant properties that account for the sedation, somnolence, ataxia, and respiratory and cardiovascular suppression in higher doses.

Diazepam

Diazepam is primarily an antianxiety agent. It blocks the electroencephalographic arousal from stimulation of brainstem reticular formation. Spinal reflexes are depressed and in turn are medicated in part by the brainstem reticular system. Diazepam has effects on the limbic system, which potentiates the effects of GABA and other inhibitory neurotransmitters.

Diazepam is widely used as a muscle relaxant, although controlled studies rarely show any advantage of any benzodiazepine over either placebo or aspirin. The CNS depressant action may account for the partial muscle relaxation.

Tizanidine

Tizanidine hydrochloride is a centrally acting muscle relaxant that has been reported to inhibit polysynaptic, rather than monosynaptic, reflexes in animal studies (29,32). It also has an analgesic property. Like clonidine, it is a centrally acting α_2- adrenergic agonist that reduces the release of noradrenaline in the CNS (32). It is suggested that some patients with tension-type headache might have an increase in central adrenergic metabolic activity (36).

Cyclobenzaprine Hydrochloride

Cyclobenzaprine is pharmacologically related to amitriptyline and imipramine (5). It relieves skeletal muscle spasm of local origin without interfering with muscle functions. Cyclobenzaprine acts primarily in the CNS at the brainstem level as opposed to the spinal cord level. It reduces the tonic somatic motor activity, influencing both τ- and α-motor systems. Like tricyclic antidepressants, cyclobenzaprine has sedative and anticholinergic effects.

Dantrolene Sodium

In isolated nerve-muscle preparation, dantrolene sodium has been shown to produce relaxation by affecting the contractile response of the skeletal muscle at a site beyond the myoneural junction, directly on the muscle itself. In skeletal muscle, dantrolene sodium dissociates the excitation–contraction coupling, probably by interfering with the release of Ca^{2+} from the sarcoplasmic reticulum. This effect appears to be more pronounced in fast muscle fibers compared with slow ones, but it generally affects both. A CNS effect occurs, with drowsiness, dizzi-

---

TABLE 2. *Classification of oral muscle relaxants*

Centrally acting
  Mephenesin-like compounds
    Methocarbamol
    Chlorphenesin carbamate
    Carisoprodol
    Chlorzoxazone
    Tolperisone Hcl
    Eperisone Hcl
  GABA-like compounds
    Baclofen
    Diazepam
  Imidazone
    Tizanidine HCl
  Cyclobenzaprine HCl
Peripherally acting
  Dantrolene Na

ness, and generalized weakness occasionally present. Although dantrolene sodium does not appear to affect the CNS directly, the extent of its indirect effect is unknown. The absorption of dantrolene sodium after oral administration in humans is incomplete and slow but consistent, and dose-related blood levels are obtained. The duration and intensity of skeletal muscle relaxation are related to the dosage and blood levels. The mean biologic half-life of dantrolene sodium in adults is 8.7 hours after a 100-mg dose. Specific metabolic pathways in the degradation and elimination of dantrolene sodium in human subjects have not been established. Table 3 lists the muscle relaxants commonly used in tension-type headache.

Clinical Trials

Controlled clinical trials are virtually nonexistent for the acute treatment of tension-type headache using muscle relaxants. On the other hand, a few studies are available that indicate the efficacy of muscle relaxants in the prophylactic treatment of CTH. Tizanidine appears to be particularly useful in this respect (11,35).

The efficacy of tizanidine in CTH was compared with placebo in a randomized, double-blind, crossover study in 37 women aged 20 to 59 years who had a history of headache for 7 months to 30 years (median, 5 years) (35). The treatment periods were 6 weeks, with an intervening 2-week washout period. Treatment began with 6 mg daily divided into three doses, and the daily dose could be increased to 18 mg, depending on the treatment response. The effect of the treatment was measured by visual analogue scale, verbal rating scale, number of headache-free days, number of analgesics needed, and the dose of trial medication needed. In all these measurements, tizanidine was statistically significantly more effective than placebo. The pretrial Beck Depression Inventory score did not predict the response to treatment, nor did the level

of electromyographic activity of the trapezium muscle. Side effects of drowsiness and dry mouth were significantly more common during tizanidine treatment, but they were usually mild. The results of this trial suggest that tizanidine is effective in the treatment of CTH in women.

The absence of correlation between electromyographic levels and clinical response may indicate that tizanidine may act through its central α_2-agonist action, reducing the release of noradrenaline in the CNS. Shimomura and colleagues (36) reported higher levels of plasma 3-methoxy4-hydroxyphenylglycol (MHPG) in tizanidine responders. Levels of MHPG decreased significantly after treatment with tizanidine.

Eperisone hydrochloride, a centrally acting muscle relaxant, has been shown to decrease the muscle spasm in patients with tension-type headache (17). It was not clear from the report whether any corresponding decrease in headache occurred in patients who demonstrated reduction in muscle spasms. Both tizanidine and eperisone will require more well-controlled clinical trials before they can be recommended for clinical use.

Nonsteroidal Antiinflammatory Drugs

Even though NSAIDs are used frequently for symptomatic relief for headache, no studies have been reported that showed significant benefit of long-term use for CTH. Because long-term use may result in gastric and renal dysfunction, these agents should be instituted with caution.

Miscellaneous Agents

A number of other agents have been used in the treatment of chronic headaches, usually the mixed variety of migraine and CTH. In an open trial, a significant success was reported with the use of propranolol or a combina-

TABLE 3. *Muscle relaxants commonly used in tension-type headache[a]*

Medication	Dose	Comments
Mephenesin-like		
Methocarbamol (Robaxin)	1–2 g by mouth, repeat up to 3 times	Longer action than mephenesin
Carisoprodol (Soma)	350 mg, repeat up to 3 times	
Chlorzoxazone (Parafon)	250 mg, repeat up to 3 times	
GABA-like		
Baclofen (Lioresal)	10 mg, 3 times a day	Drowsiness a major side effect
Diazepam (Valium)	10 mg, up to a total of 30 mg per acute attack	Dependency may develop
Imidazone		
Tizanidine (Ternelin:Zanaflex)	6–18 mg/day	Found useful in prophylaxis of chronic tension-type headache
Other agents		
Cyclobenzaprine Hydrochloride (Flexeril)	10 mg. up to 3 mg/day	

[a]No satisfactory controlled data are available for any of these compounds.

tion of propranolol plus amitriptyline (23). Valproic acid in doses of 1,000 mg to 2,500 mg was reported to be effective in the treatment of mixed migraine and CTH in an open trial of 30 subjects (24). In this study, a 67% improvement in the headache index and a 30% improvement in headache-free days per month were found after 3 months on valproic acid therapy. Because these were open studies, further confirmation with double-blind studies are necessary.

THERAPEUTIC USE

In general, the initial approach to prophylactic therapy of CTH is through the use of tricyclic antidepressants. It is important that patients are informed that these medications are antidepressant agents but have an independent action on pain. Amitriptyline is the best studied medication and the standard by which other therapies are measured. Amitriptyline should be started at low dosages (10–25 mg/day) and titrated by 10 to 25 mg weeklly until the patient has either good therapeutic effect or side effects are encountered. Low starting doses are particularly important for elderly patients, who may be sensitive to the adverse effects of the tricyclic antidepressants. The maintenance dose is usually 50 to 75 mg daily administered 2 to 3 hours before bedtime to help to circumvent any sedative adverse effects. Occasionally, patients will benefit from higher doses (up to 200 mg/day). In such cases, monitoring of blood levels should be done to ensure that the patient does not devlop toxicity to the medication. A significant effect of amitriptyline may be observed already in the first week on the therapeutic dose (4). It is therefore advisable to change to other prophylactic therapy if the patient does not respond after 3 to 4 weeks on maintenance dose.

The side effects of amitriptyline include dry mouth, drowsiness, dizziness, obstipation, weight gain, slowing of urination, orthostatic hypotension, and blurred vision. The most serious side effects include cardiac arrhythmia, glaucoma, and urinary retention. In a recent study (4), dry mouth was observed in 75% and drowsiness in 53% of patients. Adverse effects are usually mild, however, and amitriptyline is generally well tolerated (4). Some tolerance may develop to the sedative and, to a lesser extent, to the anticholinergic side effects. Amitriptyline should be administered with caution in patients with prostatic hypertrophy, glaucoma, constipation, impaired liver function, or cardiovascular disease and should be avoided in patients who have heart block or arrhythmias and should not be administered immediately after myocardial infarction, in patients with urinary retention or severe liver disease, or during pregnancy and breastfeeding.

If the patient does not respond to amitriptyline, other antidepressants could be attempted; however, no controlled studies have examined whether a headache patient who does not respond to amitriptyline may benefit from other antidepressants. If a patient does not tolerate the tricyclic antidepressants, the SSRIs could be considered; scientific evidence indicates, however, that these agents have no, or only a moderate, effect (4,31). As mentioned, the efficacy of the more recently developed antidepressants in the prophylaxis of CTH has not been investigated.

The centrally acting muscle relaxant tizanidine appears to have some promise in the prophylactic treatment of CTH. Further large placebo controlled, double-blind studies are necessary. In the meantime, the clinician may try this medicine in patients who do not respond to antidepressants. Most of the centrally acting muscle relaxant agents cause drowsiness, which limits their clinical use, even though there may be an occasional patient who does well on such medications. Peripherally acting agents, like dantrolene sodium, offer no significant benefit in CTH.

How long should prophylactic agents be continued? There is no definite answer to this question. It is a common practice to attempt to discontinue agents after 6 months. Withdrawal must be gradual. Many patients continue to maintain improvement for a long time, but many revert to experiencing CTH. It is not uncommon for a significant number of patients with CTH to be on prophylaxis for an indefinite time. Concomitant use of daily analgesics should be avoided.

REFERENCES

1. Anderson CD, Franks RD. Migraine and tension headache: is there a physiological difference? *Headache* 1981;21:63–71.
2. Ansink BJJ, Hartman JW, Smakman JGJ. Ritanserin is not effective in tension headache. *Headache* 1992;32:314–314.
3. Baldessarini RJ. Drugs and the treatment of psychiatric disorders. In: Gilman AG, Goodman LS, Gilman A, eds. *The pharmacological basis of therapeutics*, 6th ed. New York: McMillan, 1980:418–427.
4. Bendtsen L, Jensen R, Olesen J. A non-selective (amitriptyline), but not a selective (citalopram), serotonin reuptake inhibitor is effective in the prophylactic treatment of chronic tension-type headache. *J Neurol Neurosurg Psychiatry* 1996;61:285–290.
5. Bianchine JR. Drugs for Parkinson's disease: centrally acting muscle relaxants. In: Gilman AG, Goodman LS, Gilman A, eds. *The pharmacological basis of therapeutics*, 6th ed. New York: McMillan, 1980: 488–493.
6. Bryson HM, Wilde MI. Amitriptyline: a review of its pharmacological properties and therapeutic use in chronic pain states. *Drugs Aging* 1996;8:459–476.
7. Diamond S, Baltes BJ. Chronic tension headache—treated with amitriptyline—a double-blind study. *Headache* 1971;11:110–116.
8. Eisenach JC, Gebhart GF. Intrathecal amitriptyline acts as an *N*-methyl-D-aspartate receptor antagonist in the presence of inflammatory hyperalgesia in rats. *Anesthesiology* 1995;83:1046–1054.
9. Drummond PD. Scalp tenderness and sensitivity to pain in migraine and tension type headache. *Headache* 1987;27:45–50.
10. Fogelholm R, Murros K. Maprotiline in chronic tension-type headache: a double-blind cross-over study. *Headache* 1985;25:273–275.
11. Fogelholm R, Murros K. Tizanidine in chronic tension-type headache: a placebo controlled double-blind crossover study. *Headache* 1992;32: 509–513.
12. Glaum SR, Proudfit HK, Anderson EG. Reversal of the antinociceptive effects of intrathecally administered serotonin in the rate by a selective 5-HT3 receptor antagonist. *Neurosci Lett* 1988;95:313–317.
13. Göbel H, Hamouz V, Hansen C, et al. Chronic tension-type headache: amitriptyline reduces clinical headache-duration and experimental pain sensitivity but does not alter pericranial muscle activity readings. *Pain* 1994;59:241–249.

14. Holroyd KA, Nash JM, Pingel JD, Cordingley GE, Jerome A. A comparison of pharmacological (amitriptyline HCL) and nonpharmacological (cognitive-behavioral) therapies for chronic tension headaches. *J Consult Clin Psychol* 1991;59:387–393.

15. Hyttel J. Citalopram—pharmacological profile of a specific serotonin uptake inhibitor with antidepressant activity. *Prog Neuropsychopharmacol Biol Psychiatry* 1982;6:277–295.

16. Jung AC, Staiger T, Sullivan M. The efficacy of selective serotonin reuptake inhibitors for the management of chronic pain. *J Gen Intern Med* 1997;12:384–389.

17. Kitagawa Y, Okayasu H, Ebihara S, Horikawa M, Sakai F. Effect of eperisone hydrochloride on tension-type headache: assessment with a pressure-displacement transducer. *Cephalalgia* 1991;11:335–336.

18. Lance JW, Curran DA. Treatment of chronic tension headache. *Lancet* 1964;1:1236–1239.

19. Langemark M, Olesen J. Pericranial tenderness in tension headache. *Cephalalgia* 1987;7:249–255.

20. Langemark M, Loldrup D, Bech P, Olesen J. Clomipramine and mianserin in the treatment of chronic tension headache: a double-blind, controlled study. *Headache* 1990;30:118–121.

21. Langemark M, Olesen J. Sulpiride and paroxetine in the treatment of chronic tension-type headache: an explanatory double-blind trial. *Headache* 94;34:20–24.

22. Manna V, Bolino F, DiCicco L. Chronic tension-type headache, mood depression and serotonin; therapeutic effects of fluvoxamine and mianserin. *Headache* 1994;34:44–49.

23. Mathew NT. Prophylaxis of migraine and mixed headache: a randomized controlled study. *Headache* 1981;21:105–109.

24. Mathew NT, Ali S. Valproate in the treatment of persistent chronic daily headache. An open label study. *Headache* 1991;31:71–74.

25. Max MB, Lynch SA, Muir J, Shoaf SE, Smoller B, Dubner R. Effects of desipramine, amitriptyline, and fluoxetine on pain in diabetic neuropathy. *N Engl J Med* 1992;326:1250–1256.

26. Morland TJ, Storli OV, Mogstad TE. Doxepin in the prophylactic treatment of mixed "vascular" and tension headache. *Headache* 1979;19:382–383.

27. Nakashima K, Takahashi K. Exteroceptive suppression of the masseter, temporalis and trapezius muscles produced by mental nerve stimulation in patients with chronic headaches. *Cephalalgia* 1991;11:23–28.

28. Nappi G, Sandrini G, Granella F, et al. A new 5-HT2 antagonist (ritanserin) in the treatment of chronic headache with depression: a double-blind study vs amitriptyline. *Headache* 1990;30:439–444.

29. Ono H, Satoh M, Fukuda H. Alpha$_2$-agonist-induced reduction of noradrenaline release from descending noradrenergic terminals in rat spinal cord: functional relation to spinal motor system. *Biomed Res* 1988;9:169–176.

30. Pfaffenrath V, Diener HC, Isler H, Meyer C, et al. Efficacy and tolerability of amitriptylinoxide in the treatment of chronic tension-type headache: a multicentre controlled study. *Cephalalgia* 1994;14:149–155.

31. Saper JR, Silberstein SD, Lake III AE, Winters ME. Double-blind trial of fluoxetine: chronic daily headache and migraine. *Headache* 1994;34:497–502.

32. Sayers AC, Burki HR, Eichenberger E. The pharmacology of 5-chloro-4-(2-imidazolin-2-yl-amino)-2,1,3-benzothiodazole (DS 103-282), a novel myotonolytic agent. *Drug Res* 1980;30:793–803.

33. Schoenen J, Jamart BA, Gerard P, et al. Exteroceptive suppression of temporalis muscle activity in chronic headache. *Neurology* 1987;37:1834–1836.

34. Schoenen J, Bottin D, Hardy F, Gerard P. Cephalic and extracephalic pressure pain thresholds in chronic tension-type headache. *Pain* 1991;47:145–149.

35. Shimomura T, Awaki E, Kowa H, Takahashi K. Treatment of tension-type headache with tizanidine hydrochloride: its efficacy and relationship to plasma MHPG concentration. *Headache* 1991;31:601–604.

36. Shimomura T, Awaki E, Takahashi K. Treatment of tension-type headache with tizanidine hydrochloride; relationship between plasma MHPG concentration and clinical effects. *Cephalalgia* 1991;11(Suppl 11):333–334.

37. Watanabe Y, Saito H, Abe K. Tricyclic antidepressants block NMDA receptor-mediated synaptic responses and induction of long-term potentiation in rat hippocampal slices. *Neuropharmacology* 1993;32:479–486.

38. Yates AJ. *Biofeedback and modification of behavior.* New York: Plenium Press, 1980:90–92.

The Headaches, Second Edition,
edited by J. Olesen, P. Tfelt-Hansen, and K.M.A. Welch.
Lippincott Williams & Wilkins, Philadelphia © 2000.

Tension-Type Headache, Cluster Headache, and Miscellaneous
Primary Headaches

CHAPTER 89

Cluster Headache: Introduction

Gian Camillo Manzoni and Antonio Prusinski

CLASSIFICATION AND SHORT DESCRIPTION

Cluster headache (CH) falls into group 3 of the International Headache Society (IHS) classification (CH and chronic paroxysmal hemicrania) and is coded 3.1 (6) (Table 1). In the Tenth Revision of the International Classification of Diseases (ICD-10) of the World Health Organization (WHO), it is coded G44.0 (episodic CH-G44.01, chronic CH-G44.02) (21).

Cluster headache is characterized by attacks of strictly unilateral, severe pain with orbital, supraorbital, or temporal location. Attacks last 15 to 180 minutes and usually occur one or several times per day, especially at night. They are accompanied by ipsilateral conjunctival injection, lacrimation, rhinorrhea or nasal congestion, eyelid edema, miosis, and low grade ptosis. There is a clear male preponderance.

Two main clinical forms of CH may be diagnosed: *episodic* and *chronic*. The most common form is the episodic form, which affects 80% to 90% of patients. It is characterized by periods of attacks (bouts, cluster) and periods of remission. In the cluster period, the patient experiences from one to eight attacks per day (days without headache may occur); this period may last from 7 days to 1 year. Between cluster periods, patients are usually completely pain free, but short-lasting pain periods with isolated, short attacks may occur.

The chronic form lacks the remissions and is diagnosed after 1 year without remission or if remissions have lasted less than 14 days. The patient may suffer from the

TABLE 1. *IHS classification of cluster headache and chronic paroxysmal hemicrania*

3.1 Cluster headache
3.1.1 Cluster headache periodicity undetermined
3.1.2 Episodic cluster headache
3.1.3. Chronic cluster headache
3.1.3.1 Unremitting from onset
3.1.3.2 Evolved from episodic
3.2 Chronic paroxysmal hemicrania
3.3 Cluster headache-like disorder not fulfilling above criteria

IHS, International Headache Society.
From Headache Classification of the International Headache Society (6).

chronic form from the beginning of the disease (chronic CH unremitting from onset), or it may develop from the episodic form (chronic CH evolved from episodic).

Studies conducted on the natural history of CH after the IHS classification have shown that over the years a chronic form of CH occasionally may evolve into an episodic form (11,15). Therefore, future reviews of the IHS classification should include a fourth diagnostic level for episodic CH (i.e., 3.1.2.1 episodic from onset; 3.1.2.2 evolved from chronic).

Apart from these main clinical forms of CH, which affect the vast majority of patients, there are atypical cases, coded 3.3 in the IHS classification. These patients present some CH symptoms but differ in clinical course, additional signs, or both. These forms constitute the borderland of CH (also called *variants*).

OTHER TERMS

Previously used terms include *erythroprosopalgia of Bing*, *ciliary* or *migrainous neuralgia* (Harris), *erythro-*

G. C. Manzoni: Department of Neurology, University of Parma, 43100 Parma, Italy.
A. Prusinski: Department of Neurology, Medical Academy, 90-153 Lodz, Poland.

melalgia of the head, Horton's headache, histaminic cephalgia, petrosal neuralgia (Gardner), *sphenopalatine, Vidian and Sluder's neuralgia,* and *hemicrania periodica neuralgiformis.* The term *cluster headache* was introduced relatively recently, in 1952, by Kunkle and colleagues (12). By then, CH certainly had been known for a long time under other names, as demonstrated by the striking similarities between this condition and most other syndromes listed in Table 2.

The abundance of eponyms and synonyms used in the past to describe the same form may have been indirectly responsible for the late recognition of CH as such. In fact, according to Koehler (9), the first report on CH dates to 1641, when Nicolaas Tulp, a famous Dutch physician, published his *Observationes Medicae,* in which he describes the case of Isaak van Halmaal, who "... in the beginning of the summer season, was afflicted with a very severe headache, occurring and disappearing daily on fixed hours. For rarely it lasted longer than two hours. This recurring pain lasted until the fourteenth day...." Another probable case from the seventeenth century was described by Thomas Willis, who, in *De anima brutorum,* mentioned a headache whose attacks tended to recur more severely at the time of the sun's solstice and equinox, although in most cases it struck people in between, at preferred hours during the 24-hour day (16). Nappi and Manzoni (16) also argued that CH and chronic paroxysmal hemicrania were both described in 1747 when Oppermann, in his doctoral dissertation on "hemicrania horologica," described the case of a 35-year-old woman, who since the age of 29 years had been suffering from daily 15-minute attacks every hour of the day and night with such regularity as to tell the hour more accurately than the clock in the city square.

In 1822, Hutchinson, in his book *Cases of Neuralgia Spasmodica,* edited in London, described a hemicrania that, after recurring for several hours daily for long periods, departs suddenly. Also, Hall (*Principles of the Theory and Practice of Medicine,* 1834) saw similar cases, calling them *hemicrania intermittens* or *brow ague* (17).

Most of the definitions listed in Table 2 are of merely historical interest, because they were commonly used for only brief periods. Among them, however, some are worthy of mention, namely, Harris's *migrainous neuralgia* (5), a term that is still quite popular. Thus, Ekbom (2) used *chronic migrainous neuralgia* as the title for his chapter on chronic CH, and *Horton's headache* (8) was used for many years and still is considered of great interest in that the name is from the author who, more than any other, played a prominent role in investigating CH in the 1940s and 1950s. As for Sluder's *sphenopalatine ganglion neuralgia* (19), also listed in Table 2, it is still an open question whether it should be considered an equivalent form of CH or an autonomous clinical syndrome, as suggested by Sjaastad (18).

EPIDEMIOLOGY

The prevalence of CH is still a controversial subject. Table 3 reports previously published prevalence estimates, which vary considerably. The variations probably reflect different methodologies rather than real differences in frequency between the populations studied. For instance, the percentage reported by Hardman and Hopkins (4), in a study conducted among general practitioners, is probably an underestimation, because physicians who are not actually neurology specialists may have overlooked a number of cases. Also, at the time of the study (1966), the boundary between CH and migraine was not as clear as it is today, and some cases may have been misclassified as migraine.

In contrast, the prevalence rate reported by Ekbom and colleagues (3), who used a highly accurate study design, seems much closer to the actual rate. This rate, however, applied only to a limited population sample, namely, 18-year-old male subjects, and to a comparatively small number of patients (nine of 9,803 subjects).

Using a complex extrapolation from these data from Ekbom and colleagues (3) and a distribution of CH by age and sex among his own patients, Kudrow (10) argued

TABLE 2. *Cluster headache synonyms and related syndromes*

Previous terms	Authors	Year
Red migraine	Moellendorf	1867
Angioparalytic hemicrania	Eulenburg	1883
Sphenopalatine ganglion neuralgia	Sluder	1910
Erythrosopalgia	Bing	1913
Syndrome de vasodilatation hemicéphalique d'origine sympathique	Vallery-Radot and Blamoutier	1925
Ciliary neuralgia	Harris	1926
Syndrome du nerf nasal	Charlin	1931
Vidian neuralgia	Vail	1932
Autonomic faciocephalalgia	Brickner and Riley	1935
Migrainous neuralgia	Harris	1936
Erythromelalgia	Horton et al.	1939
Greater superficial petrosal neuralgia	Gardner et al.	1947
Histaminic cephalgia	Horton	1952

TABLE 3. *Prevalence of cluster headache*

Authors (year)	Country	Prevalence (‰)	Method
Hardman and Hopkins (1966)	England	0.05	Investigation among GPs
Heyck (1976)	Germany	0.4	Extrapolation
Ekbom et al. (1978)	Sweden	0.9	Investigation of 18-year-old males
Kudrow (1980)	United States	2.4	Extrapolation
D'Alessandro et al. (1980)	San Marino	0.7	Investigation of the general population
Zhao et al. (1)	China	0.06	Door-to-door investigation
Manzoni et al. (1998)	Italy	0.8	Investigation of patients in headache center

that approximately 400,000 men (0.4%) and 90,000 women (0.08%) were suffering from CH in the United States, accounting for 0.24% of the general population.

Heyck (7), too, obtained his data by extrapolating from a 6% average prevalence of migraine in the general population. Knowing that about one third of the sufferers saw a doctor and that in Heyck's own practice there was on average a CH sufferer for every 50 migraine patients, Heyck concluded that the CH prevalence in the general population was 0.4 per thousand.

The study by D'Alessandro and colleagues (1) may offer more reliable data, because it was done as a survey of the general population. These authors found 15 CH cases (0.069%) among the inhabitants of the Republic of San Marino (population, 21,792). This finding is interesting, even though the population sample was not large enough to provide reliable indications about the prevalence of a low-frequency disease, such as CH.

In a recent review of CH cases referred to his own headache center, Manzoni (14) reported on 143 CH patients living in the city of Parma (population, 173,991), Italy, or 0.82% of the total. Of course, this is a conservative estimate, because not all CH sufferers are referred to a headache center. Based on the currently available data, it can be reasonably assumed that the actual CH prevalence in the general population is about one per thousand or slightly higher but hardly lower.

The only study on CH incidence was conducted by Swanson and associates (20) involving 6,476 Olmsted County, Minnesota, residents; the overall age- and sex-adjusted incidence was 9.8 per 100,000 person-years. This figure is probably an overestimation, however, because in their survey the authors also considered people who had only one attack, and CH diagnosis was based on clinical records but was not confirmed through clinical interviews.

Cluster headache cases have been reported by authors from various continents, and it is therefore reasonable to assume that this type of headache occurs everywhere in the world. An epidemiologic study carried out in the People's Republic of China by Zhao and colleagues (22) reported only 14 CH cases of 246,812 inhabitants (0.006%). In this study, however, the prevalence of migraine (0.7%) also was found to be markedly lower than commonly reported in the literature for the general population. It is likely, therefore, that the findings of

Zhao et al. were influenced by methodologic factors as well as a possibly lower prevalence of all primary headaches in the Chinese population.

According to Kudrow (10), CH is more prevalent in the black population, with a less marked predominance of men compared with women than in the white population. As to the gender ratio, it was recently suggested that its well-known predominance in men versus women was progressively decreasing over the years (13).

REFERENCES

1. D'Alessandro R, Gamberini G, Benassi G, Morganti G, Cortelli P, Lugaresi E. Cluster headache in the Republic of San Marino. *Cephalalgia* 1986;6:159–162.
2. Ekbom K. Chronic migrainous neuralgia. In: Rose CF, ed. *Handbook of clinical neurology*, vol 48, *Headache*. Amsterdam: Elsevier Science Publishers, 1986:247–255.
3. Ekbom K, Ahlborg B, Schele R. Prevalence of migraine and cluster headache in Swedish men of 18. *Headache* 1978:18:9–19.
4. Hardman RA, Hopkins EJ. A survey of migrainous neuralgia. *Journal of the College of General Practitioners* 1966;11:195–200.
5. Harris W. Ciliary (migrainous) neuralgia and its treatment. *BMJ* 1936; 1:457–460.
6. Headache Classification Committee of the International Headache Society. Classification and diagnostic criteria for headache disorders, cranial neuralgias and facial pain. *Cephalalgia* 1988;8(Suppl 7):1–96.
7. Heyck H. Cluster Kopfschmerz (Bing-Horton syndrome?). *Fortschr Neurol Psychiatr* 1976;44:37–50.
8. Horton BT. Histaminic cephalgia. *Lancet* 1952;2:92–98.
9. Koehler PJ. Prevalence of headache in Tulp's *Observationes Medicae* (1641) with a description of cluster headache. *Cephalalgia* 1993;13: 318–320.
10. Kudrow L. *Cluster headache:* mechanisms and management. New York: Oxford University Press, 1980.
11. Kunkel RS, Frame JR. Chronic cluster headache: long-term follow-up. In: Olesen J, ed. *Headache classification and epidemiology.* New York: Raven Press, 1994:113–116.
12. Kunkle EC, Pfeiffer JR, Wilhoit WM, Hamrich LW. Recurrent brief headaches in cluster pattern. *Trans of the Amer Neurological Assoc* 1952;77:240–243.
13. Manzoni GC. Male preponderance of cluster headache is progressively decreasing over the years. *Headache* 1997;37:588–589.
14. Manzoni GC. Gender ratio of cluster headache over the years: a possible role of changes in lifestyle. *Cephalalgia* 1998;18:138–142.
15. Manzoni GC, Micieli G, Granella F, Tassorelli C, Zanferrari C, Cavallini A. Cluster headache: course over ten years in 189 patients. *Cephalalgia* 1991;11:169–174.
16. Nappi G, Manzoni GC. *Primary headaches:* clinical approach and management. London: Smith-Gordon and Company Limited, 1996.
17. Olivarius de Fine B. Migraine variants [Letter]. *BMJ* 1971;2:49–50.
18. Sjaastad O. *Cluster headache syndrome:* major problems in neurology, vol 23, London: WB Saunders, 1992.
19. Sluder G. The syndrome of sphenopalatine ganglion neuralgia. *Am J Med Sci* 1910;140:868–878.

20. Swanson JW, Yanagihara T, Stang PE, O Fallon WM, Beard CM, Melton III LJ, Guess HA. Incidence of cluster headaches: a population-based study in Olmsted County, Minnesota. *Neurology* 1994;44: 433–437.

21. World Health Organization by the International Headache Society. ICD-10 guide for headaches: guide to the classification, diagnosis and assessment of headaches in accordance with the thent revision of the international classification of diseases and related health problems and its application to neurology. *Cephalalgia* 1997;17(Suppl 19):1–82.

22. Zhao F, Tsay J-Y, Cheng X, et al. Epidemiology of migraine: a survey in 21 provinces of the Peoples Republic of China, 1985. *Headache* 1988;28:558–565.

The Headaches, Second Edition,
edited by J. Olesen, P. Tfelt-Hansen, and K.M.A. Welch.
Lippincott Williams & Wilkins, Philadelphia © 2000.

Tension-Type Headache, Cluster Headache, and Miscellaneous
Primary Headaches

CHAPTER 90

Genetics of Cluster Headache

Michael Bjørn Russell

The etiology of cluster headache remains largely unknown, and it has not previously been considered to be inherited (16, 38).

POSITIVE FAMILY HISTORY

Several studies reported a positive family history of cluster headache (2,18,20,25). A positive family history is imprecise, however, because it does not specify the number of affected family members, the size of the family, or the relation to the proband of each affected person; nor does it include a direct interview of the relatives by a

TABLE 1. *Positive family history*

	No. of affected first-degree relatives	No. of probands
Ekbom (1947)	0	23
Symonds (1956)	0	17
Robinson (1958)	0	20
Bickerstaff (1959)	1	30
Schiller (1960)	1	51
Duvoisin et al. (1961)	1	32
Eadie et Sutherland (1966)	1	42
Ekbom (1970)	2	105
Lance et Anthony (1971)	0	60
Kudrow (1980)	23	495
Manzoni et al. (1983)	12	180
Andersson (1985)	6	127
Total	47	1182

From Russell (32).

M.B. Russell: Department of Neurology, Glostrup Hospital, University of Copenhagen, DK-2600 Glostrup, Copenhagen, Denmark.

physician. Studies specifying the number of probands and affected first-degree relatives are more informative. Table 1 shows that 47 first-degree relatives were reported to be affected by 1,182 probands (1,4,9–12,17,20,22, 30,37,42). Because cluster headache occurs in about 1 of 1,500 (7), with a male-to-female ratio of 5.4:1 (32), the frequent positive family history suggests an increased familial risk of cluster headache, even though each family had numerous first-degree relatives.

GENETIC EPIDEMIOLOGIC SURVEYS

Two family studies of cluster headache provide more complete information about the relatives. A Danish genetic epidemiologic survey included 370 probands from a neurologic clinic and two departments of neurology (34,35). The probands all had a positive family history, and all possibly affected relatives alive were interviewed by a neurological resident. The probands and the closest relatives were interviewed about possibly affected deceased relatives. Compared with the general population, first-degree relatives had a 14.1-fold significantly increased risk of cluster headache after standardization for age and gender. Second-degree relatives had a 2.3-fold significantly increased risk of cluster headache (Fig. 1). The population relative risk was not influenced by generation or by gender of the probands. An American survey included 300 mainly Caucasian probands from a clinic population (17). The probands reported on their possibly affected first-degree relatives, but the diagnosis was not confirmed by interview. Compared with the general population, first- degree relatives had a 45.6-fold significantly increased risk of cluster headache after standardization for gender. Both the Dan-

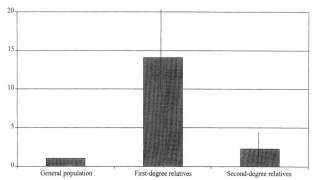

FIG. 1. Age and gender standardized risk of cluster headache among first- and second-degree relatives of probands with cluster headache relative to the population risk. The vertical lines represent the 95% confidence intervals.

ish and the American survey selected probands from clinic populations, which could affect the representativeness of the study population (3); however, most likely the manner of selection would have only minor significance: 92% (24 of 26) of affected relatives alive had at some time consulted a physician or a neurologist or both because of cluster headache (35). This rate is much higher rate than that found among migraineurs (56%) and tension-type headache sufferers (16%) (28). The familial occurrence of cluster headache in the Danish survey may be slightly underestimated because probands may fail to report some affected relatives. The American survey most likely overestimates the familial occurrence of cluster headache because the diagnosis was not confirmed by a interview of the possibly affected first-degree relatives (35). The significantly increased familial risk of cluster headache strongly suggests a genetic cause for cluster headache. Theoretically, a shared environment can produce relative risks of the magnitude observed for cluster headache only under extreme conditions (15).

TWIN CASE REPORTS

Cluster headache was reported in five pairs of monozygotic twins (6,29,40). All these twin pairs were concordant for cluster headache, supporting the importance of genetic factors, although publication itself introduces selection bias (23).

GENETIC HETEROGENEITY

A Danish family study analyzed the clinical intrafamilial and interfamilial variability of cluster headache in 31 men and 13 women from 18 families (33). Distinctive patterns of symptoms were found in three families. Two probands with chronic cluster headache unremitting from onset each had a male relative who experienced episodic cluster headache with up to eight attacks per day. A third proband had episodic cluster headache, and the son had chronic cluster headache evolving from episodic headache. Children had a significantly lower age of onset than parents (p = 0.018), which might be anticipated. This reseult probably is biased because children are one generation younger than parents, and therefore only children with a relatively early onset were included in the analysis. Another family with cluster headache in three generations is suggestive of anticipation; in this family, the age of onset declined and symptoms worsened in each successive generation (41). Episodic cluster headache and chronic cluster headache unremitting from onset may change over the years, and different forms of cluster headache may occur within the same family (8,13,21, 24,31,33,41), suggesting a common etiology of the three forms of cluster headache. In one family the proband lacked autonomic symptoms, whereas the second-degree relative had autonomic symptoms. A common etiology of cluster headache-like disorder without autonomic symptoms and cluster headache is likely (35). Cluster headache was associated with primary hyperlipidaemia in one family (27), possibly caused by the linkage of two genes.

TABLE 2. *Results of complex segregation analysis for cluster headache*

Model	Heritability	Gene Z	Displacement between two homozygous frequency	Degree of means	$-2 \times 1nL +$ dominance	constant
Sporadic	0^a	—	0	—	—	−140.90
Multifactorial	0.61	1	0	—	—	−222.15
Multifactorial with generational difference	0.55	1.7	0	—	—	−222.84
Recessive major locus	0^a	1	1.83×10^{-2}	2.85	0^a	−217.05
Additive major locus	0^a	1	7.21×10^{-5}	5.09	0.5^a	−228.39
Dominant major locus	0^a	1	7.09×10^{-5}	2.55	1^a	−228.38

[a]Z parameter that takes intergenerational differences in heritability into account, 1nL, natural logarithm of the likelihood, and fixed parameter.

Reproduced from Russell et al. (36).

TABLE 3. *Penetrance and contribution of the major dominant locus for the different gender and age group of cluster headache*[a]

Gender	Age (yr)	P(disease|genotype) AA' or A'A'	P(genotype|disease) AA	P(genotype|disease) AA' or A'A'
Men	0–19	0.17	0.91	0.09
	20–39	0.30	0.96	0.04
	40–59	0.34	0.97	0.03
	≥60	0.34	0.97	0.03
Women	0–19	0.10	0.82	0.18
	20–39	0.17	0.90	0.10
	40–59	0.21	0.93	0.07
	≥60	0.21	0.93	0.07

[a]The major locus is assumed to have two alleles, A and A', producing three genotypes AA, AA', A'A'.
From Russell et al. (37).

At present, genetic heterogeneity of cluster headache is not likely on clinical grounds.

MODE OF INHERITANCE

A complex segregation analysis of cluster headache (Table 2) resulted in the sporadic model, with no family resemblance and a poor fit compared with the multifactorial model (36). Among the three models that incorporated a major locus, the *recessive* model did not explain the observed segregation pattern as well as the *additive* and *dominant* models did. The additive and dominant models were equally likely with corresponding estimated parameters, a result of the low frequency of the susceptibility allele and the resulting low probability that any of the affected patients were homozygous. No families had both parents affected. Table 3 shows the characteristics of the major dominant locus. The penetrance was lower in women than in men. The gene is responsible for the cluster headache phenotype in 3% to 4% of men and in 7% to 10% of women. The results suggest that an autosomal dominant gene has a role in some families with cluster headache.

MOLECULAR GENETIC STUDIES

A point mutation in mitochondrial transfer RNA$^{Leu(UUR)}$ gene at nucleotide pair 3243 was reported in a Japanese man with cluster headache and no family history of mitochondrial myopathy, encephalopathy, lactic acidosis, and strokelike episodes (MELAS syndrome) or cluster headache (40). The failure to detect the mutation in Italian subjects excludes a significant role in the etiology of cluster headache in Italy (6). Whether it is important in the etiology of cluster headache in Japanese subjects remains uncertain and will require detection of the point mutation in other Japanese subjects who have cluster headaches or in familial cases of cluster headache. Multiple deletions of mitochondrial DNA was reported in a Japanese man with cluster headache and chronic progressive external ophthalmoplegia (CPEO) (26). This patient did not fulfil the International Headache Society criteria for cluster headache, however, because the duration of attacks was 7 to 8 hours (14). As mentioned, to conclude that a causal relationship exists between multiple deletions of mitochrondrial DNA and cluster headache, it is necessary to study more than one case of such an association. Furthermore, an increased frequency of cluster headache would be expected among persons with CPEO.

REFERENCES

1. Andersson PG. Migraine in patients with cluster headache. *Cephalalgia* 1985;5:11–16.
2. Balla JI, Walton JN. Periodic migrainous neuralgia. *Br Med J* 1964; 1:219–221.
3. Berkson J. Limitations of the application of fourfold table analysis to hospital data. *Biometrics* 1947;2:47–53.
4. Bickerstaff ER. The periodic migrainous neuralgia of Wilfred Harris. *Lancet* 1959;1:1069–1071.
5. Cortelli P, Zacchini A, Barboni P, Malpassi P, Carelli V, Montagne P. Lack of association between mitochondrial tRNA (Leu(UUR)) point mutation and cluster headache [Letter]. *Lancet* 1995;345:1120–1121.
6. Couturier EG, Hering R, Steiner TJ. The first report of cluster headache in identical twins. *Neurology* 1991;41:761.
7. D'Alessandro R, Benassi G, Lenzi PL, et al. Epidemiology of headache in the Republic of San Marino. *J Neurol Neurosurg Psychiatry* 1988; 51:21–27.
8. D'Amico D, Leone M, Moschiano F, Bussone G. Familial cluster headache: report of three families. *Headache* 1996;36:41–43.
9. Duvoisin RC, Parker GW, Kenoyer WL. The cluster headache. *Arch Intern Med* 1961;108:111–116.
10. Eadie MJ, Sutherland JM. Migrainous neuralgia. *Med J Aust* 1966;1: 1053–1057.
11. Ekbom KA. Ergotamine tartrate orally in Horton's "histaminic cephalgia" (also called Harris's "ciliary neuralgia"). *Acta Psychiatr Neurol Scand* 1947;46:105–113.
12. Ekbom K. A clinical comparison of cluster headache and migraine. *Acta Neurol Scand* 1970;46:1–48.
13. Ekbom K. Evaluation of clinical criteria for cluster headache with special reference to the classification of the International Headache Society. *Cephalalgia* 1990;10:195–197.
14. Headache Classification Committee of the International Headache Society. Classification and diagnostic criteria for headache disorders, cranial neuralgias and facial pain. *Cephalalgia* 1988;8:1–96.
15. Khoury MJ, Beaty TH, Liang K-Y. Can familial aggregation of disease be explained by familial aggregation of environmental risk factors? *Am J Epidemiol* 1988;127:674–683.
16. Kudrow L. *Cluster headache mechanisms and management.* Oxford: Oxford University Press, 1980.
17. Kudrow L, Kudrow DB. Inheritance of cluster headache and its possible link to migraine. *Headache* 1994;34:400–407.
18. Kunkle EC, Pfeiffer Jr JB, Wilhoit WM, Hamrick Jr LW. Recurrent brief headache in "cluster" pattern. *Transactions of the American Neurological Association* 1952;77:240–243.
19. Lance JW, Anthony M. Migrainous neuralgia or cluster headache? *J Neurol Sci* 1971;13:401–414.
20. Maendly R, Mumenthaler M, Martinez Lage JM. Die Erythroprosopalgie. Übersicht mit Einschluss 224 eigener Beobachtungen. *Dtsch Med Wochenschr* 1982;107:186–191.
21. Manzoni GC, Micieli G, Granella F, Tassorelli C, Zanferrari C, Cavallini A. Cluster headache—course over ten years in 189 patients. *Cephalalgia* 1991;11:169–174.

22. Manzoni GC, Terzano MG, Bono G, Micieli G, Martucci N, Nappi G. Cluster headache—clinical findings in 180 patients. *Cephalalgia* 1983;3:21–30.

23. Motulsky AG. Biased ascertainment and the natural history of diseases. *N Engl J Med* 1978;298:1196–1197.

24. Nappi G, Micieli G, Cavallini A, Zanferrari C, Sandrini G, Manzoni GC. Accompanying symptoms of cluster attacks: their relevance to the diagnostic criteria. *Cephalalgia* 1992;12:165–168.

25. Nieman EA, Hurwitz LJ. Ocular sympathetic palsy in periodic migrainous neuralgia. *J Neurol Neurosurg Psychiatry* 1961;24:369–373.

26. Odawara M, Tamaoka A, Mizusawa H, Yamashita K. A case of cluster headache associated with mitochondrial DNA deletions [Letter]. *Muscle Nerve* 1997;20:394–395.

27. Olesen J. Cluster headache associated with primary hyperlipidemia. *Acta Neurol Scand* 1977;56:461–464.

28. Rasmussen BK, Jensen R, Olesen J. Impact of headache on sickness absence and utilisation of medical services: a Danish population study. *J Epidemiol Community Health* 1992;46:443–446.

29. Roberge C, Bouchard JP, Simard D, Gagne R. Cluster headache in twins. *Neurology* 1992;42:1255–1256.

30. Robinson BW. Histaminic cephalalgia. *Medicine (Baltimore)* 1958;37:161–180.

31. Russell D. Cluster headache: severity and temporal profiles of attacks and patient activity prior to and during attacks. *Cephalalgia* 1981;1:209–216.

32. Russell MB. Genetic epidemiology of migraine and cluster headache. *Cephalalgia* 1997;17:683–701.

33. Russell MB, Andersson PG. Clinical intra- and interfamilial variability of cluster headache. *Eur J Neurol* 1995;1:253–257.

34. Russell MB, Andersson PG, Thomsen LL. Familial occurrence of cluster headache. *Genet Epidemiol* 1994;11:305–306 (abst).

35. Russell MB, Andersson PG, Thomsen LL. Familial occurrence of cluster headache. *J Neurol Neurosurg Psychiatry* 1995;58:341–343.

36. Russell MB, Andersson PG, Thomsen LL, Iselius L. Cluster headache is an autosomal dominantly inherited disorder in some families: a complex segregation analysis. *J Med Genet* 1995;32:954–956.

37. Schiller F. Prophylactic and other treatment for "histaminic," "cluster," or "limited" variant of migraine. *JAMA* 1960;173:1907–1911.

38. Sørensen SA, Araki S. Genetics. In: Olesen J, Tfelt-Hansen P, Welch KMA, eds. *The headaches.* New York: Raven Press, 1993:21–27.

39. Shimomura T, Kitano A, Marukawa H, et al. Point mutation in platelet mitochondrial tRNA$^{(Leu(UUR))}$ in patient with cluster headache [letter; comment]. *Lancet* 1994;27:625.

40. Sjaastad O, Shen JM, Stovner LJ, Elsas T. Cluster headache in identical twins. *Headache* 1993;33:214–217.

41. Spierings EL, Vincent AJ. Familial cluster headache: occurrence in three generations. *Neurology* 1992;42:1399–1400.

42. Symonds C. A particular variety of headache. *Brain* 1956;79:217–232.

The Headaches, Second Edition,
edited by J. Olesen, P. Tfelt-Hansen, and K.M.A. Welch.
Lippincott Williams & Wilkins, Philadelphia © 2000.

Tension-Type Headache, Cluster Headache, and Miscellaneous Primary Headaches

CHAPTER 91

Anatomy and Pathology of Cluster Headache

Jan Erik Hardebo and Norihiro Suzuki

The location of maximal pain in cluster headache (CH) is strikingly similar in almost every sufferer: it is felt deep in or behind the orbit on one side. The signs of disturbed autonomic function in the eye, nose, and facial skin are also closely linked to the pain, both spatially and temporally. This points to deep orbital or retroorbital structures as being affected in the disease. The tendency to develop CH on the other half of the pace is 200 times higher than for an individual to develop the disease at all (38). This indicates that a structure with anatomic connections over the midline is involved.

Cluster headache persists, and may also arise, after ipsilateral enucleation (22). Likewise, CH may even arise after ipsilateral orbital exenteration (6,27). This demonstrates that CH may arise after an operation in this area but that the pain of CH does not originate in the eye, and that intact structures in the orbit are not necessary for the formation of attacks. Thus, pain appears to originate from retroorbital structures.

PATHOLOGY OF IDIOPATHIC CASES

Epidemiologic studies reveal a marked correlation between CH and prior head trauma (19,26,45). Narrow nasal passages, such as a deviated nasal septum, are often found on the painful side in CH sufferers (3,24,29). Surgical resections in this area, to eliminate narrow conditions, are sometimes beneficial (3). Craniometric measures suggest narrowness of the cavernous sinus region in

CH (1). These findings may represent constitutional predisposing factors for CH. Tentatively, an obstructed drainage from ethmoidal sinuses and a disturbed venous outflow from deep nasal and orbital structures may facilitate the establishment of upper airway infections in these deeper structures.

Orbital phlebography has demonstrated signs suggestive of an obliterating process in the superior ophthalmic vein and cavernous sinus during periods of CH, particularly on the painful side (Fig. 1) (11,12). Likewise, during periods of CH an uptake of gallium, indicative of inflammation, is found in this area (7), as are inflammatory signs in cerebrospinal fluid and blood (10,16). The signs fade when the period is over (7,10). No pathologic-anatomic study of these vessels has been conducted, but the inflammatory signs indicate that the obliterating process may be a venous vasculitis. Investigations with magnetic resonance imaging of the cavernous sinus region outside of CH attacks has not revealed any pathologic changes (39).

PATHOLOGY OF SYMPTOMATIC CASES

Several symptomatic cases have been described in which CH-like attacks have evolved secondary to the growth of an intracranial expansive process, ipsilaterally or in the midline: orbitosphenoidal aspergillus infection (17), parasellar meningioma (10), adenoma of the pituitary gland (10,44), calcified lesion in the region of the third ventricle (31), aneurysm of the anterior communicating artery (9), dilated ipsilateral and aneurysmatic contralateral internal carotid artery (ICA) (9), epidermoid tumor in the clivus expanding rostrally to the suprasellar cistern (23), large arteriovenous malforma-

J.E. Hardebo: Neurologic Institution, University Hospital of Lund, S-22185 Lund, Sweden.

N. Suzuki: Department of Neurology, Kitasato University, Sagamihara, Kanagawa 228-8555, Japan.

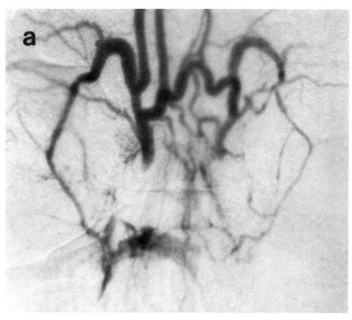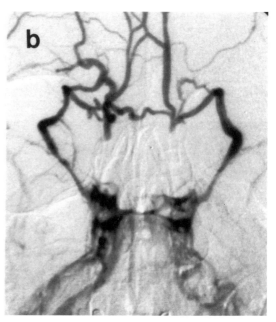

FIG. 1. a: Orbital phlebogram in a patient with episodic cluster headache, showing narrowing of the superior ophthalmic vein and partial occlusion of the cavernous sinus, most evident on the painful side (right side of photo). **b:** Normal phlebogram for comparison. Reproduced from Hannerz et al. (12).

tions in the ipsilateral frontal, temporal, parietotemporal or occipital lobes (8,18,25,30), tentorium cerebelli meningioma (42), and upper cervical meningioma (22). Thus, when restricted to a small area, most of these processes are located near the midline in the cavernous sinus region.

THE CAVERNOUS SINUS REGION: ANATOMIC CONSIDERATIONS

To understand why a process in the cavernous sinus region can cause CH, with accompanying symptoms indicative of sympathetic hypofunction and parasympathetic hyperfunction, a detailed knowledge about the local anatomy including pathways of autonomic and sensory pain fibers is important.

Pharmacologic tests have shown that during the period of attacks most CH sufferers have a partial lesion of the sympathetic fibers to the eye and forehead skin, ipsilateral to pain and sometimes bilateral, as well as disturbed melatonin production, indicative of a sympathetic lesion of fibers to the epiphysis. The sympathetic fibers to the internal carotid artery (ICA) tree, dural sinuses and veins, eye, and epiphysis leave the superior cervical ganglion at the internal carotid nerve to run along the surface of ICA in the neck and through the carotid canal. Branches form a delicate plexus to innervate the ICA wall and its branches as the artery becomes intracranial, whereas a further branching of the internal carotid nerve takes place after the ICA has entered the cavernous sinus region. Here branches are issued to (a) the ophthalmic nerve via

a short course with the abducent nerve to reach the eye and forehead skin (Fig. 2) (32), (b) the oculomotor nerve to reach the smooth muscle portion of the levator palpebrae muscle, (c) the tentorial nerve to reach the epiphysis and the dural sinuses and veins (21,35,41), and probably (d) the cavernous sinus wall and its tributary superior ophthalmic vein (Fig. 2). A tentative explanation for the sympathetic hypofunction in CH is that the presumed vasculitis in the cavernous sinus lesions the sympathetic fibers on their course through the region.

Internal carotid artery dissection as well as carotid thrombendarterectomy often lesions the sympathetic fibers in the ICA wall on their course to the ICA vascular tree and to the ocular region. CH can start in connection with an ICA dissection (34). CH-like attacks are sometimes present during the first few weeks after carotid thrombendarterectomy (5). CH can reappear after several years in silence following carotid thrombendarterectomy (2). These observations further emphasize that a disturbed local sympathetic nerve function is of crucial importance for developing CH.

Conjunctival injection, lacrimation, rhinorrhea, and nasal congestion on the painful side during attacks may indicate parasympathetic hyperfunction. Sphenopalatine ganglion blockade is sometimes beneficial in CH (29,37). Parasympathetic fibers to the intracranial ICA and its branches reach the ICA wall through (a) the deep petrosal nerve from a ganglion along the greater superficial petrosal nerve and (b) rami orbitales from the sphenopalatine ganglion and aberrant microganglia along this pathway, which runs through the supraorbital fissure to the

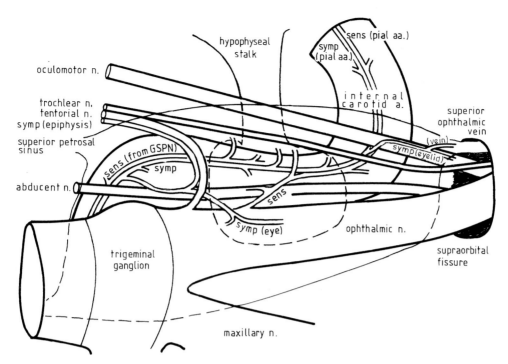

FIG. 2. Schematic illustration of sympathetic *(symp)* and sensory *(sens)* nervous pathways through the cavernous sinus region on the right side from a lateral aspect. Limits of the cavernous sinus are indicated together with its extensions into the superior ophthalmic vein and the superior and inferior petrosal sinuses. The location of the hypophysis is shown. Within the connective tissue between the vessels forming the cavernous sinus, as well as on the surface of the throughpassing internal carotid artery, the sympathetic and sensory fibers converge with parasympathetic fibers from the greater superficial petrosal nerve *(GSPN)* and sphenopalatine ganglion (not shown). Thereafter the various branches accompany the ophthalmic, abducent, trochlear, and oculomotor nerves and the internal carotid artery to their targets. An inflammatory process, presumed to be present during CH period in the walls of the cavernous sinus and the superior ophthalmic vein, causes a lesion of the throughpassing sympathetic fibers and possibly also of pain fibers from the ophthalmic trigeminal division.

cavernous region, as studied in monkeys and humans (14, 15,36,40).

Pain is intense in CH and usually located within the distribution area of the ophthalmic division of the trigeminal nerve. The pain threshold is reduced within this area during CH periods (13). Sensory fibers to the intracranial ICA and its branches in humans are mainly derived from the ophthalmic trigeminal division, leaving the ophthalmic trunk shortly distal to the ganglion and running a short course through the cavernous sinus region (40). Some of the fibers join and follow the abducent nerve to innervate the basilar artery and branches (see Fig. 2) (36,40). In monkeys a contribution from the maxillary division has been found, as has an aberrant trigeminal microganglia in the cavernous region (36). The greater superficial petrosal nerve also contributes with sensory fibers to the ICA tree in humans and monkeys (see Fig. 2) (14,40).

It is highly likely that the trigeminal and facial sensory fibers also innervate the walls of the cavernous sinus. Other dural sinuses are densely innervated by pain fibers from the tentorial nerve (20,28). The sympathetic, para-

sympathetic, and sensory fibers gather as a plexus in the connective tissue of the cavernous sinus region before they follow each other to the various destinations (14,35, 36,40). The carotid canal segment of ICA in monkeys is not equipped with pain fibers (36), but mechanoreceptors have been identified in this segment in humans (4).

REFERENCES

1. Áfra J, Proietti-Cecchini A, Schoenen J. Craniometric measures suggest narrowness of the cavernous sinus region in cluster headache. Cephalalgia 1997;7:360.
2. Björne A, Hindfelt B, Havelius U. Recurrence of cluster headache after carotid thrombendarterectomy. *Headache* 1994;34:230–233.
3. Bonaccorsi P. Revaluation of ethmoido-sphenectomy in some cephalalgic syndromes. *Res Clin Stud Headache* 1972;3:343–377.
4. Cochet B. Contribution à l etude du plexus tympanique. *Arch Anat Histol Embryol* 1967;50:1–46.
5. De Marinis M, Zaccaria A, Faraglia V, Fiorani P, Maira G, Agnoli A. Post-endarterectomy headache and the role of the oculosympathetic system. *J Neurol Neurosurg Psychiatry* 1991;54:314–317.
6. Evers S, Sörös P, Brilla R, Gerding H, Husstedt IW. Cluster headache after orbital exenteration. *Cephalalgia* 1997;17:680–682.
7. Gawel MJ, Krajewski A, Luo YM, Ichise M. The cluster diathesis. *Headache* 1990;30:652–655.
8. Gawel MJ, Willinsky RA, Krajewksi A. Reversal of cluster headache

side following treatment of arteriovenous malformation. *Headache* 1989;29:453–454.

9. Greve E, Mai J. Cluster headache-lika headaches: a symptomatic feature? *Cephalalgia* 1988;8:79–82.

10. Hannerz J. A case of parasellar meningioma mimicking cluster headache. *Cephalalgia* 1989;9:265–269.

11. Hannerz J. Orbital phlebography and signs of inflammation in episodic and chronic cluster headache. *Headache* 1991;31:540–542.

12. Hannerz J, Ericson K, Bergstrand G. Orbital phlebography in patients with cluster headache. *Cephalalgia* 1987;7:207–211.

13. Hardebo JE. How cluster headache is explained as an intracavernous inflammatory process lesioning sympathetic fibers. *Headache* 1994; 34:125–131.

14. Hardebo JE, Arbab MAR, Suzuki N, Svendgaard NA. Origins and pathways of cerebrovascular parasympathetic and sensory nerves in monkey. *Stroke* 1991;22:331–342.

15. Hardebo JE, Arbab MAR, Suzuki N, Svendgaard NA. Sensory and parasympathetic innervation by the greater superficial petrosal-Vidian nerve of the internal carotid and maxillary arteries and their branches in monkey. Importance for vascular headache. In: Clifford Rose F, ed. *New advances in headache research 2.* London: Smith-Gordon, 1991: 235–238.

16. Hardebo JE, Ryberg B. CSF findings in cluster headache indicative of inflammatory reaction or disease. *Cephalalgia* 1989;9[Suppl 10]: 301–302.

17. Heidegger S, Mattfeldt T, Rieber A, et al. Orbito-sphenoidal *Aspergillus* infection mimicking cluster headache; a case report. *Cephalalgia* 1997; 17:676–679.

18. Hindfelt B, Olivecrona H. Cerebral arteriovenous malformation and cluster-like headache. *Headache* 1989;31:514–517.

19. Italian Cooperative Study Group on the Epidemiology of Cluster Headache. Case-control study of the epidemiology of cluster headache. I. Etiological factors and associated conditions. *Neuroepidemiology* 1995;14:123–127.

20. Keller JT, Marfurt CF. Peptidergic and serotoninergic innervation of the rat dura mater. *J Comp Neurol* 1991;309:1–20.

21. Kenny GCT. Structural and ultrastructural analysis of the pineal of primates; its innervation. In: Mess B, Rúzsás C, Tima L, Pévet P, eds. *The pineal gland. Current state of pineal research.* Amsterdam: Elsevier, 1985;341–345.

22. Kuritzky A. Cluster headache-like pain caused by an upper cervical meningioma. *Cephalalgia* 1984;4:185–86.

23. Levyman C, Dagua Filho ASP, Volpato MM, Settanni FAP, Lima WC. Epidermoid tumour of the posterior fossa causing multiple facial pain—a case report. *Cephalalgia* 1991;11:33–36.

24. Loisy C. Is cluster headache a disease of endonasal origin? *Cephalalgia* 1985;5[Suppl 3]:280–281.

25. Mani S, Deeter J. Arteriovenous malformation of the brain presenting as a cluster headache—a case report. *Headache* 1982;22:184–185.

26. Manzoni GC, Terzano MG, Bono G, Micieli G, Martucci N, Nappi G. Cluster headache—clinical findings in 180 patients. *Cephalalgia* 1983; 3:21–30.

27. McKinney AS. Cluster headache developing following ipsilateral orbital exenteration. *Headache* 1983;23:305–306.

28. McNaughton FL. The innervation of the intracranial blood vessels and dural sinuses. *Assoc Res Nerv Ment Dis Proc* 1937;18:178–200.

29. Meyer JS, Binns PM, Ericsson AD, Vulpe M. Sphenopalatine ganglionectomy for cluster headache. *Arch Otolaryngol* 1970;92: 475–484.

30. Molins A, López M, Codina A, Titus F. Cefalea agregada (cluster headache) sintomática? A propósito de quatro observaciones. *Med Clin (Barc)* 1989;92:181–183.

31. Narbone MC, D'Amico D, Di Maria F, Arena MG, Longo M. Cluster-like headache and a median intracranial calcified lesion: case report. *Headache* 1991;31:684–685.

32. Parkinson D. Further observations on the sympathetic pathways to the pupil. Anat Rec 1988;220:108–109.

33. Rogado AZ, Graham JR. Through a glass darkly. *Headache* 1979; 19:58–62.

34. Rosebraugh CJ, Griebel DJ, DiPette DJ. A case report of carotid artery dissection presenting as cluster headache. *Am J Med* 1997;102: 418–419.

35. Ruskell GL. The tentorial nerve in monkeys is a branch of the cavernous plexus. *J Anat* 1988;157:67–77.

36. Ruskell GL, Simons T. Trigeminal nerve pathways to the cerebral arteries in monkeys. *J Anat* 1987;155:23–27.

37. Sanders M, Zuurmond WWA. Efficacy of sphenopalatine ganglion blockade in 66 patients suffering from cluster headache: a 12- to 70-month follow-up evaluation. *J Neurosurg* 1997;87:876–880.

38. Sjaastad O. Cluster headache: the possible significance of midline structures. *Cephalalgia* 1988;8:229–236.

39. Sjaastad O, Rinck P. Cluster headache: MRI studies of the cavernous sinus and the base of the brain. *Headache* 1990;30:350–351.

40. Suzuki N, Hardebo JE. Anatomical basis for a parasympathetic and sensory innervation of the intracranial segment of the internal carotid artery in man. *J Neurol Sci* 1991;104:19–31

41. Tamamaki N, Nojyo Y. Intracranial trajectories of sympathetic nerve fibers originating in the superior cervical ganglion in the rat: WGA-HRP anterograde labeling study. *Brain Res* 987;437:387–392.

42. Taub E, Argoff CE, Winterkorn JMS, Milhorat TH. Resolution of chronic cluster headache after resection of a tentorial meningioma: case report. *Neurosurgery* 1995;37:319–321.

43. Testa D, Frediani F, Bussone G. Cluster headache-like syndrome due to an arteriovenous malformation. *Headache* 1988;28:36–38.

44. Tfelt-Hansen P, Paulson OB, Krabbe AA. Invasive adenoma of the pituitary gland and chronic migrainous neuralgia. A rare coincidence or a causal relationship? *Cephalalgia* 1982;2:25–28.

45. Turkewitz LJ, Wirth O, Dawson GA, Casaly JS. Cluster headache following head injury: a case report and review of the literature. *Headache* 1992;32:504–506.

The Headaches, Second Edition,
edited by J. Olesen, P. Tfelt-Hansen, and K.M.A. Welch.
Lippincott Williams & Wilkins, Philadelphia © 2000.

Tension-Type Headache, Cluster Headache, and Miscellaneous Primary Headaches

CHAPTER 92

Biochemistry, Circannual and Circadian Rhythms, Endocrinology, and Immunology of Cluster Headache

Elisabet Waldenlind and Gennaro Bussone

BIOCHEMISTRY

Histamine and Mast Cells

Horton (55) suggested that cluster headache was associated with an unusual histamine sensitivity. The histamine levels have been reported to be higher during than between attacks in whole blood (3) but not in urine (122). Increased numbers of mast cells, the main source of histamine, have been found in skin biopsy specimens from the painful temporal region both during and between cluster periods (5,113) but also from the pain-free side compared with control individuals. The mast cells were typically localized perivascularly, but in cluster headache they were also found near cutaneous nerves (84). Increased degranulation, possibly as the response of an axon reflex, both during and between cluster periods (5), a few hours after cluster attacks (59), and between attacks (24), as well as a normal degree of degranulation (18,64), has been observed. In basophils from cluster patients, increased degranulation after nitroglycerin challenge *in vitro* has been shown, a response that was normalized after incubation with lithium solution (115).

Prostaglandins and Leukotrienes

Prostaglandins, leukotrienes, and other eicosanoids have been proposed as possible mediators in the pathogenesis of vascular headache. Prostaglandins are local hormones that are produced at their site of action and have vasoactive properties. Although a tendency toward higher serum levels of prostaglandin E_2-like substances during cluster attacks compared with basal values has been shown (104), which might be consistent with vasodilation, nonsteroidal antiinflammatory drugs generally have no therapeutic effect in cluster headache and prostaglandins are not believed to be of primary pathogenetic importance. The leukotriene B_4 (LTB_4) has the ability to induce hyperalgesia and to enhance vascular permeability, but leukotrienes also have been reported to reduce nociceptive responses to bradykinins (119). During attacks, increased plasma levels of LTB_4 analyzed by radioimmunoassay have been reported compared with the pain-free state (120), but with high-performance liquid chromatography the concentration of leukotrienes in cluster patients during and between attacks was below the detection limit of the method (68). During remission, the induced release of LTB_4 and LTC_4 from circulating basophils was significantly reduced (93) in cluster headache patients compared with healthy controls.

Metenkephalin and β-endorphin

Plasma, cerebrospinal fluid (CSF), and platelet concentrations of metenkephalin-like (MET) and β-endor-

E. Waldenlind: Department of Neurology, Karolinska Institute, and Department of Neurology, Huddinge University Hospital, S-14186 Huddinge, Sweden.

G. Bussone: Third Department of Clinical Neurology, Istituto Nazionale Neurologico "Carlo Besta," 20133 Milan, Italy.

phin–like activities have been studied in patients during different phases of cluster headache and in controls. CSF MET has been reported to be lower during (2,50,51) and between (51) attacks of cluster headache or not to differ (135) compared with control patients. A decrease of CSF MET during attacks may reflect altered antinociceptive functions in cluster headache. Low levels of CSF MET are probably not caused by increased degradation because the activities of enkephalinase and angiotensin-converting enzyme (ACE) in CSF at the lumbar level were not altered in cluster headache patients compared with controls (123). In chronic cluster headache plasma MET levels have been found to be lower during and after attacks than before the attack (98). In episodic cases higher levels of MET in plasma have been reported during attacks (36,51), and higher (51) or normal levels were found between attacks and during remission (36). The increase in plasma MET during pain may be secondary to sympathetic activation because MET in circulation is derived mainly from the adrenals, where it is stored with catecholamines. It also may be derived from neutrophils, in which a decrease of MET has been observed parallel to the increase in plasma (37).

As regards β-endorphin concentrations in CSF at the lumbar level, no alterations have been found in samples obtained during and between attacks of cluster headache (51). In plasma, β-endorphin has been reported to be increased during attacks (4) or normal (51) but without a normal circadian rhythmicity in several subjects (41,102). Beta-endorphin in plasma is released mainly from the pituitary gland, where it is synthesized from the same precursor as adrenocorticotropin (ACTH) and β-lipotropin. Lymphocytic β-endorphin is reviewed later in this chapter.

Neuropeptides

Much attention has been focused on the innervation of the cranial vasculature (see Chapter 9). In short, the large intra- and extracerebral vessels including the venous sinuses are supplied by the trigeminal nerve marked by calcitonin gene–related peptide (CGRP), substance P, and neurokinin A (NKA); sympathetic nerve fibers marked by norepinephrine (NE), neuropeptide Y (NPY), and adenosine triphosphate (ATP); and parasympathetic nerve fibers marked by acetylcholine, vasointestinal peptide (VIP), and nitric oxide. The primary afferents of the trigeminal nerve not only transmit nociceptive information but also have efferent properties with the ability to dilate blood vessels, cause extravasation, and release from mast cells.

Local release of neuropeptides from the ipsilateral external jugular vein has been studied in cluster headache. During spontaneous cluster headache attacks CGRP and VIP levels were elevated, whereas there were no changes in NPY or substance P compared with a

matched control group (25,46). The CGRP concentrations decreased to normal values within 15 minutes after administration of sumatriptan and oxygen as treatment but remained elevated after pethidine, although there was pain relief. The results indicate that sumatriptan, oxygen, and pethidin relieve pain by different mechanisms. The plasma levels of CGRP also have been reported to be elevated between cluster attacks and to be further increased during nitroglycerin-induced attacks but not by nitroglycerin per se (Fig. 1) (32,33) (see also Chapter 95).

Substance P can induce pain when combined with bradykinin, serotonin, or prostaglandins that lower the pain threshold. Activation of substance P fibers of trigeminal or facial nerve origin might explain the pain and the autonomous signs of cluster headache and would be expected to cause an increase of CSF substance P levels, but in samples of spinal fluid from the lumbar level the substance P concentration has been reported to be normal both during (51,121) and between (43,51) attacks.

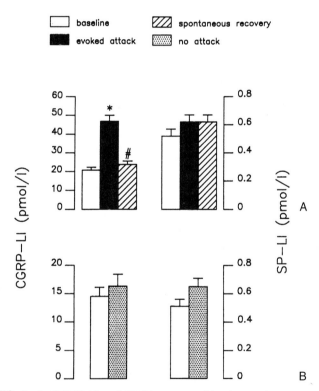

FIG. 1. A: CCRP-LI and SP-LI measured in plasma from the external jugular vein of 12 cluster patients in an active period before nitroglycerin (*open columns*), at the peak of the provoked headache (*solid columns*), and after spontaneous remission (*dashed columns*). **B:** CCRP-LI and SP-LI measured in plasma from the external jugular vein of 12 cluster patients in remission period before (*open columns*) and 40 minutes after (*dotted columns*) nitroglycerin. The columns denote the means ± SEM. Statistical significance (Duncan's test): *$p < 0.01$ versus values before nitroglycerin and #$p < 0.01$ versus values at the peak of the attack. Reprinted with permission from ref. 33.

In plasma, substance P is reported to be decreased and its degrading enzyme enkephalinase to be increased during cluster attacks (121). In saliva, CGRP, VIP, and substance P concentrations have been found to be higher during than between attacks, and CGRP and VIP were higher both during and between attacks compared with controls (107).

Somatostatin is an inhibitory transmitter peptide found in sympathetic ganglia and in some primary afferent neurons, where it may inhibit substance P release from the C fibers. Somatostatin concentrations in plasma have been shown to be lower during (121) and between (13,121) cluster attacks as well as during remission (13) compared with controls. An injection of somatostatin appeared to relieve cluster headache pain (121). Somatostatin has venoconstrictive properties (13), which may be of importance for its therapeutic effect. Due to rapid tachyphylaxis, somatostatin is not likely to become a choice for cluster headache treatment.

In cluster headache there is an increased morbidity from peptic ulcer and a marked increase of gastric acid secretion during the attack phase. *Gastrin* levels in plasma have been studied in men between and during cluster periods. When compared with healthy controls, the gastrin levels were significantly higher in cluster headache patients free of peptic ulcer symptoms (105).

Vasopressin has been shown to increase during cluster headache attacks without any concomitant variation of plasma osmolality (40). Pain is one of several inducers of vasopressin secretion via catecholaminergic afferents from the brainstem to the hypothalamus. Serotonin also may trigger vasopressin release. As a potent vasoconstrictor, the increase of vasopressin has been suggested to counteract the vasodilatation associated with the attack (40).

Monoamines

Spontaneous cluster attacks often seem to be preceded by a shift of vegetative tone, indicative of increased parasympathetic or decreased sympathetic activity as during relaxation after meals or the working day or in relation to rapid eye movement (REM) sleep. Physical exercise has been shown to reduce the pain of induced attacks, and NE infusion also appeared to alleviate the pain (28). Nitroglycerin-induced attacks seemed to occur after an initial increase of plasma NE had reversed to basal values (57). A further increase in NE occurred during both spontaneous and induced attacks, maybe as a response to vasodilation. Because posture affects NE levels, the evaluation of results during attacks may be difficult (85). When examined before and after 5 minutes of standing, plasma concentrations of NE and epinephrine did not differ between patients in remission and controls, indicating normal postural responses (56). During cluster period, contradictory results with both increased plasma

concentrations of conjugated NE and epinephrine in plasma (83) and decreased concentrations of NE in the morning and at night in comparison with healthy controls were reported (126). The same researchers also found lowered CSF concentrations of vanillyl mandelic acid, homovanillic acid, 5-hydroxyindoleacetic acid, and NE in the active period (126).

Monoamine oxidase (MAO) activity in platelets has been documented in several studies to be lowered during and between cluster periods both in men and women, and when smoking habits are considered, but with no further decrease during cluster attacks (99). The decrease in MAO activity was explained by fewer enzyme molecules (127) and lowered Vmax (capacity) with no change in Km (affinity) (133). The enzyme is also more thermostable in cluster headache patients than in controls (133). Because platelet MAO is of the B type, it does not metabolize NE, epinephrine, or serotonin (5-HT), but it may affect these amines indirectly by its decreased ability to catabolize dopamine, tyramine, and other trace amines. MAO is localized in the outer membrane of the mitochondria.

Succinate dehydrogenase (SDH), another membrane-bound mitochondrial enzyme, and the cytoplasmatic enzyme *phenolsulphotransferase M* (PST M) were analyzed in the same platelets as MAO (86). The SDH activity was significantly lowered in cluster headache, whereas the PST M activity did not differ between patients and healthy controls. In the lowest range of MAO there was an inverse correlation between the activities of MAO and PST M, which was interpreted as a possible control mechanism compensating for a deficiency of one enzyme by another enzyme acting on the same substrates, for instance, dopamine and tyramine. Other platelet functions such as release of β-*thromboglobulin* and *platelet factor 4* were decreased during cluster headache attacks, contrasting with migraine, where increased release is known to occur during headache (20). The *fibrinogen-binding properties* of platelets from episodic and chronic cluster patients did not differ from those in controls (63). As regards *5-HT uptake* into platelets, lowered Vmax and lowered Km (132) or no difference (48) in the kinetic parameters were reported in cluster headache patients compared with controls. Factors such as time of the year (90,132) and medication may explain some differences in the results.

Membranes and Phospholipids

Because a number of membrane-bound functions such as MAO B, SDH and PST M enzyme activities and 5-HT uptake in platelets are altered in cluster headache as compared with healthy individuals, it is of interest to examine membrane composition and membrane transduction properties. Therefore, *erythrocyte choline* concentrations were measured in erythrocytes from cluster headache patients and found to be depressed both during and between cluster periods to values about 50% of those found in controls (21), probably reflecting an abnormality in phospholipid metabolism. Thus, the *phosphatidylcholine* (PC) content of erythrocyte membranes, from which choline is derived, is increased, suggesting that the decreased concentration of choline could be explained by decreased PC turnover (23). Lithium treatment is known to increase the choline content of erythrocytes. Accordingly, a 12-week course of lithium treatment normalized the choline content in cluster headache (21), which may be of importance for the prophylactic effect of lithium in cluster headache. Altered receptor-mediated membrane transduction function involving the *adenylate cyclase* and the polyphosphoinositide (PPI) systems also have been demonstrated in cluster headache (22). Adenylate cyclase, which is linked to surface receptors, is dependent on phospholipid constituents of the membranes for its activity. Accordingly, a significantly lower increase of the second messenger cyclic adenosine monophosphate has been shown in lymphocytes from cluster headache patients than from controls after *in vitro* stimulation of high-affinity prostaglandin receptors, and a similar trend was shown after stimulation of β-adrenoceptors (23). The PPI system in platelets stimulated with thrombin has been shown to have enhanced activity in untreated patients and normal activity in lithium-treated patients as compared with controls (22). It has been suggested that the prophylactic effect of lithium could be related to dampening of the activated PPI system in order to balance the reduced adenylate cyclase activity.

Further alterations in phospholipid metabolism involve a decreased ability to incorporate $1\text{-}^{14}C$-arachidonic acid and $1\text{-}^{14}C$-oleic acid into phosphatidylcholine and an increased ability to incorporate these fatty acids into phosphatidylserine and phosphatidylethanolamine, respectively (38,39). This also may affect membrane function because phosphatidylserine is required to bind the cytoplasmatic enzyme protein kinase C to the membrane during transmembrane signaling. Phosphatidylserine is also a source for polyunsaturated fatty acids in the synthesis of prostaglandins and leukotrienes.

Phosphorus magnetic resonance spectroscopy (^{31}P-MRS) is a noninvasive method by which it is possible to measure high-energy phosphates and the efficacy of ATP production. A defect of brain mitochondrial respiration has been shown in cluster headache both during and after a cluster headache period compared with matched healthy volunteers (88,97). ^{31}P-MRS of resting gastrocnemius muscle did not differ between patients and healthy controls, but after exercise phosphocreatin recovery was abnormally slow in the patients. The mechanism responsible for the multisystemic mitochondrial impairment is not known. It is suggested that the altered energy metabolism might render the patients more susceptible to metabolic demands during stressful conditions.

Excitatory Amino Acids

Platelets have been studied because they take up *glutamate* and *aspartate* by an energy-dependent mechanism similar to that occurring in neurons. Glycine levels in platelets were significantly lower in cluster headache patients than in healthy controls, whereas the levels of aspartate and glutamate did not differ (19), contrasting with the findings in migraine with aura, where the concentrations of all three amino acids were increased. There was no difference in glycine levels during and between cluster attacks.

CIRCANNUAL AND CIRCADIAN PERIODICITY OF CLUSTER HEADACHE

The remitting course was clearly described by K.A. Ekbom, Sr. (29), and a seasonal variation was noted by Horton (55). In certain patients cluster periods recur at regular intervals or fixed seasons, a pattern that suggests a relationship to environmental or internal factors such as day length and light intensity (67) or changes in stress (psychological and physical) or activity, which can affect autonomous tone, including vascular regulation. The occurrence of the pain attacks after 1 to 2 hours of sleep, in the early morning, during relaxation periods (91), or with clockwise regularity (27) for at least part of the period are well known phenomena. They suggest a central disturbance of circadian rhythm regulation affecting homeostasis of vascular and autonomic tone, nociception, and the synchronization of internal and environmental temporal clues. According to this paradigm, a cluster period would occur when there is desynchronization of these rhythms and would last as long as the time needed for resynchronization. An alteration in the circadian rhythm of plasma melatonin in cluster headache indicates desynchronization of biological rhythms. Melatonin, the main product of the pineal gland, is a marker of the circadian system. Its endogenous circadian secretory rhythm is driven by an oscillator in the hypothalamic suprachiasmatic nuclei, which are entrained to temporal variations of illumination via a retinohypothalamic norepinephric pathway. In humans plasma melatonin levels are high at night and low during the day.

Reduced 24-hour plasma levels of melatonin, as well as phase shifts (advanced or delayed) in melatonin peaks are observed during the cluster period (14,76–78,131). Stress increases melatonin secretion (134), and because the melatonin levels do not correlate with duration of illness, duration of headache in course, time since last attack, or attack frequency in cluster headache (78), it is unlikely that lowered melatonin levels are due only to pain-induced stress (73).

In a multicenter study, urine melatonin was examined every month for up to 14 months in episodic cluster headache patients (Fig. 2) (129); the 12-month mean levels of

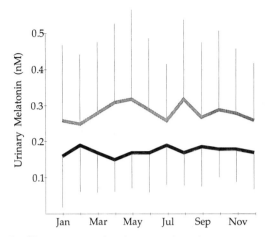

FIG. 2. Chronogram of urinary melatonin concentrations covering 12 months in 29 episodic cluster headache patients (■) and in 29 healthy controls (▨) matched to sex, nationality, and age. The effect of disease was significant ($p < 0.05$) but not the effect of time (ANOVA with repeated measurements; values are means ± SD). Reprinted with permission from ref. 133.

urinary melatonin were significantly lower in patients than controls, and no clear difference was found between cluster and remission periods (133). Similarly, nocturnal urinary excretion of 6-sulphatoxymelatonin, the chief metabolite of melatonin, is reduced in both illness phases (77). In some cluster headache patients in remission period, the circadian melatonin secretion is disrupted (typical rhythm lost). A similar melatonin disruption could also be present during the cluster period, but reduced melatonin levels would mask this. Reduced metabolism and availability of serotonin for melatonin synthesis have been invoked to explain the reduced melatonin in cluster period (131).

Reduced levels of melatonin could play a role in the pathophysiology of cluster headache via several mechanisms: modulation of $GABA_a$ synapses in the central nervous system (7); modulation of the cellular distribution of calcium ions through binding of ^3H-melatonin to calmodulin, thereby affecting the circadian variation of cell activity (6); involvement of melatonin receptors present in the main cerebral arteries (124); modulation of $5\text{-}HT_2$ receptor–mediated neurotransmission (26) (a property shared by the cluster headache prophylactic methysergide); and inhibition of synthesis of prostaglandin E_2 (69), involved in activating sterile perivascular inflammation in the trigeminovascular system. Oral melatonin administration has shown some efficacy as a cluster headache prophylactic (74,75).

Serotonin, a precursor of melatonin, has a circannual variation with respect to platelet uptake (90). Plasma levels of NE and epinephrine show a circadian variation, with peak levels in the morning; this is in part a response to posture and sleep but probably also to a circadian oscillator (85). In healthy individuals, there is also a circadian

rhythm of basal vascular tone due in part or entirely to increased sympathetic vasoconstrictor activity in the morning (109). This has not been studied in cluster headache. Circadian variation in sensitivity to experimentally induced pain in the pericranial muscles (47) as well as of the flexion reflex (R III threshold) has been shown in healthy individuals. The R III threshold is lowest in the early morning and highest around midnight (118), but in cluster headache during cluster period the spontaneous physiologic variation of this threshold is lost, and by cosinor analysis there is no significant circadian rhythm (103). In addition, there is a lack of circadian rhythm of β-endorphin and β-lipotropin levels in blood in cluster headache patients. These phenomena may support the hypothesis of cyclical failure of pain control in cluster headache (101). In chronic cluster headache there is no circadian rhythm of oral temperature or systolic and diastolic blood pressure, and in episodic cases a phase delay of these three variables is reported (103).

ENDOCRINOLOGY AND HORMONAL RHYTHMS

The Hypothalamic-Pituitary-Adrenal Axis: ACTH, Cortisol, β-endorphin, and β-lipotropin

The circadian production of cortisol is altered during cluster periods and in chronic cluster headache (34,131). Moreover, a marked shift in the morning peak (acrophase) of the hormone characterizes these patients (14,101). Similar alterations are found in patients undergoing lithium treatment (15). Hyperactivity of the hypothalamic-pituitary-adrenal (HPA) axis in cluster period is indicated by the finding that 24-hour cortisol production and morning levels are increased (14,77,78,126,131). Increased morning plasma cortisol is also seen in other head pain conditions (72,125). Morning cortisol levels are also high during the remission phase of cluster headache (75), indicating that HPA axis overactivity is not simply a stress response. The reduced response of cortisol to the ovine corticotropin-releasing hormone test, observed in both remission and cluster periods, strongly suggests a condition of HPA axis hyperactivity (downregulation of the adrenal corticotrophic cells) that is not related to pain stress (79). On the other hand, blood cortisol is suppressed normally by the dexamethasone suppression test in both phases of cluster headache (42,76), suggesting that the feedback mechanisms regulating blood cortisol are normal. A reduced response of blood cortisol and ACTH to the insulin-induced hypoglycemia test is reported both in cluster and in remission periods (79), suggesting that the hypothalamus may be hyporesponsive to hypoglycemia; the finding of reduced autonomic NE response to this test supports this (79). The finding of a reduced cortisol response to the $5\text{-}HT_{1A/2C}$ agonist m-chlorophenylpiperazine in both cluster headache phases (70,71) indicates that the reduced responsiveness of the hypothalamic pituitary adrenal axis in cluster headache is mainly due to a hypothalamic 5-HTergic dysfunction. In addition, investigation of the proopiomelanocortin-related peptides β-endorphin and β-lipotropin has revealed anomalies in their circadian production during cluster headache (41,101).

Prolactin

The diurnal rhythm of prolactin has been reported to be normal (14,34) or altered (35,112) in the cluster period. That prolactin regulatory mechanisms are in fact compromised in cluster headache is indicated by the finding that prolactin production over 24 hours is reduced in both phases of the illness (130). This reduction does not seem to be secondary either to sleep alterations or to the pain episodes. Altered central dopaminergic regulation of prolactin in cluster headache is indicated by a smaller than normal increase in prolactin levels following stimulation with the D_2 antagonist metoclopramide (61). A response of this type indicates that the lactotrophic cells of the hypophysis are downregulated. Downregulation by thyrotropin-releasing hormone (TRH) also could explain the reduced response of prolactin to the TRH test found in female patients in both phases of cluster headache and in chronic cluster headache (130). The lack of prolactin increase after morphine administration (9) indicates that opioid regulation of the hormone also may be compromised in cluster headache and further suggests that the activation threshold for the mechanisms concerned with response to stress stimuli may be altered in cluster headache, as is also indicated by the blunted cortisol and ACTH responses to the insulin test (75). The increased prolactin response to the $5\text{-}HT_{1A/2C}$ agonist m-chlorophenylpiperazine only during cluster period is probably due to $5\text{-}HT_{1A}$ hypersensitivity as indicated by the normal PRL response both to the $5\text{-}HT_{2C}$ receptor antagonist cyproheptadine (62) and the $5\text{-}HT_3$ antagonist quipazine (111). This response is not specific and is probably a pain-induced stress phenomenon (78,83).

Testosterone and Sex Hormones

Several studies have reported reduced morning levels of testosterone in cluster headache (31,60,62,65,100,106,114,130). Lowered production over 24 hours (31) and a phase shift of the morning peak (31,130) also have been described. These changes do not seem to stem from luteinizing hormone (LH) changes (130), although fewer LH peaks are seen in cluster headache patients (96). Nor can they be explained by changes in testosterone metabolism or by an altered sleep-waking cycle, although the latter is found in some patients with nocturnal pain crises (130). Possibly lowered testosterone levels in cluster headache are secondary to the increased plasma cortisol

levels (130). Estrogens, progesterone, and their metabolites are normal in cluster headache (100,130).

Luteinizing Hormone and Follicle-Stimulating Hormone

There is no circadian rhythm of luteinizing hormone (LH) or follicle-stimulating hormone (FSH) in healthy controls or in cluster headache patients; serum levels are also normal (130) but fewer and more prolonged LH peaks over 24 hours are observed in the cluster period (96). The regulation of gonadotropin production has been investigated by means of various tests. A reduced response of LH to luteinizing hormone–releasing hormone (LHRH) challenge, associated with increased FSH response, has been observed in the cluster period and in chronic cluster headache patients (100). This type of response is also observed in prepubescent and postmenopausal subjects, in whom central control of sex hormones (as occurs in fertile adults) is lacking. However, other studies have not confirmed altered secretion of LH in response to challenge with LHRH (30). Opioid and serotoninergic control of hypophyseal gonadotropins appears normal in cluster headache patients when probed by the naloxone (30) and quipazine (111) tests.

Growth Hormone

The circadian rhythm of growth hormone (GH) also has been found to be altered in cluster period (15). Pain attacks and GH levels are not clearly correlated (8,14), suggesting that stress is not implicated in the genesis of GH alterations. Challenge with metoclopramide (a dopamine antagonist) (61), but not with L-dopa (a dopamine agonist) (8) induces an excessive GH response in cluster headache patients. This response appears to be specific to cluster headache because in other pain conditions metoclopramide challenge produces the same response as in healthy subjects (61). The finding that the GH response to insulin-induced hypoglycemia is normal in cluster headache (8) contrasts with the reduced responses of ACTH, cortisol, and NE to this challenge reported by others (75). This discrepancy is probably due to different activation thresholds (to hypoglycemia) of the two hypothalamic systems controlling the release of GH and ACTH. Serotoninergic regulation of GH is normal on challenge with quipazine (111) and cyproheptadine (62).

Thyrotropin Stimulating Hormone

Basal thyrotropin stimulating hormone (TSH) levels are normal in cluster headache (10,130), but a reduced TSH response to the TRH test characterizes patients during the cluster period (10,80). This alteration persists even when prophylactic treatment completely controls the pain crises (11). A blunted TSH response to the TRH test is also found in patients suffering from endogenous depression (89), again pointing to a central origin for these abnormalities in cluster headache.

IMMUNOLOGY

There is growing interest in the relationship between the central nervous system and the immune system. It is known, for instance, that lesions to certain brain areas, particularly the hypothalamus and hippocampus, can induce specific modifications in immune system activity, probably mediated by changes in autonomic outflow to lymphoid organs (16). Animal studies have shed light on the role played by the central nervous system in immune system modulation. For instance, an immune response can be evoked by conditioning of behavior in the rat (1); thus, it is evident that changes in the immune system may reflect altered cerebral signaling to lymphoid organs.

Lymphocyte Subpopulations

Natural killer and monocyte cell populations are increased in cluster period compared with remission phase (44,52). However, stress is known to influence immune system parameters (108), and to evaluate the influence of pain on these changes, immune parameters in cluster headache patients and low back pain patients have been compared. Increased monocytes and reduced $CD3^+$ (all T-lymphocytes) and $CD4^+$ (T-helper) cells were observed both in cluster period and in low back pain patients (12). Because the number of natural killer cells in cluster period patients was similar to that in controls, immune alteration in cluster headache is partly secondary to pain-induced stress. However, monocyte and natural killer cell levels are also reduced during remission (whereas CD3 and CD4 are within the normal range) (12), and because these patients are not pain stressed, the possibility arises that the alterations are an expression of deranged central monoaminergic modulation to the immune system (12).

Cytokines

An increase in the lymphokine-activated killer (LAK) cell phenomenon induced *in vitro* by adding interleukin-2 has been described in both phases of cluster headache (45). This is likely to be caused by an increase in the number of cells bearing the interleukin-2 receptor. Interleukin-1α, and interleukin-1 levels, on the other hand, are reported to be normal in cluster headache (12).

Immunoglobulins and Complement

Concentrations of circulating immune complexes and of immunoglobulins are normal in cluster headache patients (136); similarly, anticardiolipin antibodies are absent and the venereal disease research laboratory reaction is negative in cluster headache sufferers (54). Both the classical and the alternative activation pathways of the complement system are also normal (136).

HLA

It is known that histocompatibility antigens are implicated in the regulation of testosterone in mice (58), and studies on the HLA system in cluster headache were prompted by the finding that testosterone levels are reduced in cluster headache patients (66). Increased levels of HLA A1 (17), B35, and DR5 (44), and reduced levels of A3 (92), B14 (44,92), and B21 (92) have been reported. However, none of these modifications has been corroborated by other researchers, and some researchers report different HLA alterations.

Lymphocyte β-endorphin

It was discovered only recently that β-endorphin is normally present in peripheral blood lymphocytes (53). The mRNA for the β-endorphin precursor proopiomelanocortin is also present, indicating that β-endorphin is produced endolymphocytically, a conclusion further supported by the observation that lymphocytes are unable to take up β-endorphin from the extracellular medium. Lymphocytic β-endorphin is modulated by serotonin, dopamine, and GABA in much the same way that these neurotransmitters regulate β-endorphin levels in the hypothalamus (87,95,116,117). It also has been noted that in certain brain pathologies, for example, schizophrenia, alterations in lymphocyte peptides are associated with closely analogous changes in CSF (110). These observations suggest that monitoring lymphocytic β-endorphin can provide indirect information on β-endorphin levels in the brain. Lymphocytic β-endorphin is markedly reduced in cluster headache patients, both in the cluster period and remission (82). This alteration is unrelated to the pain attacks and may indicate a diffuse opioid system derangement in this illness, but does not seem specific for cluster headache (81).

ACKNOWLEDGMENTS

Particular thanks are due to Dr. Massimo Leone for invaluable suggestions on the sections dealing with endocrinology, hormonal rhythm, and immunology.

REFERENCES

1. Ader R. Cohen N. Behaviorally conditioned immunosuppression and murine systemic lupus erythematosus. *Science* 1982:215:1534.
2. Anselmi B, Baldi E, Casacci F, Salmon S. Endogenous opioids in cerebrospinal fluid and blood in idiopathic headache sufferers. *Headache* 1980;20:294–299.
3. Anthony M, Lance JW. Histamine and serotonin in cluster headache. *Arch Neurol* 1971;25:225–231.

4. Appenzeller 0, Atkinson RA. Standefer JC. Serum β-endorphin in cluster headache and common migraine. In: Clifford Rose F, Zilkha E, eds. *Progress in migraine.* London: Pitman, 1981:106–109.

5. Appenzeller 0, Becker WJ, Ragaz A. Cluster headache. Ultrastructural aspects and pathogenetic mechanisms. *Arch Neurol* 1981;38:302–306.

6. Benitez-King G, Huerto-Delgadillo L, Anto-Tay F. Binding of ^{3}H-melatonin to calmodulin. *Life Sci* 1993;53:201–207.

7. Biella G, Panara C, Stankov B, Ferini-Strambi L, Zucconi M, Fraschini F. Melatonin-induced modulation of GABAa synapses in the central nervous system. A model and a new theory. In: Smirne S, Fraschini F, Ferini-Strambi L, Zucconi M, eds. *Sleep hormones and immunological system. Proceedings of the Third Milano International Symposium on Sleep.* Milan: Masson, 1991:177–186.

8. Boiardi A, Bussone G, Martini A, et al. Endocrinological responses in cluster headache. *J Neurol Neurosurg Psychiatry* 1983;46:956–958.

9. Boiardi A, Bussone G, Tansini E, Merati B, Di Giulio A, Panerai AE. Prolactin response to morphine in migraine headache and cluster headache [Abstract]. 12th World Congress of Neurology, Kyoto, September 1981. *Excerpta Medica* 1981:170–171.

10. Bussone G, Frediani F, Leone M, Grazzi L, Lamperti E, Boiardi A. TRH test in cluster headache. *Headache* 1988;28:462–464.

11. Bussone G, Leone M, Frediani F, Valentini S, Parati EA. TRH-test in cluster headache: pathogenetic considerations. In: Clifford Rose F, ed. *New advances in headache research 2.* London: Smith Gordon, 1991:265–269.

12. Bussone G, Salmaggi A, Leone M, Valentini S, Dufour A, Nespolo A. Immunological alterations in cluster headache during during remission and cluster period. *Cephalalgia* 1992;12:250–253.

13. Caleri 0, Marabini S, Panconesi A, Pietrini LJ. A pharmacological approach to the analgesic mechanism of somatostatin in cluster headache. *Ricerca Clin Lab* 1987;17:155–162.

14. Chazot G, Claustrat B, Brun J, Jordan D, Sassolas G, Schott B. A chronobiological study of melatonin, cortisol, growth hormone and prolactin secretion in cluster headache. *Cephalalgia* 1984;4:213–220.

15. Chazot G. Claustrat B, Brun J, Zaidan R. Effects on the patterns of melatonin and cortisol in cluster headache of a single administration of lithium at 7.00 p.m. daily over one week: a preliminary report. *Pharmacopsychiatry* 1987;20:222–223.

16. Cross RJ, Markesbery WR, Brooks WH, Roszman TL. Hypothalamic-immune interaction I. The acute effect of anterior hypothalamic lesions on the immune response. *Brain Res* 1980;196:79–87.

17. Cuypers J, Altenkirch H. HLA antigens in cluster headache. *Headache* 1979;19:228–229.

18. Cuypers J, Westphal K, Bunge S. Mast cells in cluster headache. *Acta Neurol Scand* 1980;61:327–329.

19. D'Andrea G, Cananzi AR, Joseph R, et al. Platelet glycine, glutamate and aspartate in primary headache. *Cephalalgia* 1991;11:197–200.

20. D'Andrea G, Cananzi AR, Toldo M, Ferro-Milone F. Platelet activity in cluster headache. *Cephalalgia* 1986;6:163–167.

21. de Belleroche J, Clifford Rose F, Das I, Cook GE. Metabolic abnormality in cluster headache. *Headache* 1984;24:310–312.

22. de Belleroche J, Gardiner IM, Howley P, et al. Membrane transduction in migraine and cluster headache: studies of G-protein activation. In: Clifford Rose F, ed. *New advances in headache research 2.* London: Smith Gordon, 1991:171–173.

23. de Belleroche J, Kilfeather S, Das I, Clifford Rose F. Abnormal membrane composition and membrane-dependent transduction mechanisms in cluster headache. *Cephalalgia* 1986;6:147–153.

24. Dimitridou V, Henry P, Mathiau P, Aubineau P, Brochet B. Interrelations entre mastocytes et nerfs de l'adventice de l'artere temporale chez des sujets atteints de cluster headache. In: *Societe Francais d'etude de migraine et cephalees.* Paris: Book of Abstracts, 1989:4.

25. Edvinsson L, Goadsby PJ. Neuropetides in migraine and cluster headache. *Cephalalgia* 1994;14:320–327.

26. Eisen AS, Freeman RP, Guss VB, et al. Melatonin agonists modulate 5-HT$_{2A}$-receptor-mediated neurotransmission: behavioral and biochemical studies in the rat. *J Pharmacol Exp Ther* 1995;273:304–308.

27. Ekbom K. Patterns of cluster headache with a note on the relations to angina pectoris and peptic ulcers. *Acta Neurol Scand* 1970;46:225–237.

28. Ekbom K, Lindahl J. Effect of induced rise of blood pressure on pain in cluster headache. *Acta Neurol Scand* 1970;46:585–600.

29. Ekbom KA. Ergotamine tartrate orally in Horton's "histaminic cephalgia." *Acta Psychiatr Scand* 1947:46(suppl):106–113.

30. Facchinetti F, Martignoni E, Gallai V, et al. Neuroendocrine evaluation of central opiate activity in primary headache disorders. *Pain* 1988;34:29–33.

31. Facchinetti F, Nappi G, Cicoli C, et al. Reduced testosterone levels in cluster headache: a stress-related phenomenon? *Cephalalgia* 1986;6:29–34.

32. Fanciullacci M, Alessandrini M, Figini M, Geppetti P, Michelacci S. Increase in plasma calcitonin gene-realated peptide from the extra-cerebral circulation during nitroglycerine-induced cluster headache attack. *Pain* 1995;60:119–123.

33. Fanciullacci M, Alessandri M, Sicuteri R, Marabini S. Responsiveness of the trigeminovascular system to nitroglycerine in cluster headache patients. *Brain* 1997;120:283–288.

34. Ferrari E, Canepari C, Bossolo PA, et al. Changes of biological rhythms in primary headache syndromes. *Cephalalgia* 1983:1:58–68.

35. Ferrari E, Nappi G, Vailati A, Martignoni E, Bossolo PA, Polleri A. Circadian periodicity of plasma prolactin in some neurological diseases. *Int J Chronobiol* 1979:6:231–242.

36. Figuerola M de L, Vindrola O, Barontini MB, Leston JA. Increase in plasma methionine-enkephalin levels during the pain attack in episodic cluster headache. *Cephalalgia* 1990;10:251–257.

37. Figuerola M de L, Vindrola O, Barontini MB, Leston JA. Changes in neutrophil metenkephalin containing peptides in episodic cluster headache. *Headache* 1991:31:406–408.

38. Fragoso YD, Seim A, Stovner LJ, Mack M, Bjerve KS, Sjaastad O. Cluster headache: increased incorporation of (1-14C) arachidonic acid into phosphatidylserine in polymorphonuclear cells. *Cephalalgia* 1989;9:213–220.

39. Fragoso YD, Stovner LJ, Bjerve KS, Sjaastad O. Cluster headache: incorporation of (1-14C) oleic acid in phosphatidylserine in polymorphonuclear cells. *Cephalalgia* 1989;9:207–211.

40. Franceschini R, Leandri M, Cataldi A, et al. Raised plasma arginin-vasopressin concentrations during cluster headache attacks. *J Neurol Neurosurg Psychiatry* 1995;59:381–383.

41. Franceschini R, Leandri M, Gianelli MV, et al. Evaluation of β-endorphin secretion in patients suffering from episodic cluster headache. *Headache* 1996;36:603–607.

42. Frediani F, Lamperti E, Leone M, Boiardi A, Grazzi L, Bussone G. Cluster headache patients' responses to dexamethasone suppression test. *Headache* 1988;28:130–132.

43. Geppetti P, Frilli S, Spillantini MC, et al. Evaluation of CSF neuropeptides and peptidase activities in primary headaches. *Cephalalgia* 1987;7(suppl 6):43–45.

44. Giacovazzo M, Martelletti P, Valeri M, Piaza A, Monaco PI, Casciani CU. Variations in the Leu7+ and LeuM3+ leukocyte subpopulations observed in cluster headache are dependent on HLA-DR antigens. *Headache* 1987:27:35–38.

45. Giacovazzo M, Stirparo G, De Stefano L, Martelletti P, Rinaldi-Garaci G. Lymphokine-activated killer (LAK) cell phenomenon in cluster headache "in vitro" activation by recombinant interleukin-2. *Headache* 1989;29:177–179.

46. Goadsby PJ, Edvinsson L. Human in vivo evidence for trigemino-vascular activation in cluster headache. Neuropeptide changes and effects of acute therapies. *Brain* 1994;117:427–434.

47. Göbel H, Cordes P. Circadian variation in pain sensitivity in pericranial musculature. *Headache* 1990;30:418–422.

48. Hannah P, Jarman J, Clover V, Sandler M, Davies PTG, Clifford Rose F. Kinetics of platelets 5-hydroxytryptamine uptake in headache patients. *Cephalagia* 1991:11:141–145.

49. Deleted in proofs.

50. Hardebo JE, Ekman R, Eriksson M, Holgersson S, Ryberg B. CSF opioid levels in cluster headache. Effect of acupuncture. In: Clifford Rose F, ed. *Migraine: proceedings of the 5th international migraine symposium.* Basel: Karger, 1985:79–85.

51. Hardebo JE, Ekman R. Substance P and opioids in cluster headache. In: Sicuteri F, et al., eds. *Trends in cluster headache.* Amsterdam: Elsevier Science, 1987:145–157.

52. Hardebo JE, Ryberg B. CSF findings in cluster headache indicative of inflammatory reaction or disease. *Cephalalgia* 1989;10(suppl):301–302.

53. Heijnen CJ, Kavellars A, Pallieux RE. Beta-endorphin: cytokine and neuropeptide. *Immunol Rev* 1991;119:41–61.

54. Hering R, Couturier EGM, Asherson RA, Steiner TJ. Anti-cardiolipin antibodies in cluster headache. *Cephalalgia* 1991;2:101–102.

55. Horton BT. Histaminic cephalgia: differential diagnosis and treatment. *Mayo Clin Proc* 1956:31:325–333.

56. Igarashi H, Sakai F, Suzuki S, Tazaki Y. Cerebrovascular sympathetic nervous activity during cluster headaches. *Cephalalgia* 1987;7(suppl 6):87–89.

57. Igarashi H, Sakai F, Tazaki Y, Kanda T. The role of the sympathetic nervous system in the pathogenesis of cluster headache. *Cephalalgia* 1985:5(suppl 3):362–363.

58. Ivanyi P, Hampl R, Starka L,Mickova M. Genetic association between H2 gene and testosterone metabolism in mice. *Nature (New Biol)* 1972;238:280–281.

59. Joseph R, Dhital K, Adams J, Burnstock G, Appenzeller O, Clifford Rose F. Cluster headache: a new approach using fluorescent histochemistry of nerves in temple skin. In: Clifford Rose F, ed. *Migraine: proceedings or the 5th International Migraine Symposium.* Basel: Karger, 1985:162–165.

60. Klimek A. Plasma testosterone levels in patients with cluster headache. *Headache* 1982;22:162–164.

61. Klimek A. Growth hormone and prolactin levels in the course of metoclopramide test in headache patients. *Endokrynol Polska* 1985: 36:20–27.

62. Klimek A. Durko A, Gluszcz-Zielinska A. Hormonal status in cluster headache. In: Clifford Rose F. ed. *Progress in migraine research 2.* London: Pitman, 1984:215–231.

63. Kozubski W, Davies PTJ, Steiner T, Prusinski A, Clifford Rose F. Platelet fibrinogen-binding sites in patients with classical migraine and cluster headache. In: Clifford Rose F, ed. *New advances in headache research.* London: Smith-Gordon, 1989:213–219.

64. Krabbe AA, Rank F. Histological examinations of the superficial temporal artery in patients suffering from cluster headache. *Cephalalgia* 1985:5(suppl 3):282–283.

65. Kudrow L. Plasma testosterone levels in cluster headache. Preliminary result. *Headache* 1976;16:28–31.

66. Kudrow L. HLA antigens in cluster headache and classical migraine. *Headache* 1978;18:167–168.

67. Kudrow L. The cyclic relationship of natural illumination to cluster period frequency. *Cephalalgia* 1987;7(suppl 6):76–77.

68. La Mancusa R, Pulcinelli FM, Ferroni P, et al. Blood leukotrienes in headache: correlation with platelet activity. *Headache* 1991;31: 409–414.

69. Leach CM. A comparison on the inhibitory effect of melatonin and indomethacin on platelet aggregation and thromboane release. *Prostaglandins* 1980;20:51–55.

70. Leone M, Attanasio A, Croci D, et al. The *m*-chlorophenylpiperazine test in cluster headache: a study on central serotoninergic activity. *Cephalalgia* 1997;17:666–672.

71. Leone M, Attanasio A, Grazzi L, et al. Investigation of central serotoninergic involvement in cluster headache and migraine by means of *m*-CPP. *Cephalalgia* 1997;17:361.

72. Leone M, Biffi M, Leone F, Bussone G. Leucocyte subsets and cortisol serum levels in patients with migraine with aura and chronic tension headache. *Cephalalgia* 1994;14:139–142.

73. Leone M, Bussone G. A review of hormonal findings in cluster headache. Evidence for hypothalamic involvement. *Cephalalgia* 1993;13: 309–317.

74. Leone M, Bussone G. Melatonin in cluster headache: rationale for use and possible therapeutic potential. *CNS Drugs* 1998;9:7–16.

75. Leone M, D'Amico D, Moschiano F, Fraschini F, Bussone G. Melatonin vs placebo in the prophylaxis of cluster headache: a double-blind pilot study with parallel group. *Cephalalgia* 1996;16:494–496.

76. Leone M, Frediani F, D'Amico D, et al. Dexamethasone suppression test, melatonin and TRH-test in cluster headache. *Ital J Neurol Sci* 1992:13:227–232.

77. Leone M, Lucini V, D'Amico D, et al. Alterations in the circadian production of melatonin and cortisol in cluster headache. In: Clifford Rose F, ed. *New advances in headache research 4.* London: Smith-Gordon, 1994:211–219.

78. Leone M, Lucini V, D'Amico D, et al. Twenty four-hour melatonin and cortisol plasma levels in relation to timing of cluster headache. *Cephalalgia* 1995;15:224–229.

79. Leone M, Maltempo C, Gritti A, Bussone G. The insulin tolerance test and ovine corticotrophin-releasing-hormone test in episodic cluster headache II: comparison with low back pain patients. *Cephalalgia* 1994;14:357–364.

80. Leone M, Patruno G, Vescovi A, Bussone G. Neuroendocrine dysfunction in cluster headache. *Cephalalgia* 1990;10:235–239.

81. Leone M, Sacerdote P, D'Amico D, Panerai AE, Bussone G. β-endorphin concentraton in peripheral blood mononuclear cells in migraine and tension headache. *Cephalalgia* 1992:12:155–157.

82. Leone M, Sacerdote P, D'Amico D, Panerai AE, Bussone G. β-endorphin levels are reduced in peripheral blood mononuclear cells of cluster headache patients. *Cephalagia* 1993;13:413–416.

83. Leston J. Barontini M, Mancini A, Rocchi V, Herskovits T. Free and conjugated plasma catecholamines in cluster headache. *Cephalalgia* 1987:7(supp; 6):331–332.

84. Liberski PP, Mirecka B. Mast cells in cluster headache: ultrastructure, release pattern and possible pathogenetic significance. *Cephalalgia* 1984;4:101–106.

85. Linsell CR, Lightman SL, Mullen PE, Brown MI, Causon RC. Circadian rhythms of epineophrine and norepinephrine in man. *J Clin Endocrinol Metab* 1985;60:1210–1215.

86. Littlewood J, Glover V, Sandler M, Peatfield R, Petty R, Clifford Rose F. Low platelet monoamine oxidase activity in headache: no correlation with phenolsulphotransferase, succinate dehydrogenase, platelet preparation method or smoking. *J Neurol Neurosurg Psychiatry* 1984: 47:338–343.

87. Locatelli V, Petraglia F, Penalva A, Panerai AE. Effect of dopaminergic drugs on hypothalamic and pituitary immunoreactive β-endorphin concentrations in the rat. *Life Sci* 1983:33:1711–1717.

88. Lodi R, Kemp GJ, Montagna P, et al. Quantitative analysis of skeletal muscle bioenergetics and proton efflux in migraine and cluster headache. *J Neurol Sci* 1997;146:73–80.

89. Loosen PT, Prange AJ Jr. Serum thyrotropin response to thyrotropin-releasing hormone in psychiatric patients. *Am J Psychiatry* 1982;139: 405–411.

90. Malmgren R. The central serotoninergic system. *Cephalalgia* 1990; 10:199–204.

91. Manzoni GC, Terzano MG, Bono G, Micieli G, Martucci N, Nappi G. Cluster headache-clinical findings in 180 patients. *Cephalalgia* 1983; 3:21–30.

92. Martelletti P, Romiti A, Gala MF, et al. HLA-B14 antigen in cluster headache. *Headache* 1984;24:152–154.

93. Martelletti P, Adriani E, Bonini S, et al. Basophil histamine release and leukotriene (LTB4-LTC4) production in cluster headache. *Headache* 1989;29:46–49.

94. Martelletti P, Granata M, Giacovazzo M. Serum interleukin-1β is increased in cluster headache. *Cephalalgia* 1993;13:343–345.

95. Martini A, Sacerdote P, Mantegazza P, Panerai AE. Antiepileptic drugs affect hypothalamic β-endorphin concentrations. *J Neurochem* 1984; 43:871–873.

96. Micieli G, Facchinetti F, Martignoni E, Manzoni GC, Cleva M, Nappi G. Disordered pulsatile LH release in cluster headache. *Cephalalgia* 1987;7(suppl 6):79–81.

97. Montagna P, Lodi R, Cortelli P, et al. Phosphorus magnetic resonance spectroscopy in cluster headache. *Neurology* 1997;48:113–118.

98. Mosnaim AD, Diamond S, Freitag F, Chevesich J, Wolf ME, Solomon J. Plasma and platelet methionine-enkephalin levels in chronic cluster patients during an acute headache episode. *Headache* 1987;27: 325–328.

99. Mosnaim AD, Huprikar S, Wolf ME, Freitag F, Diamond S. Studies of platelet monoaminooxidase activity during an acute cluster headache attack. *Cephalalgia* 1991;11(suppl 11):254–255.

100. Murialdo G, Fanciullacci M, Nicolodi M, et al. Cluster headache in the male: sex steroid pattern and gonadotropic response to luteinizing hormone releasing hormone. *Cephalalgia* 1989;9:91–98.

101. Nappi G, Facchinetti F, Bono G, et al. Lack of β-endorphin and β-lipotropin circadian rhythmicity in episodic cluster headache: a model for chronopathology. In: Pfaffenrath V, Lundberg PO, Sjaastad O, eds. *Updating in headache.* Berlin: Springer Verlag, 1985:269–275.

102. Nappi G, Facchinetti F, Martignoni E. et al. Endorphin patterns within the headache spectrum disorders. *Cephalalgia* 1985;5(suppl 2):201–210.

103. Nappi G, Micieli G, Facchinetti F, Sandrini G, Martignoni E. Changes in rhythmic temporal structure in cluster headache. In: Sicuteri F, et al., eds. *Trends in cluster headache.* Amsterdam: Elsevier Science, 1987:351–359.

104. Nattero G, Franzone JS, Savi L, Cirillo R. Serum prostaglandin-like substances in cluster headache and common migraine. In: Clifford

Rose F, ed. *Progress in migraine research 2*. London: Pitman, 1984: 199–204.

105. Nattero G, Savi L, Piantino P. Gastrin in cluster headache. In: Sicuteri F, et al., eds. *Trends in cluster headache*. Amsterdam: Elsevier Science, 1987:371–377.

106. Nelson RF. Testosterone levels in cluster and non-cluster migrainous headache patients. *Headache* 1978;18:265–767.

107. Nicolodi M, Del Bianco E. Sensory neuropeptides (substance P, calcitonin gene-related peptide) and vasoactive intestinal polypeptide in human saliva: their pattern in migraine and cluster headache. *Cephalalgia* 1990;10:30–50.

108. Oshida Y, Yamanouchi K, Hayamizu S, Sato I. Effect of acute physical exercise on lymphocyte subpopulations in trained and untrained subjects. *Int J Sports Med* 1988;9:137–140.

109. Panza JA, Epstein SE, Quyyumi AA. Circadian variation in vascular tone and its relation to α-sympathetic vasoconstrictor activity. *N Engl J Med* 1991;325:986–990.

110. Panza G, Monzani E, Sacerdote P, Penati G, Panerai AE. β-endorphin, vasoactive intestinal peptide and cholecystokinin in peripheral blood mononuclear cells from healthy subjects and schizophrenic patients free of drugs and during treatment with haloperidol. *Acta Psychiatr Scand* 1992;85:207–210.

111. Parati EA, Zanardi P, Cocchi D, Caraceni T, Muller EE. Neuroendocrine effects of quipazine in man in health state or with neurological disorders. *J Neural Transm* 1980;47:273–297.

112. Polleri A, Nappi G, Murialdo G, Bono G, Martignoni E, Savoldi F. Changes in the 24-hour prolactin pattern in cluster headache. *Cephalalgia* 1982;2:1–7.

113. Prusinski A, Liberski PO. Is the cluster headache local mastocytic diaethesis? *Headache* 1979;19:102.

114. Romiti A, Martelletti P, Gallo MF, Giacovazzo M. Low plasma testosterone levels in cluster headache. *Cephalalgia* 1983;3:41–44.

115. Rozniecki JJ, Kuzminska B, Prusinski A. Lithium *in vitro* influence on basophil degranulation in cluster headache. *Cephalalgia* 1987;7(suppl 6):349–350.

116. Sacerdote P, Brini A, Mantegazza P, Panerai AE. A role for serotonin and β-endorphin in the analgesia induced by some tricyclic antidepressant drugs. *Pharmacol Biochem Behav* 1987:26:153–158.

117. Sacerdote P, Rubboli F. Locatelli L, Ciciliato I, Mantegazza P, Panerai AE. Pharmacological modulation of neuropeptides in peripheral mononuclear cells. *J Neuroimmunol* 1991;32:35–41.

118. Sandrini G, Alfonsi E, Bono G, Facchinetti F, Montalbetti L, Nappi G. Circadian variation of human flexion reflex. *Pain* 1986;25:403–410.

119. Schweizer A. Leukotrienes reduce nociceptive responses to bradychinin. *Eur J Pharmacol* 1985;105:105–112.

120. Selmaj K, de Belleroche J, Das I, Clifford Rose F. Leukotriene B4 generation by polymorphonuclear leukocytes: possible involvement in the pathogenesis of headache. *Headache* 1986;26:460–464.

121. Sicuteri F, Fanciullacci M, Geppetti P, Renzi P, Caleri D, Spillantini MG. Substance P mechanism in cluster headache: evaluation in plasma and cerebrospinal fluid. *Cephalalgia* 1985;5:143–149.

122. Sjaastad O, Sjaastad ØV. Urinary histamine excretion in migraine and cluster headache. *J Neurol* 1977;216:91–104.

123. Spillantini MC, Geppetti P, Marchionni A, et al. "Enkephalinase" and converting enzyme activities in human CSF: their relation with pain and various pathologies. In: Sicuteri F, et al., eds. *Trends in cluster headache*. Amsterdam: Elsevier Science, 1987:159–165.

124. Stankov B, Capsoni S, Lucini V, et al. Autoradiographic localization of putative melatonin receptors in the brains of the two Old World primates: *Cercopithecus aethiops* and *Papio ursinus*. *Neuroscience* 1993; 52:459–468.

125. Strittmatter M, Grauer MT, Fischer C, Hamann G, Hoffmann KH, Blaes F, Schimrigk K. Autonomic nervous system and neuroendocrine changes in patients with idiopathic trigeminal neuralgia. *Cephalalgia* 1996;16:476–480.

126. Strittmatter M, Hamann GF, Grauer M, Fischer C, Blaes F, Hoffmann KH, Schimrigk K. Altered activity of the sympathetic nervous system and changes in the balance of hypophyseal, pituitary and adrenal hormones in patients with cluster headache. *Neuroreport* 1996;7:1229–1234.

127. Summers KM, Brown GK, Craig IW, et al. Platelet monoamine oxidase: specific activity and turnover numbers. *Clin Chim Acta* 1982; 121:134–146.

128. Sutherland JM, Eadie MJ. Cluster headache. *Res Clin Stud Headache* 1972;3:92–125.

129. Waldenlind E, Ekbom K, Wetterberg L, et al. Lowered circannual urinary melatonin concentrations in episodic cluster headache. *Cephalalgia* 1994;14:199–204.

130. Waldenlind E, Gustafsson SA. Prolactin in cluster headache: diurnal secretion, response to thyrotropin-releasing hormone and relation to sex steroids and gonadotropins. *Cephalalgia* 1987:7:43–54.

131. Waldenlind E, Gustafsson SA, Ekbom K, Wetterberg L. Circadian secretion of cortisol and melatonin in cluster headache during active cluster periods and remission. *J Neurol Neurosurg Psychiatry* 1987: 50:207–213.

132. Waldenlind E, Ross SB, Sääf J, Ekbom K, Wetterberg L. Concentration and uptake of 5-hydroxytryptamine in platelets from cluster headache and migraine patients. *Cephalalgia* 1985:5:45–54.

133. Waldenlind E, Sääf J, Ekbom K, Ross SB, Wahlund LO, Wetterberg L. Kinetics and thermolability of platelet monoamine oxidase in cluster headache and migraine. *Cephalalgia* 1984;4:125–134.

134. Vaughan GM, McDonald SD, Jordan RM, et al. Melatonin concentration in human blood and cerebrospinal fluid: relationship to stress. *J Clin Endocrinol Metab* 1978;47:220–223.

135. Vecchiet L, Geppetti P, Marchionni A. et al. Cerebrospinal fluid (methionin 5)-, enkephalin-, substance P-, and somatostatin-like immunoreactivities in painful and painless human diseases. In: Sicuteri F, et al., eds. *Trends in cluster headache*. Amsterdam: Elsevier Science, 1987:135–143.

136. Visintini D, Trabattoni G, Manzoni GC, Lechi A, Bortone L, Behan PO. Immunological studies in cluster headache and migraine. *Headache* 1986:26:398–402.

The Headaches, Second Edition,
edited by J. Olesen, P. Tfelt-Hansen, and K.M.A. Welch.
Lippincott Williams & Wilkins, Philadelphia © 2000.

Tension-Type Headache, Cluster Headache, and Miscellaneous Primary Headaches

CHAPTER 93

Neurophysiology, Hemodynamics, Trigger Factors, Cerebrospinal Fluid, and Psychological Factors in Cluster Headache

David Russell and Marcello Fanciullacci

NEUROPHYSIOLOGY

Several methods have been used to assess the function of central and peripheral neural pathways that may be involved in the pathophysiology of cluster headache. A few of these entail modification of brain electric activity, whereas most neurophysiologic investigations have been performed directly on target organs that are affected unilaterally during attacks. These study methods would appear to be an appropriate approach, because they allow comparison between affected and unaffected structures.

Evoked Potentials and Electroencephalography

Traditional electrophysiologic techniques provide some data that suggest a disturbance of central sensory pathways. Somatosensory evoked potentials, recorded after stimulation of the median nerve contralateral to the pain, have shown a decreased N1–P2 amplitude during histamine-induced attacks (10). Brainstem auditory-evoked potentials, outside and during attacks, exhibit on the symptomatic side a decreased conduction time for impulses through the auditory pathways (2). Electroencephalographic studies have demonstrated abnormalities in activity in few patients (15).

D. Russell: Department of Neurology, The National Hospital University of Oslo, N-0027 Oslo, Norway.

M. Fanciullacci: Institute of Internal Medicine and Therapeutics IV, Headache Centre, University of Florence School of Medicine, 50139 Florence, Italy.

Pupillary Responses to Exteroceptive Stimulation

Miosis is a typical sign during cluster headache attacks. The pupil has both sensory and autonomic innervation, and the level of activity of these respective systems may be assessed by studying this organ.

Dark and Light Adaptation

During and between attacks, both pupils constrict more rapidly and markedly to light and dilate more slowly and weakly in darkness compared with normal responses. These abnormalities are more evident during attacks on the symptomatic side, where they also persist in the remission phase (5,24).

Nociceptive Stimulation

Percutaneous painless electric stimulation of the sural nerve produces bilateral reflex pupillary dilatation, which most probably is due to central sympathetic activation. When the stimulation is painful, it also elicits a contraction of the biceps femoris muscle (RIII reflex), which is an objective physiologic correlate of pain sensation.

In cluster-headache patients who underwent examination during a headache-free interval, reduced mydriasis to sural-nerve stimulation could be observed on the symptomatic side only following a painful stimulus. This finding is also present in the nonsymptomatic eye in patients with chronic symptoms (24).

Infratrochlear Nerve Stimulation

Cluster headache-related miosis may be due to trigeminal afferent impulses acting through an antidromic release of substance P and neurokinin A, which directly causes pupillary constriction. This mechanism is also probably responsible for the noncholinergic unilateral miosis elicited by painless high-intensity transcutaneous electric stimulation of the infratrochlear nerve. This response is reduced on the symptomatic side in episodic cluster headache patients when they are examined outside of attacks (Fig. 1). This deficit disappears during remission periods (8).

The impaired pupillary responses elicited by both dark and light adaptation and by sural nociceptive stimulation may be due to a sympathetic deficit to the eye. The bilaterality of findings suggests a possible lesion of central sympathetic pathways that is unmasked by painful stimulation; however, the reduced unilateral miosis to trigeminal electric stimulation suggests involvement of iris sensory fibers in cluster headache-related miosis.

Pain Perception

During headache-free intervals, there is a bilateral lowering of the pain threshold to corneal electric stimulation, which is more evident on the symptomatic side. This alteration is restricted to cluster periods (Table 1). On the other hand, the bilateral blinking response that accompanies painful electric stimulation is normal (30). In headache-free patients, cutaneous and deep hyperalgesia is prevalent in the hemisoma homolateral to cluster attacks (26).

The assessment of pain perception in cluster headache may therefore indicate an increased excitability of trigeminal nociceptive neurons, at least at the corneal level. In addition, the lateralized hyperalgesia could be due to facilitation in the central nervous system (CNS) or activation of reflex arcs.

Pharmacologic Stimulation of the Iris and Sweat Gland Sympathetic Junctions

Experimental studies revealed derangement of the iris sympathetic junction when it is stimulated pharmacologically. Bilateral instillation of indirect sympathomimetic eyedrops, such as tyramine and hydroxyamphetamine, provokes in headache-free patients who are in an active phase a reduced mydriasis on the symptomatic side that persists during remissions in a subgroup of patients (9,29). An increased mydriasis to the direct sympathomimetic agent phenylephrine also was shown in the symptomatic eye of cluster-headache patients who have a permanent miosis (29).

Iris sympathetic hypofunction may coexist with sweating abnormalities. Forehead sweating induced by heat or exercise during attack-free periods is diminished, especially on the painful side (31). In addition, parenterally

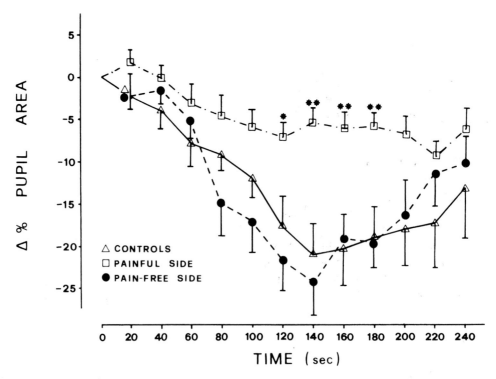

FIG. 1. During the active phase, cluster-headache sufferers show a defective miotic response after transcutaneous electric stimulation of the infratrochlear nerve. No difference appears between the pain-free side and the control eye. Each value is mean ± SEM; *$p < 0.05$, **$p < 0.01$, versus control eye.

TABLE 1. *Pain threshold to corneal electrical stimulation in cluster headache patients during active and remission periods and in a control group*

Group	Side	Pain threshold
Active phase	P	1.7 ± 0.5[a],*
	PF	2.4 ± 0.7[b]
Remission phase	P	3.1 ± 0.9
	PF	3.2 ± 1.2
Control group		3.4 ± 0.7

P, pain side; PF, pain-free side. Values (mA) are mean ± SD.

[a] $p < 0.001$ versus P and PF in remission phase.
[b] $p < 0.002$ versus control group.
* $p < 0.01$ versus PF in active phase (analysis of variance, one-way).

administered pilocarpine causes a bilateral increase in sweating that is more marked on the symptomatic side (31). These findings have been interpreted as a structural or functional lesion of sympathetic fibers that may induce a postsynaptic receptor supersensitivity. Although these autonomic tests usually suggest a third-neuron lesion, it should be noted that a similar supersensitivity to phenylephrine and pilocarpine was demonstrated in patients with Horner's syndrome as a result of brainstem damage (28). These findings may support the hypothesis of a central dysfunction in cluster headache.

TRIGGER FACTORS

Attacks of cluster headache may be provoked by histamine, nitroglycerin, or alcohol. These substances have in common their vasodilatory effect. Provocation is only possible, however, when patients are in a cluster period, not when they are in a remission period without attacks.

Histamine provokes attacks in most patients (25,16). Horton (16) used 0.3 mg of histamine base subcutaneously, which after 1.5 minutes usually caused a bifrontal pulsating headache lasting 5 to 10 minutes. Approximately 20 to 40 minutes later, most patients developed a headache attack that was similar to a spontaneous attack.

Nitroglycerin appears to be the most effective agent for provoking attacks of cluster headache (6,7,25); however, attacks may not be provoked for some hours after a previous attack (refractory period), and provocation of an attack also may postpone the arrival of the next expected spontaneous attack. After nitroglycerin administration, headache patients and nonheadache subjects may experience a bilateral diffuse throbbing headache during the first 3 to 10 minutes. These symptoms correspond to the maximum vasodilatory effect of nitroglycerin (4). A headache attack similar to the patient's spontaneous cluster headache usually develops 30 to 50 minutes later (6,7).

Small amounts of alcohol provoke attacks during cluster periods in about 50% of patients (16). After alcohol ingestion, there is also a latency period of 30 to 50 minutes before the onset of attacks. Some patients report that consumption of a large amount of alcohol may postpone attacks for 1 or 2 days. This period, however, may be followed by a rebound period of 1 to several days in which attacks arrive with increased frequency and intensity.

At present, we do not have an explanation of why there is a latency period after administration of the above substances to the onset of provoked attacks. The onset of attacks does not correspond to the maximum vasodilatory effect. On the contrary, Dahl and colleagues (4) found that provoked attacks began when the intracranial vasodilatory effect of nitroglycerin was beginning to decrease.

Kudrow (19) suggested that hypoxia may induce attacks of cluster headache. This hypothesis was based on observations that attacks are more common at night and at high altitudes. Sleep apnea also seems to be more frequent in patients who have cluster headaches (21). Furthermore, such headaches may be terminated using oxygen therapy (18). Kudrow also suggested that the carotid body may be involved in the pathogenesis of cluster headache, because this is the most sensitive chemoreceptor for hypoxia.

In a later study (20), Kudrow and Kudrow found that patients with active cluster headaches differed from remission and control groups with regard to oxygen desaturation following nitroglycerin. The magnitude of oxygen desaturation was greater and lasted longer in patients with active cluster headaches, all of whom developed a provoked attack. The authors therefore suggested that the active period of cluster headache may be characterized by an impaired mechanism to autoregulate and thus to compensate for hypoxemia. They furthermore suggested that persistence of hypoxemia and onset of a cluster attack may show a common mechanism coupling the two events and that abnormal central or peripheral chemoreceptor activity may be responsible for these events.

Zhao and colleagues (35) tested the effect of hypoxia on attack generation and found that attacks generally did not start during moderate hypoxia. They also studied oxygen saturation before nitroglycerin-provoked attacks (36). In this study, there was usually no major oxygen desaturation during the 5 minutes before headache onset.

CEREBROSPINAL FLUID

Central neural disturbances have been proposed in cluster headache, but knowledge is limited because of difficulties in directly assessing CNS function. The study of cerebrospinal fluid (CSF) offers a partial solution to these problems, because it is in constant exchange with the extracellular fluid of the CNS tissue. A pioneer study by Kunkle (22) showed acetylcholine-like activity in the CSF of some cluster-headache patients in an active phase, which may suggest involvement of the central parasympathetic system in the pathogenesis of cluster headache.

Other studies demonstrated decreased plasma levels of catecholamines corresponding to decreased levels of norepinephrine (NE), vanillyl mandelic acid (VMA), homovanillic acid (HVA), and 5-hydroxyindoleacetic acid (5-HIAA) in the CSF of patients during the cluster-headache period (34). These findings support the hypothesis of a probable activation of both systems (parasympathetic and sympathetic) and central involvement in the pathogenensis of cluster headache.

During the past decade, the development of methods for measuring neurotransmitters of peptidergic central pathways involved in pain modulation led to the identification of markers for the functional activity of these systems in the CSF. Therefore, recent studies attempted to probe the neurochemistry of pain transmission in the CSF of patients who have cluster headaches both during and outside attacks.

Opioid Peptides during Headache-free Intervals of Cluster Periods

The possibility that cluster headache may be at least partly due to an impaired central endogenous opioid system led to the assessment of opiate peptides in CSF. Measurements of β-endorphin-like activity revealed no difference in levels found in patients who had suffered from minor neurologic symptoms but were asymptomatic at the time of sampling. Acupuncture did not induce an increased inactivity (14).

Unlike patients suffering from nonpainful neurologic disorders, cluster headache patients showed CSF enkephalin concentrations that were reduced to an unde-

tectable level by radioreceptor assay (1). A subsequent study using the radioimmunoassay technique confirmed low CSF metenkephalin levels in cluster-headache patients (Fig. 2) and also established that these levels are increased by acupuncture (14).

The activity of enkephalinase, the enzyme that specifically degrades metenkephalin, also has been measured fluorimetrically. It did not differ from that in patients suffering from nonpainful neurologic diseases (see Fig. 2) (32).

Sensory Neuropeptides during Headache-free Intervals of Cluster Periods

Cerebrospinal fluid levels of substance P, the major sensory peptide in the processing of nociceptive information and calcitonin gene-related peptide, the powerful vasodilator of the trigeminal vascular system, did not differ from those observed in control groups (13,32). Somatostatin, the peptide that inhibits the release of substance P from sensory afferents, was also in the control range (32).

Neuropeptides during Attacks

The small amounts of CSF that have been collected toward the end of a spontaneous cluster headache attack have shown that the levels of β-endorphin, metenkephalin (see Fig. 2), substance P, and somatostatin are not different from those obtained outside attacks (32). Cerebrospinal fluid substance P levels also were unchanged during a histamine-induced attack of moderate intensity (32).

The data available on current neurochemistry research in the lumbar CSF of cluster headaches are too few to allow definite conclusions; however, virtually no changes in CSF levels of many pain-related neuropeptides were

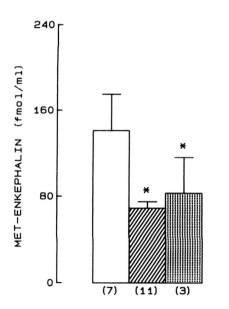

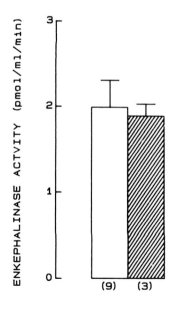

FIG. 2. Metenkephalin levels and enkephalinase activity in lumbar cerebrospinal fluid of cluster headache patients in active phase during (*dotted bars*) and outside (*striped bars*) of attacks and in control groups (*open bars*). The number of subjects is shown in parentheses. Mean ± SEM. *$p < 0.05$ versus control group (Student's t test for unpaired data).

seen, and the attack does not modify the neuropeptide pattern observed in headache-free intervals. The only marker of a putative involvement of central opioid mechanisms in cluster headache seems to be the low levels of metenkephalin. Because CSF enkephalinase activity is not enhanced, an accelerated degradation of enkephalins is unlikely. This abnormality therefore suggests an impaired enkephalinergic activity, which may be related to a primary lowered enkephalinergic tonus in the CNS or to an overstimulation resulting from the stress of the cluster period. Because longitudinal data are difficult to obtain, more extensive study is clearly needed to clarify the exact pattern of changes in the biologic markers of the pain systems in cluster headache.

The neurochemistry of CSF is influenced by a number of factors that limit the possibility of using this fluid as a predictor of neuronal activity. In cluster headache, measurements should be performed close to the neuronal pathways that regulate pain and the autonomic systems of the head. Because CSF usually is sampled at the lumbar level, it tends to reflect processes of the spinal cord rather than the brain. Thus, unaltered lumbar CSF levels do not exclude the possibility of altered neuronal activity in cluster headache.

PSYCHOLOGICAL ASPECTS

Graham (12) described certain physical characteristics of male sufferers of cluster headache as almost hypermasculine, contrasting with their rather weak personality. Facial features of a ruddy complexion, deep-furrowed, thick and orange-peel skin, broad chin and skull together with a tall, trim, and rugged general appearance constituted a hypermasculine leonine look. According to Graham, these physical characteristics did not match their psychological structure. Graham described the cluster patient as dependent, helpless, and tense. He summarized his clinical impression as the "leonine mouse" syndrome, thus depicting a weak and dependent personality within a body that is hypermasculine in appearance.

Friedman and Mikropoulos (11) described their patients as ambitious, efficient, and overconscientious, striving for perfection and having a strong tendency toward compulsive behavior.

Kudrow (17) used the Cattell 16PF personality inventory and found that cluster-headache patients differed from controls with regard to five scales. They described themselves as reserved and detached, conscientious and persevering, self-sufficient, controlling, and tense.

The Minnesota Multiphasic Personality Inventory (MMPI) was used by Steinhilber and associates (33), who compared 50 cluster-headache patients with 50 control subjects who had headaches of various types other than cluster headache. Both groups scored significantly higher on the hypochondriasis and hysteria scales and low on the depression scale.

Rogado and colleagues (27) used the MMPI profile to compare cluster-headache and migraine patients. Both groups scored significantly higher on hysteria, psychoasthenia (obsessive–compulsive), and hypochondria scales than a control group, but they did not differ from controls with regard to depression.

Cuypers and colleagues (3) compared cluster-headache and migraine patients in the Freiburg Personality Inventory, which is similar to the MMPI. Similar results were found in the two headache groups, although cluster headache patients had moderately elevated scores for anxiety and slightly diminished scores for masculinity.

Levi and associates (23) studied 49 cluster-headache patients using two personality inventories, the Karolinska Scales of Personality and the Heart and Lifestyle Type A Measure. Compared with nonheadache controls, the cluster-headache patients were significantly more anxiety prone, less successfully socialized, and had a more hostile attitude toward others.

In summary, personality variables seem to differ between cluster-headache patients and nonheadache controls. It is uncertain, however, whether cluster-headache patients differ in this respect compared with other headache groups.

REFERENCES

1. Anselmi B, Baldi E, Casacci F, Salmon S. Endogenous opioids in cerebrospinal fluid and blood in idiopathic headache sufferers. *Headache* 1980;20:294–299.1A.
2. Bussone G, Sinatra MG, Boiardi A, et al. Brainstem auditory evoked potential (BAEPs) in cluster headache (CH): new aspects for a central theory. *Headache* 1986;26:67–69.
3. Cuypers J, Altenkirch H, Bunge S. Personality profiles in cluster headache and migraine. *Headache* 1981;21:21–24.
4. Dahl A, Russell D, Nyberg-Hansen R, Rootwelt K. Cluster headache: transcranial Doppler ultrasound and rCBF studies. *Cephalalgia* 1990;10:87–94.
5. Drummond P. Autonomic disturbances in cluster headache. *Brain* 1988;111:1199–1209.
6. Drummond PD, Anthony M. Extracranial vascular responses to sublingual nitroglycerin and oxygen inhalation in cluster headache patients. *Headache* 1985;25:70–74.
7. Ekbom K. *Studies on cluster headache.* Stockholm: Solna tryckeri, 1970.
8. Fanciullacci M, Fusco BM, Alessandri M, Campagnolo V, Sicuteri F. Unilateral impairment of pupillary response to trigeminal nerve stimulation in cluster headache. *Pain* 1989;36:185–191.
9. Fanciullacci M, Pietrini U, Gatto G, Boccuni M, Sicuteri F. Latent dysautonomic pupillary lateralization in cluster headache: a pupillometric study. *Cephalalgia* 1982;2:135–144.
10. Firenze C, Del Gatto F, Mazzotta G, Gallai V. Somatosensory evoked potential study in headache patients. *Cephalalgia* 1988;8:157–162.
11. Friedman AP, Mikropoulos HE. Cluster headaches. *Neurology* 1958;8:653–663.
12. Graham JR. Some physical, physiological and psychological characteristics of patients with cluster headache. Londoon: *Proceedings of the 3rd International Symposium of the Migraine Trust.* 1969:38–52.
13. Hardebo JE, Ekman R. Substance P and opioids in cluster headache. In: Sicuteri F, Vecchiet L, Fanciullacci M, eds. *Trends in cluster headache.* Amsterdam: Elsevier, 1987:145–158.
14. Hardebo JE, Ekman R, Eriksson M. Low CSF met-enkephalin levels in cluster headache are elevated by acupuncture. *Headache* 1989;29:494–497.

15. Hasan Z, Sjaastad O, Lundervold A. An electroencephalographical investigation of patients with cluster headache. *Clin Electroencephalogr* 1976;7:203–207.

16. Horton BT. Histaminic cephalalgia. *JAMA* 1956;160:468–469.

17. Kudrow L. Physical and personality characteristics in cluster headache. *Headache* 1974;13:197–202.

18. Kudrow L. Response of cluster headache attacks to oxygen inhalation. *Headache* 1981;21:1–4.

19. Kudrow L. A possible role of the carotid body in the pathogenesis of cluster headache. *Cephalalgia* 1983;3:241–247.

20. Kudrow L, Kudrow DB. Association of sustained oxyhemoglobin desaturation and onset of cluster headache attacks. *Headache* 1990;30:474–480.

21. Kudrow L, McGinty DJ, Philips ER, Stevenson M. Sleep apnea in cluster headache. *Cephalalgia* 1984;4:33–38.

22. Kunkle EC. Acetylcholine in the mechanism of headache of the migraine type. *Arch Neurol Psychiatry* 1959;84:135–141.

23. Levi R, Edman GV, Ekbom K, Waldenlind E. Episodic cluster headache I: Personality and some neuropsychological characteristics in male patients. *Headache* 1992;32:119–125.

24. Micieli G, Magri M, Sandrini G, Tassorelli C, Nappi G. Pupil responsiveness in cluster headache: a dynamic TV pupillometric evaluation. *Cephalalgia* 1988;8:193–201.

25. Peters GA. Migraine: diagnosis and treatment with emphasis on the migraine tension headache, provocative tests and use of rectal suppositories. *Mayo Clin Proc* 1953;28:673–686.

26. Procacci P, Zoppi M, Maresca M, Zamponi A, Fanciullacci M, Sicuteri F. Lateralisation of pain in cluster headache. *Pain* 1989;38:275–278.

27. Rogado AZ, Harrison RH, Graham JR. Personality profiles in cluster headache, migraine and normal controls. *Arch Neurobiol* 1974;37:227–241.

28. Salvesen R, Fredriksen TA, Bogucki A, Sjaastad O. Sweat gland and pupillary responsiveness in Horner's syndrome. *Cephalalgia* 1987;7:135–146.

29. Salvesen R, Sand T, Sjaastad O. Cluster headache: combined assessment with pupillometry and evaporimetry. *Cephalalgia* 1988;8:211–218.

30. Sandrini G, Alfonsi E, Ruiz L, et al. Impairment of corneal pain perception in cluster headache. *Pain* 1991;47:299–304.

31. Saunte C, Russell D, Sjaastad O. Cluster headache: on the mechanism behind attack-related sweating. *Cephalalgia* 1983;3:175–185.

32. Sicuteri F, Fanciullacci M, Geppetti P, Renzi D, Caleri D, Spillantini MG. Substance-P mechanism in cluster headache: evaluaton in plasma and cerebrospinal fluid. *Cephalalgia* 1985;5:143–149.

33. Steinhilber RM, Peason JS, Rushton JG. Some psychological considerations of histaminic cephalalgia. *Mayo Clin Proc* 1960;35:691–699.

34. Strittmatter M, Hamann GF, Grauer M, et al. Altered activity of the sympathetic nervous system and changes in the balance of hypophyseal, pituary and adrenal hormones in patients with cluster headache. *Neuroreport* 1996;7:1229–1234.

35. Zhao J-M, Schaanning J, Sjaastad O. Cluster headache: the effect of low oxygen saturation. *Headache* 1990;30:656–659.

36. Zhao J-M, Sand T, Sjaastad O. Cluster headache: oxygen saturation and end-tidal CO_2 during and without attack. *Headache* 1992;32:126–131.

The Headaches, Second Edition,
edited by J. Olesen, P. Tfelt-Hansen, and K.M.A. Welch.
Lippincott Williams & Wilkins, Philadelphia © 2000.

Tension-Type Headache, Cluster Headache, and Miscellaneous Primary Headaches

CHAPTER 94

Neuroimaging of Cluster Headache

Arne May and Peter J. Goadsby

The most remarkable of the clinical features of cluster headache is the striking rhythm or cycling of the attacks and bouts. Cluster headache is probably the most severe pain syndrome known to humans, with female patients describing each attack as being worse than childbirth. The syndrome is well defined from a clinical point of view (34), and despite having been recognized in the literature for more than two centuries (41), its pathophysiology has been hitherto poorly understood. Recently, neuroimaging has made substantial contributions to understanding this relatively rare but important syndrome.

VASCULAR VERSUS NEUROGENIC MECHANISMS

In contrast to migraine, for which at least two experimental models have been developed and tested in clinically relevant settings by pharmacologic means (see Chapter 49), in this related, more severe form of headache, several different pathophysiologic concepts have emerged. A comprehensive model for cluster headache must explain the unilateral headache as well as sympathetic impairment and parasympathetic activation. Recent functional imaging data may allow such a model to be developed.

Despite the large number of investigations in recent years, the issue of peripheral (e.g., vessel or perivascular inflammation) versus central nervous system (e.g., hypothalamic or parasympathetic) mechanisms is still unresolved. The pathophysiologic concept of vascular headaches is based on the idea that changes in vessel diameter

or gross changes in cerebral blood flow (CBF) would trigger pain and thus explain the mechanism of action of vasoconstrictor drugs, such as ergotamine (74).

Cluster headache has been attributed to an inflammatory process in the cavernous sinus and tributary veins (32,56). Inflammation has been thought to obliterate venous outflow from the cavernous sinus on one side, thus injuring the traversing sympathetic fibers of the intracranial internal carotid artery and its branches. According to this theory, the active period ends when the inflammation is suppressed and the sympathetic fibers partially or fully recover. This theory is based substantially on abnormal findings using orbital phlebography in cluster headache patients (27,30,69) and on the fact that nitroglycerin and other vasodilators can induce an acute cluster headache attack (12).

In a study of cluster headache patients using magnetic resonance imaging (MRI), no definite pathologic changes were found in the area of the cavernous sinus (70). Using single photon emission computed tomography (SPECT), parasellar hyperactivity was present in 50% (episodic) to 80% (chronic) of cluster headache patients and in 70% of migraneurs (68). Similar findings on orbital phlebography can be seen in the cavernous region in patients with Tolosa-Hunt syndrome (29), hemicrania continua (3), short-lasting unilateral neuralgiform headache attacks with conjunctival infection and tearing (SUNCT) syndrome (31,45), and chronic paroxysmal hemicrania (3, 28), suggesting that the changes are not specific for cluster headache. Moreover, given the circadian rhythm of attacks and the cycling of bouts (33,48,49), a purely vasogenic cause cannot explain the entire picture of cluster headache (23). In view of the striking relapsing–remitting course (49), its seasonal variation (49), and the clockwise regularity (13),

A. May: Klinik für Psychiatrie und Psychotherapie, D-45147 Essen, Germany.

P. J. Goadsby: The National Hospital for Neurology and Neurosurgery, London WC1N 3BG, United Kingdom.

the concept of a central origin of cluster headache merits consideration (13,46).

HEMODYNAMICS

Transcranial Doppler

Because cluster headache has been regarded as a vascular headache and cluster headache attacks may be provoked by the vasodilators histamine, nitroglycerin, and alcohol, several Doppler studies were carried out to examine possible diameter changes in large intracerebral arteries (Table 1). Most studies demonstrated a bilateral decrease in blood flow velocity (BFV) in the middle cerebral artey and the anterior cerebral artery during the attack compared with the headache-free interval (1,9,47, 64,67). Three studies used the elegant combination of Doppler and blood flow measurement using SPECT. Dahl and colleagues (9) and Afra and associates (1) demonstrated a decrease in BFV during acute cluster headache attack in frontal arteries but failed to show any blood flow changes. Gawel and colleagues (20) measured the CO_2 reactivity of the major intracranial vessels and showed that the CO_2 reactivity was significantly lower during the cluster period but only in the ipsilateral anterior cerebral artery to the headache side. Using gallium SPECT, they described a lesion in the region of the cavernous sinus in three of six patients during the active cluster period; the lesion faded as the patient moved out of the active period. These authors suggested that this finding may represent the cavernous sinus plexus lesion, which is postulated as the central defect in cluster headache.

In summary, transcranial Doppler studies have shown decreased velocity in the middle cerebral artery after nitroglycerin administration and in the acute cluster headache attack. It was also shown that this vasodilation did not alter blood flow to the brain.

Cerebral Blood Flow

Studies of CBF in cluster headache are relatively few. Most have been done using SPECT, and the results of this semiquantitative method have been quite heterogeneous, probably as a result of methodologic differences (Table 2); some studies have reported an increase (43,58,61,62, 73), some a decrease (59, 73), and some no differences in cortical blood flow (1,9,35,36,44,63). The recent study by Di Piero and co-workers (11) studied cluster headache patients out of the active period and normal volunteers by using the cold-water pressor test. They found changes in pain transmission systems that bear more detailed examination. The fact that the alterations are also present outside the active period of the disease suggests a possible involvement of central tonic pain mechanisms in the pathogenesis of cluster headache.

Functional Neuroimaging

Positron emission tomography (PET) may represent the best currently available technique for visualizing *in vivo* changes in regional cerebral blood flow (rCBF) in humans. Modern high-resolution PET scanning allows the detection of subtle changes in rCBF during defined behavioral tasks and provides an index of synaptic activity relating networks of regions to tested brain functions (17,18). Attacks of cluster headache can be elicited using nitroglycerin during the active cluster period without significant side effects (12). Clinical and experimental data show nitroglycerin-provoked and spontaneous cluster attacks to be comparable (15,22), and nitroglycerin does not alter rCBF significantly (39,44). The headache can be rapidly and effectively aborted by administration of sumatriptan. This approach allows the detection of brain regions with increased blood flow during nitroglycerin-induced cluster attacks, focusing interest on the hypothalamic region.

In 1996 the first PET study in cluster headache was reported (39). The authors investigated only four patients, and their findings supported their earlier work (38), suggesting a preference for the nondominant hemisphere, especially the anterior cingulate cortex, in affective processing of chronic ongoing pain syndromes. These interesting results contribute to understanding central pain

TABLE 1. *Doppler studies different headache types*

Author	Year	Diagnosis	Study population (attack/interval)	Number of patients	BFV changes		
					Increase	Decrease	No change
Afra et al. (1)	1995	CH	Attack/interval	19		X	
Dahl et al. (9)	1990	CH	Attack	25		X	
Kudrow (47)	1979	CH	Attack/Interval	26		X	
Schroth et al. (64)	1983	CH	Attack	6	X		
Shen (65)	1993	CPH	Attack	3		X	
Shen et al. (67)	1993	CH	Attack/interval	14		X	
Shen and Johnson (66)	1994	SUNCT	Interval	4			X

BFV, blood flow velocity; CH, cluster headache; CPH, chronic paroxysmal hemicrania; SUNCT, short-lasting unilateral neuralgiform headache attacks with conjunctival injection and and tearing.

TABLE 2. *Single photon emission computerized tomography (SPECT) studies in cluster headache (CH)*

Author	Year	Diagnosis	Method	n	CBC changes		
					Increase	Decrease	No change
Afra et al. (1)	1995	CH	^{99m}TC-HMPAO	19			X
Dahl et al. (9)	1990	CH	^{133}Xenon	25			X
Henry et al. (35)	1978	CH	^{135}Xenon	3			X
Hering et al. (36)	1991	CH	^{99m}TC-HMPAO	14			X
Kobari et al. (43)	1990	CH	^{133}Xenon	5	X		
Krabbe et al. (44)	1984	CH	^{133}Xenon	18			X
Nelson et al. (58)	1980	CH	^{133}Xenon	26	X	X	
Norris et al. (59)	1976	CH	^{133}Xenon	1			X
Sakai and Meyer (62)	1978	CH	^{133}Xenon	9	X		
Schlake et al. (63)	1990	CH	^{99m}TC-HMPAO	5			X
Wesseling et al. (73)	1989	CH	^{99m}TC-HMPAO	8	X	X	

transmission systems but, given the small subject numbers, require confirmation.

In our recent studies of more than 20 cluster headache patients in and outside of the" bout," we observed, by using PET, areas of activation in acute cluster headache that fall into two broad groups: areas known to be involved in pain processing or responses to pain (e.g., cingulate, insula cortex, thalamus) and areas activated specifically in cluster headache but not in other causes of head pain, notably the hypothalamic gray area (51). These data suggest that primary headache syndromes share some processing pathways but can be distinguished on a functional neuroanatomic basis by areas of activation specific to the clinical presentation.

AREAS OF ACTIVATION COMMON TO PAIN

Activation of the anterior cingulate cortex has been reported repeatedly in PET studies on the sensation of somatic or visceral pain and has been attributed to the emotional response to pain (5,39,42,60). Activations in the insula have been demonstrated in previous studies after the application of heat (5,8,55), subcutaneous injection of ethanol (40), somatosensory stimulation (4), and during cluster headache (39) and atypical facial pain (10). Given its anatomic connections, the insula has been suggested to be a relay of sensory information into the limbic system and is known to play an important role in the regulation of autonomic responses (54). Painful stimuli are significantly effective in activating the anterior insula, a region heavily linked with both somatosensory and limbic systems. Such connections may provide one route through which nociceptive input is integrated with memory to allow full appreciation of the meaning and dangers of painful stimuli. The thalamus is a site where activations certainly would be expected in the acute pain state. Activation of the contralateral thalamus as a result of pain is known to occur from experimental studies in animals (26) and from functional imaging studies in humans

(5,60). The acute pain in cluster headache induces activation bilaterally in the cerebellar hemispheres and in the vermis. There appears to be no direct nociceptive input to the cerebellum (14), and there is no clinical evidence that cerebellar lesions or stimulation affect pain sensation in humans (5). Some PET studies, however, found activation in this area during experimental pain (5,38).

Areas of Activation in Cluster Headache Compared with other Forms of Head Pain

PET studies in primary headaches are few (Table 3). In contrast to migraine (72), no brainstem activation was found during the acute attack compared with the resting state. This finding is remarkable because migraine and cluster headache often are discussed as related disorders; identical relatively headache-specific compounds, such as ergotamine and sumatriptan, are currently used in the acute treatment of both types of headache. These data suggest that whereas primary headaches, such as migraine and cluster headache, may share a common pain pathway (i.e., the trigeminovascular innervation), the underlying pathogenesis differs significantly, as may be inferred from the different patterns of presentation and responses to preventative agents (25).

Areas of Activation Related to Cluster Headache

Significant areas of activation in PET attributable to cluster headache were observed in the ipsilateral hypothalamic gray area compared with the headache-free state (51). Just as it is striking that no brainstem activation occurs, in contrast to acute migraine (72), no hypothalamic activation was seen to occur in experimental pain induced by capsaicin injection into the forehead (53). Injection of the forehead would activate the first (ophthalmic)-division afferents, which traverse the trigeminal division responsible for pain activation in cluster headache. Thus, two other types of first-division trigemi-

TABLE 3. *Positron emission tomography (PET)-studies in headache*

Author	Year	Headache type	No. of patients	Cingulate cortex	Insulae	Thalamus	Brainstem	Hypothalamus
Derbyshire et al. (10)	1994	A-fp	6	√	√	√	×	×
Hsieh et al. (39)	1996	Cluster headache	4	√	√	×	×	×
Weiller et al. (72)	1995	MO	9	√	×	×	√	×
May et al. (53)	1998	Capsaicin	7	√	√	√	×	×
May et al. (51)	1999	Cluster headache	9	√	√	√	×	√
Andersson et al. (2)	1997	MA, MO	11	No global blood flow changes				
Chabriat et al. (6)	1995	MA,MO	9	No change in 5-HT$_2$ receptor distributions				
Sachs et al. (61)	1986	MA,MO	4	Reserpine changes glucose metabolism in migraine				

afp, atypical facial pain; MO, migraine without aura; MA migraine with aura; CH, cluster headache; Capsaicin, experimental head pain using capsaicin injection; √ demonstrated; ×, not demonstrated.

nal nerve pain, while sharing neuroanatomic pathways with cluster headache, do not give rise to hypothalamic activation. Moreover, in eight cluster headache patients not experiencing an attack after nitroglycerin administration, the rCBF in the region of the hypothalamic gray area was not increased. This finding clearly implies that the activation in the hypothalamic gray area we observed is involved in the pain process in a permissive or triggering manner rather than simply as a response to first-division nociception per se.

The functional imaging data are consistent with the known biology of cluster headache. The striking circadian rhythm of cluster headache led to the suggestion of a central origin for its initiation (13,46). Significantly lowered levels of plasma testosterone in men during cluster headache provided the first evidence of hypothalamic involvement in cluster headache (57) and was supported by the finding of a reduced response to thyrotropin-releasing hormone (50) and a range of other circadian irregularities that have been reported in cluster headache patients (7,16). Melatonin in particular is a marker of the circadian system, and a blunted nocturnal peak in melatonin level and a complete loss of circadian rhythm have been reported in cluster headache patients (7,71). The endogenous circadian rhythm is run by an oscillator in the suprachiasmatic nuclei in the ventral hypothalamus and is entrained to temporal environmental cues by light conditions through a retinohypothalamic pathway (37). Clinical observations thus suggest the hypothalamus or a closely related structure as a candidate for triggering the acute attack of cluster headache.

Vessels

Using PET, an activation pattern clearly outside the brain parenchyma was observed bilaterally in midline structures over several planes (from –32 mm to –20 mm with respect to the anterior comissure–posterior comissure line), anterior to the brainstem and posterior to the

region of the optic chiasm region. Superimposed on an MRI template, the location of the activation corresponded to the intracranial arteries bilaterally and the region of the cavernous sinus (51,52). This holds true in two group studies as well as in 15 out of 17 single subject analyses. Bilateral activation in this region might be an indication of increased venous inflow from the superior ophthalmic vein draining the ophthalmic artery. Another possibility is that the observed increase in activation might be due to bilateral dilatation of the internal carotid artery. Both spontaneous and glyceryl trinitrate (nitroglycerin)-provoked attacks are reported to be accompanied by a bilateral decrease in middle cerebral artery BFV, indicating vasodilation (9). It is difficult to assess the contribution of these two sources to the activation, particularly because it is beyond the spatial resolution of scanning to distinguish venous from arterial vessels in the cavernous sinus. Using magnetic resonance angiography (MRA) and the same experimental design as in the PET study, it was demonstrated that dilatation of the basilar artery and both internal carotid arteries occurred compared with the status in the headache-free resting state (52). Using PET, significant activity in the region of the cavernous sinus was described in cluster patients (39); however, given that we have observed vasodilatation in large vessels after capsaicin injection to the forehead, again in a PET study (53), in a condition without the influence of a systemic vasodilator and without the pathophysiologic background of cluster headache, it seems likely that the vascular changes are an epiphenomenon of activation of the trigeminovascular system (21). In healthy controls, a pain-provoking application of capsaicin to the nasal mucosa induced vasodilation in the internal carotid, whereas middle cerebral arteries and the basilar artery were narrowed (19). With this background, our data raise the possibility that vasodilation or increase in flow, or both, in the cavernous region is not specific to cluster headache or does not form a significant part of the pathophysiology of the acute attack of cluster headache. Our data suggest that activation of the trigeminal system as such is sufficient to trigger vasodilation of these vessels.

CONCLUSION

Cluster headache, like migraine, is still recognized as a vascular headache, even though in both conditions a central cause has been suggested. Functional imaging studies with positron emission tomography (PET) in cluster headache patients in the active period and when the subject is headache free underline the need to focus the scientific approach on the central nervous system. In the acute cluster headache attack, but not in the patients not having an attack, the ipsilateral inferior hypothalamic grey area was activated, which in view of the clinical data strongly suggests that this area plays a significant role in the pathophysiology of cluster headache.

Additionally, activation in the region of the major basal arteries was observed, probably as a result of vasodilation of these vessels. This vasodilation was caused in part by nitroglycerin but more significantly by headache during the acute pain-attack as opposed to the headache-free state in cluster headache. Vasodilatation was observed in experimental trigeminal transmitted pain as well; therefore, we conclude that the observed dilatation of these vessels in trigeminal pain is not, as was implied, inherent to a specific headache syndrome. Clinical and animal data rather suggest that the observed vasodilation is not specific to the cause but is rather an effect of a trigemino-parasympathetic reflex (24). The known physiology and pathophysiology of the system involved suggest that these disorders should be regarded collectively as neuro-vascular headaches to emphasize the interaction between nerves and vessels, which is the underlying characteristic of these syndromes.

REFERENCES

1. Afra J, Ertsey C, Jelencsik H, Dabasi G, Panczel G. SPECT and TCD studies in cluster headache patients. *Funct Neurol* 1995;10:259–264.
2. Andersson JL, Muhr C, Lilja A, Valind S, Lundberg PO, Langstrom B. Regional cerebral blood flow and oxygen metabolism during migraine with and without aura. *Cephalalgia* 1997;17:570–579.
3. Antonaci F. Chronic paroxysmal hemicrania and hemicrania continua: orbital phlebography and MRI studies. *Headache* 1994;34:32–34.
4. Burton H, Videen TO, Raichle ME. Tactile vibration activated foci in insular and parietal opercular cortex studied with positron emission tomography. *Somatosens Mot Res* 1993;3:297–308.
5. Casey KL, Minoshima S, Berger KL, Koeppe RA, Morrow TJ, Frey KA. Positron emission tomographic analysis of cerebral structures activated specifically by repetitive noxious heat stimuli. *J Neurophysiol* 1994;71:802–807.
6. Chabriat H, Tehindrazanarivelo A, Vera P, et al. 5HT2 receptors in cerebral cortex of migraineurs studied using PET and 18F-fluorosetoperone. *Cephalalgia* 1995;15:104–108.
7. Chazot G, Claustrat B, Brun J, Jordan D, Sassolas G, Schott B. A chronobiological study of melatonin, cortisol, growth hormone and prolactin secretion in cluster headache. *Cephalalgia* 1984;4:213–220.
8. Coghill RC, Talbot JD, Evans AC, et al. Distributed processing of pain and vibration by the human brain. *J Neurosci* 1994;14:4095–4108.
9. Dahl A, Russell D, Nyberg Hansen R, Rootwelt K. Cluster headache:

10. transcranial Doppler ultrasound and rCBF studies. *Cephalalgia* 1990; 10:87–94.
10. Derbyshire SW, Jones AK, Devani P, et al. Cerebral responses to pain in patients with atypical facial pain measured by positron emission tomography. *J Neurol Neurosurg Psychiatry* 1994;57:1166–72.
11. Di Piero V, Fiacco F, Tombari D, Pantano P. Tonic pain: a SPET study in normal subjects and cluster headache patients. *Pain* 1997;70:185–191.
12. Ekbom K. Nitroglycerin as a provocative agent in cluster headache. *Arch Neurol* 1968;19:487–493.
13. Ekbom K. Patterns of cluster headache with a note on the relations to angina pectoris and peptide ulcer. *Acta Neurol Scand* 1970;46:225–237.
14. Ekerot CF, Garwicz M, Schouenborg J. Topography and nociceptive receptive fields of climbing fibres projecting to the cerebellar anterior lobe in the cat. *J Physiol (Lond)* 1991;441:257–274.
15. Fanciullacci M, Alessandri M, Figini M, Geppetti P, Michelacci S. Increases in plasma calcitonin gene-related peptide from extracerebral circulation during nitroglycerin-induced cluster headache attack. *Pain* 1995;60:119–123.
16. Ferrari E, Canepari C, Bossolo PA, et al. Changes of biological rhythms in primary headache syndromes. *Cephalalgia* 1983;3:58–68.
17. Fox PT, Mintun MA. Noninvasive functional brain mapping by change-distribution analysis of averaged PET images of H215O tissue activity. *J Nucl Med* 1989;30:141–149.
18. Frackowiak RS, Friston KJ. Functional neuroanatomy of the human brain: positron emission tomography—a new neuroanatomical technique. *J Anat* 1994;184:211–225.
19. Fusco BM, Fiore G, Gallo F, Martelletti P, Giacovazzo M. "Capsaicin-sensitive" sensory neurons in cluster headache: pathophysiological aspects and therapeutic indication. *Headache* 1994;34:132–137.
20. Gawel MJ, Krajewski A, Luo YM, Ichise M. The cluster diathesis. *Headache* 1990;30:652–655.
21. Goadsby PJ, Duckworth JW. Effect of stimulation of trigeminal ganglion on regional cerebral blood flow in cats. *Am J Physiol* 1987;253:270–274.
22. Goadsby PJ, Edvinsson L. Human *in vivo* evidence for trigeminovascular activation in cluster headache: neuropeptide changes and effects of acute attacks therapies. *Brain* 1994;117:427–434.
23. Goadsby PJ, Lance JW. Brainstem effects on intra- and extracerebral circulations: relation to migraine and cluster headache. In: Olesen J, ed. *Basic mechanisms of headache*. Amsterdam: Elsevier Science Publishers, 1988:413–427.
24. Goadsby PJ, Lipton RB. A review of paroxysmal hemicranias, SUNCT syndrome and other short-lasting headaches with autonomic feature, including new cases. *Brain* 1997;120:193–209.
25. Goadsby PJ, Silberstein SD. *Headache*. New York: Butterworth-Heinemann, 1997.
26. Goadsby PJ, Zagami AS, Lambert GA. Neural processing of craniovascular pain: a synthesis of the central structures involved in migraine. *Headache* 1991;31:365–371.
27. Hannerz J. Orbital phlebography and signs of inflammation in episodic and chronic cluster headache. *Headache* 1991;31:540–542.
28. Hannerz J, Ericson K, Bergstrand G. Chronic paroxysmal hemicrania: orbital phlebography and steroid treatment: a case report. *Cephalalgia* 1987;7:189–192.
29. Hannerz J, Ericson K, Bergstrand G. A new etiology for visual impairment and chronic headache: the Tolosa-Hunt syndrome may be only one manifestation of venous vasculitis. *Cephalalgia* 1986;6:59–63.
30. Hannerz J, Ericson K, Bergstrand G. Orbital phlebography in patients with cluster headache. *Cephalalgia* 1987;7:207–211.
31. Hannerz J, Greitz D, Hansson P, Ericson K. SUNCT may be another manifestation of orbital venous vasculitis. *Headache* 1992;32:384–389.
32. Hardebo JE. How cluster headache is explained as an intracavernous inflammatory process lesioning sympathetic fibres. *Headache* 1994; 34:125–131.
33. Harris W. Ciliary (migraneous) neuralgia and its treatment. *BMJ* 1936; 1:475–460.
34. Headache Classification Committee of the International Headache Society. Classification and diagnostic criteria for headache disorders, cranial neuralgias and facial pain. *Cephalalgia* 1988;8:1–96.
35. Henry PY, Vernhiet J, Orgogozo JM, Caille JM. Cerebral blood flow in migraine and cluster headache: compartmental analysis and reactivity to anaesthetic depression. *Research Clinical Studies in Headache* 1978;6:81–88.
36. Hering R, Couturier EGM, Davies PTG, Steiner TJ. 99mTC-HMPAO

study during cluster headache period and in acute cluster attacks. In: *Frontiers in headache research,* vol. 1. New York: Raven Press, 1991: 297–299.

37. Hofman MA, Zhou JN, Swaab DF. Suprachiasmatic nucleus of the human brain: an immunocytochemical and morphometric analysis. *J Comp Neurol* 1996;305:552–556.

38. Hsieh JC, Belfrage M, Stone Elander S, Hansson P, Ingvar M. Central representation of chronic ongoing neuropathic pain studied by positron emission tomography. *Pain* 1995;63:225–36.

39. Hsieh JC, Hannerz J, Ingvar M. Right-lateralised central processing for pain of nitroglycerin-induced cluster headache. *Pain* 1996; 67:59–68.

40. Hsieh JC, Stahle Backdahl M, Hagermark O, Stone Elander S, Rosenquist G, Ingvar M. Traumatic nociceptive pain activates the hypothalamus and the periaqueductal gray: a positron emission tomography study. *Pain* 1996;64:303–314.

41. Isler H. Episodic cluster headache from a textbook of 1745: Van Swieten's classic description. *Cephalalgia* 1993;13:172–174.

42. Jones AK, Friston K, Frackowiak RS. Localization of responses to pain in human Cerebral cortex. *Science* 1992;255:215–216.

43. Kobari M, Meyer JS, Ichijo M, Kawamura J. Cortical and subcortical hyperperfusion during migraine and cluster headache measured by Xe CT-CBF. *Neuroradiology* 1990;32:4–11.

44. Krabbe AA, Henriksen L, Olesen J. Tomographic determination of cerebral blood flow during attacks of cluster headache. *Cephalalgia* 1984;4:17–23.

45. Kruszewski P. Shortlasting, unilateral, neuralgiform headache attacks with conjunctival injection and tearing (SUNCT syndrome): V. Orbital phlebography. *Cephalalgia* 1992;12:387–389.

46. Kudrow L. The cylic relationship of natural illumination to cluster period frequency. *Cephalalgia* 1987;7:76–78.

47. Kudrow L. Thermographic and Doppler flow asymmetry in cluster headache. *Headache* 1979;19:204–208.

48. Kunkle EC. Clues in the tempos of cluster headache. *Headache* 1982; 22:158–161.

49. Kunkle EC, Pfieffer J, Wilhoit WM, Hamrick J. Recurrent brief headache in cluster pattern. *Transactions of the American Neurological Association* 1952;27:240–243.

50. Leone M, Patruno G, Vescovi A, Bussone G. Neuroendocrine dysfunction in cluster headache. *Cephalalgia* 1990;10:235–239.

51. May A, Bahra A, Büchel C, Frackowiak RSJ, Goadsby PJ. First direct evidence for hypothalamic activation in cluster headache attacks. *Lancet* 1998;352:275–278.

52. May A, Büchel C, Bahra A, Goadsby PJ, Frackowiak RSJ. Intra-cranial vessels in trigeminal transmitted pain: a PET study. *Neuroimage* 1999;9:453–460.

53. May A, Kaube H, Buechel C, et al. Experimental cranial pain elicited by capsaicin: a PET-study. *Pain* 1998;74:61–66.

54. Mesulam MM, Mufson EF. The insula of Reil in man and monkey. In: *Architectonics, connectivity and function.* New York: Plenum, 1985:179–226.

55. Minoshima S, Morrow TJ, Koeppe RA, Casey KL. Involvement of the insular cortex in central autonomic regulation during painful thermal stimulation. *J Cereb Blood Flow Metab* 1995;15:859.

56. Moskowitz MA. Cluster headache: evidence for a pathophysiologic focus in the superior pericarotid cavernous sinus plexus. *Headache* 1988;28:584–586.

57. Nelson RF. Testosterone levels in cluster and non-cluster migrainous patients. *Headache* 1978;18:265–267.

58. Nelson RF, du Boulay GH, Marshall J, Russell RW, Symon L, Zilkha E. Cerebral blood flow studies in patients with cluster headache. *Headache* 1980;20:184–189.

59. Norris JW, Hachinski VC, Cooper PW. Cerebral blood flow changes in cluster headache. *Acta Neurol Scand* 1976;54:371–374.

60. Rosen SD, Paulesu E, Frith CD, et al. Central nervous pathways mediating angina pectoris. *Lancet* 1994;344:147–150.

61. Sachs H, Wolf A, Russell JA, Christman DR. Effect of reserpine on regional cerebral glucose metabolism in control and migraine subjects. *Arch Neurol* 1986;43:1117–1123.

62. Sakai F, Meyer JS. Regional cerebral hemodynamics during migraine and cluster headaches measured by the ^{133}Xe inhalation method. *Headache* 1978;18:122–132.

63. Schlake HP, Bottger IG, Grotemeyer KH, et al. Single photon emission computed tomography with technetium-^{99}m hexamethyl propylenamino oxime in the pain-free interval of migraine and cluster headache. *Eur Neurol* 1990;30:153–156.

64. Schroth G, Gerber WD, Langohr HD. Ultrasonic Doppler flow in migraine and cluster headache. *Headache* 1983;23:284–288.

65. Shen JM. Transcranial Doppler sonography in chronic paroxysmal hemicrania. *Headache* 1993;33:493–496.

66. Shen JM, Johnsen HJ. SUNCT syndrome: estimation of cerebral blood flow velocity with transcranial Doppler ultrasonography. *Headache* 1994;34:25–31.

67. Shen JM, Johnsen HJ, Juul R. Cluster headache: transcranial Doppler assessment of dynamic cerebral circulatory changes during hypocapnia and attack. *Headache* 1993;33:488–492.

68. Sianard-Gainko J, Milet J, Ghuysen V, Schoenen J. Increased parasellar activity on gallium SPECT is not specific for active cluster headache. *Cephalalgia* 1994;14:132–133.

69. Sjaastad O. Cluster Headache Syndrome. In: *Major problems in neurology.* London: WB Saunders, 1992:191–193.

70. Sjaastad O, Rinck P. Cluster headache: MRI studies of the cavernous sinus and the base of the brain. *Headache* 1990;30:350–351.

71. Waldenlind E, Gustafsson SA, Ekbom K, Wetterberg L. Circadian secretion of cortisol and melatonin in cluster headache during active cluster periods and remission. *J Neurol Neurosurg Psychiatry* 1987; 50:207–213.

72. Weiller C, May A, Limmroth V, et al. Brain stem activation in spontaneous human migraine attacks. *Nat Med* 1995;1:658–660.

73. Wesseling P, Suess E, Koch G, Woeber C, Deecke L. SPECT (99M)TC-HMPAO Findings in acute headache and during synptom free interval. *Cephalalgia* 1989;9:62–63.

74. Wolff HG. *Headache and other head pain,* 3rd ed. New York: Oxford University Press, 1963.

The Headaches, Second Edition,
edited by J. Olesen, P. Tfelt-Hansen, and K.M.A. Welch.
Lippincott Williams & Wilkins, Philadelphia © 2000.

Tension-Type Headache, Cluster Headache, and Miscellaneous Primary Headaches

CHAPTER 95

Synthesis of Cluster Headache Pathophysiology

Elisabet Waldenlind and Peter D. Drummond

Cluster headache is a distinct syndrome, rarely causing any diagnostic problems when applying the International Headache Society (IHS) diagnostic criteria. However, the etiology of cluster headache is still unknown, and there is no unifying pathogenetic model explaining all the various findings of cluster headache. Some challenging issues are the relapsing-remitting course with clusters of severe periorbital, unilateral pain attacks associated with local autonomic symptoms, the circannual periodicity of the cluster periods, the clockwise regularity of the headache attacks, and the male preponderance (10). Cluster headache is categorized as a vascular headache based on findings of vasodilation during attacks and relief by vasoconstrictive drugs, but the knowledge of how cluster headache pain is generated is incomplete. However, progress concerning craniovascular innervation, neuroendocrinology and chronobiology, neurochemistry, functional neuroimaging, neurogenetics, and neuropharmacology has contributed to an increased understanding of the pathophysiology in cluster headache.

UNILATERALITY OF PAIN

One of the main diagnostic criteria for cluster headache attacks is the strict unilaterality, suggesting a locus, either constitutional or acquired, where pain is generated or to which it is referred. Rarely does a cluster headache shift sides for a complete cluster period. The risk of having a cluster period on the previously asymptomatic side

is about 200 times higher (48) than the overall incidence. This may indicate an increased vulnerability in subjects already suffering from cluster headache. Alternatively, cluster headache may be a manifestation of pathology affecting midline structures (48) such as the cavernous sinus (39,22,17). Infections, trauma, or toxic effects have been put forward as possible initiators of cluster headache, but there are no studies characterizing the events that precede the debut of cluster headache. Neither are there any studies of the cluster headache symptomatology during the very first episode of cluster headache.

PAIN CHARACTER

The maximum intensity of pain is generally localized behind the eye, radiating toward the temple or to the upper cheek. It is described as excruciating, almost intolerable, as if the eye is pushed out of the orbit or a knife is being turned around. During pain most patients prefer to stand up or walk about. Attacks of kidney stone or intensive tooth ache, which both are examples of locked-in pain processes, resemble cluster headache with respect to pain character and behavior during pain. The ophthalmic, anterior cerebral, and middle cerebral arteries dilate during attacks of cluster headache (12,19,51). Vascular dilatation together with lowering of the pain threshold by sensitization of pain receptors is likely to contribute to pain; vascular pain, however, would be expected to have a throbbing character, which is rather uncommon in cluster headache (11). Alternatively, pain may be caused by dilated and edematous vessels pressing against surrounding tissues in narrow passages such as the bony carotid canal and the pterygo-palatine fossa, or by obstructed venous outflow from the cavernous sinus. Symptoms

E. Waldenlind: Department of Neurology, Karolinska Institute, and Department of Neurology, Huddinge University Hospital, S-14186 Huddinge, Sweden.

P. D. Drummond: Department of Psychology, Murdoch University, Perth, Western Australia 6150, Australia.

mimicking cluster headache have been described in patients with tumors of the middle fossa, but in cluster headache no structural process has been identified other than dilatation of vessels. Cluster headache has been proposed to be caused by a remitting venous phlebitis in the cavernous sinus based on pathologic orbital phlebograms (17) and inflammatory signs in blood (17) and cerebrospinal fluid (24) in some patients during the cluster period. However, it has not been possible to demonstrate any consistent correspondence between phlebopathic signs and the symptomatic side, and similar phlebopathic findings have been reported in patients with other headache syndromes and in healthy controls (1).

AUTONOMIC DISTURBANCES IN CLUSTER HEADACHE

Opinions diverge over the source of autonomic disturbances in cluster headache. According to some researchers, autonomic dysregulation originates centrally in association with a hypothalamic disturbance that compromises inhibitory pain control mechanisms. Others hold that venous stasis or an inflammatory process in the cavernous sinus accounts for the cyclical pain and associated autonomic symptoms. Another possibility is that many of the autonomic disturbances are secondary to trigeminal discharge, and are not directly involved in the production of pain.

DISTURBANCES IN BLOOD PRESSURE AND HEART RATE

Blood pressure typically increases, whereas heart rate decreases during attacks of cluster headache. Bradycardia is sometimes preceded by transient tachycardia at the onset of the attack. To investigate whether dysregulation of sympathetic vasoconstrictor outflow might contribute to these cardiovascular disturbances, Nordin et al. (41) recorded sympathetic traffic in the peroneal nerve during attacks of cluster headache. Corresponding increases in blood pressure and pulse-synchronous bursts of sympathetic activity indicated that an increase in sympathetic vasoconstrictor outflow to muscles contributed to the increase in blood pressure. This response is almost certainly secondary to pain because the same relationship between bursts of sympathetic activity in the peroneal nerve and blood pressure was observed during eye pain induced by the installation of soapy water (40). Pain or the anticipation of pain also might account for transient tachycardia at the onset of attacks. Cardiac arrhythmias develop during cluster headache attacks in some patients (36), possibly in association with changes in autonomic balance (44) or breathing patterns during intense pain.

The mechanism of bradycardia in cluster headache is uncertain. Spectral analysis of heart rate fluctuations suggests that sympathetic activation causes mild tachycardia at the start of the attack; however, a parasympa-

thetic influence develops later on that produces relative bradycardia (2). Perhaps the parasympathetic response forms part of a normal baroreflex mechanism that attempts to reduce blood pressure; alternatively, activation of trigeminal depressor or oculocardiac reflexes might contribute to bradycardia. A decrease in arterial oxygen saturation precedes attacks of cluster headache, suggesting that hypoxemia may trigger attacks during active cluster periods (30). The bradycardia during attacks of cluster headache is unlikely to be due to this decrease in arterial oxygen saturation because heart rate increases normally in cluster headache patients during oxygen deprivation (47).

Other cardiovascular reflexes also seem to be grossly normal in cluster headache patients during the headache-free interval. Kruszewski et al. (29) reported that decreases in diastolic blood pressure were marginally greater in cluster headache patients than in controls after head-up tilt, but this trend did not achieve statistical significance. Increases in heart rate and decreases in systolic blood pressure did not differ between patients and controls during this test. Respiratory sinus arrhythmia, an index of vagal modulation of heart rate, was lower in patients than in controls, but within normal limits in most cases (28); furthermore, respiratory sinus arrhythmia did not change consistently during attacks of cluster headache.

OCULAR DISTURBANCES

A lesion compromising the peripheral part of the ocular sympathetic pathway appears to be responsible for ocular sympathetic deficit in cluster headache. In patients with a central or preganglionic sympathetic lesion, the symptomatic pupil dilates normally in response to tyramine or hydroxyamphetamine eyedrops, which release noradrenaline from the terminal projections of postganglionic sympathetic fibers. However, pupillary dilatation is impaired in patients with a postganglionic sympathetic lesion and in cluster headache patients with signs of ocular sympathetic deficit (8), presumably because the postganglionic sympathetic fibers are injured or dead.

Micieli et al. (38) reported that pupillary dilatation in response to painful corneal stimulation was attenuated bilaterally in cluster headache patients during the active phase of their headache cycle, but more so on the symptomatic side. The mydriatic response is mediated by sympathetic activation, whereas the miosis that follows this brief mydriatic response is mediated by parasympathetic activity or by the peripheral release of neuropeptides from sensory nerve terminals. Pupillary dilatation in response to painful electrical stimulation of the sural nerve was also attenuated on the symptomatic side in cluster headache patients during bouts (37), but did not differ from control values during the remission period between bouts. It is difficult to reconcile these findings with those of Havelius et al. (25), who reported that bilateral pupillary dilatation induced by painful stimulation of the neck was greater in asymptomatic cluster headache patients than in controls. Havelius et al. (26) subsequently reported that pupillary dilatation in response to neck pain was unrelated to mydriasis after installation of tyramine or phenylephrine eyedrops in asymptomatic cluster headache patients, seemingly ruling out a peripheral adrenergic influence on the size of the pupillary response. Importantly, however, dilatation was impaired on the symptomatic side in patients with persistent signs of ocular sympathetic deficit, consistent with injury to postganglionic sympathetic fibers (25). The occasional presence of ocular sympathetic deficit on the nonsymptomatic side (3) or bilaterally in patients with cluster headache (27) raises questions about the mechanism and site of lesion in these unusual cases. However, in the vast majority of cluster headache patients, persistent signs of ocular sympathetic deficit on the symptomatic side seem to be due to postganglionic sympathetic deficit.

FACIAL FLUSHING AND SWEATING

Thermoregulatory flushing and sweating are impaired on the symptomatic side of the forehead in cluster headache patients with persistent signs of ocular sympathetic deficit (8), but, paradoxically, sweating and blood flow often increase in this region during attacks (7,49). Our studies suggest that cross-innervation of denervated blood vessels and sweat glands by parasympathetic lacrimal fibers may account for this paradoxical response. In particular, we found that painful stimulation of the eye induced sweating and flushing on the sympathetically denervated side of the forehead in patients with a postganglionic lesion, including patients with cluster headache (8); importantly, sweating was symmetrical in most patients with a central or preganglionic sympathetic lesion. If lacrimal fibers sprout collaterally into vacant peripheral sympathetic pathways to establish functional connections with sweat glands, the forehead would sweat when the eye waters, both during painful ocular stimulation and during attacks of cluster headache.

A trigeminal-parasympathetic vasodilator reflex increases forehead blood flow during painful stimulation of the eye (4). This response was greater on the symptomatic side of the forehead than contralaterally in patients with ocular sympathetic deficit (including patients with cluster headache), irrespective of the site of lesion (8). The forehead sweat glands of cluster headache patients are supersensitive to cholinergic substances, presumably in response to denervation (46). Denervation also may induce vascular supersensitivity to other sympathetic neurotransmitters and neuromodulators; if so, vascular supersensitivity might contribute to vasodilatation during attacks of cluster headache.

A central sympathetic lesion usually interrupts sweating and releases sympathetic vasoconstrictor tone in the symptomatic upper limb (31). Thus, if a central sympa-

thetic lesion were responsible for ocular sympathetic deficit in cluster headache, the lesion should also block sweating and vascular activity in the hand. We found that sudomotor responses were symmetrical in patients with cluster headache but were diminished on the symptomatic side of patients with a central or preganglionic cervical sympathetic lesion (6); thus, a central origin of sympathetic deficit in cluster headache seems unlikely.

LACRIMATION, NASAL SECRETION, AND SALIVATION

The lacrimation, nasal stuffiness, and nasal secretion that develop on the symptomatic side during attacks are probably secondary to primary trigeminal discharge, although release of sympathetic vasocontrictor tone during attacks also might contribute to nasal stuffiness. Interruption of parasympathetic pathways in the greater superficial petrosal nerve prevents lacrimation during attacks (15), indicating that the trigeminal-parasympathetic lacrimal reflex mediates this response. Neuropeptides released peripherally from trigeminal nerve endings also might play a minor role in this response or in other signs of autonomic disturbance, such as miosis, eyelid swelling, and conjunctival injection (20). Unlike the sympathetic innervation of the face, trigeminal-parasympathetic reflexes function normally without evidence of denervation supersensitivity in cluster headache patients (45).

Minor increases in sweating, lacrimation, and nasal secretion on the nonsymptomatic side during attacks of cluster headache have prompted speculation that these responses are mediated by a central disturbance (48). When one side of the nose is pinched, corneal moisture increases substantially on the stimulated side (5); however, corneal moisture also increases slightly in the other eye, indicating minor crossover of the trigeminal-parasympathetic lacrimal reflex in the brain stem. This crossover probably accounts for the presence of minor sweating and lacrimation on the nonsymptomatic side during attacks of cluster headache.

Salivation decreases on both sides of the mouth during attacks of cluster headache (45), presumably because sympathetic activation in response to pain overrides reflex trigeminal-parasympathetic salivation due to trigeminal discharge. The sympathetic innervation of salivary glands follows branches of the external carotid artery and trigeminal nerve to the periphery, thus bypassing possible intracranial sites of injury.

POSSIBLE MECHANISMS OF AUTONOMIC DISTURBANCE IN CLUSTER HEADACHE

Most evidence points to a peripheral source of autonomic disturbances in cluster headache. Vasodilatation of the internal carotid artery or swelling of the arterial wall in the carotid canal during attacks might injure the plexus of sympathetic fibers that follow the artery to the periphery (12); alternatively, an inflammatory process in the cavernous sinus may compromise sympathetic fibers en route to the eye and forehead (23). As argued above, activation of trigeminal-parasympathetic reflexes probably mediates lacrimation, nasal secretion, forehead sweating, and vasodilatation during attacks of cluster headache. Thus, in our view, both sympathetic and parasympathetic disturbances are secondary to a primary trigeminal discharge in cluster headache. In support of this view, surgical treatments that target the trigeminal ganglion block recurrent attacks of cluster headache and associated autonomic disturbances (21). Although autonomic disturbances are probably secondary to a primary trigeminal discharge in cluster headache, vascular disturbances might facilitate pain. For example, vasodilatation or swelling of the internal carotid artery in the carotid canal could cause pain because of entrapment of sensory fibers that supply the arterial wall; alternatively, the swollen artery might compress the trigeminal ganglion directly (21).

VASCULAR REGULATION

Vascular events appear to be crucial for the evolution and termination of a cluster headache attack and for the onset of bouts of cluster headache. The three major neural systems regulating cranial vascular tone are the trigeminovascular, the parasympathetic, and the sympathetic systems (see Chapters 11 and 17). The trigeminovascular system uses calcitonin gene–related peptide (CGRP) and substance P as transmitters. The trigeminal innervation of cranial vessels has both afferent and efferent functions because it conveys sensory input from the vessels but also causes vasodilation by antidromic activation of the primary afferents. Cranial parasympathetic vasodilator fibers originate in the brain stem; travel with the facial and glossopharyngeal nerves to synapse in the otic ganglia, sphenopalatine ganglia, and internal carotid miniganglia; and, among other actions, cause vasodilation and increased cerebral blood flow. Vasoactive intestinal peptide (VIP) is a marker for the parasympathetic system. The sympathetic system uses norepinephrine, neuropeptide Y (NPY) and possibly adenosine triphosphate (ATP) as transmitters. It arises in the hypothalamus, passes to the intermediolateral cell column of the spinal cord, and synapses before passing to the superior cervical ganglion, then forms a nerve plexus around the carotid artery. Its effect on intracranial vessels is mainly vasoconstrictive.

A recent breakthrough in understanding of cluster headache pathophysiology was the finding that CGRP and VIP concentrations increase in plasma from the external jugular vein on the symptomatic side both during spontaneous (16) and nitroglycerin-induced (14) headache attacks. Furthermore, the CGRP plasma levels decrease to within the normal range concomitant with pain relief after treatment with oxygen inhalation or subcutaneous injection of sumatriptan but not after injection of pethidine (16). Nitroglycerin-induced attacks generally do not start until the first painless phase of vasodilatation is about to end. A most challenging issue is to clarify the mechanism leading to the painful second phase of vasodilation and the parallel increase of CGRP and VIP, and to identify why this occurs only during the active cluster period (14). One hypothesis is that nitroglycerin may trigger a cluster attack by stimulating trigeminal nociceptive fibers to release CGRP (13). This view seems unlikely because the CGRP levels do not increase until the attack is well established (14).

Calcitonin gene–related peptide in external jugular venous blood remains higher than normal between attacks of cluster headache (14), possibly because of repeated discharge of the trigeminovascular system during attacks or because of abnormal cyclical activation of the trigeminovascular system (14,33). The increase in CGRP levels appears to be a marker for the peculiar pathophysiologic state of active cluster headache during which nitroglycerine can trigger attacks. Raised plasma levels of CGRP and VIP in the cranial venous blood also may reflect activation of a brain stem reflex, the afferent arm of which is the trigeminal nerve and the efferent the parasympathetic outflow from the VIIth nerve (16). This, however, does not clarify the starting point for the cluster headache process.

Peptide markers of sympathetic activity are not altered during cluster headache attacks (16). This is not surprising because, as discussed above, some of the autonomic signs in cluster headache indicate lowered rather than increased sympathetic activity, at least regionally. Accordingly, in the morning and at night when cluster headache attacks frequently occur, lowered plasma norepinephrine levels as well as lowered spinal fluid levels of norepinephrine and catecholamine metabolites also have been observed compared with healthy controls (50). In contrast, muscular sympathetic activity in the ipsilateral peroneal nerve is increased both during the initial painless phase of vasodilatation after nitroglycerin administration and during induced and spontaneous cluster headache pain (41). This indicates that the systemic vascular sympathetic regulation of blood pressure is normal in cluster headache.

TEMPORAL PATTERN OF CLUSTER HEADACHE

The temporal pattern of attacks and cluster periods may provide clues about the pathogenesis of cluster headache. Thus, a local disturbance within the central nervous system (35), presumably in the hypothalamus, might explain the circadian cycle of attacks and the apparent vulnerability of vascular regulation in these patients. As described in detail in Chapter 92, cluster headache appears to have a temporal relationship with the dark–light cycle, the sleep–wake cycle, and the activity–

relaxation cycle. Cluster periods tend to occur at regular intervals and with an increased incidence during autumn and spring and sometimes can be interrupted after changing work schedules or traveling across time zones. Cluster headache attacks often develop at certain hours, after about an hour of sleep or in the early morning, and can be postponed by staying awake. In Italy cluster headache attacks often start in the early afternoon (32), a pattern not seen in Scandinavian countries (43), where there is no *siesta*. Altered 24-hour secretory patterns for melatonin, cortisol, testosterone, β-endorphin, and norepinephrine indicate involvement of central neural pathways, as does the phase delay or advance of melatonin, cortisol and β-endorphin during the active cluster period, the decreased prolactin nocturnal secretion during remission, and altered responses to inhibitory or stimulatory neuroendocrine tests (52). Twenty-four hour data regarding melatonin, cortisol, and β-endorphin concentrations in blood, blood pressure, body temperature, or pain sensitivity data have shown that more patients than controls lack a significant circadian rhythm when the data are analyzed by cosinor rhythmometry. This method implies fitting of the data to a particular cosinor function, which is a mathematical approximation of several circadian rhythms. The circannual nocturnal urinary secretion of melatonin is permanently depressed (for details and references, see Chapter 92). Although some pathologic neuroendocrine

findings may be partially related to pain, stress, or interrupted sleep, others, such as the blunted nocturnal prolactin secretion, are also present during remission and are believed to reflect the pathophysiology of cluster headache. Evidence of direct involvement of the hypothalamus in cluster headache has recently been reported (34): a positron emission tomographic study using H_2-^{15}O as a marker showed increased activity in the ipsilateral hypothalamus during attacks of cluster headache induced by nitroglycerin but not during the cluster period between attacks, after a negative nitroglycerin provocation, or when patients were in remission. This is in opposition to the finding in migraine (53), where activation in the brain stem was seen both during and after the migraine attack had subsided. Hypothalamic activation has not been observed in other types of cranial pain (34). Thus, this study lends further support for involvement of central structures in the vicinity of rhythm-generating centers in cluster headache pathogenesis.

In summary, the first of two main hypotheses of cluster headache pathogenesis favors a pathologic focus within the cavernous sinus, a proposed venous phlebitis (Fig. 1). According to this hypothesis, pain is produced by obstructed venous outflow, which could be triggered in the prone position or by intermittent dilatation of arteries and veins whose sympathetic innervation has been compromised by the phlebitis (22). The second hypothe-

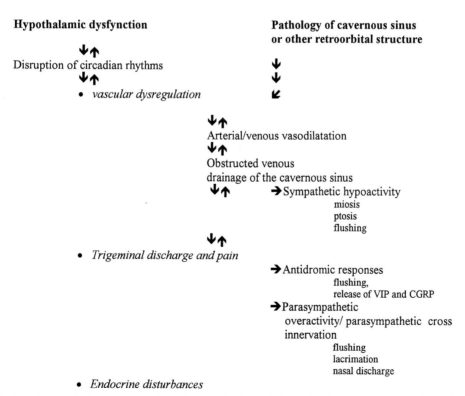

FIG. 1. The two main hypotheses of cluster headache aetiology. A primary hypothalamic dysfunction and a local retro-orbital lesion, as related to the cluster headache symptomatology, are schematically illustrated.

sis favors a disturbance of rhythm regulation as essential for the periodicity of attacks and cluster periods, for pain regulation, and for autonomic and vascular control. According to this view, the pain process involves retro-orbital structures, and the unilaterality is due to local anatomic factors (42). The presence of a peripheral sympathetic third neuron lesion in cluster headache is not an argument against the central hypothesis and may be considered a complication of cluster headache.

The two theories, the peripheral and the central, may appear to be contradictory at present, but there seems to be evidence in favor of both. Thus, a unifying theory that acknowledges both central and peripheral involvement would probably account for more findings than either theory alone. For example, cyclical ultradian factors might influence the recurrence of an inflammatory process in the cavernous sinus, which in turn could initiate endocrine disturbances that influence the timing of individual attacks. The final common pathway for these attacks may be a recurrent activation of the trigeminovascular system with secondary parasympathetic recruitment. The rapid escalation of pain from a niggling sensation to intense pain suggests that the pain-producing mechanism quickly builds upon itself, perhaps in a positive loop. For example, trigeminal activation by an inflammatory process might provoke local swelling of intracranial vessels, which in turn facilitates trigeminal discharge and further vascular swelling until the trigeminovascular response fatigues and pain subsides.

REFERENCES

1. Bovim G, Jenssen G, Ericson K. Orbital phlebography: a comparison between cluster headache and other headaches. *Headache* 1992;32:408–412.
2. de Marinis M, Strano S, Granata M, et al. Sympathetic-parasympathetic activation during spontaneous attacks of cluster headache: evaluation by spectral analysis of heart-rate fluctuations. *Cephalalgia* 1995;15:504–510.
3. Drummond PD. Dissociation between pain and autonomic disturbances in cluster headache. *Headache* 1990;30:505–508.
4. Drummond PD. The mechanism of facial sweating and cutaneous vascular responses to painful stimulation of the eye. *Brain* 1992;115:1417–1428.
5. Drummond PD. Lacrimation and cutaneous vasodilatation in the face induced by painful stimulation of the nasal ala and upper lip. *J Auton Nerv Syst* 1995;51:109–116.
6. Drummond PD. The site of sympathetic deficit in cluster headache. *Headache* 1996;36:3–9.
7. Drummond PD, Lance JW. Thermographic changes in cluster headache. *Neurology* 1984;34:1292–1298.
8. Drummond PD, Lance JW. Pathological sweating and flushing accompanying the trigeminal lacrimal reflex in patients with cluster headache and in patients with a confirmed site of cervical sympathetic deficit: evidence for parasympathetic cross-innervation. *Brain* 1992;115:1429–1445.
9. Ekbom K. Nitroglycerine as a provocative agent in cluster headache. *Arch Neurol* 1968;19:487–493.
10. Ekbom K. Patterns of cluster headache with a note on the relation to angina pectoris and peptic ulcer. *Acta Neurol Scand* 1970;46:225–237.
11. Ekbom K. A clinical comparison of cluster headache and migraine. *Acta Neurol Scand* 1970;46[Suppl 41]:1–48.
12. Ekbom K, Greitz T. Carotid angiography in cluster headache. *Acta Radiol Diagn* 1970;10:177–186.
13. Fanciullacci M, Alessandri M, Figini M, Geppetti P, Michelacci S. Increase in plasma calcitonin gene-related peptide from the extracerebral circulation during nitroglycerine induced cluster headache attacks. *Pain* 1995;60:119–123.
14. Fanciullacci M, Alessandri M, Sicuteri R, Marabini S. Responsiveness of the trigeminovascular system to nitroglycerine in cluster headache patients. *Brain* 1997;120:283–288.
15. Gardner WJ, Stowell A, Dutlinger R. Resection of the greater superficial petrosal nerve in the treatment of unilateral headache. *J Neurosurg* 1947;4:105–114.
16. Goadsby P, Edvinsson L. Human *in vivo* evidence for trigeminovascular activation in cluster headache. Neuropeptide changes and effects of acute attack treatments. *Brain* 1994;117:427–434.
17. Hannerz J. Orbital phlebography and signs of inflammation in episodic and chronic cluster headache. *Headache* 1991;31:540–542.
18. Hannerz J, Ericson K, Bergstrand G. Orbital phlebography in patients with cluster headache. *Cephalalgia* 1987;7:207–211.
19. Hannerz J, Hellström G, Klum T, Wahlgren NG. Cluster headache and dynamite headache. Blood flow velocities in the middle cerebral artery. *Cephalalgia* 1990;10:31–38.
20. Hardebo JE. The involvement of trigeminal substance P neurons in cluster headache. An hypothesis. *Headache* 1984;24:294–304.
21. Hardebo JE. On pain mechanisms in cluster headache. *Headache* 1991;31:91–106.
22. Hardebo JE. How cluster headache is explained as an intracavernous inflammatory process lesioning sympathetic fibres. *Headache* 1994;34:125–131.
23. Hardebo JE, Elner Å. Nerves and vessels in the pterygopalatine fossa and symptoms of cluster headache. *Headache* 1987;27:528–532.
24. Hardebo JE, Ryberg B. Cerebrospinal fluid findings in cluster headache indicative of inflammatory reaction or disease. *Cephalalgia* 1989;9[Suppl 10]:301–302.
25. Havelius U, Heuck M, Milos P, Hindfelt B. Ciliospinal reflex response in cluster headache. *Headache* 1996;36:568–573.
26. Havelius U, Heuck M, Milos P, Hindfelt B. The enhanced ciliospinal refex in asymptomatic patients with cluster headache is due to preganglionic sympathetic mechanisms. *Headache* 1997;37:496–498.
27. Khurana RK. Bilateral Horner's syndrome in cluster type headaches. *Headache* 1993;33:449–451.
28. Kruszewski P. Respiratory sinus arrhythmia in cluster headache syndrome. *Headache* 1993;33:98–104.
29. Kruszewski P, Bordini C, Brubakk AO, Sjaastad O. Cluster headache: responses to head-up tilt. *Headache* 1995;35:465–469.
30. Kudrow L. The pathogenesis of cluster headache. *Curr Opin Neurol* 1994;7:278–282.
31. List CF, Peet MM. Sweat secretion in man. V. Disturbances of sweat secretion with lesions of the pons, medulla and cervical portion of the cord. *Arch Neurol Psychiatry* 1939;42:1098–1127.
32. Manzoni GC, Terzano MG, Bono G, Micieli G, Martucci N, Nappi G. Cluster headache: clinical findings in 180 patients. *Cephalalgia* 1981;3:21–30
33. Mathiau P, Brochet B, Boulan P, Henry P, Aubineau P. Spontaneous and 5HT-induced cyclic concentrations in superficial temporal arteries from chronic and episodic cluster headache patients. *Cephalalgia* 1994;14:419–429.
34. May A, Bahra A, Buchel C, Frackowiak RSJ, Goadsby PJ. Hypothalamic activation in cluster headache attacks. *Lancet* 1998;352:275–278.
35. Medina JL, Diamond S, Fareed J. The nature of cluster headache. *Headache* 1979;19:309–322.
36. Micieli G, Cavallini A, Bosone D, et al. Imbalance of heart rate regulation in cluster headache as based on continuous 24-h recordings. *Clin Auton Res* 1993;3:291–298.
37. Micieli G, Magri M, Sandrini G, Tassorelli C, Nappi G. Pupil responsiveness in cluster headache: a dynamic TV pupillometric evaluation. *Cephalalgia* 1988;8:193–201.
38. Micieli G, Tassorelli C, Ruiz L, Sandrini G, Nappi G. The trigemino-pupillary response in cluster headache. *Cephalalgia* 1993;13:338–342.
39. Moscowitz MA. Cluster headache: evidence for a pathophysiologic focus in the superior pericarotid cavernous plexus. *Headache* 1988;28:584–586.
40. Nordin M, Fagius J. Effect of noxious stimulation on sympathetic vasoconstrictor outflow to human muscles. *J Physiol (Lond)* 1995;489:885–894.
41. Nordin M, Fagius J, Waldenlind E. Sympathetic vasoconstrictor out-

flow to extremity muscles in cluster headache. Recordings during spontaneous and nitroglycerin-induced attacks. *Headache* 1997;37: 358–367.

42. Proietti-Cecchini A, Schoenen J. Craniometric measures suggest narrowness of the cavernous sinus region in cluster headache. *Cephalalgia* 1997;17:360.

43. Russell D. Cluster headache: severity and temporal profiles of attacks and patients activity prior to and during attacks. *Cephalalgia* 1981;1: 209–216.

44. Russell D, Storstein L. Cluster headache: a computerized analysis of 24 h holter ECG recordings and description of ECG rhythm disturbances. *Cephalalgia* 1983;3:83–107.

45. Saunte C. Autonomic disorders in cluster headache, with special reference to salivation, nasal secretion and tearing. *Cephalalgia* 1984; 4:57–64.

46. Saunte C, Russell D, Sjaastad O. Cluster headache: on the mechanism behind attack-related sweating. *Cephalalgia* 1983;3:175–185.

47. Shen JM, Schaanning J. Cluster headache: pulse rate changes evoked by hyperoxia and hypoxia. *Headache* 1994;34:79–82.

48. Sjaastad O, Saunte C, Fredriksen TA. Bilaterality of cluster headache. An hypothesis. *Cephalalgia* 1985;5:55–58.

49. Sjaastad O, Saunte C, Russell D, Hestnes A, Marvik R. Cluster headache: the sweating pattern during spontaneous attacks. *Cephalalgia* 1981;1:233–244.

50. Strittmatter M, Hamann GF, Grauer M, Fischer C, Blaes F, Hoffman KH, Schimrigk K. Altered activity of the sympathetic nervous system and changes in the balance of hypophyseal, pituitary and adrenal hormones in patients with cluster headache. *Neuroreport* 1996;7: 1229–1234.

51. Waldenlind E, Ekbom K, Torhall J. MR-angiography during spontaneous attacks of cluster headache: a case report. *Headache* 1993;33: 291–295.

52. Waldenlind E, Ekbom K, Wetterberg L. Evidence for hypothalamic involvement in cluster headache. In: Nappi G et al, eds. *Headache and depression: serotonin pathways as a common clue.* New York: Raven, 1991:145–151.

53. Weiller C, May A, Limmroth V, et al. Brain stem activation in spontaneous human migaraine attacks. *Nat Med* 1995;1:658–660.

The Headaches, Second Edition,
edited by J. Olesen, P. Tfelt-Hansen, and K.M.A. Welch.
Lippincott Williams & Wilkins, Philadelphia © 2000.

Tension-Type Headache, Cluster Headache, and Miscellaneous Primary Headaches

CHAPTER 96

Symptomatology of Cluster Headache

Giuseppe Nappi and David Russell

DEFINITION OF CLUSTER HEADACHE

IHS code and diagnosis: 3.1 Cluster headache.
WHO code and diagnosis: G44.0 Cluster headache syndrome.
Short description (Headache Classification Committee, 1988): Attacks of severe strictly unilateral pain orbitally, supraorbitally, and/or temporally, lasting 15 to 180 minutes and occurring from once every other day to eight times a day. Are associated with one or more of the following: conjunctival injection, lacrimation, nasal congestion, rhinorrhea, forehead and facial sweating, miosis, ptosis, and eyelid edema. Attacks occur in series lasting for weeks or months (so-called cluster periods) separated by remission periods usually lasting months or years. About 10% of patients have chronic syndromes.
Other terms: Erythroprosopalgia of Bing, ciliary or migrainous neuralgia (Harris), erythromelalgia of the head, Horton's headache, histaminic cephalalgia, petrosal neuralgia (Gardner), sphenopalatine, Vidian and Sluder's neuralgia, hemicrania periodica neuralgiformis.

The IHS diagnostic criteria for cluster headache (Headache Classification Committee, 1988) is provided as follows (5):

A. At least five attacks fulfilling B through D.
B. Severe unilateral orbital, supraorbital, and/or temporal pain lasting 15 to 80 minutes untreated.
C. Headache is associated with at least one of the following signs, which have to be present on the pain side:

1. Conjunctival injection
2. Lacrimation
3. Nasal congestion
4. Rhinorrhea
5. Forehead and facial sweating
6. Miosis
7. Ptosis
8. Eyelid edema

D. Frequency of attacks: from one every other day to eight per day.
E. At least one of the following:

1. History and physical and neurologic examinations do not suggest one of the disorders listed in groups 5 through 11.
2. History and/or physical and/or neurologic examinations do suggest such disorder, but it is ruled out by appropriate investigations.
3. Such disorder is present, but cluster headache does not occur for the first time in close temporal relation to the disorder.

Cluster headache is characterized by a clinical profile that is so typical that a clinical diagnosis can be made without additional investigations. Although the episodic form seems to have a different age distribution at onset in males (24,29), it has the same clinical characteristics as chronic cluster headache. We shall therefore describe the clinical features of the two forms of cluster headache together in the following paragraphs.

PRODROMA AND PREMONITORY SYMPTOMS

Warning symptoms may be reported by cluster headache patients and can be divided into prodromes that start minutes before the pain and premonitory symptoms

G. Nappi: Department of Neurology, University of Rome La Sapienza, 00185 Rome, and C. Mondino Foundation, 27100 Pavia, Italy.

D. Russell: Department of Neurology, The National Hospital University of Oslo, N-0027 Oslo, Norway.

(4). Prodroma may be characterized by sensations in the head and neck, alimentary or cerebral symptoms, and mood alterations. Patients also may experience sensations in the area of subsequent pain, including awareness, twinge, pressure and tingling, and pulsation and throbbing distinct from ache or pain. Premonitory symptoms preceding a bout may occur from 1 to 8 weeks before.

CHARACTERISTICS OF INDIVIDUAL ATTACKS

As a function of the cyclical occurrence of the disease, cluster attacks usually have their onset once or twice a day, usually in the same hours in many patients, at least for particular time intervals (1–2 weeks). When plotting the most common hours of onset for the patients described by Manzoni et al. (31), sharp peaks were found between 1 and 2 a.m. and between 1 and 3 p.m., with a third peak reached around 9 p.m. Therefore, the main "entraining" factors of cluster attacks can be considered to be some phases of sleep (REM, in particular) (32) and the time of meals, as well as all the events that occur in the time span considered (activity rest cycle, working hours, and so forth).

In Russell's study (37), 51% of attacks began when patients were asleep, the peak frequency being from 4:00 a.m. to 10:00 a.m. (Fig. 1). The average time asleep per 24 hours for patients during the study did not exceed 6.9 hours, so that the relative frequency of attacks was increased during sleep. There is also a tendency for day-

time attacks to begin during naps or periods of physical activity. It is of interest that Manzoni et al. (31) found an increased frequency of attacks between 1:00 p.m. and 3:00 p.m. However, as they point out, this may be explained by the different living habits of their patients, the majority of whom stopped working during this period.

Pain attacks are typically unilateral, extremely severe, and often accompanied by local ipsilateral symptoms and signs of autonomic dysfunction. In the majority of cases, pain starts in the orbital and periorbital regions (i.e., around or above one eye), but it may radiate to the forehead, temporal region, upper or lower jaw, nostril, ear, half of the head, and, in some cases, the neck or shoulder on the same side (Fig. 2).

The attack often begins as a vague discomfort and rapidly increases to excruciating pain. The quality of pain is constant, boring, pressing, or burning when reaching its peak. During attacks and more rarely between attacks, patients may be supersensitive to touch in the symptomatic area. In some patients a slight discomfort persists in the symptomatic area between attacks. This is usually described as an ache or slight pressure behind the eye on the symptomatic side.

A minority (30%) describe the pain as throbbing or pulsating. However, sometimes it cannot be described or classified, and in some other cases it may have a mixed quality (throbbing and "neuralgic"). Sudden jabs of intense pain lasting 1 to 2 seconds also may be experi-

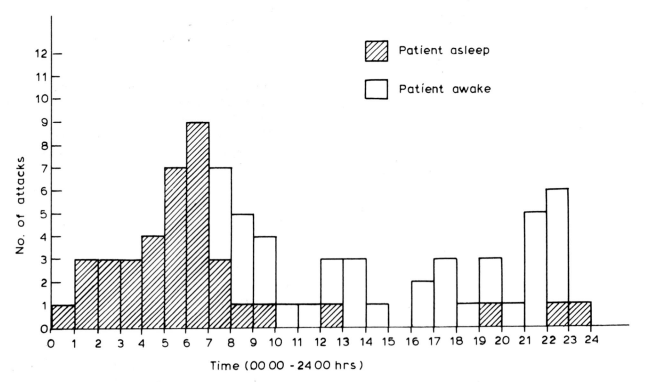

FIG. 1. Time of onset of cluster headache attacks. Reproduced from Russell (37).

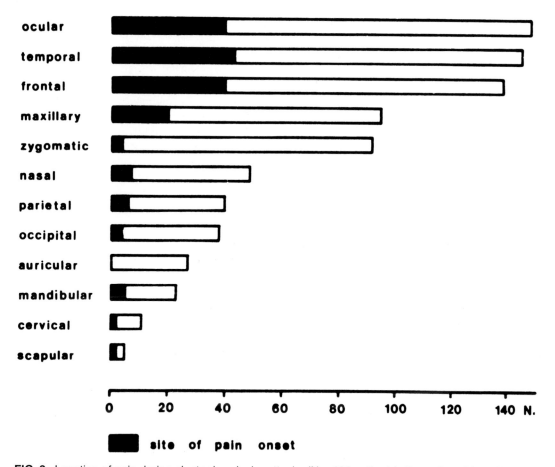

FIG. 2. Location of pain during cluster headache attacks (N = 180 patients). Reproduced from Manzoni et al. (31).

enced in the symptomatic area during the attack. The severity of attacks usually increases (together with the frequency) in the first few days or weeks and is most severe in the middle phase of the cluster period, but even then patients may occasionally experience milder attacks (37). In the great majority of patients the pain of cluster headache always affects the same side of the head. However, in some cases it can change sides from one cluster period to another or, more rarely, within the same cluster period (31).

Usually cluster attacks last between 15 minutes and 2 hours, generally being shorter at the beginning and end of each cluster period. According to the diagnostic criteria of the IHS classification, each attack should last not more than 3 hours if untreated. In a prospective study of 77 attacks (37), total duration was less than 30 minutes in 29%, less than 45 minutes in 62%, and less than 1 hour in 78% of patients (Fig. 3). In the same study, the pain reached its peak in less than 10 minutes in almost all cases, maximal pain intensity lasted less than 30 minutes, and the pain subsided in less than 40 minutes. The severity and duration of nocturnal and daytime attacks were similar.

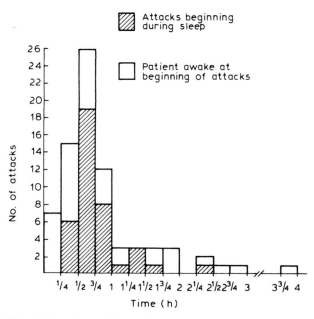

FIG. 3. Duration of cluster headache attacks. Reproduced from Russell (37).

The attack frequency is usually one or two per 24 hours, although the IHS diagnostic criteria suggest a minimum of one attack every other day and a maximum of eight per day. It is noteworthy that, in the evaluation of the outcome of the disease made by Manzoni et al. (30), the frequency of attacks showed a dichotomic evolution in primary episodic and primary chronic cluster headache patients. In the former condition the attacks tended to increase in frequency, whereas in the latter they tended to decrease during the course of the disease. The duration of each attack tended to lengthen in all groups.

PRECIPITATING FACTORS

Alcohol intake during cluster periods (but not during remission) is known to precipitate cluster attacks. However, according to Kudrow (24), Ekbom (11), and Klimek (21), only small quantities of alcohol trigger attacks, whereas larger amounts can have an opposite (or, in some cases, protective) effect on the daily occurrence of the painful crisis. Klimek reported that in some patients suffering from chronic cluster headache the attacks were reduced after the intake of a large amount of alcohol, the length of their remission being related to the quantity of alcohol consumed.

Interestingly, drugs that are known to treat cluster periods successfully cannot prevent the attack induced by alcoholic drinks. Among the precipitating factors of cluster headache crisis, some drugs should be cited, such as histamine, administered intravenously or subcutaneously, and sublingual nitroglycerin. Both of these drugs can be used as diagnostic tools in order to induce more or less typical attacks in the absence of adequate catamnestic data (7).

ALLEVIATING FACTORS

Factors and procedures alleviating headache symptomatology are reported only anecdotally by patients, and systematic studies are lacking. Ekbom (9) in 1975 found that the compression of the ipsilateral superficial temporal artery can reduce the pain of spontaneous or trinitrine-induced attacks. In some cases the digital compression of the common carotid artery may have the same effect. It is interesting to note that some patients alleviate the pain symptomatology through short-lasting, intense, physical activity.

ASSOCIATED SIGNS AND SYMPTOMS

Accompanying signs and symptoms, mostly described on the pain side and suggesting a disturbance in the function of the autonomic nervous system, are typical for cluster headache attacks and have been considered as significant as the pain itself for the diagnosis by the recent IHS classification. However, there are considerable variations with regard to their reported frequency. This fact presumably depends on whether information was obtained by patient interviews or by personal observation (8,12,27,31,44).

The typical patient behavior has been described in detail (3). During the attacks there are typical patterns during walking, sitting, kneeling, lying, and standing, the awareness of which will help the patient to learn that bizarre behavioral responses are not a mark of insanity.

The frequency and degree of the associated symptoms are usually considered as dependent on the severity of attacks. Among the local signs of autonomic involvement, lacrimation is the most common, being reported in 82% to 84% of cases, followed by injection of the conjunctiva on the side of pain (58%–84%). A partial Horner's syndrome, with a slight ipsilateral ptosis or miosis, or a combination of both, is often present during attacks (57%–69%) and may persist between attacks in later stages of the disease in some patients. Nasal stuffiness or rhinorrhea experienced by most patients during attacks (68%–76%) is usually ipsilateral to the headache, but rarely may be bilateral. Nasal stuffiness in some cases may precede the onset of pain, later in the attack being replaced by rhinorrhea (38). Increased forehead sweating can be measured during severe attacks, especially on the symptomatic side. This sign can be clinically observed, however, in only a minority of patients (43). A few patients report generalized sweating during attacks. Cardiovascular findings accompanying cluster attacks include the following heart rate changes: increase in heart rate at the onset of attacks; relative decrease in heart rate after attacks; and rhythm disturbances (39). These consist of frequent premature ventricular beats, transient episodes of atrial fibrillation (Fig. 4), and first-degree atrioventricular block or sinoatrial block. Moreover, both diastolic and systolic blood pressures may be increased (40). Gastrointestinal symptoms are not typical of cluster headache attacks. Nausea was experienced during severe attacks in 40% of the patients in the series described by Manzoni et al. (31), but vomiting was rare. In many patients nausea may be due to drug ingestion. A few patients have reported increased salivation or diarrhea during attacks. Photo- and phonophobia are frequently described during attacks, as are erythema of the eyelid or of a circumscribed area of the face or forehead. Contralateral carpal spasm, seizures, contralateral paresthesias, vertigo, and mild ataxia (20,27,38,41,44) have been reported during attacks in a few isolated cases.

Regarding the accompanying autonomic signs and symptoms of cluster attacks, it is noteworthy that recent contributions debate their role in diagnosis and physiopathology. In a large series of consecutive patients, Ekbom (12) found that in 3% of cases the diagnostic criteria were not fulfilled because of the absence of local autonomic signs during cluster attacks. In the series described by Nappi et al. (35), regarding attacks that were not personally observed, 3% had never experienced local symptoms during cluster headache crisis (Fig. 5). It may

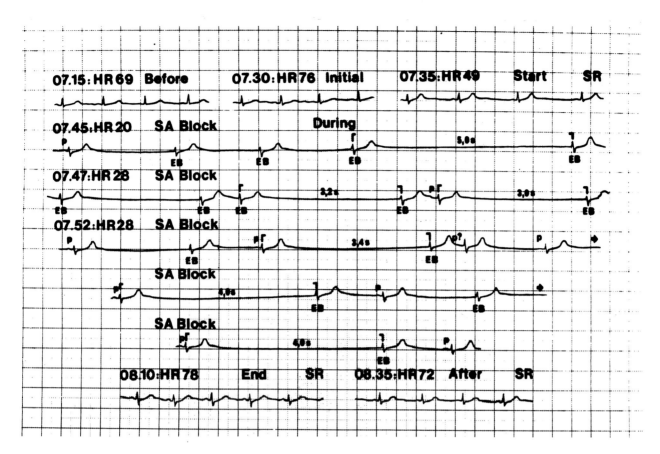

FIG. 4. Patient no. 5. During attacks, the electrocardiogram showed bradycardia and sinoatrial block (*SA block*) with nodal or ventricular escape beats (*EB*). *SR*, sinus rhythm. Reproduced from Russell and Storstein (39).

Episodic CH
202 (97.1%)

PRESENT: 244 (97.2%)

Chronic CH
42 (97.7%)

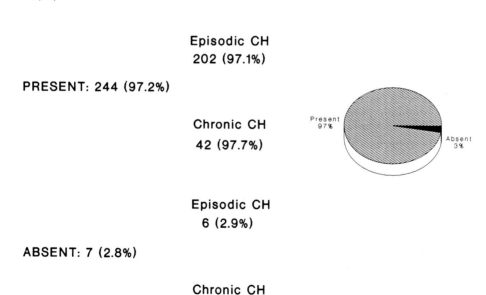

Episodic CH
6 (2.9%)

ABSENT: 7 (2.8%)

Chronic CH
1 (2.3%)

FIG. 5. Local autonomic signs during cluster headache attacks. Reproduced from Nappi et al. (35).

be assumed that the impairment of autonomic functions in these cases was present to a mild degree that was not clinically manifest but would have required advanced laboratory studies for sheer detection. Finally, the cluster attack profile is characterized by a typical patient behavior. Subjects prefer to isolate themselves; they look restless and agitated, and feel an impulse to move around and change body position in the hope that this may bring pain relief. This behavior appears to be dependent on the severity of the pain during attacks (37).

FAMILY HISTORY

A family history for cluster headache is rare and was not present in more than 3% to 4% of patients (women 7%–8%, men 2%–5%) reported by Kudrow (24). Manzoni and co-workers found a positive family history in only 5 (0.8%) of 590 cases examined in the Headache Centers of Pavia and Parma (I) (34).

The prevalence of migraine in parents and siblings of cluster headache patients appears to differ little from control populations (1,27,44) but may be more frequent in females with cluster headache (5).

SEX

Cluster headache represents the only form of primary headache that prevails among males, with females representing only 10% to 30% of those affected. The sex ratio is apparently the same in episodic and chronic cluster headache (31).

PAST MEDICAL HISTORY

The past medical history of cluster headache patients is usually unremarkable. However, several researchers have reported an increased incidence of previous head trauma (15,27,31) and peptic ulcer (16,18,23). In the posttraumatic patients described by Manzoni et al. (31), who suffered from unilateral head injury with loss of consciousness, the traumatized cluster headache side was the one subsequently affected by cluster headache. A personal history of both cerebrovascular disease and hypertension has not been found to be statistically different from that of controls, whereas a higher incidence of coronary heart disease has been found in some reports among cluster headache patients (27).

AGE OF ONSET

The mean age of onset was 28.0 years in the series of Friedman and Mikropoulos (15), 27.5 years in the series of Ekbom (10), 29.6 years in that of Kudrow (24), and 28.9 years in that of Manzoni et al. (31). Although cluster headache may appear at any age, its onset is usually later compared with that of migraine. Cluster headache is uncommon in children. Only 17.7% of the cases

described by Zanferrari et al. had their onset prior to 18 years of age, and only 2.2% prior to 10 years (45).

LIFE HABITS AND PERSONALITY PROFILE

Alcohol and cigarette use were higher in cluster headache patients compared with controls in two studies (10,24), but were no higher than in patients with migraine or tension-type headache (31). If only heavy drinkers are considered, the difference is statistically significant for cluster headache, the subjects with a daily consumption of at least 1 liter of wine (or equivalent) being much more frequent among the cluster headache cases. The percentage of smokers, particularly heavy smokers (more than 20 cigarettes per day), also is significantly higher in cluster headache when compared with other primary headaches (31). However, no significant correlation was demonstrated between the withdrawal from alcoholic drinks or smoking and changes in the course of cluster headache. It seems likely, however, that giving up drinking can favor the onset of a remission period in some cases (30). Moderate or severe stress may precede the onset of a cluster period, and an exaggerated life habit profile seems to characterize cluster headache patients (33).

Graham (16) first described male subjects with cluster headache as having a leonine appearance. He hypothesized that they were usually very insecure, were dependent on their wives' decisions, and had strong traits of hysteria (17). According to other researchers (15,22), the typical patient suffering from cluster headache is ambitious, is hard working, has obsessive personality traits, but also has feelings of inadequacy and dependency (42).

In contrast, cluster headache patients did not differ essentially from other headache groups with regard to psychological status (6). Using the Minnesota Multiphasic Personality Inventory, cluster headache subjects had a personality profile similar to that observed in migraine (2,26,36).

ACTIVE PHASES AND REMISSIONS

The most striking feature of cluster headache is the cyclical, almost regular occurrence of cluster periods and attacks. The active phases of the disease (cluster periods) usually last from 1 to 2 months (28,31), but they also may last from a few days to a year. When the cluster periods last more than 12 months, the disease is usually classified as chronic (13). Most patients experience one to two cluster periods per year. A seasonal occurrence of cluster periods has been found by Ekbom in a series of patients examined in 1970 (8) and by Kudrow (24) who found an increased number of cluster periods in February and June, whereas August and November had the lowest number of cluster periods. More recently, the same researcher found that the frequency of onset of cluster headache phases parallels the increase (and/or decrease) of light hours of daylight (Fig. 6); he identified two peaks of the cluster onset

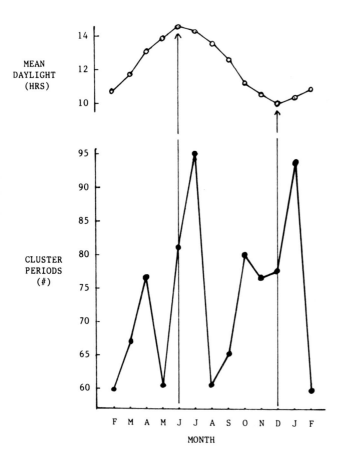

MEAN DAYLIGHT (HRS)

CLUSTER PERIODS (#)

F M A M J J A S O N D J F

MONTH

FIG. 6. Daylight changes and cluster onset. Reproduced from Kudrow (25).

occurring 7 to 10 days before the longest and the shortest days of the year (25). A possible influence of light and dark cycles for cluster headache is now under investigation in a long-term, multinational study involving different countries at different latitudes and hemispheres (33).

Remissions usually last between 6 months and 2 years. Although they are often relatively constant in individual patients, there are considerable interpatient variations. In the series of 428 patients described by Kudrow (24), remissions lasted 1 year or less in 67% and 2 years or less in 81% of patients. Rarely they may last as long as 25 years (19). A remission period is sometimes experienced by female patients during pregnancy, with the attacks often returning shortly after delivery (14). Occasionally patients report the occurrence of a few mild attacks during a period when they are otherwise asymptomatic.

REFERENCES

1. Andersson PG. Migraine in patients with cluster headache. *Cephalalgia* 1985;5:6–11.
2. Andrasik F, Blanchard EB, Arena JG, Teders SJ, Rodichok LD. Cross validation of the Kudrow Sutkus MMPI classification system for diagnosis headache type. *Headache* 1980;20:2–5.
3. Blau JN. Behaviour during a cluster headache. *Lancet* 1993;342:723–725.
4. Blau JN, Engel HO. Premonitory and prodromal symptoms in cluster headache. *Cephalalgia* 1998;18:91–93.
5. Classification and diagnostic criteria for headache disorders, cranial neuralgias and facial pain of the Headache Classification Committee of the IHS. *Cephalalgia* 1988;8(suppl 7):1–96.
6. Cuypers J, Attenkirch H, Bunge S. Personality profile in cluster headache and migraine. *Headache* 1981;21:21–24.
7. Ekbom K. Nitroglycerin as a provocative agent in cluster headache. *Arch Neurol* 1968;19:487–493.
8. Ekbom K. A clinical comparison of cluster headache and migraine. *Acta Neurol Scand* 1970;46(suppl 41):1–48.
9. Ekbom K. Some observations on pain in cluster headache. *Headache* 1975;14:219–225.
10. Ekbom K. Pattern of cluster headache with a note on the relation to angina pectoris and peptic ulcer. *Acta Neurol Scand* 1981;46:225–256.
11. Ekbom K. Pathogenesis of cluster headache. In: Blau JN, ed. *Migraine. Clinical, therapeutic, conceptual and research aspects*. London: Chapman & Hall, 1987:433–448.
12. Ekbom K. Evaluation of clinical criteria for cluster headache with special reference to the classification of the International Headache Society. *Cephalalgia* 1990;10:195–197.
13. Ekbom K, De Fine Olivarius B. Chronic migrainous neuralgia: diagnostic and therapeutic aspects. *Headache* 1971;11:97–101.
14. Ekbom K, Waldenlind E. Cluster headache in women: evidence of hypofertility (?): headaches in relation to menstruation and pregnancy. *Cephalalgia* 1981;1:167–174.
15. Friedman AP, Mikropoulos HE. Cluster headache. *Neurology* 1958;8:653–663.
16. Graham JR. Cluster headache. *Headache* 1972;11:175–185.
17. Graham JR, Rogado AZ, Rahman M, Gramer IV. Some physical, physiological, and psychological characteristics of patients with cluster headache. In: Cochrane AL, ed. *Background to migraine*. London: Heinemann, 1970:38–51.
18. Heyck H. *Headache and facial pain*. Stuttgart: Thieme, 1981.
19. Hornabrook RW. Migrainous neuralgia. *N Z Med J* 1964;63:774–779.
20. Horton BT. Histaminic cephalalgia (Horton's headache or syndrome). *Md Med J* 1961;10:178–203.
21. Klimek A. Chronic cluster headache and alcohol. *Headache* 1978;18:102–103.
22. Kudrow L. Physical and personality characteristics in cluster headache. *Headache* 1973;13:197–201.
23. Kudrow L. Lithium prophylaxis for chronic cluster headache. *Headache* 1977;17:15–18.
24. Kudrow L. *Cluster headache: mechanisms and management*. New York: Oxford University Press, 1980.
25. Kudrow L. The cyclic relationship of natural illumination to cluster period frequency. *Cephalalgia* 1987;7(suppl):76–78.
26. Kudrow L, Sutkus BJ. MMPI pattern specificity in primary headache disorders. *Headache* 1979;19:18–24.
27. Lance JW, Anthony M. Migrainous neuralgia or cluster headache? *J Neurol Sci* 1971;13:401–414.
28. Lovshin LL. Clinical caprices of histaminic cephalalgia. *Headache* 1961;1:3–6.
29. Manzoni GC, Micieli G, Granella F, Martignoni E, Farina S, Nappi G. Cluster headache in women: clinical findings and relationship with reproductive life. *Cephalalgia* 1988;8:37–44.
30. Manzoni GC, Micieli G, Granella F, Tassorelli C, Zanferrari C. Cluster headache: course over ten years in 189 patients. *Cephalalgia* 1991;11:169–174.
31. Manzoni GC, Terzano MG, Bono G, Micieli G, Martucci N, Nappi G. Cluster headache: clinical findings in 180 patients. *Cephalalgia* 1981;3:21–30.
32. Manzoni GC, Terzano MG, Moretti G, Cocchi M. Clinical observation on 76 cluster headache cases. *Eur Neurol* 1981;20:88–94.
33. Micieli G, Sjaastad O, Leston JA, et al. Cluster headache temporal patterns and environmental changes: a prospective, multinational, multicentric study. Preliminary results. In: Nappi G, et al., eds. *Headache and depression: serotonin pathways as a common clue*. New York: Raven, 1991.
34. Nappi G, Manzoni GC. *Primary headaches. Clinical approach and management*. London: Smith-Gordon, 1996.
35. Nappi G, Micieli G, Cavallini A, Zanferrari C, Sandrini G, Manzoni GC. Accompanying symptoms of cluster attacks: their relevance to the diagnostic criteria. *Cephalalgia* 1992;3:165–168.
36. Rogado A, Harrison RH, Graham JR. Personality profiles in cluster

headache, migraine and normal controls. Presented at the 10th International Congress of World Federation of Neurology, 1973.

37. Russell D. Cluster headache: severity and temporal profiles of attacks and patients' activity prior to and during attacks. *Cephalalgia* 1981;1: 209–216.

38. Russell D. Clinical characterization of the cluster headache syndrome. In: Olesen J, Edvinsson L, eds. *Basic mechanisms of headache: pain research and clinical management.* Vol. 2. New York: Elsevier, 1988:15–22.

39. Russell D, Storstein L. Cluster headache: a computerised analysis of 24 h Holter ECG recordings and description of ECG rhythm disturbances. *Cephalalgia* 1983;3:83–107.

40. Russell D, Von der Lippe A. Cluster headache: heart rate and blood pressure changes during spontaneous attacks. *Cephalalgia* 1982;2:61–70.

41. Sjaastad O. So-called "vascular headache of the migraine type": one or more nosological entities? *Acta Neurol Scand* 1976;54:125–139.

42. Sjaastad O. Cluster headache. In: Clifford F, ed. *Handbook of clinical neurology.* Vol 4. No. 48. Headache. Amsterdam: Elsevier, 1986:13–22.

43. Sjaastad O, Saunte C, Russell D, Hestnes A, Marvik R. Cluster headache: the sweating pattern during spontaneous attacks. *Cephalalgia* 1981;1:233–244.

44. Sutherland JM, Eadie MJ. Cluster headache. In: Friedman AP, ed. *Research and clinical studies in headache.* Vol 3. Basel: Karger, 1972: 92–125.

45. Zanferrari C, Granella F, Bisi M, Alfieri M, Dadatti A, Manzoni GC. Cluster headache in childhood. In: Lanzi G, et al., eds. *Headache in children and adolescents.* Amsterdam: Elsevier, 1989:95–100.

The Headaches, Second Edition,
edited by J. Olesen, P. Tfelt-Hansen, and K.M.A. Welch.
Lippincott Williams & Wilkins, Philadelphia © 2000.

Tension-Type Headache, Cluster Headache, and Miscellaneous Primary Headaches

CHAPTER 97

Diagnosis, Differential Diagnosis, and Prognosis of Cluster Headache

Karl Ekbom and Giuseppe Nappi

DIAGNOSIS

Most patients with cluster headache seek medical help between attacks, and it is in fact relatively seldom that the physician has an opportunity to witness an actual attack of headache. With the exception of a possible partial Horner syndrome on the symptomatic side, the results of a physical and neurologic examination are negative. Consequently, the diagnosis is based mainly on the history of the patient. The interview should be performed as soon as possible after an attack and also eventually during an actual attack of headache. If there is only a short history of disease, the diagnosis may be difficult, but if the patient has suffered previously from several identical periods of headache, it is easy to establish a correct diagnosis. Most patients seen at a specialized clinic have had many series of headache attacks and are thus most commonly able to give a detailed and reliable anamnesis.

Some features of the pain of cluster headache are of special diagnostic importance: (a) strict unilaterality, (b) severe intensity, (c) orbital localization, and (d) short duration. In addition there is a peculiar temporal pattern of the attacks that helps to distinguish cluster headache from other types of head pain. The clinical picture in most cases is so clear-cut that there are really no diagnostic difficulties. However, in less typical cases, pain is

only vaguely described, may have a long duration, or may alternate between both sides of the head. Some patients may at times suffer from sporadic attacks having neither cluster nor chronic patterns, and in all these situations it can be helpful to observe the patient directly in the hospital ward. The physician can obtain valuable information of the attacks and their time pattern if the patient keeps a record during one or more cluster periods. The intensity, duration, and time of day of the attacks should be recorded, along with the effects of any medication.

Clinical examination during spontaneous or provoked attacks is an additional valuable aid to diagnosis. An attack is readily provoked by giving nitroglycerin during an active cluster headache period (1). A prerequisite for provocation is that the patient has not had a spontaneous attack within the previous 8 hours and has not taken any vasoconstricting agent for the past 18 hours. Nor should the patient have taken any prophylactic medication. After at least 15 minutes of rest in the recumbent position, the patient is given 1 mg of nitroglycerin sublingually. The test result is accounted positive if a pain attack is induced with clinical features identical to those of a spontaneous attack. An attack is usually preceded by a lag of 30 to 50 minutes after administration and is followed by a refractory phase lasting a few hours. The test reproducibility is good, attacks being provoked repeatedly on different occasions with an identical dose. In the quiescent remission period, however, nitroglycerin fails to induce an attack. During an attack the patient is often restless, and cannot remain still. Instead, the patient turns and twists in bed, or sits up and rocks the body to and fro, or wanders restlessly back and forth across the floor. Ipsilateral con-

K. Ekbom: Department of Neurology, Huddinge University Hospital at the Karolinska Institute, S-14186 Huddinge, Sweden.

G. Nappi: Department of Neurology, University of Rome La Sapienza, 00185 Rome, and C. Mondino Foundation, 27100 Pavia, Italy.

junctival injection is seen as a rule, with lacrimation, rhinorrhea, and often miosis, ptosis, and frontal sweating. In a few patients, however, attacks of cluster headache are never accompanied by these autonomous symptoms or signs (3,9). Nausea and vomiting are unusual in cluster headache, in contrast to the typical migraine attack. In common with migraine patients, however, cluster headache patients are often photophobic during attacks. Facial flush has been considered a characteristic phenomenon, although it is not a consistent finding. Digital compression of the superficial temporal artery usually eases the temporal ache, but may exacerbate the periorbital pain (2). Compression of the carotid artery in the upper neck commonly alleviates or eliminates the orbital ache, whereas a rotatory head jolt is without effect in most cases. The Valsalva maneuver usually has no effect on the pain. Some patients manifest pronounced bradycardia and increased blood pressure during attacks.

Routine Investigations

The diagnosis of cluster headache is thus mainly based on clinical criteria, and there is generally no indication for a radiologic investigation if the history and neurologic examination are unremarkable. Special investigations are, however, occasionally necessary in the following conditions: (a) an onset of first headaches in the elderly patient; (b) a short history of illness (e.g., in cases when the periodicity of headaches is still undetermined); (c) an atypical clinical picture (e.g., in cases with longstanding or even continuous headache); (d) a protracted course of disease and especially when the headache is progressively worsening; (e) a headache that is accompanied by confusion, loss of consciousness, or convulsions; and (f) any significant pathologic findings at neurologic examination or in laboratory tests.

As mentioned above, unilateral signs of miosis, ptosis, or both may be recorded in a substantial number of cases, but in clinical practice it is not necessary to perform a special ophthalmologic examination. Some cases may require particular provocation tests such as nitroglycerin sublingually or histamine subcutaneously (4) or intramuscularly. In the active phases of the disease, histamine administration may provoke a typical cluster attack with the usual accompanying symptoms within 15 to 50 minutes. In diagnosing structural brain lesions, computed tomography (CT) or magnetic resonance imaging (MRI) are the imaging procedures of first choice. Even small tumors or vascular malformations may be detected. MRI has a better sensitivity than CT in searching for an eventual pituitary or skull base tumor that, although only rarely, may be suspected in atypical cases of chronic cluster headache (13). An otologic examination and x-rays of the paranasal sinuses may occasionally be necessary in cases where a sinusitis has to be excluded. Such laboratory procedures as lumbar puncture, evoked responses, or electroencephalography have no place in the routine investigation of cluster headache.

Cluster headache appears to be characterized by a disruption of internal chronoorganization, particularly during the active phases of the disease (10). An altered biorhythmic activity might have a predictive value of therapeutic effects of some drugs (lithium, verapamil) and procedures (sleep deprivation, daily schedule shifts, etc). So far, however, there is no single or combined set of biochemical, neuroendocrinologic, or physiologic tests that has high enough sensitivity and specificity to secure the diagnosis except for the pharmacologic provocations described above.

Research Investigations

In some centers, biochemical, endocrinologic, or electrophysiologic tests are performed as additional parts of the routine examinations, but their clinical value is limited, and they should mainly be considered as being tools of research (see Chapters 92 and 93). Investigations of autonomic parameters are represented by, for example, the evaluation of corneal indentation pulse and intraocular pressure, pupillometry, quantification of sweating, salivation, and lacrimation. Neurophysiologic and hemodynamic parameters are also studied (see Chapter 93).

DIFFERENTIAL DIAGNOSIS

Today, cluster headache is considered a distinct clinical entity, the most common differential diagnoses being migraine and trigeminal neuralgia (Table 1).

Migraine and cluster headache differ from each other in such respects as incidence, hereditary factors, and sex and age distribution, as well as the nature, intensity, duration, and frequency of the pain. Patients with cluster headache will be restless and typically pace the floor during the headache attack. This is in contrast to the behavior of the migraine patient. Another important difference lies in the timing of the attacks.

In migraine the pain sometimes starts on one side of the head, but may subsequently spread to the contralateral side, and may ultimately extend throughout the greater part of the head; this is not the case in cluster headache. The absence of visual or other focal cerebral symptoms in conjunction with cluster headache attacks is striking. If a patient with cluster headache reports scintillating scotoma (teichopsia), for instance, it should be borne in mind that migraine is common and that it may be a question of coincidence.

Trigeminal neuralgia (tic douloureux) is characterized by brief attacks of pain most commonly limited to the distribution of the second or third divisions of the trigeminal nerve. The pain is paroxysmal, with instant peak intensity, and lasts from seconds to a couple of minutes. In contrast to cluster headache, it can be provoked by stim-

TABLE 1. *A clinical comparison of cluster headache, migraine and trigeminal neuralgia*

	Cluster headache	Migraine	Trigeminal neuralgia
Sex	Male (80–90%)	Female (60–70%)	Female:male 2:1
Age (years) at onset (mean)	20–40	10–20	50–60
Aura	0	Scintillating scotoma (10%)	0
Pain			
Localization	Always unilateral, ocular, frontal, temporal, maxillar	Often unilateral, upper part of the head	Unilateral, within distribution of maxillar and mandibular nerves
Quality	Excruciating, boring, burning	Severe, boring, throbbing	Excruciating, stabbing, electric-like
Associated symptoms/signs	Conjunctival injection, lacrimation, rhinorrhea, miosis	Photophobia, phonophobia, nausea, vomiting	Tic douloureux
Duration of attack	15–180 min	4–72 hours	Seconds to 1/2 min
Frequency of attacks (mean)	1–2 per day	Varies, often 1–3 per month	Several per day
Time pattern	Often at night	Often early in the morning	Early in the morning, at meals
Remission periods	Months to years	Varies, notably during pregnancy	Varies
Provocative factors	Alcohol	Stress, cheese, red wine, chocolate, menstruations	Stimulation of trigger zones

ulation of limited areas in the facial skin or the oral mucosa, so-called trigger zones. Carbamazepine provides immediate relief, another difference from cluster headache.

Chronic paroxysmal hemicrania (CPH) is characterized by brief attacks of unilateral headache, recurring periodically, at least 15 times a day, which is a greater frequency than in cluster headache. Attacks of CPH can be induced by rotation or bowing of the head, or powerful continuous pressure behind and below the mastoid process or on the transverse process at C4–C5 and pressure on the greater occipital nerve, none of which occurs in cluster headache. The pain disappears promptly with indomethacin, an important diagnostic criterion.

Pericarotid syndrome is an alternative diagnosis to be considered in cases of unilateral headache and signs of oculosympathetic paralysis (14). In contrast to cluster headache, the pain is generally continuous, and there is evidence of local ipsilateral anhidrosis of the forehead. When the patient's history of the condition is brief, caution is to be recommended in diagnosis in that the syndrome may have its origin in various pathologic processes in or around the carotid artery, for example, in symptomatic or asymptomatic dissection or occlusion of the internal carotid artery, aneurysms, or aneurysmal dilatation. Unilateral headache may occur after endarterectomy.

Sinusitis, usually bilateral, is rarely characterized by pain as intense as in cluster headache. The painful sensation of sinusitis is localized in the supraorbital or zygomatic regions, is continuous, and in many cases associated with purulent nasal secretion, not fluidlike as in cluster headache. Rarely, lacrimation is an accompanying symptom of sinusitis.

Glaucoma and other ocular disorders should be included in the differential diagnosis. The pain of acute glaucoma is continuous (sometimes bilateral) and is associated with visual impairment, ipsilateral pupillary dilatation, photophobia, and increased intraocular pressure (up to 40 mm Hg). Major problems of differential diagnosis can derive from the chronic form of glaucoma, which is characterized by intermittent, sometimes intense pain. The typical temporal profile of cluster headache and its local accompanying symptoms (lacrimation, rhinorrhea, etc.) are absent in glaucoma. Recurrent corneal erosions (corneitis) can simulate the symptomatology of cluster headache because of the unilaterality of the pain, the local accompanying phenomena (lacrimation, "red eye"), and the temporal pattern characterized by the frequent onset during the night hours and the short duration of each attack (<1 hour). However, it is possible to demonstrate a corneal lesion. Furthermore, the pain is very localized and frequently associated with blepharospasm. A similar clinical picture may occur in posterior scleritis, but the pain is more continuous.

PROGNOSIS

Knowledge on the natural history and the prognosis of cluster headache has increased in recent years. Kudrow (7) contacted patients who had not returned for follow-up visits for periods from 3 to 8 years (so called drop-outs). Information was obtained from 149 of 178 patients. Seventy-five of them, or 50.3% reported no change in head-

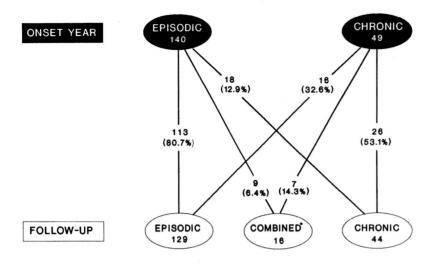

FIG. 1. Outcome of 189 consecutive cluster headache patients (8) referred to Pavia and Parma Headache Centers (1976–1986) suggests new categories for the IHS classification: 3.1.2 Episodic cluster headache; 3.1.2.1 episodic from onset; 3.1.2.2 evolved from chronic; 3.1.4 combined cluster headache; 3.1.4.1 evolved from episodic; 3.1.4.2 evolved from chronic. Alternation of cluster (remission) periods longer or shorter than 1 year (15 days).

ache. Eleven (7.4%) had experienced a shift in headache type, that is, from chronic to episodic or episodic to chronic, equally. Fifty-one (34.2%) had experienced a prolonged remission, and 12 (8.1%) had died. Sacquegna et al. (12) studied the course of episodic cluster headache in 72 patients seen from 1977 to 1986. Sixty-two patients (86.1%) showed a regular frequency of cluster periods per year, whereas 4 (5.6%) reported an increase and 6 (8.3%) a decrease in cluster frequency. Krabbe (6) got information on 260 of 290 patients registered between 1976 and 1989. The length of the disease varied from 2 to 58 years. Thirteen patients had died, whereas 27 had lost their cluster headache for 1 to 9 years. Seventeen had developed typical cluster periods and remission phases, having previously suffered for several years from chronic cluster headache.

Detailed data on the prognosis have been presented by Manzoni et al. (8) in a series of 189 consecutive patients having a disease duration of over 10 years. Based on the temporal course of onset during the year, patients were classified as suffering from either episodic (n = 140) or chronic (n = 49) cluster headache. Episodic patients maintained the episodic form in about 80% of cases, shifted toward a chronic form (secondary chronic) in 12.9% of cases, or shifted toward an intermediate pattern (combined form) in a little over 6% of cases (Fig. 1). Chronic cluster headache was still chronic (primary chronic form) after 10 years or more in 53.1% of cases, whereas it had turned into episodic in 32.6% and into a combined form in 14.3% of cases. Nineteen patients (10%) had not had any attack for the past 3 years.

The results of a follow-up study of 123 patients with episodic and 9 patients with chronic cluster headache first seen between 1967 and 1982 were presented by Pearce (11). It showed a significant but low remission rate in both patient groups and confirmed that some patients change from episodic to chronic pattern, and that occasionally chronic clusters may become episodic.

Igarashi and Sakai (5) reported on the course of disease in 68 of 94 patients seen at an outpatient clinic between 1972 and 1990. Attacks did not change in severity, frequency, or duration during the follow-up period. The remission periods tended to change at the age of 42 years, either becoming longer or shorter.

Thus, it seems that in all its forms cluster headache is a chronic disease lasting in most cases for many years or even for the rest of the patient's life. However, it is also striking that active cluster headache is seldom seen after the age of 75. Episodic cluster headache tends to worsen from year to year, but the opposite pattern also may be experienced. The prognosis of the chronic form appears to be better than previously thought, changing in many patients into an episodic form (6,8). Pharmacotherapy (especially lithium) may be a reason for a change from chronic into episodic cluster headache, but does not otherwise influence the outcome. A late onset, male gender, and history of episodic cluster headache for more than 20 years seem to be related to a negative course.

REFERENCES

1. Ekbom K. Nitroglycerin as a provocative agent in cluster headache. *Arch Neurol* 1968;19:487–493.
2. Ekbom K. Some observations on pain in cluster headache. *Headache* 1975;14:219–225.
3. Ekbom K. Evaluation of clinical criteria for cluster headache with special reference to the classification of the International Headache Society. *Cephalalgia* 1990;10:195–197.
4. Horton BT. Histaminic cephalgia: differential diagnosis and treatment. *Mayo Clin Proc* 1956;31:325–333.
5. Igarashi H, Sakai F. Natural history of cluster headache [Abstract XI Migraine Trust International Symposium, London, September 9–12, 1996]. *Cephalalgia* 1996;16:42–43.
6. Krabbe A. The prognosis of cluster headache. In: Clifford Rose F, ed. *New advances in headache research* 2. London: Smith Gordon, 1991: 289–291.
7. Kudrow L. Natural history of cluster headache-part 1. Outcome of drop-out patients. *Headache* 1982;22:203–206.
8. Manzoni GC, Micieli G, Granella F, Tassorelli C, Zanferrari C, Cavallini A. Cluster headache-course over ten years in 189 patients. *Cephalalgia* 1991;11:169–174.

9. Nappi G, Micieli G, Cavallini A, Zanferrari C, Sandrini G, Manzoni GC. Accompanying symptoms of cluster attacks: their relevance to the diagnostic criteria. *Cephalalgia* 1992;12:165–168.
10. Nappi G, Micieli G, Facchinetti F, Sandrini G, Martignoni E. Changes in rhythmic temporal structure in cluster headache. In: Sicuteri F, Vecchiet L, Fanciullacci M, eds. *Trends in cluster headache*. Amsterdam: Excerpta Medica, 1987:351–359.
11. Pearce JMS. Natural history of cluster headache. *Headache* 1993;33: 253–256.
12. Sacquegna T, de Carolis P, Agati R, de Capoa D, Baldrati A, Cortelli P. The natural history of episodic cluster headache. *Headache* 1987;27:370–371.
13. Tfelt-Hansen P, Paulson OB, Krabbe A. Invasive adenoma of the pituitary gland and chronic migrainous neuralgia: a rare coincidence or a causal relationship? *Cephalalgia* 1982;2:25–28.
14. Vijayan N, Watson C. Raeder's syndrome, pericarotid syndrome and carotidynia. In: Vinken PG, Bruyn GW, Klawans HL, Clifford Rose F, eds. *Handbook of clinical neurology*, vol 4 (48). Amsterdam: Elsevier, 1986:329–341.

The Headaches, Second Edition,
edited by J. Olesen, P. Tfelt-Hansen, and K.M.A. Welch.
Lippincott Williams & Wilkins, Philadelphia © 2000.

Tension-Type Headache, Cluster Headache, and Miscellaneous
Primary Headaches

CHAPTER 98

Management of Cluster Headache

Karl Ekbom and Seymour Solomon

GENERAL APPROACH TO TREATMENT

Frequent attacks of excruciating pain that seem to have no cause and are often misdiagnosed lead to fear, bewilderment, and anxiety. Discussion of the clinical features of cluster headache and their mechanism will reassure the patient that this condition is self-limiting and is not associated with and will not lead to structural disease. The first step is to assure the patient that, for the vast majority, treatment is available to quickly abort attacks and prevent the frequent bouts. Treatment options are reviewed with the patient, particularly with regard to timing of therapy, the probable need for changing dosages, and potential adverse effects. The temporal pattern of attacks should be carefully noted, and it is particularly helpful if the patients keep a diary of their headaches. Cooperation between patient and physician is essential to implement or change therapeutic strategies.

As with migraine, treatment can be divided into (a) acute symptomatic treatment of individual attacks and (b) prophylactic treatment.

Sumatriptan by subcutaneous injection and oxygen inhalation are the treatments of choice for the acute attack of cluster headache. Dihydroergotamine by injection can be useful. Anesthetic blocks of the sphenopalatine ganglion by nose drops of lidocaine or cocaine are less effective.

Because attacks occur daily, pharmacologic prophylactic treatment is almost always necessary. As a first-

line drug we recommend verapamil. In severe cases it may be combined with steroids for 10 to 14 days of the cluster period. Ergotamine may be used in divided doses on a regular basis or in single doses prior to the anticipated attack. Lithium can be effective, especially in chronic cluster headache, but requires monitoring of blood levels. Methysergide is a potent prophylactic agent but rarely causes fibrotic reactions. Other medications include pizotifen (not available in the United States) and valproic acid, neither of which have been extensively studied.

Efficacy may not be apparent until the drug has been used for several weeks. In addition, one must not assume that the prophylactic drug is ineffective until dosages are increased, sometimes beyond standard recommendations. The increase in dosage is limited primarily by the advent of side effects.

NONPHARMACOLOGIC TREATMENT

Most patients with cluster headache recognize that alcoholic beverages trigger attacks during cluster periods; these agents should, of course, be avoided. Other foods causing vasodilation also may precipitate attacks, but their actions may be less obvious than alcohol. In contrast to migraine, other dietary factors are not important in patients with cluster headache. Similarly, such measures as biofeedback and acupuncture have little place in cluster headache therapy. A surprisingly large number of people with cluster headache are heavy smokers. Cessation of this habit is always warranted, but there is no immediate effect on attacks of cluster headache. Afternoon naps should be avoided because they can elicit an attack.

K. Ekbom: Department of Neurology, Huddinge University Hospital at the Karolinska Institute, S-14186 Huddinge, Sweden.

S. Solomon: Department of Neurology, Albert Einstein College of Medicine, and Headache Unit, Department of Neurology, Montefiore Medical Center, Bronx, New York 10467.

If all other therapeutic measures fail and cluster headaches are chronic, or remissions brief, lesioning of the trigeminal nerve may be considered as a last resort treatment (10,68).

PHARMACOLOGIC TREATMENT

Acute Treatment

Oxygen

Oxygen inhalation is commonly used as a standard abortive treatment of cluster headache not only at the emergency clinic but also at the patient's home office. Patients can rent an oxygen tank and regulator from suppliers.

Horton (46) was the first to discover that 100% oxygen inhalation at the onset of cluster attacks alleviates the cluster headache. Friedman and Mikropoulus (35) also reported on its favorable effect. Kudrow (56,57) systematically evaluated the symptomatic response to oxygen inhalation administered at a rate of 7 L per minute for 15 minutes in 55 consecutive patients with cluster headache. The best responders were patients with the episodic type of cluster headache under 50 years of age. A favorable aspect of oxygen inhalation was the rapidity with which it offered significant pain relief. Headache relief occurred 62% of the time within the first 7 minutes of oxygen inhalation, 31% within 8 to 10 minutes, and 7% within 10 to 15 minutes. Kudrow also emphasized that oxygen inhalation causes no side effects and, unlike ergotamine, is not contraindicated by cardiovascular, peripheral vascular, pulmonary, hepatic, or renal diseases. A double-blind comparison of oxygen versus air inhalation in 19 patients confirmed the value of the former as a symptomatic treatment of cluster headache (32).

Oxygen has vasoconstricting properties, but this quality is unlikely to be the sole mechanism. Hemodynamic studies during oxygen inhalation for cluster headache fail to show an increase in brain oxygenation (48). Nevertheless, increased arterial oxygen pressure is thought to have a direct effect on cranial blood vessels. Brain hyperperfusion occurs with cluster headache, and oxygen abolishes the hyperperfusion; cerebral vasoconstriction then occurs (51). After nitroglycerin-induced cluster headache there is greater and more prolonged oxygen desaturation than normal (58). During the cluster period, patients have less reduction in oxygen saturation than controls when hypoxia is induced and during nitroglycerin-induced attacks (100). These studies postulate abnormal chemoreceptor sensitivity in patients with cluster headache. Oxygen therapy may redress this defect.

Hyperbaric oxygen (HBO) has been claimed to be effective in treating patients with cluster headache (18). However, a recent double-blind placebo-controlled and cross-over trial in 16 patients (4 chronic) showed that HBO was no better than placebo (75). HBO may act by decreasing immunoreactivity of substance P and suppressing neurogenic inflammation (19). Serotonin binding to mononuclear cells before and after HBO treatment in 14 patients with chronic cluster headache suggested that HBO might act through serotonergic pathways (20).

Ergot

The first to describe the effects of *ergotamine tartrate* in acute attacks of cluster headache was Horton (44). He reported on a female patient with severe nocturnal attacks of histaminic cephalalgia; although she had taken as many as 24 aspirin tablets (300 mg) in one night without obtaining relief, intravenous administration of 0.2 to 0.3 mg of ergotamine tartrate (Gynergen) during an attack provided relief. In 1952, Kunkle et al. (59) reported the rapid termination of attacks in four patients by intravenous injection of ergotamine tartrate. Horton et al. (47) used ergotamine tartrate in the form of Cafergot tablets (ergotamine tartrate 1 mg and caffeine 100 mg) for the symptomatic treatment of acute attacks. The average dose was two tablets administered at the onset of an attack. An excellent effect was reported in 10 of 14 patients, and substantial reduction of subjective symptoms in 3 patients. Friedman and Mikropoulos (35) reported the most effective relief to be obtained by early and adequate administration of ergotamine and caffeine preparations, alone or combined with antiemetics or sedatives. Without reporting any details they noted a beneficial effect in 30 of 35 patients.

Ergotamine may ameliorate and cut short an attack of headache if given orally or rectally early during the attack, although experimental findings suggest inhalation to be more effective (26). Ergotamine inhalation in cluster headache was first described by Speed (86), who reported its effect to be excellent in 11 of 13 patients. It also was found to be successful in giving relief to another small series of patients (21) and comparable in rapidity of effect to intramuscular injection. In 12 patients treated by Graham et al. (41), ergotamine inhalation gave relief from pain within half an hour in 71% of 114 attacks, and Kudrow (56) reported that 79 of 100 patients obtained significant relief from sublingual or inhalant ergotamine preparations. However, there have been no clinical studies on ergotamine inhalation for cluster headache during recent years.

Dihydroergotamine (DHE 45) given intramuscularly or intravenously has been recommended as an excellent method of aborting an attack and also has been said to produce fewer side effects than ergotamine tartrate. Occasionally, some patients experience mild pains in their legs, although blood pressure is unaffected.

Dihydroergotamine administered by a nasal spray (1 mg) was compared with placebo in 25 patients in a double-blind cross-over study (2). There was no difference in the duration of the attacks, but a significantly better effect on the intensity of individual attacks.

Sumatriptan

In a pilot study of sumatriptan in patients with cluster headache, Krabbe (53) reported that four of six patients obtained marked relief after a subcutaneous injection of either 3 or 6 mg. In a double-blind, placebo-controlled, cross-over study comprising 49 patients, one dose of sumatriptan (6 mg subcutaneously) was given to treat one attack and one dose of placebo to treat another, the order being randomized (90). Response to treatment was defined as complete relief from headache (no pain = grade 0) or almost complete relief (residual mild pain = grade 1) within 15 minutes after administration. Evaluable data were obtained from 39 patients who completed the study according to the protocol. Sumatriptan was significantly more effective than placebo in relieving headache: 74% of sumatriptan-treated attacks responded by 15 minutes after administration, as compared with 26% of placebo-treated attacks. Thirty-six percent of the patients given sumatriptan were pain-free within 10 minutes, as compared with 3% of those given placebo, and 46% and 10%, respectively, by 15 minutes (Fig. 1). Both differences were highly significant. Functional disability and an ipsilateral conjunctival injection were significantly improved in the sumatriptan-treated group as compared with the placebo-treated group. The resolution of the classic autonomic sign of conjunctival injection suggested that sumatriptan may interrupt basic processes underlying cluster headache rather than merely act as a suppressor of pain. There were no serious side effects.

A second large randomized controlled study also has been performed (29) using a higher dosage. This was a double-blind, three-treatment, two-period, cross-over trial. All patients were hospitalized for the duration of the study and received subcutaneous sumatriptan 6 mg, 12 mg, or placebo for the treatment of an attack of at least moderate severity. The efficacy population consisted of all 134 patients who received treatment for two cluster

headache attacks. Subcutaneous sumatriptan 12 mg did not produce a clinically significant increase in either headache relief or rate at which attacks were relieved, compared with the 6-mg dose. It also was associated with more adverse events. The recommended dose of sumatriptan for the acute treatment of cluster headache is therefore 6 mg by subcutaneous injection.

Long-term results of acute treatment of cluster headache have been reported in a multinational open clinical trial (27). Patients treated up to two cluster headache attacks per day at home, each with a 6-mg subcutaneous injection of sumatriptan at the earliest onset of symptoms. In an interim review of 3-month data, 138 patients had treated 6,353 attacks with a median of 31 attacks per patient (range 1–182). Sumatriptan was generally well tolerated. The incidence and nature of adverse events were similar to those reported in long-term migraine studies. There was no evidence of any increased incidence of adverse events in patients who used sumatriptan frequently. There were no significant treatment effects on vital signs, laboratory, or electrocardiographic (ECG) parameters. During the 3-month study period, effective headache relief was reported by 96% of patients (median) 15 minutes after treatment with sumatriptan. Eighty-nine percent of patients rated the treatment as good or excellent, and 94% of patients would take sumatriptan again. Efficay was not changed when comparing the results in the first and second halves of attacks treated (Fig. 2). There was thus no evidence of any tachyphylaxis over the 3 months. Excellent long-term results also have been reported by others (39,93).

A multinational, randomized, double-blind, placebo-controlled, parallel-group study investigated the effect of 1 week's preemptive treatment with oral sumatriptan (73). One hundred sixty-eight patients treated a single attack at home with 6 mg subcutaneous sumatriptan and were then randomized to take 100 mg oral sumatriptan or placebo three times daily for 1 week. Oral sumatriptan given in

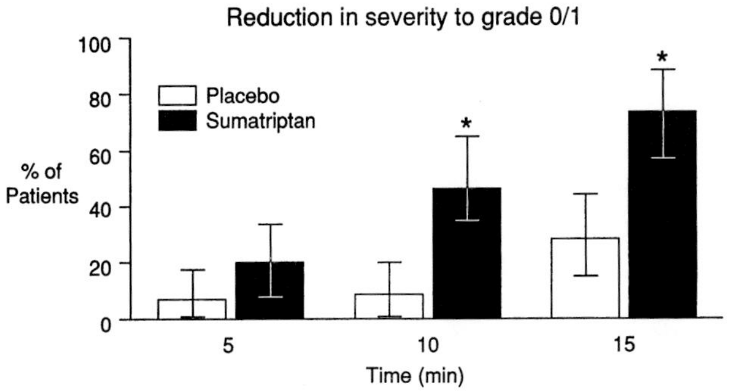

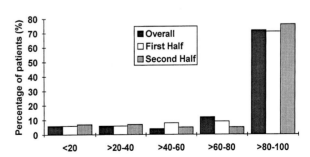

FIG. 1. Response of cluster headache (n = 39) to treatment with sumatriptan 6 mg subcutaneously (90). The reduction in the mean score for the severity of headache was significantly larger after the injection of sumatriptan than after placebo at both 10 and 15 minutes.

FIG. 2. An open long-term trial (n = 138) of sumatriptan 6 mg subcutaneously for acute attacks of cluster headache (27). Percentage of attacks that were grade 0 or 1 at 15 minutes after sumatriptan, overall and split by first and second halves of attacks. Reproduced from Ekbom et al. (27).

this dose regimen did not reduce the number, severity, or duration of cluster headache attacks.

Ottervanger et al. (76) reported on a 47-year-old woman with an acute transmural myocardial infarction after the administration of sumatriptan 6 mg subcutaneously for cluster headache. She had had no history of any underlying ischemic heart disease or Prinzmetal's angina. Another two patients with cluster headache had transitory ischemic ECG changes following subcutaneous injection of sumatriptan (1,99). However, in both of these patients evident contraindications to the use of sumatriptan were not taken into consideration before treatment. None of 200 cluster headache patients who were treated in the randomized studies described above displayed any ECG abnormalities indicating myocardial ischemia following sumatriptan administration.

In rare cases, sumatriptan is not sufficiently efficacious, and this unresponsiveness has tentatively been attributed to an absence of an increase of 5-HT receptor expression during the attack (89).

Prioritization

Oral administration of analgesics and ergotamine tartrate is of limited value in the treatment of acute attacks. Sublingual or inhaled ergotamine are seldom used and have not been studied in clinical trials during recent years. In some quarters dihydroergotamine is recommended via intramuscular (or intravenous) injection for the abortion of acute attacks. However, inhalation of 100% oxygen is a more convenient alternative, easy to administer, often effective within a few minutes and with no side effects. It is used both in ambulant care and in the hospital.

At present, sumatriptan 6 mg subcutaneously appears to constitute the most effective therapy of cluster headache attacks (25,98). For many patients sumatriptan injections are more practical to handle than oxygen inhalation. Sumatriptan is well tolerated and, with rare exceptions, has no serious side effects. There is no evidence of any tachyphylaxis during long-term treatment. Generally, more than two injections should not be given a day, although in rare cases it has been administered up to four times daily during short periods.

Intranasal application of cocaine (6) or lidocaine for anesthesia of the sphenopalatine foramen region has not gained widespread acceptance.

Prophylactic Treatment

Ergotamine

The first to use ergotamine tartrate for prophylactic treatment of cluster headache was K.A. Ekbom (30). Sixteen patients were given ergotamine tartrate (Gynergen) in 1-mg tablets twice or (in three patients) three times daily. Treatment was continued for one to four weeks. Thirteen patients were considerably improved. It was

pointed out that the disease may manifest a capricious course and that spontaneous remissions must be taken into consideration when judging the therapeutic response.

Horton (45) reported that a rectal suppository of 2 mg of ergotamine tartrate and 100 mg of caffeine at bedtime frequently prevented nocturnal attacks. Rectal administration was said to be more effective than the oral administration. Others have confirmed the prophylactic effect of ergotamine tartrate in cluster headache. Excellent results have been obtained with intramuscular or subcutaneous injections of 0.25 to 0.5 mg ergotamine at bedtime to prevent nocturnal attacks (7,82,91). In some instances, it was necessary to give an additional injection of 0.25 mg on rising.

Many experienced clinicians still recommend ergotamine orally for the prophylactic treatment of cluster headache. The dosage is 3 to 4 mg daily, divided into two or more doses. Treatment should be continued for several weeks, or until the attacks have ceased. Side effects are few.

Lithium

Ever since its introduction for the treatment of manic-depressive disorders and periodic depression, lithium has been tried in various psychiatric, neurologic, and medical diseases. Its effect in cases of cluster headache sheds new light on the pathogenesis of this condition.

Pharmacology

Lithium is readily and almost completely absorbed from the gastrointestinal tract, but passage through the blood–brain barrier is slow (5). Peak plasma concentrations occur within 2 to 4 hours of an oral dose; and with daily administration, equilibrium between absorption and excretion is reached in about 5 days. The therapeutic range is narrow, and adverse effects may occur even at the higher upper range of the treatment window (0.8–1.2 mM). Serum lithium concentrations should be measured in the morning, 12 hours after the last oral dose. Lithium interacts with such drugs as indomethacin, diclofenac, thiazides, and thiazide-related diuretics. It displaces intracellular sodium. Dehydration may quickly increase lithium levels.

Review of Trials

Ekbom (23) was the first to report the effect of lithium in cluster headache. Three of five patients with chronic cluster headache obtained immediate partial remission with lithium, the headaches increased again in intensity and frequency upon withdrawal of the drug. A second course of treatment produced a more definite improvement. Placebo was without effect. These findings were soon confirmed by Kudrow (55), Mathew (68), and others.

A review of the literature and preliminary results of long-term treatment were reported by Ekbom (24).

To date, a total of 28 clinical trials comprising 468 patients have been published. Lithium has been effective against chronic cluster headache in 236 (78%) of 304 patients in 25 trials. It also works against episodic cluster headache, although to a lesser degree, an overall remission rate of 63% having been obtained in a total of 164 patients treated. In a meticulous investigation by Manzoni et al. (66), 90 patients were treated, of whom 22 had the chronic form of the disease. Of those taking lithium carbonate 900 mg per day, 11 of the 22 patients with chronic cluster showed a definite, constant improvement both in the short and long term (average duration of treatment 22 months, range 3–48). Upon interruption of treatment, chronic cluster headache may turn into the episodic variant (24).

One double-blind cross-over study compared verapamil and lithium (9). Thirty patients received either verapamil (360 mg daily) or lithium carbonate (900 mg daily), and both drugs were found to be effective. Verapamil caused fewer side effects and was also said to result in more rapid headache improvement than lithium. In another double-blind comparison of matched parallel groups, episodic cluster headache patients received either slow-release lithium carbonate or placebo (88). Lithium gave rise to a subjective substantial improvement rate of 62% to 70%, but the trial was stopped after planned sequential analysis of the 27th patient (13 on lithium, 14 on placebo) because superiority over placebo could not be demonstrated.

Lithium may give rise to side effects, especially tremor, polyuria, and diarrhea. Renal and thyroid functions should be checked before and during treatment. Lithium has been shown to be effective at rather low serum concentrations, between 0.3 and 0.8 mM (66). Most patients benefit from a daily dose of 600 to 900 mg of lithium carbonate.

The benefits of lithium therapy probably has to do with its ability to alter ions in the central nervous system, affecting metabolism of biogenic amines (5). Lithium inhibits polypeptides implicated in the trigeminovascular concept of perivascular inflammation. It inhibits responses to substance P and vasoactive intestinal polypeptide but not to calcitonin gene–related peptide (95). Lithium appears to modulate nerve transmission by altering sodium transport and catecholamine reuptake, thus enhancing their inactivation (5). It inhibits depolarization-provoked and calcium ion–dependent release of dopamine and norepinephrine (but not serotonin) from nerve terminals. However, it may enhance the release of serotonin, especially in the hippocampus (5). Lithium affects serotonin metabolism, as noted by its effect on neurotransmitter metabolism (50) and platelet serotonin transport (12). It may act by modulating normal serotonergic tone (9). Lithium interferes with sleep patterns, a factor that may explain the suppression of cluster headache that commonly occurs during sleep (54). Changes in hormonal circadian rhythms in patients with cluster headache may be shifted toward normal by lithium therapy.

In summary, lithium has a role in the prophylaxis of both chronic and episodic cluster headaches. It is widely used in clinical practice, but it should be borne in mind that, with the exception of the two studies mentioned above, results have been derived solely from open clinical trials. Lithium has many potential side effects, especially if the therapeutic level is exceeded. It is important that the patient be well informed as to the need for periodic lithium blood level determinations and the adverse as well as beneficial effects.

Steroids

Pharmacology

Prednisone and its congeners are readily absorbed from the gastrointestinal tract. Most of the compound is protein bound. The half-life of prednisone, the most commonly used steroid for cluster headache, is 12 to 36 hours. The pharmacologic effects are widespread (83). Adrenocortical steroids maintain homeostasis by influencing metabolism of proteins, carbohydrates, and fats; water and electrolyte balance; and function of the neuromuscular systems and virtually all other major systems. These agents also influence actions of other hormones.

Review of Trials

Jammes (49) performed a double-blind controlled study in 19 patients with a single cross-over. Compared with placebo, a single oral dose of prednisone 30 mg produced "sustained improvement" in 17 patients and "permanent freedom of symptoms" for at least 60 days in 14 patients. However, this study has methodologic weaknesses. Cough and Ziegler (13) retrospectively studied 19 patients; prednisone was given in daily doses of 10 to 80 mg. Good results were obtained in 14 patients, but initial doses of 40 mg or more were apparently needed to induce a persistent remission. Recurrence was common when the dosage was tapered off. In an open trial, Kudrow (56) found that prednisone provided marked relief in 77% of 77 episodic cluster patients, and partial improvement in another 12%. In contrast, only 40% of 15 chronic cluster headache patients manifested marked improvement. Prednisone was also found to be significantly better than methysergide in either episodic or chronic cluster headache groups. Prusinski et al. (78) reported beneficial effects of dexamethasone administered orally or intravenously in 12 and 9 patients, respectively. This, too, was an open study, and only short-term results were reported. Anthony and Daher (4) treated 15 patients who had episodic cluster headache with dexamethasone within 3 days of the onset of the cluster headache period. The dose was 4 mg twice daily for 2 weeks, followed by 4 mg daily for 1 week. Once the dose of dexamethasone was reduced to below 4 or 3 mg daily, the attacks of cluster headache returned. The authors often used brief courses of steroids for 2 or 3 weeks to suppress bouts of cluster headaches.

Scientific documentation of efficacy has thus not been rigorous, perhaps because the beneficial effects of steroids are so rapid (within 24 to 48 hours) and obvious. These attributes have placed prednisone as one of first-line therapies for severe cases of cluster headache. Sixty milligrams per day may be given for 10 days, then the medication is tapered off over the next week. Prednisone may be started at the same time as verapamil, and verapamil continued for the duration of the cluster period.

The reason for steroid efficacy is speculative. Suppression of the presumptive perivascular inflammation is the most obvious mechanism. Steroid therapy may modify the defects in the hypothalamic-pituitary-adrenal axis that are manifested by altered basal cortisol levels and blunted cortisol responses to hormonal challenges in patients with cluster headache (61,63). An increase in neutrophil metenkephalin–containing peptides is noted after prednisone therapy; thus, steroids may act by stimulating the opioid system (31). If serotonergic mechanisms are important in patients with cluster headache, corticosteroids may act by exerting tonic control on serotonergic transmission (in the rat) (17).

Calcium Antagonists

Pharmacology

Verapamil is almost completely absorbed but is highly bound to plasma proteins (77). Depolarization and contraction of vascular smooth muscle is dependent on influx of calcium ions. Calcium channel blockers prevent vascular contraction and relax arterial smooth muscle. Although its physiologic effect is rapid, verapamil's maximal clinical effect may be delayed for weeks.

Review of Trials

The only double-blind trial with this group of drugs compared lithium and verapamil with placebo in chronic cluster headache (9). Of 24 patients who completed the study, both active agents were associated with significant reduction in attacks. Other studies of calcium channel blockers for cluster headache have been open trials. Meyer et al. (72) reported responses of patients with cluster headache to calcium channel blockers (nimodipine, nifedipine, verapamil), but the study was mainly designed to evaluate the hemodynamic effects of these agents. They found that the calcium channel antagonists decreased the frequency of cluster attacks. De Carolis et al. (11) found that treatment with nimodipine was followed by disappearance of attacks in 7 of 13 patients with

episodic cluster headache. Gabai and Spierings (38) studied 48 patients treated with verapamil. In 33, cluster headache frequency was reduced by more than 75%; only 9 patients did not benefit. Doses of verapamil as high as 1,200 mg per day were used. Only 3 patients discontinued treatment because of gastrointestinal symptoms or bradycardia. Constipation is common, and edema of the ankles sometimes occurs with use of verapamil, but other adverse effects are rare even with long-term therapy.

It is unlikely that verapamil and similar agents act by evoking vasodilation. For example, intravenous verapamil can abort nitroglycerin-induced attacks of cluster headache (8). There is little correlation between changes in cerebral blood flow and clinical efficacy (8,72). The calcium channel blockers may act on the nociceptive system by interfering with the calcium-dependent release of substance P from sensory nerve terminals. In addition, these agents may modify the action of other polypeptides associated with nociceptors. Bussone et al. (9) postulate that verapamil acts by influencing serotonergic, dopaminergic, noradrenergic, and other receptors within the central nervous system as well as by modifying hypothalamic-noradrenergic activity.

Methysergide

Methysergide is a congener of LSD. It is metabolized to methylergonovine, the presumptive active component (94). Its action can be evident within 1 or 2 days. Methysergide is a serotonin antagonist inhibiting the vasoconstrictor and pressor effects of serotonin. Although it has only weak vasoconstrictor action by itself, methysergide may potentiate the vasoconstricting effects of norepinephrine.

Methysergide is a potent prophylactic agent, but its use has been restricted by fear of rare fibrotic reactions (retroperitoneal, pleuropulmonary, and endocardial). These conditions clear with the discontinuation of drug. It is recommended that methysergide use be terminated before 6 months and resumed after a 4-week drug holiday. Whether this prevents the fibrotic complications is debatable because the complication appears to be idiosyncratic (79). The short-term use of methysergide would suit most cases of episodic cluster headache because cluster periods usually do not last 6 months.

Early studies by Friedman and Elkind (34) and Graham (40) found methysergide to be effective in 50% to 70% of cases. Curran et al. (14) reviewed all studies prior to 1967, totaling 451 patients; improvement occurred in 73%. Kudrow (56), on the other hand, studying 15 patients with chronic cluster headache, noted its efficacy in only 20%, and Krabbe (52) similarly noted an efficacy of 25% to 30%. The dosage range is 4 to 10 mg per day, but dosages as high as 16 mg per day have sometimes been necessary (79).

The effectiveness of methylergonovine, the major metabolite of methysergide, was evaluated in a retrospective uncontrolled study of 20 patients with episodic cluster headache (74). Methylergonovine was added to concomitant prophylactic medications that had not evoked satisfactory relief. In 19 of 20 patients there was a decrease in frequency of attacks of 50% or more. The dose was 0.2 mg three to four times per day. The most common adverse effects are gastrointestinal upset, leg muscle cramps, and dizziness.

Valproate

Valproate is a new addition to the preventive therapy of chronic recurrent headache. Hering and Kuritzky (43) in an open trial found that sodium valproate was effective in 11 of 15 patients with cluster headache. In 9 of the 11 there was complete cessation of attacks. Dosage ranged from 600 to 2,000 mg per day.

Valproate induces an increase in the central nervous system of the inhibitory transmitter gamma amino butyric acid (GABA) (70). Circadian rhythms are disrupted in patients with cluster headache, and GABA may affect these rhythms. GABA is thought to suppress migraine by its action on serotonergic centers (43).

Pizotifen

Sicuteri et al. (84) were the first to report the beneficial effects of pizotifen in seven cases of cluster headache. During the period 1969 to 1970 a number of open studies of pizotifen were performed (87), and although the series were small, a "definite improvement" was obtained in about 50% of cases.

In the only single-blind trial of pizotifen in cluster headache (22), 28 patients were assessed as having a remaining cluster period of at least 4 weeks. Placebo was given for 5 days, after which pizotifen was administered in successively increasing doses, and the maintenance dose was usually 3 mg daily. The mean duration of treatment was 5 weeks. Of 28 patients, 6 (21%) became free of attacks, and 10 (36%) manifested better than 50% improvement. Both the frequency and the intensity of the headache attacks were significantly reduced during treatment with pizotifen as compared with placebo. The most common side effects were drowsiness and weight increase.

To sum up, valproate and pizotifen may be tried as alternatives in the prevention of cluster headache, particularly in cases where the patient does not respond to ergotamine or when the latter is contraindicated. It should be noted, however, that documentation of the effects of valproate and pizotifen has been based almost exclusively on open trials. Pizotifen is not available in the United States

Other Treatments

A decrease of nocturnal serum melatonin has been reported in cluster headache. Leone et al. (62) compared 10 mg melatonin orally with placebo in 20 cluster headache patients for 14 days in a double-blind pilot study comprising parallel groups. Headache frequency was significantly reduced, and there were strong trends toward reduced analgesic consumption in the active treatment group. Responders improved within 3 days after beginning melatonin. No side effects occurred.

Clonidine was administered transdermally (5–7.5 mg) for 1 week to 13 patients suffering from cluster headache as a short-term open pilot study (16). Mean weekly frequency, as well as intensity and duration of attacks, decreased during the observation period. It was suggested that clonidine might act in cluster headache via its sympathetic inhibition. In another similar open trial, clonidine was given transdermally for 2 weeks (60). In contrast to the former study, only 5 of 15 patients improved, and some of the patients may have spontaneously reached the final phase of their cluster headache periods.

Tizanidine is structurally similar to clonidine and is mainly used as an adjunct to the management of spasticity and painful muscle spasm. Positive results have been reported (15) in four of five consecutive patients with chronic cluster headache treated in an open fashion for 8 to 12 weeks. However, our experience in a few patients has been negative (Ekbom, unpublished observations).

Topical application of capsaicin to the nasal mucosa for 5 consecutive days significantly reduced the frequency of attacks in 20 patients with cluster headache (85). Only treatment of the ipsilateral nostril gave positive results (37). Fusco et al. (36) evaluated the long-term effects of nasal capsaicin in 25 patients (17 episodic and 8 chronic). In 65%, a beneficial effect was noted with repeated administration. Others also noted the effectiveness of topical capsaicin (67). It may act in cluster headache by desensitization of those sensory neurons involved in the pathogenetic process.

Although most interesting from both clinical and pathogenetic aspects, the results summarized above are mainly based on open, short-term trials in a limited number of selected patients. There are no data on long-term treatment. Further confirmation is needed before a judgment can be made on the practical value of the respective treatments in everyday clinical practice.

In order to facilitate high-quality controlled clinical trials, official guidelines recently have been published (64). Many issues have to be considered, such as patient selection, trial design, selection of endpoints, evaluation of results, and data analyses. The unforseeable length of the remaining cluster period and spontaneously occurring remissions must be taken into consideration when evaluating treatment results.

Prioritization

Drugs of choice are listed in Table 1, which contains our recommendations for the prophylactic treatment. The drugs are ranked based on our experience and available data in the literature.

TABLE 1. *Prophylactic treatment of cluster headache*

Episodic cluster headache
  Verapamil
  Prednisone (eventually a combination of both verapamil
    and prednisone)
  Ergotamine tartrate
  Methysergide
  Pizotifen
  Lithium carbonate
Chronic cluster headache
  Lithium carbonate
  Verapamil
  Methysergid
  Pizotifen

TABLE 2. *Criteria for surgical therapy*

Total resistance to pharmacotherapy (ineffectiveness or
  serious adverse effects of, or contraindications to
  pharmacotherapy)
Headache locked to the same side
Pain mainly in the distribution of the ophthalmic division of
  the trigeminal nerve
Psychologically stable individuals, particularly the absence
  of an addicting personality

SURGICAL THERAPY

Many sites have been surgically attacked in an attempt to terminate cluster headaches. The parasympathetic pathways have been interrupted by sectioning the nervus intermedius (80), the greater superficial petrosal nerve (97), and the sphenopalatine ganglion (71). In most of these cases relief was inconsistent and, when effective, recurrences were reported. The recurrence of cluster headache was attributed to nerve regeneration. Anesthetic blocks of the sphenopalatine ganglion by intranasal application of blocking agents such as cocaine and lidocaine can abort acute attacks (6). Results of anesthetic blocks by direct injection in early years were reported in terms of "highly satisfactory" and "significantly relieved." These early treatments were performed at a time when cluster headaches were not well defined and the occurrence of spontaneous remissions was not universally recognized.

Recently, the sphenopalatine ganglion was lesioned by radiofrequency (81) in 66 patients with medically refractory cluster headache (episodic in 56 patients, chronic in 10). Complete relief was reported in 34 patients with episodic cluster headache and in 3 with chronic cluster headache; partial relief was noted in 14 and 3 patients, respectively. The mean follow-up periods were at least 2 years.

In another recent series of patients with chronic cluster headache, microvascular decompression of the trigeminal nerve was performed alone (n=9) or with microvascular decompression of the nervus intermedius (n=3) or with section of the nervus intermedius (n=10). Excellent results were reported in about half of this group during a follow-up period averaging 5.3 years (65).

Occipital nerve blocks have been advocated for the treatment of cluster headache (3). Benefit may be derived by steroids administered with the anesthetic agent or the nonspecific reduction of somatic sensory impulses into central pathways.

The ophthalmic and maxillar divisions of the trigeminal nerve carry the pain impulses of cluster headache, and the most consistent benefits of surgical therapy have followed the lesioning of these afferent pathways. Taha and Tew (92) reviewed reports of radiofrequency gangliorhizolysis in a total of 97 patients. Good results (cessation of cluster headaches) occurred in 50% to 60% of patients. Most recently gamma knife radiosurgery was used to lesion the trigeminal nerve root (33). Excellent results were noted in four of six patients. Glycerol injections in the trigeminal cistern has been reported as a treatment for cluster headache in a relatively few cases (28, 42,96). This procedure was not associated with as high a percentage of good to excellent results as radiofrequency lesioning of the trigeminal nerve roots (69). The efficacy of these surgical procedures also appears to be related to the degree of sensory loss; total analgesia is associated with highest percentage of efficacy.

A summary of clinical criteria for surgery is given in Table 2. Poor results are mainly associated with inadequate analgesia in the area of pain. Personality defects, particularly addiction-prone individuals, have a poor prognosis. Keratitis, anesthesia dolorosa, and recurrence of cluster headache on the opposite side are additional causes of dissatisfaction.

REFERENCES

1. Abrahamsen B, Christiansen BD. Angina pectoris after administration of sumatriptan. *Ugeskr Laeger* 1992;154:3602–3603.
2. Andersson PG, Jespersen LT. Dihydroergotamine nasal spray in the treatment of attacks of cluster headache *Cephalalgia* 1986;6:51–54.
3. Anthony M. Arrest of attacks of cluster headache by local steroid injection of the occipital nerve. In: Clifford Rose F, ed. *Migraine.* Basel: Karger, 1985:169–173.
4. Anthony M, Daher BN. Mechanism of action of steroids in cluster headache. In: Clifford Rose F, ed. *New advances in headache research 2.* London: Smith-Gordon, 1992:271–274.
5. Baldessarini RJ. Depression and mania. In: Hardman JG, Limbird LE, Molinoff PB, Ruddon RW, Gilman AG, eds. *Goodman & Gilman's the pharmacological basis of therapeutics,* 9th ed. New York: McGraw-Hill 1996:446–447.
6. Barré F. Cocaine as an abortive agent in cluster headache. *Headache* 1982;22:69–73.
7. Bickerstaff ER. The periodic migrainous neuralgia of Wilfred Harris. *Lancet* 1959;1:1069–1071.
8. Boiardi A, Gemma M, Peccarisi PE, Bussone G. Calcium entry blocker: treatment in acute pain in cluster headache patients. *Ital J Neurol Sci* 1986;7:531–534.
9. Bussone G, Leone M, Peccarisi C et al. Double blind comparison of lithium and verapamil in cluster headache prophylaxis. *Headache* 1990;30:411–417.
10. Campbell JK. Cluster headache: the treatment resistant patient. In: Mathew NT, ed. *Cluster headache.* Lancaster: Spectrum Publications, 1984:127–133.

11. Carolis de P, Baldrati A, Agati R, de Capoa D, D'Alessandro R, Sacquegna T. Nimodipine in episodic cluster headache: results and methodological considerations. *Headache* 1987;27:397–399.

12. Coppen A, Swade C. Lithium restores abnormal platelet 5-HT transport in patients with affective disorders. *Br J Psychiatry* 1980;136: 235–238.

13. Couch JR, Ziegler DK. Prednisone therapy for cluster headache. *Headache* 1978;18:219–221.

14. Curran DA, Hinterberger H, Lance JW. Methysergide. *Res Clin Stud Headache* 1967;1:74–122.

15. D'Alessandro R, Granella F. Tizanidine for chronic cluster headache. *Arch Neurol* 1996;53:1093.

16. D'Andrea G, Perini F, Granella F, Canazi A, Sergi A. Efficacy of transdermal clonidine in short-term treatment of cluster headache. *Cephalalgia* 1995;15:430–433.

17. De Kloet ER, Sybesma H, Reul HMHM. Selective control by corticosterone of serotonin S receptor activity in raphe-hippocampal systems. *Neuroendocrinology* 1986;42:513–521.

18. Di Sabato F, Fusco BM, Pelaia P, Giacovazzo M. Hyperbaric oxygen therapy in cluster headache. *Pain* 1993;52:243–245.

19. Di Sabato F, Giacovazzo M, Cristalli G, Rocco M, Fusco BM. Effect of hyperbaric oxygen on the immunoreactivity to substance P in the nasal mucosa of cluster headache patients. *Headache* 1996;36: 221–223.

20. Di Sabato F, Rocco M, Martelletti P, Giacovazzo M. Hyperbaric oxygen in chronic cluster headaches: influence on serotonergic pathways. *Undersea Hyperbaric Med* 1997;24:117–122.

21. Duvoisin RC, Parker GW, Kenoyer WL. The cluster headache. *Arch Intern Med* 1961;108:711–716.

22. Ekbom K. Prophylactic treatment of cluster headache with a new serotonin antagonist, BC 105. *Acta Neurol Scand* 1969;45:601–610.

23. Ekbom K. Litium vid kroniska symptom av cluster headache. *Opusc Med* 1974;19:148–156.

24. Ekbom K. Lithium for cluster headache: review of the literature and preliminary results of long-term treatment. *Headache* 1981;21: 132–139.

25. Ekbom K. Sumatriptan in the management of cluster headache. *Rev Contemp Pharmacother* 1994;5:311–318.

26. Ekbom K, Aebelholt-Krabbe A, Paalzow G, Paalzow L, Tfelt-Hansen P, Waldenlind E. Optimal routes of administration of ergotamine tartrate in cluster headache patients. A pharmacokinetic study. *Cephalalgia* 1983;3:15–20.

27. Ekbom K, Krabbe A, Micieli G, et al. Cluster headache attacks treated for up to three months with subcutaneous sumatriptan (6 mg). *Cephalalgia* 1995;15:230–236.

28. Ekbom K, Lindgren L, Nilsson BY, Hardebo JE, Waldenlind E. Retro-Gasserian glycerol injection in the treatment of chronic cluster headache. *Cephalalgia* 1987;7:21–27.

29. Ekbom K, Monstad I, Prusinski A, Cole J, Pilgrim AJ, Noronha D. Subcutaneous sumatriptan in the acute treatment of cluster headache: a dose comparison study. *Acta Neurol Scand* 1993;88:63–69.

30. Ekbom KA. Ergotamine tartrate orally in Horton's "Histaminic cephalgia" (also called Harris's "ciliary neuralgia"). *Acta Psychiatr Scand* 1947;[Suppl 46]:106–113.

31. Figuerola M de L, Levin G, Leston J, Barontini M. Opioid and sympathetic nervous system activity in cluster headache under verapamil or prednisone treatment. *Headache* 1994;34:257–260.

32. Fogan L. Treatment of cluster headache. A double-blind comparison of oxygen v air inhalation. *Arch Neurol* 1985;42:362–363.

33. Ford RG, Ford KT, Swaid S, Young P, Jennelle R. Gamma knife treatment of refractory cluster headache. *Headache* 1998;38:3–9.

34. Friedman AP, Elkind AH. Appraisal of methysergide in treatment of vascular headache of migraine-type. *JAMA* 1963;184:125–128.

35. Friedman AP, Mikropoulos HE. Cluster headaches. *Neurology* 1958; 8:653–663.

36. Fusco BM, Fiore G, Gallo F, Martelletti P, Giacovazzo M. Capsaicin-sensitive sensory neurons in cluster headache: pathophysiological aspects and therapeutic indication. *Headache* 1994;34:132–137.

37. Fusco BM, Marabini S, Maggi CA, Fiore G, Geppetti P. Preventative effect of repeated nasal applications of capsaicin in cluster headache. *Pain* 1994;59:321–325.

38. Gabai IJ, Spierings ELH. Prophylactic treatment of cluster headache with verapamil. *Headache* 1989;29:167–168.

39. Göbel H, Lindner V, Heinze A, Ribbat M, Peuschl G. Acute therapy

40. Graham JR. Methysergide for prevention of headache: experience in five hundred patients over three years. *N Engl J Med* 1964;270:67–72.

41. Graham JR, Malvea BP, Gramm HF. Aerosol ergotamine tartrate for migraine and Horton's syndrome. *N Engl J Med* 1960;263:802–804.

42. Hassenbusch SJ, Kunkel RS, Kosmorsky GS, Covington EC, Pillay PK. Trigeminal cisternal injection of glycerol for treatment of chronic intractable cluster headaches. *Neurosurgery* 1991;29:504–508.

43. Hering R, Kuritzky A. Sodium valproate in the treatment of cluster headache: an open trial. *Cephalalgia* 1989;9:195–198.

44. Horton BT. The use of histamine in the treatment of specific types of headaches. *JAMA* 1941;116:377–383.

45. Horton BT. Histaminic cephalgia. *Lancet* 1952;2:92–98.

46. Horton BT. Histaminic cephalgia: differential diagnosis and treatment. *Mayo Clin Proc* 1956;31:325–333.

47. Horton BT, Ryan R, Reynolds JL. Clinical observations of the use of E.C. 110, a new agent for the treatment of headache. *Mayo Clin Proc* 1948;23:105–108

48. Igarashi H, Sakai F, Kanda T, Tazaki Y, Saitoh Y. The mechanism by which oxygen interrupts cluster headache. *Cephalalgia* 1991;11[Suppl 11]:238–239.

49. Jammes JL. The treatment of cluster headaches with prednisone. *Dis Nerv Syst* 1975;36:375–376.

50. Judd A, Parker J, Jemmer FA. The role of noradrenaline, dopamine and 5-hydroxytryptamine in the hyperactivity response resulting from the administration of tranylcypromine to rats pretreated with lithium or rubidium. *Psychopharmacologia* 1975;1:73–78.

51. Kawamura J, Meyer JS, Terayama Y, Weathers S. Cerebral hyperemia during spontaneous cluster headaches with excessive cerebral vasoconstriction to hyperoxia. *Headache* 1991;31:222–227.

52. Krabbe A. Limited efficacy of methysergide in cluster headache. A clinical experience. *Cephalalgia* 1989;9[Suppl 10]:404–405.

53. Krabbe A. Early clinical experience with subcutaneous GR43175 in acute cluster headache attacks. *Cephalalgia* 1989;9[Suppl 10]: 406–407.

54. Kripke DF, Judd LL, Hubbard B, Janowsky DS, Huey LY. The effect of lithium carbonate on the circadian rhythm of sleep in normal human subjects. *Biol Psychol* 1979;14:545–548.

55. Kudrow L. Lithium prophylaxis for chronic cluster headache. *Headache* 1977;17:15–56.

56. Kudrow L. *Cluster headache. Mechanisms and management.* Oxford: Oxford University Press, 1980.

57. Kudrow L. Response of cluster headache attacks to oxygen inhalation. *Headache* 1981;21:1–4.

58. Kudrow L, Kudrow DB. Association of sustained oxyhemoglobin desaturation of onset of cluster headache attacks. *Headache* 1990;30: 474–480.

59. Kunkle EC, Pfeiffer JB Jr, Wilhoit WM, Hamrick LW Jr. Recurrent brief headaches in cluster pattern. *Trans Am Neurol Assoc* 1952;77: 240–243.

60. Leone M, Attanasio A, Grazzi L, et al. Transdermal clonidine in the prophylaxis of episodic cluster headache: an open study. *Headache* 1997;37:559–560.

61. Leone M, Bussone G. A review of hormonal findings in cluster headache. Evidence for hypothalamic involvement. *Cephalalgia* 1993;13:309–317.

62. Leone M, D Amico D, Moschiano F, Fraschini F, Bussone G. Melatonin versus placebo in the prophylaxis of cluster headache: a double-blind pilot study with parallel groups. *Cephalalgia* 1996;16: 494–496.

63. Leone M, Zappacosta BM, Valentini S, Colangelo AM, Bussone G. The insulin tolerance test and the ovine corticotrophin-releasing hormone test in episodic cluster headache. *Cephalalgia* 1991;11: 269–274.

64. Lipton RB, Micieli G, Russell D, Solomon S, Tfelt-Hansen P, Waldenlind E. Guidelines for controlled trials of drugs in cluster headache. *Cephalalgia* 1995;15:452–462.

65. Lovely TJ, Kotsiakis X, Jannetta PJ. The surgical management of chronic cluster headache. *Headache* 1998; 38:590–594.

66. Manzoni GC, Bono G, Lanfranchi M, Micieli G, Terzano MG, Nappi G. Lithium carbonate in cluster headache: assessment of its short- and long-term therapeutic efficacy. *Cephalalgia* 1983;3:109–114.

67. Marks DR, Rapoport A, Padla D, et al. A double-blind placebo-con-

for cluster headache with sumatriptan: findings of a one-year long-term study. *Neurology* 1998;51;908–911.

trolled trial of intranasal capsaicin for cluster headache. *Cephalalgia* 1993;13:114–116.

68. Mathew NT. Clinical subtypes of cluster headache and response to lithium therapy. *Headache* 1978;18:26–30.

69. Mathew NT, Hurt W. Percutaneous radiofrequency trigeminal gangliorhizolysis in intractable cluster headache. *Headache* 1988;28: 328–331.

70. McNamara JO. Drugs effective in the therapy of the epilepsies. In: Hardman JG, Limbord LE, Molinoff PB, Ruddon RW, Gilman AG, eds. *Goodman & Gilman's the pharmacological basis of therapeutics,* 9th ed. New York: McGraw-Hill, 1996:476–477.

71. Meyer JS, Binns PM, Ericsson AD, Vulpe M. Sphenopalatine ganglionectomy for cluster headache. *Arch Otolaryngol* 1970;92:475–484.

72. Meyer JS, Nance M, Walker M, Zetusky WJ, Dowell RE. Migraine and cluster headache treatment with calcium antagonists supports a vascular pathogenesis. *Headache* 1985;25:358–367.

73. Monstad I, Krabbe A, Micieli G, et al. Preemptive oral treatment with sumatriptan during a cluster period. *Headache* 1995;35:607–613.

74. Mueller L, Gallagher RM, Ciervo CA. Methylergonovine maleate as a cluster headache prophylactic: a study and review. *Headache* 1997; 37:437–442.

75. Nilsson-Remahl AIM, Ansjön A, Lind F, Waldenlind E. No prophylactic effect of hyperbaric oxygen during active cluster headache: a double-blind placebo-controlled cross-over study. *Cephalalgia* 1997; 17:456.

76. Ottervanger JP, Paalman HJA, Boxma GL, Stricker BHCH. Transmural myocardial infarction with sumatriptan. *Lancet* 1993;341: 861–862.

77. Peroutka S. The pharmacology of calcium channel antagonists: a novel class of anti-migraine agents? *Headache* 1983;23:278–283.

78. Prusinski A, Kozubski W, Szulc-Kuberska J. Steroid treatment in the interruption of clusters in cluster headache patients. *Cephalalgia* 1987; 7[Suppl 6]:332–333.

79. Raskin HH. *Headache*, 2nd ed. New York: Churchill Livingstone, 1988.

80. Sachs E Jr. Further observations on surgery of the nervus intermedius. *Headache* 1969;9:159–161.

81. Sanders M, Zuurmond WWA. Efficacy of sphenopalatine ganglion blockade in 66 patients suffering from cluster headache: a 12- to 70-month follow-up evaluation. *J Neurosurg* 1997;87:876–880.

82. Schiller F. Prophylactic and other treatment for "histaminic," "cluster," or "limited" variant of migraine. *JAMA* 1960;173:1907–1911.

83. Schimmer BP, Parker KL. Adrenocorticotropic hormone; adrenocortical steroids and their synthetic analogs. In: Hardman JG, Limbird LE, Molinoff PB, Ruddon RW, Gilman AG, eds. *Goodman & Gilman's the pharmacological basis of therapeutics*, 9th ed. New York: McGraw-Hill, 1996:1465–1475.

84. Sicuteri F, Franchi G, Del Bianco PL. An antaminic drug, BC 105, in the prophylaxis of migraine. *Int Arch Allergy* 1967;31:78–93.

85. Sicuteri F, Fusco BM, Marabini S, et al. Beneficial effect of capsaicin application to the nasal mucosa in cluster headache. *Clin J Pain* 1988; 5:49–53.

86. Speed WG III. Ergotamine tartrate inhalation: a new approach to the management of recurrent vascular headaches. *Am J Med Sci* 1960; 240:327–331.

87. Speight TM, Avery GS. Pizotifen (BC-105); a review of its pharmacological properties and its therapeutic efficacy in vascular headaches. *Drugs* 1972;3:159–203.

88. Steiner TJ, Hering R, Couturier EGM, Davis PTG, Whitmarsh TE. Double-blind placebo-controlled trial of lithium in episodic cluster headache. *Cephalalgia* 1997;17:673–675.

89. Stirparo G, Fusco BM, Giacovazzo M, Rinaldi C, Martelletti P. Is the unresponsiveness to sumatriptan in cluster headache related to an alteration in the 5-HT receptors? *Int J Clin Pharm Res* 1993;13: 247–253.

90. The Sumatriptan Cluster Headache Study Group. Treatment of acute cluster headache with sumatriptan. *N Engl J Med* 1991;325:322–326.

91. Symonds C. A particular variety of headache. *Brain* 1956;79: 217–232.

92. Taha JM, Tew JM. Long-term results of radiofrequency rhizotomy in the treatment of cluster headache. *Headache* 1995;35:193–196.

93. Tehindrazanarivelo A, Lutz G, Massiou H, Bousser M-G. Sumatriptan in chronic cluster headache: a long term follow up. *Cephalalgia* 1993; 13[Suppl 13]:205.

94. Tfelt-Hansen P, Bredberg U, Eyjolfsdottir GS, Paalzow L, Tfelt-Hansen V. Kinetics of methysergide and its main metabolite, methylergometrine, in man. *Cephalalgia* 1985;5[Suppl 3]:54–55.

95. Vincent MB. Lithium inhibits substance P and vasoactive intestinal peptide-induced relaxations on isolated porcine ophthalmic artery. *Headache* 1992;32:335–339.

96. Waltz TA, Dalessio DJ, Ott KH, Copeland B, Abbott G. Trigeminal cistern glycerol injections for facial pain. *Headache* 1985;25: 354–357.

97. Watson CP, Morley CP, Richardson JC, Schutz H, Tasker RR. The surgical treatment of chronic cluster headache. *Headache* 1983;23: 289–295.

98. Wilkinson M, Pfaffenrath V, Schoenen J, Diener H-C, Steiner TJ. Migraine and cluster headache—their management with sumatriptan: a critical review of the current clinical experience. *Cephalalgia* 1995; 15:337–357.

99. Willett F, Curzen N, Adams J, Armitage M. Coronary vasospasm induced by subcutaneous sumatriptan. *Br Med J* 1992;304:1415.

100. Zhao JM, Schaanning J, Sjaastad O. Cluster headache: the effect of low oxygen saturation. *Headache* 1990;30:656–659.

The Headaches, Second Edition,
edited by J. Olesen, P. Tfelt-Hansen, and K.M.A. Welch.
Lippincott Williams & Wilkins, Philadelphia © 2000.

Tension-Type Headache, Cluster Headache, and Miscellaneous Primary Headaches

CHAPTER 99

Chronic Paroxysmal Hemicrania

David Russell and Maurice Vincent

DEFINITION OF CHRONIC PAROXYSMAL HEMICRANIA

IHS code and diagnosis: 3.2 Chronic paroxysmal hemicrania

WHO code and diagnosis: G44.03 Chronic paroxysmal hemicrania

Short description: Attacks with largely the same characteristics of pain, associated symptoms and signs as cluster headache, but they are shorter lasting, more frequent, occur mostly in females, and respond absolutely to indomethacin (22).

Other terms: Sjaastad syndrome

EPIDEMIOLOGY

Prevalence

Chronic paroxysmal hemicrania (CPH) is a rare syndrome, but the number of diagnosed cases is increasing steadily. Many cases still may be overlooked. There are reports regarding several cases throughout the world among different races and in different countries (4,26,57), including Norway, Czechoslovakia, Denmark, Italy, France, Mexico, the United Kingdom, Canada, Sweden, Australia, Germany, Poland, India, Spain, Brazil, South Africa, and New Zealand. The number of cases diagnosed is probably much higher because all new cases are no longer being published. The prevalence of CPH is

not known, but the relative frequency compared with cluster headache is reported to be approximately 1% to 3% (4). Prevalences estimated in cluster headache vary from 0.09% to 0.7% of the population (12,52).

Sex Distribution

Chronic paroxysmal hemicrania was originally considered to be a disease of women. However, cases in men have been reported in increasing numbers (40,42). By 1979 there was a female:male ratio of 7:1. Among the 84 patients reviewed in 1989, the sex distribution was 59 females (70%) and 25 males (30%), a female:male ratio of 2.36:1 (4,63). It is therefore possible that future observations may reduce the female predominance in CPH.

Age of Onset

Chronic paroxysmal hemicrania usually begins in adulthood, with a mean age of onset of 34 years (4,62). However, it may begin at any age. The youngest patient described was 6 years old and the oldest (4,28). In the reviewed material from 1989, the mean age at diagnosis was 47 years and the mean illness duration 13 years. As far as the different stages are concerned, the nonchronic, remitting form of CPH seems to occur earlier (mean age of onset 27 years) than does the unremitting form (mean age of onset 37 years) (4).

GENETICS

There is no positive family history of CPH. Parents or siblings do not have an increased incidence of cluster headache or migraine compared with the general population (4,26).

D. Russell: Department of Neurology, The National Hospital University of Oslo, N-0027 Oslo, Norway.

M. Vincent: Department of Neurology, Faculdade de Medicina, Universidade Federale do Rio de Janeiro, and Headache Sector, Servico de Neurologia, Hospital Universitário Clementino Fraga Filho, Rio de Janeiro, RJ 21949-590, Brazil.

PATHOGENESIS

The pathogenesis of CPH is unknown. Important features must, however, be taken into consideration, such as (a) the unilaterality and pain intensity, (b) ocular findings, (c) autonomic symptoms and signs, and (d) the absolute indomethacin effect.

ANATOMY AND PATHOLOGY

The pain in CPH is strictly unilateral. However, the autonomic involvement and ocular signs may be bilateral, but more pronounced on the symptomatic side. The bilateral ocular signs would seem to exclude the existence of a single lesion in the peripheral nervous system. A possibility is that they are due to one lesion in the central nervous system if the latter involves midline structures (e.g., hypothalamus, cavernous sinus) (36,55).

The pain is CPH cannot be explained by a disturbance in the autonomic nervous system alone. This is based on the observations that autonomic signs may precede the development of pain in precipitated attacks and that pharmacologic suppression of autonomic signs does not influence the pain pattern during attacks (58). Besides, the clinical picture does not fit with any classic sympathetic or parasympathetic syndrome.

PATHOPHYSIOLOGY

The pathophysiologic mechanisms responsible for the pain in CPH remain unknown. It has been suggested that the ipsilateral distribution of trigeminal fibers in the trigeminovascular system may explain the unilaterality of the pain (32), and evidence of trigeminoparasympathetic activation during a CPH attack has emerged (18).

The ocular findings in CPH patients have been studied in detail using dynamic tonometry (23,64). Normally there are pulse synchronous changes in intraocular pressure (IOP), which depend on the volume of the pulsatile part of ocular blood flow (24). The pulse synchronous changes in IOP are reflected by the corneal indentation pulse (CIP) amplitudes, which are measured in micrometers using dynamic tonometry (23). The corresponding changes in intraocular volume in cubic milliliters can be calculated using conversion tables. In CPH there is a significant attack-related increase in CIP amplitudes, ocular blood flow, and IOP that is bilateral but more pronounced on the symptomatic side (44,64) (Fig. 1). The attack-related increase in IOP cannot be solely explained by changes in aqueous humor dynamics because the increased volume exceeds turnover of aqueous humor and the IOP changes occur so rapidly (<30 seconds). These findings are probably the result of an acute vasodilatation, which increases intraocular volume due to a neurogenic impulse and vasoactive neuropeptide release (51,57).

Because changes in IOP and CIP may indicate local abnormal hemodynamics, spontaneous CPH attacks were

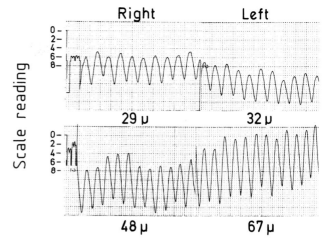

FIG. 1. Dynamic tonometry results obtained just prior to **(upper)** and during **(lower)** a typical headache attack. A marked attack-induced increment in corneal indentation pulse amplitudes from 32 to 67 µm on the symptomatic (i.e., left) side may be seen. Reproduced from Russell et al. (44).

studied using transcranial Doppler ultrasonography (50). During attack, there was hyperventilation, reduction of the end-tidal P_{CO_2}, and decrease in blood flow velocity in all insonated arteries, in both symptomatic and nonsymptomatic sides. In the anterior cerebral artery, the reduction was significantly smaller on the symptomatic side. There was no major difference between patients and controls regarding reduction of flow during hypocapnia, indicating that there is a normal vascular reactivity in CPH.

Corneal temperature has been found to be increased on the symptomatic side during attacks, a finding that also may be due to increased ocular blood flow following vasodilatation (14,57).

Evidence regarding the pathogenesis of CPH is mostly limited to study of the autonomic nervous system. In this respect there are coexisting autonomic phenomena of both sympathetic and parasympathetic origin (i.e., sweating and lacrimation). The abruptness with which the accompanying signs occur in mechanically precipitated attacks suggests that they may be mediated by a neurogenic impulse. This would involve neuropeptide-containing perivascular axons of the trigeminovascular system with its connection to the cavernous sinus plexus and brainstem (32). The release of vasoactive peptides from sensory fibers, which are running in close relationship to other autonomic fibers, also may lead to miosis, increased IOP, and other autonomic disturbances observed in CPH (5,57). Levels of calcitonin gene–related peptide, which is released from trigeminal fibers, and vasoactive intestinal peptide [VIP], a parasympathetic peptide, have been found to be abnormally high during a CPH attack (18). Values returned to basal levels following indomethacin treatment. This is similar to the peptides' profiles found in cluster headache (17), suggesting that this disorder and CPH may share some pathophysiologic mechanisms. It is possible that the clinical picture in CPH results from the interaction between neurotransmitters and neuromodulators released from sympathetic, parasympathetic, and sensory fibers at the frontal area and local autonomic and vascular mediators.

The ocular vascular findings (increased IOP, conjunctival injection) also may be explained by autonomic changes (i.e., a vasodilatation caused by a decreased sympathetic activity). The situation seems to be more intricate because experiments show that the IOP increase is inhibited by an alpha-blocking agent (thymoxamine) as well as stellate ganglion blockade (58). This observation together with increased sweating and decreased salivation on the symptomatic side during CPH attacks may signify sympathetic stimulation (47,48). The sweat anomaly observed in some patients (66,69) suggests a direct sympathetic stimulation rather than a supersensitivity reaction, which has been found in cluster headache (52,54). Increased tearing, nasal secretion, and miosis, on the other hand, may be due to a parasympathetic stimulation during attacks (47,51,58).

Heart rate and electrocardiographic changes during attacks show no typical pattern and differ therefore from those observed during cluster headache attacks (46). However, there is a tendency toward marked variations in heart rate in association with attacks of CPH (Fig. 2). Attack-related heart rhythm disturbances have been observed in a few patients: bradycardia and sinoatrial block, bundle branch block with episodes of atrial fibrillation, multiple extrasystoles, and bradycardia (Fig. 3) (38,46,63). These findings may indicate a dysfunction in the central control of the autonomic nervous system during CPH attacks, which affects both sympathetic and parasympathetic systems.

Pain pressure threshold (PPT), nociceptive flexion reflex (RIII), corneal reflex, and blink reflex have been studied in few CPH cases (3). The PPT and the subjective pain perception following sural nerve stimulation were reduced in CPH, and so was the RIII reflex threshold on the symptomatic side as compared with controls. Blink reflexes were normal, and the corneal reflex thresholds were found to be reduced bilaterally, irrespective of indomethacin intake. Interestingly, the RIII threshold was not affected by indomethacin, but the subjective pain perception was significantly more asymmetric in CPH on this drug than in controls.

The Indomethacin Effect

The mechanism behind the absolute indomethacin effect and the reason why equipotent cyclooxygenase inhibitors are not as effective remain unknown. It does not seem to be due to its effect on prostaglandin synthesis because other NSAIDs with an even more potent antiprostaglandin effect have little or no effect in CPH (64). Both indomethacin and acetylsalicylic acid block neurogenic inflammation (10).

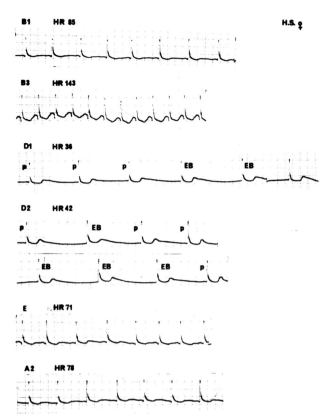

FIG. 2. Patient with normal sinus rhythm *(B1)* that changed into sinus tachycardia with a heart rate of 143 beats/min and showed ST-T changes *(B3)*. During the attack *(D1, D2)* the patient developed bradycardia and sinoatrial block with nodal escape beats *(EB)*. At the end *(E)* and after the attack *(A2)*, the heart rhythm was normalized *(sinus rhythm)*. HR, heart rate. Reproduced from Russell et al. (46).

Indomethacin reduces cerebral blood flow (76), but its effect on peptide-induced vasodilatation on isolated ophthalmic arteries is not different from that induced by other nonsteroidal antiinflammatory drugs. It is possible that indomethacin effects on vessels occur via a non–prostaglandin-related phenomenon (16,41). It is still not known how and at which level indomethacin works. The effect would seem to be symptomatic rather than curative because symptoms recur after the discontinuation of the drug.

The mechanism behind precipitation of attacks may be due to reflex mechanisms involving connections between the trigeminovascular system and brainstem. However, local pathologic findings in the neck structures have not been found.

In conclusion, the pathologic mechanisms behind the CPH syndrome are incompletely understood. However, based on the available information, the occurrence of both unilateral and bilateral symptoms may suggest a primary central triggering mechanism and a secondary involvement of peripheral factors, probably mediated by neurogenic impulses.

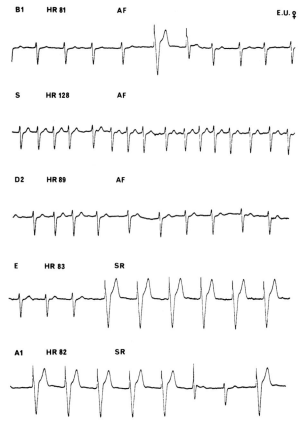

FIG. 3. Patient with atrial fibrillation *(AF)* before *(B1)*, at the start *(S)*, and during *(D2)* an attack that changed into regular sinus rhythm *(SR)* with bundle branch block at the end *(E)* and after *(A1)* the attack. HR, heart rate. Reproduced from Russell et al. (46).

CLINICAL FEATURES

IHS diagnostic criteria for chronic paroxysmal hemicrania (Headache Classification committee, 1988 (22)):

A. At least 50 attacks fulfilling B–E
B. Attack frequency above 5 per day for more than half of the time (periods with lower frequency may occur)
C. Attack frequency above 5 a day for more than half of the time (periods with lower frequency may occur).
D. Pain is associated with at least one of the following signs/symptoms on the symptomatic side:

  1. Conjunctival injection
  2. Lacrimation
  3. Nasal congestion
  4. Rhinorrhea
  5. Ptosis
  6. Eyelid edema

E. Absolute effectiveness of indomethacin (150 mg/day or less).
F. At least one of the following:

  1. History, physical, and neurologic examinations do not suggest one of the disorders listed in groups

5–11, that is, organic headaches, headaches associated with drug withdrawal, metabolic disorders, and so forth.
  2. History and/or physical and/or neurologic examination do suggest such a disorder, but it is ruled out by appropriate investigations.
  3. Such a disorder is present, but CPH does not occur for the first time in close relation to the disorder.

Pain

The pain is unilateral and always affects the same side. However, a few exceptions have been reported, including one possible bilateral case, a possible side shift from the nonchronic to the chronic stage, a case in which the pain was felt slightly beyond the midline at its maximum, and a case with primary side-locked attacks that started to occur nonsimultaneously on the contralateral side (21, 28,39,64). The pain is usually most severe in the oculotemporal area, the forehead, and above or behind the ear, and it may spread to involve the ipsilateral shoulder, arm, and neck. The intensity of the pain has been described as "excruciating" during severe attacks and it has a "clawlike," throbbing, boring, or pulsating character. Between attacks patients usually sit quietly or they may "curl up in bed" (62,64,73), which contrasts with the usually increased patient activity during attacks of cluster headache.

Frequency and Duration of Attacks

In CPH attacks occur every day with a high maximum attack frequency. This usually exceeds 15 per 24 hours and may range from 2 to more than 30 per 24-hour period (62). Attacks usually last between 2 and 25 minutes, occasionally up to 46 to 60 minutes (7,43,57). In a prospective study of 105 attacks, we found a mean attack duration of 13 minutes (range 3–46) and a mean attack frequency of 14 per 24 hours (range 4–38). In mild attacks the frequency ranged from 4 to 8, and in severe attacks the mean was 22 with a range of 13 to 38 per 24 hours (43). In a retrospective study consisting of 84 patients, the mean duration of attacks was 21 minutes, with a range of 2 to 120 minutes and a mean attack frequency of 11 per 24 hours (range 2–40). The minimum attack frequency was 8 (range 2–14) and the maximum 15 (range 6–40) (4). There may occasionally be short-lasting attacks of less than 1 minute duration associated with CPH due to the so-called jabs-and-jolts syndrome described by Sjaastad (62).

Nocturnal Attacks

Attacks occur regularly throughout the 24-hour period without a preponderance of attacks at night as in cluster headache (52,62,64). In our study (43), where 105 attacks were exactly timed, about one third of the attacks occurred during sleep (32 attacks occurred between midnight and 8 A.M., whereas 33 began between 8 A.M. and 4 P.M., 40 attacks between 4 P.M. and midnight) (Fig. 4). Nocturnal attacks in association with rapid eye movement (REM) phase sleep also have been described (27).

Trigger Mechanisms

In some patients (approximately 10%) attacks may be precipitated mechanically, either by bending or by rotating the head (4,68). Attacks also may be provoked by external pressure against the transverse process of C4–C5, C2 root, or the greater occipital nerve (67). The onset of an attack usually occurs within a few seconds (range 5–60). and they may be precipitated in succession without refractory periods (58,67,68). The attack pattern of provoked attacks seems to be similar to that of spontaneous attacks and shows different inter- and intraindividual clinical expressions (47,48). This is probably dependent on the severity of symptoms at this time. Attacks are more easily precipitated during periods with severe symptoms (58,67,68).

Hormonal Factors

The probable female predominance of CPH suggests that the female hormonal cycle may be of importance. In several patients with CPH, attacks have disappeared or improved during pregnancy and then returned after delivery (37,62,73). In others, the onset of symptoms occurred immediately after delivery (62). Menstruation may have a positive or negative influence on attacks (4,62). Birth control pills do not seem to influence attack frequency. We do not at present have sufficient information regarding the effects of menopause (57). Female preponderance, however, also occurs in other headache disorders. Therefore, from the pathophysiologic point of view, this should be regarded as nonspecific.

Previous Medical History

The previous medical history of CPH is usually unremarkable. Although head or neck trauma is reported by approximately 20% of patients (4), these findings do not differ significantly from those for cluster headache or migraine (29,57).

Clinical Signs and Symptoms

The majority of patients (62%) have lacrimation from the eye on the symptomatic side during attacks. This may be observed bilaterally but is more pronounced on the side with the pain. Conjunctival injection on the symptomatic side is another frequent sign accompanying attacks (36%), as are ipsilateral nasal congestion (42%) and rhinorrhea (36%) (Table 1) (4,57,62–64). Occasionally there is eyelid edema on the symptomatic side during attacks. This may explain the clinical impression of ptosis observed by some patients (33%) (4,57). Slight ipsilateral miosis may be present during attacks in some cases (14,38,63). In one patient who had typical CPH attacks, autonomic phenomena also occurred on the usually symptomatic side, but with mild (10%) or no pain (36). This indicates that pain and autonomic phenomena may be partially independent. It is emphasized, however, that there is no definite evidence of latent or attack-related Horner-like syndrome, as described for cluster headache (11,12,51,54). Photophobia may accompany attacks, but gastrointestinal symptoms are extremely unusual (63). Increased forehead sweating is observed in a few patients, especially on the symptomatic side. Generalized sweating also has been reported (66,69).

The modified cluster pattern has been used to describe the temporal pattern of attack frequency in CPH because it bears some resemblance to that in cluster headache (62,63). There is considerable intraindividual variation between mild and severe periods, with a varying attack frequency from 2 to more than 30 per 24 hours. These periods last from several weeks to months, and the transition from a period with severe symptoms to a period with mild symptoms usually takes place over several days (Fig. 5) (62). It is important to recognize the sometimes extremely slight headaches that may be present during milder periods in those patients with chronic symptoms. On the other hand,

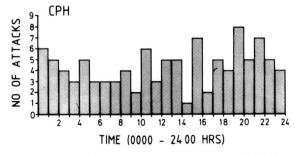

FIG. 4. The 24-hour distribution of attacks in CPH. Reproduced from Russell (43).

TABLE 1. *Accompanying symptoms during attacks of CPH*

Symptom	Incidence (%)
Lacrimation	62
Nasal stenosis	42
Conjunctival injection	36
Rhinorrhea	36

Data from ref. 1.

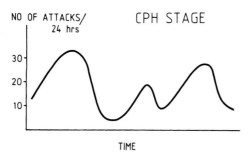

FIG. 5. Constant transition between periods with severe symptoms (more frequent attacks) and milder symptoms (fewer attacks). Reproduced from Joubert et al. (26).

during severe periods patients may feel a "constant headache" because of the high attack frequency and sometimes persisting tenderness in the symptomatic area between attacks (62,63). It is therefore very important to establish the presence of well-defined but extremely frequent attacks.

Supplementary Investigation

Neuroimaging is usually normal in CPH patients. Magnetic resonance (MR) scans were performed in six patients, and no abnormality was found (1). However, MR should be part of the routine examination of such individuals because secondary cases may occur. Reports include patients with infarcts, arteriovenous malformation (33), a frontal lobe tumor (although indomethacin was not used in this case, the clinical picture could resemble CPH), and a collagen vascular disorder (31). One patient with a gangliocytoma growing from within the sella turcica was also reported (75). It is noteworthy that this patient, with relatively short attacks, was treated with indomethacin only after surgery, when the pain recurred. In another case, an MR scan showed a meningioma originating in the roof of the cavernous sinus on the symptomatic side (72). This patient had unremitting CPH, sometimes requiring indomethacin at high doses, up to 350 mg per day, which could be reduced after surgery. Indomethacin requirements also were reduced after a herniated disk producing a C7 root compression was surgically removed (72). It is possible that patients who need comparatively high indomethacin doses should preferably undergo an MR investigation.

Orbital phlebography may be abnormal in some patients, either uni- or bilaterally (1,20), but the interpretation of such findings is still questionable in terms of sensitivity and specificity. Electroencephalography, brain mapping, and skull radiography should not be required for typical CPH patients.

Stages

CPH may be present in a nonchronic or a chronic form, the latter being four times more common than the former

(4,56). Sjaastad coined the term "chronic paroxysmal hemicrania" based on the first two patients, who had lasting, daily (hence chronic), solitary, limited attacks (hence paroxysmal) of strictly unilateral headache that did not shift sides (hence hemicrania) (64). It later became clear that before the development of chronic symptoms, many of the patients (42%) had passed through a nonchronic stage with headache attacks separated by intervals with complete remission (4,30,62,73) (Fig. 6). These attacks, also abolished by indomethacin, are similar but may be less severe and less frequent than attacks in the chronic stage (62). The term "pre-CPH stage" was chosen assuming that all cases would develop chronic symptoms. However, approximately 20% of patients appear to remain nonchronic for longer periods, up to 34 years (6). Sjaastad followed a case with indomethacin response in both stages from the remitting to the unremitting form (60). The nonchronic stage may therefore represent a subgroup entity. In terms of the different stages it would be appropriate, as suggested by Sjaastad, to divide CPH into an (a) unremitting (chronic) form, either unremitting from onset or evolved from the remitting form, and (b) remitting form (56,60).

Differential Diagnosis

Cluster headache is the most important differential diagnosis for CPH (51,57). The differentiation has considerable therapeutic consequences because CPH can be completely abolished by indomethacin therapy. Both headaches are unilateral with extremely severe attacks of pain, mainly in the ocular area. The attacks are accompanied by ipsilateral autonomic symptoms. However, CPH differs from cluster headache in several important respects (Table 2). In CPH there is no male preponderance as in cluster headache (52). CPH has a higher maximum attack frequency (usually >15 per 24 hours), and they are shorter lasting (2–25 minutes) compared with cluster headache, which has an attack frequency of 1 to 4 (maximum 8) per 24 hours (7,45,52,62). Each attack usually lasts 15 to 60 minutes. Finally, the absolute response to indomethacin characteristic of CPH is not seen in cluster headache. It may sometimes be difficult to distinguish

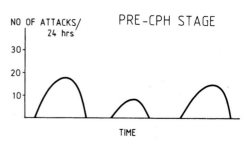

FIG. 6. Patterns of headache attacks before onset of the chronic stage of CPH. Reproduced from Russell et al. (45).

TABLE 2. *Differential diagnostic criteria of CPH and cluster headache (CH)*

Criterion	CPH	CH
Sex distribution	male:female = 1:2	male:female = 8:1
Attack frequency	4 to greater than 30/24 h	1 to 8/24 h
Attack duration	2–25 min	15–60 min
Therapy	Indomethacin, effect absolute	Usually no effect of indomethacin

between CPH and chronic cluster headache. The gender of the patient, as well as the frequency and duration of attacks and the temporal pattern, may help in this respect.

Concomitant CPH and cluster headache features were reported in two patients (74), including the response to specific treatments. The crucial factor in the differential diagnosis is the absolute response to indomethacin. Associations of CPH with trigeminal neuralgia (CPH-tic syndrome) (19) and migraine (34) also have been reported.

Hemicrania continua is a disorder described by Sjaastad characterized by unilateral indomethacin-responsive hemicrania (71). The pain is comparatively mild, lasts for longer time or may be continuous, and the autonomic phenomena, if present, are less intense. Similar to CPH, a noncontinuous form may rarely occur (8). In SUNCT (the acronym for *s*hortlasting, *u*nilateral, *n*euralgiform headache attacks with *c*onjunctival injection, *t*earing, and subclinical forehead sweating), the pain, usually in the frontal and periocular area, is much shorter. There is a male preponderance, and the indomethacin effect is absent (65,70).

PROGNOSIS

When the chronic stage of CPH is reached, the therapy may be lifelong but with a decreased indomethacin requirement. Long-lasting remission periods may reflect a nonchronic stage but are also present in established chronic CPH. There is one report on recurrence of attacks after a drug-free period of 1.5 years in a chronic case (59). This suggests that indomethacin has a symptomatic effect but does not modify the underlying pathologic mechanism

MANAGEMENT

The treatment of CPH is prophylactic. Indomethacin, the drug of choice, has an absolute effect on the symptoms. When a relatively high attack frequency is present in a unilateral headache (i.e., >4 attacks per 24 hours), a drug trial should be considered according to Sjaastad (53). The trial dosage should be increased to at least 150 mg per 24 hours for 3 to 4 days. The beneficial effect is seen within 48 hours (a few hours to 5 days). Six of 11 CPH patients became pain free within 7 hours after indomethacin, and in only one was the time before relief

longer than 24 hours (35). The maintenance dosage is usually 25 to 100 mg/day but may vary inter- and intraindividually between 12.5 and 300 mg/day, depending on the fluctuation in attack severity (51). On discontinuation, symptoms usually reappear within 12 hours to a few days (1 to 14 days) (62). However, long-lasting remission periods up to years have been described (25,30,58). Indomethacin requirements usually vary with time, and many patients find that the minimum effective dose varies from one moment to the next.

In about 10% of the cases, an indomethacin side effect may be expected (4). The potentially most serious side effect of indomethacin is dyspepsia and the development of a bleeding peptic ulcer. In order to prevent these side effects, antacids or H_2 blockers should be considered when indomethacin is being given over longer periods. Nausea, vomiting, vertigo, and purpura also have been reported during indomethacin use (4,9,62). Suppositories of indomethacin may help if gastric intolerance is a major problem, or when the dose eventually needs to be increased up to higher doses, such as 300 mg/day.

Other Drugs

No drug tested so far has an effect as good as indomethacin, if any. There are reports of partial effects with verapamil (15) and acetylsalicylic acid, especially in the early stages of CPH (49,63,64). Two of six CPH patients obtained complete relief with piroxicam beta-cyclodextrin, and one had a moderate effect (61). Because CPH attacks are relatively short, testing the effect of acute drugs may be particularly difficult. However, except for some reports (15,21), sumatriptan and oxygen are considered noneffective (13). Prophylactic drugs should be tested preferably in nonremitting cases because an eventual "response" may correspond to the natural fluctuation of the disease. Anecdotal reports on the efficacy of various drugs may be related to unobservance of this fact. Lithium, carbamazepine, and other anticonvulsants are ineffective. Anesthetic blockades of the greater occipital nerve, supraorbital nerve, and minor occipital nerve are ineffective (2).

Surgical and Nonpharmacologic Treatment

There is no evidence of efficacy of surgical treatment, chiropractic manipulation, or acupuncture (4,57).

REFERENCES

1. Antonaci F. Chronic paroxysmal hemicrania and hemicrania continua: orbital phlebography and MRI studies. *Headache* 1994;34:32–34.
2. Antonaci F, Pareja JA, Caminero AB, Sjaastad O. Chronic paroxysmal hemicrania and hemicrania continua: anaesthetic blockades of pericranial nerves. *Funct Neurol* 1997;12:11–15.
3. Antonaci F, Sandrini G, Danilov A, Sand T. Neurophysiological studies in chronic paroxysmal hemicrania and hemicrania continua. *Headache* 1994;34:479–483.

4. Antonaci F, Sjaastad O. Chronic paroxysmal hemicrania (CPH): a review of the clinical manifestations. *Headache* 1989;29:648–656.
5. Bill A, Stjernschantz J, Mandahl A, Brodin E, Nilsson G. Substance P: release on trigeminal nerve stimulation, effects in the eye. *Acta Physiol Scand* 1979;106:371–373.
6. Blau JN, Engel H. Episodic paroxysmal hemicrania: a further case and review of the literature. *J Neurol Neurosurg Psychiatry* 1990;53:343–344.
7. Bogucki A, Szymanska R, Braciak W. Chronic paroxysmal hemicrania: lack of pre-chronic stage. *Cephalalgia* 1984;4:187–189.
8. Bordini C, Antonaci F, Stovner LJ, Schrader H, Sjaastad O. "Hemicrania continua": a clinical review. *Headache* 1991;31:20–26.
9. Brant T, Paulus W, Pollmann W. Clusterkopfschmerz und chronisch paroxysmale Hemikranie: aktuelle Therapie. *Nervenarzt* 1991;62:329–339.
10. Buzzi MG, Sakas DE, Moskowitz MA. Indomethacin and acetylsalicylic acid block neurogenic plasma protein extravasation in rat dura mater. *Eur J Pharmacol* 1989;165:251–258.
11. Carvalho DS, Salvesen R, Sand T, Smith SE, Sjaastad O. Chronic paroxysmal hemicrania. 13. The pupillometric pattern. *Cephalalgia* 1988;8:219–229.
12. D'Allessandro R, Gamberini G, Benassi G, Morganti G, Cortelli P, Lugaresi E. Cluster headache in the republic of San Marino. *Cephalalgia* 1986;6:159–162.
13. Dahlöf C. Subcutaneous sumatriptan does not abort attacks of chronic paroxysmal hemicrania (CPH). *Headache* 1993;33:201–202.
14. Drummond PD. Thermographic and pupillary asymmetry in chronic paroxysmal hemicrania. *Cephalalgia* 1985;5:133–136.
15. Evers S, Husstedt IW. Alternatives in drug treatment of chronic paroxysmal hemicrania. *Headache* 1996;36:429–432.
16. Feigen LP, King LW, Beckett W, Kadowitz PJ. Differential effects of ibuprofen and indomethacin in the regional circulation of the dog. *J Pharmacol Exp Ther* 1981;219:679–684.
17. Goadsby PJ, Edvinsson L. Human *in vivo* evidence for trigeminovascular activation in cluster headache. Neuropeptide changes and effects of acute attacks therapies. *Brain* 1994;117:427–434.
18. Goadsby PJ, Edvinsson L. Neuropeptide changes in a case of chronic paroxysmal hemicrania—evidence for trigemino-parasympathetic activation. *Cephalalgia* 1996;16:448–450.
19. Hannerz J. Trigeminal neuralgia with chronic paroxysmal hemicrania: the CPH-tic syndrome. *Cephalalgia* 1993;13:361–364.
20. Hannerz J, Ericson K, Bergstrand G. Chronic paroxysmal hemicrania: orbital phlebography and steroid treatment. A case report. *Cephalalgia* 1987;7:189–192.
21. Hannerz J, Jogestrand T. Intracranial hypertension and sumatriptan efficacy in a case of chronic paroxysmal hemicrania which became bilateral (the mechanism of indomethacin in CPH). *Headache* 1993;33:320–323.
22. Headache Classification Committee of the International Headache Society. Classification and diagnostic criteria for headache disorders, cranial neuralgias and facial pain. *Cephalalgia* 1988;8[Suppl 7]:1–96.
23. Horven I. Dynamic tonometry. 2. Methods of corneal indentation pulse registration. *Acta Ophthalmol* 1970;48:23–38.
24. Horven I, Russell D, Sjaastad O. Ocular blood flow changes in cluster headache and chronic paroxysmal hemicrania. *Headache* 1989;29:373–376.
25. Jensen NB, Joensen P, Jensen J. Chronic paroxysmal hemicrania: continued remission of symptoms after discontinuation of indomethacin. *Cephalalgia* 1982;2:163–164.
26. Joubert J, Powell D, Djikowski J. Chronic paroxysmal hemicrania in a South African black. A case report. *Cephalalgia* 1987;193:196.
27. Kayed K, Godtlibsen OB, Sjaastad O. Chronic paroxysmal hemicrania. 4. "REM sleep locked" nocturnal headache attacks. *Sleep* 1978;1:91–95.
28. Kudrow DB, Kudrow L. Successful aspirin prophylaxis in a child with chronic paroxysmal hemicrania. *Headache* 1989;29:280–281.
29. Kudrow L. *Cluster headache: mechanisms and management.* New York: Oxford University Press, 1980.
30. Kudrow L, Esperança P, Vijayan N. Episodic paroxysmal hemicrania? *Cephalalgia* 1987;7:197–201
31. Medina JL. Organic headaches mimicking chronic paroxysmal hemicrania. *Headache* 1992;32:73–74.
32. Moskowitz MA. Basic mechanisms in vascular headache. *Neurol Clin* 1990;8:801–815.
33. Newman LC, Herskovitz S, Lipton RB, Solomon S. Chronic paroxysmal headache: two cases ith cerebrosvascular disease. *Headache* 1992;32:75–76.
34. Pareja J. Chronic paroxysmal hemicrania coexisting with migraine.

35. Pareja J, Sjaastad O. Chronic paroxysmal hemicrania and hemicrania continua. Interval between indomethacin administration and response. *Headache* 1996;36:20–23.
36. Pareja JA. Chronic paroxysmal hemicrania: dissociation of the pain and autonomic features. *Headache* 1995;35:111–113.
37. Pelz M, Merskey H. A case of pre-chronic paroxysmal hemicrania. *Cephalalgia* 1982;2:47–50.
38. Petty RG, Clifford Rose F. Chronic paroxysmal hemicrania: first reported British case. *Br Med J* 1983;286:438.
39. Pollmann W, Pfaffenrath V. Chronic paroxysmal hemicrania: the first possible bilateral case. *Cephalalgia* 1986;6:55–57.
40. Price RW, Posner JB. Chronic paroxysmal hemicrania: a disabling headache syndrome responding to indomethacin. *Ann Neurol* 1978;3:183–184.
41. Quintana A, Raczaka E, Giralt MT, Quintana MA. Effects of aspirin and indomethacin on cerebral circulation in the conscious rat: evidence for a physiological role of endogenous prostaglandins. *Prostaglandins* 1983;25:549–556.
42. Rapoport AM, Sheftell FD, Baskin SM. Chronic paroxysmal hemicrania: case report of the second known definite occurrence in a male. *Cephalalgia* 1981;1:67–69.
43. Russell D. Chronic paroxysmal hemicrania: severity, duration and time of occurrence of attacks. *Cephalalgia* 1984;4:53–56.
44. Russell D, Christoffersen B, Horven I. Chronic paroxysmal hemicrania: a case report. *Headache* 1978;18:99–100.
45. Russell D, Sjaastad O. Chronic paroxysmal hemicrania. In: Pfaffenrath V, Sjaastad O, Lundberg PO, eds. *Updating in headache.* Berlin: Springer-Verlag, 1984:1–6.
46. Russell D, Storstein L. Chronic paroxysmal hemicrania: heart rate changes and ECG recordings. A computerized analysis of 24 ambulatory ECG recordings. *Cephalalgia* 1984;4:135–144.
47. Saunte C. Chronic paroxysmal hemicrania: salivation, tearing and nasal secretion. *Cephalalgia* 1984;4:25–32.
48. Saunte C, Russell D, Sjaastad O. Chronic paroxysmal hemicrania. 9. On the mechanism of attack-related sweating. *Cephalalgia* 1983;3:191–199.
49. Schlake HP, Bottger IG, Grotemeyer KH. Single photon emission computed tomography with technetium-99m hexamethyl propylennamino oxime in the pain-free interval of migraine and cluster headache. *Eur Neurol* 1990;30:153–156.
50. Shen JM. Transcranial doppler sonography in chronic paroxysmal hemicrania. *Headache* 1993;33:493–496.
51. Sjaastad O. Chronic paroxysmal hemicrania. In: Vinken PJ, Bruyn GW, Klawans HL, Clifford Rose F, eds. *Handbook of clinical neurology.* Volume 48: Headache. Amsterdam: Elsevier, 1986:257–266.
52. Sjaastad O. Cluster headache. In: Vinken PJ, Bruyn GW, Klawans HL, Clifford Rose F, eds. *Handbook of clinical neurology.* Volume 48: Headache. Amsterdam: Elsevier, 1986:217–246.
53. Sjaastad O. Chronic paroxysmal hemicrania: recent developments. *Cephalalgia* 1987;7:179–188.
54. Sjaastad O. Cluster headache and its variants. *Headache* 1988;28:667–668.
55. Sjaastad O. Cluster headache: the possible significance of midline structures. *Cephalalgia* 1988;8:229–236.
56. Sjaastad O. Chronic paroxysmal hemicrania (CPH): nomenclature as far as the various stages are concerned. *Cephalalgia* 1989;9:1–2.
57. Sjaastad O. Chronic paroxysmal hemicrania. In: Sjaastad O, ed. *Cluster headache syndrome.* London: WB Saunders, 1992:291–392.
58. Sjaastad O, Aasly J, Fredriksen T, Wysocka Bakowska MM. Chronic paroxysmal hemicrania. 10. On the autonomic involvement. *Cephalalgia* 1986;6:113–124.
59. Sjaastad O, Antonaci F. Chronic paroxysmal hemicrania: a case report. Long-lasting remission in the chronic stage. *Cephalalgia* 1987;7:203–205.
60. Sjaastad O, Antonaci F. Chronic paroxysmal hemicrania (CPH) and hemicrania continua: transition from one stage to another. *Headache* 1993;33:551–554.
61. Sjaastad O, Antonaci F. A piroxicam derivative partly effective in chronic paroxysmal hemicrania and hemicrania continua. *Headache* 1995;35:549–550.
62. Sjaastad O, Apfelbaum R, Caskey W, et al. Chronic paroxysmal hemicrania (CPH): the clinical manifestations—a review. *Uppsala J Med Sci* 1980;[Suppl 31]:27–33.

63. Sjaastad O, Dale I. Evidence for a new (?) treatable headache entity. *Headache* 1974;14:105–108.

64. Sjaastad O, Dale I. A new (?) clinical headache entity "chronic paroxysmal hemicrania" 2. *Acta Neurol Scand* 1976;54:140–159.

65. Sjaastad O, Kruszewski P. Trigeminal neuralgia and "SUNCT" syndrome: similarities and differences in the clinical pictures. An overview. *Funct Neurol* 1992;7:103–107.

66. Sjaastad O, Russell D, Saunte C. Chronic paroxysmal hemicrania. 8. The sweating pattern. *Cephalalgia* 1983;3:45–52.

67. Sjaastad O, Russell D, Saunte C, Hørven I. Chronic paroxysmal hemicrania. 6. Precipitation of attacks. Further studies on the precipitation mechanisms. *Cephalalgia* 1982;2:211–214.

68. Sjaastad O, Saunte C, Graham JR. Chronic paroxysmal hemicrania. 7. Mechanical precipitation of attacks: new cases and localization of trigger points. *Cephalalgia* 1984;4:113–118.

69. Sjaastad O, Saunte C, Russell D, Hestness A, Mårvik R. Cluster headache. The sweating pattern during spontaneous attacks. *Cephalalgia* 1981;1:233–244.

70. Sjaastad O, Saunte C, Salvesen R, et al. Shortlasting, unilateral neuralgiform headache attacks with conjunctival injection, tearing, sweating, and rhinorrhea. *Cephalalgia* 1989;9:147–156.

71. Sjaastad O, Spierings ELH. "Hemicrania continua": another headache absolutely responsive to indomethacin. *Cephalalgia* 1984;4:65–70.

72. Sjaastad O, Stovner LJ, Stolt Nielsen A, Antonaci F, Fredriksen TA. CPH and hemicrania continua: requirements of high indomethacin dosages—an ominous sign? *Headache* 1995;35:363–367.

73. Stein HJ, Rogado AZ. Chronic paroxysmal hemicrania: two new patients. *Headache* 1980;20:72–76.

74. Tehindrazanarivelo AD, Visy JM, Bousser MG. Ipsilateral cluster headache and chronic paroxysmal hemicrania: two case reports. *Cephalalgia* 1992;12:318–320.

75. Vijayan N. Symptomatic chronic paroxysmal hemicrania. *Cephalalgia* 1992;12:111–113.

76. Wennmalm A, Carlsson A, Edlund S, Erikson L, Kaijser L, Nowak J. Central and peripheral haemodynamic effects of non-steroidal anti-inflammatory drugs in man. *Arch Toxicol* 1984;[Suppl 7]:350–359.

The Headaches, Second Edition,
edited by J. Olesen, P. Tfelt-Hansen, and K.M.A. Welch.
Lippincott Williams & Wilkins, Philadelphia © 2000.

Tension-Type Headache, Cluster Headache, and Miscellaneous Primary Headaches

CHAPTER 100

Miscellaneous Headaches Unassociated with a Structural Lesion

James W. Lance and Peter J. Goadsby

The syndromes described in this chapter are benign in the sense that no structural lesion can be held responsible and the prognosis is favorable. Because of the association of similar symptoms with the presence of space-occupying intracranial lesions, aneurysms, or cerebral atherosclerosis in some instances, clinical judgment is required to determine the extent of investigation required for each individual. Rasmussen (75) assessed the lifetime prevalence of headache in 1,000 people between the ages of 25 and 64 years. Idiopathic stabbing headache was reported by 2%, external compression headache by 4%, and cold stimulus headache by 15%. Hangover headache had been experienced by 72%, fever headache by 63%, and benign cough headache, benign sexual headache, and headaches associated with sexual activity each by 1%.

IDIOPATHIC STABBING HEADACHE

Definition of Idiopathic Stabbing Headache

IHS code and diagnosis: 4.1 Idiopathic stabbing headache

WHO code and diagnosis: G44.800 Idiopathic stabbing headache

Other terms: icepick-like pains (74), "jabs and jolts" syndrome (82), and ophthalmodynia (37)

J. W. Lance: Department of Neurology, University of New South Wales, and Institute of Neurological Sciences, Prince of Wales Hospital, Sydney, New South Wales 2031, Australia.

P. J. Goadsby: The National Hospital for Neurology and Neurosurgery, London WC1N 3BG, United Kingdom.

Short description: Transient stabs of pain in the head that occur spontaneously in the absence of organic disease or underlying structures or of the cranial nerves

Pathophysiology

Although the mechanism of these transient pains is unknown, the lancinating quality of the pain resembles that of trigeminal neuralgia and suggests a paroxysmal neuronal discharge. The localization of stabbing pains to the habitual site of migraine or cluster headache may be a pointer to the pathophysiology of these conditions. Although it is possible that there is a source of irritation in the peripheral branches of the trigeminal or other nerves, it would seem more likely that there is an intermittent deficit in central pain control mechanisms that permits the spontaneous synchronous discharge of neurons receiving impulses from the area to which stabbing pain is referred.

Clinical Features

Diagnostic criteria of idiopathic stabbing headache (27):

A. Pain is confined to the head and exclusively or predominantly felt in the distribution of the first division of the trigeminal nerve (orbit, temple, and parietal area).

B. Pain is stabbing in nature and lasting for a fraction of a second; occurs as single stabs or series of stabs.

C. It recurs at irregular intervals (hours to days).

D. Diagnosis depends on the exclusion of structural changes at the site of pain and in the distribution of the affected cranial nerve.

Icepick-Like Pains

Raskin and Schwartz (74) described sharp, jabbing pains about the head resembling a stab from an icepick, nail, or needle. They compared the prevalence of such pains in 100 migrainous patients (20 men, 80 women) and 100 headache-free controls (53 men, 47 women). Only three of the control subjects had experienced icepick pains compared with 42 of the migraine patients, of whom 60% had more than one attack per month. The pains affected the temple or orbit more often than the parietal and occipital areas and often occurred before or during migraine headaches. Drummond and Lance (19) obtained a history of icepick pains in 200 of 530 patients with recurrent headache (migraine and tension headache). The sites of the icepick pains were recorded for 92 patients and coincided with the site of the patients' habitual headache in 37 (19 unilateral and 18 bilateral). This was most apparent when the icepick pains were restricted to one eye or temple.

Icepick pains also have been described in conjunction with cluster headaches, experienced in the same area as the cluster pain. Three of 60 patients studied by Lance and Anthony (34) and 11 of 33 patients examined by Ekbom (20) described icepick pains during the cluster headache attack, becoming more frequent as the attack abated. Similar lancinating pains have been reported with temporal arteritis (74), but we have not encountered this. Pareja and colleagues (62) studied 38 patients diagnosed over a 1-year period. The mean age at onset was 47 years and the female:male ratio was 6:1. The frequency varied from 1 attack per year to 50 episodes daily. Indomethacin 75 mg daily gave partial relief in the 17 patients for whom it was prescribed, thereby distinguishing the condition from jabs and jolts mentioned in the title of their article.

There have been some reports at variance with the IHS definition cited above. Soriani and colleagues (88) reported 83 juvenile patients whose stabbing pains lasted as long as a few minutes in some instances, usually not associated with other types of headache. Dangond and Spierings (12) commented that the duration of stabbing headache was several seconds in four of their patients, rather than a fraction of a second. The site of pain need not necessarily be limited to the distribution of the trigeminal nerve because Martins and colleagues (45) reported six patients whose pains affected the retroauricular and occipital region yet responded promptly to indomethacin.

Jabs and Jolts Syndrome

Sjaastad (82) first referred to sharp pains associated with chronic paroxysmal hemicrania (CPH) in 1979. He describes jabs and jolts as sharp, knifelike pains, less than 1 minute in duration, occurring in patients with tension headache, migraine, or cluster headache as well as in headache-free individuals. It is probable that these sensations are a variation on icepick pains but last longer and must be distinguished from episodes of CPH, which have a minimal duration of 3 minutes. Confusion with the SUNCT syndrome (short-lasting unilateral neuralgiform headache with conjunctival injection and tearing, discussed later in this chapter) is more likely. SUNCT syndrome does not respond to indomethacin, a clinical feature it shares with jabs and jolts. Medina and Diamond (49) reported multiple jabbing pains with episodic headaches that they regarded as a cluster variant.

Ophthalmodynia

Sudden stabbing pain in the eye has been described as *ophthalmodynia periodica*. Lansche (37) reported that over 60% of patients with this syndrome were migraine sufferers.

Management of Idiopathic Stabbing Headache

Mathew (48) reported that five patients with this syndrome improved substantially while being treated with indomethacin 50 mg three times daily and did not respond to aspirin or placebo. Medina and Diamond (49) found that 20 patients who were subject to frequent jabbing pains (unilateral in 13 cases) in association with atypical vascular headaches responded well to indomethacin, whereas Sjaastad (82) stated that the response of jabs and jolts to indomethacin was partial or lacking.

EXTERNAL COMPRESSION HEADACHE

Definition of External Compression Headache

IHS code and diagnosis: 4.2 External compression headache

WHO code and diagnosis: G44.801 External compression headache

Other terms: Swim-goggle headache (69)

Short description: Headache resulting from continued stimulation of cutaneous nerves by the application of pressure, for example, by a band around the head, a tight hat, or goggles worn for the protection of eyes during swimming

Pathophysiology

The mechanism responsible is compression of branches of trigeminal or occipital nerves.

Clinical Features

Diagnostic criteria for external compression headache (27):

A. Results from application of external pressure to the forehead or the scalp
B. Is felt in the area subjected to pressure
C. Is a constant pain
D. Is prevented by avoiding the precipitating cause
E. Is not associated with organic cranial or intracranial disease

Management: Avoiding the stimulus.

COLD STIMULUS HEADACHE

Definition of Cold Stimulus Headache

IHS code and diagnosis: 4.3 Cold stimulus headache
WHO code and diagnosis: G44.802 Cold stimulus headache
Short description: Headache resulting from the exposure of the head to low temperatures

External Application of a Cold Stimulus

IHS code and diagnosis: 4.3.1 External application of a cold stimulus
WHO code and diagnosis: G44.802 Cold stimulus headache
Short description: Generalized headache following exposure of the unprotected head to a low environmental temperature as in subzero weather or in diving into cold water

Pathophysiology

Exposure of the bare head to subzero temperatures or diving into cold water will cause headache, presumably from excessive stimulation of temperature-sensitive receptors in the face and scalp. Pain induced by dipping the top of the head into cold water reaches a peak in 60 seconds and spreads from the vertex to the temples and occiput (97).

Clinical Features

Diagnostic criteria for external application of a cold stimulus:

A. Developing during external exposure to cold
B. Is bilateral
C. Varying in intensity with the severity and duration of the cold stimulus
D. Is prevented by avoiding exposure to cold
E. Is not associated with organic cranial or intracranial disease.

Management: Avoiding exposure of the head to cold.

Ingestion of a Cold Stimulus

IHS code and diagnosis: 4.3.2 Ingestion of a cold stimulus

WHO code and diagnosis: G44.82 Cold stimulus headache
Previously used term: Ice cream headache
Short description: Ice cream headache is a pain produced in susceptible individuals by the passage of cold material, solid or liquid, over the palate and posterior pharyngeal wall.

Pathophysiology

Wolff (96) found that applying ice to the palate referred pain to the frontal region and that cooling the posterior pharynx caused pain behind the ears. Odell-Smith (55) reported on his own sensations. Discomfort in the temples appeared 20 to 30 seconds after the application of ice and ceased 10 to 20 seconds after the stimulus was removed. He attributed the pain to local vasoconstriction. A direct effect on cold receptors in the oropharynx would seem to be a more likely explanation, although Mumford (52) demonstrated a decrease in forehead temperature of 1°C during ice cream headache. The fact that ice cream headache is more common in migrainous patients and is often referred to the part of the head afflicted by the patient's customary headache suggests that there may be a segmental disinhibition of central pain pathways in migrainous patients responsible for undue susceptibility of an afferent volley of impulses from the excitation of cold receptors in the oropharynx.

Clinical Features

Diagnostic criteria of ingestion of a cold stimulus (27):

A. Developing during ingestion of a cold food or drink
B. Lasting for less than 5 minutes
C. Is felt in the middle of the forehead, except in people subject to migraine, in which case the pain may be referred to the area habitually affected by migraine headache
D. Is prevented by avoiding rapid swallowing of cold food or drinks
E. Is not associated with organic disease

In 1850, Drake (18) commented on the possible injurious effects of eating ice cream: "First, swallowing it before the ice has dissolved in the mouth, when it sometimes raises an acute pain in the pharynx, and gives a sense of coldness and sinking in the stomach; second, eating it when the stomach is torpid and inactive from dyspepsia, and the individual is inclined, at the time, to sick headache."

Holding ice or ice cream in the mouth or swallowing a cold food or drink as a bolus may cause discomfort in the palate and throat. It also may refer pain to the forehead or temple by the trigeminal nerve and to the ears by the glossopharyngeal nerve. Raskin and Knittle (73)

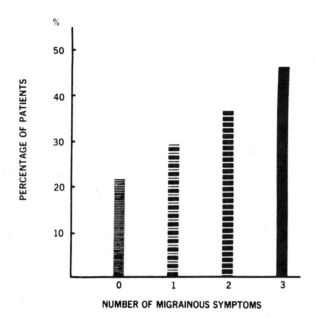

FIG. 1. Prevalence of ice cream headache in 530 headache patients grouped according to the number of migrainous characteristics (unilateral headache, focal neurologic symptoms, and gastrointestinal disturbance) experienced by each. It can be seen that the prevalence increases progressively from 20% in tension-type headache (no migrainous symptoms) to almost 50% in typical migraine headache (all three groups of migrainous symptoms). Reproduced from Drummond and Lance (19).

found that 15 of 49 subjects not normally prone to headache had experienced infrequent, mild ice cream headache at some time in their lives. In contrast, 50 of 55 migraineurs were subject to such headaches, which were frequent and severe in 46. Most patients felt the pain in the midfrontal region, but eight referred it to the occiput. Drummond and Lance (19) reported that 189 (36.7%) of 530 patients attending a headache clinic had experienced ice cream headache. The prevalence of such headaches increased in direct proportion to the number of migrainous symptoms associated with the patient's customary headache (Fig. 1). Although the headache was usually midline or bilateral, the pain was localized to one side of the head for 18 of the 90 patients in whom the site had been documented. In 13 of these 18, and in 17 of the 72 patients with bilateral headache, the site of the ice cream headache coincided with the area habitually affected by their headache.

Management: Caution in ingesting cold substances is the only sensible management.

BENIGN COUGH HEADACHE

IHS code and diagnosis: 4.4 Benign cough headache
WHO code and diagnosis: G44.803 Benign cough headache
Short description: Headache precipitated by coughing in the absence of any intracranial disorder

Pathyphysiology

Williams (94) recorded cerebrospinal fluid (CSF) pressures from the cisterna magna and lumbar region during coughing. He found that there was a phase in which lumbar pressure exceeded cisternal pressure, followed by a phase in which the pressure gradient was reversed. He postulated that cough headache may be caused by a valvelike blockage at the foramen magnum, which interferes with the downward or rebound pulsation. Williams (95) followed up this observation by studying two patients with cough headache whose cerebellar tonsils descended below the foramen magnum without any obvious obstruction and confirmed a severe craniospinal pressure dissociation during the rebound after a Valsalva maneuver. Decompression of the cerebellar tonsils relieved the headache and eliminated the steep pressure gradient upon coughing. Williams (95) commented that coughing increased intrathoracic and intraabdominal pressure, which was transmitted to the epidural veins, causing a pressure wave and CSF to move rostrally. The headache was presumably caused by temporary impaction of the cerebellar tonsils when the subject relaxed and the pressure gradient then reversed. Whether this explanation applies to those patients without an Arnold-Chiari type 1 malformation remains uncertain. The possibility of a sudden increase in venous pressure being sufficient by itself to cause headache must be considered. Lance (33) reported the case of a man with a goiter sufficiently large to cause sudden headache when his arms were elevated and the jugular veins distended. Calendre et al. (10) suggested the term "benign Valsalva's maneuver-related headache" to cover headaches provoked by coughing, straining, or stooping, but "cough headache" is more succinct and unlikely to be displaced.

Clinical Features

Diagnostic criteria of benign cough headache (27):

A. Is a bilateral headache of sudden onset, lasting less than 1 minute, precipitated by coughing
B. May be prevented by avoiding coughing
C. May be diagnosed only after structural lesions such as posterior fossa tumor have been excluded by neuroimaging

The presence of an Arnold-Chiari malformation or any lesion causing obstruction of CSF pathways or displacing cerebral structures must be excluded before cough headache is assumed to be benign. Cerebral aneurysm (87), carotid stenosis (8,76), and vertebrobasilar disease (89) also may present with cough or exertional headache as the initial symptom.

Sharp pain in the head upon coughing, sneezing, straining, laughing, or stooping has long been regarded as a symptom of organic intracranial disease, commonly associated with obstruction of the CSF pathways.

Symonds (91) presented the case histories of six patients in whom cough headache was a symptom of a space-occupying lesion in the posterior fossa or of basilar impression from Paget's disease. He then described 21 patients with the same symptom in whom no intracranial disease became apparent. Cough headache disappeared in nine patients and improved spontaneously in another six patients. Two patients died of heart disease, and four were lost to follow-up. Symonds (91) concluded that there was a syndrome of benign cough headache, which he attributed to the stretching of a pain-producing structure in the posterior fossa, possibly the result of an adhesive arachnoiditis. Of Symonds' 21 patients, 18 were men, and ages ranged from 37 to 77 years, with an average age of 55 years (91).

Ekbom (21) cited an earlier description in the French literature by Tinel from 1932 concerning four patients whose headaches were brought on by coughing, nose blowing, breath holding, and bending the head forward. He also quoted observations by Nick concerning 15 patients, 12 of whom were men, ranging in age from 19 to 73 years.

Rooke (77) considered cough headache as a variety of exertional headache and recorded his experiences with 103 patients who experienced transient headaches upon running, bending, coughing, sneezing, lifting, or straining at stool in whom no intracranial disease could be detected and who were followed for 3 years or more. During the follow-up period, reinvestigation discovered structural lesions such as Arnold-Chiari malformations, platybasia, subdural hematoma, and cerebral or cerebellar tumor in 10 patients. Of the remaining 93, 30 were free of headache within 5 years, and 73 were improved or free of headache after 10 years. This type of headache was found more often in men than in women, at a ratio of 4:1. Rooke observed that this form of headache may appear for the first time after a respiratory infection with cough and that some patients reported an abrupt recovery after the extraction of abscessed teeth, which had also been noted by Symonds (91). We prefer to maintain the separation between benign cough headache and benign exertional headache (which is more common in a younger age group), although there is obvious overlap between the two. This view is supported by Pascual and colleagues (65), who reported that the average age of their patients with benign cough headache was 43 years older than their patients with exertional headache.

Management

Mathew (48) reported two patients with benign cough headache (one of whom had proved unresponsive to ergotamine, propranolol, and methysergide) who improved with indomethacin 50 mg three times daily. When this therapy was compared with placebo, the reduction in cough headache with the active drug was 95% in one case

and 85% in the other, whereas the reductions on placebo medication were 0% and 18%, respectively. One patient who had particularly severe cough headaches unresponsive to indomethacin responded completely to the intravenous injection of dihydroergotamine (26), but this has not been our experience. Raskin (72) has reported that some patients with cough headache are relieved by lumbar puncture, which is a simple option when compared with prolonged use of indomethacin. The mechanism of this response remains unclear.

BENIGN EXERTIONAL HEADACHE

IHS code and diagnosis: 4.5 Benign exertional headache
WHO code and diagnosis: G44.804 Benign exertional headache
Short description: Headache precipitated by any form of exercise. Subvarieties, such as weightlifter's headache (66), are recognized.

Pathophysiology

The acute onset of headache with straining and breath holding, as in weightlifter's headache, is most likely explained by acute venous distension, similar to the patient with thoracic outlet obstruction from goiter mentioned above (33). The development of headache after sustained exertion, particularly on a hot day, is more likely to be caused by arterial dilatation, but objective evidence is lacking. Anginal pain may be referred to the head, probably by central connections of vagal afferents and may present as exertional vascular headache (25,36,39,92). Frontal hypoperfusion was demonstrated by single photon emission computed tomography (SPECT) in a boy with benign exertional vascular headache by Basoglu and colleagues (6), but the significance of this is uncertain.

Clinical Features

Diagnostic criteria of benign exertional headache (27):

A. Is specifically brought on by physical exercise
B. Is bilateral and throbbing in nature at onset and may develop migrainous features in those patients susceptible to migraine
C. Lasting from 5 minutes to 24 hours
D. Is prevented by avoiding excessive exertion, particularly in hot weather or at high altitude
E. Is not associated with any systemic or intracranial disorder

Pheochromocytoma occasionally may be responsible for exertional headache (68). Intracranial lesions or stenosis of the carotid arteries may have to be excluded, as discussed for benign cough headache. Headache may be precipitated by any form of exercise and often has the pulsatile quality of migraine. Credit must be given to

Hippocrates (2) for first recognizing this syndrome when he wrote, "one should be able to recognize those who have headache from gymnastic exercises, or walking, or running, or any other unseasonable labor, or from immoderate venery."

Dalessio (11) drew attention to this form of headache in an editorial in which he cited running, rowing, tennis, and wrestling as possible causes and mentioned that heat, high humidity, lack of training, and performance at high altitudes (such as the Olympic games in Mexico City) were contributing factors. Massey (46) presented three cases of headaches resembling migraine, one with visual disturbance and mild hemiparesis, precipitated by running short or long distances. Sudden severe headache also can be precipitated by swimming (28) and weightlifting (66). Paulson (66) considered strain or stretch of cervical ligaments as a possible cause of weightlifter's headache, but the sudden onset and persisting sensitivity to coughing, sneezing, and straining suggest acute venous distension as a possible mechanism.

Walk headache is a rare variant. The problem of one patient with this symptom was explained by Vernay et al. (92) as an ischemic phenomenon because it disappeared after a few minutes of rest and returned after the patient walked for another 1 to 2 minutes. In this 71-year-old man, the onset of headache was associated with depression of ST segments in the electrocardiogram (ECG) and was relieved by vasodilator drugs. A number of papers have documented exertional vascular headaches as the presenting symptom of cardiac ischemia (25,36,39).

Management

The most logical form of treatment is to take exercise gradually and progressively whenever possible. Lambert and Burnet (31) described how a prescribed warm-up period prevented swimmer's headache. Diamond and Medina (16) reported that 9 of 11 patients were relieved of exertional headache with the administration of indomethacin over a follow-up period of 3 to 18 months. A similar successful outcome with indomethacin 50 mg three times daily (with an antacid) was recorded by Mathew (48). Diamond (15) described 15 patients 8 to 54 years of age with exertional headaches lasting for an average of 4 hours. Indomethacin at daily doses varying from 25 to 150 mg controlled the headache almost completely in 13 patients. We have found that ergotamine tartrate 1 to 2 mg orally, ergotamine by inhalation, and methysergide 1 to 2 mg orally given 30 minutes before exercise are useful prophylactic measures.

HEADACHE ASSOCIATED WITH SEXUAL ACTIVITY

IHS code and diagnosis: 4.6 Headache associated with sexual activity

WHO code and diagnosis: G44.805 Headache associated with sexual activity

Other terms: benign sex headache, coital cephalalgia

Short description: Headache precipitated by masturbation or coitus, usually starting as a dull bilateral ache while sexual excitement increases and suddenly becoming intense at orgasm, in the absence of any intracranial disorder

Pathophysiology

There are three kinds of headache associated with sexual activity. The first is a dull headache, commonly bilateral and occipital in location, that comes on as sexual excitement mounts (IHS classification 4.6.1). It is probably related to excessive contraction of head and neck muscles because it can be prevented or relieved by deliberate relaxation of these muscle groups. The second type of headache, more severe and explosive in onset, appeared immediately before or at the moment of orgasm (IHS classification 4.6.2), presumably caused by the severe increase in blood pressure at this time. A third type, which we have not encountered, was described by Paulson and Klawans (67) in 3 of their 14 patients with headache arising during coitus. This form of headache (IHS classification 4.6.3) was worse on standing up and thus resembles the low-pressure headache following lumbar puncture, leading them to postulate that a dural leak may have developed during enthusiastic sexual intercourse.

Muscle contraction appears to be a major feature in the milder headache that becomes more severe as sexual excitement increases. Of 21 patients (32), 10 stated that they were subject to headache at times of emotional tension unrelated to sexual activity. The tension headache was similar to but milder than the headache as experienced with intercourse in several patients. Five patients stated that they were aware of excessive muscle contraction, particularly involving the jaw and neck muscles, and found that they could reduce the intensity of the headache by deliberately relaxing those muscles while continuing with intercourse or masturbation. The headache seemed to be related to the degree of sexual excitement and not to physical exertion. If patients with such muscle contraction headache continued to orgasm, the headache usually became very intense and persisted for up to 48 hours afterward. Masters and Johnson (47) have commented on the excessive contraction of facial, jaw, and neck muscles as sexual excitement mounts.

The vascular aspect of sex headaches may be superimposed on the tension-type headache or may occur without warning at orgasm. It is abrupt in onset, occipital or generalized, frequently throbbing, and sometimes associated with palpitations, resembling the headache of pheochromocytoma (35). Masters and Johnson (47) observed that blood pressure increased by 40 to 100 mm Hg systolic and 20 to 50 mm Hg diastolic during orgasm, comparable with the paroxysms caused by pheochromocytoma. Littler et al. (40) recorded similar increases of up to 214/135 mm Hg. One of our patients experienced a headache, comparable in severity with her sex headache, after taking a tablet of the sympathomimetic drug pseudoephedrine (32), supporting the concept that a sudden increase in blood pressure at orgasm may be responsible for the explosive nature of these headache. An interesting example of a pressor response causing coital cephalgia was provided by Staunton and Moore (90). A patient with obstruction of the lower aorta who presented with this problem developed a blood pressure of 250/130 mm Hg after 3 minutes of exercise on a bicycle ergometer. After successful aortic-iliac bypass, his coital headache disappeared.

Multiple areas of cerebral arterial spasm were found in a 30-year-old man after a coital headache that exertion had exacerbated (81). Similar areas of segmental cerebral artery constriction were demonstrated angiographically in a 55-year-old woman 10 days after the onset of a headache with orgasm (30), but the relationship of these structural changes to the headache is dubious in that some of the narrowed areas were still present 8 months later. If cerebral arterial spasm is a feature of the explosive orgasmic headache, it is not surprising that strokes result on some occasions. It may be concluded that an acute pressor response with or without preexisting hypertension and arterial disease is responsible for the thunder-clap headache that may occur at the moment of orgasm.

Clinical Features

Diagnostic criteria of headache associated with sexual activity (27):

A. Is precipitated by sexual excitement
B. Is bilateral at onset
C. Is prevented or eased by ceasing sexual activity before orgasm
D. Is not associated with any intracranial disorder such as an aneurysm

4.6.1 Dull type
Diagnostic criteria: a dull ache in the head and neck that intensifies as sexual excitement increases.
4.6.2 Explosive type
Diagnostic criteria: a sudden severe (explosive) headache occurring at orgasm.
4.6.3 Postural type
Diagnostic criteria: postural headache resembling that of low CSF pressure developing after coitus

Hippocrates (2) included immoderate venery, defined by the Oxford English Dictionary as "the practice or pursuit of sexual pleasure or indulgence of sexual desire," as a cause of exertional headache, but this is not necessarily the case because benign sex headache can arise with little or no physical exertion by the participant (32).

Headaches developing at the time of orgasm are not always benign. Subarachnoid hemorrhage was precipitated by sexual intercourse in 3 (4.5%) of 66 cases reported by Fisher (22) and in six (12%) of 50 cases studied by Lundberg and Osterman (41). Cerebral or brainstem infarction has been reported by Lance (32), Levy (38), and Martinez and colleagues (44). One young man developed a brainstem thrombosis (32) and another a left hemisphere infarction (38). Martinez et al. (44) described three patients whose neurologic deficits began at the moment of orgasm. A 50-year-old woman developed confusion and amnesia lasting 3 days with a right Babinski sign for 20 days; a 40-year-old man had a right hemisensory defect for 24 hours, and a 36-year-old man had a left homonymous hemianopia, which cleared over 2 weeks. Cerebral angiography was normal in the first two patients but showed poor filling of the right posterior cerebral artery in the third. Another three cases were described by Nick and Bakouche in 1980 (44).

The recognition that most headaches occurring during sexual activity are not associated with an underlying vascular malformation and have a benign prognosis may be attributed to Wolff (96), but Kriz later reported 25 cases from Czechoslovakia in 1970, cited by Martin (43), who related the histories of five men subject to severe headache toward the end of intercourse, three of whom had a history of migraine. Paulson and Klawans (67) reported 14 patients with this condition as "benign orgasmic cephalgia," but this term does not cover those patients whose headache begins before orgasm.

Sex headache affects men more often than women and may occur at any time during the years of sexual activity. It is capricious in that it may develop on several occasions in succession and then not trouble the patient again, although there is no obvious change in sexual technique. Of 21 patients in our series (32), 16 were men and 5 were women, ranging in age from 18 to 58 years. Three patients experienced headache with masturbation, two of whom also complained of similar headaches during sexual intercourse. The headaches of the remaining patients were confined to sexual intercourse. Those patients who desisted from sexual activity when headache was first noticed found that it subsided within a period of 5 minutes to 2 hours. Those who proceeded to orgasm reported that a severe headache persisted for 3 minutes to 4 hours and a milder headache lingered for 1 to 48 hours afterward (32). Only four of these patients had previously suffered from migraine, and two had experienced exertional headache. Seven were hypertensive. The headaches were more likely to occur when intercourse was attempted for a second time after a brief interval. One young man complained of headache at orgasm while he was on holiday for a month, indulging in sexual intercourse two or three times daily. When the holiday was over and the frequency of intercourse declined to once daily, he remained free of headache. Carotid or vertebral angiography was performed in nine of our patients (32) with this syndrome, yielding completely normal results. As familiarity with the syndrome increased, this investigation can be reserved for those patients in whom there is a suspected underlying lesion and is being replaced by magnetic resonance angiographic techniques.

What is the relationship between sex headaches and physical exertion? Silbert et al. (80) found that 18 of their 45 patients subject to acute vascular headaches during sexual intercourse also had experienced headaches on exertion. Nine patients described a close link between the two sorts of headache, with one following the other within a few days and a dull, generalized headache persisting between the two acute events. During follow-up for an average of 6 years, two fifths of them had recurrences of their sex headaches, usually at times of fatigue or stress. Pascual et al. (65) also found an association between benign sex headaches with exertional but not with cough headache. Ostergaard and Kraft (57) followed 26 patients for up to 14 years. Half of the patients had lost their headaches after periods of 6 weeks to 6 months, but half had recurrences after freedom for up to 6 years. Selwyn (78) reported that, of 32 patients with headache related to coitus who replied to a questionnaire, 11 had experienced similar headache after both exercise and sexual intercourse. Nine of the 32 patients had a history of hypertension and 15 a background of migraine. Among 10 patients whose headaches developed at the time of orgasm, five had previously suffered from migraine. Taking into account all 32 patients, 21 had a history of migraine and 11 of hypertension. Two patients had experienced such headache with masturbation and one after a nocturnal emission following dreaming during sleep.

Johns (29) summarized 110 cases recorded in the literature at that time, 86 male and 24 female. Five had a low CSF pressure syndrome after intercourse, 17 had a muscle contraction type of headache, and the remaining headache had vascular features, with 40 occurring at orgasm. Johns (29) also described four sisters with this syndrome. Headaches of explosive onset may be caused by the ingestion of sympathomimetic drugs or tyramine-containing foods while a patient is taking monoamine oxidase inhibitors and can also be a symptom of pheochromocytoma (35).

This type of headache was called thunderclap headache by Day and Raskin (13), who reported a woman with three such episodes who was found to have an unruptured aneurysm of the internal carotid artery, with adjacent areas of segmental vasospasm. The relationship between thunderclap headache and aneurysm in the absence of computer tomography (CT) scan or CSF evidence of subarachnoid hemorrhage was questioned by Abbott and van Hille (1), who described 14 patients, six of whom underwent normal four-vessel cerebral angiography. Wijdicks and colleagues (93) observed 71 patients whose CT scans and CSF findings were negative for an average of 3.3 years. Twelve patients had additional headaches, and 31 (44%) later had regular episodes of migraine or tension-type headaches. Factors identified as precipitating the headache were sexual intercourse in 3 cases, coughing in 4, and exertion in 12, whereas the remainder had no obvious cause. A history of hypertension was found in 11 patients and a history of previous headache in 22. Markus (42) compared the presentation of 37 patients with subarachnoid hemorrhage and 189 with a similar thunderclap headache but normal CSF examination results and could not discern any characteristic to distinguish the two conditions on clinical grounds.

It may be concluded that the investigations for thunderclap headache unrelated to coitus should include a CT scan and CSF examination but that cerebral angiography is usually unnecessary. When a typical explosive headache occurs at orgasm, particularly if it is preceded by an escalating tension-type headache, investigation could be limited to CT scanning unless other features such as neck stiffness make a CSF examination mandatory.

Management

Benign sex headaches are usually irregular and infrequent in recurrence, so management can often be limited to reassurance and advice about ceasing sexual activity if a milder, warning headache develops. When the condition recurs regularly or frequently, it can be prevented by the administration of propranolol, but the dosage required varies from 40 to 200 mg daily (70). Beta-blockers presumably act by limiting the surge of blood pressure at orgasm. One patient was successfully treated with the calcium channel-blocking agent diltiazem 60 mg three times daily (3). Ergotamine (1–2 mg) or indomethacin (25–50 mg) taken about 30 minutes prior to sexual activity also can be helpful.

OTHER MISCELLANEOUS SYNDROMES NOT YET CLASSIFIED

Hemicrania Continua

IHS code and diagnosis: ? to be added as 4.7.1
Short description: New daily persistent headache that is unilateral and responsive to indomethacin

Pathophysiology

The mechanism is unknown, but associated autonomic features resemble those of cluster headache. Pressure pain threshold is reduced, particularly on the symptomatic side (5).

Clinical Features

In 1984 Sjaastad and Spierings (86) reported two patients, a woman of 63 and a man of 53, who developed unilateral headache without obvious cause. One of these patients noticed redness, lacrimation, and sensitivity to light in the eye on the affected side, and the other also described jabs and jolts. Both patients were relieved slightly by aspirin but completely by indomethacin. Other nonsteroidal antiinflammatory drugs (NSAIDs) were of little or no benefit. Newman et al. (54) reviewed the 24 previously reported cases and added 10 of their own, some with pronounced autonomic features resembling cluster headache. They divided their case histories into remitting and unremitting forms. Of the 34 patients reviewed, 22 were women and 12 men, with the age of onset ranging from 11 to 58 years. Jabs and jolts were experienced by 25 patients, and 19 were subject to nocturnal attacks. The symptoms were controlled by indomethacin 75 to 150 mg daily.

Goadsby and Lipton (23) contrasted the clinical presentation of hemicrania continua with that of chronic and episodic paroxysmal hemicrania, cluster headache, SUNCT syndrome, and hypnic headache under the general heading of trigeminal-autonomic cephalgias. Magnetic resonance imaging has not shown any abnormalities. Silberstein et al. (79) proposed that patients with hemicrania continua be subdivided into those with and without medication overuse. Some reports of so-called hemicrania continua have not been consistent with the original definition in that the headache may have alternated sides, become bilateral, have remitted, and have not responded to indomethacin (56). The case for recognition of hemicrania continua as a distinct entity requires elaboration.

Management

Sjaastad and Antonaci (83) regard responsiveness to indomethacin as being essential for the diagnosis. Antonaci et al. (4) proposed the indotest by which the intramuscular injection of 50 mg of indomethacin could be used as a diagnostic tool. In hemicrania continua, pain was relieved in 73 ± 66 minutes and the pain-free period was 13 ± 8 hours. The time elapsed between the oral administration of 25 to 50 mg three times daily and relief varied from 30 minutes to 48 hours (58). Some patients also may respond to piroxicam and other NSAIDs (83).

Suggested diagnostic criteria for hemicrania continua:

A. Headache present for at least 1 month
B. Unilateral headache
C. Pain has the following qualities
  1. Continuous but fluctuating
  2. Moderate severity
  3. Lack of precipitating mechanisms
D. Headache must have either one of
  1. Complete response to indomethacin
  or
  2. One of the following autonomic features in association with exacerbations of pain:

    a. Conjunctival injection
    b. Lacrimation
    c. Nasal congestion
    d. Rhinorrhea
    e. Ptosis
    f. Eyelid edema

HYPNIC HEADACHE

IHS code and diagnosis: ? to be added as 4.7.2
Short description: a brief nocturnal headache occurring in older patients, awakening them from sleep—pathophysiology unknown

Clinical Features

This syndrome was first described by Raskin (71) in patients 67 to 84 years of age who had headache of a moderately severe nature that typically came on a few hours after going to sleep. These headaches last from 15 to 30 minutes, are typically generalized [although they may be unilateral (24,51)], and can be throbbing (53). Patients may report falling back to sleep only to be awoken by a further attack a few hours later with up to three repetitions of this pattern over the night. In a large series of 19 patients, 16 (84%) were female and the mean age at onset was 61 ± 9 years (17). Headaches were bilateral in two thirds and unilateral in one third and in 80% of cases mild or moderate. Three patients reported similar headaches when falling asleep during the day. None had photophobia or phonophobia (17).

Management

Patients with this form of headache generally respond to a bedtime dose of lithium carbonate (200–600 mg) (53,71); if lithium carbonate is not tolerated, verapamil or methysergide at bedtime may be alternative strategies. Two patients who responded to flunarizine 5 mg at night have now been reported (51). Dodick and colleagues (17) reported that one to two cups of coffee or caffeine 60 mg orally at bedtime was helpful. Other strategies are important because in the age group affected by the condition lithium may have significant side effects.

Suggested Diagnostic Criteria

4.7 Hypnic headache
Diagnostic criteria:

A. Headaches occur at least 15 times per month for at least 1 month
B. Headaches awaken patient from sleep
C. Attack duration of 5 to 60 minutes
D. Pain is bilateral or unilateral
E. Pain **not** associated with autonomic features

A rapid clinical response to lithium at bedtime is usually expected.

SHORT-LASTING UNILATERAL NEURALGIFORM HEADACHE WITH CONJUNCTIVAL INJECTION AND TEARING (SUNCT SYNDROME)

IHS code and diagnosis: ? to be added as 3.3

Short description: This form of headache is among the rarest of headache syndromes and is characterized by frequent paroxysms of short-lasting unilateral eye pain and marked ipsilateral autonomic features.

Pathophysiology

The mechanism is unknown but is presumably related to that of trigeminal neuralgia and cluster headache. It has been discussed with other trigeminal-autonomic cephalgias by Goadsby and Lipton (23).

Clinical Features

The condition was described by Sjaastad et al. (85). The patients are mostly men (63), with a gender ratio of 17:4 (64). The paroxysms of pain usually last between 5 and 250 seconds (61), although longer duller interictal pains have been reported, as have attacks of up to 2 hours in two patients (59). Patients may have up to 30 episodes an hour, although usually they number 5 to 6 per hour. The frequency may also vary in bouts. A systematic study of attack frequency demonstrated a mean of 28 attacks per day with a range of 6 to 77 (59). The conjunctival injection seen with SUNCT syndrome is often the most prominent autonomic feature, and tearing also may be obvious. Other less prominent autonomic stigmata include sweating of the forehead and rhinorrhea. The attacks may become bilateral, but the most severe pain remains unilateral.

Secondary SUNCT Syndrome and Associations

There have been several reported patients with SUNCT syndromes secondary to homolateral cerebellopontine angle and brainstem arteriovenous malformations diagnosed on MRI (9,14). One patient had a cavernous hemangioma of the cerebellopontine angle seen only on MRI (50), so that MRI of the brain should be part of the investigation of this syndrome when it is recognized.

Management

Unlike some of the other short-lasting headache syndromes, such as the paroxysmal hemicranias that are highly responsive to indomethacin, SUNCT syndrome is remarkably refractory to treatment, including indometha-

cin (60). The relationship between trigeminal neuralgia and SUNCT syndrome remains unclear (84). There is a single report of a patient with trigeminal neuralgia who developed a SUNCT syndrome (7), which may have relevance to these questions. Rarely do these patients respond to carbamazepine.

Suggested Diagnostic Criteria

3.3 Short-lasting unilateral neuralgiform headache with conjunctival injection and tearing (SUNCT syndrome)

Comment: This section will replace the current unclassified section which then is renumbered.

Diagnostic criteria:

A. At least 30 attacks fulfilling B–E
B. Attacks of unilateral moderately severe orbital or temporal stabbing or throbbing pain lasting from 15 to 120 seconds
C. Attack frequency from 3 to 100/day
D. Pain is associated with at least one of the following signs or symptoms of the affected side, with feature 1 being present most often and very prominent:
   1. Conjunctival injection
   2. Lacrimation
   3. Nasal congestion
   4. Rhinorrhea
   5. Ptosis
   6. Eyelid edema
E. At least one of the following:
   1. There is no suggestion of one of the disorders listed in groups 5–11.
   2. Such a disorder is suggested but excluded by appropriate investigations.
   3. Such a disorder is present, but the first headache attacks do not occur in close temporal relation to the disorder.

The literature suggests that the most common secondary cause of SUNCT syndrome would be a lesion in the posterior fossa.

REFERENCES

1. Abbott RJ, van Hille P. Thunderclap headache and unruptured cerebral aneurysm. *Lancet* 1986;2:1459.
2. Adams F. *The genuine works of Hippocrates.* London: Sydenham Society, 1848. Baltimore: Williams & Wilkins, 1939, 94.
3. Akpunonu BE, Ahrens J. Sexual headaches: case report, review, and treatment with calcium blocker. *Headache* 1991;31:141–145.
4. Antonaci F, Pareja JA, Caminero AB, Sjaastad O. Chronic paroxysmal hemicrania and hemicrania continua. Parenteral indomethacin: the "Indotest." *Headache* 1998;38:122–128.
5. Antonaci F, Sandrini G, Danilov A, Sand T. Neurophysiological studies in chronic paroxysmal hemicrania and hemicrania continua. *Headache* 1994;34:479–483.
6. Basoglu T, Ozbenli T, Bernay I, et al. Demonstration of frontal hypoperfusion in benign exertional headache by technetium 99m. *J Nucl Med* 1996;37:1172–1174.
7. Bouhassira D, Attal N, Esteve M, Chauvin M. SUNCT syndrome. A

case of transformation from trigeminal neuralgia. *Cephalalgia* 1994; 14:168–170.

8. Britton TC, Guiloff RJ. Carotid artery disease presenting as cough headache. *Lancet* 1988;1:1406–1407.

9. Bussone G, Leone M, Volta GD, Strada L, Gasparotti R. Short-lasting unilateral neuralgiform headache attacks with tearing and conjunctival injection: the first symptomatic case. *Cephalalgia* 1991;11:123–127.

10. Calendre L, Hernandez L-A, Lopez-Valdez E. Benign Valsalva's maneuver–related headache: an MRI study of six cases. *Headache* 1996;36:251–253.

11. Dalessio DJ. Effort migraine [Editorial]. *Headache* 1974;14:53.

12. Dangond F, Spierings ELH. Idiopathic stabbing headaches lasting a few seconds. *Headache* 1993;33:257–258.

13. Day JW, Raskin NH. Thunderclap headache: symptom of unruptured cerebral aneurysm. *Lancet* 1986;2:1247–1248.

14. De Benedittis G. SUNCT syndrome associated with cavernous angioma of the brain stem. *Cephalalgia* 1996;16:503–506.

15. Diamond S. Prolonged benign exertional headache: its clinical characteristics and response to indomethacin. *Headache* 1982;22:96–98.

16. Diamond S, Medina JL. Benign exertional headache: successful treatment with indomethacin. *Headache* 1979;19:249.

17. Dodick DW, Mosek AC, Campbell JK. The hypnic ("alarm clock") headache syndrome. *Cephalalgia* 1998;18:152–156.

18. Drake D. *A systematic treatise, historical, epidemiological and practical, on the principal diseases of the interior valley of North America, as may appear in the Caucasian, African and Indian and Esquimaux varieties of its population.* Cincinnati: WB Smith & Co, 1850.

19. Drummond PD, Lance JW. Neurovascular disturbances in headache patients. *Clin Exp Neurol* 1984;20:93–99.

20. Ekbom K. Some observations on pain in cluster headache. *Headache* 1975;14:219–225.

21. Ekbom K. Cough headache. In: Rose FC, ed. *Headache.* Handbook of clinical neurology, Vol. 4. Amsterdam: Elsevier, 1986:367–371.

22. Fisher CM. Headache in cerebrovascular disease. In: Vinken PJ, Bruyn GW, eds. *Handbook of clinical neurology, Vol. 5.* Amsterdam: Elsevier, 1968:124–126.

23. Goadsby PJ, Lipton RB. A review of paroxysmal hemicranias, SUNCT syndrome and other short-lasting headaches with autonomic features, including new cases. *Brain* 1997;120:193–209.

24. Gould JD, Silberstein SD. Unilateral hypnic headache: a case study. *Neurology* 1997;49:1749–1751.

25. Grace A, Horgan J, Breathnach K, Staunton H. Anginal headache and its basis. *Cephalalgia* 1997;17:195–196.

26. Hazelrigg RL. IV DHE-45 relieves exertional cephalgia. *Headache* 1986;26:52.

27. The Headache Classification Committee of the International Headache Society. Classification and diagnostic criteria for headache disorders, cranial neuralgias and facial pain. *Cephalalgia* 1988;8:1–96.

28. Indo T, Takahashi A. Swimmer's migraine. *Headache* 1990;30: 485–487.

29. Johns DR. Benign sexual headache within a family. *Arch Neurol* 1986; 43:1158–1160.

30. Kapoor R, Kendall BE, Harrison MJG. Persistent segmental cerebral artery constrictions in coital cephalgia. *J Neurol Neurosurg Psychiatry* 1990;53:266–270.

31. Lambert RW, Burnet DL. Prevention of exercise induced migraine by quantitative warm-up. *Headache* 1985;25:317–319.

32. Lance JW. Headaches related to sexual activity. *J Neurol Neurosurg Psychiatry* 1976;39:1226–1230.

33. Lance JW. Solved and unsolved headache problems. *Headache* 1991; 31:439–445.

34. Lance JW, Anthony M. Migrainous neuralgia or cluster headache? *J Neurol Sci* 1971;13:401–414.

35. Lance JW, Hinterberger H. Symptoms of pheochromocytoma, with particular reference to headache, correlated with catecholamine production. *Arch Neurol* 1976;33:281–288.

36. Lance JW, Lambros J. Headache associated with cardiac ischemia. *Headache* 1998;38:315–316.

37. Lansche RK. Ophthalmodynia periodica. *Headache* 1964;4:247–249.

38. Levy RL. Stroke and orgasmic cephalalgia. *Headache* 1981;21:12–13.

39. Lipton RB, Lowenkopf T, Bajwa ZH, et al. Cardiac cephalgia: a treatable form of exertional headache. *Neurology* 1997;49:813–816.

40. Littler WA, Honour AJ, Sleight P. Direct arterial pressure, heart rate and electrocardiogram during human coitus. *J Reprod Fertil* 1974;40: 321–331.

41. Lundberg PO, Osterman PO. The benign and malignant forms of orgasmic cephalgia. *Headache* 1974;14:164–165.

42. Markus HS. A prospective follow-up of thunderclap headache mimicking subarachnoid haemorrhage. *J Neurol Neurosurg Psychiatry* 1991; 54:1117–1125.

43. Martin EA. Severe headache accompanying orgasm. *BMJ* 1973;4:44.

44. Martinez JM, Roig C, Arboix A. Complicated coital cephalgia. Three cases with benign evolution. *Cephalalgia* 1988;8:265–268.

45. Martins IP, Parreira E, Costa I. Extratrigeminal ice-pick status. *Headache* 1995;35:107–110.

46. Massey EW. Effort headache in runners. *Headache* 1982;22:99–100.

47. Masters WH, Johnson VE. *Human sexual response.* Boston: Little, Brown, 1966.

48. Mathew NT. Indomethacin-responsive headache syndromes. *Headache* 1981;21:147–150.

49. Medina JL, Diamond S. Cluster headache variant: spectrum of a new headache syndrome. *Arch Neurol* 1981;38:705–709.

50. Morales F, Mostacero E, Marta J, Sanchez S. Vascular malformation of the cerebellopontine angle associated with SUNCT syndrome. *Cephalalgia* 1994;14:301–302.

51. Morales-Asin F, Mauri JA, Iniguez C, Espada F, Mostacero E. The hypnic headache syndrome: report of three new cases. *Cephalagia* 1998; 18:157–158.

52. Mumford JM. Thermography and ice cream headache. *Acta Thermogr* 1979;4:33–37.

53. Newman LC, Lipton RB, Solomon S. The hypnic headache syndrome: a benign headache disorder of the elderly. *Neurology* 1990;40: 1904–1905.

54. Newman LC, Lipton RB, Solomon S. Hemicrania continua: ten new cases and a review of the literature. *Neurology* 1994;44:2111–2114.

55. Odell-Smith R. Ice cream headache. In: Vinken PJ, Bruyn GW, eds. *Handbook of clinical neurology, Vol. 5.* Amsterdam: Elsevier, 1968: 188–191.

56. Olesen J, Rasmussen BK. The International Headache Society classification of chronic daily or near daily headaches: a critique of the criticism. *Cephalalgia* 1996;16:407–411.

57. Ostergaard JR, Kraft M. Natural course of benign coital headache. *BMJ* 1992;305:1129.

58. Pareja J, Sjaastad O. Chronic paroxysmal hemicrania and hemicrania continua. Interval between indomethacin administration and response. *Headache* 1996;36:20–23.

59. Pareja JA, Joubert J, Sjaastad O. SUNCT syndrome. Atypical temporal patterns. *Headache* 1996;36:108–110.

60. Pareja JA, Kruszewski P, Sjaastad O. SUNCT syndrome: trials of drugs and anesthetic blockades. *Headache* 1995;35:138–142.

61. Pareja JA, Ming JM, Kruszewski P, Caballero V, Pamo M, Sjaastad O. SUNCT syndrome: duration, frequency and temporal distribution of attacks. *Headache* 1996;36:161–165.

62. Pareja JA, Ruiz J, Deisla C, Alsabbah H, Espejo J. Idiopathic stabbing headache (jabs and jolts syndrome). *Cephalalgia* 1996;16:93–96.

63. Pareja JA, Sjaastad O. SUNCT syndrome in the female. *Headache* 1994;34:217–220.

64. Pareja JA, Sjaastad O. SUNCT syndrome. A clinical review. *Headache* 1997;37:195–202.

65. Pascual P, Iglesias F, Oterino A, Vazquez-Barquero A, Berciano J. Cough, exertional, and sexual headache. *Neurology* 1996;46: 1520–1524.

66. Paulson GW. Weightlifter's headache. *Headache* 1983;23:193–194.

67. Paulson GW, Klawans HL. Benign orgasmic cephalgia. *Headache* 1974;13:181–187.

68. Paulson GW, Zipf RE, Beekman JF. Pheochromocytoma causing exercise-related headache and pulmonary edema. *Ann Neurol* 1979;5: 96–99.

69. Pestronk A, Pestronk S. Goggle migraine. *N Engl J Med* 1983;308: 226–227.

70. Porter M, Jankovic J. Benign coital cephalgia. Differential diagnosis and treatment. *Arch Neurol* 1981;38:710–712.

71. Raskin NH. The hypnic headache syndrome. *Headache* 1988;28: 534–536.

72. Raskin NH. The cough headache syndrome: treatment. *Neurology* 1995;45:1784.

73. Raskin NH, Knittle SC. Ice cream headache and orthostatic symptoms in patients with migraine headache. *Headache* 1976;16:222–225.

74. Raskin NH, Schwartz RK. Icepick-like pain. *Neurology* 1980;30:203–205.

75. Rassmussen BK. Epidemiology of headache. *Cephalalgia* 1995;15:45–68.

76. Rivera M, del Real MA, Teruel JL, Gobernado JM, Ortuno J. Carotid artery disease presenting as cough headache in a patient on haemodialysis. *Postgrad Med J* 1991;67:702.

77. Rooke E. Benign exertional headache. *Med Clin North Am* 1968;52:801–808.

78. Selwyn DL. A study of coital related headaches in 32 patients. *Cephalalgia* 1985;5(Suppl 3):300–301.

79. Silberstein SD, Lipton RB, Sliwinski M. Classification of daily and near-daily headaches: a field study of revised IHS criteria. *Neurology* 1996;47:871–875.

80. Silbert PL, Edis RH, Stewart-Wynn EG, Gubbay SS. Benign vascular sexual headache and exertional headache: interrelationships and long term prognosis. *J Neurol Neurosurg Psychiatry* 1991;54:417–421.

81. Silbert PL, Hankey GJ, Prentice DA, Apsimon HT. Angiographically demonstrated arterial spasm in a case of benign sexual headache and benign exterioral headache. *Aust N Z J Med* 1989;19:466–468.

82. Sjaastad O. *Cluster headache syndrome.* London: WB Saunders, 1992.

83. Sjaastad O, Antonaci F. A piroxicam derivative partly effective in chronic paroxysmal hemicrania and hemicrania continua. *Headache* 1995;35:549–550.

84. Sjaastad O, Pareja JA, Zukerman E, Jansen J, Kruszewski P. Trigeminal neuralgia. Clinical manifestations of first division involvement. *Headache* 1997;37:346–357.

85. Sjaastad O, Saunte C, Salvesen R, et al. Shortlasting unilateral neuralgiform headache attacks with conjunctival injection, tearing, sweating, and rhinorrhea. *Cephalalgia* 1989;9:147–156.

86. Sjaastad O, Spierings EL. Hemicrania continua: another headache absolutely responsive to indomethacin. *Cephalalgia* 1984;4:65–70.

87. Smith WS, Messing RO. Cerebral aneurysm presenting as cough headache. *Headache* 1993;33:203–204.

88. Soriani S, Battistella PA, Arnaldi C, et al. Juvenile idiopathic stabbing headache. *Headache* 1996;36:565–567.

89. Staikov IN, Mattle HP. Vertebrobasilar dolicoectasia and exertional headache. *J Neurol Neurosurg Psychiatry* 1994;57:1544.

90. Staunton HP, Moore J. Coital cephalgia and ischaemic muscular work of the lower limbs. *J Neurol Neurosurg Psychiatry* 1978;41:930–933.

91. Symonds C. Cough headache. *Brain* 1956;79:557–568.

92. Vernay D, Deffond D, Fraysse P, Dordain G. Walk headache: an unusual manifestation of ischemic heart disease. *Headache* 1989;29:350–351.

93. Wijdicks EFM, Kerkhoff H, van Gijn J. Long-term follow up of 71 patients with thunderclap headache mimicking subarachnoid haemorrhage. *Lancet* 1988;2:68–70.

94. Williams B. Cerebrospinal fluid pressure changes in response to coughing. *Brain* 1976;99:331–346.

95. Williams B. Cough headache due to craniospinal pressure dissociation. *Arch Neurol* 1980;37:226–230.

96. Wolff HG. *Headache and other head pain.* New York: Oxford University Press, 1963.

97. Wolff S, Hardy JD. Studies on pain. Observations on pain due to local cooling and on factors involved in the "cold pressor" effect. *J Clin Invest* 1941;20:521–533.

The Headaches, Second Edition,
edited by J. Olesen, P. Tfelt-Hansen, and K.M.A. Welch.
Lippincott Williams & Wilkins, Philadelphia © 2000.

The Secondary Headaches

CHAPTER 101

The Secondary Headaches: Introduction

Jes Olesen

There are only four main types of *primary* headaches: migraine, tension-type headache, cluster headache, and a miscellaneous group. In contrast, the causes of *secondary* or *symptomatic* headaches are numerous. In the headache classification of the International Headache Society (IHS classification), they have been ordered in seven groups (1) (Table 1). Among the most common causes of headache are alcohol overuse (hangover), infections, trauma, and fasting (3). Quite often, secondary headaches have the same characteristics as migraine or tension-type headache. Therefore, it is sometimes difficult to determine whether the headache is secondary or primary. The IHS classification chose a close temporal relationship as the decisive factor. If a headache occurs for the first time in close temporal proximity to an organic disorder, it is coded as a secondary headache. If it occurs a long time after the organic disorder, it is not accepted as a secondary headache. Preexisting headaches that are merely aggravated by an organic disorder are not secondary but primary. In most cases, the analysis of temporal relationships is easy and unequivocal; however, in others the temporal relationship is difficult or impossible to establish. If, for example, a patient has suffered from rare migraine attacks for years, and a cerebral arteriovenous malformation (AVM) is disclosed in association with increasing attack frequency, are the two disorders then causally related? We cannot know this, because AVMs may be silent for many years. Similar problems often are encountered with meningiomas. The answer is more obvious if attacks disappear after an operation. Within each group of secondary headaches listed in Table 1, a hierarchical subclassification has been given by the IHS using up to four digits (1). These subclassifications are listed in the relevant chapters of the present book.

The level of evidence required by the Headache Classification Committee to accept an organic disorder as a cause of headache was not defined. All published evidence, of course, was considered, but the scarcity of such material made it necessary also to use the clinical experience of committee members. The level of general use of a symptomatic headache diagnosis also was taken into account. Unfortunately, primary headaches are so prevalent that the coexistence of headache and an organic disorder often is due to chance (2). Thus, it was previously generally accepted that arterial hypertension causes headache. Only relatively recent epidemiologic studies with suitable control groups made it clear that this association simply reflects the high prevalence of both disorders. Only diastolic blood pressures above 120 mm Hg are associated with increased headache prevalence (see Chapter 109). In virtually every drug trial, headache is recorded as a side effect. In double-blind, placebo-controlled trials, however, headache usually occurs equally in the placebo group and in the actively treated group. To be absolutely sure that an organic factor can cause headache, it is therefore necessary to have a comparable control group; but it is impossible to devise a proper control group for most organic disorders, such as cerebrovascular accidents, tumors, and other conditions. Is headache associated with stroke attributable to the emotional trauma of stroke or to the ischemic event itself? The answer has been uncertain, but several studies now have shown a relation between the location of the ischemic lesion and the location of headache, indicating that it is the lesion itself that directly causes the headache (see Chap. 104).

Among patients with brain tumors, some have headache and some do not. Is headache due to the size, location, and other characteristics of the tumor, or is it due to the premorbid constitution of the individual patient, that is, to a preset low headache threshold? Relatively recent studies

J. Olesen: Department of Neurology, Glostrup Hospital, University of Copenhagen, DK-2600 Glostrup, Copenhagen, Denmark.

TABLE 1. *Groups of secondary headaches according to the International Headache Society*

5	Headache associated with head trauma
6	Headache associated with vascular disorders
7	Headache associated with nonvascular intracranial disorder
8	Headache associated with substances or their withdrawal
9	Headache associated with noncephalic infection
10	Headache associated with metabolic disorder
11	Headache or facial pain associated with disorder of cranium, neck, eyes, ears, nose, sinuses, teeth, mouth, or other facial or cranial structures

TABLE 2. *Types of secondary headaches according to the International Headache Society*

0. Headache is as described in the diagnostic criteria for the particular disorder *Comment: For some disorders in groups 5–11 headache characteristics are not part of the diagnostic criteria; for some they are; fourth digit 0 applies only to the latter*
1. Migraine
   Fulfilling criteria for 1.1 or 1.2 with the exception that migraine occurs for the first time in close temporal relation to one of the disorders listed in groups 5–11
2. Tension-type headache
   Fulfilling criteria for 2.1 or 2.2 with the exception that tension-type headache occurs for the first time in close temporal relation to one of the disorders listed in groups 5–11
3. Cluster headache
   Fulfilling criteria for one form of cluster headache or chronic paroxysmal hemicrania with the exception that cluster headache or chronic paroxysmal hemicrania occurs for the first time in close temporal relation to one of the disorders listed in groups 5–11
4. Increased intracranial pressure type (prototype: brain tumor headache)
   A. Crescendo time profile over 3 mo or less
   B. Bilateral of moderate or severe intensity
   C. Occurs in the morning or after napping and remits or improves spontaneously after rising
   D. Is present at least 50% of all mornings
5. Decreased intracranial pressure type (prototype: postlumbar puncture headache)
   A. Bilateral
   B. Absent or mild in the recumbent position, occurs or worsens markedly in the upright position
6. Local lesion type (prototype: pain from bone metastasis)
   A. Headache is nonpulsating and constantly present
   B. Pain has a distinct maximum in a circumscribed area of 5 cm or less but may irradiate to surroundings or refer to more distant areas
7. Vasodilator type (prototype: nitroglycerine-, histamine-, and prostacyclin-induced headache)
   A. Bifrontotemporal pulsating pain
   B. No aura, nausea, or voming
8. Stabbing type (icepick type)
   A. Stabbing head pains lasting <1 s
   B. Occur as single stabs or series of stabs
   C. Each stab or series of stabs occurs in a small, sharply localized area
9. Other type (specify)
10. Two or more types (specify)

indicate that both factors are involved (Chapter 113). The exact characteristics of the various symptomatic headaches still are not sufficiently and clearly documented. The IHS Headache Classification Committee has tried to advance the situation by listing the number of different types of headache that can be caused by organic disorders. The fourth digit is used to code for this (Table 2). A vast number of infections exist, most of which can cause headache. The same is true of the large number of noninfectious intracranial disorders. All these are not listed separately in the IHS classification (1), or in this book, because there are no known distinctive features of the accompanying headaches; nor do the various etiologies imply different treatment strategies for the headaches.

To write about the secondary headaches is a challenge. Until we see the advent of prospective, controlled studies, evidence often must be pieced together from articles dealing with the primary disorders in general, and not with the headache caused by these disorders. In such articles, headache data can be extracted only with difficulty and uncertainty in many cases. The focus in this book is strictly on the headache itself, and other features of the underlying disorders are covered only when necessary for understanding the headache. Secondary headaches are sometimes the first symptom of an organic disorder and thus may represent an important differential diagnostic problem. Disorders in which this can happen receive more attention in this book than disorders in which headache is a late phenomenon accompanying many other symptoms. A secondary headache also may be an important therapeutic problem. A meningioma, for instance, may be radically excised, but the associated headache may continue as a therapeutic problem. Finally, a secondary headache may be important because it illuminates one or more basic headache mechanisms. Benign intracranial hypertension, for example, is interesting not only from the perspective of diagnosis and management but also because further study of this disorder is likely to help in understanding the interrelationships between increased intracranial pressure and headache.

In conclusion, the secondary headaches should receive much more attention in the future. They are an important element in neurologic differential diagnosis, may be key to our understanding of headache mechanisms, and often are troublesome not only to the patient but also to the physician who lacks good treatment options.

REFERENCES

1. Headache Classification Committee of the International Headache Society (Jes Olesen, Chairman). Classification and diagnostic criteria for headache disorders, cranial neuralgias and facial pain. *Cephalalgia* 1988;8(Suppl 7):1–96.
2. Rasmussen BK, Olesen J. Symptomatic and non-symptomatic headaches in a general population. *Neurology* 1992;42:1225–1231.
3. Rasmussen BK, Jensen R, Schroll M, Olesen J. Epidemiology of headache in a general population—a prevalence study. J Clin Epidemiol 1991;44:1147–1157.

The Headaches, Second Edition,
edited by J. Olesen, P. Tfelt-Hansen, and K.M.A. Welch.
Lippincott Williams & Wilkins, Philadelphia © 2000.

The Secondary Headaches

CHAPTER 102

Acute Posttraumatic Headache

Matthias Keidel and Nabih M. Ramadan

IHS code:

5.1 Acute posttraumatic headache
5.1.1 with significant head trauma and/or confirmatory signs
5.1.2 with minor head trauma and no confirmatory signs
WHO code:
None

Headache is the cardinal symptom of the posttraumatic syndrome following head trauma (HT) and cervical spine whiplash injury (WI). The knowledge of the different types of the posttraumatic headache (PTH) is of particular clinical importance for early recognition of the trauma history, initiation of a headache-specific treatment, avoiding chronification of the headache, supporting the remission of the posttraumatic syndrome, and improving the clinical outcome of the patient. This chapter provides an overview of the definition, epidemiology, classification, pathogenesis, clinical picture, diagnosis, course, and treatment of the acute PTH. Chronic PTH is discussed in the subsequent chapter.

As indicated in the IHS classification, PTH is defined by a close temporal relationship between HT or WI of varying severity, the pathologic and neuroinvestigational findings, and the onset and length of the headache. In contrast to former suggestions (2,14), the IHS classification does not recognize late-acquired headaches, occurring up to 3 months after a traumatic event, to be PTH.

M. Keidel: Department of Neurology, University of Essen, D-45122 Essen, Germany.

N. M. Ramadan: Eli Lilly and Company, Indianapolis, Indiana 46285.

EPIDEMIOLOGY

Posttraumatic headache is not uniform in its epidemiology. The clinical phenomenology of PTH is varied. Headaches characteristic of tension-type headache, migraine, cluster headache, cervicogenic headache, headache of intracranial hemorrhage, or elevated intracranial pressure headache all have been described following HT.

The frequency of the different types of PTH is as follows: tension-type headache 85% (21,25–27); cervicogenic headache 8% (female:male ratio of 3:2) (19); and migrainelike headache 2.5% (more common in children and teenagers) (24,63,65). The lifetime prevalence of a HT-associated migraine is 1.4% (58). The exact frequency of posttraumatic clusterlike headache is not known. This type of headache remains a rare event (56,64). Anecdotally described are a basilar migrainelike PTH (27,30) and a PTH associated with sexual activity (21). Analgesic overuse is described in 19% of all cases of chronic PTH and in 25% of chronic posttraumatic tension-type headache (27).

Head trauma has an incidence of 180 to 220 per 100,000 in North America and of about 350 per 100,000 in Europe (22). The incidence of HT is comparable with that of cerebrovascular ischemia; it is 10 times more frequent than Parkinson's disease (20 of 100,000), 100 times more frequent than Guillain-Barré syndrome (2 of 100,000), and 500 times more frequent than myasthenia gravis (0.4 of 100,000) (41,42). In the United States, about 2 million HTs occur per year; 80% are mild, 10% moderate, and 10% severe (35,41,42).

The frequency of headaches has been reported as 31% in one series (48), 36% in Cartlidge's study (13), over 71% by Levin et al. (43), and up to 90% in another study (15). This implies that the relative incidence of acute PTH is up to 200 of 100,000 in the United States and 315 of

100,000 in Europe (specifically, Germany). The absolute rates of newly diagnosed PTH per year are estimated as 1,800,000 (chronic PH as 400,000) in the United States and 270,000 (chronic PH as 60,000) in Germany.

The acceleration injuries of the cervical spine (i.e., WI) are the most common mechanisms of cervical trauma in traffic accidents (61). In one study, 88% of patients complained of headache after a mild WI without bony injuries or accompanying neurologic deficits (31). In others, the incidence varied between 40% and 97% (37). In 49% of patients, the headache is accompanied by a feeling of heaviness in the head. Exact figures for the incidence of PTH following moderately severe WI (with bony cervical spine injuries or neurologic deficits) or severe WI (with osseous lesions and neurologic deficits) are not available because of inadequacies in reporting the severity of the injury and difference in patient populations.

PATHOPHYSIOLOGY

The exact pathophysiology of acute PTH is unknown. Different mechanisms of pain are likely to play a role in acute PTH because the clinical presentation could mimic migraine, tension-type headache, or other forms of primary headaches. The mechanism(s) of primary headache may help us understand the corresponding subtype of acute PTH.

Acute posttraumatic cervicogenic headache (following WI or an HT combined with neck sprain) is likely the result of the multisegmental pain impulses generated from nociceptive afferents in stretched muscles, ligaments, and intervertebral disks as well as from sympathetic nerve fibers of the arterial vessels entering the cervical spinal cord via C fibers of the C2–C5 dorsal rami (51,52). The convergence between these upper cervical roots and the spinal nucleus of the trigeminal nerve provides a pathway for referral of posttraumatic neck pain to the frontal region (and vice versa; 11, 40). Rarely, direct traumatic compression of C2 fibers in the lateral atlantoaxial joint as another explanation for cervicogenic headache is possible as demonstrated postmortem (9). Sympathetic vertebral nerve irritation (6) and ischemia of the vertebral artery (4,5) as causes of posttraumatic cervicogenic headache are postulated, although not confirmed (10), mechanisms of posttraumatic cervicogenic headache.

An alteration of the anti-nociceptive inhibitory temporalis reflex in acute PTH of the tension type following WI suggests a transient dysfunction in central pain processing with an impairment of the serotonergic descending inhibitory pain system (38). Similar reflex abnormalities also have been described for the idiopathic tension-type headache (62). Acute PTH of tension type is accompanied by a varying degree of increase in general pain sensitivity (49). Subsequent chronification of the acute posttraumatic pain syndrome may be related to a wind-up

phenomenon of central pain sensitization. The impact of the accompanying vegetative disturbances, subjective impediment, or of disturbances in mood and well-being on pain intensity and duration is not fully elucidated (31,34,39).

In head injury, a variety of posttraumatic neurochemical, neurohumoral and neuroelectrical changes are described (68). They include elevated extracellular K^+ and intracellular Na^+, Ca^+, and Cl^-, reduced intracellular and total brain Mg, influx of extracellular Ca^{2+} (in axolemmas), accumulation of platelet-derived 5-hydroxytryptamine in the central nervous system, increased release of excitatory amino acids (e.g., glutamate), cortical spreading depression, increased levels of endogenous opioids, and increased nitric oxide activity (50,68). Young and Packard consider this altered neurochemical environment responsible for the acute manifestation of PTH or aura (50,68). Because of the similarity between the biochemical changes in primary migraine and those observed after head injury, Packard suggests that a comparable cascade of biochemical and bioelectrical events underlies the posttraumatic migrainelike headache (68).

Animal models and functional brain imaging studies in HT and WI show various structural, blood flow, and metabolic changes, which do not necessarily translate into mechanisms of the acute PTH. Factors likely to be involved in the pathophysiology include:

1. Referred pain from nociceptive input caused by lesions of musculoskeletal, discoligamentous, and other soft-tissue structures (including vessels, perivessel sheets, and nerves).
2. Activation of meningeal nociceptive afferents due to traumatic epidural, subdural, and subarachnoidal bleeding.
3. Stretching of pain-sensitive intracranial structure from increased intracranial pressure.
4. Intracranial hypotension (55).
5. Activation of the trigeminovascular system by posttraumatic sinus venous thrombosis.

CLINICAL FEATURES

The IHS diagnostic criteria (5.1.1) for acute PTH with significant head trauma and/or confirmatory signs (Headache Classification Committee, 1988) (28) are as follows:

A. Significance of head trauma documented by at least one of the following:
   1. Loss of consciousness
   2. Posttraumatic amnesia lasting more than 10 minutes
   3. At least two of the following showing relevant abnormality:
      a. Clinical neurologic examination
      b. X-ray of skull

c. Neuroimaging
d. Evoked potentials
e. Cerebrospinal fluid examination
f. Vestibular function test
g. Neuropsychological testing

B. Headache occurs less than 14 days after regaining consciousness (or after trauma if there has been no loss of consciousness)
C. Headache disappears within 8 weeks after regaining consciousness (or after trauma if there has been no loss of consciousness)

The IHS diagnostic criteria (5.1.2) for acute PTH with minor head trauma and no confirmatory signs (Headache Classification Committee, 1988) (28):

A. Head trauma that does not satisfy 5.1.1 criterion A
B. Headache occurring less than 14 days after injury
C. Headache disappearing within 8 weeks after injury

Headache (with or without accompanying neck pain) is the cardinal symptom of the posttraumatic syndrome. In the acute phase, it is characterized by vegetative symptoms (dizziness, nausea, vomiting, orthostatic dysregulation, and thermodysregulation), a neurasthenic depressive syndrome (subjectively reduced cognitive performance sometimes with overt neuropsychological deficits, mood alteration, nervousness, and irritability), and a sensory syndrome characterized by excessive sensitivity to light and noise.

The clinical features of PTH overlap with those of the primary headache disorders (i.e., migraine, cluster, tension, etc.) (Table 1). Posttraumatic tension-type headache (90%) is characterized by a dull-pressing, dragging, or pulling pain, which is mainly holocephalic, bandlike or helmetlike, usually nuchooccipital, seldom episodic, and often continuous. The clinical features are identical to those of primary tension-type headache (27). Tension-type PTH must be differentiated from posttraumatic cervicogenic headache [8% after WI (19)] which is mainly occipitonuchal and typically dragging. The pain of posttraumatic cervicogenic headache radiates from occipital to frontal. It is not holocephalic, strongly unilateral without side change, and commonly associated with limited mobility of the cervical spine. The pain can be triggered by turning the head, sometimes in a position resulting in pressure on the occipital nerve entry points. The diagnosis is confirmed by a trauma-related bony injury of the cervical spine and by pain relief after local anaesthetic infiltration of the tender greater occipital nerve or C2 root (52).

Posttraumatic migrainelike headache (2.5%) (25–27, 66,67) is mainly felt as a pulsating, hemicranial, side-changing headache. Accompanying vegetative complaints such as nausea, vomiting, dizziness, photophobia, and phonophobia are common. Posttraumatically isolated aura symptoms also may occur. Rarely, posttraumatic basilary migraine is described with vertigo, nausea, vomiting, and cranial nerve disorders of variable severity

TABLE 1. *Type, incidence, characteristics, and differential diagnosis of posttraumatic headache following HT and WI*

Type	Incidence	Localization	Characteristics	Differential diagnosis	Differentiating features
Tension-type headache	90%	Holocephalic, mainly occipital	Dull-pressing, dragging	Increased intracranial pressure	Level of consciousness, vegetative signs
				Subarachnoid bleeding	Signs of meningeal irritation, focal neurologic signs
				Drug-induced (analgesia) headache	History of medication, drug abuse
				Intracerebral bleeding	Unilateral preponderance, focal neurologic signs
Cervicogenic headache	8%	Nuchal, unilateral	Dragging, triggerable	Vertebral artery dissection	Brainstem symptoms (also transient)
				Prolapsed disk	Brachialgia, radicular signs and symptoms
				Subarachnoid bleeding	Bilateral neck pain, signs of meningeal irritation, altered mentation
Migraine-like	2,5%	Hemicranial, side changing	Pulsating	Head contusion	Circumscript, cranial vault localization
				Cranial vault fracture	X-ray
				Scalp injury (subgaleal hematoma)	Clinical inspection, cranial computer tomography
				Unilateral intracranial bleeding	Focal signs, cranial computer tomography
Cluster-type	Unknown	Periorbital, frontotemporal	Stabbing, pulsating, dragging	Facial skull fracture	Hematoma, x-ray
				Carotid artery dissection	Cervical/facial pain

TABLE 2. *Characteristics of posttraumatic headache following mild whiplash injury*

Occurrence	88%
Onset	5 hrs 13 min
Localization	Mainly occipital (67%)
Character	Dull, pressing, dragging (77%)
Frequency	Initially 8 hrs/day
Daily distribution	Evening maximum
Duration	3 weeks (max. 64 days)

Data from Keidel and Diener (31) and Keidel and Pearce (37).

(27,30). Cluster-type PTH does not differ clinically from primary cluster headache (56,64). The clinical picture is characterized by unilateral periorbital and frontotemporal pressing, stabbing or throbbing head or facial pain, accompanied by local autonomic signs such as ptosis, miosis, enophthalmus, lacrimation, rhinorrhea, and conjunctival injection.

Clinically important—because it is often misdiagnosed as posttraumatic tension-type headache—is drug-induced persisting headache, which can develop after HT or WI due to prolonged intake of analgesics. Drug-induced headache occurs daily, is prominent in the morning, has a dull-pressing character and holocephalic distribution, and is exacerbated by physical activity (17). Clinically, it is best differentiated from chronic PTH or tension-type headache only after successful withdrawal of analgesic intake.

Following WI, the PTH is associated with a feeling of heaviness of the head in almost half of the patients. It usually follows a complaint-free interval of a few hours to 1 day (37). The headache is mainly occipital, dull pressing, or dragging and reaches maximum intensity in the evening (31,32,37). Headaches of the tension type following head or neck (i.e., WI) injury have similar features (27) (Table 2). Some patients with the posttraumatic stress disorder (PTSD) report headache shortly after the trauma (a mild or trivial head injury in some cases). The DSM IV diagnostic criteria for PTSD do not include headache as a prominent symptom (3). Furthermore, acute PTH and PTSD are distinct in temporal profile despite the overlap in vegetative symptomatology. Acute PTH usually resolves within 3 weeks (32,33,34,36). In contrast, PTSD is only diagnosed safely when symptoms persist for more than 2 months.

DIAGNOSIS

The investigation of first choice following head injury is cranial computer tomography (CCT) including a bone window technique used to screen for any fracture (vault or base of skull) and to identify potential sequelae of intracranial trauma, such as hematoma, focal contusion, or hydrocephalus. The CCT is sufficient for deciding whether a neurosurgical operative procedure is necessary.

Cranial MRI is more sensitive for showing nonhemorrhagic focal contusions. In HT with accompanying cervical spine distortions or in isolated WI, plain cervical spine multiplanar x-rays are necessary to identify fracture, luxation, or kinking of the spine. In addition, functional x-rays with cervical spine flexion and extension views help to delineate indirect signs of a ligamentous lesion or traumatic structural damages such as spondylolisthesis. A dens fracture, luxation, or atlantodental loosening can be excluded with supplementary dens views. Further investigational studies could be conducted depending on the symptom complex and the neurologic signs that accompany PTH (37). Repeated studies may be necessary if the character of the headache or its localization change, there is a change or appearance of new, nonheadache symptoms, and new focal neurologic signs emerge.

PROGNOSIS

Most young patients with a mild cerebral concussion (e.g., without loss of consciousness but with vegetative symptoms and PTH) fully recover within a few days (7). The classic cerebral concussion patient with a momentary loss of consciousness and amnesia of less than 60 minutes duration generally recovers completely within 6 to 12 weeks (23,43). The posttraumatic syndrome after a severe cerebral concussion (e.g., with loss of consciousness greater than 10 minutes and a loss of memory greater than 4–6 hours) usually recovers within months to years (29,57). In an investigation of its course, Denker (15) showed that 90% of patients suffered from PTH within the first months following mild HT, 35% still after 1 year, 22% after 2 years, and only 20% after 3 years. After 6 months, over 80% of patients were headache free (15). These figures are supported by numerous other studies (8,13,16,20,43–45,48,59,60). Prevalence rates of PTH at 6 and 24 months are reported as 27% and 24% after head injury (14) and as 27% and 15% after WI (53, 54). Up to 15% of patients show an incomplete remission from the posttraumatic syndrome (12,18,46,47,60). Details of chronic PTH are provided in the following chapter.

The average length of PTH after mild WI without neurologic deficits or bony cervical spine injuries is 3 weeks. In this group the headache generally disappears within 3 months (31–33,36,37). A delayed remission of PTH following WI is found in those patients with an initially severe headache, with marked limitation of passive cervical spine mobility (particularly flexion), in patients with poor general well-being and depressive mood with somatic-vegetative complaints, and in the elderly (32). Posttraumatic *de novo* cervicogenic headache after WI is rare and has a good prognosis. The prevalence decreases from 8.3% within the first 6 weeks to 4.5% after 6 months and to 3.5% 1 year following WI (19).

MANAGEMENT

The treatment of acute PTH varies according to the type of headache and depending on the duration. The treatment guidelines are based on clinical experience and controlled studies (36). First-choice treatment for the acute posttraumatic tension-type headache are analgesics such as acetylsalicylic acid (ASA; 500–1,000 mg daily, maximum 1,500 mg daily after excluding intracranial hemorrhage) or paracetamol (500–1,000 mg, maximum 1,500 mg daily). Alternatively, ibuprofen in retard form (400–600 mg daily) or naproxen (500–1,000 mg daily) can be used. The use of combination preparations is discouraged. Should the headache continue for longer than 4 weeks, no further analgesics should be given because of the danger of developing drug-induced persisting headache.

The posttraumatic migraine-type headache is treated during the attack, with an analgesic (e.g., ASA 1,000 mg in effervescent tablet form) together with an antiemetic (e.g., domperidone or metoclopramide, 10–20 mg orally). In the case of severe, long-lasting, or frequent migraine-like attacks, prophylactic drug treatment with an adrenergic beta-blocker such as metoprolol or propranolol could be used. Migrainelike PTH responds to propranolol or amitriptyline (25–150 mg daily) as monotherapy or in combination. The seldom seen PTH of the cluster type is treated in the same way as primary cluster headache (see Chapter 98).

Acute posttraumatic (cervico)cephalic pain following WI is treated with a temporary and short-term cervical collar to limit movements of the neck. To avoid atrophy of the neck musculature from inactivity, the collar should be worn for less than 14 days. When neck and head pain is stronger in the morning, wearing a support collar at night is recommended to avoid the additional cervical soft-tissue straining with head movement in deep sleep due to nocturnal-dependent hypotonia of the neck musculature.

Supplementary physical measures with heat applications are indicated. Dry heat (infrared light, arc light, warm air, and heat pillows) or moist heat (hydrocollator packs) have all proved useful (personal observation). If there is no therapeutic benefit from physical measures, additional therapy with muscle relaxants, antiinflammatories/antirheumatics, and if necessary analgesics may be necessary (37). In order to prevent medication overuse and subsequent drug-induced headache, the drug treatment of acute PTH following WI should include strict control of medication intake.

Acute PTH following HT or WI should not be treated, as a rule, with opioid analgesics, because of the possibility of dependency and substance overuse. Similarly, prolonged use of benzodiazepines as muscle relaxants should be avoided. Although the short-term use of a peripherally acting analgesic is reasonable in the initial acute stages, longer use (i.e., longer than 4 weeks) should be disallowed in order to avoid drug-induced headache. Similarly, drug-induced headache also can develop with regular use of combination analgesics. Other obsolete therapies for the pain of acute PTH include antihistamines, steroids, neuroleptics, barbiturates, and ergot preparations. Manual traction or pulling of the cervical spine with Glisson slings in the acute phase of the cervicocephalic pain syndrome following cervical spine distorsion are obsolete. The same is true for immobilization with a plaster collar (minerva plaster). Nonbeneficial and often pain- intensifying maneuvers include massage of the stretched musculature and reflex zone; locally invasive anesthetic measures such as subcutaneous, perineural, or intraarticular infiltration; neural therapy; acupuncture; and acupressure. Fresh cell and ozone therapy are obsolete in posttraumatic tension-type headache. The benefit of local unguent treatment for the nuchal pain that often accompanies the headache is not proven. Prolonged bed rest after cerebral contusion may increase the risk of delayed remission; a 24-hour clinical observation period is usually sufficient.

REFERENCES

1. Alexander MP. Mild traumatic brain injury: pathophysiology, natural history and clinical management. *Neurology* 1995;45:1253–1260.
2. Alves WM, Colohan ART, O'Leary TJ, Rimel RW, Jane JA. Understanding post-traumatic symptoms after minor head injury. *J Head Trauma Rehabil* 1986;1:1–12.
3. American Psychiatric Association. *Diagnostic and statistical manual of mental disorders,* 4th ed. Washington, DC: American Psychiatric Association, 1994.
4. Bärtschi-Rochaix W. *Migraine cervicale, das encephale Syndrom nach Halswirbelsäulentrauma.* Bern, Switzerland: Huber, 1949.
5. Bärtschi-Rochaix W. Headache of cervical origin. In: Vinken PJ, Bruyn GW, eds. *Handbook of clinical neurology,* Vol 5. Headache. Amsterdam: North-Holland Publishing, 1968:192–203.
6. Barre N. Sur un syndrome sympathique cervical posterieur et sa cause fréquente, l'arthrite cervical. *Rev Neurol (Paris)* 1926;33:1246–1248.
7. Barth JT, Alves WM, Ryan TV, et al. Mild head injury in sports: neuropsychological sequelae and recovery of function. In: Levin HS, Eisenberg HM, Benton AL, eds. *Mild head injury.* New York: Oxford University Press, 1989:257–273.
8. Binder LM. Persisting symptoms after mild head injury: a review of the postconcussive syndrome. *J Clin Exp Neuropsychol* 1986;8:323–346.
9. Bogduk N. The anatomy of occipital neuralgia. *Clin Exp Neurol* 1980; 17:167–184.
10. Bogduk N. The clinical anatomy of the cervical dorsal rami. *Spine* 1982;7:319–330.
11. Bogduk N. Cervical causes of headache. *Cephalalgia* 1989;9(Suppl 10):172–173.
12. Bohnen N, Twijnstra A, Jolles J. Post-traumatic and emotional symptoms in different subgroups of patients with mild head injury. *Brain Injury* 1992;6:481–487.
13. Cartlidge NE. Postconcussional syndrome. *Scott Med J* 1978;23:103.
14. Cartlidge NE, Shaw DA. *Head injury.* London: WB Saunders 1981: 106–108.
15. Denker PG. The postconcussion syndrome. Prognosis and evaluation of the organic factors. *NY State J Med* 1994;44:379–384.
16. Denny-Brown D. Disability arising from closed head injury. *JAMA* 1945;127:429–436.
17. Diener HC, Wilkinson M, eds. *Drug induced headache.* New York: Springer, 1988.
18. Dikmen SS, Temkin N, Armsden G. Neuropsychological recovery: relationship to psychosocial functioning and postconcussional com-

plaints. In: Levin HS, Eisenberg HG, Benton AL, et al. *Mild head injury.* New York: Oxford University Press, 1989:229–241.

19. Drottning M, Staff PH, Sjaastad O. Cervicogenic headache after whiplash injury [Abstract]. *Cephalalgia* 1997;17:288.

20. Edna T-H. Disability 3–5 years after minor head injury. *J Oslo City Hosp* 1987;37:41–48.

21. Evans RW. The postconcussion syndrome and the sequelae of mild head injury. *Neurol Clin* 1992;10:814–847.

22. Frommelt P. Neurologische Erkrankungen. In: VdR, ed. *Sozialmedizinische Begutachtung in der gesetzlichen Rentenversicherung.* Stuttgart: Fischer, 1995:409–451.

23. Gronwall D, Wrightson P. Delayed recovery after mild head injury. *Lancet* 1974;2:605–609.

24. Guthkelch AN. Benign post-traumatic encephalopathy in young people and its relation to migraine. *Neurosurgery* 1977;1:101–105.

25. Haas DC. Acute posttraumatic headache. In: Olesen J, Tfelt-Hansen P, Welch KMA, eds. *The headaches.* New York: Raven, 1993:623–627.

26. Haas DC. Chronic posttraumatic headache. In: Olesen J, Tfelt-Hansen P, Welch KMA, eds. *The headaches.* New York: Raven, 1993:629–637.

27. Haas DC. Chronic PTHs classified and compared with natural headaches. *Cephalalgia* 1996;16:486–493.

28. Headache Classification Committee of the International Headache Society. Classification and diagnostic criteria for headache disorders, cranial neuralgias and facial pain. *Cephalalgia* 1988;8(Suppl 7):1–96.

29. Hugenholtz H, Stuss DT, Stethem LL, Richard MT. How long does it take to recover from a mild concussion? *Neurosurgery* 1988;22:853–868.

30. Jacome DE. Basilar artery migraine after uncomplicated whiplash injuries. *Headache* 1986;26:515–516.

31. Keidel M, Diener HC. Headache and acceleration trauma of the cervical spine. *News Headache* 1993;3:1.

32. Keidel M, Diener HC. Der posttraumatische Kopfschmerz. *Nervenarzt* 1997;68:769–777.

33. Keidel M, Eisentraut R, Baume B, Yagüez L, Diener HC. Prospective analysis of acute headache following whiplash injury. *Cephalalgia* 1993;13(Suppl 13):177.

34. Keidel M, Eisentraut R, Diener HC. *Predictors for prolonged recovery from posttraumatic headache in whiplash injury.* Seattle: IASP Publications, 1993:12.

35. Keidel M, Miller JD. Head trauma. In: Brandt T, Caplan LR, Dichgans J, Diener HC, Kennard C, eds. *Neurological disorders: course and treatment.* San Diego: Academic, 1996:531–544.

36. Keidel M, Neu I, Langohr HD, Göbel H. Management of posttraumatic headache after head trauma and whiplash injury. Recommendations of the German Migraine and Headache Society [in German]. *Schmerz* 1998;12:352–372.

37. Keidel M, Pearce JMS. Whiplash injury. In: Brandt T, Dichgans J, Diener HC, Caplan LR, Kennard C, eds. *Neurological disorders: course and treatment.* San Diego: Academic, 1996:65–76.

38. Keidel M, Rieschke P, Jüptner M, Diener HC. Pathologischer Kieferöffnungsreflex nach HWS-Beschleunigungsverletzung. *Nervenarzt* 1994;65:241–249.

39. Keidel M, Yagüez L, Wilhelm H, Diener HC. Prospektiver Verlauf neuropsychologischer Defizite nach zervikozephalem Akzelerationstrauma. *Nervenarzt* 1992;63:731–740.

40. Kerr FWL. Central relationships of trigeminal and cervical primary afferents in the spinal cord and medulla. *Brain Res* 1972;43:561–572.

41. Kraus JF, Nourjah P. The epidemiology of mild uncomplicated brain injury. *J Trauma* 1988;28:1637–1643.

42. Kurtzke JF, Kurland LT. The epidemiology of neurologic disease. In: Joynt RJ, ed. *Clinical neurology review.* Philadelphia: JB Lippincott, 1993.

43. Levin HS, Mattis S, Ruff RM, et al. Neurobehavioral outcome following minor head injury. A three-center study. *J Neurosurg* 1987;66:234–243.

44. Marshall LF, Ruff RM. Neurosurgeon as victim. In: Levin HS, Eisenberg HM, Benton AL, eds. Mild head injury. New York: Oxford University Press, 1989:276–280.

45. Mazzuchi A, Cattelani R, Missale G, et al. Head-injured subjects aged over 50 years: correlations between variables of trauma and neuropsychological follow-up. *J Neurol* 1992;239:256–260.

46. McLean A, Temkin NR, Dikmen S, et al. The behavioral sequelae of head injury. *J Clin Neuropsychol* 1983;5:361–376.

47. Middleboe T, Andersen HS, Birket-Smith M, et al. Minor head injury: impact on general health after 1 year. A prospective follow-up study. *Acta Neurol Scand* 1992;85:5–9.

48. Minderhoud JM, Boelens MEM, Huizenga J. Treatment of minor head injuries. *Clin Neurol Neurosurg* 1980;82:127–140.

49. Nebe J, Keidel M, Lüdecke Ch, Diener HC. Schmerzquantifizierung nach HWS-Schleudertrauma mittels Computer-interaktiver Druckalgesimetrie. *Nervenarzt* 1998;69:924–928

50. Packard RC, Ham LP. Pathogenesis of posttraumatic headache and migraine: a common headache pathway. *Headache* 1997;37:142–152.

51. Pfaffenrath V, Dandekar R, Pöllmann W. Cervicogenic headache —the clinical picture, radiological findings and hypotheses on its pathophysiology. *Headache* 1987;27:495–499.

52. Pöllmann W, Keidel M, Pfaffenrath V. Headache and the cervical spine: a critical review. *Cephalalgia* 1997;17:801–816.

53. Radanov BP, Di Stefano G, Schnidrig A, Aljinovic M. Factors influencing recovery from headache after common whiplash. *BMJ* 1993;307:652–655.

54. Radanov BP, Sturzenegger M, Di Stefano G. Long-term outcome after whiplash injury. A 2-year follow-up considering features of injury mechanism and somatic, radiologic and psychosocial findings. *Medicine* 1995;74:281–297.

55. Ramadan NM. Headache caused by raised intracranial pressure and intracranial hypotension. *Curr Opin Neurol* 1996;9:214–218.

56. Reik L. Cluster headache after head injury. *Headache* 1987;27:509–510.

57. Rimel RW, Giordani B, Barth JT, et al. Disability caused by minor head injury. *Neurosurgery* 1981;9:221–228.

58. Russell MB, Olesen J. Migraine associated with head trauma. *Eur J Neurol* 1996;3:424–428.

59. Rutherford WH. Concussion symptoms: relationship to acute neurological indices, individual differences and circumstances of injury. In: Levin HS, Eisenberg HM, Benton AL, eds. *Mild head injury.* New York: Oxford University Press, 1989:217–228.

60. Rutherford WH, Merrett JD, McDonald JR. Symptoms at one year following concussions from minor head injuries. *Injury* 1978;10:225–230.

61. Schmidt G. Zur Biomechanik des Schleudertraumas der Halswirbelsäule. *Versicherungsmedizin* 1989;4:121–125.

62. Schoenen J, Jamart B, Gerard P, Lenarduzzi P, Delwaide PJ. Exteroceptive suppression of temporalis muscle activity in chronic headache. *Neurology* 1987;37:1834–1836.

63. Snoek JW, Minderhout JM, Wilmink JT. Delayed deterioration following mild head injury in children. *Brain* 1984;107:15–36.

64. Turkewitz LJ, Wirth O, Dawson GA, Casaly JS. Cluster headache following head injury: a case report and review of the literature. *Headache* 1992;32:504–506.

65. Vohanka S, Zouhar A. Benign posttraumatic encephalopathy. *Acta Nerv Super* 1990;32:179–183.

66. Weiss HD, Stern BJ, Goldberg J. Post-traumatic chronic migraine precipitated by minor head or neck trauma. *Headache* 1991;31:451–456.

67. Winston KR. Whiplash and its relationship to migraine. *Headache* 1987;27:452–445.

68. Young WB, Packard RC. Posttraumatic headache and posttraumatic syndrome. In: AASH, ed., The 39th Annual Scientific Meeting of the American Association for the Study of Headache (AASH), New York. Abstract Volume, 1997:63–99.

The Headaches, Second Edition,
edited by J. Olesen, P. Tfelt-Hansen, and K.M.A. Welch.
Lippincott Williams & Wilkins, Philadelphia © 2000.

The Secondary Headaches

CHAPTER 103

Chronic Posttraumatic Headache

Nabih M. Ramadan and Matthias Keidel

IHS Code:

5.2 Chronic posttraumatic headache
5.2.1 With significant head trauma or confirmatory signs
5.2.2 With minor head trauma and no confirmatory signs

WHO Code:

G44.3 Chronic posttraumatic headache

SHORT DESCRIPTION

Headache resulting from head injury was described many centuries ago. Posttraumatic headache (PTH) follows head and sometimes neck injury without a direct head impact. Headaches that start hours to days after the insult and persist for less than 2 months are called *acute PTH* by International Headache Society (IHS) criteria (described elsewhere in this book). Sometimes, PTH becomes chronic, lasting months to several years. Although the IHS criteria indicate that the onset of chronic headache is within 2 weeks of the head trauma, delayed-onset chronic PTH has been described.

Chronic PTH can have features of migraine, tension-type headache, or both. Rarely, headaches mimicking cluster headache, idiopathic jabbing headache, and facionuchal neuralgias are described.

Posttraumatic headache is a cardinal symptom of the postconcussion syndrome (PCS) (Table 1), which encompasses a constellation of complaints, most notably dizziness, memory loss, fatigue, impaired concentration, irritability, anxiety, insomnia, and phonophobia. The PCS

N.M. Ramadan: Eli Lilly and Company, Indianapolis, Indiana 46285.

M. Keidel: Department of Neurology, University of Essen, D-45122 Essen, Germany.

follows mild head injury (MHI), with or without loss of consciousness. MHI is defined as occurring when direct head trauma is associated with a 13 to 15 score on the Glasgow Coma Scale (GCS) [the range of GCS scores is from zero (no eye opening response, no verbal response, no motor response) to 15 (spontaneous eye opening, oriented, obeys commands)] (Table 2).

Chronic PTH follows MHI and severe head injury. The latter is the result of structural lesions, such as subdural or epidural hematoma, and is easily differentiated from PTH of MHI by neuroradiologic studies. This chapter focuses on headaches that follow MHI.

Chronic PTH has long been considered a functional disorder. More than a hundred years ago, the role of financial compensation in the genesis and perpetuation of

TABLE 1. *Features of the postconcussion syndrome*

Symptoms	Frequency (%)
Headache	Up to 90
Dizziness	Up to 53
Blurred vision	14
Anosmia	5
Photophobia	7
Phonophobia	15
Psychosomatic complaints	Up to 85
Fatigue	
Disturbed sleep	
Memory loss	
Poor concentration	
Impaired libido	
Apathy	
Anger	
Personality changes	
Depression	
Anxiety	
Irritability	

From Evans (19).

771

TABLE 2. *Glasgow Coma Scale (GCS)*

Test	Response	Score
Eye opening	Spontaneous	4
	To sound	3
	To pain	2
	Never	1
	Obeys commands	6
	Localizes pain	5
	Normal flexion	4
Best motor response	Abnormal flexion	3
	Extension	2
	No response	1
Best verbal response	Oriented	5
	Confused	4
	Inappropriate words	3
	Incomprehensible sounds	2
	None	1

posttraumatic symptoms was emphasized (48). This contention was challenged recently, however. Arguments defending both views are presented in the sections that follow.

EPIDEMIOLOGY

Mild head injury accounts for more than 75% of brain injuries (38). The annual incidence of MHI varies from 131 to 511 per 100,000 subjects (19). Posttraumatic headache follows head trauma and whiplash injury in 30% to 90% of patients (18,32). The reported incidence of chronic PTH also varies from one study to another, in part because of disagreement on the duration of symptoms from the time of injury. The IHS defined chronic PTH as involving symptoms that persist beyond 2 months of the original insult (27). This arbitrary definition of chronicity was suggested by Brenner and colleagues many years ago (10) but was challenged recently. Indeed, Packard and Ham argue that PTH becomes chronic when patients continue to report headaches 6 months or longer after injury (50). Packard coined the term *permanent PTH* as headache persisting longer than 1 year postinjury or for 6 months with 3 months or more of a plateau with an adequate trial of treatment (49). Up to 32% of patients with head injury report persistent headaches 6 months after trauma, and approximately one in four continues to report headache at 4 years (Table 3) (10,11,17,32,56).

The IHS criteria require the onset of PTH to be within 2 weeks of head trauma (27). Late-acquired headaches

TABLE 3. *Chronicity of posttraumatic headache*

Duration	Incidence (%)	References
Up to 6 mo	26–32	10,11,56
Up to 1 yr	18	11
Up to 2 yr	24	11
Up to 4 yr	20–24	17,32

have been recognized, however, in children (40) and in adults (11,15). These studies indicate that late-acquired headaches (starting more than 2 weeks after the trauma) are as common (11,40), or more common (15), than those of early onset.

RISK FACTORS (TABLE 4)

Jensen and Nielson conducted a study to examine the risk factors for chronic PTH (30). They found that patients with preexisting headaches (i.e., before head trauma) had a similar incidence of chronic PTH to those who reported no history of headache before the accident. Of note is that the prevalence of headache increased in that cohort from 40% pretrauma to 64% after the injury. Most of the increase was in significant headaches, that is, those occurring 1 to 2 days per week or more. Also, Jensen and Nielsen found that more women (49%) than men (30%) developed chronic PTH (relative risk = 1.6) (30), confirming the results of an earlier study indicating an increased incidence of chronic PTH in women 2 years posttrauma but not at 6 months (11). Neither of these studies noted whether the headaches began in the early posttraumatic period or later. Posttraumatic migraine was equally frequent in men and women in one study of 13 patients (5) and three times as frequent in another study of 35 patients (70). Older age was not a risk factor for chronic PTH in one study (30) but was associated with slower and incomplete recovery in two subsequent studies (9,43).

A commonly held view is that chronic PTH is more common in people who sustain mild injury compared

TABLE 4. *Determinants of chronic headache following mild closed head injury. (?) indicates factors that are either controversial or that have been demonstrated in some studies but not in others*

Demographics
  Females
  Older age
  Lower socioeconomic status
  Lower degree of education
Severity of injury
  Mild
  No, or lesser degree of, amnesia
  No, or minimal duration of, loss of consciousness
History of recurrent headache (?)
Prior head injury
Psychological and psychiatric factors
  Posttraumatic depression
  Posttraumatic stress disorder
  Premorbid personality traits
  Immediate premorbid adverse events
  Lower IQ
Social factors
  Unstable preinjury work history
  Skilled/unskilled labor
  Desire for financial compensation (?)

with those who suffer a major insult; that is, there is an inverse relationship between the severity of the head injury and the occurrence of chronic PTH (18,48,50). Brenner and associates (10) noted that headaches lasting longer than 2 months after accidents affected 10% of 20 patients who were merely dazed by their trauma and 34% of 175 patients rendered unconscious. Within the latter group, however, the incidence of headache did not differ appreciably in patients who were unconscious for less than 10 minutes, for 10 to 60 minutes, or for longer than 1 hour (10).

Cartlidge and Shaw found that, among 372 patients, chronic headaches were more common in those whose posttraumatic amnesia had a duration of less than an hour than in those who had more prolonged amnesia (11). At 6 months, 34% of patients with short-duration amnesia and 19% of those with prolonged amnesia reported headache; at 1 year, 21% and 14%; and at 2 years, 24% and 19%, respectively. In agreement with these findings are those of Jensen and Nielsen, who interviewed patients 9 to 12 months after their head injuries (30). They observed chronic PTH in 42% of 48 patients who had not lost consciousness, in 38% of 74 patients unconscious for less than 15 minutes, and in 23% of 30 patients unconscious for 15 minutes to 24 hours. In determining the relationship between the incidence of posttraumatic headache and the severity of head trauma, these studies did not separate the headaches into early onset and late onset.

Two recent studies further support the belief in an inverse relationship between the severity of head trauma and chronic PTH. In the first, Yamaguchi found that 46 of 64 patients (72%) with mild injury and 19 of the 57 severely injured (33%) complained of severe headache ($p < 0.001$) (72). Also, headache was more common ($p < 0.01$) in the group who had a normal cranial computed tomography (CT) (21 of 32, 66%) than in those whose CT was abnormal (14 of 48, 29%). *Abnormal* was not defined further, however. In the second study, Haas evaluated 48 patients with chronic PTH and reported that 40 (83%) sustained a MHI (24). The remaining eight patients developed posttraumatic amnesia of varied duration.

POSTTRAUMATIC MIGRAINE: INCIDENCE AND ONSET

Head injury from playing soccer, boxing, American football, rugby, basketball, wrestling, volleyball, and whiplash injury all have been reported to trigger migrainous headache (18,19). These headaches are appropriately termed *trauma-triggered migraines* (23). A family history of migraine may be a predisposing factor to these trauma-induced migraines (19). Alternatively, recurrent posttraumatic migrainelike headaches have been well documented in the literature (5,6,70,71). The studies of Behrman (5) and Weiss and colleagues (70) indicate that

migrainelike headache is the most common type of posttraumatic headache, but Haas did not confirm these observations when he reported that 75% of 48 patients with chronic PTH had IHS-defined chronic tension-type headache and only 21% complained of headaches that were migraine without aura by IHS criteria (24).

Posttraumatic migraines can begin either shortly after head injuries or much later. Behrman reported that, among 13 patients, the time interval between trauma and the first attack of migraine varies from 18 hours to 10 weeks (5). Weiss and colleagues defined trauma-induced migraine as headaches with migrainous features that occur within hours to days of the injury (70). Migraine-like headache with late onset was excluded from that series of 35 patients.

CHRONIC HEADACHES FOLLOWING WHIPLASH INJURIES

It is estimated that one million whiplash injuries occur yearly in the United States (20). One study indicated that the frequency of headache after whiplash injury is 82% within 4 weeks of the insult, and 73% of the 180 patients continue to suffer recurrent headaches at 3 months (3). Most recently, Schrader and colleagues reported that, compared with 202 control subjects, patients with whiplash injury had similar incidence of headaches ($p < 0.1$) 1 to 3 years after the accident (59). Infrequent headaches (less than 1 day per month), those recurring more than 7 days per month, and chronic daily headaches were distributed equally among patients and controls.

Stovner (63) reviewed the literature on the whiplash syndrome and reported that pretrauma headaches, insurance claim, neurologic findings, and degenerative changes on initial radiologic studies correlated highly ($p < 0.001$) with chronic complaints posttrauma, including headache (63).

PATHOPHYSIOLOGY

The mechanisms of headache following MHI are varied. Axonal injury, soft-tissue damage, cerebral metabolic derangements, and altered cerebral hemodynamics have been implicated in the genesis of symptoms, including headache, following head trauma (11,19,22,51,52). In a review of the literature, Evans described reports of parenchymatous lesions on cranial magnetic resonance imaging (MRI) that decrease in size 1 to 3 months postinjury, decreased gray matter blood flow on single-photon emission computed tomography (SPECT), reduced metabolic rate of glucose utilization on positron emission tomography (PET), and asynchronous theta and delta activity on electroencephalography (EEG) (19). Drake and colleagues recently reported significant attenuation and latency prolongation of middle-latency, auditory-evoked responses of 20 patients with postconcussive syndrome compared with 25 neurologically intact controls, suggesting that cortical dysfunction plays an etiologic role in those patients with neuropsychiatric sequelae but no objective findings in previous evaluations (16); the time that elapsed between the head injury and the evoked potential studies was not specified. Two recent regional cerebral blood flow (rCBF) studies using ^{133}Xe-inhalation (22) and technetium-99 (^{99m}Tc) HMPAO (1) indicate that abnormally asymmetric rCBF and focal areas of cerebral hypoperfusion could be observed in patients with posttraumatic symptoms up to 3 years after the head injury. Many of these studies support an organic basis for acute posttraumatic symptoms, including headache, but do not establish irrevocably an organicity to the persistent complaints following head trauma. Abnormal rCBF (1,22) and derangements in middle-latency auditory-evoked potentials (16) argue for deranged cortical function long after head injury in patients with MHI. Furthermore, some authors, most notably Taylor (64) and then Kelly (34,35), believe that postconcussion symptoms result in part from lesions to the brainstem and white matter, similar to those demonstrated in experimental animals subjected to concussions. This hypothesis is, however, inconsistent with the considerable data showing an inverse relationship between the occurrence of postconcussion symptoms, including headache, and the severity of head trauma (described under the section entitled Risk Factors).

Relation of Symptoms to Various Psychosocial Factors (see Table 4)

Cartlidge and Shaw studied 372 survivors of head injury and found that depression plays an important role in causing PTH, particularly of the late-acquired type (11). The role of depression in chronic PTH was confirmed subsequently (12). Other contributors to PTH include posttraumatic stress disorder (PTSD) (12,28); suppressed anger (12); significant psychopathology on psychological measures (26); certain preexisting personality traits, including neuroticism (2,10,37); a lower IQ (19); and adverse life events in the year preceding the trauma (19). Whereas it could be argued that the performance of patients on neuropsychological testing may be influenced by headache during testing, Tsushima and Newbill demonstrated that the scores on the Luria-Nebraska Neuropsychological Battery (LNNB) and the Minnesota Multiphasic Personality Inventory (MMPI) were independent of the presence or absence of headache (65).

Complex psychological disturbances may be responsible for posttraumatic symptoms, including headache, even in the absence of direct head trauma (4,8,53). The study of Parker is particularly interesting, because chronic headaches were more prevalent among patients who did not sustain head injuries than among those who did (53).

Many social factors are implicated in the development of chronic posttraumatic symptoms (19). These factors include lower educational level, lower socioeconomic status, unstable preinjury work history, skilled and unskilled labor compared with executive and managerial jobs, and lower household income.

Relation of Symptoms to Desire for Financial Compensation

Whether a relation exists between the desire for financial compensation and the occurrence of posttraumatic headache and other symptoms has been debated for many years. Many physicians and lawyers are convinced of the conclusions of Miller, who in 1961 studied 200 consecutive patients with MHI and argued that accident neurosis (headache, dizziness, irritability) was not related to the accident but a manifestation of hope for financial compensation (45). The author based his opinion on the observation that almost 25% of patients had psychoneurotic complaints. He stated that gross exaggeration of disability is a common feature of accident neurosis and believed that malingering was more common than generally recognized. Miller proceeded to state that posttraumatic syndrome is closely related to extraneous factors, among which the circumstances of the injury and the possibility of financial gain loom large, a previous history of headache, and personal inadequacy or psychoneurotic predisposition only slightly less so (46). Miller reported almost identical descriptions of accident neurosis and postconcussion syndrome; yet he considered them as separate entities. The author seemed puzzled by the consistency of symptoms among patients with the postconcussion syndrome and suggested a structural or at least a pathophysiologic basis (45). Finally, Miller's extreme position regarding the relation of posttraumatic symptoms to compensation claims was based on evaluations of 200 MHI patients who were referred to him for medicolegal assessment; therefore, the cohort was not representative of head-injured patients in general.

Miller's view of a relationship between compensation claims and work absenteism were substantiated by Cook, who observed that patients seeking compensation had more prevalent and more prolonged symptoms (including headache) and returned to work later than those who were not seeking compensation for injury (13). On the other hand, Brenner and colleagues (10) and Kelly (33,34) reached a different conclusion. They independently reported that posttraumatic symptoms persist despite compensation settlement. Kelly's review of the subject (34) indicates that (a) most patients with posttraumatic headache return to work before financial settlement (76% of 110 patients in one prospective study [33]); (b) many (24 of 34; 71% in one series [36]) are not involved in a claim situation; and (c) some remain symptomatic despite settlement of the compensation claim.

Cartlidge and Shaw further dissected the issue of a relationship between financial compensation and posttraumatic symptoms in a study comparing compensation claims in patients with posttraumatic headache of both early and late onset (11). Six months after head trauma, 83% of late-onset posttraumatic headache patients and 20% of the early-onset headache group sought financial compensation. The authors concluded from this observation that an organic basis for the late-acquired posttraumatic headache is difficult to accept.

Relation of Postconcussion Symptoms to Expected Symptoms

Mittenberg and colleagues sought to determine whether postconcussion symptoms are related to patients' expectations of symptoms (47). They presented a 30-symptom checklist to 223 volunteers without a history of head injury and to 100 patients at an average interval of 1.7 years after head injury. The volunteers marked the symptoms they would expect to have 6 months after a motor-vehicle accident, and the patients recorded their current symptoms. No statistically significant group difference was found in the affirmative answers to the symptoms checklist. Also, the answers for the two groups showed significant rank-order correlation. Based on these results, Mittenberg and colleagues concluded that commonly held expectations of postconcussion symptoms play an etiologic role in their development (47). These conclusions seem too strong because (a) presenting a list of symptoms could have biased the volunteers to form their expectations; (b) 19 of 30 items could have led the volunteers to answer "yes" as they began with either forgets or losses; and (3) an awareness of postconcussion symptoms is not a necessary cause to their development.

Synthesis of Ideas about the Etiology of Chronic PTH

To date, the cause of chronic PTH remains unknown. Advances in electrophysiologic, hemodynamic, and neuroimaging techniques are hinging toward establishing an organic etiology for PCS and chronic PTH. Cortical dysfunction with resultant alteration in neuronal threshold for pain, axonal injury with subsequent dysregulation of brainstem nociceptive pathways, and unstable cerebral hemodynamics may provide the basis for the organicity of chronic PTH. The inverse relationship between the severity of the injury and the persistence of chronic symptoms and the psychosocial risk factors outlined in Table 4 speak against the hypothesis of an organic basis for the chronic symptoms that follow a head injury. We believe that an intricate interplay between the physical injury of the brain, however minimal; psychological disturbances generated by the physical and emotional stresses of the accident and perpetuated by persistent individual concerns regarding the injury suffered and the ability to work; and the patient's premorbid disposition all contribute to chronic PTH. The desire for financial compensation may play a role in some cases but not in all.

Pathophysiology of Posttraumatic Migraine

It is fairly accepted that migrainelike headaches develop following MHI (19,50,51). Packard and Ham (50,51) and Solomon (61) drew a parallel between the cascade of events implicated in migraine and those reported with MHI. Neurochemical and hemodynamic factors that may be common to both conditions include (a) cortical spreading depression subsequent to ionic shifts across neuronal membranes or excessive release of excitatory aminoacids, (b) reduced levels of magnesium, (c) increased nitric oxide activity; (d) changes in endogenous opioids, (e) unstable serotonergic or noradrenergic neurotransmission, and (f) cerebral hemodynamic instability. Admittedly, these comparisons are tenuous and await further research before firm conclusions can be drawn.

Sometimes transient hemiparesis and headache are seen following MHI, particularly in children and adolescents. This observation and that of hemiplegic attacks triggered by MHI in patients with familial hemiplegic migraine may point to a genetic susceptibility to posttraumatic migraine, perhaps an inherited channelopathy.

CLINICAL FEATURES

The IHS divides chronic PTH into those associated with significant head trauma and headaches caused by MHI (27).

5.2.1 Chronic posttraumatic headache with significant head trauma and/or confirmatory signs
    A. Significance of head trauma documented by at least one of the following:
        1. Loss of consciousness
        2. Posttraumatic amnesia lasting 10 minutes or longer
        3. At least two of the following exhibit relevant abnormality: clinical neurologic examination, radiography of the skull, neuroimaging, evoked potentials, spinal fluid examination, vestibular function test, neuropsychological testing
    B. Headache occurring 14 days or less after regaining consciousness (or after trauma if there has been no loss of consciousness)
    C. Headache continuing for longer than 8 weeks after regaining consciousness (or after trauma if there has been no loss of consciousness)
5.2.2 Chronic posttraumatic headache with minor head trauma and no confirmatory signs

A. Head trauma that does not satisfy 5.2.1 criterion A
B. Headache occurs less than 14 days after injury
C. Headache continues longer than 8 weeks after injury

The IHS criteria for PTH address the severity of the head trauma, the temporal relationship to the injury, and the duration of the headaches. The clinical features of PTH are considered under a fourth-digit coding. For example, a 5.2.2.1 code represents a patient with chronic PTH following MHI and headaches that fulfill the criteria for migraine. This schema implies that posttraumatic headaches do not have unique features that would distinguish them from primary headaches (e.g., migraine, tension-type headache). Indeed, many headache descriptions have been reported in the literature (Table 5), although Russell argues that the type of headache was remarkably constant among 141 patients interviewed at an average interval of 6 months after their head injuries. It was a dull pain referred to the frontal and temporal regions, often throbbing in nature (56). It was usually worse when the head was lowered, as when the patient went to bed at night, but in many cases it was worse on waking in the morning. It was usually aggravated by physical exertion or by excitement. In some cases, it could be brought on by shaking the head, and in more than a few, it was more noticeable in dull, wet weather. A gradual reduction of the degree of pain was the rule, but in some cases the headaches continued with considerable severity and were seriously incapacitating (56).

Chronic PTH could recur from one to three times a month (44% according to reference 15) to daily (14). One study indicates that the intensity of the pain of PTH is mild in 30%, moderate in 52%, and severe in the remaining 18% of patients (15).

Our clinical experience is in agreement with the observations that PTH has no special clinical features. An exception may be dysautonomic cephalalgia, a condition characterized by unilateral frontotemporal headache and ipsilateral facial sweating and mydriasis after a traumatic injury to the region of the carotid sheath (67).

Features of Posttraumatic Migraines

Posttraumatic migraines, as described by Behrman (5) and by Weiss annd colleagues (70), meet the criteria of the IHS (27) for migraine either with or without aura. Most of the 35 patients reported by Weiss and associates (70) experienced two or three severe throbbing headaches weekly, and ten of these patients had visual symptoms (including scintillating scotoma), hemisensory symptoms, vertigo, or confusion with some attacks. Many patients with posttraumatic migraine also suffer frequent generalized headaches resembling chronic tension-type headaches (70), although some of these headaches might be analgesic-overuse headaches, as suggested by Weeks (69) and Warner and Fenichel (68). The role of analgesic overuse in perpetuating chronic PTH has been challenged, however (24,25,62).

Features of Whiplash Headaches

Headache occurs in 50% to 90% of patients within 1 month of a whiplash injury, and 8% to 30% continue to complain of headache 6 months later (63). Schrader and associates argue that the incidence of headache in an unselected population with WI, outside the medicoloegal context, is similar to that of naturally occurring primary headaches (59).

Similar to chronic PTH, there are no distinguishing features of headache after WI (Table 6). Morning headaches, headaches with features of migraine (with aura, without aura, basilar) or tension-type headache, and cervicogenic headaches all have been described (4,20,29, 63,70,71).

Cervical pain is a prominent symptom of the whiplash syndrome. In a recent review, Stovner reported that neck

TABLE 5. *Clinical descriptions of chronic posttraumatic headache*

Type of headache	Headache classification	References
Any type, and of variable severity, duration, and frequency	Unspecified	10
Chronic scalp muscle contraction (42%); migraine (28%); mixed (12%); others (10%)	1980 Wolff's Headache and Other Head Pain	15
Tension-type (75%); migraine (21%); others (4%)	IHS	24
Chronic daily headache indistinguishable from idiopathic headache	Unspecified	14
Headaches with features similar to those of increased intracranial pressure and spontaneous low pressure	IHS	54,60
Clusterlike	Unspecified	19,52
Temporomandibular joint-related headache	Unspecified	19,52
Supraorbital and infraorbital neuralgia	Unspecified	19
Cervicogenic headache	Unspecified	19
Dysautonomic cephalalgia	Unspecified	67
Analgesic overuse headache	Unspecified	68,69

IHS, International Headache Society.

TABLE 6. *Clinical features of chronic headaches related to whiplash injury*

Features	Descriptors	References
Chronicity	Up to 30% at 6 mo	63
Frequency	Constant in >50%; weekly in 40%	4
Type	Morning headache	4
	Muscle contraction (50%)	4
	Migraine like (with or without aura)	20,29,70,71
	Cervicogenic	4,20,63
	Greater occipital neuralgia	20,42
	Third occipital	7

pain remained the most common chronic symptom (≥6 months) after WI (63). The author emphasized, however, that up to 80% of patients are asymptomatic at that stage. Symptoms of the greater occipital neuralgia type also can follow WI (42). A direct blow to the suboccipital region or an entrapment by the semispinalis capitis is a suggested mechanism of these symptoms (20). Finally, headache after WI can develop in the distribution of the third occipital nerve, hence the term third occipital headache (7). These headaches are associated with C2–3 facet joint tenderness.

Symptoms Associated with Chronic Posttraumatic Headache

Headache is not the only symptom that follows head trauma, although it is the most common. The PCS consists of somatic complaints such as dizziness, blurred vision, anosmia, photophobia and phonophobia, and psychosomatic symptoms such as impaired concentration, memory loss, depression, anxiety, and insomnia (see Table 1). The reported incidence of each of these symptoms varies in relation to the composition of the group studied, the timing of the study, and the method of data collection. In an early study, Russell (56) evaluated 141 patients at an average interval of 6 months after head trauma. Excluding 14 patients who were involved in compensation, the author reported that 32% of the patients complained of PTH since their hospitalization; dizziness, memory loss, and nervousness were present in 24%, 20%, and 20%, respectively (56). Rutherford and colleagues (57) found that 8% of 131 patients were complaining of headache 1 year after MHI. Dizziness and irritability each were reported by 5% of patients, anxiety by 4%, memory loss by 4%, loss of concentration by 3%, insomnia by 2%, and fatigue by 2% (57). Cartlidge and Shaw (11) reported frequencies of posttraumatic symptoms similar to those found by Russell (56) and Rutherford and colleagues (57). Six months after head trauma, headache was the most prevalent symptom, followed by dizziness, depression, anxiety, irritability, impaired con-

centration and memory, and fatigue. When spontaneous symptoms were recorded, headache was present in 9% of the patients, dizziness in 8%, depression in 3%, and anxiety in 2%. On the other hand, as expected, the frequencies of these symptoms were higher on direct questioning; headache was found in 27%, dizziness in 22%, and depression in 18%. Finally, Rimel and associates reported persistent headaches 3 months after MHI in 78% of 424 patients and impaired memory in 59% (55).

Various combinations of the posttraumatic symptoms are observed. Cartlidge and Shaw found that dizziness was equally associated with early-onset and late-onset headaches 6 months after head injury (11). One and 2 years after injury, dizziness appeared more frequently with the early-onset headache group. Dizziness was early or late in onset after MHI, and it did not correlate with the time of onset of headaches. Both depression and anxiety were strongly associated with the late-onset headaches at 6 months, 1 year, and 2 years after head trauma.

Postconcussion Syndrome

Some investigators, such as Kay and associates, consider the PCS as merely a descriptive term (31). Lewin stated that these symptoms (the postconcussion symptoms) have various explanations and do not necessarily occur together (41); he also stated that it is of little service and does not advance the care of the patient to label him or her as suffering from PCS (41). Accord to Rutherford and colleagues, in a syndrome, one expects groupings of interrelated symptoms but found no such groupings (57). Cartlidge and Shaw believed that the syndrome itself was misconceived and that the search for a unitary hypothesis was therefore ill fated (11). They based their view on the observation that their patients symptoms varied markedly, were associated inconstantly, and began after extremely variable posttraumatic intervals. Parker denied the validity of PCS not only as a meaningful constellation of symptoms but also as an entity particular to head injuries (53). He evaluated 750 accident litigants, of whom only 163 had suffered a head injury, and found that individual symptoms and their clustering varied too much to warrant the concept of a syndrome. Also, Parker reported that headache was more prevalent among those who had not sustained a head injury (53). Finally, headache after accidents not causing head or neck injury was common in one series of 82 patients who had sustained back injuries (3).

On the other hand, some investigators believe that PCS is a valid clinical entity (6,34,46). Miller stated that the consistency of the postconcussional syndrome of headache, postural dizziness, irritability, failure of concentration, and intolerance of noise argues a structural or at the least a pathophysiologic basis (46). Binder reached a similar conclusion (6). Also, Kelly referred to the syndrome as a devastating illness (34).

PROGNOSIS

Most patients who report PTH for longer than 8 weeks after the injury continue with these headaches for at least 1 to 2 years (11,19) (see Table 4). Several studies, however, indicate that the prognosis could be improved by thorough individualized treatment programs consisting primarily of preventive medications and psychotherapy (see section entitled Management). Posttraumatic migraines tend to recur for months or years unless they are recognized as migraine and treated appropriately. The success rate of therapy is similar to that for regular migraine (70).

The risk factors detailed in Table 4 not only predict the development of chronic symptoms following head trauma but also may have some prognostic values. Higher levels of education and employment and greater income predict a better chance of return to work (55). Although older age may be a risk factor for the development of chronic PTH, older people are more likely to return to work than younger ones (55). Neuropsychological testing is helpful to evaluate cognitive impairment in patients with PTH but may not predict the extent of recovery following head injury (9).

MANAGEMENT

The treatment of patients with chronic PTH should be individualized (Table 7). Pharmacologic therapies should be specific to the type of headache that the patient suffers. For example, the patient with frequent migraine headaches after head trauma would be treated with prophylactic migraine therapies (discussed elsewhere in this volume), such as beta-blockers, divalproex, or tricyclic antidepressants (TCAs). Randomized, placebo-controlled, and double-blind studies have not been conducted to scientifically establish, or disprove, the value of any pharmacological intervention in chronic PTH. Whereas some nonrandomized, placebo-controlled trials (39,66) indicate that up to 90% of patients with chronic PTH improve with TCAs such as amitriptyline (25–250 mg per day) or maprotyline (25–50 mg per day) (39,66), others failed to demonstrate a benefit with TCAs (amitriptyline) (58). Some physicians advocate the use of nortriptyline

over amitriptyline because of better tolerability of the latter (48). Packard prefers the newer antidepressants (selective serotonin reuptake inhibitors) because of fewer side effects than those associated with the tricyclics and advocates the combination of amitriptyline and propranolol for posttraumatic migraine (52). Finally, Young and colleagues recently reported the benefit of repeated doses of intravenous dihydroergotamine (DHE), similar to the regimen used for refractory nontraumatic headaches, in treating patients with unrelenting PTH (73).

Similar to the case of preventive treatment for chronic PTH, no rigorously performed studies have been done to evaluate the value of commonly used headache-abortive therapies. Analgesics may help symptomatically; their judicious use may prevent rebound headache (68). One study indicated that subcutaneous sumatriptan may be helpful (21).

Posttraumatic greater occipital neuralgia could be treated with greater occipital nerve blocks, nonsteroidal antiinflammatory drugs, muscle relaxants, transcutaneous electrical nerve stimulation, or physical therapy (19). Evans recommends carbamazepine for posttraumatic paroxysms of shooting pain (19).

Kelly drew a connection between treatment in general and symptomatic recovery from his study of 129 patients whose posttraumatic syndrome was the subject of a compensation claim (33,34). Among these patients, persistence of the syndrome correlated with inadequate treatment, often from an unsympathetic physician, whereas recovery correlated with early and continuous treatment. Kelly did not specify what the treatment was, but a brief description of one patient's recovery indicates that it was primarily supportive counseling directed toward a graduated return to full employment. The value of nonpharmacologic therapy for patients with chronic PTH is further supported by a promising recent study (44). Medina provided intensive multifaceted, individualized treatment to 20 patients with disabling daily PTH. Preventive medications (including beta-blockers and antidepressants), education about headache and stress, and biofeedback therapy were the core of the program. Patients were seen one to three times a week for an average of 9 weeks (range, 3—12 weeks). This therapeutic program resulted in improvement in 17 patients (85%) enough to enable them

TABLE 7. *Management of chronic posttraumatic headache (see text for references)*

Treatment	Specific recommendations
Aborting acute pain	Simple or combination analgesics; avoid excessive use that may lead to "rebound" headache. Sumatriptan. Dihydroergotamine for severe and unrelenting pain
Preventative medications	TCAs (amitriptyline, maprotyline, nortriptyline). SSRIs, NSAIDs, muscle relaxants, carbamazepine. amitriptyline, and propranolol
Nonpharmacological therapy	Counseling, education, biofeedback, stress management, physical therapy, occipital nerve blocks, transcutaneous electric stimulation

NSAIDs, nonsteroidal antiinflammatory drugs; SSRIs, selective serotonin uptake inhibitors; TCAs, tricyclic antidepressants.

to return to work within an average of 111 days (range, 21–224 days) (44). These preliminary observations are encouraging and need confirmation in a controlled study.

In summary, the treatment of PTH should be designed for the particular patient. A sympathetic physician, even when financial compensation is an issue, would establish a much needed rapport between the patient and the healer. An honest explanation of the condition and reassurance to the patient that a progressive disease is unlikely may have a calming effect and may prevent repeated, often unnecessary diagnostic testing. Encouraging the gradual resumption of normal activities is indicated. Biofeedback is an innocuous therapy that could be used adjunctively. Symptomatic pain relief with analgesics should be limited and preventative treatments preferentially used. Amitriptyline seems to be a good therapy, particularly when depression is present.

ACKNOWLEDGMENT

The structure and many components of this chapter were adapted from the Chronic Posttraumatic Headache chapter in *The Headaches* (First Edition), which was authored by Dr. D. C. Haas.

REFERENCES

1. Abdel-Dayem HM, Abu-Judeh H, Kumar M, et al. SPECT brain perfusion abnormalities in mild or moderate traumatic brain injury. *Clin Nucl Med* 1998;23:309–317.
2. Andrasik F, Wincze JP. Emotional and psychological aspects of mild head injury. *Semin Neurol* 1994;14:60–66.
3. Balla JI, Moraitis S. Knights in armor: a follow-up study of injuries after legal settlement. *Med J Aust* 1970;2:355–361.
4. Balla J, Karnaghan J. Whiplash headache. *Clin Exp Neurol* 1987;23:179–182.
5. Behrman S. Migraine as a sequella of blunt head injury. *Injury* 1977;9:74–76.
6. Binder LM. Persisting symptoms after mild head injury: a review of the postconcussive syndrome. *J Clin Exp Neuropsychol* 1986;8:323–346.
7. Bogduk N, Marsland A. On the concept of third occipital headache. *J Neurol Neurosurg Psychiatry* 1986;49:775–780.
8. Bohnen N, Twijnstra A, Jolles J. Posttraumatic and emotional symptoms in different subgroups of patients with mild head injury. *Brain Injury* 1992;6:481–487.
9. Bohnen N, Jolles J, Twijnstra A. Neuropsychological deficits in patients with persistent symptoms six months after head injury. *Neurosurgery* 1992;30:692–696.
10. Brenner C, Friedman AP, Merritt HH, Denny-Brown DE. Posttraumatic headache. *J Neurosurg* 1944;1:379–391.
11. Cartlidge NEF, Shaw DA. Posttraumatic headache. In: *Head injury.* London: WB Saunders, 1981:95–154.
12. Chibnall JT, Duckro PN. Posttraumatic stress disorder in chronic post-traumatic headache patients. *Headache* 1994;34:357–361.
13. Cook JB. The post-concussional syndrome and factors influencing recovery after minor head injury admitted to hospital. *Scand J Rehabil Med* 1972;4:27–30.
14. Couch JR, Swann M, Sarah S. Chronic daily headache (CDH) as a result of head injury (HI) and comparison to CDH of idiopathic origin (abstract). *Headache* 1998;38:379.
15. De Benedittis G, De Santis A. Chronic post-traumatic headache: clinical, psychopathological features and outcome determinants. *J Neurosurg Sci* 1983;27:177–186.
16. Drake ME, Weate SJ, Newell SA. Auditory evoked potentials in postconcussive syndrome. *Electromyogr Clin Neurophysiol* 1996;36:457–462.
17. Edna TH, Cappelen J. Late postconcussional symptoms in traumatic head injury. An analysis of frequency and risk factors. *Acta Neurochir* 1987;86:12–17.
18. Evans RW. The postconcussion syndrome and the sequelae of mild head injury. *Neurol Clin* 1992;10:815–847.
19. Evans RW. The postconcussion syndrome and the sequelae of mild head injury. In: Evans RW, ed. *Neurology and trauma.* Philadelphia: WB Saunders, 1996:91–116.
20. Evans RW. Whiplash injuries. In: Evans RW, ed. *Neurology and trauma.* Philadelphia: WB Saunders, 1996:439–457.
21. Gawel MJ, Rothbart P, Jacobs H. Subcutaneous sumatriptan in the treatment of acute episodes of post-traumatic headache. *Headache* 1993;33:96–97.
22. Gilkey SJ, Ramadan NM, Aurora TK, Welch KMA. Cerebral blood flow is abnormal in chronic posttraumatic headache. *Headache* 1997;37:583–587.
23. Haas DC, Lourie T. Trauma-triggered migraine: an explanation for common neurologic attacks following mild head injury. *J Neurosurg* 1988;68:181–188.
24. Haas DC. Chronic posttraumatic headaches classified and compared with natural headaches. *Cephalalgia* 1996;16:486–493.
25. Haas DC. Posttraumatic headache [Letter to the Editor]. *Neurology* 1997;47:1735.
26. Ham LP, Andrasik F, Packard RC, Bundrick CM. Psychopathology in individuals with posttraumatic headache and other pain types. *Cephalalgia* 1994;14:118–126.
27. Headache Classification Committee of the International Headache Society. Classification and diagnostic criteria for headache disorders, cranial neuralgias and facial pain. *Cephalalgia* 1988;8(Suppl 7):1–96.
28. Hickling EG, Alanchard EG, Schwartz SP, et al. Headaches and motor vehicle accidents: results of the psychological treatment of post-traumatic headache. *Headache Quarterly* 1992;3:285–289.
29. Jacome DE. Basilar artery migraine after uncomplicated whiplash injuries. *Headache* 1986;26:515–516.
30. Jensen OK, Nielsen FF. The influence of sex and pre-traumatic headache on the incidence and severity of headache after head injury. *Cephalalgia* 1990;10:285–293.
31. Kay DWK, Kerr TA, Lassman LP. Brain trauma and the post-concussional syndrome. *Lancet* 1971;2:1052–1055.
32. Keidel M, Diener HC. Post-traumatic headache. *Nervenartzt* 1997;68:769–777.
33. Kelly R. The post-traumatic syndrome: an iatrogenic disease. *Forensic Sci Int* 1975;6:17–24.
34. Kelly R. Posttraumatic headache. In: Rose FC, ed. *Handbook of clinical neurology.* Amsterdam: Elsevier, 1985:48:383–390.
35. Kelly R. The post-traumatic syndrome. *J R Soc Med* 1981;74:242–245.
36. Kelly R, Smith BN. Post-traumatic syndrome: another myth discredited. *J R Soc Med* 1981;74:275–277.
37. Keshavan MS, Channabasavanna SM, Narayana Reddy GN. Post-traumatic psychiatric disturbances: patterns and predictors of outcome. *Br J Psychiatry* 1981;138:157–160.
38. Kraus JF, Nourjah P. The epidemiology of mild uncomplicated brain injury. *J Trauma* 1988;28:1637–1643.
39. Label LS. Treatment of post-traumatic headache: maprotiline or amitriptyline? (abstract). *Neurology* 1991;41 (Suppl 1):247.
40. Lanser JBK, Jennekens-Schinkel A, Peters ACB. Headache after closed head injury in children. *Headache* 1988;28:176–179.
41. Lewin W. Rehabilitation needs of the brain-injured patient. *Proc R Soc Med* 1970;63:28–32.
42. Magnusson T. Extracervical symptoms after whiplash injury. *Cephalalgia* 1994;14:223–227.
43. McClelland RJ, Fenton GW, Rutherford W. The postconcussion syndrome revisited. *J R Soc Med* 1994;87:508–510.
44. Medina JL. Efficacy of an individualized outpatient program in the treatment of chronic post-traumatic headache. *Headache* 1992;32:180–183.
45. Miller H. Accident neurosis. *BMJ* 1961;1:919–925, 992–998.
46. Miller H. Posttraumatic headache. In: Vinken PJ, Bruyn GW, eds. *Handbook of clinical neurology.* Amsterdam: North-Holland, 1968:178–184.
47. Mittenberg W, DiGiulio DV, Perrin S, Bass AE. Symptoms following mild head injury: expectation as etiology. *J Neurol Neurosurg Psychiatry* 1992;55:200–204.
48. Moore KL. Headache associated with head trauma. *Neurobase*, 3rd ed. San Diego: Arbor Publishing Co., 1997.

49. Packard RC. Posttraumatic headache: permanency and relationship to legal settlement. *Headache* 1992;32:496–500.
50. Packard RC, Ham LP. Posttraumatic headache: determining chronicity. *Headache* 1993;33:133–134.
51. Packard RC, Ham LP. Pathogenesis of posttraumatic headache and migraine: a common headache pathway. *Headache* 1997;37:142–152.
52. Packard RC. Mechanisms of injury and headache type. *Seminars in Headache Management* 1997;2:1–13.
53. Parker N. Accident litigants with neurotic symptoms. *Med J Aust* 1977; 2:318–322.
54. Ramadan NM. Headache caused by raised intracranial pressure and intracranial hypotension. *Curr Opin Neurol* 1996;9:214–218.
55. Rimel RW, Giordani B, Barth JT, Boll TJ, Jane JA. Disability caused by minor head injury. *Neurosurgery* 1981;9:221–228.
56. Russell WR. Cerebral involvement in head injury: a study based on the examination of 200 cases. *Brain* 1932;55:549–603.
57. Rutherford WH, Merrett JD, McDonald JR. Symptoms at one year following concussion from minor head injuries. *Injury* 1979;10: 225–230.
58. Saran A. Antidepressants not effective in headache associated with minor closed head injury. *Int J Psychiatry Med* 1988;18:75–83.
59. Schrader H, Obelieniene D, Bovim G, Surkiene D, Miseviciene I, Sand T. Natural evolution of late whiplash syndrome outside the medicolegal context. *Lancet* 1996;347:1207–1211.
60. Silberstein SD, Marcelis J. Headache associated with changes in intracranial pressure. *Headache* 1992;32:84–94.
61. Solomon S. Chronic posttraumatic headache. In: Mathew NT, ed. *Headaches in adults.* Minneapolis: American Academy of Neurology, 1998:8FC.004-81–8FC.004-88.
62. Sternberg PE. Posttraumatic headache [Letter to the Editor]. *Neurology* 1997;47:1735.
63. Stovner LJ. The nosologic status of the whiplash syndrome: a critical review based on a methodological approach. *Spine* 1996;21:2735–2746.
64. Taylor AR. Post-concussional sequelae. *BMJ* 1967;3:67–71.
65. Tsushima WT, Newbill W. Effects of headache during neuropsychological testing of mild head injury patients. *Headache* 1996;36:613–615.
66. Tyler GS, McNeely HE, Dick ML. Treatment of post-traumatic headache with amitriptyline. *Headache* 1980;20:213–216.
67. Vijayan N. A new post-traumatic headache syndrome. *Headache* 1977; 17:19–22.
68. Warner JS, Fenichel GM. Chronic posttraumatic headache often a myth? *Neurology* 1996;46:915–916.
69. Weeks RE. Analgesic overuse/rebound: a treatment variable and not an outcome variable. *Headache* 1991;32:157–158.
70. Weiss HD, Stern BJ, Goldberg J. Post-traumatic migraine: chronic migraine precipitated by minor head or neck trauma. *Headache* 1991; 31:451–456.
71. Winston KR. Whiplash and its relation to migraine. *Headache* 1987;27: 452–457.
72. Yamaguchi M. Incidence of headache and severity of head injury. *Headache* 1992;32:427–431.
73. Young WB, Hopkins MM, Janyszek B, Primavera JP. Repetitive intravenous DHE in the treatment of refractory posttraumatic headache (abstract). *Headache* 1994;34:297.

The Headaches, Second Edition,
edited by J. Olesen, P. Tfelt-Hansen, and K.M.A. Welch.
Lippincott Williams & Wilkins, Philadelphia © 2000.

The Secondary Headaches

CHAPTER 104

Headache Associated with Ischemic Stroke and Intracranial Hematoma

Troels Staehelin Jensen and Philip B. Gorelick

The occurrence of headache in vascular disorders has been known for centuries. Headache in cerebrovascular disease was described by Thomas Willis in 1664 and, according to Edmeads (10), has been described several times by others, for example, Richard Bright, Sir Charles Symonds, and Miller Fisher (7,13,40). Because stroke is so common (the third leading cause of death in the Western world) and headache may be a presenting feature of stroke, it is important to understand headache in ischemic and hemorrhagic stroke.

Headache may be an important but often neglected symptom of stroke, probably because it is overshadowed by other dramatic symptoms, such as hemiplegia, hemianopia, aphasia, and cognitive dysfunction. The importance of headache in ischemic stroke is apparent in the fact that headache not only may accompany or follow stroke, but it also may precede the apoplectic episode by days or even weeks (5,8,17,41). Headaches associated with stroke are also important to recognize because this symptom may be a warning of a serious, life-threatening condition.

This chapter reviews headache that follows ischemic stroke, transient cerebral ischemia, intracerebral hematoma, and epidural and subdural hematoma.

T. S. Jensen: Department of Neurology F, Århus Kommunehospital, DK-8000 Århus C, Denmark.

P. B. Gorelick: Department of Neurological Sciences, Rush University Medical College, and Center for Stroke Research, Chicago, Illinois 60612.

HEADACHE IN ISCHEMIC CEREBROVASCULAR DISEASE

IHS code and diagnosis: 6.1 Headache associated with acute cerebrovascular disease. 6.1.1 Transient cerebral ischemia; 6.1.2 Thromboembolic stroke.

WHO code and diagnosis: 44.81. Headache associated with other vascular disorders.

Short description: Headache occurring in close connection with transient cerebral ischemia, or ischemic stroke.

The reported frequency of headache in ischemic cerebrovascular disease varies considerably from one study to another. The type of stroke, study design, and populations are some of the variables that may explain the different figures obtained in previous studies. It appears that headache is most common in large-artery occlusive disease but less common in lacunar infarction. In addition, headache is more common with stroke in the vertebrobasilar circulation compared with stroke in the carotid circulation.

Epidemiology

The reported frequency of headache in ischemic vascular disease varies among studies, most of which are retrospective studies and represent selected cases. Table 1 shows the frequency of headache in cerebral infarction, including lacunar infarcts. The study populations and data collection methods from which the frequency data in Table 1 were determined differ from one study to the next. Mohr and colleagues (32) reported data originating

TABLE 1. *Frequency of headache in cerebral infarction, lacunar stoke, and intracerebral hematoma in selected studies*

Study (reference)	Year of publication	Frequency of headache (%)		
		Large cerebral infarction	Lacunar infarction	Intracerebral hematoma
Mohr et al. (32)	1978	11[a]	3	33
Portenoy et al. (36)	1985	29	17	57
Gorelick et al. (17)	1986	17	6	55
Koudstaal et al. (23)	1991	29	13	—[b]
Vestergaard et al. (41)	1993	26	15	50
Jørgensen et al. (19)	1994	25	—[b]	49
Arboix et al. (3)	1994	32	23	65
Ferro et al. (12)	1995	34	7–9	—[b]
Kumral et al. (24)	1995	16	9	36
Melo et al. (31)	1996	—[b]	—[b]	57

[a]Includes cases with large artery thrombosis and cerebral emboli.
[b]No figures available.

from a stroke register that included referral hospitals in Boston, and Gorelick and associates (17) used data derived from a stroke register at two inner-city referral hospitals in Chicago. In the latter two studies, the stroke registry questionnaires served as the means for ascertaining information about headache characteristics in stroke. Portenoy and co-workers' (36) data were from consecutive patients who experienced cerebrovascular events at two teaching hospitals in New York City, and the data reported by Koudstaal and colleagues (23) were from patients entered into the Dutch TIA (transient ischemia attack) Trial. The study by Vestergaard aand colleagues (41) was a community-based, prospective study of 25- to 80-year-old people. The study by Jørgensen and associates (19) was also a community-based, prospective study, but it was not designed primarily for headache assessment. On the basis of the few prospective studies that have been reported, the frequency of headache in cerebral infarction is in the order of 25%.

Pathophysiology of Pain in Stroke

The cause of headache in ischemic stroke and transient cerebral ischemia (TIA) is not clear; however, knowledge about the physiology of pain in migraine and tension-type headache has provided important information about underlying mechanisms (34).

The nociceptive innervation of the meninges and the intracranial vasculature originates from the trigeminal system (see Chapter 127), but the brain itself is devoid of nociceptive innervation. Several clinical findings (Table 2) suggest that the pain in ischemic vascular disorders is related to the specific innervation of the brain and the cerebral vascular system: (a) headache is more common in patients with vertebrobasilar stroke than in patients with carotid stroke and is consistent with a more dense trigeminovascular innervation of the posterior circulation; (b) according to some, but not all, studies, headache is more common in major than in minor strokes; (c) it is

also more common with cortical than with subcortical lesions, the latter of which has a less dense trigeminal innervation; (d) according to most studies, headache is ipsilateral to the lesion, suggesting that the pain originates from or in the vicinity of the lesion and in ipsilateral trigeminal innervation (38). Exactly how the trigeminal system is activated is not clear. We have suggested that the heavy nociceptive innervation of the posterior circulation may play a role in the higher frequency of headache in stroke confined to the posterior circulation (41). Furthermore, it has been suggested that ipsilateral headaches are related to ipsilateral activation of nociceptive fibers in the vicinity of the cerbral lesion (41). This idea was later also proposed by Jørgensen et al. (19) in their multivariate analysis of 867 stroke patients in Copenhagen.

TABLE 2. *Factors associated with headache in stroke*

Factor	Yes (references)	No (references)
More frequent in women	19,31,36	24,41
Related to age	19,24,31,41	
More frequent on side of brain injury	17,19,31,41	
More frequent in posterior than anterior stroke	19,23,24,31, 42	17
More frequent in major than in minor stroke	19,23,24,26, 27,31,41	
More frequent in cortical than subcortical stroke	19,23,27,31, 42	17,19
Headache more frequent in hemorrhagic than ischemic stroke	17,19,23,24, 42	
More frequent in stroke patients with heart disease	19,23,28	24,41
More frequent in smokers		24,41
More frequent in migraineurs	24	19,41
Relation between infarct size and headache severity		19,41

Along these lines, it has been suggested that headache is due to dilatation of pain-sensitive vessels induced by the release of vasoactive substances such as substance P, calcitonin gene-related peptide (CGRP), and other peptides from nerve terminals, which together with cytokines, nitrogen oxide released from tissue, and bradykinins released from vessels contribute to an increased nociceptive input to the nervous system (9) and hence pain.

Study of release products from nerve terminals, tissue, and vasculature in vascular headache represents a way to increase our understanding of the pathophysiology of headache in stroke. Research on the trigeminal and the sympathetic and the parasympathetic innervation of intracranial vessels has provided considerable new insight into the role of neurotransmitters in migraine and cluster headache (for review see reference 11). These studies have shown that there is an association between release of CGRP and headache. Further research into release of CGRP and other chemical transmitters in secondary headaches holds promise for elucidating the mechanism of headache in ischemic cerebrovascular disease.

Clinical Features

The IHS diagnostic criteria for headache associated with acute ischemic cerebrovascular disease (Headache Classification Committee, 1988):

A. Focal central nervous system symptoms or signs developed within 48 hours.
B. Appropriate investigations indicate acute ischemic vascular disorder.

Headache as a new symptom or of a new type occurs in close temporal relation to onset of the vascular disorder. In transient ischemic attacks (6.1.1), central nervous system symptoms clear within 24 hours, whereas in thromboembolic stroke (6.1.2) symptoms persist longer than 24 hours.

Location

It is debated whether the location of headache provides useful information about the vascular site and mechanism in ischemic cerebrovascular disease. Fisher (13) noted that lateralized headache accompanying carotid artery occlusion usually was located in the ipsilateral frontal region and involved the forehead or eye. In middle cerebral artery thrombosis, pain was located behind, in, and above the corresponding eye; and in middle cerebral artery embolism, the pain was above the temple. In one of our studies (17), lateralized onset headache in internal carotid artery occlusive disease and middle cerebral artery embolism was located in the orbit or frontal region, whereas onset headache in middle cerebral artery thrombosis was nonlateralized in some cases. Portenoy and colleagues (36) found that headache location did not vary

with the type of vascular event and did not predict the location of stroke, and the incidence of headache did not differ significantly between cerebrovascular events in the anterior or posterior circulations. Koudstaal and colleagues (23) found that patients with cortical infarcts on cranial computed tomography (CT) more frequently had headaches than those with small, deep infarcts. Similar findings were noted by Vestergaard and associates (41). Furthermore, in their study, headache was more frequent with infarcts in the posterior circulation than with those confined to the anterior circulation, even after accounting for a lower frequency of small, deep infarcts in the posterior circulation. Jørgensen and co-workers (17) found that 37% with posterior infarcts had headache, whereas 26% with infarcts in the carotid circulation had headache. Most studies show that in lacunar infarction headache is rare (10,17,23,26,32,36,41).

Intensity and Quality

Usually, the pain in ischemic vascular disease is described as dull and throbbing, but there is a relative paucity of information about the quality of headache. In contrast to subarachnoid hemorrhage and intraparenchymal hemorrhage, in which the intensity of head pain or discomfort is reported as severe (13), the headache intensity in ischemic stroke ranges from barely noticeable to mild or moderate (10). Headache severity is not related to the size of the infarction but is more severe in posterior infarcts than in those localized in the anterior circulation (41). Portenoy and co-workers (36) found that about 50 % of onset headaches were throbbing, with no distinction by lesion type or location. In the study by Koudstaal and colleagues (23), the nature of headache was mostly continuous and not throbbing, regardless of the main symptom or findings on CT. In the study by Vestergaard and associates (41), most patients had a pressing headache, some had throbbing, and some had a stabbing pain. By classifying headache according to IHS criteria, these authors found that the most common type was a tension-type headache (49%), whereas 28% had a migraine-like headache.

Transient Ischemic Attacks (TIA)

Headache may occur in association with TIA. The reported frequency in TIA ranges from 6% to 44% (13,17,18,23,25,30). In a retrospective study, Grindal and Toole (18) reviewed medical records of 240 TIA patients and concluded that (a) there were no distinguishing demographic or medical risk factors or arteriographic or prognostic features among patients whose TIAs were accompanied by headache compared with those without headache; (b) frontal headache was more characteristic of carotid-territory TIA, whereas occipital-nuchal headache was more common in vertebrobasilar TIA; (c) nonlocalized headache occurred frequently in both carotid and vertebrobasilar territory TIAs; (d) headache usually accompanied or followed TIA but rarely preceded other neurologic symptoms, and the character and duration of pain did not differ remarkably between the carotid and vertebrobasilar territories; (e) headache was more likely to be a constant feature in cases with more than one vertebrobasilar TIA; and (f) headache was sometimes reported in amaurosis fugax and subclavian steal syndrome. In amaurosis fugax, pain was localized to the orbit of the affected eye in three patients, described as severe and stabbing in two, and localized to the ipsilateral temporal region and generalized in one.

Loeb and colleagues (25) reported headache in 30% of 90 patients with TIA, and headache was more common in vertebrobasilar than in carotid TIAs. Medina and associates (30) studied 34 TIA patients who had follow-up for 1 to 24 months. Of these 34 patients, 22 had carotid-territory TIA, and 12 had vertebrobasilar TIA. Episodic headaches occurred during, immediately before, or after TIA in 15 patients. Episodic headaches lasted an average of 2 hours, were of mild or moderate intensity, and when associated with carotid-territory TIA were usually unilateral and frontal and described as throbbing or pressure-like. A second type of headache, late-onset vascular headaches, started in middle or late life, occurred independently of TIA, and preceded TIA in 38% of patients.

In carotid TIA, Gorelick and associates (17) observed onset headache in 6%, and in each case it was ipsilateral to the symptomatic vessel site and of mild or moderate severity. In the series by Loeb and associates (25), onset headache occurred in 13%. In 7%, headache followed the neurologic symptoms, and in 10% headache was a prodromal symptom of TIA.

Koudstaal and colleagues (23) reported headache in 16% of all patients with TIA and in 16% of patients with transient monocular blindness. These findings are in contrast to the those of Fisher and co-workers (14), who found that either none or only one of 58 patients with amaurosis fugax had headache (13,16). Furthermore, Koudstaal and co-workers (23) found no relationship between the occurrence of headache and the nature of the visual symptoms.

In summary, for large infarcts, headache occurs in approximately 20% to 25% and is usually ipsilateral to the symptomatic vascular territory. Headache is generally less common when in association with TIA but may be more common when TIAs are in the vertebrobasilar than in the carotid circulation.

Sentinel Headache

Premonitory headache, also termed *sentinel headache*, which is a well-known feature in aneurysmal subarachnoid hemorrhage (5,8,22), also has been described in association with cerebral ischemic stroke or TIA. Airing and Merritt (1) noted premonitory symptoms that included headache in patients with cerebral embolism. Wells (43) reported that headache was the most common premonitory symptom in cerebral embolism. It occurred unilaterally on the side of subsequent cerebral infarction and within hours of infarction in many patients. Premonitory headache also was reported by Fisher and co-workers (14) and by Mohr and colleagues (35) as occurring in large-artery occlusive disease.

In the study by Gorelick and colleagues (17), premonitory headache occurred in 10% of 151 ischemic stroke patients. It was usually unilateral, focal, and lasted longer than 24 hours. Portenoy and co-workers (36) reported that 11% of their study patients had a history of episodic throbbing headache, and Vestergaard and associates (41) found that 43% had headache preceding stroke and that in 13% the headache began more than 3 days before the stroke.

The relationship between migraine or periodic headache and aneurysm or ischemic stroke was reviewed in detail by Fisher (13,15), and Edmeads (10). It was concluded by consensus that typical periodic headache or migraine occurring years before the detection of aneurysm or ischemic stroke is probably independent of the stroke mechanism. Most headaches that precede hemorrhagic or ischemic stroke by a reasonably short time, however, are thought to be related to cerebrovascular disease (13).

Relation of Headache in Ischemic Cerebrovascular Disease to Other Factors

Koudstaal and colleagues (23) prospectively studied headache features in 3,126 patients with acute cerebral ischemia or retinal ischemia who entered a multicenter treatment trial. The aim of the study was to relate the occurrence and nature of headache to the presence of vascular risk factors, the probable site of origin of the neurologic symptoms, the time course of the attack, and the CT findings. The key results were that (a) patients with headache had ischemic heart disease more frequently; (b) headache was less frequent in patients with hypertension, small deep infarcts, and infarcts in the anterior circulation, but it was more frequent in patients with cortical infarcts and infarcts in the posterior circulation; and (c) headache occurrence was not related to the mode of onset, mode of disappearance, duration of the attack, or gender. Portenoy and colleagues (36), however, reported that of patients with cerebrovascular disease, women developed headache more often than men. Similar findings were reported Jørgensen and colleagues (19), whereas Kumral and associates (24) found that men complained of headache more frequently. Table 2 summarizes factors that have been or have not been associated with headache in both ischemic and hemorrhagic stroke.

TABLE 3. *Headache and other characteristics predictive of stroke subtype*

Stroke subtype	Predictor variables[a]
Subarachnoid hemorrhage	Onset headache Vomiting Younger age
Intraparenchymal hemorrhage	Onset headache Higher systolic and diastolic blood pressures
Ischemic stroke	Absence of onset headache Absence of vomiting Lower systolic blood pressures Older age

[a]Determined by stepwise logistic regression analysis. From ref. 17, with permission.

Headache and Other Characteristics as Predictors of Stroke Subtype

An important question relates to the prediction of stroke subtype based on headache and other clinical characteristics. Gorelick and associates (17) explored this issue by using logistic regression analysis and categoric data-modeling techniques. By stepwise logistic regression analysis, it was shown that (Table 3) (a) onset headache, vomiting, and younger age were factors that favored a diagnosis of subarachnoid hemorrhage; (b) onset headache and higher systolic and diastolic blood pressures favored a diagnosis of intraparenchymal hemorrhage; and (c) the absence of onset headache, lower systolic blood pressure, absence of vomiting, and older age favored a diagnosis of ischemic stroke. By categoric data-modeling techniques, it was shown that (a) the joint absence of onset headache, vomiting, and sentinel headache was predictive of ischemic stroke; (b) the joint presence of vomiting and onset headache was predictive of subarachnoid hemorrhage; and (c) vomiting in the absence of either sentinel headache or onset headache was predictive of intracerebral hemorrhage. In contrast, Portenoy and colleagues (36) concluded that neither the occurrence of headache nor its characteristics predicted lesion type or location.

HEADACHE IN INTRACEREBRAL HEMATOMA, SUBDURAL HEMATOMA, AND EPIDURAL HEMATOMA

Intracerebral Hematoma

IHS code and diagnosis: 6.2.1 Headache associated with intracerebral hematoma.
WHO code and diagnosis: Headache associated with other vascular disorders.

The following discussion of headache in intracerebral hematoma is limited to hemorrhages in the brain paren-chyma. Headache associated with subarachnoid hemorrhage is reviewed in Chapter 105.

Epidemiology

The frequency of headache in intracerebral hematoma varies from 8% to 80% of patients (1,2–4,6,13,17,19,20, 24,32,36,39,41), depending on both the type of study and the anatomic location of the hematoma. Table 1 summarizes the frequency of headache in intraparenchymal hemorrhage in a series of recent studies. Headache frequency is higher than in ischemic stroke, and the frequency is highest in cerebellar and occipital lobar hemorrhages (10,27,31,41). Overall, most studies report a headache frequency in the range of 40% to 60%. When the intraparenchymal hemorrhage is small, headache may not be present.

Pathophysiology

As for ischemic stroke, the mechanism underlying headache is not exactly known. It is commonly held that headache in intraparenchymal hemorrhage and extracerebral hemorrhage is related to the blood mass that causes local distention, distortion, deformation, or stretching of pain-sensitive intracranial structures (10,31). The organization of the trigeminovascular system explains the ipsilateral and sometimes bilateral location of pain and the high frequency of headacahe in occipital and cerebellar heamatomas (33).

Clinical Features

IHS diagnostic criteria for headache associated with intracranial hematoma (Headache Classification Committee, 1988)

A. Focal central nervous system symptoms or signs developed within 24 hours
B. Intracerebral hematoma diagnosed by appropriate investigations
C. Headache as a new symptom or of a new type occurs in close temporal relation to the neurologic symptoms

Ropper and Davis (39) found that the location and features of headache might be useful in identifying specific lobar hematoma sites. In a series of 289 intracerebral hematomas, Melo and associates (31) found that headache was significantly more common on the hematoma side than contralaterally and that occipital headache usually was associated with cerebellar or occipital hematomas. Headache is reported to be more frequent in lobar heamatomas than in basal-ganglia heamatomas (27).

Several studies have reported the presence of premonitory (sentinel) headache in intraparenchymal hemorrhage (17) and occurred in 14% of patients with intraparenchymal hemorrhage (19). However, its pathophysiology and significance remain to be clarified. According to Melo and associates (31), meningeal signs, a posterior location, transtentorial herniation, and female gender can predict headache in intracerebral haematoma (Table 4).

Subdural Hematoma

IHS code and diagnosis: 6.2.2 Headache associated with subdural hematoma.
WHO code and diagnosis: 44.81 Headache associated with other vascular disorders.

Epidemiology

Headache is a frequent accompaniment of subdural hematoma (29,37). In 100 consecutive patients with subdural hematoma who were examined by a neurosurgical service, Voris (42) reported that 62 had headache. A definite history of antecedent head injury was found in 96 patients, and the time between the injury and operation ranged from a few hours to 6 months. In McKissock's review of 389 cases of subdural hematoma (29), which included 82 acute, 91 subacute, and 216 chronic hematomas, 231 patients had headache. Headache occurred in nine of 82 patients (11%) with acute subdural hematoma, 48 of 91 patients (53%) with subacute hematoma, and 174 of 216 patients (81%) with chronic hematoma. As in other reports, the frequency of patients in McKissock's (29) series with disturbances of consciousness was substantial. Accordingly, ascertainment of headache may be difficult, and the proportions reported may be underestimated.

Clinical Features

Although headache is a prominent feature of subdural hematoma, no headache features can differentiate an acute subdural hematoma from cerebral contusion or laceration. Kelly (21) concluded that headache associated with subdural hematoma does not differ from that seen with other space-occupying lesions. Headache can be paroxysmal, irregular, and occur on and off throughout the day, sometimes lasting only a few minutes at a time

TABLE 4. *Predictors of headache in intracerebral haematoma*

Predictor[a]
Meningeal signs
Cerebellar or lobar hematoma localisation
Transtentorial herniation
Female gender
Age <70 yr

[a]Determined by multiple logistic regression analysis.
From ref. 31, with permission.

and accompanied by autonomic symptoms. Headache in subdural hematoma may be moderate or mild, but it is often reported as persistent and troublesome. In some patients with chronic subdural hematoma, headache may not elicit any attention from patients or from their relatives.

In McKissock's series (29), 19 patients gave a clear history of unilateral headache, and in all these patients the subdural hematoma was ipsilateral to the headache. In patients with frontoparietal hematomas, headaches usually are referred to the same region, whereas subdural hematomas in the posterior fossa causes occipital headache and neck stiffness.

Epidural Hematoma

IHS code and diagnosis: 6.2.3 Headache associated with epidural hematoma.
WHO code and diagnosis: 44.81 Headache associated with other vascular disorders.

Headache may be a prominent and early symptom associated with an epidural hematoma (21). This type of extracerebral hematoma may be associated with an asymptomatic, lucid interval following head injury. After the lucid interval, headache may reappear, with disturbances of consciousness and focal neurologic symptoms and signs. Headache may be due to separation of the dura from the skull, with stretching and distortion of pain-sensitive vascular structures.

TREATMENT

In general, headache associated with stroke is self-limited or responds to surgical treatment when there is intracranial hemorrhage, and when surgical intervention (e.g., hematoma evacuation, shunting in hydrocephalus) is used as the primary treatment for the hemorrhage. Data about the treatment of headache in ischemic and hemorrhagic stroke is scarce. Ischemic stroke patients with headache may respond to mild analgesics, including aspirin, acetaminophen, nonsteroidal antitinflammatory drugs (NSAIDs). When severe head pain is associated with stroke, more centrally acting analgesics may be necessary; however, adverse effects of these agents, including nausea, respiratory depression, increased cerebrospinal fluid pressure, and alteration of mental status, may occur, especially in elderly patients. Thus, these agents should be administered only with careful scrutiny. Aspirin and other antiplatelet agents are contraindicated in intracranial hemorrhage.

REFERENCES

1. Airing CD, Merritt HH. Differential diagnosis between cerebral hemorrhage and cerebral thrombosis: a clinical and pathological study of 245 cases. *Arch Intern Med* 1935;56:435–456.
2. Anderson CS, Chakera TMH, Stewart-Wynne EG, Jamrozik KD. Spec-

trum of primary intracerebral haemorrhage in Perth, Western Australia, 1989–90: incidence and outcome. *J Neurol Neurosurg Psychiatry* 1994; 57:936–940.

3. Arboix A, Massons J, Oliveres M, Arribas MP, Titus F. Headache in acute cerebrovascular disease: a prospective clinical study in 240 patients. *Cephalalgia* 1994;14:37–40.

4. Auerbach SH, Butler RB, Levine HL. Headache in cerebral embolism. *Stroke* 1981;12:367–369.

5. Ball MJ. Pathogenesis of the sentinel headache preceding berry aneurysm rupture. *Can Med Assoc J* 1975;112:78–79.

6. Barraquer-Bordas L, Illa I, Escartin A, Ruscalleda J, Marti-Valalta JL. Thalamic hemorrhage: a study of 23 patients with diagnosis by computed tomography. *Stroke* 1981;12:524–527.

7. Bright R. Cases illustrative of the effects produced when the arteries of the brain are diseased, selected chiefly with a view to the diagnosis in such affections. *Guy's Hospital Reports* 1836;1:9–40.

8. Calvert JM. Premonitory symptoms and signs of subarachnoid hemorrhage. *Med J Aust* 1966;1:651–657.

9. Dray A. Agonists and antagonists of nociception. In: Jensen TS, Turner JA, Wiesenfeld-Hallin Z, eds. *Proceedings of the 8th* World Congress on Pain, *Progress in Pain Research and Management*, vol 8, Seattle: IASP Press, 1997:279–292.

10. Edmeads J. Headache in cerebrovascular disease: In: Vinken PJ, Bruyn GW, Klawans HL, eds. *Handbook of clinical neurology: headache.* New York: Elsevier, 1986:273–290.

11. Edvinsson L, Goadsby PJ. Neuropeptides in headache. *Eur J Neurol* 1998;5:329–341.

12. Ferro JM, Melo TP, Oliveiro AV, Crespo M, Canhao P, Pinto AN. A multivariate study of headache associated with ischemic stroke. *Headache* 1995;35:315–319.

13. Fisher CM. Headache in acute cerebrovascular disease: In: Vinken PJ, Bruyn GW, eds. *Handbook of clinical neurology, headaches and cranial neuralgias*, vol 5. New York: John Wiley and Sons, 1968:124–156.

14. Fisher CM, Picard EH, Polak A, Dalal P, Ojemann RG. Acute hypertensive cerebellar hemorrhage: diagnosis and surgical treatment. *J Nerve Ment Dis* 1965;140:38–57.

15. Franke CL, van Swieten JC, Algra A, van Gijn J. Prognostic factors in patients with intracebral haematoma. *J Neurol Neurosurg Psychiatry* 1992;55:653–657.

16. Goodwin J, Gorelick PB, Helgason Cm. Symptoms of amaurosis fugax in atherosclerotic carotid artery disease. *Neurology* 1987;37:829–823.

17. Gorelick PB, Hier DB, Caplan LR, Langenberg P. Headache in acute cerebrovascular disease. *Neurology* 1986;36:1445–1450.

18. Grindal A, Toole JF. Headache and transient ischemic attacks. *Stroke* 1974;5:603–606.

19. J rgensen HS, Jespersen HF, Nakayama H, Raaschou HO, Olsen TS. Headache in stroke: the Copenhagen stroke study. *Neurology* 1994;44:1793–1797.

20. Kase CS, Williams JP, Wyatt DA, Mohr JP. Lobar intracerebral hematomas: clinical and CT analysis of 22 cases. *Neurology* 1982;32:1146–1150.

21. Kelly R. Headache after cranial trauma. In: Hopkins A, ed. Headache. *Problems in diagnosis and management.* Philadelphia: WB Saunders, 1988:1–220.

22. King RB, Saba MI. Forewarnings of major subarachnoid hemorrhage. *NY State J Med* 1974;74:638–639.

23. Koudstaal PJ, van Gijn J, Kappelle LJ, for the Dutch TIA Study Group. Headache in transient or permanent cerebral ischemia. *Stroke* 1991;22:754–759.

24. Kumral E, Bogousslavsky J, Melle GV, Regli F, Pierre P. Headache at stroke onset: the Lausanne Stroke Registry. *J Neurol Neurosurg Psychiatry* 1995;58:490–492.

25. Loeb C, Gandolfo C, Dall`Agata D. Headache in transient ischemic attacks (TIA). *Cephalalgia* 1985;5(Suppl 2):17–19.

26. Loeb C, Gandolfo C, Dall`Agata D. Headache in lacunar syndromes: a very unusual symptom. *Stroke* 1986;17:777–778.

27. Massaro AD, Sacco RL, Mohr JP, et al. Clinical discriminators of lobar and deep hemorrhages: the Stroke Data Bank. *Neurology* 1991;41:1881–1885.

28. McDowell FH. Cerebral embolism. In: Vinken PJ, Bruyn GW, eds. *Handbook of clinical neurology:* vascular diseases of the nervous system, vol 11. New York: Elsevier, 1972:386–404.

29. McKissock W. Subdural hematoma: a review of 389 cases. *Lancet* 1960;1:1365–1370.

30. Medina J, Diamond S, Rubino FA. Headache in patients with transient ischemic attacks. *Headache* 1975;15:194–197.

31. Melo TP, Pinto AN, Ferro JM. Headache in intracerebral hematomas. *Neurology* 1996;47:494–500.

32. Mohr JP, Caplan LR, Melski JW, et al. The Harvard Cooperative Stroke Registry: a prospective registry. *Neurology* 1978;28:754–762.

33. Moskowitz MA. The neurobiology of vascular head pain. *Ann Neurol* 1984;16:157–168.

34. Olesen J. Clinical and pathophysiological observations in migraine and tension-type headache explained by vascular, supraspinal and myofascial inputs. *Pain* 1991;46:125–132.

35. Okawara S-H. Warning signs prior to a rupture of an intracranial aneurysm. *J Neurosurg* 1973;38:575–580.

36. Portenoy RK, Abissi CJ, Lipton RB. Headache in cerebrovascular disease. *Stroke* 1984;15:1009–1012.

37. Putnam TJ, Cushing H. Chronic subdural hematoma: its pathology, its relation to pachymeningitis hemorrhagica and its surgical treatment. *Arch Surg* 1975;11:329–393.

38. Ray BS, Wolff HG. Experimental studies on headache: pain sensitive structures of the head and their significance in headache. *Arch Surg* 1940;41:813–856.

39. Ropper AH, Davis KR. Lobar cerebral hemorrhages: acute clinical syndromes in 26 cases. *Ann Neurol* 1980;8:141–147.

40. Symonds SC. The circle of Willis. *BMJ* 1955;1:119–121.

41. Vestergaard K, Andersen G, Nielsen MI, Jensen TS. Headache in stroke. *Stroke* 1993;24:1621–1624.

42. Voris HC. Subdural hematoma. *JAMA* 1946;132:686–692.

43. Wells CE. Premonitory symptoms of cerebral embolism. *Arch Neurol* 1961;5:44–50.

The Headaches, Second Edition,
edited by J. Olesen, P. Tfelt-Hansen, and K.M.A. Welch.
Lippincott Williams & Wilkins, Philadelphia © 2000.

The Secondary Headaches

CHAPTER 105

Unruptured Vascular Malformation and Subarachnoid Hemorrhage

John R. Østergaard and Nabih M. Ramadan

DEFINITION OF UNRUPTURED VASCULAR MALFORMATION AND SUBARACHNOID HEMORRHAGE

IHS code: ICD-10 code:
6.3 Subarachnoid hemorrhage G44.810
6.4 Unruptured vascular malformation G44.811
6.4.1. Arteriovenous malformation G44.811
6.4.2. Saccular aneurysm G44.811

Short Description

Subarachnoid hemorrhage (SAH) occurs when blood leaks between the layers of the pia-arachnoid membrane. Arteries and veins passing through this potential space are both possible sources of bleeding. The majority of SAHs arise from ruptured saccular aneurysms or arteriovenous malformations (AVMs) (33). Miscellaneous causes include cavernous and venous malformations and capillary telangectasias. The headache of SAH typically is abrupt in onset, and is often described as the worst ever experienced. The headache is usually followed by pain radiating into the occipital or cervical region and is often accompanied by blunting of consciousness, vomiting, phono- and photophobia, and neck stiffness. The headache remains severe for hours and then clears over several days to a few weeks.

Patients with AVMs usually present with either an intraparenchymal hemorrhage or seizures (5,68). In a

subgroup of patients with SAH (perimesencephalic or pretruncal SAH) in which no saccular aneurysms or AVMs can be demonstrated, the headache may be explosive but the course of the illness is generally benign (67).

Saccular aneurysms and AVMs produce headache either through rupture (i.e., SAH) or as part of their natural history, which of necessity does not involve rupture. Unruptured saccular aneurysms often remain asymptomatic for many years but may suddenly produce warning symptoms because of either impending rupture (21,43) or progressive enlargement, leading to compression of neighboring structures such as the oculomotor nerve (43). Unruptured AVMs may mimic migraine (8,27). Epilepsy is the most common clinical presentation of cavernous malformations (52) followed by signs and symptoms of cerebral hemorrhage. Venous malformations are incidental findings in patients presenting with seizures or headache. In the majority, a causal relationship between the angioma and the presenting symptoms is not established (46).

EPIDEMIOLOGY

The true prevalence of saccular aneurysms and other intracranial vascular malformations is not precisely known. Venous malformations are thought to have a low risk of bleeding or causing symptoms by other mechanisms, and they are often found incidentally at autopsy, as are capillary telangectasias (68). They occur in some 2.6% of subjects (68).

The prevalence of cavernous malformations is 0.5% on autopsy series and 0.4% to 0.9% on serial magnetic resonance (MR) studies (53). Epilepsy is the most common

J.R. Østergaard: Department of Pediatrics, University of Århus, and Department of Pediatrics A, Skejby Hospital, DK-8200 Århus N, Denmark.

N.M. Ramadan: Eli Lilly and Company, Indianapolis, Indiana 46285.

clinical presentation of these vascular malformations (52). They affect both sexes with equal frequency.

Most cavernous malformations appear as solitary lesions; however, they have been reported in association with other vascular lesions such as capillary telangectasias, AVMs, and venous malformations (53). The prevalence of cavernous malformations range between 0.02% on some autopsy series to as high as 0.9% on MR studies (35).

Postmortem studies of consecutive autopsies indicate that approximately 5% of the population may harbor one or more saccular aneurysm (9,58). In these studies, more than half of the demonstrated aneurysms were unruptured and unrecognized prior to death. Long-term follow-up studies of patients harboring incidentally discovered cerebral aneurysms suggest that the vast majority never rupture or cause any symptoms (65).

Twenty to thirty percent of patients with cerebral aneurysms have multiple lesions (aneurysms), usually two or three (43,50). Arterial hypertension and multiple aneurysms highly positively correlated and, considering both experimental and epidemiologic studies, it seems reasonable to conclude that arterial hypertension is a risk factor for aneurysm formation (43). The significance of hypertension for aneurysmal rupture, however, is less conclusive (40).

Overall, aneurysmal SAH is more common in women than in men (34,62). However, in considering the gender difference by decade, a 4:1 male:female ratio is encountered in the first decade of life, which becomes 1:1 by the fifth decade of life (64). The increased incidence of aneurysmal SAH in women is most probably related to their greater susceptibility to aneurysm formation, rather than an increased risk of aneurysmal rupture (43,63). In contrast, there is a modest male preponderance among patients with AVMs (68).

The cause of AVMs is uncertain, but it is probably related to a disturbance of normal embryonic development. Coexistence of an AVM and a saccular aneurysm occurs in approximately 10% of patients with an AVM. Because the associated aneurysms have predilection to the AVM feeding arteries, it is believed that increased blood flow is a major factor in the formation of the saccular aneurysm (68).

Estimates of the annual incidence of SAH depend on the population surveyed, the methods used for analysis, and the accuracy and extent of the investigations. Reports can be divided into series from epidemiologic studies and those arising from referral centers or large-scale cooperative studies. Epidemiologic studies include not only hospitalized patients, but also those 15% to 20% of individuals with SAH who died before receiving medical treatment. In the Western countries, the average annual incidence of SAH is estimated at 12 per 100,000 population, with variations for age, sex, and geographic locations (54). Saccular aneurysms account for approxi-

mately 75% of SAH; AVMs constitute approximately 10% of SAH, and the cause is undetermined in the remaining 15% (33). Patients with angiographically negative SAH (e.g., perimesencephalic or pretruncal hemorrhage) have an excellent prognosis and are unlikely to rebleed (67). Rupture of a dilated vein or venous malformation in the prepontine or interpeduncular cistern is believed to be responsible for the majority of these cases (50).

Up to 50% of patients with saccular aneurysms who are admitted to neurosurgical departments experience warning symptoms in the form of minor bleeding episodes, days or even several months before a major hemorrhage (21,43,62). Headache is the most common symptom of this warning leak (43), occurring in 9 of 10 patients. Minor leaks occur with AVM as well, as evidenced by pathologic documentation of hemosiderin adjacent to the malformation (68). At surgery, at least 10% of AVMs show evidence of minor bleeding episodes. Small AVMs are more likely to cause minor bleeding than large ones (68).

GENETICS

There is no significant genetic predisposition to the development of AVMs (68). In contrast, the existence of a familial form of cavernous malformations, characterized by multiple lesions and an autosomal-dominant inheritance pattern, is well documented (69). Furthermore, a recent study indicates that a gene responsible for familial cavernous malformations is mapped to chromosome 7q (13). Also, considerable evidence supports the role of genetic factors in the pathogenesis of intracranial aneurysms. The two main lines of evidence are the association of intracranial aneurysms with inherited connective-tissue disorders (e.g., autosomal polycystic kidney disease, Ehlers-Danlos syndrome type IV, Marfan syndrome) and their familial occurrence (54). In contrast to sporadic aneurysms, familial ones (a) occur less often on the anterior communicating artery; (b) rupture at a younger age; and (c) are smaller in size at rupture (30). In a segregation analysis of published pedigrees, several possible patterns of inheritance of saccular aneurysms were identified, with autosomal transmission being the most likely (55). This suggests that genetic heterogeneity is an important feature of intracranial saccular aneurysms (54).

ANATOMY AND PATHOLOGY

After a hemorrhage, the subarachnoid space contains a variable mixture of cerebrospinal fluid (CSF) and clotted and liquid blood. The extent of dissemination varies considerably. Bleeding on the surface of the brain spreads out and collects later at the base, whereas a hemorrhage at the base initially fills the cisterns. In cases of severe SAH, the blood rapidly (within minutes) spreads over the convexities of the cerebral hemispheres. The average SAH releases 7 to 10 mL of blood into the CSF. A red blood cell (RBC) count of $10^5/mm^3$ indicates that 3 mL of blood entered the CSF. Following the initial hemorrhage, the RBC count decreases, and RBCs remain detectable in the fluid only for 4 to 21 days. The average survival of RBCs in CSF is much shorter than in the circulation. It has been suggested that RBCs in the subarachnoid space lose their cellular integrity, resulting in an immune mediated hemolysis (47).

Red blood cell lysis liberates pigments (oxyhemoglobin, methemoglobin, and bilirubin), causing the supernatant of the centrifuged CSF to stain yellow (xanthochromia). By spectrophotometry, oxyhemoglobin can be detected as early as 2 hours after the bleeding, but usually it takes a few hours or more for RBCs to lyse and for xanthochromia to develop. In a large series of patients with SAH, it was shown that xanthochromia could be detected in all patients in whom the CSF was examined within the initial 2 weeks and at least 12 hours after the hemorrhage (60).

In the subarachnoid space, extravasated blood causes an aseptic inflammatory reaction (19). The meningeal reaction is evident within 2 hours of the hemorrhage and begins as an outpouring of polymorphonuclear leukocytes, followed by the appearance of lymphocytes and large mononuclear phagocytes. This cellular reaction is transient and persists only as long as blood or products of the breakdown of blood are demonstrated in the subarachnoid space. Thickening and pigmentation of the pia and arachnoid occur, and hemosiderin-containing adhesions are forced among these membranes, the blood vessels, the nerves, and the brain. In case of aneurysmal SAH, the process is most marked at the base of the brain. If the exit foraminae of the fourth ventricle are affected, obstructive hydrocephalus may occur. Hydrocephalus is more common after SAH in the territory of the anterior communicating artery, probably because blood is directed into the basal subarachnoid space. Hydrocephalus is also common in patients with multiple episodes of SAH because of the functional impairment of the arachnoid villi and increasing leptomeningeal fibrosis.

Cerebral vasospasm is one of the most important causes of death and disability in patients surviving the first critical days of SAH. Cerebral vasospasm is a syndrome of ischemic consequences of an angiographically proven, time-dependent, transient cerebral arterial narrowing. It is rarely pronounced before day 4 following the initial hemorrhage and peaks at approximately day 7. At that time, 40% to 70% of patients will have some reduction in the caliber of one or more of the arteries of the circle of Willis or its branches (10,24). The clinical symptoms of delayed cerebral ischemia are characterized by an insidious onset of confusion and decreased level of con-

sciousness, followed by focal motor and speech impairment (10,24). Manifest neurologic deficits related to delayed cerebral vasospasm occur in 20% to 30% of patients with aneurysmal SAH, whereas they occur much less frequently in patients with SAH due to AVMs (24).

PATHOPHYSIOLOGY

Following SAH, the initial pain results from local distention, distortion, deformation, and stretching of the cerebral vessel and its adjacent arachnoid. It is a referred pain due to stimulation of arteries in the circle of Willis, which derive their innervation from the fifth, ninth, and tenth cranial nerves, and the upper cervical spinal nerves. Sensory fibers are directly stimulated by subarachnoid blood with the resultant release of neuropeptides such as substance P and initiation of head pain (15,32,39). Levels of calcitonin gene–related peptide (CGRP) are low in patients who die after SAH (16,17). Furthermore, there is increased release of CGRP following SAH (22), analogous to what is demonstrated in migraine. To this is added an element of increased intracranial pressure headache. Later, headache related to development of hydrocephalus and delayed cerebral ischemia may evolve.

Distention of an aneurysmal sac may produce pain through pressure on the free edge of the tentorium, with pain referred through trigeminal nerve fibers, or by direct pressure on the first branch of the fifth cranial nerve. Enlargement of aneurysms arising from the internal carotid artery near the take-off of the posterior communicating artery or the distal part of the basilar artery may produce incomplete or complete oculomotor nerve palsy. This is the most common nonhemorrhagic presentation of an intracranial aneurysm and is almost always accompanied by pain (48). Because cranial nerve III carries no pain-sensitive fibers, distention of the arterial wall is the most likely pain mechanism. The pain is almost always ipsilateral to the aneurysm and usually is periorbital or retroorbital in location (2).

Aneurysms of the intracavernous portion of the internal carotid artery, which constitute approximately 2% to 3% of all intracranial aneurysms, rupture only rarely. If they do so, they do not bleed into the subarachnoid space but produce a carotid-cavernous fistula with exophthalmos, congestion of conjunctival and fundus veins, and often a bruit audible over the ipsilateral eye and the skull. Carotid-cavernous fistulas are dural arteriovenous shunts that cause predominantly orbital and periorbital pain and discomfort, largely related to pressure build-up and compression of neighboring pain-sensitive structures. When not associated with a carotid-cavernous fistula, intracavernous saccular aneurysms can produce pain along the first and second divisions of the trigeminal nerve (probably from direct compression of these structures or their branches), and palsies of the third, fourth, or sixth cranial nerves (62). Sometimes, if the pressure in the cavernous sinus is sufficiently increased, patients develop an acute cavernous sinus syndrome with paresis of muscles of ocular movement, secondary to compression of cranial nerves III, IV, or VI, and severe pain (61).

Generalized or localized headache episodes may be due to warning symptoms of impending subarachnoid hemorrhage. Minor leakage of blood into the subarachnoid space stimulates the sensory nerve endings both mechanically and chemically. Alternatively, the pain could be caused by hemorrhage confined to the aneurysmal wall or a sudden expansion of the aneurysm (43).

Unruptured AVMs are often discovered during investigations of patients complaining of headache (7). The literature is abundant with isolated cases and small case series implicating AVMs in migraine (37). However, because the majority of people have headaches, it is difficult to evaluate whether the association between an AVM and headache is coincidental, contributory, or causative. Bruyn reviewed the relationship between AVMs and migraine and argued that, based on prevalence and incidence figures of both conditions, the relationship between AVMs and migraine is causal (8). The mechanisms of AVM-related migraine headaches were not discussed.

Clusterlike headaches have recently been linked to unruptured middle cerebral artery AVMs (40). Muñoz and colleagues argued that the relationship between the headache and the AVMs is likely causal because both patients experienced no further cluster headache symptoms after excision of the lesions. Furthermore, they speculated that blood flow alteration in the intracavernous portion of the internal carotid artery sets a pericarotid neurogenic focus, leading to cluster headache.

Patients with headache and documented cavernous or venous malformations are considered asymptomatic (35,46). A recent report challenges that concept (12). De Benedittis reported the case of a 62-year-old man who presented with a cluster headache variant (SUNCT) and later was found to have a cavernous angioma on MRI. De Benedittis postulated that the pontine lesion could involve the trigeminal root entry zone and irritate fibers of the first division of the trigeminal nerve as well as the greater superficial petrosal nerve, thus causing head and facial pain with dysautonomic symptoms (12).

CLINICAL FEATURES

Headache and Subarachnoid Hemorrhage

The IHS diagnostic criteria for headache with SAH (Headache Classification Committee, 1988) are:

6.3 Subarachnoid hemorrhage
A. Present or past subarachnoid bleeding demonstrated by CSF examination or computed tomography (code 6.2 if hematoma is present)

B. Headache of sudden onset (<60 minutes) if it is an aneurysm, <12 hours if it is an AVM
C. At least one of the following:
1. Severe headache intensity
2. Bilateral headache location
3. Stiff neck
4. Increased body temperature

A sudden headache that has never been previously experienced and that is accompanied by depressed consciousness and neck stiffness is the hallmark of SAH. The most common cause of SAH is a ruptured saccular aneurysm; bleeding AVMs are distant seconds (33). Descriptive terms of the headache include "worst ever," "tremendous," "bursting," "exploding," and "unbearable." Although it could be initially focal and lateralized, SAH-related headaches rapidly generalize and radiate into the occipitonuchal region. With blood seeping into the spinal subarachnoid space, back pain, meningismus and radicular symptoms follow (26).

The headache of aneurysmal SAH commonly, although not always, peaks instantly. Indeed, Linn et al. prospectively evaluated 102 patients with sudden severe headache and reported that only 50% of the 42 patients with aneurysmal SAH complained of an instantly severe headache (31). The researchers also found that some patients (35%) with pretruncal nonaneurysmal hemorrhage and many with benign thunderclap headache (68%) complained of instantly severe headache.

The duration of SAH-related headache varies from 2 to 3 days, usually with the minor hemorrhages, and up to several days (average 8 days) with large hemorrhages. The excruciating headache that usually drives the patient to seek medical care is shorter lived, however, lasting 1 to 2 hours.

Various neurologic signs and symptoms accompany the headache of SAH (Table 1). Neck stiffness, disorientation, photophobia, nausea, and altered mentation are common. Unconsciousness for greater than 1 hour is

TABLE 1. *Neurological symptoms and signs of SAH*

Signs and symptoms	Frequency (%)
Headache	85–95
Neck stiffness	74–84
Disorientation	48
Nausea, vomiting	45
Altered mentation	43
Focal motor deficits	20
Seizures, convulsions	15
Coma	14
Cranial nerve palsy	13
Papilledema	13
Ocular hemorrhage	12
Homonymous hemianopsia	9
Paresthesia	5

Adapted from refs. 25 and 62.

associated with a high mortality rate. If consciousness is lost slowly or supervenes after a lucid period, then secondary hemorrhage or acute hydrocephalus should be suspected. Photophobia is part of the meningism that occurs in up to 60% of patients (62). Neuroophthalmologic findings include homonymous hemianopsia, papilledema, and intraocular hemorrhage (subhyaloid, vitreous, subretinal). Finally, systemic signs and symptoms that are often encountered in patients with SAH include elevated temperature, hypertension, chest pain, arrhythmias, abnormalities on ECG, and rarely cardiopulmonary arrest (25,62). In some patients, the time course of the elevated temperature has a close correlation with the onset of signs of delayed ischemia (63).

Prior to a definitive aneurysmal SAH, about half of patients experience warning symptoms, particularly headache, due to minor leakage of blood into the subarachnoid space or caused by aneurysmal expansion without actual subarachnoid hemorrhage (4,11,28,42,62). This so-called warning leak occurs days to several months before the major hemorrhage (43). In about two thirds of patients, the headache has associated signs and symptoms such as nausea and vomiting (20%), neck stiffness or pain (30%) visual disturbances like blurred or decreased vision and visual defects (15%), and motor or sensory disturbances (15%–20%) (43). Photophobia rarely occurs. The headache is most often characterized as unusual in severity and location, being similar to but less intense than that of the major bleed. It usually subsides over 1 or 2 days, but in some cases it is unremitting for as long as 2 weeks or until a subsequent major hemorrhage occurs (28). Overall, the site of the headache seems to be a poor localizing symptom for the aneurysm, with the exception of those on the posterior communicating artery, in which the headache is often ipsilateral and retroorbital. The warning headache of aneurysmal origin is so unusual that 40% to 75% of patients seek medical advice (14,28). Unfortunately, the attacks of headache are too often misinterpreted as migraine, tension headache, the flu, or sinusitis, and patients are discharged without appropriate investigations (23,42). In a 5-year study from Denmark, 15% of over 1,000 patients with SAH volunteered a history of sudden headache with neck pain, dizziness, vomiting, or drowsiness (20). Almost two thirds of the patients were misdiagnosed by physicians, and 43% were dead in 2 years. A more recent study from the United Kingdom indicates that only the minority of patients (one third) with warning leaks are referred for appropriate care (59).

Due to the abrupt and instantaneous onset of the intense headache, Day and Raskin compared the warning headache of cerebral aneurysms to a clap of thunder and called it thunderclap headache, even in the absence of SAH (11). Bleeding within the aneurysm wall or vasospasm was considered a potential cause of that warning headache pattern.

A history of thunderclap headache should always prompt an investigation for cerebral aneurysm. This catastrophic headache presentation, however, could be encountered in other conditions as well (Table 2).

Slivka and Philbrook suggested classifying thunderclap headaches into asymptomatic (with or without neurological signs or symptoms) and symptomatic (of an intracranial disorder) varieties (56). These researchers and others (66) have argued that thunderclap headache may represent a benign condition when the appropriate neuroinvestigational studies (CT scan with or without lumbar puncture [LP]) do not reveal any evidence of SAH. They have stressed, however, that benign thunderclap headache is a diagnostic exclusion. This leaves us with the question, how often do patients with a thunderclap headache have SAH? In the study of Duffy (14), 71 patients with severe headache of sudden onset suggestive of SAH were admitted to a local neurosurgical department. All patients underwent cranial computed tomography (CT) and angiography. If SAH was not demonstrated on CT, lumbar puncture was performed. Forty-six of the 63 patients with a proven SAH had an aneurysm (73%). In 8 patients, no SAH was demonstrated either on CT or at lumbar puncture. Angiography was performed in these patients in view of the suggestive history. No aneurysms or other vascular malformations were found, and none of the patients had recurrence of symptoms during follow-up periods of at least 6 months. The more recent prospective study of Linn et al. indicated that 65 of 102 patients (64%) who present with sudden and severe headache are found to have SAH; 42 had aneurysmal and 23 had pretruncal nonaneurysmal SAH (31).

Subarachnoid hemorrhage or a warning leak of a saccular aneurysm or AVMs should be suspected in any patient who presents with a severe, unusual, and unremitting headache of abrupt onset or an unusual pain in the head or face, particularly if it is hemicranial or hemifacial. The suspicion of SAH should be heightened when the headache is associated with vomiting, neck stiffness, or altered mentation. In those patients presenting with only sudden and severe headache, the probability of SAH

TABLE 2. *Some conditions that can cause thunderclap headache*

Condition	References
Aneurysmal SAH	25
Non-aneurysmal pretruncal SAH	68,32,50
Warning headache of unruptured cerebral aneurysms	3,11,14,20, 21,28,43,44
Intracerebral hemorrhage	36
Pituitary apoplexy	64
"Crash migraine"	18
Sexual headaches	45
Cough and exertional headaches	45
Benign thunderclap headaches	14,67,32

is increased when the pain is associated with exertion or when the headache is preceded by transient focal symptoms, an episode of loss of consciousness, vomiting, or seizures (31).

Figure 1 shows a flow chart of operational diagnostic procedures in patients with sudden onset of a severe and unusual headache ("the worst headache"). Modern CT scanning is the first-line investigation for these patients because it can sufficiently exclude 97% of SAHs (38). However, the CT may fail to detect subarachnoid blood resulting from a minor leak, and a lumbar puncture is recommended when SAH is still suspected. If xanthochromic staining of the CSF is seen or if there are RBCs on CSF microscopy after an atraumatic puncture, then cerebral angiography should be performed. If, on the other hand, the CT scan and the CSF are normal, it is generally accepted that the headache can be regarded as a benign symptom, and cerebral angiography is not indicated (14). MRI is of less use in the acute stage of SAH (25) because leakage of blood into CSF causes only small changes in MRI signal characteristics. When the initial SAH is missed or if the diagnosis is delayed, an MRI may indicate evidence of prior bleeding (an abnormally high signal intensity due to conversion of oxyhemoglobin into methemoglobin) or could detect the aneurysm or the AVM.

Headache and Unruptured Vascular Malformation

The IHS diagnostic criteria for headache with unruptured vascular malformation are (Headache Classification Committee, 1988):

6.4.1 Unruptured arteriovenous malformation: unruptured arteriovenous malformation diagnosed by CT, MR, and/or angiography.
6.4.2 Unruptured saccular aneurysm: unruptured saccular aneurysm diagnosed by CT, MR, and/or angiography.

Patients with unruptured AVMs can present with headaches that mimic migraine (37) or cluster headache (40). The argument whether these headaches are directly caused by the vascular malformation or are merely coincidental is still open. Headache is a frequent complaint of patients who harbor cavernous or venous angiomas, but the lesions are not believed to be pathophysiologically related (35,46). Epilepsy followed by hemorrhage are the two most common clinical presentations of cavernous angiomas (35). Venous angiomas are largely asymptomatic lesions that are found on autopsy or during radiologic investigations of patients with various neurologic complaints, including headache (46).

Headache is reported in approximately 18% of patients with unruptured cerebral aneurysms (57); cerebral

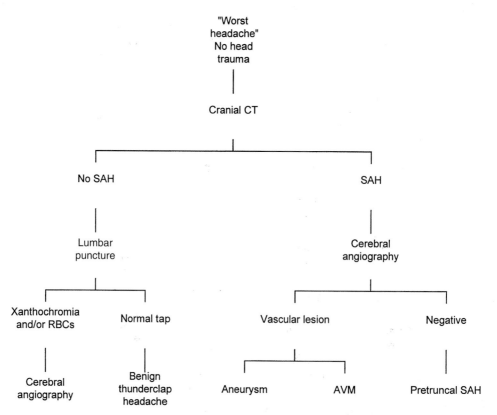

FIG. 1. Diagnostic approach to patients with worst headache.

ischemic symptoms and seizures are less frequent. No specific clinical features of headaches are related to unruptured cerebral aneurysms. They could be focal or diffuse, unilateral or bilateral, frontal or occipital or ocular, acute in onset or gradual (3,48). Cranial nerve palsies from aneurysmal compression can accompany the headaches of unruptured cerebral aneurysms. Palsy of eye movement and facial pain mimicking trigeminal neuralgia can occur with aneurysms of the carotid-cavernous sinus (29). On the other hand, aneurysms of the posterior communicating artery cause cranial nerve III palsy, whereas those located on the anterior inferior cerebellar artery or the basilar artery can result in abducens nerve palsy (29,62).

PROGNOSIS

Nearly one in five patients with SAH dies before they reach the hospital (6,25). The prognosis of the patients who make it to the hospital is not good. Overall, approximately 50% die following an SAH, and 50% of the survivors are left more or less disabled (1,6,49). These morbidity and mortality data have not changed in recent decades despite recent advances in the management of complications of SAH (e.g., vasospasm). This is primarily because the diagnosis is still usually established only after a major hemorrhage. Among survivors of SAH, a disabling headache may occur in every fourth patient (49).

MANAGEMENT

Headache and restlessness should be controlled with appropriate analgesics and moderate sedation. Aspirin is relatively contradicted because it could increase the risk of bleeding by (a) enhancing the fibrinolytic activity of the blood; (b) increasing the bleeding time; and (c) impairing platelet aggregation. Instead, acetaminophen or codeine is recommended. Narcotics can be used judiciously. In many centers nimodipine, a calcium channel antagonist, is administered intravenously and later orally for a total of 14 days to reduce the delayed cerebral ischemia of SAH (1,25).

REFERENCES

1. Ausman JI, Diaz FG, Malik GM, Andrews BT, McCormick PW, Balakrishnan G. Management of cerebral aneurysms: further facts and additional myths. *Surg Neurol* 1989;32:21–35.
2. Bartleson JD, Trautmann JC, Sundt TM Jr. Minimal oculomotor nerve paresis secondary to unruptured intracranial aneurysm. *Arch Neurol* 1986;43:1015–1020.
3. Bartolomei JC, Harris D, Awad IA. Unruptured cerebral aneurysms. In: *Neurobase 1997*, 3rd ed. San Diego: Arbor Publishing Corp., 1997.
4. Bassi P, Bandera R, Loiero M, et al. Warning signs in subarachnoid hemorrhage: a cooperative study. *Acta Neurol Scand* 1991;84:277–281.
5. Bills DC, Rosenfeld JV, Phelan EM, Klug GL. Intracranial arteriovenous malformations in childhood—presentation, management and outcome. *J Clin Neurosci* 1996;3:220–228.
6. Bonita R, Thomson S. Subarachnoid hemorrhage: epidemiology, diagnosis, management, and outcome. *Stroke* 1985;16:591–594.
7. Brown RD, Weibers DO, Forbes G, et al. The natural history of unruptured intracranial arteriovenous malformations. *J Neurosurg* 1988;68:352–357.
8. Bruyn GW. Intracranial arteriovenous malformation and migraine. *Cephalalgia* 1984;4:191–207.
9. Chanson JL, Hindman WM. Berry aneurysms of the circle of Willis. *Neurology* 1958;8:41–44.
10. Chyatte D, Sundt Jr TM. Cerebral vasospasm after subarachnoid hemorrhage. *Mayo Clin Proc* 1984;59:498–505.
11. Day JW, Raskin NH. Thunderclap headache: symptoms of unruptured cerebral aneurysm. *Lancet* 1986;2:1247–1248.
12. De Benedittis G. SUNCT syndrome associated with cavernous angioma of the brain stem. *Cephalalgia* 1996;16:503–506.
13. Dubovsky J, Zabramski JM, Kurth J, et al. A gene responsible for cavernous malformations maps to chromosome 7q. *Hum Mol Genet* 1995;4:453–458.
14. Duffy GP. The warning leak in spontaneous subarachnoid hemorrhage. *Med J Aust* 1983;1:514–516.
15. Edvinsson L, Delgado-Zygmunt T, Ekman R, Jansen I, Svendgaard N-A, Uddman R. Involvement of perivascular sensory fibres in the pathophysiology of cerebral vasospasm following subarachnoid haemorrhage. *J Cereb Blood Flow Metab* 1990;10:602–607.
16. Edvinsson L, Juul R, Jansen I. Perivascular neuropeptides (NPY, VIP, CGRP and SP) in human brain vessels after subarachnoid haemorrhage. *Acta Neurol Scand* 1994;90:324–340.
17. Edvinsson L, Juul R, Jansen I, McCulloch J, Mortensen A, Uddman R. Reduced levels of calcitonin gene-related in human brain vessels after subarachnoid haemorrhage. *Neurosci Lett* 1991;121:151–154.
18. Fisher CM. Painful states: a neurological commentary. *Clin Neurosurg* 1984;31:32–53.
19. Hammes EM. Reaction of the meninges to blood. *Arch Neurol Psychiatry* 1944;52:505–514.
20. Hauerburg J, Andersen BB, Eskesen V, Rosenom J, Schmidt K. Importance of the recognition of a warning leak as a sign of a ruptured intracranial aneurysm. *Acta Neurol Scand* 1991;83:61–64.
21. Jakobsson KE, Saveland H, Hillman J, et al. Warning leak and management out in aneurysmal subarachnoid hemorrhage. *J Neurosurg* 1996;85:995–999.
22. Juul R, Hara H, Gisvold SE, et al. Alteration in perivascular dilatory neuropeptides (CGRP, SP, VIP) in the external jugular vein and in cerebrospinal fluid following subarachnoid haemorrhage in man. *Acta Neurochir* 1995;132:32–41.
23. Kassel NF, Kongable GL, Torner JC, Adams HP Jr, Mazuz H. Delay in referral of patients with ruptured aneurysms to neurosurgical attention. *Stroke* 1985;16:587–590.
24. Kassel NF, Sasaki T, Colohan ART, Nazar G. Cerebral vasospasm following aneurysmal subarachnoid hemorrhage. *Stroke* 1985;16:562–572.
25. Khajavi K, Chyatte D. Subarachnoid hemorrhage. In: *Neurobase 1997*, 3rd ed. San Diego: Arbor Publishing Corp., 1997.
26. Kopitnik TA, Samson DS. Management of subarachnoid hemorrhage. *J Neurol Neurosurg Psychiatry* 1993;56:947–959.
27. Kowacs PA, Werneck LC. Atenolol prophylaxis in migraine secondary to an arteriovenous malformation. *Headache* 1996;36:625–627.
28. Leblanc R. The minor leak preceding subarachnoid hemorrhage. *J Neurosurg* 1987;66:35–39
29. Leblanc R. Unruptured aneurysms, multiple aneurysms, familial aneurysms, and aneurysms in pregnancy. In: Awad IA, ed. *Current management of cerebral aneurysms*. Park Ridge, IL: American Association of Neurological Surgeons, 1993:277–295.
30. Leblanc R. Familial cerebral aneurysms. *Can J Neurol Sci* 1997;24:191–199.
31. Linn FHH, Rinkel GJE, Algra A, van Gijn J. Headache characteristics in subarachnoid haemorrhage and benign thunderclap headache. *J Neurol Neurosurg Psychiatry* 1998;65:791–793.
32. Linnik MD, Sakas DE, Uhl GR, Moskowitz MA. Subarachnoid blood and headache: altered trigeminal tachykinin gene expression. *Ann Neurol* 1989;25:179–184.
33. Locksley HB. Report on the cooperative study of intracranial aneurysms and subarachnoid hemorrhage. Section V, Part I. Natural history of subarachnoid hemorrhage, intracranial aneurysms, and arteriovenous malformations. *J Neurosurg* 1966;25:219–239.
34. Longstreth WT Jr, Nelson LM, Koepsell TD, van Belle G. Clinical

course of spontaneous subarachnoid hemorrhage: a population-based study in King County, Washington. *Neurology* 1993;34:712–718.

35. Maraire JN, Awad IA. Cavernous malformations. In: *Neurobase 1997*, 3rd ed. San Diego: Arbor Publishing Corp., 1997.
36. Mitsias P. Head pain and stroke. *Semin Headache Manage* 1997;2:2–7.
37. Mohr JP, Stein BM, Hilal SK. Arteriovenous malformations. In: Vinken PJ, Bruyn GW, Klawans HL, Toole JF, eds. *Handbook of clinical neurology*. Part II. Vascular diseases. Amsterdam: Elsevier, 1989:361–393.
38. Morgenstern LB, Lunagonzales H, Huber JC, et al. Worst headache and subarachnoid hemorrhage—prospective, modern computed tomography and spinal fluid analysis. *Ann Emerg Med* 1998;32:297–304.
39. Moskowitz MA, Buzzi MG, Sakas DE, Linnik MD. Pain mechanisms underlying vascular headaches. *Rev Neurol* 1989;145:181–193.
40. Muñoz C, Díez-Tejedor E, Frank A, Barreiro P. Cluster headache associated with middle cerebral artery arteriovenous malformation. *Cephalalgia* 1996;16:202–205.
41. Østergaard JR. Risk factors in intracranial saccular aneurysms. Aspects of the formation and rupture of aneurysms, and the development of cerebral vasospasm [Thesis]. *Acta Neurol Scand* 1989;80:81–98.
42. Østergaard JR. Warning leak in subarachnoid hemorrhage. All too often the diagnostic importance of a warning headache is missed. *BMJ* 1990;301:190-191.
43. Østergaard JR. Headache as a warning symptom of impending aneurysmal subarachnoid hemorrhage. *Cephalalgia* 1991;11:53–55.
44. Østergaard JR, Høg E. Incidence of multiple intracranial aneurysms. Influence of arterial hypertension and gender. *J Neurosurg* 1985;63:49–55.
45. Pascual J, Iglesias F, Oterino A, Vásquez-Barquero A, Berciano J. Cough, exertional, and sexual headache. *Neurology* 1996;46:1520–1524.
46. Patwardhan R, Martin N. Venous angiomas. In: Welch KMA, Caplan LR, Reis DJ, Seisjö BK, Weir B, eds. *Primer on cerebrovascular diseases*. San Diego: Academic, 1997:520–525.
47. Peterson JW, Kwun B-D, Teramura A, et al. Immunological reaction against the aging human subarachnoid erythrocyte. *J Neurosurg* 1989;71:718–726.
48. Raps EC, Rogers JD, Galetta SL, et al. The clinical spectrum of unruptured intracranial aneurysms. *Arch Neurol* 1993;50:265–268.
49. Rasmussen P, Bush H, Haase J, et al. Intracranial saccular aneurysms. Results of treatment in 851 patients. *Acta Neurochir* 1981;53:1–17.
50. Rinkel GJE, van Gijn J, Wijdicks EFM. Subarachnoid hemorrhage without detectable aneurysm: a review of the causes. *Stroke* 1993;24:1403–1409.
51. Rinne J, Hernesniemi J, Puranen M, Sari T. Multiple intracranial aneurysms in a defined population: prospective angiographic and clinical study. *Neurosurgery* 1994;35:803–808.
52. Robinson JR, Awad IA, Little JR. Natural history of the cavernous angioma. *J Neurosurg* 1991;75:709–714.
53. Robinson JR, Awad IA, Masaryk TJ, Estes ML. Pathological heterogeneity of angiographic occult vascular malformations of the brain. *Neurosurgery* 1993;33:547–554.
54. Schievink WI. Intracranial aneurysms. *N Engl J Med* 1997;336:28–40.
55. Schievink WI, Schaid DJ, Rogers HM, Piepgras DG, Michels VV. On the inheritance of intracranial aneurysms. *Stroke* 1994;25:2028–2037.
56. Slivka A, Philbrook B. Clinical and angiographic features of thunderclap headache. *Headache* 1995;35:1–6.
57. Solomon RA, Fink ME, Pike-Spellman J. Surgical management of unruptured intracranial aneurysms. *J Neurosurg* 1994;80:440–446.
58. Stehbens WE. Aneurysms and anatomical variation of cerebral arteries. *Arch Pathol* 1963;75:45–64.
59. Tolias CM, Choskey MS. Will increased awareness among physicians of the significance of sudden agonizing headache affect the outcome of subarachnoid hemorrhage. *Stroke* 1996;27:807–812.
60. Vermeulen M, van Gijn J. The diagnosis of subarachnoid hemorrhage. *J Neurol Neurosurg Psychiatry* 1990;53:365–372.
61. Wecht DW, Awad IA. Carotid cavernous and other dural arteriovenous fistulas. In: Welch KMA, Caplan LR, Reis DJ, Seisjö BK, Weir B, eds. *Primer on cerebrovascular diseases*. San Diego: Academic, 1997:541–548.
62. Weir B. Headache from aneurysms. *Cephalalgia* 1994;14:79–87.
63. Weir B, Disney L, Grace M, Roberts P. Daily trends in white blood cell count and temperature after subarachnoid hemorrhage from aneurysm. *Neurosurgery* 1989;25:161–165.
64. Weir BKA. *Aneurysms affecting the nervous system*. Baltimore: Williams & Wilkins, 1987:74–82.
65. Wiebers DO, Whisnant JP, Sundt TM Jr, O'Fallon WM. The significance of unruptured intracranial saccular aneurysms. *J Neurosurg* 1987;66:23–29.
66. Wijdicks EFM, Kerkhoff H, van Gijn J. Long-term follow-up of 71 patients with thunderclap headache mimicking subarachnoid hemorrhage. *Lancet* 1988;2:68 70.
67. Wijdicks EFM, Schievink WI, Miller GM. Pretruncal nonaneurysmal subarachnoid hemorrhage. *Mayo Clin Proc* 1998;73:745–752.
68. Wilkins RH. Natural history of intracranial vascular malformations: a review. *Neurosurgery* 1985;16:421–430.
69. Zabramski JM, Wascher TM, Spetzler RF, et al. The natural history of familial cavernous malformations: results of an ongoing study. *J Neurosurg* 1994;80:59–68.

The Headaches, Second Edition,
edited by J. Olesen, P. Tfelt-Hansen, and K.M.A. Welch.
Lippincott Williams & Wilkins, Philadelphia © 2000.

The Secondary Headaches

CHAPTER 106

Arteritis

Michael Wall and James John Corbett

Arteritis causes headache by inflammation of dural and cerebral arteries. Arteritis is thought to be due to immune complex deposition in vessel walls. Of the many causes of arteritis, this chapter concentrates on giant cell arteritis, systemic lupus erythematosus (SLE), and primary central nervous system (CNS) vasculitis.

GIANT CELL ARTERITIS

Definition of Giant Cell Arteritis

IHS code and diagnosis: 6.5.1 Headache associated with giant cell arteritis

WHO code and diagnosis: G44.81 Headache associated with other vascular disorders

Short description: Giant cell arteritis is a polysymptomatic disease of the elderly characterized by granulomatous inflammation of aortic origin vessels. Prominent symptoms are headache and other cranial pains, jaw claudication, visual loss, hip and shoulder girdle stiffness, and constitutional symptoms.

Other terms: Temporal arteritis, Horton's disease, cranial arteritis

Giant cell arteritis (GCA), also called *cranial* or *temporal arteritis*, was first described by Ali ibn Isâ in the tenth century (48), who noted heat and inflammation in the temporalis muscles associated with loss of sight. Hutchinson in 1890 described a man who had symmetric, painful red streaks on his head that prevented him from wearing his hat; he ascribed the disorder to the pressure of the hat on the temples (27). In 1932, Horton and col-

leagues reported on two patients with a characteristic clinical presentation for GCA. They performed the first temporal artery biopsies that showed the well-known pathologic findings (25). Jennings in 1938 emphasized the blinding ocular complications and the associated musculoskeletal symptoms now known as *polymyalgia rheumatica* (28).

Epidemiology

The incidence of the disease is 3 per 100,000/year in Rochester, Minnesota (16), and 9 per 100,000/year in Goteborg, Sweden (5). It has been found in 1.7% of 889 postmortem examinations (1). The incidence rises dramatically with increasing age after age 50 (17.4 of 100,000) (26); it is nine times as frequent in the ninth decade as the sixth (5). The mean age at diagnosis is about 70 years. Rarely are patients reported to be younger than 50 years, but the diagnosis in these cases of GCA is seldom confirmed (22). This disease is found in white patients but is rare in Orientals and African Americans. It appears to be most common in northern geographic areas, especially in persons of British or Scandinavian heritage (33). A slight predominance of women patients is found. Ninet and colleagues summarized the data for a genetic basis for GCA (37), and they concluded that a genetic predisposition is probable because of the higher frequency in whites and reports of familial forms (familial cases appear to be uncommon). In addition, there is an association with human leukocyte antigen (HLA) DR4 antigen.

Pathology

The presence of granulomatous arteritis is the *sine qua non* for the diagnosis of GCA. The histologic fea-

M. Wall: Departments of Neurology, Ophthalmology, and Visual Sciences, University of Iowa, Iowa City, Iowa 52242.

J. J. Corbett: University of Mississippi School of Medicine, and Department of Neurology, University of Mississippi Medical Center, Jackson, Mississippi 39216-4505.

tures usually include (a) patchy, granulomatous inflammation involving the media of the vessel with an inflammatory reaction consisting mostly of lymphocytes; epithelioid cells and histiocytes must be present, whereas giant cells often are seen but are not necessary for the diagnosis; (b) fragmentation of the internal elastic lamina; (c) the vessel lumen may be occluded with thrombus or marked subintimal edema and cellular proliferation; (d) areas of subintimal fibromuscular hyperplasia and lymphocytic and plasma cell infiltration of the adventitia are often present, but their presence is nondiagnostic (3).

"Skip" areas are a major cause of false-negative biopsies; thus, a segment of artery of at least 1 inch should be obtained and serial sectioned at least every 1 mm throughout its length. Direct immunofluorescence microscopy using antibodies to IgG, IgM, IgA, complement, and fibrinogen is usually abnormal but is not more sensitive than light microscopy (46). Humoral immunity is abnormal with the presence of circulating immune complexes in the serum and deposition of immunoglobulins in arteries. Cellular immunity also appears to be abnormal with a decrease in OKT 8 in the blood.

Autopsies of GCA patients show a high incidence of involvement of superficial temporal, posterior ciliary, ophthalmic, and vertebral arteries (47) that parallels the amount of elastic tissue in the media and adventitia of the arteries of the head and neck. The internal and external carotid and central retinal arteries and anterior ciliary arteries are less commonly involved. Involvement of arteries after they penetrate the dura is rare. The pathologic process is similar to that of Takayasu's arteritis, which led to the suggestion that Takayasu's arteritis may be a related or biphasic manifestation of a similar pathogenic process.

Clinical Features

IHS diagnostic criteria for giant cell arteritis (Headache Classification Committee, 1988):
A. One or more of the following:
  1. Swollen and tender scalp artery (usually superficial temporal artery)
  2. Elevated RBC sedimentation rate
  3. Disappearance of headache within 48 hr of steroid therapy
B. Temporal artery biopsy demonstrating GCA.
C. Headache as a new symptom or of a new type occurs in close temporal relation to onset of giant cell arteritis.

Symptoms

Giant cell arteritis is a disease that may be expressed in numerous ways (Table 1). Headache, jaw claudication, throat pain, and other head and neck pains are usually present. The presence of jaw claudication or neck pain markedly increases the likelihood of a positive biopsy (18). Constitutional symptoms, nontender shoulder and hip girdle aching and stiffness, diplopia, and hair loss may be present before the occurrence of visual loss. Although postmortem studies usually show involvement of the vertebral artery, stroke is uncommon. Patients uncommonly present with few or no symptoms, a condition that is called *occult giant cell arteritis*. In this form, presentation is purely visual (anterior ischemic optic neuropathy, ocular motor palsies, or central retinal artery occlusion), with no systemic symptoms. This occult form also may represent a failure on the part of patient or physician to recognize symptoms (21).

Hutchinson's original patient had headache that worsened when he wore a hat and had scalp ischemia with

TABLE 1. *Cranial symptoms of giant cell arteritis*

Symptoms	Temporal arteritis	Temporal arteritis and PMR	Total
Headache	23	20	43
Diffuse headache	3	5	8
Unilateral temporal headache	4	2	6
Bilateral temporal headache	10	13	23
Forehead pain	4	1	5
Occipital pain	2	1	3
Neck pain	9	13	22
Ear pain	8	4	12
Throat pain	4	4	8
Jaw claudication	4	0	4
Severe scalp tenderness	1	2	3
Facial pain	1	0	1
Eye pain	1	0	1
Gum pain	0	1	1

PMR, polymyalgia rheumatica.
From the prospective study of Bengtsson and Maimvall (5), n = 95.

gangrene. Headache is present in up to 90% of patients, often localized to one or both temporal regions or the forehead, but it may be holocranial, spare the temple, or occur in any location (41). In about half of patients, the pain is constant, and in the other half the pain is intermittent (41). The pain is often described as throbbing (41) or superficial and burning with a superimposed lancinating quality (5), but it may be a boring sensation (30); its intensity ranges from mild to severe (5). The headache may be a relatively minor feature in the background of generalized aches and pains of polymyalgia rheumatica. It may be so far in the background as to be recognized only by its absence after therapy is started. Head soreness, an unusual feature of other types of headache, is an important complaint of these patients. These patients find that the skin and hair is sensitive to touch, brushing, combing, or pressure such as laying the head on a pillow. With severe granulomatous inflammation, frank scalp necrosis can occur (Fig. 1).

The visual loss in GCA may be transient (*amaurosis fugax*), unilateral, or bilateral (19). When visual loss is permanent, it is due to granulomatous inflammation of the posterior ciliary arteries with anterior ischemic optic neuropathy. Jaw or masticatory claudication is almost pathognomonic; it does not occur with atherosclerosis. The pain produced by chewing is an aching cramp in the jaw or the temporalis muscle and should be differentiated from temporomandibular joint disease, which is preauricular (anterior to the tragus) in location and often occurs immediately on chewing. Tongue pain or infarction of the tongue also can occur.

Polymyalgia rheumatica (PMR) is a syndrome of synovial inflammation that accompanies many cases of GCA. Biopsy of the synovium shows nonspecific inflammatory changes without changes of granulomatous arteritis. Patients have chronic stiffness of the shoulder girdles with common involvement of the sternoclavicular joint. Thickened synovium can be palpated in the sternoclavicular joint in about 40% of patients. The hip girdle is less commonly affected. The pain and stiffness are especially prominent in the morning. Proximal muscle pain may occur, but muscle biopsies are normal; the pain is thought to be referred from joints, tendons, and ligaments. The erythrocyte sedimentation rate (ESR) is greater than 50 mm per hour, and there is dramatic relief of symptoms within 4 days with a daily dose of 10 mg of prednisone. At least 20% of patients (possibly many more) with GCA appear to have a PMR-like prodrome (15). About half of patients with PMR later develop GCA; about one fourth have serious visual or neurologic complications (30). Patients with PMR may have positive temporal artery biopsies but, according to some investigators, if they do not have any symptoms of GCA, they appear to be at low risk for visual loss. Also, low-dose corticosteroids do not protect patients from developing GCA. A number of questions remain regarding the relationship of GCA and PMR, largely because of the lack of large, long-duration, prospective studies.

Signs

Many of the signs of GCA are visual. Anterior ischemic optic neuropathy resulting from granulomatous inflammation of the posterior ciliary arteries is common. Patients characteristically develop pale, swollen optic discs (Fig. 2) with accompanying blinding visual loss. Diplopia, when present, is likely due to ischemia of the extraocular muscles (4) as a result of involvement of muscular branches of the anterior ciliary arteries. Ischemia of the third, fourth, or sixth cranial nerves probably also occurs but is rare (19). Prominent (Fig. 3) tender, nonpulsatile, noncompressible, or beaded temporal arteries may be present, but the artery may be normal to palpation.

Differential Diagnosis

The diagnostic criteria of the IHS were presented earlier (21). Patients present with a typical clinical course or have a characteristic temporal artery biopsy. Biopsies should show interruption of the internal elastic membrane with infiltration of mononuclear cells in the arterial wall. The presence of giant cells is not required.

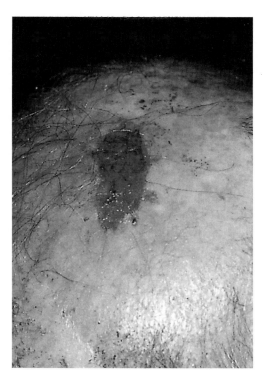

FIG. 1. Scalp necrosis in a case of giant cell arteritis. (Courtesy of Mr. Roger Hitchings, Moorefields Eye Hospital.)

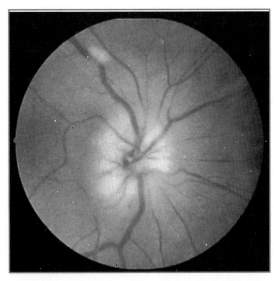

FIG. 2. Pallid disk edema in giant cell arteritis. When this much pallor is present associated with disk edema in a case of anterior ischemic optic neuropathy, one should consider giant cell arteritis as a cause. (Courtesy of Sohon S. Hayreh, MD, PhD.)

A 77-year-old woman presented with a 2-week history of temporal headache, fever, myalgias and fatigue, and anorexia. The ESR was 125 mm per hour. At surgery, the left temporal artery was thickened. The first biopsy specimen, shown in Figure 4, showed evidence of resolution: so-called healed arteritis. A biopsy on the other side (Fig.

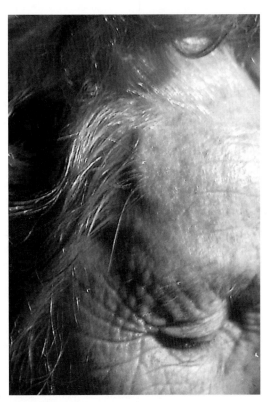

FIG. 3. Prominent temporal artery in a case of giant cell arteritis.

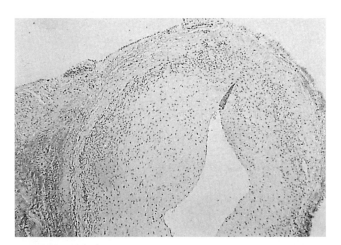

FIG. 4. Pathologic changes of giant cell arteritis. A normal temporal artery is present with granulomatous inflammation present in a branch of the artery (example of skip areas). The high magnification view (B) shows transmural inflammation consistent with arteritis. (Courtesy of Robert Folberg, Educational Resources Group, Department of Ophthalmology, University of Iowa.)

5) demonstrates an area of granulomatous inflammation adjacent to normal artery.

Bengtsson and Malmvall propose that biopsy-negative patients with GCA are identified by at least one of the following characteristic symptoms and signs: temporal ache, scalp tenderness, jaw claudication, anterior ischemic optic neuropathy, or abnormal temporal arteries (5). In addition, an ESR above 40 mm per hour (Westergren) and an age of 50 years or more are required, as is rapid and lasting relief of symptoms after institution of corticosteroid therapy. Only a few well-documented, otherwise typical cases of GCA in patients younger than 50 years have been reported.

It is well established that the temporal artery may be uninvolved despite GCA lesions elsewhere in the arterial system (45). It is equally well known that the changes can appear interspersed with normal arterial segments (Fig. 4), the so-called skip lesions. Therefore, a second biopsy on the opposite side may be rewarding (13,18). The differential diagnosis of headache in the elderly patient includes GCA, brain tumor, carcinomatous meningitis, and aneurysm. Most other types of vasculitis that present with headache have other organ systems affected and have no association with PMR. Characteristic findings on temporal artery biopsy clearly distinguish GCA.

Patients presenting with anterior ischemic optic neuropathy may have a "nonarteritic" type. Cranial pain, diplopia, or amaurosis fugax are not present, and no constitutional symptoms are noted. Patients usually have systemic arterial hypertension or diabetes mellitus and have a small or absent optic cup in the uninvolved eye. ESR and C-reactive protein are normal in nonarteritic ischemic optic neuropathy.

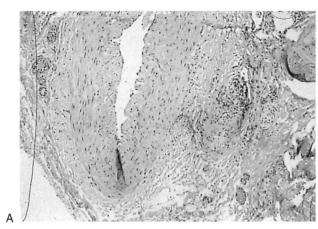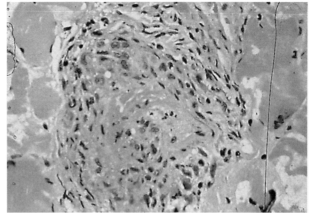

A   B

FIG. 5. Healed arteritis. There is asymmetric intimal thickening with concomitant focal disruption and scarring of the media. (Courtesy of Robert Folberg, Educational Resources Group, Department of Ophthalmology, University of Iowa.)

Laboratory Findings

The ESR is the most frequently used test for the diagnosis of GCA. Other useful tests include elevated acute-phase reactants, such as C-reactive protein and von Willebrand's factor, fibrinogen, and anemia of chronic disease as well as abnormal liver-function studies. Also, thrombocytosis, leukocytosis, lymphocytosis, and elevation of $\alpha 1-$, $\alpha 2-$, $\beta -$, and γ-globulins occur. Serum haptoglobin may rise, as may total complement, C3, and C4. The ESR is a measure of the size and number of red blood cell aggregations. The more the red cells adhere to each other, the higher the sedimentation rate, because large-volume masses sediment faster than small ones. Factors that increase the sedimentation rate are fibrinogen, globulins (especially a and b), pregnancy, hypercholesterolemia, macrocytosis, and anemia. Thus, the ESR must be corrected for anemia (Wintrobe, not Westergren).

The normal values for the Westergren sedimentation rate are less than 10 mm per hour in men and less than 20 mm per hour in women. In patients aged over 60, many use 40 mm per hour as indicative of disease. Elevated ESRs, even greater than 80 mm per hour, may be found in apparently normal (especially elderly) subjects. Sedimentation rates greater than 100 may be seen in monoclonal gammopathies, polyclonal hyperglobulinemias, hyperfibrinogenemia, connective-tissue diseases, leukemias, lymphomas, carcinomas, and sarcomas. This rate also may be exceeded in collagenoses, acute bacterial infections, portal or biliary cirrhosis, and ulcerative colitis. The mean ESR during the acute phase of GCA is 91 mm per hour. The ESR is greater than 50 mm per hour in 89% and is more than 100 mm per hour in 41% (5). It is well known that the ESR may be in the normal range in this disorder in about 1% to 2% of cases (5,19). The ESR decreases with corticosteroid therapy and is used by some as a management guide. Relapses may occur with a nor-

mal sedimentation rate, and resolution of the disease can occur with a mildly to moderately elevated rate (about 40 mm per hour).

C-reactive protein, an acute-phase plasma protein, may be more specific for detecting inflammation. It is not elevated by anemia, altered red blood cell morphology, or the level of a number of plasma proteins. C-reactive protein in our experience is a more useful parameter than the ESR for diagnosis and following disease activity. It appears to be as sensitive and more specific than the ESR and may correlate with symptoms better than the ESR (17, 18). It may be elevated in GCA when the ESR is normal (17,18). In the extensive experience with CGA of Hayreh and colleagues, no case of active GCA without an elevated C-reactive protein has been seen (18).

Prognosis

Many cases of GCA are chronic and need treatment for years. Recurrences also have been noted years later. The time between the first symptom and subsequent visual loss varies, usually weeks to several months but occasionally longer. The time between visual loss in the first eye and visual loss in the second eye is usually within the first week and nearly always within a month; uncommonly it is longer than 2 months. It appears that after first-eye involvement, if the second eye is to be involved, it will nearly always be within 2 months (28,31).

Ross Russell reported 13 patients treated with salicylates alone during the headache phase of GCA; five developed visual loss (40). Of the ten patients in his study treated with steroids, none developed visual loss. In Palm's series, 14 of 16 untreated cases became blind bilaterally as opposed to 1 of 8 treated with steroids (38). No evidence has been reported that GCA shortens the life span; however, the side effects of corticosteroids can be fatal, especially in elderly patients.

Management

The headache of GCA responds rapidly to treatment with steroids. Doses of steroids should be high initially and megadose (1 g methylprednisolone twice daily) in selected cases, for example, patients who have had unilateral visual loss of less than 1 week's duration or episodes of amaurosis. Even with large doses of steroids, vision eventually may be lost in the second eye; if this occurs, it is nearly always within the first week after institution of therapy.

Follow-up of patients with GCA includes serial Westergren sedimentation rates and we also use the C-reactive protein. Because there is diurnal variation of the ESR, it is useful to have the ESR drawn at the same time of the day at each return visit. Patients must be asked specifically about steroid side effects, and the patient's visual and masticatory symptoms and headache should be reviewed. Ideally, the ESR and C-reactive protein should fall and stay low, and symptoms should improve. Steroids then can be tapered gradually. If the ESR increases by more than 10 mm per hour, if the C-reactive protein becomes abnormal, or if symptoms reappear, the dose of steroids should be increased and then gradually tapered again. Steroid reduction responses vary; it is common for patients to be on low doses of steroids for years.

OTHER SYSTEMIC ARTERIDITIES: SYSTEMIC LUPUS ERYTHEMATOSUS

Definition of Other Systemic Arteritides

IHS code and diagnosis: 6.5.2 Other systemic arteritides
WHO code and diagnosis: G44.81 Headache associated with other vascular disorders
Short description: Systemic lupus erythematosus is a chronic autoimmune inflammatory disease of unknown etiology. Like multiple sclerosis, it is characterized by exacerbations and remissions. The incidence of headache is difficult to determine. Many confounding factors such as the frequency of headache in the general population, presence of systemic arterial hypertension, increased intracranial pressure, and uremia make the headache due to lupus difficult to isolate and characterize.

Epidemiology

Lupus occurs at any age. Women are affected three times as often as men. Most often, SLE begins between puberty and 40 years. In this age range, more than 90% are women. Blacks outnumber whites 3:1. The prevalence

of lupus is 51 of 100,000; the incidence is 3 to 27 of 100,000 per year. In black women, the incidence is 1:245 per year (11). CNS involvement occurs in about 60%. There is a slightly increased risk for those with family history of lupus. There is about two-thirds concordance in identical twins (92% concordance for autoantibodies); dizygotic twins are discordant (12). The frequency of lupus in first- and second-degree relatives is 5% to 12%. HLA-DR antigens have been shown to be associated with cases of lupus.

Pathology

Small parenchymal and leptomeningeal vessels show fibrinoid and hyaline degeneration and endothelial proliferation with occlusion and perivascular lymphocytic infiltrations or microhemorrhages. Later, mononuclear infiltration with deposition of eosinophilic material and hematoxylin bodies (nuclear fragments) is found. There is immunoglobulin and complement deposition in vessels. Although the presence of inflammatory cells within blood vessels, a cardinal feature of vasculitis, is rare within the CNS in lupus cases, perivascular inflammatory infiltrates are common (10,26).

Clinical Features

IHS diagnostic criteria for other systemic arteritides (Headache Classification Committee, 1988): Headache with evidence of systemic arteritis.

Symptoms

Symptoms are variable and initially are commonly nonspecific. The symptoms and their frequencies are found in Table 2. The neurologic manifestations are seizures, cranial nerve palsies, long-tract signs, movement disorders, pseudotumor cerebri, meningitis, psychosis, and headache. Maida and Horvatits reported that

TABLE 2. *Common clinical abnormalities in patients with systemic lupus erythematosus rounded to the nearest 10%*

Abnormality	Approximate frequency (%)
Constitutional	
Fatigue	90
Fever	80
Weight loss, anorexia	60
Musculoskeletal	
Arthritis, arthralgia	90
Myalgia, myositis	30
Central nervous system	
Personality disorders	50
Seizures	20
Psychoses	20
Stroke or long-tract signs	10
Migraine headaches	10

From ref. 39, with permission.

headache occurs in one third of patients with CNS involvement (34). The headache is said to be similar to migraine with hemicrania and fortification scotoma (31,40). Until a controlled study is performed, the headache attributed to lupus will remain unclear.

Signs

On examination, CNS findings may be focal or diffuse. There may be signs of stroke, pseudotumor cerebri, a multiple sclerosis-like presentation with involvement of long tracts, or encephalopathy dementia.

Diagnostic Criteria

The IHS does not have specific criteria for systemic lupus erythematosus. The American Rheumatologic Association criteria are found in Table 3 (40). Lupus should be suspected if any of these findings are present and unexplained.

Laboratory Findings

There is no single test diagnostic for lupus. High titers of antinuclear antibodies are 95% sensitive and 86% specific. A battery of tests of specifically reactive antigens are most useful (e.g., Sm, SS-A, SS-B, native DNA—Table 4). Patients with antibodies to Ro (SS-A) or La (SS-B) have a higher incidence of sicca syndrome, muscle disease, and lung disease with little or no renal disease. Also, anti-Ro is associated with skin lesions and heart block. Anti-DNA antibodies are thought to cause damage by forming antigen–antibody complexes in the circulation with deposition in various organs. Antiribosomal protein antibodies are present in about 12% of lupus patients; their presence appears to be highly correlated

TABLE 3. *American Rheumatologic Association diagnostic criteria for systemic lupus erythematosus*[a]

Malar rash
Discoid rash
Photosensitivity
Arthritis without deformity
Serositis (pleuritis or pericarditis)
Oral or nasopharyngeal ulceration
Kidney disease (proteinuria, cellular casts)
CNS manifestations (seizures or psychosis)
Hemolytic anemia, leukopenia, lymphopenia, or thrombocytopenia
Positive LE prep or anti-DNA antibody, or anti-Sm antibody or false-positive serological test of syphillis
Antinuclear antibody

CNS, central nervous system; LE, lupus erythematosus.
[a]The presence of 4 or more of the above 11 criteria is required.
From ref. 43, with permission.

TABLE 4. *Diagnostic criteria for primary CNS vasculitis*

Clinical pattern of headaches and multifocal neurological deficits for at least 6 months unless the onset is with a severe deficit.
Cerebral angiography showing areas of segmental arterial narrowing.
No evidence of systemic inflammation, infection, or vasculitis.
Leptomeningeal or parenchymal biopsy characterized by vascular inflammation and exclusion of alternate diagnoses (infection, atherosclerosis, and neoplasia).

CNS, central nervous system.
From ref. 35, with permission.

with lupus psychosis. The SLE cell is found in about 80% of patients. Anemia and leukopenia are common, and the ESR is usually elevated.

Prognosis

With treatment, organ system function can be preserved for prolonged periods in many cases.

Management

Therapy for SLE is beyond the scope of this text. Corticosteroids and immunosuppressives (azothiaprine and cyclophosphamide) are commonly used. Plasmapheresis may be useful.

Antiphospholipid Antibodies and Migraine

Antiphospholipid antibodies occur with SLE and other autoimmune diseases or as an isolated syndrome. Antiphospholipid antibodies are immunoglobulins (usually IgG) directed against any negatively charged phospholipid. They may be found by their reaction with cardiolipin (anticardiolipin antibodies) or by prolonging phospholipid-dependent coagulation tests (lupus anticoagulants); however, *in vivo* this group of antibodies appears to contribute to disease by immune-mediated thrombosis. There is also an apparent association with spontaneous abortion. There is debate over the pathogenetic role of these antibodies in stroke (29).

Petri and associates (39) reported lupus anticoagulant in SLE in 6.5% of cases and by anticardiolipin assay in 25%; controls were 0 and 2.5%. Reviews of combined series show respective frequencies of 34% and 44%, but not all studies have adequate controls. Many patients have been reported with an association of antiphospholipid antibodies and migraine, but other studies have shown no association.

A study of 94 consecutive patients with migraine concluded that there was no association between lupus anticoagulant and migraine (20). A prospective study of 500 lupus patients also found no association of anticardiolipin antibodies and migraine (2). The link between migraine and antiphospholipid antibodies appears tenuous at best.

PRIMARY CNS VASCULITIS (GRANULOMATOUS ANGIITIS)

Definition of Primary Intracranial Arteritis

IHS code and diagnosis: 6.5.3 Primary intracranial arteritis

WHO code and diagnosis: G44.81 Headache associated with other vascular disorders

Short description: Primary CNS vasculitis is a noninfectious recurrent angiopathy confined to the CNS. It is usually fatal if untreated. Patients are adults and they usually present with headache and recurrent stroke.

Other terms: Granulomatous angiitis and isolated angiitis of the nervous system

Epidemiology

Age at onset ranges from 3 to 78 years (mean, 49 years) (14). Men are affected more frequently than are women (1.8:1). Particles like mycoplasma were observed in two necropsies. Interestingly, a condition such as primary CNS vasculitis occurs in turkeys infected with *Mycoplasma gallisepticum* (41). The cause of primary CNS vasculitis is unknown. According to Moore, the presence of granulomas and the absence of antibodies or immune complexes in the vessel walls suggest that it is a disorder of cell-mediated immunity (35). There is no apparent genetic predisposition. Particles resembling viruses have been described; however, they can also be found in apparently normal brains.

Pathology

There is segmental necrotizing granulomatous involvement of vessel walls with a predilection for small blood vessels. Inflammatory infiltrates are present with varying degrees of granuloma formation. The inflammation is characterized by the presence of mononucleocytes, polymorphonucleocytes, epithelioid-appearing histiocytes, and multinucleated giant cells with granulomas. Leptomeningeal vessels more often are involved than parenchymal vessels. Any vessel of the brain or spinal cord can be involved. Any portion of the vessel wall can be affected, but the media appears to be less involved than the adventitia or intima. Granulomatous angiitis is a variable finding; hence the disease is more appropriately termed *primary* or *primary CNS vasculitis*.

Clinical Features

IHS diagnostic criteria for primary intracranial arteritis (Headache Classification Committee, 1988): Head-ache with angiographic signs of arteritis or biopsy demonstrating arteritis.

Symptoms

The most common presenting symptom is headache, which occurs in about two thirds of cases and is usually severe (32). Headaches can be generalized or localized and are usually pulsatile (9). Onset may be acute, or progression may be stepwise. Patients may present with a low-grade fever, weight loss, confusion, or visual loss or have an apoplectic onset. Although encephalopathy is present in about half, focal or multifocal neurologic deficits develop in more than 90% of patients (9). Nonconstitutional symptoms such as arthritis or skin involvement are absent. Seizures occur in one third. Mental symptoms occur in two thirds and often predominate. Patients with spinal cord involvement may present with back pain.

Signs

On examination, patients have signs of stroke with cortical and long-tract signs, or encephalopathy may be present. Signs of generalized increased intracranial pressure (i.e., papilledema with resultant visual loss and sixth-nerve palsies) may be present. Meningismus is occasionally present. Myelopathy is a less common finding.

Diagnostic Criteria

Moore proposed the diagnostic criteria listed in Table 4 (35). Unfortunately, biopsy is only diagnostic in about three quarters of patients because of patchy involvement.

Differential Diagnosis

The differential diagnosis of primary CNS vasculitis includes the many types of vasculitis that can affect the CNS. Polyarteritis nodosa commonly affects the peripheral nervous system, but CNS involvement is rare. Rheumatoid vasculitis and lupus are differentiated by systemic involvement and laboratory abnormalities of collagen vascular disease. Lymphomatoid granulomatosis is characterized by infiltration of lymphoid and plasmacytoid cells with granulomatous inflammation. It primarily involves the lungs but may involve the skin, kidneys, and CNS. It has some aspects of a lymphoproliferative disease and is usually fatal. The chest radiography almost always shows bilateral infiltrates. Malignant angioendotheliosis is another rare fatal disease characterized by malignant cell deposition in small vessels in several organs. It may be a variant of lymphoma.

Giant cell arteritis rarely affects arteries after they penetrate the dura. Some of the reported cases with intracranial involvement actually may be cases of primary CNS vasculitis. Temporal artery biopsy is negative in isolated primary CNS vasculitis.

Infectious angiitis (herpes zoster) and the vasculitis associated with Hodgkin's disease, although histologically similar, are distinguished by a lack of systemic involvement. In the case of zoster, there is, of course, a preceding infection. Sarcoidosis can be differentiated by its nodular-enhancing lesions involving the base of the brain, noncaseating granulomata, and system involvement. Wegener's granulomatosis is a necrotizing granulomatous vasculitis and is differentiated by its common involvement of the upper and lower respiratory tracts and kidney (glomerulonephritis). Less commonly, the orbit, skin, and CNS are involved. Lyme disease and syphilis yield characteristic abnormal serologic tests; involvement outside the CNS is common. Headache and upper-extremity claudication may be prominent features of Takayasu's (pulseless) disease, an obliterative arteritis of the aorta and medium-sized arteries that primarily affects young women.

Laboratory Findings

The ESR is usually normal or mildly elevated in primary CNS vasculitis; rarely, it is markedly elevated. In the review by Hankey, the ESR mean was reported to be 27 mm per hour (range, 2–95) (14). A leukocytosis greater than 10,000/mm^3 without eosinophilia is present in one half of cases. Lumbar puncture may show increased intracranial pressure, and elevated protein occurs in three quarters with a mild lymphocytic pleocytosis. The cell count is seldom greater than 400 (6). There is blood in the cerebrospinal fluid (CSF) in about one fourth of cases. CSF protein often is elevated and may be greater than 100 mg%. CSF glucose is usually normal, but it can be less than 45 mg%. Although there may be elevation of CSF IgG, oligoclonal bands are absent. The CSF can be normal.

The electroencephalogram (EEG) shows generalized or localized slowing. Neuroimaging is nonspecific with signs of multifocal ischemia; evidence of cerebral edema may be present. Laboratory findings of collagen vascular disease are notoriously absent. Cerebral arteriography is abnormal in about three fourths of cases and has no pathognomonic features. It shows segmental arterial narrowing of medium-sized vessels (sausage pattern) in about half of the cases. Other findings are vascular occlusions, vascular shifts, vascular channels, and avascular areas. These "vasculitic" patterns, however, may be seen in atherosclerosis, heroin and amphetamine abuse, and infection. Cerebral angiography may be normal in spite of pathologic confirmation of the disease. Biopsy is abnormal in only three fourths of patients studied because of patchy involvement (8). There is frequent involvement of leptomeninges.

Prognosis

The clinical course can be rapidly progressive over weeks or "smolder" for months. There may be a fluctuating course with periods of stability. If it goes untreated, primary CNS vasculitis usually results in death within 3 years. Although no controlled trials of treatment have been reported, of the 26 survivors described in the literature, one third became asymptomatic with treatment and one half had mild deficits (14). Patients with isolated focal deficits have a better prognosis than those with encephalopathy, thus implying a more diffuse process.

Management

Patients suspected of the diagnosis should have leptomeningeal and temporal tip biopsy that includes a longitudinally oriented surface vessel. When the diagnosis is confirmed, patients should be treated with a combination of prednisone 40 to 60 mg and cyclophosphamide 100 mg/day.

REFERENCES

1. Ainsworth RW, Gresham GA, Balmforth GV. Pathological changes in temporal arteries removed from unselected cadavers. *J Clin Pathol* 1961;14:115–119.
2. Alarcon-Segovia D, Deleze M, Oria CV. Antiphospholipid antibodies in the Antiphospholipid syndrome in systemic lupus erythematosus. *Medicine* 1989;68:353–365.
3. Albert DM, Searl SS, Craft JL. Histologic and ultrastructural characteristics of temporal arteritis. *Ophthalmology* 1982;89:1111–1126.
4. Barricks ME, Traveisa DB, Glaser JG, Levy IS. Ophthalmoplegia in cranial arteritis. *Brain* 1977;100:209–221.
5. Bengtsson B-Å, Malmvall B-E. Giant cell arteritis. *Acta Med Scand* 1982;658:1–102.
6. Biller J, Adams HP. Noninfectious granulomatous angiitis of the central nervous system. In: Vinken PV, Bruyn GW, Klawans HL, eds. *Handbook of clinical neurology*, vol 2. Amsterdam: Elsevier, 1988:387–400.
7. Brandt KD, Lessell S, Cohen AS. Cerebral disorders of vision in systemic lupus erythematosus. *Ann Intern Med* 1975;83:163–169.
8. Calabrese LH, Mallek JA. Primary angiitis of the central nervous system: report of eight new cases, review of the literature, and proposal for diagnostic criteria. *Medicine* 1987;67:20–39.
9. Cupps TR, Moore PM, Fauci AS. Isolated angiitis of the central nervous system: prospective diagnostic and therapeutic experience. *Am J Med* 1983;74:97–105.
10. Ellis SG, Verity MA. Central nervous system involvement in systemic lupus erythematosus: a review of neuropathic findings in 57 cases 1955–1977. *Semin Arthritis Rheum* 1982;12:68–76.
11. Fessel MB. Systemic lupus erythematosus in the community. Incidence, prevalence, outcome and first symptoms: the high prevalence in black women. *Arch Intern Med* 1974;134:1027–1035.
12. Goldstein R, Arnett FC. The genetics of rhematic disease in man: immunology of the rheumatic diseases. *Rheum Dis Clin North Am* 1987;13:487–510.
13. Hall SH, Hunder GG. Is temporal artery biopsy prudent? *Mayo Clin Proc* 1984;59:793–796.
14. Hankey GJ. Isolated angiitis/angiopathy of the central nervous system. *Cerebrovascular Diseases* 1991;1:2–15.
15. Harrison MJH, Bevan AT. Early symptoms of temporal arteritis. *Lancet* 1967;2:638–640.
16. Hauser KA, Ferguson RH, Holley KE, et al. Temporal arteritis in Rochester, Minnesota, 1951–1967. *Mayo Clin Proc* 1971;46:597–602.
17. Hayreh SS. Ophthalmic features of giant cell arteritis. In: *Clinical rheumatology*, vol 5, 1991:431–459.
18. Hayreh SS, Podhajsky PA, Raman RI, Zmmeman B. Giant cell arteri-

tis: validity and reliability of various diagnostic criteria. *Am J Ophthalmol* 1997;123:285–296.

19. Hayreh SS, Podhajsky PA, Zimmerman B. Ocular manifestations of giant cell arteritis. *Am J Ophthalmol* 1998;125:509–520.

20. Hayreh SS, Podhajsky PA, Zimmerman B. Occult giant cell arteritis: ocular manifestations. *Am J Ophthalmol* 1998;125:521–526.

21. Headache Classification Committee of the International Headache Society. Classification and diagnostic criteria for headache disorders, cranial neuralgias and facial pain. *Cephalalgia* 1988;8:1–96.

22. Healy LA, Wilske KR. *The systemic symptoms of temporal arteritis.* New York: Grune and Stratton, 1978.

23. Hering R, Couturier EGM, Steiner TJ, et al. Anticardiolipin antibodies in migraine. *Cephalalgia* 1991;11:19–21.

24. Hollenhorst RW, Brown JR, Wagener HP, Shick RM. Neurologic aspects of temporal arteritis. *Neurology* 1960;10:490–498.

25. Horton BT, Magath TB, Brown GE. An undescribed form of arteritis of the temporal vessels. *Mayo Clin Proc* 1932;7:700–701.

26. Huston KA, Hunder GG, Lie JT, et al. Temporal arteritis: a 25-year epidemiologic clinical and pathologic study. *Ann Intern Med* 1978;88:162–167.

27. Hutchinson J. Disease of the arteries: on a peculiar form of thrombotic arteritis of the aged which is sometimes productive of gangrene. *Arch Surg* 1890;1:323–329.

28. Jennings GH. Arteritis of the temporal arteries. *Lancet* 1938;1:424–428.

29. Johnson RT, Richardson EP. The neurological manifestations of systemic lupus erythematosus. *Medicine* 1968;47:337–369.

30. Jones JG, Hazelman JL. Prognosis and management of polymyalgia rheumatica. *Ann Rheum Dis* 1981;40:1–5.

31. Keltner JL. Giant cell arteritis. *Ophthalmology* 1982;89:1101–1110.

32. Levine SR, Welch KMA. Antiphospholipid antibodies. *Ann Neurol* 1989;26:386–389.

33. Liang GC, Simkin PA, Hunder CC, et al. Familiar aggregation of polymyalgia rheumatica and giant cell arteritis. *Arthritis Rheum* 1974;17:19–24.

34. Maida E, Horvatits E. Neurological manifestations. In: Smolen JS, Zielinski, eds. *Systemic lupus erythematosus:* clinical and experimental aspects. Berlin: Springer-Verlag, 1987:251–269.

35. Moore PM. Diagnosis and management of isolated angiitis of the central nervous system. *Neurology* 1989;39:167–173.

36. Moskowitz N. Systemic lupus erythematosus of the central nervous system: I. Classification, epidemiology, pathology, diagnosis and therapy. *Mt Sinai J Med* 1988;55:147–152.

37. Ninet J, Gebuhrer L, Betuel H, et al. Immunogenetique de la maladie de Horton et de la pseudo-polyarthrite rhizomelique. *J Mal Vasc* 1989; 14:128–136.

38. Palm E. The ocular crisis of temporal arteritis syndrome (Horton). *Acta Ophthalmol* 1958;36:208–243.

39. Petri M, Rheinschmidt M, Whiting-O'Keefe Q, Hellmann D, et al. The frequency of lupus anticoagulant in systemic lupus erythematosus. *Ann Intern Med* 1987;106:524–531.

40. Ross Russell RW. Giant cell arteritis: a review of 35 cases. *QJM* 1959; 28:471–489.

41. Solomon S, Cappa KG. The headache of temporal arteritis. *J Am Geriatr Soc* 1987;35:163–165.

42. Steinberg AD, Systemic lupus erythematosus. In: Wyngaarden JB, Smith LH, Bennett JC, eds. *Cecil textbook of medicine*, 19th ed. Philadelphia: WB Saunders, 1992.

43. Tam EM, Cohen AS, Fries JF, et al. The 1982 revised criteria for the classification of systemic lupus erythematosus. *Arthritis Rheum* 1982; 25:1271–1277.

44. Thielen KR, Wydicks EFM, Nichols DA. Giant cell (temporal) arteritis: involvement of the vertebral and internal carotid arteries. *Mayo Clin Proc* 1998;73:444–446.

45. Thomas L, Davidson M, McClusky RT. Studies of PPLO infections. I. The production of cerebral polyarteritis by *Mycoplasma gallisepticum* in turkeys. *J Exp Med* 1966;123:897–912.

46. Wells KK, Folberg R, Goeken JA, Kemp JD. Temporal artery biopsies. Correlation of light microscopy and immunofluorescence microscopy. *Ophthalmology* 1989;86:1058–1064.

47. Wilkinson IMS, Russell RWR. Arteries of the head and neck in giant cell arteritis. *Arch Neurol* 1972;27:378–391.

48. Wood CA. *Memorandum book of a tenth century oculist* (a translation of the *Tadkivat of Ali ibn Isâ)*. Chicago: Northwestern University Press, 1936.

The Headaches, Second Edition,
edited by J. Olesen, P. Tfelt-Hansen, and K.M.A. Welch.
Lippincott Williams & Wilkins, Philadelphia © 2000.

The Secondary Headaches

CHAPTER 107

Carotid or Vertebral Artery Pain

Valérie Biousse and Panayiotis Mitsias

HEADACHE IN CERVICAL ARTERIAL DISSECTION

Definitions

IHS code and diagnosis: 6.6.1 Carotid or vertebral dissection.

WHO code and diagnosis: G44.81 Headache associated with other vascular disorders.

Short Description

Dissection of the cervical cerebral arteries is a relatively uncommon disorder in which blood enters into the wall of the artery, presumably through a tear on the endothelial surface. It is increasingly recognized as an important cause of stroke, especially in young persons (7,11,14,21,29). In recent reports, dissection accounted for up to 20% of ischemic strokes in patients under the age of 40 (14). The internal carotid artery is affected more often than the vertebral artery, and the location of the dissection is more often in the extracranial than in the intracranial segments (14,21).

The etiology of cervical cerebral arterial dissection remains largely unknown. It is often classified as spontaneous or traumatic. The contributory role of minor neck trauma and unusual neck torsion or extension is suggested by clinical anecdote as well as by the frequent location of the dissection at specific points of the arteries (14,21,29), but the importance of these findings remains unclear. In the so-called spontaneous cases, observational data suggest an association with migraine, oral contraceptive use, chronic arterial hypertension, recent infection, or with an underlying disorder of the arterial wall, such as fibromuscular dysplasia, more subtle intimal abnormalities, or arterial elastic tissue disease (12,14,21).

Epidemiology

The annual incidence of spontaneous internal carotid artery dissection is at least 2.6 per 100,000 population (21,29); between 0.5 and 2.5 cases of vertebral dissection per year are reported from large referral-based hospitals (22). The overall frequency of head pain is extremely high, ranging from 60% to 95% in carotid artery dissections (5,11,19,21,29) and 69% in vertebral artery dissections (29). Pain is the most frequent inaugural symptom of both carotid and vertebral dissections (5,20,21,29), potentially leading to recognition of the condition before the occurrence of ischemic signs.

Pathophysiology

The pain of cervical arterial dissections is a referred pain to the face, head, and neck originating from the dissected artery. In carotid artery dissection, the pain is referred to ipsilateral cephalic and facial regions, the location of which follows the patterns outlined during electric stimulation of the carotid bifurcation (10) or during balloon inflation in the distal carotid artery (24). In vertebral artery dissection, the location of pain at the posterior neck and also to anterior head regions is likely to be explained on the basis of innervation of these arteries by the upper cervical roots and the convergence of those with descending trigeminal impulses (19,20,23).

The pain mechanisms remain largely undetermined. Proposed potential mechanisms include mechanical stim-

V. Biousse: Department of Neurology, Hôpital Lariboisière, 75475 Paris, France.

P. Mitsias: Department of Neurology, Case Western Reserve University, School of Medicine, Cleveland, Ohio 44109, and Acute Stroke Unit, Department of Neurology, Henry Ford Hospital, Detroit, Michigan 48202.

ulation of the pain-sensitive receptors in the vessel wall as a result of dilatation or distention of the artery and ischemia of the perivascular pain-sensitive nerve fibers resulting from direct mechanical injury and occlusion of the vasa nervorum. The variability of the observed head pain patterns, including whether it occurs or not, the various localizations, the different degrees of severity, the types (i.e., quality) of pain, is not explained adequately by any of the proposed explanations. Thus, the pain mechanisms are poorly understood as yet.

Clinical Features

The IHS diagnostic criteria (Headache Classification Committee, 1988) include:

A. At least one of the following:
  1. Transient ischemic attack (TIA) or ischemic stroke in territory of affected artery
  2. Horner's syndrome, arterial bruits, or tinnitus
B. Dissection demonstrated by appropriate investigations or surgery
C. Headache and cervical pain ipsilateral to arterial dissection

Pain Characteristics

Frequency

Headache is experienced by about 68% of patients with carotid artery dissection, whereas isolated orbital or facial pain is reported by 10% of the patients (29). Similarly, 69% of patients with vertebral artery dissection report headache, and 46% report neck pain, either isolated or in conjunction with headache (22,29).

Timing in Relation to Other Neurologic Manifestations

Headache is often (45%) the initial symptom of carotid dissection, with other manifestations appearing with a delay ranging from 1 hour to 90 days (mean, 9 days) (7,29). Rarely, headache develops after the appearance of other manifestations, with a delay ranging from 1 to 96 hours. In the remaining cases, headache appears simultaneously with other clinical symptoms and signs, such as those of cerebral ischemia (7,29).

In almost two thirds of patients with vertebral dissection (61%), headache occurs simultaneously with the signs of vertebrobasilar ischemia or cranial nerve dysfunction (22,29), and in one third the head pain may precede those by a variable interval ranging from 1 hour to 14 days (29).

Mode of Onset

In carotid dissection, the onset of pain is occasionally sudden, severe, and with thunderclap qualities raising suspicion of subarachnoid hemorrhage (4,5,11,14,19, 21,29). Contrary to common belief, however, the most frequently reported pattern is that of a gradual-onset pain, mentioned by 85% of patients (29). Similarly, many patients with vertebral dissection (72%) report head pain of gradual onset, and only 22% report a sudden-onset headache (29). Occasionally, a gradual onset of pain is followed by sudden escalation (29).

Location

The headache of carotid dissection is almost always (91%) ipsilateral to the affected side; generalized or bifrontal headache is uncommon, but it can occur even if the dissection is unilateral (5,29). It is more often localized than diffuse and has a predilection for the frontal and temporal areas (4,5,11,14,19,21,29), although any part of the head may be affected, either in isolation or in combination. Facial pain, including ear pain, and orbital pain may accompany the dissection in 48% and 61% of cases, respectively (29). Facial or orbital pain may occur in isolation, that is, in the absence of headache. Neck pain at the lateral cervical regions is reported by 26% of patients at the time of dissection.

Almost half of patients with vertebral artery dissection (44%) report a unilateral occipital or parieto-occipital pain (19,29). Less often, a bilateral occipital, unilateral frontal, or generalized headache is reported. When the pain has an occipital location, it frequently is felt medially rather than laterally, even when dissection is unilateral (19). About 46% of patients report neck pain, usually unilateral, involving the upper and midposterior cervical areas.

Quality

The pain of carotid dissection is perceived as a constant, steady aching by two thirds of patients, as throbbing by 25%, and infrequently as a steady, sharp pain (29). In vertebral dissection, most patients report the head pain as either steady, pressurelike or throbbing; only a few patients report the pain as being sharp (29). The severity of the pain is highly variable, ranging from a mild sensation of tenderness to an excruciating headache simulating subarachnoid hemorrhage (4,5,29).

Duration

Often, published series do not mention the duration of the pain. In the vast majority of patients (90%), the head pain of carotid dissection resolves within 1 week (5,12, 29). In vertebral dissection, the headache may last up to 5 weeks (29). In rare cases, however, the headache may last for years after the dissection, particularly in patients who develop pseudoaneurysms (12,21,29).

In summary, a unilateral cervical pain of sudden onset, radiating to the ipsilateral eye or ear, is suggestive of carotid artery dissection. This condition can occur almost as frequently with other varieties of head and neck pain, however, and it can mimic migraine, cluster headache, carotidynia, subarachnoid hemorrhage, or even Raeder's syndrome (32).

Associated Clinical Manifestations

Carotid Artery Dissection

The most often associated signs are those related to retinal or cerebral ischemia. In these cases, there is no diagnostic difficulty. A unilateral head or neck pain in a patient presenting with amaurosis fugax (7,11,14,23, 27,30), TIA, or stroke (5,7,21,29) strongly suggests the possibility of internal carotid artery dissection (5,7,11,14, 19–21,29). In almost half of the cases, the presence of ipsilateral local signs associated with the cephalic pain is a key to the diagnosis. Horner's syndrome is the most frequent local sign and has long been recognized as a sign suggestive of internal carotid artery dissection (5,7,11,14, 21,29). Painful Horner's syndrome has been found in up to 58% of patients (5,7,11,21,29), and in about 10% it is the only clinical manifestation of carotid dissection (5,7, 11,21,29). Other manifestations include pulsatile tinnitus, dysgeusia, tongue paresis, and diplopia (5,7,11,14,21, 26,29). The absence of both ischemic and local signs is unusual; occasional case reports have described patients presenting only with head or neck pain (4,13).

Vertebral Artery Dissection

The usual associated signs are those of brainstem or cerebellar ischemia and those of ischemia to more remote areas, such as the occipital lobes, as a result of artery-to-artery embolism (22). Of the recognizable syndromes, Wallenberg's syndrome is the single most often reported syndrome (22). Consequently, an occipital or posterior neck pain associated with signs of either vertebrobasilar territory ischemia, especially with Wallenberg's syndrome, in a young patient, strongly points to the diagnostic possibility of vertebral artery dissection (19,20,29). Rarely, dissection may result in spinal cord ischemia (2).

As previously indicated, ischemic signs often are delayed, occasionally up to 1 month after the onset of pain (6,19,26). It is thus crucial to maintain a high index of suspicion and recognize the arterial dissection before a stroke occurs.

Management

The presence of any of the aforementioned symptoms should prompt diagnostic investigations that should be performed as soon as possible and always within the first few days after the onset of pain, given the facts that progression of the neurologic deficit regularly occurs in the days following onset and rapid recanalization and resolution of the radiologic signs of the dissection are known to occur, obscuring the diagnosis if investigations are delayed (7,14,21,29). The diagnostic investigations should include noninvasive vascular studies such as extracranial Duplex ultrasound scanning, magnetic resonance imaging (MRI) and angiography (MRA) (Figs. 1 and 2), and, if necessary, conventional cerebral angiography. Noninvasive vascular studies have become reasonably reliable in suggesting the diagnosis and are useful tools for following the vascular response to treatment. It should be kept in mind, however, that each of the noninvasive investigations can give false-negative results, even at an early stage.

Treatment of cervical artery dissections revealed only by the presence of headache is aimed at prevention of ocular and cerebral infarction. Because of the unpredictable risk of hemodynamic stroke in dissections with occlusion or severe stenosis, initial therapy should include immediate strict bed rest, hydration, and prevention of hypotension until recanalization of the artery or effective collateral circulation can occur. The value of each of these treatment modalities has not been established.

Despite the lack of controlled studies on any treatment modality in cervical artery dissection, empiric treatment with anticoagulants usually is prescribed to prevent complete occlusion of the dissected artery or artery-to-artery embolization. Careful monitoring with noninvasive vascular studies, such as extracranial duplex scanning, transcranial Doppler sonography, and MRA, are extremely helpful to assess the adequacy of the intracranial circulation and should be used to monitor these patients to prevent subsequent ocular or brain infarction (7,14).

Cervical Artery Dissections and Migraine

The relation between migraine and carotid artery dissection is complex and not clearly defined. It has been suggested that migraine is a predisposing factor for cervical artery dissection. This notion was confirmed only by one case–control study of 50 patients with nontraumatic carotid or vertebral dissection, which indicated that migraine was present significantly more frequently in patients with dissection compared with controls (1). Other authors dispute this association, however (29).

In addition, dissection can present with features of an attack of migraine with or without aura (7,11,14,26,29). Indeed, some cases of so-called migrainous infarcts have angiographic features typical of internal carotid artery dissection. The reverse also can occur in which in migraineurs vascular spasm during cerebral angiography may be mistaken for dissection. As a result, the nature of the link that seems to exist between these two conditions remains obscure.

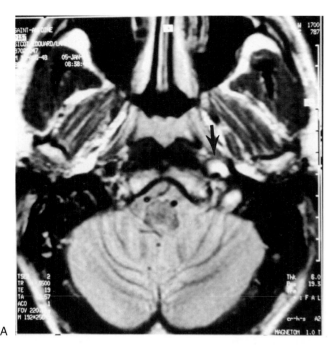
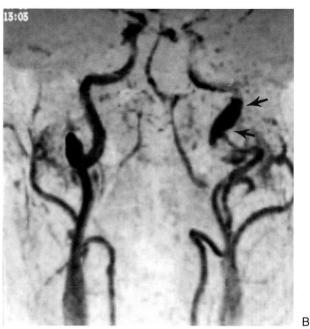

FIG. 1. Dissection localized to the petrous segment of the left extracranial internal carotid artery. **A**: Axial T2-weighted imaging of the brain demonstrating a typical eccentric hyperintense signal of the internal carotid artery corresponding to the mural hematoma *(arrow)* surrounding the residual lumen. **B**: Magnetic resonance angiography showing a left internal carotid artery stenosis associated with a subpetrous hematoma *(arrows)* with increased external diameter typical of dissection.

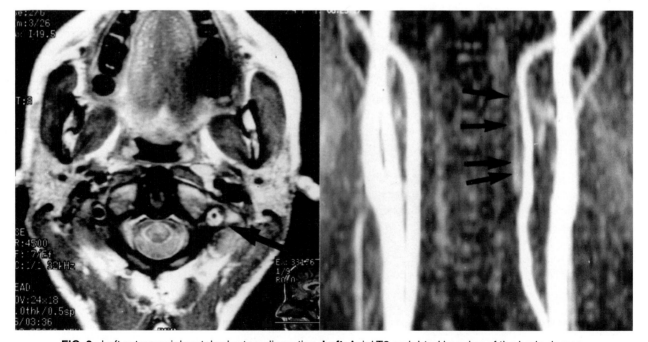

FIG. 2. Left extracranial vertebral artery dissection. **Left**: Axial T2-weighted imaging of the brain demonstrating an hyperintense signal of the left vertebral artery corresponding to the mural hematoma *(arrow)* surrounding the residual lumen. **Right**: Magnetic resonance angiography showing a signal corresponding to the mural hematoma *(arrows)* with increased external diameter consistent with a dissection.

CAROTIDYNIA

Definition

IHS code and diagnosis: 6.6.2 Carotidynia.
WHO code and diagnosis: G44.81 Headache associated with other vascular disorders.

Short Description

Fay (10) was the first to use the term *carotidynia* in 1927 to refer to tenderness of the carotid bifurcation, occasionally observed in patients with atypical facial pain. He believed that the pain arose from the sheath of the common carotid artery and reported the satisfactory remission of symptoms following carotid sheath resection and cervical sympathectomy. In its early description, the term carotidynia was used to refer to the physical sign of local carotid arterial tenderness, later called the *Fay sign* (32).

Over the years, the definition of carotidynia evolved as a name for a distinct syndrome characterized by two cardinal signs: (a) unilateral neck pain, and (b) tenderness of the carotid artery. The literature, especially from the 1960s and 1970s, includes several hundreds of reported cases of carotidynia, from which one can distinguish two main types: acute and chronic. Acute idiopathic carotidynia was even accepted as a valid entity by the International Headache Society (IHS). In the last 10 years, however, carotidynia seems to have vanished almost completely from the medical literature.

Clinical Features

IHS diagnostic criteria (Headache Classification Committee, 1988):

A. At least one of the following overlying the carotid artery:
   1. Tenderness
   2. Swelling
   3. Increased pulsations
B. Appropriate investigations do not reveal any structural abnormality
C. Pain over the affected side of the neck; may project to the ipsilateral side of the head.
D. A self-limiting syndrome of less than 2 weeks' duration.

In the comment, it is emphasized that organic disease of the carotid artery may cause a similar picture; it is therefore clear that appropriate investigations should rule out conditions such as hemorrhage in an atherosclerotic plaque, fibromuscular dysplasia, and carotid artery dissection, all of which have been recognized as possible causes of carotidynia (6,32). These investigations include extracranial Duplex ultrasound scanning, MRI, aand MRA. They should be performed in the first few days after symptom onset because of the possibility of missing important diagnostic features, as is the case in carotid dissection, where rapid recanalization is known to occur. In the hundreds of cases of carotidynia published in earlier decades (6,32), angiography usually was not performed or reported. In recent years, however, carotidynia seems to have completely vanished from the literature, and we were unable to find even a single case report of idiopathic carotidynia (as defined by the IHS) with normal diagnostic investigations. This finding would suggest either that the IHS diagnostic criteria are too restrictive or that idiopathic carotidynia is not a specific entity and that modern neuroimaging techniques almost always lead to discovery of some type of underlying vascular pathology.

Carotidynia: a Nonvalidated Entity

Thus, critical review of the relevant literature reveals that carotydinia is not a valid entity (6). The two clinical signs on which the diagnosis is based (neck pain and carotid artery tenderness) are neither constant nor specific, and there is no consistent pattern or temporal profile. What has been reported under this term in the literature is a "potpourri" of various conditions. Recurrent attacks of carotidynia with headache lasting a few days are likely related to migraine. Attacks lasting for a few minutes suggest chronic paroxysmal hemicrania, and regular daily attacks of 1 to 2 hours' duration point to cluster headache. A viral etiology has been postulated in the acute varieties with a self-limited course. As indicated, carotid dissection should be ruled out in such cases. Chronic varieties with a permanent background pain probably have an important psychological component. Numerous other causes have been reported, including various forms of carotid artery pathology (occlusion, fibromuscular dysplasia, giant cell arteritis, or following carotid endarterectomy) but also carotid body tumors, lymphadenitis, pharyngitis, dental infection, local aphthous ulcers, or malignant infiltration (6,32).

In conclusion, the present state of knowledge suggests that idiopathic carotidynia is not a valid nosological entity and that carotidynia is a syndrome consisting of unilateral neck pain and local arterial tenderness caused by a variety of vascular and nonvascular disease processes, not necessarily implying a vascular origin.

POST-CAROTID ENDARTERECTOMY HEADACHE

Definition

IHS code and diagnosis: 6.6.3 Postendarterectomy headache.
WHO code and diagnosis: G44.81 Headache associated with other vascular disorders.

Short Description

Postendarterectomy headache is defined as headache ipsilateral to the side of the procedure, beginning within 2 days of carotid endarterectomy, and where appropriate diagnostic studies fail to reveal occlusion or dissection of the carotid artery

Clinical Features

IHS diagnostic criteria (Headache Classification Committee, 1988):

A. Thromboendarterectomy or other surgery of the extracranial carotid artery
B. Patent carotid artery without dissection as demonstrated by appropriate investigations
C. Headache that begins within 2 days after surgery and is ipsilateral

   Comment: The headache usually disappears after days, but it may persist for months.

Most reported studies on this variety of headache (3,9,15–18,25,31) did not use these diagnostic criteria, because carotid angiography or ultrasonography were not systematically performed to assess the internal carotid artery patency, and several studies included patients with bilateral headache or headache occurring more than 2 days after the operation. Taking into account all patients in whom headache occurs within 1 month after carotid surgery, with either no past history of headache or previous headache of clearly different type and with a patent internal carotid artery as assessed by angiography or ultrasonography, the following varieties can be described:

1. Headache accompanying a postoperative ischemic or hemorrhagic stroke occurring in the absence of carotid occlusion or dissection. This type of headache, which is always associated with focal neurologic deficits or alteration of the level of consciousness, should not be included in postcarotid endarterectomy headache.

2. Clusterlike headache is considered rare by some (17,18,26) and common by other researchers (18). It is ipsilateral to the surgical side, occurs 12 to 120 hours after the operation, and consists of attacks lasting 2 to 3 hours and occurring once or twice daily. There are no prodromal symptoms. The pain is pulsating, moderate or severe, and located mainly in the retro-orbital and temporoparietal regions. Occasionally, the headache is accompanied by ipsilateral conjunctival injection, lacrimation, rhinorrhea, nasal stuffiness, and Horner's syndrome. The pain usually resolves spontaneously in 2 to 25 days in most cases (18). In patients with this type of headache, decreased activity of the oculosympathetic system was found, based on pharmacologic pupillary testing (17), suggesting that direct surgical damage to the pericarotid sympathetic plexus is an essential element for its production.

3. The severe unilateral headache of the cerebral hyperperfusion syndrome is rare and is observed mainly after correction of a high-grade stenosis in patients with long-lasting, severe, chronic cerebral ischemia (3,8,9, 16,28). This type of headache is severe, unilateral, and throbbing. It starts postoperatively after a headache-free latent interval of about 3 days. It is often preceded by an increase in systemic blood pressure and is accompanied by seizures and contralateral focal deficits (3,8,9,15, 16,28). This symptom complex may herald the occurrence of cerebral hemorrhage (3,28) but has been reported mainly in the absence of stroke (16,28). Computed tomography (CT) scan of the brain is often normal, but it may demonstrate diffuse or patchy cerebral edema consistent with hyperperfusion. This syndrome requires careful management. A high index of suspicion will lead to prompt diagnostic evaluation with invasive or noninvasive vascular studies to exclude the possibility of carotid or other major cerebral vessel occlusion and thus avoid the unnecessary use of potentially dangerous treatment modalities, such as anticoagulants. Acute hypertension, usually unresponsive to propranolol, responds to prazosyn (9). Heavy sedation and assisted ventilation are necessary for seizure control (28).

4. The most frequent type of headache after carotid endarterectomy is a mild, diffuse, nonspecific headache that is not associated with focal deficits, seizures, or an increase in systemic blood pressure (30). It is reported in up to 60% of cases (30). It occurs in the first 5 days following surgery, particularly in the first 2 days (30). It is more often bilateral than unilateral and preferentially affects the frontal regions. It is usually of mild or moderate intensity, described as a sensation of pressure or heaviness, and requires no treatment (30). The temporal profile is variable, either continuous or intermittent, and the average duration is about 3 days. Although it has been previously acknowledged (18,19), this variety of headache is rarely mentioned, probably because of its benign, mild, self-limiting nature and the lack of specific characteristics. The fact that it can occur in patients with no past history of headache suggests a direct relation to the surgical procedure, although this relation might be nonspecific and would be best evaluated in a case–control study that includes patients undergoing other types of arterial surgery.

5. A single case of gustatory pain following carotid endarterectomy has been reported (31). It was a paroxysmal pain in the right preauricular region beginning within several hours after surgery, occurring only with gustatory stimuli, and eventually disappearing within 1 year. Asymmetric, early parotid vasodilatation and sympathetic dysfunction in cutaneous areas overlaying the gland was documented. It is likely that this type of pain is due to interruption of sympathetic vasoconstrictor fibers to the parotid gland, resulting in unopposed parasympathetic-mediated vasodilation in response to gustatory stimuli.

6. Other types of headache, such as severe hemicrania, delayed cluster headache, chronic paroxysmal hemicrania, carotidynia, and Eagle's syndrome also have been reported to occur after carotid endarterectomy (18,25). In all these cases, however, any past history of headache, the time course of the pain, and assessment of carotid patency were poorly documented; consequently no firm conclusions about their direct connection with the carotid surgery can be reached.

In summary, analysis of the existing, and rather confusing, literature does not permit isolation of a single group of patients who satisfy the diagnostic criteria set forth by the IHS for postendarterectomy headache (30), suggesting that it is not a single nosological entity. Three main types have been documented. The most frequent one is a mild, diffuse, self-limiting, nonspecific headache beginning within the first 5 days after surgery. The second is an ipsilateral clusterlike pain attributed to surgical damage of the pericarotid sympathetic plexus. The third is a severe unilateral throbbing headache, frequently accompanied by arterial hypertension, seizures, and focal neurologic deficits. The last type is rare and may herald cerebral hemorrhage.

REFERENCES

1. D'Anglejan-Chatillon J, Ribeiro V, Mas JL, Youl BD, Bousser MG. Migraine: a risk factor for dissection of cervical arteries. *Headache* 1989;29:560–561.
2. Bergqvist CAG, Goldberg HI, Thorarensen O, Bird SJ. Posterior cervical spinal cord infarction following vertebral artery dissection. *Neurology* 1997;48:1112–1115.
3. Bernstein M, Fleming JFR, Deck JHN. Cerebral hyperperfusion after carotid endarterectomy: a cause of cerebral hemorrhage. *Neurosurgery* 1984;15:50–56.
4. Biousse V, Woimant F, Amarenco P, Touboul PJ, Bousser MG. Pain as the only manifestation of extracranial internal carotid artery dissection. *Cephalalgia* 1992;12:314–317.
5. Biousse V, D'Anglejan-Chatillon J, Massiou H, Bousser MG. Head pain in non-traumatic artery dissection: a series of 65 patients. *Cephalalgia* 1994;14:33–36.
6. Biousse V, Bousser MG. The myth of carotidynia. *Neurology* 1994;44:993–995.
7. Biousse V, D'Anglejan-Chatillon J, Touboul PJ, Amarenco P, Bousser MG. Time course of symptoms in extracranial carotid artery dissections: a series of 80 patients. *Stroke* 1995;26:235–239.
8. Breen JC, Caplan LR, DeWitt LD, Belkin M, Mackey WC, O'Donnell TP. Brain edema after carotid surgery. *Neurology* 1996;46:175–181.
9. Dolan JG, Mushlin AI. Hypertension, vascular headaches, and seizures after carotid endarterectomy. *Arch Intern Med* 1984;144:1489–1491.
10. Fay T. Atypical facial neuralgia. *Arch Neurol Psychiatry* 1927;18:309–315.
11. Fisher CM. The headache and pain of spontaneous carotid dissection. *Headache* 1982;22:60–65.
12. Grau A, Brandt T, Forsting M, Winter R, Hacke W. Infection-associated cervical artery dissection. *Stroke* 1997;28:453–455
13. Guillon B, Biousse V, Massiou H, Bousser MG. Isolated long lasting facial pain due to internal carotid artery dissection. *Cephalalgia* 1998;18:222–224.
14. Guillon B, Levy C, Bousser MG. Internal carotid artery dissection: an update. *J Neurol Sci* 1998;153:146–158.
15. Ille O, Woimant F, Pruna A, Corabianu O, Idatte JM, Haguenau M. Hypertensive encephalopathy after bilateral carotid endarterectomy. *Stroke* 1995;26:488–491.
16. Leviton A, Caplan L, Salzman E. Severe headache after carotid endarterectomy. *Headache* 1975;15:207–209.
17. De Marinis M, Zaccaria A, Faraglia V, Fiorani P, Maira G, Agnoli A. Post endarterectomy headache and the role of the oculo-sympathetic system. *J Neurol Neurosurg Psychiatry* 1991;54:314–317.
18. Messert B, Black JA. Cluster headache, hemicrania, and other head pains : morbidity of carotid endarterectomy. *Stroke* 1978;9:559–562.
19. Mitsias P, Ramadan N. Headache in ischemic cerebrovascular disease. Part I: clinical features. *Cephalalgia* 1992;12:269–274.
20. Mitsias P, Ramadan N. Headache in ischemic cerebrovascular disease. Part II: mechanisms and predictive value. *Cephalalgia* 1992;12:269–274.
21. Mokri B, Sundt TM, Houser OW, Piepgras DG. Spontaneous dissection of the cervical internal carotid artery. *Ann Neurol* 1986;19:126–138.
22. Mokri B, Houser WO, Sandok BA, Piepgras DG. Spontaneous dissections of the vertebral arteries. *Neurology* 1988;38:880–885.
23. Moskowitz M. Sensory connections to cephalic blood vessels and their possible importance to vascular headaches. In: Rose C, ed. *Advances in headache research*. John Libbey, 1987:81–93.
24. Nichols FT, Mawad M, Mohr JP, Stein B, Hilal S, Michelsen J. Focal headache during balloon inflation in the internal carotid and middle cerebral arteries. *Stroke* 1990;21:555–559.
25. Pearce J. Headache after carotid endarterectomy. *BMJ* 1976;2:85–86.
26. Ramadan NM, Tietjen GE, Levine SR, Welch KMA. Scintillating scotomata associated with internal carotid artery dissection: report of three cases. *Neurology* 1991;41:1084–1087.
27. Reigel MM, Hollier LH, Sundt TM, Piepgras DG, Sharbrough FW, Cherry KJ. Cerebral hyperperfusion syndrome: a cause of neurologic dysfunction after carotid endarterectomy. *J Vasc Surg* 1987;5:628–634.
28. Schoser BG, Heesen C, Eckert B, Thie A. Cerebral hyperperfusion injury after percutaneous transluminal angioplasty of extracranial arteries. *J Neurol* 1997;244:101–104.
29. Silbert PL, Mokri B, Schievink WI. Headache and neck pain in spontaneous internal carotid and vertebral artery dissections. *Neurology* 1995;45:1517–1522.
30. Tehindrazanarivelo A, Lutz G, PetitJean C, Bousser MG. Headache following carotid endarterectomy : a prospective study. *Cephalalgia* 1991;11(Suppl 11):353.
31. Truax BT. Gustatory pain: a complication of carotid endarterectomy. *Neurology* 1989;39:1258–1260.
32. Vijayan N, Watson C. Raeder's syndrome, pericarotid syndrome and carotidynia. In: Vinken PJ, Bruyn GW, Rose FC eds. *Handbook of clinical neurology*, vol 4. *Headache*. Amsterdam: Elsevier Science Publishers, 1986:329–341.

The Headaches, Second Edition,
edited by J. Olesen, P. Tfelt-Hansen, and K.M.A. Welch.
Lippincott Williams & Wilkins, Philadelphia © 2000.

The Secondary Headaches

CHAPTER 108

Cerebral Venous Thrombosis

Marie-Germaine Bousser and Karl Einhäupl

DEFINITION OF CEREBRAL VENOUS THROMBOSIS

IHS code and diagnosis: 6.7 Venous thrombosis.
WHO code and diagnosis: G 44.81 Headache associated with other vascular disorders.
Short description: Recognized since the early part of the nineteenth century, cerebral venous thrombosis (CVT) has long been considered a rare and severe disease characterized by headache, papilledema, seizures, bilateral focal deficits, coma, and death (16). In the last 20 years, the widespread use of angiography, computerized tomography (CT) of the brain, magnetic resonance imaging (MRI), and magnetic resonance angiography (MRA) have allowed early diagnosis of CVT, completely modifying our knowledge of this condition. More common than previously thought, CVT is remarkable by its variety of causes, its wide spectrum of clinical presentations (with headache as its most frequent sign), and its unpredictable but usually favorable outcome; MRI is nowadays the best diagnostic tool, and heparin the treatment of choice.

EPIDEMIOLOGY

The incidence of CVT is totally unknown in the absence of population-based epidemiologic studies. The recent publication of large clinical series and the present low mortality rate (4) suggest that CVT is much more frequent than classically thought, with three to four new cases each year in neurology departments belonging to a general hospital. All age groups are concerned—from the neonate to the very old—with a slight preponderance in young women because of specific causes such as oral contraceptives, pregnancy, and postpartum.

GENETICS

In itself, CVT is not a hereditary condition, but among its numerous causes, congenital thrombophilia are increasingly recognized: antithrombin, protein C and protein S deficiencies, factor V Leiden (Arg 506 gn mutation), and mutation 20210 A of the prothrombin gene.

PATHOLOGY AND PATHOPHYSIOLOGY

Pathologic findings vary depending on the site of thrombosis and the interval between the onset of symptoms and death. Superior sagittal sinus (SSS) and lateral sinuses are involved most frequently, followed by cortical veins, the deep venous system, and cerebellar veins. In about 75% of cases, multiple veins or sinuses (1,4,12) are involved. In autopsy series, extensive thrombosis of SSS and its tributary veins is the most frequent finding, with massive edema and bilateral hemorrhagic infarcts located in the superior and internal part of both hemispheres. Such cases are now rare and the most frequent parenchymal consequence of CVT is a reversible edema, explaining the usually good recovery.

CLINICAL FEATURES

IHS diagnostic criteria for venous thrombosis (Headache Classification Committee, 1988):

A. At least one of the following :
   1. Raised intracranial pressure

M.-G. Bousser: Department of Neurology, Lariboisière Medical Faculty, Paris VII University, and Department of Neurology, Hôpital Lariboisière, 75475 Paris, France.

K. Einhäupl: Department of Neurology, Universtätsklinikum Charité, D-10117 Berlin, Germany.

2. Focal neurologic deficit
3. Seizures

B. Venous occlusion demonstrated by appropriate investigations

C. Headache is located to affected area or is diffuse

Headache Characteristics

Alhough CVT presents with a remarkably wide spectrum of signs, as illustrated in our series of 150 patients (Table 1), headache is, in all series, the most frequent symptom (80% of cases) and often the initial one (1–4,6,8,12). Mainly described in superior sagittal sinus thrombosis, headache has no topographic value; in our series, it was as common in other situations, such as lateral sinus or cerebral vein thrombosis. Most often diffuse, headache can be unilateral, localized to any region of the head, or even limited to the neck. The severity is again highly variable, ranging from a mild sensation of heaviness to a severe "thunderclap" headache. The mode of onset also varies from patient to patient. Most frequently, the onset of headache is subacute (more than 48 hours but less than 30 days), but it also can be sudden or, by contrast, progressive over several weeks. In the vast majority of cases, headache is persistent, but it can be intermittent, particularly initially, and it sometimes it occurs in attacks. Thus, headache in CVT has no typical clinical characteristic or specific temporal profile. The only suggestive feature is the presence, in more than 95% of cases, of associated signs (1–4,6,8,12).

Associated Signs

Headache can be associated with any of the signs indicated in Table 1, either in isolation or in combination. Taking into account all varieties of associated signs and different modes of onset, four main patterns can be distinguished, to which a number of unusual presentations should be added.

Headache with Isolated Intracranial Hypertension

This pattern of presentation is the most homogeneous. Headache is progressive over days or weeks and is asso-

TABLE 1. *Cerebral venous thrombosis: main neurological signs and symptoms*

Sign/symptom	Incidence (n = 50)
Headache	121 (80.6%)
Papilledema	76 (50.6%)
Seizures	63 (42%)
Focal deficits (motor, sensory, aphasia)	57 (38%)
Drowsiness, mental changes, confusion, or coma	45 (30%)
Multiple cranial nerve palsies	17 (11.3%)
Bilateral cortical signs	6 (4%)
Cerebellar incoordination	4 (2.6%)

ciated with bilateral papilledema and, less frequently, with sixth-nerve palsy, tinnitus, and transient visual obscurations. Such a presentation is that of so- called benign intracranial hypertension (pseudotumor cerebri) and accounts for 40% of our 150 patients. Despite the fact that superior sagittal sinus and lateral sinus thrombosis have long been recognized as one of its leading causes, benign intracranial hypertension has in numerous reports been diagnosed purely on clinical, cerebraospinal fluid (CSF), and CT findings. Because CVT can mimic all the features of benign intracranial hypertension, normal MRI and MRA should be added to the classic diagnostic criteria of this syndrome (1,4). In a prospective study of 24 consecutive patients presenting with all the characteristics of benign intracranial hypertension, MRA disclosed CVT in six (25%) (24).

Headache with Focal Signs

This presentation occurs the most frequently, accounting for roughly 75% of published cases, but it is a heterogeneous one, depending on the mode of onset of focal signs, their nature (deficits, seizures, or both), and their possible association with altered consciousness and signs of raised intracranial pressure. Acute cases simulate an arterial stroke, chronic ones simulate tumors, and subacute cases mimic abscess.

Subacute Encephalopathy

This misleading presentation is characterized by diffuse headache and a depressed level of consciousness with occasional deficits or seizures but without recognizable features of raised intracranial pressure. The differential diagnosis includes encephalitis, disseminated intravascular coagulation, and cerebral vasculitis.

Cavernous Sinus Thrombosis

Cavernous sinus thrombosis has a distinctive clinical picture that includes, in classic acute cases, chemosis, proptosis, and painful ophthalmoplegia, initially unilateral but frequently becoming bilateral. Cavernous sinus thrombosis can also take a more indolent and misleading form (either spontaneously or because of the masking effect of an inadequate antibiotic regimen), with only mild frontal headache, chemosis, and proptosis (4,17).

Unusual Presentations

The grouping of signs of CVT into the preceding four main patterns does not account for every case, and isolated headache can be the only symptom of CVT (7 of 150 in our series). It is particularly misleading when it simulates other conditions. Cases of CVT have been reported of a postural headache after lumbar puncture or epidural anesthesia mimicking a postdural puncture headache, a classic differential diagnosis during the postpartum period (15, 29). Other cases present with a sudden severe headache and CT scan or lumbar puncture evidence of subarachnoid hemorrhage simulating a ruptured intracranial aneurysm, making it necessary to carefully look at the venous system in a patient with subarachnoid hemorrhage (SAH) without arterial causes (4,9). Thunderclap headache (4) and migraine attack (19) (with or without aura) also may be the presenting symptoms of CVT. Other varieties of headache, particularly in patients with lateral sinus thrombosis are unclassifiable: One of our patients presented with unilateral hearing loss and diffuse headache (7), another with an isolated sharp monocular pain as the only sign of ipsilateral lateral sinus thrombosis.

PROGNOSIS

The prognosis of CVT is much better than classically thought but remains unpredictable. In recent large series, mortality still ranks from 33% (6) to 4% (6 of 150 in our series). The three main causes of death are the following:

1. The brain lesion itself, particularly when there is a massive hemorrhagic infarct
2. Intercurrent complications, such as sepsis, uncontrolled seizures, or pulmonary embolism
3. The underlying condition itself, such as carcinoma, leukemia, septicemia, paroxysmal nocturnal hemoglobinuria, heart failure

Most patients survive, with an excellent prognosis in terms of recovery of function. In the most recent series, more than 70% of patients recovered completely (1–4,6, 8,12,25). Headache has not been documented as a sequelae of CVT, whereas focal deficits or seizures can persist in up to 10% to 30% of cases (21).

MANAGEMENT

Given the extremely variable and often misleading signs of CVT, it must be considered in all the aforementioned clinical presentations, particularly when there is an underlying condition known to increase the risk of venous thrombosis (e.g., puerperium, postoperative, posttraumatic, cardiac failure, Behçet's disease). Thus, any recent headache, regardless of its severity, location, and associated signs, should raise suspicion and prompt appropriate investigations.

Today the best diagnostic tools for CVT are MRI, the only investigation to visualize the thrombus itself (Fig. 1) appearing as an increased signal both on T1 and T2 images, and MRA (28) (Fig. 2) (22). The increased signal in MRI is usually obvious between days 5 to 30 after the onset of symptoms (11,18,20,25). In unclear cases, conventional intraarterial angiography is still necessary. The

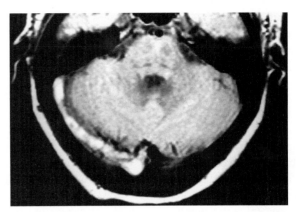

FIG. 1. Magnetic resonance imaging in T1-weighted sequence: hyperintense signal in the right transverse sinus indicating thrombosis.

role of the CT scan is mainly to rule out, on an emergency basis, the numerous conditons that CVT can mimic, such as arterial stroke, abscess, tumor, encephalitis, or subarachnoid hemorrhage. In about 20% of cases, CT can be diagnostic by showing on plain images the spontaneous hyperdensity of the thrombosed sinus and, after contrast, the empty triangle sign (or delta sign) typical of SSS thrombosis (5,27). CSF examination still may be useful when meningitis or encephalitis is suspected or in the patient with isolated intracranial hypertension to measure CSF pressure and to improve vision rapidly when the patient experiences transient or permanent visual loss (3,4). Once the diagnosis of CVT is established, an extensive workup is needed to try to find one of the numerous

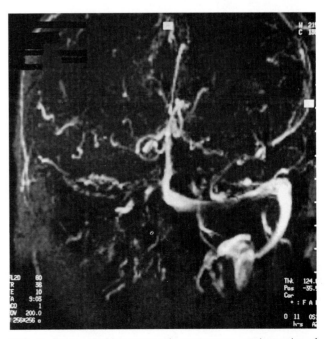

FIG. 2. Flow sensitive magnetic resonance angiography of the same patient: lack of flow signal in the superior sagittal and right transverse sinus.

causative or predisposing conditions (1,3,10). In this respect, headache is not indicative, although in our series it was slightly more frequent when CVT was related to Behçet's disease, oral contraceptive use, pregnancy, and the postpartum period.

Anticoagulation is now a generally accepted therapy, and intravenous full-dose heparin treatment should be started as soon as possible (1,3,4,13,26). After an initial bolus of 3,000 to 5,000 IU, 1,200 to 1,400 IU of heparin should be given hourly until the pretreatment partial thromboplastin time (PTT) is at least doubled. Heparin should be associated, whenever necessary and possible, with an etiologic treatment such as antibiotics in septic cases or steroids in Behçet's disease and systemic lupus erythematosus. Treatment must be continued until remission of the acute stage of the disease (e.g., resolution of headache, remission or stable improvement of focal deficits, normal level of consciousness). At this stage, overlapping transition to oral anticoagulation with warfarin should be initiated, but heparin therapy must be resumed if clinical deterioration occurs. Management of patients with CVT further includes adequate control of seizures, which occur in 30% to 50% of all cases, and reduction of an elevated intracranial pressure.

In the rare patient with extensive sinus thrombosis whose clinical condition deteriorates despite optimal anticoagulation and symptomatic treatment, local thrombolysis with urokinase or recombinant tissue plasminogen activator (rt-PA) is worth trying (14,23). The routine use of fibrinolytics in patients with CVT is not recommended because considerable experience and good results with heparin therapy as well as the risks of fibrinolytic therapy and the lack of randomized trials favor anticoagulation.

REFERENCES

1. Ameri A, Bousser MG. Cerebral venous thrombosis. *Neurol Clin* 1992; 10:87–111.
2. Barinagarrementeria F, Cantu C, Arredondo H. Aseptic cerebral venous thrombosis: proposed prognostic scale. *J Stroke Cerebrovasc Dis* 1992; 2:34–39.
3. Bousser MG, Chiras J, Sauron B, Bories J, Castaigne P. Cerebral venous thrombosis: a review of 38 cases. *Stroke* 1985;16:199–213.
4. Bousser MG, Ross Russell R. Cerebral venous thrombosis. *Major problems in neurology*, vol 1. London: WB Saunders, 1997 175 pp.
5. Buonanno FS, Moody DM, Ball RM. CT scan findings in cerebral sinovenous occlusion. *Neurology* 1982;12:288–292.
6. Cantu C, Barinagarrementeria F. Cerebral venous thrombosis associated with pregnancy and puerperium: review of 67 cases. *Stroke* 1993; 24:1880–1884.
7. Crassard I, Biousse V, Bousser MG, Meyer B, Marsot-Dupuch K. Hearing loss and headache revealing lateral sinus thrombosis in a patient with Factor V Leiden mutation. *Stroke* 1997;28:876–877.
8. Daif A, Awada A, Al-Rajeh S, et al. Cerebral venous thrombosis in adult: a study of 40 cases from Saudi Arabia. *Stroke* 1995;26: 1193–1195.
9. De Bruijn SFTM, Stam J, Kappelle LJ for CVST study group: thunderclap headache as first symptom of cerebral venous sinus thrombosis. *Lancet* 1996;348:1623–1625.
10. Deschiens MA, Conard J, Horellou MH, et al. Coagulation studies, Factor V Leiden, antiphospholipid antibodies in 40 cases of cerebral venous thrombosis. *Stroke* 1996;27:1724–1730.
11. Dormont D, Anxionnat R, Evrard S, et al. MRI in cerebral venous thrombosis. *J Neuroradiol* 1994;21:81–99.
12. Einhäupl KM, Masuhr F. Cerebral venous and sinus thrombosis. An update : *Eur J Neurol* 1994;1:109–126.
13. Einhäupl KM, Villringer A, Meister W, et al. Heparin treatment in sinus venous thrombosis. *Lancet* 1991;338:597–600.
14. Horowitz M, Purdy P, Unwin H, et al. Treatment of dural sinus thrombosis using elective catheterization and urokinase. *Ann Neurol* 1995;38: 58–67.
15. Hubbert CH. Dural puncture headache suspected, cortical vein thrombosis diagnosed. *Anesth Analg* 1987;66:285.
16. Kalbag RM, Woolf AL. *Cerebral venous thrombosis.* University Press. London: Oxford University Press, 1967.
17. Levine SR, Twyman RE, Gilman S. The role of anticoagulation in cavernous sinus thrombosis. *Neurology* 1988;38:517–521.
18. Mattle H, Edelkman RR, Reis MA, Atkinson DJ. Flow quantification in the superior sagittal sinus using magnetic resonance. *Neurology* 1990; 40:813–815.
19. Newman DS, Levine SR, Curtis VL, Welch KMA. Migraine like visual phenomena associated with cerebral venous thrombosis. *Headache* 1989;29:82–85.
20. Padayachee TS, Bingham JB, Grave MJ, Colcheter AC, Cow TC. Dural sinus thrombosis: diagnosis and follow-up by magnetic resonance angiography and imaging. *Neuroradiology* 1991;33:165–167.
21. Preter M, Tzourio C, Ameri A, Bousser MG. Long term prognosis in cerebral venous thrombosis: a follow-up of 77 patients. *Stroke* 1996;27: 243–246.
22. Rippe DJ, Boyko OB, Spritzer CE, et al. Demonstration of dural sinus occlusion by the use of MR angiography. *AJNR Am J Neuroradiol* 1990; 11:199–201.
23. Smith TP, Higashida R, Barnwell S, et al. Treatment of dural sinus thrombosis by urolinase infusion. *AJNR Am J Neuroradiol* 1994;15: 801–807.
24. Tehindfazanarivelo AD, Evrard S, Schaison M, et al. Prospective study of cereral sinus venous thrombosis in patients presenting with benign intracranial hypertension. *Cerebrovasc Dis* 1992;2:22–27.
25. Tsai FY, Wang AM, Matovich V, et al. MR staging of acute dural sinus thrombosis : correlation with venous pressure measurements and implications for treatment and prognosis. *AJNR Am J Neuroradiol* 1995;16: 1021–1029.
26. Villringer A, Meraein S, Einhäupl KM. Treatment of sinus venous thrombosis-beyond the recommendation of anticoagulation. *J Neuroradiol* 1994;21:72–80.
27. Virapongse C, Cazenave C, Quisling R, Sarwar M, Hunter S. The empty delta sign: frequency and significance in 76 cases of dural sinus thrombosis. *Radiology* 1987;162:779–785.
28. Vogl TJ, Bergman C, Villringer A, et al. Dural sinus thrombosis: value of venous MR angiography for diagnosis and follow-up. *AJR Am J Roentgenol* 1994;162:1191–1198.
29. Wilder-Smith E, Kothbauer-Margreiter I, Lämmle B, et al. Dural puncture and activated protein C resistance : risk factors for cerebral venous sinus thrombosis. *J Neurol Neurosurg Psychiatry* 1997;63:351–356.

The Headaches, Second Edition,
edited by J. Olesen, P. Tfelt-Hansen, and K.M.A. Welch.
Lippincott Williams & Wilkins, Philadelphia © 2000.

The Secondary Headaches

CHAPTER 109

Arterial Hypertension

Svend Strandgaard and Patrick Henry

International Headache Society (IHS) Classification

6.8.1 Acute pressor response to exogenous agent
6.8.2 Pheochromocytoma
6.8.3 Malignant (accelerated) hypertension (including hypertensive encephalopathy)
6.8.4 Preeclampsia and eclampsia

WHO code and diagnosis: G44.81 Headache associated with other vascular disorders

Short description: Headache caused by a rather severely elevated blood pressure or a sudden rise in blood pressure, most likely of vascular origin. Tension-type headache may be caused by anxiety over hypertension. Finally, some antihypertensive drugs have headache as a side effect.

EPIDEMIOLOGY

Hypertension is defined as a sustained diastolic blood pressure at or above 90 mm Hg or a systolic blood pressure at or above 140 mmHg (18). This definition of hypertension includes 10% to 20% of the population in the developed world and is considered meaningful because of the increased cardiovascular morbidity and mortality associated with even moderately raised blood pressures. Because so many people are hypertensive, the association between common forms of headache and hypertension is coincidental in most cases.

Three types of studies have dealt with the incidence and prevalence of headache in hypertension: large-scale epidemiologic studies in the general population and studies in samples of varying size of headache patients or hypertensive patients. In an American study from 1972 comprising 6,672 subjects, the prevalence of headache was about 25% and was unrelated to the level of blood pressure. Retinopathy was associated with a slight, significant increase of the prevalence of headache, irrespective of the blood pressure level (20). Likewise, in a British population study from 1971 of 414 subjects, no association was found between headache and blood pressure (19).

In a Danish population study of 975 subjects, 11% had a blood pressure at hypertensive levels or were in antihypertensive treatement. No difference was found in the incidence of headache in the subjects who were categorized as hypertensive and the normotensive participants in the study (14). This latter study, the first of its kind to use the headache classification of the IHS, documented that neither migraine, tension headache, nor other types of headache were overrepresented in the hypertensive subgroup of the population sample. It was found, however, that women with migraine had a slightly but significantly elevated diastolic blood pressure compared with nonmigrainous women.

In a U.S. study of 508 young women with migraine and 3,192 without migraine, no association was found between migraine and hypertension (4). In the Italian Longitudinal Study of Aging (ILSA), investigation of a subgroup of 312 elderly persons from a community near Milan showed an association of migraine and secondary headaches with hypertension (8).

Studies of headache in samples of hypertensive patients usually include a subgroup with severely elevated blood pressure. Badran et al. (2) compared 100 hypertensive patients to 100 controls. The prevalence of

S. Strandgaard: Department of Nephrology, Herlev Hospital, DK-2730 Herlev, Denmark.

P. Henry: Service de Neurologie, Hôpital Pellegrin, 33076 Bordeaux, France.

headache was 39% in normotensive patients, and 36% in mildly to moderatley hypertensive patients. With diastolic blood pressures above 130 mmHg, the prevalence of headache was higher, around 50%. Bulpitt et al. (3) found headache in approximately 31% of untreated, moderately severe hypertension, as compared with 15% in treated patients and normal controls.

In a survey of no less than 11,710 hypertensive patients, Cooper et al. (5) found that headache was common and was related to the blood pressure level. The incidence of headache could be reduced by antihypertensive treatment, even though treatment with calcium antagonists appeared to be an independent cause of headache in these patients. In controlled trials of antihypertensive treatment, the reported incidence of headache is rather varying. Sometimes, it is identical in the treatment and placebo groups, sometimes it appears to be lowered by treatment. On the other hand, the incidence of headache is very high, above 80%, in paroxystic hypertension secondary to pheochromocytoma (17).

In an Italian study of 449 patients with hypertensive crisis (diastolic blood pressure at or above 120 mm Hg), 108 were classified as emergencies (with target-organ damage) and 341 as urgencies (without target-organ damage). Headache was reported in 22% of hypertensive emergencies and in 3% of hypertensive urgencies (21).

PATHOPHYSIOLOGY

Headache in severe hypertension as listed in the IHS classification probably is of vascular origin and is caused by hypertensive dilatation or stretching of the resistance vessels. The evidence favoring this origin, however, is of an indirect nature. For example, in one study, which was published before the advent of modern antihypertensive therapy, intravenous injection of aminophylline, a cerebral vasoconstrictor, as well as caffeine would constrict stretched hypertensive resistance vessels in the brain (16). Possibly, hypertensive headache may be related to failure of autoregulation and the formation of brain edema, which are instrumental in the pathogenesis of acute hypertensive encephalopathy (Fig. 1). Intracranial pressure often is raised in malignant hypertension (13), probably because of a low-grade chronic brain edema, which may be implicated in the pathogenesis of headache in these patients.

CLINICAL FEATURES

IHS diagnostic criteria for the four subgroups of headache associated with severe hypertension (Headache Classification Committee, 1988) (10):
1. Acute pressor response to exogenous agent
   A. Headache occurs with acute rise (greater than 25%) of diastolic blood pressure
   B. Evidence of appropriate toxin or medication

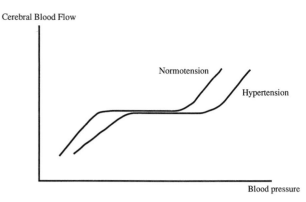

FIG. 1. Autoregulation of cerebral blood flow in normotension and chronic untreated hypertension. Autoregulation maintains a constant blood flow during rather wide variations of blood pressure by varying the degree of constriction of the smaller cerebral resistance vessels. Both the lower and upper blood pressure limits of autoregulation are shifted toward higher blood pressure in hypertension. Nonetheless, autoregulation may fail when the blood pressure is quite high, and localized brain edema may develop, which may be the cause of the headache seen in patients with severe hypertension. Controlled lowering of blood pressure leads to prompt relief of the headache.

   C. Headache disappears within 24 hours after normalization of blood pressure
2. Pheochromocytoma
   A. Headache occurs with acute rise (greater than 25%) of diastolic blood pressure
   B. At least one of the following:
      1. Sweating
      2. Palpitation
      3. Anxiety
   C. Pheochromocytoma proved by biologic and imaging tests or surgery
   D. Headache disappears within 24 hours after normalization of blood pressure
3. Malignant (accelerated) hypertension (including hypertensive encephalopathy)
   A. Headache associated with grade 3 or 4 retinopathy
   B. Diastolic blood pressure persistently above 120 mm Hg
   C. Appropriate investigations rule out vasopressor toxins, medication, or pheochromocytoma as causative factors
   D. Headache is temporarily related to an increase in blood pressure and disappears within 2 days after reduction of blood pressure. If hypertensive encephalopathy is present, headache may persist for up to 7 days after reduction of blood pressure.
4. Preeclampsia and eclampsia
   A. Headache during pregnancy
   B. Edema or proteinuria and a blood pressure increase from a prepregnant level (not necessarily markedly increased but at least mean elevation of 15 mm Hg or diastolic of 90 mm Hg)

C. Appropriate investigations rule out vasopressor toxins, medication, or pheochromocytoma as causative factors

D. Headache occurs with an increase in blood pressure and disappears within 7 days after blood pressure reduction or after termination of pregnancy

The literature on headache in hypertension is relatively sparse, and only a few studies have attempted to apply the IHS classification. Hence, it is not always possible to infer from published studies whether an increased incidence of headache in hypertension, if present, is of tension-type or of vascular origin.

The type of headache described in patients with diastolic blood pressure above 130 mm Hg is frequently diffuse, present when the patient wakes in the morning, and subsides over the following hours. In this disease, paroxystic throbbing headache often wakes the patient from sleep. The intensity of pain increases within minutes and then subisdes over several minutes. This brief duration is an important feature of pheochromocytoma-related headache (10).

Whether some patients with mild to moderate hypertension suffer from headache caused by elevated blood pressure is quite uncertain. Hence, it is hardly possible to categorize any other type of hypertensive headache than the vasogenic type seen in the more severely hypertensive patients. In some patients with hypertension, headaches are tensive in nature and probably are not directly related to hypertension but rather to the anxiety of being conscious of an elevated blood pressure. Indeed, headaches are more frequent in hypertensive patients who are aware of their elevated pressure than in those unaware of it (7).

REACTIVE RISE IN BLOOD PRESSURE DURING SEVERE HEADACHE

Pain and distress of whatever origin often tend to increase blood pressure. This effect, which may be prominent, for example, during an attack of angina pectoris, is apparently not common in headache. Thus, Krogh-Rasmussen (14) found that the blood pressure was not influenced by point headache, that is, headache coinciding with a structured health interview. Blood pressure may be transiently increased during a migraine attack (9) and during cluster headache (1). Some authors, however, report that the incidence of hypertension in cluster headache is slightly although insignificantly lower than in controls (15).

HEADACHE AS A SIDE EFFECT OF ANTIHYPERTENSIVE TREATMENT

Lowering of a severely elevated blood pressure sometimes relieves concomitant headache. Headache unrelated to blood pressure obviously persists. Some antihypertensive drugs may produce headache as an adverse effect. This type of headache is seen primarily with the use of vasodilators, most notably the calcium antagonists (6,11) and hydralazine. These drugs tend to raise intracranial pressure by dilating cerebral resistance vessels (12). Headache caused by cerebral vasodilatation may respond to dose reduction, making discontinuation of the drug unnecessary.

MANAGEMENT AND PROGNOSIS OF HYPERTENSIVE HEADACHE

Treatment of hypertensive headache is first and foremost the lowering of blood pressure. In most cases, this step has a relieving effect within 24 hours. With full-blown hypertensive encephalopathy, headache may persist for some days after pressure control, presumably as brain edema is cleared. As noted, cerebral vasoconstrictors such as aminophylline and caffeine may relieve hypertensive headache. Coincidental headache in hypertension, unrelated to high blood pressure, obviously will persist during blood pressure lowering. The same applies to tension-type headache caused by hypertension-related anxiety. As noted, the occasional headache may be induced by antihypertensive vasodilator drugs.

CONCLUSION

Contrary to common belief, hypertension is not an important cause of headache. In the developed world, uncontrolled severe hypertension is rare, and the occurrence of headache and hypertension in the same patient often is coincidental. Patients complaining of headache nonetheless should have their blood pressure measured, which may lead to the occasional recognition of severe hypertension otherwise undiagnosed. Finally, it should be kept in mind that vasodilating antihypertensive drugs sometimes have headache as a side effect.

REFERENCES

1. Attanasio A, Capria A, Quatrana M, et al. Sinus bradycardia, functional rhythm and blood pressure during repeated cluster headache attacks. *Headache* 1990;30:509–510.
2. Badran RH, Weir RJ, McGuiness JB. Hypertension and headache. *Scand Med J* 1970;15:48–51.
3. Bulpitt CJ, Dollery CT, Carne S. Change in symptoms of hypertension patients after referral to hospital clinic. *Br Heart J* 1976;38:121–128.
4. Chen TC, Leviton A, Edelstein S, Ellenberg JH. Migraine and other diseases of women of reproductive age: the influence of smoking on observed associations. *Arch Neurol* 1987;44:1024–1028.
5. Cooper WD, Glover DR, Hormbrey JM, Kimber GR. Headache and blood pressure: evidence of a close relationship. *J Hum Hypertens* 1989;3:41–44.
6. Dougall HT, McLay J. A comparative review of the adverse effects of calcium antagonists. *Drug Safety* 1996;15:91–106.
7. Fisher CM. Headache in cerebrovascular disease. In: Vinken PJ, Bruyn GW, eds. *Handbook of clinical neurology, vol 5. Headaches and cranial neuralgias.* Amsterdam: North Holland, 1968:124–156.
8. Franseschi M, Colombe B, Rossi P, Canal N. Headache in a population-based elderly cohort: an ancillary study to the Italian Longitudinal Study of Aging (ILSA). *Headache* 1997;37:79–82.
9. Freitag FG, Diamond M. Emergency treatment of headache. *Med Clin North Am* 1991;75:749–761.

10. Headache Classification Committee of the International Headache Society: Classification and diagnostic criteria for headache disorders, cranial neuralgias and facial pain. *Cephalalgia* 1988;8:(Suppl 8):1–96.

11. Hedner T. Calcium channel blockers: Spectrum of side effects and drug interactions. *Acta Pharmacol Toxicol* 1986;58(suppl 12):119–130.

12. Johansson BB, Auer LM, Trummer UG. Pial vascular reaction to intravenous dihydralazine in the cat. *Stroke* 1975;6:402–404.

13. Kincaid-Smith P, McMichael J, Murphy EA. The clinical course and pathology of hypertension with pilloedema (malignant hypertension). *QJM* 1958;27:117–153.

14. Krogh-Rasmussen B, Olesen J. Symptomatic and non-symptomatic headaches in a general population. *Neurology* 1992;42:1225–1231.

15. Kudrow L. *Cluster headache:* mechanisms and management. New York: Oxford University Press, 1980.

16. Moyer JH, Tashnek AB, Miller SI, Snyder H, Bowman RO. The effect of theophylline with ethylenediamine (aminophylline) and caffeine on cerebral hemodynamics and cerebrospinal fluid pressure in patients with hypertensive headaches. *Am J Med Sci* 1952;224:377–385.

17. Raskin NH, Appenzeler O. *Headache.* Philadelphia: WB Saunders, 1980:12–15.

18. The Sixth Report of the Joint National Committee on Prevention, Detection, Evaluation, and Treatment of High Blood Pressure. *Arch Intern Med* 1997;157:2413–2446.

19. Waters WE. Headache and blood pressure in the community. *BMJ* 1971;1:142–143.

20. Weiss NS. Relation of high blood pressure to headache, epistaxis, and selected other symptoms. *N Engl J Med* 1972;287:631–633.

21. Zampaglione B, Pascale C, Marchisio M, Cavallo-Perin P. Hypertensive urgencies and emergencies: prevalence and clinical presentation. *Hypertension* 1996;27:144–147.

The Headaches, Second Edition,
edited by J. Olesen, P. Tfelt-Hansen, and K.M.A. Welch.
Lippincott Williams & Wilkins, Philadelphia © 2000.

The Secondary Headaches

CHAPTER 110

High Cerebrospinal Fluid Pressure

Per Soelberg Sørensen and James John Corbett

IDIOPATHIC INTRACRANIAL HYPERTENSION (BENIGN INTRACRANIAL OR PSEUDOTUMOR CEREBRI)

IHS code and diagnosis: 7.1.1 Benign intracranial hypertension.

WHO code and diagnosis: G44.82 Headache associated with other intracranial disorders.

Short Description: Idiopathic intracranial hypertension (IIH), or benign intracranial hypertension, is defined as increased intracranial pressure (ICP) in the absence of an intracranial mass or hydrocephalus. The syndrome is characterized by headache, papilledema, no localizing neurologic signs, and normal cerebrospinal fluid (CSF) composition. Rarely, it occurs in the absence of papilledema.

Other Terms: Serous meningitis, pseudotumor cerebri, meningeal hydrops, otitic hydrocephalus, toxic hydrocephalus, intracranial hypertension without ventriculomegaly, and benign intracranial hypertension. Because the condition does not always run a self-limiting course, but is often a chronic disorder or leaves the patient with variably severe visual loss, the term benign is certainly a misnomer, and the term *idiopathic intracranial hypertension* is preferred.

Epidemiology

Idiopathic intracranial hypertension is a relatively common neurologic disease that has been reported from most parts of the world with an annual incidence of 1 to 2 per 100,000. The annual incidence in the general population was reported to be 0.9 per 100,000 persons in Iowa and Louisiana in the United States (14) and 1.7 per 100,000 in northeastern Libya (37). The syndrome occurs in both children and adults. No sex difference is seen in children, whereas the female-to-male ratio in most series of adult patients is between 3:1 and 10:1 (5,14,48,60,61). The condition occurs most commonly in obese women of childbearing age, in whom the incidence has been reported to be as high as 19 per 100,000 (14). Familial occurrence has been encountered in siblings and in mother and son (3,41,56).

Pathophysiology and Etiology

The pathophysiology of intracranial hypertension is controversial. In the absence of a space-occupying lesion or hydrocephalus, a number of mechanisms have been suggested as possible explanations of increased ICP: increased brain volume caused by increased brain water content (20), increased blood volume (11), increased ICP transmitted from elevated intraabdominal and intrathoracic pressure in obese persons (53), increased rate of CSF formation (12), or a decreased rate of CSF absorption at the site of the arachnoid villi (28). Only insignificant increments in cerebral blood volume have been reported by some investigators studying IIH (1,32), and recently a normal CSF production rate was found using magnetic resonance (MR) techniques for indirect calculations of CSF production (19).

Hence, the two prevailing hypotheses of the pathophysiologic mechanisms are increased brain water content or increased resistance to CSF outflow. Indirect evidence of increased brain volume has been provided by computerized tomography (CT) and MR showing

P.S. Sørensen: University of Copenhagen, and Department of Neurology, Copenhagen University Hospital, Righospitalet, DK-2100 Copenhagen, Denmark.

J.J. Corbett: University of Mississippi School of Medicine, and Department of Neurology, University of Mississippi Medical Center, Jackson, Mississippi 39216–4505.

decreased CSF volume in ventricles and sulci (38). MR imaging (MRI) of brain water self-diffusion has indicated increased brain water content, particularly in the periventricular white matter, in patients with IIH (20). Johnston and Paterson (28) suggested increased resistance to CSF outflow across the arachnoid villi as the underlying cause of IIH, and many investigators have convincingly demonstrated an increased resistance to CSF outflow using spinal infusion or perfusion tests (18,28,46,49). Unfortunately, abnormal spinal infusion tests do not differentiate clearly between impairment of CSF absorption and decreased intracranial compliance resulting from an increase in brain volume. These two hypotheses are not necessarily mutually exclusive, however. Increased resistance to CSF outflow causes an excessive amount of CSF in the brain; because no ventricular enlargement or increased subarachnoid space is found in IIH, an expanded brain extracellular space may simulate a form of brain edema. On the other hand, a primary intracellular brain water accumulation would reduce the subarachnoid space over the hemispheres and increase the resistance to CSF outflow. The mutual dependence of these two mechanisms remains unclear, and the demonstration of increased brain water content or increased resistance to CSF outflow do not allow one to conclude which of these two are the primary defect and which is a secondary phenomenon.

No common etiology of intracranial hypertension has been found in patients with IIH. Many diseases and conditions have been associated with the syndrome, some of which have been claimed to be causal. Some of the most frequently mentioned are listed in Table 1. Many of these proposed etiologic factors are common conditions that probably occur by chance in patients with IIH. The only consistent finding seems to be a predilection for obese women of childbearing age (27,61). Further, many patients report a recent substantial weight gain (21,43,59). These observations have led to speculations of hypothalamic–pituitary disturbances in patients with IIH, but conventional tests of endocrine functions have disclosed only inconsistent and insignificant abnormalities in the function of the pituitary or the peripheral target glands (39,48). A number of other conditions can produce a clinical picture resembling IIH, that is, increased ICP in the absence of a mass lesion or hydrocephalus. These disorders, some of which are listed in Table 2, should not be included under the term IIH.

Clinical Features

Diagnostic criteria of benign intracranial hypertension are:

1. Increased ICP (>200 mm H_2O) measured by epidural, intraventricular, or lumbar subarachnoid pressure monitoring or by lumbar puncture

TABLE 1. *Possible etiologic factors in idiopathic intracranial hypertension*

Endocrine disturbances
  Pituitary disorders
    Acromegaly
    Growth hormone therapy
    Pituitary adenoma
    Empty sella syndrome
  Pituitary-adrenal disturbances
    Cushing's disease
    Corticosteroid therapy
    Corticosteroid withdrawal
    Addison's disease
  Gonadal dysfunction
    Menstrual irregularities
    Pregnancy
    Oral contraceptives
    Turner's syndrome
  Thyroid disease
    Hyperthyroidism
    Hypothyroidism
  Parathyroid disorders
    Hypoparathyroidism
    Pseudohypoparathyroidism
Overweight
Drugs
  Vitamin A overuse, isotretionin, all-trans-retinoic acid
  Tetracyclines, nitrofurantoin, nalidixic acid, sulphonamides
  Indomethacin, phenytoin, cyclosporine
Hematologic disorders
  Anemia
  Polycythemia
  Coagulation abnormalities
Head injury
Infections
Others
  Vitamin A deficiency
  Collagen disorders, antiphospholipid antibody syndrome, Behcet's disease

2. Symptoms and signs of ICP but an absence of any localizing signs
3. No mass lesion and no ventricular enlargement on neuroimaging
4. Normal or low protein concentration and normal cell count in CSF
5. No clinical or neuroimaging suspicion of venous sinus thrombosis

The most prominent symptom is headache, which is a presenting symptom in 75% to 100% of patients (2,21,43,49,58). The headache is usually gradual in onset, but some patients experience acute severe headache (49). In most patients, the headache occurs daily and is of moderate intensity, although 93% of the patients examined by Wall using a questionnaire reported that the headache of IIH was their severest headache ever (58). The localization and quality of pain show no specific pattern. The headache can be holocranial or one-sided, and a few patients report bouts of lightening pain in a localized area of the scalp. The headache can be throbbing or pressing

TABLE 2. *Condition that may produce papilledema with no focal signs and normal neuroimaging*

Neoplasms
  Primary cerebral lymphoma (gliomatosis cerebri)
  Gliomas
  Meningeal carcinomatosis
  Spinal cord tumors
Vascular diseases
  Venous sinus thrombosis
  Arteriovenous malformation
Infectious diseases
  Chronic encephalitis
  Chronic meningitis
  HIV associated meningoradiculitis
CSF hyperviscosity
  Guillain-Barré syndrome
  Spinal cord tumor
Others
  Chronic respiratory disease (CO_2 retention)
  Obstructive sleep apnea syndrome

CSF, cerebrospinal fluid; HIV, human immunodeficiency virus.

and worsens with Valsalva maneuvers or postural changes (47). Retroocular pain aggravated by eye movement is described in some patients (2,58). In patients with migraine, the intracranial hypertension may worsen the condition (57), and refractory transformed migraine type of chronic daily headache has been reported in patients with IIH, even in the absence of papilledema (33).

Artificial production of elevated spinal fluid pressure using saline infusion usually produces frontal and temporal headaches but may be associated with unilateral or holocranial head pain of any kind. Some patients sense no pain despite rapid rises in CSF pressure during the infusion tests (16). Thus, there is little specific to identify a headache as being caused by high spinal fluid pressure.

Nausea is an accompanying symptom in about half of these patients, and vomiting is less common (49,58,61). Neck stiffness has been recognized in a high proportion of patients by some investigators (42,58). In addition to headaches that are attributed to high CSF pressure in patients with IIH, other factors related either to chronicity of increased ICP or to treatment may confound the picture further. After lumbar puncture, the headache is frequently relieved but may be complicated by the addition of a headache due to CSF leak. Spontaneous CSF rhinorrhea through the cribriform plate or through an empty sella may result in low CSF pressure and a low-pressure headache. Furthermore, after lumbar–peritoneal shunt, the patient may become shunt dependent or tonsillar herniation can occur with a new type of headache, known as the *hindbrain herniation headache* (35).

Aside from headache, visual complaints are the most important feature of IIH. Transient visual obscurations are seconds-long spells of loss of vision caused by transient ischemia of the visual pathways. Most patients with IIH (50%–75%) experience transient visual obscurations (8,43,49,60) that occur several times a day and are provoked by postural changes. Permanent blurring of vision with normal visual acuity and photopsias are additional nonspecific visual complaints. Double vision, sometimes intermittent, is usually horizontal because of a sixth-nerve palsy and occurs in 16% to 38% of patients with IIH as a false localizing sign (8,49,60). Intracranial noises or tinnitus, both objective and subjective, which can be unilateral or bilateral, are common but often ignored signs or symptoms in IIH. The noises are more often a pulsatile bruitlike sound than the high-frequency ringing sound in typical tinnitus (60). The noises have been attributed variously to the intensified vascular pulsations of the CSF resulting from the high ICP and to turbulence in the venous sinuses. Less common symptoms in IIH are radicular pain and paresthesias in the arms and legs, low-back pain, unsteadiness or vertigo, and difficulties with concentration and memory (2,5,21,42,50).

The ophthalmologic signs in IIH are papilledema, visual-field defects, loss of visual acuity, and sixth-nerve palsy. Bilateral papilledema is considered almost obligatory for the diagnosis, but cases with unilateral or absent papilledema have been reported (31,33,34,51), a finding that may be explained by anatomic variations in the extension of the subarachnoid space in the optic-nerve sheath of the optic canal. Splinters or subretinal hemorrhages are commonly seen around the disk. With long-standing papilledema, the disk may become pale, gliotic, and flat. These changes make it difficult to evaluate recurrent swelling of the disk (8,49). Blind-spot enlargement almost always is seen in IIH. Generalized constriction of the visual field and a lower nasal visual field loss are the other most commonly reported defects (8,43,49,60). Field defects are found with increasing frequency (up to 90%) when static perimetry is used (60). Visual acuity is normal in most patients at the initial presentation of the disease, but the risk of visual impairment increases with longer duration of papilledema. The visual loss can progress gradually or stepwise into blindness of one or both eyes, but some patients experience acute loss of vision. The risk of blindness is between 4% and 10%. Systemic hypertension and increased intraocular pressure increase the hazard (8).

The ICP is usually moderately increased to 18 to 25 mm Hg (normal pressure is <15 mm Hg), but in some cases steady-state pressures of 30 to 50 mm Hg have been measured. Virtually all patients have abnormal pressure waves, B waves (increments from this steady-state pressure of one or two waves per minute with an amplitude of 5 to 15 mm Hg). About half of the patients show typical plateau waves of 5 to 15 minutes' duration, with a peak pressure of 40 to 70 mm Hg (28,49) (Fig. 1). There is poor correlation between the clinical symptoms and the ICP and no clear relationship between the height of the CSF pressure and the severity of the headache (28).

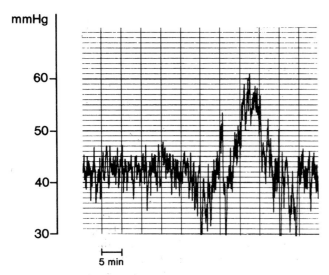

FIG. 1. Epidural pressure recording from a patient with idiopathic intracranial hypertension (*IIH*) showing increased steady-state pressure, B-wave activity, and a plateau wave.

Diagnosis

The diagnosis of IIH should not be made without neuroimaging of the brain by MRI or CT, examination of the CSF, and measurement of the ICP. MRI of the brain indicating saggital T1-weighted images and MR angiography must be normal. Diffusion-weighted images on MRI show increased water diffusion periventricularly and in some cases in the whole brain (20). MRI of the optic nerves may show an enlarged, elongated subarachnoid space around the optic nerve (18). Ultrasonography of the optic nerves also may be helpful as a noninvasive evaluation of increased ICP in children. The CSF should show a normal or low protein level, a normal glucose concentration, and a normal cell count. At lumbar puncture, the CSF pressure should be elevated (>200 mm H_2O, equivalent to 15 mm Hg). Opening spinal fluid pressures between 200 and 250 mm H_2O are, however, not diagnostic and may be seen in normal persons. Preferably, the CSF pressure should be monitored for at least 30 to 60 minutes by an epidural intracranial or a subarachnoid lumbar transducer. As a minimum, the pressure should be measured carefully using a lumbar puncture performed with the patient relaxed and the head and legs extended. Monitoring the ICP with a transducer allows calculation of the mean steady-state pressure and characterization of abnormal increments from this steady-state pressure. Measuring the opening pressure does not always give the true steady-state pressure because of fluctuations in ICP seen in all patients with IIH (22,28). Demonstration of an increased resistance to CSF outflow at a spinal infusion test helps to corroborate the diagnosis but is rarely done (22). Ophthalmologic examination should include fundus photographs and repeated quantitative visual fields with either static or kinetic perimetry. Blind-spot measurement alone and measurement of visual acuity are not helpful in monitoring these patients.

Prognosis

Idiopathic intracranial hypertension is usually regarded as a self-limiting disease, but CSF pressure measurements over many years have shown it to be a chronic condition (8,49). Spontaneous remission of the papilledema is common, but recurrence is seen in 10% of cases. Visual loss is common in IIH, but milder degrees of visual-field defects are often reversible. Permanent serious visual loss occurs in 10% to 25% of patients, and blindness develops in 4% to 10% (8,60). The symptoms of increased ICP, headache, and transient visual obscurations usually decrease on treatment of the intracranial hypertension, but spontaneous disappearance of headache and nausea before any treatment is begun is not uncommon. Three months after the start of treatment, about one half of patients have only minor headache and visual complaints (49). With the exception of permanent visual loss, the prognosis is considered excellent in the most patients. In a smaller proportion of patients, however, the condition runs a protracted course with long-standing complaints of headache, visual disturbances, and mild impairment of concentration and memory (49). Rare complications include CSF rhinorrhea and the development of acquired Arnold-Chiari malformation (type I) with cervical syrinx following a lumbar peritoneal shunt. In some patients, visual function deteriorates despite medical and even surgical treatment of the increased pressure (8,60).

In spite of the disappearance of symptoms of intracranial hypertension, prospective studies of ICP in IIH have shown that many patients develop chronic intracranial hypertension for many years (8,49). Therefore, patients with papilledema will be at continuous risk of visual deterioration, and all patients with IIH should be checked at regular intervals by ophthalmologic examinations. Repeated quantitative perimetry is the cornerstone of long-term follow-up of IIH patients, whereas the grades of papilledema, visual acuity, and visual evoked potentials correlated less reliably to the visual outcome (8,9,60). About 10% of patients have recurrence of the clinical symptoms of intracranial hypertension.

In conclusion, the previously used term *benign intracranial hypertension* is misleading, because a high proportion of the patients develop permanent visual impairment and about 25% have a chronic disease that limits their capacity to work and enjoy a social life (49).

Management

No causal treatment yet is known for IIH. Weight loss should be recommended for every obese patient, but weight control and guidance of a dietitian often fail to effect weight loss. Weight loss is, nonetheless, an effective treatment (54). Symptomatic treatment includes measures to lower the ICP, management of the headache, and procedures to protect the optic nerves. Medical treatment with the carbonic anhydrase inhibitor acetazolamide (in doses of 1 to 2 g daily) to decrease CSF production, alone or combined with a loop diuretic such as furosemide (doses of 40 to 120 mg daily), is usually the first therapeutic measure for lowering the ICP within 1 to 6 weeks (44). Corticosteroids have been widely used, but their mechanism of action remains unclear, the side effects are disagreeable (especially in already obese women), and tapering of therapy implies a potential risk of a rebound effect on the ICP. Other drugs have been tried in a limited number of patients; these drugs include glycerol, thiazides, and digoxin (9). Repeated lumbar punctures have been used to lower the ICP, but this approach is usually not acceptable to the patient.

Aspirin or paracetamol is usually an adequate analgesic for control of headache. Ergots are of little value in IIH. Prophylactic migraine drugs are useful in the treatment of headache from intracranial hypertension, especially beta-blockers and naproxen. Tricyclics, valproate, and flunarizine should be avoided because they may cause weight gain. Headache disappears in many patients for several days to weeks after a diagnostic lumbar puncture.

In patients with impending visual loss or who have prolonged incapacitating symptoms of intracranial hypertension despite medical therapy, surgical intervention is indicated. A ventricular–peritoneal or a lumbar–peritoneal shunt operation is an effective measure to lower the ICP, ameliorate the headache, and prevent further visual loss (22,49); however, these procedures are not without complications. Shunt revision is required in a substantial number of patients (40); in particular, patients with a lumbar–peritoneal shunt are inclined to develop sciatica, postural low-pressure headache, and shunt dependency. Optic-nerve sheath fenestration, an old procedure, has reemerged in the past years as a procedure for relief of papilledema and, in some cases, restoration of visual loss. Strangely, unilateral fenestration is effective in relieving papilledema in both eyes in more than half of the cases. Headache relief, first reported in patients treated surgically in 1872, occurs in about two thirds of patients who have optic-nerve sheath fenestration (7,45). The operation probably forms a functioning fistula into the orbit, the tissues of which act as the CSF absorptive surface. CSF pressures measured after optic nerve sheath fenestration have not been found to be universally normal, but it is likely that mean CSF pressure is lowered (7,45).

HIGH-PRESSURE HYDROCEPHALUS

IHS code and diagnosis: 7.1.2 High-pressure hydrocephalus.

WHO code and diagnosis: G44.82 Headache associated with other intracranial disorders.

Short Description: Hydrocephalus means water in the head. It is caused by an obstruction to the flow of CSF from the ventricular system to the site of absorption, which occurs primarily into the pacchionian granulations and the arachnoid villi and the vessels of the subarachnoid space over the hemispheres. Because of the blockade to CSF outflow, the ventricles enlarge and the ICP increases. Hydrocephalus should be considered a complication of a number of malformations or acquired diseases of the central nervous system rather than a disease itself. In acquired hydrocephalus caused by a nonprogressive disease, the hydrocephalus may stabilize, and eventually the ICP will fall to normal or nearly normal.

Hydrocephalus can be classified as high-pressure hydrocephalus or normal-pressure hydrocephalus. For practical reasons, high-pressure hydrocephalus may be divided into congenital or infantile hydrocephalus and adult hydrocephalus.

Other Terms: *Obstructive hydrocephalus* and *tension hydrocephalus* are other terms for high-pressure hydrocephalus. Hydrocephalus can be of the communicating or the noncommunicating type, depending on whether the ventricular system is in communication with the subarachnoid space. The distinction between the two types is not useful because all forms of hydrocephalus are obstructive. The term *acquired hydrocephalus* specifies that the condition is caused by a disease developed after birth, contrary to *prenatally determined hydrocephalus*.

Epidemiology

The incidence of congenital or infantile hydrocephalus is 50 to 100 per 100,000 births, with considerable variation according to the incidence of intrauterine infections and the use of prenatal diagnosis of central nervous system malformations (52).

Pathophysiology and Etiology

Hydrocephalus can be caused by obstruction of the normal flow of the CSF at several sites. Occlusion of the foramen of Monro causes dilatation of the lateral ventricle, compression of the third ventricle makes both lateral ventricles dilate, and if the aqueduct of Sylvius is occluded, dilatation then includes the third ventricle. Occlusion of the foramina of Magendie and Luschka or of the subarachnoid space in the cisterns around the midbrain and brainstem provokes enlargement of the entire ventricular system. Obstruction of the resorption of CSF over the hemispheres, at the site of the arachnoid villi or in the venous sinuses, can cause either high-pressure of normal-pressure hydrocephalus. Ventricular enlargement develops because the CSF pressure in the ventricles is greater than the pressure applied on the outer surface of the hemispheres. The pressure gradient leads to an expansion of the ventricular system at the expense of the brain parenchyma and with damage to the ependyma.

In children, hydrocephalus occurs in many disorders (Table 3) (62). In adults, spontaneous subarachnoid hemorrhage, usually from a ruptured aneurysm, is a common cause of hydrocephalus. About 10% of patients surviving a subarachnoid hemorrhage develop hydrocephalus because of blockage of the CSF outflow (63). Head injury with traumatic subarachnoid hemorrhage and meningitis are other important underlying disorders in adult hydrocephalus. Tumors in the posterior fossa or in relation to the third ventricle may block the CSF pathways.

Clinical Features

The following are the operational diagnostic criteria of high-pressure hydrocephalus:

1. Ventricular enlargement on neuroimaging
2. Increased ICP (>200 mm H_2O) measured by intraventricular or epidural pressure monitoring

The following are the operational diagnostic criteria of normal pressure hydrocephalus:

1. Ventricular enlargement on neuroimaging
2. Clinical symptoms of progressive dementia, gait disturbances, and urinary incontinence
3. Normal ICP (<200 mm H_2O) and increased resistance to outflow of CSF

The clinical picture of high-pressure hydrocephalus varies with age of onset. If the condition develops before the age of 4 to 5 years, the head will enlarge because the fusion of the cranial bones is incomplete or because the high ICP will separate the sutures. The child shows increasing head circumference, a tense anterior fontanelle,

TABLE 3. *Etiology of hydrocephalus in children*

Congenital defects
Chiari malformation
Dandy-Walker cyst
Porencephaly, arachnoid cyst
Aqueduct stenosis
Encephalocele
Infection
Neonatal meningitis
Toxoplasmosis
Viral infections
Intraventricular hemorrhage
Neonatal
AV malformation
Tumor
Trauma
Obstetrical trauma
Postnatal trauma

A-V, arteriovenous.

splayed sutures, and scalp-vein distension. Headache and vomiting are the most common symptoms (30%–50%), but many children are asymptomatic. The headache can occur at night after waking from a period of rapid eye movement (REM) sleep associated with increased cerebral blood flow and increased ICP (4). Change in behavior, including irritability, is a common but nonspecific symptom (30). Tonic downward gaze, the sunset sign or loss of upward gaze, and pathologic lid contraction are classic signs of hydrocephalus seen in some but not all patients (55). Papilledema and pupillary abnormalities are other ophthalmologic signs of hydrocephalus (6).

In older children and adults, the symptoms of high-pressure hydrocephalus are dominated by typical symptoms and signs of increased ICP: headache, vomiting, diplopia, dysequilibrium of stance and gait, and papilledema (25). Headache in hydrocephalic patients can be episodic and may resemble migraine with or without aura (13,26) or may be related to exertion and provoked by cough, sneeze, strain, or physical activity. The latter type of headache, which also can be seen in patients with type I Arnold-Chiari malformation without hydrocephalus (29,30), is a severe throbbing pain in the occipital region or vertex that evolves over seconds and lasts for minutes (35). An acute disturbance in CSF circulation with episodic impaction of the cerebellar tonsils in the foramen magnum may be the underlying factor (57).

A special problem in treated hydrocephalic children and adolescents is shunt dysfunction. Whereas most patients with shunt malfunction show ventricular enlargement and other symptoms and signs of intracranial hypertension, some shunt-dependent patients develop intermittent or chronic headache as the only manifestation of shunt dysfunction. These patients show a normal-sized ventricular system or slit ventricles. Resistance to ventricular dilatation and increased brain water causes intermittent neurologic dysfunction (6). The headache may occur as episodic bilateral severe pain lasting for days or weeks or may become progressively more severe and constant. It may be accompanied by vomiting, behavioral changes, and reappearance of signs of the dorsal midbrain syndrome (6,10,15).

Normal-pressure hydrocephalus is characterized by the clinical triad of progressive dementia, gait disturbances, and urinary incontinence (24). Headache is usually not a complaint in this disorder.

Prognosis

About one half of children with untreated high-pressure hydrocephalus die, and 25% have mental deficiencies. Motor impairment of various severity is common, and only 10% to 20% are normal or nearly normal (23). In hydrocephalus resulting from tumor growth, the prognosis is determined by the nature of the underlying tumor.

Management

A ventricular–peritoneal shunt operation is the management of choice in both children and adults with hydrocephalus. Other extracranial CSF diverting shunts used today include ventriculoatrial and lumboperitoneal devices. The complications of shunt operations are subdural hygroma or hematoma, shunt infections and meningitis, ventricular catheter occlusion, and distal shunt obstructions.

Medical treatments of hydrocephalus include carbonic anhydrase inhibitors, acetazolamide, furosemide, fluid restriction, and, rarely today, osmotic diuretic agents like mannitol, urea, and glycerol. Few patients with high-pressure hydrocephalus seem to benefit from medical treatment alone. In patients with hydrocephalus caused by tumor, surgical removal is, of course, the therapy of choice.

Arachnoidal Cysts

Arachnoidal cysts are intracranial leptomeningeal malformations, most commonly located in the middle cranial fossa. The highest incidence is in the first two decades of life, and there is a predilection for the male sex (17).

Many cysts are asymptomatic, but symptomatic cases present with cranial deformities, symptoms of elevated ICP, and focal epilepsy. Mental retardation, behavioral problems, and focal symptoms reflecting the anatomic location of the cyst are often seen. Arachnoid cysts may be associated with other abnormalities, for example, aqueduct stenosis, agenesis of corpus callosum, and Chiari I malformation (36). The cysts are susceptible to trauma, which may cause bleeding either in the cyst or into the subarachnoid space. Headache is related to cysts producing increased ICP and often is combined with other symptoms of increased ICP.

The diagnosis and need of a surgical procedure are established by CT and MRI. Surgical treatment for middle cranial fossa cysts include craniotomy with excision of the cyst walls and perforation into the basal cisterns or cystoperitoneal shunting (17).

REFERENCES

1. Brooks DJ, Beaney RP, Leenders KL, Marshall J, Thomas DJ, Jones T. Regional cerebral oxygen utilization, blood flow, and blood volume in benign intracranial hypertension studied by positron emission tomography. *Neurology* 1985;35:1030–1034.
2. Bulens C, De Vries WA, van Crevel H. Benign intracranial hypertension: a retrospective and follow-up study. *J Neurol Sci* 1979;40: 147–157.
3. Coffey CE, Ross DR, Massey EW, Olanow CW. Familial benign intracranial hypertension and depression. *Can J Neurol Sci* 1982;9: 45–47.
4. Cooper R, Hulme A. Intracranial pressure and related phenomena during sleep. *J Neurol Neurosurg Psychiatry* 1966;29:564–577.
5. Corbett JJ. The 1982 Silversides lecture. Problems in the diagnosis and treatment of pseudotumor cerebri. *Can J Neurol Sci* 1983;10:221–229.
6. Corbett JJ. Neuro-ophthalmologic complications of hydrocephalus and shunting procedures. *Semin Neurol* 1986;6:119–123.
7. Corbett JJ, Nerad JA, Tse DT, Anderson RL. Results of optic nerve sheath fenestration for pseudotumor cerebri: the lateral orbitotomy approach. *Arch Ophthalmol* 1988;106:1391–1397.
8. Corbett JJ, Savino PJ, Thompson HS, et al. Visual loss in pseudotumor cerebri: follow-up of 57 patients from five to 41 years and a profile of 14 patients with permanent severe visual loss. *Arch Neurol* 1982;39: 461—474.
9. Corbett JJ, Thompson HS. The rational management of idiopathic intracranial hypertension. *Arch Neurol* 1989;46:1049–1051.
10. Dahlerup B, Gjerris F, Harmsen A, Sorensen PS. Severe headache as the only symptom of long-standing shunt dysfunction in hydrocephalic children with normal or slit ventricles revealed by computed tomography. *Childs Nerv Syst* 1985;1:49–52.
11. Dandy WE. Intracranial pressure without brain tumor. *Ann Surg* 1937; 106:492–513.
12. Donaldson JO. Cerebrospinal fluid hypersecretion in pseudotumor cerebri. *Transactions of the American Neurological Association* 1979; 104:196–198.
13. Donaldson MG. Migraine due to hydrocephalus. *Headache* 1984;24: 272–273.
14. Durcan FJ, Corbett JJ, Wall M. The incidence of pseudotumor cerebri: population studies in Iowa and Louisiana. *Arch Neurol* 1988;45:875–877.
15. Epstein F, Marlin AE, Wald A. Chronic headache in the shunt-dependent adolescent with normal ventricular volume: diagnosis and treatment. *Neurosurgery* 1978;3:351–355.
16. Fay T. A new test for the diagnosis of certain headaches: the cephalogram. *Diseases of the Nervous System* 1940;1:312–315.
17. Galassi E, Gaist G, Giuliani G, Pozzati E. Arachnoid cysts of the middle cranial fossa: experience with 77 cases treated surgically. *Acta Neurochir Suppl (Wien)* 1988;42:201–204.
18. Gass A, Barker GJ, Riordan EP, et al. MRI of the optic nerve in benign intracranial hypertension. *Neuroradiology* 1996;38:769–773.
19. Gideon P, Sorensen PS, Thomsen C, Stahlberg F, Gjerris F, Henriksen O. Assessment of CSF dynamics and venous flow in the superior sagittal sinus by MRI in idiopathic intracranial hypertension: a preliminary study. *Neuroradiology* 1994;36:350–354.
20. Gideon P, Sorensen PS, Thomsen C, Stahlberg F, Gjerris F, Henriksen O. Increased brain water self-diffusion in patients with idiopathic intracranial hypertension. *AJNR Am J Neuroradiol* 1995;16:381–387.
21. Giuseffi V, Wall M, Siegel PZ, Rojas PB. Symptoms and disease associations in idiopathic intracranial hypertension (pseudotumor cerebri): a case–control study. *Neurology* 1991;41:239–244.
22. Gjerris F, Soelberg Sorensen P, Vorstrup S, Paulson OB. Intracranial pressure, conductance to cerebrospinal fluid outflow, and cerebral blood flow in patients with benign intracranial hypertension (pseudotumor cerebri). *Ann Neurol* 1985;17:158–162.
23. Hadenius AM, Hagberg B, Hytnäs-Bensch K, Sjögren K. The natural prognosis of infantile hydrocephalus. *Acta Paediatr Scand* 1962;51: 117–118.
24. Hakim S, Adams RD. The special clinical problem of symptomatic hydrocephalus with normal cerebrospinal fluid pressure. Observations on cerebrospinal fluid hydrodynamics. *J Neurol Sci* 1965;2:307–327.
25. Honig PJ, Charney EB. Children with brain tumor headaches. *J Dis Child* 1982;136:121–124.
26. James HE, Nowak TP. Clinical course and diagnosis of migraine headaches in hydrocephalic children. *Pediatr Neurosurg* 1991;17:310–316.
27. Johnston I, Paterson A. Benign intracranial hypertension. I. Diagnosis and prognosis. *Brain* 1974;97:289–300.
28. Johnston I, Paterson A. Benign intracranial hypertension. II. CSF pressure and circulation. *Brain* 1974;97:301–312.
29. Khurana RK. Headache spectrum in Arnold-Chiari malformation. *Headache* 1991;31:151–155.
30. Kirkpatrick M, Engleman H, Minns RA. Symptoms and signs of progressive hydrocephalus. *Arch Dis Child* 1989;64:124–128.
31. Marellis J, Silberstein SD. Idiopathic intracranial hypertension without papilledema. *Arch Neurol* 1991;48:392–399.
32. Mathew NT, Meyer JS, Ott EO. Increased cerebral blood volume in benign intracranial hypertension. *Neurology* 1975;25:646–649.
33. Mathew NT, Ravishankar K, Sanin LC. Coexistence of migraine and idiopathic intracranial hypertension without papilledema. *Neurology* 1996;46:1126–1230.

34. Maxner CE, Freedman MI, Corbett JJ. Asymmetric papilledema and visual loss in pseudotumor cerebri. *Can J Neurol Sci* 1987;14:593–596.
35. Nightingale S, Williams B. Hindbrain hernia headache. *Lancet* 1987;1:731–734.
36. Pascual-Castroviejo I, Roche MC, Martinez Bermejo A, Arcas J, Garcia Blazquez M. Primary intracranial arachnoidal cysts: a study of 67 childhood cases. *Childs Nerv Syst* 1991;7:257–263.
37. Radhakrishnan K, Sridharan R, Ashok PP, Mousa ME. Pseudotumor cerebri: incidence and pattern in North-Eastern Libya. *Eur Neurol* 1986;25:117–124.
38. Reid AC, Teasdale GM, Matheson MS, Teasdale EM. Serial ventricular volume measurements: further insights into the aetiology and pathogenesis of benign intracranial hypertension. *J Neurol Neurosurg Psychiatry* 1981;44:636–640.
39. Reid AC, Thomson JA. Absence of significant endocrine deficiencies in benign intracranial hypertension. *J Neurol Neurosurg Psychiatry* 1981;44:731–734.
40. Rsenberg ML, Corbett JJ, Smith C, et al. Cerebrospinal fluid diversion procedures in pseudotumor cerebri. *Neurology* 1993;43:1071–1072.
41. Rothner AD, Brust JC. Pseudotumor cerebri: report of a familial occurrence. *Arch Neurol* 1974;30:110–111.
42. Round R, Keane JR. The minor symptoms of increased intracranial pressure: 101 patients with benign intracranial hypertension. *Neurology* 1988;38:1461–1464.
43. Rush JA. Pseudotumor cerebri: clinical profile and visual outcome in 63 patients. *Mayo Clin Proc* 1980;55:541–546.
44. Schoeman JF. Childhood pseudomotor cerebri: clinical and intracranial pressure response to acetazolamide and furosemide treatment in a case series. *J Child Neurol* 1994;9:130–134.
45. Sergott RC, Savino PJ, Bosley TM. Optic nerve sheath decompression: a clinical review and proposed pathophysiologic mechanism. *Aust N Z J Ophthalmol* 1990;18:365–373.
46. Sklar FH, Beyer CWJ, Ramanathan M, Cooper PR, Clark WK. Cerebrospinal fluid dynamics in patients with pseudotumor cerebri. *Neurosurgery* 1979;5:208–216.
47. Solomon SK, Wisoff H, Thorpy M. Symptoms of vascular headache triggered by intracranial hypertension. *Headache* 1983;23:307–312.
48. Sorensen PS, Gjerris F, Svenstrup B. Endocrine studies in patients with pseudotumor cerebri: estrogen levels in blood and cerebrospinal fluid. *Arch Neurol* 1986;43:902–906.
49. Sorensen PS, Krogsaa B, Gjerris F. Clinical course and prognosis of pseudotumor cerebri: a prospective study of 24 patients. *Acta Neurol Scand* 1988;77:164–172.
50. Sorensen PS, Thomsen AM, Gjerris F. Persistent disturbances of cognitive functions in patients with pseudotumour cerebri. *Acta Neurol Scand* 1986;73:264–268.
51. Spence JD, Amacher AL, Willis NR. Benign intracranial hypertension without papilledema: role of 24-hour cerebrospinal fluid pressure monitoring in diagnosis and management. *Neurosurgery* 1980;7:326–336.
52. Stevenson AC, Johnson HA, Golding DR, Stewart MIP. World Health Organization comparative study of congenital malformations. Medical Research Council of Great Britain, Population Genetic Research Unit, London, 1966.
53. Sugerman HJ, DeMaria EJ, Felton WL, Nakatsuka M, Sismanis A. Increased intra-abdominal pressure and cardiac filling pressures in obesity-associated pseudotumor cerebri. *Neurology* 1997;49:507–511.
54. Sugerman HJ, Felton WL, Salvant JB Jr, Sismanis A, Kellum JM. Effects of surgically induced weight loss on idiopathic intracranial hypertension in morbid obesity. *Neurology* 1995;45:1655–1659.
55. Swash M. Disorders of ocular movement in hydrocephalus. *Proc R Soc Med* 1976;69:480–489.
56. Traviesa DC, Schwartzman RJ, Glaser JS, Savino P. Familial benign intracranial hypertension. *J Neurol Neurosurg Psychiatry* 1976;39:420–423.
57. Van Alpern HAM. Migraine, a result of increased CSF pressure: a new pathophysiological concept. *Neurosurg Rev* 1986;9:121–124.
58. Wall M. The headache profile of idiopathic intracranial hypertension. *Cephalalgia* 1990;10:331–335.
59. Wall M. Idiopathic intracranial hypertension. *Neurol Clin* 1991;9:73–95.
60. Wall M, George D. Idiopathic intracranial hypertension. A prospective study of 50 patients. *Brain* 1991;114:155–180.
61. Weisberg LA. Benign intracranial hypertension. *Medicine (Baltimore)* 1975;54:197–207.
62. Welch K. The etiology and classification of hydrocephalus in childhood. *Z Kinderchir* 1980;31:331–335.
63. Yasargil MG, Yonekawa Y, Zumstein B, Stahl H-J. Hydrocephalus following spontaneous subarachnoid hemorrhage: clinical features and treatment. *J Neurosurg* 1973;39:474–479.

The Headaches, Second Edition,
edited by J. Olesen, P. Tfelt-Hansen, and K.M.A. Welch.
Lippincott Williams & Wilkins, Philadelphia © 2000.

The Secondary Headaches

CHAPTER 111

Low Cerebrospinal Fluid Pressure

Steinar T. Vilming and J. Keith Campbell

DEFINITION OF POSTLUMBAR PUNCTURE HEADACHE (PPH)

IHS code and diagnosis: 7.2.1 Postlumbar puncture headache.

WHO code and diagnosis: G44.88 Headache associated with other specified disorders.

Short description: Bilateral headache that develops within 7 days after lumbar puncture and disappears within 14 days after lumbar puncture. Headache occurs or worsens in the upright position and disappears or improves after resuming the recumbent position.

Other terms: Neurologists usually use the term *postlumbar puncture headache*, anesthesiologists use *postdural headache*, and radiologists *postmyelogram headache*; but other synonyms also are in use.

Since W. Essex Wynter in 1889 and H. Quincke in 1891 performed the first dural punctures, the distressing headache that may ensue has been the subject of a vast number of scientific papers. PPH is unique because of its postural character, occurring or worsening when the patient assumes the erect posistion.

Pathophysiology

Although the etiology of PPH is still being debated, most authors favor the "leakage theory" proposed at the beginning of this century (66). The theory implies that after-leakage of cerebrospinal fluid (CSF) through the dural rent leads to a decreased CSF pressure (CSFP) and volume, whereby the cerebral veins dilate and the brain is deprived of its CSF cushion. The consequent gravity-dependent downward sagging of the brain causes traction on the distended and distorted anchoring veins (the sagittal sinus and its tributary veins) and pressure on the large arteries at the skull base and the tentorium (Fig. 1). All these structures are pain sensitive (81). Several facts support this theory.

The *dural rent* caused by a Quincke-cut needle has the form of a nearly opened tin lid hinged on one side (Fig. 2), and a complete sealing may take more than 14 days (18). Small rents caused by thin needles heal more rapidly than larger rents, and rents made through the thickest parts of the dura retract more readily than rents in the thinner parts (18,25). It has been suggested that a rent created by an oblique needle insertion, a penetration through a richly vasculated area of the dura (53), or parallel with the dural fibers (25) might be more likely to heal, but this suggestion has not been proved.

The CSF is normally produced at a rate of about 0.3 mL per minute, but despite this great renewal capacity, a low CSF volume and pressure may be maintained by *the leakage of CSF*. A continuous leakage of CSF has been observed by direct inspection and isotope studies after weeks and even months. The CSF lost epidurally seems to be absorbed through the intervertebral foramina (25). The CSFP closely parallels the venous pressure at all levels of the intracraniospinal system. In the erect human, the intracranial CSFP is negative at the vertex, approximately -150 mm H_2O. In the human in the horizontal position, the intracranial CSFP is positive at all levels, normally 50 to 180 mm H_2O. Removal of 30 mL CSF regularly induces headache in the erect position concomitant with a reduction of the vertex CSFP down to -220 to -290 mm of water. The headache is ameliorated by restoration of the CSF volume or tilting toward the horizontal position and augmented by jugular compression (38,81). In some PPH patients with repuncture, the CSFP is zero or low (53,73),

S. T. Vilming: Department of Neurology, Ullevaal Hospital, University of Oslo, 0407 Oslo, Norway.

J. K. Campbell: Department of Neurology, Mayo Clinic and Mayo Medical School, Rochester, Minnesota 55905.

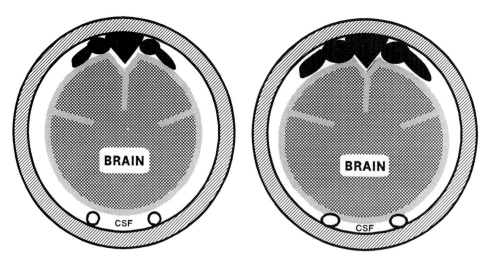

FIG. 1. A schematic presentation of intracranial structures before (**left**) and after (**right**) withdrawal of cerebrospinal fluid explaining the mechanism of postlumbar puncture headache (*PPH*). The loss of volume is compensated for by a significant distention of the pain-sensitive sagittal sinus and its tributary veins. The downward sagging of the brain causes traction on these veins and pressure on the large arteries at the skull base.

and intrathecal infusion of saline relieves the headache by restoring the CSFP (57). In a controlled clinical study, the average reduction in CSFP after lumbar puncture (LP) was significantly greater for patients with headache compared with patients without headache (82). In another study, however, only three of five PPH patients with repuncture after 24 hours had a low CSFP, and a low CSFP was found in 7 of 37 patients who had not developed PPH (46). Thus, the association between PPH and a low CSFP is not invariable, and other factors may play a part.

The CSF serves to buoy about 97% of the weight of the slightly denser brain (58). By magnetic resonance imaging (MRI), it has been shown that the CSF volume is significantly reduced in nearly all patients 24 hours after LP and that there is a trend toward a greater reduction in those who develop PPH than in controls (30). This loss of CSF causes the thin-walled veins to distend, which has been observed directly through a cranial window in cats (23); also, the brain appeared edematous and cyanotic, and the arteries constricted slightly. This finding is in accordance with the Monro-Kellie doctrine with Burrow's modification, which has been confirmed experimentally (29), stating that the blood and CSF volumes are reciprocally interrelated: Blood volume increases when the CSF volume is reduced and vice versa. The increased blood volume is due exclusively to a venous dilatation, because the venoarterial reflex, which occurs within seconds of CSF removal, causes the arteries to constrict to keep the cerebral blood volume unaltered.

Clinical Features

IHS diagnostic criteria for postlumbar puncture headache (Headache Classification Committee, 1988):

A. Bilateral headache develops less than 7 days after LP.
B. Headache occurs or worsens less than 15 minutes after assumption of the upright position, and disappears or improves less than 30 minutes after resumption of the recumbent position.
C. Headache disappears within 14 days after LP (if duration exceeds 14 days, consider 7.2.2).

First onset of PPH occurs within 2 days after LP in about 90% of patients (77), ranging between a few minutes and several days. It usually lasts about a week, but a duration of several weeks or even months has been reported (38,57,70,73,77), probably because of persisting fistula. PPH with early onset seems to last longer and

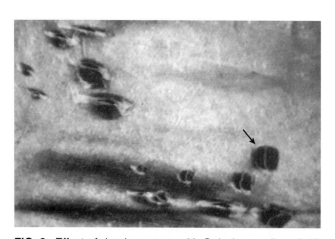

FIG. 2. Effect of dural puncture with Quincke needles of different sizes from 20 to 29G. The typical "tin-lid effect" is visualized, and one example is given (*arrow*). From Dittmann et al. (18).

tends to be more severe than PPH with a later onset (31,75). PPH is posture dependent, usually starting to increase within 20 seconds when the patient assumes an upright position, reaching its maximum within another 30 seconds, and when the patient lies down, it subsides within 20 seconds (Fig. 3) (77). The time variables have a wide range, however (77). In the individual patient, the time course of PPH is fairly stable, but during the last couple of days, the headache severity will start to subside, and the patient's mobility will increase; the time required for headache to develop on rising increases significantly the last day (78). The headache usually is described as aching, dull, deep, constricting, or throbbing, and it is most frequently frontal but often occipital, frontooccipital, or generalized (1,38,70,73). More than half of PPH patients have associated symptoms, and the more severe the PPH, the more frequently the symptoms occur. Dizziness and nausea, occasionally with vomiting, are most prevalent. Auditory difficulties and tinnitus are not rare and may be caused by leakage of perilymphatic fluid from the cochlea to the cerebrospinal space through a cochlear aqueduct, which is functionally open in about 50% of adults (47,79), resulting in a Ménière-like syndrome. Blurred vision and other visual disturbances are quite infrequent; in solitary cases, lesions of cranial nerves, usually the abducens nerve, have been reported (1,70,73,75).

The results of clinical studies of PPH are conflicting. After thorough literature studies, Tourtellotte and colleagues in 1961 (70) and Hilton Jones in 1985 (35) stated that there is an appalling lack of randomized controlled studies and that most of what has been written is anecdotal. The incidence of PPH may depend on how the patients are questioned, and care should be taken not to ask "leading questions" (70). Also, results of diagnostic LP and spinal anesthesia (SA) are not comparable, because patients often are kept in bed for several days after SA, which may hide cases of short-lasting PPH; also, the consequence of introducing chemicals intrathecally in SA and myelography is unclear. Most studies show a significantly lower incidence of PPH in SA than after diagnostic LP (70). In recent years, only a few well-designed studies have been published. This chapter gives emphasis mainly to studies that meet the minimum requirements of being randomized, controlled if necessary, blinded if possible, and containing a sufficient number of patients to permit an adequate statistical analysis.

Female sex and *young age* seem to predispose to PPH. Review of older studies, which include a great number of patients (70,73), and a recent study (75) convincingly shows that the frequency of PPH is highest among younger patients with the exception of prepubertal patients. It seems that children aged under 10 years do not develop PPH (80). Some authors report a decreased incidence of PPH above the age of 40 years, others above the age of 50 or 60 years, but the conclusions are dependent on the study design, and factors such as sex have generally not been taken into account (70). The reduced incidence of PPH in older patients may be explained by the decreased elastisity of vessels (73) or a narrowed epidural space, which is the escape route for the leaking CSF (72). Many reports, most of them not designed for the purpose of studying the role of sex, concluded that there is a higher incidence of PPH in females compared with males (15,20,70,71,73,75,82). In a study of 300 patients, the incidence of PPH was assessed separately in different age groups for the two sexes (75). Although a tendency toward a decreased incidence of PPH with increasing age was found both for men and women, it was pronounced only for women. The increased incidence of PPH in women was explained nearly exclusively by a high incidence in women of childbearing age (Fig. 4). Younger females with a lower body mass index have the highest risk of developing PPH (39). It is pertinent that prevalence studies of PPH are well balanced for age and sex.

Many investigators have stated that the incidence of PPH decreases with a smaller *needle size*, possibly because of reduced leakage through smaller rents. During the last two decades, several well-designed controlled studies have been conducted (Table 1) (22,27,37,54,71). Even though minor shortcomings in design may be pointed out, these studies convincingly show that needle size is of major importance. From a theoretic point of view, an oblique penetration of the dura might leave a rent more susceptible to sealing (33), but this has not been confirmed clinically (51); nor has any study with an acceptable design proved the effect of inserting the nee-

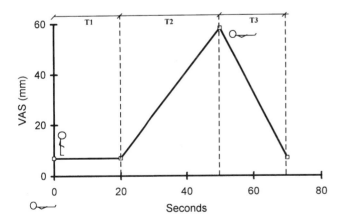

FIG. 3. Headache severity on a 100-mm visual analogue scale (*VAS*) related to time; median values from 79 patients. The body position of the patient is indicated. The pain is minimal when the patient is in the recumbent position, but pain starts to increase after 20 seconds when the patient is in the upright position (*T1*). The time to maximal pain is 30 seconds (*T2*). When the patient lies down, the pain decreases to its lowest level within 20 seconds (*T3*). From Vilming and Kloster (77).

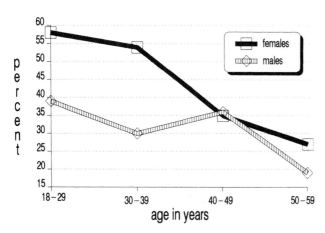

FIG. 4. Incidence of postlumbar puncture headache (*PPH*) related to age for 150 men and 150 women. There was a significantly higher incidence of PPH in women ($p < 0.025$) and in patients younger than 40 years ($p < 0.005$). A significant difference between the two age groups is only shown for women ($p < 0.005$), and the incidence of PPH is significantly different for the two sexes only below the age of 40 years ($p < 0.01$). From Vilming et al. (75).

dle with the bevel parallel instead of perpendicular to the dural fibers. Several studies have shown that atraumatic (blunt-tipped) needles reduce the incidence of PPH (24, 42,56), and the 20-gauge needle is recommended for diagnostic LP (12). Its favorable effect was not confirmed in two well-designed studies, however (9,44).

No evidence has been found to show that *body position* during LP is important. The position after LP, however, has been the subject of discussions since Sicard in 1902 stated that in his experience headache after LP almost never occurred if the patient stayed in bed for 24 hours, preferably with the head tilted down for some hours (66). Tourtellotte and investigators (70) found no evidence that these procedures were of any use. Well-designed studies comparing immediate mobilization with bed rest for dif-

ferent lengths of time were published recently (3,11,13,69, 74) (Table 2) and showed that bed rest after LP has no prophylactic effect. Some studies conclude that early mobilization may be preferable (3,74). Thus, remaining in bed after LP is meaningless or obsolete. Brocker (8) in a 1958 study of questionable design found that resting prone for 3 hours after LP nearly completely prevented PPH, but subsequently several well-designed studies disproved this effect (32,70,74). Lying with the head tilted down after LP does not seem to be of any use (32,68).

Contrary to widely held belief, patients considered apprehensive do not seem to be more likely to develop PPH than those who are not apprehensive (70). Several investigators have commented on the role of neuroticism in PPH, but the results are conflicting. In a recent study, the profiles based on the Minnesota Multiple Personality Inventory were strikingly similar for patients with and without PPH (76). Kaplan (36) found that headache occurred almost as frequently after sham LP as after real LP, but he did not distinguish between PPH and unspecific headache, and there are also other shortcomings in this study. The role of psychology in PPH awaits further clarification. PPH incidence in relation to a diagnosis such as multiple sclerosis and syphilis has been considered, but no definite conclusions can be drawn because no prospective controlled study has been performed. The following factors have not been shown to influence the incidence of PPH: race, the quantity of CSF removed, a bloody tap, multiple perforations of the dura, and the qualifications of the person performing the LP (70).

Management

No standard therapeutic concept for PPH has had universal agreement. Hilton-Jones emphasized that PPH is a benign and self-limiting condition and that the treatment should not have more side effects than the symptom being treated (35). It is usually sufficient to advise the

TABLE 1. *Well-designed controlled studies regarding the significance of needle size[a]*

Author	Design					Number of patients	% PPH					
	Year	R	B	A	S		20G	22G	23G	25G	26G	29G
Tourtellotte et al. (71)	1972[b]	+	DB	+	−	100		36			12	
Nestvold (54)	1978[b]	+	−	+	+	99	48	27				
Kovanen and Sulkava (37	1986[b]	−	−	+	−	300	52	37	28			
Flaatten et al. (22)	1989[c]	+	−	+	−	149					7	0
Geurts et al. (27)	1990[c]	+	DB	+	−	80				25		0

+, yes; −, no, or not stated; R, randomized; B, blinded; DB, double blind; A, groups congruent for age; S, groups congruent for sex; n, number of patients; G, gauge.
[a]The table shows details concerning the design of different studies and the incidence of PPH in relation to needle size.
[b]Diagnostic LP.
[c]Spinal anesthesia.

TABLE 2. *Well-designed controlled studies regarding the significance of body position after LP[a]*

Author	Design						% PPH				
	Year	R	B	A	S	n	0h	2h	4h	6h	24h
Carbaat et al. (11)	1981[b]	-	-	+	-	100	38				36
Andersen et al. (3)	1986[b]	+	-	+	+	112		11			14
Vilming et al. (74)	1988[b]	+	+	+	+	300	35			39	
Cook et al. (13)	1989[c]	+	+	+	-	102		12			12
Spriggs et al. (69)	1992[b]	+	+	+	-	110	32		31		

h, hours; +, yes; –, no or not stated; R, randomized; B, blinded; A, groups congruent for age; S, groups congruent for sex; n, number of patients; PPH, postlumbar puncture headache; LP, lumbar puncture; ???

[a]The table shows details concerning the design of different studies and the incidence of PPH in relation to bed rest for different lengths of time. No statistically significant differences are observed in any of the studies.
[b]Diagnostic LP.
[c]Spinal anesthesia.

patient to lie down as long as the PPH lasts and to use mild analgesics if necessary.

The clinical practice of advising patients to increase their daily fluid intake after LP is ineffective (16). Many investigators argue that restoring the CSFP by installing saline intrathecally gives immediate relief, but this procedure implies that a second dural puncture is performed and is not recommended. Although no well-designed study exists, several reports maintain that lumbar *epidural saline* given as a single injection (10–60 mL) gives immediate relief and only in a few cases does recurrence within a few hours occur (60,72). It also may be given as a slow infusion of 15 to 30 mL per hour, 700 mL in total. Most investigators report a success rate of 70% to 100%. The side effects are insignificant with a slow infusion rate, or backache, dizziness, nausea, tachypnea, or ocular-frontal pain may occur. Injection of as little as 10 mL of saline epidurally in the lumbar region raises both the epidural and CSF pressure significantly, but the pressure returns to previous values within 3 to 10 minutes (72). The beneficial effect may be explained by ameliorated conditions for sealing the rent (60,72), but the exact mechanism is obscure.

The *epidural blood patch* (EBP) was introduced by J.B. Gormley in 1960 and came into common use after the publication of DiGiovanni et al. in the mid seventies (17). Most researchers recommend a slow injection of 10 to 20 mL (1 mL/2 seconds) near the rent and bed rest thereafter for 1 hour. The indication for this therapy may be incapacitating pain or PPH lasting longer than 5 days. Anesthesiologists often use this method at an early stage, neurologists only if the headache proves intractable. EBP is contraindicated by fever, local infection, and coagulopathies (1). Only a couple of controlled studies that have included few patients have been carried out (5,65), but a considerable number of studies conclude that EBP gives immediate relief in about 90% of treated patients, and after a second EBP almost all patients are relieved. EBP is more effective than epidural saline injection (5). A prophylactic EBP with 4 to 8 mL of blood seems to reduce the incidence of

PPH (34). The immediate effect of EBP probably results from the focal compression of the the the thecal sac (6), but then a gelatinous tamponade is created (17); when in contact with the CSF and the bare epithelium and collagen of the rent, the blood rapidly coagulates and seals it (61). EBP may be effective for PPH that has lasted several months. The side effects may be troublesome in a few cases. During the injection, some patients experience pain locally in the neck, shoulder, or occipitally, but such pain may be avoided by a slow injection rate. Meningism may follow an accidental dural puncture. A third of the patients report backache, usually for some days but in a few cases for weeks or months. Others report irradiating pain or paresthesias during the injection for days or weeks afterward (1). No evidence has been reported that EBP prevents a successful epidural anesthesia at a later stage, which was originally feared. Single reports have described the immediate success of clipping or suturing of an open dural rent, even several months after LP.

The cerebral vasoconstrictors caffeine and theophyllamine have been effective in well-conducted studies; 0.5 mg of caffeine sodium benzoate in 2 mL of saline (64) or as an infusion in 1 L of Ringer's solution (19), alternatively USP 300 mg anhydrous caffeine powder orally in a single dose has been used (10). Theophyllamine 282 mg three times daily has been shown to have better results than placebo (21). The efficacy of these drugs are not impressive, however, and their long-term effect has not been established.

DEFINITION OF CSF FISTULA HEADACHE

IHS code and diagnosis: 7.2.2 Cerebrospinal fluid fistula headache.

WHO code and diagnosis: G44.88 Headache associated with other specified disorders.

Short description: Headache occurs or worsens shortly after assuming the upright position and improves or disappears after resuming the recumbent position. It is caused by a cerebrospinal fistula, the existence of which may or may not be proven, and disappears within 14 days after successful closure of a fistula.

Other terms: None.

IHS diagnostic criteria for CSF fistula headache (Headache Classification Committee, 1988):

A. Posttraumatic, postoperative, or idiopathic CSF leak demonstrated by measurement of glucose concentration in leaking fluid or by leakage of spinally injected dye or radioactive tracer
B. Headache characteristics of 7.2.1 (postlumbar puncture headache)
C. Headache disappears within 14 days after effective treatment of fistula

CSF fistula headaches are due to CSF leaks, which are secondary to major trauma, neurosurgery, or erosive lesions. Primary (idiopathic) CSF hypotensive states are included in this category, although it is not certain whether these conditions are always caused by leaks.

Primary Intracranial Hypotension

The clinical picture of primary intracranial hypotension (PIH) is more or less identical to that of PPH (43,49). By definition, there should be no evidence of a major trauma, but it may be associated with a trivial trauma, such as a fall onto the buttocks, a sudden strain, a sudden cough or sneeze, and with orgasm (43,49).

Other Terms

The first reference to this rare condition was made by Schaltenbrand in 1938, and in 1940 he reported three cases with spontaneous aliquorrhea (62,63). Subsequently, it also has been referred to as *spontaneous hypoliquorrhea*, *spontaneous intracranial hypotension*, *essential aliquorrhea*, and *low-pressure headache syndrome*.

Pathophysiology

The pathogenesis of PIH remains obscure. Three possible mechanisms have been proposed: a diminished production of CSF by the choroid plexus, hyperabsorption of CSF, or leakage of CSF through small tears in the dura. Some evidence supports the last two causes. Isotope cisternography may be normal, but in several cases a rapid reabsorption of the isotope has been demonstrated with no signs of leakage (41,45,50). This finding has been interpreted as evidence of a hyperabsorption by the arachnoid villi, but it does not rule out the possibility of small dural tears (41,43,49). Rents in the dural sleeves of lumbar, thoracic, and cervicothoracic nerve roots have been demonstrated by isotope and contrast media investigations and are the most frequent cause of PIH in the opinion of some investigators (43,49). Demonstration of the leak can be difficult and may require isotope cisternography and computed tomography (CT) myelography.

Clinical Features

Onset of PIH headache may be sudden or gradual and typically disappears within 2 to 16 weeks. It is far more frequent in women than in men. The headache mimics PPH, being postural, usually severe and throbbing, and located in the frontal or occipital area. It may be associated with nausea or vomiting, pallor, sweating, faintness, dizziness or vertigo, diplopia, photophobia, anorexia, and generalized malaise. It is usually not relieved by analgesics. Mental confusion and seizures may occur. Subdural hematomas have complicated PIH in a few cases (14,40,67), and subdural collections of fluid have been identified on CT or MRI in up to 69% of patients with PIH (49). The physical examination may reveal mild neck stiffness, and the headache is usually increased with forward flexion of the neck. A unilateral or bilateral abducens nerve palsy may be present. Bradycardia (*vagus pulse*) may be recorded (63).

Management

The diagnosis is made in patients with a history of an orthostatic headache and the demonstration of a low CSFP (<60 mm H_2O) in the lateral recumbent position. After a period of recumbency, the pressure may approach normal values; therefore, LP should be performed as soon as PIH is suspected. The CSFP may be negative, in which case air may be aspirated when the stylette is removed from the needle after dural puncture. The pachymeninges are thickened with increased vascularity and a variable degree of fibrosis, and the examination of the CSF may reveal a slightly elevated protein content and a slight pleocytosis. Mild xanthochromia and a few red cells may be present. A diffuse thickening and gadolinium enhancement of the supratentorial and infratentorial pachymeninges may be shown by MRI. These changes develop some weeks after the onset of PIH and may persist for several months after its resolution (49,48). A cerebral CT scan may show "slit ventricles" and tight basal cisterns, possibly caused by interstitial edema (50,52), and a subdural hygroma or hematoma in a few cases. MRI may show similar changes but also a descent of the brain and hindbrain with tonsillar herniation, flattening of the basis pontis, and bowing of the optic chiasm over the pituitary gland (Fig. 5A) (48). These changes sometimes resemble those of an Arnold-Chiari malformation. Figure 5B shows a return to normal appearance following surgery.

Determination of the cause of PIH may be difficult. Isotope cisternography may reveal leakage of the tracer outside the normal confines of the neuraxis but rarely pinpoints the actual site of a leak. Myelography with CT images of the area identified by the isotope study may provide greater resolution in locating the defect in the meninges. Spinal MRI occasionally will reveal a collection of extraarchnoid CSF, but it rarely identifies the exact source of the leak.

The experience with therapy for PIH is limited, but the therapeutic approach should be the same as described for PPH. Bed rest is sufficient in most cases for this self-limiting condition. Oral caffeine may give slight symptomatic benefit (45). High doses of steroids have been recommended (52) but may fail (45). Also, relief from an epidural blood patch (4,26,45) and epidural saline infusion (14,28) has been reported, probably as a result of the volume effect, but recurrences are not unusual. Surgical repair of a ruptured root sleeve, meningeal diverticulum, or Tarlov cyst occasionally is required if conservative management fails (43,49).

Secondary CSF Leakage, non-PPH

Traumatic Fistulas

The leaks are most frequently located at the skull base, where the meninges are in close contact with weak parts of the bone. The cribiform plate, where the meninges follow the olfactory rootlets through the perforations, is particularly vulnerable. The fistulas occur in 2% to 3% of all patients with head injuries, but anterior basal skull fractures are associated with a fistula in 25% to 50% of cases. No correlation between the severity of the head injury and the risk of developing a fistula seems to exist. Only a few patients develop symptoms immediately. In 90% of patients, the symptoms appear within 3 months, but occasionally symptoms are delayed for several years. The clinical characteristics of the headache do not differ from those of PPH and PIH. Most fistulas present with rhinorrhea or otorrhea. Rhinorrhea may be provoked by flexion of the head in the erect posistion. The definite diagnosis is made by analysis of the nasal fluid, a CT scan after the intrathecal injection of a water soluble contrast medium (2), or by

isotope cisternography, which must be performed with numbered cotton pledgets in the nose (43). The condition is complicated by meningitis in about 25% of cases.

Postoperative Low CSFP

CSF leaks are frequently seen after cranial surgery, but headache resulting from low CSFP is usually not a major problem; however, the treatment of hydrocephalus with ventricular shunts has been associated with many complications, one of which is a low CSFP induced by valvular overdrainage. The clinical picture is characterized by an intermittent or chronic postural headache and may be associated with nausea, vomiting, diplopia, paresis of upward gaze, and lethargy. Bed rest gives immediate relief. The diagnosis is based on the documentation of small or slit ventricles by CT scan, meningeal enhancement on MRI, and slow refill of the palpable valve mechanism (59).

Erosive Lesions

Fistulas are created either directly by erosion of meninges and bone or indirectly via pressure on fragile areas of the skull base. Erosions may be due to congenital anomalies, inflammations, or hydrocephalus, but more than half of the cases are caused by tumors, most frequently pituitary adenomas (55). CSF rhinorrhea often is associated with the empty sella syndrome. Most of these cases are caused by adenoma necrosis (7). The normal CSF pulse and normal fluctuations in CSFP may exert a continuous erosive effect, ultimately leading to CSF leakage into the sphenoid sinus, the nose, and the nasopharynx.

REFERENCES

1. Abouleish E, de la Vega S, Blendinger I, Tio T-O. Long-term follow-up of epidural blood patch. *Anesth Analg* 1975;54:459–463.
2. Ahmadi J, Weiss MH, Segall HD, et al. Evaluation of cerebrospinal

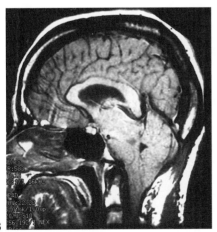
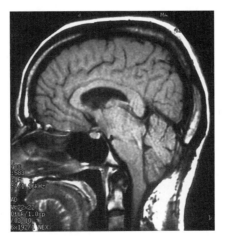

A,B

FIG. 5. A: Magnetic resonance imaging sagittal view demonstrating descent of the brain with crowding of the posterior fossa structures, resembling a Chiari type I malformation. **B**: Return to normal posterior fossa appearance with ascent of the brain, following surgical repair of the cerebrospinal fluid leak.

fluid rhinorrhea by metrizamide computed tomographic cisternography. *Neurosurgery* 1985;16:54–60.

3. Andersen APD, Wanscher MCJ, Hüttel MS. "Postspinaler" Kopfschmerz. Ist die 24-stündige flache Bettruhe eine Prophylaxe? *Reg Anesth* 1986;9:15–17.

4. Baker CC. Headache due to spontaneous low spinal fluid pressure. *Minn Med* 1983;66:325–328.

5. Bart AJ, Wheeler AS. Comparison of epidural saline placement and epidural blood placement in the treatment of post-lumbar-puncture headache. *Anesthesiology* 1978;48:221–223.

6. Beards SC, Jackson A, Griffiths AG, Horsman EL. Magnetic resonance imaging of extradural blood patches: appearances from 30 min to 18 h. *Br J Anaesth* 1993;71:182–188.

7. Bjerre P. The empty sella: a reappraisal of etiology and pathogenesis. *Acta Neurol Scand* 1990;82(Suppl):3–24.

8. Brocker RJ. Technique to avoid spinal-tap headache. *JAMA* 1958;168:261–263.

9. Büttner J, Wresch KP, Klose R. Bietet eine konisch geformte Kanülenspitze Vorteile bei der Spinal-anaesthesie? *Reg Anesth* 1990;13:124–128.

10. Camann WR, Murray RS, Mushlin PS, Lambert DH. Effects of oral caffeine on postdural puncture headache: a double-blind, placebo-controlled trial. *Anesth Analg* 1990;70:181–184.

11. Carbaat PAT, van Crevel H. Lumbar puncture headache: controlled study on the preventive effect of 24 hours' bed rest. *Lancet* 1981;2:1133–1135.

12. Carson D, Serpell M. Choosing the best needle for diagnostic lumbar puncture. *Neurology* 1996;47:33–37.

13. Cook PT, Davies MJ, Beavis RE. Bed rest and postlumbar puncture headache. The effectiveness of 24 hours' recumbency in reducing the incidence of postlumbar puncture headache. *Anesthesia* 1989;44:389–391.

14. Diamond S, Baltes BJ. Headache associated with low spinal fluid pressure syndrome. *Ill Med J* 1973;144:560–561, 601.

15. Dieterich M, Brandt T. Is obligatory bed rest after lumbar puncture obsolete? *Eur Arch Psychiatry Neurosci* 1985;235:71–75.

16. Dieterich M, Brandt T. Incidence of post-lumbar puncture headache is independent of daily fluid intake. *Eur Arch Psychiatry Neurosci* 1988;237:194–196.

17. DiGiovanni AJ, Galbert MW, Wahle WM. Epidural injection of atologous blood for postlumbar-puncture headache. II. Additional clinical experiences and laboratory investigation. *Anesth Analg* 1972;51:226–232.

18. Dittmann M, Schäfer HG, Ulrich J, Bond-Taylor W. Anatomical re-evaluation of lumbar dura mater with regard to postspinal headache. *Anesthesia* 1988;43:635–637.

19. Dodd JE, Efird RC, Rauck RL. Cerebral blood flow changes with caffeine therapy for postdural headaches. *Anesthesiology* 1989;71:A679.

20. Eckstein K-L, Rogacev Z, Vicente-Eckstein A, Grahovac Z. Prospektiv vergleichende Studie postspinaler Kopfschmerzen bei jungen Patienten (<51 Jahre). *Reg Anesth* 1982;5:57–61.

21. Feuerstein TJ, Zeides A. Theophylline relieves headache following lumbar puncture: placebo-controlled, double-blind pilot study. *Klin Wochenschr* 1986;64:216–218.

22. Flaatten H, Rodt SÅ, Vamnes J, Rosland J, Wisborg T, Koller ME. Postdural puncture headache: a comparison between 26- and 29-gauge needles in young patients. *Anaesthesia* 1989;44:147–149.

23. Forbes HS, Nason GI. The cerebral circulation: vascular responses to (A) hypertonic solutions and (B) withdrawal of cerebrospinal fluid. *Arch Neurol Psychiatry* 1935;34:533–547.

24. Fox RTG, Reiche W, Kiefer M, Hagen T, Huber G. Inzidenz des Postmyelographiesyndroms (PMS) und postmyelographischer Beschwerden nach lumbaler Punktion mit der Bleistiftförmigen Nadel nach Sprotte im Vergleich zur Nadel nach Quincke. *Radiologie* 1996;36:921–927.

25. Franksson C, Gordh T. Headache after spinal anesthesia and a technique for lessening its frequency. *Acta Chir Scand* 1946;94:443–454.

26. Gaukroger PB, Brownridge P. Epidural blood patch in the treatment of spontaneous low CSF pressure headache. *Pain* 1987;29:119–122.

27. Geurts JW, Haanschoten MC, van Wijk RM, Kraak H, Besse TC. Postdural puncture headache in young patients: a comparative study between the use of 0.52 mm (25-gauge) and 0.33 mm (29-gauge) spinal needles. *Acta Anesthesiol Scand* 1990;34:350–353.

28. Gibson BE, Wedel DJ, Faust RJ, Petersen RC. Continuous epidural

29. Grant R, Condon B, Patterson J, Wyper DJ, Hadley MDM, Teasdale GM. Changes in cranial CSF volume during hypercapnia and hypocapnia. *J Neurol Neurosurg Psychiatry* 1989;52:218–222.

30. Grant R, Condon B, Hart I, Teasdale GM. Changes in intracranial CSF volume after lumbar puncture and their relationship to post-LP headache. *J Neurol Neurosurg Psychiatry* 1991;54:440–442.

31. Göbel H, Schenkl S. Post-lumbar puncture headache: the relation between experimental suprathreshold pain sensitivity and a quasi-experimental clinical pain syndrome. *Pain* 1990;40:267–278.

32. Handler CE, Smith FR, Perkin GD, Clifford Rose F. Posture and lumbar puncture headache: a controlled trial in 50 patients. *J R Soc Med* 1982;75:404–407.

33. Hatfalvi BI. The dynamics of post-spinal headache. *Headache* 1977;17:64–66.

34. Heide W, Diener HC. Epidural blood patch reduces the incidence of post lumbar puncture headache. *Headache* 1990;30:280–281.

35. Hilton-Jones D. What is postlumbar puncture headache and is it avoidable? In: Warlow C, Garfield J eds. *Dilemmas in the management of the neurological patient.* London: Churchill Livingstone 1984:144–157.

36. Kaplan G. The psychogenic etiology of headache post lumbar puncture. *Psychosom Med* 1967;29:376–379.

37. Kovanen J, Sulkava R. Duration of postural headache after lumbar puncture: effect of needle size. *Headache* 1986;26:224–226.

38. Kunkle EC, Ray BS, Wolff HG. Experimental studies on headache. Analysis of the headache associated with changes in intracranial pressure. *Arch Neurol Psychiatry* 1943;49:323–358.

39. Kuntz KM, Kokmen E, Stevens JC, Miller P, Offord KP, Ho MM. Postlumbar puncture headaches: experience in 501 consecutive procedures. *Neurology* 1992;42:1884–1887.

40. Labadie EL, Glover D. Chronic subdural hematomas: concepts of physiopathogenesis—a review. *Can J Neurol Sci* 1974;1:222–225.

41. Labadie EL, van Antwerp J, Bamford CR. Abnormal lumbar isotope cisternography in an unusual case of spontaneous hypoliquorrheic headache. *Neurology* 1976;26:135–139.

42. Lambert DH, Hurley RJ, Hertwig L, Datta S. Role of needle gauge and tip configuration in the production of lumbar puncture headache. *Reg Anesth* 1997;22:66–72.

43. Lay CL, Campbell JK, Mokri B. Low cerebrospinal pressure headache. In: Goadsby PJ, Silberstein SD, eds. *Headache. Blue books of practical neurology.* Boston: Butterworth-Heinemann, 1997:355–367.

44. Lenaerts M, Pepin JL, Tombu S, Schoenen J. No significant effect of an atraumatic needle on incidence of post-lumbar puncture headache or traumatic tap. *Cephalalgia* 1993;13:296–297.

45. Marcelis J, Silberstein SD. Spontaneous low cerebrospinal fluid pressure headache. *Headache* 1990;30:192–196.

46. Marshall J. Lumbar-puncture headache. *J Neurol Nerosurg Psychiatry* 1950;13:71–74.

47. Michel O, Brusis T. Hearing loss as a sequel of lumbar puncture. *Ann Otol Rhinol Laryngol* 1992;101:390–394.

48. Mokri B, Krueger BR, Miller GM, Piepgras DG. Meningeal gadolinium enhancement in low-pressure headaches. *Ann Neurol* 1991;30:294–295(Abst).

49. Mokri B, Piepgras DG, Miller GM. Syndrome of orthostatic headaches of diffuse pachymeningeal gadolinium enhancement. *Mayo Clin Proc* 1997;72:400–413.

50. Molins A, Alvárez J, Sumalla J, Titus F, Codina A. Cisternographic pattern of spontaneous liquoral hypotension. *Cephalalgia* 1990;10:59–65.

51. Morrow JI, McAuley A, Patterson VH. Failure of oblique needle insertion to prevent post-lumbar puncture headache. *Arch Neurol* 1987;44:795.

52. Murros K, Fogelholm R. Spontaneous intracranial hypotension with slit ventricles. *J Neurol Neurosurg Psychiatry* 1983;46:1149–1151.

53. Nelson MO. Postpuncture headaches. A clinical and experimental study on the cause and prevention. *Arch Dermatol Syph* 1930;21:615–627.

54. Nestvold K. The influence of lumbar puncture needle size on postpuncture complications particularly with regard to patients under daycare and fully hospitalized patients. *Tidsskr Nor Laegeforen* 1978;98:569–570.

55. Ommaya AK, Di Chiro G, Baldwin M, Pennybacker JB. Non-traumatic cerebrospinal fluid rhinorrhoea. *J Neurol Neurosurg Psychiatry* 1968;31:214–225.

56. Pedersen ON. Use of a 22-gauge needle to reduce the incidence of side

effects after lumbar myelography: a prospective randomised study comparing Whitacre and Quincke spinal needles. *Eur Radiol* 1996;6; 184–187.

57. Pickering GW. Lumbar puncture headache. *Brain* 1948;71:274–280.

58. Plum F, Siesjö BK. Recent advances in CSF physiology. *Anesthesiology* 1975;42:708–730.

59. Pudenz RH, Foltz EL. Hydrocephalus: overdrainage by ventricular shunts. A review and recommendations. *Surg Neurol* 1991;35:200–212.

60. Rice GG, Dabbs CH. The use of peridural and subarachnoid injections of saline solution in the treatment of severe postspinal headache. *Anesthesiology* 1950;11:17–23.

61. Rosenberg PH, Heavner JE. *In vitro* study of the effect of epidural blood patch on leakage through a dural puncture. *Anesth Analg* 1985; 64:501–504.

62. Schaltenbrand VG. Neuere Anschauungen zur Pathophysiologie der Liquorzirkulation. *Zentralbl Neurochir* 1938;3:290–299.

63. Schaltenbrand VG. Die akute Aliquorrhoe. *Verh Dtsch Ges Inn Med* 1940;52:473–481.

64. Sechzer PH, Abel L. Post-spinal anesthesia headache treated with caffeine. Evaluation with demand method. Part I. *Curr Ther Res* 1978;24: 307–312.

65. Seebacher J, Ribeiru V, LeGuillou JL, et al. Epidural blood patch in the treatment of post dural puncture headache: a double blind study. *Headache* 1989;29:630–632.

66. Sicard JA. *Le liquide céphalo-rachidien.* Paris: Masson et Gautier-Villars, 1902.

67. Sipe JC, Zyroff J, Waltz TA. Primary intracranial hypotension and bilateral isodense subdural hematomas. *Neurology* 1981;31:334–337.

68. Smith FR, Perkin GD, Clifford Rose F. Posture and headache after lumbar puncture. *Lancet* 1980;1:1245.

69. Spriggs DA, Burn DJ, French J, Cartlidge NEF, Bates D. Is bed rest useful after diagnostic lumbar puncture? *Postgrad Med J* 1992;68: 581–583.

70. Tourtellotte WW, Haerer AF, Heller GL, Somers JE. *Post-lumbar puncture headaches.* Springfield, IL: Charles C Thomas, 1964.

71. Tourtellotte WW, Henderson WG, Tucker RP, Gilland O, Walker JE, Kokman E. A randomized, double-blind clinical trial comparing the 22 versus 26 gauge needle in the production of the post-lumbar puncture syndrome in normal individuals. *Headache* 1972;12:73–78.

72. Usubiaga JE, Usubiaga LE, Brea LM, Goyena R. Effect of saline injections on epidural and subarachnoid space pressures and relation to post-spinal anesthesia headache. *Anesth Analg* 1967;46:293–296.

73. Vandam LD, Dripps RD. Long-term follow-up of patients who received 10,098 spinal anesthetics. *JAMA* 1956;161:586–591.

74. Vilming ST, Schrader H, Monstad I. Post-lumbar-puncture headache: the significance of body posture. A controlled study of 300 patients. *Cephalalgia* 1988;8:75–78.

75. Vilming ST, Schrader H, Monstad I. The significance of age, sex, and cerebrospinal fluid pressure in post-lumbar-puncture headache. *Cephalalgia* 1989;9:99–106.

76. Vilming ST, Ellertsen B, Troland K, Schrader H, Monstad I. MMPI profiles in post-lumbar puncture headache. *Acta Neurol Scand* 1997; 95:184–188.

77. Vilming ST, Kloster R. Post-lumbar puncture headache: clinical features and suggestions for diagnostic criteria. *Cephalalgia* 1997;17: 778–784.

78. Vilming ST, Kloster R. The time course of post-lumbar puncture headache. *Cephalalgia* 1998;18:97–100.

79. Wang LP, Schmidt JF. Central nervous side effects after lumbar puncture: a review of the possible pathogenesis of the syndrome of postdural puncture headache and associated symptoms. *Dan Med Bull* 1997;44:79–81.

80. Wee LH, Lam F, Cranston AJ. The incidence of post dural puncture headache in children. *Anesthesia* 1996;51:1164–1166.

81. Wolff HG. Headache mechanisms. *Int Arch Allergy* 1955;7:210–278.

82. Yu-Lin H, Chia-Erh C. Headache following spinal anesthesia. *Chin Med J* 1951;69:251–257.

The Headaches, Second Edition,
edited by J. Olesen, P. Tfelt-Hansen, and K.M.A. Welch.
Lippincott Williams & Wilkins, Philadelphia © 2000.

The Secondary Headaches

CHAPTER 112

Headache Associated with Intracranial Infection

Milena De Marinis and K. Michael A. Welch

DEFINITION OF HEADACHE ASSOCIATED WITH INTRACRANIAL INFECTION

IHS code and diagnosis: 7.3 Intracranial infection.
WHO code and diagnosis: G44.82 Headache associated with other intracranial disorders.
Short description: Headache occurs at the onset of intracranial infection and disappears after successful treatment of the intracranial infection.
Other terms: None.

IHS diagnostic criteria for headache associated with intracranial infection (Headache Classification Committee, 1988):

A. Symptoms or signs of intracranial infection
B. Confirmation by appropriate investigations
C. Headache as a new symptom or of a new type occurs temporally related to intracranial infection

Headache is common in intracranial infections, including meningitis, encephalitis, brain abscess, subdural empyema, and acquired immunodeficiency syndrome (AIDS). Headache also may be associated with these infections as a manifestation of the infectious disease syndrome that includes fever, chills, malaise, myalgia, arthralgia, and asthenia.

BACTERIAL MENINGITIS

Headache is the most common symptom of bacterial meningitis. It may be the first symptom to appear and the only symptom to remain as a long-term complication (18). A variety of agents may cause primary and secondary meningitis (19,30,65) (Table 1).

Pathologically, the inflammation spreads throughout the subarachnoid space of the brain and spinal cord. The cerebrospinal fluid (CSF) space is filled with purulent exudate, and the cortical veins and meningeal vessels are congested and dilated. The purulent exudate over the brain cortex is most marked in the frontal and parietal regions, but the bulk of the exudate is found at the base, where it fills the great cisterns and the interpeduncular space and passes upward along the middle and anterior cerebral arteries.

Microscopically, the leptomeninges show inflammatory cell infiltration of polymorphonuclear cells and in the later stages lymphocytes and plasma cells. The vessels are greatly dilated, and microhemorrhage may be seen.

Meningococcus and other forms of acute suppurative meningitis produce the characteristic pathological picture. Pneumococcal meningitis is complicated by the formation of fibrous exudate that causes obstructive hydrocephalus. Tuberculous meningitis is characterized by an abundant greenish, creamy, or cheesy exudate that settles to the base of the brain, causing adhesions of all surfaces and usually obstructive hydrocephalus. Microscopically, the meningitic reaction is partly inflammatory and partly tuberculous.

Physiopathology

The physiopathology of headache associated with meningitis has a number of different mechanisms that are

M. De Marinis: Department of Neurological Sciences, University of Rome "La Sapienza," 00185 Rome, Italy.

K. M. A. Welch: Department of Neurology, University of Kansas School of Medicine, University of Kansas Medical Center, Kansas City, Kansas, 66106.

TABLE 1. *Primary and secondary bacterial meningitis*

Type of meningitis	Bacteria involved
Primary: direct infection of the meninges	
Healthy subjects	*Meningococcus, Pneumococcus, Hemophilus influenzae, Streptococcus, Staphylococcus, Escherichia coli,* and *Mycobacterium tuberculosis*
Immunosuppressed patients receiving chemotherapy or patients with lymphoma, leukemia, malnutrition, and AIDS	Unusual pathogens (*Nocardia, Listeria monocytogenes*), *Cryptococcus,* and *M tuberculosis*
Secondary: complication of other diseases (by diffusion or septicemia)	
Cranial diseases: skull fracture, osteitis of the cranial bones, mastoiditis, sinus infections (especially the frontal sinus), scalp infections, and thrombophlebitis of the intracranial venous sinuses	
Focal infection elsewhere in the body: pneumonia, empyema, osteomyelitis, erysipelas, military tuberculosis, and infective endocarditis by similar mechanisms	

AIDS, acquired immunodeficiency syndrome.

based essentially on the interaction of inflammation and pain transmission (Fig. 1). These mechanisms also are involved in headache associated with other intracranial infections and headache associated with noncephalic infections (see Chapter 116).

Hyperalgesia and prolonged spontaneous pain are due to increased sensitivity of peripheral nociceptors (primary hyperalgesia) and to facilitated second sensory neuron transmission (secondary hyperalgesia, receptive field expansion, and allodynia). Hyperexcitability of second sensory neurons (dorsal horn neurons) is triggered first by an increased barrage of sensory discharge into the central nervous system (CNS) (windup), and later by retrograde chemical influences from peripheral inflammation (central sensitization) (see Fig. 1).

Meningeal irritation with direct stimulation of the sensory terminals localized in meninges and meningeal vessels usually accounts for the earliest onset of headache. At this level, nociceptors can be activated (primary hyperalgesia) by mediators of inflammation, such as bradykinin, histamine, and prostaglandins, and also by tissue acidosis and release of oxygen radicals, nitric oxide, and endothelin-1. Kinins (e.g., bradykinin) are commonly released at sites of injury and inflammation and produce sensitization of afferents through the activation of B2 bradykinin receptors that stimulate other proinflammatory mediators, including prostanoids and cytokines. Cytokines are soluble proteins secreted by cells of the immune system that principally regulate inflammatory and immune responses (see Fig. 1).

Second sensory neuron excitability also is increased (secondary hyperalgesia) by two mechanisms. Inflammatory processes act as a conditioning stimulation of C fibers that generates a gradual increase in reflex magnitude (*windup*), followed by a period of reflex hyperexcitability (*first mechanism*). Nociceptors themselves contain substance P and calcitonin gene-related-peptide, which are antidromically released by peripheral stimulation (*second mechanism*) and act as hyperalgesia sensitizing factors.

Activation of chemosensitive afferents by inflammatory substances also releases glutamate, which activates NMDA receptors that induce hyperalgesia and pain. NMDA receptors mediate windup, postsynaptic neuronal discharge, and generation of nitric oxide. Nitric oxide is involved in the spinal transmission of nociceptive information, particularly after peripheral inflammation has developed.

Peripheral tissue injury resulting from inflammation causes change, not only in the excitability of the second sensory (spinal dorsal horn) neurons but also in central sensitization and hyperalgesia. Central transmission and hyperexcitability are mediated by excitatory amino acids (aspartate and glutamate) and by tachykinins (substance P). Driven by descending projections from brainstem sites, the net effect of the activity in a complex network of inhibitory neurons in the spinal cord (*gate control*) is to dampen and counteract spinal cord hyperexcitability induced by tissue or nerve injury. Thus, peripherally evoked pain and headache impulses pass through a filtering process involving gamma-aminobutyric acid, glycine, and enkephalin neurotransmission. The activity of these substances in the spinal cord usually attenuates and limits the duration of pain.

Headache also may be secondary to increased intracranial pressure in meningitis, caused by an accumulation of purulent exudate in the subarachnoid space of the brain and spinal cord, which obstructs the CSF circulation. This situation is worsened by edema complicating the inflammatory process. Abnormality of CSF circulation becomes extreme when hydrocephalus occurs as a result of inflammatory adhesions in the basal cisterns and foramina of the fourth ventricle, particularly in tuberculous meningitis. Finally, headache may be a generalized response to the fever of infection (see Chapter 116).

Clinical Features

Bursting headache, rapidly increasing in severity over minutes, is usually the initial symptom of acute bacterial

Peripheral inflammation

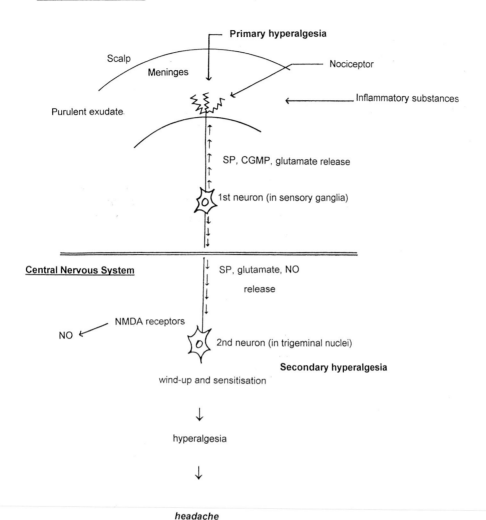

FIG. 1. Mechanisms involved in hyperalgesia, pain, and headache due to meningitis.

meningitis (18). It may be generalized or frontal and usually radiates down the neck and into the spinal region, even to the limbs. Vomiting and photophobia are frequent, especially in the early stages of infection. The patients adopt a flexed, curled-up posture and exhibit reflex protective spasm of the neck and spine with rigidity, head retraction, and Kernig's and Brudzinski's signs. Movement of the eyes may be painful, and oculoparesis may be present. Cognitive function varies according to the stage and progress of the disease. Delirium, drowsiness, stupor, coma, and seizures may occur. These features of acute bacterial meningitis are typified by meningococcal infection (20,59).

Other clinical patterns of bacterial meningitis and associated headache depend on such factors as the responsible microorganism, age of patients, and the presence of malnutrition, immunosuppression, or AIDS (19). For example, in elderly persons or infants, the features of meningitis are frequently atypical; headache, irritability or lethargy, and

fever may be the only symptoms (19). A rare recurrent or chronic meningitis caused by meningococcus may be characterized by fever, daily occipital headache, shoulder pain, and muscle weakness lasting up to 3 months (47). Less commonly, severe headache associated with fever, malaise, and positive CSF culture, without meningeal or focal neurologic signs, has been described, for example, in sepsis following *Escherichia coli* urinary tract infection (22). Headache with nonspecific symptoms such as myalgia, low-grade temperature, and low white cell count may be the only manifestation of *Brucella* menigitis (10).

Chronic meningitis is typified by tuberculosis (TB). TB meningitis usually is associated with severe, unrelenting generalized headache that usually presents subacutely, but chronic headache (lasting months) and fever may be the only clinical expression. Eventually, headache together with vomiting and impaired consciousness may occur as a consequence of hydrocephalus, even without obvious symptoms of raised intracranial pressure (8).

Headache lasting from weeks to months and increasing in severity from day to day in subjects without fever or other neurologic findings is the most common presenting symptom of cryptococcal meningitis (58). In this condition, chronic headache may be due to meningeal irritation, increased intracranial pressure, and hydrocephalus (13,29,60). Generally, the duration of the headache depends on complications of the meningitis itself; for example, hydrocephalus may be a consequence of intracranial cryptococcal granulomata (13,29).

Subacute or chronic meningitis also may develop in immunosuppressed patients. For example, the typical presentation in a series of patients with *Nocardia* infection was subacute to chronic meningitis characterized by headache, fever, and nuchal rigidity in 55% to 70% of patients (7). An associated brain abscess was present in 43% of the patients. Meningitis associated with leukemia or most of the non-T-cell lymphomas is likely to be from *Listeria* infection. Patients with Hodgkin's disease, AIDS, or patients treated with steroids or receiving chemotherapy are more likely to have cryptococcal or tuberculous meningitis (19,64) (see Table 1).

The investigation of meningitis includes spinal puncture and examination of the CSF to identify the nature of the inflammatory reaction and to identify the organism by appropriate testing, including culture and sensitivity studies. Imaging studies of the head and sometimes the spine may be required to evaluate complications such as obstructive hydrocephalus, abscess, or subdural empyema. The management of headache and meningitis in the active phase consists of appropriate antibiotic or antifungal therapy and support with fluids, analgesics, and antipyretics. Corticosteroids, in the case of TB, and frequent lumbar punctures may be helpful to relieve persistent raised intracranial pressure. A ventricular shunt may be needed if obstructive hydrocephalus develops. Once the acute event has been managed successfully, the long-term prognosis is dependent on the neurologic complications that develop during active infection, including cerebral infarction from inflammatory endarteritis, cranial nerve paresis, obstructive hydrocephalus, spinal cord compression, and, in the long term, communicating hydrocephalus. The last of these may present as a generalized headache years after meningitis has been cured.

ASEPTIC MENINGITIS (NONBACTERIAL)

Aseptic meningitis also should be suspected in meningitis that fails to respond to antibiotic therapy. Severe headache of rapid onset over hours, fever, malaise, anorexia, fever, phonophobia, photophobia, and nuchal rigidity are the main symptoms of aseptic meningitis. The course of the disease is generally benign. A lymphocytic pleocytosis with a total cell count in the low hundreds, a normal or mildly elevated protein (usually <100 mg%), and a normal CSF plasma:glucose ratio are helpful diagnostic findings (14,36). Episodes of throbbing and bilateral headache (lasting hours), frequently preceded by transient neurologic deficits (lasting hours), have been described in patients with lymphocytic pleocytosis who may have had a viral-like illness up to 3 weeks before the onset of the syndrome (23). Enteroviruses *Coxsackie* A and B account for most cases of aseptic meningitis (53). Others include mumps, herpes simplex, adenovirus, cytomegalovirus, rubella, herpes zoster, Epstein-Barr, influenza, and parainfluenza. Arboviruses are geographic in distribution and seasonal in outbreak.

Epstein-Barr and *Coxsackie* viruses occasionally run a subacute or chronic course (14). Severe episodic headache has been reported in recurrent herpes virus type 2 (HSV-2) and in Epstein-Barr-virus–induced meningitis (4,57). Episodic headache also can occur during recrudescence of genital lesions in patients with previous HSV meningitis (4).

Lyme disease is an endemic tick-borne illness that lasts for months and has a typical neurologic involvement consisting of aseptic meningitis, cranial neuropathy, and radiculoneuritis, alone or in combination (41). This *Borrelia* infection frequently presents with distinct stages characterized by intermittent attacks of severe headache, mild meningism, and a predominantly lymphocytic pleocytosis (42). In the early stage (erythema migrans), headache is reported in 42% of cases, associated with systemic symptoms such as fatigue in 54%, arthralgia in 44%, myalgia in 44%, and fever in 39% (38). After a few weeks to months, some patients (15%) develop frank neurologic symptoms that can recur (stage 2). Months to years after onset of the disease (stage 3), patients develop symptoms of intermittent or chronic arthritis (51). In children, chronic headache, loss of appetite, fatigue, and low-grade fever may be the only presenting symptoms (39).

A rare form of aseptic meningitis ascribed to Mollare is of unknown cause is characterized by CSF pleocytosis with large epithelioid cells. Headache is a prominent feature with signs of meningism and low-grade fever. Meningitis may recur every few days or weeks and follow a protracted course of recurrent episodes over months to years.

On rare occasions, a syndrome resembling migraine, particularly migraine with prolonged aura, may present with fever, neck stiffness, and cellular reaction in the CSF suggesting aseptic meningitis (2,49,54). This condition is described more completely in the section on CSF.

ENCEPHALITIS

A specific virus is identified in fewer than half of the cases of encephalitis. Arborvirus and mumps are common causes of encephalitis, whereas enterovirus-induced encephalitis is uncommon. Herpes simplex virus is another prominent cause of encephalitis. Encephalitis may occur with influenza, adenovirus, Epstein-Barr virus, toxoplasmosis, and herpes zoster. Measles, mumps, and chickenpox also can cause a postinfectious illness as well as encephalitis.

Pathologically, the brain and cord are swollen and congested. Microscopically, the most common feature is chromatolysis followed by necrosis and neuronophagia, microglial proliferation, neuronal and glial inclusion bodies, perivascular cellular infiltration, and meningeal inflammation.

The mechanisms of the head pain include meningeal irritation and increased intracranial pressure. In addition, headache may be a general reaction to fever or the toxic products of the infecting agent (see Chapter 116).

Clinical Features

The characteristic signs of encephalitis include confusion, delirium, stupor, and coma with additional signs of focal neurologic deficit. Headache is frequently present in acute encephalitis and commonly associated with fever and meningism. Abrupt and severe headache may occur early and may be the only manifestation of encephalitis. Occasionally, a prodrome of less severe but constant headache associated with malaise, mild fever, and myalgia may precede the onset of the neurologic deficit by several days. The clinical picture may reflect the organism, for example, mild as in mumps encephalitis, to catastrophic as in herpes simplex encephalitis.

One of the most common nonepidemic viral encephalitides is HSV. It is usually an acute fulminant infection with high mortality. Generalized headache of rapid onset with confusion occurs in over 50% of cases in association with fever (about 39 °C) in 50% to 80% of patients, meningism in 40% to 60%, deep coma in up to 40%, focal neurologic signs in 80% to 90%, and seizures in 45% to 60% (31,32). [Epstein-Barr virus also may induce acute infections in children (17).] Localized headache may occur when there is mass effect due to tissue necrosis and edema that commonly involves the temporal cortex. A subacute or chronic course has been described. Some patients may suffer from a chronic encephalopathy that progresses over 4 to 5 months characterized by headache, fatigue, lethargy, mild confusion, and even psychosis, with or without focal signs. The symptoms may recur after antiviral therapy in some instances (15,48).

Headache is also a prominent symptom according to reports on other, less common encephalitides. For example, headache, a common symptom in *Coxiella burnetii* infection, may be the presenting symptom when the CNS is involved (6). *Listeria* monocytogenes encephalitis may have a biphasic clinical pattern with a prodromal phase characterized by headache, nausea, fever, and leukocytosis and subsequent lower cranial nerve paresis, ataxia, respiratory insufficiency, and coma (9,33).

An influenza-like illness with severe headache, fever, chills, abdominal pain, myalgia, and arthralgia may be the only manifestation of St. Louis encephalitis (43). In Japanese encephalitis, headache was reported in 76% of patients, together with altered consciousness, fever, convulsions, and vomiting, meningeal signs, hemiplegia, papilledema, and other cranial nerve palsies occurred in 20% to 60% of these patients (44).

Transient episodes of bifrontal headache, aphasia, and unilateral sensory symptoms preceded by several days of malaise and fever occur in cytomegalovirus encephalitis. Cytomegalovirus infection frequently develops in immunosuppressed and AIDS patients (45).

BRAIN ABSCESS

Brain abscess arises from a contiguous focus of infection, direct implantation due to trauma, or hematogenous spread from a remote site (11,12,25,34). The most common organisms isolated from brain abscess include streptococci, *Staphylococcus aureus*, *Bacteroides* species, and *Enterobacter*. Infections of paranasal sinuses (11), ears (34), lungs, and jaw are predisposing factors in about 70% of cases (12,25). Congenital heart disease complicated by infective endocarditis causes brain abscess in up to 19% of cases. Anaerobic streptococci are generally involved (21).

Pathologically, there is a focal encephalitis without pus formation in the early stage. When pus develops, a capsule forms to localize the abscess. Headache may be the first symptom of brain abscess in 46% of cases (63). Direct compression and irritation of the meningeal structures and increased intracranial pressure are the mechanisms that commonly cause headache.

Clinical Features

Headache, vomiting, focal neurologic signs, and depressed level of consciousness are the main symptoms of brain abscess. Headache is usually the first manifestation (63), unless it is preceded by symptoms arising from the primary infection. Fever and leukocytosis are often absent. In fact, headache may be the predominant clinical feature of brain abscess with acute or chronic evolution. Nausea and vomiting generally begin around 1 week after the onset of headache (12). With a chronic abscess, headache is paroxysmal and is increased by exertion, having the features of headache that results from increased intracranial pressure. In more acute cases, headache may be persistent and severe. In cerebellar abscess, headache is predominantly suboccipital, and pain may radiate into the neck with associated cervical rigidity.

In brain abscess resulting from ear infections, headache is generally preceded by chronic otitis and pain in the temporal region (34). In brain abscesses originating from the sinuses, there is frequently a history of frontal headache. In these patients, acute frontal headache, particularly unilateral, may suggest brain abscess even in the absence of nausea or vomiting (34). An abscess of hematogenous origin complicating pyemia or bacteremia may present with headache developing slowly and insidiously in a course that is clinically indistinguishable from that of intracranial tumor. In brucellosis, headache and papilledema may be the only clinical features of single or multiple brain abscesses (24). In patients with immunosuppression, leukemia, or recipients of renal transplants, chronic headache may be the presenting symptom of *Listeria* infection (55).

The diagnosis of abscess is generally made late in the illness. The abscess is confirmed by computerized tomography (CT) or magnetic resonance imaging (MRI). Many cases require confirmation by surgical biopsy. Blood cultures are positive in about 11% of cases. Lumbar puncture rarely provides data from which a diagnosis can be established. Optimal management consists of intensive antibiotic therapy. Aggressive surgical treatment is required for patients who do not respond to antibiotics. Neurologic deficit may recur in up to 60% of cases (25). The incidence and mortality associated with cerebral abscess have changed little in the last 25 years despite improvements in diagnostic imaging, surgical technique, and antibiotic therapy (11).

SUBDURAL EMPYEMA

Severe headache, fever, and meningism are common presenting symptoms of subdural empyema. This intracerebral infection is frequently secondary to sinusitis or middle ear infection. The bacteria involved stem from the upper respiratory tract (particularly *Streptococcus milleri*). Subdural empyema also may be a rare complication of meningitis.

An initial diagnosis of viral or bacterial meningitis often is made based on presenting symptoms; however, alteration in the level of consciousness and focal neurologic deficit rapidly follows. In certain cases, symptoms may be mild and linked to those of the original infection. In other cases, neurologic symptoms are preceded by headache and vomiting lasting 1 to 2 weeks (37). Headache is caused by fever, meningeal irritation, increased intracranial pressure, or a combination of all three. Morbidity and mortality are minimized by early diagnosis, which is best made by CT or MRI. Appropriate management consists of surgical drainage and antibiotic administration (27,50).

AIDS

Headache is an important symptom in the following AIDS-related conditions: acute human immunodeficiency virus (HIV) infection, HIV-associated aseptic meningitis, HIV-associated encephalopathy, secondary cerebral toxoplasmosis, secondary meningitis (cryptococcal, tuberculous), and secondary encephalitis (cytomegalovirus).

Headache is a part of the acute HIV infection that generally lasts from a few days to 3 weeks and includes fever, sore throat, myalgia, arthralgia, rash, and lymphadenopathy. Headache associated with photophobia has a reported prevalence that ranges from 60% to 100% (16). Recurrent migrainelike episodes, associated or not with transient neurologic deficit, have been described in HIV-infected patients without an apparent structural lesion of the cerebral structures; in these patients, anticardiolipin antibodies were present (46). Headache is also a common symptom in association with the primary encephalopathy and aseptic meningitis of HIV (5). Aseptic meningitis with lymphocytic pleocytosis may occur either at the time of seroconversion or sporadically. Patients suffer recurrent acute onset of headache and fever, at times accompanied by nausea and meningeal signs, lasting less than 4 weeks. In other patients, chronic headache and pleocytosis, with or without fever or signs of meningeal irritation, persist for months (28).

Toxoplasma gondii is a common pathogen in patients with AIDS (40). Multiple abscesses surrounded by inflammation and vascular proliferation are found at autopsy. Headache is a major complaint that develops either at the same time as other neurologic manifestations or, less frequently, preceding them by up to 4 weeks. The headache is characteristically bilateral, but in certain cases it is unilateral, severe, and persistent, frequently awakening the patient at night. Headache responds poorly to analgesics. The diagnosis can be made by CT or MRI. Brain biopsy sometimes is indicated for differential diagnosis, particularly if the abscess is solitary.

Cryptococcal meningitis has a prevalence of 5% to 10% in AIDS patients (62) (see Table 1). The main presenting features in more than 80% of cases are headache, fever, and nausea. Meningism and mental changes are frequently absent or rare. CSF examination for cryptococcal antigen or culture will confirm the diagnosis.

OTHER TYPES OF CNS INVOLVEMENT

Sarcoidosis

Headache associated with intracranial sarcoidosis and other noninfectious inflammatory diseases is coded to group 7.4 of the International Headache Society (IHS) classification (26). Neurosarcoidosis occurs in fewer than 10% of all cases of sarcoidosis. Headache occurs in association with chronic meningitis as a result of granulomatous infiltration of the leptomeninges. At this stage, the headache may be indolent in onset, chronic, of mild to moderate severity, and more often localized posteriorly. Occasionally, meningitis can present abruptly. Obstruction of the foramina of Lushka and Magendie may cause hydrocephalus with acute worsening of the headache due to raised intracranial pressure. Tonsillar herniation may be a complicating feature, causing severe occipital pain and neck stiffness. Headache is first localized and later generalized on the rare occasions when an intraparenchymal mass develops. Cranial nerve paresis, particularly facial, is a common presentation of sarcoid. Local optical nerve involvement may cause papilledema with or without localized pain but without generalized headache typical of intracranial pressure. Trigeminal nerve involvement may cause facial pain. Treatment is usually with corticosteroids, but surgical shunt placement may be necessary when hydrocephalus occurs.

Chemical Meningitis

Headache associated with chemical meningitis is coded to group 7.5.2. of the IHS classification. Chemical meningitis may result from the release of irritative substances into the subarachnoid space, for example, after removal or spontaneous rupture of dermoid and epidermoid cysts or craniopharyngiomas containing material rich in cholesterol, keratin, and lipids (3). Neoplasia will present rarely with such a complication (8). Violent headache, vomiting, high fever, and nuchal rigidity can precede loss of consciousness and coma (35).

Multiple complications have been reported after metrizamide myelography, including a high incidence of headache, meningeal irritation, confusion, seizures, and occasionally focal neurologic deficit occurring several hours after the injection of metrizamide, it usually resolving within 48 hours (1). Drug reactions may take the form of acute or recurrent meningitis. Severe frontal headache, vomiting, fever, nuchal rigidity, and CSF mononuclear pleocytosis have been described in patients after intravenous infusion of immunoglobulin (61). Carbamazepine may cause headache, fever, rash, peripheral eosinophilia, aseptic meningitis, and myoclonus (52). Severe headache followed by fever, chills, nuchal rigidity, and nausea has been described as a complication of nonsteroidal antiinflammatory drugs (NSAIDs), particularly in patients with autoimmune disease (56). The mechanism of drug-induced meningitis is presumed to be an acute hypersensitivity reaction limited to meninges, without systemic anaphylaxis.

REFERENCES

1. Baker FJ, Gosson G, Bortoni JM. Aseptic meningitis; complications of metrizamide myelography. *AJNR Am J Neuroradiol* 1982;3:662–663.
2. Bartleson JD, Swanson JW, Whisnant JP. A migrainous syndrome with cerebrospinal fluid pleocytosis. *Neurology* 1981;31:1257–1262.
3. Becker WJ, Watters GV, de Chadarévian JP, Vanasse M. Recurrent aseptic meningitis secondary to intracranial epidermoids. *Can J Neurol Sci* 1984;1:387–389.
4. Bergström T, Vahlne A, Alestig K, Jeansson S, Forsgren M, Lycke E. Primary and recurrent herpes simplex virus type 2-induced meningitis. *J Infect Dis* 1990;162:322–330.
5. Brew BJ, Miller J. Human immunodeficiency virus-related headache. *Neurology* 1993;43:1098–1100.
6. Brooks RG, Licitra CM, Peacock MG. Encephalitis caused by *Coxiella burnetii. Ann Neurol* 1986;20:91–93.
7. Bross JE, Gordon G. Nocardial meningitis: case reports and review. *Rev Infect Dis* 1991;13:160–165.
8. Brown IA, Peyton WT. Brain tumors simulating meningitis. *J Neurosurg* 1951;8:459–468.
9. Callea L, Donati E, Faggi L, Scalzini A, Callea F. Pontomedullary encephalitis and basal meningitis due to *Listeria* monocytogenes: report of a case. *Eur Neurol* 1985;254:217–220.
10. Challoner KR, Riley KB, Larsen RA. Brucella meningitis. *Am J Emerg Med* 1990;8:40–42.
11. Chalstrey S, Pfleiderer AG, Moffat DA. Persisting incidence and mortality of sinogenic cerebral abscess: a continuing reflection of late clinical diagnosis. *J R Soc Med* 1991;84:193–195.
12. Chun CH, Johnson JD, Hofstetter M, Raff MJ. Brain abscess: a study of 45 consecutive cases. *Medicine* 1986;65:415–431.
13. Cochius JI, Burns RJ, Willoughby JO. CNS cryptococcosis: unusual aspects. *Clin Exp Neurol* 1989;26:183–191.
14. Dalton M, Newton RW. Aseptic meningitis. *Dev Med Child Neurol* 1991;33:446–458.
15. Davis LE, McLaren LC. Relapsing herpes simplex encephalitis following antiviral therapy. *Ann Neurol* 1983;13:192–195.
16. Denning DW. The neurological features of acute HIV infection. *Biomed Pharmacother* 1988;42:11–14.
17. Domachowske JB, Cunningham CK, Cummings DL, Crosley CJ, Hannan WP, Weiner LB. Acute manifestations and neurologic sequelae of Eptein-Barr virus encephalitis in children. *Pediatr Infect Dis J* 1996;15:871–875.
18. Drexler ED. Severe headaches: when to worry, what to do. *Postgrad Med* 1990;87:164–170, 173–180.
19. Francke E. The many causes of meningitis. *Postgrad Med* 1987;82:175–178, 181–183, 187–188.
20. Gedde-Dahl TW, Lettenstrom GS, Bovre K. Coverage for meningococcal disease in the Norwegian morbidity and mortality statistics. *NIPH Ann* 1980;3/2:31–35.
21. Ghosh S, Chandy MJ, Abraham J. Brain abscess and congenital heart disease. *J Indian Med Assoc* 1990;88:312–314.
22. Gilmore RL, Lebow R, Berk SL. Spontaneous *Escherichia coli* K1 meningitis in an adult. *South Med J* 1983;76:1202–1203.
23. Gomez-Aranda F, Canadillas F, Marti-Masso JF, et al. Pseudomigraine with temporary neurological symptoms and lymphocytic pleocytosis. *Brain* 1997;120:1105–1113.
24. Guvenc H, Kocabay K, Okten A, Bektas S. Brucellosis in a child complicated with multiple brain abscesses. *Scand J Infect Dis* 1989;21:333–336.
25. Harris LF, Maccubbin DA, Triplett JN, Haws FP. Brain abscess: recent experience at a community hospital. *South Med J* 1985;78:704–707.
26. Headache Classification Committee of the International Headache Society. Classification and diagnostic criteria for headache disorders, cranial neuralgias and facial pain. *Cephalalgia* 1988;(Suppl 7):52–53.
27. Hodges J, Anslow P, Gillet G. Subdural empyema: continuing diagnostic problems in the CT scan era. *QJM* 1986;59:387–393.
28. Hollander H, Stringari S. Human immunodeficiency virus-associated meningitis. Clinical course and correlations. *Am J Med* 1987;83:813–816.
29. Hutchinson DO, Anderson NE, Ingram RJ, et al. Cryptococcal meningitis in Auckland 1969–89. *N Z Med J* 1991;104:57–59.
30. Jones HR, Siekert RG. Neurological manifestations of infective endocarditis. *Brain* 1989;112:1295–1315.
31. Kennedy PG. Retrospective analysis of 46 cases of herpes simplex encephalitis seen in Glasgow between 1962 and 1985. *QJM* 1988;68:533–540.
32. Kennedy PG, Adams IH, Graham DI, Clements GB. A clinico-pathological study of herpes simplex encephalitis. *Neuropathol Appl Neurobiol* 1988;14:395–415.
33. Kohler J, Winkler T, Wakhloo AK. *Listeria* brainstem encephalitis: two own cases and literature review. *Infection* 1991;19:36–40.
34. Kulay A, Ozatik N, Topcu I. Otogenic intracranial abscesses. *Acta Neurochir (Wiren)* 1990;107:140–146.
35. Lunardi P, Missori P, Fraioli B. Chemical meningitis: unusual presentation of a cerebellar astrocytoma: case report and review of the literature. *Neurosurgery* 1989;25:264–270.

36. Mak SC, Jeng JE, Jong JY, Chiang CH, Chou LC. Clinical observations and virological study of aseptic meningitis in the Kaohsiung area. *Taiwan I Hsueh Hui Twa Chih* 1990;89:868–872.
37. McIntyre PB, Lavercombe PS, Kemp RJ, McCormack JG. Subdural and epidural empyema: diagnostic and therapeutic problems. *Med J Aust* 1991;154:653–657.
38. Nadelman RB, Nowakowski J, Forseter G, et al. The clinical spectrum of early Lyme borreliosis in patients with culture-confirmed erythema migrans. *Am J Med* 1996;100:502–508.
39. Naglo AS, Wide K. *Borrelia* infection in children. *Acta Paediatr Scand* 1989;78:918–922.
40. Navia BA, Petito CK, Gold JWM, Cho E-S, Jordan BD, Price RW. Cerebral toxoplasmosis complicating the acquired immune deficiency syndrome: clinical and neuropathological findings in 27 patients. *Ann Neurol* 1986;19:224–238.
41. Pachner AR, Steere AC. Neurological findigns of Lyme disease. *Yale Biol Med* 1984;57:481–483.
42. Pachner AR, Steere AC. The triad of neurologic manifestations of Lyme disease: meningitis, cranial neuritis, and radiculoneuritis. *Neurology* 1985;35:47–53.
43. Pinheiro FP, LeDuc JW, Travassos da Rosa PA, Leite OF. Isolation of St. Louis encephalitis virus from a patient in Belem, Brazil. *Am J Trop Med Hyg* 1981;30:145–148.
44. Poneprasert B. Japanese encephalitis in children in northern Thailand. *Southeast Asian J Trop Med Public Health* 1989;20:599–603.
45. Richert JR, Potolicchio S, Garagusi VF, et al. Cytomegalovirus encephalitis associated with episodic neurologic deficits and OKT-8-pleocytosis. *Neurology* 1987;37:149–152.
46. Rinaldi R, Manfredi R, Azzimondi G, et al. Recurrent "migrainelike" episodes in patients with HIV disease. *Headache* 1997;37:443–448.
47. Rosen MS, Lorber B, Myers AR. Chronic meningococcal meningitis. An association with C5 deficiency. *Arch Intern Med* 1988;148:1441–1442.
48. Saged JI, Weinstein MP, Miller DC. Chronic encephalitis possibly due to herpes simplex virus: two cases. *Neurology* 1985;35:1470–1472.
49. Schraeder PL, Burns RA. Hemiplegic migraine associated with an aseptic meningeal reaction. *Arch Neurol* 1980;37:377–379.
50. Sellik JA. Epidural abscess and subdural empyema. *J Am Osteopath Assoc* 1989;89:806–810.
51. Sigal LH, Taylor E, Malawista SE. Clinical manifestations of Lyme diseases. *Zentralbl Bakteriol Mikrobiol Hyg* 1986;263:201–205.
52. Simon LT, Hsu D, Adornato BT. Carbamazepine-induced aseptic meningitis. *Ann Intern Med* 1990;112:627–628.
53. Singer JI, Maur PR, Riley JP, Smith PB. Management of central nervous system infections during an epidemic of enteroviral aseptic meningitis. *J Pediatr* 1980;96:559–563.
54. Stamboulis E, Spengos M, Rombos A, Haidemenos A. Aseptic inflammatory meningeal reaction manifesting as a migrainous syndrome. *Headache* 1987;27:439–441.
55. Stamm AM, Dismuke WE, Simmons BP, et al. Listeriosis in renal transplant recipients; report of an outbreak and review of 102 cases. *Rev Infect Dis* 1982;4:665–682.
56. Sylvia LM, Forbenza SW, Brocavich JM. Aseptic meningitis associated with naproxen. *Drug Intell Clin Pharm* 1988;22:399–401.
57. Takeuchi M, Yamane K, Kobayashi I, Maruyama S. A case of recurrent Epstein-Barr virus meningitis. *Rinsho Shinkeigaku* 1989;29:85–88.
58. Tjia Tl, Yeow YK, Tan CB. Cryptococcal meningitis. *J Neurol Neurosurg Psychiatry* 1985;48:853–858.
59. Tonjum T, Nilsson F, Bruun JN, Haneberg B. The early phase of meningococcal disease. *NIPH Ann* 1983;6:175–181.
60. Waterston JA, Gilligan BS. Cryptococcal infections of the central nervous system: a ten year experience. *Clin Exp Neurol* 1987;23:127–137.
61. Watson JDG, Gibson J, Joshua DE, Kronenberg H. Aseptic meningitis associated with high dose intravenous immunoglobulin therapy. *J Neurol Neurosurg Psychiatry* 1991;54:275–276.
62. Weinke T, Rogler G, Sixt C, et al. Cryptococcosis in AIDS patients: observations concerning CNS involvement. *J Neurol* 1989;236:38–42.
63. Yen PT, Chan ST, Huang TS. Brain abscess: with special reference to otolaryngologic sources of infection. *Otolaryngol Head Neck Surg* 1995;113:15–22.
64. Yu YL, Lau YN, Woo E, Wong KL, Tse B. Cryptococcal infection of the nervous system. *QJM* 1988;66:87–96.
65. Zhang SR, Zhang YS, Zhao XD. Tuberculous meningitis with hydrocephalus: a clinical and CT study. *Chung Hua Nei Ko Tsa Chih* 1989;28:202–204.

The Headaches, Second Edition,
edited by J. Olesen, P. Tfelt-Hansen, and K.M.A. Welch.
Lippincott Williams & Wilkins, Philadelphia © 2000.

The Secondary Headaches

CHAPTER 113

Intracranial Neoplasms

Peter A. Forsyth and Jerome B. Posner

DEFINITION OF INTRACRANIAL NEOPLASMS

IHS code and diagnosis: 7.6 Intracranial neoplasm.
WHO code and diagnosis: G44.82 Headache associated
with other intracranial disorders.
Short Description: Headache occurs in approximately
50% of patients with primary or metastatic brain
tumors. The headaches are usually not severe or characteristic. Tension-type headaches are the most common and are seen in 75% of patients, migraine in about
10%, and other types in 15%. The typical headache is
a dull ache, pressure, or sinus pain, located bifrontally
and worse ipsilateral to the tumor. Unlike true tension-
type headaches, brain tumor headache is worsened by
bending over in a third of patients and is associated
with nausea or vomiting in about half of patients. In
15% of patients, brain tumor headache may be similar
to the patient's prior headaches but is more severe,
more frequent, or associated with abnormal neurologic
signs. Factors associated with a brain tumor headache
are (a) increased intracranial pressure (ICP), (b) larger
enhancing tumor and greater midline shift, (c) a history of previous headache.

Headache is a common symptom in otherwise healthy
people. In a few persons, however, headache is the presenting symptom of cancer. The physician's role is to
identify those few patients whose headache is caused by
a brain tumor and to reassure the remainder. The purpose
of this chapter is to describe the characteristics of

P. A. Forsyth: Departments of Neurosciences and Oncology,
University of Calgary and Tom Baker Cancer Centre, and Depart-
ment of Clinical Neurosciences, Foothills Hospital, Calgary,
Alberta T2N 4N2, Canada.
J. B. Posner: Department of Neurology, Cornell University Med-
ical College, and Department of Neurology, Memorial Sloan-
Kettering Cancer Center, New York, New York 10021.

headaches in patients with brain tumors (primary or
metastatic), to identify the factors that cause these
headaches, and to provide a diagnostic and management
approach. Some features of headache in patients with
brain tumor may aid the clinician in differentiating
benign headaches from those requiring further investigation.

FREQUENCY

The frequency of headache in patients with brain
tumors ranges from 36% to 80% (Table 1), depending on
tumor type (Table 2). These estimates may be inaccurate,
because most studies were retrospective, lacked pathologic confirmation, were performed before the era of
modern imaging, and were institution based with marked
selection bias. One prospective study at a large cancer
hospital (23) found headaches to be present in 48% of
patients with brain tumors and were equally common in
primary and metastatic brain tumors. Others report similar estimates (46,54,70). Suwanwela and colleagues (78)
found that 72% of patients with primary and 67% of
patients with metastatic brain tumors had headache. The
incidence of headache in brain tumors may be higher in
children (69%), presumably related to the increased incidence of posterior fossa tumors (38).

Headache is a common complaint in systemic cancer.
One study found that 15.4% of patients with systemic
cancer had headache. Causes of headache in cancer
patients include fever (38%), migraine (13%), tension-
type headache (4%), side effects of therapy (3%),
postlumbar puncture headache (2%), parenchymal and
leptomeningeal metastasis (21%), base of skull metastasis (9%), intracranial bleed (6%), upper cervical metastasis (2%), and primary brain tumor (1%). Thus, nonstruc-
tural causes were responsible for 61% and structural

TABLE 1. *Frequency of headaches in brain tumor patients*

Type	Kunkle et al., 1942 (46)	Northfield 1938 (54)	Rushton and Rooke, 1962 (70)	Honig and Charney, 1982 (38)	CBTC, 1991 (82)	Forsyth and Posner, 1992 (23)
Overall	90	36	60	69	62	48
Supratentorial	—	34	58	—	58	40
Infratentorial	—	48	64	—	70	82

CBTC, The Childhood Brain Tumor Consortium.

causes for 39% of headaches in patients with systemic cancer (13).

The incidence of headache in central nervous system (CNS) metastasis is about 50% (23,56,63,65,75,98), but this figure is probably an overestimate, because many metastases are asymptomatic and discovered only at autopsy (86). Metastases to the leptomeninges (28,65) cause headache in 30% to 75% of patients (1,2,51,55, 84,93). About one third of patients who have rare primary meningeal tumors have headaches (37,48,62,85,97). Headaches are common in patients with skull-base tumors, whether primary or metastatic, presumably because of irritation of the dura. For example, 83% of patients with nasopharyngeal carcinoma have headache (12), and 27% of patients with skull-base chordomas have headache (25); breast, lung, or prostate cancer with base of skull metastases commonly (44%) present with headache (29).

The incidence of headache in primary brain tumors is related to both the *rate of growth* and *location*. Slow growing, low-grade supratentorial tumors are more likely to cause seizures than to cause headaches (14,26,43,45, 61,95), whereas the faster growing malignant gliomas cause headaches in about half of patients (92). Tumors that obstruct cerebrospinal fluid (CSF) pathways, such as infratentorial tumors, are commonly associated with headache (23,78); headaches are present in 90% of patients with medulloblastoma. Brain tumors presenting as isolated headache were most common with posterior fossa tumors causing hydrocephalus (88); even subependymomas, which are usually asymptomatic, may cause headaches if CSF flow is obstructed (52). Meningioma and acoustic neuroma have a lower incidence of headache

TABLE 2. *Frequency of headache in different tumors*

Tumor type	Frequency of headache (%)
Primary brain tumor (adults)	50–72
Primary brain tumor (children)	64
CNS parenchymal metastasis	50–67
Leptomeningeal metastasis	33–76
Skull-base metastasis	44
Primary meningeal tumors	33
Nasopharyngeal carcinoma	83
Skull-base chordoma	27

CNS, central nervous system.

(78). Acoustic neuromas cause headache in about a third of patients (35,91,94), but headache is rare in tumors smaller than 2 cm. The mechanism of headache in these tumors is also likely to be obstructive hydrocephalus from compression of the brainstem and fourth ventricle.

PATHOPHYSIOLOGY

Brain tumors cause headaches by directly or indirectly stimulating intracranial pain-sensitive structures, including (a) cerebral arteries at the base of the brain, (b) dural arteries, (c) great venous sinuses and their tributaries, (d) regions of dura at the base of the brain, and (e) intracranial portions of the trigeminal, glossopharyngeal, vagus, and upper cervical nerves.

Ray and Wolff (68) reported that stimulation of the superior surface of the tentorium refers pain to the ipsilateral forehead and eye, whereas stimulation of pain-sensitive structures in the posterior fossa refers pain to the ipsilateral ear (by way of the recurrent meningeal branch of the vagus nerve) and the lower occipital and upper cervical region (by way of the upper three cervical roots). Wirth and Van Buren (96), however, reported a much less consistent pattern of referral and concluded that the pain of dural origin had poor localizing value.

The mechanism of headache (46) has been proposed to be local traction on pain-sensitive structures by the tumor mass itself or distant traction by mass effect or hydrocephalus. Local traction is likely to be responsible for exclusively unilateral headaches with tumors on the ipsilateral side and with dura-based tumors (77). Distant traction is probably responsible in patients with an elevated ICP whose headaches are bilateral (24).

Increased ICP alone may not be reliably associated with headache. Artificially raising ICP above 800 mm H_2O does not cause headache (73) in headache-free subjects, and many brain-tumor patients normally have an ICP much lower than this level. Plateau waves may account for the headache in these patients. A significant number of patients with increased ICP did not have headache (46,54,70), including 14% of patients in one prospective study (23). On the other hand, patients with pseudotumor cerebri commonly have headache that is relieved by lowering ICP. The cause of headache in pseudotumor is unknown, but it does not appear to be traction on pain-sensitive structures.

CLINICAL FEATURES

IHS diagnostic criteria for headache associated with intracranial neoplasm (Headache Classification Committee, 1988):

1. Symptoms or signs of intracranial neoplasm
2. Confirmation by appropriate investigation
3. Headache as a new symptom or a new type temporally related to intracranial neoplasm

Few studies of the clinical features of headache in patients with brain tumors have been reported. In this section, the clinical features in patients with primary or metastatic brain tumors (usually intraparenchymal metastases) are presented together.

Type of Headache

The most common type of brain tumor headache is a tension-type headache, seen in 77% of patients and usually described as a "dull ache," a "pressure," or being "like a sinus headache." Migrainelike headaches are the second most common type of headache, seen in 9% of patients in one series (23). These headaches were throbbing, developed gradually over several minutes to a half an hour, and were accompanied by nausea but no other signs or symptoms. No tumor type or location consistently identified patients with migrainelike tumor headache, and there was no fixed association with increased ICP.

"Classic" migraine headaches have been reported in patients with brain tumor. Pepin (59) described a patient with a parietal lobe cerebral metastasis who had a 5-month history of progressively more severe migraine with a visual prodrome of "colored stars." Cala and Mastaglia (9) described a patient with glioblastoma multiforme who had a classic history of migraine with teichopsia for 2 years. Verma and colleagues (90) described an occipital lobe tumor that presented as migraine with aura and met the IHS criteria for migraine.

Migrainelike headache may be common in patients with intraventricular tumors (17). Several patients with brain tumors and migrainelike headaches improved with antimigraine medication, suggesting that a response to therapy should not mislead the clinician into assuming that there is no underlying etiology. Clusterlike headaches have been reported as a symptom of brain metastases (80) and of primary CNS lymphoma (16).

Timing and Duration

Brain-tumor headaches are usually intermittent and tend to develop and resolve over several hours (23). One study reported that 78% of these headaches were intermittent (78). Brain-tumor headache is worse in the morning in only 36% of patients; 32% complained that the headache worsened with bending, and for 23% headache was worse with the Valsalva maneuver. The headache roused patients from sleep or interfered with sleep in 32%. Another study found nocturnal headache present in 71% of patients, and 18% had early morning headache severe enough to awake from sleep. Headache also was precipitated by changing body position, particularly rising from bed. Straining and movement worsened headache in 18.0% and 7.4%, respectively (78).

Site of Headache

Unilateral headache is present in 25% to 30% of headache patients. Unilateral headaches accurately predict ipsilateral tumor (23,78). A bifrontal headache was the most common location of headache even without increased ICP (Fig. 1). Bifrontal headaches also may be seen with bilateral or midline tumors. Dura-based tumors produce headache locally over the tumor site. The most common headache location is frontal or frontotemporal, particularly in patients with a supratentorial tumor or increased ICP. Occipital and diffuse headaches also commonly occur. Neck pain accompanies the headache in patients with infratentorial tumors or increased ICP (Fig. 2).

Severity

The headaches can be of mild, moderate, or severe intensity (median of 7 on a scale of 1–10) (23). Headaches are the worst symptom in only 45% of patients. About half of the patients with brain tumors have experienced headache relief with simple analgesics. A severe headache in a cancer patient is likely due to obstructive or communicating hydrocephalus producing increased ICP. This headache often causes nausea and vomiting and is resistant to common analgesics. Of patients with increased ICP (due to communicating or obstructive hydrocephalus), 86% had evidence of headache (23). The increased ICP headache is usually severe and described as "the worst pain I have had" or like "my head is blowing off." The headache is usually constant (61%), not relieved by common analgesics (72%), worse in the morning (37%), and worse with the Valsalva maneuver (33%). Headaches are usually frontal (44%), in the neck and bifrontal region or neck and top of the head (33%), and on the top of the head in 6% of patients. Headaches associated with supratentorial tumors and no increased ICP were less severe and more likely to be mistaken for benign headaches. The "classic" brain tumor headache, which occurs only in the morning and is progressive, was found in 17% to 18% of patients. The headache caused by cerebral metastasis is more commonly a subacute progressive headache (23,63).

Associated Signs and Symptoms

Headache as the sole manifestation of brain tumor is uncommon in patients with a normal neurologic exami-

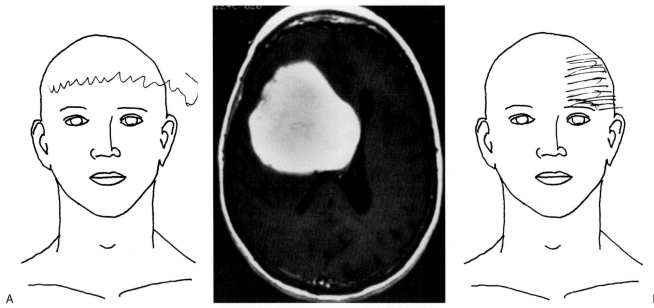

A

B, C

FIG. 1. A bifrontal headache was the most common location of headache in patients with supratentorial tumors without increased intracranial pressure even if the tumor was unilateral. This 65-year-old woman (**A**) with no prior diagnosis of cancer had 2 1/2 months of a dull, aching headache, the same character as her headaches of 20 years' duration but more frequent and slightly more severe. It was easily relieved with simple analgesics but became constant. She underwent imaging after an episode of confusion and disorientation at work. MRI scan with contrast (**B**) shows a large, enhancing, unilateral supratentorial tumor that was resected and found to be an adenocarcinoma. The second most common location of headache with supratentorial tumors without increased intracranial pressure was frontal but unilateral and ipsilateral to the brain tumor, as in this 41-year-old man (**C**) with 2 months of a progressive aching, throbbing headache and light-headedness. The headache was intermittent, moderately severe, relieved by common analgesics, and worse in the afternoon. A large, enhancing glioblastoma multiforme ipsilateral to the headache was resected (not shown).

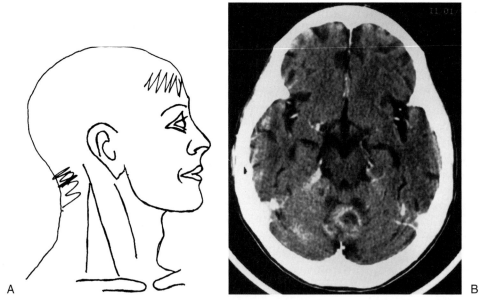

A

B

FIG. 2. Often patients with increase intracranial pressure resulting from a posterior fossa mass have at least some component of their headache in the neck, as shown in this 31-year-old woman with a history of acquired immunodeficiency syndrome (*AIDS*) and prior lymphoma affecting her cauda equina. She had 6 days of progressive, constant headache, which she described as a pressure. She described it as the worst pain of her life, unrelieved by common analgesics, worse with bending over, coughing, and at night. It was located bifrontally and in her neck (**A**). Her examination showed papilledema, somnolence, and gait ataxia. The head computed tomography (*CT*) scan shows an enhancing lesion in the posterior fossa that obstructs the fourth ventricle (at lower cuts) and dilated temporal horns (**B**) consistent with obstructive hydrocephalus. Given the patient's history of lymphoma and the radiographic appearance, this posterior fossa lesion was believed to be a lymphoma.

nation and no history of systemic cancer. One study (77) found a brain tumor in only two of 207 (1%) such patients. Evans (20) reviewed the literature on imaging including 1,282 patients with chronic headaches and a normal neurologic examination; only one had a brain tumor. Elderly patients with a new headache are more likely to harbor a brain tumor (57). Burton and colleagues (7) reviewed the records of 696 children who visited an emergency department for headache; one meningeal tumor but no cases of brain tumor were found. Papilledema was present in 40% of brain-tumor headache patients in one study (78). Nausea and vomiting are the most common associated symptoms and are present in half of the patients with brain tumors. Transient visual obscurations are commonly (68%) reported in pseudotumor cerebri (32), but their incidence in brain-tumor headache is not known. Headache from brain tumor without other symptoms is uncommon, reported in only 8% of patients in one study (88). Few brain-tumor headaches last more than 10 weeks without other symptoms developing. Patients with brain tumors and headache have a longer duration of symptoms preceding diagnosis (median time, 3.5 weeks), because patients presenting with seizures or rapidly progressive hemiparesis tend to be imaged more quickly than patients with headaches alone (23).

Factors Associated with an Increased Incidence of Brain Tumor Headache

We identified (23) four factors associated with an increased incidence of headache in patients with primary or metastatic brain tumors. (a) *Increased intracranial pressure* (ICP): 18 of 21 (86%) of patients with ICP had headache. (b) *Location of the brain tumor*: 82% of infratentorial tumors and 75% of leptomeningeal tumors caused headache due to obstruction of the CSF pathways. (c) *Size of the enhancing lesion, degree of midline shift,* and *amount of edema* (Fig. 3): Larger tumors with more midline shift and edema tended to cause headaches. The mean size of brain tumors without headache was 9.3 cm^2 compared with 18.3 cm^2 in patients with headache. The midline shift was 2.7 mm in patients without headache but 6.1 mm in patients with headache. The amount of edema without headache was 26.1 cm^2 but with headache was 33.9 cm^2. (d) *History of headache:* Patients with a previous history of headache were more susceptible to headache associated with brain tumor; 78% of patients with prior headaches had headaches with their brain tumor. Several patients had headaches with the same characteristics as the patient's prior headaches. In every case, however, the headache was more severe, frequent, or associated with other symptoms (e.g., seizures, confusion, prolonged nausea, abnormal signs). Other researchers have reported that a change in severity or frequency of headache or abnormal signs may signal the presence of brain tumor in patients with chronic headache, even if the quality of the headache was unchanged (9,42,70).

Headache Caused by Tumor Involving Other Structures

In patients with systemic cancer, metastases to other intracranial structures (see Table 2), such as the skull, dura, and venous structures, occur and may cause headache, but these are not well studied. Headaches as referred pain, caused by tumors affecting extracranial structures, are also discussed in the following section.

Base of Skull Metastases

Greenberg and colleagues (29) characterized five distinctive syndromes attributable to base of skull metastases that commonly cause headache; their recognition helps to localize the metastasis and direct further therapy: (a) *The orbital syndrome* is caused by metastases to the orbit (usually from breast, lung, prostate, lymphoma, or neuroblastoma) and consists of a dull supraorbital ache followed by diplopia, proptosis, V1 sensory loss, and decreased visual acuity. (b) *The parasellar syndrome* is caused by metastases to the sella that erode into the cavernous sinus (usually from carcinoma of breast, lung, or prostate) and produces unilateral frontal headache, ocular paresis, and V1 sensory loss. Striking periorbital edema may occur related to compression of veins draining into the cavernous sinus. (c) *The gasserian ganglion syndrome* consists of trigeminal nerve distribution pain and numbness (usually seen with breast, lung, or head and neck cancer invading the gasserian ganglion). The pain is a dull ache in the cheek, jaw, or forehead. Trigeminal neuralgia-like pain can occur. Sensory changes usually begin close to the midline in the chin or lip and spread laterally. Motor involvement is usually late. (d) The *jugular foramen syndrome* from metastases to the jugular foramen (usually from breast, lung, prostate, or head and neck cancer) causes a dull, unilateral, aching pain behind one ear, hoarseness, and dysphagia. Weakness of the vocal cords, palate, and spinal accessory muscles may develop. Papilledema from jugular vein compression may occur. (e) *The occipital condyle syndrome* is caused by metastasis to the occipital condyle (usually from breast, lung, or prostate cancer) and consists of severe unilateral occipital headache, often worse with neck flexion. About half of the patients complain of dysarthria and dysphagia. Ipsilateral tongue atrophy is common (29,64).

Leptomeningeal Metastases

These produce headaches in about one third to one half of patients (2,93) and are usually nonspecific in location

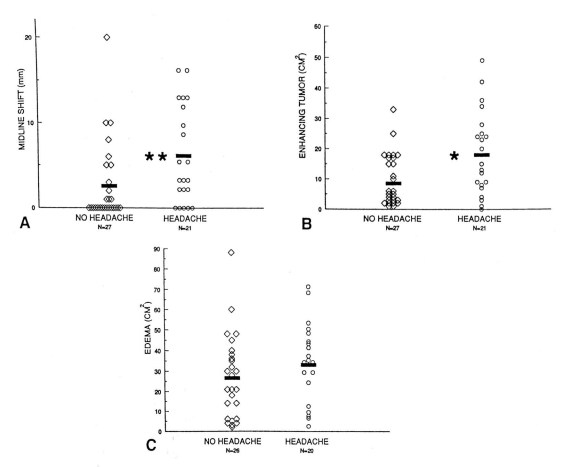

FIG. 3. The association of headache with the amount of midline shift (**A**), enhancing tumor size (**B**), and edema (**C**). Patients with headache had significantly more midline shift (**$p < 0.05$) and larger tumors (*$p < 0.02$) than patients without headache. Patients with headache also tended to have more edema than patients without headache. *Thick horizontal bar,* is average value. From Forsyth and Posner (23).

and timing. Headaches may be progressive and accompanied by nausea, vomiting, and changes in mental status that reflect an elevated ICP or meningeal irritation. Cranial nerve involvement and spinal dysfunction are common.

Head and Neck Tumors

Pain is experienced by 40% to 80% of patients with head and neck cancers (31). Tumors in this location are in close proximity to many pain-sensitive structures (e.g., mucosa, bone, nerves). Head pain associated with head and neck tumors can be quite severe. Nociceptive pain caused by A-delta and C-fiber stimulation is the most common type of pain. Often this pain is the result of tumor, tumor recurrence, or inflammation. Neuropathic pain is also common, usually as a result of nerve damage from neck dissection (89) or other therapies. Furthermore, the advanced cancers often have more than one cause of pain (11).

Venous Sinus Thrombosis

In this rare but serious cause of headache in the cancer patient, patients develop sagittal sinus thrombosis either from external compression (from an adjacent metastases) or a hypercoagulable state (e.g., induced by L-asparaginase) (8,21,66,67). Headache is almost universal, may be mild, and may not be accompanied by other symptoms or signs (64). Papilledema is common (74).

Uncommon Headache Syndromes in Patients with Brain Tumors

Uncommon headache syndromes have been described in patients with a variety of brain tumors.

Paroxysmal headache is a distinctive headache associated with colloid cysts of the third ventricle or other pedunculated tumors that can block the flow of CSF (27,36,44). These headaches have sudden onset, peak in intensity within seconds, are of brief duration (minutes to a few hours), and terminate quickly. The headaches are precipitated by changes in posture and may be associated with loss of consciousness, sudden weakness in the legs ("drop attacks"), vertigo, and sudden death. Patients often have gait imbalance between episodes. These paroxysmal headaches originally were thought to result from intermittent obstruction of the foramen of Munro by a "ball valve" action of the tumor. A more recent explanation is that the symptoms are those of plateau waves caused by sudden increases in ICP superimposed on chronic increased ICP (6). The plateau waves probably develop because of the sudden dilatation of intracranial small vessels, resulting in increased cerebral blood flow and volume (53).

Benign cough or benign exertional headache consists of transient, severe headache precipitated by coughing, sneezing, straining at stool, laughing, stooping, lifting, or running. The duration of headache is brief and without a characteristic location. Symonds (79) found intracranial masses in 11% of patients with "cough headaches," and Rooke (69) found brain tumors in 2% of 303 patients with "exertional headaches."

De Angelis and Payne (16) described a patient with atypical *cluster headache* as a presentation of leptomeningeal lymphoma. The atypical features were that the patient was a woman, she had no nocturnal attacks, the pain was moderate to severe but not excruciating, the first attack was at age 50, and the only autonomic symptom was lacrimation. Headaches fulfilling the diagnostic criteria for episodic or chronic cluster headache also have been reported in acoustic neuroma (30,83), sphenoid ridge (49), cavernous sinus (33), and foramen magnum meningiomas (47) and metastases (80). Taub and colleagues (81) described a patient with chronic cluster headache for 20 years. After a trochlear nerve palsy developed, neuroimaging was performed and showed a meningioma of tentorium cerebelli. Surgical removal of the meningioma led to resolution of the headaches.

An unusual *atypical facial pain* was reported in 26 patients with *nonmetastatic lung cancer* (2–5,10,19,41). An often debilitating unilateral facial pain was located mainly around the ear but also involving the temple, jaw, cheek or eye has been described. The character of the pain is a constant aching, unlike the sharp, jabbing pain of trigeminal or glossopharyngeal neuralgia of metastatic infiltration of these nerves that is occasionally reported. In all cases, the facial pain was ipsilateral to the lung cancer. No evidence of metastasis to the brain, leptomeninges, or skull base was found. Many patients also had weight loss and digital clubbing. The most plausible explanation is local invasion or compression of the vagus nerve within the thorax; the vagus nerve contains somatic and visceral afferents necessary for referred pain. A right-sided predominance is likely a result of the close anatomic relationship of the right vagus nerve to the trachea and mediastinal lymph nodes. Radiation or local tumor resection improved facial pain in most cases,

sometimes dramatically. A chest radiograph in all patients who smoke and report unexplained facial pain is recommended.

APPROACH TO HEADACHE IN A CANCER PATIENT

Intracranial metastases are common and occur in about 25% of cancer patients (60,65). Therefore, brain imaging with magnetic resonance imaging (MRI) or computed tomography (CT) with contrast usually is warranted in a cancer patient who is experiencing a new or different headache. MRI or CT also may help to identify other frequent causes of headache, such as hemorrhage, arterial infarction, or venous thrombosis. A history and physical examination are indispensable in determining which other laboratory investigations are needed to differentiate between the many possible causes (some quite rare) of headache in cancer patients (Table 3).

A headache history determines which patients require imaging, how quickly it needs to be done, and which structures should be visualized. There is no single feature that is uniquely characteristic of a headache caused by a brain tumor. In general, however, cancer patients who experience any of the worrisome features listed in Table 4 should undergo imaging. Careful questioning may be required, and interviewing the family may be particularly useful. In some cases, a history alone may render the diagnosis, as is the case when there is a close temporal relationship between the use of an agent such as ondansetron or retinoic acid, both of which commonly cause headache, with the onset of the headache. A physical examination is similarly important in determining the cause of the headache (see Table 3).

A MRI scan is the best diagnostic test for brain metastasis. If a carefully done MRI with contrast is negative, it effectively rules out brain metastasis. MRI with gadolinium is preferable to a CT scan because it is more sensitive; it can reveal smaller lesions not detected by CT, particularly in the brainstem or cerebellum; show enhancement from leptomeningeal disease; or show involvement of cranial nerves or blood vessels or thrombosis of the venous sinuses. It also may help with therapy if resection of a single brain metastasis is planned or if focal radiotherapy is contemplated.

Other laboratory tests should be used as clinically indicated by the history and physical examination. A CT scan with bone windows and fine cuts through the region of interest or a bone scan may be superior to MRI in a patient with metastasis to the calvarium or base of the skull. Epidural or subdural metastases are best imaged by MRI scans. Evidence of leptomeningeal metastasis may be seen with meningeal enhancement or communicating hydrocephalus; a spinal fluid examination is critical to establishing the diagnosis, but the lumbar puncture should follow, not precede, the scan because the lumbar puncture may cause meningeal enhancement (58). All

TABLE 3. *Causes of a new headache in cancer patients*

Intracranial metastases
    Skull-calvarium, base of skull
    Meninges-epidural, subdural, leptomeningeal
    Brain (parenchymal)
    Cranial nerves or vessels (invasion or compression)
Nonmetastatic causes
    Vascular hemorrhage (intratumoral, subdural, SAH) infarction, venous thrombosis
    Infectious (abscess, meningitis, vasculitis, etc.)
Side effects of therapy
    Chemotherapy
        Hormones (e.g. tamoxifen)
        Differentiation agents (retinoic acid)
        Antibiotics (e.g. trimethoprim-sulfamethoxazole)
        Reverse transcriptase inhibitors (e.g. AZT, DDI)
        Conventional agents (e.g. L-asparaginase, procarbazine, PCNU, fludarabine, fazarabine, caracemide, gallium nitrate)
        Cytokines (e.g., tumor necrosis factor, OKT_3, interferons, interleukins, levamisole, GM-CSF)
        Intrathecal therapy (e.g., methotrexate, Ara-C)
    Supportive therapies:
        Corticosteroids, cimetidine, ondansatron, narcotics (withdrawal), metoclopramide, anticoagulants (intratumoral hemorrhage), dipyridamole, ibuprofen (aseptic meningitis)
    Radiotherapy
        Acute edema (early), delayed radionecrosis (late) radiation-induced neoplasm (late), radiation-induced atherosclerosis causing stroke
    Surgery
        Hemorrhage, vascular injury, perioperative stroke, cerebrospinal fluid leak
Other causes:
    Fever
    Metabolic
        Hypoxemia, hypercarbia and hypoglycemia.
    Referred pain from extracranial structures (cervical metastasis, lung tumors)
    Postlumbar puncture

SAH, subarachnoid hemorrhage; Ara-C, cytosine arapinoside; AZT, azidothymadine; DDI, didanosine; GM-CSF, granulocyte-macrophage colony-stimulating factor; PCNU, 1-(2-chlorethyl)-3-(2,6-dioxo-3-piperidyl)-1-nitrosourea.

patients with suspected meningeal disease should be considered for a lumbar puncture done with an opening pressure, cell count, protein and glucose concentrations, and a cytologic examination. Other special spinal fluid studies may include biochemical and cellular markers, flow cytometry, or cell-surface markers.

Headache also may be a side effect of cancer treatment, such as the acute edema seen early in the course of radiotherapy, or from surgical complications such as hemorrhage, vascular injury, or CSF leaks. Certain chemotherapy or supportive therapies also commonly cause headaches (e.g., retinoic acid or ondansetron); headache occurs in up to 14% of patients (22). Cytokines and biologic modifiers also commonly cause headache (see Table 3).

Management of Headache in Cancer

The management of headache in cancer is straightforward. Prior to the histologic diagnosis, if the headache is not severe, analgesics such as acetaminophen should be tried first. To prevent liver damage, the dose of acetaminophen should not exceed 4 to 6 g per day. Aspirin or other nonsteroidal antiinflammatory drugs (NSAIDs)

should be avoided if surgical intervention is likely because of the increased risk of bleeding. If an NSAID is used, the patient must be monitored closely for gastropathy, renal failure, and hepatic dysfunction (50). Misoprostol at a dose of 200 µg twice a day is effective in preventing NSAID-induced gastric ulceration (87). NSAIDs are particularly effective in pain associated with bone metastasis, soft-tissue infiltration, and recent surgery (50).

If pain persists despite nonopioid treatment, an opioid drug should be added. Codeine is the best option because it is prepared in fixed combinations with nonopioid analgesics. An increased incidence of side effects occurs at doses above 1.5 mg per kilogram of body weight (50).

TABLE 4. *Headache features in a cancer patient that suggest a structural cause*

Any change in prior headache pattern
Headaches unresponsive to previous therapy
Any focal motor, sensory, or visual symptoms or signs
Change in memory, personality, or mentation
Vomiting
Worse with bending over, cough, sneeze, or valsalva maneuver

Patients who have a deficiency of CYP2D6 enzyme or patients taking inhibitors of CYP2D6, such as quinidine, cimetidine, or fluoxetine, may not be able to convert codeine to morphine and therefore have no analgesic effect (18,76).

Strong opioids such as morphine, hydromorphone, or fentanyl may be useful adjuvants in the treatment of severe headache that does not respond to nonopioid and codeine therapy. Opioids theoretically may induce increased ICP by precipitating hypercapnea and subsequent vasodilation (40). This is an acceptable risk, however, considering the morbidity associated with undertreatment of severe headache. Morphine is the most commonly used opioid. The controlled-release formulations allow oral administration once every 12 hours. Hydromorphone also may be used, which has increased solubility and potency, allowing smaller injections or infusion volumes when parental opioids are required. Fentanyl transdermal patches can control pain for up to 72 hours and are particularly useful in patients who cannot take pain medications orally. Meperidine should not be prescribed because of the short half-life and toxic metabolite produced. Mixed-opioid agonists–antagonists, such as pentazocine and butorphanol, also should not be prescribed because of the potential for reverse analgesia and lack of efficacy (50). Methadone offers some advantages over other opioids in that it is well absorbed enterally but has a long half-life.

If a significant amount of edema is seen on imaging studies and is thought to be causing the headache or other symptoms and signs, dexamethasone 4 mg two to four times daily is usually effective. Higher doses of dexamethasone (40–100 mg daily in two doses) also can be administered safely if necessary. Corticosteroids are useful for pain associated with acute nerve compression, soft-tissue infiltration, and leptomeningeal metastasis (39,50). If CNS lymphoma is a consideration, dexamethasone should be avoided prior to biopsy. Lymphoma is exquisitely sensitive to corticosteroids, and a biopsy could yield normal, necrotic, or nondiagnostic tissue and delay definitive diagnosis and treatment (15).

Tricyclic antidepressant drugs should be considered in neuropathic pain. Desipramine and nortriptyline cause fewer side effects and facilitate upward titration. Anticonvulsants such as carbamazepine and clonazepam are also useful in neuropathic pain (50), particularly if a stabbing or lancinating quality is present (31).

Management of head and neck tumors can be especially difficult. Patients often have difficulty with swallowing or psychosocial problems (excessive alcohol, smoking, or substance abuse). Dysphagia and psychosocial problems are common in this population. Anti-tumor directed therapy may be beneficial. Neurolytic or neurosurgical procedures for headache management are not preferred as severe side effects are common and pain relief is of limited duration. Pharmacotherapy is again the mainstay of treatment. Usually several attempts at treatment are required before relief is achieved. Diagnosing the cause of pain (nociceptive or neuropathic) will lead to appropriate and effective treatment (31). Enteral or transdermal routes of administration are preferred even if nasogastric or gastrostomy is required as this route allows for prolonged analgesia, avoids toxicity, and causes less restriction in patients activities. Multiple drug regimens are often required. A four drug regimen of: 1. methadone, 2. acetaminophen or NSAID, 3. tricyclic antidepressant, and 4. hydroxyzine was very effective in one study (11).

Brain tumor headaches from primary brain tumors usually resolve with surgical or radiotherapeutic treatment. In our experience these are usually not difficult to control once definitive treatment of the tumor has begun. Resolution of headache is especially dramatic in patients who undergo surgical procedures that decrease raised ICP. Patients with acoustic neuromas seem to be especially at risk of having postoperative headaches. One study found that 82% of patients had continuous headaches postoperatively and another 40% of patients who were without headaches preoperatively developed headaches postoperatively (91). Headache may be more frequent and severe after retrosigmoid surgery than after translabyrinthine surgery (71,72). Cranioplasty with methylmethacrylate performed at the end of retrosigmoid surgery resulted in a reduction in postoperative headache (34). Radiotherapy may induce headache initially, presumably by increased edema, but this reduction is usually transient and well controlled with corticosteroids. Maintenance of appropriate levels of steroid for the first 2 weeks of radiotherapy is advised (39).

REFERENCES

1. Amer MH, Al-Sarraf M, Baker LH, Vaitkevicius VK. Malignant melanoma and central nervous system metastases. *Cancer* 1978;42:660–668.
2. Balm M, Hammack J. Leptomeningeal—presenting features and prognostic factors. *Arch Neurol* 1996;53:626–632.
3. Bindoff LA, Heseltine D. Unilateral facial pain in patients with lung cancer: a referred pain via the vagus? *Lancet* 1988;1:812–815.
4. Bongers KM, Willigers HMM, Koehler PJ. Referred facial pain from lung carcinoma. *Neurology* 1992;42:1841–1842.
5. Broux R, Moonen G, Schoenen J. Unilateral facial pain as the first symptom of lung cancer: report of three cases. *Cephalalgia* 1991;11(Suppl 11):319–320.
6. Brun A, Egund N. The pathogenesis of cerebral symptoms in colloid cysts of the third ventricle: a clinical and pathoanatomic study. *Acta Neurol Scand* 1973;49:525–535.
7. Burton LJ, Quinn B, Pratt-Cheney JL, Pourani M. Headache etiology in a pediatric emergency department. *Pediatr Emerg Care* 1997;13:1–4.
8. Cairo MS, Lazarus K, Gilmore RL, Baehner RL. Intracranial hemorrhage and focal seizures secondary to use of L-asparaginase during induction therapy of acute lymphocytic leukemia. *J Pediatr* 1980;97:829–833.
9. Cala LA, Mastaglia FL. Computerized axial tomography findings in a group of patients with migrainous headaches. *Proceedings of the Australian Association of Neurology* 1976;13:35–41.
10. Capobianco DJ. Facial pain as a symptom of nonmetastatic lung cancer. *Headache* 1995;33:581–585.

11. Carrol EN, Fine E, Ruff RL, Stepnick D. A four-drug pain regimen for head and neck cancers. *Laryngoscope* 1994;104:694–700.

12. Chen MS, Lin FJ, Tang SG, Leung WM, Leung W. Clinical significance of cranial nerve deficit in the therapy of nasopharyngeal carcinoma. *Br J Radiol* 1989;62:739–743.

13. Clouston PD, DeAngelis LM, Posner JB. The spectrum of neurological disease in patients with systemic cancer. *Ann Neurol* 1992;31:268–273.

14. Daumas-Duport C, Scheithauer BW, Chodkiewicz JP, Laws Jr ER, Vedrenne C. Dysembryoplastic neuroepithelial tumor: a surgically curable tumor of young patients with intractable partial seizures: report of thirty-nine cases. *Neurosurgery* 1988;23:545–556.

15. De Angelis LM. Primary central nervous system lymphoma: a new clinical challenge. *Neurology* 1991;41:619–621.

16. De Angelis LM, Payne R. Lymphomatous meningitis presenting as atypical cluster headache. *Pain* 1987;30:211–216.

17. Debryne J, Crevits L, Vander Eecken H. Migraine-like headache in intraventricular tumors. *Clin Neurol Neurosurg* 1982;84:51–57.

18. Desmeules J, Gascon MP, Dayer P, Magistris M. Impact of environmental and genetic factors on codeine analgesia. *Eur J Clin Pharmacol* 1991;41:23–26.

19. Des Prez, RD, Freemon FR. Facial pain associated with lung cancer: a case report. *Headache* 1983;23:43–44.

20. Evans RW. Diagnostic testing for the evaluation of headaches. *Neurol Clin* 1996;14:1–26.

21. Feinberg WM, Swenson MR. Cerebrovascular complications of L-asparaginase therapy. *Neurology* 1988;38:127–133

22. Finn AL. Toxicity and side effects of ondansetron. *Semin Oncol* 1992; 19(4 suppl 10):53–60.

23. Forsyth PA, Posner JB. Headaches in patients with brain tumors: a study of 111 patients. *Neurology* 1993;43:1678–1683.

24. Forsyth PA, Posner JB. Intracranial neoplasms. In: Olesen J, Tfelt-Hansen P, Welch KMA, eds. *The headaches.* New York: Raven Press, 1993:705–714.

25. Forsyth PA, Cascino TL, Shaw EG, et al. Intracranial chordomas: a clinicopathologic and prognostic study of 51 cases. *J Neurosurg* 1993; 78:741–747.

26. Forsyth PA, Shaw EG, Scheithauer BW, O'Fallon JR, Layton Jr DD, Katzmann JA. Supratentorial pilocytic astrocytoma: a clinicopathologic, prognostic, and flow-cytometric study of 51 patients. *Cancer* 1993;72:1335–1342.

27. Gassel MM, Davies H. Meningiomas in the lateral ventricles. *Brain* 1961;84:605–627.

28. Gonzales JC, Garcia-Bunuel R. Meningeal carcinomatosis. *Cancer* 1976;37:2906–2911.

29. Greenberg HS, Deck MD, Vikram B, Chu FC, Posner JB. Metastasis to the base of the skull: clinical findings in 43 patients. *Neurology* 1981; 31:530–537.

30. Greve E, Mai J. Cluster headache-like headaches: a symptomatic feature? A report of three patients with intracranial pathologic findings. *Cephalalgia* 1988;8:79–82.

31. Grond S, Zech D, Lynch J, Diefenbach C, Schug SA, Lehmann KA. Validation of World Health Organization guidelines for pain relief in head and neck cancer. *Ann Otol Rhinol Laryngol* 1993;102:342–348.

32. Guiseffi V, Wall M, Siegel PZ, Rojas PB. Symptoms and disease associations in idiopathic intracranial hypertension (pseudotumor cerebri): a case–control study. *Neurology* 1991;41(Suppl 2):239–244.

33. Hannerz J. A case of parasellar meningioma mimicking cluster headache. *Cephalalgia* 1989;9:265–269.

34. Harner SG, Beatty CW, Ebersold MJ. Impact of cranioplasty on headache after acoustic neuroma removal. *Neurosurgery* 1995;36: 1097–1100.

35. Harner SG, Laws ER. Clinical findings in patients with acoustic neuromas. *Mayo Clinic Proc* 1983;58:721–728.

36. Harris W. Paroxysmal and postural headaches from intraventricular cysts and tumors. *Lancet* 1944;2:654–655.

37. Ho KL, Hoschner JA, Wolfe DE. Primary leptomeningeal gliomatosis: symptoms suggestive of meningitis. *Arch Neurol* 1981;38:662–666.

38. Honig PJ, Charney EB. Children with brain tumor headaches. *Am J Dis Child* 1982;136:121–124.

39. Jaeckle KA. Causes and management of headaches in cancer patients. *Oncology* 1993;7:27–32.

40. Jaffe JM, Martin WR. Opioid analgesics and antagonists. In: Gilman A, Goodman LS, Rall TW, Murad F, eds. *Goodman and Gilman's pharmacologic basis of therapeutics.* New York: MacMillan 1985;497–502.

41. Jones MT, Lawson RAM. Unilateral facial pain as a rare presentation of bronchial carcinoma. *Br J Clin Pract* 1987;41:1025–1026.

42. Joseph R, Cook GE, Steiner TJ, Rose FC. Intracranial space occupying lesions in patients attending a migraine clinic. *Practitioner* 1985;229: 477–481.

43. Kaylan-Raman UP, Olivero WC. Ganglioglioma: a correlative clinicopathological and radiological study of ten surgically treated cases with follow-up. *Neurosurgery* 1987;20:428–433.

44. Kelley R. Colloid cysts of the third ventricle. *Brain* 1951;74:23–65.

45. Kepes JJ, Rubinstein LJ, Eng LF. Pleomorphic xanthoastrocytoma: a distinctive meningocerebral glioma of young subjects with relatively favorable prognosis: a study of 12 cases. *Cancer* 1979;44:1839–1852.

46. Kunkle EC, Bronson SR, Wolff HG. Studies on headache: the mechanisms and significance of the headache associated with brain tumor. *Bull NY Acad Med* 1942;18:400–422.

47. Kuritzky A. Cluster headache-like pain caused by an upper cervical meningioma. *Cephalalgia* 1984;4:185–186.

48. Lachance DH, O'Neill BP, MacDonald DR, et al. Primary leptomeningeal lymphoma: report of 9 cases, diagnosis with immunocytochemical analysis and review of the literature. *Neurology* 1991;41: 95–100.

49. Lefevre JP, Simmat G, Bataille B, et al. Algies vasculaires de la face dues a un meningiome: deux observations [Letter]. *Presse Med* 1984; 13:2323.

50. Levy MH. Pharmacologic treatment of cancer pain. *N Engl J Med* 1996;335:1124–1132.

51. Little JR, Dale AJ, Okasaki H. Meningeal carcinomatosis: clinical manifestations. *Arch Neurol* 1974;30:138–143.

52. Lobato RD, Sarabia M, Castro S, et al. Symptomatic subependymomas: report of four new cases studied with computed tomography and review of the literature. *Neurosurgery* 1986;19:594–598.

53. Newell DW, Aaslid R, Stooss R, Reulen HJ. The relationship of blood flow velocity fluctuations to intracranial pressure B waves. *J Neurosurg* 1992;76:415–421.

54. Northfield DWC. Some observations on headache. *Brain* 1938;61: 133–162.

55. Olson ME. Infiltration of leptomeninges by systemic cancer. *Arch Neurol* 1974;30:122–137.

56. Paillas JE, Pellet W. Brain metastases. In: Vinken PJ, Bruyn GW, eds. *Handbook of clinical neurology.* Amsterdam: North-Holland, 1975; 201–232.

57. Pascual J, Berciano J. Experience in the diagnosis of headaches that start in elderly people. *J Neurol Neurosurg Psychiatry* 1994;57: 1255–1257.

58. Panullo SC, Reich JB, Krol G, et al. MRI changes in intracranial hypotension. *Neurology* 1993;43:919–926.

59. Pepin EP. Cerebral metastasis presenting as migraine with aura. *Lancet* 1990;336:127–128.

60. Pickren, JW, Lopez G, Tsukada Y. Brain metastases: an autopsy study. *Cancer Treatment Symposia* 1983;2:295–313.

61. Piepmeier JM. Observations on the current treatment of low grade astrocytic tumors of the cerebral hemispheres. *J Neurosurg* 1987;67: 177–181.

62. Polmeteer FF, Kernohan JW. Meningeal gliomatosis: a study of 42 cases. *Arch Neurol Psychiatry* 1947;57:593–616.

63. Posner JB. Management of central nervous system metastases. *Semin Oncol* 1977;4:81–91.

64. Posner JB. Cancer involving cranial and peripheral nerves. In: *Neurologic complications of cancer.* Philadelphia: FA Davis, 1995:174–184.

65. Posner JB, Chernik NL. Intracranial metastases from systemic cancer. *Adv Neurol* 1978;19:575–592.

66. Priest JR, Ramsay NKC, Latchaw RE, et al. Thrombotic and hemorrhagic strokes complicating early therapy for childhood acute lymphoblastic leukemia. *Cancer* 1980;46:1548–1554.

67. Priest JR, Ramsay NKC, Steinherz PG, et al. A syndrome of thrombosis and hemorrhage complicating L-asparaginase therapy for childhood acute lymphoblastic leukemia. *J Pediatr* 1982;100:984–989.

68. Ray BS, Wolff HG. Experimental studies on headache: pain sensitive structures of the head and their significance in headache. *Arch Surg* 1940;41:813–856.

69. Rooke ED. Benign exertional headache. *Med Clin North Am* 1968;52: 801–808.

70. Rushton JG, Rooke ED. Brain tumor headache. *Headache* 1962;2: 147–152.

71. Schessel DA, Nedzelski JM, Rowed DW, Feghali JG. Headache and local discomfort following surgery of the cerebellopontine angle. In: Tos M, Thomsen J, eds. *Proceedings of the First International Conference on Acoustic Neuroma.* New York: Kugler Publications, 1992: 899–904.

72. Schessel DA, Nedzelski JM, Rowed DW, Feghali JG. Pain after surgery for acoustic neuroma. *Otolaryngol Head Neck Surg* 1992;107:424–429.

73. Schumacher GA, Wolff HG. Experimental studies on headache. *Arch Neurol Psychiatry* 1941;45:199–214.

74. Sigsbee B, Deck MD, Posner JB. Nonnmetastatic superior sagittal sinus thrombosis complicating systemic cancer. *Neurology* 1979;29:139–146.

75. Simionescu MD. Metastatic tumors of the brain: a follow-up study of 195 patients with neurosurgical consideration. *J Neurosurg* 1960;17: 363–373.

76. Sindrup SH, Arendt-Nielsen L, Brosen K, et al. The effect of quinidine on the analgesic effect of codeine. *Eur J Clin Pharmacol* 1992;42: 587–591.

77. Sotaniemi KA, Rantala M, Pyhtinen J, Myllyla VV. Clinical and CT correlates in the diagnosis of intracranial tumors. *J Neurol Neurosurg Psychiatry* 1991;54:645–647.

78. Suwanwela N, Phanthumchinda K, Kaoropthum S. Headache in brain tumor: a cross-sectional study. *Headache* 1994;34:435–438.

79. Symonds C. Cough headache. *Brain* 1956;79:557–568.

80. Tajti J, Sas K, Szok D, Voros E, Vecsei L. Clusterlike headache as a first sign of brain metastases of lung cancer. *Headache* 1996;36:259–260.

81. Taub E, Argoff CE, Winterkorn JMS, Milhorat TH. Resolution of chronic cluster headache after resection of a tentorial meningioma: case report. *Neurosurgery* 1995;37:319–322.

82. The Childhood Brain Tumor Consortium. The epidemiology of headache among children with brain tumor. *J Neuro–Oncol* 1991,1:31–46.

83. Tfelt-Hansen P, Paulson OB, Krabbe AA. Invasive adenoma of the pituitary gland and chronic migrainous neuralgia: a rare coincidence or a causal relationship? *Cephalalgia* 1982;2:25–28.

84. Theodore WH, Gendelman S. Meningeal carcinomatosis. *Arch Neurol* 1981;38:696–699.

85. Thibodeau LL, Ariza A, Piepmeier JM. Primary leptomeningeal sarcomatosis. *J Neurosurg* 1988;68:802–805.

86. Tsukada Y, Fouad A, Pickren JW, Lane WW. Central nervous system metastasis from breast carcinoma: autopsy study. *Cancer* 1983;52: 2349–2354.

87. Valentini M, Cannizzaro R, Poletti M, et al. Nonsteroidal antiinflammator drugs for cancer pain: comparison between misoprostol and ranitidine in prevention of upper gastrointestinal damage. *J Clin Oncol* 1995;13:2637–2642.

88. Vasquez-Barquero A, Ibanez FJ, Herrera S, Izquierdo JM, Berciano J, Pascual J. isolated headache as the presenting clinical manifestation of intracranial tumors: a prospective study. *Cephalalgia* 1994;14: 270–272.

89. Vecht CJ, Hoff AM, Kansen PJ, De Boer MF, Bosch DA. Types and Causes of pain in cancer of the head and neck. *Cancer* 1991;70: 178–184.

90. Verma A, Rosenfeld V, Forteza A, Sharma KR. Occipital lobe tumor presenting as migraine with typical aura. *Headache* 1996;36:49–52.

91. Vijayan, N. Headache after acoustic neuroma. *Notes of the Acoustic Neuroma Association* 1991;39:3–4.

92. Walker MD, Green SB, Byer DP, et al. Randomized comparisons of radiotherapy and nitrosureas for the treatment of malignant glioma after surgery. *N Engl J Med* 1980;303:1323–1329.

93. Wasserstrom WR, Glass JP, Posner JB. Diagnosis and treatment of leptomeningeal metastases from solid tumors: experience with ninety patients. *Cancer* 1982;49:759–772.

94. Weigand DA, Fickel V. Acoustic neuroma-the patients's perspective: subjective assessment of symptoms, diagnosis, therapy and outcome in 541 patients. *Laryngoscope* 1989;99:179–187.

95. Whitton AC, Bloom HJG. Low grade glioma of the cerebral hemispheres in adults: a retrospective analysis of 88 cases. *Int J Radiat Oncol Biol Phys* 1990;18:783–786.

96. Wirth FP, Van Buren JM. Referral of pain from dural stimulation in man. *J Neurosurg* 1971;34:630—642.

97. Yung WA, Horten BC, Shapiro WR. Meningeal gliomatosis: a review of 12 cases. *Ann Neurol* 1980;8:605–608.

98. Zimm S, Wampler GL, Stablein D, Hazra T, Young HF. Intracerebral metastases in solid-tumor patients: natural history and results of treatment. *Cancer* 1981;48:384–394.

The Headaches, Second Edition,
edited by J. Olesen, P. Tfelt-Hansen, and K.M.A. Welch.
Lippincott Williams & Wilkins, Philadelphia © 2000.

The Secondary Headaches

CHAPTER 114

Single Use of Substances

José M. Pereira Monteiro and Carl G. H. Dahlöf

DEFINITION OF HEADACHE ASSOCIATED WITH SINGLE USE OF SUBSTANCES

IHS code and diagnosis: 8 Headaches associated with substances use or withdrawal.

WHO code and diagnosis: G44.4 Drug-induced headache.

Short description: A headache or a new form of headache (including migraine, tension, or cluster-type headaches) that develops in close temporal relation to single substance use or withdrawal; however, effective doses and temporal relationships have not yet been determined for most substances.

Other terms: toxic headaches, chemical headaches, drug-induced headaches, substance-induced headaches.

Since Hippocrates (460 B.C.) and Cornelius Celsus (25–50 A.D.), we have known of substances that can induce headaches, especially in susceptible persons. The substances involved are many: drugs, chemical products, alcoholic drinks, vapors, and others. Drugs are the most widely cited, and their effects have been studied the most thoroughly. The headaches they induce can be of different types: vascular and neurovascular headaches (including migraine), headache secondary to an increase in the intracranial pressure, or unclassified headaches. The descriptions of headaches induced by substances are generally not precise. Most commonly, these headaches are generalized, persistent, and at times throbbing; they

intensify with increased dosage of substances but only to a certain point.

EPIDEMIOLOGY

There is no population-based epidemiologic data on the incidence of substance-induced headaches. The data available come from bibliographic references on the adverse effects of certain substances (5,56,57,59). The incidence of drug-induced headaches can be gathered from data supplied to the World Health Organization (WHO) Collaborating Centre for International Monitoring in Uppsala by the 27 member countries between 1972 and 1987. These data comprise 10,506 reports, 9,733 of which were of unclassified headaches, 611 migraine-type headaches or worsening of a preexisting migraine, and 162 attributable to intracranial hypertension (4). In this study, the ten most reported drugs associated with headaches were indomethacin, nifedipine, cimetidine, atenolol, trimethoprim-sulphamethoxazole, zimelidine, glyceryl trinitrate, isosorbide dinitrate, zomepirac, and ranitidine. Most of these drugs are nonsteroidal antiinflamatory drugs (NSAIDs), peripheral vasodilators, calcium channel blockers, beta-receptor blockers, histamine-receptor blockers, or angiotensin-converting enzyme (ACE) inhibitors. Oral contraceptives were the most common cause of migraine (4). Other common precipitants of migraine-type headaches were atenolol, cimetidine, danazol, diclofenac, ethinylestradiol, indomethacin, nifedipine, and ranitidine (4). As a cause of intracranial hypertension tetracyclines, isotretinoin and trimethoprim-sulphamethoxazole were the most reported (4). If we analyze the frequency of headaches in relation to the volume of sales from the data of Sweden between 1972 and 1987, the

---

J. M. P. Monteiro: Department of Neurology, Instituto de Ciencias Biomedicas Abel Salazar, Porto University, and Department of Neurology, Hospital Santo Antonio, 4050 Porto, Portugal.

C. G. H. Dahlöf: Department of Clinical Pharmacology, Sahlgrenska University Hospital, and Gothenburg Migraine Clinic, S-41117 Göteborg, Sweden.

drugs most often mentioned (4) were zimeldine, nalidixic acid, trimethoprim, griseofulvin, ranitidine, and nifedipine (4).

GENETICS

There is no record of any genetic studies on the families of persons who suffer from substance-induced headaches, but the susceptibility of certain persons is a recognized fact; therefore, a genetic study is justified, such as has been done in studying alcoholism (14).

PATHOPHYSIOLOGY

Why certain substances cause headaches is still uncertain, although specific mechanisms have been suggested, such as vasodilatation and cerebral edema. Vasodilatation is the oldest concept. Schumacher, Ray, and Wolff (66) showed that intracranial vasodilatation was responsible for headaches induced by histamine and that the trigeminal nerve section blocked the occurrence of histaminic headache but only along the area of the selected nerve. They concluded that dilatation of intracranial arteries was responsible for the headache and that the afferent impulses were transported by the trigeminal nerve. The drugs implicated most frequently in the origin of headaches are vasoactive and do not penetrate the blood–brain barrier, which led some investigators to suggest that the mechanism of action was extracranial and vascular. In light of present knowledge of the vasomotor regulation capacity of the central nervous system, however, a central action also may be accepted. Cerebral edema as a cause of headaches is less well documented. Headaches occur in situations associated with cerebral edema, such as hypertensive encephalopathy (72,75) and mountain sickness (35). Drugs that may have caused some degree of cerebral edema and intracranial hypertension are beclomethasone, cimetidine, indomethacin, isotretinoin, monocycline, methylprednisolone, nalidixic acid, nitrofurantoin, prednisolone, tamoxifen, tetracycline, and trimethoprim-sulfamethoxazole (4,23).

Other, so far unidentified, mechanisms must be involved because certain drugs such as NSAIDs, hormones, and other substances do not have a vascular effect and do not cause cerebral edema. Some drugs related to unspecified headaches are atenolol, benoxaprofen, captopril, cimetidine, diclofenac, glyceryltrinitrate, indomethacin, isosorbide dinitrate, isotretinoin, methyldopa, metoprolol, metronidazole, nifedipine, piroxicam, propranolol, ranitidine, terfenadine, trimethoprim-sulfamethoxazole, zimeldine, and zomepirac (4,23). The affirmation that some drugs are able to influence the various mechanisms mentioned (e.g., cimetidine, indomethacin, ranitidine) could mean that a relation between these diverse facts exists and allows us to speculate that substance-induced headaches are the result of a primary cerebral neuronal action, triggering off a vascular reaction, which by its nature or intensity may bring on the headache. The possibility that substance-use headaches result from direct chemically mediated irritative effects on trigeminal afferents has been presented, but this hypothesis requires further investigation (24).

CLINICAL FEATURES

Headache induced by acute substance use or exposure

IHS code and diagnosis: 8.1.
WHO code and diagnosis: G44.40.
Short description: Headache related with the use or exposure to a particular substance.
Other terms: Drug-induced headache.

It is not easy to know whether a particular headache is causally related to the acute use or exposure to a specific substance or combination of substances. To prove it, double-blinded, placebo-controlled experiments are necessary. Two studies of patients who reported headaches after dark chocolate and aspartame, respectively, demonstrated such a need (26). In both studies, headache occurred with equal frequency after placebo. The first step to establish whether a substance really induces a particular type of headache is to determine whether it fulfills the diagnostic criteria proposed by the International Headache Society (IHS) for substance-induced headache given in Table 1 (27). These general criteria should be fulfilled for all headaches to ensure that they are caused by the acute use of a substance. Additional criteria required for each substance are presented herein. These additional criteria do not replace the general criteria. Headaches induced by the following substances are included: nitrates or nitrites, monosodium glutamate, carbon monoxide, alcohol, opiates, and other substances.

Nitrate/Nitrite-induced Headache

This type of headache is related to the acute use and absorption of nitrates or nitrites. Diagnosis of this type of headache should be established when it occurs within 1 hour after absorption of nitrate/nitrite (IHS diagnostic criteria) (27). It includes headaches associated with the contact or use of nitroglycerine (nitroglycerine headache

TABLE 1. *IHS diagnostic criteria for substance-induced headache (Headache Classification Committee, 1988)*

Occurs within a specified time after substance intake
A certain required minimum dose should be indicated
Has occurred in at least 50% of exposures and at least three times
Disappears when substance is eliminated or within a specified time thereafter

IHS, International Headache Society.
From ref. 27, with permission.

or dynamite headache), nitrates, or nitrites (hot-dog headache).

Nitroglycerin

Workers explosives factories suffered from this type of headache in the middle of the last century. It was the first headache of chemical origin to be well defined. The headache occurred within a period of minutes to an hour of exposure to dynamite. It was bilateral, frontotemporally located, and pulsating, occasionally preceded by monocular amaurosis or temporary double vision, and worsened considerably with physical effort. Nitroglycerin (NTG), the main component of dynamite, was later included as a cause of headaches (67). Pharmacologic doses of NTG caused headache episodes that lasted hours. The minimum dose needed to result in a headache could be rapidly reduced by consumption of alcohol. Migraine sufferers are more susceptible to NTG, as are cluster-headache sufferers during cluster episodes. Headaches among patients taking NTG for angina have been described, even when long-acting or topical formulations are used and when the patient has no history of migraine (71). The peak of the peripheral and central vasodilator effect occurs 3 to 4 minutes after administration and disappears about 30 minutes later (30). The fact that the headache in some cases is preceded by loss of vision and in others takes more than an hour to appear suggests that other factors are involved in the origin of the headache besides vasodilatation (58). Headache associated with chronic exposure to NTG is dealt with in Chapter 115. The experimental use of nitroglycerine to induce headache or migraine is discussed in Chapter 24.

Nitrates and Nitrites

Some people cite variable-intensity headaches minutes or hours after eating sausages or other cured meats and fish, such as frankfurters, bacon, ham, salami, pepperoni, corned beef, pastrami, and lox (28) These headaches are usually bilateral, frontal, or temporal as well as frequently pulsating, and sometimes are accompanied by facial flushing. This type of headache has become known as the "hot-dog headache" (28) and is related to the nitrates or nitrites added to these foods. Sodium nitrite is used as food coloring, to impart a cured flavor, and to prevent botulism. The use of amyl nitrate in the treatment of angina frequently causes a pulsating bilateral headache of variable intensity and duration related to the dosage. This type of headache is usually of short duration (less than 15 minutes) (12) and is attributable to its vasodilator effect (37). Nitrates normally become toxic only under conditions in which they are, or may be, reduced to nitrites (65). Toxicity of nitrites is due primarily to their interaction with blood pigment to produce methemoglobinemia (3). Usually the authorities limit the use of nitrites in cured meat (to 200 mg/kg). Storing and cooking reduces the nitrite content (i.e., to 50–130 mg/kg) (60). The headaches induced by these substances are usually bilateral, frontal, or temporal; moderately severe as well as frequently pulsating; and sometimes accompanied by facial flushing. The use of amyl nitrate in the treatment of angina frequently causes a pulsating bilateral headache of variable intensity and duration related to the dosage. This type of headache is usually of short duration (less than 15 minutes) (12) and attributable to its vasodilator effect (37). Other substances in the same group, such as cyclandelate, dipyridamole, erythrityl tetranitrate, isosorbide dinitrate, mannitol hexanitrate, nimodipine, papaverine hydrochloride, pentaerythritol tetranitrate, tolazoline hydrochloride, and trolnitrate phosphate, also can cause headaches of the same types, particularly in susceptible patients (58).

Monosodium Glutamate-induced Headache

Monosodium glutamate (MSG) is a substance that is used as a flavor enhancer in Chinese cooking, especially in soy sauce (63). Almost 30% of people who eat Chinese food mention disagreeable effects (61): a hot flush in the chest, neck, and shoulders; abdominal discomfort associated with tightening of the chest, face, and head (bifrontal or bitemporal); and pulsating headache that occurs 20 to 25 minutes after consumption of Chinese food (63). Nevertheless, some controversy has arisen about these symptoms, which constitute a clinical picture known as the *Chinese restaurant syndrome* attributed to MSG (25,63). Over the past decades, the use of MSG has become far more prevalent in canned, packaged, and prepared foods under the labels of flavor, natural flavor, or hydrolyzed vegetable protein (HVP) additives, according to Food and Drug Administration (FDA) labelling codes. Flavors and HVP additives contain large amounts of MSG (10%–30%) and can trigger symptoms better referred to as *MSG symptom complex* according to FDA recommendations (68,80). To make the diagnosis of Chinese restaurant syndrome, the IHS diagnostic criteria included in Table 2 should be fulfilled (27). The Chinese restaurant

TABLE 2. *IHS diagnostic criteria for glutamate-induced headaches (Headache Classification Committee, 1988)*

Occurs within 1 hr after ingestion of monosodium glutamate.
Associated with at least two of the other symptoms of this syndrome:
Pressure in the chest
Pressure and tightness in the face
Burning sensation in the chest, neck, or shoulders
Flushing of the face
Dizziness
Abdominal discomfort

IHS, International Headache Society.
From ref. 27, with permission.

syndrome was studied in a general population in whom a 12.8% prevalence of one or more symptoms of this syndrome was found, but only 2.3% of the study population believed they had experienced it (34). Clinical evidence of the effects of MSG is still a controversial topic. In 1972 Kenney and Tidball, who performed placebo-controlled studies of reactions to an oral solution of MSF concluded that large doses (> 150 mL) or high concentrations (3.33%) of MSG will provoke a variety of sensations in 32% of a tested population, thereby removing any doubt about the validity of the Chinese restaurant syndrome (33). Furthermore, he stated that at a level of 1.5%, only a few persons will be affected and that concentrations lower than 0.75% are extremely unlikely to cause symptoms, even in sensitive persons (33). In 1993, however, Tarasoff and Kelly (53) studied the effects of 1.5, 3.0, and 3.15 g give to each of 77 healthy subjects compared with those given placebo but did not find any significant difference between the symptoms presented by subjects on MSG (15%) and those on placebo (14%). Recently, Yang et al. performed a double-blind, placebo-controlled, randomized study of MSG in 61 subjects; these investigators found a nonsignificant difference ($p = 0.324$) between the response to MSG (36.1%) and to placebo (24.6%). However, the severity of symptoms was significantly greater ($p = 0.018$) in MSG-sensitive subjects than in placebo-sensitive subjects, and an apparent effect threshold of 2.5 g of MSG was revealed (80).

Oral MSG can produce symptoms in about 20 minutes with a dosage of 3 g or less, that is, throughout the MSG content of 200 mL of wonton soup. The previous consumption of food delays the absorption, whereas simultaneous consumption of alcohol may exacerbate symptoms. MSG-sensitive and MSG-nonsensitive persons reach the same MSG plasma levels. The glutamate is present in high concentrations throughout the whole body and is synthesized in the brain and retina. The mechanism of MSG-induced headache is unclear, but arterial effects have been suggested. In the study performed by Merrit and Williams (48), a direct vasoconstrictor effect was obtained with high doses. Another possible mechanism of action of the MSG syndrome is that it activates a neurotransmission pathway mediated by nitric oxide, which results in the release of nitric oxide in endothelial cells, which in turn acts on neighboring vascular smooth-muscle cells to induce vasodilation (65). Furthermore, the peripheral vascular effects of MSG were demonstrated by Herndon and Coyle (29) and by Seltzer (69), who showed that the administration of MSG to rodents causes degeneration of neurons in the inner layer of the retina and the hypothalamus, which strongly suggests that glutamate is also a neurotoxic substance causing depolarization of neurons (66,67). The exact mechanisms involved in MSG syndrome are largely unknown, however. Whatever the dosage necessary and the mechanisms involved, it seems clear that avoidance of MSG is helpful in patients who report this syndrome.

Carbon Monoxide-induced Headache

This type of headache is associated with exposure to carbon monoxide. The headache caused by carbon monoxide intoxication constitutes a model of toxic or metabolic headache (46), the clinical characteristics of which are shown in Table 3. Headache caused by carbon monoxide is often a dull, continuous bilateral discomfort or a pain with an intensity related to the severity of the carbon monoxide intoxication, at least up to a certain point. Mild headache or dizziness may occur in heavy smokers or in persons using gas for cooking food or in those exposed to automobile exhaust (54).

Alcohol-Induced Headache

IHS code number: 8.1.4.
WHO code number: G44.83.F10.
Short description: This type of headache is associated with the single ingestion of alcohol-containing drinks, foods, or drugs.
Other terms: Alcoholic drinks and other products containing alcohol can cause headaches in susceptible patients. The alcohol-induced headache, also known as *cocktail headache*, generally occurs 30 to 45 minutes after consumption of alcohol, which corresponds to the time needed for alcohol to be absorbed fully (22). Alcohol has little or no effect on vascular smooth-muscle or cerebral blood flow (73); so the headache probably is not a result of intracranial or extracranial vasodilatation caused by alcohol. Alcohol impairs cerebral autoregulation (1) and depresses cerebral serotonin turnover, which probably offers the best explanation for its mechanism (52). Hypomagnesemia and the effects of additives also have been suggested to be involved. Combining alcohol with other substances, such as monoamine oxidase inhibitors, tyramine, disulfiram, metronidazol, furazolidone, chloramphenicol and moxalactam disodium, tolbutamide, or chlorpropamid, also may cause headache (69). To diagnose a alcohol-induced headache, it is necessary that the headache occur within 3 hours after the ingestion of alcohol to fulfill the IHS criteria.

TABLE 3. *Characteristics of carbon monoxide headache*

Characteristic	CO level (%)
Holocranial and suboccipital headache	
Sustained, progressively intense, and pounding	
Mild, without GI or neurologic symptoms	10–20
Moderate, pounding, irritability	20–30
Severe nausea, vomiting, blurred vision	30–40
Confusion and obnubilation	40–50
Coma	50–60
Death	80

CO, carbon monoxide; GI, gastrointestinal.

Food Components and Additives

This type of headache includes those associated with the use of specific food components (e.g., phenylethylamine and tyramine) or food additives (e.g., aspartame). They sometimes are described as *dietary headaches.*

Phenylethylamine

Phenylethylamine is a substance found in various foods such as chocolate and cacao (62). Phenylethylamine causes the release of vasoactive amines, such as serotonin and catecholamine, particularly in patients suffering from migraine provoked by food (dietary migraine) who have reduced monoamine oxidase B (MAOB) activity and thus are unable to metabolize phenylethylamine rapidly. Phenylethylamine readily crosses the blood–brain barrier and thus could be a mediator of cerebrovascular disturbances (45). Two clinical trials tested the capacity of chocolate to cause migraine attacks. In the first, chocolate produced headaches in 50% (62), and in the second study, 30% (49). These results suggest that chocolate and, indirectly, phenylethylamine can precipitate migraine in susceptible persons. In a more recent double-blind study of the effects of biogenetic amines in 27 healthy volunteers, however, it could not be confirmed that phenylethylamine causes headaches (42), although this study did not exclude the possibility of phenylethylamine to be the cause of headache in susceptible persons.

Tyramine

Tyramine is an amine derived from tyrosine and was first extracted from cheese at the beginning of the century. It causes arterial hypertension and headaches when ingested orally or administered parenterally. In 1968, Hannington and Harper found this substance in foods mentioned by patients with dietary migraine (26). In 1970 Smith and colleagues (50) carried out a trial on a tyramine- sensitive migraine population and succeeded in precipitating a migraine-type attack after ingestion of 125 mg of tyramine in 80% of cases, although neither the population of nondietary migraine sufferers nor the control population complained of any significant headache. These results were confirmed in part by Bonnet and Nepveux (7) and by Ghose and colleagues (20) but were contested by Moffett and co-workers (49), who studied eight patients and by Shaw and colleagues, who studied nine patients with dietary migraine and were not able to demonstrate a reaction to tyramine (70). Gibb and associates, in 1991, tested 20 migraine sufferers who reported attacks after the consumption of chocolate. They gave the subjects a 40 g chocolate bar or placebo bar in double-blind fashion, with the flavor of each disguised by carob. Five of the 12 patients tested with chocolate and none of the eight in the placebo group developed a migraine headache within 24 hours period (21). Marcus and colleagues, in 1997, tested 63 women with chronic headaches (50% migraine, 37.5% tension-type, and 12.5% combined forms) with a double-blind provocative trial using two samples of chocolate and two of carob presented in random order after 2 weeks of restricted vasoactive-rich foods. They demonstrated that chocolate was not more likely to provoke headache than carob was in any of the headache diagnostic groups (5,44). These data contradict the common belief of patients and doctors.

Aspartame

Aspartame is a dipeptide sweetener that is 180 to 200 times sweeter than sugar. The widespread use of aspartame after the authorization of its use in 1981 provoked the appearance of various reports on reactions attributed to sensitivity to the substance (10). The U.S. Centers for Disease Control and Prevention (CDC) investigated the complaints of 517 consumers and found that 67% cases involved neurologic or behavioral symptoms, especially headaches. The CDC studies suggested the need to carry out clinical trials to prove a possible relationship with the substance. Schiffmann and colleagues carried out a double-blind study that included 40 patients who reported having repeated headaches after ingestion of products containing aspartame and concluded that in the population studied aspartame did not cause more headaches than placebo (64). Other investigators also documented the safety of long-term administration of 75 mg/kg of aspartame per day evaluated in a randomized, double-blind, placebo-controlled, parallel-group trial in 108 volunteers of both sexes who failed to show significant differences in symptoms (38); however, these conclusions were contested by other authors (5). More recently, a double-blind crossover study using volunteers with self-identified headaches after using aspartame was performed by van den Eeden and colleagues (78) and included 32 subjects randomized to receive aspartame (approximately 30 mg/kg daily) or placebo in a two-treatment, four-period crossover design. This experiment provided evidence that, among persons with self-reported headaches after ingestion of aspartame, a subset of this group reports more headaches when tested under controlled conditions. It appears that some people are particularly susceptible to headaches caused by aspartame and may need to limit their consumption (78).

Illicit Drugs

IHS code number: 8.1.5.
WHO code number: G44.83.
Short description: Includes headaches associated with single use of drugs, particularly illicit drugs (e.g., cocaine, crack, marijuana).
Other terms: Rebound headache.

Headaches can occur as a consequence of the use of several illicit drugs, such as central nervous system

(CNS) stimulants (e.g., amphetamines, cocaine, designer drugs), barbiturates, sedatives, or opiates. The headaches may be associated with either acute use or chronic use and occur during withdrawal from these substances. Here we discuss only headaches induced by the acute use of illicit drugs; headaches associated with chronic use of these substances are discussed in Chapter 115.

Cocaine

Cocaine leads to a rapid block of presynaptic norepinephrine reuptake with potent sympathomimetic effects and acute constriction of vascular smooth muscle and produces a migrainelike headache, usually with a benign course (15). The adverse and pharmacologic effects of cocaine, namely, addiction and abuse, have been known for longer than a century, but little has been written about the acute neurologic complications arising from its use, which include generalized or partial epileptic seizures, ischemic or hemorrhagic strokes, visual loss caused by retinal artery occlusion or optic neuropathy, extrapyramidal symptoms (tics, dystonia), cardiac events (myocardial infarction, dysrhythmias, aortic dissection), pregnancy disturbances (pre-eclampsia or eclampsia), psychiatric disturbances (agitation, anxiety, depression, psychosis, paranoia, suicidal ideation), and headaches (9,41,76,79). Cocaine occasionally triggers a syndrome that resembles hemiplegic migraine (40). Cocaine as well as amphetamine-induced headaches are frequent, begin immediately after drug ingestion, and usually are not associated with nervous system pathology. If prolonged and accompanied by focal neurologic signals, they are often due to hemorrhagic or ischemic stroke or vasculitis (47). There does not seem to be any correlation between the previous use, amount, route of administration, and appearance of neurologic complications (11). The mechanism of these headaches is largely unknown (41) but may be related to the sympathomimetic or vasoconstrictive effects of cocaine (15).

Crack

The growing use of crack (the alkaloid form of cocaine prepared with sodium bicarbonate), which is cheaper, fast acting, and highly potent, frequently provokes significant adverse effects, including ischemic or hemorrhagic events and headaches (9,39,40). Levine and colleagues, in 1990, studied a group of 28 patients who had strokes temporally related with the use of "crack" (during or within 72 hours of use) and found the following types of cerebral infarction: 18 cerebral infarction (one fatal) of middle cerebral artery ($n = 10$), anterior cerebral artery ($n = 3$), posterior cerebral artery ($n = 1$), vertebrobasilar arteries ($n = 4$), subarachnoid hemorrhage ($n = 5$), intraparenchymal hemorrhage ($n = 4$), and primary intraven-

tricular hemorrhage ($n = 1$). Eighteen patients (64%) had acute neurologic symptoms immediately or within 1 hour of using cocaine. Fifteen patients (45%) had severe headache as an early symptom (40). Cocaine-related stroke occurs mainly in young people and probably has many causes. A thorough history focusing on the use of cocaine or its alkaloid form and toxicologic screening of urine and serum should be done (39). Sometimes the effects of crack are lethal when it is prepared along with toxic solvents (79).

Marijuana

Marijuana is a drug prepared by drying the flowering tops of plants of *Cannabis sativa*. Its medicinal use began in India around 1,000 B.C. and in Western medicine during the nineteenth century. It was extensively used as an analgesic, nocturnal sedative, and hypnotic and, less frequently, to treat dysmenorrhea, neuralgia including tic douloureux, muscle spasms, and migraine (18). The use of marijuana was found to be the cause of mild and frontal headaches in five of ten patients observed by Ames. In these cases, headaches were accompanied by other symptoms, such as dryness of the mouth, paresthesia, sensation of warmth, and suffusion of the conjunctivae (2). Most reports are about migrainelike or tension-type headaches associated with discontinuation of long-term marijuana use. Because cannabinoids have been reported to have both a peripheral vasoconstrictor effect and an ability to inhibit platelet serotonin release, they may have a specific migraine prophylactic effect, and abrupt interruption of chronic marijuana intake may lead to a withdrawal syndrome (13,18,19).

Headache Induced by Withdrawal of Acute Use of Substances

IHS code and diagnosis: 8.3.
WHO code and diagnosis: G44.83.
Short description: Headache from acute use substance withdrawal.
Other terms: Withdrawal headache.

Diagnosis of this particular type of headaches should not be made without fulfilling the following IHS diagnostic criteria included in Table 4.

Alcohol Withdrawal Headache

Alcohol withdrawal headache is the headache associated with withdrawal of a single abundant ingestion of alcohol. The full clinical picture is also called *hangover syndrome*. The IHS diagnostic criteria for alcohol withdrawal headache is the following: The headache may be preceded by intake of sufficient alcohol to have made the particular person drunk (27).

TABLE 4. *IHS diagnostic criteria for headache from substance withdrawal (acute use) (Headache Classification Committee, 1988)*

A Follows acute use of a substance.
B A certain required minimum dose should be indicated.
C Occurs when the substance is largely or completely eliminated, but may last longer.
D Is relieved or improved by renewed intake of the substance.

IHS, International Headache Society.
From ref. 27, with permission.

The hangover syndrome is characterized by headaches, dry mouth, paleness, nausea, dizziness, and hyperexcitability, which occur several hours after the interruption of the ingestion of alcohol and when the tissue level of the alcohol is low or nil. Headaches are a common but not a constant feature of the syndrome. They are generally throbbing and aggravated by body movements, coughing, and rapid head movements. The syndrome usually lasts 5 to 10 hours after the alcohol has been metabolized (6,16,17,43,51,56,74). The immediate reduction of symptoms with a fresh ingestion of alcohol indicates that the hangover may be a slight withdrawal syndrome. A delay in the clearance of metabolic products has been suggested as a cause of the hangover syndrome. Ogata and colleagues (57) found high pyruvate levels in the blood but not acetaldehyde or lactate in sufferers of hangover syndrome. The fact that pilots often get relief from the hangover syndrome by inhaling oxygen is consistent with the hypothesis that the this syndrome is due to a delay in the metabolic recovery of the redox state modified by ingestion of alcohol (55,57). A close interrelationship and involvement of the hormonal, peptidergic, and opiate systems in the pathogenesis of the acute withdrawal syndrome were suggested by Kokkanenko (36).

Other Substances

A high incidence of headaches has been reported in connection with withdrawal from opiates and other addictive substances (13). Different types of headache have been reported, mainly tension-type or migrainelike headaches. The withdrawal symptoms associated with the use of many of these agents generally are characterized by rebound effects in those physiologic systems that were initially modified by the substance (31). The mechanism of action is unknown but in some cases may be related to drug-induced alterations in the serotoninergic system (15) or to the abrupt decrease in the levels of endorphins (13).

Headache Associated with Substances but with Uncertain Mechanism

IHS code number: 8.5.
WHO code number: G44.408.

Short description: Includes many other organic and inorganic substances.

Birth Control Pill or Estrogens

This subject is discussed extensively in Chapter 32.

Other Substances

Intoxication with a number of organic and inorganic substances is associated with headaches (4,55). Generally, headache is not dealt with in great detail in the literature on intoxication, but headache is most often the diffuse toxic–metabolic type already mentioned. The following list of substances is not exhaustive but contains those most commonly encountered. *Inorganic compounds* are arsenic, borate, bromate, chlorate, copper, iodine, lead, lithium, and mercury. *Organic compounds* (4,55) include alcohols (long-chain), amphetamine, aniline, atropine, balsam, camphor, carbon disulfide, carbon tetrachloride, clordecone, digitalis, disulfiram, EDTA, heptachlor, histamine, hydralazine, hydrogen sulfide, imipramine, kerosene, methyl alcohol, methyl bromide, methyl chloride, methyl iodine, naphthalene, nicotine, organophosphorus compounds (parathion, pyrethrum), nitrogen oxides (NO; NO_2; N_2O_3; N_2O_4).

PROGNOSIS

The prognosis of headaches associated with the acute use of substances in general is good, because symptoms fade spontaneously after exposure ceases. The development of chronic headache is rare, but headache can appear on renewed contact with the substance. Excessive exposure to carbon monoxide might be lethal as can excessive use of illicit drugs, particularly those containing contaminants or combinations with other substances such as crack or amphetamine analogues like "ecstasy."

MANAGEMENT

It is important to identify the clinical syndrome and to stop further exposure to the substance immediately. Specific measures may be necessary, for example, pure or hyperbaric oxygen in case of carbon monoxide intoxication.

Patients need to be advised that contact with the specific substance or substances should be avoided in the future. If this is not possible, symptomatic medication may be indicated. Ergotamine can abort 40% of headaches induced by NTG (67), but pretreatment with a daily dose (80–160 mg) of propranolol does not prevent headaches. NSAIDs may be used to prevent alcohol withdrawal headaches (56,77). Transdermic clonidine is an effective treatment for the relief of the main symptoms and signs of acute alcohol withdrawal syndrome, namely, headache, dizziness, fatigue, cognitive disturbances, arterial hypertension, accelerated heart rate, and diarrhea (6). Buspirone may be useful in the management of acute severe alcohol and opiate withdrawal syndromes (8,32).

REFERENCES

1. Altura BM, Altura BT, Gebrewold A. Alcohol induced spasm of cerebral blood vessels. *Science* 1983;220:331–333.
2. Ames F. A clinical and metabolic study of acute intoxication with *Cannabis sativa* and its role in the model psychoses. *Journal of Mental Sciences* 1958;104:972–999.
3. Askew Gl, Finelli L, Genese CA, Sorhage FE, Sosin DM, Spitalny HC. Bouillabaisse: an outbreak of methemoglobinemia in New Jersey in 1992. *Pediatrics* 1994;94:381–384.
4. Askmark H, Lundberg PO, Olsson S. Drug related headache. *Headache* 1989;29:441–444.
5. Atkins FM. A critical evaluation of clinical trials in adverse reactions to foods in adults. *J Allergy Clin Immunol* 1986;78:174–182.
6. Baumgartner GR, Rowen RC. Transdermal clonidine versus chlordiazepoxide in alcohol widrawal: a randomized, controlled clinical trial. *South Med J* 1991;84:312–321.
7. Bonnet GF, Nepveux P. Migraine due to tyramine. *Sem Hop* 1971;47:2441–2445.
8. Bonvalot T, Boulenger JP, Zarifian E. Buspirone: pharmacological and clinical properties of the first member of a new anxiolytic drug family. *Rev Med Interne* 1988;1:97–103.
9. Catalano G, Catalano MC, Rodriguez R. Dystonia associated with crack cocaine use. *South Med J* 1997;90:1050–1052.
10. Council of Scientific Affairs. Aspartame: review of safety issues. *JAMA* 1985;254:400–402.
11. Cregler LL, Mark H. Medical complications of cocaine abuse. *N Engl J Med* 1986;315:1495–1501.
12. Dalessio DJ. Toxic vascular headache. In: Dalessio DJ, ed. *Wolff's headache and other head pain*, 3rd ed. New York: Oxford University Press, 1972;198–219.
13. De Marinis M, Janiri L, Agnoli A. Headache in the use and withdrawal of opiates and other associated substances of abuse. *Headache* 1991;31:159–163.
14. Devor EJ, Cloninger CR. Genetics of alcoholism. *Annu Rev Genet* 1989;23:19–36.
15. Dhuna A, Pascual-Leone A, Belgrade M. Cocaine-related vascular headaches. *J Neurol Neusurg Psychiatry* 1991;54:803–806.
16. Dick P, Costa C, Fayolle K, Grandjean ME, Khoshbeen A, Tissot R. DSIP in the treatment of withdrawal syndromes from alcohol and opiates. *Eur Neurol* 1984;23:364–371.
17. Dogherty RJ, Gates RR. The role of buspirone in the management of alcohol withdrawal: a preliminary investigation. *J Subst Abuse Treat* 1990;7:189–192.
18. El-Mallakh RS. Marijuana and migraine. *Headache* 1987;27:442–443.
19. El-Mallakh RS, Kranzler HR, Kamanitz JR. Headaches and psychoactive substance use. *Headache* 1991;31:584–587.
20. Ghose K, Carrol JD. Mechanism of tyramine-induced migraine: similarities with dopamine and interactions with disulfiran and propranolol in migraine patients. *Neuropsychobiology* 1984;12:2–3, 122–126.
21. Gibb CM, Davies PTG, Glover V, Steiner TJ, Clifford Rose F, Sandler M. Chocolate is a migraine-provoking agent. *Cephalalgia* 1991;11:93–95.
22. Gillespie JA. Vasodilator properties of alcohol. *BMJ* 1967;2:274–277.
23. Giuseffi V, Michel W, Siegel PZ, Rojas PB. Symptoms and disease associations in idiopathic intracranial hypertension (pseudotumor cerebri) a case–control study. *Neurology* 1991;41:239–244.
24. Goadsby PG. Headache associated with acute substance use or exposure. In: Gilman S, Goldstein GW, Waxman SG, eds. *Neurobase*. San Diego: Arbor Publishing, 1998.
25. Gore ME, Salmon PR. Chinese restaurant syndrome: fact or fiction. *Lancet* 1980;1:251–252.
26. Hannington E, Harper AM. The role of tyramine in the aetiologie of migraine and related studies on the cerebral and intercerebral circulations. *Headache* 1968;8:84–97.
27. Headache Classification Committee of the International Headache Society. Classification and Diagnostic criteria for headache disorders, cranial neuralgias and facial pain. *Cephalalgia* 1988;7(Suppl 8):1–96.
28. Henderson WR, Raskin NH. "Hot-dog" headache: individual susceptibility to nitrite. *Lancet* 1972;2:1162–1163.
29. Herndon RM, Coyle JT. Selective destruction of neurons by a transmitter agonist. *Science* 1977;198:71–72.
30. Horowitz LD, Herman MV, Gorlin R. Clinical response to nitroglycerine as a diagnostic test for coronary artery disease. *Am J Cardiol* 1972;29:149–153.
31. Jaffe JH, Martin WR. Opioid analgesics and antagonists. In: Gilman AG, Rall TW, Nies AS, eds. *Goodman and Gilman's the pharmacological basis of therapeutics*, 8th ed. New York: Pergamon Press, 1990:485–521.
32. Jann MW. Buspirone: an update on a unique anxiolytic agent. *Pharmacotherapy* 1988;8:100–116.
33. Kenney RA, Tidball CS. Human susceptibility to oral monosodium l-glutamate. *Am J Clin Nutr* 1972;25:140–146.
34. Kerr GR, Wu-lee M, El-lozy M, Mcgandy R, Stare F. Prevalence of the "Chinese Restaurant Syndrome." *J Am Diet Assoc* 1979;75:29–33.
35. King AB, Robinson SM. Vascular headache of acute mountain sickness. *Aerospace Medicine* 1972;43:849–851.
36. Kokkanenko EM. Participation of the peptidergic and endogenous opiate system in the pathogenesis of early manifestations of the alcohol abstinence syndrome. *Probl Endokrinol (Moskva)* 1988;34:24–29.
37. Lance JW. *Mechanism and management of headache*. London: Butterworth, 1982;198–200.
38. Leon AS, Hunninghake DB, Bell C, Rassin DK, Tephly TR. Safety of long-term doses of aspartame. *Arch Intern Med* 1989;149:2318–2324.
39. Levine SR, Brust JC, Futrell N, et al. Cerebrovascular complications of the use of the crack form of alkaloidal cocaine. *N Engl J Med* 1990;323:699–704.
40. Lipton RB, Choy-Kwong M, Solomon S. Headaches in hospitalized cocaine users. *Headache* 1989;29:225–228.
41. Lowenstein DH, Massa SM, Rowbotham MC, et al. Acute neurologic and psychiatric complications associated with cocaine abuse. *Am J Med* 1987;83:841–846.
42. Lüthy J, Schlatter C. Biogenic amines in food: effects of histamine, tyramine and phenylethylamine in the human. *Z Lebensm Unters Forsch* 1983;177:439–443.
43. Mannix LK, Frame JR, Solomon GD. Alcohol, smoking and caffeine use among headache patients. *Headache* 1997;37:572–576.
44. Marcus DA, ScharffL, Turk D, Gourley LM. A double-blind provocative study of chocolate as a trigger of headache. *Cephalalgia* 1997;17:855–862.
45. McCullock J, Harper AM. Phenylethylamine and the cerebral circulation. In: *Current concepts in migraine research*. New York: Raven Press, 1978:85–88.
46. Meigs JL, Hughes JPW. Acute carbon monoxide poisoning: an analysis of 105 cases. *AMA Archives of Industrial Hygiene and Occupational Medicine* 1952;6:344–356.
47. Merkel PA, Koroshetz WJ, Irizarry MC, Cudkovicz ME. Cocaine-associated cerebral vasculitis. *Semin Arthritis Rheum* 1995;25:172–183.
48. Merrit JE, Williams PB. Vasospasm contributes to monosodium glutamate-induced headache. *Headache* 1990;30:575–580.
49. Moffet AM, Swash M, Scott DF. Effect of chocolate in migraine: a double blind study. *J Neurol Neurosurg Psychiatry* 1974;37:445–448.
50. Smith I, Kellow AH, Hannington E. Clinical and biochemical correlation between tyramine and migraine headache. *Headache* 1970;10:43–52.
51. Murphree AB, Greenberg LA, Carrol RB. Neuropharmacological effects of substances other than ethanol in alcoholic beverages. *Fed Proc* 1967;26:1468–1473.
52. Myers RD, Melchior CL. Alcohol and alcoholism: role of serotonin. In: Essman WB, ed. *Serotonin in health and disease*, vol 2. New York: Spectrum, 1978:373–430.
53. Tarasoff L, Kelly MF. Monosodium L-glutamate: a double-blind study and review. *Food Chem Toxicol* 1993;31:1019–1035.
54. Nattero G, Enrico A. Outdoor pollution and headache. *Headache* 1996;36:243–245.
55. Norton S. Toxicology of the central nervous system. In: Casarett LJ, Doult J, eds. *Toxicology*. New York: Macmillan, 1975:151–169.
56. Olesen J. Management of acute nonvascular headache: the Danish experience. *Headache* 1990;30(Suppl 2):540–543.
57. Ogata S, Hosoi T, Saji H. Studies on acute alcohol intoxication. *Japanese Journal of Studies of Alcohol* 1966;1:67–79.

58. Pereira Monteiro JM. Headache associated with single use of substances. In: Olesen J, Tfelt-Hansen P, Welch KMA, eds. *The headaches.* New York: Raven Press, 1993:715–720.

59. Pereira Monteiro JM. Drug abuse in headache: epidemiology. *Funct Neurol* 1992;7(Suppl 6):7–10.

60. Raskin NH. Ice-cream, ice pick and chemical headaches. In: Vinken PJ, Bruyn GW, Klawans HL, eds. *Handbook of clinical neurology*, vol 48. Amsterdam: Elsevier, 1986:441–448.

61. Reif-Lehrer L. A questionnaire study of the prevalence of chinese restaurant syndrome. *Fed Proc* 1977;36:1617–1623.

62. Sandler M, Youdim MBH, Hannington E. A phenylethylamine oxidizing defect in migraine. *Nature* 1974;250:335–337.

63. Schaumburg HH, Byck R, Gerstl R, Mashman JH. Monosodium L-glutamate: its pharmacology and role in the Chinese restaurant syndrome. *Science* 1969;163:826–828.

64. Schiffmann SS, Buckley CE, Sampson HA, et al. Aspartame and susceptibility to headache. *N Engl J Med* 1987;317:1181–1185.

65. Scher W, Scher BM. A possible role for nitric oxide in glutamate (MSG)-induced Chinese restaurant syndrome, glutamate induced asthma, "hot-dog headache," pugilistic Alzheimer's disease, and other disorders. *Med Hypotheses* 1992;38:185–188.

66. Schumacher GA, Roy BS, Wolf HE. Experimental studies on headache and its pain pathways. *Arch Neurol Psychiatry* 1940;44:701–717.

67. Schwartz AM. The cause, relief and prevention of headaches arising from contact with dynamite. *N Engl J Med* 1946;235:541–544.

68. Scopp AL. MSG and hydrolysed vegetable protein induced headache review and case studies. *Headache* 1991;31:107–110.

69. Seltzer S. Foods and drug combinations, responsible for head and neck pain. *Cephalalgia* 1982;2:111–124.

70. Shaw SWJ, Johnson RH, Keogh HG. Oral tyramine in dietary migraine sufferers. In: *Current concepts in migraine research.* New York: Raven Press, 1978:31–39.

71. Shively M, Riegel B. Effect of nitroglycerin ointment placement on headache and flushing in healthy subjects. *Int J Nurs Stud* 1991;28:153–161.

72. Skinhoj E, Strandgaard S. Pathogenesis of hypertensive encephalopathy. *Lancet* 1973;1:461–462.

73. Sokoloff L. The action of drugs on the cerebral circulation. *Pharmacol Rev* 1959;11:1–85.

74. Solovov AV. Neurological and neurophysiological aspects of the alcohol abstinence syndrome. *Zh Nevropatol Psikhiatr Im S S Korsakova* 1995;95:57–59.

75. Standgaard S, Olesen J, Skinhoj E, Lassen NA. Autoregulation of brain circulation in severe arterial hypertension. *BMJ* 1973;1:507–510.

76. Towers CV, Pircon RA, Nageotte MP, Porto M, Garite TJ. Cocaine intoxication presenting as preeclampsia and eclampsia. *Obstet Gynecol* 1993;81:545–547.

77. Wallgreen H, Barry A. Drug actions in relation to alcohol effects. In: *Actions of alcohol.* New York: Elsevier, 1970:621–714.

78. Van den Eeden SK, Koepsell TD, Longstreth WT Jr, Van Belle G, Daling JR, McKnight B. Aspartame ingestion and headaches: a randomized crossover trial. *Neurology* 1994;44:1787–93.

79. Van Viet H, Chevalier P, Sereni C, et al. Accidents neurologiques liaises a l'usage de la cocaine. *Presse Med* 1990;19:1045–1049.

80. Yang WH, Drouin MA, Herbert M, Mao Y, Kursh J. The monosodium glutamate symptom complex: assessement in a double blind, placebo controlled, randomized study. *J Allergy Clin Immunol* 1997;99:757–762.

The Headaches, Second Edition,
edited by J. Olesen, P. Tfelt-Hansen, and K.M.A. Welch.
Lippincott Williams & Wilkins, Philadelphia © 2000.

The Secondary Headaches

CHAPTER 115

Headache Associated with Chronic Use of Substances

Hans-Christoph Diener and Carl G. H. Dahlöf

DEFINITION OF HEADACHE ASSOCIATED WITH CHRONIC USE OF SUBSTANCES

IHS code and diagnosis:

8.2 Headache induced by chronic substance use or exposure.

8.4 Headache from substance withdrawal (chronic use).

WHO code and diagnosis: G44.4 Drug-induced headache.

Short description: Headache occurring during daily use of symptomatic headache medication or chronic intake of other substances as well as headache occurring in the withdrawal phase after such substance use. The headache is daily or almost daily and disappears within a few weeks after withdrawal.

Other terms: None.

Inappropriate use of headache medication may contribute to the development of chronic daily headache that is refractory to most treatments. Physicians who are experienced in the treatment of migraine and other headaches are well aware that the daily intake of antipyretic or anti-inflammatory analgesics, ergotamine, dihydroergotamine (DHE), the "triptans," and opioids may result in chronic daily headache. Conversely, if a patient complains of chronic daily headache and takes pain medication every day, this headache is most likely to be caused and sus-

tained by the medication and will vanish or improve with discontinuation of the drug use. Little experimental work has been done in this field, and the following information is based mainly on clinical series describing patients presenting at headache clinics with this problem, with subsequent treatment and follow-up.

EPIDEMIOLOGY

Prevalence and incidence rates of chronic drug-induced headache are not available. Most headache centers report that between 5% and 10% of the patients they see fulfill the criteria of drug-induced headache (3–6,27,47). Micieli and colleagues (49) observed an incidence of 4.3% in 3,000 consecutive headache patients. Because headache centers and clinics see a negative selection of headache sufferers, the true prevalence is estimated to be 0.5% to 1% of patients with migraine and 0.3% to 0.5% of patients with chronic tension-type headache. Higher numbers of patients who have a combination of both migraine and tension-type headache are seen. Patients with cluster headache rarely develop drug-induced headache. A survey of family doctors showed that drug-induced headache was the third most common cause of headache (55).

Some additional studies give hints about the prevalence of regular intake of analgesics. Interviews of a representative sample of the Swiss population revealed that 4.4% of men and 6.8% of women take analgesics at least once a week (28); 2.3% reported taking these drugs daily. Inpatient records from 1974 through 1977 from several departments of psychiatry in Switzerland showed dependency on analgesics to be more common than dependency on tranquilizers, hypnotics, and stimulating drugs

H.-C. Diener: Department of Neurology, University of Essen, and Department of Neurology, University Hospital Essen, D-45122 Essen, Germany.

C. G. H. Dahlöf: Department of Clinical Pharmacology, Sahlgrenska University Hospital, and Gothenburg Migraine Clinic, S-41117 Göteborg, Sweden.

(36). Calculations from the number of tablets sold indicate that possibly 1% of the German population take up to ten pain tablets every day (62). Taken together, these studies indicate that drug-induced headache is a major health problem. Considering the side effects of chronic intake of analgesics and ergotamine (see the following), this problem must be considered serious.

PATHOPHYSIOLOGY

Some researchers who doubt that drug-induced headache exists cite several facts. People who take DHE because of arterial hypotension or who take nonsteroidal antiinflammatory drugs (NSAIDs) or acetylsalicylic acid daily because of chronic rheumatism, low-back pain, or for prophylaxis of stroke or myocardial infarction develop daily headache only at a rate of 2% to 5% (7,38). Improvement during the acute withdrawal phase and afterward often can be attributed to corresponding behavioral or medical therapy of migraine or tension-type headache. Double-blind studies of drug withdrawal compared with continuous intake have not been undertaken; however, most headache experts agree that patients with migraine and tension-type headache have a higher potential for drug-induced headache. The basis for this potential could be genetic, or it could result from the fact that migraine pain is more severe than joint pain.

In two studies (13,16), hospitalized patients were withdrawn from ergotamine and analgesics without further therapy, and migraine prophylaxis was delayed for at least 3 months after the withdrawal. More than 60% of these patients no longer had daily headache, although about 40% still had migraine attacks. Different mechanisms probably contribute to the transition from the original headache to drug-induced headache. Psychological factors include the reinforcing properties of pain relief by drug consumption, a powerful component of positive conditioning. Many patients report taking migraine drugs prophylactically because they worry about losing a working day (or, inevitably, the job) or missing an important social event (e.g., dinner, theater). More importantly, patients often fear an imminent headache and take analgesics or specific migraine drugs prophylactically. Often patients are instructed by their physician or by the instructions supplied with the medication to take the migraine drug as early as possible at the start of either the aura or the headache phase of a migraine attack.

Withdrawal headache is an additional factor. Whenever the patient tries to stop or reduce the medication, the preexisting headache worsens. Barbiturates are contained in drugs used for the treatment of tension-type headache; these drugs have a high potency for addiction and can cause headache. The psychotropic side effects of analgesic or migraine drugs, such as sedation or mild euphoria, and their stimulating action may lead to drug dependency. Bar-biturates, codeine, other opioids, and caffeine are the most likely substances to produce this effect. Caffeine increases vigilance, relieves fatigue, and improves performance and mood. The typical symptoms of caffeine withdrawal, such as irritability, nervousness, restlessness, and especially "caffeine-withdrawal headache" (1,66,72), which may last several days, encourage patients to continue the abuse. Despite the fact that caffeine may enhance the analgesic action of acetylsalicylic acid and acetaminophen (39,41), it should be removed from analgesics. Similarly, caffeine and meprobamat, the main metabolite of carisoprodol, should be removed from ergotamine-containing formulations.

Some reports have described physical dependence on codeine and other opioids in headache patients (24,74). No studies have been conducted to investigate the effects of codeine intake over periods as long as 10 years, although many headache patients have done so. It should be remembered that up to 10% of codeine is metabolized to morphine (46).

Ergotamine and DHE certainly may lead to physical dependency (60). Many patients who feel a migraine attack may take ergotamine as prophylactic treatment. Professional women (e.g., teachers) are particularly likely to do this (13). The withdrawal headache confirms the patient's belief that she or he is better off with than without the drugs. The reason for the physical dependency on ergotamine remains obscure. Verhoeff and colleagues (73) observed no upregulation of D_2-receptors in the brains of patients with ergotamine abuse. Ergotamine abusers react similarly to other migraine patients to the vasoconstrictor effect of ergotamine (70). In one study, the tyramine-induced mydriasis after ergotamine administration was increased during abuse but not after withdrawal of ergotamine, indicating a central inhibition of pupillary sympathetic activity during abuse (23). Thus, a possible central nervous system effect of ergotamine can be observed after chronic use but not after a single dose of the drug. Other studies investigating the effect of chronic use of ergotamine on the regulation of the autonomic nervous system by the central nervous system are needed.

It is more difficult to explain why aspirin and paracetamol can lead to chronic headache. Both drugs act preferentially on peripheral receptors. The chronically suppressed afferent information from trigeminal fibers could lead to an increase in the central threshold for pain perception (as with deafferentation pain).

CLINICAL FEATURES

IHS diagnostic criteria for headache associated with chronic use of substances (29):

8.2 Headache induced by chronic substance use or exposure
    A. Occurs after daily doses of a substance for longer than 3 months

B. A certain required minimum dose should be indicated

C. Headache is chronic (15 days or more a month).

D. Headache disappears within 1 month after withdrawal of the substance

8.2.1 Ergotamine-induced headache

A. Preceded by daily ergotamine intake (oral >2 mg, rectal >1 mg).

B. Diffuse, pulsating, and distinguished from migraine by absent attack pattern or absent associated symptoms

Comment: The diagnosis can be made only after withdrawal of ergotamine resulting in relief from ergotamine-induced headache (but usually not from the primary headache)

8.2.2 Analgesics abuse headache

One or more of the following:

1. More than 50 g of aspirin a month or the equivalent of other mild analgesics

2. More than 100 tablets a month of analgesics combined with barbiturate or other nonnarcotic compounds

3. One or more narcotic analgesics

Comment: The diagnosis can be made only after withdrawal of substance resulting in relief from substance-induced headache (but usually not from the primary headache).

8.4.1 Headache from substance withdrawal (chronic use)

A. Occurs after a high daily dose (specified when possible under each substance) of a substance for more than 3 months

B. Occurs within hours after elimination of the substance

C. Relieved by renewed intake of the substance

D. Disappears within 14 days after withdrawal of the substance

8.4.1 Ergotamine-withdrawal headache

A. Preceded by daily ergotamine intake (oral >2 mg, rectal >1 mg)

B. Occurs within 48 hours after withdrawal of ergotamine

8.4.2 Caffeine-withdrawal headache

A. Patient has consumed caffeine daily and >15 g/month

B. Occurs within 24 hours after last caffeine intake

C. Relieved within 1 hour by intake of 100 mg of caffeine

8.4.3 Narcotics-abstinence headache

8.4.4 Other substances (specify)

This classification urgently needs revision, which will occur with the edition of diagnostic criteria. More adequate definitions of drug-induced headache can be found in Diener (14) and Silberstein and Lipton (63) and Silberstein and colleagues (64).

For the purpose of this chapter, a metanalysis was performed summarizing 29 studies comprising a total of 2,612 patients with chronic drug-induced headache (3–6,13,16,20,27,30,32,34) (Table 1). Sixty-five percent of patients reported migraine as primary headache, 27% of patients reported tension-type headache, and 8% of patients reported mixed or other headaches (e.g., cluster headache). Women were more likely to experience drug-induced headache than men (3.5:1; 1,533 women, 442 men). This ratio is slightly higher than could be expected from the gender differences in the frequency of migraine. The mean duration of primary headache was 20.4 years. The mean admitted time of frequent drug intake was 10.3 years in one study (16), and the mean duration of daily headache was 5.9 years.

TABLE 1. *Chemical components contained in drugs taken by patients with drug-induced headache*

Chemical agent	Patients taking the agent (%)		
	Baumgartner et al. (6) (n = 54)	Diener et al. (13) (n = 30)	Micieli et al. (48) (n = 128)
Caffeine	100	94	87
Pyrazolone derivatives	77	44	71
Barbiturates	63	72	47
Ergotamine	80	61	24
Dihydroergotamine		42	
Para-aminophenol derivatives	48	45	22
Indomethacin			13
Phenothiazines			12
Salicylates	43	20	8
Other analgesics		8	26
Codeine	26	34	
Opiates		3	9
Minor tranquilizers	26	10	22

Data from Baumgartner et al (6) and Micieli et al (48).

TABLE 2. *Critical cumulative doses (mg) taken per month and interval of overlap*

Substance	Dose limit (mg)	Critical interval[a]	
		A	B
Caffeine	1,350	1,200	1,700
Ergotamine	20	8	20
Dihydroergotamine	28	16	70
Barbiturates	840	840	840
Pyrazolone	4,100	2,100	4,400
Codeine	240	240	240
Paracetamol	7,500	4,800	9,200
Acetylsalicylic acid	7,000	7,000	7,000

[a]A, <5% of patients with daily headache; B, <5% of patients with migraine.
From Diener et al. (15).

The drugs leading to chronic drug-induced headache vary considerably in the different series, depending probably on both the selection of patients (e.g., "pure" ergotamine abusers being reported) (3,4,20,31,32,40, 42,53,57,69) and cultural factors. Potentially each component contained in analgesics or drugs for the treatment of migraine attacks probably could induce headache. This is also true for acetylsalicylic acid and paracetamol (30,44,56). It is, however, difficult to identify a single substance, because about 90% of patients take more than one compound simultaneously. Table 2 shows data from three studies (6,15,49) regarding the frequency of the chemical compounds of drugs used. Sumatriptan also can lead to drug-induced headache, as first observed in patients who abused ergotamine (8,35). Later, *de novo* cases were reported (25,26,54). As a result of the delay between frequent intake of triptans and the development of drug-induced headache, similar cases are now observed with zolmitriptan, naratriptan, and rizatriptan. The risk appears to be particularly high in headache patients with a history of misuse of analgesics or ergotamine.

Results from headache diaries show that the number of tablets or suppositories taken per day averages 4.9 (range 0.25–25). Patients take on average 2.5 to 5.8 different pharmacologic components simultaneously (range, 1–14).

In our experience, patients with migraine as the primary headache report two different kinds of headaches:

- A constant, diffuse, dull headache without associated symptoms is experienced (see 8.2.1 and 8.2.2).
- Often patients who take ergotamine or a triptan daily also experience a throbbing, pulsating headache in the early morning, sometimes combined with nausea. The headache disappears between 30 and 60 min after the intake of ergotamine or a triptan. This headache is probably a minor withdrawal headache (see 8.4.1).

In addition to the diffuse, daily headache, patients may experience migraine attacks with intensified unilateral headaches and associated symptoms. Patients with chronic tension-type headache or posttraumatic headache as the primary headache most often are not able to discriminate the characteristics of their primary headache and chronic drug-induced headache.

- The withdrawal headache (8.4.1) experienced after stopping medication resembles a severe and prolonged migraine attack in patients with migraine as primary headache.

The psychological examination reveals a high prevalence of depression, as observed in many patients with chronic pain (45,59).

Dynamite headache, that is, headache associated with withdrawal of nitroglycerine (NTG) after chronic exposure to the substance (8.4.4) is interesting as a curiosity. Blasting workers who frequently handle dynamite report that they suffer from a severe pounding headache as soon

TABLE 3. *Complications of chronic intake of migraine drugs and analgesics*

Substance	Complication	Reference
Acetylsalicylic gastric ulcer acid (ASA)	Thrombozytopenia	
ASA + paracetamol	Renal failure	62
Analgesics	Tumors of the kidney and urinary tract, anemia, death from cardiovascular disorders	51
		21
Ergotamine and Dihydroergotamine	Acrocyanosis, muscle cramps, abdominal pain, nausea, intermittent claudication, paresthesia, ischemic neuropathy, dorsal column lesion, hypertension, angina pectoris	4,7,28
		31,32
		43,69,70
Nonsteroidal antirheumatics	Erosive gastritis, peptic ulcer	
Phenacetin	Renal failure	50
		68
Pyrazolone derivatives	Aplastic anemia Agranulocytosis	

as they are not exposed to dynamite. The unofficial way of treating this disabling NTG-withdrawal headache is to handle a piece of dynamite, which they carry around in their pockets. During vacation periods, these patients normally need about a week before the NTG-withdrawal headache disappears and the patients are headache free. Nitrate/nitrite-induced headache (8.1.1) is dealt with in Chapter 114.

Complications

In addition to the chronic headache, other symptoms and disorders may be associated with chronic intake of migraine drugs and analgesics, for example, symptoms of ergotamine toxicity, overt ergotism, nephropathy, and gastrointestinal, cardiovascular, and hematologic disorders (12,21,22) (Table 3). The best known complication of chronic intake of analgesics is nephropathy (9,10,52, 67). A significant percentage of patients (between 0.9% and 32.5%) requiring hemodialysis or renal transplantation are abusers of analgesics (28). There is new evidence that NSAIDs may cause chronic renal failure (2).

Concerning the intensity and duration of ergotamine headache, there is, however, a low correlation between ergotamine headache, the plasma levels of ergotamine measured, and the occurrence of clinical symptoms of ergotamine toxicity in single subjects (3), as would be expected from the low and variable bioavailability of ergotamine (33) and variability among subjects to the pharmacodynamic effects of ergotamine (71).

PROGNOSIS

The success rate of withdrawal therapy within a time window of 1 to 6 months is 72.4% (17 studies, n = 1,101 patients). Success is defined as no headache at all or an improvement of more than 50% in terms of headache days. Three studies had a longer observation period of between 9 and 35 months (6,16,69). The success rates in these studies were 60%, 70%, and 73%, respectively. A 5-year follow-up study found a relapse rate of 40% (61). Whereas Baumgartner and colleagues (6) could not identify prognostic factors that predicted a favorable outcome, Diener and colleagues (16) reported that migraine patients responded better than patients with tension-type headache or patients with both. Regular intake of ergotamine for less than 10 years was also a positive prognostic factor.

MANAGEMENT

A careful history is necessary in the evaluation of chronic headache patients. These patients commonly take several different substances daily, despite the fact that the effect is negligible. The mechanism behind this behavior is merely an attempt to avoid a disabling withdrawal headache. The present and prior use of prescription drugs, nonprescription compounds, and caffeine intake should be recorded. Many patients also abuse other substances, such as tranquilizers, opioids, decongestants, and laxatives (11,34,37). In addition, it is often helpful to allow the patient to keep a diagnostic headache diary for 1 month to register the headache pattern and drug use (58). History and examination also should search for possible complications of regular drug intake, for example, recurrent gastric ulcers, anemia, and ergotism (for details, see the preceding). A good indicator is the number of physicians consulted by the patient and the number of previous unsuccessful therapies. Thus, in one study (16), headache patients had consulted an average of 5.5 physicians each, who had prescribed 8.6 different therapies.

Abrupt drug withdrawal seems to be the first treatment of choice for drug-induced headache. There are, however, no prospective and randomized trials comparing continuation of drug intake and drug withdrawal. A survey of 22 studies dealing with the therapy of drug-induced headache shows that most centers use drug withdrawal as the primary therapy (19). Clinical experience indicates that medical and behavioral headache treatment fails as long as the patient continues to take symptomatic drugs daily. The typical withdrawal symptoms last 2 to 10 days (average, 3.5 days) and include withdrawal headache, nausea, vomiting, arterial hypotension, tachycardia, sleep disturbances, restlessness, anxiety, and nervousness. Seizures or hallucinations were observed only rarely, even in patients abusing barbiturate-containing migraine drugs.

Drug withdrawal is performed differently by different physicians. Most prefer inpatient programs. Hering and Steiner (30) abruptly withdraw the offending drugs on an outpatient basis by adequate explaining the disorder, having regular follow-up, and administering amitriptyline (10 mg at night) and naproxen (500 mg) for the relief of headache symptoms. A consensus paper by the German Migraine Society (18) recommends outpatient withdrawal for patients who do not take barbiturates or tranquilizers with their analgesics and who are highly motivated. Inpatient treatment is recommended for patients who take tranquilizers, codeine, or barbiturates who have failed to withdraw the drugs as outpatients or who have a high depression score.

Treatment

Treatment recommendations for the acute phase of drug withdrawal vary considerably in the 22 studies mentioned herein. They include fluid replacement, analgesics, tranquilizers, neuroleptics, amitriptyline, valproate, intravenous DHE, oxygen, and electric stimulation (65). A double-blind study showed a single subcutaneous dose of sumatriptan to be superior to placebo in the treatment of ergotamine-withdrawal headache, but the headache reappeared within 12 hours (17). An open randomized study indicated that naproxen was better than symptomatic treatment with antiemetics and analgesics (45). Further double-blind controlled trials are needed. In contrast, Dichgans and associates (13) favor giving no replacement therapy at all during the first days of withdrawal, with the intention of reversing the previously learned conditioning response. In this way, patients experience headache improvement without taking any medication.

If more than three migraine attacks per month continue after withdrawal, medical and behavioral prophylaxis should be initiated. The clinical experience shows that many patients respond to prophylactic treatment, for example, with beta-blockers or flunarizine, after drug withdrawal, despite the fact that these drugs seemingly had been unsuccessful previously. Ergotamine, triptans, and possibly analgesics counteract the action of prophylactic therapy and will not improve drug-induced headache. The same phenomenon can be observed for the action of amitriptyline (37) and behavioral therapy (48) in patients with tension-type headache.

Prevention

The most important preventive measure is proper instruction and appropriate surveillance of patients. The migraine patients at risk often have a mixture of migraine and tension-type headaches and should be instructed carefully to use specific antimigraine drugs only for migraine attacks and to treat the other headaches as described in Chapter 83. This point was emphasized in 1951 by Peters and Horton concerning ergotamine abuse; that is, complications can be avoided by taking enough time to give the patient proper instructions to be able to distinguish between vasodilating and nondilating headache (53).

Restricting the dose of ergotamine per attack (4 mg) per week (no more than twice per week) and per month (no more than 20 mg ergotamine) is also helpful in avoiding dependency. In a similar way, the number of doses of triptans should be limited per attack and per month. Migraine drugs that contain barbiturates, codeine, or tranquilizers as well as mixed analgesics should be avoided. An early start of migraine prophylaxis, either by medical or behavioral treatment, can be a preventive measure to avoid drug-induced headache.

REFERENCES

1. Abbott PJ. Caffeine: a toxicological overview. *Med J Aust* 1986;145:518–521.
2. Adams DH, Michael J, Bacon PA, Howie AJ, McConkey B, Adu D. Non-steroidal anti-inflammatory drugs and renal failure. *Lancet* 1986;1:57–59.
3. Ala-Hurula V, Myllylae V, Hokkanen E. Ergotamine abuse: results of ergotamine discontinuation, with special reference to the plasma concentrations. *Cephalalgia* 1982;2:189–195.
4. Andersson PG. Ergotamine headache. *Headache* 1975;15:118–121.
5. Andersson PG. Ergotism—the clinical picture. In: Diener HC, Wilkin-son M, eds. *Drug-induced headache.* Heidelberg: Springer, 1988:16–19.
6. Baumgartner C, Wessely P, Bingöl C, Maly J, Holzner F. Longterm prognosis of analgesic withdrawal in patients with drug-induced headaches. *Headache* 1989;29:510–514.
7. Bowdler I, Kilian J, Gänsslen-Blumberg S. The association between analgesic abuse and headache—coincidental or causal? *Headache* 1988;28:494.
8. Catarci T, Fiacco F, Argentino C, Sette G, Cerbo R. Ergotamine-induced headache can be sustained by sumatriptan daily intake. *Cephalalgia* 1994;14:374–375.
9. De Broe ME, Elseviers MM. Analgesic nephropathy—still a problem? *Nephron* 1993;64:505–513.
10. De Broe ME, Elseviers MM. Analgesic nephropathy. *N Engl J Med* 1998;338:446–452.
11. De Marinis M, Janiri L, Agnoli A. Headache in the use and withdrawal of opiates and other associated substances of abuse. *Headache* 1991;31:159–163.
12. Dichgans J, Diener HC. Clinical manifestations of excessive use of analgesic medication. In: Diener HC, Wilkinson M, eds. *Drug-induced headache.* Heidelberg: Springer, 1988:8–15.
13. Dichgans J, Diener HC, Gerber WD, Verspohl EJ, Kukiolka H, Kluck M. Analgetika-induzierter Dauerkopfschmerz. *Dtsch Med Wschr* 1984;109:369–373.
14. Diener HC. A personal view on the classification and definition of drug dependence headache. *Cephalalgia* 1993;13:68–71.
15. Diener HC, Bühler K, Dichgans J, Geiselhart S, Gerber WD, Scholz E. Analgetikainduzierter Dauerkopfschmerz: Existiert eine kritische Dosis? *Arzneimitteltherapie* 1988;6:156–164.
16. Diener HC, Dichgans J, Scholz E, Geiselhart S, Gerber WD, Bille A. Analgesic-induced chronic headache: long-term results of withdrawal therapy. *J Neurol* 1989;236:9–14.
17. Diener HC, Haab J, Peters C, Ried S, Dichgans J, Pilgrim A. Subcutaneous sumatriptan in the treatment of headache during withdrawal from drug-induced headache. *Headache* 1990;31:205–209.
18. Diener HC, Pfaffenrath V, Soyka D, Gerber W. Therapie des medikamenteninduzierten Kopfschmerzes. *Münch Med Wschr* 1992;134:159–162.
19. Diener HC, Tfelt-Hansen P. Headache associated with chronic use of substances. In: Olesen J, Tfelt-Hansen P, Welch KMA, eds. *The headaches.* New York: Raven Press, 1993:721–727.
20. Dige-Petersen H, Lassen NA, Noer J, Toennesen KH, Olesen J. Subclinical ergotism. *Lancet* 1977;i:65–66.
21. Elkind AH. Drug abuse in headache patients. *Clin J Pain* 1989;5:111–120.
22. Elkind AH. Drug abuse and headache. *Med Clin North Am* 1991;75:717–732.
23. Fanciullacci M, Alessandri M, Pietrini U, Briccolani-Bandini E, Beatrice S. Long-term ergotamine abuse: effect on adrenergically induced mydriasis. *Clin Pharmacol Ther* 1992;51:302–307.
24. Fisher MA, Glass S. Butorphanol (Stadol): a study in problems of current drug information and control. *Neurology* 1997;48:1156–1160.
25. Gaist D, Hallas J, Sindrup SH, Gram LF. Is overuse of sumatriptan a problem? A population-based study. *Eur J Clin Pharmacol* 1996;3:161–165.
26. Gaist D, Tsiropoulus I, Sindrup SH, Hallas J, Rasmussen BK, Kragstrup J. Inappropriate use of sumatriptan: population based register and interview study. *Br J Med* 1998;316:1352–1353.
27. Granella F, Farina S, Malferrari GC. Drug abuse in chronic headache; a clinico-epidemiologic study. *Cephalalgia* 1987;7:15–19.
28. Gutzwiller F, Zemp E. Der Analgetikakonsum in der Bevölkerung und sozioökonomische Aspekte des Analgetikaabusus. In: Mihatsch MJ, ed. *Das analgetikasyndrom.* Stuttgart: Thieme, 1986:197–205.
29. Headache Classification Committee of the International Headache Society. Classification and diagnostic criteria for headache disorders, cranial neuralgias and facial pain. *Cephalalgia* 1988;8(Suppl 7):1–93.
30. Hering R, Steiner TJ. Abrupt outpatient withdrawal of medication in analgesic-abusing migraineurs. *Lancet* 1991;337:1442–1443.
31. Hokkanen E, Waltimo O, Kallanranta T. Toxic effects of ergotamine used for migraine. *Headache* 1978;18:95–98.
32. Horton BT, Peters GA. Clinical manifestations of excessive use of ergotamine preparations and management of withdrawal effect: report of 52 cases. *Headache* 1963;3:214–226.
33. Ibraheem JJ, Palzow L, Tfelt-Hansen P. Low bioavailability of ergota-

mine tartrate after oral and rectal administration in migraine patients. *Br J Clin Pharmacol* 1983;16:695–699.

34. Isler H. Die Behandlung der Kopfschmerzen. *Schweiz Med Wochenschr* 1984;114:1174–1180.

35. Kaube H, May A, Diener HC, Pfaffenrath V. Sumatriptan. *BMJ* 1994; 308:1573–1574.

36. Kielholz P, Ladewig D. Probleme des Medikamentenmißbrauches. *Schweiz Ärztezeitung* 1981;62:2866–2869.

37. Kudrow L. Paradoxical effects of frequent analgesic use. In: Critchley M, Fridman AP, Gorini S, Sicuteri F, eds. *Advances in neurology*, vol 33. New York: Raven Press, 1982:335–341.

38. Lance F, Parkes C, Wilkinson M. Does analgesic abuse cause headache de novo? *Headache* 1988;38:61–62.

39. Laska EM, Sunshine A, Mueller F, Elvers WB, Siegel C, Rubin A. Caffeine as an analgesic adjuvant. *JAMA* 1984;251:1711–1718.

40. Lippman C. Characteristic headache resulting from prolonged use of ergot derivates. *J Nerv Ment Dis* 1955;121:270–273.

41. Lipton RB, Stewart WF, Ryan RE, Saper J, Silberstein S, Sheftell F. Efficacy and safety of acetaminophen, aspirin, and caffeine in alleviating migraine headache pain—three double-blind, randomized, placebo-controlled trials. *Arch Neurol* 1998;55:210–217.

42. Lucas RN, Falkowski W. Ergotamine and methysergide abuse in patients with migraine. *Br J Psychiatry* 1973;122:199–203.

43. Ludolph AC, Husstedt IW, Schlake HP, Grotemeyer KH, Brune GG. Chronic ergotamine abuse: evidence of functional impairment of long ascending spinal tracts. *Eur Neurol* 1988;28:311–316.

44. MacGregor EA, Vorah C, Wilkinson M. Analgesic use: a study of treatments used by patients for migraine prior to attending the City of London migraine clinic. *Headache* 1990;30:571–574.

45. Mathew NT, Kurman R, Perez F. Drug induced refractory headache—clinical features and management. *Headache* 1990;30:634–638.

46. Meadows B. Codeine combinations in clinical practice. *Curr Ther Res* 1984;35:501–510.

47. Medina JL, Diamond S. Drug dependency in patients with chronic headaches. *Headache* 1977;17:12–14.

48. Michultka DM, Blanchard EB, Appelbaum KA, Jaccard J, Dentinger MP. The refractory headache patient. II. High medication consumption (analgesic rebound) headache. *Behav Res Ther* 1989;27:411–420.

49. Micieli G, Manzoni GC, Granella F, Martignoni E, Malferrari G, Nappi G. Clinical and epidemiological observations on drug abuse in headache patients. In: Diener HC, Wilkinson M, eds. *Drug-induced headache*. Berlin: Springer, 1988:20–28.

50. Mihatsch MJ, Hofer HO, Gutzwiller F, Brunner FP, Zollinger HU. Phenacetinabusus I. Häufigkeit, Pro-Kopf-Verbrauch und Folgekosten. *Schweiz Med Wochenschr* 1980;110:108–115.

51. Mihatsch MJ, Knüsli C. Phenacetin abuse and malignant tumors. *Klin Wochenschr* 1982;60:1339–1349.

52. Mihatsch MJ, Schmidlin P, Brunner FP, Hofer HO, Zollinger HU. Phenacetinabusus II. Die chronische renale Niereninsuffizienz im Basler Autopsiegut. *Schweiz Med Wochenschr* 1980;110:116–124.

53. Peters GA, Horton BT. Headache: with special reference to the excessive use of ergotamine preparations and withdrawal effects. *Mayo Clin Proc* 1951;26:153–161.

54. Pini LA, Trenti T. Case report: does chronic use of sumatriptan induce dependence? *Headache* 1994;34:600–601.

55. Rapoport A, Stang P, Gutterman DL, et al. Analgesic rebound headache in clinical practice: data from a physician survey. *Headache* 1996;36:19–19.

56. Rapoport A, Weeks R, Sheftell F. Analgesic rebound headache: theoretical and practical implications. In: Olesen J, Tfelt-Hansen P, Jensen K, eds. *Proceedings of the Second International Headache Congress*. Copenhagen, 1985:448–449.

57. Rowsell AR, Neylan C, Wilkinson M. Ergotamine induced headaches in migrainous patients. *Headache* 1973;13:65–67.

58. Russel MB, Rasmussen BK, Brennum J, Iversen HK, Jensen RA, Olesen J. Presentation of a new instrument: the diagnostic headache diary. *Cephalalgia* 1992;12:369–374.

59. Saper JR. Daily chronic headache. *Neurol Clin* 1990;8:891–901.

60. Saper JR, Jones JM. Ergotamine tartrate dependency: features and possible mechanisms. *Clin Neuropharmacol* 1986;9:244–256.

61. Schnider P, Aull S, Baumgartner C, et al. Long-term outcome of patients with headache and drug abuse after inpatient withdrawal: five year follow-up. *Cephalalgia* 1996;16:481–485.

62. Schwarz A, Faber U, Glaeske G, et al. Daten zu Analgetika-Konsum und Analgetika-Nephropathie in der Bundesrepublik. *Öffentliches Gesundheitswesen* 1985;47:298–300.

63. Silberstein SD, Lipton RB. Chronic daily headache. In: Goadsby PJ, Silberstein SD, eds. *Headache*. Boston: Butterworth-Heinemann, 1997: 201–225.

64. Silberstein SD, Lipton RB, Solomon S, Mathew NT. Classification of daily and near-daily headaches: proposed revisions to the IHS criteria. *Headache* 1994;34:1–7.

65. Silberstein SD, Silberstein JR. Chronic daily headache: long-term prognosis following inpatient treatment with repetitive i.v. DHE. *Headache* 1992;32:439–445.

66. Silverman K, Evans SM, Strain EC, Griffiths RR. Withdrawal syndrome after the double-blind cessation of caffeine consumption. *N Engl J Med* 1992;327:1109–1114.

67. Spühler O, Zollinger HU. Die chronisch interstitielle Nephritis. *Helv Med Acta* 1950;17:564–567.

68. Tfelt-Hansen P. Ergotamine headache. In: Pfaffenrath V, Lundberg P, Sjaastad O, editors. *Updating in headache*. Berlin: Springer, 1985: 169–172.

69. Tfelt-Hansen P, Krabbe AA. Ergotamine abuse. Do patients benefit from withdrawal? *Cephalalgia* 1981;1:29–32.

70. Tfelt-Hansen P, Olesen J. Arterial response to ergotamine tartrate in abusing and non-abusing migraine patients. *Acta Pharmacol Toxicol* 1981;48:69–72.

71. Tfelt-Hansen P, Paalzow L. Intramuscular ergotamine: plasma levels and dynamic activity. *Clin Pharmacol Ther* 1985;37:29–35.

72. van Dusseldorp M, Katan MB. Headache caused by caffeine withdrawal among moderate coffee drinkers switched from ordinary to decaffeinated coffee: a 12 week double blind trial. *BMJ* 1990;300: 1558–1559.

73. Verhoeff NPLG, Visser WH, Ferrari MD, Saxena PR, van Royen EA. Dopamine D2 receptor imaging with 123-I-iodobenzamide SPECT in migraine patients abusing ergotamine: does ergotamine cross the blood brain barrier? *Cephalalgia* 1993;13:325–329.

74. Ziegler DK. Opiate and opioid use in patients with refractory headache. *Cephalalgia* 1994;14:5–10.

The Headaches, Second Edition,
edited by J. Olesen, P. Tfelt-Hansen, and K.M.A. Welch.
Lippincott Williams & Wilkins, Philadelphia © 2000.

The Secondary Headaches

CHAPTER 116

Noncephalic Infection

Milena De Marinis and K. Michael A. Welch

DEFINITION OF HEADACHE ASSOCIATED WITH NONCEPHALIC INFECTION

IHS code and diagnosis:

9.   Headache associated with noncephalic infection
   9.1.   Viral infection
      9.1.1.   Focal noncephalic
      9.1.2.   Systemic
   9.2.   Bacterial infection
      9.2.1.   Focal noncephalic
      9.2.2.   Systemic (septicemia)
   9.3.   Headache related to other infection

WHO code and diagnosis: G44.88. Headache associated with other specific disorders.

Short description: Headache is a new symptom or a new type that occurs concomitantly with a noncephalic infection and disappears less than one month after successful treatment or spontaneous remission of the infection (10).

Other terms: Fever-related headache, headache caused by microorganisms, toxemic headache, septicemic headache, headache as part of the infectious disease syndrome.

EPIDEMIOLOGY

Although commonly reported in the medical history of patients suffering from infectious diseases, there is relatively little information concerning the nature and prevalence of headache associated with noncephalic infections.

M. De Marinis: Department of Neurological Sciences, University of Rome "La Sapienza," 00185 Rome, Italy.

K. M. A. Welch: Department of Neurology, University of Kansas School of Medicine, University of Kansas Medical Center, Kansas City, Kansas, 66106.

This headache type, being a secondary complaint of a common primary disorder, is too complex to lend itself easily to epidemiologic study. In particular, the incidence of headache associated with any one infectious disease is generally unpredictable, with wide variation in reported rates. For example, headache occurs in common infections such as influenza as well as in rare conditions such as malaria, brucellosis, and leptospirosis. The epidemiology of these infections varies widely, depending on the season of the year, geographic location, and individual pattern of disease. The complexity of the problem is further illustrated in the instance of human immunodeficiency virus (HIV)-related headaches, which can occur anytime during the infection, not necessarily as a result of direct intracranial infection. HIV-1 itself, opportunistic conditions, HIV-specific medications, and intracranial complications all may cause headache.

ANATOMY AND PATHOLOGY

By definition, no structural or pathological involvement of intracranial structures is present in this headache type. Nevertheless, certain physiopathologic changes occur in the central nervous system (CNS) that underlie the mechanism of headache.

PATHOPHYSIOLOGY

The mechanisms causing headache associated with noncephalic infection can be considered *direct* or *indirect*. In the former, headache mechanisms are dependent on intrinsic characteristics of microorganisms and, in the latter, headache depends on mechanisms induced by fever. Both involve the interaction of inflammatory mechanisms with pain transmission, however. In particular, localized and systemic inflammatory processes can induce primary hyperalgesia by peripheral nociceptor stimulation and secondary hyperalgesia by increased excitability of spinal second sensory neurons. At the CNS level, inflammation generates a gradual increase in pain reflex magnitude (windup), which is followed by reflex hyperexcitability and central sensitization (see Chap. 112). These phenomena are responsible for the development of diffuse pain (e.g., myalgias, arthralgia) and headache in infectious diseases.

Fever-related Headache

The headache of noncephalic infectious disease is most commonly coincident with fever. Fever can be stimulated exogenously by pyrogens, such as inflammatory mediators and toxins, or directly by microorganisms or fragments of microorganisms that act through intermediary compounds or endogenous pyrogens. For example, endogenously produced antigen–antibody complexes, complement components, and some lymphocyte products induce fever. Endogenous pyrogens release additional pyrogens from stimulated leukocytes or induce interleukin 1 (IL-1), interferon, and tumor necrosis factor (TNF). IL-1 also is produced by monocytes and macrophages, and its targets include neutrophils, fibroblasts, striated muscle cells, and hepatocytes. Intravenous administration of IL-1 and interferon to patients directly induces headache. IL-1 is known to activate serotonergic brainstem nuclei responsible for the sleep disturbances of fever, which is the same brainstem system implicated in headache induction. It also mobilizes amino acids from muscle (through prostaglandin E1, or PGE_1) to induce myalgias that accompany fever, through which it contributes to a tension-type component of the headache indirectly caused by fever. Endothelin-1 seems to participate in the development of fever, possibly through activation of a prostanoid-independent endothelin receptor-mediated mechanism downstream from IL-1β in the fever cascade (7) (Fig. 1). TNF also induces headache when given to patients, although the mechanisms of action remain to be determined.

Pyrogens induce increases in arachidonic acid metabolites, such as the cyclooxygenase-derived prostaglandins prostacyclin and thromboxane. Prostaglandin E_2 (PGE_2) acts directly on the hypothalamus and can initiate fever independent of endogenous pyrogen production. PGE_2 has vasoactive properties and could be indirectly implicated in any vascular component of headache. Endothelin-1 may participate in this process by increasing cyclooxygenase expression and PGE_2 production via endothelin receptors in macrophages (see Fig. 1).

Nitric oxide, possibly involved in migraine (20), also plays an important role in thermoregulation and production of fever. This gas is a mediator of IL-1–induced fever and is involved in pyrogenic fever through nitric oxide synthase–cyclooxygenase pathways. Its increase during

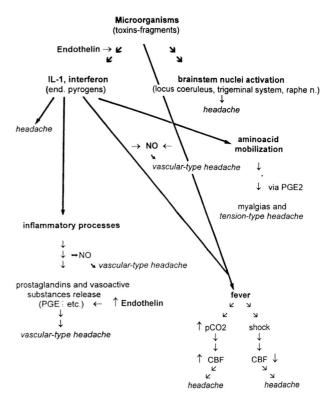

FIG. 1. Physiopathologic mechanisms of headache associated with noncephalic infection.

infections can induce headache with vascular features (see Fig. 1).

Cerebral blood flow (CBF) abnormalities can be produced by shifts in pCO_2 as the respiratory centers participate in the thermoregulatory reflexes of fever. Headache can be secondary to either an increase or a decrease in CBF but most commonly to increased CBF produced by high pCO_2. Hypotension resulting from shock can induce a decrease in CBF and possibly headache (see Fig. 1).

Headache Caused Directly by Microorganisms

These mechanisms may be active during fever but cannot be distinguished from those indirectly due to fever. Some infective agents have a particular tropism for the CNS. They may invade brainstem nuclei, such as the locus ceruleus, trigeminal nuclei, and raphe nuclei, where the release of toxins or the toxic properties of cellular fragments activate headache mechanisms (see Fig. 1). Microorganism-infected cells, especially activated macrophages, release IL-1 and interferon. Besides acting as pyrogens and mediating inflammatory responses, IL-1 and interferon, directly or through nitric oxide, induce headache. The inflammatory response induced by infected cells is also potentiated by these compounds. Activation of the enzymes cyclooxygenase and lipooxygenase leads to the further synthesis and release of pain-sensitizing vasoactive compounds such as prostaglandins, peptides, and amines.

Cyclooxygenase and prostaglandin E_2 production also may be increased by endothelin-1 through activation of endothelin receptors localized in macrophages (see Fig. 1). Plasma protein extravasation and painful vasodilation are induced in the arteries, veins, and meninges supplied by the trigeminal system. Some microorganisms, particularly gram-negative bacteria, provoke platelet activation and degranulation. The release of compounds from platelets, for example, serotonin, has been implicated in the pathogenesis of headache, although some investigators consider this an epiphenomenon. Nitric oxide synthase--cyclooxygenase pathways, which are activated in pyrogenic fever (11), also can contribute to the development of headaches with vascular features.

CLINICAL FEATURES

IHS diagnostic criteria for headache associated with noncephalic infection (Headache Classification Committee, 1988):

A. Symptoms or signs of noncephalic infection
B. Laboratory diagnosis of systemic or focal noncephalic infection
C. Headache as a new symptom or of a new type occurs concomitantly with infection
D. Headache disappears less than 1 month after successful treatment or spontaneous remission of infection

There is little information concerning the characteristics of headache from the available literature. Headache is often reported without specific descriptive features as part of the "infectious disease syndrome" that includes fever, chills, malaise, myalgia, arthralgia, and asthenia. The headache is usually bilateral and diffuse; but in certain cases, occipital, frontotemporal, or distinctive retroocular pain has been reported. The pain is of variable intensity, described as throbbing, pulsatile, or steady, and can be worsened by head movement, coughing, or straining. Apart from symptoms particular to the infection or specifically caused by fever, or both, there may be associated symptoms such as photophobia, phonophobia, conjunctival injection, neck guarding, nausea, and vomiting. The pain may be acute or chronic, outlasting symptoms of active infection. Occasionally, recurrent headaches are experienced. When other neurologic symptoms develop, direct involvement of cerebral structures (e.g., meningitis, encephalitis, brain abscess) should be suspected.

In infectious diseases, headache commonly coexists with fever and is strictly dependent on it, but headache can occur in the absence of fever. Under different circumstances, the pain may have different mechanisms. Thus, the presence or absence of fever may be used in the differential classification of headache, which is rein-forced by the lack of specific headache patterns for any infectious disease. The following alternative categorization may be helpful (5):

1. Headache associated with fever
   a. Headache during fever
   b. Headache persisting after fever
2. Headache not associated with fever
3. Delayed or recurrent headache
4. Migraine, cluster, and tension-type headache occurring in association with noncephalic infection

TYPES OF HEADACHE

Headache Associated with Fever

Headache during Fever

In this classification, fever is considered the cause of headache, which in turn must be time-locked with fever. In viral influenza, headache accompanies fever with an incidence ranging from 68% to 100%. A distinctive retroorbital pain has been described in 26% of patients. In a case series of epidemic adenovirus infection, headache had an incidence of 83% and associated conjunctival injection of 51% (21). A reported epidemic of Oropouche virus illness was characterized by headache, retroorbital pain, and photophobia in the presence of fever. Retroorbital pain, photophobia, nausea, vomiting, skin rash, and severe headache have been reported in dengue fever (16).

In infections caused by *Rickettsiaceae* species, the pathogenic agents of *Ehrlichia canis*, Mediterranean spotted fever, Rocky Mountain spotted fever, and Q fever, headache coexists with fever in a high percentage of patients. In Q fever, 68% of patients have been reported to suffer from severe headache (19). In *E canis* infection, headache, fever and fatigue were reported in 94% of patients (17). A lower prevalence of headache (69%) has been reported in Mediterranean spotted fever (8). Severe retroorbital headache also has been described in association with fever to 104 °F in this illness.

In *Legionella pneumophila* and *Mycoplasma pneumoniae*, headache parallels fever, fatigue, arthralgia, myalgia, cough, and breathlessness. In leptospirosis, which also presents with severe kidney and liver damage sometimes associated with meningeal involvement, headache occurs in 97% of cases and fever in 70% (15). Gastrointestinal infectious diseases may be associated with headache although less predictably. Besides diarrhea and abdominal cramps, which are the most prominent symptoms, coexisting fever is of variable incidence.

There are a number of diseases in which, although headache is coincident with fever, the incidence is low. For example, headache accompanies brucellosis in 23% of cases (13). Daily persistent headaches (mean duration of about 13 days) associated with a low prevalence of fever (34%) have been described in patients who have a variety of other systemic infections, for example, gastrointestinal *Salmonella*, urinary *Coli*, *Streptococcus*, and Epstein-Barr virus (18).

Headache Persisting after Fever

In the acute stage of malaria, fever has been found in 94% of patients and severe headache in 33.5%; however, shivering and headache are the main symptoms in the chronic phases of this disease. A persistent headache lasting beyond the acute fever has been described in Semliki Forest infection (14). Headache is closely associated with erythema and fever in 88% of patients suffering from borreliosis in the acute stages, but radicular pain and cranial neuritis also have been observed in 58% of the cases within 2 weeks and up to 4 months from the onset. Headache duration of about 3 weeks beyond fever has been reported (1).

Headache without Fever

Only a few reports of this category are found in the literature. In trypanosomiasis, headache does not coincide with fever. A long-lasting headache (about 3 months) was found in 73% to 75% of patients, whereas fever was present in only 30% to 36% (3). Other investigators have described a shorter duration of headache (1 week) in this disease. Chronic headaches have been described in *Xylohypha bantiana* infection (6). The fact that this fungal disease was followed later by fever and hemiparesis, however, raises the possibility that the initial headache might have been caused by direct CNS involvement.

Headaches frequently occur independently of fever in HIV-seropositive patients. The presence of headache is higher in women (12) and seems to be correlated with the degree of immunosuppression (2). Headache resembling chronic tension-type headache may precede Lyme neuroborreliosis by months and years in patients who are asymptomatic (4).

Delayed or Recurrent Headache

Meningeal involvement associated with headache is generally present in patients suffering from septicemia, but severe headache that recurs when high fever ends may be the early expression of a delayed septicemia (23). Among the viral illness, herpes simplex and Epstein-Barr virus seem particularly related to the occurrence of delayed or recurrent headaches. For example, chronic headache is the prominent symptom of herpes simplex-induced chronic fatigue syndrome. Moreover, an increased frequency of Epstein-Barr virus excretion has been found in patients with daily persistent headache; so some investigators recommend a search for Epstein-Barr virus infection in patients with "chronic benign daily headache" (22).

Migraine, Cluster, and Tension-Type Headache

Migraine, cluster, and tension-type headache may be induced by noncephalic infections, most probably the fever that occurs in such infections, in patients who have an established history of these disorders. An association of herpes simplex and possibly Epstein-Barr virus has been drawn with the occurrence of cluster headache, although the association between Epstein-Barr virus and cluster headache is uncertain; however, a relationship has been suggested between herpes simplex and cluster headache (9).

PROGNOSIS

Overall, the prognosis for headache depends on successful resolution of systemic infection. When headache occurs during fever, its duration is strictly related to the duration of the acute phase of illness. The persistence of headache lasting months after the resolution of fever and infection is a long-term complication with a good prognosis. If headache occurs with systemic infection and no fever, its course is usually benign, and it terminates spontaneously. The prognosis of delayed or recurrent headache as the expression of a delayed septicemia is adverse and depends on the evolution of the systemic infection itself (fever and toxemia). In some instances of herpes simplex and Epstein-Barr virus infections, headache may either persist or relapse with chronic episodes.

MANAGEMENT

In general, the management of headache associated with noncephalic infections consists of the following procedures: control of fever, specific treatment for the infection, support for the general condition, and bed rest, particularly when fever is high and the infection is severe. Antibiotics, analgesics, antipyretics, and appropriate supportive therapy with intravenous fluids may be needed when headache occurs with fever or when headache recurs as a manifestation of a delayed septicemia. Specific antibiotics may be required when headache persists after fever if this is symptomatic of chronicity of the infectious disease. In headache as a long-term complication after fever and in headache without fever, simple analgesics or nonsteroidal antiinflammatory drugs (NSAIDs) are suggested until the headache resolves. Simple analgesics and NSAIDs are recommended as symptomatic therapy in delayed or recurrent headache. Besides antipyretics and analgesics, specific treatment for migraine, cluster, and tension-type headache are recommended when these preexisting primary headaches are triggered by the infectious disorder. The association of certain drugs is, however, contraindicated. Ergotamine derivatives and serotonin-acting drugs, for instance, cannot be given together with erythromycin.

REFERENCES

1. Asbrink E, Olsson I. Clinical manifestations of erythema chronicum migrans Afzelius in 161 patients: a comparison with Lyme disease. *Acta Dermatol Venereol* 1985;65:43–52.
2. Berger JR, Stein N, Pall L. Headache and human immunodeficiency virus infection: a case control study. *Eur Neurol* 1996;36:229–233.
3. Boa YF, Traore MA, Doua F, Kouassi-Traore MT, Kouassi BE, Giordano C. The different present-day clinical picture of human African trypanosomiasis caused by *T.b. gambiense*: analysis of 300 cases from a focus in Daloa, Ivory Coast. *Bull Soc Pathol Exot* 1988;81:427–444.
4. Brinck T, Hansen K, Olesen J. Headache resembling tension-type headache as a single manifestation of Lyme neuroborreliosis. *Cephalalgia* 1993;13:207–209.
5. De Marinis M, Welch KMA. Headache associated with non-cephalic infections: classification and mechanisms. *Cephalalgia* 1992;12:197–201.
6. Dixon DM, Walsh TJ, Merz WG, McGinnis MR. Infections due to Xylohypha bantiana (*Cladosporium trichoides*). *Rev Infect Dis* 1989;11:515–525.
7. Fabricio AS, Silva CA, Rae GA, D'Orleans-Juste P, Souza GE. Essential role for endothelin ET(B) receptors in fever induced by LPS (E. coli) in rats. *Br J Pharmacol* 1998;125:542–548.
8. Font-Creus B, Bella-Cueto F, Espejo-Arenas E, et al. Mediterranean spotted fever: a cooperative study of 227 cases. *Rev Infect Dis* 1985;7:635–642.
9. Hardebo JE. An association between cluster headache and herpes simplex. *N Engl J Med* 1986;314:316.
10. Headache Classification Committee of the International Headache Society. Classification and diagnostic criteria for headache disorders, cranial neuralgias and facial pain. *Cephalalgia* 1988;8(Suppl 7):57–58.
11. Holloway RG, Kieburtz KD. Headache and the human immunodeficiency virus type 1 infection. *Headache* 1995;35:245–255.
12. Kelleher P, Cox S, McKeogh M. HIV infection: the spectrum of symptoms and disease in male and female patients attending a London hospice. *Palliat Med* 1997;11:152–158.
13. Lulu AR, Araj GF, Khateeb MI, Mustafa MY, Yusuf AR, Fenech FF. Human brucellosis in Kuwait: a prospective study of 400 cases. *QJM* 1988;66:39–54.
14. Mathiot CC, Grimaud G, Garry P, et al. An outbreak of human Semliki Forest vurus infection in Central Africa Republic. *Am J Trop Med Hyg* 1990;42:386–393.
15. Park SK, Lee SH, Rhee YK, et al. Leptospirosis in Chonbuk Province of Korea in 1987: a study of 93 patients. *Am J Trop Med Hyg* 1989;41:345–351.
16. Ramirez-Ronda CH, Garcia CD. Dengue in Western Hemisphere. *Infect Dis Clin North Am* 1994;8:107–128.
17. Rohrbach BW, Harkess JR, Ewing SA, Kudlac J, McKee GL, Istre GR. Epidemiologic and clinical characteristics of persons with serologic evidence of E. canis infection. *Am J Public Health* 1990;80:442–445.
18. Santoni JR, Cantoni-Williams CJ. Headache and painful lymphadenopathy in extracranial or systemic infection: etiology of new daily persistent headaches. *Intern Med* 1993;32:530–532.
19. Smith DL, Ayres JG, Blair I, et al. A large Q fever outbreak in the West Midlands: clinical aspects. *Respir Med* 1993;87:509–516.
20. Thomsen LL, Olesen J. Nitric oxide thory of migraine. *Clin Neurosci* 1998;5:28–33.
21. Turner M, Istre GR, Beauchamp H, Baum M, Arnold S. Community outbreak of adenovirus type 7a infections associated with a swimming pool. *South Med J* 1987;80:712–715.
22. Vanast WJ, Diaz-Mitoma F, Tyrrell DLJ. Hypothesis—Epstein-barr virus-related syndromes: implications for headache research. *Headache* 1987;27:321–324.
23. Westerink MA, Amsterdam D, Petell RJ, Stram MN, Apicella MA. Septicemia due to DF-2. Cause of a false-positive cryptococcal latex agglutination result. *Am J Med* 1987;83:155–158.

The Headaches, Second Edition,
edited by J. Olesen, P. Tfelt-Hansen, and K.M.A. Welch.
Lippincott Williams & Wilkins, Philadelphia © 2000.

The Secondary Headaches

CHAPTER 117

Metabolic and Endocrine Disorders

Peter J. Goadsby

DEFINITION OF HEADACHE ASSOCIATED WITH METABOLIC OR ENDOCRINE DISORDERS

IHS code and diagnosis: 10 Headache associated with metabolic disorders.

WHO code and diagnosis: G44.88 Headache associated with other specified disorders.

Short description: Headache occurring during a metabolic disturbance and disappearing within 7 days after normalization of the metabolic state.

Other terms: None.

IHS diagnostic criteria for headache associated with metabolic or endocrine disorders (Headache Classification Committee, 1988):

A. Symptoms or signs, or both, of metabolic disorder
B. Confirmation by laboratory investigations when specific
C. Headache intensity or frequency, or both, related to variations in metabolic disorder with a specified time lag
D. Headache disappears within 7 days after normalization of metabolic state

The headaches included in this chapter are those that arise *de novo* in close relationship to a metabolic disorder and do not include preexisting headaches worsened by a metabolic perturbation. The main subcategories are discussed individually, and an expanded classification is proposed. Many patients in a variety of situations complain of headache as well as complaining about the medical problem that confronts the physician. Often the headache is ignored as the physician deals with the

P. J. Goadsby: The National Hospital for Neurology and Neurosurgery, London WC1N 3BG, United Kingdom.

patient's primary disorder. These headaches have two levels of importance: To the physician, they are a discomfort that, with recognition, may be treated and certainly will resolve as the patient's primary disorder is managed; they also may provide interesting insights into some of the nociceptive systems that are activated and the sensitivities of these systems to a broad range of insults. It has been suggested that this group of secondary headaches is particularly common in elderly patients and always should be considered in geriatric practice (39).

HYPOXIA

Headache associated with hypoxia is one of the best recognized headache syndromes in this category. It may be caused by either environmental circumstances or disease and can, in the situation of disease, be difficult to ameliorate.

High-Altitude Headache

IHS code and diagnosis: 10.1.1 High-altitude headache.
WHO code and diagnosis: G44.88.

IHS diagnostic criteria for high-altitude headache (Headache Classification Committee, 1988):

A. Occurs within 24 hours after sudden ascent to altitudes above 3,000 m
B. Associated with at least one other symptom typical of high altitude:
  1. Cheyne-Strokes respiration at night
  2. Desire to overbreathe
  3. Exertional dyspnea

One of the best described forms of hypoxic headache is high-altitude headache (1). Interest in this form of headache has been fueled by the expansion of air travel, although its best described phenomenology involves mountainous environments. It is said to have been first described by Jose De Acosta in 1569 after riding a donkey at about 12,500 feet (2). Other clinical features seen in association with headache include nausea, vomiting, vertigo, palpitations, and impaired vision (1,36). Headache is said to be the most common clinical manifestation of altitude sickness and becomes of itself more common as the patient ascends (31). Reasonable population-based data now exist to establish that altitude commonly induces headache, but it does not alter the prevalence of migraine (21). The clinical features of the headache are that it may be pounding (24) and is often frontal. It may be unilateral in up to 25% of patients (31). The pounding feature led to the description of a vascular altitude headache (25), which only represents a subgroup of these headaches and is probably best not subclassified because, at high altitude, migraine is no more common than at sea level (21). Altitude headache is seen commonly in decompression sickness in military aviation, where headache is present in 42% of patients (40).

Altitude headache is worsened by exertion or straining and may be improved by intake of either cold fluids or carbohydrates, although its best treatment is return of the patient to normal altitude. Headache may be associated with cerebral edema or raised cerebrospinal fluid pressure in a more malignant setting (16). Therapeutically, dexamethasone has been trialed against placebo in the setting of altitude headache. Given as 4 mg every 6 hours at the onset of symptoms, it was more effective than placebo (34). This dose cannot be used in a prolonged setting, but it should not be stopped abruptly because to do so this will result in the return of symptoms. In less controlled settings, acetazolamide also has been used in mountain sickness (11,30) but this awaits confirmation. Aspirin has been shown to be effective as a prophylaxis for high-altitude headache in a double-blind, placebo-controlled study that used aspirin 320 mg (9). Oral sumatriptan has been reported to improve high-altitude headache (5), although in a subsequent study ibuprofen 600 mg was effective and sumatriptan 100 mg was not effective (10). From a mechanistic viewpoint, it is likely that the headache is related to the hypoxia directly rather than to any stress that may be attendant with altitude exposure, because endocrine measures of stress are not seen in controlled exposure (37).

Hypoxic Headache

IHS code and diagnosis: 10.1.2 Hypoxic headache (low-pressure environment, pulmonary disease causing hypoxia).

WHO code and diagnosis: G44.88.

HIS diagnostic criteria for hypoxic headache (Headache Classification Committee, 1988): Occurs within 24 hours after acute onset of hypoxia with PaO_2 of 70 mm Hg or less or in chronic hypoxic patients with PaO_2 persistently at or below this level.

For hypoxic headache, the International Headache Society (IHS) classification lists a P_aO_2 of 70 mm Hg or lower as the working level, which seems a reasonable point for its purpose, which is largely nosological. Patients who have reproducible headache at higher levels but with a clear association with the reduced P_aO_2 should also be classified and managed in this group. Hypoxia may be seen in a number of settings, and these are reflected in the more usual setting of the differential diagnosis of hypoxia in Table 1. Although sleep apnea headache has been classified under a separate subheading in the current classification system, its basic pathophysiology would seem not to differ from that of other hypoxic conditions. Contrary to this view, it has been proposed that neck movements during sleep may play a role in headache associated with sleep apnea (6). This concept is not widely held or experimentally validated, however.

The basis for hypoxia leading to headache is not entirely clear, although some useful comprehension may be gleaned from the current understanding of the interaction of hypoxia with cerebral circulatory physiology. Hypoxia leads to increased cerebral blood flow, presumably through a direct metabolic influence (14). This increase in cerebral blood flow is achieved by vasodilatation, which has been thought to be painful, with the stretching of the vessel exciting trigeminal sensory afferents, thus innervating large pain-producing cranial vessels (for review of the trigeminal innervation of the cerebral circulation, see Chap. 9). Many questions remain unanswered concerning this hypothesis, such as, Does hypoxia alter trigeminal firing independent of any effect on the vessels? For the moment, there is some evidence that the reaction on cerebral vessels, whether monitored clinically (33) or in the trigeminal system of experimental animals (15,17), will induce pain or cell firing; thus, the vessel wall concept is attractive by virtue of its simplicity.

Many conditions can lead to hypoxia, some of which are listed in Table 1. Few hypoxic conditions have been studied independently in relationship to the headache they produce, but it would be a reasonable clinical observation that

TABLE 1. *Headache associated with hypoxia (alternative classification)*

Reduced ambient O_2
Altitude-associated headache
Normal altitude, low-O_2 environments
Normal ambient O_2
Pulmonary disease
Disorders of oxygen delivery
Anemia
Cardiac failure
Carbon monoxide intoxication
Cellular hypoxia, such as cyanide poisoning

the method of hypoxia induction is not the chief factor in whether the patient will experience headache. Hypoxia can result from either inadequate pulmonary exchange, such as that seen in pulmonary disease of many etiologies (3), to inadequate tissue or cellular delivery. Carbon monoxide poisoning is now recognized to be associated with a severe, often pounding headache (23) that, in this author's experience, responds to hyperbaric oxygen treatment. Although sleep apnoea is listed in the IHS classification as a hypoxia-associated cause of headache and its clinical cause studied carefully (13,22), modern understanding of the disease with recordings of end-expiratory CO_2 and O_2 saturation would indicate that both are altered; therefore, it should be included in the mixed hypoxia/hypercapnia category. In practice, this does not effect either understanding of the condition or its management, which is the management of the airway obstruction.

Hypercapnia and Mixed Hypoxia and Hypercapnia

IHS code and diagnosis:

10.2 Hypercapnia.
10.3 Mixed hypoxia and hypercapnia.

WHO code and diagnosis: G44.88.

IHS diagnostic criteria for hypercapnia and mixed hypoxia and hypercapnia (Headache Classification Committee, 1988):

102.2 Hypercapnia: Arterial pCO_2 increased above 50 mmHg in the absence of hypoxia.
10.3 Mixed hypoxia and hypercapnia: None.

Hypercapnia, considered significant with a P_aCO_2 of greater than 50 mm Hg, is certainly a powerful cause of headache in many persons. Its mechanism is presumed to be similar to that outlined for hypoxia. The cerebral vasodilating ability of hypercapnia is well recognized and exploited, particularly in the clinical setting of raised intracranial pressure, where it is used in reverse, and hyperventilation is used to lower CO_2, thereby causing cerebral vasoconstriction. This mechanism of the action of hypercapnia is thought to be direct by its generation of H^+ ions that dilate cerebral vessels (14); however, it is unclear what the final mediator is. Hypercapnic vasodilatation depends on the generation of nitric oxide (NO), by activation of NO synthase (NOS) (29), because hypercapnic vasodilatation is blocked in the presence of NOS inhibitors (18), which seems to serve a facilitatory role in the vasodilator process (19). This provides the exciting prospect of a link between the well-characterized experimental headache generated by nitrates that Olesen used to model migraine in humans (20), the treatment of acute migraine by NOS inhibitors (27,28), and a well-recognized and simple headache associated with hypercapnia.

Clinically, hypercapnic headaches are often pounding and generalized. They usually worsen with worsening hypercapnia and always are readily reversed when the hypercapnia is reversed. There are no consistent associations, and they generally respond poorly if not recognized for what they are and treated by analgesics. Mechanistically and clinically, there is little to distinguish mixed hypoxic and hypercapnic headache from simple hypercapnic headache. Their clinical features are indistinguishable, except correction of hypercapnia in the few instances that this occurs tends to leave a duller, generalized, less severe discomfort than that seen before intervention.

HYPOGLYCEMIA

IHS code and diagnosis: 10.4 Hypoglycemia.
Who code and diagnosis: G44.88.
IHS diagnostic criteria for hypoglycemia (Headache Classification Committee, 1988): Blood glucose reduced to below 2.2 mmol/L.

The recognition that reduced blood sugar may have some precipitant or aggravating role in migraine is not new (12). It is a robust clinical observation that skipping meals can trigger headache in susceptible persons and indeed may trigger migraine, particularly in young persons (26). Explanation of this fact to the patient and advice to ensure that lunch is taken can prove invaluable in controlling attacks. Moreover, it can be useful to consider this factor when establishing the time of onset of attacks, because analgesic preparations often may be more successful if given with a small meal. The pathophysiologic basis for these hypoglycemic headache is unclear. The headaches can occur in diabetes (7); however, they do seem different or even necessarily more severe than those seen with much less hypoglycemia. Curiously, headache also has been reported with the use of glucagon to treat hypoglycemia (38); so the simple measure of carbohydrate intake remains superior. The requirement for headaches of a migrainous type would seem to be that there is the basic migrainous diathesis, the genetic component (see elsewhere in this volume), perturbed by the change in blood sugar. The mechanisms may have some relationship to the near absolute requirement of the brain for glucose as a metabolic fuel. Perhaps with a relatively small change, the slightly dysfunctioning cranial pain system inherited by the migraine sufferer is affected sufficiently to release the trigeminal system, with the end result being headache. This question requires further study and, given the lack of well-established methods for studying central pain pathways, may yield some understanding of the condition as a whole.

HEMODIALYSIS

IHS code and diagnosis: 10.5 Dialysis.
Who code and diagnosis: G44.88.

HIS diagnostic criteria for dialysis (Headache Classification Committee, 1988):

A. Onset during hemodialysis and termination within 24 hours after dialysis

B. Occurred during at least half of hemodialyses and at least three times

C. Can be prevented by changing dialysis parameters.

The large water and electrolyte shifts seen in dialysis are well recognized to produce headache (4). Because significant changes could alter many factors, such as the blood–brain barrier, venous side vascular volume, or even cellular neuronal event by virtue of the water changes, it is difficult to achieve a clear understanding of the problem. This problem is important to recognize nonetheless, because it can be important to the patient. It is always amenable to change in the conduct of the dialysis, such as sodium ramping (35) or altering treatment time (8), again suggesting a biophysical basis.

OTHER METABOLIC CONDITIONS

Definition of Other Metabolic Conditions

IHS code and diagnosis: 10.6 Headache related to other metabolic abnormality.

WHO code and diagnosis: G44.88.

IHS diagnostic criteria for headache related to other metabolic abnormality (Headache Classification Committee, 1988): None; syndromes not sufficiently validated.

Several other possible causes of metabolic disturbance have been linked to headache in less convincing ways. Indeed, symptomatic headache is relatively common in the community. Olesen's group has clarified this issue. Some events are so common in their causation of headache that they may be put aside, whereas more sinister causes are sought. It is useful to note that the lifetime prevalence of hangover headache in Denmark is 72%, whereas that for fever-associated headache is 63% (32). Headache is common, and many associations are drawn that should be regarded with caution until they are well established.

In summary, this chapter has attempted to set out and describe some of the main causes of metabolically linked headache. These are interesting and diverse, with the common theme that alterations in the biochemical milieu can have profound and rapid clinically recognizable effects in headache. Many of these syndromes require simple recognition so that their biochemical basis can be corrected and the patient rendered headache free.

REFERENCES

1. Appenzeller O. Altitude headache. *Headache* 1972;12:126–130.
2. Appenzeller O. Cerebrovascular aspects of headache. *Med Clin North Am* 1978;62:467–480.
3. Austen FK, Carmichael MW, Adams RD. Neurologic manifestations of chronic pulmonary insufficiency. *N Engl J Med* 1957;257:579–590.
4. Bana DS, Yap AU, Graham JR. Headache during hemodialysis. *Headache* 1972;112:1–14.
5. Bartsch P, Maggi S, Kleger GR, Ballmer PE, Baumgartner RW. Sumatriptan for high-altitude headache. *Lancet* 1994;344:1445.
6. Biber MP. Nocturnal neck movements and sleep apnea in headache. *Headache* 1988;28:673–674.
7. Blau JN, Pyke DA. Effect of diabetes on migraine. *Lancet* 1970;2:241–243.
8. Brunet P, Saingra Y, Leonetti F, Vacher Coponat H, Ramananarivo P, Berland Y. Tolerance of haemodialysis: a randomized cross-over trial of 5-h versus 4-h treatment time. *Nephrol Dial Transplant* 1996;8:46–51.
9. Burtscher M, Likar R, Machbauer W, Philadelphy M. Aspirin for prophylaxis against headache at high altitudes: randomised, double blind, placebo controlled trial. *BMJ* 1998;316:1057–1058.
10. Burtscher M, Likar R, Nachbauer W, Schaffert W, Philadelphy M. Ibuprofen versus sumatriptan for high-altitude headache. *Lancet* 1995;346:254–255.
11. Coote JH. Medicine and mechanisms in altitude sickness. Recommendations. *Sports Med* 1995;20:148–159.
12. Critchley M, Ferguson FR. Migraine. *Lancet* 1933;1:123–126.
13. Dexter JD. Headache as a presenting complaint of sleep apnea syndrome. *Headache* 1984;24:171.
14. Edvinsson L, MacKenzie ET, McCulloch J. *Cerebral blood flow and metabolism.* New York: Raven Press, 1993.
15. Goadsby PJ, Hoskin KL. The distribution of trigeminovascular afferents in the non-human primate brain *Macaca nemestrina*: a *c-fos* immunocytochemical study. *J Anat* 1997;190:367–375.
16. Hamilton AJ, Cymmerman A, Black PM. High altitude cerebral edema. *Neurosurgery* 1986;19:841–849.
17. Hoskin KL, Kaube H, Goadsby PJ. Sumatriptan can inhibit trigeminal afferents by an exclusively neural mechanism. *Brain* 1996;119:1419–1428.
18. Iadecola C. Does nitric oxide mediate the increases in cerebral blood flow elicited by hypercapnia? *Proc Natl Acad Sci U S A* 1992;89:3913–3916.
19. Iadecola C, Zhang F. Permissive and obligatory roles of NO in cerebrovascular responses to hypercapnia and acetylcholine. *Am J Physiol* 1996;271:R990–1001.
20. Iversen HK, Olesen J, Tfelt-Hansen P. Intravenous nitroglycerin as an experimental headache model: basic characteristics. *Pain* 1989;38:17–24.
21. Jaillard AS, Mazetti P, Kala E. Prevalence of migraine and headache in a high-altitude town of Peru: a population-based study. *Headache* 1997;37:95–101.
22. Kales A, Vela-Bueno A, Kales JD. Sleep disorders: sleep apnea and narcolepsy. *Ann Intern Med* 1987;106:434–443.
23. Kales SN. Carbon monoxide intoxication. *Am Fam Physician* 1993;48:1100–1104.
24. Kassirer MR, Such RV. Persistent high-altitude headache and aguesia without anosmia. *Arch Neurol* 1989;46:340–341.
25. King AB, Robinson SM. Vascular headaches of acute mountain sickness. *Aerospace Medicine* 1972;43:849–851.
26. Lance JW, Goadsby PJ. *Mechanism and management of headache,* 6th ed. London: Butterworth-Heinemann, 1998.
27. Lassen LH, Ashina M, Christiansen I, et al. Nitric oxide synthesis inhibition: a new principle in the treatment of migraine attacks. *Cephalalgia* 1998;18:27–32.
28. Lassen LH, Ashina M, Christiansen I, Ulrich V, Olesen J. Nitric oxide synthesis inhibition in migraine. *Lancet* 1997;349:401–402.
29. Moncada S, Palmer RMJ, Higgs EA. Nitric oxide: physiology, pathophysiology, and pharmacology. *Pharmacol Rev* 1991;43:109–142.
30. Mountain RD. Treatment of acute mountain sickness [Letter]. *JAMA* 1983;250:1392.
31. Raskin NH. *Headache.* New York: Churchill-Livingstone, 1988.
32. Rasmussen BK, Olesen J. Symptomatic and nonsymptomatic headaches in a general population. *Neurology* 1992;42:1225–1231.
33. Ray BS, Wolff HG. Experimental studies on headache: pain sensitive structures of the head and their significance in headache. *Arch Surg* 1940;41:813–856.
34. Rock PB, Johnson TS, Cymerman A, Burse RL, Falk LJ, Fulco CS.

Effect of dexamethasone on symptoms of acute mountain sickness at Pikes Peak, Colorado (4,300 m). *Aviat Space Environ Med* 1987;58: 668–672.

35. Sang GL, Kovithavongs C, Ulan R, Kjellstrand CM. Sodium ramping in hemodialysis: a study of beneficial and adverse effects. *Am J Kidney Dis* 1997;29:669–677.

36. Singh I, Khanna PK, Srivastava MC. Acute mountain sickness. *N Engl J Med* 1969;280:175–184.

37. Vaernes RJ, Owe JO, Myking O. Central nervous reactions to a 6.5-hour altitude exposure at 3048m. *Aviat Space Environ Med* 1984;55: 921–926.

38. Vukmir RB, Paris PM, Yealy DM. Glucagon: prehospital therapy for hypoglycemia. *Ann Emerg Med* 1991;20:375–379.

39. Warner JJ. Headaches in older patients: Ddx and Tx of common non-vascular causes. *Geriatrics* 1985;40:69–76.

40. Wirjosemito SA, Touhey JE, Workman WT. Type II altitude decompression sickness (DCS): U.S. Air Force experience with 133 cases. *Aviat Space Environ Med* 1989;60:252–262.

The Headaches, Second Edition,
edited by J. Olesen, P. Tfelt-Hansen, and K.M.A. Welch.
Lippincott Williams & Wilkins, Philadelphia © 2000.

The Secondary Headaches

CHAPTER 118

Disorders of the Skull and Cervical Spine

Hartmut Göbel and John G. Edmeads

HEADACHE ASSOCIATED WITH THE SKULL

IHS code and diagnosis: 11.1 Cranial bone.
WHO code and diagnosis: G44.84 Headache or facial pain associated with disorders of cranium, cranial and facial structures, cranial nerves, neck, and spine. G44.840 Headache associated with disorders of the cranial bone (M80-M89.8).

Anatomy and Pathophysiology

The Skull as a Cause of Headache

The bone of the skull has limited sensitivity to pain because only a few nerve fibers enter it from the overlying periosteum. The periosteum is more pain sensitive, and skull lesions therefore produce headache chiefly by involving it (Fig 1). The lesions of the skull most likely to do this are those that are rapidly expansile, aggressively osteoclastic, or have an inflammatory component.

Most skull lesions are asymptomatic (32) and are discovered as incidental findings on roentgenograms or other imaging procedures done to investigate unrelated complaints, including fibrous dysplasia, osteomas, epidermoid cysts, metastatic cancers, hemangiomas, eosinophilic granulomas, and Paget's disease of the skull. Some of these lesions, notably hemangiomas and eosinophilic granulomas and the rare aneurysmal bone cysts, may present with a tender swelling on the calvarium but not with spontaneous headache.

H. Göbel: Kiel Pain Clinic, University of Kiel, D-24149 Kiel, Germany.
J.G. Edmeads: Department of Medicine, Sunnybrook Health Science Center, University of Toronto, Toronto, Ontario M4N 3M5, Canada.

Relatively few skull lesions produce headache. Multiple myeloma often presents with bone pain anywhere in the body, and skull deposits are sometimes a source of such pain. The multiplicity of the deposits and the proclivity of tbe myeloma cells to produce osteoclast activating factor likely account for the production of head pain by this particular bone tumor. Osteomyelitis produces spontaneous head pain because of its rapid evolution and its inflammatory component. Although most cases of Paget's disease of the skull are asymptomatic, remodeling of bone, by producing basilar invagination, may cause headache either through traction on the upper cervical nerve roots or by the production of cerebrospinal fluid pathway distortion with hydrocephalus.

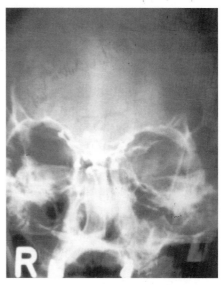

FIG. 1. Headache due to skull fractures after a horse kick.

HEADACHES ASSOCIATED WITH DISORDERS OF THE CERVICAL SPINE

IHS code and diagnosis: 11.2 Neck. 11.2.1 Cervical spine. 11.2.2 Retropharyngeal tendinitis.

WHO code and diagnosis: G44.841 Headache associated with biomechanical lesions of cervical spine (M99.x1). G44.842 Headache associated with retropharyngeal tendinitis (M79.8).

Short description: Cervical headaches are associated with movement abnormalities in cervical intervertebral segments. The disorder may be located in the joints or ligaments. The abnormal movement may occur in any component of intervertebral movement and manifests during either active or passive examination of the movement.

Other terms: Cervicogenic headache.

Anatomy and Pathophysiology

The Neck as a Cause of Headache

To implicate diseases or dysfunctions of the neck as a cause of headache, three conditions should apply (8):

1. The cervical structures held to be the source of the headache must be pain sensitive.
2. They must be located in an area where the "hard wiring" of the neural network permits referral of pain from that cervical focus to the head.
3. The disease or dysfunctions involving those structures must be identifiable and verifiable.

Following some amplification of these criteria, the various entities that have been cited as examples of headache arising from the neck will be assessed in terms of how well they fulfill them.

Numerous cervical structures contain nociceptors (1): the joints, periosteum, and ligaments of the cervical spine; the muscles around the cervical spine; the cervical nerve roots and nerves; and the vertebral arteries that travel in intimate relationship to the cervical spine (Table 1). Pathways through which nociceptive impulses origi-

TABLE 1. *Pain-sensitive structures of the neck*

Vertebral column
Apophyseal joints
Atlantooccipital (condylar) joints
Annulus fibrosus
Spinal ligaments
Vertebral periosteum
Cervical muscles
Cervical nerve roots and nerves
Vertebral arteries
Carotid arteries

From ref. 8, with permission.

nating in these structures may be referred to the head include the following:

1. The C2 sensory root and its extensions, the greater and lesser occipital nerves; stimulation of these produces pain in the back of the head.
2. The C1 sensory root (although by some authorities believe it to be nonexistent or inconsequential); stimulation produces pain in the vertex or frontal head region (17).
3. Connections between the tentorial branches of the ophthalmic division of the trigeminal nerve and posterior fossa branches of C2 may allow referral of pain from C2-innervated structures to the front of the head.
4. The spinal tract of the trigeminal nerve descends to the level of C2–4; intermingling of impulses from the upper cervical segments with those from VI may allow referral of pain from these segments to the head (18).

It would appear that nociceptive impulses originating in the rostral three or four cervical segments, or at the craniovertebral junction, can be referred to the head; there seems to be no known physiologic basis for cephalic referral of pain originating from the lower cervical segments.

The *cervical causes of headaches* are listed in Table 2. Among these are *developmental anomalies* of the craniovertebral junction and upper cervical spine, which frequently cause headaches. McRae (22) reported occipital or suboccipital pain as the presenting complaint in 26% of anomalies such as basilar invagination, congenital atlantoaxial dislocation, and separate odontoid; in cases such as these, stretching of upper cervical nerve roots can be seen at surgery. The common Klippel-Feil anomaly does not produce head or neck pain in isolation but may do so when excessive mobility occurs between vertebrae rostral to this congenital fusion, with secondary facet joint changes. The even more common spina bifida is also usually asymptomatic, but associated soft-tissue anomalies, such as Arnold-Chiari malformation, with or without hydrocephalus, may cause headaches (Fig 2). Whereas there is nothing specific about headaches from craniovertebral anomalies, they tend to exhibit some suggestive features, such as posterior location, triggering by flexing of the neck or by coughing and straining, and sometimes a pronounced postural component that may mimic low-pressure headaches (19). Depending on what neural anomalies are associated, there may be complaints of vertigo, facial numbness, limb weakness, or ataxia, as well as neurologic findings related to the upper cervical nerve roots, lower brainstem, or upper cervical cord.

Acquired lesions of the craniovertebral junction and upper cervical spine, such as primary tumors (meningioma, schwannoma, ependymoma), Paget's disease of the

TABLE 2. *Cervical causes of headache*

Accepted causes	Developmental anomalies of the craniovertebral junction and upper cervical spine
	Tumors of craniovenebral junction and upper cervical spine (primary, and multiple myeloma)
	Paget's disease of the skull with secondary basilar invagination
	Osteomyelitis of the upper cervical vertebrae
	Rheumatoid arthritis of the upper cervical spine
	Ankylosing spondylitis of the upper cervical spine
	Traumatic subluxation of the upper cervical vertebrae
	Retropharyngeal tendinitis
	Craniocervical dystonias
Controversial causes	Cervical disk disease and spondylosis
	"Whiplash" injuries[a]
Currently unaccepted causes	Posterior cervical sympathetic syndrome of Barré
	Migraine cervicale syndrome of Bartschi-Rochaix

[a]Bogduk's "third occipital headache" and Sjaastad's "cervicogenic headache" are not specific disease entities but rather syndromes or reaction patterns said to result from a variety of lesions.

skull with secondary basilar invagination, osteomyelitis of the upper cervical vertebrae, and multiple myeloma of the skull base or upper cervical vertebrae may produce headache by erosion of the pain-sensitive structures or traction on upper cervical nerve roots (Fig 3). Blows to the head or even forceful sneezing may produce rotatory subluxation of the atlas, which, through irritation of synovial joints, causes persistent occipital headache. Rheumatoid arthritis of the upper cervical spine produces headaches through a variety of mechanisms, including inflammation of the synovial atlantooccipital and atlantoaxial joints and stretching of upper cervical ligaments and nerve roots caused by atlantoaxial subluxation secondary to attenuation of the transverse ligament of the odontoid (this also may occur in ankylosing spondylitis). As with the congenital atlantoaxial and upper cervical anomalies, these acquired disorders tend to produce occipital headaches that are worsened or triggered by neck movements or straining, although often the postural element of the headache is not so evident. In addition, aids to diagnosis include the stigmata of the underlying diseases encountered in the history, examination, and investigations. When examining patients with rheumatoid arthritis who have headache, care should

be taken when the patient is asked to flex the neck, because occasional fatalities have resulted from compression of the medulla by the odontoid, which, no longer bound to the atlas by the transverse ligament, fails to move away from the brainstem on anteflexion of the cervical spine.

Cervical spondylosis and *cervical disc* disease are not universally accepted as cervical causes of headache, first because they are almost ubiquitous in persons over the age of 40 years, and, second, because they typically involve the lower cervical discs and vertebrae, where it would be difficult to explain, physiologically, referral of pain to the head. Possibly, the restriction of movement in these lower cervical regions leads to excessive "play" in the rostral apophyseal joints, for example, at C2–3 or C3–4, and this could refer pain to the head. This explanation is plausible, but the evidence is incomplete, and the issue is unresolved. Researchers who teach that cervical spondylosis is an important cause of headache describe the headache of cervical disc disease as being posterior, often unilateral, sometimes constant, nonthrobbing, and aggravated by neck movements and occasionally by coughing and straining (23).

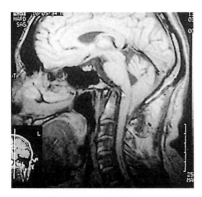

FIG. 2. Arnold-Chiari malformation with persistent movement-dependent neck pain.

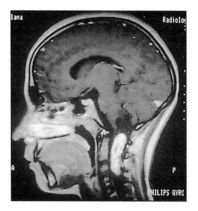

FIG. 3. Intraspinal tumor (cervical ependymoma) with increasing cervicogenic headache.

Trauma, including "whiplash" injuries to the neck, also has met with a mixed reception as a cause of headache. Clearly, many people with an extension–flexion injury of the neck do experience self-limited neck, occipital, and occasionally frontal pain, which clears within days or a few weeks; likely, this pain results from injury to the upper cervical ligaments and muscles. More chronic headaches, lasting months or years, are more difficult to explain. Some investigators (4), noting the frequency of litigation in such cases, ascribe them to psychological factors, and others (13) postulate that other mechanisms, such as compression of the C1 or C2 sensory nerve roots between the occiput and the atlas or the atlas and the axis, respectively, are responsible. Still others believe that shearing injuries of the long axons in the brainstem and upper cord may disrupt central pain and other regulatory mechanisms, allowing the emergence of headache; such a mechanism could account for the typical migraine that has followed some whiplash injuries and that has responded well to prophylactic antimigraine medication despite ongoing litigation (32). It may be that such subtle brainstem or cervical cord trauma leads to the full-blown whiplash syndrome, which, in addition to the posterior, often unilateral headache worsened by neck movements, also comprises dizziness, anxiety, visual disturbances, loss of stamina, and a host of other symptoms that lend a "neurotic coloring" to the clinical picture. This coloring, in combination with the usual failure to detect objective physical, neurophysiologic, or roentgenographic changes, contributes to the disrepute accorded this entity by some authorities.

Pain arising from *craniocervical dystonia* is either due to continuous contraction of muscles, or it may occur as a result of secondary irritation of neural structures, for example, at the emergence of the occipital nerves, induced by the muscular hyperactivity (20). If the condition persists for a long time, it may in some cases give rise to degenerative changes in the skeletal system of the cervical spine, mandibular joint, or dentition, which may cause additional local pain. The continuous contraction may lead to hypertrophy of the affected muscles.

Dystonia is not a disease in itself, but like spasticity or headache, a syndrome diagnosis. Dystonia is a syndrome characterized by continuous muscle contractions, which cause rotatory and repeated movements or abnormal postures. The involuntary movements may be phasal, tonic, or rhythmic and may occur to varying degrees and at various speeds. As in headache conditions, a distinction is made between primary (*idiopathic*) and secondary (*symptomatic*) forms.

In recent decades, the focal dystonias occurring in the head and neck region have been described by various collective names (cranial, cervicofacial, oromandibular), which often have been used as synonyms. Certainly, there is no controversy about the distinction between *cranial dystonia* (blepharospasm, spasmodic dysphonia, mandibu-lar, or lingual dystonia) and the *cervical dystonias* (torticollis). In view of the similarities between these two groups, it would seem sensible to use the term *craniocervical dystonia* (CCD). Here, too, distinction should be made between primary (idiopathic) and secondary (symptomatic) CCD. The individual forms of CCD occur with an incidence of 5 to 15 per million (13).

Clinical Features

Cervical spine disorders are not infrequently seen as one of the most common causes of headache, because the pain often is localized in the occipital and nuchal region. Moreover, degenerative changes in the cervical vertebral column are found in almost everyone over the age of 40 years (7,8). In view of the localization of the identifiable degenerative changes, it is logical to assume that spondylosis or osteochondrosis are responsible for the headache. Large-scale controlled studies have shown, however, that cervical spine changes are as widespread in patients without headache and neck pains. In other words, spondylosis or osteochondrosis cannot be taken as an explanation of the headache.

The following are the *general diagnostic criteria for headache associated with disorders of the skull or neck* (14):

A. Clinical or laboratory evidence of disorder in cranium.
B. Headache located in the affected cranial structure and radiating to its surroundings. Pain may or may not be referred to more distant areas of the head.
   1. Headache disappears within 1 month after successful treatment or spontaneous remission of the underlying disorder.

The following are the diagnostic criteria for headache associated with disorders of the cervical spine:

A. Pain is localized to the neck and occipital region. May project to forehead, orbital region, temples, vertex, or ears.
B. Pain is precipitated or aggravated by special neck movements or sustained neck posture.
C. At least one of the following occurs:
   1. Resistance to or limitation of passive neck movements.
   2. Changes in neck muscle contour, texture, tone, or response to active and passive stretching and contraction.
   3. Abnormal tenderness of neck muscles.
D. Radiological examination reveals at least one of the following:
   1. Movement abnormalities in flexion and extension.
   2. Abnormal posture.
E. Fractures, congenital abnormalities, bone tumors, rheumatoid arthritis, or other distinct pathology (not spondylosis or osteochondrosis).

A diagnosis of headache caused by the cervical spine requires the satisfaction of specific criteria. These relate in the first instance to the headache symptoms, which must occur in the *nuchal and occipital region*; radiation to other parts of the head or neck is possible. The headache may occur either *unilaterally* or *bilaterally.*

The second major criterion is that it must be possible to provoke the pain by means of *particular neck movements* or particular positions (Table 3). This provocation is due to manifestation of a motility disorder of intervertebral segments of the cervical spine. The functional disorder may be localized either in the ligaments or in the joints. To provoke the pain, it is necessary to make active and passive movements in every conceivable intervertebral movement component. Whereas a large number of headache syndromes involve occipital and nuchal headache localization, pain provocation by means of particular neck movements in particular positions is possible in onlly a minority of headache types (25,33).

Certain additional clinical criteria also must be satisfied as an important condition. The examination must reveal evidence of the following:

- Restricted movement when testing passive motility or
- Changes in structure, contour, or tone of cervical muscles or
- Increased sensitivity to pain on palpation

As a further condition, the radiologic diagnosis must reveal at least one of the following findings:

- Motility problems on flexion and extension
- Abnormal posture of the cervical spine
- Fractures, congenital malformation, bone tumors, rheumatoid arthritis, or other marked change (but not spondylosis or osteochondrosis)

Retropharyngeal tendinitis is an uncommon condition of unknown etiology that is characterized by the acute onset of upper cervical and occipital pain, aggravated by neck movements (especially extension) and accompanied by pain on swallowing and, in the early stages, tenderness in the sides of the upper neck, mild to moderate fever, and often an increased erythrocyte sedimentation rate. Radiographs of the cervical spine show increased thickness of the C1–4 prevertebral soft tissue, sometimes with calcification (computerized tomography may show this better); the symptoms and the prevertebral swelling subside over several days, although resolution may be accelerated by using nonsteroidal antiinflammatory drugs (NSAIDs) (9,10).

The following are the *diagnostic criteria for retropharyngeal tendinitis*

A. Pain is in the back of the neck radiating to the back of the head or to the whole head.
B. Pain is nonpulsating, unilateral or bilateral, and aggravated severely by bending the head backward.

C. Prevertebral soft tissues in adults measure more than 7 mm at the level between C1 and C4 (special radiographic technique may be required).
D. Alleviation within 2 weeks of treatment with NSAIDs in recommended doses.

Focal dystonias and *especially CCDs* are conditions encountered in middle-aged adults (Table 4). If they occur in children, the possibility of incipient focal development of a generalized dystonia or a symptomatic CCD should be considered.

The common central symptom of focal dystonia is the abnormal movement or defective position of the affected parts of the body. The underlying muscular hyperactivity may be tonic and therefore give rise to a *slow, smooth movement* or a *fixed defective position*; it may be *phasal*, thereby causing *jerky, repetitive movements* (*myoclonic dystonia*), or it may have a *rhythmic movement* character, which frequently makes it difficult to distinguish from various forms of tremor.

Craniocervical dystonias can be classified on the basis of the musculature affected. Both isolated dystonias of individual muscle areas served by cranial nerves, and combinations of various types of focal dystonia may occur. Table 4 summarizes the main clinical characteris-

TABLE 3. *Examination of cervical spine functions*

Normal findings for motility of cervical spine
Forward inclination
chin–sternum distance <2 cm
Backward inclination
chin–sternum distance >20 cm
Rotation in upright head position at least 60 degrees to each side
Rotation at maximum forward inclination at least 45 degrees to each side
Rotation at maximum backward inclination at least 40 degrees to each side
Lateral inclination at least 45 degrees to each side
Radiologic evidence of motility disorders of cervical spine
Increased excursion on flexion or extension
Formation of angulation of spine with increased motility of a segment
Subluxation with spondylolisthesis
Reduced motility or blockage of a single segment with failure to reach the following normal values
C0/C1: 15 degrees
C1/C2: 14 degrees
C2/C3: 11 degrees
C3/C4: 17 degrees
C4/C5: 21 degrees
C5/C6: 22 degrees
C6/C7: 17 degrees
Possible defective positions of cervical spine (normal: physiologic lordosis)
Stretched posture
Kyphosis
Scoliosis

From ref. 11, with permission.

TABLE 4. *Main clinical characteristics of focal dystonias of the head and neck accompanied by pain*

Form	Main clinical characteristics	Pain criteria
Mandibular dystonia	Dystonia of the jaw closing or jaw opening muscles. The principal symptoms are the defective jaw position and the painful spasms of the masticatory muscles. Patients may bite their own tongue. In severe cases, dystonia of the jaw-closing muscle in particular leads to heavy wear of the teeth, or even loss of teeth due to their breaking out	Owing to hypercontracted muscles, pain is frequent and often involves great suffering; as a secondary symptom, a mandibular joint syndrome or oromandibular dysfunction may occur and maintain pain; pain often corresponds to tension-type headache
Pharyngeal dystonia	Pharyngeal dystonia or spasmodic dysphagia occurs very rarely as isolated focal dystonia. More frequently it is a symptom of the Meige syndrome, or it accompanies lingual and laryngeal dystonia. Even if it dominates the overall clinical picture, dystonia of other muscle groups will also be found as a rule	Very annoying sensation of cramp and tension
Torticollis spasmodicus (TS)	The main symptom is the abnormal movement or position of the head; depending on the dominant direction of movement, a distinction is made between rotatory TS (the most common variant), laterocollis, and retrocollis or anterocollis. Combinations of these positions are found in about 66% of patients	Pain in neck region: pain is often a principal symptom of the condition; the pain is caused by local contractions and secondary vertebragenic changes, in rare cases going as far as vertebra luxation with paraplegia; responds well to botulinum toxin and nonsteroidal antirheumatics
Lingual dystonia	Involuntary sticking-out of tongue; continual rolling movements of the tongue, which can be observed particularly well with the mouth open; sometimes accompanying oral movements	Occasionally accompanied by pain
Segmental craniocervical dystonia	Combinations of the cranial and cervical dystonias described above; a combination of blepharospasm with an oromandibular dystonia is most common (Meige syndrome)	

tics of focal dystonias accompanied by pain arranged in order of the cranial nerve regions affected (20).

SYNDROMES NOT GENERALLY ACCEPTED

The third occipital headache of Bogduk (5) is controversial. The third occipital nerve, which is the superficial medial branch of the C3 dorsal ramus, supplies the C3 dermatome, part of the semispinalis capitis muscle, and the C2–3 zygapophyseal joint. Bogduk and Marsiand, in a group of patients with occipital headaches radiating frontally and at least one feature that could suggest a cervical origin for the pain (e.g., history of neck injury, triggering of pain by neck movement) blocked this nerve and recorded relief of headache in two thirds of patients. He postulated that disease of the C2–3 zygapophyseal joints could produce headaches with pain transmitted by the third occipital nerve (6). There was no radiologic evidence of any such disease, however. An alternative explanation is that the nerve blocks relieved headache in a nonspecific fashion by interrupting normal afferent impulses

that, along with other impulses, were helping to reduce the stimulation threshold of the trigeminal system in the upper cervical cord. A crucial physiologic point, often overlooked by advocates of cervicogenic head pain syndromes, is that relief of pain following nerve block does not mean necessarily that the pain emanates from a structure supplied by that nerve.

Most modern researchers no longer support the validity of the posterior cervical sympathetic syndrome of Barré (2) or of the "migraine cervicale" syndrome of Bartschi-Rochaix (3). These are closely related concepts. In the former, symptoms of headache, neck pain, dizziness, visual blurring, emotional and cognitive disturbances, and so forth were ascribed to osteophytes irritating the sympathetic nerve plexus around the vertebral artery. In the latter, similar symptoms were believed to be due to actual compression of the vertebral artery by osteophytes. In both, trauma was believed to be a major precipitating factor. The physical findings were said to be the same in suboccipital tenderness, spasm of neck muscles, limitation of neck movements, aggravation of headache by neck movement, and occasionally C2 sensory changes. The similarity of these syndromes to the whiplash syndrome is apparent, and the mutual identity of these three entities is likely but, of course, renders the situation no less unclear.

Currently, there is debate about the frequency and validity of the concept of cervicogenic headache as promulgated by Sjaastad and colleagues (3,26–29). These investigators indicated that many patients report a fairly uniform headache profile that suggests that the neck is the origin of the headache (8,30). The profile includes unilateral pain (always on the same side) beginning in the neck and eventually spreading to the oculofrontotemporal areas, where the maximum pain often is "located"; the headache is moderate and nonthrobbing, of variable duration, or continuous and is provoked by neck movements or sustained awkward head postures or by pressure over the posterior neck or occiput. It may be accompanied by vague, nonradicular neck, shoulder, and arm pain and by a reduced range of motion in the cervical spine (33). Sjaastad and colleagues believe that female gender, a history of head or neck trauma, and transient relief by anesthetic blockade of the major occipital nerve or the C2 root are important diagnostic criteria. As optional extras, they cite the occurrence of nausea, vomiting, phonophotophobia, edema, or flushing about the eye, blurred vision of the eye ipsilateral to the pain, and difficulty swallowing.

The Sjaastad school carefully stipulates (26–29) that "cervicogenic headache" is not a disease entity but rather a reaction pattern, nor do they maintain that the headache emanates for any one single structure or process in the neck; rather, it may originate in any cervical bony or soft tissue. Thus, in a sense, the concept of cervicogenic headache simply reiterates what has been known for many years and what has been reviewed in this chapter: that some headaches may result from dysfunction or disease of the neck and that these headaches may exhibit clinical characteristics that suggest their origin in the neck. None of this is controversial. Sjaastad and colleagues have drawn criticism, however, because of their position that cervicogenic headache may be extremely common and that, given the similarity between some of the clinical features of migraine without aura and those of cervicogenic headache, in all probability several cervicogenic headache cases at present are being classified as cases of migraine without aura. Also criticized is their consideration of relief by neural blockade as a major diagnostic criteria for cervicogenic headache; as noted above, the physiologic basis of this conclusion is doubtful.

Further impeding general acceptance of this particular concept of cervicogenic headache is the association that has grown between it and other concepts not in the mainstream of current scientific thought, such as the occurrence of myofascial trigger points (16) and the finding of other soft-tissue changes (21), such as thickening of the skin (the so-called pinch-and-roll sign). Elicitation of these signs seems to be a subjective art, with poor interobserver agreement; even should these signs be verified, they may be nonspecific accompaniments of pain rather than markers of some cervical process. "Harder" investigations of cervical function failed to yield consistent abnormal findings in cervicogenic headache. For example, Sjaastad and associates (26–29) found no differences between radiographs of the cervical spine of patients with cervicogenic headache and those of age- and sex-matched controls. Pfaffenrath and colleagues (24) found mobility in the upper cervical spine to be decreased more in cervicogenic patients than in controls; however, from a qualitative point of view, there were no changes in the cervicogenic headache patients that could not be found in some control patients.

The International Headache Society (IHS) has adopted a more conservative view of cervicogenic headache. These somewhat more stringent criteria form a more acceptable basis for considering a headache to originate in the neck (30), but the current controversy is far from settled.

MANAGEMENT

Therapy always starts with a thorough diagnostic investigation to identify *symptomatic forms* and, insofar as possible, treat the causes. Ipsilateral blockades of the C2 root or greater occipital nerve, in the opinion of some investigators, may allow differentiation between cervicogenic headache due to irritation of the C2 root and primary headache syndromes, such as migraine or tension-type headache, but whether it does or not, the therapeutic results are of short duration; in any event, the differential diagnosis can be made through history and clinical examination. Neither symptomatic pharmacologic nor surgical nor chiropractic procedures lead to significant improvement or remission. The side effects of analgesics, antiphlogistics, and muscle relaxants preclude long-term treatment. Additional physiotherapy, including muscle relaxation techniques (Jacobson) and psychotherapy, can provide some relief.

Currently, no specific therapy for craniocervical dystonia has achieved general recognition. Dopa-sensitive dystonic syndromes and symptomatic forms, in particular Wilson's disease (hepatolenticular degeneration), must be detected as early as possible. Whereas in the past the focus has been on systemic (oral) pharmacotherapy, in recent years, local injections of botulinum toxin have brought a decisive improvement in CCD treatment (12,15,20). The success rate is more than 60% and can be increased further by targeted myographic selection of the dystonic muscles. In cases of multifocal or segmental dystonia, administration of botulinum toxin often has a favorable effect on the untreated muscle groups as well; the reason for this phenomenon is unclear. Specific side effects may be produced by excessive weakening of the treated muscle or diffusion into adjacent muscles, which, depending on the injection site, may result in double vision, swallowing problems, reduced head control, and other effects. These and the nonspecific side effects (tiredness, dizziness) are relatively rare and also completely reversible. Therapeutic control of the pain is particularly successful, being achieved in nearly all patients. The actual motility disorder, by contrast, is less easy to influence effectively (blepharospasm and spasmodic dysphonia in approximately 90%, torticollis spasmodicus in approximately 80%).

Physiotherapy is a crucial mainstay of therapy for torticollis. Psychotherapeutic methods have been suggested and sometimes can be used with success. Opinions about the effect of biofeedback and hypnosis differ.

In cases of craniocervical dystonia that are otherwise untreatable, serious consideration should be given to surgical methods in the individual case. In the past, stereotactic thalamotomies in particular have been suggested; however, complications (especially dysarthria) were a frequent occurrence with bilateral operations. For this reason, nerve resection is preferred today.

REFERENCES

1. Bansevicius D, Pareja JA, Sjaastad O. "Skin roll" ('pinch and roll') test: skinfold thickness and tenderness. *Headache* 1997;37:281–285.
2. Barré JA. Sur un syndrome sympathique cervical posterjeur et sa cause frequent, l'arthrite cervicale. *Rev Neurol* 1926;33:1246–1248.
3. Bartschi-Rochaix W. Headache of cervical origin. In: Vinken PJ, Bruyn GW, eds. *Handbook of clinical neurology*, vol 5, *Headache*. Amsterdam: North-Holland, 1968:192–203.
4. Berry H. Psychological aspects of chronic neck pain following hyperextension–flexion strains of the neck. In: Morley TP, ed. *Current controversies in neurosurgery*. Philadelphia: WB Saunders, 1976:51–61.
5. Bogduk N, Marsiand A. On the concept of third occipital headache. *J Neurol Neurosurg Psychiatry* 1986;49:775–780.
6. Bogduk N, Marsland A. The cervical zygapophyseal joints as a source of neck pain. *Spine* 1988;13:610–617.
7. Bono G, Antonaci F, Ghirmai S, Sandrini G, Nappi G. The clinical profile of cervicogenic headache as it emerges from a study based on the early diagnostic criteria. *Funct Neurol* 1998;13:75–77.
8. Edmeads J. The cervical spine and headache. *Neurology* 1988;38:1874–1878.
9. Fahlgren H. Retropharyngeal tendinitis: three probable cases with an unusually low epicenter. *Cephalalgia* 1988;8:105–110.
10. Fahlgren R. Retropharyngeal tendinitis. *Cephalalgia* 1986;6:169–174.
11. Göbel H. Die Kopfschmerzen. *Ursachen, mechanismen, diagnostik und therapie in der praxis*. Berlin: Springer-Verlag, 1997:1–901.
12. Hallett M, Glocker FX, Deuschl G. Mechanism of action of botulinum toxin. *Ann Neurol* 1994;36:449–450.
13. Hawkins GW. Flexion and extension injuries of the cervicocapital joints. *Clin Orthop* 1962;24:22–33.
14. Headache Classification Committee of the International Headache Society. Classification and diagnostic criteria for headache disorders, cranial neuralgias and facial pain. *Cephalalgia* 1988;8(suppl 7):1–96.
15. Hobson DE, Gladish DF. Botulinum toxin injection for cervicogenic headache. *Headache* 1997;37:253–255
16. Jaeger B. Are "cervicogenic" headaches due to myofascial pain and cervical spine dysfunction? *Cephalalgia* 1989;9:157–164.
17. Kerr FWL, Olafson RA. Trigeminal and cervical volleys. *Arch Neurol* 1961;5:171–178.
18. Kerr FWL. A mechanism to account for frontal headaches in cases of posterior fossa tumors. *J Neurosurg* 1961;18:605–609.
19. Khurana R. Headache spectrum in Arnold-Chiari malformation. *Headache* 1991;31:151–155.
20. Lobbezoo F, Tanguay R, Thon MT, Lavigne GJ. Pain perception in idiopathic cervical dystonia (spasmodic torticollis). *Pain* 1996;67:483–491.
21. Maigne R. *Douleur d'origine vertebrale et traitment par manipulation*, 3rd ed. Paris: Expansion Scientifique, 1977.
22. McRae DL. Bony ahnormalities at the craniospinal junction. *Clin Neurosurg* 1969;16:356–375.
23. Peterson D, Austin G, Dayes L. Readaches associated with discogenic disease of the cervical spine. *Bulletin of the Los Angeles Neurol Soc* 1975;40:96–100.
24. Pfaffenrath V, Dandekar R, Mayer E, Hermann G, Pollmann W. Cervicogenic headache: results of computer-based measurements of cervical spine mobility in 15 patients. *Cephalalgia* 1988;8:45–48.
25. Pollmann W, Keidel M, Pfaffenrath V. Headache and the cervical spine: a critical review. *Cephalalgia* 1997;17:801–816.
26. Sjaastad O, Bovim G. Cervicogenic headache: the differentiation from common migraine. An overview. *Funct Neurol* 1991;6:93–100.
27. Sjaastad O, Fredriksen TA, Pfaffenrath V. Cervicogenic headache: diagnostic criteria. *Headache* 1990;30:725–726.
28. Sjaastad O, Fredriksen TA, Stolt-Nielsen A, et al. Cervicogenic headache: a clinical review with special emphasis on therapy. *Funct Neurol* 1997;12:305–317.
29. Sjaastad O, Salvesen R, Jansen J, Fredriksen TA. Cervicogenic headache: a critical view on pathogenesis. *Funct Neurol* 1998;13:71–74.
30. Soyka D. Zervikogener Kopfschmerz. *Nervenheilkunde* 1990;9:265–267.
31. Voorhies RM, Sundaresan N. Tumors of the skull. In: Wilkins RH, Rengachary SS, eds. *Neurosurgery*. New York: McGraw-Hill, 1985:984–1001.
32. Weiss RD, Stern BJ, Goldberg J. Post-traumatic migraine: chronic migraine precipitated by minor head or neck trauma. *Headache* 1991;31:451–456.
33. Zwart JA. Neck mobility in different headache disorders. *Headache* 1997;37:6–11.

The Headaches, Second Edition,
edited by J. Olesen, P. Tfelt-Hansen, and K.M.A. Welch.
Lippincott Williams & Wilkins, Philadelphia © 2000.

The Secondary Headaches

CHAPTER 119

Ocular Disorders

Hartmut Göbel and Timothy J. Martin

Most patients who present with head pain from ocular disorders have obvious signs (red eye), symptoms (decrease in vision), or history (eye trauma) that implicate the eye as the origin of pain. Occasionally, however, the headache caused by ocular disease is accompanied by more subtle findings. This chapter focuses on these less obvious disorders of the globe and orbit and discusses the role of refractive errors and strabismus in headache. Many excellent reviews of this subject, have been done (2,3,6,16,24,25). The ophthalmic manifestations of other headache syndromes, such as ophthalmic migraine, are discussed elsewhere in this volume.

ACUTE GLAUCOMA

IHS code: 11.3.1.
WHO code: G44.84; H40.
Short description: Glaucoma is a broad term, describing a large array of clinical disorders that are characterized by damage to the optic nerve with visual-field defects, generally (but not always) associated with elevated intraocular pressure. Pain in glaucoma is entirely a function of the rate of rise of intraocular pressure, so only acute forms of glaucoma are likely to be painful.

Epidemiology

The incidence of glaucoma is about 1.5%. Estimates of the worldwide prevalence predict that 67 million people will suffer from glaucoma by the year 2000 (11). The

H. Göbel: Kiel Pain Clinic, University of Kiel, D-24149 Kiel, Germany.
T. J. Martin: Department of Ophthalmology, Wake Forest University School of Medicine, Winston-Salem, North Carolina 27157-1033.

overwhelming majority of these patients *do not* have pain as a component of their glaucoma.

Anatomy and Pathophysiology

Aqueous humor is produced by the ciliary body in the posterior chamber; it flows through the pupillary aperture and exits the anterior chamber through the trabecular meshwork in the anterior chamber angle (Fig. 1). Disorders of elevated intraocular pressure are divided logically into two types: *open angle* (i.e., the aqueous has access to the trabecular meshwork) and *closed angle* (i.e., the iris or some other structure is physically blocking access to the trabecular meshwork). These types are further subdivided into *primary* and *secondary* forms (2–4,6,16,24,25).

Clinical Features

IHS diagnostic criteria:
Acute glaucoma diagnosed by appropriate investigations. Pain in the eye and behind or above it.

Primary Open-Angle Glaucoma

By far, the most common type of glaucoma is *primary open-angle glaucoma*, a multifactional disorder that is often genetically determined. This entity is characterized by a normal-appearing trabecular meshwork (as viewed by an ophthalmologist through a gonioprism), moderately elevated intraocular pressure (usually 22–35 mm Hg), and cupping of the optic nerve with visual-field loss. Although generally a bilateral disorder, it may be asymmetric. Patients with primary open-angle glaucoma may slowly achieve chronic, marked elevations in intraocular pressure without ocular discomfort, as the pain is thought to be directly related to the rate of change and the persis-

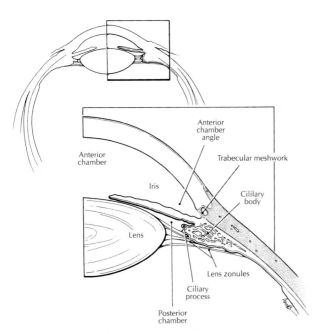

FIG. 1. Anatomy of the anterior segment.

TABLE 1. *Characteristics of acute-angle-closure glaucoma*

Symptoms	Blurred vision (from corneal edema) often with "halos" around lights; Pain often severe, localized to the eye, or radiating to teeth, ear, sinuses, forehead; episodes frequently precipitated by dilation of the pupil from physiologic (in a dark movie theater, emotional stress) or pharmacologic (dilated ocular examination) means
Signs	Red eye with ciliary injection (dilated episcleral vessels radiating from the limbus)
	Cloudy appearing cornea
	Dilated, unresponsive pupil
	Narrow angle configuration in both eyes (see Fig. 2)
	Marked elevation of intraocular pressure (globe is firm to the touch when compared to an uninvolved side)

tence of the abnormal pressure (10). Thus, this diagnosis alone is rarely a cause of head or eye pain; however, the miotic eyedrops (e.g., pilocarpine) commonly prescribed for this disorder are known to produce browache similar to the asthenopic symptoms discussed subsequently herein, which presumably is secondary to traction on the scleral spur (17).

Angle-closure Glaucoma

Although acute primary angle-closure glaucoma is far less common than open-angle glaucoma, it generates the most anxiety among physicians who treat head pain. Because the aqueous does not have free passage through the pupil, a pressure difference between the posterior and anterior chambers is created, which balloons the iris forward to occlude the trabecular meshwork. The pain may be intense, may radiate widely, and often is associated with nausea and vomiting. Tooth extractions have been performed for this diagnosis as well as laparotomies for the accompanying gastrointestinal complaints (17). A patient may experience intermittent, self-aborting episodes or present with unrelenting pain. The key features of this syndrome are summarized in Table 1. Prompt diagnosis is crucial, because urgent referral to an ophthalmologist is required not only to save the vision in the affected eye but also to prevent a similar occurrence in the fellow eye. Laser iridotomy (creating a hole in the iris) may stop an attack and prevent recurrence. The potential for diagnostic confusion between acute glaucoma, iritis, and cluster headache must be recognized. Although cluster headache may present with pain, nau-

sea, and a red eye, the vision is not affected and the pupil generally is small and associated with a ptosis (from an oculosympathetic paresis) (12). Intermittent angle-closure glaucoma may present more subtly and should be suspected in patients who experience a decline in vision with intermittent eye, brow, or frontal pain, especially if a narrow angle is suspected (22) (Fig. 2).

Low-tension Glaucoma

In low-tension glaucoma, glaucomatous optic atrophy and visual field loss progress despite normal or low intraocular pressures. An association between this disorder and headache has been made, but its significance is unknown (19). Although the pressure readings are in the

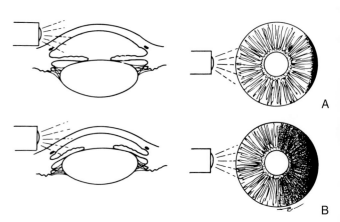

FIG. 2. Penlight examination for estimating the depth of the anterior chamber. **A**: When the anterior-chamber angle is normal, a penlight directed from the side illuminates the entire iris. **B**: Forward bowing of the iris casts a shadow with side illumination in the anterior chamber with a narrow angle. From Shields (22).

normal range, treatment is indicated to lower the pressure further to avoid progressive optic nerve damage and visual-field loss.

Secondary Glaucoma

Increased intraocular pressure may occur as a postoperative complication or as a result of trauma. Lens displacement, hemorrhage into the anterior chamber, lacerations, and contusions can disrupt the flow pattern of aqueous humor. Encroachment by a rapidly growing tumor and chronic use of topical corticosteroids also may produce the symptoms of open-angle glaucoma. Some secondary forms of open-angle glaucoma may promote a more acute rise of intraocular pressure and thus cause pain. In the patient with pigmentary glaucoma, exercise may liberate the iris pigment into the aqueous and clog the trabecular meshwork, thereby rapidly elevating the intraocular pressure. These patients generally are young, near-sighted male patients, and they may present with exercise-induced headache and blurred vision (22).

A common mechanism of secondary angle-closure glaucoma involves neovascularization of the iris, in which new blood vessels form in the angle and close the trabecular meshwork. This process is often the result of ischemic ocular disorders such as diabetic retinopathy or carotid insufficiency. The pain that invariably accompanies this problem is deep, boring, and unrelenting and associated with a red eye and poor vision (22).

Characteristics of Acute Angle-Closure Glaucoma

Symptoms: Blurred vision (from corneal edema), often with "halos" around lights

Pain: Often severe, localized to the eye, or radiating to teeth, ear, sinuses, forehead; episodes frequently precipitated by dilation of the pupil from physiologic (in a dark movie theater, emotional stress) or pharmacologic (dilated ocular examination) means.

Signs: Red eye with ciliary injection (dilated episcleral vessels radiating from the limbus);

Cloudy appearing cornea

Dilated, unresponsive pupil

Narrow-angle configuration in both eyes (see Fig. 2)

Marked elevation of intraocular pressure (globe is firm to the touch compared with uninvolved side)

Management

The diagnosis and treatment of glaucoma are complex (11). Patients in whom glaucoma is suspected should be referred to an ophthalmologist. Treatment decisions are based on the degree and progression of optic disc cupping, visual field loss, and intraocular pressure.

OCULAR INFLAMMATORY DISORDERS

IHS code: None.

WHO code: Scleritis H15.0, episcleritis H15.1, ceratoscleritis A18.5- H19.2*, chorioretinitis H30.9, photoretinitis H31.0, zoster B02.3- H58.8*, neuritis optica G36.0.

Short Description: *Ocular inflammation* takes many forms and may be categorized variously by anatomic site (i.e., iritis, cyclitis, pars planitis, choroiditis), course (acute, subacute, chronic), presumed cause (infectious agents that are endogenous or exogenous, lens related, traumatic), or by type of inflammation (granulomataus, nongranulomatous). The last of these four categories is most useful in describing ocular causes of pain.

Clinical Features

Granulomatous ocular inflammation is characterized by a slow, indolent, chronic, smoldering course and can present with a relatively normal-appearing eye. On slit-lamp examination, characteristic large "mutton-fat" precipitates on the corneal endothelium are noted. Visual decline may be modest, and pain is usually minimal. Causes include sarcoidosis and tuberculosis (18).

The *acute nongranulomatous type* is more common. Patients present with a red eye (ciliary injection) and pain ranging from a minimal ache to overwhelming agony. The pain may be related to the inflammation or to a secondary elevation in the intraocular pressure. The patient may complain of earache, toothache, or sinus pain, and tearing and blepharospasm are common (24). Photophobia is prominent, as traction on the inflamed ciliary body with the pupillary light reflex causes pain. Unfortunately, photophobia is a common complaint among ordinary headache sufferers (26). A unique characteristic of the light-induced pain with unilateral inflammation is that a light stimulus to the fellow eye will cause pain in the involved eye (1). Ophthalmic examination will reveal cells and protein (*flare*) in the anterior segment. Unlike in acute glaucoma, the pupil tends to be small. Posterior inflammation (retinitis, choroiditis) is more likely to present as a decline in vision rather than as discomfort. Occasionally, an inflammatory exudate manifests as a decrease in the red reflex of the involved eye.

Scleritis generally is evident as a nodular or diffuse area of redness on the sclera, with overlying injection of conjunctival vessels. A posterior scleritis can occur with pain and decreased vision, without any lesion or abnormality being visible anteriorly.

The pain of *herpes zoster* often precedes the cutaneous signs and may overshadow potentially serious corneal and uveitic involvement. Oral acyclovir may be effective in preventing ocular involvement if it is started soon after the appearance of the cutaneous signs (8).

MISCELLANEOUS OCULAR DISORDERS

Corneal abrasion or the presence of a *superficial foreign body* gives a characteristic "foreign body" sensation referred to the upper lid. Dry eye problems may present with variable discomfort and blurred vision, usually worsening throughout the day. *Corneal ulcers, conjunctivitis,* and *inflammatory disorders of the lids* all may cause pain locally or with radiation to other head structures and generally are associated with a red eye. *Orbital disorders* ranging from inflammatory pseudotumor to orbital metastasis may present pain and a few ocular signs. *Optic neuritis* may present with pain on eye movement; the mechanism is believed to be secondary to the close attachments of the rectus muscles to the optic nerve sheath at the orbital apex (15).

Every clinician who sees patients with head pain should be equipped to assess visual acuity and confrontation visual fields, to perform a penlight examination of the adnexa and anterior segment, to examine the pupil for anisocoria or relative afferent papillary defects, to judge abnormalities of ocular motility, and to view the optic nerve head using an ophthalmoscope. Tonometry and Shirmer's testing also are helpful. By using these basic tools, few significant ocular causes of head pain will be missed.

REFRACTIVE ERRORS

IHS code: 11.3.2.
WHO code: G44.84; H52.

Epidemiology

Refractive errors are extremely common in the general population, including those corrected with lenses and those that remain uncorrected (21). In 1993 a screening of visual acuity, refractive error, oculomotor balance, and axial length was performed on Chinese schoolchildren (7). The prevalence of myopia was 37% in the 6- to 12-year age group and 50% in the 13- to 18-year age group. Approximately 63% of the sample population had unaided visual acuity of 6/6 or better, and 24% had unaided acuity of 6/12 or worse, and 625 students (33%) failed the vision screening test and were referred for further examinations. The group who failed the vision screening test and had the highest rate of referral (46%) was the 11- to 12-year-old age group. The most common visual disorder was uncorrected myopia, accounting for 38% of the referrals (235 students). Only 26% of total sample population were wearing a spectacle correction.

Despite the high incidence of refractive errors in all populations (13), refractive errors are unlikely to be the cause of severe headache but may be associated with a mild ache above the brow called *asthenopia*, defined as head pain associated with visual effort. Classically, it presents as a bilateral brow ache that may radiate to the frontal or occipital areas and is initiated by extended reading or concentration, especially with closeup tasks. The patient often perceives that a "strain on the eyes" is required to clear a blurred image (17). Cameron (5) helped to establish the relative frequency of eye-strain–induced headache by examining 50 patients with headache referred to his ophthalmology practice. Only five patients had symptoms that could be related to visual effort; of these, only two had relief of their symptoms after correction of their refractive error (5).

Clinical Features

IHS diagnostic criteria:

A. Uncorrected refractive errors (e.g., hypermetropia, astigmatism, presbyopia, wearing of incorrect glasses)
B. Mild headaches in the frontal region and in the eyes themselves
C. Pain absent on awakening and aggravated by prolonged visual tasks at the distance or angle where vision is impaired

Ideally, the ciliary body is at rest when an emmetropic subject is attentive on a distant object. This circular structure pulls radially on the lens by way of the zonular fibers to create an appropriately shaped refractive element for distant focus (see Fig. 1). If the object of regard approaches, the ciliary body contracts, loosening the zonules and allowing the lens to assume a more convex (i.e., a more "plus") configuration. *Hyperopic subjects* (those who need "plus" lenses in their spectacles) may have to activate the ciliary muscle at all times to see clearly, even when viewing distant objects. Attempts to focus on nearby objects require even greater effort. Whether the resulting asthenopic discomfort is due to fatigue of the ciliary muscles, traction on the scleral spur (14), or the action of "accessory" facial muscles (5) is uncertain. This type of eye pain is rarely a problem in hyperopic children because their accommodative reserve is tremendous. *Myopic subjects* (those who need "minus" lenses in their spectacles) do not experience typical asthenopia because they require less accommodative effort than normal; however, subjects with undercorrected myopia may develop tension-type headaches with distance viewing because they often "squint" to clear distant images (using the pinhole effect).

Although there is a steady decline in accommodative potential with age, it is unusual for this normal aging process to cause ocular discomfort or headache (17). Cameron (5) noted that among 50 patients with *"new"* presbyopia (aged 40–50 years), only six had headache with near tasks and, of these, three had improvement with correction (reading aids). Occasionally, *medications* that have an anticholinergic action may induce a pharmacologic pseudopresbyopia, but this generally manifests as blur, not as pain. *Aniseikonia* (a spectacle-induced magnification disparity between the two eyes) and *astigmatism* are even more unlikely to cause significant headache (17).

Patients with headache attributable to refractive error or muscle imbalance constitute only a tiny percentage of all headache patients (2,5,6,12,24,27). True asthenopia requires a reasonable amount of visual effort. Instant pain on glancing at printed material is a sign of a nonphysiologic head pain (17).

Management

Headache attributable to refractive error should disappear promptly with the correct refraction (17). Beware of patients with many pairs of "incorrect" eyeglasses (24).

HETEROPHORIA OR HETEROTROPIA

IHS code: 11.3.3.
WHO code: G44.84; H50.

Epidemiology

Convergence disorders are the most common eye alignment problems implicated in head pain and are often complex because of the "linkage" between convergence and accommodation. In a survey of about 60,000 eye examinations, each with orthoptic assessment, 5% of patients were found to have a binocular vision anomaly. Of 3,075 binocular anomalies, 74% had concomitant strabismus, 10% were paretic, 8% had decompensated heterophoria, and 6% had convergence insufficiency. (23). In another clinical study, the prevalence and clinical implications of general binocular dysfunctions (nonstrabismic) in a population of university students with heavy near visual demands were determined (20): 32.3% of the subjects showed general binocular dysfunctions; in 10.8% of cases, accommodative excess was present; 7.7% had convergence insufficiency with accommodative excess; 6.2% showed accommodative insufficiency; 3.1% had basic exophoria; and convergence excess with accommodative insufficiency, basic esophoria, and fusional convergence dysfunction all showed the same prevalence of 1.5%.

Although any ocular muscle imbalance may "overwork" certain muscles and cause discomfort, it is often stated that the small deviations that allow fusion with effort are more likely to cause pain than the large deviations that preclude fusion (3). Eckhardt and colleagues (9) demonstrated that browache, head pain, and irritability were common features in normal subjects who wore prisms to simulate a muscle imbalance.

Anatomy and Pathophysiology

When viewing infinity, the optical axes of the two eyes are essentially parallel; however, as an object moves closer, the optical axis of each eye must turn in (*converge*) to keep the image on both foveas. The convergence and accommodation mechanisms are linked to a third mechanism (*miosis*) to complete the near-synkinetic triad. For example, in convergence insufficiency, there is too little convergence for the required amount of accommodation, and the result is double vision. In this frustrating situation, the patient may be able to help the diplopia by overaccommodating, but this results in a blurred single image. Conversely, hyperopic persons may require an extra accommodative effort, which may be linked to too much convergence and thus to diplopia and eye fatigue (14). Convergence spasm is usually a disorder of young, anxious students; it presents with *esotropia* (excessive convergence), blurred vision (excessive accommodation), small pupils, and discomfort. Pharmacologic "relaxation" of this near spasm with cycloplegia may be necessary for relief (25).

Clinical Features

IHS diagnostic criteria:

A. Demonstrated eterophoria or heterotropia
B. Mild to moderate constant headache in the frontal region
C. At least one of the following:
   1. Headache occurring or worsening during a visual task, especially when tiring
   2. Intermittent blurred vision or diplopia
   3. Difficulty adjusting focus from near to distant objects or vice versa
   4. Relief or improvement of symptoms by closing one eye.

Management

The etiology of any ocular imbalance (e.g., myasthenia gravis, Graves' disease) must be determined before correction with prisms or surgery is attempted. Convergence insufficiency presents a unique problem, because often it is found in the setting of hyperopia or presbyopia, and refractive correction may make the muscle imbalance worse. Full correction of the muscle imbalance with prism glasses may reduce the patient's ability to converge and make him or her totally dependent on the prism glasses. Orthoptic exercises that help to build convergence amplitudes may lessen, but rarely correct, this frustrating entity.

In summary, the patient with headaches who has a history of strabismus, high refractive error, diplopia, blurred vision, or a history suggestive of asthenopia should be examined by an ophthalmologist. The ophthalmologist must look carefully for refractive errors (using a cycloplegic examination to evaluate hyperopia) and perform alternate cover testing to measure the amount of phoria or tropia both at a distance and near.

REFERENCES

1. Au Y-K, Henkind P. Pain elicited by consensual pupillary reflex: a diagnostic test for acute iritis. *Lancet* 1981;2:1254–1255.
2. Behrens MM. Headaches associated with disorders of the eye. *Med Clin North Am* 1978;62:507–521.
3. Bellows JG. Headaches and the eye. *Headache* 1968;7:165–170.
4. Burton H. Somatosensory features of the eye. In: Moses RA, Hart WM Jr, eds. *Adler's physiology of the eye:* clinical application, 8th ed. St. Louis: Mosby, 1987;60–88.
5. Cameron ME. Headaches in relation to the eyes. *Med J Aust* 1976;1: 292–294.
6. Carlow TJ. Headache and the eye. In: Dalessio DJ, ed. *Wolff's headache and other head pain.* New York: Oxford University Press, 1987;304.
7. Chung KM, Mohidin N, Yeow PT, Tan LL, O'Leary D. Prevalence of visual disorders in Chinese schoolchildren. *Optom Vis Sci* 1996;73: 695–700.
8. Cobo LM, Foulks GN, Liesegang T, et al. Oral acyclovir in the treatment of acute herpes zoster ophthalmicus. *Ophthalmology* 1986;93: 763–770.
9. Eckhardt LB, McLean JM, Goodell H. Experimental studies on headache: the genesis of pain from the eye. *Res Publ Assoc Res Nerv Ment Dis* 1943;23:209.
10. Epstein DL. *Chandler and Grant's glaucoma*, 3rd ed. Philadelphia: Lea & Febiger, 1986:4–5.
11. Flanagan JG, Glaucoma update: epidemiology and new approaches to medical management. *Ophthalmic Physiol Opt* 1998;18:126–132.
12. Hedges TR. An ophthalmologist's view of headache. *Headache* 1979; 19:151–155.
13. Katz J, Tielsch JM, Sommer A. Prevalence and risk factors for refractive errors in an adult inner city population. *Invest Ophthalmol Vis Sci* 1997;38:334–340.
14. Leigh RJ, Zee DS. *The neurology of eye movements*, 3rd ed. Philadelphia: FA Davis Co, 1999.
15. Lepore FE. The origin of pain in optic neuritis: determinants of pain in 101 eyes with optic neuritis. *Arch Neurol* 1991;48:748–749.
16. Meythaler H. Der Gesichtsschmerz aus augenarztlicher Sicht. In: Soyka D, ed. *Der Gesichtsschmerz.* Stuttgart: Springer-Verlag, 1973:117–135.
17. Miller N. *Walsh and Hoyt's clinical neuro-ophthalmology*, vol II, 5th ed. Baltimore: Williams & Wilkins, 1998.
18. Nussenblatt RB, Palestine AG. *Uveitis:* fundamentals and clinical practice. Chicago: Mosby–Year Book, 1995.
19. Phelps CD, Corbett JJ. Migraine and low-tension glaucoma: a case–control study. *Invest Ophthalmol Vis Sci* 1985;26:1105–1108.
20. Porcar E, Martinez-Palomera A, Prevalence of general binocular dysfunctions in a population of university students. *Optom Vis Sci* 1997;74: 111–113
21. Quinn GE, Dobson V, Kivlin J, et al. Prevalence of myopia between 3 months and 5 1/2 years in preterm infants with and without retinopathy of prematurity. *Ophthalmology* 1998;105:1292–1300
22. Shields MB. *Textbook of glaucoma*, 2nd ed. Baltimore: Williams & Wilkins, 1997.
23. Stidwill D, Epidemiology of strabismus. *Ophthalmic Physiol Opt* 1997; 17:536–539.
24. Stafford WR. Headache of ophthalmic origin. In: Ryan RE Sr, Ryan RE Jr, eds. *Headache and head pain: diagnosis and treatment.* St. Louis: Mosby, 1978:279–289.
25. Tomsak RL. Ophthalmologic aspects of headache. *Med Clin North Am* 1991;75:693–706.
26. Vincent AJP, Spierings ELH, Messinger HB. A controlled study of visual symptoms and eye strain factors in chronic headache. *Headache* 1989;29:523–527.
27. Waters WE. Headache and the eye: a community study. *Lancet* 1970;2: 1–4.

The Headaches, Second Edition,
edited by J. Olesen, P. Tfelt-Hansen, and K.M.A. Welch.
Lippincott Williams & Wilkins, Philadelphia © 2000.

The Secondary Headaches

CHAPTER 120

Disorders of Ear, Nose, and Sinus

Hartmut Göbel and Robert W. Baloh

EARS

IHS code and diagnosis: 11.4 Headache associated with ear disease.

WHO code and diagnosis: G44.844 Headache associated with disorders or diseases of the ear and mastoid process.

H60:   Otitis externa
H61:   Other disorders of external ear
H62*:   Disorders of external ear in diseases classified elsewhere
H65:   Nonsuppurative otitis media
H66:   Suppurative and unspecified otitis media
H68:   Eustachian salpingitis and obstruction
H69:   Other disorders of eustachian tube
H70:   Mastoiditis and related conditions
H71:   Cholesteatoma of middle ear
H75*:   Other disorders of middle ear and mastoid in diseases classified elsewhere
H92:   Otalgia and effusion of ear
H92.0: Otalgia

Epidemiology

No systematic population-based studies of the epidemiology of the different forms of pain associated with diseases of the ears are known. Only studies of individual clinical cases exist. A Spanish study analyzed the epidemiology of acute otitis media in 20,532 schoolchildren over a 6-month period (4). The study was based on a question-

naire sent to all Spanish pediatricians. The most frequent symptom of otitis media, in 92.7% of cases, was earache. In 45.6% of cases, the symptoms occurred on both sides.

In general, earache is a frequent symptom, especially in children. An analysis of the most frequent symptoms in the emergency department of a university pediatric clinic showed that five symptoms were responsible for 40% of all consultations: high temperature, vomiting or diarrhea (or both), infection of the upper respiratory tract, earache, and skin rashes (21). An Austrian study investigated symptoms in children in connection with swimming in lakes open for public bathing. At 32.4%, otalgia was the most common symptom. The study also found a significant correlation with rhinitis, conjunctivitis, coughing, and sore throat (36.5%) (6). Otitis media is thus one of the most frequent causes of earache.

Earache, otorrhea, and otorrhea with bleeding are the principal symptoms of patients with tumors of the middle ear (12). A study that analyzed the symptoms of nasopharyngeal carcinomas revealed that deafness and earache, encountered in 85% of cases, were the most common symptoms besides swelling of the throat. The earache had been present for as long as 9 months before a correct diagnosis was made (22). The most common cause of intracranial abscesses, with a frequency of 73%, was chronic infection of the middle ear. The clinical symptoms are characterized by chronic otitis with otorrhea, earache, headache in the region of the temples, high temperature, nausea, and vomiting (13).

Anatomy and Pathology

Local structural lesions in the region of the pinna, external ear canal, tympanic membrane, and middle ear may give rise to primary otalgia. Only about 50% of all earaches are due to structural lesions of the external or

H. Göbel: Kiel Pain Clinic, University of Kiel, D-24149 Kiel, Germany.

R. W. Baloh, Department of Neurology/Head and Neck Surgery, U.C.L.A. Medical School, and Division of Neurotology, Department of Neurology, U.C.L.A. Hospital, Los Angeles, California 90095-1769.

middle ear. Disorders outside this region may lead to referred otalgia as a result of radiation of pain into the ear region. Sensory fibers of the fifth, seventh, ninth, and tenth cranial nerves project into the auricle, external auditory canal, tympanic membrane, and middle ear (Table 1). For this reason, referred pain from remote structural lesions in these anatomic regions can be felt as referred otalgia.

Pathophysiology

Primary Otalgia

Pinna

Primary pinna pain in the first instance may be caused by injuries or traumas, which may result in laceration, burns, frostbite, infections, or abscesses. In the case of persistent minor lesions, a biopsy should be performed, because these lesions may obscure a malignant new growth, especially a basal cell carcinoma, a squamous cell carcinoma, or small benign growths.

External Ear Canal

The external ear canal is a particularly common source of primary earache. External otitis arises from an acute inflammatory process after an ear trauma, inadequate cleansing of the external ear canal, or lengthy contact with liquid in bacterially contaminated water, especially in bathing lakes or swimming pools (swimmer's ear). External otitis, however, may occur on the basis of a chronic middle ear infection or as a result of a malignant new growth in the external ear canal. Malignant external otitis may be observed, particularly in patients with diabetes mellitus or an immune deficiency. In addition to strong earache with reddening of the pinna and inflammation of the periauricular region, there is great sensitivity to pain, swelling of the pinna, and swelling of the mastoidale. A general feeling of malaise and elevated temperature also may occur.

Ear wax also may be responsible for earache and pressure in the ear. The same applies to foreign bodies in the ear canal. Removal of such objects must be undertaken with the utmost care and precision to avoid injuring the external ear canal and the tympanic membrane. Another cause of earache may be benign or malignant new growths in the external ear canal. In case of doubt, a biopsy should be performed. New growths are rare and in most cases take the form of a squamous cell carcinoma or adenocarcinoma.

Middle Ear and Mastoid

An acute infection of the mucous membrane of the middle ear in the form of acute otitis media usually stems from an infection of the upper air passages with dysfunction of the eustachian tube. Rhinitis and adenoid inflammation also may be causal factors of acute otitis media. The disease usually is accompanied by an elevated temperature and increasing infection of the upper respiratory tract. Examination reveals reddening and swelling of the tympanic membrane. Occasionally, a purulent discharge is present.

If otitis media is not treated properly, acute mastoiditis may occur as a complication. Typically, a highly sensitive and swollen mastoidale is present. Obstruction of the pinna, a reddened and bulging tympanic membrane, and purulent otorrhea are typical examination findings. An initial slight ache increases sharply with the purulent inflammation and radiates into the entire neck and head area.

Petrositis

If the inflammation spreads to the petrous bone, further complications of meningitis or an intracranial or

TABLE 1. *Sources of referred otalgia*

Nerve	Location of lesion	Common disorders
Fifth cranial nerve, Mandibular division (auriculotemporal branch)	Teeth	Pulpitis, periapical dental abscess, third molar impaction
	Oral cavity	Glossitis, osteitis, intraoral abscess, benign or malignant growth
	Sinus	Inflammation, malignant or benign growth
	Temporomandibular joint (TMJ)	Dental malocclusion, arthritic process
Seventh cranial nerve (Nervus intermedius branch)	Middle ear	Ramsey-Hunt syndrome (herpes zoster oticus)
Ninth cranial nerve (Jacobson's nerve)	Nasopharynx, eustachian tube, palatine tonsils, tongue	Inflammation, benign or malignant growth
Tenth cranial nerve (Arnold's branch)	Hypopharynx, larynx, nasopharynx	Benign or malignant growth
Second and third cervical roots (Greater auricular nerve and lesser occipital nerve)	Base of skull	Abscess, inflammation and tumor, thyroid carcinoma, lesions of nasopharynx and oropharynx
Cranial neuralgia	See Chapter 123	

extradural abscess may occur. Strong pains typically occur in the temporoparietal, retroorbital, and temporal regions. Lesions of the cranial nerves also may be observed. Paresis of the sixth cranial nerve, otorrhea, and otalgia are defined as the *Gradenigo syndrome*, which occurs in advanced clinical stages and has a mortality rate of 20%.

Acoustic Neuroma

Acoustic neuroma is a benign tumor of the neural sheath of the eighth cranial nerve. Peak incidence is mostly between the ages of 30 and 40. Women are affected more frequently than men. Tinnitus and hearing loss are early symptoms. A tingling sensation and a deep pain in the ear are also initial indications of the disorder. Over time, these symptoms may be joined by vertigo. As the pressure of the tumor on the inner ear canal increases and the tumor spreads to the posterior cranial fossa and the cerebellopontine angle, including the fifth and seventh cranial nerves, numbness of the facial region and paresis of the facial nerve may occur. Cerebellar symptoms with speech disorders, ataxia, and coordination problems also may be observed on compression of the adjacent cerebellum. Obstruction of the circulation of the cerebrospinal fluid may give rise to headache with elevated intracranial pressure with nausea, vomiting, and neuropsychological deficits.

Traumas

Trauma of the tympanic membrane may be caused by direct mechanical damage with fracture of the temporal bone or by an external compression trauma. Foreign bodies also may give rise to traumatic perforation of the tympanic membrane. Rupture of the tympanic membrane also may occur as a result of increased pressure in the external ear canal, especially as a result of a slap on the ear with an open hand or by compression of the cylindric body of air in the external ear canal. Earache and hearing loss occur as typical symptoms.

A barotrauma is caused by elevated pressure in the external ear canal, for example, by sudden changes of pressure in an airplane or during diving activities. Symptoms include localized or radiating pain in the region of the middle ear but also along the fifth, ninth, and tenth cranial nerves. Hematotympanum and conduction deafness also may occur.

A trauma of the temporal bone most commonly leads to a longitudinal fracture, which may result in rupture of the tympanic membrane. Depending on its course, the fracture may lead to paralysis of the seventh cranial nerve. Pain radiates into the area of distribution of the fifth, ninth, and tenth cranial nerves. In addition, conduction deafness or facial paralysis may be observed. Given appropriate localization, drainage of cerebrospinal fluid

or blood from the external ear canal also may occur. An ecchymosis over the mastoid is an indication of a fracture of the base of the skull.

In a transverse fracture, there may be no rupture of the tympanic membrane, depending on the course of the fracture line. If the internal auditory canal is involved, lesions of the seventh and eighth cranial nerves may occur with sensory–neural hearing loss, vertigo, and facial paralysis.

Benign and Malignant New Growths in the Middle Ear

New growths in the middle ear are rare but always should be considered a possibility if a chronic middle ear infection or a polypoid lesion does not respond to adequate treatment and chronic pain continues. The pain is typically localized, but it may radiate into the areas of distribution of the fifth, ninth, and tenth cranial nerves. Examination reveals local ulceration, which should be subjected to biopsy.

Secondary or Referred Otalgia

Referred otalgia may arise from structural lesions in the region of the branches of the fifth, seventh, ninth, and tenth cranial nerves and of the second and third cervical roots. The common causes of referred otalgia are described in Table 1.

Clinical Features

IHS diagnostic criteria for headache associated with ear disease:

A. Clinical or laboratory evidence of ear disorders
B. Headache located to ear or its surroundings
C. Headache disappears within 1 month after successful treatment or spontaneous remission of ear disorders

Headache associated with ear disease is experienced as fullness in the ear, throbbing, pressure, tenderness, phonophobia, burning, or itching. The pain can radiate to vertex and temples and can involve half of the head or even the global head. Pain intensity may vary from mild to quite severe. The character is described as dull, aching, or lancinating. Associated symptoms may be tinnitus, hearing loss, or vestibular disorders. Pathologic changes are often visible by examination, and manipulation may increase the pain intensity. Retroauricular or subauricular lymphadenitis is a possible marker of a pathologic situation and can increase pain and pressure.

Management

Treatment of the referred otalgia must be targeted specifically to the relevant local causes (see Table 1). Treatments for the various causes of primary otalgia must focus on the specific lesion (Table 2).

TABLE 2. *Sources of primary otalgia*

Source of primary otalgia	Lesion
Pinna	Abscess and Infection
	Frostbite
	Burns
	Laceration
External ear canal	External otitis
	Furunculosis
	Malignant external otitis
	Cerumenosis
	Foreign bodies
	Malignant (squamous cell carcinoma, adenocarcinoma) or benign growths
Mastoid and middle ear	Acute otitis media
	Chronic serous otitis media
	Acute mastoiditis
Tympanic membrane	Perforation
	Barotrauma
Internal auditory cana	Acoustic neuroma
	Fractures

NOSE

IHS code and diagnosis: 11.5.2 Other diseases of nose or sinuses.

WHO code and diagnosis: G44.845 Headache associated with disorders or diseases of the respiratory system: other disorders of nose and nasal sinuses (J34).

Short description: Other conditions that may cause headache are nasal passage abnormality due to septal deflection (J34.2), hypertrophic turbinates (J34.3), and atrophic sinus membrane (J34.8). These conditions are not sufficiently validated as being causes of headache.

Epidemiology

A study in Israel investigated the incidence of nasal septal deflection in about 4,000 consecutive newborn infants over a period of 2 years. They found an incidence of 0.93% for anterior nasal septal cartilaginous dislocation (18). In another study, 100 consecutive computed tomography (CT) scans for evaluation of diseases of the nasal sinuses were compared with 82 consecutive scans for evaluation of diseases of the orbital cavity with regard to the frequency of concha pollosa, paradoxical middle turbinate, and septal deviation. In patients with diseases of the nose and nasal sinuses, abnormal findings of the osteomeatal complex were significantly more frequent. Whereas the data showed clearly that paradoxical turbinates were not associated with a disorder of the nasal sinuses, a clear link was found between concha pollosa or septum deviation and a disorder of the nasal sinuses (2).

A study in Finland investigated the effect of sulfur fumes from pulp mills with regard to the induction of irritation of the eyes, respiratory symptoms, and headache in children. A control group comprised children from a rural region where air pollution was not found. Symptoms were more than twice as common in children from the region with the malodorous sulfur fumes (15).

The prevalence of the sick-building syndrome, characterized by a pattern of nasal, ocular, and mucous membrane symptoms with lethargy, dry skin, and headache, was investigated in employees working in various office facilities (7). The offices had complete air conditioning, an air-recirculation system, or natural ventilation. A highly significant increase was found in the frequency of sick-building syndrome in the fully air-conditioned offices compared with the naturally ventilated buildings (7).

Numerous studies on the prevalence of allergic rhinitis have shown a marked increase in frequency over the last 30 years. The prevalence of allergic rhinitis and the increase were most marked in children and young adults. Allergic rhinitis occurs in about 20% of people (of all ages) worldwide. If there is a family history of rhinitis, the risk compared with those without such a prior history is two to six times greater (14). Worldwide, the frequency of allergic rhinitis in various countries varies by a factor of 20 to 60 (10).

Anatomy and Pathology

Pain sensations from the nasal region are mediated by the first and second branch of the trigeminal nerve (Fig. 1). Autonomous innervation of the nasal cavity takes place through the sphenopalatine ganglion with parasympathetic branches of the facial nerve, which take the same course as the greater superficial petrosal nerve. The parasympathetic fibers innervate the glands and blood vessels of the nose. The sympathetic fibers take the same course as the deep petrosal nerve and the seventh cranial nerve.

Pathophysiology and Clinical Features

Nasal Septum

Deviation of the nasal septum may find expression in symptoms of nasal obstruction. Particularly marked symptoms are found if the deviation is in the region of the nasal valve. An obstruction of the nasal air passages may be responsible for the development of an acute disease of the nasal sinuses that leads to facial pain. As a result of the nasal obstruction, the mucous membrane exerts pressure on the lateral wall of the nasal cavity. Inadequate constriction of the nasal mucous membrane results in squeezing of the nasal septum, which may lead to facial pain. A further consequence may be secondary development and persistence of acute or chronic sinusitis. In a clinical study of the success of operations to correct the nasal septum in 392 patients, conducted as part of an external quality-control program by a health insurance

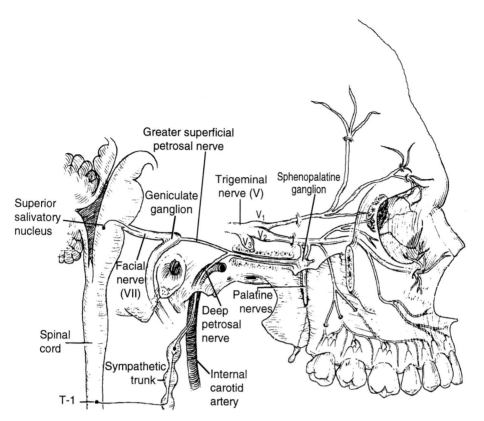

FIG. 1. Innervation of the nasal and paranasal regions.

fund, in 31% of the subjects, headache was the main reason for the operation along with impeded breathing through the nose and blocked nose (1). Complete remission of the symptoms was found in only 10.6% of the respondents; 7.9% displayed no improvement; and postoperative complications such as adhesions, perforations, and such conditions occurred in 29.9%. Deflection of the nasal septum plays only a minor role as a possible cause of headache and should therefore be regarded as an operation indication in exceptional cases only (20).

Septal Hematoma and Septal Abscess

Hematoma of the nasal septum or an abscess of the nasal septum express themselves in a purulent and swollen nasal septum. The associated pain is clearly localized and quite strong, and marked sensitivity to local pressure and reddening of the tip of the nose are noted. In particular, an abscess of the nasal septum may be present in cases of granulomatous disease and polychondritis or other immunologic disorders.

Inflammatory Rhinitis

The disease is accompanied by rhinorrhea, elevated temperature, pain affecting the middle part of the face and the area of distribution of the first and second trigem-

inal branches, and symptoms of an infection of the upper respiratory tract. The nasal mucous membrane is reddened and swollen and may display a purulent discharge. In terms of differential diagnosis, a nasal swab exhibits larger quantities of neutrophils in cases of inflammatory rhinitis, whereas an increase in eosinophilic leucocytes is found in cases of allergic rhinitis.

Allergic Rhinitis

As a rule, allergic rhinitis does not involve primary pain, but it may give rise to acute sinusitis, with facial pain as a secondary development. Allergic rhinitis is typically seasonal. Symptoms include nasal obstruction, nasal pain, and rhinorrhea. By contrast with inflammatory rhinitis, the nasal mucous membrane exhibits a bluish discoloration in allergic rhinitis.

Vasomotor Rhinitis

Vasomotor rhinitis is characterized by excessive reactivity of the mucous membrane, which may be due to a wide variety of factors. The nasal discharge is clear, and the nasal mucous membrane is swollen and displays a slight reddening compared with inflammatory rhinitis. The causal factors have not been definitively clarified, and the clinical picture is regarded as attributable to multiple factors. Environmental factors, hormones, stress, emotions, and medication play a part here.

Atrophic Rhinitis

Atrophic rhinitis is characterized by reduced reactivity of the nasal mucous membrane. Mucus production is reduced, and the nasal mucous membrane is dry, encrusted, inflamed, and irritated.

Management

Acute inflammatory rhinitis is treated with detumescent nose drops, moist inhalations, and antibiotics. Treatment of allergic rhinitis primarily involves identifying the allergens responsible. The main elements here are the case history and skin tests. Allergen avoidance or desensitization may alleviate the symptoms. Antihistamines can be used for seasonal episodes. A topically applied nasal steroid also may alleviate allergic rhinitis. In the treatment of vasomotor rhinitis, the first priority is to seek to eliminate the causal factors. Occasionally, operative intervention may be necessary. Atrophic rhinitis may be treated by topical application of nasal steroids and moistening of the nasal mucous membrane by means of nasal sprays or inhalations. Application of vasoconstrictive nasal sprays over long periods should be avoided, because to do so can cause medication-induced rhinitis with rebound phenomena.

NASAL SINUSES

IHS code and diagnosis: 11.5.1 Acute sinus headache.
WHO code and diagnosis: G44.845 Headache associated
   with disorders or diseases of the respiratory system:
Acute sinusitis headache (J01)
Acute maxillary sinusitis (J01.0)
Acute frontal sinusitis (J01.1)
Acute ethmoidal sinusitis (J01.2)
Acute sphenoidal sinusitis (J01.3)
Acute pansinusitis (J01.4)
Other acute sinusitis (J01.5)
Acute sinusitis unspecified (J01.9)
Chronic sinusitis (J32)

Epidemiology

A 45% prevalence of sinusitis was found in magnetic resonance tomograms of children examined primarily for neurologic reasons but who were without clinical symptoms of sinusitis (8). In another study, the prevalence of abnormal radiologic findings in the region of the nasal sinus was recorded in adults who had undergone magnetic resonance tomography for neurologic disorders. In 49.2% of the patients examined, at least one or more abnormal findings within the nasal sinus were noted, although without any clinical relevance. The most common of these abnormalities was swelling of the mucous membrane of the nasal sinus. The ethmoidal cells exhibited the most changes (3). This study offers impressive evidence that inflammatory changes of the nasal sinus can occur in large numbers without necessarily being associated with any clinically relevant symptoms. Furthermore, reversible radiologic signs of sinusitis are common with any viral upper respiratory tract infection (9). Inflammatory changes in the region of the nasal sinuses, like headaches, are extremely frequent. This does not, however, mean a causal connection exists in the sense of etiologic causation of the headache by the inflammatory changes (17).

Pathophysiology

When discussing inflammations of the nasal sinuses, it is important to distinguish between acute and chronic inflammations.

Acute Sinusitis

Acute sinusitis is characterized by acute inflammation symptoms of the nasal membrane and nasal sinuses and their vicinity. Patients' complaints focus mainly on the nasal sinus that is primarily affected, but frequently several nasal sinuses are affected. In acute inflammation of the nasal sinuses, a purulent discharge into the nose is present. Headache also occurs simultaneously with the start of the nasal sinusitis. Previously existing headaches must not be attributed to the acute inflammation of the nasal sinus. Acute sinusitis typically occurs after an infection of the upper respiratory tract with rhinitis and swelling of the nasal mucous membrane. The result is obstruction of the orifices of the nasal sinuses with blockade of normal drainage and ventilation.

Inflammation of the mucous membrane also disturbs the nasal ciliary action. This, too, causes a reduction in drainage. If an obstructive lesion is present in the region of the nasal cavity, normal drainage also is altered. The same applies to an obstruction of the middle meatus by nasal polyps. Maxillary sinusitis also may be caused by inflammations of dental origin, such as periapical abscesses or of iatrogenic origin as a result of dental surgery. Allergies, hypothyroidism, and cystic fibrosis also may favor the occurrence of sinusitis. The same applies to immune suppression and the existence of diabetes mellitus. Inflammation of the nose with swelling and blockade of sinus drainage may be due to nasotracheal intubation or nasogastral tube feeding. Traumatic impacts on the nasal sinus with fractures also may give rise to nasal sinusitis. Finally, hypertrophy of the adenoids or tonsils may induce nasal sinusitis as a result of reduced ventilation.

Chronic Sinusitis

Chronic sinusitis is characterized by chronic inflammation of the mucous membrane of the nasal sinus. The mucous membrane becomes hypertrophic, resulting in a permanent disturbance of nasal ciliary action. The function of the mucous glands also is affected. Symptoms of chronic nasal sinusitis or hypertrophic nasal concha are not validated as causes of headache. Nearly 50% of the population exhibit chronic inflammatory alteration of the mucous membrane of the nasal sinus without suffering from headaches or continuous headaches (14). There is no causal connection between symptoms of chronic nasal sinusitis and primary headache disorders. Exact determination of the symptoms of the primary headache disorder permits a reliable distinction from the headache associated with acute nasal sinusitis. Headache based on acute nasal sinusitis takes the form of a dull, oppressive headache in the region of the inflamed nasal sinus. There is no nausea or vomiting. Owing to the changed fluid level in the nasal sinus, the intensity of the pain increases as the head is bent forward. The same applies to shaking the head.

A transillumination examination can reveal pus levels in sinusitis. Plain radiographs of the nasal sinuses may show shadows or fluid levels. It is not possible to differentiate chronic from acute sinusitis by means of radiologic examination; this must be done on the basis of clinical features and the examination findings. A CT or magnetic resonance tomogram may be helpful in differentiating between a cystic and a solid lesion or a fluid level (Fig. 2).

Clinical Features

IHS diagnostic criteria for acute sinus headache:

A. Purulent discharge in the nasal passage, either spontaneous or by suction
B. Pathologic findings in one or more of the following tests:
   1. Radiographic examination
   2. CT
   3. Transillumination
C. Simultaneous onset of headache and sinusitis
D. Headache location
   1. In acute frontal sinusitis, headache is located directly over the sinus and may radiate to the vertex or behind the eyes.
   2. In acute maxillary sinusitis, headache is located over the antral area and may radiate to the upper teeth or forehead.
   3. In acute ethmoiditis, headache is located between and behind the eyes and may radiate to the temporal area.
   4. In acute sphenoiditis, headache is located in the occipital area, the vertex, the frontal region or behind the eyes.
E. Headache disappears after treatment of acute sinusitis

Chronic sinusitis is not validated as being a cause of headache or facial pain unless it relapses into an acute stage. For postoperative chronic pain resulting from nerve damage, see group 12 of the IHS Classification. Migraine and tension-type headache often are confused with true sinus headache because of the similarity of their location. To diagnose sinus headache, these criteria must be strictly fulfilled.

Maxillary Sinusitis

In acute maxillary sinusitis, the pain is usually felt most strongly over the nasal sinus affected. The pain may radiate into the neighboring ear or the teeth. The affected nasal sinus is sensitive to palpation or percussion. The same applies to the neighboring teeth. There is a mucous or purulent discharge from the middle meatus. The sense of smell is limited, and there is sensitivity to pain and pressure in the region of the maxilla along the upper row of teeth.

In chronic maxillary sinusitis, unspecific symptoms are found. There is rhinorrhea with nasal obstruction. Typically, facial pain and headache do not occur.

Frontal Sinusitis

The headache in acute frontal sinusitis typically is located behind the eyes and around the center of the forehead. Patients report strong local pressure. The pain is strongest on waking in the morning and is eased by get-

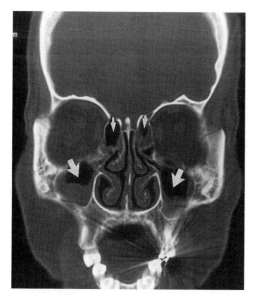

FIG. 2. Computed tomography showing chronic sinusitis involving maxillary (*large arrows*) and ethmoid (*small arrows*) sinuses. The patient was asymptomatic.

ting up. The frontal sinus region is sensitive to percussion, and the supraorbital nerve is highly sensitive to pain. A purulent discharge comes from the nasofrontal duct. In the event of complete obstruction, the purulent discharge may not be observed.

In chronic inflammation of the frontal sinus, there may be slight pain above the affected nasal sinus. The nasofrontal duct may be obstructed by a mucocele.

Ethmoidal Sinusitis

In acute ethmoidal sinusitis, the pain is retroorbital, radiating to the temples. The eyes are sensitive to pressure, and there is bilateral blockage of the nose. The eye examination is normal. Nasopharyngeal examination reveals purulent drainage at the rear pharyngeal wall. If the orbits are involved, there may be swelling of the eyelids with chemosis. An orbital abscess may develop with time.

Sphenoidal Sinusitis

In acute sphenoidal sinusitis, the headache is localized in the orbital region and the vertex region. The pain also may radiate to the forehead, ear, and mastoid. There is a purulent discharge from the sphenoid orifice.

Management

Acute inflammation of the nasal sinuses calls for the use of antibiotics. In addition, oral decongestants are used. Detumescent nasal drops are used for a maximum of 3 days to improve drainage in the region of the nasal concha and the orifices of the nasal sinuses. Infrared treatment and hot compresses in the region of the nasal sinus may reduce the pain, as may analgesics. Moist inhalations or hot aerosol vapors should be inhaled to improve mucus drainage.

Treatment embraces facilitating drainage from the congested nasal sinus and eliminating the pathogenic bacteria. Drainage can be improved by clearing the orifices by means of detumescent measures and local corticosteroids. The pathogenic bacteria can be eliminated by irrigating the nasal sinuses with saline solution and by antibiotic therapy. In patients with continual recurrences of sinusitis, it may be necessary to apply topical corticoid therapy over a lengthy period. Most patients can be treated effectively with this medication therapy and do not require invasive treatment. Surgery aims to achieve an improvement in sinus drainage by enlarging the orifices and by removing obstructive anatomic structures (11).

Rhinitis can be treated with topical corticosteroids, mastoid cell stabilizers, or antihistamines, either as monotherapy or in combination. Nasal secretion can be improved by steam inhalation or by irrigating the nose with saline solution. If conservative measures do not prove sufficiently effective, operative therapy may be necessary. Removal of nasal polyps, reduction of the lower nasal concha, or cor-

rection of septal deviation may be necessary. In some cases, endoscopic ethmoidectomy and middle meatal antrostomy are necessary. Complications that may arise from acute or chronic sinusitis are intraorbital or intracranial infections. Such diseases require urgent imaging diagnosis using CT, intravenous administration of broad-spectrum antibiotics, and, if necessary, operative drainage (5).

Because of the high complication rate, the Caldwell-Luc procedure, formerly used for treating maxillary sinusitis, should no longer be used. The preferred method for operative treatment today is endoscopy (16,19).

REFERENCES

1. Bitzer EM, Döning H, Schwartz FW. Clinical outcome of septal surgery. *Laryngorhinootologie* 1996;75:649–656.
2. Calhoun KH, Waggenspack GA, Simpson CB, Hokanson JA, Bailey BJ. CT evaluation of the paranasal sinuses in symptomatic and asymptomatic populations. *Otolaryngol Head Neck Surg* 1991;104:480–483.
3. Collins JG. Prevalence of selected chronic conditions: United States, 1990–1992. *Vital Health Stat* 1997;194:1–89.
4. Del Castillo F, Corretger JM, Medina J, Rosell J, Cruz M. Acute otitis media in childhood: a study of 20,532 cases. *Infection* 1995;23(Suppl 2):p70–p73.
5. Evans KL. Recognition and management of sinusitis. *Drugs* 1998;56: 59–71.
6. Feenstra O, Pridnig G, Schmidt D, Marth E. Bathing water related diseases: the Carinthian Sentinel Project as the source of epidemiological data. *Zentralbl Hyg Umweltmed* 1995;198:165–-171.
7. Finnegan MJ, Pickering CA, Burge PS. The sick building syndrome: prevalence studies. *BMJ* 1984;289:1573–1575.
8. Gordts F, Clement PA, Destryker A, Desprechins B, Kaufman L. Prevalence of sinusitis signs on MRI in a non-ENT paediatric population. *Rhinology* 1997;35:154–157.
9. Gwaltney JM, Phillips CD, Miller RD, Riker DK. Computed tomographic study of the common cold. *N Engl J Med* 1994;6;330:25–30.
10. The International Study of Asthma and Allergies in Childhood (ISAAC) Steering Committee. Worldwide variation in prevalence of symptoms of asthma, allergic rhinoconjunctivitis, and atopic eczema: ISAAC. *Lancet* 1998;351:1225–1232.
11. Kaliner M. Medical management of sinusitis. *Am J Med Sci* 1998;316: 21–28.
12. Kawana M, Nonomura N, Okura T, Nakano Y, Ikarashi F. Twenty-one cases of malignant tumor of the external auditory canal or middle ear. *Nippon Jibiinkoka Gakkai Kaiho* 1996;99:645–652.
13. Kulai A, Ozatik N, Topcu I. Otogenic intracranial abscesses. *Acta Neurochir (Wien)* 1990;107:140–146.
14. Lundback B. Epidemiology of rhinitis and asthma. *Clin Exp Allergy* 1998;28(Suppl 2):3–10.
15. Marttila O, Jaakkola JJ, Vilkka V, Jappinen P, Haahtela T. The South Karelia Air Pollution Study: the effects of malodorous sulfur compounds from pulp mills on respiratory and other symptoms in children. *Environ Res* 1994;66:152–159.
16. Orlandi RR, Kennedy DW. Surgical management of rhinosinusitis. *Am J Med Sci* 1998;316:29–38.
17. Patel K, Chavda SV, Violaris N, Pahor AL. Incidental paranasal sinus inflammatory changes in a British population. *J Laryngol Otol* 1996; 110:649–651.
18. Podoshin L, Gertner R, Fradis M, Berger A. Incidence and treatment of deviation of nasal septum in newborns. *Ear Nose Throat J* 1991;70: 485–487.
19. Romagnoli R, Aimetti M, Secco F, Brucoli M. The Caldwell-Luc procedure in the management of maxillary sinusitis: long-term results. *Minerva Stomatol* 1998;47:143–147.
20. Rudert H. Editorial. *Laryngorhinootologie* 1996;75:656–659.
21. Villarreal SF, Berman S, Groothuis JR, Strange V, Schmitt BD. Telephone encounters in a university pediatric group practice: a 2-year analysis of after-hour calls. *Clin Pediatr (Phila)* 1984;23:456–458.
22. Woollons AC, Morton RP. When does middle ear effusion signify nasopharyngeal cancer? *N Z Med J* 1994;107:507–509.

The Headaches, Second Edition,
edited by J. Olesen, P. Tfelt-Hansen, and K.M.A. Welch.
Lippincott Williams & Wilkins, Philadelphia © 2000.

The Secondary Headaches

CHAPTER 121

Oromandibular Structures

Steven B. Graff-Radford and Rigmor Jensen

The association of headache and oromandibular structures may be considered in two forms: those in which the headache arises in the oromandibular structures and is referred to the head and those in which the headache is perceived in the oromandibular structures. There is an artificial division of the head by the occulotragus line, with neurologists principally treating above the line and dentists below the line. This division has resulted in little exploration of the relationship between oromandibular structures and headache. This chapter attempts to review what is known of the relationship and to suggest what is lacking.

TEETH, JAWS, AND RELATED STRUCTURES

IHS code and diagnosis: 11.6 Teeth, jaws, and related structures.
WHO code and diagnosis: None.

The pathology associated with dental disease is not a common cause of headache. Dental disease may be summarized as *pulpal* or *periodontal*. Pulpal pain may be characterized as an irreversible pulpitis, in which death of the pulpal tissue is inevitable and which requires root-canal therapy. In reversible pulpitis, the inflammation has reached a point at which removal of the pathology (e.g., caries) will allow the pulpal tissue to return to normal. Periodontal disorders involve the supporting structures of the teeth: the bone, periodontal ligament, and cementum. Inflammation of these tissues produces pain and often swelling in the area of disease. When acute pain occurs in

the dental structures, patients often complain of referred pain and tenderness to adjacent structures, including headache. The frequency and epidemiology of headache and tooth pain are unknown. Headache is usually a secondary phenomenon that does not pose a significant diagnostic dilemma. Possibly, pericoronitis is the most frequent periodontal inflammation to cause headache. This pain results from infection or traumatic irritation around a partially erupted tooth, usually a wisdom tooth.

The dental problems are managed best by using conventional dental therapies and rarely produce any long-term or significant disability. Chronic dental pains are different, however. Atypical odontalgia (AO) has been linked with headache and described as possibly being secondary to a migrainous etiology (34,41). Unfortunately, *atypical facial pain* has become a "wastebasket" term for all pains in the face that are not readily diagnosed. AO does have the significance of a site that can be localized; it was first described by Harris as a subcategory of atypical facial pain, in which the pain was perceived as being in a tooth or tooth site. Graff-Radford and Solberg (17) define AO as pain in a tooth or tooth site where no organic cause is obvious. They emphasize that before making a diagnosis, positive inclusive criteria are required rather than arriving at the diagnosis by exclusion. Suggested diagnostic criteria for AO are summarized in Table 1.

Recently, Sicuteri and colleagues described the relationship of AO with headache, suggesting a neurovascular etiology (43). Further evaluation of this relationship is required before a cause and effect statement can be made. Graff-Radford and Solberg have data supporting a deafferentation mechanism, most likely sympathetically maintained pain, as the cause of AO (20,21). The high frequency of associated trauma, the equivocal effect of somatic block, and the positive effects of sympathetic block are the bases for these claims (21). The relationship between psy-

S.B. Graff-Radford: Department of Diagnostic Sciences, U.C.L.A., and The Pain Center, Cedars-Sinai Medical Center, Los Angeles, California 90048.
R. Jensen: Department of Neurology, Glostrup Hospital, University of Copenhagen, DK-2600 Glostrup, Copenhagen, Denmark.

TABLE 1. *Suggested diagnostic criteria for atypical odontalgia*

Major criteria
  Dentoalveolar pain with no local cause
  Continuous pain
  Duration greater than 4 mo
  Hyperesthesia
  Somatosensory block equivocal
Minor criteria
  Sympathetic block effective
  Thermogram positive
  History of trauma

chopathology and AO also was explored by Graff-Radford and Solberg, but no positive relationship was found (19).

TEMPOROMANDIBULAR DISORDERS

IHS Code and diagnosis: 11.7 Temporomandibular joint disease.

WHO Code and diagnosis: None.

Functional disorders and pain in the anatomic region of the temporomandibular joint (TMJ) and associated musculature are referred to as temporomandibular disorders (TMD) (9).

Other terms: Other names have included *Costen's syndrome* (8), *craniomandibular disorders*, *oromandibular disorders*, and *temporomandibular joint dysfunction syndrome*.

Epidemiology

Epidemiologic studies of TMD have not specifically differentiated headache from facial pain. Cross-sectional epidemiologic studies of nonpatient populations show that about 75% have at least one sign of joint dysfunction, and about 33% have at least one symptom (37,38). The problem with the epidemiologic studies is that there has been little conformity to diagnostic criteria and terminology in data collection. The American Academy of Orofacial Pain (9) developed a classification system that conforms to the format of the International Headache Society Classification (6). It is the intention that this classification evolve to allow more controlled and comparable research. Of the 70% of patients with signs of TMD, it is estimated that only 5% require treatment (11,22,34, 36) and fewer have headache.

Genetics

At present, no clinical or scientific evidence for a possible genetic factor in TMD has been found.

Anatomy and Pathology

The TMJ is a diarthroidial synovial joint characterized by having two compartments separated by fibrous discs. The movements in the joint are both rotational and translational. The first 25 mm of the mouth opening involves rotation of the condyle within the fossa. The second 25 mm involves translation of the disc condyle complex along the articular eminence. The TMDs are classified into joint-related problems (*arthrogenous*) and muscle disorders (*myogenous*). Usually, these problems occur in combination but may present as isolated problems. Figure 1 shows a magnetic resonance imaging (MRI) of a normal TMJ to review the anatomy.

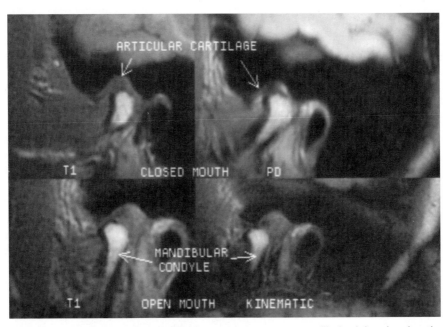

FIG. 1. Magnetic resonance imaging (*MRI*) of a normal temporomandibular joint showing the condyle and cartilage dividing the joint into an upper and lower joint space.

Pathophysiology

Pain of the TMJ is secondary to inflammation within the joint and is complicated by dysfunctions of the intracapsular parts (ligaments and disc). The etiology of muscle disorders is not understood, although suggestions of central nervous system mechanism have been proposed (29,36). By far, the most frequent cause of pain appearing to arise from the TMJ is myofascial as a result of the basic mechanisms described in the sections on tension-type headache (70,72,73).

The association of muscle tenderness is viewed by some investigators as the cause of headache (9,18,24,28), although the cause-and-effect relation has not been clarified. Increased tenderness in pericranial muscles is the most prominent clinical finding in patients with tension-type headache, and the degree of tenderness increases with increasing frequency of tension-type headache (24). In migraineurs, tenderness is not related to the frequency of migraine but only to the frequency of coexisting tension-type headache (26,35). In TMDs, tenderness and pain in masticatory muscles are also the most frequently reported symptoms and signs and are included in the diagnostic criteria for TMD (9). Travell and Simons popularized the term myofascial pain (45), but the pathophysiology behind local as well as generalized myofascial pain and its role in TMD is still not clear. The previously suggested mechanism of local ischemia was never confirmed. On the basis of numerous experimental animal studies, the present hypothesis of myofascial pain is either a local mechanical or chemical trauma that led to local sensitization of peripheral nociceptors, thereby causing increased peripheral nociceptive input (7,23,31). In predisposed subjects, prolonged and continuous peripheral input may lead to a central sensitization at the spinal dorsal horn or trigeminal level (7,23,31). This hypothesis of central sensitization, which was confirmed in several animal models and indirectly in human pain conditions as fibromyalgia and chronic tension-type headache (2,3,25,30), can explain the refractory chronic pain condition in these patients. Whether this is the explanation in TMD is as yet unknown, although it is considered likely, based on experimental studies in animal models (44,46,47) and because these TMD patients have many clinical and paraclinical features in common with patients with chronic tension-type headache. (For further discussion, see Chapters 73, 76, 80, 81, and 82).

Other common suggested etiologic factors for headache associated with TMD include bruxism, trauma, occlusal interferences, and emotional stressors (1,14,32,39). Berlin and colleagues reported a reduction in the incidence of headache in a group of patients with bruxism. They addressed their treatment toward functional disturbances of the masticatory system and suggested that in so doing they changed the forces produced by bruxism on the musculoskeletal system, thereby decreasing pain. Because bruxism is so common a problem, it is difficult to attribute its action to the cause of pain (41,42). Although parafunctional habits have been implicated in TMD (32,40) their relationship to headache is unknown. Occlusal interferences are by far the most controversial aspects of the cause and treatment of TMD and related headache. In a recent review based on a series of studies, Seligman and Pullinger described little, if any, relationship of occlusal factors, when taken together, with TMD (41,42). The literature has some studies (13,32) stating that occlusion is an important etiologic factor in headache based on treatment outcome. Certainly, more data are required before a final conclusion to this story can be established.

Inflammation of the TMJ may occur in conjunction with internal derangements or incoordinations of disc condyle and temporal bone. When joint noise is present on movement, it may be due to anatomic changes to any of the articulating surfaces secondary to remodeling from microtraumas or macrotraumas. Additionally, noise may be present when the disc is displaced (usually anteriorly and laterally). In these situations, there is rotation of the condyle (up to 25 mm of interincisal opening); at this point, the patient experiences catching caused by binding of the disc against the eminence. Manipulation or movement of the mandible by the patient will result in a "clicking" or "popping" noise as the condyle moves under the disc; then the jaw will translate. In these situations, a noise again can be noted on closing as the teeth come back together. This condition is called an *anterior displaced disc with reduction*. Usually, these situations are painful if there is associated intracapsular inflammation. Joint injection with local anesthetic or steroid will decrease the pain and helps in localizing the pathology. In cases where the mandible cannot move beyond the displaced disc, the condition is called a closed-lock or *anterior displaced disc without reduction*. Pain is associated only with local inflammation. Treatment of the closed lock may require manual manipulation with local anesthetic or arthroscopic intervention.

Inflammation of the TMJ is associated primarily with degenerative changes seen on bony imaging. Rarely is there the presence of inflammation secondary to systemic arthritides. Rheumatoid arthritis and psoriatic arthritis do affect the TMJ, and standard serology for these conditions can help to confirm the diagnosis.

Clinical Features

IHS diagnostic criteria for temporomandibular joint disease. (Headache Classification Committee, 1988):

At least two of the following:

1. Pain of the jaw precipitated by movement or clenching
2. Decreased range of movement

3. Noise during joint movements
4. Tenderness of the joint capsule
5. Positive radigraphic or isotope scintigraphic findings
6. Mild to moderate pain located to the TMJ or radiating from it

The most frequent presenting symptom is pain, usually localized in the muscles of mastication, the preauricular area, or the TMJ. The pain is characteristically aggravated by jaw function. Additional characteristics are limited or asymmetric jaw movements as well as joint noise on movement or locking on opening. Headache is a common associated complaint of TMD, and some studies report it to be the most common symptom of dysfunction (16). The association of TMD and headache is described by some to be directly related to the pathology of the TMJ (13,32,39). An alternate hypothesis is that headache in the presence of TMD is an associated symptom, possibly triggered but not etiologically related.

Prognosis

Patients with TMD are well treated, and long-term residual problems are few. It is reassuring to inform TMD patients that these problems are rarely present beyond the fourth decade of life. Patients who are non-responsive to physical medicine approaches should not automatically become surgical candidates; rather, any behavioral factors perpetuating the disorder should be considered.

Management

In general, treatment outcome studies of headache related to TMD use various methods of assessing pain reduction, seldom with the same outcome variables. One of the greatest problems is the generalization that if headache is decreased by treatment of the TMD, then the etiology of the pain is the TMD (1,12,32). Little comment is ever made of the role of the central nervous system or behavioral factors. The therapies described here may reduce headache that is aggravated by the coexistence of the TMD, but care should be exercised in making a cause-and-effect "leap" when patients respond.

The general principles of management include decreasing pain, decreasing adverse loading, resuming function, and resuming normal activity. These goals may be achieved through a structured, time-limited program that addresses the physical disorder and the perpetuating factors. Often, as in other musculoskeletal disorders, TMD is self-limiting, resolving without serious long-term problems. Thus, overtreatment should be avoided; the need for conservative management is emphasized. The five basic areas that should be considered are summarized in Table 2.

TABLE 2. *Basic principles of management of temporomandibular disorders*

Patient education and self-care
Cognitive behavioral interventions
Pharmacologic management
e.g., Analgesics, antiinflammatories, muscle relaxants, sedatives, antidepressants
Physical therapies
e.g., Posture training, stretching exercises, mobilization, physical modalities, appliance therapy, occlusal therapy
Surgery

Patient Education and Self-Care

The overall effect of patient education is to develop a rapport and treatment compliance. It should include an explanation of the diagnosis, an outline of the therapy, and an explanation of the goals as well as the patient's role in treatment. In the patient for whom compliance is expected to be an issue, a written treatment agreement may serve well. Details in the explanations should include modifications in function, if needed (e.g., soft diet, not clenching during the day) and explanations regarding the role habits play and how to break them. The use of visual reminders (e.g., colored sticky dots) may be helpful. This aspect of treatment should not be minimized; if the patient understands what the therapy is about, compliance may be enhanced.

Cognitive-Behavioral Intervention

Although simple habits may be modified when patients are made aware of them, changing persistent habits and problems with lifestyle issues may require a structured approach involving a well-trained behavioral therapist. The behavior modification is often best accompanied by progressive relaxation training, hypnosis, or biofeedback. Treatment should be individualized to deal specifically with each patient's problems, preferences, and lifestyle. More comprehensive programs may be better than individual physical or behavioral modalities.

Pharmacologic Management

When dealing with the pain and disability of TMD, it may be useful to administer adjuvant therapy with medication given orally or injected into the joint. The most effective pharmacologic agents used in TMD management include analgesics (narcotic and nonnarcotic), nonsteroidal antiinflammatory agents, corticosteroids (often injected), sedatives, muscle relaxants, antidepressants, and anticonvulsants. Patients should be monitored carefully, especially patients who have chronic conditions; long-term use of medications always must be assessed carefully.

Physical Therapy

Physical therapy is aimed at reducing pain and restoring normal function, which are best accomplished by altering sensory input; reducing inflammation; decreasing, coordinating, and strengthening muscle activity; and promoting the repair and regeneration of tissues. The usual program requires a series of posture, stretching, and strengthening exercises, often accompanied by the use of modalities such as fluorimethane spray and stretch, trigger-point injections, hot packs, ice, ultrasound, or other stimulating techniques.

The purpose of these modalities is to reduce inflammation and decrease pain so the patient may carry out an exercise program in less pain. Often the therapist will be better able to mobilize the joint without reflex muscle spasm.

Orthopedic appliances in the form of stabilization appliances or anterior repositioning appliances are also a mainstay of TMD therapy. The stabilization appliance should cover all the maxillary or mandibular teeth. They are intended to provide joint stabilization, protect the teeth, redistribute forces, relax the elevator muscles, and decrease parafunctional behavior. It is suggested the appliances be worn at night only and that behavioral modification be used during the day to keep the teeth apart. The anterior repositioning appliance holds the jaw forward of the normal muscle-contacting position and usually is used in acute joint pain situations in which the noise can be eliminated by anterior positioning of the jaw. Because these appliances may alter the structural relationship of the jaw, patients must be aware that this therapy may progress to orthodontic or prosthetic therapy to correct the change in the teeth relationship. Short-term response with this therapy is good, but long-term outcome is uncertain. If anterior repositioning therapy is used, it should be short term (less than 3 months), and the patient should wear the appliance only at night to ensure that significant occlusal or jaw changes do not take place.

Occlusal Therapy

The topic of occlusion is controversial. Occlusion is not often a causative factor in TMD. Many studies suggest a positive outcome in treatment of TMD with modification of occlusion; however, review of placebo-controlled studies shows that little if any benefit is derived from this therapy. Although it is useful from a dental point of view to maintain the occlusion stable, correction of an occlusion that has been present for years before the onset of TMD probably will not be useful.

Surgery

Surgery for TMD is effective therapy for specific articular disorders; the more progressive pathology may require surgical intervention. The least invasive technique involves *arthrocentesis*, or intraarticular irrigation and lavage of the joint. This procedure usually is indicated in acute closed-lock situations. In some cases, *arthroscopy*, which allows direct vision and directed therapy, may be required. In rare cases, *arthrotomy*, or open surgical interventions is required. The cases are usually complex and include but are not limited to ankylosis, neoplasm, severe degeneration, and disc displacement or perforation. Many cases require total joint replacement, usually following multiple failed surgeries resulting from complications of alloplastic prostheses.

HEADACHE PROBLEMS PRESENTING IN OROMANDIBULAR STRUCTURES

Often the clinician is faced with a patient who has pain in the oromandibular structures, but no local cause is obvious. These difficult to explain problems often result in numerous unnecessary treatments, including irreversible dental and sinus procedures. The clinician dealing with facial pain should consider the common headache problems that are often present in the lower half of the head.

Migraine

Lovshin was first to describe migraine as a facial-pain problem that could occur in the absence of headache (27). Raskin and Prusiner also described this problem as being associated with tenderness of the carotid on the ipsilateral side and suggest that dental trauma may be the precipitating factor (36). Moncada and Graff-Radford described a case of exertional migraine presenting as a toothache. This patient was treated successfully with indomethacin (29).

Cluster Headache

Brooke described cluster headache presenting as facial pain under the diagnosis of *periodic migrainous neuralgia*. Of the patients described by Brooke, 100% had pain in the oromandibular region, 53% with toothache, 47% with jaw pain (5). Bittar and Graff-Radford described 42 patients with cluster headache, of whom 65% received unnecessary dental treatments because of the facial presentation (4).

Chronic Paroxysmal Hemicrania (CPH)

Delchano and Graff-Radford described two patients with CPH who presented with the pain primarily in the tooth but radiating to the maxillotemporal regions of the face. Both patients were well controlled with indomethacin (10).

Trigeminal Neuralgia and Pretrigeminal Neuralgia

Although not headache problems, trigeminal neuralgia and pretrigeminal neuralgia are often misdiagnosed as being dental problems. Merrill and Graff-Radford described 61 patients, 19 with pretrigeminal and 42 with trigeminal neuralgia who received more than 100 unnecessary dental treatments before an appropriate diagnosis and treatment (33) were made. Pretrigeminal neuralgia is more likely to be misdiagnosed because of its "toothache-like" presentation. The pain is longer lasting and often dull or aching (15,33).

CONCLUSION

Because headache is a major source of suffering and lost work, better epidemiologic studies are needed to clarify the role of TMD and headache. TMD is believed to be an aggravating factor in headache and the cause only if clearly related to clinical signs and symptoms involving the masticatory system. Until proof of headache mechanisms relating to TMD is available, the association may be coincidental, which should in no way deter clinicians from treating headache using proven treatments aimed at the tempormandibular structures; rather, caution is indicated before drawing conclusions that if treatment is effective, then the cause is the TMD. There is still much to be learned about the relationship between oromandibular disorders and headache; it is hoped that with time the devolopment of classification criteria and treatment guidelines will lead to a better understanding of the clinical problem and, in turn, translate into development of models for the mechanism and thereby better treatment of these disorders.

REFERENCES

1. Agerberg D, Carlsson GE. Late results of treatment of functional disorders of the masticatory system: a follow-up by questionnaire. *J Oral Rehabil* 1974;1:309–316.
2. Bendtsen L, Jensen R, Olesen J. Qualitatively altered nociception in chronic myofascial pain. *Pain* 1996;65:259–264.
3. Bendtsen L, Nørregaard J, Jensen R, Olesen J. Evidence of qualitatively altered nociception in patients with fibromyalgia. *Arthritis Rheum* 1997;40:98–102.
4. Bittar G, Graff-Radford SB. Cluster Headache. *Oral Surg Oral Med Oral Pathol* 1992;73:519–525.
5. Brooke RI. Periodic migrainous neuralgia: a cause of dental pain. *Oral Surg Oral Med Oral Pathol* 1978;46:511–515.
6. Classification and Diagnostic Criteria for headache disorders, cranial neuralgias and facial pain. Headache classification committee of the International Headache Society. *Cephalalgia* 1988;8(Suppl 7):1–96.
7. Coderre TJ, Katz J, Vaccarino AL, Melzack R. Contribution of central neuroplasticity topathological pain: review of clinical and experimental evidence. *Pain* 1993;52:259–285.
8. Costen JB. A syndrome of ear and sinus symptoms dependent upon disturbed function of the temporomandibular joint. *Ann Otolaryngol Chir Cervicofac* 1934;43:1–7.
9. *Craniomandibular disorders:* guidelines for evaluation, *diagnosis and management*, 2nd ed. Charles McNeill, ed. Quintessence, 1992.
10. Delcanho R, Graff-Radford SB. Chronic paroxysmal hemicrania presenting as toothache. *Journal of Orofacial Pain* 1993;75:579–582.
11. Dworkin SF, LeResche LR, Von Korff M, Howard J, Truelove E, Sommers E. Epidemiology of signs and symptoms in temporomandibular disorders: 1. Clinical signs in cases and controls. *J Am Dent Assoc* 1990;120:273–281.
12. Forssell H, Kangasniemi P. Mandibular dysfunction in patients with migraine. *Proc Finn Dent Soc* 1984;80:211–216.
13. Forssell H, Kirveskari P, Kangasniemi P. Changes in headache after treatment of mandibular dysfunction. *Cephalalgia* 1985;5:229–236.
14. Forssell H, Kirveskari P, Kangasniemi P. Distinguishing between headaches responsive and irresponsive to treatment of mandibular dysfunction. *Proceedings of the Finnish Dental Society* 1986;82:219–222.
15. Fromm GH, Graff-Radford SB, Terrence CF, Sweet WH. Pretrigeminal neuralgia. *Neurology* 1990;40:1493–1495.
16. Gelb H, Tarte J. A two year clinical dental evaluation of 200 cases of chronic headache: the cranio-cervical mandibular syndrome. *J Am Dent Assoc* 1975;91:1230–1236.
17. Graff-Radford SB, Solberg WK. Atypical odontalgia. *CDA* 1986;14:27–31.
18. Graff-Radford SB, Reeves JL, Jaeger B. Management of head and neck pain: effectiveness of altering factors perpetuating myofascial pain. *Headache* 1987;27:186–190.
19. Graff-Radford SB, Solberg WK. Is atypical odontalgia a psychological problem? *Oral Surg Oral Med Oral Pathol* 1993;75:579–582.
20. Graff-Radford SB, Solberg WK. Differential neural blockade in atypical odontalgia. *Cephelalgia* 1991;(Suppl 11):289–291.
21. Graff-Radford SB, Solberg WK. Atypical odontalgia. *J Craniomandib Disord Oral Facial Pain* 1992;6:260–266.
22. Green CS, Marbach JJ. Epidemiologic studies of mandibular dysfunction: a critical review. *J Prosth Dent* 1982;48:184–190.
23. Hoheisel U, Koch K, Mense S. Functional reorganization in the rat dorsal horn during an experimental myositis. *Pain* 1994;59:111–118.
24. Jensen R, Rasmussen BK, Pedersen B, Olesen J. Muscle tenderness and pressure pain thresholds in headache: a population study. *Pain* 1993;52:193–199.
25. Jensen R, Bendtsen L, Olesen J. Muscular factors are important in tension-type headache. *Headache* 1998;38:10–17.
26. Jensen K, Tuxen C, Olesen J. Pericranial muscle tenderness and pressure pain threshold in the temporal region during common migraine. *Pain* 1988;35:65–78.
27. Lovshin LL. Carotidynia. *Headache.* 1977;17:192–195.
28. Lund JP, Donga R, Widmer CG, Stohler CS. The pain-adaption model: a discussion of the relationship between chronic musculoskeletal pain and motor activity. *Can J Physiol* 1991;69:683–694.
29. Moncada E, Graff-Radford SB. Cough headache presenting as a toothache: a case presentation. *Headache* 1993;33:240–243.
30. Mense S. Considerations concerning the neurobiological basis of muscle pain. *Can J Physiol Pharmacol* 1991;9:610–616.
31. Mense S. Nociception from skeletal muscle in relation to clinical muscle pain. *Pain* 1993;54:241–289.
32. Magnusson T, Carlsson GE. Changes in recurrent headache and mandibular dysfunction after various types of dental treatment. *Acta Odontol Scand* 1980;38:311–320.
33. Merrill RL, Graff-Radford SB. Trigeminal neuralgia: how to rule out the wrong treatment. *J Am Dent Assoc* 1992;123:63–68.
34. Nilner M, Lassing SA. Prevalence of functional disturbances and diseases of the stomatognathic system in 7–14 year olds. *Swed Dent J* 1981;5:173–187.
35. Olesen J. Some clinical features of the acute migraine attack: an analysis of 750 patients. *Headache* 1978;18:268–271.
36. Raskin NH, Prusiner S. Carotodynia. *Neurology* 1977;27:43–46.
37. Rugh JD, Solberg WK. Oral health status in the United States: temporomandibular disorders. *J Dent Educ* 1985;49:398–404.
38. Schiffman E, Fricton JR. Epidemiology of TMJ and craniofacial pain. In Fricton JR, Kroening RJ, Hathaway KM, eds. *TMJ and craniofacial pain:* diagnosis and management. St Louis: IEA Publishers, 1988:1–10.
39. Schiffman E, Fricton JR, Haley D, Shapiro BL. The prevalence and treatment needs of subjects with temporomandibular disorders. *J Am Dent Assoc* 1989;120:295–304.
40. Sessel BJ, Hu JW. Mechanisms of pain arising from articular tissues. *Can J Physiol Pharmacol* 1991;69:617–626.
41. Seligman DA, Pullinger AG. The role of functional occlusal relationships in temporomandibular disorders. *J Craniomandib Disord* 1991;5:231–238.

42. Seligman DA, Pullinger AG. The role of intercuspal occlusal relationships in temporomandibular disorders: a review. *J Craniomandib Disord* 1991;5:96–106.

43. Sicuteri F, Nicolodi M, Fusco BM, Orlando S. Idiopathic headache as a possible risk factor for phantom tooth pain. *Headache* 1991;31:577–581.

44. Svensson P, Arendt-Nielsen L, Houe L. Sensory-motor interactions of human experimental unilateral jaw muscle pain: a quantitative analysis. *Pain* 1996;64:241–249.

45. Travell JG, Simons D. *Myofascial pain and dysfunction:* the *trigger point manual.* Baltimore: Williams & Wilkins, 1988.

46. Yu XM, Sessle BJ, Hu JW. Differential effects of cutaneous and deep application of inflammatory irritant on the mechanoreceptive field properties of trigeminal brain stem nociceptive neurons. *J Neurophysiol* 1993;70:1704–1707.

47. Yu XM, Sessle BJ, Vernon H, Hu JW. Effects of inflammatory irritant application to the rat temporomandibular joint on jaw and neck muscle activity. *Pain* 1995;60:143–149.

The Headaches, Second Edition,
edited by J. Olesen, P. Tfelt-Hansen, and K.M.A. Welch.
Lippincott Williams & Wilkins, Philadelphia © 2000.

The Secondary Headaches

CHAPTER 122

Pain of Cranial Nerve and Cervical Nerve Origin Other than Primary Neuralgias

Nikolai Bogduk

The cranial and upper cervical spinal nerves can be involved in mediating either neurogenic or nociceptive pain that is perceived as headache. Neurogenic pain arises when the axons or cell bodies of nerves are directly affected by intrinsic or extrinsic disorders; this pain manifests clinically as *neuralgia*. Nociceptive pain arises when nerve endings are stimulated by lesions in structures that the nerve innervates. The cranial neuralgias are described in Chapter 123, and nociceptive pain mediated by cranial nerves occurs in the context of headaches associated with disorders of the eye (Chapter 119) and the ear, nose, and sinuses (Chapter 120). Nociceptive pain mediated by cervical spinal nerves is considered in Chapter 118. This leaves a miscellany of relatively uncommon disorders that are neither neuralgias of the cranial nerves nor nociceptive disorders of the cervical spine. These are the conditions of painful ophthalmoplegia involving the trigeminal nerve and C2 neuralgia as well as neck–tongue syndrome involving the upper cervical spinal nerves. To this collection can be added acute and chronic pain associated with herpes zoster infection.

C2 OR C3 NERVE COMPRESSION

IHS code and diagnosis: 12.1.1 Compression or distortion of the second or third cervical nerve roots.
WHO code and diagnosis: G44.848.

N. Bogduk: Department of Anatomy and Musculoskeletal Medicine, University of Newcastle, and Newcastle Bone and Joint Institute, Royal Newcastle Hospital, Newcastle, New South Wales 2300, Australia.

Short description: Headaches caused by a lesion that compresses or otherwise compromises the C2 or C3 spinal nerves or their roots. Most reported cases, however, have involved the C2 nerve.
Other terms: C2 neuralgia.

Anatomy and Pathology

The C3 spinal nerve occupies a typical intervertebral foramen and is vulnerable to any of the causes of foraminal stenosis: disc herniation, spondylosis, zygapophysial osteoarthrosis, and others. Such disorders are relatively uncommon at the C2–3 level, however.

The C2 spinal nerve is relatively immune to entrapment or compression because, unlike the typical spinal nerves, it does not run in an intervertebral foramen. Consequently, it is not subject to the hazards of intervertebral disc herniation or spondylosis; nor is it vulnerable to compression during extension injuries of the neck, because the height of the articular pillars of C1 and C2 protect it from compression by the posterior arch of the atlas (6). The C2 nerve runs behind the lateral atlantoaxial joint, resting on its capsule (7,8) (Fig. 1). Inflammatory or other disorders of the joint may result in the nerve becoming incorporated in the fibrotic changes of chronic inflammation (35,59)

Otherwise, the C2 spinal nerve and its roots are surrounded by a sleeve of dura mater and a plexus of epiradicular veins, lesions of which can compromise the nerve. These include meningioma (44) and neurinoma (35), but most reported cases have involved vascular abnormalities ranging from single to densely interwoven, dilated veins surrounding the C2 spinal nerve and its roots (34) to U-shaped arterial loops or angiomas com-

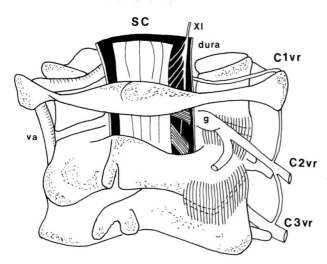

FIG. 1. A posterior view of the right atlantoaxial region showing the relationship of the C2 ganglion (*g*) and ventral ramus (*vr*) to the posterior aspect of the lateral atlantoaxial joint. The dural sac has been opened posteriorly to show the upper end of the spinal cord (*SC*), the C2 and C3 nerve roots, and the roots of the accessory nerve (*XI*). The vertebral artery (*va*) is shown on the left.

pressing the C2 dorsal root ganglion (28,34,35). Nerves affected by vascular abnormalities exhibit a variety of features indicative of neuropathy, such as myelin breakdown, chronic hemorrhage, axon degeneration and regeneration, and increased endoneurial and pericapsular connective tissue (34). It is not clear, however, whether the vascular abnormality causes these neuropathic changes or is only coincident with them.

Pathophysiology

The pathophysiology of C2 neuralgia is unknown, but the neuralgic quality of pain strongly implies a neurogenic basis. Ectopic, nociceptive impulses could be generated by ischemia or mechanical compression of the dorsal root ganglion.

Clinical Features

C2 neuralgia is a distinctive condition characterized by intermittent, lancinating pain in the occipital region associated with lacrimation and ciliary injection. The pain typically occurs in association with a background of dull occipital pain and dull, referred pain in the temporal, frontal, and orbital regions. Most often, this latter pain is focused on the frontoorbital region but encompasses all three regions when severe. The distinguishing feature of this condition is a cutting or tearing sensation in the occipital region, which is the hallmark of its neurogenic basis.

The frequency of attacks varies from four to five per day to two to seven per week, alternating with pain-free intervals of days, weeks, or months (34,35). About 75%

of patients suffer the associated features of ipsilateral conjunctival and ciliary injection and lacrimation (34,35). Blurred vision, rhinorrhea, and dizziness are less common accompaniments. Neurologic examination is normal. In particular, hypoesthesia in the territory of the trigeminal or cervical nerves is not present.

C2 neuralgia is distinguished from occipital neuralgia and referred pain from the neck by its neurogenic quality, its periodicity, and its association with lacrimation and ciliary injection. The latter association has attracted the appellation of *clusterlike headache* (44).

The cardinal diagnostic feature is complete relief of pain following local anesthetic blockade of the suspected nerve root, typically the C2 spinal nerve but occasionally the C3 nerve. These blocks are performed under radiologic control and employ discrete amounts (0.6–0.8 mL) of long-acting local anesthetic to block the target nerve selectively (35).

Plain radiographs, computed tomography (CT), myelo-CT, or myelography reveal no suggestion of these lesions. No provocative test reveals arterial lesions (34), but in most patients with venous lesions, challenge with 0.8 mg of nitroglycerin provokes an attack of pain; conversely, inhalation of 100% O_2 at 10 L per minute for 5 minutes relieves the pain (34).

Management

There is no evidence that C2 neuralgia responds to pharmacotherapy (34). Surgery appears to be the only definitive means of treatment. Nerves entrapped by scarring may be liberated (59); meningiomas may be excised (44). With respect to vascular lesions, resection of the vascular abnormality alone does not reliably relieve the pain; resection or thermocoagulation of the nerve appears to be necessary to guarantee relief of pain (34).

ACUTE HERPES ZOSTER

IHS code and diagnosis: 12.1.4.1 Herpes zoster.
WHO code and diagnosis: G53.000.
Short description: Pain in the head or face associated with acute herpes zoster infection.

Epidemiology

With an incidence of 131 per 100,000 person-years, the disease can affect any age group, but it occurs more frequently in elderly persons (61,63) and in patients with lymphoma or Hodgkin's disease or who are under immune suppression (61).

Anatomy and Pathology

Herpes zoster is a disease of dorsal root ganglia characterized by a vesicular eruption in the affected dermatome. It is a reactivation of a latent infection by the varicella virus (49,61). The thoracic nerve roots are most commonly affected (61), but about 12% of presentations involve the cervical spinal nerves, and 13% involve the trigeminal nerve (63). The ophthalmic division is affected in 80% of trigeminal presentations. The pathology of the disease involves inflammation, hemorrhage, and necrosis of the affected ganglion and dorsal horn with intranuclear inclusion bodies in satellite cells and ganglion cells (49).

Pathophysiology

The mechanism of pain is unknown but possibly involves ectopic discharges from the affected dorsal root ganglion cells (61).

Clinical Features

IHS diagnostic criteria for herpes zoster

A. Pain is followed by a herpetic eruption in the distribution of the affected nerve within 1 week of onset.
B. Pain subsides within 6 months after onset of the rash.

The onset of acute herpes zoster usually is heralded by pain that precedes the vesicular eruption by a few days. When the trigeminal or C2 ganglion is affected, the pain occurs in the forehead or occipital region; however, no practical method has been found to establish the diagnosis while pain is the only feature. The condition declares itself once the vesicular eruption occurs. In rare instances, the geniculate ganglion can be affected, presenting with otalgia or facial pain before the eruption of vesicles in the external auditory meatus and palate (30).

Prognosis

The usual course of herpes zoster infection is that the vesicles dry out within about 1 week and heal within about 1 month (49,61). The cardinal complication is postherpetic neuralgia, which ensues in about 10% of patients (63). When the nasociliary nerve is affected uveitis, keratitis and iridocyclitis are complications that may threaten vision as well as cause ocular pain.

Management

A variety of interventions have been advocated, but few have survived scientific scrutiny (36,61). The confounding factor in the treatment of acute herpes zoster is that the disease is self-limiting with a short, natural course. Consequently, many forms of therapy may appear to work, and stringent, controlled trials are required to establish the true efficacy.

A variety of topical therapies have been advocated (11,38,39,49,50,61). Oral acyclovir (and the newer agents, famciclovir and valaciclovir) arrest the formation of new lesions, promote healing, shorten the period of infectivity, reduce pain, and shorten the period of pain;

but they do not prevent postherpetic neuralgia (36,53,54,58,61,93). Guidelines (36,37) recommend that these drugs be used in patients of any age presenting with ophthalmic involvement within the first 72 hours after onset of rash and in any patients with active zoster affecting the neck, limbs, and perineum.

Other measures, such as analgesics, tricyclics, or opiates, may be used in an effort to palliate symptoms but are not of proven benefit (49,61). Sympathetic nerve blocks are advocated by some, but the literature is devoid of sufficiently powerful controlled trials and remains divided (2,36,49,61).

The classic mainstay for acute herpes zoster, particularly ophthalmic herpes, has been systemic steroids (16,46), but their effects are uncertain because of inadequacies of trial designs (62). One double-blind, controlled study, however, showed that triamcinolone reduced the duration of pain but only in patients over the age of 60 years; the disease was too short-lived to establish significance in younger patients (14). Other controlled trials have shown steroids, when combined with acyclovir, to afford some benefits in terms of reduction of pain and quality of life (92,94); however, no form of therapy reliably prevents postherpetic neuralgia (17,36,62,69,92,93).

POSTHERPETIC NEURALGIA

IHS code and diagnosis: 12.1.4.2 Chronic postherpetic neuralgia.
WHO code and diagnosis: G53.001.
Short description: Postherpetic neuralgia is a neuralgic pain that persists in the affected dermatome long after the vesicular eruption of acute herpes zoster has healed.

Epidemiology

In patients under the age of 40, postherpetic neuralgia does not usually follow acute herpes zoster; but of patients aged over 60, more than 60% of patients develop pain, and up to 50% or more suffer pain lasting more than a year (61,86).

Anatomy and Pathology

The pathology of postherpetic neuralgia involves atrophy of the dorsal horn and cell loss, axon loss, and demyelination with fibrosis in the dorsal root ganglion (89). These changes appear to be specific for patients with pain, whereas demyelination and axon loss in the affected peripheral nerve occur in patients both with and without pain (89).

Pathophysiology

The pathophysiology of postherpetic pain is unknown but may involve central deafferentation rather than mechanisms in the peripheral nerves or sensory ganglia (61). The notion that postherpetic pain arises as a result of selective loss of large-diameter afferents with loss of inhibition of small-diameter, nociceptive afferents is inconsistent with the results of pathology studies that found no difference in fiber loss when comparing patients with pain and patients without pain (49).

Clinical Features

IHS diagnostic criteria for chronic postherpetic neuralgia (Headache Classification Committee 1988):

A. Pain is restricted to the distribution of the affected cranial nerves or divisions thereof.
B. Pain persists more than 6 months after the onset of herpetic eruption.

The pain is archetypal of neuralgia, characterized by constant burning and aching with superimposed jabs of shooting or lancinating pain. The skin of the affected dermatome is hypoesthetic but may involve zones of hyperesthesia from which attacks of pain may be triggered by light touch or brushing (86). Midthoracic dermatomes and the first-division trigeminal nerve are most commonly affected (86).

Prognosis

Follow-up studies reveal that at 2 years, 25% of patients have a good outcome with no therapy; 22% benefit from therapy; but 53% have a poor outcome despite therapy (88).

Management

Postherpetic neuralgia is one of the most refractory of pain problems. No single therapy has been validated, but a vast armamentarium of suggestions exists from which a physician might choose (36,49,61,85,86).

Topical therapies to palliate the cutaneous sensitivity include local anaesthetic creams (10,41,65,67,76), dry ice (77), aspirin in chloroform (39), and aspirin in diethyl ether (11). The use of capsaicin creams (4,87) has been validated by a controlled trial (91). Baclofen, diphenylhydantoin, carbamazepine, and valproic acid have been advocated but are unsupported by controlled trials (49,55,85) and are frequently not helpful (86). Postherpetic neuralgia is usually unresponsive to opiates, although patients resistant to other therapies may benefit from slow-release morphine or oxycodone (57). Ophthalmic postherpetic neuralgia is relieved temporarily by somatic blocks but not by sympathetic blocks (56,86).

Of all the drugs that have been advocated for postherpetic neuralgia, amitriptyline has emerged as the most consistently worthwhile (61,86); its effectiveness has been verified in placebo-controlled and comparison trials (52,83,84,90). The optimal dose is 75 mg at night, achieved by building up the dose over 10 days after an initial dose of 25 mg. Adding fluphenazine may improve the response in some patients who do not respond to amitriptyline alone (49,61,80,86). Similarly, combining a tricyclic with an anticonvulsant may be an advantage (26,61). Desipramine is also effective although in fewer patients than is amitriptyline (40). The selective serotonin reuptake inhibitors (e.g., zimelidine) have little effect on postherpetic neuralgia (36,84,90). Analgesics such as acetaminophen provide some relief to patients refractory to other measures (36,86). Intravenous local anesthetics have been advocated, particularly for intractable trigeminal post-herpetic neuralgia (46,71) and has been shown to be equipotent to intravenous morphine and superior to placebo (66).

Acupuncture is distinctly unsuccessful for postherpetic neuralgia (48). Transcutaneous electric nerve stimulation is palliative in some patients, but response cannot be predicted (49,61,86). Various surgical interventions have been advocated for trigeminal postherpetic neuralgia, including trigeminal rhizotomy, avulsion, alcohol injection or cryocoagulation of the supraorbital nerve, alcohol injection of the trigeminal ganglion, and trigeminal tractotomy; but none of these procedures has been found to work consistently or to achieve prolonged relief of pain (49,61). Thalamic stimulation is claimed to offer excellent pain relief in properly selected patients (49), and about 70% of patients with ophthalmic neuralgia are said to derive long-term benefit from nucleus caudalis dorsal root entry zone (DREZ) lesions (3) or stereotactic nucleotomy (70).

PAINFUL OPHTHALMOPLEGIA

IHS code and diagnosis: 12.1.5 Painful ophthalmoplegia.
WHO code and diagnosis: G44.850.
Short description: Orbital pain or headache associated with some degree of ophthalmoplegia.
Other terms: *Painful ophthalmoplegia* comprises conditions that have previously been referred to as *superior orbital fissure syndrome, orbital apex syndrome, cavernous sinus syndrome, parasellar syndrome, Collier's syndrome*, and *Tolosa-Hunt syndrome*.

Anatomy and Pathology

The anatomic basis for painful ophthalmoplegia lies in the density of relationships in the cavernous sinus between the internal carotid artery; the trigeminal nerve; the third, fourth, and sixth cranial nerves; and the parasympathetic and sympathetic nerves of the eye. Painful ophthalmoplegia arises when a pain-producing lesion also involves one or more of these nerves. Such lesions may be vascular, neurologic, space-occupying,

TABLE 1. *Differential diagnosis of painful ophthalmoplegia*

Cause	Diagnostic test
Vascular	
Internal carotid aneurysm	Angiography
Carotico cavernous fistula	Ocular features
Cavernous sinus thrombosis	
Temporal arteritis	ESR, biopsy
Neurologic	
Diabetic neuropathy	Blood glucose
Ophthalmoplegic migraine	
Neoplastic	
Nasopharyngeal tumors	CT, MRI
Tumors of skull base	
Parasellar meningioma	
Metastases	
Pituitary tumors	
Chondroma	
Chordoma	
Retrobulbar tumors	CT, angiography
Infectious	
Actinomycosis	Biopsy, serology
Aspergillosis	
Tuberculosis	
Infiltrative	
Systemic lupus erythematosus	Serology
Lymphoma	Biopsy
Sarcoid	Serology, biopsy
Syphilis	Serology
Miscellaneous	
Pseudotumour of the orbit	CT, angiography
Sphenoid sinus mucocoele	CT
Epidermoid tumor	CT

CT, computed tomography; ESR, erythrocyte sedimentation rate; MRI, magnetic resonance imaging.

inflammatory, or infiltrative (Table 1). Different clinical manifestations arise, depending on whether the causative lesion affects the sinus extensively or the lesion is focal and located anteriorly or posteriorly in the sinus.

Pathophysiology

Orbital pain or headache arises presumably as a result of inflammation or distension of the meningeal walls of the cavernous sinus or as a result of irritation of the frontal branch of the trigeminal nerve. Ophthalmoplegia arises as a result of compression or ischemia of the third, fourth, or sixth cranial nerves.

Clinical Features

IHS diagnostic criteria for painful ophthalmoplegia:

A. Episode or episodes of unilateral orbital pain for an average of 8 weeks if untreated

B. Association with paralysis of one or more of the third, fourth, or sixth cranial nerves, which may coincide with the onset of the pain or follow it by a period of up to 2 weeks

C. Pain relieved within 72 hours after initiation of corticosteroid therapy

D. Exclusion of other causative lesions by neuroimaging and (not compulsory) carotid angiography

The third nerve is involved in about 90% of presentations; in 40%, the fourth or sixth nerves also are involved or affected alone (31,51). The third-nerve involvement manifests most obviously by paralysis or paresis of the ocular muscles it supplies. Parasympathoplegia is not overt but may be evident as a sluggish pupillary light reflex (1,31,51). Involvement of the ocular sympathetic fibers is evident in the form of ptosis and poor mydriasis (1,31,51). Involvement of the frontal nerve manifests by depression of the corneal reflex and periorbital hypoesthesia (1,51,73). About 10% of patients may have involvement of the optic nerve in the form of diminished visual acuity, but papilloedema or venous congestion of the optic disc is not a feature (31,33,51). Optic-nerve involvement suggests anterior extension of the causative lesion from the cavernous sinus. Posterior extension may involve the second division of the trigeminal nerve (72).

Clinical examination alone is insufficient to elucidate the causative lesion of painful ophthalmoplegia. Resolution of the diagnosis relies on biochemical and serologic investigations to confirm or exclude diabetic neuropathy, immunological disorders, and infection; carotid angiography is required to confirm or exclude internal carotid aneurysm; CT or magnetic resonance imaging (MRI) is required to identify space-occupying and infiltrative lesions (see Table 1). Even comprehensive application of such studies may fail to reveal the actual cause, however.

No firm guidelines are available to distinguish painful ophthalmoplegia from ophthalmoplegic migraine. Indeed, the distinction has been questioned, because some patients diagnosed as suffering from ophthalmoplegic migraine have been found on investigation to have structural lesions (13).

Painful ophthalmoplegia is distinguishable from *pseudotumor of the orbit* because the latter typically involves chemosis, proptosis, and inflammatory symptoms, and typically it spares the fifth nerve (1,51,72). It has been suggested, however, that painful ophthalmoplegia and pseudotumor of the orbit may only be anatomic variants of the same basic condition (64).

Temporal arteritis is distinguished by an elevated erythrocyte sedimentation rate and typically affects elderly patients with an average age of 70 (73), whereas patients with painful ophthalmoplegia have an average age of 41 (1,51,73). Also, temporal arteritis rarely affects the sixth nerve (73), and temporal artery biopsy should confirm the diagnosis.

Certain variants of painful ophthalmoplegia have attracted specific appellations but constitute no more than examples of lesions in particular locations. Thus,

Gradenigo's syndrome is a variant that involves a sixth-nerve palsy caused by lesions at the apex of the petrous temporal bone. *Raeder's paratrigeminal neuralgia* is a not a distinct entity; the term has been applied to painful ophthalmoplegia involving sympathoplegia of the eye ascribed inconsistently to various lesions of the internal carotid artery or its relations in the cavernous sinus. Because of the lack of pathologic specificity and consistency the term is no longer credited (27,46).

Historically, *Tolosa-Hunt syndrome* has been regarded as a distinctive variant of painful ophthalmoplegia that is ostensibly caused by granulomatous infiltration of the cavernous sinus (31,33). The criteria for its diagnosis were failure to identify a structural cause, a response to steroids, and a relapsing course. Whereas these criteria were attractive when the syndrome was first described, they are now either untenable or have been refuted.

Previous reports of granulomatous tissue in this condition can be questioned on the grounds that epithelioid cells, which are the *sine qua non* of granulomata, had not been recorded properly in Tolosa-Hunt syndrome; rather, what had been described was either ambiguous or not more than chronic inflammation (9). Angiographic and phlebographic abnormalities thought to be consistent with arteritis or occlusion of the cavernous sinus are exceptions rather than the rule in apparent Tolosa-Hunt syndrome and are not specific for this condition (23–25,31,51,73,79).

Although dramatic, the response of Tolosa-Hunt syndrome to systemic steroids is not specific. A response to steroids has been reported in cases of painful ophthalmoplegia caused by tumors (74,81), lymphoma (9,74,81), aneurysm (19,43,74,81), nasopharyngeal carcinoma (74), pituitary adenoma (43), parasellar epidermoid tumor (42), metastases (74), and actinomycosis (13).

Modern imaging techniques permit a more thorough investigation of patients with painful ophthalmoplegia to identify structural lesions (74). Even so, some patients remain in whom a distinctive lesion cannot be identified. Occasionally, CT scanning may reveal enhancing lesions in the cavernous sinus or orbital apex (9,20,21,45,82), but more often there is no abnormality characteristic of Tolosa-Hunt syndrome (20–23,60,68,78]. Thickening of the lateral wall or infiltration of the cavernous sinus has been found by using MRI (12,21,45,95), which is consistent with previous notions of a granulomatous aetiology of Tolosa-Hunt syndrome, but MRI does not disclose the nature of this tissue.

One study, however, of a patient with Tolosa-Hunt syndrome using CT-guided needle biopsy of the cavernous sinus has raised a challenging observation (68). CT revealed an enhancing lesion at the orbital apex and anterior cavernous sinus. Biopsy of the lesion revealed inflammatory tissue and frequent epithelioid cells, the latter satisfying the criterion for granuloma. Further study of the specimen revealed hyphae, however, which

were shown to be those of aspergillus. This case suggests that what may have been regarded as idiopathic granulomata in previously recorded cases of Tolosa-Hunt syndrome could have been unrecognized fungal infections.

On the other hand, some evidence suggests that Tolosa-Hunt syndrome may be but one manifestation of a wider spectrum of disorders involving multiple cranial nerves. Some instances of Tolosa-Hunt syndrome also involve the seventh cranial nerve (23,78), and an entity has been described that involves not only the cranial nerves of the cavernous sinus but also the first, seventh, eighth, ninth, tenth, or twelfth cranial nerves (29,32,75). The anatomic separation of these nerves denies a single focal cause such as those known for painful ophthalmoplegia and suggests a systemic or idiosyncratic basis. Thus, what has been regarded as Tolosa-Hunt syndrome may be a subset of a more general disorder of cranial nerves and not necessarily a condition that uniquely affects the cavernous sinus.

NECK–TONGUE SYNDROME

IHS code and diagnosis: 12.1.6 Neck–tongue syndrome.
WHO code and diagnosis: G44.851.
Short description: Neck–tongue syndrome is an uncommon but distinct condition characterized by attacks of occipital pain precipitated by sudden rotation of the head and associated with a subjective sensation of numbness in the ipsilateral half of the tongue (5,15, 18,47).

Anatomy and Pathology

The C2 spinal nerve lies behind the lateral atlantoaxial joint, which is innervated by the C2 ventral ramus (7). During rotation of the atlas, its ipsilateral, inferior articular process subluxates backward. If the range of movement is excessive, the capsule of the joint is strained and the C2 nerve may be impacted by the edge of the inferior articular process and stretched around it (8).

Neck–tongue syndrome usually occurs in otherwise normal individuals (47), but it has been reported in patients with rheumatoid arthritis or congenital joint laxity (5). Hypomobility in the contralateral, lateral atlantoaxial joint may predispose to the condition (5).

Pathophysiology

If the lateral atlantoaxial joint temporarily subluxates, stretching of its capsule produces joint pain that is perceived in the occipital region (8). Numbness of the tongue arises because of impingement, or stretching, of the C2 ventral ramus against the edge of the subluxated articular process (8) (Fig. 2) and is produced by compression of proprioceptive afferents from the tongue, which pass from the ansa hypoglossi into the C2 ventral ramus (47).

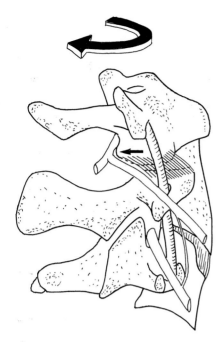

FIG. 2. A lateral view of a right atlantoaxial joint in which the atlas has rotated to the right. Its inferior articular process impacts and stretches the C2 spinal nerve and ventral ramus (*arrow*).

Clinical Features

IHS diagnostic criteria for neck–tongue syndrome:

A. Pain and numbness in the distribution of the lingual nerve and the second cervical root
B. Precipitation by sudden turning of the head

Management

Some investigators have found immobilization by a soft collar to be adequate therapy (18); others have resorted to atlantoaxial fusion (5) or resection of the C2 spinal nerves (15). Operative findings have confirmed that the syndrome involves compression of the C2 spinal nerves by the lateral atlantoaxial joint (15).

REFERENCES

1. Aaron-Rosa D, Doyan D, Salamon G, Michotey P. Tolosa-Hunt syndrome. *Ann Ophthalmol* 1978;10:1161–1168
2. Ali NM. Does sympathetic ganglionic block prevent postherpetic neuralgia [Review]? *Reg Anesth* 1995;20:227–233.
3. Bernard EJ, Nashold BS, Caputi F, Moossy JJ. Nucleus caudalis DREZ lesions for facial pain. *Br J Neurosurg* 1987;1:81–91.
4. Bernstein JE, Korman NJ, Bickers DR, et al. Topical capsaicin treatment of chronic postherpetic neuralgia. *J Am Acad Dermatol* 1989;21:265–270.
5. Bertoft ES, Westerberg CE. Further observations on the neck-tongue syndrome. *Cephalalgia* 1985;5(Suppl 3):312–313.
6. Bogduk N. The anatomy of occipital neuralgia. *Clin Exp Neurol* 1980;17:167–184.
7. Bogduk N. Local anaesthetic blocks of the second cervical ganglion: a technique with application in occipital headache. *Cephalalgia* 1981;1:41–50.
8. Bogduk N. An anatomical basis for neck tongue syndrome. *J Neurol Neurosurg Psychiatry* 1981;44:202–208.
9. Campbell RJ, Ikazaki H. Painful ophthalmoplegia (Tolosa-Hunt variant): autopsy findings in a patient with necrotizing intracavernous carotid vasculitis and inflammatory disease of the orbit. *Mayo Clinic Proc* 1987;62:520–526.
10. Collins PD. EMLA cream and herpetic neuralgia. *Med J Aust* 1991;155:206–207.
11. De Benedittis G, Besana F, Lorenzetti A. A new topical treatment for acute herpetic neuralgia and post-herpetic neuralgia: the aspirin/diethyl ether mixture. An open-label study plus a double-blind controlled clinical trial. *Pain* 1992;48:383–390.
12. Desai SP, Carter J, Jinkins JR. Contrast-enhanced MR imaging of Tolosa-Hunt Syndrome: a case report. *AJNR Am J Neuroradiol* 1991;12:182–183.
13. Dornan TL, Espir MLE, Gale EAM, Tattersall RB, Worthington BS. Remittant painful ophthalmoplegia: the Tolosa-Hunt syndrome? *J Neurol Neurosurg Psychiatry* 1979;42:270–275.
14. Eaglestein WH, Katz R, Brown JA. The effects of early corticosteroid therapy on the skin eruption and pain of herpes zoster. *JAMA* 1970;211:1681–1683.
15. Elisevich K, Stratford J, Bray G, Finlayson M. Neck tongue syndrome: operative management. *J Neurol Neurosurg Psychiatry* 1984;47:407–409.
16. Elliot FA. Treatment of herpes zoster with high doses of prednisone. *Lancet* 1970;2:1065–1066.
17. Esmann V, Geil JP, Kroon S, et al. Prednisolone does not prevent post-herpetic neuralgia. *Lancet* 1987;2:126–129
18. Fortin CJ, Biller J. Neck tongue syndrome. *Headache* 1985;25:255–258.
19. Fowler TJ, Earl CJ, McAllister VL, MacDonald WI. Tolosa-Hunt syndrome: the dangers of an eponym. *Br J Ophthalmol* 1975;59:149–154.
20. Goadsby PJ, Lance JW. Clinicopathological correlation in a case of painful ophthalmoplegia: Tolosa-Hunt syndrome. *J Neurol Neurosurg Psychiatry* 1989;52:1290–1293
21. Goto Y, Hosokawa S, Goto I, Hirakata R, Hasuo K. Abnormality in the cavernous sinus in three patients with Tolosa-Hunt syndrome: MRI and CT findings. *J Neurol Neurosurg Psychiatry* 1990;55:231–234.
22. Hannerz J. Pain characteristics of painful ophthalmoplegia (the Tolosa-Hunt syndrome). *Cephalalgia* 1985;5:103–106.
23. Hannerz J. Recurrent Tolosa-Hunt syndrome. *Cephalalgia* 1992;12:45–51.
24. Hannerz J, Ericson K, Bergstrand G. Orbital phlebography in patients with Tolosa-Hunt's syndrome in comparison with normal subjects. *Acta Radiol* 1984;25:457–463.
25. Hannerz J, Ericson K, Bergstrand G. Orbital phlebography in patients with cluster headache. *Cephalalgia* 1987;7:207–211.
26. Hatangdi VS, Boas RA, Richards EG. Postherpetic neuralgia: management with antiepileptic and tricyclic drugs. In: Bonica JJ, Albe-Fessard D, eds. *Advances in pain research and therapy*, vol 1. New York: Raven Press, 1976:583–587.
27. Headache Classification Committee of the International Headache Society. Classification and diagnostic criteria for headache disorders, cranial neuralgias and facial pain. *Cephalalgia* 1988;8 (Suppl 7):1–96.
28. Hildebrandt J, Jansen J. Vascular compression of the C2 and C3 roots—yet another cause of chronic intermittent hemicrania? *Cephalalgia* 1984;4:167–170.
29. Hokkanen E, Haltia T, Myllyla VV. Recurrent multiple cranial neuropathies. *Eur Neurol* 1978;17:32–37.
30. Hunt JR. On herpetic inflammations of the geniculate ganglion: a new syndrome and its complications. *J Nerv Ment Dis* 1907;34:73–96.
31. Hunt WE. Tolosa-Hunt syndrome: one cause of painful ophthalmoplegia. *J Neurosurg* 1976;44:544–549.
32. Hunt WE, Brightman RP. The Tolosa-Hunt syndrome: a problem in differential diagnosis. *Acta Neurochir (Wien)* 1988;42:248–252.
33. Hunt WE, Meagher JN, Lefever HE, Zeman W. Painful ophthalmoplegia: its relation to indolent inflammation of the cavernous sinus. *Neurology* 1961;11:56–62.
34. Jansen J, Bardosi A, Hildebrandt J, Lucke A. Cervicogenic, hemicranial attacks associated with vascular irritation or compression of the cervical nerve root C2: clinical manifestations and morphological findings. *Pain* 1989;39:203–212.
35. Jansen J, Markakis E, Rama B, Hildebrandt J. Hemicranial attacks or

permanent hemicrania—a sequel of upper cervical root compression. *Cephalalgia* 1989;9:123–130.

36. Johnson RW. Aspects of postherpetic neuralgia: can we zap Z-ap? *Pain Reviews* 1996;3:117–135.

37. Johnson RW, Mandal BK. Guidelines for the management of shingles: report of a working group of the British society for the study of Infection. *J Infect* 1995;30:193–200.

38. Juel-Jensen BE, MacCallum FO, McKenzie AMR, Pike MC. Treatment of zoster with idoxuridine in dimethyl sulphoxide: results of two double-blind controlled trials. *BMJ* 1970;4:776–780.

39. King RB. Concerning the management of pain associated with herpes zoster and postherpetic neuralgia. *Pain* 1988;33:73–78.

40. Kishmore-Kumar R, Max MB, Schafer SC. Desipramine relieves postherpetic neuralgia. *Clin Pharmacol Ther* 1990;47:305–312.

41. Kissin I, McDonal J, Xavier AV. Topical lidocaine for relief of superficial pain in postherpetic neuralgia. *Neurology* 1989;39:1132–1133.

42. Kline LB, Galbraith JG. Parasellar epidermoid tumour presenting as painful ophthalmoplegia. *J Neurosurg* 1981;54:113–117.

43. Koppel BS. Steroid responsive painful ophthalmoplegia is not always Tolosa-Hunt. *Neurology* 1987;37:544.

44. Kuritzky A. Cluster headache-like pain caused by an upper cervical meningioma. *Cephalalgia* 1984;4:185–186.

45. Kwan ESK, Wolpert SM, Hedges TR, Laucella M. Tolosa-Hunt syndrome revisited: not necessarily a diagnosis of exclusion. *AJNR Am J Neuroradiol* 1987;8:1067–1072.

46. Lance JW. *Mechanism and management of headache*, 5th ed. Oxford: Butterworth, 1993:257–258.

47. Lance JW, Anthony M. Neck tongue syndrome on sudden turning of the head. *J Neurol Neurosurg Psychiatry* 1980;43:97–101.

48. Lewith GT, Field J, Machin D. Acupuncture compared with placebo in post-herpetic pain. *Pain* 1983;17:361–368.

49. Loeser JD. Herpes zoster and postherpetic neuralgia. *Pain* 1986;25:149–164

50. Mandal BK, Dunbar EM, Ellis ME, Ellis J, Dowd P. A double-masked, placebo-controlled trial of acyclovir cream in immunocompetent patients with herpes zoster. *J Infect* 1988;17:57–63.

51. Matthew NT, Chandy J. Painful ophthalmoplegia. *J Neurol Sci* 1970;11:243–256.

52. Max MB, Schafer SC, Culnane M, et al. Amitriptyline, but not lorazepam, relieves postherpetic neuralgia. *Neurology* 1988;381:1427–1432.

53. McKendrick MW, McGill JI, White JE, Wood MJ. Oral acyclovir in acute herpes zoster. *BMJ* 1986;293:1529–1532.

54. McKendrick MW, McGill JI, Wood MJ. Lack of effect of acyclovir on postherpetic neuralgia. *BMJ* 1989;298:431.

55. McQuay H, Carroll D, Jadad AR, Wiffen P, Moore A. Anticonvulsant drugs for the management of pain: a systematic review. *BMJ* 1995;311:1047–1052.

56. Nurmikko T, Wells C, Bowsher D. Pain and allodynia in postherpetic neuralgia: a role of somatic and sympathetic nervous systems. *Acta Neurol Scand* 1991;84:146–152.

57. Pappagallo M, Campbell JN. Chronic opioid therapy as alternative treatment for post-herpetic neuralgia. *Ann Neurol* 1994;35:54–56.

58. Peterslund NA. Management of varicella zoster infections in immunocompetent hosts. *Am J Med* 1988;85(Suppl 2A):75–78.

59. Poletti CE, Sweet WH. Entrapment of the C2 root and ganglion by the atlanto-epistrophic ligament: clinical syndrome and surgical anatomy. *Neurosurgery* 1990;27:288–291.

60. Polsky M, Janicki PC, Gunderson CH. Tolosa-Hunt syndrome with sellar erosion. *Ann Neurol* 1979;6:129–131.

61. Portenoy RK, Duma C, Foley KM. Acute herpetic and postherpetic neuralgia: clinical review and current management. *Ann Neurol* 1986;20:651–664.

62. Post BT, Philbrick JT. Do corticosteroids prevent postherpetic neuralgia? *J Am Acad Dermatol* 1988;18:605–610.

63. Ragazzino MW, Melton IJ, Kurland LT, et al. Population-based study of herpes zoster and its sequelae. *Medicine* 1982;61:310–316.

64. Rosenbaum DH, David MJ, Song IS. The syndrome of painful ophthalmoplegia: a case with intraorbital mass and hypervascularity. *Arch Neurol* 1979;36:41–43.

65. Rowbotham MC, Fields HL. Topical lignocaine reduces pain in postherpetic neuralgia. *Pain* 1989;39:297–301.

66. Rowbotham MC, Reisner-Keller LA, Fields HL. Both intravenous lidocaine and morphine reduce the pain of postherpetic neuralgia. *Neurology* 1991;41:1024–1028.

67. Rowbotham MC, Miller KV, Davies P. Topical lidocaine for post-herpetic neuralgia pain: results of a double-blind, vehicle controlled trial. *Neurology* 1992;42:390.

68. Rowed DW, Kassel EE, Lewis AJ. Transorbital intracavernous needle biopsy in painful ophthalmoplegia. *J Neurosurg* 1985;62:776–780

69. Schmader KE, Studenski S. Are current therapies useful for the prevention of postherpetic neuralgia? *J Gen Intern Med* 1989;4:83–89.

70. Schvarcz JR. Craniofacial postherpetic neuralgia managed by stereotactic spinal trigeminal nucleotomy. *Acta Neurchir Suppl (Wien)* 1989;46:62–64.

71. Shanbrom E. Treatment of herpetic pain and postherpetic neuralgia with intravenous procaine. *JAMA* 1961;176:1041–1043.

72. Smith JL, Taxdal DSR. Painful ophthalmoplegia: the Tolosa-Hunt syndrome. *Am J Ophthalmol* 1966;61:1466–1472.

73. Sondheimer FK, Knapp J. Angiographic findings in the Tolosa-Hunt Syndrome: painful ophthalmoplegia. *Radiology* 1973;106:105–112.

74. Spector RH, Fiandaca MS. The "sinister" Tolosa-Hunt syndrome. *Neurology* 1986;36:198–203.

75. Steele JC, Vasuvar A. Recurrent multiple cranial nerve palsies: a distinctive syndrome of cranial polyneuropathy. *J Neurol Neurosurg Psychiatry* 1970;33:828–832.

76. Stow PJ, Glynn CJ, Minor B. EMLA cream in the treatment of postherpetic neuralgia. Efficacy and pharmacokinetic profile. *Pain* 1989;39:301–305.

77. Suzuki H, Ogawa S, Nakagawa H, et al. Cryocautery of sensitized skin areas for the relief of pain due to post-herpetic neuralgia. *Pain* 1980;9:355–362.

78. Swerdlow B. Tolosa-Hunt syndrome: a case with associated facial nerve palsy. *Ann Neurol* 1980;8:542–543

79. Takeoka T, Gotoh F, Fukuchi V, Inagaki Y. Tolosa-Hunt syndrome: arteriographic evidence of improvement in carotid narrowing. *Arch Neurol* 1978;35:219–223.

80. Taub A. Relief of postherpetic neuralgia with psychotropic drugs. *J 20Neursurg* 1973:39:235–239.

81. Thomas DJB, Charlesworth MC, Afshar F, Galton DJ. Computerised axial tomography and magnetic resonance scanning in the Tolosa-Hunt syndrome. *Br J Ophthalmol* 1988;72:299–302.

82. Thomas JE, Yoss RE. The parasellar syndrome: problems in determining etiology. *Mayo Clin Proc* 1970;45:617–623.

83. Watson CPN, Evans RJ, Reed K, Merskey H, Goldsmith, Warsh J. Amitriptyline versus placebo in postherpetic neuralgia. *Neurology* 1982;32:671–673.

84. Watson CPN, Evans RJ. A comparative trial of amitriptyline and zimelidine in post-herpetic neuralgia. *Pain* 1985;28:387–394.

85. Watson CPN, Evans RJ. Postherpetic neuralgia. *Arch Neurol* 1986;43:836–840.

86. Watson CPN, Evans RJ, Watt VR, Birkett N. Post-herpetic neuralgia: 208 cases. *Pain* 1988;35:289–297.

87. Watson CPN, Evans RJ, Watt VR. Post-herpetic neuralgia and topical capsaicin. *Pain* 1988;33:333–340.

88. Watson CPN, Watt VR, Chipman M, Birkett N, Evans RJ. The prognosis of postherpetic neuralgia. *Pain* 1991;46:195–199.

89. Watson CPN, Deck JH, Morshead C, Van der Kooy D, Evans RJ. Postherpetic neuralgia: further post-mortem studies of cases with and without pain. *Pain* 1991;44:105–117.

90. Watson CPN, Chipman M, Reed K. Evans RJ, Birkett N. Maprotiline is postherpetic neuralgia: a randomized double-blind, crossover trial. *Pain* 1992;48:29–36.

91. Watson CPN, Tyler KL, Bicers DR, Millikan LE, Smith S, Coleman E. A randomized vehicle-controlled trial capsicin in the treatment of postherpetic neuralgia. *Clin Ther* 1993;15:510–526.

92. Whitley RJ, Weiss W, Guann J et al., and the NIAID Collaborative Antiviral Study Group. The efficacy of steroids and acyclovir therapy of herpes zoster in the elderly. *Antiviral Res* 1995;26:A303.

93. Wood MJ, Ogan PH, McKendrick MW, et al. Efficacy of oral acyclovir treatment of acute herpes zoster. *Am J Med* 1988;85(Suppl 2A):79–83

94. Wood MJ, Johnson RW, McKendrick MW, Taylor J, Mandal BK, Crooks J. A randomized trial of acyclovir for 7 days of 21 days with and without prednisolone for treatment of acute herpes zoster. *N Engl J Med* 1994;330:896–900.

95. Yousem DM, Atlas SW, Grossman RI, Sergott RC, Savino PJ, Bosley TM. MR imaging of Tolosa-Hunt syndrome. *AJNR Am J Neuroradiol* 1989;10:1181–1184

The Headaches, Second Edition,
edited by J. Olesen, P. Tfelt-Hansen, and K.M.A. Welch.
Lippincott Williams & Wilkins, Philadelphia © 2000.

The Secondary Headaches

CHAPTER 123

Trigeminal Neuralgia and Other Facial Neuralgias

Christopher F. Terrence and Troels Staehelin Jensen

TRIGEMINAL NEURALGIA

IHS code and diagnosis: 12.2 Trigeminal Neuralgia
WHO code and diagnosis: G50.0 Trigeminal Neuralgia
IHS code and diagnosis: 12.2.1 Idiopathic trigeminal neuralgia
WHO code and diagnosis: G50.0 Idiopathic trigeminal neuralgia
Short description: Trigeminal neuralgia is a painful unilateral affliction of the face, characterized by brief electric shock–like (lancinating) pains limited to the distribution of one or more divisions of the trigeminal nerve. Pain is commonly evoked by trivial stimuli, including washing, shaving, smoking, talking, and brushing the teeth, but may also occur spontaneously. The pain is abrupt in onset and termination and may remit for varying periods.
Other terms: Tic douloureux, tic

Epidemiology

Although published prior to superior imaging techniques, the best prevalence figures are those of John Penman (68). He estimated a prevalence per 1 million population as 107.5 and 200.2 for men and women, respectively. The annual incidence rates for men and women was 4.67 and 7.15, respectively. Interestingly, the reported average age at onset was the same in both the men and the women, 50 years. This female preponderance and relatively late onset has been supported by many other researchers (37,67).

Anatomy, Pathology, and Pathophysiology

As noted in Figure 1, compression, distortion or stretching of the trigeminal roots by arteries, vascular malformation, or slowly growing tumors can cause the pain of trigeminal neuralgia. Meningiomas and epidermoids can present with the typical pain of trigeminal neuralgia and can be missed at the neurologic examination. Vascular compression appears to be a very frequent and perhaps indeed the most frequent cause (43). Computed tomographic (CT) scanning and magnetic resonance imaging (MRI) are imperative in all cases to exclude underlying mass lesions (52,60).

The rare central causes are multiple sclerosis, syringobulbia, and sequelae of brainstem infarction (95). Of the central etiologies, multiple sclerosis is the only one to occur with any real frequency. In the few autopsy cases of trigeminal neuralgia associated with multiple sclerosis, the plaques usually involve the pons at the trigeminal root entry zone. Thus, even in multiple sclerosis, these cases represent the peripheral pathology typical of trigeminal neuralgia.

Despite the almost exclusive peripheral pathology, trigeminal neuralgia has many characteristics of a centrally mediated process such as a seizure (19,23):

1. There is a measurable latent period between the onset of the stimulus to its trigger point and the onset of the attack of trigeminal neuralgia.
2. The attacks are self-sustained once they have started.

C. F. Terrence: Department of Neuroscience, New Jersey Medical School, Newark, New Jersey 07102, and VA New Jersey Health Care System, East Orange, New Jersey 07019-1095.

T. S. Jensen: Department of Neurology F, Århus Kommunehospital, DK-8000 Århus C, Denmark.

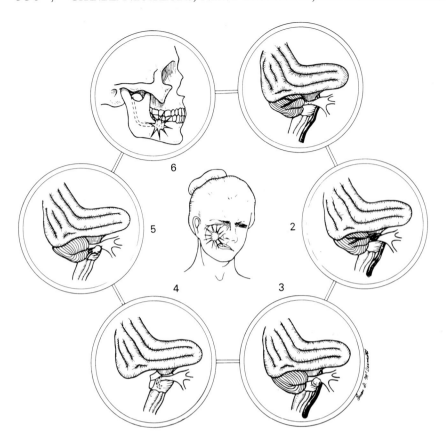

FIG. 1. Various lesions that have been implicated as a cause of trigeminal neuralgia: (*1*) arterial loop; (*2*) vascular malformation; (*3*) epidermoid cyst; (*4*) multiple sclerosis plaque; (*5*) acoustic neuroma; (*6*) chronic oral or dental disease. Drawing by B.D. McDermott.

3. The attacks are followed by a refractory period, during which it is not possible to trigger another attack.
4. The attacks are most readily evoked by non-noxious stimuli.
5. The pain radiates outside the stimulated area, and in some cases the painful paroxysm is only experienced in an entirely different division of the trigeminal nerve than the location of the trigger point.
6. The efficacy of central acting drugs such as baclofen.

Faced with the conundrum of a pain syndrome that has an almost exclusive reliance on a peripheral pathology somewhere along the course of the trigeminal nerve but clinical pharmacologic and biochemical features most consistent with a central type of disease, it would be best to summarize trigeminal neuralgia as a pain syndrome with a peripheral etiology but a central pathogenesis (71,87). Pathologic findings associated with trigeminal neuralgia caused by vascular compression include focal loss of myelin, close opposition of demyelinated axons, and few inflammatory cells. Trigeminal neuralgia occurs when disease of the trigeminal primary afferents causes increased firing in these fibers as well as impairment of the efficacy of the inhibitory mechanism in the trigeminal brainstem complex that normally controls its level of activity. When the ensuing paroxysmal burst of activity in the wide dynamic range neurons of the nucleus caudalis reach the firing level usually elicited by noxious stimuli, the affected individual experiences the excruciating attack of trigeminal neuralgia (24,32). Unfortunately there is no good animal model for trigeminal neuralgia, so confirmation of the exact pathophysiology will have to wait for a suitable model.

Clinical Features

Diagnostic criteria:

A. Paroxysmal attacks of facial or frontal pain that last a few seconds to less than 2 minutes.
B. Pain has at least four of the following characteristics:
    1. Distribution along one or more divisions of the trigeminal nerve
    2. Sudden, intense, sharp, superficial, stabbing, or burning in quality
    3. Pain intensity severe
    4. Precipitation from trigger areas, or by certain daily activities such as eating, talking, washing the face, or cleaning the teeth
    5. Between paroxysms the patient is entirely asymptomatic
C. No neurologic deficit.
D. Attacks are stereotyped in the individual patient.
E. Exclusion of other cases of facial pain by history, physical examination, and special investigation when necessary.

The lightning-like pains of trigeminal neuralgia are incredibly intense and painful (Fig. 2) and the unilateral grimaces of pain so characteristic of trigeminal neuralgia (25,29,69) led to the designation *tic douloureux*. Such descriptions as "like a firecracker going off in my cheek" to "having a dental drill being briefly applied to exposed nerve endings, one at a time" explain why in 1853 Trousseau (100) suggested the term "epileptiform neuralgia" for this condition.

In contradistinction to other types of pain, there is almost no placebo response. In placebo-controlled studies, the placebo response has ranged from 0 to 1 in 10 (31,88), the lowest placebo response in any similar pain syndrome study (5). The pain comes in repetitive flashes of sharp, stabbing pain, usually lasting seconds. Between clusters of pain the patient is usually pain free, but the patient lives in dread of the future pain. With especially long duration or intense clusters of pain, there may be a dull aching confined to the trigeminal division lasting a few minutes. Continuous dull aching pain punctuated by flashes of pain is atypical of idiopathic trigeminal neuralgia and would suggest a mass lesion etiology (93).

Trigger zones have been reported in two large series to be present in 91% of cases (109). These zones are areas innervated by the trigeminal nerve that when stimulated by non-noxious stimuli cause the onset of flashes of pain. These zones are usually in the central part of the face around the nose and lips, and on some occasions the trigger zone is in a different division of the trigeminal nerve than the elicited pain (93).

It is of interest that light touch and vibratory stimuli are more effective in eliciting the pain than a pinch or pinprick. In an elegant study by Kugelberg and Linblom, touch and vibration were found to be the best stimuli (49,50). The latency between onset of vibratory stimulus to onset of pain could be shortened by increasing the frequency or amplitude. Clinically, patients frequently report that electric shavers, talking, chewing, washing the face, or even a light breeze on the face can trigger a paroxysm of pain (93).

Probably the most interesting feature of trigeminal neuralgia that sets it off from other types of pain is the relative refractory phase following a paroxysm of pain. Patients find that after a paroxysm of pain there is a period of time that can last up to several minutes during which stimulation of the trigger zone will not elicit a paroxysm of pain. The duration of the relative refractory period is usually proportional to the length and intensity of the attack.

Spontaneous remission is a common feature. Ruston and MacDonald reported on 155 persons with trigeminal neuralgia, of which 78 had a spontaneous remission of at least 6 months in duration during the course of their illness (76). Of special note is the 38 patients who had a spontaneous remission of 1 year or longer. Not surprisingly, patients who have a history of long-term spontaneous remissions of trigeminal neuralgia are the least willing to undergo surgery. Spontaneous remissions in trigeminal neuralgia associated with multiple sclerosis is rare. Because spontaneous remissions are such a frequent occurrence in trigeminal neuralgia, any study—be it surgical or medical—must take into account that relief observed may be the result of a spontaneous remission rather than therapy.

For years, dentists and oral surgeons have been the butt of unfair criticism for failing to diagnose "obvious cases of trigeminal neuralgia." Many of these cases undoubtedly represent cases of pretrigeminal neuralgia (81). The first cogent description of pretrigeminal neuralgia was made by Symonds in 1949 (91). A number of years later, Mitchell reported on 38 persons who were initially thought to have dental pain but went on to develop typical trigeminal neuralgia weeks to months later. In 1990, 18 patients who had pretrigeminal neuralgia pain described as toothache or sinusitis-like discomfort were reported (27). In 8 of 18 patients the pain was brought on by chewing, drinking liquids, brushing the teeth, yawning, or talking. Classical trigeminal neuralgia pain appeared within a few months to as many as 12 years later in the tysame branch of the trigeminal nerve in all cases. In two thirds of patients the pain evolved directly into trigeminal neuralgia, whereas the rest experienced a pain-free interval of up to 11 months before the onset of trigeminal neuralgia. As with trigeminal neuralgia, the typical age at onset was in the fifties, with a similar female:male preponderance.

When the clinician is faced with an older patient who demonstrates no abnormalities after a detailed neurologic

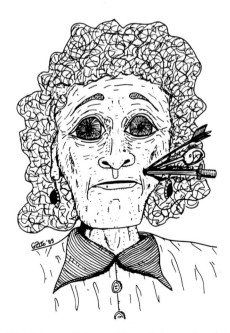

FIG. 2. Physician artist rendition of the pain of trigeminal neuralgia. Drawing by Dr. G. Zito.

and dental evaluation with appropriate radiologic evaluation that includes CT or MRI of the posterior and middle fossa, a trial of carbamazepine or baclofen may aid in making a diagnosis of pretrigeminal neuralgia. Pretrigeminal neuralgia must be carefully differentiated from small tumors causing pain, atypical odontalgia or atypical facial pain, facial or "lower half" migraine, toothache of pulpal origin, sinusitis, and temporomandibular dysfunction (28). As noted by Forthergill (22) and Pujol (70), it is important to distinguish trigeminal neuralgia and pretrigeminal neuralgia from dental disease pain to avoid "the useless and unnecessary extraction of entire rows of healthy teeth."

Medical Management

Phenytoin

The first effective therapy for trigeminal neuralgia was brought forward by Bergouignan (8) when he used phenytoin. Only about 25% of trigeminal neuralgia patients are relieved of their pain with phenytoin alone. The usual maintenance dose is 300 to 400 mg/day in two divided doses. A total loading dose of 1,000 mg can be given orally over a 24-hour period in divided doses. When using a loading dose in older patients it is important to monitor for side effects such as drowsiness, dizziness, and ataxia. Some 5% to 10% of patients on maintenance dosage may have significant side effects even with subtherapeutic phenytoin levels.

Carbamazepine and Oxcarbazepine

The results of Blom's study on the use of carbamazepine have been confirmed by numerous investigators (9,98). Carbamazepine therapy must be initiated gradually and carefully, especially in older patients, who are the ones most commonly affected by trigeminal neuralgia. The usual starting dosage is 100 to 300 mg twice daily. The total daily dose should be increased by 200 mg every other day until the patient is pain free or side effects occur. Typically, the paroxysms come under control in the first 48 to 72 hours of therapy. The usual maintenance dosage is 600 mg to 1,200 mg/day.

Because of the need to stop the excruciating attacks of trigeminal neuralgia, it is sometimes difficult to avoid initial side effects such as drowsiness, unsteadiness, nausea, and anorexia. It is important to remember that although they occur in up to 40% of patients, the side effects usually subside in a few weeks on maintenance therapy. Only in 10% of patients must carbamazepine be stopped due to side effects. It is important for the physician to warn the patient of these side effects and take precautions accordingly.

Although rare, aplastic anemia has been reported in patients taking carbamazepine. Prior to initiating therapy with carbamazepine, baseline complete blood counts as well as hepatic and renal function tests should be performed. Subsequent monitoring should be performed as recommended by the drug manufacturer. Patients should be warned to notify their physician immediately should fevers, sore throat, stomatitis, easy bruisability, or petechiae develop. The appearance of congestive heart failure or water intoxication due to inappropriate secretion of antidiuretic hormone have been reported in patients taking carbamazepine (96).

Oxcarbazepine is an alternative to carbamazepine. The dosage is one third higher, and the drug should be initiated gradually, with a starting dose of 300 mg and followed by increments of 300 mg every other day until pain subsides. A lowering of plasma sodium is obligatory during oxcarbazepine therapy, and cardiac patients or patients treated with diuretics should have their sodium values checked carefully (21,99).

One of the most difficult decisions facing a physician who treats a patient with trigeminal neuralgia is: "The patient is pain free on medication—when do I stop the drugs." Like epilepsy, there are no hard and fast rules for the timing of discontinuation of drug after pain relief has been achieved. If the patient has been pain free for 6 to 8 weeks, then gradual tapering of medication would be appropriate. If the patient is on more than one drug for trigeminal neuralgia, only one drug at a time should be tapered (13).

Baclofen

The most consistent neurophysiologic effects of the antineuralgic drugs carbamazepine, oxcarbazepine, and phenytoin are to facilitate segmental inhibition by blocking sodium channels peripherally and centrally (86). The antispasticity drug baclofen depresses excitatory transmission in the trigeminal nucleus complex (26,30). An open-label pilot trial of efficacy showed baclofen to be an effective drug for trigeminal neuralgia either alone or in combination with carbamazepine. A subsequent more rigorous double-blind crossover trial confirmed the initial study (31). As of today, there have been reported over a half-dozen trials of baclofen in trigeminal neuralgia, all showing efficacy (2,39,58,85).

Baclofen has great promise for the initial treatment of patients with trigeminal neuralgia because it lacks any of the rare life-threatening side effects of carbamazepine. Another major advantage of baclofen is its strong synergistic action with carbamazepine and phenytoin.

Baclofen is rapidly absorbed after oral administration. Its biologic half-life is about 3 to 4 hours, and it is excreted primarily by the kidney with little metabolic change. Because of its renal excretion, it is important that dosage be altered if there is any renal impairment.

The starting dose for baclofen is 5 to 10 mg given three times a day. This daily dosage should be increased by 10 mg every other day until the patient is pain free or side effects develop. The usual maintenance dose is 50 to

60 mg/day. Because of its relatively short half-life, baclofen dosing may need to be every 4 hours in difficult to control cases. The combination of baclofen with carbamazepine (or phenytoin) is much more effective than either drug alone (31) and should be tried in those patients who do not respond to monotherapy.

Like carbamazepine and oxcarbazepine, the frequency and severity of side effects can be reduced by a more gradual dosage ascension. The most common side effects include drowsiness, dizziness, and gastrointestinal upset. About 10% of patients are not able to tolerate baclofen due to various side effects. Unlike carbamazepine and phenytoin, the abrupt withdrawal of baclofen after months of usage should be avoided. Hallucinations and seizures have been reported after abrupt cessation of long-term therapy (97). Baclofen should be tapered over 10 to 14 days. If withdrawal symptoms do develop, the highest symptom-free dosage should be reinstituted, and tapering should be restarted by 5 to 10 mg per week.

Other Drug Therapies

One double-blind placebo-controlled study showed that lamotrigine was superior to placebo in trigeminal neuralgia (111). Of the most recent anticonvulsants brought to market, gabapentin seems to be particularly useful in the treatment of trigeminal neuralgia. Valzania and colleagues reported gabapentin to be effective in 83% of first therapy patients and 57% of patients previously treated with carbamazepine (101). The mean gabapentin dosage was 1,107 mg/day, with a range of 600 to 2,000 mg/day. Thus, there is a need for a controlled trial on this promising drug.

Surgical Management

The history of surgical treatment of trigeminal neuralgia is probably best thought of as a linear history, the line being the trigeminal nerve and its central connections (168). The approaches have been many, ranging from peripheral injections of alcohol and treatment of tooth pulp cavities to trigeminal tractotomy. To paraphrase Penman (68), we will confine this review to a summary of current surgical techniques and an appraisal of their success, limitation, and complications. About 30% of patients suffering from trigeminal neuralgia fail to respond to medical therapy (18).

Alcohol Injection

Various sites have been used for alcohol injection. These sites include the supraorbital or infraorbital nerve, the mandibular division at the foramen ovale, the maxillary division at the sphenopalatine fossa, and the trigeminal cistern. As will be discussed later with radiofrequency rhizotomy, the best results tend to be related to persistent anesthesia in the trigger zone.

Success rates reported for alcohol injection vary widely. The longer lasting successes are usually seen with the more proximal injections. Henderson reported that only about 2% of patients were pain free 5 years after infraorbital injection (37). He also reported a 10% pain-free experience with foramen ovale injections. In a large series of gasserian ganglion injection, Harris reported a success rate of almost 70% at 3 years and 21% at up to 10 years (36). The major side effects of this procedure are the sensory loss. Dysesthesias occur in almost half the cases. Falconer and Harris noted a 4% incidence of anesthesia dolorosa, a complaint that many patients find almost as bad as trigeminal neuralgia. Because of the side effects and poor long-term cure rate, alcohol injections are not a popular procedure for trigeminal neuralgia, but they do have potential for the elderly frail individual who is not a good surgical candidate for more invasive procedures.

Radiofrequency Gangliolysis and Retrogasserian Glycerol Injection

Like alcohol injection, radiofrequency gangliolysis is not a very invasive procedure, and it relies on destruction of nerve fibers (63,66). Browne reported 100% immediate pain relief with a technically adequate radiofrequency lesion (12). The 2-year recurrence rate was 13%. As with alcohol injections, the best results are noted when there is anesthesia in the trigger zone area. Side effects reported were meningitis, herpes simplex, local infection, corneal anesthesia, diplopia, and ear discomfort postulated as being due to paresis of the tensor tympani muscle. A temporally distant side effect was dysesthesis, which interestingly occurred most often in those patients who were destined to have recurrent pain. Nugent has reported a second procedure rate of 27% for late recurrences (65). The use of glycerol in the treatment of trigeminal neuralgia is one of the many examples of serendipity in medicine. As pointed out by Hakanson (34), "glycerol was used as a vehicle to deposit tantalum dust as a marker in the trigeminal cistern . . . Quite unexpectedly, the glycerol injection alone abolished pain completely in several patients for long periods in spite of markedly well-preserved facial sensation."

Hakanson reported 75 patients, and all but one was pain free after the first injection. Eighty-six percent were pain free after 17 months (33). Mild facial numbness was common, but painful dysesthesias were rare, and most importantly the absence of anesthesia dolorosa was noted. Another advantage of this procedure over radiofrequency gangliolysis is that it can be done without general anesthesia (35,44,45); an important plus in this aged patient population. It would also seem to be a useful form of therapy in multiple sclerosis–related trigeminal neuralgia. In multiple sclerosis patients who fail medical therapy, glycerol rhizotomy in one study showed a 75% good to excellent response rate (46,47).

Microvascular Decompression

The most invasive surgical treatment for trigeminal neuralgia discussed thus far is the microvascular decompression procedure popularized by Jannetta (43). Except for dental pathology treatments, this procedure is the only surgical treatment of trigeminal neuralgia that purports to address directly the underlying cause of the paroxysmal pain. The results of the procedure are impressive. Janetta reported that 79% of the patients were pain free after surgery. Another 19% either stopped spontaneously after a short period or required small doses of medication. The long-term results are equally impressive with 73% being pain free with a mean duration of follow-up of 78.4 months. Major complications occurred in less than 3% of cases. Burchiel in his review of the literature of microvascular decompression cited a figure of 22% recurrence for long-term follow-up. He also suggested that after 2 years of being pain free, the patient who had microvascular decompression had the greatest likelihood of remaining pain free as compared with patients undergoing less invasive procedures. Thus, it would seem that if a patient fails on drug therapy and is a good anesthesia and surgical risk, then microvascular decompression would be the procedure of choice.

Gamma Knife Radiosurgery

Two recent articles have proposed a new and radical treatment of trigeminal neuralgia (48,110). Not since Gocht in 1897 has one suggested using ionizing radiation for the treatment of trigeminal neuralgia. Young et al. reported an almost 81% pain free group with a mean follow-up of 16.3 months following a radiosurgical maximum dose of 70 Gy delivered to the trigeminal nerve root adjacent to the pons.

GLOSSOPHARYNGEAL NEURALGIA

IHS code and diagnosis: 12.3 Glossopharyngeal neuralgia
WHO code and diagnosis: G52.1 Disorders of glossopharyngeal nerve
IHS code and diagnosis: 12.3.1 Idiopathic glossopharyngeal neuralgia
WHO code and diagnosis: G52.1 Disorders of Glossopharyngeal nerve
Short description: Glossopharyngeal neuralgia is a severe transient stabbing pain experienced in the ear, base of the tongue, tonsillar fossa or beneath the angle of the jaw. The pain is therefore felt in the distribution of the auricular and pharyngeal branches of the vagus nerve as well as that of the glossopharyngeal nerve. It is commonly provoked by swallowing, talking, and coughing, and may remit and relapse in the fashion of trigeminal neuralgia.

Diagnostic criteria:

A. Paroxysmal attacks of facial pain that last a few seconds to less than 2 minutes
B. Pain has at least four of the following characteristics:
  1. Unilateral location
  2. Distribution within the posterior part of the tongue, tonsillar fossa, pharynx, or beneath the angle of the lower jaw, or in the ear
  3. Sudden, sharp, stabbing, or burning in quality
  4. Pain intensity severe
  5. Precipitation from trigger areas or by swallowing chewing, talking, coughing, or yawning
C. No neurologic deficit
D. Attacks are stereotyped in the individual patient
E. Other causes of pain ruled out by history, physical, and special investigation

Glossopharyngeal neuralgia (vagoglossopharyngeal neuralgia) is in many ways similar to trigeminal neuralgia. Its incidence when compared with trigeminal neuralgia ranges from 1 in 70 to 1 in 100 (77). Like trigeminal neuralgia, its average age of onset is about 50. The attacks of pain come in paroxysms and are lightening like. The pain occurs in the region of the base of the tongue, tonsillar fossa, under the angle of the jaw, or in the ear. The usual triggers are talking, chewing, or swallowing. In addition to the sharp pains, Rushton noted other sensation such as clicking, scratching, or foreign body sensations in the throat. Spontaneous remissions are common in glossopharyngeal neuralgia. Glossopharyngeal neuralgia may be associated with severe bradycardia or asystole, resulting in syncope or convulsions.

As with trigeminal neuralgia, the diagnosis of glossopharyngeal neuralgia is based on a history of the characteristic paroxysms of pain in a patient where neurologic, dental, and imaging studies are normal. Some unfortunate individuals have been found to have combined trigeminal and glossopharyngeal neuralgia. In the 217 cases of glossopharyngeal neuralgia reported by Rushton, 25 had the combination. Only 9 cases presented simultaneously with the two pain syndromes. Like trigeminal neuralgia, medical therapy of glossopharyngeal neuralgia consists of carbamazepine, oxcarbazepine, baclofen, phenytoin, or perhaps lamotrigine either alone or in combination (111). Microvascular decompression also has been reported as a useful surgical alternative if medical management fails (73).

POST-HERPETIC NEURALGIA

IHS code and diagnosis: 12.1.4.2 Chronic post-herpetic neuralgia

WHO code and diagnosis: G53.0 Postzoster neuralgia
Short description: Facial pain developing during the acute phase of herpes zoster and persisting for more than 6 months thereafter

Diagnostic criteria:

A. Pain is restricted to the distribution of the affected cranial nerves or divisions thereof.
B. Pain persists for more than 3 to 6 months after the onset of herpetic eruption.

About 25% of patients with post-herpetic neuralgia have involvement of one division of the trigeminal nerve, with a slight left versus right predominance (107). Of the cases with trigeminal nerve involvement, a large majority will involve the first division. Herpes zoster is more common in elderly and immunosuppressed patients, and these patients are at higher risk for the development of post-herpetic neuralgia (56).

The diagnosis of post-herpetic neuralgia is based on the occurrence of pain along the course of a nerve following herpes zoster and persisting beyond 1 month, the time it usually takes the rash to heal (107). The pain has three different components, which patients experience in varying combination: (a) a constant, deep burning or gnawing pain; (b) a paroxysmal flickering, shooting, or shocking pain; and (c) a sharp, radiating pain elicited by light mechanical stimulation (allodynia) (75).

The acute phase of the herpes zoster infection is characterized by hemorrhagic inflammation of the dorsal root ganglion, nerve root, and distal nerve, which sometimes also involves the leptomeninges and spinal cord (102, 106). Fibrosis occurs in the involved neural elements following the acute infection. In addition, there is degeneration in the ipsilateral posterior column that can extend over several segments, even though the damage is restricted to one ganglion. As first suggested by Livingston, pain caused by damage to the nervous system is probably due to deafferentation-induced changes in the central nervous system, even when the lesion is in the peripheral nervous system (54,55). Peripheral nerve injury leads to an impairment of segmental or afferent inhibition and a sensitization of wide–dynamic range neurons that mimic the response to noxious stimuli (19,74,80). The fact that peripheral nerve injuries that produce neuropathic-like pain in experimental animals cause the degeneration of presumed inhibitory interneurons supports this notion, as do clinical observations suggesting that neuropathic pain is due to dysfunction in the central nervous system secondary to peripheral nerve injury (3,4,89,90).

Unlike other pain syndromes we have discussed, the potential exists to prevent the onset of pain by medical therapeutic intervention. Some drugs [acyclovir (60) and famciclovir (41,42)] have demonstrated either accelerated healing or a decrease in the time it takes for the pain to disappear. The oral dosage of acyclovir is 800 mg five times per day for 7 days (41,42); the oral dosage of famciclovir is 500 mg three times daily (40).

Although post-herpetic neuralgia usually subsides in a month, a small minority, usually the elderly, have persistent pain (32). The most commonly used drugs for persistent pain are the tricyclic antidepressants amitriptyline and imipramine (59,103,105). One must be careful in prescribing these drugs in the typical frail elderly population. The topically applied drug capsacin recently has been shown to be beneficial in the treatment of post-herpetic neuralgia (6,7).

POSTTRAUMATIC NEURALGIA

IHS code and diagnosis: 12.7.1 Anesthesia dolorosa
WHO code and diagnosis: G50.9 Disorder of trigeminal nerve, unspecified
Short description: Painful anesthesia or dysesthesia, often related to surgical trauma of the trigeminal ganglion, evoked most frequently after rhizotomy or thermocoagulation has been performed for treatment of idiopathic trigeminal neuralgia. Anesthesia dolorosa may also follow upon trauma to the trigeminal complex and, rarely, after vascular lesions of the central trigeminal pathways.

Diagnostic criteria:

A. Pain or dysesthesia is limited to the distribution of one or more divisions of the trigeminal nerve.
B. Sensation to pinprick is diminished over the affected area.
C. Symptoms follow a lesion of the trigeminal nerve or its central projections.

Damage to the supraorbital and infraorbital nerves is a common consequence of craniofacial trauma (32). During the initial phase following injury the area innervated by the injured nerve usually is anesthetic (79). With regeneration and return from the acute insult, the area that was previously anesthetic now may have paresthesias, dysesthesias, or constant burning pain. As in the case with post-herpetic neuralgia, the pathophysiology of the pain in posttraumatic neuralgia would be damage to peripheral nerves causing changes in the central nervous system.

Of all the pain syndromes discussed in this chapter, the treatment of pain due to posttraumatic neuralgia is probably one of the most frustrating, both for the physician and the patient. This pain does not respond to opiates and other analgesic agents (17,94). Sectioning of the nerve and other surgical procedures are not effective in the long term. Some patients may get initial relief of the pain with sectioning, but it is all too common for the pain to return (64). There have been encouraging reports on the efficacy of electric stimulation of the gasserian ganglion relieving this type of pain (75). Tricyclic antidepressants may be effective in dosages used for the treatment of post-herpetic neuralgia. Early treatment with repeated blocks appears to improve long-term outcome (104), as do stellate ganglion blocks (57), but controlled trials are lacking. Lastly, psychological and behavioral approaches are important adjuncts to the management of this pain syndrome (17).

ATYPICAL FACIAL PAIN

IHS code and diagnosis: 12.8 Facial pain not fulfilling criteria in groups 11 and 12
WHO code and diagnosis: G50.1 Atypical facial pain
Short description: Persistent facial pain that does not have the characteristics of the cranial neuralgias classified above and is not associated with physical signs or a demonstrable organic cause

Diagnostic criteria:

A. Is present daily and persists for most or all of the day.
B. Is confined at onset to a limited area on one side of the face. May spread to the upper or lower jaws or a wider area of the face or neck. Is deep and poorly localized.
C. Is not associated with sensory loss or other physical signs.
D. Laboratory investigations including x-ray of face and jaws do not demonstrate relevant abnormality.

A number of patients complain of face pain that does not fit into any of the disease categories described so far, and in whom there is no clinical, imaging, or laboratory evidence of pathology. The term "atypical facial pain" has been applied to this group of patients (16,83,84,91). The distribution of the pain does not correspond to the anatomic boundaries of the trigeminal or cervical nerves and is often not well localized. Although these patients complain of excruciating pain, they do not appear to be in severe pain (83). Atypical facial pain is much more common in women than in men, and these patients are often depressed and anxious. The pain is refractory to analgesics, nerve blocks, and surgical procedures, but these patients nevertheless often take excessive amounts of medication and repeatedly seek surgical intervention. Atypical odontalgia (72,82) and burning mouth or burning tongue syndrome (84) are probably localized variants of atypical facial pain. Most psychological studies of patients suffering from atypical facial pain have found evidence of significant psychopathology. Depression and anxiety have been the most common and indeed almost universal psychiatric symptoms in these patients (15,20, 53,83).

Before making the diagnosis of atypical facial pain, it is imperative to rule out all possible organic causes of facial pain by a careful physical, neurologic, and dental examination, as well as MRI studies and appropriate laboratory tests. Dental disease, chronic sinusitis, and nasopharyngeal tumors can all cause poorly defined orofacial pain, and even intracranial tumors occasionally can mimic dental or facial pain (62,78).

Conventional analgesic drugs, including opiates, are generally ineffective, as are nerve blocks and acupuncture. Surgical procedures often aggravate the pain and should be studiously avoided (51,84,91). The tricyclic antidepressants and psychotherapy are the mainstays of therapy but are far from being consistently effective.

REFERENCES

1. Arner S, Meyerson BA. Lack of analgesic effect of opioids on neuropathic and idiopathic forms of pain. *Pain* 1988;33:11–23.
2. Baker KA, Taylor JW, Lilly GE. Treatment of trigeminal neuralgia: use of baclofen in combination with carbamazepine. *Clin Pharm* 1985;4:93–96.
3. Baron R, Haendler G, Schulte H. Afferent large fiber polyneuropathy predicts development of postherpetic neuralgia. *Pain* 1997;73:231–238.
4. Baron R, Saguer M. Mechanical allodynia in postherpetic neuralgia: evidence for central mechanisms depending on nociceptive C-fiber degeneration. *Neurology* 1995;45[Suppl]:63–65.
5. Benson H, Epstein, MD. The placebo effect. *JAMA* 1975;232:1255–1258.
6. Bernstein JE, Bickers DR, Dahl MV, Roshal JY. Treatment of chronic postherpetic neuralgia with topical capsaicin. *Dermatology* 1987;17:93–96.
7. Bernstein JE, Korman NJ, Bickers DR, Dahl MV, Millikan LE. Topical capsaicin in chronic postherpetic neuralgia. *J Am Acad Dermatol* 1989;21:265–270.
8. Blom S. Trigeminal neuralgia: its treatment with a new anti-convulsant drug (G32883). *Lancet* 1962;1:839–840.
9. Bouquot JE, Christian J. Long-term effects of jawbone curettage on the pain of facial neuralgia. *J Oral Maxillofac Surg* 1995;53:387–397.
10. Bowsher D. Postherpetic neuralgia and its treatment: a retrospective survey of 191 patients. *J Pain Symptom Management* 1996;12:290–299.
11. Browne L. Radiofrequency lesioning of the trigeminal ganglion for the treatment of trigeminal neuralgia. *Irish Med J* 1985;78:68–71.
12. Bucci FA, Gabriels CF, Kreohel CB. Successful treatment of postherpetic neuralgia with capsacin. *Am J Ophthalmol* 1988;106:758–759.
13. Court JE, Kase CS. Treatment of tic douloureux with a new anticonvulsant (clonazepam). *J Neurol Neurosurg Psychiatry* 1976;39:297–299.
14. Dalessio DJ. The major neuralgias, postinfectious neuritis, intractable pain, and atypical facial pain. *Wolff's headache and other head pain*. New York: Oxford University Press, 1980.
15. Dalessio DJ. Diagnosis and treatment of cranial neuralgias. *Med Clin North Am* 1991;75:605–615.
16. Davar G, Maciewicz RJ. Deafferentation pain syndromes. *Neurol Clin* 1984;7:289–304.
17. Diamond S, Dalessio DJ. *The practicing physician's approach to headache*. Baltimore: Williams & Wilkins, 1982.
18. Dubner R, Sharav Y, Gracely RH, et al. Idiopathic trigeminal neuralgia: sensory features and pain mechanisms. *Pain* 1987;31:23–33.
19. Dworkin SF, Burgess JA. Orofacial pain of psychogenic origin: current concepts and classification. *J Am Dent Assoc* 1987;115:565–571.
20. Farago F. Trigeminal neuralgia: its treatment with two new carbamazepine analogues. *Eur Neurol* 1987;26:73–83.
21. Fothergill J. Of a painful affection of the face. *Medical Observations and Inquiries by a Society of Physicians London* 1773;5:129–142.
22. Fromm GH, Terrence CF, Chattha AS, Glass JD. Baclofen in trigeminal neuralgia. Its effect on the spinal trigeminal nucleus: a pilot study. *Arch Neurol* 1980;37:768–771.
23. Fromm GH. Medical treatment of patients with trigeminal neuralgia. In: Fromm GH, Sessle BJ, eds. *Trigeminal neuralgia current concepts regarding pathogenesis and treatment*. Boston: Butterworth-Heinemann, 1991:131–140.

24. Fromm GH. Neuralgia of the face and oral cavity. *Pain Digest* 1991; 1:67–77.

25. Fromm GH. Pathophysiology of trigeminal neuralgia. In: Fromm GH, Sessle BJ, eds. *Trigeminal neuralgia current concepts regarding pathogenesis and treatment.* Boston: Butterworth-Heinemann, 1991: 105–122.

26. Fromm GH, Chattha AS, Terrence CF, Glass JD. Role of inhibitory mechanisms in trigeminal neuralgia. *Neurology* 1981;31:683–687.

27. Fromm GH, Graff-Radford SB, Terrence CF, et al. Pre-trigeminal neuralgia. *Neurology* 1990;40:1493–1495.

28. Fromm GH, Sessle BJ. Introduction and historical review. In: Fromm GH, Sessle BJ, eds. *Trigeminal neuralgia current concepts regarding pathogenesis and treatment.* Boston: Butterworth-Heinemann, 1991: 1–26.

29. Fromm GH, Shibuya T, Terrence CF. Comparison of L-baclofen and racemic baclofen in trigeminal neuralgia. *Neurology* 1987;37: 1725–1728.

30. Fromm GH, Terrence CF, Chattha AS. Baclofen in the treatment of trigeminal neuralgia: double-blind study and long-term follow-up. *Ann Neurol* 1984;15:240–244.

31. Fromm GH, Terrence CF, Maroon JC. Trigeminal neuralgia: current concepts regarding etiology and pathogenesis. *Arch Neurol* 1984;41: 1204–1207.

32. Galbraith AW. Prevention of post-herpetic neuralgia by amantadine hydrochloride (Symmetrel). *Br J Clin Pract* 1983;37:304–306.

33. Hakanson S. Trigeminal neuralgia treated by injection of glycerol into the trigeminal cistern. *Neurosurgery* 1981;9:638–646.

34. Hakanson S. Surgical treatment: retrogasserian glycerol injection. In: Fromm GH, Sessle BJ, eds. *Trigeminal neuralgia: current concepts regarding pathogenesis and treatments.* Boston: Butterworth-Heinemann, 1991:185–204.

35. Harding SP, Porter SM. Oral acyclovir in herpes zosters ophthalmicus. *Curr Eye Res* 1991;10[Suppl]:177–182.

36. Harris W. An analysis of 1,433 cases of paroxysmal trigeminal neuralgia (trigeminal tic) and the end-results of gasserian alcohol injection. *Brain* 1940:63:209–224.

37. Henderson WR. Trigeminal neuralgia: the pain and its treatment. *BMJ* 1967;1:7–15.

38. Hering R, Kuritzki A, Bechar M. Baclofen in trigeminal neuralgia-case report. *Harefuah* 1982;102:63–64.

39. Hilton DA, Love S, Gradidge T, et al. Pathologic findings associated with trigeminal neuralgia caused by vascular compression. *Neurosurgery* 1994;35:299–303.

40. Huse DM, Schainbaum s, Kirsch AJ, et al. Economic evaluation of famciclovir in reducing the duration of postherpetic neuralgia. *Am J Health Systems Pharm* 1997;54:1180–1184.

41. Jackson JL, Gibbons R, Meyer G, et al. The effect of treating herpes zoster with oral acyclovir in preventing postherpetic neuralgia. A meta-analysis. *Arch Intern Med* 1997;157:909–912.

42. Jannetta PJ. Surgical treatment; microvascular decompression. In: Fromm GH, Sessle BJ, eds. *Trigeminal neuralgia current concepts regarding pathogenesis and treatment.* Boston: Butterworth-Heinemann, 1991:145–157.

43. Jensen TS, Rasmussen P, Reske-Nielsen E. Association of trigminal neuralgia with multiple sclerosis: clinical and pathological features. *Acta Neurol Scand* 1982;65:182–189.

44. Jho HP, Lunsford LD. Percutaneous retrogasserian glycerol rhizotomy. Current technique and results. *Neurosurg Clin North Am* 1997;8:63–74.

45. Keczkes K, Basheer AM: Do corticosteriods prevent postherpetic neuralgia? *Br J Dermatol* 1980:102:551–555.

46. Kondziolka D, Flickinger JC, Lunsford LD, et al. Trigeminal neuralgia radiosurgery: the University of Pittsburgh experience. *Stereotact Funct Neurosurgery* 1996;66[Suppl 1]:343–348.

47. Kondziolka D, Lunsford LD, Bissonette DJ. Long-term results after glycerol rhizotomy for multiple sclerosis-related trigeminal neuralgia. *Can J Neurol Sci* 1994;21:137–140.

48. Kugelberg E, Lindblom U. The mechanism of the pain in trigeminal neuralgia. *J Neurol Neurosurg Psychiatry* 1959;22:36–43.

49. Kugelberg E, Lindblom U. Studies on the mechanism of pain in trigeminal neuralgia. In: Wolstenholme GEW, O'Connor M, eds. *Pain and itch: nervous mechanisms.* Boston: Little, Brown, 1959: 98–107.

50. Kuhner A. The value of destructive surgery of the trigeminal nerve in atypical facial pain. *Neurochirurgia* 1988;31:210–212.

51. Kuroiwa T, Matsumoto S, Kato A, et al. MR imaging of idiopathic trigeminal neuralgia: correlation with non-surgical therapy. *Radiat Med* 1996;14:235–239.

52. Lehmann HJ, Buchholz G. Atypical facial neuralgia or depressive facial pain. Diagnostic aspects of a well-demarcated form of masked depression. *Fortschr Neurol Psychiatry* 1986;54:154–157.

53. Lindblom U, Verrillo RT. Sensory functions in chronic neuralgia. *J Neurol Neursurg Psychiatry* 1979;42:422–435.

54. Livingston WK. *Pain mechanisms: a physiological interpretation of causalgia and its related states.* New York: MacMillan, 1943.

55. Loeser JD. Herpes zoster and postherpetic neuralgia. *Pain* 1986;25: 149–164.

56. Loh L, Nathan PW. Painful peripheral states and sympathetic blocks. *J Neurol Neurosurg Psychiatry* 1978;41:664–671.

57. Maertens de Noordhout A, Schoenen J. Les algies faciales. *Rev Med Liege* 1986;41:342–348.

58. Majoie CB, Hulsmans FJ, Verbeeten B, et al. Trigeminal neuralgia; comparison of two MR imaging techniques in the demonstration of neurovascular contact. *Radiology* 1997;204:455–460.

59. Max BM, Schafer SC, Culnane M, et al. Amitriptyline, but not lorazepam, relieves postherpetic neuralgia. *Neurology* 1988;38: 1427–1432.

60. McKendrick MW, McGill JI, White JE, et al. Oral acyclovir in acute herpes zoster. *BMJ* 1986;293:1529–1532.

61. Monaghan AM, McKinlay KP. An intracranial tumor causing dental pain. *Br Dent J* 1991;171:249–250.

62. Muroli R, Rovit RL. Are peripheral neurectomies of value in the treatment of trigeminal neuralgia? *J Neurosurg* 1996;85:435–437.

63. Noordenbos W, Wall PD. Implications of the failure of nerve resection and graft to cure chronic pain produced by nerve lesions. *J Neurol Neurosurg Psychiatry* 1981;44:1068–1073.

64. Nugent GR. Surgical treatment: radiofrequency gangliolysis and rhizotomy. In: Fromm GH, Sessle BJ, eds. *Trigeminal Neuralgia Current Concepts Regarding Pathogenesis and Treatment.* Boston: Butterworth-Heinemann, 1991:159–184.

65. Oturai AB, Jensen K, Eriksen J, et al. Neurosurgery for trigeminal neuralgia: comparison of alcohol block, neurectomy, and radio frequency coagulation. *Clin J Pain* 1996;12:311–315.

66. Patrick HT. The symptomatology of trifacial neuralgia. *JAMA* 1914; 62:1519–1525.

67. Penman J. Trigeminal neuralgia. In: Vinken PJ, Bruyn GW, eds. *Handbook of clinical neurology,* Vol. 5. Amsterdam: North Holland, 1968:296–322.

68. Probst C. Treatment of atypical post-traumatic and postoperative facial neuralgias by chronic stimulation. Apropos of 2 cases, with review of the literature. *Neurochirurgie* 1988;34:106–109.

69. Pujol M. *Essai sur la maladie de la face nomme le tic douloureux.* Paris: Theophile Barrois, 1787.

70. Rappaport ZH, Devor M. Trigeminal neuralgia: the role of self sustaining discharge in the trigeminal ganglion. *Pain* 1994;56:127–138.

71. Reik L. Atypical odontalgia: a localized from of atypical facial pain. *Headache* 1984;24:222–224.

72. Resnick DK, Jannetta PJ, Bissonnette D, et al. Microvascular decompression for glossopharyngeal neuralgia. *Neurosurgery* 1995;36: 64–68.

73. Roberts WJ. A hypothesis on the physiological basis for causalgia and related pains. *Pain* 1986;24:297–311.

74. Rowbotham MC, Fields HL. Post-herpetic neuralgia: the relationship of pain complaint, sensory disturbance, and skin temperature. *Pain* 1989;39:129–144.

75. Rushton JG, MacDonald HNA. Trigeminal neuralgia: special consideration of non-surgical treatment. *JAMA* 1957;165:437–440.

76. Rushton JG, Stevens C, Miller RH. Glossopharyngeal (vagoglossopharyngeal) neuralgia. *Arch Neurol* 1981;38:201–205.

77. Schnetler J, Hopper C. Intracranial tumours presenting with facial pain. *Br Dent J* 1989;166:80–83.

78. Selby G. Disease of the fifth cranial nerve. In: Dyck PJ, Thomas PK, Lambert EH, Bunge R, eds. *Peripheral neuropathy,* 2nd ed. Philadelphia: WB Saunders, 1984:1224–1265.

79. Sessle BJ. The neurobiology of facial and dental pain: present knowledge, future directions. *J Dent Res* 1987;66:962–981.

80. Shankland WE. Osteocavitational lesions (Ratner bone cavities): frequently misdiagnosed as trigeminal neuralgia a case report. *Cranio* 1993;11:232–236.

81. Slobber WK, Graff-Radford. Orodental considerations in facial pain. *Semin Neurol* 1988;8:318–323.

82. Solomon S, Lipton RB. Atypical facial pain: a review. *Semin Neurol* 1988;8:332–338.

83. Solomon S, Lipton RB. Facial pain. *Neurol Clin* 1990;8:913–928.

84. Steardo L, Leo A, Marano E. Efficacy of baclofen in trigeminal neuralgia and some other painful conditions. *Eur Neurol* 1984;23: 51–55.

85. Stookey BP, Ransohoff J. *Trigeminal neuralgia: its history and treatment*. Springfield, IL: Charles C. Thomas, 1959.

86. Strittmatter M, Grauer M, Isenberg E, et al. Cerebrospinal fluid neuropeptides and monoaminergic transmitters in patients with trigeminal neuralgia. *Headache* 1997;37:211–216.

87. Sturman RH, O'Brien FH. Non-surgical treatment of tic douloureux with carbamazepine (#G32883). *Headache* 1969;9:88–91.

88. Sugimoto T, Bennett GJ, Kajander KC. Strychnine-enhanced transsynaptic degeneration of dorsal horn neurons in rats with an experimental painful neuropathy. *Neurosci Lett* 1989;98:139–143.

89. Sugimoto T, Bennett GJ, Kajander KC. Transsynaptic degeneration in the superficial dorsal horn after sciatic nerve injury: effects of a chronic constriction injury, transaction, and strychnine. *Pain* 1990;42: 205–213.

90. Symonds Sir C. Facial pain. *Ann R Coll Surg Engl* 1949;4;206–212.

91. Tasker RR. Deafferentation. In: Wall PD, Melzack R, eds. *Textbook of pain*. Edinburgh: Churchill Livingstone, 1984:119–132.

92. Terrence CF. Differential diagnosis of trigeminal neuralgia. In: Fromm GH, ed. *Medical and surgical management of trigeminal neuralgia*. New York: Futura, 1987:43–60.

93. Terrence CF. History of trigeminal neuralgia. In: Fromm GH, ed. *Medical and surgical management of trigeminal neuralgia*. New York: Futura, 1987:1–6.

94. Terrence CF, Costa R, Fromm GH. An unusual case of paroxysmal face pain. *J Neurol* 1979;221:73–76.

95. Terrence CF, Fromm GH. Congestive heart failure during carbamazepine therapy. *Ann Neurol* 1980;8:200–201.

96. Terrence CF, Fromm GH. Complications of baclofen withdrawal. *Arch Neurol* 1981;38:588–589.

97. Terrence CF, Sax M, Fromm GH, et al. Effect of baclofen enantiomorphs on the spinal trigeminal nucleus and steric similarities of carbamazepine. *Pharmacology* 1983;27:85–94.

98. Thomson T, Bertilsson L. Potent therapeutic effect of carbamazepine 10, 11-epoxide in trigeminal neuralgia. *Arch Neurol* 1984;41:598–601.

99. Trousseau A. De la neuralgia epileptiforme. *Arch Gen Med* 1853;1: 33–44.

100. Valzania F, Strafella AP, Massetti SA, et al. Gabapentin in idiopathic trigeminal neuralgia. *Neurology* 1998;50[Suppl 4]:A379.

101. Wang JK, Johnson KA, Ilstrup DM. Sympathetic blocks for reflex sympathetic dystrophy. *Pain* 1985;23:13–17.

102. Watson CPN. Postherpetic neuralgia. *Neurol Clin* 1989;7:231–248.

103. Watson CPN, Evans RJ. A comparative trial of amitriptyline and zimelidine in post-herpetic neuralgia. *Pain* 1985:23:387–394.

104. Watson CP, Evans RJ, Reed K, et al. Amitriptyline versus placebo in postherpetic neuralgia. *Neurology* 1982;32:671–673.

105. Watson CPN, Evans RJ, Watt VR. Postherpetic neuralgia and topical capsaicin. *Pain* 1988;33:333–340.

106. Watson CPN, Morshead C, Van de Kooy D, et al. Post-herpetic neuralgia: post-mortem analysis of a case. *Pain* 1988;34:129–138.

107. Wepsic, JG. Tic douloureux. Etiology, refined treatment. *N Engl J Med* 1973;288:680–681.

108. White JC, Sweet WH. *Pain and the neurosurgeon. A forty year experience*. Springfield, IL: Charles C. Thomas, 1969.

109. Young RF, Vermeulen SS, Grimm P, et al. Gamma knife radiosurgery treatment of trigeminal neuralgia: idiopathic and tumor related. *Neurology* 1997;48:608–614.

110. Zakrzewska J, Chaudhry Z, et al. Latrigine (Lamictal) in refractory trigeminal neuralgia: results from a double-blind placebo controlled cross over trial. *Pain* 1977;73:223–230.

111. Zakrzewska J, Patsalos PN. Oxcarbamazepine: a new drug in the management of intractable trigeminal neuralgia. *J Neurol Neurosurg Psychiatry* 1989;52:472–476.

The Headaches, Second Edition,
edited by J. Olesen, P. Tfelt-Hansen, and K.M.A. Welch.
Lippincott Williams & Wilkins, Philadelphia © 2000.

The Secondary Headaches

CHAPTER 124

Central Pain in the Face and Head

Jörgen Boivie and Kenneth L. Casey

IHS code and diagnosis:
12.7.1 Anesthesia dolorosa
12.7.2 Thalamic pain
12.2.2.2 Central lesions
(12.2.2 Symptomatic trigeminal neuralgia)
WHO code and diagnosis: G 52.9 cranial nerve disorder
  unspecified

OTHER TERMS

The term *thalamic pain* is often used in a general sense to refer to all central pain. The expression *pseudothalamic pain* is then sometimes used for central pain caused by extrathalamic lesions. *Central poststroke pain* denotes central pain resulting from a cerebrovascular lesion (CVL). In the IHS classification of headache, thalamic pain (12.7.2) is used as a general term to denote central pain caused by a CVL affecting the "quintothalamic pathway or thalamus." Some researchers use the term *dysesthetic pain* to refer to central pain with a predominantly dysesthetic character. Such pain can have either central or peripheral causes. It is recommended that the general term *central pain* be used in most instances; only central pain caused by lesions in the thalamus should be labeled thalamic pain.

The term *anesthesia dolorosa* denotes pain in a region with decreased sensibility after lesions in the central or peripheral nervous system. This term is not restricted to pain of certain causes, but it has been used chiefly for head and face pain, and particularly as a name for the

neurogenic pain that sometimes develops after neurosurgical lesions of the trigeminal nerve or ganglion, or after destructive nerve blocks performed to treat trigeminal neuralgia (see Chapter 123). It also has been used for central pain in an anesthetic region caused by neurosurgical brain lesions for treatment of severe pain. The term *deafferentation pain* is used for similar conditions, but it is more commonly used in patients with lesions of spinal nerves.

SHORT DESCRIPTION

The International Association for the Study of Pain (IASP) has defined central pain as pain caused by a lesion or dysfunction in the central nervous system (CNS) (26). Note that the cause shall be a primary process in the CNS. Thus, peripherally induced pain with central mechanisms is not central pain, even if the central mechanisms are prominent.

EPIDEMIOLOGY

There are large differences in the prevalence of central pain among the disorders that may lead to such pain (Tables 1 and 2) (8,33). To some extent the prevalence figures are estimates, because few epidemiologic studies have been conducted. Such estimates are difficult to make because it is sometimes difficult to distinguish central pain from other possible causes of pain. This, for instance, is the case in many patients with pain after spinal injury and multiple sclerosis (MS). Nevertheless, the figures given in Table 2 are probably in the right range, which means that even if pain in epilepsy and Parkinson's disease are excluded, about 278,000 Americans have central pain, that is, a prevalence of about 115 per 100,000 individuals.

J. Boivie: Department of Neurology, University Hospital, S-581 85 Linköping, Sweden.

K. L. Casey: Department of Neurology, University of Michigan, and Department of Neurology, Veteran's Affairs Medical Center, Ann Arbor, Michigan 48105.

TABLE 1. *Causes of central pain*

Vascular lesions in the brain and spinal cord
   Infarct
   Hemorrhage
   Vascular malformation
Multiple sclerosis
Traumatic spinal cord injury
   Cordotomy
Traumatic brain injury
Syringomyelia and syringobulbia
Tumors
Abscesses
Inflammatory diseases other than MS
   Myelitis caused by viruses, syphilis
Epilepsy
Parkinson's disease

The only prospective epidemiologic study that has been conducted concerns central poststroke pain (1). In this study 191 patients were followed for 12 months after stroke onset with regard to sensory abnormalities and the development of spontaneous and evoked central pain. Sixteen of these patients developed central pain (8.4%), which is a much higher incidence than had previously been suspected. Among patients with somatosensory deficits (42% of all stroke patients), the incidence of central pain was 18%. The corresponding figure in a mainly retrospective study of central pain in 63 patients with brainstem infarcts was 44% (25). In this study the overall incidence for central poststroke pain was 25%.

A study of the prevalence of central pain in 371 patients with MS found that 28% of MS patients experience, or have experienced, central pain (Österberg and Boivie, manuscript in preparation). This includes 5% who had trigeminal neuralgia, which in this context is considered to be a central pain condition because it is caused by an inflammatory lesion located in the CNS. In two studies of central poststroke pain, 33% of 27 patients and 37% of 111 patients had facial pain, in addition to pain at other sites (10,23). In a mixed material of 73 patients with "central pain of brain origin," 11% had facial pain (33).

TABLE 2. *Estimated prevalences of major disorders with central pain in the United States (population around 250 million)*

Disease	Total no. of patients	Patients with CP	% Patients with CP
Spinal cord injury	225,000	68,000	30
Multiple sclerosis	150,000	42,000	28
Stroke	2,000,000	168,000	8.4
Epilepsy	1,600,000	44,800	2.8
Parkinsons disease	500,000	50,000	10

Data from Bonica (8), Andersen et al. (1), and Österberg Boivie (from a study of central pain in MS).

Brain tumors seldom cause central pain (27,33). It is not known whether pain has any particular features in such patients.

About 3% of patients with spinal anterolateral cordotomy develop late-onset central pain, usually of a dysesthetic nature (18,27,33). The corresponding lesions in the brainstem (i.e., mesencephalic and pontine tractotomy) have been reported to carry a high risk of causing central pain (31).

From the scanty information in the literature, it would appear that the incidence of central head pain, including central face pain, is low, the only exceptions being stroke and surgical tractotomies for severe pain, which seem to carry a considerable risk of causing central pain.

GENETICS

No information about the genetics of central pain seems to have been published. However, because apparently similar lesions lead to the development of central pain in some, but not all, patients, a genetic factor cannot be ruled out, but there is no evidence to support or refute the idea. Studies on rats suggest that a genetic factor could be important for the development of peripheral neurogenic pain that follows the induction of experimental nerve lesions in some rat strains, but not in others (15).

PATHOPHYSIOLOGY

Which diseases or lesions can induce central pain? This is the cardinal question regarding the pathophysiology of central head pain. These states are listed in Table 1. Most kinds of disease processes affecting the CNS can lead to central pain. They include rapidly and slowly developing lesions such as parenchymal hemorrhage and the inflammatory demyelinating lesions of MS. However, the incidence of central pain differs in different diseases, and it is therefore reasonable to suspect that differences in the lesions are important factors. Unfortunately, little is known about these factors at the cell level, including what happens to transmitter receptors.

The location of the lesions is important for the incidence of central pain. Several investigators have reported results indicating that central pain develops as a result of lesions that affect the spino- and quintothalamic pathways, that is, the pathways that are most important for the sensibility of pain and temperature (4,8,32,38). These reports also show that the lesion can be located at any level of these pathways along the neuraxis, from the origin in the spinal trigeminal nucleus or the spinal dorsal horn to the cerebral cortex.

Studies on stroke patients have yielded information about the lesions that cause central pain. The first central pain condition to be described in detail was the thalamic pain of Dejerine and Roussy (14). It was viewed as one component of the thalamic syndrome. The thalamic syndrome is usually caused by a thalamic infarction or hemorrhage (16), but in many cases the lesion causing thalamic pain extends considerably laterally to the thalamus.

The term "thalamic pain" has focused attention about the mechanisms of central pain on the thalamus itself. However, thalamic involvement by the lesion is not even necessary in central poststroke pain. Some computed tomographic and magnetic resonance imaging studies have indicated that at most about half of stroke patients with central pain have lesions involving the thalamus (11,23). Both supra- and infrathalamic lesions, including cortical lesions, can cause central pain. For instance, there is good evidence that the lesions involving the parietal cortex and the insular and adjacent perisylvian cortex can produce loss of pain and temperature sensibility (3). Brainstem strokes of the Wallenberg type, that is, infarctions in the region of the posterior inferior cerebellar artery, are well known to cause central pain in some patients. In one study, 8 of 27 consecutive patients with central poststroke pain had such lesions (23). The risk of developing central pain may be higher with brainstem lesions affecting the quintothalamic pathways than with suprathalamic lesions (25).

Thalamic lesions can undoubtedly cause central pain, but evidence indicates that central pain develops only if the ventroposterior region is involved (9,23). The incidence of central pain after such lesions was about 17% (9).

On the basis of findings in stroke patients with central pain, it has been concluded that this pain occurs independently of nonsensory symptoms (Table 3) (7,10,11,23, 31). Using quantitative sensory tests it has been found that all such patients have abnormal sensibility to temperature and pain, whereas many have normal thresholds to touch, vibration, and kinesthesia (Table 3).

In accordance with the outcome of cordotomy, studies of neurosurgical lesions of the quintothalamic tract in the treatment of intractable head pain have shown that lesions of this pathway in the pons and midbrain also can lead to central pain (18,31). Some of these patients develop central pain, often with a dysesthetic quality several months after the operation.

TABLE 3. *Diagnostic criteria for central pain*

History of disease in the brain or spinal cord
Laboratory examinations showing CNS disease including
   x-ray, MRI, CSF assays
Pain starting after the onset of CNS disease; onset of pain
   often delayed
Pain with a regional distribution, rather than corresponding
   to individual nerves
Pain quality compatible with central pain, which can be of
   many different kinds, often more than one quality
Sensory abnormality, including abnormal sensibility to
   temperature and pain, and commonly hyperesthesia
   and dysesthesia
Non-sensory symptoms and signs may or may not be
   present

In syringobulbia the lesion involves the spinal trigeminal nucleus, demonstrated by the dissociated sensory loss in such patients (2). Central pain is common in MS, but why some patients with MS develop central pain is unclear (6). The location of the demyelinating lesion is probably a crucial factor. The increased incidence of trigeminal neuralgia in MS (5%) is well documented (see Chapter 123).

Current knowledge supports the hypothesis that central pain occurs in patients with lesions that impair temperature and pain sensibility (i.e., that affect the quinto- and spinothalamic pathways), including the thalamocortical projections (4,7,10,33). This hypothesis is contrary to the older, often cited hypothesis, according to which central pain is produced by lesions affecting the medial lemniscal pathways, thereby removing inhibition exerted via these pathways on thalamic and cortical centers (i.e., a result of disinhibition).

Two general pathophysiologic processes have been hypothesized as possible causes of the severe spontaneous central pain and the painful overreactions to somatic stimulation that often accompany central pain:

1. An "irritative lesion" hypothesis that hyperactive cells at or adjacent to the lesion site produced increased activity in otherwise normal nociceptive pathways
2. A "denervation or hypersensitivity" hypothesis that neurons remote from the lesion, but within nociceptive processing pathways become hyperactive and hypersensitive because they have lost normal synaptic inputs (20)

These hypothetical mechanisms are not mutually exclusive. Both may participate, to varying degrees, in the pathophysiology of central pain in different patients.

In Head's disinhibition hypothesis, it was assumed that pathways mediating tactile sensations normally exert a tonic inhibitory influence on a separate population of pain-mediating neurons (20), and that central pain was produced when this inhibition was removed by a lesion in the lemniscal pathways. Modern research has shown, however, that lesions in the lemniscal pathways are not necessary for central pain to appear.

Craig has presented a new version of the thalamic disinhibition hypothesis based on results from experimental studies in cats, monkeys, and humans (12). The hypothesis states that "central pain is due to the disruption of thermosensory integration and the loss of cold inhibition of burning pain" (12). This disruption is, according to the hypothesis, caused by a lesion somewhere along the spinothalamic projections to the thalamus (to the ventroposterior, posterior, and mediodorsal nuclear regions—nuclei VPI, VMpo, MDvc). These projections are thought to tonically inhibit nociceptive thalamocortical neurons, which by the lesion increase their firing and produce pain. The pathway is activated by cold receptors in the periphery.

Recent experimental studies on the mechanisms behind neurogenic pain induced by lesions of the spinal cord and peripheral nerves indicate that excitatory amino acids, particularly glutamate and its effects via N-methyl-D-aspartate (NMDA) receptors, play an important role in the development of hyperactive and hyperexcitable neuron pools in the CNS (36). Injection of NMDA antagonists during the critical period can apparently prevent the development of neurogenic pain. One may hope that in the future it will prove possible to prevent the development of central pain with the use of drugs. However, then it will be necessary to be able to identify the patients at risk of developing such pain. Detailed analysis of the sensory abnormalities, including quantitative sensory testing, would appear to be helpful in this identification.

CLINICAL FEATURES

Both the pain and the neurologic symptoms and signs vary greatly in patients with central pain, which may make diagnosis difficult. Some patients experience intense pain, and this can differ greatly in character and location from patient to patient. Some patients have severe motor and sensory symptoms, whereas others have only mild pain and minor neurologic symptoms. The diagnosis of central pain must therefore be based on the total clinical picture, in which history, symptoms, and signs indicate a disease process in the CNS, and with pain the characteristics of which are compatible with central pain. The diagnostic criteria are summarized in Table 3. Because no specific investigations appear to have been performed specifically of the clinical features of central head pain, this section will mainly summarize the current knowledge about central pain in general.

Studies on patients with central poststroke pain have identified the characteristics of central pain, which, apart from the location of the pain, seem to be shared by central pain in other diseases (6,7,11,23,31).

The pain is usually a hemipain and includes the face in about 33% to 50% of all patients. In some patients with brainstem strokes the pain is located to the lesion side in the face and to the contralateral side in the rest of the body. An example of this is shown by a patient who had aching, pricking, and shooting pain in the left side of the face and in the right leg and foot, where there was also burning pain, as a result of a brainstem infarct of the Wallenberg type (23). Most patients experience more than one pain quality, the most common being burning, aching, pricking, lacerating, and lancinating pain, with some differences depending on where the lesion is located.

The intensity of the pain varies between patients, from excruciating to low-intensity pain. Even if the intensity, as assessed for instance with the visual analogue scale (VAS) is low, it causes much suffering, because of its very irritating and unpleasant qualities. The pain is commonly increased by external and internal stimuli, such as light touch, cold, movements, and emotional distress. It is usually constant, but intermittent attacks, spontaneous or evoked, may occur.

The onset of central pain is commonly delayed. In 13 of 27 patients the delay was at least 1 month, the longest being 34 months (23). The onset of pain often coincides with the return of some sensibility after a period of deep numbness.

Because central pain is a result of CNS disease, it is important to know whether it is accompanied by other neurologic symptoms. Also in this respect the best information is available from central poststroke pain. In this group the only feature common to all patients with central pain, apart from the pain, was abnormal somatic sensibility (Fig. 1) (23). The most prominent sensory signs in central poststroke pain are abnormal temperature and pain sensibility, dysesthesia, and hyperesthesia (Table 4). Quantitative sensory tests showed that all 27 patients had abnormal thresholds to temperature and pain, whereas at most half had abnormal thresholds to touch, vibration, and joint movements (7,10). Of patients examined by traditional clinical tests, which are less sensitive, not all with central pain showed such sensory abnormalities (31). However, there are patients with central pain in whom not even quantitative tests have shown sensory loss (Boivie, Bowsher, and Leijon, unpublished observations).

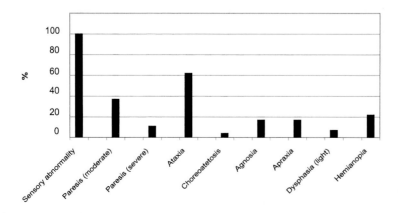

FIG. 1. Symptoms in patients with central poststroke pain. Percentages of 27 patients. Reproduced from Leijon et al. (23).

TABLE 4. *Sensory abnormalities in central poststroke pain*

	BS	TH	SE	UI	All
Vibration	1/8	7/9	3/6	0/4	11/27 (40%
Touch	2/8	8/9	2/6	2/4	14/27 (52%)
Innocuous temp.	8/8	9/9	6/6	4/4	27/27 (100%)
Temp. pain	7/8	9/9	5/6	4/4	25/27 (93%)

Proportion of patients with threshold abnormalities as shown by quantitative sensory tests.

Abbreviations show location of CVL. BS, brain stem; TH, includes thalamus; SE, supratentorial, extrathalamic; UI, location unidentified.

From Boivie and Leijon (7).

All eight patients with brainstem infarcts and central pain had dissociated sensory loss, that is, severely abnormal sensibility to temperature and pain and normal or almost normal tactile sensibility ipsilaterally in the face and contralaterally in the extremities (7). However, only three of them had facial pain, which in one patient was on the same side as the extremity pain.

Most patients with central poststroke pain have hyperesthesias, often of a hyperpathic nature, with painful overreactions to touch, cold (i.e., touch and cold allodynia), and pinprick (i.e., hyperalgesia) (6,7,11). These hyperesthesias hamper the patients considerably in their activity. Spontaneous dysesthesias are also common.

Syringobulbia can cause central pain in the face (17), but this has not been specifically studied. Syringobulbia is usually present together with syringomyelia, in which central pain is common (5,16; J. Boivie, unpublished observations). In seven of a series of 25 patients with syringomyelia, the syrinx extended into the medulla oblongata (J. Boivie, unpublished observations). Two of these had neck pain that probably formed part of their central pain, but none had facial pain. About half of all patients had central pain. This would appear to be the highest prevalence of central pain reported in any neurologic disease. In this group too the central pain was accompanied by abnormal temperature and pain sensibility, which is characteristic of syringomyelia.

As reported in the section on epidemiology, a recent study on 371 MS patients found that 28% of the patients had central pain (Österberg and Boivie, manuscript in preparation). This included 5% who have trigeminal neuralgia. The other central pain was dominant in the lower extremities (90% of all patients) and the upper extremities (36%). Four of the 18 patients with trigeminal neuralgia also had pain in the legs. The pain in the extremities was not found to be caused by spasticity. It was almost solely constant pain.

PROGNOSIS

Central pain is almost always chronic, commonly lasting for many years, and not infrequently for the rest of life. In stable lesions such as those in stroke, the pain is usually stable and does not change character with time, but in MS new demyelinating lesions can modify the pain. Central pain also can spontaneously and gradually subside in stroke and MS (22). In a recently reported case with central pain after a thalamic infarct, the pain disappeared when the patient was struck 7 years later by a second infarct located ipsilaterally at the internal capsule (30). It is not known whether presently available drug treatments affect the natural course of central pain.

MANAGEMENT

Ideally, patients at risk should receive treatment that prevents the development of central pain. Such patients would have to be identified, the pathophysiology should be known, and effective modes of treatment should be available. Research on experimental models (36,38) and on patients (7,10,24,32) may yield the necessary information in coming years, but until such information is available, treatment remains empirical.

Most current treatment for central pain can be assigned to one of four categories:

1. Peripheral and central electrical stimulation of the afferent systems to counteract the pathologic brain activity
2. Drugs that reduce the hyperactivity in the CNS, namely, as membrane-stabilizing agents such as carbamazepin, lidocaine, or mexiletine, or GABAergic agents affecting the inhibitory neurons, including clonazepam, valproate, gabapentine, NMDA antagonists, or baclofen
3. Drugs that are believed to increase the activity in the endorphinergic systems by influencing the reuptake of serotin, including antidepressant drugs
4. Drugs that influence adrenoreceptors, such as the α_2-agonist clonidine.

The list of treatments that have been tried for central pain is long, but few have been evaluated in controlled clinical trials. Table 5 lists the most common and most interesting forms of treatment.

The question whether or not neurogenic pain responds to analgesics is controversial. Some researchers claim that their findings indicate that neuropathic pain in general responds poorly or not at all. Others report experience to the contrary. Apparently most clinicians agree that neurogenic pain in general responds less well to analgesics than does most nociceptive pain, and that many patients do not respond at all to opioids. A reasonable conclusion from the evidence available seems to be that a few central pain patients may benefit from analgesics, and that it is important to evaluate these effects carefully in each individual before prescribing them for long-term use. If the patient reports that the opioid clearly reduces the pain, and thereby the suffering significantly, then he or she should not be denied this relief.

TABLE 5. *Treatment modalities for central pain*

Transcutaneous electrical nerve stimulation[a]
Brain stimulation
Sympathetic block
Antidepressant drugs[a]
Antiepileptic drugs[a]
Baclofen
α_2-adrenergic agonists (clonidine)
Local i.v. anesthetics
Antiarrhythmic drugs
Naloxone
Neuroleptic drugs
Analgesics

[a]First-choice therapies.

Before giving a drug it is worthwhile to try transcutaneous electrical nerve stimulation (TENS). Electrical stimulation in the brain, for instance, in the ventroposterior thalamic region and internal capsule, also has been tried with varying success. Recent reviews suggest that deep brain stimulation, or destructive lesions in the brain, should only be considered if other treatments have failed and if the pain is severe (18,31). Excellent results were reported following surface stimulation of the motor cortex in central pain (28,35,37).

If TENS is unsuccessful, the next step is to try an antidepressant drug. The only drugs so far tested in controlled studies are amitriptyline [central poststroke pain (21)] and trazodon [central pain after spinal cord injury (13)]. It is widely agreed that antidepressant drugs relieve central pain in many patients, irrespective of the etiology, but further controlled trials are needed, notably to evaluate the newer antidepressants. From comparisons with studies on peripheral neurogenic pain, and particularly painful diabetic polyneuropathy, one would expect that drugs such as clomipramine, desipramine, doxepin, imipiramine, nortriptyline, and others might be roughly as effective as amitriptyline in central pain, but this remains to be shown. The specific serotonin reuptake inhibitors (e.g., fluoxetine, paroxetine) appear to have weaker pain-relieving effects than the tricyclic antidepressants, and the new antidepressants with mixed serotinergic and noradrenergic effects have not yet been studied systematically with respect to their possible effects on central pain or other neuropathic pains.

Undoubtedly antidepressants cause problems in some patients, but with careful management and with the new drugs with fewer side effects, they can often be kept under control. It has been suggested that the effect of antidepressants can be enhanced by combining the antidepressant with propranolol (34) or with cholinesterase inhibitor (19,29), but controlled trials are needed. Neuroleptic drugs are sometimes used for central pain, alone or in combination with antidepressants. Their effect on neurogenic and nociceptive pain has not been docu-

mented in controlled trials, and their potentially irreversible, severe side effects must be borne in mind.

In the only controlled study on antiepileptic drugs in the treatment of central pain, 3 of 15 patients were responders to carbamazepine [statistically not significant (21)]. These patients had no paroxysmal pain attacks, so other kinds of pain might also respond to such therapy. The only neurogenic pain conditions in which antiepileptic drugs have been convincingly demonstrated to be effective are tic douloureux and paroxysmal painful seizures in MS. In other neuralgias and central pain conditions, the reports are of an anecdotal, retrospective character.

REFERENCES

1. Andersen G, Vestergaard K, Ingeman-Nielsen M, Jensen TS. Incidence of central post-stroke pain. *Pain* 1995;61:187–193.
2. Barnett JM, Stein BM, Mohr JP, Yatsu FM. *Stroke, pathophysiology, diagnosis and management.* New York: Churchill Livingstone, 1986.
3. Bassetti RD, Bogousslavsky J, Regli F. Sensory syndromes in parietal stroke. *Neurology* 1993;43:1942–1949.
4. Beric A, Dimitrijevic MR, Lindblom U. Cortical evoked potentials and somatosensory perception in chronic spinal cord injury patients. *J Neurol Sci* 1987;80:333–342.
5. Boivie J. Hyperalgesia and allodynia in patients with CNS lesions. In: Willis WDJ, ed. *Hyperalgesia and allodynia.* New York: Raven, 1992: 363–373.
6. Boivie J. Central pain. In: Wall PD, Melzack R, eds. *Textbook of pain.* New York: Churchill Livingstone, 1994:871–902.
7. Boivie J, Leijon G, Johansson I. Central post-stroke pain—a study of the mechanisms trough analyses of the sensory abnormalities. *Pain* 1989;37:173–185.
8. Bonica JJ. Introduction: semantic, epidemiologic, and educational issues. In: Casey KL, ed. *Pain and central nervous system disease: the central pain syndromes.* New York: Raven, 1991:13–29.
9. Bougosslavsky J, Regli F, Uske A. Thalamic infarcts: clinical syndromes, etiology and prognosis. *Neurology* 1988;38:837–848.
10. Bowsher D. Central pain: clinical and physiological characteristics. *J Neurol Neurosurg Psychiatry* 1996;61:62–69.
11. Bowsher D, Leijon G, Thuomas K-Å. Central post-stroke pain: correlation of magnetic resonance imaging with clinical pain characteristics and sensory abnormalities. *Neurology* 1998;51:1352–1358.
12. Craig AD. A new version of the thalamic disinhibition hypothesis of central pain. *Pain Forum* 1998;7:1–14.
13. Davidoff G, Guarrachini M, Roth E, Sliwa J, Yarkony G. Trazodone hydrochloride in the treatment of dysesthetic pain in traumatic myelopathy: a randomized, double-blind, placebo-controlled study. *Pain* 1987;29:151–161.
14. Dejerine J, Roussy G. La syndrome thalamique. *Rev Neurol (Paris)* 1906;14:521–532.
15. Devor M, Raber P. Heritability of neuropathic pain: evidence from an experimental model. In: Bond MR, ed. *Proceedings of the Vth world Congress on Pain.* Amsterdam: Elsevier, 1991:343–347.
16. Garcin R. Thalamic syndrome and pain central origin. In: Soulairac A, Cahn J, Charpentier J, eds. *Pain.* London: Academic, 1968:521–541.
17. Garcin R, Lapresle J. Syndrome sensitif de type thalamiq et à topograpiecheiro-orale par lèsion localisèe du thalamus. *Rev Neurol* 1954; 90:124–129.
18. Gybels JM, Sweet WH. *Neurosurgical treatment of persistent pain.* Basel: Karger, 1989.
19. Hampf G, Bowsher D. Distigmine and amitriptyline in the treatment of chronic pain. *Anesth Prog* 1989;36:58–62.
20. Head H, Holmes G. Sensory disturbances from cerebral lesions. *Brain* 1911;34:102–254.
21. Leijon G, Boivie J. Central post-stroke pain—a controlled trial of amitriptyline and carbamazepine. *Pain* 1989;36:27–36.
22. Leijon G, Boivie J. Central post-stroke pain (CPSP)—a longterm follow up. In: *Abstracts of the 8th World Congress on Pain.* Seattle: IASP Press, 1996:380.

23. Leijon G, Boivie J, Johansson I. Central post-stroke pain—neurological symptoms and pain characteristics. *Pain* 1989;36:13–25.
24. Lenz FA, Dougherty PM. New version of the thalamic disinhibition hypothesis may explain some clinical features of central pain syndromes. *Pain Forum* 1998;7:20–23.
25. MacGowan DJL, Janal MN, Clark WC, et al. Central post-stroke pain and Wallenberg's lateral medullary infarction: frequency, character, and determinants in 63 patients. *Neurology* 1997;49:120–125.
26. Mersky H, Bogduk N. *Classification of chronic pain*, 2nd ed. Seattle: IASP Press, 1994.
27. Pagni C. *Central pain. A neurosurgical challange.* Torino, Italy: Edizioni Minerva Medica, 1998.
28. Peyron R, Garcia-Larrea L, Deiber MP, et al. Electrical stimulation of precentral cortical area in the treatment of central pain: electrophysiological and PET study. *Pain* 1995;62:275–286.
29. Schott GD, Loh L. Anticholinesterase drugs in the treatment of chronic pain. *Pain* 1984;20:201–206.
30. Soria ED, Fine EJ. Disapperance of thalamic pain after parietal subcortical stroke. *Pain* 1991;44:285–288.
31. Tasker R. Pain resulting from central nervous system pathology (central pain). In: Bonica JJ, ed. *The management of pain.* Philadelphia: Lea & Febiger, 1990:264–280.
32. Tasker RR. Can we explain how strokes cause pain? *Pain Forum* 1998; 7:18–19.
33. Tasker RR, de Carvalho G, Dostrovsky JO. The history of central pain syndromes, with observations concerning pathophysiology and treatment. In: Casey KL, ed. *Pain and central nervous disease: the central pain syndromes.* New York: Raven, 1991:31–58.
34. Tourian AY. Treatment of central pain with combination of Doxepin and Inderal. *Neurology* 1987;37:239.
35. Tsubokawa T. Motor cortex stimulation for deafferentation pain relief in various clinical syndromes and its possible mechanisms. In: Besson JM, Guildbaud G, Ollat H, eds. *Forebrain areas involved in pain processing.* Paris: John Libby Eurotext, 1995:261–276.
36. Wiesenfeld-Hallin Z, Hao J-X, Xu X-J. Mechanisms of central pain. In: Jensen TS, Turner JA, Wiesenfeld-Hallin Z, eds. *Progress in pain research and management.* Seattle: IASP Press, 1997:575–588.
37. Yamamoto T, Latayama Y, Hirayama T, Tsubokawa T. Pharmacological classification of central post-stroke pain: comparison with the results of chronic motor cortex stimulation therapy. *Pain* 1997;72: 5–12.
38. Yezierski RP, Liu S, Ruenes GL, Kajander KJ, Brewer KL. Excitotoxic spinal cord injury: behavioral and morphological characteristics of a central pain model. *Pain* 1998;75:141–155.

The Headaches, Second Edition,
edited by J. Olesen, P. Tfelt-Hansen, and K.M.A. Welch.
Lippincott Williams & Wilkins, Philadelphia © 2000.

Special Problems in the Headaches and Their Management

CHAPTER 125

Headache in the Elderly

John Edmeads

"Old age," said the poet Bion (300 B.C.E.), "is the harbour of all ills." A merciful exception is headache, which visits the elderly less. The nineteenth century poet Ralph Waldo Emerson wrote that "at fifty years . . . afflicted citizens lose their sick headaches," and an eminent clinician, Moritz Romberg (28), stated in the first textbook of neurology (1853), that "hemicrania generally diminishes in advanced age." Modern epidemiologists agree.

EPIDEMIOLOGIC ASPECTS

Community surveys reveal that headache is extremely prevalent in the general population. Taking all ages together, about 75% of men and 80% of women have had a headache within the past year (22,40). Headache prevalence declines, however, with age. In Waters' series (40), for example, whereas 92% of women and 74% of men between the ages of 21 and 34 years had had a headache in the preceding year, the prevalence decreased to 66% and 53%, respectively, in the group 55 to 74 years of age, and only 55% of women and 22% of men over the age of 75 years had headaches. Other series (6,14,31,36) indicate that the prevalence of headache in those over the age of 70 ranges from 53% to 14%, the prevalence of frequent headaches in this age group is 17% to 11%, and only 10% of women and 5% of men in this age group report having severe headaches. One of the most common symptoms in the young, headache declines in old age to become only the 10th most common symptom of elderly women, and the 14th of elderly men (14). Even so, headache in the elderly creates a heavy burden. In a British survey (29) of an arbitrarily defined "all age population" of 100,000, headache caused 1,560 people over the age of 65 to consult their physicians within a 1-year period; in the United States even more old people go to their doctors for headaches (7).

CAUSES OF HEADACHE IN THE ELDERLY

As in the younger age groups, benign dysfunctional headaches such as migraine, tension-type headaches, and cluster headaches still account for most of the headaches that afflict the elderly. An important difference between the two age groups is that headaches due to disease is much more common in the aged than in youths, constituting a significant minority (10%–20%) of cases in the elderly (18,34). Table 1 lists some of the toxic, metabolic,

TABLE 1. *Causes of headache in the elderly*

Benign dysfunctional headaches
  Migraine
  Tension-type headache
  Cluster headaches
  Hypnic headache
Toxic and metabolic headaches
  Medications (including rebound syndromes)
  Chronic respiratory disease
  Hypercalcemia
  Hyponatremia
  Chronic renal failure
  Anemia, polycythemia
Structural lesions
  Cervical spondylosis and disc disease
  Giant cell arteritis
  Atherothrombotic cerebrovascular disease
  Hypertension
  Intracranial mass lesions, including
    hydrocephalus and hematomas
  Meningeal irritation: hemorrhage and infection

J.G. Edmeads: Department of Medicine, Sunnybrook Health Science Center, University of Toronto, Toronto, Ontario M4N 3M5, Canada.

and structural diseases that may present with headache; all are distinctly more common in older people. One conclusion to be drawn from this is that the clinical approach to headache, always requiring care, requires more attention in the older patient, with correspondingly readier recourse to laboratory investigation and neuroimaging.

Although older people are more likely than the younger to suffer the various cranial neuralgias, these syndromes seldom are described as "headache," and thus are not discussed here (see Chapters 122–124).

BENIGN DYSFUNCTIONAL HEADACHES IN THE ELDERLY

Migraine

Migraine attenuates and sometimes disappears with age, but even so, a significant number of the elderly remain troubled by this condition. Indeed, some (2%–3%, experience migraine for the first time in their lives after the age of 50 (30). The prevalence of migraine in the elderly has been variously estimated at between 2.9% (34) and 10.5% (31), with more women than men affected, and prevalence declining with advancing age. Migraine with aura was less common in the aged than the young in all series, reflecting the well-known clinical observation that people tend to lose their auras as they get older.

The converse may occur; that is, patients who have had migraine with aura when younger may lose their headaches as they age and have only recurrent painless auras (39). These episodic focal disturbances may be confused with transient ischemic attacks, particularly if the prior history of migraine has not been elicited. Fisher (11) has provided guidelines that may help to distinguish these essentially harmless transient migrainous accompaniments from the more ominous transient ischemic attacks (TIAs).

Various conditions that occur in old age, or sometimes the medications taken for these conditions, may aggravate migraine or make it more resistant to treatment. For example, high blood pressure may make coexistent migraine difficult to treat (38). Some of the drugs used to treat hypertension are useful as migraine prophylactics (e.g., beta-blockers and calcium channel blockers), but others (e.g., methyldopa) may make migraine worse. Ischemic heart disease, common in the elderly, does not in itself worsen migraine, although very rarely it may present primarily as migrainelike headaches (4), which are usually accompanied by less conspicuous chest or left arm discomfort. These "anginal headaches" tend to clear with nitrates, whereas in the much more typical situation, a patient with anginal chest pain who takes nitrates will precipitate a headache that, in the case of a migraine sufferer, may be overtly migrainous.

Treatment of migraine thus presents special problems in the elderly. Coincidental disease may prohibit the use of some migraine medications. For example, vascular disease in general contraindicates the use of ergotamine, dihydroergotamine, and the triptans; depression militates against the use of beta-blockers and flunarizine; the beta-blockers and calcium channel blockers should not be used in heart failure; and prostatism, glaucoma, and heart disease make the use of tricyclics problematic. Moreover, even when these contraindications do not exist, older patients are more likely than younger ones to develop adverse effects from migraine medications. For example, the elderly are especially prone to have sedation and confusion from tricyclics, and their decreased renal reserve makes them vulnerable to kidney failure with nonsteroidal antiinflammatory drugs (NSAIDs).

Managing the older migraine patient calls for thorough familiarity with that individual's general health status, a wide practical knowledge of pharmacology, and, most important, caution (7).

Tension-Type Headache

The prevalence of tension-type headache appears to decline in the elderly, but not nearly as much as migraine. The various epidemiologic surveys are not strictly comparable, mostly because the diagnostic criteria for tension headaches differed from study to study, particularly with regard to so-called mixed or tension-vascular headaches; but with this caveat, the prevalence of tension-type headache in the healthy elderly ranges from 18.3% (35) to 51.8% (31). Most series did not distinguish between episodic and chronic tension-type headaches, but in those that did, more people had the episodic type. While most of the aged who have tension-type headaches have had them since youth or middle age, they begin for the first time after the age of 50 in about 10% of tension-type headache patients (17); when this occurs, a special search should be made for concomitant and often masked depression (5,13,35).

Even in apparently nondepressed people with tension headaches, tricyclic antidepressants are useful in treatment, although in the elderly there may be increased contraindications to these drugs and more adverse effects from them.

Cluster Headaches

The elderly with cluster headaches nearly always have had them since youth or middle age [the mean age of onset of cluster headache over a number of series is 31.5 years (32)], but they can begin for the first time after the age of 70 (37). Cluster headache is quite uncommon in random population surveys of the healthy elderly (31), but in a study of elderly patients presenting to a major headache clinic (34) it accounted for 4% of that population, suggesting that when it does occur it may be a severe problem.

As with migraine and tension-type headaches, the treatment of cluster headache in the elderly is complicated by the specters of comorbid disease and increased liability to adverse effects. Although probably the most effective treatment for the individual attacks of cluster headache, sumatriptan (and other triptans in a formulation suitable for this purpose) must be used with great caution in the elderly, and only after excluding cardiovascular disease, a process that substantially reduces the number who can take these medications. Oxygen inhalation, although safer, is less effective. All of the prophylactic medications can cause special problems in old people, but of these, verapamil is probably the least dangerous.

Hypnic Headaches

In 1988 Raskin (27) described six patients, all over 65, who for years had awoken from sleep once or twice a night, nightly or almost every night, with bilateral headaches lasting 30 to 60 minutes each, associated in half the patients with nausea, but with no other autonomic symptoms or signs. Clearly these were not cluster headaches. All six were unresponsive to amitriptyline and propranolol; all six responded to lithium carbonate 300 to 600 mg at bedtime. Raskin hypothesized that these evidently benign dysfunctional headaches might be related to perturbation of the biologic clock. Subsequently, Newman et al. (23), Queiroz and Coral (26), Skobieranda et al. (33), Gould and Silberstein (12), and Morales-Asin et al. (21) reported a total of 12 new patients, three of whom had unilateral headaches (12,21). Most recently, Dodick et al. (8) have reported 19 new cases. In their series, although the mean age of onset was 60.5 years, some patients were as young as 40; women outnumbered men; some patients had unilateral headaches; half had had other types of headache (usually migraine) in the past; only one of four patients given lithium obtained relief, but the drug had to be stopped in all four because of adverse effects; only two could successfully abort their attacks (one with sumatriptan 50 mg and a cup of coffee, one with acetylsalicylic acid 400 mg plus caffeine 40 mg); and only four could successfully prevent their headaches (one with caffeine at bedtime, one with acetylsalicylic acid and caffeine at bedtime, one with atenolol 25 mg at bedtime, and one with a tablet of egotamine tartrate 60 mg, phenobarbital 40 mg, and belladonna 0.2 mg at bedtime). Morales-Asin et al. (21) found that two of their three patients responded to flunarizine 5 mg at bedtime.

HEADACHES OCCURRING IN THE ELDERLY AS A SYMPTOM OF UNDERLYING DISEASE

Cerebrovascular Disease

As already noted, *hypertension* of any degree may aggravate migraine, but only severe hypertension (diastolic >120 mm Hg) can produce headache *de novo*. In mild to moderate hypertension, the prevalence of headache is no greater than in normal controls (2), and those headaches that do occur are mostly tension-type or migraine without aura. In severe hypertension, two types of headaches may result. The more common is a dull occipital ache, present on awakening in the morning and clearing within 1 hour or so of getting up and moving about. Rarer is the explosive, extremely intense headache that may result from sudden increases in blood pressure to extreme levels, as may occur in people on monoamine oxidase inhibitors for depression (or migraine) who eat tyramine-rich foods or take sympathomimetic medication for colds (see Chapter 109).

Atherothrombotic cerebrovascular disease, in some as yet undefined fashion, may produce headaches (see Chapter 104). Fully 25% of patients who experience TIAs or completed strokes, either from atherothrombotic carotid or vertebrobasilar disease or from cardiogenic embolism, have headaches with or between these cerebrovascular events. Usually these are brief (up to a few hours), ipsilateral to the ischemic part of the brain, and mild; they have the vascular characteristics of pulsatility and worsening with activity (9). People who had migraine when younger are perhaps more likely to experience them. There is nothing specific about these headaches. As a new-onset headache in the elderly, they may give warning of mischief brewing in the cerebral vasculature.

The majority of people with *hemorrhagic cerebrovascular disease* suffer headaches, but not all do, and especially not those with small intraparenchymal hemorrhages that do not leak into the ventricular system (see Chapter 104).

Temporal (or giant cell) arteritis is almost unheard of in the young but becomes increasingly common with advancing age, so much so that it becomes one of the major considerations to be entertained in any patient who presents with headache onset after the age of 50 years. Its prevalence in people in their fifties is 6.8 per 100,000, increasing to 73 per 100,000 in people in their eighties. At one major headache clinic (34) temporal arteritis was diagnosed in 15% of its patients who were over 65. This progressively obliterative vasculitis is capable of causing not just headache, but catastrophic consequences such as blindness and stroke, and therefore must be considered as a diagnostic possibility in any older person with the new onset of headache. Although biopsy-proven temporal arteritis can occur with a normal erythrocyte sedimentation rate (ESR) (41), this is uncommon enough that the ESR can be used as a reasonably reliable screen; it should be determined in all old people with new headaches (see Chapter 106).

Intracranial Lesions

The incidence of intracranial disease increases with age. This holds true for metastatic tumors, some primary brain tumors, communicating hydrocephalus, and, especially, chronic subdural hematomas. The onset of headaches associated with these conditions may be quite insidious and the headaches themselves quite nonspecific, and, especially with the more slowly evolving lesions, the neurologic examination may be normal. A high index of suspicion is necessary when dealing with recent onset headaches in the elderly, and there should be little hesitation about resorting to imaging procedures. This is not to suggest that mass lesions are a common cause of headaches in old people—in fact they are rare—but they must not be missed.

Diseases of the Neck, Eyes, and Teeth

Cervical spondylosis increases with age, and some authorities claim that it is one of the most common and important causes of headache beginning in and after middle age (25). Others, pointing to the fact that most people over the age of 50 have some radiologic evidence of cervical spondylosis but only a few have symptoms, disagree (10), holding that the majority of headaches occurring in those with cervical spondylosis are tension-type headaches. The fact that the treatments for cervical spondylosis and tension-type headache may be similar (analgesics, NSAIDs, rest, physiotherapy) does nothing to resolve the issue.

Temporomandibular joint disease also is said to produce headaches in the elderly, especially in those in whom loss of teeth has led to misalignment of the jaw. Again, however, there is dispute.

Glaucoma, common in the elderly, is alleged to produce headaches, although it is doubtful that this occurs in the absence of a red eye.

Metabolic Headaches

Many diseases of the aged incorporate metabolic aspects that may cause headaches. For example, chronic obstructive lung disease produces hypercarbia and hypoxia, both of which, through increasing cerebral blood flow, may produce dull diffuse throbbing headaches. Often, because of decreased ventilatory efficiency through the night, these headaches are particularly evident first thing in the morning and tend (like the headaches of hypertension and increased intracranial pressure) to clear as the patient gets up and about. These headaches may be aggravated by the secondary polycythemia sometimes present in chronic respiratory disease. Also, many of the bronchodilators and some of the antibiotics prescribed for these patients may precipitate or aggravate headaches.

Similar dull diffuse headaches may attend anemia of any cause, provided that the anemia is profound enough. Chronic renal failure, sometimes because of the associated anemia but more often for unknown reasons, may be associated with dull headaches; dialysis, of course, may produce headaches, likely through osmotic mechanisms.

Hypercalcemia, usually associated in the elderly with malignancy (often myeloma), may cause headaches, as may hyponatremia.

Parkinson's disease, a neurodegenerative condition believed to be on a metabolic basis, may be associated with headaches. In one series (24) headaches occurred in 41.2% of patients with Parkinson's disease and in only 13.4% of age- and gender-matched controls. In an uncontrolled series (15) 35.2% of parkinsonian patients had headaches. However, in another controlled study (19) there was no difference in headache prevalence between those with and those without Parkinson's disease. In some of these studies it is not clear that headaches caused by antiparkinson medications such as amantadine and levodopa were not confounding the issue, although Indo and Takahashi (16) reported that the headaches of their parkinsonian patients in fact cleared with levodopa treatment. The cause of the Parkinson's headaches (assuming they exist) is not known; Meco et al. (20) attributed them to increased muscle contraction, anxiety, and depression, whereas Indo and Takahashi felt that central nociceptive dysfunction was the cause.

MEDICATION HEADACHES

The illnesses that attend old age sometimes require medication, some of which can cause headaches (1). Table 2 lists some of these. These drug-induced headaches are usually mild to moderate, diffuse, at times throbbing, and of variable duration; in short, they are totally nonspecific. They are also quite common. Many

TABLE 2. *Medications causing headaches in the elderly*

Disease	Medications
Central nervous system	Sedatives (barbiturates, benzodiazepines, alcohol, hypnotics)
	Stimulants (caffeine, methylphenidate)
	Antiparkinson (levodopa, amantadine)
Cardiovascular	Vasodilators (nitroglycerin, isosorbide dinitrate, dipyridamole, nicotinic acid)
	Hypotensives (atenolol, nifedipine, methyldopa, reserpine, enalapril)
	Antiarrhythmics (quinidine, digoxin)
Musculoskeletal	Nonsteroidal antiinflammatory drugs
Gastrointestinal	H$_2$ blockers (ranitidine, cimetidine)
Respiratory	Bronchodilators (theophylline, aminophylline, pseudoephedrine)
Infections	Antibiotics (trimethoprim-sulfamethoxazole, tetracyclines)
Oncologic	Chemotherapeutics (tamoxiphen, cyclophosphamide)
Reproductive	Hormones (estrogens)
	Erectogenic agents (sidenafil)

patients do not regard over-the-counter drugs as "real medications" because they are not prescribed, and will not mention them unless asked. Contrary to common belief, herbal remedies are not always harmless, and some may cause headache (see Chapter 48). Also, many patients do not know that caffeine and alcohol are pharmacologically active and can, in either the toxic or withdrawal mode, cause headaches. When dealing with mysterious headaches in any age group, but especially the elderly, it is often useful to have the patient stop taking any medication that is not absolutely necessary.

The elderly suffer the same analgesic, ergot, and triptan rebound headaches that beset the younger age groups. When withdrawing the elderly from these substances, it is prudent to do so gently because the aging cardiorespiratory system can be quite intolerant of acute withdrawal symptoms.

APPROACH TO THE OLD PERSON WITH NEW HEADACHES

Most old patients with headaches have had them since their youth. It is distinctly unusual for benign dysfunctional headaches such as migraine, tension-type headaches, and cluster headaches to begin de novo after the age of 60. Therefore, old people with new headaches are likelier than younger patients to have a structural or metabolic lesion causing their headaches. They are also much more likely than younger patients to harbor "coincidental" diseases that can confound diagnosis and therapy of their headaches. Accordingly, older headache patients require special care, which includes readier than usual recourse to investigations, special awareness of the patient's general medical condition, and extra caution with medications.

REFERENCES

1. Askmark H, Lundberg PO, Olsson S. Drug related headache. *Headache* 1989;29:441–444.
2. Badran RH, Weir RJ, McGuiness JB. Hypertension and headache. *Scott Med J* 1970;15:48–51.
3. Bengtsson BA. Incidence of giant cell arteritis. *Acta Med Scand* 1982;58[Suppl 6]:15–17.
4. Bowen J, Oppenheim G. Headache as a presentation of angina: reproduction of symptoms during angioplasty. *Headache* 1993;33:238–239.
5. Chung MK, Kraybill DE. Headache: a marker of depression. *J Fam Pract* 1990;31:360–364.
6. Cook NR, Evans DA, Funkenstein H, et al. Correlates of headache in a population-based cohort of elderly. *Arch Neurol* 1989;46:1338–1346.
7. Cyprus BK. Patients' reasons for visiting physicians. National ambulatory medical care survey. US 1977–8. Vital and Health Statistics Series 13, No. 56. DHSS Publication No 82-1717. Washington: US Government Printing Office, 1981.
8. Dodick DW, Mosek AC, Campbell JK. The hypnic ("alarm clock") headache syndrome. *Cephalalgia* 1998;18:152–156.
9. Edmeads J. The headaches of ischemic cerebrovascular disease. *Headache* 1979;19:345–349.
10. Elias F. Roentgen findings in the asymptomatic cervical spine. *NY State J Med* 1958;58:300–303.
11. Fisher CM. Late-life migraine accompaniments as a cause of unexplained transient ischemic attacks. *Can J Neurol Sci* 1980;7:9–18.
12. Gould JD, Silberstein SD. Unilateral hypnic headache: a case study [Abstract]. *Cephalalgia* 1997;17:310.
13. Hale WE, May FE, Marks RG, Moore MT, Stewart RB. Headache in the elderly: an evaluation of risk factors. *Headache* 1987;27:272–276.
14. Hale WE, Perkins LL, May FE, Marks RG, Stewart RB. Symptom prevalence in the elderly. *J Am Geriatr Soc* 1986;34:333–340.
15. Indo T, Naito A, Sobue I. Characteristics of headache in Parkinson's disease. *Headache* 1983;23:211–212.
16. Indo T, Takahashi A. Early morning headache in Parkinson's disease: a hitherto unrecognized symptom? *Headache* 1987;27:151–154.
17. Lance JW, Curran DA, Anthony M. Investigations into the mechanism and treatment of chronic headache. *Med J Aust* 1965;2:909–912.
18. Lipton RB, Pfeffer D, Newman L, Solomon S. Headaches in the elderly. *J Pain Sympt Mgmt* 1993;8:87–97.
19. Lorentz IT. A survey of headache in Parkinson's disease. *Cephalalgia* 1989;9:83–86.
20. Meco G, Frascarelli M, Pratesi L, Linfante I, Rocchi L, Formisano R. Headache in Parkinson's disease. *Headache* 1988;28:26–29.
21. Morales-Asin F, Mauri JA, Iniguez C, Espada F, Mostacero E. The hypnic headache syndrome: a report of three new cases. *Cephalalgia* 1998; 18:157–158.
22. Newland CA, Illes LS, Robinson PK, Batchelor BG, Waters WE. A survey of headache in an English city. *Res Clin Stud Headache* 1978;5: 1–20.
23. Newman LC, Lipton RB, Solomon S. The hypnic headache syndrome: a benign headache disorder of the elderly. *Neurology* 1990;40: 1904–1905.
24. Nishikawa S, Harada H, Takahashi K, Shimomura T. Clinical study on headache in patients with Parkinson's disease. *Clin Neurol Neurosurg* 1982;22:403–408.
25. Poser CM. The types of headache that affect the elderly. *Geriatrics* 1976;31:103–106.
26. Queiroz LP, Coral LC. The hypnic headache syndrome—a case report [Abstract]. *Cephalalgia* 1997;17:303.
27. Raskin NH. The hypnic headache syndrome. *Headache* 1988;28: 534–536.
28. Romberg M. *A manual of the nervous diseases of man,* Vol. 1 [translated by Sieveking EH]. London: The Sydenham Society, 1853:177.
29. Royal College of Practitioners, Office of Population Consensus and Surveys, and Department of Health and Social Security. Morbidity statistics from general practice: second national study 1970–71. Studies on medical and population subjects, No. 26. London: HMSO, 1974.
30. Selby G, Lance JW. Observations on 500 cases of migraine and allied vascular headache. *J Neurol Neurosurg Psychiatry* 1960;23:23–32.
31. Serratrice G, Serbanesco F, Sanbuc R. Epidemiology of headache in elderly. Correlations with life conditions and socio-professional environment. *Headache* 1985;25:85–89.
32. Sjaastad O. Cluster headache. In: Vinken PJ, Bruyn GW, Klawans H, Rose FC, eds. *Handbook of clinical neurology,* Vol. 4, No. 48. Headache. Amsterdam: Elsevier, 1986:217–246.
33. Skobieranda PG, Lee TG, Solomon GD. The hypnic headache syndrome: six additional patients [Abstract]. *Cephalalgia* 1997;17:304.
34. Solomon GD, Kunkel RS, Frame J. Demographics of headaches in elderly patients. *Headache* 1990;30:273–276.
35. Srikiathachorn A. Epidemiology of headache in the Thai elderly: a study in the Bangkae Home for the Aged. *Headache* 1991;31:677–681.
36. Stewart WF, Lipton RB, Celentano D, Reed ML. Prevalence of migraine headache in the United States. *JAMA* 1992;267:64–69.
37. Sutherland JM, Eadie MJ. Cluster headache. *Res Clin Stud Headache* 1972;3:92–125.
38. Walker CH. Migraine and its relationship to hypertension. *BMJ* 1959;2: 1430–1433.
39. Waters WE. The Pontypridd headache survey. *Headache* 1974;14: 81–90.
40. Wilkinson M. Clinical features of migraine. In: Vinken PJ, Bruyn GW, Klawans H, Rose FC, eds. *Handbook of clinical neurology,* Vol. 4. No. 48. Headache. Amsterdam: Elsevier, 1986:117–133.
41. Wong RL, Korn JH. Temporal arteritis without an elevated erythrocyte sedimentation rate. Case report and review of the literature. *Am J Med* 1986;80:959–964.

The Headaches, Second Edition,
edited by J. Olesen, P. Tfelt-Hansen, and K.M.A. Welch.
Lippincott Williams & Wilkins, Philadelphia © 2000.

Special Problems in the Headaches and Their Management

CHAPTER 126

Headache in the Abuse-Prone Individual

Joel R. Saper and Fred D. Sheftell

The patient with severe, recurring headache is often poorly understood and inadequately treated. And because pain is a compelling and motivating symptom, one that cannot be ignored when severe, it powerfully incites a variety of behaviors in search of relief. Restraint in the use of medicines is often lacking.

Compounding the tendency to overuse treatment to control pain is that when medications—from acetaminophen to the triptans to the opioids—are used excessively, they can promote increasingly frequent headaches, as well as toxic, untoward effects. Moreover, patients with exclusive responsiveness to one or only a few agents, perhaps understandably, persist in their demands to obtain that medication.

This chapter considers the approach to headache patients who have traditionally been called abuse prone. A wide spectrum of dynamics and circumstances confound simple characterization of the patient or his or her treatment. The underlying therapeutic principles include:

- Severe pain requires effective treatment
- All medications can be abused when used excessively
- Pain when severe enough will prompt excessive drug-taking behaviors
- "Abuse" may reflect iatrogenic dynamics related to the inadequacy of care and thus can be adaptive, prompted primarily by the need to cope and carry on

J. R. Saper: Michigan Head Pain and Neurological Institute, Ann Arbor, Michigan 48104-5199.

F. D. Sheftell: Department of Psychiatry, New York Medical College, Valhalla, New York 10595, and New England Center for Headache, Stamford, Connecticut 06902.

PREVALENCE

It is difficult to delineate the prevalence of overuse, misuse, or abuse in the headache population. In general, 6% to 15% of the U.S. population has a substance use disorder of some type, and nearly one third of the U.S. population has used illicit drugs (7,18). The incidence of medication overuse in patients with pain would be expected to be much higher. Sixty-five percent of patients hospitalized for pain rehabilitation were misusing drugs (15) and 89.7% of patients on an inpatient substance abuse treatment unit had headaches (4). In patients with known medication dependence, as many as 75% complain of headache (27). Saper (22) noted that over 50% of patients attending a tertiary center for headache used medications excessively, and Mathew (16) confirmed that 66% to 87% of patients with chronic headache overused medications. Many such patients require inpatient-level care (13,26) and fulfill current IHS codes and diagnoses reflecting headaches related to medication usage or withdrawal from substances (8).

Unfortunately, patients who have pain and have been diagnosed (accurately or not) with a drug-taking problem are often denied the very treatment necessary to allow them to escape from the self-defeating behavior. The challenge is thus to identify the presence and the origin of the problem and institute effective pain control and other measures that address the overuse phenomena.

DRUGS OF SPECIAL CONCERN

Any medication used excessively may prove troublesome. However, some are more likely than others to be overused by patients with headache and pain. Mixed analgesics and ergotamine tartrate medications have been

TABLE 1. *Drugs frequently overused/misused by headache patients*

Primary analgesics	Benzodiazepines	Mixed analgesics	Special headache medications
Propoxyphene	Diazepam	Vicodin	Ergotamine tartrate
Codeine	Chlordiazepoxide	Vicodin ES	"Triptans"
Oxycodone	Lorazepam	Fiorinal	
Hydrocodone	Alprazolam	Fiorinal no. 3	
Morphine	Clonazepam	Esgic	
Meperidine	Flurazepam	Esgic Plus	
Hydromorphone	Temazepam		
Oxymorphone	Triazolam		
Methadone			
Fentanyl			
Pentazocine			
Butorphanol			
Tramadol			

Modified from Swanson (27).

cited most often as troublesome for headache patients (2,21,24,26). Table 1 lists common medications that are often overused by patients with headache (27).

Benzodiazepines and Barbiturate-Containing Analgesics

The benzodiazepines, like the barbiturates, have clear reinforcing qualities because they are rapidly absorbed into the brain (27). Drugs with a shorter half-life, such as alprazolam, are more likely to lead to withdrawal symptoms. Physical dependence is a risk in all patients, but particularly those who have frequent headaches, obsessive drug-taking tendencies, or a history of substance overusage.

Excessive use of barbiturate-containing mixed analgesics (Fiorinal [Novartis], Esgic) has long been recognized as problematic in a headache patient. That they are effective in controlling the pain of patients with headache is not disputed. Appropriate and quantitative prescribing, along with vigilant monitoring, are at the heart of safe administration.

Meperidine

Generally opioids can be avoided in the treatment of acute headache. They are relatively short acting and often contribute to nausea. Numerous parenteral alternatives exist (25). Nonetheless, a large number of individuals with acute migraine seek meperidine administration. Many patients are persistent in their pursuit of this drug and insist that this drug and this drug alone is required to relieve their acute headache. The mere request, rightly or wrongly, prompts emergency department staff to consider possible abusive patterns.

Unanswered is whether a person who is not rebounding may nonetheless be exclusively responsive to this drug and none others. Unlike other opioids, meperidine has an active metabolite, normeperidine, that has central stimulant actions. This may explain its "added value" for migraine. Normeperidine, unlike its parent product, has a prolonged half-life of 15 to 40 hours and accumulates in the central nervous system (1).

Because the analgesic effect is relatively short lived, repeated dosages of the analgesic are often requested and administered. Because the stimulant metabolite has a longer half-life than that of the parent product, repetitive administration of meperidine leads to accumulation of normeperidine, particularly in the presence of renal impairment (28). Accumulation of normeperidine causes central nervous system (CNS) toxicity (seizures, myoclonus, excitability, etc.) (12). Initially, meperidine's depressant activity masks the excitatory effects of normeperidine. When administration ceases, the suppressing parent drug dissipates first, leaving the longer half-lived stimulant by-product (normeperidine) unopposed. Naloxone is not effective in treating meperidine toxicity and may even exacerbate normeperidine's untoward effects (5).

Butorphanol Nasal Spray

The overuse of butorphanol nasal spray has gained national attention in the United States. Butorphanol is a synthetic agonist/antagonist opioid analgesic that exerts its effect on mu, kappa, and sigma opioid receptors. Its analgesic effect appears to be exerted primarily through the agonist action of the kappa receptor and mixed agonist/antagonist activities of the mu receptor. Because it is antagonistic at the mu receptor, butorphanol is reported to have less respiratory depression, euphoria, or potential for physical dependence than that occurring with pure opioid analgesics. However, increasing numbers of patients have presented to tertiary centers with frank physical (and emotional) dependency on butorphanol (personal observations). Usage patterns exceeding a bottle or more of butorphanol a day are not uncommon. Patients describe increasing headaches and drug use (rebound), euphoria (or perhaps dysphoria), and an irresistible desire for more medication. Many of the patients encountered by us had problems of overuse or misuse with other products and were given the butorphanol by physicians who mistakenly believed that the drug did not produce dependency. The U.S. Food and Drug Administration (FDA) has just recently categorized butorphanol as a schedule IV analgesic.

Withdrawal from butorphanol has proven difficult and at times dramatic. Escalation of drug-seeking behaviors, aggravation of preexisting personality disorders, hallucinations, and other frank abstinence symptomatology can occur. Many of the patients required extended hospitalizations to treat the rebound period. At least one patient described to the one of the authors (J.R.S.) a "Stadol hunger" for months after complete detoxification.

Recent work suggests that withdrawal from butorphanol results in focal increases in extracellular levels of glutamate within the locus ceruleus and may act through the N-methyl-D-aspartate glutamate receptor (11). If valid, this implies a novel aspect to the neuropharmacology of opioid dependence as it applies to the role of kappa opioid receptors.

Tramadol

Tramadol is an oral analgesic and currently not scheduled by the FDA. It is partially mediated via the mu opioid receptor system and exerts an antidepressant effect through inhibition of a reuptake mechanism for norepinephrine and serotonin. Reports suggest a significant opioid-type dependency (6). A manufacturer's "Dear Doctor" letter in March 1996 warned of the possibility of drug abuse, seizures, and anaphylactic-type reactions with tramadol.

Propoxyphene

Like meperidine, propoxyphene also has an active metabolite, norpropoxyphene, that has a half-life of 30 to 36 hours. This is much longer than its parent product. Like normeperidine, norpropoxyphene accumulates and can cause CNS toxicity. Both meperidine and propoxyphene metabolites increase in patients with disease of the liver or kidneys (17).

EVALUATING THE PATIENT FOR OVERUSE OR MISUSE

Assessment for excessive usage is necessary, as part of the general examination for headache, particularly when frequent. The examiner should be nonbiased and nonjudgmental, extending to the patient the sense that questions are relevant to the problem of diagnosis and treatment, and not inquisitional. Among the key variables are:

- All medications and other substances used, including caffeine, nicotine, alcohol, vitamins, recreational drugs, herbs, supplements, etc.
- Pattern and frequency of use by the day and by the week
- Dosage and duration of usage of each of the medications and substances
- Past history of physical dependency, toxicity, withdrawal, adverse sequelae, or substance abuse treatment
- The sources of each of the medications (when relevant, the names of the physicians and pharmacists)

In cases where suspicion is warranted, the following must also be assessed:

- Attitude toward medication usage (too casual, argumentative, defensive, assignment of blame, reluctance to discuss, etc.)
- School or work absences or impairment due to medication usage
- The presence of axis I (primary psychiatric illness) and axis II (characterologic) disturbances

The patient's attitude toward medication is important. Is it minimized, rationalized, denied, or discussed defensively? Is blame for overusage assigned to others or rationalized inappropriately?

Obtaining collateral information is critical. This should begin by gaining the patient's permission to communicate with family members, physicians, and pharmacists involved in the care. Refusal to allow this communication or failure to identify all relevant parties represents important warning signs.

Table 2 identifies the warning behaviors (red flags) that may indicate potential problems.

TABLE 2. *Specific warning behaviors of substance misuse and abuse*

Unauthorized dose escalations
Frequent phone calls, particularly after hours or on weekends, for more medication
"Doctor shopping" or obtaining medications from other physicians, including emergency departments (even if new "justification" occurs)
Losing or reporting prescription as stolen, ruined, melted, washed down the drain, etc.
More frequent (often premature) visits than anticipated (usually for more medication)
Resistance or unwillingness to accept efforts to reduce treatment or to use alternate medications
Assignment of blame to others for overuse
Threatening suicide with medications
Refusal to allow gathering of collateral information from family, physicians, and others
Usage for reasons other than pain control (sedation, control anxiety, etc.)

WHO IS REALLY AT RISK?

Saper (22), based on a series of patients with daily chronic headache, suggested that those most vulnerable to overuse appeared to belong to families with a history of alcoholism, other substance abuse, or depression. A positive dexamethasone suppression test was also noted to be higher in that group (ergot-dependent) than in controls. Patients with borderline personalities may be more prone to headache than initially believed. Hegarty (9) noted that 60% of patients diagnosed with borderline personality disorder suffered from severe headache. Medication overuse, suicidal gestures, and other dynamics are characteristic of this and other personality disorders.

The presence of comorbidity appears to markedly increase the risk for misuse/abuse (perhaps to control anxiety, depression, etc.), as does a previous history of polysubstance abuse (4). Mathew (16) has noted that relapse following detoxification is most likely in patients whose behavioral, psychological, and neuroendocrine features are different than those who showed improvement. Alcoholism and physical, emotional, and sexual abuse were distinctively higher in those with relapse than in those without.

Is it prudent to administer drugs of high abuse potential to a patient with a previous history of "substance abuse"? Would a patient with a previous history of substance abuse be given drugs of risk for severe headache? The answers are uncertain. However, from the general pain literature, it appears that successful long-term opioid therapy can be given to patients even if a history of abuse or addiction is present (3,14,18). Dunbar (3), in a retrospective review of 20 patients with nonmalignant pain and a prior history of substance abuse who had been treated with opioid therapy in a pain clinic setting, found that those who did well had a well-functioning family or outside support system, including a substance abuse support group. Patients who had a history of only alcohol abuse generally did well. Those with a history of polysubstance abuse did not.

Portenoy and Foley (19) evaluated patients who used chronic opioids for pain of nonmalignant origin for up to 7 years. They reported only occasional examples of inappropriate dose escalation. Saper and associates (23) reported their interim findings from a 5-year study of patients using scheduled, daily opioids for proven intractable headache. Rigorous criteria for entry into the tightly controlled, structured program were established. Thus far the researchers have noted little in the way of "abusive" behavior. Interestingly, by 2 years into the program, approximately half of those who entered were no longer taking opioids, and only 25% to 30% of those who were originally entered noted substantial benefit.

MANAGEMENT RECOMMENDATIONS

Despite previous history of misuse or vulnerability to it, patients with severe headaches require effective treatment. Effective treatment in and of itself may help control overuse and misuse behaviors. The recommendations and guidelines that follow are based on the experience of the authors, both of whom practice in tertiary headache centers. Although some of the recommendations imply or encourage the use of a team of professionals, many are easily managed by a one-on-one physician/patient relationship.

Guidelines for Treatment of Patients at Risk for Misuse

The following guidelines are offered to assist in the management of patients who are at risk for overuse or misuse but also apply to the use of medications in any patient with frequent pain. In general, the intensity of medical supervision must be consistent with the treatment needs and usage patterns of patients and the type of medication prescribed. The patient must have sufficient supplies of medication to cover the treatment interval, but excessive amounts must be avoided. During visits, patients should have medication usage quantified. Timing of visits must be coordinated with the type of medication used, frequency of prescribed usage, and frequency of attacks. As mentioned, it is desirable but not always possible to treat high-risk patients within the perspective of an interdisciplinary, therapeutic team. Capable and diligent physicians who spend adequate time with their high-risk patients can often achieve the same or even better results, but not always. The presence of comorbidity (20), past history of substance abuse, or the presence of one or more warning signs for misuse (see Table 2) must not be ignored.

Limit-Setting and Principles of Care

A delineation of boundaries and guidelines for usage are required. Reasonably strict limitations on frequency of use must be established for all patients taking medications for symptomatic control of frequent headaches, but are particularly important for patients at high risk. The following guidelines are recommended:

1. Properly match patient clinical profile and diagnosis with medication choice.
2. Establish clear and appropriate guidelines for administration.
   a. For abortive medications that can cause rebound or dependency, usage no more than two or three times a week must be agreed to.
   b. Prescription quantities and use directives must be coordinated with and reconciled to frequency of

anticipated usage and limitations that have been established.

3. The frequency of visits must be consistent with the severity of the headache, its frequency, and the amount of medications allowed and used. (The use of a patient-maintained headache calendar, which also contains guidelines for medication use, is an aid in monitoring and controlling usage patterns.)

4. Refilling prescriptions between visits, at night, or on holidays should be limited or avoided altogether.

5. If medications are not effective or if need is greater than the limits established for usage, then a restructuring of treatment must take place.

6. Alternate means of pain control must be established, including self-help interventions and pain rescue techniques.

7. One physician (or team) and pharmacy. Patients with the potential for excessive use must be prescribed medications from one physician (or team) and one pharmacy. This must be clear to the patient at the outset, and violation must be effectively confronted.

Use of a Multidisciplinary Team

If used, a treatment team assists in assessment, monitoring, and administering treatment. Team members play a critical role in evaluation and treatment of comorbid, substance overuse, and behavioral disturbances that increase noncompliance and the risk of overuse, misuse, or abuse. A physician practicing alone can at times be overwhelmed by the demands of monitoring, requests for treatment, and educational responsibilities for patients with severe pain and at high risk. Treatment intensity must be increased when comorbidity is present. In addition to regular physician visits, at which time medical assessment occurs, other team members must be consulted and evaluate the patient regularly. They must obtain collateral information from family members and others, as well as provide additional perspective as to compliance and functional stability of the patient.

Education

The patient must be thoroughly educated regarding the implications of symptomatic medication usage and overuse and the consequences that are likely if it occurs. Acts of noncompliance must be considered serious infringements upon the patient-doctor relationship. Patients must be given the means to endure pain without resorting to excessive medication use, and this requires both educational as well as therapeutic and behavioral interventions.

Emergency Department Use

From time to time emergency department needs arise. Patients must be instructed to request of the emergency staff that they call the attending physician prior to administration of medication. Sufficient options exist to allow the general avoidance of drugs of special abuse potential (if possible), such as meperidine and others. Neuroleptic medications, dihydroergotamine, sumatriptan, and ketorolac are alternate agents that are often effective in the control of headache in the emergency department setting (25).

Monitoring and Surveillance

Periodic evaluation of urine for drugs other than those prescribed is an optional tool for monitoring. Periodic communications to other treating physicians or collateral information gathered from spouse, friend, or family members aid in the oversight task.

PROGNOSIS

The primary headache disorders and substance-related disorders are chronic conditions. They are frequently characterized by periods of improvement and exacerbations. Review of available outcome studies on the treatment of patients with daily chronic headache and overuse syndromes (2,10,13,16,26) demonstrate that at least 25% to 50% of patients may relapse, even with appropriate treatment and monitoring. Appropriate and effective treatment, strategic prescribing practices, careful monitoring, vigilance, and interdisciplinary services may enhance outcome. Hospitalization programs (2,10,13, 16,26) as well as formal substance abuse treatment programs, including at times 12-step programs, and the use of nonmedical treatment such as physical therapy, biofeedback, and others, may all enhance pain control and limit the likelihood of excessive use.

REFERENCES

1. Armstrong PJ, Bersten A. Normeperidine toxicity. *Anesth Analg* 1986; 65:536–538.
2. Diener HC, Dichgans J, Scholz E, et al. Analgesic-induced chronic headache. Long-term results of withdrawal therapy. *J Neurol* 1989; 236:9–14.
3. Dunbar SA, Katz NP. Chronic opioid therapy for non-malignant pain in patients with a history of substance abuse: report of 20 cases. *J Pain Symptom Mgmt* 1996;11:163–171.
4. el Mallakh RS, Kranzler HR, Kamanitz JR. Headaches and psychoactive substance use. *Headache* 1991;31:584–587.
5. Gilbert PE, Martin WR. Antagonism of the convulsant effects of heroine, d-propoxyphene, meperidine, normeperidine, and thebaine by naloxone in mice. *J Pharmacol Exp Ther* 1975;192:538–541.
6. Goeringer KE, Logan PK, Christian GD. Identification of tramadol and its metabolites in blood from drug-related deaths and drug-impaired drivers. *J Anal Toxicol* 1997;21:529–537.
7. Groerer J, Brodsky M. The incidence of illicit drug use in the United States 1962–1989. *Br J Addiction* 1992;87:1345–1351.

8. Headache Classification Committee of the International Headache Society. Classification and diagnostic criteria for headache disorders, cranial neuralgias, and facial pain. *Cephalalgia* 1988;8[Suppl 7]:1.

9. Hegarty AM. The prevalence of migraine in borderline personality disorder [Abstract]. *Headache* 1993;33:291.

10. Henry P, Dartigues JF, Benetier MP, et al. Ergotamine- and analgesic-induced headache. In: Rose FC, ed. *Migraine: Clinical and research advances.* Karger: Basel, 1985;186–196.

11. Hoshi K, Ma T, Oh S, Ho IK. Increased release of excitatory amino acids in rat locus ceruleus in kappa-opioid antagonist-dependent rats precipitated by nor-binaltorphimine. *Brain Res* 1997;753:63–68.

12. Kaiko RF, Foley KM, Grabinski PY, et al. Central nervous system excitatory effects of meperidine in cancer patients. *Ann Neurol* 1983;13:180–185.

13. Lake AL, Saper JR, Madden SF, Kreeger C. Comprehensive inpatient treatment for intractable migraine: a prospective long-term outcome study. *Headache* 1993;33:55–62.

14. Macaluso D, Weinberg D, Foley KM. Opioid abuse and misuse in a cancer pain population. *J Pain Symptom Mgmt* 1988;3[Suppl]:24.

15. Maruta T, Swanson DW, Finlayson RE. Drug abuse and dependency in patients with chronic pain. *Mayo Clin Proc* 1979;54:241–244.

16. Mathew NT, Reuveni U, Perez F. Transformed or evolutive migraine. *Headache* 1987;27:102–106.

17. Pappagallo M. Ethical issues on the management of chronic non-malignant pain. *Semin Neurol* 1997;17:203–211.

18. Passik SD, Portenoy RK. Substance abuse issues in palliative care. In: Berger A, Portenoy R, Weissman D, eds. *Principles and practice of supportive oncology.* Philadelphia: JB Lippincott, 1998:513–530.

19. Portenoy RK, Foley KM. Chronic use of opioid analgesics in nonmalignant pain. Report of 38 cases. *Pain* 1986;25:171–186.

20. Rapoport AM, Sheftell FD. Psychiatric aspects of primary headache disorders. In: *Headache disorders: a management guide for practitioners.* Philadelphia: WB Saunders, 1996.

21. Rapoport AM, Weeks RE, Sheftell FD. Analgesic rebound headache: theoretical and practical implications. *Cephalalgia* 1985;5[Suppl 3]:448–450.

22. Saper JR. Headache disorders: current concepts and treatment strategies. Littleton, MA: Wright-PSG Publishers, 1983.

23. Saper JR, Jones JM. Ergotamine tartrate dependency: features and possible mechanisms. *Clin J Neuropharmacol* 1986;9:244–256.

24. Saper JR, Lake AE III, Madden SF, Kreeger C. Tertiary care for headache: a 6-month prospective outcome [Abstract]. *Headache* 1998;38:402.

25. Saper JR, Silberstein SD, Gordon CD, Hamel RL. Handbook of headache management. Baltimore: Williams & Wilkins, 1998.

26. Schnider P, Aull S, Baumgartner C, et al. Long-term outcome of patients with headache and drug abuse after inpatient withdrawal: 5-year follow-up. *Cephalalgia* 1996;16:481–485.

27. Swanson DW. Medication abuse. In: Olesen J, Tfelt-Hansen P, Welch KMA, eds. *The headaches.* New York: Raven, 1993:815–819.

28. Szeto HH, Inturrisi CE, Houde R, et al. Accumulation of normeperidine, an active metabolite of meperidine, in patients with renal failure or cancer. *Ann Intern Med* 1977;86:738–741.

The Headaches, Second Edition,
edited by J. Olesen, P. Tfelt-Hansen, and K.M.A. Welch.
Lippincott Williams & Wilkins, Philadelphia © 2000.

Special Problems in the Headaches and Their Management

CHAPTER 127

Headache in the Psychiatrically Ill

Harold Merskey and Richard C. Peatfield

The medical literature has long reflected the belief among many researchers that pain could be attributable to the state of the mind. This belief gained more supporters in the 1920s and thereafter, but probably reached a peak by about 1970, after which greater emphasis was placed on the role of physical illness in causing chronic pain (17). Since then, the emotional changes seen in patients with chronic pain have been discussed in terms of their relationship to the disruptive effects of headache. These effects include persistent suffering, the difficulty of working in the face of pain, loss of employment, loss of income, and loss of status. This is not to say that psychological factors are no longer important etiologically, or in exacerbating pain. Every comprehensive clinic emphasizes the importance of looking at concomitant psychological events such as marital changes and independent stress. However, the emphasis is shifting toward recognizing the primacy of physical illness, so that it is no longer acceptable to diagnose a psychological cause of pain only because a sound physical cause cannot be found.

The incidence of depressive illness in the general population is 6% to 8%; among people with chronic pain in the general population this rate increases to 14% to 15% (15); and in clinic studies this rate increases further, to 30% to 70% depending on the study, but may be even higher (22) because of the tendency for patients with more severe illnesses to be referred to specialist centers. It is generally supposed that some painful illnesses are produced by depression and some cause depression, but the extent to which each of these factors contributes is still an open topic. Recent evidence for other types of pain (3,14) suggests that with physical conditions, even states as broadly defined as low-back pain or irritable bowel syndrome, the effect of an existing physical illness is the more prominent factor.

More than half of psychiatric patients tend to complain of pain spontaneously (10,19), and when those who mention pain on being asked about it are included as well, this proportion generally increases to two thirds. This is almost as high as the proportions reported by medical clinics (19). Typically, headache has been the most common cause of pain in psychiatric patients (16) and general practice (4). Among patients with acute pain, headache was also more common than low-back pain in the general population, although low-back pain was slightly more common among those with chronic complaints (9).

This chapter addresses the important minority of patients in whom psychological causes appear to be the principal factors in the origin or maintenance of chronic pain.

PSYCHIATRIC CATEGORIES

We can relate headache to psychological mechanisms (e.g., stress at work causing muscle contraction) or to psychiatric categories (e.g., anxiety state, depressive illness, etc.). Both forms of explanation are necessary for a complete understanding of all cases, although they vary in importance from individual to individual. The diagnostic categories used currently in psychiatry have a number of subdivisions, but only four broad groupings are important in discussing headache in psychiatric illness. These are anxiety disorders, depressive disorder, hysterical and hypochondriacal conditions, and schizophrenia. The tenth revision of the International Classification of Diseases (ICD-10) (11) describes as dissociative (conversion) most conditions formerly called hysterical, except for those

H. Merskey: Department of Psychiatry, University of Western Ontario, and Department of Psychiatry, London Health Sciences Centre, London, Ontario N6A 5A5, Canada.

R. C. Peatfield: Charing Cross Hospital, London W6 8RF, United Kingdom.

associated with pain, which are now grouped under the term "somatoform disorders," as is hypochondriasis. The most relevant diagnosis in the somatoform group, besides hypochondriasis, is persistent somatoform pain disorder. This is modeled on an earlier formulation used by the American Psychiatric Association (APA). The categories used by the ICD-10 are largely similar to those of the *Diagnostic and Statistical Manual of Mental Disorders*, 4th edition (DSM-IV) of the APA. The latter volume uses a set of standard criteria for diagnosis that is not a feature of ICD-10. However, by design, the two systems and their descriptions largely correspond with each other, and ICD-10 also has been adapted to incorporate categories for migraine and tension-type headache that resemble those of classification by the International Headache Society.

The ICD-10 category of persistent somatoform pain disorder is reserved for persistent pain with the following features: it is severe and distressing, it lacks a physical or physiologic explanation, it is not due to conditions of anxiety or depression, and there is sufficient associated evidence of emotional conflict or psychosocial problems to lead to the conclusion that these problems are the main causative influence. These criteria impose fairly stringent limitations on efforts to account for headache, among other pains, on the grounds of psychological conflict and motivation, the traditional basis for a diagnosis of hysteria. The DSM-IV system (9) is similar but no longer uses the word "somatoform" in the title of the category for pain, which is now only described as "pain disorder," although it is listed under the general section of somatoform conditions and allows for two types of cases: those in which psychological conflict alone is the principal factor and those in which both physical conditions and psychological influences contribute to the etiology.

In this chapter we review the treatment of headache falling into aforementioned categories. We do not discuss the relationship between psychiatric illness and some headache syndromes with psychiatric aspects, for example, tension-type headache, migraine, and the group of headaches related to cluster headache.

PRIMARY PSYCHIATRIC ILLNESSES

Anxiety Disorders

Anxiety is the most common psychiatric disorder. A substantial proportion of the population have occasional isolated phobias such as fear of heights, snakes, mice, or spiders. More troublesome problems arise with such fears as claustrophobia or agoraphobia, even when these too are isolated. Women are more prone to these symptoms. When anxiety occurs not only as a phobia but also in a more generalized fashion with diffuse uneasiness or tension, pains usually are reported among the symptoms. These include chest pain and gastrointestinal discomfort. Most of all, headache appears in individuals who suffer

from sustained anxiety. When anxiety is acute or chronic, the pain of headache often seems to have the features of a tension-type headache and is eased by relaxation, sedatives, and supportive or interpretive psychotherapy. It is not clear, however, that these types of headache are attributable to the obvious mechanisms of tension-type headache. Alternative types of muscle dysfunction such as myofascial tender points and bands may be relevant, together with the spread of pain to adjoining areas. Whatever the mechanism, even chronic headache associated with anxiety may respond to the usual treatments for anxiety but does not tend to respond to analgesic measures.

In individuals who have headache with anxiety, the therapeutic approach is the same as for anxiety in general and for most of the nonpsychotic psychiatric illnesses. Management begins with history taking. A full psychiatric history is necessary—at least in more protracted cases—in order to build a knowledge base of the background of the individual, the liability to anxiety symptoms, and the existence of current events that may be relevant. Therefore, in taking the history the psychiatrist will ordinarily look for evidence of a family history of psychological illness that might have contributed either by hereditary or by engendering difficult conditions for the patients in childhood; the childhood history also may be important because of events such as bereavement or other misfortune. The quality of care given in childhood is liable to be relevant in understanding the patient's personality and his or her responses to whatever current stresses may be identified. The temperament that was evident in childhood also helps to determine what is expected of the adult. Individuals who were anxious from childhood are likely to be more anxious in adult life. If someone presents with anxiety without such a background there should either be a very prominent stressful cause or an alternative diagnosis of which anxiety is a part. Anxiety is often part of other diagnoses, particularly severe depressive illnesses and schizophrenia, which override attention to it. This aspect will be discussed further below. It is also important to make sure that the illness is not a complication of a physical state such as the rare phenomenon of panic attacks due to pheochromocytoma, or the occasional pituitary tumor, or, perhaps most often among organic causes, occult thyrotoxicosis.

Some current specific causes, such as bereavement, loss of a job, or the loss of a relationship, cannot be altered. These usually tend to produce both anxiety and depression. They can be remedied to some extent by encouraging feelings that help the patient adapt to the situation: that the deceased parent was truly loved and suitably appreciated; that there are still constructive tasks to undertake in life; and that alternative jobs can be found, as well as an alternative friend of the opposite (or same) sex. Other problems giving rise to continuing anxiety and headache therefrom may still be current and hang over the head of the individual like the sword of Damocles, including the critical illness of a relative; threat of discipline for inadequate performance at work, or simply the threat of loss of employment because of redundancies; or the outcome of a lawsuit. Here also it is necessary to try to help the individual to adapt to the situation. Occasionally a continuing problem at work or in the home can be resolved by the patient's getting out of the intractable situation. Many physicians have seen patients whose symptoms appeared to persist endlessly until they reached retirement age and gave up a job that really did not suit them, and then reappeared much better in the doctor's office. Sometimes it can be helpful to the individual, in making up his or her mind on what to do, to point to the relationship between the symptom and the stress. Physicians are wise to avoid telling patients what decisions to make for themselves. This particularly applies to the rupture or maintenance of a marital relationship or the relinquishing of a job. However, most patients will recognize the trend of thought even if specific instruction is not given on how to act.

Besides specific measures, general measures are often useful. One of the first is simply reassurance and validation of the patient's complaints. Reassurance involves indicating, after appropriate physical and psychological examination, that the symptoms have no important physical basis and that the pain seems to be a consequence of anxiety, producing headache. This, in turn, enables the patient to see the pain in a different light and to regard it with less fear. Once there is less fear there is likely to be less pain. The teaching of relaxation exercises and cognitive methods of distancing oneself from headache also can be helpful for patients with chronic headache. Relaxation and active coping with alternative concerns seem to be the best ways to diminish headache of any type when it is not due to a powerful overriding physical mechanism, for example, cluster headache.

Medications

Analgesics are not particularly helpful for the pain of anxiety or depression unless they have a placebo effect. Antidepressants are useful in both groups of disorders. Amitriptyline is favored for patients with pain because it is known to have prophylactic effects in vascular headaches, especially migraine, and to have analgesic effects independent of depression. However, in patients with anxiety or depression it may not be the best choice. Maprotiline also has analgesic effects and may be used, as may desipramine, but on the whole the physician should aim at using an antidepressant with which he or she is familiar and which is known to be relatively effective for anxiety. In general this means choosing a drug with moderate sedative powers and not too many side effects. Chapters 60 and 88 discuss this topic in more detail.

Besides the tricyclic antidepressants, there is a common inclination to use benzodiazepines. These do not help pain directly. They may be useful in the short term for anxiety, but often the problem in controlling pain in patients with anxiety is to get them off benzodiazepines, which may be provoking withdrawal effects. Drugs with a long half-life, such as diazepam, may need more than a week or two to be completely eliminated from the blood and are best stopped by gradual withdrawal. The possibility of an increase in headache when medication is stopped exists both with analgesics and with benzodiazepines in patients who are using them for pain. The increase may be evidence of a rebound beyond the initial level of suffering (12). On the whole, benzodiazepines are best avoided; however, occasionally there may be a need to use them. Among the benzodiazepines, alprazolam has some reputation as an antidepressant and as a possible partner with ibuprofen in the treatment of fibromyalgia (23). Clonazepam also has been recommended for chronic pain but more often for pain that has a stabbing quality, which is not often the case with anxiety headache (see also Chapter 87).

Neuroleptics (see Chapter 54) occasionally are used for pain because they have analgesic effects (20) and sometimes are also used for anxiety, although they are often not particularly good for that purpose. However, one neuroleptic is recognized in a number of countries as an antidepressant or anxiolytic drug when used in small quantities. This is flupenthixol, which is used in western Europe for these purposes. In North America flupenthixol is more commonly used (in larger doses) for the treatment of schizophrenia. Flupenthixol 0.5 mg at breakfast and lunch is often an effective treatment for anxiety or depression. It has some unusual features. It can of course cause parkinsonism or tardive dyskinesia but in the dose recommended those effects are rare in patients under the age of 60. However, like most antidepressants, flupenthixol has a tendency to cause increased appetite and unwelcome weight gain for many patients. Fluoxetine (Prozac, Lilly) is an antidepressant that is licensed in most countries and does not as a rule cause weight gain, but rather the opposite. Unfortunately, fluoxetine is less likely to help anxiety, making some patients tense.

Buspirone (Buspar, Bristol Myers) might be a good choice, if it is available, because it is a serotonin reuptake inhibitor marketed in a number of countries for the treatment of anxiety. It presumably also could be used for depression and, theoretically, pain, although we have observed no apparent alleviation of pain with buspirone, particularly that resulting from an organic lesion. Like other drugs, buspirone must be titrated carefully to ensure that it will work. Buspirone 10 mg three times daily is a full dose that may relieve anxiety, but it should almost never be the starting dose. It is generally best to start with just half a tablet (i.e., 5 mg) twice daily for a few days, increasing to 5 mg three times daily, then waiting 1 or 2 weeks to get some indication of its effect. If signs of improvement begin to emerge in that time, this dosage may be sufficient, or the clinician may elect to increase the dosage to 10 mg twice daily, then perhaps to 10 mg three times daily after another week or two. If the dosage is increased too early in treatment, acute headache may become a complication on top of the chronic headache, and postural hypotension also may become a significant problem. Occasionally buspirone can produce disinhibited aggressive behavior, and one should take care to monitor this possibility. This side effect seems to be more likely to occur in patients who are already tense or anxious. Monoamine oxidase inhibitors (MAOIs) (e.g., phenelzine) also may be used in the treatment of anxiety.

These are the principal measures that may benefit patients with chronic headache due to anxiety. For further details on the use of tricyclic antidepressants and MAOIs, the reader is referred to in Chapters 54, 60, and 88 in this volume, as well as to regular textbooks on psychiatry and psychopharmacology.

Depression

Traditionally two types of depression have been recognized: endogenous and reactive. This distinction is no longer made as often, but it is still inherent in identifying the depressive states associated with manic illness and that form part of a bipolar pattern (bipolar affective disorder). Such depressions usually have a classic endogenous pattern. Typically, the patient wakes early, broods, has much guilt, is unable to concentrate or undertake daily affairs, and presents a suicidal risk. Headache also may appear. These "endogenous" mood patterns also occur with agitation and even delusional beliefs. In general the delusions involve self-blame, and if they are persecutory there is a feeling that the persecution is justified. They are often pain free. With the exception of one patient who experienced pain like a "crown of thorns" and probably had a combined schizoaffective disorder, we have not seen a convincing example of delusional headache in patients with this type of depression, but we have seen delusions of other pains in endogenous depression, for example, a patient believing that the devil was punishing her per vaginam with a trident for her misdeeds. However, a number of patients with endogenous depression have headache, which is usually symmetrical, produces symptoms similar to those of tension headache, and clears up with the treatment of the depression. More will be said about this shortly.

Endogenous depressive illnesses, whether retarded or agitated, are often precipitated by stressful events such as bereavement but seem to have a degree of autonomy once they have started. There is also a subgroup of patients with apparent endogenous depression who tend to be guilty and to sleep more and gain weight, whereas the typical patient with endogenous depression tends to lose weight.

Reactive depression is somewhat more in proportion (although not wholly so) to external events when compared with endogenous depression. There is less tendency to wake early and more tendency to have difficulty in falling asleep, and there is less tendency to exacerbation in the morning. As with endogenous depression there may be self-blame, but it is less pronounced and there is more anger. As in endogenous depression, concentration, memory, energy, and zest are impaired, but there is more fluctuation, and sometimes intervals of improvement occur when matters seem more hopeful. However, none of these rules serves as a hard-and-fast distinction because patients with endogenous depression also often fluctuate quite unaccountably and have quick switches into improvement of mood that may be brief or quite prolonged. In reactive depression there are more often human and personal conflicts, and as a result it is sometimes called neurotic depression.

The system of the APA has departed from these distinctions somewhat, relying instead on three major methods of classifying depressive responses. One is to link them with manic-depressive illness in what is called bipolar affective disorder; another is to give a broad description of "major depressive disorder," which applies to most patients with depression without other complicating features; and the third is to recognize adjustment disorder with depressed mood, for which there are similar categories in the ICD-10 system.

It is worth noting that the description of a major depressive episode given in the APA system has features that are found in many types of depression. A major depressive episode should normally have been present for at least 2 weeks with the occurrence of at least five out of the set of nine symptoms to be specified. The symptoms should not include those that are clearly attributable to physical conditions or to phenomena that may be linked to schizophrenia, such as mood-incongruent delusions or hallucinations. They must include either depressed mood or a loss of interest or pleasure. The list of nine symptoms then includes depressed mood for most of the day nearly every day, markedly diminished interest or pleasure in almost all activities, significant weight loss or weight gain when not dieting, insomnia or hypersomnia nearly every day, psychomotor agitation or retardation nearly every day, fatigue or loss of energy nearly every day, feelings of worthlessness or excessive or inappropriate guilt nearly every day, diminished ability to think or concentrate or indecisiveness nearly every day, and recurring thoughts of death, suicidal ideation, or suicide attempts. For the full criteria, the reader is referred to DSM-IV (1).

The mechanism of headache with depression is unsettled. First, there is a speculation that some pain that occurs without overt depression may be related to similar changes at serotonin or other receptors to those in depression. The evidence in favor of this view is limited to a small amount of information that suggests similarities between some types of pain without depression and some types of depression (13). Second, because of the prominent association of depression with anxiety and because of evidence of agitation and tension in patients with depression, it may be supposed that some patients with depression have pain resulting from muscle contraction. However, as previously noted, this is less well regarded as an explanation for chronic headache than formerly. Third, it is possible that a hysterical conversion mechanism occurs concomitantly with depression and is responsible for some of the symptoms that accompany it. Fourth, some of it could be delusional. No mechanism is well defined in this context, and the treatments remain empirical. Fortunately, the treatments for depression are frequently more effective than regular analgesics, even if those analgesics most prone to abuse are avoided. It is possible that antidepressants serve to break the vicious circle of pain producing depression and vice versa. Nevertheless, understanding the mechanism is usually less important than recognizing depression and knowing its treatments.

The most effective treatment for severe depression is electroconvulsive therapy (ECT). It is also very effective for other less severe forms of depression whenever there is an endogenous pattern. ECT is used much less frequently now, however, because of the availability of antidepressant medication.

Medications

Antidepressant drugs have become the mainstay of treatment in patients with a combination of headache and depression. Amitriptyline is the treatment of choice; it is known to be effective in both migraine (8) and tension-type headache (25), regardless of whether the patient is clinically depressed or not. Amitriptyline's sedative properties are often of great clinical value, but dothiepin or nortriptyline may be more suitable for patients without a preceding sleep disturbance. MAOIs also have proved effective (2).

Of the more recent antidepressants, mianserin has proved effective in headache patients (21), but there have not yet been adequate trials of, for example, lofepramine or viloxazine. The principal metabolite of trazodone metochlorophenylpiperazine has been found to cause headache in at least a proportion of migrainous subjects (7), so this drug is also probably best avoided.

The tricyclic group of drugs not only blocks serotonin reuptake but also antagonize some subtypes of 5-HT$_2$ receptor in therapeutic concentrations, and the recent finding that selective serotonin reuptake inhibitors, although undoubtedly effective in depression, may be less valuable in migraine prophylaxis (5) is evidence that the older drugs have a specific antimigraine action that may be pharmacologically distinct from its antidepressant action. Whether this can be related only to it action on 5-HT$_2$ receptors is open to debate.

The side effects of medication that may occur with depression are the same as those for anxiety and have been discussed above. If patients do not respond to tricyclic antidepressants after a due trial of two different such medications, the MAOIs combined with lithium or L-tryptophan can be very helpful in persistent depression, but this requires special experience in psychopharmacology.

Other Therapies

Apart from treatment with medication, cognitive therapy is often effective. This cannot be described in detail here. Briefly, it attempts to modify the self-deprecatory thoughts that commonly occur in depressed patients, and to improve the patient's perception of self and the environment. It may be useful in moderate or mild depression, particularly where there are questions as to whether the patient can or will take medication.

Relaxation is less important in patients with depression because the response to medication is good in up to 80% of suitable chosen patients who do not have continuing causes of stress or conflict.

All patients need psychological support and, as is the case in those with anxiety, some will benefit from exploratory psychotherapy. But, except for support, psychotherapy should take second place to the choice of effective antidepressant medication that may quickly relieve suicidal ideation and reduce suicidal risk. There is a phase when some patients, after improving from depression, become more suicidal because they become more mobile. Once this has passed, the trend is toward improvement in the depression, and if headache is found with the depression, that too will improve as the depression remits. Social management of patients with depression can be quite important, particularly in relieving continuing causes of stress.

Hysterical and Hypochondriacal Disorders

There is a tendency to describe symptoms that affect the body and that appear to be related to psychological dysfunction as evidence of "somatization." This confuses different possibilities that may be inherent in somatic symptoms with psychological illness. Some chronic headache may be due to muscle contraction, even if not in a large number of cases. This forms the basis for the idea that overactive physiologic changes in the voluntary musculature or the autonomic nervous system may produce pain through a psychophysiologic mechanism. This is very different from the notion—now much questioned—that pain might be due to an unconscious resolution of a conflict. For example, if a patient unconsciously develops pain as an attempt to solve an emotional conflict that itself becomes repressed out of consciousness, this would constitute a psychodynamic solution to the problem, albeit one bought at a price. In this case, the pain is due to thoughts, not to a psychophysiologic mechanism, and has to be seen as a different type of effect. It will not respond to treatment for reducing muscle tension. Instead it will resolve, in theory, either through the passage of time and spontaneous resolution of the conflict, or through measures taken to unearth the conflict from the patient's unconscious mind and assist him or her in resolving it. In addition, there is the concern over physical symptoms, usually called *hypochondriasis,* that is marked by both a fear of having a disease manifest by a particular symptom and an uneasy conviction that one really has got that symptom and disease despite what the doctor states after examination. These three mechanisms are distinct, although they can occur together. Furthermore, there is an additional condition in which the patient has multiple hypochondriacal complaints with more contentment of the hysterical type and less concern of the hypochondriacal type. This has been called *somatization disorder* (1) for the purpose of delimiting a special group of patients who might be studied for their strong presentation of somatic symptoms that are not based on recognizable physical processes. All of these patients will be included haphazardly under the word "somatization," so it is best avoided, but the category of somatization disorder can be useful.

The idea that headache and other pain might be a conversion symptom has a long history, dating back to the seventeenth century and possibly, although less certainly, to earlier researchers of hysteria. It has been said to have been recognized in the Kahun papyrus, which is about 3,500 years old, but the justification for regarding this text as describing hysteria is questionable (18). Breuer and Freud in their *Studies on Hysteria* (6), which inaugurated psychoanalytic theory and practice, described a number of patients with facial pain who were thought to have the pain as a means of resolving a conflict. We might doubt the validity of some of those interpretations because the possibility that the pains were related to muscle tension or to depression was not well excluded. At one time it appeared that in the absence of alternative diagnoses in psychiatry a high proportion of psychiatric patients might be diagnosed as having pain due to hysterical conversion (16). This view was reinforced by findings with, for example, the Minnesota Multiphasic Personality Inventory (MMPI) of increased scores on hysteria and hypochondriasis scales in patients with chronic pain.

This conclusion is no longer tenable. Although the diagnoses that supported the notion of hysteria were made according to the standards of the day, they lacked positive evidence, which is hard to find for pain due to hysteria, and in only a few instances was it proven by further psychological exploration that the symptoms resulted from conflict and could be dispelled when the conflict was partly or wholly resolved. In any case, although these diagnoses could be made for research purposes, for the sake of group comparisons they were rarely available to offer to patients, and those who were offered such a diagnosis rarely understood it. Such diagnoses are harder to prove and still harder to treat if found.

Meanwhile, the MMPI itself has lost credibility as a method for diagnosing the psychological phenomena associated with pain. The principal diagnostic patterns for pain depended on increased scores for hypochondriasis, depression, and hysteria, all of which rely considerably on a symptom count in which pains, fatigue, and insomnia could figure as part of the complaints leading to the psychiatric diagnosis. However, the MMPI was not meant to be used as evidence of hypochondriasis of hysteria unless physical disease had been excluded. In fact, its common application in pain clinics did not incorporate this precaution, so any patient in a medical department who had some physical complaints would automatically be at risk for scoring higher on the MMPI than would a patient who was physically well. Hence, a significant proportion of the patterns that had been attributed to hysteria or hypochondriasis in patients in pain clinics, and patients in psychiatric care who have chronic pain, were unjustified, and the MMPI has proved misleading. Not surprisingly, it is no longer as popular as it was formerly, and it is now preferred as a guide to symptom clusters and predictive patterns rather than as proof of psychogenesis.

The so-called somatization disorder is another way in which hysterical phenomena have presented (1). This is defined on the basis of a number of symptoms presenting before the age of 30 and not based on physical illness but leading the patient to take treatment or consult a doctor. This method of definition breaks off one portion of a continuum and treats it as a separate category. It is probably justified because of the usefulness of the category in determining phenomena that are associated with severe forms of hysterical or hypochondriacal complaints.

The treatment of patients with conversion headaches, on the rare occasions when they are found, is by psychotherapy and perhaps suggestion. There is a vulgar error that confuses pain in individuals involved in litigation with so-called secondary gain. If pain occurs in people who are pursuing litigation, and if the pain is due to an emotional conflict in which at least some of the feelings concerned with the litigation are repressed, so that the pain itself is a problem-solving symptom, then this pain does not reflect secondary gain but is rather a consequence of the patient achieving primary gain, which is abolishing or quelling anxiety as a result of making a particular conflict unconscious. In that situation, secondary gain may appear not because financial benefits are being paid but because the individual is recognized as sick and treated accordingly by others. Flowers, sympathy, relief from the burden of work, and so forth are secondary gains for a patient, whether or not the pain has a physical basis. It can be argued further that financial compensation for actual losses is not secondary gain but simply the replacement of something that should ordinarily be present. In general, the diagnosis of hysterical pain should only be made with great circumspection, and treatment initiated tentatively and with care.

Hypochondriacal phenomena can be managed directly. It is possible to hold discussions with patients and to indicate to them that they have reasons to be concerned about their body but the reasons are out of proportion. This can be treated both by reassurance and by cognitive therapy. However, some patients with hypochondriacal conditions are resistant to cognitive therapy and to argument. They may still benefit from a sympathetic relationship that recognizes that they have not abandoned their ideas but treats the patient in a supportive fashion. Many cases of hypochondriasis also may be recognized as being due to other illnesses, for example, depression, schizophrenia, or organic brain changes affecting the mood and reactions of the individual. In these cases a relevant etiologic treatment for depression or schizophrenia may prove successful, and the hypochondriasis will then vanish.

A somewhat similar approach in terms of support and acceptance is appropriate for patients with somatization disorder who can be kept from undue investigation if maintained in a friendly, unambitious relationship with the physician. In those cases cure is not realizable, but continued attention may help to keep the patient from seeking out more damaging treatments.

Schizophrenia

Lastly, a few words should be devoted to schizophrenia. This is an important illness that affects almost 1% of the population but is rarely a problem with respect to chronic pain or headache. Patients with schizophrenia have pain less often than other psychiatric patients (10). Rarely do they have a headache that is clearly delusional or hallucinatory, and this is of theoretical importance. However, we have only encountered one such case of headache, and that was in the patient with a schizoaffective disorder who complained of pain like a "crown of thorns" and believed she was Jesus. A number of schizophrenic patients describe dull headaches that are not well characterized. At most, about 10% of schizophrenic patients have this sort of headache (24), and the topic has not been well investigated. Whatever the complaint of pain, if it is related to schizophrenia, the treatment is the same as that of the psychiatric illness (i.e., the use of neuroleptics in most cases with psychological and social sup-

port). Because this is a serious and troublesome illness, it usually requires specialist advice at some stage.

REFERENCES

1. American Psychiatric Association. *Diagnostic and statistical manual of mental disorders,* 4th ed, revised. Washington, DC: Author, 1994.
2. Anthony M, Lance JW. Monoamine oxidase inhibition in the treatment of migraine. *Arch Neurol* 1969;21:263–268.
3. Atkinson JH, Slater MA, Patterson TI, et al. Prevalence, onset and risk of psychiatric disorders in men with chronic low back pain: a controlled study. *Pain* 1991;45:111–121.
4. Baker JW, Merskey H. Pain in general practice. *J Psychosom Res* 1967;10:383–387.
5. Bendtsen L, Jensen R, Olesen J. A non-selective (amitriptyline), but not a selective (citalopram), serotonin reuptake inhibitor is effective in the prophylactic treatment of chronic tension-type headache. *J Neurol Neurosurg Psychiatry* 1996;61:285–290.
6. Breuer J, Freud S. *Studies on hysteria. Complete psychological works of Freud,* Vol. 2 (1893–1895), standard edition. London: Hogarth Press, 1966.
7. Brewerton TD, Murphy DL, Mueller EA, Kimerson DC. Induction of migraine-like headaches by the serotonin agonist *m*-chlorophenylpiperazine. *Clin Pharmacol Ther* 1988;43:605–609.
8. Couch JR, Hassanein RS. Amitriptyline in migraine prophylaxis. *Arch Neurol* 1979;36:695–699.
9. Crook J, Rideout E, Browne G. The prevalence of pain complaints in a general population. *Pain* 1984;18:299–314.
10. Delaplaine R, Ifabumuyi OI, Merskey H, et al. Significance of pain in psychiatric hospital patients. *Pain* 1978;4:361–366.
11. The ICD-10. *Classification of mental and behavioural disorders,* 10th ed. Geneva: World Health Organization, 1992.
12. Kudrow L. Paradoxical effects of frequent analgesic use. *Adv Neurol* 1982;33:335–341.
13. Magni G. On the relationship between chronic pain and depression when there is no organic lesion. *Pain* 1987;31:1–21.
14. Magni G, Bernosconi G, Mauro P, et al. Psychiatric diagnosis in ulcerative colitis, a controlled study. *Br J Psychiatry* 1991;158:413–415.
15. Magni G, Caldieron C, Rigatti-Luchini S, Merskey H. Chronic musculoskeletal pain and depressive symptoms in the general population. An analysis of the first national health and nutrition examination survey data. *Pain* 1990;43:299–307.
16. Merskey H. The characteristics of persistent pain in psychological illness. *J Psychosom Res* 1965;9:291–298.
17. Merskey H. Psychological aspects of pain relief; hypnotherapy; psychotropic drugs. In: Swerdlow M, ed. *Relief of intractable pain.* New York: Excerpta Medica, 1974.
18. Merskey H, Potter P. The womb lay still in ancient Egypt. *Br J Psychiatry* 1989;154:751–753.
19. Merskey H, Spear FG. *Pain: psychological and psychiatric aspects.* London: Bailliere, Tindall & Cassell, 1967.
20. Monks R. Psychotropic drugs. In: Wall PD, Melzack R, eds. *Textbook of pain,* 3rd ed. London: Churchill Livingstone, 1994:963–989.
21. Monro P, Swade C, Coppen A. Mianserin in the prophylaxis of migraine: a double-blind study. *Acta Psychiatr Scand* 1985;72:98–103.
22. Romano JM, Turner JA. Chronic pain and depression: does the evidence support a relationship? *Psychol Bull* 1965;97:18–34.
23. Russell IJ, Fletcher EM, Michalek JE, et al. Treatment of primary fibrositis; fibromyalgia syndrome with ibuprofen and alprazolam. *Arthritis Rheum* 1991;34:552–560.
24. Watson GD, Chandarana PC, Merskey H. Relationships between pain and schizophrenia. *Br J Psychiatry* 1981;138:33–36.
25. Zagami AS. Chronic tension-type headache: rational drug treatment options. *CNS Drugs* 1995;4:90–98.

The Headaches, Second Edition,
edited by J. Olesen, P. Tfelt-Hansen, and K.M.A. Welch.
Lippincott Williams & Wilkins, Philadelphia © 2000.

Special Problems in the Headaches and Their Management

CHAPTER 128

Headache and Sleep

Teresa Paiva and Rachel Hering-Hanit

The complex links between sleep, sleep disturbances (SD), and headaches have been known for many years (21,22); the International Classification of Sleep Disorders (73) even specifies the item "sleep-related headaches," encompassing chronic paroxysmal hemicrania (CPH), cluster headache (CH), and migraine. Headache specialists are well acquainted with the importance of sleep in triggering or relieving these headaches, and in the International Classification of Headache (30) a subitem of "headache association with metabolic disorder with hypoxia" focuses on sleep apnea headache. Sleep complaints are frequent in chronic headache patients (25,49,69), and it has been shown that they significantly affect the quality of life in migraineurs, tension headache patients, and those with combined headaches, with their scores significantly higher than those of controls (55,64). Indeed, when investigated by questionnaires, chronic headache patients presented a moderate degree of insomnia, associated with other sleep complaints such as hypnagogic startles, pain, or discomfort during the night (51).

Nevertheless, several aspects remain open to research because physiologic, genetic, epidemiologic, and physiopathologic links are sometimes unclear and some results remain controversial.

SLEEP AND HEADACHE: FUNCTIONAL LINKS

Sleep is an all-body recurrent phenomena, during which a complex set of functions occur that promote tissue repair (1): for example, thermoregulation (53), im-

mune function (24,44), regulation of noradrenergic sensitivity (70), and maintenance of memory (16). Nevertheless, many sleep functions are either incompletely understood or still unknown (42). Sleep researchers usually focus on the brain/body restorative effects of sleep. These effects are achieved by a sophisticated organization of nocturnal sleep, which implies a recurrent alternation of two basic sleep states intermixed with small amounts of the awake state. Awake is expressed in terms of transient awakenings or brief arousals; the two basic sleep stages are rapid eye movement sleep (or REM sleep) and non-REM (NREM) sleep. Minimal SDs, as well as more severe disturbances, arise whenever an imbalance of these states occurs. Increased awakenings induce initiation, maintenance, and early morning insomnia or a fragmented sleep due to an increased number of arousals. Lack of the deep phases of NREM sleep (phases III and IV) affects the restorative function, with tiredness, lack of concentration, and performance difficulties the next morning, whereas increased amounts of these stages may be associated with an abnormal arousal function, and consequently with some of the parasomnias, such as somnambulism and sleep terrors. Abnormalities in REM sleep occur often in depression and in narcolepsy, with reduced REM latency and abnormal distribution of REM during the night. A set of examples is shown in Figure 1.

The influence of sleep upon headaches is often attributed to disturbances in its restorative function.

SLEEP AND HEADACHE: PHYSIOPATHOLOGIC LINKS

The relationships between headache and sleep can be classified in two groups. First, sleep can influence a headache and vice versa (69). This relationship may be further subdivided into (a) sleep-triggered or -related

T. Paiva: Laboratory EEG/SLEEP, Centro de Estudos Egas Moniz, Hospital Santa Maria, 1600 Lisbon, Portugal.

R. Hering-Hanit: Sackler School of Medicine, Tel Aviv University, Ramat Aviv 69978, and Headache Unit, Department of Neurology, Meir General Hospital, Kfar-Sava 44281, Israel.

Normal sleep

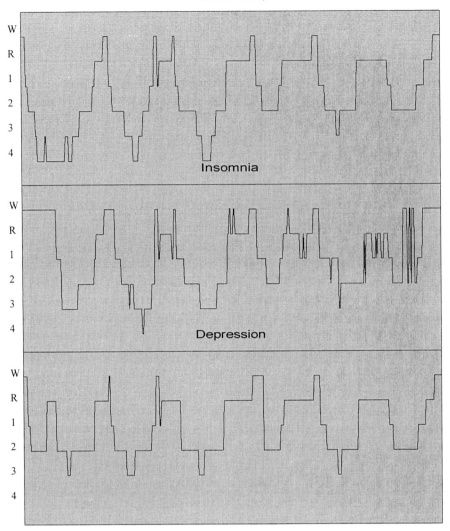

FIG. 1. The three hypnograms show the evolution of normal sleep, with REM predominating at the end of the night and slow-wave sleep at the beginning of the night. Insomnia corresponds to increased sleep latency and early morning awakening. Depression shows decreased REM latency and increased REM percentage; the increase in REM sleep at the end of the night is lacking.

headaches, namely those occurring during or after sleep; (b) sleep duration and headaches, namely episodes due to excess, lack, disruption, or change in the pattern of sleep; (c) sleep phase–related headaches, that is, headaches occurring in a specific sleep stage; (d) sleep-relieved headaches; (e) dreams and headaches; and (f) effects of headaches on sleep (69) (Fig. 2).

Second, there is the relationship between specific headache entities and specific sleep disorders. Finally, we also discuss the influence of sleep disorders in patients referred to a headache clinic.

Sleep-Triggered Headaches

The patient may be either awakened by the pain during night or is aware of an attack upon awakening in the morning (73). Headaches are classified as sleep-related when 75% of the episodes occur during sleep or upon awakening. Three headache entities currently known sometimes fulfill these requirements: migraine, CH, and CPH.

In migraine the incidence of nocturnal attacks has been described in temporal relation with REM sleep (22,23), which is associated with increased cerebral blood flow with altered autoregulation.

Several researchers have described the typical temporal profile of CH, with consensus concerning nocturnal peaks of occurrence (40,41,67). Fifty-one percent of CH attacks begin during nocturnal sleep (67); indeed, the number of nocturnal attacks per hour is 2.5 times more frequent then diurnal attacks, and the last ones are often associated with naps or periods of physical relaxation (73).

About one third of attacks in CPH occur during nocturnal sleep (68), but it must be stressed that pain paroxysms are evenly distributed throughout day and night.

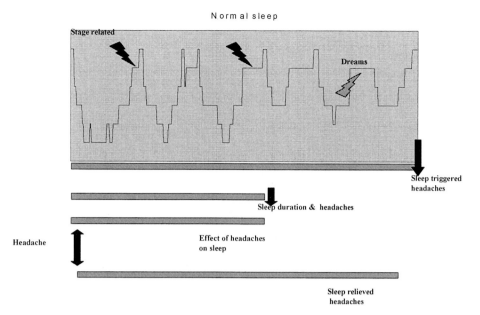

FIG. 2. The mutual influences of sleep and headache are depicted. Headaches may appear at the end of sleep, when sleep is shortened, in relation to sleep stages, associated with dream content, relieved by a sleep episode or even able to prevent normal sleep due to the intensity of the pain.

Length and Pattern of Sleep and Headache

This influence of sleep upon headache occurs even in normal subjects. After sleep deprivation one may experience a dull or pressing bilateral headache in the forehead (10). The lack of sleep is also a cause for tension headaches; it has been associated with frequent awakenings and decreased slow-wave sleep (25), yet the involved mechanisms are not fully understood (30). Migraine attacks can be precipitated by both oversleep or lack of sleep (69).

Sleep alteration pattern, namely by sleeping too little, too much, or by changing sleep schedule, are also known to precipitate headache (71), particularly migraine (56).

Adding complexity is the fact that in migraineurs a short nap may be a useful strategy to end an attack but it may also precipitate an attack (9,77).

Sleep Phase and Headache

Certain headache entities occur in relation to specific sleep stages (69). Migraine occurrence after diurnal or nocturnal sleep seems to be related to excessive percentages of stages III and IV (19). Attack onset after a nap is also associated with REM sleep (19). A significant association with REM sleep was described whenever patients awake with an attack (19,32). Unfortunately, these observations are not substantiated by systematic studies (56).

Cluster headache is often triggered by REM sleep (22,39), but NREM sleep also has been implicated (57); some researchers have proposed hypoxia, and not the sleep stage per se, as the main trigger for CH attacks (38,39). CPH has been considered a REM-locked headache (36); this characteristic has been recently questioned by polysomnographic studies of some patients, showing that the trigger was not the sleep stage but a sustained increase in blood pressure (15).

Sleep-Relieved Headaches

It is well recognized that a short nap or even nocturnal sleep often may end a migraine attack (9,77), particularly in children (7). This is also true for confusional migraine (26,54).

Dreams and Headaches

Some clinical observations suggest a relationship between unpleasant dreams and migraine headaches. In a study of 37 migraineurs, the dream contents that preceded nocturnal migraine were described: the variables contributing significantly to dreams were anger, misfortune, apprehension, and aggressive interactions (31).

Effect of Headaches on Sleep

Insomnia and sleep disruption may occur in patients with CH and CPH due to the nocturnal attacks. Abnormalities in the sleep recordings during the headache periods with normalization during remissions have been described in individual patients, but no systematic studies exist (48).

Hypnic headaches in elderly patients also induce several nocturnal awakenings (46,63). Patients with tension-type headaches also were reported to have poor sleep, with reduced sleep efficiency and reduced slow-wave sleep in a polysomnographic study of 10 patients (25).

The same researchers postulated that migraine also may transiently affect the quality of sleep (25); this was particularly so premenstrually (72).

Clinical Links between Sleep Disorders and Headaches

In clinical practice the association between headaches and SDs is frequent and must be suspected in patients with nocturnal and early morning headaches. In a specialized headache clinic 17% of the patients had awakening or nocturnal headache; 53% of them, that is, 9% of the total headache population, had a sleep disorder (50).

The relationship between headache and sleep disorder may be characterized as follows: (a) the SD is the cause of headache; (b) the headache is the cause of an SD; (c) headache and SD overlap in the same subject, due to the high incidence of both; (d) headache and SD have a common intrinsic origin; (e) headache and SD have a common extrinsic origin; and (f) headache and SD independently of their original cause mutually reinforce (48) (Fig. 3).

The Sleep Disturbance is the Cause of Headache

When treatment of the sleep disorder cures the headache, a casual relationship seems likely. Some sleep disorders may be the cause of headache complaints. It has been specially studied for obstructive sleep apnea syndrome (OSAS) (3,13,20,29,59,73), but may be present in other disorders causing apnea, such as neuromuscular disorders (6,65,75) or acromegaly (66). It also may occur in snorers (35,47) and in patients with periodic limb movements of sleep (48,50,51).

Morning headaches are a recognized symptom of OSAS (28,29,52). According to the International Classification of Sleep Disorders, the headaches are dull and bilateral, frontal or generalized (50,73), and usually last for 1 to 2 hours after awakening (73); however, other headache types have been described, namely mixed and vascular headaches (59). The incidence of morning headaches in OSAS has been reported as 24%, which was identical to their incidence in other sleep disorders (2,59). In a community study a negative correlation between morning headaches and sleep-disordered breathing was described (47). Other studies using structured questionnaires and polysomnography found that morning headaches occurred in 58% of OSAS patients (52). There is consensus concerning the effect of treatment: morning pain tends to improve or disappear after efficient treatment, either with CPAP (48,50,59) or by adequate surgery (17).

Snoring in men is also significantly associated with headaches. In a Danish community study, headache occurred in 56.1% of the 3,323 subjects investigated; in 10.7% of them a temporal profile with morning headaches was present. This association between headache and snoring was not explained by potential confounders, such as age, body mass index, alcohol consumption, and smoking (35). Self-reported snoring in 37 women 65 to 94 years of age showed a positive correlation between snoring and morning headaches (74).

Nocturnal hypoxemia together with changes in intracranial pressure and cerebrovascular tone, as well as the associated sleep fragmentation, have all been suggested as the main mechanism for morning headache in OSAS (69).

The other intrinsic sleep disorder that may provoke headaches is periodic limb movement of sleep (PLMS). According to Poceta et al., approximately 25% of PLMS patients complain of morning headache (59). Treatment of PLMS with low doses of clonazepam prevented in some patients the occurrence of headaches (48).

Headache is the Cause of Sleep Disturbance

Sleep disruption induced by CH and CPH may be due to the pain itself or to the fear of its occurrence during sleep (36,39,48). However, in chronic daily headaches sleep disruption is considered to have a psychogenic origin (69).

Headache and Sleep Disturbance Overlap at Random

The association between headaches and SD may be due to the high prevalence of both disturbances in the general population or to genetic links still not clarified. In previous work it has been shown that PLMS and migraine were found in the same patient; the temporal evolution and age of onset of both disturbances showed no correlation, and successful treatment could only be achieved when both were specifically treated (48).

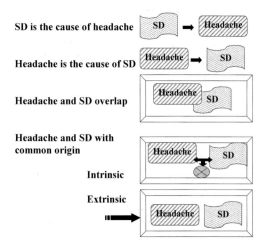

FIG. 3. The interrelationships between headaches and sleep disorders are schematically represented. SD can cause headaches and vice versa; both may overlap or have a common cause, which can be intrinsic or extrinsic to the organism.

A strong association between somnambulism and migraine often has been described (5,21,27,51,62).

Headache and Sleep Disturbances Have a Common Intrinsic Cause

Psychological and psychiatric disturbances are commonly the cause of headache and SD (48,69). The high incidence of depression in headache and in SD has been documented in several studies (43,58). This is particularly true for chronic tension-type headache.

Another cause is fibromyalgia (78). The presence of both headaches and insomnia is very high in these patients (14,48). Alpha delta sleep is a specific sleep electroencephalographic pattern common but not pathognomonic of fibromyalgia syndrome (FMS) (11,45). In a previous polysomnographic study of headache sufferers with morning headaches, FMS was suspected whenever alpha delta sleep pattern was found by polysomnography; the suspicion proved to be true when the diagnosis was latter confirmed by trained rheumatologists (48). Patients with FMS may present with tension-type or migraine headaches (14). The association between headache and SDs seems weaker in a related syndrome also coursing with headaches, namely, chronic fatigue syndrome (8,37).

Headache and Sleep Disturbances have a Common Extrinsic Cause

Chronic substance abuse, particularly of ergot derivatives and/or analgesics, is a frequent cause of daily chronic headaches; these patients also present with SDs (48). However, the underlying mechanisms are not easy to understand and are most likely complex because in some patients discontinuation of the abused substance was sufficient to treat headaches and insomnia. In other patients insomnia and headaches fluctuated (48). Chronic substance abuse may not be associated with SD.

A large set of external causes, either concerning medications, toxic agents, or infectious organisms, may induce headache as well as SDs. However, in these situations both symptoms appear among a broader spectrum of disturbance and, more likely, represent an unspecific response of the central nervous system (CNS) to external aggression. The available data do not point to other conclusions. A few examples follow.

The benzodiazepine withdrawal syndrome is characterized by a complex cluster of symptoms, which besides insomnia and headache also include irritability, anxiety, hand tremor, sweating, difficulty in concentration, nausea, weight loss, palpitations, and muscular pain (61). Abstinence of caffeine also includes headaches, decreased wakefulness, and decreased motor activity, but has no evident effects on nocturnal sleep (33). Psychoactive substance use is also associated with headache, sleep disorders, and psychiatric disturbances (4).

The exposure to organic solvents may induce CNS dysfunction, including headache sleepiness, vertigo, concentration difficulties, and mood swings (34).

Some infectious diseases, such as pertussis in adults have, besides the infectious signs and symptoms, associated SDs (52%) and headaches (14%) (60). The two symptoms were also selected—among 12 others such as fatigue, fever, imbalance, paresthesias, memory loss, cough, nausea, diarrhea, sadness, and skin problems—to integrate an index of infection with human immunodeficiency virus (76).

Posttraumatic stress following acts of violence provokes a complex behavioral disturbance involving excitability, distrust, avoidance, nightmares, difficulties in concentration, hyperfatigability, headaches, and SDs (18).

HEADACHE AS A WARNING SYMPTOM FOR SLEEP DISTURBANCES

It has been pointed out that headaches, especially when occurring predominantly in the morning or during nocturnal sleep, may be a warning of an SD. In a systematic clinical/polysomnographic investigation of 49 patients attending a headache clinic and presenting headaches as the most troublesome symptom, an important proportion of them (53%) had headaches associated with a sleep disorder. This subgroup when compared with the subgroup without sleep disorders had a high prevalence of work-related problems due to sleepiness (80%), along with also daytime sleepiness, nocturnal SD, suffocation, sleep walking, and sleep paralysis (50). Researchers were unable to distinguish between the two subgroups, but there was a predominance of men in the investigated sample, and several patients had a late onset or late worsening headache (48,50).

REFERENCES

1. Adam K, Oswald I. Protein synthesis, body renewal and the sleep wake cycle. *Clin Sci* 1983;65:561–567.
2. Aldrich MS, Chauncey JB. Are morning headaches part of obstructive sleep apnea syndrome? *Arch Intern Med* 1990;150:1265–1267.
3. Ancoli-Israel S, Klauber MR, Stepnowsky C, Estline E, Chinn A, Fell R. Sleep-disordered breathing in African-American elderly. *Am J Respir Crit Care Med* 1995;152(apt 1):1946–1949.
4. Ardila A, Bateman JR. Psychoactive substance use: some associated characteristics. *Addict Behav* 1995;20:549–554.
5. Barabas G, Ferrari M, Matthews WS. Childhood migraine and somnambulism. *Neurology* 1983;33:948–949.
6. Barb F, Quera-Salva MA, McCann C, et al. Sleep-related respiratory disturbances in patients with Duchenne muscular dystrophy. *Eur Respir J* 1994;7:1403–1408.
7. Barlow CF. Migraine in the infant and toddler. *J Child Neurol* 1994; 9:92–94.
8. Bell DS, Bell KM, Cheney PR. Primary juvenile fibromyalgia syndrome and chronic fatigue syndrome in adolescents. *Clin Infect Dis* 1994;18[Suppl 1]:21–23.
9. Blau JN. Resolution of migraine attacks: sleep and the recovery phase. *J Neurol Neurosurg Psychiatry* 1982;45:223–226.
10. Blau JN. Sleep deprivation headache. *Cephalalgia* 1990;10:157–160.
11. Branco J, Atalaia A, Paiva T. Sleep cycles and alpha-delta sleep in fibromyalgia syndrome. *J Rheumatol* 1994;21:1113–1117.

12. Breslau N, Davis GC, Schultz LR, Peterson EL. Migraine and major depression: a longitudinal study. *Headache* 1994;34:387–393.
13. Bresnitz EA, Goldberg R, Kosinski RM. Epidemiology of obstructive sleep apnea. *Epidemiol Rev* 1994;16:210–227.
14. Clauw DJ. The pathogenesis of chronic pain and fatigue syndromes, with special reference to fibromyalgia. *Med Hypotheses* 1995;44: 369–378.
15. Conelli P, Plazzi G, Pierangeli G, De Monte A, Prologo G, Lugaresi E. Cardiovascular changes in chronic paroxysmal hemicrania—a nocturnal polygraphic study. In: Rose FC, ed. *New advances in headache research.* Great Britain: Smith Gordon and Company, 1994:225.
16. Davis BD. Sleep and the maintenance of memory. *Perspect Biol Med* 1985;28:457–464.
17. Davis JA, Fine ED, Maniglia AJ. Uvulopalatopharyngoplasty for obstructive sleep apnea in adults:clinical correlation with polysomnographic results. *Ear Nose Throat J* 1993;72:63–66.
18. De Mol J. Clinical and psychometric study of post-traumatic stress disorders following acts of violence. *Rev Med Brux* 1994;15:118–123.
19. Dexter JD. The relationship between stage III-IV-REM sleep and arousals with migraine. *Headache* 1979;19:364–369.
20. Dexter JD. Headache as a presenting complaint of the sleep apnea syndrome. *Headache* 1984;24:171.
21. Dexter JD. The relationship between disorders of arousal from sleep and migraine. *Headache* 1986;26:322.
22. Dexter JD, Riley TL. Studies in nocturnal migraine. *Headache* 1975; 15:51–62.
23. Dexter JD, Weitzman ED. The relationship of nocturnal headaches to sleep stage patterns. *Neurology* 1970;20:513–518.
24. Dinges DF, Douglas SD, Hamarman S, et al. Sleep deprivation and human immune function. *Adv Neuroimmunol* 1995;5:97–110.
25. Drake ME Jr, Pakanis A, Andrews JM, Bogner JE. Nocturnal sleep recording with cassette EEG in chronic headaches. *Headache* 1990; 30:600–603.
26. Ehyai A, Fenichel GM. The natural history of acute confusional migraine. *Arch Neurol* 1978;35:368–369.
27. Giraud M, D Aghis P, Guard O, Dumas R. Migraine et somnambulisme: une enquête portant sur 122 migraineux. *Rev Neurol (Paris)* 1986;142:42–46.
28. Guilleminault C. Clinical features and evaluation of obstructive sleep apnea. In: Kryger M, Roth T, Dement WC, eds. *Principles and practice of sleep medicine,* 2nd ed. Philadelphia: WB Saunders, 1994: 667–677.
29. Guilleminault C, Hold J, Mitler MM. Clinical overview of the sleep apnea syndromes. In: Guilleminault C, Dement WC, eds. *Sleep apnea syndromes.* New York: Alan R Liss, 1978:1–12.
30. Headache Classification Committee of the International Headache Society. Classification and diagnostic criteria for headache disorders, cranial neuralgias and facial pain. *Cephalalgia* 1988;8[Suppl 7]:10–73.
31. Heather-Greener GA, Comstock D, Joyce R. An investigation of the manifest dream content associated with migraine headaches: a study of the dreams that precede nocturnal migraine. *Psychother Psychosom* 1996;65:216–221.
32. Hsu LKG, Kalucy RS, Crisp AH, Koval J, Chen CN, Carrithers M, Zikha KJ. Early morning migraine. Nocturnal plasma levels of cathecolamines, tryptophan, glucose and free fatty acids and sleep encephalograms. *Lancet* 1977;1:447–450.
33. Hufer I, Buttig K. Cardiovascular, behavioral, and subjective effects of caffeine under field conditions. *Pharmacol Biochem Behav* 1994;48: 899–908.
34. Indulski JA, Siunzuk-Walczak H, Szymczak M, Wesolowski W. Neurological and neurophysiological examinations of workers occupationally exposed to organic solvent mixtures used in the paint and varnish production. *Int J Occup Med Environ Health* 1996;9:235–244.
35. Jennum P, Hein HO, Suadicani P, Gyntelberg F. Headache and cognitive dysfunction in snorers: a cross-sectional study of 3323 men aged 54 to 74 years: the Copenhagen male study. *Arch Neurol* 1994;51:937–942.
36. Kayed K, Godtlibsen OB, Sjaastad O. Chronic paroxysmal hemicrania IV: REM sleep locked nocturnal headache attacks. *Sleep* 1973;1:91–95.
37. Komaroff AL, et al. An examination of the working case definition of chronic fatigue syndrome. *Am J Med* 1996;100:54–64.
38. Kudrow L. The pathogenesis of cluster headache. *Curr Opin Neurol* 1994;7:278–282.
39. Kudrow L, McGinty DJ, Philips ER, Stevenson M. Sleep apnea in cluster headache. *Cephalalgia* 1984;4:33–38.
40. Lance JW, Anthony M. Migrainous neuralgia or cluster headache. *J Neurol Sci* 1971;13:401–414.
41. Manzoni GC, Terzano MG, Bono G, et al. Cluster headache—clinical findings in 180 patients. *Cephalalgia* 1983;3:21–30
42. Maquet P. Sleep function(s) and cerebral metabolism. *Behav Brain Res* 1995;69:75–83.
43. Marazziti D, Toni C, Pedri S, et al. Headache, panic disorder and depression:co-morbidity or a spectrum? *Neuropsychobiology* 1995;31: 125–129.
44. Moldofsky H, Lue FA, Eisen J, et al. The relationship of interleukin-1 and immune functions to sleep in humans. *Psychosom Med* 1986;48: 309–318.
45. Moldofsky H, Saskin P, Lue FA. Sleep and symptoms in fibrositis syndrome after a febrile illness. *J Rheumatol* 1988;15:1701–1704.
46. Newman LC, Lipton RB, Solomon S. The hypnic headache syndrome: a benign headache disorder of the elderly. *Neurology* 1990;40: 1904–1905.
47. Olson LG, King MT, Hensley MJ, Saunders NA. A community study of snoring and sleep-disordered breathing. Symptoms. *Am J Respir Crit Care Med* 1995;152:707–710.
48. Paiva T, Batista A, Martins P, Martins. The relationship between headaches and sleep disturbances. *Headache* 1995;35:590–596.
49. Paiva T, Esperanza P, Martins I, Batista A, Martins P. Sleep disorders in headache patients. *Headache Q* 1992;3:438–442.
50. Paiva T, Farinha A, Martins A, Batista A, Guilleminault C. Chronic headaches and sleep disorders. *Arch Intern Med* 1997;157:1701–1705.
51. Paiva T, Martins P, Batista A, Esperanza P, Martins I. Sleep disturbances in chronic headache patients: a comparison with healthy controls. *Headache Q* 1994;5:135–141.
52. Paiva T, Vasconcelos P, Leito AN, Andrea M. Obstructive aleep apnea: clinical and laboratory studies. *Acta Med Port* 1994;7:43–50.
53. Parmeggiani PL. Interaction between sleep and thermo-regulation: an aspect of the control of behavioral states. *Sleep* 1987;10:426–435.
54. Parrino L, Pietrini V, Spaggiari MC, Terzano MG. Acute confusional migraine attacks resolved by sleep: lack of significant abnormalities in post-ictal polysomnograms. *Cephalalgia* 1986;6:95–100.
55. Passchier J, Boo M, Quaak HZA, Brienen JA. Health-related quality of life of chronic headache patients is predicted by the emotional component of their pain. *Headache* 1996;36:556–560.
56. Peatfield RC, Olesen J. Precipitating factors. In: Olesen J, Tfelt-Hansen P, Welch KMA, eds. *The headaches.* New York: Raven, 1993:241–245.
57. Pfaffenrath V, Pollmann W, Ruther E, Lund R, Hajak G. Onset of nocturnal attacks of chronic cluster headache in relation to sleep stages. *Acta Neurol Scand* 1986;73:403–407.
58. Pine DS, Cohen P, Brook J. The association between major depression and headache: result of a longitudinal epidemiologic study in youth. *J Child Adolesc Psychopharmacol* 1996;6:153–164.
59. Poceta JS, Dalessio DJ. Identification and treatment of sleep apnea in patients with chronic headache. *Headache* 1995;35:586–589.
60. Postels-Multani S, Schmitt HJ, Wirsing von Konig CH, Bock HL, Bogaerts H. Symptoms and complications of pertussis in adults. *Infection* 1995;23:139–142.
61. Potursson H. The benzodiazepine withdrawal syndrome. *Addiction* 1994;89:1455–1459.
62. Pradalier A, Guroud M, Dry J. Somnambulism, migraine and propanolol. *Headache* 1987;27:143–145.
63. Raskin NH. The hypnic headache syndrome. *Headache* 1988;28: 534–536.
64. Rasmussen BK. Migraine and tension-type headache in a general population: precipitating factors, female hormones, sleep pattern and a relation to lifestyle. *Pain* 1993;53:65–72.
65. Rochester DF, Esau SA. Assessment of ventilatory function in patients with neuromuscular disease. *Clin Chest Med* 1994;15:751–763.
66. Rosenow F, et al. Sleep apnoea in acromegaly-prevalence, pathogenesis and therapy. Report on two cases. *Presse Med* 1994;23:1203–1208.
67. Russel D. Cluster headache: severity and temporal profiles of attacks and patients activity prior to and during attacks. *Cephalalgia* 1981;1: 209–216.
68. Russel D. Chronic paroxysmal hemicrania: severity, duration and time of ocurrence of attacks. *Cephalalgia* 1984;4:53–56.
69. Sahota PK, Dexter JD. Sleep and headache syndromes: a clinical review. *Headache* 1990;30:80–84.
70. Siegel JM, Rogawski MA. A function of REM sleep: regulation of noradrenergic receptor sensitivity. *Brain Res* 1988;472:213–233.

71. Solomon S, Rose FC. General principles of management. In: Olesen J, Tfelt-Hansen P, Welch KMA, eds. *The headaches.* New York: Raven, 1993:159–164.

72. Spierings EL, Sorbi M, Haimowitz BR, Tellegen B. Changes in daily hassles, mood, and sleep in the 2 days before a migraine headache. *Clin J Pain* 1996;12:38–42.

73. The International Classification of Sleep Disorders of the American Sleep Disorders Association. *Diagnostic and coding manual.* Rochester, MN: American Sleep Disorders Association, 1997.

74. Thoman EB. Snoring, nightmares and morning headaches in elderly women: a preliminary study. *Biol Psychol* 1997;46:275–284.

75. Tsuda N, Negoro K, Fukusako T, Morimatsu M. A case of myotonic dystrophy with morning headache following sleep apnea syndrome. *No To Shinkei* 1995;47:173–176.

76. Whalen CC, Antani M, Carey J, Landfeld CS. An index of symptoms for infection with human immunodeficiency virus: reliability and validity. *J Clin Epidemiol* 1994;47:537–546.

77. Wilkinson M, Williams K, Leyton M. Observations on the treatment of actue attack of migraine. *Res Clin Study Headache* 1978;6:141–146.

78. Wolf F, Smythe H, Yunus MB, et al. The American College of Rheumatology: 1990 criteria for the classification of fibromyalgia: a report of the Multicenter Committee. *Arthritis Rheum* 1990;33:160–172.

The Headaches, Second Edition,
edited by J. Olesen, P. Tfelt-Hansen, and K.M.A. Welch.
Lippincott Williams & Wilkins, Philadelphia © 2000.

Special Problems in the Headaches and Their Management

CHAPTER 129

Headache in Patients with Medical Problems

Stephen D. Silberstein and Carl G. H. Dahlöf

Headache is such a common complaint that patients will have a wide variety of concurrent medical problems. Older patients, in particular, have more comorbid and coexistent medical illnesses (1,8), and some headache disorders, such as temporal arteritis, occur principally in the elderly. In patients 65 years of age or older with chronic medical diseases, unrelated disorders are undertreated (15). The goals of headache treatment are to relieve or prevent the pain and associated symptoms of headache disorders and to optimize the patient's ability to function normally. Drugs that are used to treat headache can be divided into two major categories: abortive and preventive. Medications are chosen from these classes based on the drug's efficacy, the patient's profile, and the presence or absence of coexisting or comorbid diseases (21).

Difficulties can arise in treating patients with coexistent medical disorders: (a) the disorder itself may be a cause of headache (the description of headache with specific organic disorders is discussed elsewhere in this book); (b) the disorder may create limitations on the use of certain classes of headache drugs or may influence drug distribution or metabolism; (c) drugs used to treat the disorder can produce headaches; and (d) drugs used to treat the disorder may interact with, prevent the use of, or decrease the effectiveness of the headache drugs. The objective of this review is to consider the management of headache disorders when they coexist with other medical conditions: cerebrovascular disease, liver and renal impair-

ment, hypertension, coronary artery disease, depression, asthma, and peptic ulcer disease.

Certain medical conditions create limitations in the use of specific migraine medications. When cerebrovascular, coronary, or peripheral vascular disease is present, the issue is potentiation of vasoconstriction and enhanced thrombosis, especially by triptans and ergots. Liver or kidney disease alters drug distribution, metabolism, and excretion, and drugs can produce further organ damage. Elderly patients have more coexistent conditions and a higher sensitivity to drugs, which complicates and limits migraine treatment options. Obesity affects drug distribution and metabolism and limits the use of drugs that produce weight gain. The triptans and ergot alkaloids (including methysergide) are contraindicated in patients with ischemic heart disease and uncontrolled hypertension. Nonsteroidal antiinflammatory drugs (NSAIDs) and aspirin must be used with caution in patients on anticoagulation therapy and those with renal or ulcer disease. The beta-blockers should be used with caution in patients with asthma, brittle diabetes, and depression. Valproate cannot be used in patients with liver disease (21).

Gender, age, and coexistent disorders may influence drug distribution or metabolism. Women often have higher plasma drug concentrations than men on the same dose, usually the result of a lower volume of distribution and reduced drug clearance (11). Differences in vascular resistance, muscle mass, and muscle composition may cause variation in absorption from intramuscular injections (17).

Aging can create treatment problems, as many elderly patients fail to take their medicine as prescribed. Over half of elderly patients make at least one drug error, and over 25% make potentially serious medication errors (16). The rate of gastric emptying is delayed, gastroin-

S. D. Silberstein: Department of Neurology, Thomas Jefferson University, and Department of Neurology, Jefferson Headache Center, Thomas Jefferson University Hospital, Philadelphia, Pennsylvania 19107-5092.

C. G. H. Dahlöf: Department of Clinical Pharmacology, Sahlgrenska University Hospital, and Gothenburg Migraine Clinic, S-41117 Göteborg, Sweden.

testinal motility is decreased, gastric pH levels increase, and active drug transport is reduced with age.

The more drugs used, the greater the possibility of undesirable pharmacokinetic and pharmacodynamic interactions. Some drugs can lower the concentrations of others by decreasing absorption. Cholestyramine and colestipol, drugs used to treat high cholesterol, can bind to and decrease the absorption of other orally administered drugs. Sucralfate (used to treat ulcer disease) can reduce phenytoin absorption. Drugs that delay gastric emptying (e.g., anticholinergics) can result in increased degradation of coadministered acid-sensitive drugs. Drugs that speed gastric emptying, such as metoclopramide, can increase the absorption of acid-unstable drugs (13) and can decrease the time-to-maximal effect of drugs that are absorbed in the small intestine. Combination headache therapy often includes metoclopramide (in combination with analgesics) to reverse the delayed gastric emptying seen with migraine.

Drugs that require active transport to reach their site of action can be blocked at their uptake site. The antihypertensive drugs guanethidine, guanadrel, and bethanidine are actively transported into adrenergic neurons by an amine transport system. Tricyclic antidepressants (TCAs), phenothiazines, and some sympathomimetic amines can interfere with this transport system and block their effects (13).

Some drugs induce a microsomal drug-metabolizing system (resulting in decreased plasma levels of hepatically metabolized drugs, such as oral contraceptives), whereas some toxins inhibit it (13). Examples of mixed function oxidase (P450) system inducers include phenobarbital, other barbiturates, phenytoin, rifampin, glutethimide, griseofulvin, ethanol, phenylbutazone, chronic smoking, some chlorinated hydrocarbons such as lindane and DDT, carbamazepine, and primidone. The metabolism of oral anticoagulants, corticosteroids, low-dose oral contraceptives, some beta-adrenergic blockers, mexiletine, and theophylline can be increased, resulting in lower plasma levels of these drugs (13).

Nonselective monoamine oxidase inhibitors (MAOIs) inhibit the metabolism of catecholamines. Serious and lethal drug reactions have resulted from interactions between MAOIs and other antidepressants, meperidine, levodopa, and oral antidiabetic drugs. Hypertensive crisis has occurred after ingestion of proscribed foods due to enhanced catecholamine release. MAOIs can also increase the plasma levels of drugs such as sumatriptan (12).

Decreased renal excretion of lithium occurs when proximal tubular reabsorption is enhanced. Dietary salt restriction, salt depletion due to diarrhea, and distally acting diuretics can reduce renal lithium excretion, producing higher lithium levels. Indomethacin and other NSAIDs also reduce lithium clearance, probably by enhancing proximal tubular reabsorption (13).

Some drug interactions are pharmacodynamic. Propranolol blocks the beta-adrenergic receptors, allowing the unopposed alpha-adrenergic effects of epinephrine, which can result in severe hypertension. Clonidine's antihypertensive effects can be blocked by TCAs. Additive negative cardiac inotropic effects of disopyramide, beta-adrenergic blockers, and calcium channel blocking drugs can produce heart failure. The additive negative chronotropic and inotropic effects of amiodarone, digoxin, beta-adrenergic blockers, and calcium channel blocking drugs can produce bradycardia, sinus arrest, or atrioventricular block.

SPECIFIC DISORDERS

See Table 1.

Cerebrovascular Disease

Stroke, subarachnoid hemorrhage, and intracranial hemorrhage are all associated with headache, and treatment is dependent on the cause of the headache. Patients with ischemic cerebrovascular disease or an unruptured aneurysm should avoid drugs that could induce vasospasm or raise blood pressure. In addition, there are anecdotal reports of migrainelike headaches due to subarachnoid headache and meningitis being successfully treated by sumatriptan and delaying the correct diagnosis. Thus, triptans, ergot alkaloids (including methysergide), and isometheptene should be avoided or used with extreme caution. NSAIDs and acetylsalicylic acid can be used with ischemic stroke but should be avoided in patients with subarachnoid or intracranial hemorrhage. Antidepressants, anticonvulsants, beta-blockers, or calcium channel blockers can be used with impunity. Pizotifen or cyproheptadine is safe, but methysergide should be used with caution, if at all (6,21,23).

Hypertension

Sudden severe increases in blood pressure can cause headache and are often life threatening. Disorders causing both headache and hypertension include malignant hypertension, pheochromocytoma, vasculitis, and vasoactive recreational drugs such as cocaine and amphetamines. Patients with controlled hypertension can be treated with most of the antimigraine medications, but overuse should be especially avoided. In patients with labile or uncontrolled hypertension, the triptans or ergot alkaloids, including methysergide, should be avoided. Beta-blockers and calcium channel blockers can be used to treat both headache and hypertension. Clonidine is useful for hypertension and opioid detoxification. Diuretics are useful for high blood pressure but not useful for headache. Angiotensin-converting enzyme (ACE) inhibitors may be useful, whereas the use of reserpine is con-

TABLE 1. *Migraine and coexistent disease*

Drug	Cerebrovascular disease		Hyper-tension	Heart disease	PVD	Asthma	Renal disease	Liver disease	PUD	Obesity	Depression
	Ischemic	Bleed									
Acute											
ASA; NSAIDS	S↑	X	S	S↑	S	C	C	S	X	S	S
Triptans	C	X	C	X	X	S	C	C	S	C	S
Ergots	C	X	C	X	X	S	C	C	S	C	S
Isometheptene	C	X	C	X	X	S	C	C	S	C	S
Butalbital	S	S	S	S	S	S	S	C	S	C	S
Opioids	S	S	S	S	S	S	S[a]	C	S	C	S
Neuroleptics	S	S	S	S	S	S	S	C	S	S	S
Preventive											
Pizotifen	S↑	S	S↑	S↑	S↑	S	S	S	S	S↓	S↓
Methysergide	C	X	C	X	X	S	C	C	S	C	S
Beta-blockers	S↑	C	S↑	S↑	S↓	C/X	S	S	S	S	S
Calcium channel blockers	S↑	S↑	S↑	S↑	S↑	S	S	S	S	S	S/X[b]
Tricyclics	S	S	S	C	S	S	S	S	S↑	S↓	S↑
SSRIs	S	S	S	S	S	S	S	S	S	S↑	S↑
Divalproex	S↑	S↑	S↑	S↑	S↑	S	S	X	S	S↓	S↑

S, safe; ↓, less likely to; ↑, most likely to; C, caution; X, contraindicated; PVD, peripheral vascular disease; PUD, peptic ulcer disease.
[a]Avoid meperidine.
[b]Avoid flunarazine.

troversial. Triptans and ergots must be used with caution, if at all, in patients with uncontrolled hypertension.

Cardiovascular Disease

Many of the drugs used to treat ischemic cardiovascular disease, particularly the nitrates and certain calcium channel blockers, can aggravate migraine. The origin of typically 5-hydroxytryptamine 1B/1D (5-HT$_{1B/1D}$) agonist-induced symptoms of tightness, heaviness, pressure, and/or pain in the chest, neck, and/or throat is still debated. Although the pathophysiology of these chest symptoms is not known, they have warranted special attention. Triptans and ergot alkaloids are contraindicated in patients with coronary artery disease because they can constrict coronary arteries. TCAs can cause alpha-adrenergic block and produce orthostatic hypotension. (This is less common with the secondary amines, nortriptyline and desipramine.) In addition, they have a quinidine-like antiarrhythmic effect and can induce conduction disturbances and need to be used with caution. Divalproex is safe in these patients, as are the selective serotonin reuptake inhibitors, which can slow cardiac conduction and may be a problem in patients with bundle branch disease (24). The beta-blockers and calcium channel blockers can be used to treat both migraine and ischemic heart disease. Cardiac patients are often treated with daily aspirin that

might preclude the use of other NSAIDs. Mitral valve prolapse, which is often associated with paroxysmal tachycardia, is frequently found in young women, who often have migraine. Beta-blockers are useful to treat both disorders (23).

Peripheral Vascular Disease

Occlusive disease of the extremities is usually due to atherosclerosis and can manifest itself by claudication, loss of pulses, and even gangrene. Raynaud's disease is attributed to vasospasm and is comorbid with migraine. Raynaud's disease is thought to be caused by increased circulating levels of the vasoconstrictor peptide endothelin-1 and impaired release of the endogenous vasodilator calcitonin gene–related peptide (3,5). In both disorders, vasoconstrictors such as ergots and triptans should be used with caution. A calcium channel blocker would be an acceptable drug in both migraine and Raynaud's.

Renal Failure

Decreased renal function produces decreased renal clearance of drugs, which may require a dosage adjustment of a renally excreted drug. The adjustment is based on the creatinine clearance and the percentage of drug cleared by the kidney. When a patient is on dialysis and the drug is removed, supplemental dosing is required. Some drugs, such as meperidine and propoxyphene (13), have active or toxic metabolites, which are normally eliminated by the kidneys. They can accumulate in patients with renal failure, producing encephalopathy. Aspirin, ergots, triptans, and NSAIDs should be avoided in patients with renal insufficiency. There is no reason to limit their use in patients who are on dialysis.

Liver Disease

Patients with liver failure often have decreased drug clearance. The liver metabolizes drugs and toxins, in part utilizing the cytochrome P450-dependent microsomal mixed function oxidase system, and conjugates them for easier elimination. Liver diseases can impair the biotransformation of exogenous substances, resulting in increased drug sensitivity (e.g., sedatives and opiates) or enhanced biologic effects. A low serum albumin level and high prothrombin time are often associated with decreased clearance of drugs metabolized by the P450 system, but with preserved elimination of drugs metabolized by conjugation. If portacaval anastomoses develop, hepatic blood flow decreases, with a possible reduction in drug clearance. Portacaval shunting can allow drugs to avoid the first-pass or presystemic elimination. If a drug is largely extracted from the blood by the liver (e.g., propranolol, metoprolol, and lidocaine), more of an orally administered dose can reach the systemic circulation (14). Divalproex should be avoided in patients with liver disease. The ergot alkaloids and acetaminophen are relatively contraindicated. Doses of acute and preventive medications that undergo hepatic metabolism need to be adjusted.

Obesity

The prevalence of obesity is high and is increasing. A link between excess weight and an increased risk of death is found in all age groups except for the elderly. Over half of American men and women over 20 years of age are now considered overweight, and one fourth are clinically obese. Being overweight is associated with an increased risk of heart disease, diabetes, and cancer (25). Patients who are markedly obese have an increased prevalence of idiopathic intracranial hypertension. The association of obesity with diabetes, hypertension, and coronary artery disease makes it a risk factor for those disorders, which must be excluded prior to the use of the vasoactive drugs. In addition, drugs that produce weight gain, such as TCAs, divalproex, cyproheptadine, and pizotifen, should be avoided. Exercise is important to prevent headache (9), to reduce weight, and to reduce the risk of death even without weight loss (25). Drugs that distribute through the total body water have a decreased volume of distribution. Drugs that are primarily distributed through the

extracellular fluid show little change in their volume of distribution. In contrast, lipid-soluble drugs (e.g., the benzodiazepines) have larger volumes of distribution due to the greater percentage of fat in elderly persons. The elimination half-life of lipid-soluble drugs is increased because of a larger volume of distribution. Elimination half-life may decrease because of decreased renal or metabolic clearance (13,21).

Peptic Ulcer Disease

Chronic peptic ulcer disease (PUD) is common, occurring with a lifetime prevalence as high as 10% in industrialized countries. PUD is now believed to be associated with *Helicobacter pylori* infections. Drugs used to treat PUD can cause headache or interact with drugs used to treat headache. The H_2 blockers can produce headache; sucralfate can interfere with drug absorption; whereas anticholinergics delay gastric emptying. NSAIDs and aspirin must be used with caution.

Asthma

Reversible airway obstruction, in part on an immune-mediated basis, is believed to be the mechanism of asthma. Asthma itself is comorbid with migraine. Some asthmatics have heightened sensitivity to acetylsalicylic acid (ASA) and other NSAIDs, which should be used with caution. The beta-blockers should be avoided because of the risk of aggravating bronchospasm. Triptans, ergots, and other preventive medications can be used safely.

Depression

Major depression has a lifetime prevalence of 5% to 20% and is comorbid with migraine. Drugs such as barbiturates, benzodiazapenes, beta-blockers, corticosteroids, and estrogen have been associated with depression and must be used with caution.

SUMMARY

The goals of treatment are to relieve or prevent the pain and associated symptoms of migraine and to optimize the patient's ability to function normally. The medications used to treat migraine can be divided into two major categories: abortive and preventive. A drug is chosen based on its efficacy, the patient's profile, and the presence or absence of coexisting or comorbid disease (Table 2). The choice of drug is made based on the best risk-to-benefit ratio for the individual patient and the side effect profile of the drug. An underweight patient would be a candidate for one of the medications that commonly produce weight gain, such as a TCA; in contrast, one would avoid these drugs in the overweight patient. Sedating tertiary TCAs

TABLE 2. *Migraine and comorbid disease*

Cardiovascular
    Hyper- or hypotension
    Raynaud's
    Mitral valve prolapse
    Angina/myocardial infarction
    Stroke
Psychiatric
    Depression
    Mania
    Panic disorder
    Anxiety disorder
Neurologic
    Epilepsy
Gastrointestinal
    Functional bowel disorders
Other
    Asthma
    Allergies

would be useful at bedtime for patients with insomnia. In the athletic patient, beta-blockers should be avoided. Medication that can impair cognitive functioning should be avoided in patients who are dependent on their wits (e.g., truck drivers) [18].

Comorbid and coexistent diseases have important implications for treatment. The presence of a second illness provides therapeutic opportunities but also imposes certain therapeutic limitations. In some instances, two or more conditions may be treated with a single drug. When migraine and hypertension or angina occur together, beta-blockers or calcium channel blockers may be effective for all conditions [22]. For the patient with migraine and depression, TCAs or selective serotonin reuptake inhibitors (SSRIs) may be especially useful [19]. For the patient with migraine and epilepsy [7,10], or migraine and manic depressive illness [2,4], divalproex sodium is the drug of choice. The pregnant migraineur who has a comorbid condition that needs treatment should be given a medication that is effective for both conditions and has the lowest potential for adverse effects on the fetus. In individuals with more than one disease, certain categories of treatment may be relatively contraindicated. For example, beta-blockers should be used with caution in the depressed migraineur, whereas TCAs, neuroleptics, or sumatriptan may lower the seizure threshold and should be used with caution in the epileptic migraineur [18].

Ergot alkaloids, triptans, and other vasoconstrictors such as isometheptane mucate (present in Midrin [Carnrick Labs, London]) [14] must be used with caution if at all in patients with cardiovascular disease, uncontrolled hypertension, and recent stroke because these drugs may cause vasoconstriction. Benzodiazepines and barbiturates may cause excessive sedation; the long-acting benzodiazepines, in particular, may cause excessive side effects due to slowed metabolic clearance in the elderly or in

patients with liver impairment. Antiemetic drugs and neuroleptics are more likely to cause tardive dyskinesia in the elderly and in men with neuroleptic malignant male syndrome. NSAIDs may cause cognitive side effects and are associated with an increased risk of gastrointestinal bleeding in the elderly and must be used with caution in patients with renal failure [21].

Preventive treatments also may cause more side effects and be less well tolerated in the presence of coexistent disease. Therefore, they should be started at a very low dose and slowly increased. The tertiary amine TCAs, such as amitriptyline and doxepin, which are potent anticholinergic agents, can delay gastric emptying and have adverse cardiac effects. They need to be used with caution in the elderly because they can exacerbate glaucoma, produce visual blurring, and cause problems with cognition. The SSRIs are safe in the elderly and in patients with cardiac disease. Antihypertensive drugs may cause more hypotension or lethargy in the elderly than in younger patients. Divalproex sodium has a particularly good benefit–to–side effect profile in the elderly. Methysergide and methylergonovine are relatively contraindicated in the elderly because they are vasoconstrictors and should be avoided, especially in patients with uncontrolled hypertension or coronary artery disease [20].

In patients with severe medical disorders, nonpharmacologic treatment is attractive because it avoids medications that may present risks or cause excessive side effects. Elimination of triggers, proper diet, regular sleep, and avoidance of excess caffeine are useful in all patients. Biofeedback may not be as effective in the elderly patient. The most important nonpharmacologic approach involves the meticulous identification and treatment of comorbid medical and psychiatric conditions. Cervical triggers and other sources of pain should be treated with physical modalities if possible. Depression is extremely common and should be addressed.

REFERENCES

1. Baumel B, Eisner LS. Diagnosis and treatment of headache in the elderly. *Med Clin North Am* 1991;75:661–675.
2. Bowden CL, Brugger AM, Swann AC. Efficacy of divalproex vs lithium and placebo in the treatment of mania. *JAMA* 1994;271: 918–924.
3. Bunker CB, Goldsmith PC, Leslie TA, Hayes N, Foreman JC, Dowd PM. Calcitonin gene-related peptide, endothelin-1, the cutaneous microvasculature and Raynaud's phenomenon. *Br J Dermatol* 1998; 134:399–406.
4. Curran DA, Hinterberger H, Lance JW. Methysergide. *Res Clin Stud Headache* 1967;1:74–122.
5. Dowd PM, Goldsmith PC, Chopra S, Bull HA, Foreman JC. Cutaneous responses to endothelin-1 and histamine in patients with vibration white finger. *J Invest Dermatol* 1998;110:127–131.
6. Goadsby PJ. Management of headache patients with medical problems. In: Olesen J, Tfelt-Hansen P, Welch KMA, eds. *The headaches.* New York: Raven, 1993:843–847.
7. Hering R, Kuritzky A. Sodium valproate has a prophylactic effect in migraine: a double-blind study vs placebo. *Cephalalgia* 1992;12:81–84.
8. Lipton RB, Pfeffer D, Newman L, Solomon S. Headaches in the elderly. *J Pain Symptom Mgmt* 1993;8:87–97.

9. Lockett DM, Campbell JF. The effects of aerobic exercise on migraine. *Headache* 1992;32:50–54.

10. Mathew NT, Saper JR, Silberstein SD, et al. Prophylaxis of migraine headaches with divalproex sodium. *Arch Neurol* 1995;52:2816.

11. Matthews HW. Racial, ethnic and gender differences in response to medicines. In: Matthews HW, ed. *Drug metabolism and drug interactions.* Freund Publishing House, 1995:77–91.

12. Medical Economics Company. *Physicians' desk reference,* 52nd ed. Montvale, NJ: Medical Economics Company, 1998:1.

13. Nies AS. Interactions between drugs. In: Wyngaarden JB, Smith LH Jr, Bennett JC, eds. *Cecil textbook of medicine,* 19th ed. Philadelphia: WB Saunders, 1991:92–99.

14. Nies AS. Principles of drug therapy. In: Wyngaarden JB, Smith LH Jr, Bennett JC, eds. *Cecil textbook of medicine,* 19th ed. Philadelphia: WB Saunders, 1991:81–91.

15. Redelmeier DA, Siew HT, Booth GL. The treatment of unrelated disorders in patients with chronic medical diseases. *N Engl J Med* 1998;338:1516–1520.

16. Schwartz D, Wang M, Geitz L. Medication errors made by elderly chronically ill patients. *Am J Public Health* 1962;52:2018–2029.

17. Silberstein SD. Drug treatments and trials in women. In: Kaplan PW, ed. *Neurologic disease in women.* New York: Demos Vermande, 1998:25–44.

18. Silberstein SD, Lipton RB. Overview of diagnosis and treatment of migraine. *Neurology* 1994;44:6–15.

19. Silberstein SD, Lipton RB, Breslau N. Migraine: association with personality characteristics and psyshopathology. *Cephalalgia* 1995;15:337–369.

20. Silberstein SD, Lipton RB, Goadsby PJ. *Headache in clinical practice.* Oxford: Isis Medical Media, 1998.

21. Silberstein SD, Young WB. Headache. In: Pathy MSJ, ed. *Principles and practice of geriatric medicine.* John Wiley & Sons, 1998:733–746.

22. Solomon GD. Management of the headache patient with medical illness. *Clin J Pain* 1989;5:95–99.

23. Solomon GD. Concomitant medical disease and headache. *Med Clin North Am* 1991;75:631–639.

24. Sutor B, Rummans TA, Jowsey SG, et al. Major depression in medically ill patients. *Mayo Clin Proc* 1998;73:329–337.

25. Wickelgren I. Obesity. How big a problem? *Science* 1998;280:1364–1367.

The Headaches, Second Edition,
edited by J. Olesen, P. Tfelt-Hansen, and K.M.A. Welch.
Lippincott Williams & Wilkins, Philadelphia © 2000.

Special Problems in the Headaches and Their Management

CHAPTER 130

Headache during Migraine, Pregnancy, and Lactation

Stephen D. Silberstein and Hélène Massiou

DRUGS AND PREGNANCY: OVERVIEW

It used to be believed that the placenta served as a barrier that protected the fetus from drugs and toxins (11). However, the recognition of the teratogenicity of aminopterin and thalidomide and the rubella epidemic of 1963 to 1964 changed this perception and resulted in the recommendation of extremely conservative drug use during pregnancy (24). In 1977 the U.S. Food and Drug Administration (FDA) developed a policy against phase I and early phase II testing in pregnant women or in women of childbearing potential, and many practitioners now avoid drug treatment in pregnancy even when it is indicated. The FDA has tested over 3,000 drugs, and only 20 are known human teratogens. There is insufficient knowledge about birth defect risks from drug exposure despite the fact that 67% of women take drugs during pregnancy and 50% take them during the first trimester (18). Most drugs cross the placenta and have the potential to adversely affect the fetus.

A negative pregnancy test is often a condition of enrollment in a study, whereas postenrollment pregnancy can lead to termination of participation. This poses a problem for pregnant women who are sick and in need of treatment. If a drug has not been tested in pregnant women during the research phase, information is lacking about the safety and efficacy of the drug for the woman as well as the fetus (14). The Institute of Medicine Committee on Research in

Women made the controversial recommendation that pregnant and lactating women be considered eligible for enrollment in clinical studies on a routine basis (14).

With more women of childbearing age participating in clinical trials, more information will be gained about the risks of birth defects, but uncertainty will still persist. However, if the medication is associated with a high level of birth defects (e.g., thalidomide), few exposures need to be followed to detect this risk; if the medication is associated with a slight increase in the overall occurrence of birth defects, approximately 300 exposed pregnancies need to be followed to detect a doubling of risk; and if the medication is associated with a rare increase of a specific defect (e.g., 1 in 1,000), approximately 10,000 exposed pregnancies need to be followed to detect a doubling of risk (1).

EPIDEMIOLOGY

The World Health Organization completed an international survey of 14,778 pregnant women on prescription drug utilization during pregnancy. Eighty-six percent of the subjects took medication, each receiving an average of 2.9 prescriptions. Of a total of 37,309 prescriptions, 73% were given by obstetricians, 12% by general practitioners, and 5% by midwives (3). In a survey of pregnant women at Parkland Memorial Hospital in Dallas, 40% took some type of medication other than iron or vitamin supplements, and up to 20% used an illicit drug or alcohol (12). The National Hospital Discharge Survey found that there was a 576% increase in discharges of drug-using parturient women and a 456% increase in discharges of drug-affected newborns in the United States between 1979 and 1990.

S. D. Silberstein: Department of Neurology, Thomas Jefferson University, and Department of Neurology, Jefferson Headache Center, Thomas Jefferson University Hospital, Philadelphia, Pennsylvania 19107-5092.

H. Massiou: Department of Neurology, Hôpital Lariboisière, 75475 Paris, France.

Adverse Effects

Adverse drug effects depend on the dose and route of administration, concomitant exposures, and the timing of the exposure relative to the period of development, which consist of the preimplantation period, embryogenesis, and fetal development. The preimplantation period lasts from conception to 1 week postconception, during which time the conceptus is relatively protected from drugs (12). Embryogenesis is the time of organogenesis, which occurs from the time of implantation to 60 days postconception (12). Most congenital malformations arise during this time. Placental transport is not well established until the 5th week after conception. This protects the embryo from maternal drugs. The final phase, fetal development, follows embryogenesis. The fetus grows mainly in size, although structural changes such as neuronal arrangement also occur. Malformations can develop at this time in normally formed organs due to their necrosis and reabsorption (12).

Death to the conceptus, teratogenicity, fetal growth abnormalities, perinatal effects, postnatal developmental abnormalities, delayed oncogenesis, and functional and behavioral changes can result from drugs or other agents (Table 1) (9). According to the Perinatal Collaborative Project, a prospective and concurrent epidemiologic study of more than 50,000 pregnancies, many drugs have little or no human teratogenic risk (2,9).

Spontaneous Abortion

Nearly half of early pregnancies spontaneously abort, most due to chromosomal abnormalities. Prior to the time of organogenesis, exposure to a potential teratogen or toxic drug has an all-or-none effect. An exposure around the time of conception or implantation may kill the con-

ceptus, but if the pregnancy continues, there is no increased risk of congenital anomalies (2).

Developmental Defects

Developmental defects may result from genetic or environmental causes, or from interactions between them. Teratogenic drug effects are generally visible anatomic malformations; they are defined as the production of a permanent alteration of an organ's structure or function due to intrauterine exposure. These effects are dose and time related, with the fetus at greatest risk during the first trimester of pregnancy. Drug exposure accounts for only 2% to 3% of birth defects: approximately 25% are genetic, and the causes of the remainder are unknown (2). The incidence of major malformations either incompatible with survival or requiring major surgery is approximately 2% to 3% in the general population. If all minor malformations are included (ear tags or extra digits), the rate may be as high as 7% to 10%. The risk of malformation after drug exposure must be compared with this background rate.

The classic teratogenic period in the human is a critical 6 weeks, lasting from approximately 31 days through 10 weeks from the last menstrual period. A teratogenic effect depends on the timing of the exposure as well as the nature of the teratogen. Exposure early in the pregnancy, when the heart and central nervous system are forming, may result in an anomaly such as congenital heart disease or neural tube defect, whereas later exposure may result in malformation of the palate or ear (2). Once the teratogenic period has passed, the major risk of congenital anomaly is gone, but other abnormalities can occur. These include fetal effects, neonatal effects, and postnatal effects.

Fetal, Neonatal, and Postnatal Effects

Fetal effects include damage to normally formed organs, damage to systems undergoing histogenesis, growth retardation, or fetal death. Growth retardation is the most common of these. Certain drugs are associated with adverse neonatal effects, such as drug withdrawal and neonatal hypoglycemia, or adverse maternal effects, such as hemostasis and uterine contracture disorders. Chronic exposure to psychoactive medications, such as alcohol, during the second and third trimesters may cause mental retardation, which may not be recognized until later in life (2). Developmental delay and long-term cognitive dysfunction have been reported in children born to mothers who took antiepileptic drugs (AEDs) during pregnancy. Delayed oncogenesis also can occur with exposure to diethylstilbestrol as late as 20 weeks' gestation and may cause reproductive organ anomalies that are not recognized until after puberty.

Drug Risk Categories

The FDA lists five categories of labeling for drug use in pregnancy (Table 2) (3,15,18). These categories are

TABLE 1. *Definitions and drug effects*

Spontaneous abortion	Death of the conceptus; mostly due to chromosomal abnormality
Embryotoxicity	The ability of drugs to kill the developing embryo
Congenital anomalies	Deviation from normal morphology or function
Teratogenicity	The ability of an exogenous agent to produce a permanent abnormality of structure or function in an organism exposed during embryogenesis or fetal life
Fetal effects	Growth retardation, abnormal histogenesis (also congenital abnormalities and fetal death); the main outcome of fetal drug toxicity during the second and third trimester of pregnancy
Perinatal effects	Effects on uterine contraction, neonatal withdrawal, or hemostasis
Postnatal effects	Drugs may have delayed long-term effects; delayed oncogenesis, and functional and behavioral abnormalities

TABLE 2. FDA risk categories

Category A	Controlled human studies show no risk
Category B	No evidence of risk in humans, but there are no controlled human studies
Category C	Risk to humans has not been ruled out
Category D	Positive evidence of risk to humans from human or animal studies
Category X	Contraindicated in pregnancy

intended to provide therapeutic guidance, weighing the risks as well as the benefits of the drug. Although this system is an improvement over previous labeling, it is still not ideal. Tricyclic antidepressants are still classified as class D, even though the evidence suggests they are safe (11). An alternate rating system is TERIS, an automated teratogen information resource wherein the rating for each drug or agent is based on a consensus of expert opinion and the literature (Table 3) (8). It was designed to assess the teratogenic risk to the fetus from a drug exposure. The FDA categories have little, if any, correlation to the TERIS teratogenic risk. This discrepancy results in part from the fact that the FDA categories were designed to provide therapeutic guidance and the TERIS ratings are useful for estimating the teratogenic risks of a drug and not vice versa (7).

Prevention

A woman's risk of having a child with a neural tube defect is associated with early pregnancy red cell folate levels in a continuous dose-response relationship (5). Low serum and red blood cell folate levels are associated with spontaneous abortion and fetal malformations in animals and in humans (6,10,17,18,21). Treatment with some drugs, including carbamazepine and barbiturates, can impair folate absorption. Valproic acid does not produce folate deficiency, but it may interfere with the production of folinic acid by inhibiting glutamate formyl transferase (25). The current guidelines suggest increasing folic acid intake by 4 mg, which would result in a 48% reduction in neural tube defects (5).

Migraine Treatment

The major concerns in the management of the pregnant migraineur are the effects of both medication and mi-

TABLE 3. TERIS risk rating

N	None (A)
N–Min	None–minimal (A)
Min	Minimal (B)
Min–S	Minimal–small (D)
S	Small ( )
S–Mod	Small–Moderate ( )
Mod	Moderate ( )
H	High (X)
U	Undetermined (C)

Equivalent FDA ratings in parentheses.

graine on the fetus. Because of the possible risk of injury to the fetus, medication use should be limited; however, it is not contraindicated during pregnancy (18,19). Because migraine usually improves after the first trimester, many women can manage their headaches with this reassurance and nonpharmacologic means of coping, such as ice, massage, and biofeedback (18,22,23). Some women, however, will continue to have severe, intractable headaches, sometimes associated with nausea, vomiting, and possible dehydration. Not only are these conditions disruptive to the patient, they may pose a risk to the fetus that is greater than the potential risk of the medications used to treat the pregnant patient (19,22).

Symptomatic treatment, designed to reduce the severity and duration of symptoms, is used to treat an acute headache attack (Tables 4–6). Individual attacks should be treated with rest, reassurance, and ice packs. For headaches that do not respond to nonpharmacologic treatment, symptomatic drugs are indicated. Nonsteroidal anti-inflammatory drugs (NSAIDs), acetaminophen (alone or with codeine), codeine alone, or other narcotics can be used during pregnancy (11). Aspirin in low intermittent doses is not a significant teratogenic risk, although large doses, especially if given near term, may be associated with maternal and fetal bleeding. Aspirin should probably be reserved unless there is a definite therapeutic need for it (other than headache). In general, NSAIDs may be taken safely for pain during the first trimester of pregnancy. However, their use should be limited during pregnancy because some NSAIDs may constrict or close the fetal ductus arteriosus (11). Byron (4) believes that the

TABLE 4. Analgesics and narcotics

	FDA	Teris	Lactation
Simple analgesics			
Aspirin	C[a]	N–Min	Caution
Acetaminophen	B	N	Compatible
Caffeine	B	N–Min	Compatible
NSAIDS			
Fenoprofen	B[a]	U	Compatible
Ibuprofen	B[a]	N–Min	Compatible
Indomethacin	B[a]	N	Compatible
Ketorolac	B[a]	U	Caution
Meclofenamate	B[a]	U	Compatible
Naproxen	B[a]	U	Compatible
Sulindac	B[a]	U	Compatible
Tolmetin	B[a]	U	Compatible
Narcotics			
Butorphanol	B[b]	N–Min	Compatible
Codeine	C[b]	N–Min	Compatible
Hydromorphone	B[b]	N–Min	Compatible
Meperidine	B[b]	N–Min	Compatible
Methadone	B[b]	N–Min	Compatible
Morphine	B[b]	N–Min	Compatible
Propoxyphene	C[b]	N–Min	Compatible

[a]D if third trimester.
[b]D if prolonged or at term.

TABLE 5. *Ergots and serotonin agonists*

	FDA	Teris	Lactation
Ergots			
Ergotamine	X	Min	Contraindicated
Dihydroergotamine	X	U	Contraindicated
Methylergonovine	C	U	Caution
Methysergide	D	U	Caution
Triptans			
Naratriptan	C	U	Caution
Rizatriptan	C	U	Caution
Sumatriptan	C	U	Caution
Zolmitriptan	C	U	Caution

most potent inhibitors of prostaglandin synthesis, such as salicylates and indomethacin, should be avoided throughout pregnancy if possible, and certainly during the last trimester. Barbiturate and benzodiazepine use should be limited. Ergotamine, dihydroergotamine, and sumatriptan should be avoided (18,23).

The associated symptoms of migraine, such as nausea and vomiting, can be as disabling as the headache pain itself. In addition, some medications that are used to treat migraine can produce nausea. Metoclopramide, which decreases the gastric atony seen with migraine and enhances the absorption of coadministered medications, is extremely useful in migraine treatment (24). Mild nausea can be treated with phosphorylated carbohydrate solution (emetrol) or doxylamine succinate and vitamin B6 (pyridoxine) (11,24). More severe nausea may require the use of injections or suppositories. Trimethobenzamide, chlorpromazine, prochlorperazine, and promethazine are available orally, parenterally, and by suppository and can all be used safely. We frequently use promethazine and prochlorper-

TABLE 6. *Neuroleptics, antiemetics, and corticosteroids*

	FDA	Teris	Lactation
Neuroleptics			
Phenothiazines			
Chlorpromazine	C	N–Min	Concern
Prochlorperazine	C	N	Compatible
Promethazine	C	N	NA
Promazine	C	U	NA
Butyrophenones			
Haloperidol	C	N–Min	Concern
Thioxanthenes			
Thiothixene	C	U	NA
Other			
Metoclopramide	B	N–Min	Concern
Antiemetics			
Emetrol	B	U	Compatible
Doxylamine and vitamin B6	B	N	NA
Trimethobenzamide	C	N–Min	NA
Corticosteroids			
Cortisone	D	N–Min	Compatible
Dexamethasone	C	N–Min	Compatible
Prednisone	B	N–Min	Compatible

azine suppositories. Corticosteroids can be used occasionally. Some use prednisone in preference to dexamethasone (which crosses the placenta more readily). Domperidone is an antiemetic used outside the United States. In the United Kingdom (13) its use is not advised during pregnancy, because of variable embryotoxic effects in animal tests. In France, on the contrary, the product summary indicates no teratogenicity in animals or humans. Minimal amounts are transferred in breast milk.

Severe acute attacks of migraine should be treated aggressively (19,20). In the United States we start intravenous (i.v.) fluids for hydration and then use prochlorperazine 10 mg i.v. to control both nausea and head pain. Intravenous narcotics or i.v. corticosteroids can supplement this. This is an extremely effective way of handling status migrainosus during pregnancy. In France, instead of neuroleptics or corticosteroids, infusions of amitriptyline are used except during the third trimester.

Preventive Treatment

Increased frequency and severity of migraine associated with nausea and vomiting may justify the use of daily prophylactic, or preventive, medication. This treatment option should be a last resort and used only with the consent of the patient and her partner after the risks have been completely explained. Preventive therapy is designed to reduce the frequency and severity of headache attacks. Prophylaxis should be considered when patients experience at least three or four prolonged, severe attacks a month that are particularly incapacitating or unresponsive to symptomatic therapy and may result in dehydration and fetal distress (23). Beta-adrenergic blockers such as propranolol have been used under these circumstances, although adverse effects, including intrauterine growth retardation, have been reported (11,24). If the migraine is so severe that drug treatment is essential, the patient should be told of the risks posed by all the drugs that are used (Tables 7 and 8) (23).

TABLE 7. *Sedatives, hypnotics, and antihistamines*

	FDA	Teris	Lactation
Antihistamines			
Cyclizine	B	U	NA
Cyproheptadine	B	U	Contraindicated
Dimenhydrinate	B	U	NA
Meclizine	B	N–Min	NA
Barbiturates			
Butalbital	C	N–Min	Caution
Phenobarbital	C	N–Min	Caution
Benzodiazepam			
Chlordiazepoxide	D	N–Min	Concern
Clonazepam	D	U	Concern
Diazepam	D	N–Min	Concern
Lorazepam	D	U	Concern
Other			
Zolpidem	B	U	Not recommended

TABLE 8. *Anticonvulsants, antidepressants, and antihypertensives*

	FDA	Teris	Lactation
Anticonvulsants			
Carbamazepine	C	S	Compatible
Gabapentin	C	U	Uncertain
Phenytoin	D	S–Mod	Compatible
Valproic acid	D	S–Mod	Compatible
Antidepressants			
Tricyclics			
Amitriptyline	D	N–Min	Concern
Doxepin	C	U	Concern
Nortriptyline	D	U	Concern
Protriptyline	C	U	Concern
SSRIs			
Fluoxetine	B	N	Caution
Paroxetine	C	U	Concern?
Sertraline	B	U	Concern?
Monoamine oxidase inhibitors			
Phenelzine	C	U	Concern
Antihypertensives			
Beta-blockers			
Atenolol	C	U	Compatible
Metoprolol	B	U	Compatible
Nadolol	C	U	Compatible
Propranolol	C	U	Compatible
Timolol	C	U	Compatible
Adrenergic blockers			
Clonidine	C	U	Compatible
Calcium channel blockers			
Verapamil	C	U	Compatible

If the patient has a coexistent illness that requires treatment, one drug should be chosen that will treat both disorders. For example, propranolol and perhaps the tricyclic antidepressants (11) can be used to treat hypertension and migraine, whereas fluoxetine can be used to treat comorbid depression.

Drug Exposure

During pregnancy, the patient's neurologist and obstetrician should work together. If a woman inadvertently takes a drug while she is pregnant or becomes pregnant while taking a drug, the dose, timing, and duration of the exposure(s) should be determined. The patient's past and present state of health and the presence of mental retardation or chromosomal abnormalities in the family should be ascertained. Using a reliable source of information (such as TERIS), it must be determined whether the drug is a known teratogen (although for many drugs this is not possible) (2,3,8,12).

If the drug is teratogenic or the risk is unknown, the obstetrician should confirm the gestational age by ultrasonography. If the exposure occurred during embryogenesis, then high-resolution ultrasonography can be performed to determine whether damage to specific organ

systems or structures has occurred. If the results of high-resolution ultrasonography are normal, it is reasonable to reassure the patient that the gross fetal structure is normal (within the 90% sensitivity of the study) (12). However, fetal ultrasonography cannot exclude minor anomalies or guarantee the birth of a normal child. Delays in achieving developmental milestones, including cognitive development, are potential risks, especially for children born to epileptics, that cannot be predicted or diagnosed prenatally. The obstetrician should discuss the results of these studies with the mother and the significant other; formal prenatal counseling may be helpful in uncertain cases (12).

Breastfeeding

Milk is a suspension of fat and protein in a carbohydrate-mineral solution. A nursing mother secretes 600 mL of milk per day containing sufficient protein, fat, and carbohydrate to meet the nutritional demands of the growing and developing infant (26). The transport of a drug into milk depends on its lipid solubility, molecular weight, degree of ionization, protein binding, and the presence or absence of active secretion. Species differences in the composition of milk can result in differences in drug transfer. Because human milk has a much higher pH (usually >7.0) than cow's milk (usually <6.8), bovine drug transfer data may not be accurate in humans.

Many drugs can be detected in breast milk at levels that are not of clinical significance to the infant. The concentration of drug in breast milk is a variable fraction of the maternal blood level. The infant dose is usually 1.2% of the maternal dose, which is usually trivial. Any exposure to a toxic drug or potential allergen may be inappropriate.

Classification of Drugs Used During Lactation

The American Academy of Pediatrics Committee on Drugs has reviewed drugs in lactation and categorized the drugs as follows (16): (a) contraindicated; (b) requires temporary cessation of breastfeeding; (c) effects unknown but may be of concern; (d) use with caution; and (e) usually compatible. When prescribing drugs to lactating women, the following procedure should be followed. First, it should be ascertained whether the drug is necessary. If so, the safest drug should be used, for example, acetaminophen instead of aspirin. If there is a possibility that a drug may present a risk to the infant (e.g., phenytoin or phenobarbital), the infant's blood level may be measured. Drug exposure to the nursing infant may be minimized by having the mother take the medication just after completing a breastfeeding.

The migraineur who is breastfeeding should avoid bromocriptine, ergotamine, and lithium, and use sumatriptan, benzodiazepam, antidepressants, and neuroleptics cautiously. Acetaminophen is compatible with breastfeeding and is preferred to aspirin. Moderate caffeine use is compatible with breastfeeding. However, accumulation may occur in infants whose mothers use excessive amounts. Opioids can be used by women who are breastfeeding. Phenobarbital has caused sedation in some nursing infants and it should be given to nursing mothers with caution.

REFERENCES

1. Andrews EB. Use of observational methods to monitor the safety of marketed medications for risks of birth defects. Proceedings from the Food and Drug Administration Conference on Regulated Products and Pregnant Women, 1994.
2. Blake DA, Niebyl JR. Requirements and limitations in reproductive and teratogenic risk assessment. In: Niebyl JR, ed. *Drug use in pregnancy,* 2nd ed. Philadelphia: Lea & Febiger, 1988:1–9.
3. Briggs GG, Freeman RK, Yaffe SJ. *Drugs in pregnancy and lactation,* 4th ed. Baltimore: Williams & Wilkins, 1994.
4. Byron MA. Prescribing in pregnancy: treatment of rheumatic disease. *BMJ* 1987;294:236–238.
5. Daly LE, Kirke PN, Molloy A, Weir DG, Scott JM. Folate levels and neural tube defects: implications for prevention. *JAMA* 1995;274: 1698–1702.
6. Dansky LV, Andermann E, Rosenblatt D, Sherwin AL, Andermann F. Anticonvulsants, folate levels, and pregnancy outcome: a prospective study. *Ann Neurol* 1987;21:176–182.
7. Friedman JM, Little BB, Brent RL, Cordero JF, Hanson JW, Shepard TH. Potential human teratogenicity of frequently prescribed drugs. *Obstet Gynecol* 1990;75:594–599.
8. Friedman JM, Polifka JE. *Teratogenic effects of drugs: a resource for clinicians (TERIS).* Baltimore: Johns Hopkins University Press, 1994.
9. Heinonen OP, Slone S, Shapiro S. *Birth defects and drugs in pregnancy.* Littleton, MA: Publishing Sciences Group, 1977.
10. Jordan RL, Wilson JG, Shumacher HJ. Embryotoxicity of the folate antagonist methotrexate in rats and rabbits. *Teratology* 1977;15: 73–80.
11. Koren G, Pastuszak A, Ito S. Drugs in pregnancy. *N Engl J Med* 1998; 338:1128–1137.
12. Little BB, Gilstrap LC. Counseling and evaluation of the drug-exposed pregnant patient. In: Gilstrap LC, ed. *Drugs and pregnancy.* New York: Elsevier, 1992:23–29.
13. MacGregor A. Treatment of migraine during pregnancy. *IHS News Headache* 1994;4:3–9.
14. Macklin, R. Ethical conflicts and practical realities. Proceedings from the Food and Drug Administration conference on regulated products and pregnant women, 1994.
15. Medical Economics Company. *Physicians' desk reference,* 52nd ed. Montvale, NJ: Medical Economics Company, 1998:1.
16. Murray L, Seger D. Drug therapy during pregnancy and lactation. *Emerg Med Clin North Am* 1994;12:129–149.
17. Ogawa Y, Kaneko S, Otani K, Fukushima Y. Serum folic acid levels in epileptic mothers and their relationship to congenital malformations. *Epilepsy Res* 1991;8:75–78.
18. Pitkin RM. Drug treatment of the pregnant woman: the state of the art. Proceedings from the Food and Drug Administration conference on regulated products and pregnant women, 1995.
19. Raskin NH. Migraine treatment. In: Raskin NH, ed. *Headache,* 2nd ed. New York: Churchill-Livingstone, 1988.
20. Rayburn WF, Lavin JP. Drug prescribing for chronic medical disorders during pregnancy: an overview. *Am J Obstet Gynecol* 1986;155:565.
21. Reynolds EH. Anticonvulsants, folic acid and epilepsy. *Lancet* 1973; 1:1376–1378.
22. Silberstein SD. Appropriate use of abortive medication in headache treatment. *Pain Mgmt* 1991;4:22–28.
23. Silberstein SD. Headaches and women: treatment of the pregnant and lactating migraineur. *Headache* 1993;33:533.
24. Silberstein SD. Migraine and pregnancy. *Neurol Clin* 1997;15:209–231.
25. Wegner C, Nau H. Alteration of embryonic folate metabolism by valproic acid during organogenesis: implications for mechanism of teratogenesis. *Neurology* 1992;42:17–24.
26. Yerby MS, Friel PN, McCormick K. Antiepileptic drug disposition during pregnancy. *Neurology* 1992;42:12–16.

The Headaches, Second Edition,
edited by J. Olesen, P. Tfelt-Hansen, and K.M.A. Welch.
Lippincott Williams & Wilkins, Philadelphia © 2000.

Special Problems in the Headaches and Their Management

CHAPTER 131

The Complex Chronic Patient

Mixed Headache and Drug Overuse

Seymour Solomon and Markus Färkkilä

THE COMPLEX CHRONIC HEADACHE

Two main overlapping groups may be considered complex chronic headaches. One is the mixed headache (particularly migraine and tension-type headache), and the other is chronic tension-type headache or chronic daily headache (CDH). Migraine and tension-type headache may occur at different times in the same patient, but this is not mixed headache. The term "mixed headache" usually refers to the coexistence of symptoms of migraine and episodic tension-type headache during the same episode of headache. Other primary headaches may occur together, but rarely: the migraine-cluster headache syndrome and the tic-cluster headache syndrome (30,31). Not uncommonly a bout of headache will begin as a tension-type headache and then evolve into migraine. A headache may start as a steady ache and become throbbing or begin on one side and become generalized. Headaches with both qualities should be coded as both migraine and episodic tension-type headache. In some instances, episodes of migraine occur on a base of chronic daily tension-type headaches. This is particularly noted in the posttraumatic/postconcussion syndrome. Treatment of the mixed headache is directed to the major component or to both features. For example, prophylaxis

of mixed migraine/tension-type headaches might consist of both a beta-blocker and tricyclic antidepressant.

Chronic tension-type headaches or CDH are among the most challenging problems in the headache field. We will use the term "chronic daily headache" instead of "chronic tension-type headache" (11). Although both terms include headaches occurring more than 15 days per month, CDH connotes the more common frequency of daily or almost daily headache. CDHs are primary headaches not secondary to other disease. The headache of a brain tumor or other structural or metabolic disease of the brain may be chronic and daily, but these headaches are excluded from this discussion, as is posttraumatic/postconcussion headache. Hemicrania continua has been discussed elsewhere in this text and can be distinguished from other CDHs by the site of pain locked to one side. Different subtypes of CDH (29) have been proposed and are listed in Table 1. Most headaches of this type seen in specialized headache clinics have evolved from migraine (19,21). In a population-based study, the CHDs usually evolved from episodic tension-type headache (4). Older longitudinal studies showed that with time migraine may lose its typical features and evolve into tension-type headache (22). As frequency increases, intensity of pain and the associated symptoms of photophobia and nausea decrease. A small number of CDHs begin *de novo* and are termed "new daily persistent headache" (38). In all forms of CDH, analgesics, ergotamines, or other medications designed to be used for episodes of headache are often overused and appear to cause or perpetuate CDH (18).

S. Solomon: Department of Neurology, Albert Einstein College of Medicine, and Headache Unit, Department of Neurology, Montefiore Medical Center, Bronx, New York 10467.

M. Färkkilä: Department of Neurology, University of Helsinki, and Department of Neurology, Meilahti Hospital, 00290 Helsinki, Finland.

TABLE 1. *Proposed headache classification for chronic daily headache*

Daily or near-daily headache lasting >4 hours/day for >15 days/month
    1.8 Transformed migraine
        1.8.1 with medication overuse
        1.8.2 without medication overuse
    2.2 Chronic tension-type headache
        2.2.1 with medication overuse
        2.2.2 without medication overuse
    4.7 New daily persistent headache
        4.7.1 with medication overuse
        4.7.2 without medication overuse
    4.8 Hemicrania continua
        4.8.1 with medication overuse
        4.8.2 without medication overuse

Data From Silberstein et al. (28).

Prevalence

Epidemiologic studies in Denmark and in Germany indicate that 3% of the population have chronic tension-type headache (8,26). In Spain, using smaller samples the incidence was 2.5% (4). Two thirds of people with CDH were classified as having chronic tension-type headache and only one third were classified as having transformed migraine. Medication overuse was recorded in 18.4% of those with chronic tension-type headache and in 40.9% of those with transformed migraine. This is in contrast to studies from headache centers in the United States and Italy where patients with CDHs had transformed from migraine in 77% and 71%, respectively (19,21). Analgesic or ergotamine overuse was noted in 52% and 59%, respectively. The discrepancies are probably due to the differences between a population-based study and those from specialized headache clinics.

Clinical Features

The clinical features of 100 consecutive patients with CDH were analyzed from an U.S. headache center (32). Patients were included in the study if they had headaches at least 6 days per week for at least 6 months. The study population was composed of 68 females and 32 males whose ages when first seen at the headache center ranged from 11 to 82 years. A steady ache was reported by half of the patients, nuchal stiffness in 53%, and throbbing pain in 29%. One third classified their pain as severe. Nausea was reported in 24% of the patients. About two thirds met the International Headache Society (IHS) criteria for chronic tension-type headache, 39% met the IHS criteria for migraine without aura except for the daily occurrence of the headache. The authors concluded that in patients selected on the basis of headache frequency alone, a heterogeneous group emerges. An Italian specialized headache center evaluated CDH in 150 consecutive patients 18 to 64 years of age (16). Patients were included in this study if they had a history of headache for a least 15 days a month during the previous 6 months. Eighty-one percent were female and 19% male. The mean age was 44.2 years. Only 17% of patients fulfilled the IHS criteria for analgesic abuse, even though almost 60% had taken analgesics on a daily basis for at least 3 months and often for several years. The patients were divided into four groups. Almost half of the total had chronic tension-type headache and coexisting migraine. The remainder were equally divided between chronic tension-type headache, migraine, and coexisting unclassifiable interval headache, and unclassifiable daily headache. In another study of 150 consecutive patients with CDH using new criteria for transformed migraine, all patients could be classified (28). Seventy-eight percent had transformed migraine, 15.3% had chronic tension-type headache, and 6.7% had either new daily persistent headache or hemicrania continua.

DRUG OVERUSE

The definition, epidemiology, and pathophysiology of headache associated with chronic use of substances was discussed in Chapter 115. In summary, the diagnosis of headache induced by chronic drug overuse is warranted in a patient who has been taking daily medication designed for acute episodes of headache for more than 3 months (11). The headache usually occurs daily or almost every day, although chronic tension-type headache may be diagnosed by as few as 15 headaches per month. According to IHS classification the headache induced by drug overuse disappears within 1 month after withdrawal of the substance. Many headache experts believe that this criterion is too rigid. Patients with CDH often have evolved from migraine (transformed migraine) (19). Exacerbations of headache within a background of CDH or chronic tension-type headache often have migraine characteristics.

Patients with CDH are commonly seen in specialized headache clinics, and the vast majority (as high as 82%) are overusing medications designed for episodic headaches (10,19). The drugs most commonly overused by headache patients are analgesics and ergotamine. In addition, barbiturates, opioids, and caffeine used singly or more often in combination may perpetuate headache if overused. But almost any medication designed for episodic use of acute headache may cause rebound headaches. The main exception to this general rule is dihydroergotamine, which when administered intravenously every 8 hours for several days usually breaks the cycle of CDH (Fig. 1) (25). There have been many observations attesting to the benefits of drug withdrawal in patients with CDH (18,23,24,37).

Drug overuse in headache therapy has the potential for many adverse events. The most serious systemic ailments affect the gastrointestinal tract, liver, and kidney. Psychological and behavioral disturbances may be triggered or aggravated, especially comorbid depression or anxiety, as well as sleep disturbances (20). Withdrawal symptoms

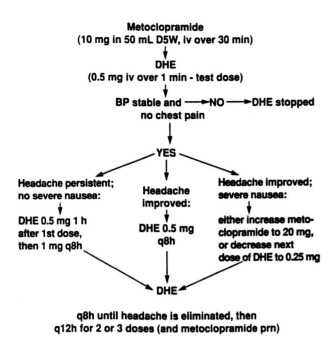

Metoclopramide
(10 mg in 50 mL D5W, iv over 30 min)

↓

DHE
(0.5 mg iv over 1 min - test dose)

↓

BP stable and ——→ NO ——→ DHE stopped
no chest pain

↓

YES

Headache persistent; | Headache | Headache improved;
no severe nausea: | improved: | severe nausea:

DHE 0.5 mg 1 h | DHE 0.5 mg | either increase meto-
after 1st dose, | q8h | clopramide to 20 mg,
then 1 mg q8h | | or decrease next
| | dose of DHE to 0.25 mg

→ DHE ←

q8h until headache is eliminated, then
q12h for 2 or 3 doses (and metoclopramide prn)

FIG. 1. Algorithm for the use of intravenous DHE. Administration of intravenous dihydroergotamine during hospitalization. Reproduced from Dalessio (5).

are similar to those associated with withdrawal of barbiturates or narcotics. Moreover, daily analgesics used to treat CDH impair the effectiveness of prophylactic medication (18).

Pathophysiology

Several mechanisms had been proposed to explain why excessive use of acute medications leads to CDH. Psychological conditioning may take place (6). Other psychological and behavioral factors include biological predisposition and comorbid depression or anxiety.

Rebound phenomena have been evoked to explain the excessive use of drugs designed to treat episodic headache. The medication initially suppresses pain, but as the blood level of the drug decreases, the pain level rebounds. Patients naturally seek recurrent pain suppression, leading to a cycle of increasing drug use. Few scientific studies have been performed in support of this concept, but in one double-blind study the discontinuation of caffeine consumption was followed by headaches (27).

There is evidence of altered central excitatory circuits in patients with CDH. The intensity of the "second pain" (the sensation following initial pain) was greater after percutaneous electric shock in patients with CDH than in patients with episodic headaches or in a control group (7). It has been suggested that chronic analgesic use lowers the pain threshold by suppressing endogenous opioid systems, allowing lesser stimuli to evoke headache (15). Analgesics that chronically suppress central nociceptive

activity upregulate postsynaptic nociceptive receptors. The increased number of nociceptive receptors may lead to increased perception of pain on withdrawal of the analgesic or decrease in its blood level (33). A similar concept has been invoked to explain the transformation from episodic migraine to CDH (34). Platelet serotonin decreased in migraineurs overusing analgesics compared with other migraine patients or a control group, suggesting that excessive use of analgesics depletes serotonin from storage sites, leading to increased headache frequency (35). In patients with analgesic-induced headache studied after 1 month of withdrawal from the acute drug, an increase in blood serotonin has been found along with decrease in headache frequency (12).

MANAGEMENT OF THE PATIENT OVERUSING MEDICATIONS

It is important to establish goals in the management of patients with chronic daily primary headaches. Patients who have had a headache every day for months or years should not expect to be completely free of headaches for the rest of their lives. The goal of therapy is to break the cycle of daily headaches, but the patient should realize that episodes of headaches will occur. Prophylactic therapy should prevent these attacks from occurring frequently, and when headaches do occur, they can be appropriately treated with acute medication.

The treatment of these patients should follow a sequential pattern. First, the offending agents should be withdrawn. The immediate withdrawal effects, including exacerbation of headache, must be treated. Prophylactic measures are necessary, nonpharmacologic as well as pharmacologic. If the headache remains uncontrolled, hospitalization may be warranted for a course of intravenous medication. Finally, after a washout period of 1 to 2 months, former medication for episodic acute attacks may be reinstituted if other agents are ineffective.

Withdrawal of Daily Acute Medication

The first step in treating patients experiencing rebound CDH is to withdraw the medications that may be fueling the fire while trying to extinguish it. Patients must be made aware of the fact that headaches may get worse during the early withdrawal period. Exacerbation of headaches, catching the patient unaware, may be disheartening and disrupt the withdrawal process. To counteract exacerbations of headache during the withdrawal period, especially the first 7 to 10 days, the following regimen may be considered. Nonsteroidal antiinflammatory drugs (NSAIDs) or phenothiazines may be used, especially if ergotamine or other vasoactive agents are the offending medications. Phenothiazines counter the anxiety and other withdrawal symptoms and have some analgesic potential as well. Dihydroergotamine, isometheptene preparations, or triptan may be considered if analgesics are being overused. It must be emphasized that virtually all of the acute therapeutic agents, including sumatriptan, may cause rebound headache, and their use must be limited to headaches that are incapacitating or nearly so (9). The alternative drugs for those being overused must not be taken daily.

The withdrawal can be abrupt if one is dealing with simple analgesics but should be gradual when dealing with drugs containing caffeine, barbiturates, benzodiazepines, or narcotics. Sudden withdrawal of a barbiturate may evoke seizures. Similarly, opioids require gradual withdrawal to avoid the nausea, vomiting, restlessness, and other features of the withdrawal syndrome. If a barbiturate is part of the overused medication, it is wise to taper off the dose by 10% per day. Alternately, 30 mg of phenobarbital may be substituted for 100 mg of the (probable) short-acting barbiturate, such as butalbital or pentobarbital. The dose is then reduced by 30 mg of phenobarbital per day. Sometimes patients grossly underestimate or lie about the amount of barbiturate they have been taking. If this is suspected, the substituted dose of phenobarbital can be calculated by initially giving the patient a sufficiently high dosage of pentobarbital to evoke toxicity and follow the protocol outlined in Table 2. For opioid withdrawal, clonidine 0.1 to 0.3 mg two or three times a day may be helpful in suppressing withdrawal symptoms (14). Other agents to counteract withdrawal effects include phenothiazines, other antinauseants, and benzodiazepines. In tapering off benzodiazepines and other agents, use the lowest dose tablets and decrease by one tablet every 3 days. Adrenocortical steroid therapy may be useful during the week or more of withdrawal. Some clinicians advocate a combination of drugs such as amitriptyline with dexamethasone; sumatriptan may be used for headache exacerbations (1). In patients who are taking analgesics, ergotamine, or sumatriptan, the withdrawal can be adjusted to the patient's tolerance. Withdrawal from ergotamine is often difficult, but abrupt withdrawal from sumatriptan is usually well tolerated (9).

Prophylactic Therapy

Although most patients notice a reduction in the frequency of headaches after withdrawal from the excessive use of acute medications, almost all will require prophylactic therapy to maintain the decreased headache frequency. Follow-up observation of the patient is essential to evaluate the frequency and type of headache recurrence. Choice of medications depends on the type of headache recurrence, usually the headaches from which the CDH evolved or the headaches that were intermittently superimposed upon the CDH. If migraine is a factor, all of the prophylactic agents for migraine would be appropriate, not only the tricyclic antidepressants but also beta-adrenergic blockers, divalproex, calcium channel blockers, or small doses of ergot alkaloids such as methyl ergonovine. Antiserotonin agents, such as cyproheptadine for children and methysergide for adults, are additional considerations.

Tricyclic antidepressants (which have analgesic actions) are often the drugs of choice. Not only do they suppress headaches and help sleep disorders, but they may also ameliorate comorbid depression. (However, the antidepressant dose is usually higher than the analgesic dose.) The beginning dose of the tricyclic antidepressant may be low, for example, 10 to 25 mg of amitriptyline or nortriptyline. If headaches are unremitting and side effects of the medication (most commonly dry mouth, sedation, weight gain) are absent or slight, the dose should be increased by 10 to 25 mg every 7 to 10 days until headaches ameliorate or side effects become troublesome. Particularly in patients of middle or later life, an electrocardiogram should be obtained to rule out cardiac conduction defects that may be aggravated by the anticholinergic effects of the tricyclic agent. In addition, other headache prophylactic therapy may be started or adjusted.

Comorbid and coexistent factors play an important role in choosing prophylactic medications. Depression and anxiety are the most important considerations (2). In some individuals the physical symptom of headache is more socially acceptable than the overt symptoms of depression or anxiety. Other signs of depression should be sought, such as fatigue on awakening, loss of spontaneity, impairment of libido, alteration of appetite, and sleep patterns. The newer selective serotonin reuptake inhibitors are less effective as headache prophylactic agents than the tricyclics but more effective as antidepressants and with superior side effect profiles.

TABLE 2. *Barbiturate challenge to determine withdrawal dosage*

Day 1: administer pentobarbital 200 mg			
Response	Severe: ataxia and dysarthria	Moderate: nystagmus	None or persistence of withdrawal symptoms
Daily need of pentobarbital	<200–300 mg	600–800 mg	1,000 mg or more

May repeat above on day 2 to establish stable dose, that is, one that evokes neither toxicity nor symptoms of withdrawal. On determination of stable dose, substitute 30 mg of phenobarbital for 100 mg pentobarbital and reduce the dose by 30 mg every 1 or 2 days.

Monoamine oxidase inhibitors (MAOIs) may be helpful for headache and associated depression but, because of the dietary and medication restrictions required when taking MAOIs, these agents are the last to be tried. The use of benzodiazepines may be required for associated anxiety; propranolol affords the double benefit of ameliorating anxiety and suppressing migraine. Another important prophylactic agent is divalproex. Open-label studies have shown its effectiveness in decreasing the frequency of CDH (17). Comorbidity of epilepsy would make divalproex the drug of choice. Such coexistent factors as hypertension, coronary artery disease or cerebrovascular disease would preclude the use of vasoconstrictor medications.

Nondrug therapy should always be considered. Healthy habits may be encouraged by recommending the cessation of nicotine and excessive alcohol, maintenance of regular hours for sleep and meals, and periodic exercise. Precipitating or aggravating factors must be sought and eliminated; a headache diary is useful in this respect. Relaxation techniques, for example biofeedback conditioning, may be tried to ameliorate pain intensity and decrease headache frequency (13).

Psychological factors are a common accompaniment of chronic pain. This is especially true of people who abuse or overuse medications to treat chronic headaches. These patients may be less able to tolerate the sleep disturbances and anxiety that may persist for weeks after withdrawal. Depression is more common than anxiety in headache sufferers, and these phenomena are more prevalent in migraineurs irrespective of the intensity or frequency of attacks (3,36).

Psychological support must be initiated and maintained. The family, employer, teacher, and sometimes the doctor of headache patients may be unsympathetic, generating anger, frustration, and hostility. These important others may have to be contacted, counseled, and educated. The patient may be helped by learning pain-coping techniques, including cognitive and behavioral therapy such as stress management. Social workers, dieticians, occupational therapists, and physical therapists may contribute to the patients favorable course. Self-help support groups may be useful in preventing recidivism. Psychological counseling is often helpful; formal psychotherapy is rarely necessary. Most important, the patient must be committed to and responsible for a plan of therapy. Finally, there is no substitute for empathetic, compassionate continuity of care.

Hospitalization

If outpatient therapy is ineffective, the patient should be hospitalized. The excessively used agent is abruptly withdrawn (unless it is a barbiturate, benzodiazepine, or narcotic) and a course of intravenous dihydroergotamine is administered following the standard algorithm (see Fig.

1) (5,25). This procedure is continued until the patient is headache free or almost so for 24 hours, usually 3 to 5 days. Exacerbations of headache or other withdrawal symptoms are treated with NSAIDs or a phenothiazine or both. Parenteral steroid therapy may be appropriate, especially if dihydroergotamine is not quickly effective (5). Intravenous or intramuscular administration of a phenothiazine may be useful. Lastly, intravenous barbiturate or benzodiazepine therapy inducing sleep or deep sedation may be appropriate.

One must plan for resumption of acute therapy for bouts of headache that occur even after the cycle of daily rebound headache has been broken. Alternatives to the withdrawn medication have been noted above, but sometimes the most effective medication is that which had been overused. Doctors are understandably reluctant to reinstitute medication formerly abused, but this can be done with a responsible, highly motivated patient. If an ergotamine preparation or analgesic combination is the only medication useful in aborting an attack of headache, it can be restarted after 1 or 2 months of withdrawal. To prevent recidivism, the physician must insist that acute medications be taken no more than 2 days per week.

REFERENCES

1. Bonucelli U, Nuti A, Lucetti C, Pavese N, Dell'Angello G, Muratorio A. Amitriptyline and dexamethasone combined treatment in drug induced headache. *Cephalalgia* 1996;16:197–200.
2. Brandt JD, Celentano W. Stewart, Linet M, Folstein MF. Personality and emotional disorder in a community sample of migraine headache sufferers. *Am J Psychiatry* 1990;147:303–308.
3. Breslau N, Merikangas K, Bowden CL. Comorbidity of migraine and major affective disorders. Neurology 1994;44[Suppl 7]:17–22.
4. Castillo J, Guitera V, Munoz P, Pascual J. Prevalence and diagnostic distribution of chronic daily headache in the general population. *Cephalalgia* 1997;17:283.
5. Dalessio DJ, Silberstein SD, eds. *Wolff's headache and other head pain,* 6th ed. New York: Oxford University Press, 1993:130–131.
6. Fordyce WE. Learning processes in pain. In: Sternbach RA, ed. *The psychology of pain,* 2nd ed. New York: Raven, 1986:49–66.
7. Fusco BM, Colantoni O, Giacovazzo M. Alteration of central excitation circuits in chronic headache and analgesic misuse. *Headache* 1997;37: 486–491.
8. Gobel H, Petersen-Braum M, Soyka D. The epidemiology of headache in Germany: a nationwide survey of a representative sample on the basis of the headache classification of the International Headache Society. *Cephalalgia* 1994;14:97–106.
9. Gobel H, Stolze H, Heinze A, Dworschak M. Easy therapeutical management of sumatriptan-induced daily headache. *Neurology* 1996;47: 297–298.
10. Granella F, Farina S, Malferrari G, Manzoni GC. Drug abuse in chronic headache: a clinico-epidemiologic study. *Cephalalgia* 1987;7:15–20.
11. Headache Classification Committee of the International Headache Society. Classification and diagnostic criteria for headache disorders, cranial neuralgias, and facial pain. *Cephalalgia* 1988;8[Suppl 7]:1–96.
12. Hering R, Glover V, Pattichis K, Catarci T, Steiner TJ. 5HT in migraine patients with medication-induced headache. *Cephalalgia* 1993;13: 410–412.
13. Holroyd KA. Psychological and behavioral techniques. In: Olesen J, Tfelt-Hansen P, Welch KMA. eds. *The headaches.* New York: Raven, 1993:515–520.
14. Jaffe JH. Substance-related disorders: opioid-related disorders. In: Kaplan HI, Sadock BJ, eds. *Comprehensive textbook of psychiatry,* 6th ed. Baltimore: Williams & Wilkins, 1995:842–863.
15. Kudrow L. Possible mechanisms and treatment of analgesic-induced

chronic headache. In: Diener HC, Wilkinson M, eds. *Drug induced headache.* Berlin: Springer-Verlag, 1988:157–161.

16. Manzoni G, Granella F, Sandrini G, Cavallini A, Zanferrari C, Nappi G. Classification of chronic daily headache by International Headache Society criteria: limits and new proposals. *Cephalalgia* 1995;15:37–43.

17. Mathew NT. Valproate in the treatment of persistent daily headache. An open label study. *Headache* 1991:31:71–74.

18. Mathew NT, Kurman R, Perez F. Drug-induced refractory headache: clinical features and management. *Headache* 1990;30:634–638.

19. Mathew NT, Reuveni U, Perez F. Transformed or evolutive migraine. *Headache* 1987;27:102–106.

20. Merikangas KR, Angst J. Headache syndrome and psychiatric disorders: association and familial transmission. *J Psychiatr Res* 1993;27:197–210.

21. Micieli G, Manzoni GC, Granella F, Martignoni E, Malferrari G, Nappi G. Clinical and epidemiological observations on drug abuse in headache patients. In: Diener HC, Wilkinson M. eds. *Drug-induced headache.* Berlin: Springer-Verlag, 1988:20–28.

22. Ostfeld A. The natural history and epidemiology of migraine and muscle contraction headache. *Neurology* 1963;13:11–15.

23. Pini L, Bigarelli M, Vitale G, Sternieri E. Headaches, associated with chronic use of analgesics: a therapeutic approach. *Headache* 1996;36:433–439.

24. Rapoport AM, Weeks RE, Sheftell FD, et al. Analgesic rebound headache: theoretical and practical implications. *Cephalalgia* 1985;5[Suppl 3]:448–449.

25. Raskin NH. Repetitive intravenous dihydroergotamine as therapy for intractable migraine. *Neurology* 1986;36:995–997.

26. Rasmussen BK, Jensen R, Schroll M, Olesen J. Epidemiology of headache in a general population—a prevalence study. *J Clin Epidemiol* 1991;44:1147–1157.

27. Silverman K, Evans SM, Strain EC, Griffith RR. Withdrawal syndrome after the double-blind cessation of caffeine consumption. *N Engl J Med* 1992;327:1109–1114.

28. Silberstein SD, Lipton RB, Sliwinski M. Classification of daily and near-daily headaches: field trial of revised IHS criteria. *Neurology* 1996;47:871–875.

29. Silberstein SD, Lipton RB, Solomon S, Mathew N. Classification of daily and near-daily headaches: proposed revisions to the IHS criteria. *Headache* 1994;34:1–7.

30. Solomon S, Apfelbaum R, Guglielmo KM. The cluster-tic syndrome and its surgical treatment. *Cephalalgia* 1985;5:83–89.

31. Solomon S, Karfunkel P, Guglielmo KM: Migraine-cluster headache syndrome. *Headache* 1985;25:236–239.

32. Solomon S, Lipton R, Newman L. Clinical features of chronic daily headache. *Headache* 1992;32:325–329.

33. Srikiatkhachorn A, Anthony M. Serotonin receptor adaptation in patients with analgesic-induced headache. *Cephalalgia* 1996;16:419–422.

34. Srikiatkhachorn A, Govitrapong P, Limthavon C. Up-regulation of 5-HT2 serotonin receptor: a possible mechanism of transformed migraine. *Headache* 1994;34:8–11.

35. Srikiatkhachorn A, Maneesri S, Govitrapong P, Kasantikul V. Derangement of serotonin system in migrainous patients with analgesic abuse headache: clues from platelets. *Headache* 1998;38:43–49.

36. Stewart W, Breslau N, Keck PE. Comorbidity of migraine and panic disorder. *Neurology* 1994;44[Suppl 7]:23–27.

37. Tfelt-Hansen P, Krabbe E. Ergotamine abuse. Do patients benefit from withdrawal? *Cephalalgia* 1981;1:29–32.

38. Vanast WJ. New daily persistent headaches: definition of a benign syndrome. *Headache* 1986;26:317.

The Headaches, Second Edition,
edited by J. Olesen, P. Tfelt-Hansen, and K.M.A. Welch.
Lippincott Williams & Wilkins, Philadelphia © 2000.

Special Problems in the Headaches and Their Management

CHAPTER 132

Headache in the Emergency Room

K. Michael A. Welch, Taruna K. Aurora, Pawan Suri, and Guy Arnold

This chapter provides a systematic approach to the diagnosis and appropriate management of a patient who presents with a headache to the emergency room (ER) or an urgent care setting. For detailed information on the pathophysiology, anatomy, diagnosis, and routine management of various types of headache, the reader is referred to other sections of this book.

There are approximately 2 million annual ER visits for headache related complaints in the United States alone (19). Headache is the most prevalent neurologic symptom associated with any disease. Proper assessment of headache is a time-consuming process, a luxury not afforded to the busy emergency physician. Nevertheless, an adequate history, physical examination, and judicious use of ancillary tests are essential to making an accurate diagnosis. When confronted with a headache patient in the ER, the clinician must assess the patient for life-threatening conditions. Fortunately most headaches are of a benign nature. Up to 90% of ambulatory patients with a complaint of headache fall into the category of tension-type headache and migraine (22). Having knowledge of the classification and differential diagnosis of headaches is an important first step in their effective management.

CLINICAL ASSESSMENT

History

To elicit a relevant history from an uncomfortable patient with a severe headache is a challenging task. A

quiet, dark room usually helps in this situation. Because most patients with a headache do not manifest positive neurologic findings on the physical examination, history taking is essential to establish a diagnosis. The clinician may find it helpful to ask four key questions in the following order:

How long have you had the headache?
What do you think caused it?
Where is the headache located?
What is it like?

How long have you had the headache? Answers to this question should provide information about the duration, onset, and frequency of the headache. Based on the response, three broad categories of patients can be recognized:

1. A patient coming to the ER with a first-time severe headache. Such a patient will have had no previous evaluation, and falls into the highest risk group for serious intracranial pathology.
2. A patient with a history of chronic headaches who has experienced a change in the frequency, character, or intensity of the headache.
3. A patient with a chronic paroxysmal headache (e.g., migraine) with attacks occurring at regular intervals. This type of patient comes to the ER primarily for pain relief after failing outpatient medications.

Information about onset of the headache provides further clues to its possible cause. Thunderclap onset may indicate a subarachnoid hemorrhage. If the patient survived, or had more than one such event, this is termed *sentinel headache*. Failure to recognize a sentinel headache should be the fear of every emergency physician. A headache of onset 5 to 6 weeks before the consultation with increasing severity may indicate elevated intracranial pressure, for example, due to a brain neo-

K. M. A. Welch: Department of Neurology, University of Kansas School of Medicine, University of Kansas Medical Center, Kansas City, Kansas 66106.

T. K. Aurora and P. Suri: Department of Emergency Medicine, Henry Ford Hospital, Detroit, Michigan 48202.

G. Arnold: Universitätsklinikum Charité, Medizinische Fakultät der Humboldt-Universität zu Berlin, Universitätsklinik und Piloklinik für Neurologie, 10117 Berlin, Germany.

plasm. Awakening with a headache indicates an organic cause and may occur in conditions as varied as obstructive sleep apnea, cluster headache, migraine, hypertension, and cerebrovascular disease. Migraine and tension headaches almost always begin before the fourth decade of life. Before attributing a first-time headache in an elderly person to migraine or tension, more serious conditions should be excluded.

What do you think caused it? Knowledge about the precipitating factors of the headache is most valuable in narrowing the diagnosis. Headache related to stress, fatigue, hunger, concentration, excitement, ingestion of chocolate, and the use of contraceptive pills or estrogens may support a diagnosis of migraine. Any recent head or neck trauma is an obvious cause for headache. Headache precipitated by activity, straining, blood pressure increase, and sudden head turning may indicate elevated intracranial pressure. A first and worst headache during sexual intercourse should alert the physician to the possibility of subarachnoid hemorrhage. A history of fever, ingestion of toxins, caffeine, alcohol, tobacco, or nitrates suggests headache of infectious, chemical, toxic, or metabolic origin. Carbon monoxide poisoning must be considered when several patients from the same location present with a headache.

Where is the headache located? Headache due to infratentorial disease will most often be localized to the occipital region. Supratentorial pathology will usually produce pain in the frontal region. Remember, however, that pain from infratentorial structures may be referred to frontal regions and vice versa. Structural lesions obstructing the flow of cerebrospinal fluid circulation in the infratentorial ventricular system also can produce frontal headache secondary to hydrocephalus of the lateral ventricles. Approximately two thirds of migraine attacks are unilateral, although the location may vary with different attacks. Chronic pain experienced over the vertex or in a bandlike distribution around the head may suggest tension-type headache. A severe, pulsatile, retroorbital pain may suggest cluster headache, inflammatory lesions of the orbital structures, or an expanding aneurysm around the circle of Willis. Some other considerations concerning headache localization are provided as follows:

1. A headache that presents unilaterally and progresses over time to become bilateral may be the result of increasing intracranial pressure.
2. Lesions that cause traction on the falx or midline structures may cause pain in either eye.
3. Cerebellopontine angle tumors produce pain behind the ear, and lesions involving the lateral sinus result in pain deep in the ear.

What is it like? The character and intensity of pain are qualitative judgments made by the patient and are only occasionally helpful in making the diagnosis. In this regard, specific information on the increasing or decreasing severity of the headache becomes important. A steady, generalized pain increasing over several weeks may indicate elevated intracranial pressure. Bending, stooping, coughing, defecation, or sexual intercourse enhances this type of headache. Headache of a pulsatile nature (corresponding to the radial/carotid pulse) is highly suggestive of vascular origin, whereas a throbbing pain is less specific. Sharp, lancinating, or a deep boring pain when localized behind the eye may suggest cluster headache. A stabbing, icepick-like pain in the distribution of the fifth cranial nerve indicates trigeminal neuralgia. A constant vicelike gripping pain, or a dull pressure pain, may indicate muscle contraction headache.

Associated Symptoms

A sudden, severe headache with loss or alteration in consciousness or a drop attack should be taken as a sign of potentially serious intracranial pathology. Symptoms of paresis, paralysis, ataxia, or sensory disturbance associated with a headache indicate structural lesions. Visual symptoms are frequently associated with an acute headache and are helpful in formulating a differential diagnosis. A scintillating scotoma, photophobia, hemianopsia, and teichopsia occur as a part of the migraine aura. Raised intracranial pressure associated with a headache and papilledema may manifest as a rapid and progressive loss of vision with a centrocecal scotoma. Persistent field defects are a serious complication of temporal arteritis. Extracranial cerebrovascular disease may present with a headache and amaurosis fugax. Vomiting may accompany a severe migraine headache and may occasionally alleviate it. Projectile vomiting is classically associated with elevated intracranial pressure. Vomiting may be a symptom of other systemic conditions likely to be associated with headache, such as fever, heat-related illness, and allergic reactions.

Head and Neck Structures

Examination of the head and neck structures may provide important clues to the diagnosis. For example, temporal arteritis may be associated with soreness and tenderness over one temple or temporomandibular joint. Neck stiffness and soreness are early signs of meningeal irritation. Localized pain in the upper quadrant of the teeth or face may indicate sinusitis. Nasal stuffiness and watery discharge along with lacrimation are usually present in cluster headache. Pain and a bloody discharge from the ear may indicate head injury and basal skull fracture.

PHYSICAL EXAMINATION

Although history contributes greatly to diagnosing the cause of a headache, positive findings on the physical examination can make the difference between initiating emergent treatment versus undertaking nonemergent, routine outpatient workup. As always, ER examination should start with a review of the vital signs. Fever always mandates a search for meningitis, encephalitis, or brain abscess. Mild increases in blood pressure and heart rate are a normal physiologic response to pain. True hypertensive headache does not occur until the diastolic blood pressure is above 130 mm Hg (2). Blood pressure is often elevated as a secondary mechanism in cases of cerebral edema or acute stroke. Tachypnea may be present in conditions such as chronic obstructive pulmonary disease exacerbation and severe anemia.

Next, a general impression of the patient should be obtained through his or her appearance and response to pain. Most patients with migraine headache will lie still with eyes closed, unwilling to talk or move. Patients with meningeal irritation due to any cause may exhibit extreme restlessness. Signs of any external trauma and head injury may be visible at first sight. Most pain-sensitive structures of the head and neck can be viewed directly or palpated. Palpating or tapping can easily identify local sources for pain over sinuses, teeth, and neck musculature. Tenderness overlying the superficial temporal artery is the hallmark of temporal arteritis. Tenderness of the internal carotid artery occurs in carotidynia. Infections in the head and neck often cause tender lymphadenopathy. An enlarging lymph node in the region of the occipital canal may entrap the occipital nerve and cause severe ipsilateral hemicranial pain. Tolosa-Hunt syndrome or painful ophthalmoplegia may be linked to enlarged tubercular nodes in the neck. In a patient with trauma, a boggy mass under the temporalis muscle may indicate the site of a ruptured middle meningeal artery and an intracranial, extradural hematoma. Trapezius muscle spasm may be the primary cause of a muscle contraction headache or occur secondarily as a result of severe head pain of a different etiology. The clinician should always test for nuchal rigidity. It indicates meningismus due to meningitis, encephalitis, severe cervical spondylosis, or a subarachnoid hemorrhage.

Ophthalmologic examination should seek the presence of redness, corneal clouding, and the ciliary flush of iritis seen in glaucoma. A tonopen can be used to easily measure the intraocular pressure. If untreated, glaucoma can rapidly progress to blindness. Errors of refraction rarely cause a headache. In the ear, the clinician should look for signs of infection or cholesteatoma, which may erode intracranially, causing a brain abscess. Presence of hemotympanum or blood in the external auditory meatus suggests a basilar skull fracture as a result of head trauma. The clinician should listen over the carotid arteries for bruits of atherosclerotic origin and over the eyes and head for bruits of arteriovenous malformations. Dermatologic examination should assess for the typical skin lesions of herpes zoster. The skin over the temporal arter-

ies may be swollen or inflamed. Needle tracks and skin popping are evidence of intravenous drug abuse.

Neurologic Examination

Every patient with a headache should undergo a complete neurologic examination. The clinician should start by assessing the higher cortical functions and conscious state. Altered mentation and confusion are signs of serious intracranial pathology. Cranial nerve abnormalities are most frequently encountered in the ocular systems. Fundoscopic examination should assess for spontaneous venous pulsations, which ensure a low intracranial pressure. The patient's pupils should not be dilated to examine the fundus because this can either mask preexistent anisocoria or precipitate angle closure glaucoma in patients with a narrow angle. Papilledema, when present, is usually bilateral and indicates elevated intracranial pressure. With hypertensive emergencies the fundus may show acute hemorrhages and exudates. Retinal and subhyaloid hemorrhages are virtually diagnostic of subarachnoid hemorrhage. Scotomas of hemianopic field defects may indicate less common causes of headache, such as a brain tumor, arteriovenous malformation, or expanding aneurysm. A bitemporal field defect in a patient with severe frontotemporal headache can be caused by an expanding pituitary adenoma. Unilateral ophthalmoplegia with sensory loss in the first division of the fifth cranial nerve in association with unilateral retroorbital headache may be due to a superior orbital fissure syndrome, painful ophthalmoplegia, or Tolosa-Hunt syndrome. Ophthalmoplegic migraine is a rare syndrome. Unilateral third nerve or bilateral sixth nerve palsies are frequently related to aneurysms of the cerebral vasculature or elevated intracranial pressure. Unilateral Horner syndrome and headache may indicate carotid arterial dissection. Miosis together with excessive sweating may indicate posttraumatic dysautonomic cephalalgia. Ischemic or hemorrhagic cerebrovascular disease may present with a headache, visual field defects, and motor weakness.

DIAGNOSTIC EVALUATION

A computed tomography (CT) scan and lumbar puncture are the most common and useful diagnostic tests in the evaluation of headache in the ER. In the absence of focal neurologic deficits or papilledema it is safe to directly proceed to lumbar puncture. Cerebrospinal fluid (CSF) findings may indicate early meningitis or a subarachnoid hemorrhage. Most other laboratory studies—such as complete blood count, ABG, and electrolyte profile—may be undertaken depending on the underlying medical problems or the need for a specific search for secondary causes of headache. For all patients over the age of 50 in whom the diagnosis of temporal arteritis is suspected, an erythrocyte sedimentation rate should be determined. A carbon monoxide level or toxicology screen may be ordered in the appropriate setting.

In the following sections we present a systematic discussion of headaches as they may present to the ER: secondary headaches of acute onset; subacute or chronic secondary headaches; and the management of primary headaches in the emergency setting.

Headaches with Sudden Onset

Subarachnoid Hemorrhage (IHS Code 6.3)

Subarachnoid hemorrhage results from ruptured berry aneurysm, trauma, or an arterovenous malformation. Most cases of subarachnoid hemorrhage occur between the ages of 20 and 40 years. An expanding aneurysm gives rise to intermittent headache in the same location. Almost 40% of patients will describe a premonitory sentinel bleed before their major subarachnoid hemorrhage. The incidence of headache in a ruptured aneurysm approaches 100%. The leading symptom is the so-called thunderclap headache, which is present in about 80% of patients. The acute onset of headache is caused by a ruptured aneurysm and the entrance of blood into the subarachnoid space, rapidly causing meningeal irritation and clinical signs of meningismus, neck pain, and stiffness. Hemorrhagic CSF also causes varying degrees of cerebral vasoconstriction that causes alteration of consciousness ranging from mild confusion to coma. Nausea, vomiting, diaphoresis, photophobia, neck pain, tachypnea, tachycardia, and hypertension are common associated symptoms and signs.

A third-generation CT scanner can accurately detect subarachnoid hemorrhage in up to 95% of cases; however, sensitivity decreases to 74% after 3 days (1). A lumbar puncture is mandatory if no blood is detected. The remainder of the cases can be detected on lumbar puncture by the presence of red blood cells that do not clear in four samples of CSF. Subarachnoid hemorrhage can be distinguished from a traumatic tap by the presence of xanthochromia in the CSF sample. Once the diagnosis of subarachnoid hemorrhage is confirmed, prompt neurosurgical consultation is required to determine if the patient qualifies for arteriography and surgical clipping. Aneurysms are best confirmed by four-vessel catheter angiography. Patients in deep coma are managed conservatively. Medical management includes intravenous hydration, control of hypertension, and nimodipine therapy to reduce vasospasm. In most countries surgery is recommended within 72 hours after headache onset, depending on the grade of the disease. For the appropriate neurosurgical management, Hunt and Hess (12) established a ranking scale ranging from headache plus nuchal pain (I) to deep coma (V). The overall mortality rate from subarachnoid hemorrhage is approximately 50%.

Cerebral Venous Thrombosis (IHS Code 6.7)

Cerebral sinus or venous thrombosis is the most important differential diagnosis of subarachnoid hemorrhage because the leading symptom in cerebral venous thrombosis is headache (>80%). Thunderclap headache is the first symptom in approximately 25% (20). In other cases the headache is dull, and waxing and waning. Cerebral sinus or venous thrombosis is most often accompanied by additional signs, especially epileptic seizures (50%) and drowsiness, somnolence, or coma (50%). Motor deficits occur in about one third of patients. In almost 50% of patients papilledema can be detected. A contrast-enhanced CT scan usually shows nonspecific signs of elevated intracranial pressure, such as small ventricles or diminished sulci. In certain circumstances the very specific delta sign is observed (20), a contrast-sparing region within the occipital part of the superior sagittal sinus or the confluence of sinuses. If the CT scan is suspicious for cerebral venous thrombosis, the diagnosis can be confirmed by magnetic resonance (MR) angiography or digital subtraction angiography when the former is unavailable. Early diagnosis is essential because heparin therapy may improve consciousness and resolve neurologic function. Recently, tPA has been used with anecdotal success. Patients with cerebral venous thrombosis should be monitored carefully because of secondary complications such as infarction, intraparenchymal bleeding, hydrocephalus, and seizures. An antiepileptic strategy should be initiated on the first day.

Headache Due to Dissection of Carotid or Vertebral Arteries (IHS Code 6.6.1)

The onset of pain is usually acute and of moderately severe intensity, often with a pulsating character. The pain might be referred to the cranium or face, or it may be located in the neck. The most frequent associated signs are those of cerebral ischemia. Ischemic signs may be delayed up to 1 month after the onset of pain, and may be due to embolism from the site of dissection (14). The combination of cervical pain, headache, and ischemic signs is characteristic and provides a strong clue to the diagnosis. One of the most common features of carotid dissection is ipsilateral Horner syndrome (40%–60%), followed by tinnitus, hemiparesis, and cervical pain. Whether there is increased frequency of carotid or vertebral dissection in migraineurs remains controversial (18). Nevertheless, when ischemic signs occur in migraineurs, the differential diagnosis of dissection must always be considered. Doppler and duplex sonography are sensitive tests for dissection, but MR angiography is the preferred investigation, or catheter angiography if this is not available. Anticoagulant therapy to prevent embolism is administered for up to 6 months, unless the dissection extends intracranially.

Hypertensive Headache

Acute, severe headache is a prominent symptom of hypertensive encephalopathy, which occurs when sustained elevation in blood pressure exceeds the upper limits of cerebral autoregulation. The rate of blood pressure increase is more important than the absolute value; nonetheless, most patients will have a blood pressure that is in the range of 250/150 mm Hg. Other symptoms of hypertensive encephalopathy include nausea, vomiting, visual disturbances, seizures, confusion, and coma. Evidence of other end-organ damage (e.g., proteinuria and azotemia), focal neurologic deficits, retinal hemorrhages, and papilledema also may be present.

One to two percent of patients with essential hypertension will progress to hypertensive emergency for unknown reasons. Arteriolar distension and interstitial extravasation produce focal vasogenic edema, which often shows up as nonspecific bilateral abnormalities in the occipital lobes and subcortical white matter (16). The therapeutic goal in the treatment of hypertensive emergency is reduction of the mean arterial pressure by 15% to 25% in the first 48 hours. Nitroprusside, administered intravenously, is the drug of choice because it can be rapidly titrated and is highly effective. Invasive blood pressure monitoring should be performed via an arterial line while infusing nitroprusside. Use of oral nifedipine has fallen out of favor due to its potential for causing a steep decrease in blood pressure and precipitating ischemic stroke.

Ischemic and Hemorrhagic Stroke

Headache is three times more common in intraparenchymal hemorrhage than in ischemic stroke. The headache is usually focal, mild to moderate in severity, and ipsilateral to the stroke. The character of the headache may vary widely, depending on the location and extent of the hemorrhage. In general, the severity of the headache does not correlate well with the size of the stroke or cortical involvement (9). In their review, Karacagil et al. reported that headache was lateralized in only 46% of patients; of those cases, 68% of headaches were ipsilateral to the stroke. When a patient presents with a headache and lateralized findings, a CT scan without contrast is the initial investigation of choice (13).

Acute Posttraumatic Headache, Associated With or Without Epidural Hematoma (IHS Codes 5.1 and 6.2.3)

Headache following head trauma is common. For example, headache is always present in epidural hematoma caused by ruptured meningeal arteries involved in skull fracture. Depending on the size of the hematoma, the patient appears to be normal during the first minutes or hours after the head injury. During this lucid interval only headache might be present. Subsequent symptoms and signs include anisocoria, deterioration of headache, nausea, and rapid loss of consciousness. If skull fracture is suspected, x-ray in at least two planes is recommended. A subsequent CT scan is mandatory (23). Immediate trepanation of the skull is the treatment of choice.

Central Nervous System Infections

Patients with central nervous system infections such as bacterial and viral meningitis, encephalitis, brain abscess, and human immunodeficiency virus (HIV) infection will often present to the ER with acute severe headache. Untreated bacterial meningitis has a high rate of mortality. Fever (95%), neck stiffness (88%), and altered consciousness (80%) are the common associated findings in meningitis (5). A CSF protein of greater than 220 mg%, cell count above 2,000/mL, and a CSF:serum glucose ratio of less than 0.23 are 99% specific for bacterial meningitis. Antibiotic therapy should not be delayed while waiting for the results of a CT scan or a lumbar puncture. Ceftriaxone or cefotaxime should be given as soon as possible. Ampicillin is added if infection with *Listeria* is suspected. Children with presumptive Hemophilus influenzae meningitis also should receive dexamethasone, 0.15 mg/kg every 6 hours for 2 to 4 days. Untreated herpes encephalitis has a 70% rate of mortality, even though it accounts for only 3% of all cases of viral encephalitis (21). Associated symptoms and signs include headache, low-grade fever, altered consciousness, vomiting, seizures, and focal neurologic deficits. A contrast-enhanced CT is only 60% sensitive in diagnosing herpes encephalitis, and MR imaging with gadolinium is the neuroimaging study of choice. A definitive diagnosis may require temporal lobe biopsy. Herpes simplex encephalitis requires immediate treatment with intravenous acyclovir, 10 mg/kg every 8 hours for at least 10 days.

Of all the patients with HIV who visit the ER, 20% do so with complaints of headache and 82% of these headaches are from secondary causes (8). Cryptococcal meningitis, toxoplasmosis, progressive multifocal leukoencephalopathy, HIV encephalitis, undiagnosed mass lesions, sepsis, and drug reactions are some of the common causes of headache in an HIV patient (15). All new headaches in patients with HIV should be evaluated with a neuroimaging study such as MR imaging and a lumbar puncture.

Acute Glaucoma

Patients with acute angle closure glaucoma usually present with severe pain localized to the eye and radiating to the ear, the sinuses, the teeth, or the forehead.

Accompanying signs are blurred vision, dilated unresponsive pupil, and ciliar injection. Nausea and vomiting are less common. Diagnosis is made by measuring intraocular pressure. Treatment is with miotics (β-receptor blocking eye drops, pilocarpine, or systemic acetazolamide).

Exercise Headache and Headache Associated with Sexual Activity (IHS Codes 4.5 and 4.6)

Recurrent headache associated with sexual activity is termed coital cephalalgia. It is categorized as explosive, similar to the thunderclap headache of subarachnoid hemorrhage. The differential diagnosis from the latter can be established if a series, even a cluster, of headache attacks under identical circumstances is reported. Often the diagnosis is helped when the headache is time locked with orgasm (orgasmic cephalalgia).

Exercise headache is also explosive in character and time locked with strenuous activity. Again, subarachnoid hemorrhage figures prominently in the differential diagnosis. Often the complaint is recurrent. All patients should have an MR imaging scan of the head, with particular attention to the posterior fossa structures, although rarely is an abnormality found to explain the headache.

Subacute and Chronic Headache of High Intensity

In these cases, focal or generalized neurologic symptoms and signs, rather than the headache itself, usually cause the patient to present to an ER. Most of the diseases that cause acute secondary headaches discussed above also may present with subacute headache, for example, cerebral venous thrombosis. In the diseases discussed below, headache is subacute in onset with growing intensity during days or weeks.

Arteritis Cranialis (Headache Associated with Giant Cell Arteritis, IHS Code 6.5.1)

Headache is the leading symptom of giant cell arteritis, present in about 80% to 90% of patients. It is described variably as unilateral or bilateral temporal headache, forehead pain, or diffuse headache. Occipital headache is rare, although occasionally patients complain about neck pain (11). Often the pain is severe and pulsating in nature and can be localized to the artery of involvement. Giant cell arteritis is associated with polymyalgia rheumatica. Additional symptoms include visual, especially transient or permanent unilateral or bilateral vision loss. An almost pathognomonic symptom is jaw or masticatory claudication. Furthermore, some patients present with tongue pain or tongue infarction. The disorder occurs in patients over 60 years of age. Neurologic examination may reveal prominent, tender, nonpulsatile temporal arteries, although both temporal arteries might be normal. Funduscopy may reveal pale, swollen optic discs, indicating visual dysfunction. In the ER, the most rapid investigative information can be obtained from the erythrocyte sedimentation rate (ESR) or results of C-reactive protein tests. The ESR might be as high as 100 mm, but may be normal. The sensitivity of this test decreases with the patient's age. Biopsy of the temporal artery is the investigation of choice but may be negative if the arterial segment involved is limited in extent. Symptoms and signs respond rapidly to steroids, usually 100 mg of oral prednisolone. To avoid visual loss, treatment with steroids should be started urgently as soon as the diagnosis is suspected and before arterial biopsy.

Chronic Posttraumatic Headache, Associated With or Without Subdural Hematoma (IHS Codes 5.2 and 6.2.2)

Subdural hematomas result from tearing of bridging veins. A history of trauma, presence of a CSF shunt catheter, or anticoagulation therapy should raise the suspicion of a subdural hematoma. Elderly persons are at high risk. Headache associated with subdural hematoma may present within as short a time as 6 hours, or after as long as 6 months. It may be a mild to moderate dull daily headache, without neurologic symptoms and only subtle neurologic signs. On the other hand, some patients report dizziness, drowsiness, disorientation, delusion, or personality changes, together with focal neurologic signs. A contrast-enhanced CT scan is the method of choice, if subdural hematoma is suspected. The management of a subdural hematoma, either conservative or surgical drainage, depends on its size and clinical signs.

Intracranial Infection (IHS Code 7.3)

Acute, severe secondary headaches associated with intracranial infections are discussed above. Certain intracranial infections and encephalitides present with more indolent forms of headache.

Meningitis caused by *Mycobacterium tuberculosis* may take a chronic course of weeks to months. Immunosuppressed patients and patients with a history of pulmonary tuberculosis or a history of tuberculosis in the neighborhood are at particular risk. Characteristically, CSF has a pleocytosis of under 100 lymphocytes/cm^3 and an elevated protein level of 100 mg%. It also may be hemorrhagic. The CSF glucose level is moderately decreased to 20 to 40 mg%. Ziehl-Nehlsen staining is negative in most cases. The sensitivity and specificity of diagnostic procedures for tuberculosis have been markedly improved by polymerase chain reaction testing. Indolent headache and clinical course are also features of cryptococcal meningitis and borelliosis. The neurologic complications are much less severe in the former. CSF india-ink or antigen tests may identify the cryptococea. Testing CSF for *Borrelia* produces variable positivity.

A specific virus is identified in less than half the cases of encephalitis; the most common virus identified is herpes simplex. No precise data exist on headache duration and localization in this disorder, but the patient's history can be short, lasting from hours to a few days. Occasionally, the headache and clinical presentation take an indolent course. Headache may be accompanied by meningism and fever (3). Other characteristic symptoms are fever, epileptic seizures, somnolence, coma, confusion, and focal neurologic deficits that localize to frontotemporal regions of the brain cortex. MRI is the first-line mode of diagnostic investigation. Mass lesions of necrotic tissue, usually in the frontal or temporal cortex, can cause elevated intracranial pressure and shift of brain structures. Lumbar puncture should be performed immediately after scanning, mass effect permitting. CSF study may reveal a predominately lymphocytic pleocytosis of up to $300/mm^3$, a slightly elevated protein level, higher if the CSF is hemorrhagic, and a moderately decreased glucose level. Electroencephalography may indicate a temporal focus. Treatment is with intravenous acyclovir.

Nasal and Sinus Headaches

Acute sinus infection often presents with moderate to severe headache and facial pain. Localization of the head pain corresponds to the affected sinus, for example, retroorbital or temporal in ethmoid sinusitis, or frontal in frontal sinusitis. Pain is often alleviated by an upright position (4). Sinusitis is typically associated with nasal obstruction, fever, and localized tenderness. Investigation with sinus x-rays or CT scanning is diagnostic. To avoid intracranial complications, immediate antibiotic and anticongestant therapy is mandatory. Severe infections and pain may be relieved by sinus drainage if appropriate, for example, maxillary sinusitus.

Headache Due to Brain Tumor or Other Causes of Elevated Intracranial Pressure

Headache is the leading symptom in brain tumors, present in 48% of patients (7) or other conditions that elevate intracranial presure. In brain tumors, headache usually takes a course of weeks to months, having a crescendo intensity. Initially, it may present only upon wakening, before becoming continuous. Headache may reflect the tumor locus, for example, posterior with cerebellar lesions, by involving contiguous pain-sensitive intracranial structures, later becoming generalized when intracranial pressure becomes elevated. Characteristically, the headache is briefly accentuated by behaviors that increase intracranial pressure such as coughing, sneezing, bending, defecation, and sexual intercourse. Patients with brain neoplasia usually present to the ER because of neurologic

complications such as seizures, confusion, and paresis. If the ER patient has a history of headache as described above and seizures, contrast-enhanced CT scanning is required to confirm the diagnosis and to estimate the degree of any mass shift and secondary hydrocephalus.

MANAGEMENT OF PRIMARY HEADACHES IN THE EMERGENCY ROOM

After a complete history and physical examination, the ER physician should have a working diagnosis of the headache. Secondary headaches are managed by treating the underlying cause. For severe head pain relief, some form of narcotic may be necessary, but preferably after the diagnosis is established. This section will focus on the therapy of primary headaches in the emergency department.

Tension-Type Headache

Patients with tension-type headache syndrome often have a chronic course and are at a higher risk for narcotic analgesic addiction. These patients are initially treated with simple nonsteroidal antiinflammatory agents such as naproxen sodium (Anaprox) and ibuprofen (Motrin). Bed rest, hot packs to the head and neck area, and complete relaxation may alleviate some of the pain. However, if the patient has used narcotic analgesics in the past, the pain of an acute exacerbation of severe muscle contraction headache may respond only to parenteral narcotics such as demerol. Narcotics should be used as a last resort and only rarely. Tranquilizers such as lorazepam or oral muscle relaxants may be attempted first. It is important that the patient follow up with a neurologist or a headache clinic.

Acute Migraine Attack and Status Migrainosus

When migraine attacks are severe, prolonged, and unresponsive to self-administered medication, patients may require treatment in the clinic or ER. If they have not already used the drugs, the patients may be treated with intramuscular or intravenous dihydroergotamine, or subcutaneous sumatriptan. Other triptans are not available by subcutaneous administration but may be used when the diagnosis of acute migraine is made for the first time in patients presenting to the ER. If these fail, metoclopramide (10 mg intravenously), prochlorperazine (10 mg intravenously), or chlorpromazine (given in three intravenous injections of 0.1 mg/kg 15 minutes apart) may be given. Less effective is intramuscular Ketorolac, given with caution in the elderly, and contraindicated in asthmatic subjects or those who use beta-blockers as migraine prophylaxis. In Europe, lysine acetylsalicylic acid (Aspisol) has been used for many years. Intravenous acetylsalicylic acid is superior to placebo but less effective than subcutaneous sumatriptan, but has fewer side effects. It provides a useful alternative to sumatriptan or dihydroergotamine when these have already been given without effect.

Major narcotic analgesic drugs, especially meperidine, are also used in the emergency treatment of migraine attacks, but should be limited to patients who have attacks that do not respond to antimigraine preparations, or patients with conditions in which antimigraine drugs are contraindicated, such as coronary artery disease and pregnancy. This is emphasized because some patients frequent ERs with regularity and accordingly are at risk of addiction. Despite these cautions, in the United States, narcotics, in combination with an antiemetic, are most frequently prescribed for acute migraine in the ER setting.

Occasionally, patients suffer pain so severe, continuous, and unresponsive to medication that hospitalization is needed. Usually patients require intravenous fluids. Dihydroergotamine intravenously given over 3 to 4 days is a popular and effective treatment regimen after discontinuation of all other drugs (17). Although not proven, some headache specialists recommend intravenous hydrocortisone, given serially up to 100 mg per day for 2 to 3 days, or in single doses of up to 1 g.

Cluster Headache

Because cluster headache attacks are short-lived, they only occasionally present to the ER, with the exception of a first attack or cluster of attacks in a previously undiagnosed patient who is concerned by pain severity and requires diagnosis. Another exception might be an escalation of the illness and pain.

Oxygen should always be administered first, even when it has been tried previously. Response to 100% O_2 also may support the diagnosis of cluster headache in new cases. Sumatriptan, given subcutaneously for a rapid result, is the most effective acute treatment (6). Although intranasal sumatriptan also has a reasonably rapid action, it is less effective than when given by the subcutaneous route (10). Intravenous dihydroergotamine is an effective alternative. If the serotonin agonists are contraindicated, then intranasal lidocaine is effective in some patients. Narcotics should not be given to these patients because of the frequency, severity, and often chronic nature of the pain. If the aforementioned medications fail, an intravenous pulse of high-dose hydrocortisone, up to 1 g, may be tried and followed by a tapered oral steroid regimen. A careful history of previous steroid use is essential because cluster headache patients are at increased risk of avascular bone necrosis caused by repeated use of steroid bursts to terminate clusters of attacks. Prophylaxis should be started immediately under the steroid cover. Verapamil is most often used as a first line of approach. If the disorder is chronic, however, lithium carbonate may be prescribed.

Hospitalization for severe unremitting cluster headache is less common than for migraine. Under these circumstances, however, the same regimen of intravenous dihydroergotamine can be instituted as described above for status migrainosus, and accompanied by intravenous hydrocortisone.

REFERENCES

1. Adams HP Jr, Kassell NF, Torner JC, Sahs AL. CT and clinical correlations in recent aneurysmal subarachnoid hemorrhage: a preliminary report of the Cooperative Aneurysm Study. *Neurology* 1983;33: 981–988.
2. Badran RH, Weir RJ, McGuiness JB. Hypertension and headache. *Scott Med J* 1970;15:48–51.
3. Bale JF Jr. Viral encephalitis. *Med Clin North Am* 1993;77:25–42.
4. Close LG, Aviv J. Headaches and disease of the nose and paranasal sinuses. *Semin Neurol* 1997;17:351–354.
5. Durand ML, Calderwood SB, Weber DJ, et al. Acute bacterial meningitis in adults. A review of 493 episodes. *N Engl J Med* 1993;328:21–28.
6. Ekbom K. Treatment of cluster headache: clinical trials, design and results. *Cephalalgia* 1995;15(Suppl):33–36.
7. Forsyth PA, Posner JB. Headaches in patients with brain tumors: a study of 111 patients. *Neurology* 1993;43:1678–1683.
8. Goldstein J. Headache and acquired immunodeficiency syndrome. *Neurol Clin* 1990;8:947–960.
9. Gorelick PB, Hier DB, Caplan LR, Langenberg P. Headache in acute cerebrovascular disease. *Neurology* 1986;36:1445–1450.
10. Hardebo JE, Dahlof C. Sumatriptan nasal spray (20 mg dose) in the acute treatment of cluster headache. Cephalalgia 1998;18:487–489.
11. Hayreh SS, Podhajsky PA, Raman R, Zimmerman B. Giant cell arteritis: validity and reliability of various diagnostic criteria. *Am J Ophthalmol* 1997;123:285–296.
12. Hunt WE, Hess RM. Surgical risk as related to time of intervention in the repair of intracranial aneurysms. *J Neurosurg* 1998;28:14–20.
13. Jorgensen HS, Jespersen HF, Nakayama H, Raaschou HO, Olsen TS. Headache in stroke: the Copenhagen Stroke Study. *Neurology* 1994;44: 1793–1797.
14. Karacagil S, Hardemark HG, Bergqvist D. Spontaneous internal carotid artery dissection [Review]. *Int Angiol* 1996;15:291–294.
15. Lipton RB, Feraru ER, Weiss G, et al. Headache in HIV-1-related disorders. *Headache* 1991;31:518–522.
16. Phillips SJ, Whisnant JP. Hypertension and the brain. The National High Blood Pressure Education Program. *Arch Intern Med* 1992;152: 938–945.
17. Raskin NH. Repetitive intravenous dihydroergotamine as therapy for intractable migraine. *Neurology* 1986;36:995–997.
18. Silbert PL, Mokri B, Schievink WI. Headache and neck pain in spontaneous internal carotid and vertebral artery dissections. *Neurology* 1995;45:1517–1522.
19. Vital and Health Statistics of the Centers for Disease Control and Prevention/National Center of Health Statistics. National Hospital Ambulatory Medical Survey: 1995 Emergency Department Summary.
20. Villringer A, Einhaupl KM. Dural sinus and cerebral venous thrombosis. *New Horiz* 1997;5:332–341.
21. Whitley RJ. Antiviral treatment of a serious herpes simplex infection: encephalitis. *J Am Acad Dermatol* 1988;18(Part 2):209–211.
22. Wolff HG. *Headache and other head pain,* 3rd ed. New York: Oxford University Press, 1972.
23. Zee CS, Go JL. CT of head trauma. *Neuroimag Clin North Am* 1998; 8:525–539.

Subject Index